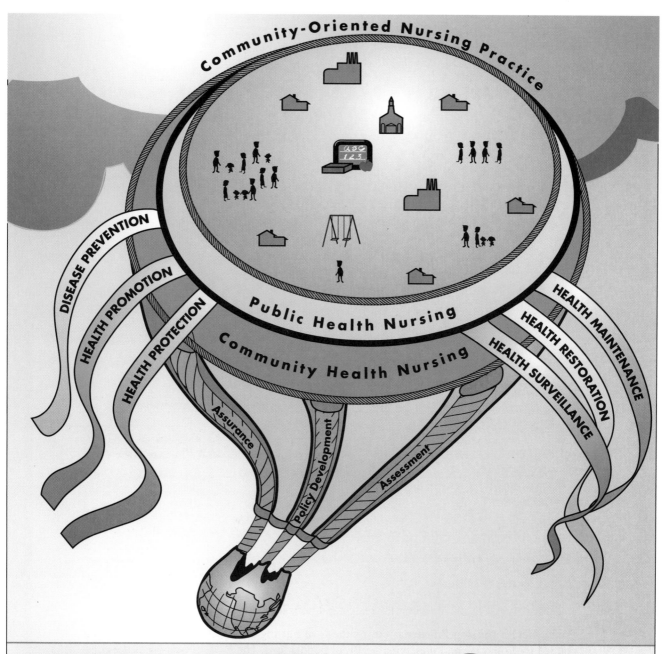

**Overarching Concept**
- Community-oriented nursing practice

**Subconcepts**
- Community health nursing
- Public health nursing

**Foundational Pillars**
- Assurance
- Assessment
- Policy development

**Settings**
- Community
- Environment
- School
- Industry
- Church
- Prisons
- Playground
- Home

**Clients**
- Individuals
- Families
- Groups
- Populations
- Communities

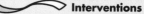

**Interventions**
- Disease Prevention
- Health Promotion
- Health Protection
- Health Maintenance
- Health Restoration
- Health Surveillance

**Services**
- Personal Health Services
- Populations/Aggregate Services
- Community Services

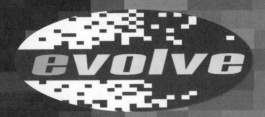

# The Latest *Evolution* in Learning.

Evolve provides online access to free learning resources and activities designed specifically for the textbook you are using in your class. The resources will provide you with information that enhances the material covered in the book and much more.

Visit the Web address listed below to start your learning evolution today!

**LOGIN:** *http://evolve.elsevier.com/Stanhope*

Evolve Student Learning Resources for Stanhope/Lancaster: *Community & Public Health Nursing,* 6th edition, offer the following features:

- **Case Studies**
  Real-life clinical situations to help you develop your assessment and critical thinking skills, with answers provided.

- **Sample Test Questions**
  Multiple-choice questions with instant scoring and feedback at the click of a button.

- **WebLinks**
  An exciting resource that lets you link to hundreds of websites carefully chosen to supplement the content of the textbook. The WebLinks are regularly updated, with new ones added as they develop.

- **Content Resources**
  Numerous resources such as immunization tables, assessment tools, practice guidelines, and many other clinical reference materials.

- **Content Updates**
  The latest content updates to keep you current with recent developments in this area of study.

- **Glossary**
  Complete definitions of key terms and other important community and public health nursing concepts.

## Think outside the book... *evolve.*

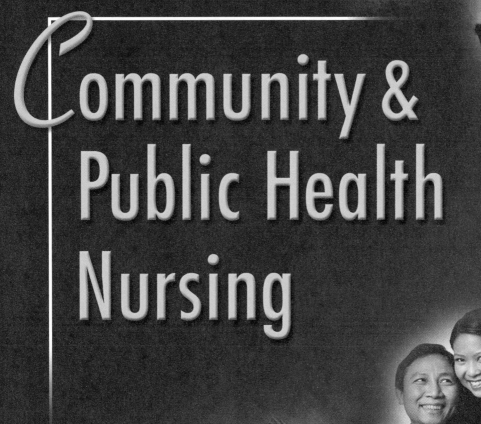

# Community & Public Health Nursing

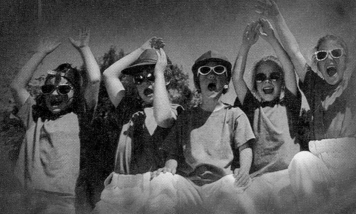

**Sixth Edition**

# Community & Public Health Nursing

**Marcia Stanhope, RN, DSN, FAAN, c**

**Associate Dean and Professor**
**Good Samaritan Chair in Community**
  **Health Nursing**
**College of Nursing**
**University of Kentucky**
**Lexington, Kentucky**

**Jeanette Lancaster, RN, PhD, FAAN**

**Dean and Sadie Heath Cabaniss Professor**
**School of Nursing**
**University of Virginia**
**Charlottesville, Virginia**



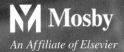

Mosby
*An Affiliate of Elsevier*

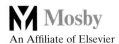
**Mosby**

An Affiliate of Elsevier

11830 Westline Industrial Drive
St. Louis, Missouri 63146

---

**Notice**

Pharmacology is an ever-changing field. Standard safety precautions must be followed, but as new research and clinical experience broaden our knowledge, changes in treatment and drug therapy may become necessary or appropriate. Readers are advised to check the most current product information provided by the manufacturer of each drug to be administered to verify the recommended dose, the method and duration of administration, and contraindications. It is the responsibility of the licensed health care provider, relying on experience and knowledge of the patient, to determine dosages and the best treatment for each individual patient. Neither the Publisher nor the editor assumes any liability for any injury and/or damage to persons or property arising from this publication.

---

Previous editions copyrighted 1984, 1988, 1992, 1996, 2000

**International Standard Book Number 0-323-02240-5**

*Executive Vice President:* Sally Schrefer
*Executive Publisher:* Darlene Como
*Executive Editor:* Loren Wilson
*Managing Editor:* Linda Thomas
*Senior Developmental Editor:* Nancy L. O'Brien
*Publication Services Manager:* John Rogers
*Project Manager:* Beth Hayes
*Design Manager:* Bill Drone

Printed in the United Sates of America

Last digit is the print number:   9   8   7   6   5   4   3   2

# About the Authors

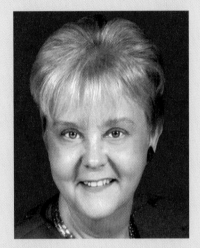

## MARCIA STANHOPE, RN, DSN, FAAN, c

Marcia Stanhope is currently Associate Dean and Professor at the University of Kentucky College of Nursing, Lexington, Kentucky. She was recently appointed to the Good Samaritan Endowed Chair in Community Health Nursing. She has practiced community and home health nursing and has served as an administrator and consultant in home health, and she has been involved in the development of two nurse-managed centers. She has taught community health, public health, epidemiology, primary care nursing, and administration courses. Dr. Stanhope formerly directed the Division of Community Health Nursing and Administration at the University of Kentucky. She has been responsible for both undergraduate and graduate courses in community-oriented nursing.

She has also taught at the University of Virginia and the University of Alabama, Birmingham. Her presentations and publications have been in the areas of home health, community health and community-focused nursing practice, and primary care nursing. Dr. Stanhope holds a diploma in nursing from the Good Samaritan Hospital, Lexington, Kentucky, and a bachelor of science from the University of Kentucky. She has a master's degree in public health nursing from Emory University in Atlanta and a doctorate of science in nursing from the University of Alabama, Birmingham. Dr. Stanhope is the co-author of four other Mosby publications: *Handbook of Community-Based and Home Health Nursing Practice*, *Public and Community Health Nurse's Consultant*, *Case Studies in Community Health Nursing Practice: A Problem-Based Learning Approach*, and *Foundations of Community Health Nursing: Community-Oriented Practice*.

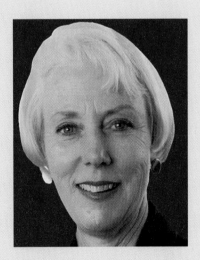

## JEANETTE LANCASTER, RN, PhD, FAAN

Jeanette Lancaster is currently the Sadie Heath Cabaniss Professor of Nursing and Dean at the University of Virginia School of Nursing in Charlottesville, Virginia. She has practiced psychiatric nursing and taught both psychiatric and community health nursing. She formerly directed the master's program in community health at the University of Alabama, Birmingham and served as dean of the School of Nursing at Wright State University in Dayton, Ohio. Her publications and presentations have been largely in the areas of community and public health nursing leadership and change and the significance of nurses to effective primary health care. Dr. Lancaster is a graduate of the University of Tennessee, Memphis, College of Nursing. She holds a master's degree in psychiatric nursing from Case Western Reserve University and a doctorate in public health from the University of Oklahoma. Dr. Lancaster is the author of another Mosby publication, *Nursing Issues in Leading and Managing Change*, and coauthor of *Foundations of Community Health Nursing: Community-Oriented Practice*.

# Dedication

In 1980, Jeanette Lancaster never dreamed that this text would be a part of her life's work. Thanks for your many contributions to this work through the years. A special thanks to the Good Samaritan Foundation Board and staff, past and present, for their contributions to making communities healthier, especially Arch Manous, Phil Harmon, and Verona Cumberledge.

**Marcia Stanhope**

It hardly seems that the work on the first edition of this text began in 1980. This sixth edition marks over two decades of colleagueship with Marcia Stanhope and with many of the contributors. I am grateful to each of you. I would like to express appreciation to my family who have changed plans and made other accommodations over these years so that I could devote time and attention to the book. Wade, Melinda, and Jennifer, thank you. A special thanks to my first school of nursing dean, Virginia Jarratt, who encouraged me to write my first book.

**Jeanette Lancaster**

# Contributors

**Brenda Afzal, MS, RN**
Program Manager
Environmental Health Education
School of Nursing
University of Maryland
Baltimore, Maryland

**Debra Gay Anderson, PhD, RNC**
Associate Professor
College of Nursing
University of Kentucky
Lexington, Kentucky

**Dyan A. Aretakis, RN, FNP, MSN**
Project Director
Teen Health Center
University of Virginia Health System
Charlottesville, Virginia

**Anne S. Belcher, DNS, RN, PNP**
Associate Professor and Director of Faculty Affairs
School of Nursing
Indiana University
Indianapolis, Indiana

**Ruth D. Berry, RN, MSN**
Professor Emeriti
College of Nursing
University of Kentucky
Lexington, Kentucky

**Virginia Trotter Betts, MSN, JD, RN, FAAN**
Commissioner, Tennessee Department of
    Mental Health and Developmental Disabilities
Nashville, Tennessee

**Linda K. Birenbaum, RN, PhD**
Professor
School of Nursing
University of Portland
Portland, Oregon

**Christine Di Martile Bolla, RN, DNSc**
Clinical Assistant Professor
Department of Nursing
San Francisco State University
San Francisco, California

**Marjorie Buchanan, RN, MS**
New Initiatives Consultant
College of Health and Human Performance
University of Maryland
College Park, Maryland

**Angeline Bushy, PhD, RN, FAAN**
Professor and Bert Fish Chair
Community Health Nursing
School of Nursing
University of Central Florida
Daytona Beach, Florida

**Jacquelyn C. Campbell, PhD, RN, FAAN**
Anna D. Wolf Endowed Professor
Associate Dean for Faculty Affairs
School of Nursing
Johns Hopkins University
Baltimore, Maryland

**Ann H. Cary, PhD, MPH, RN, A-CCC**
Director of the Institute for Research, Education
    and Consultation
American Nurses Credentialing Center
Washington, D.C.

**Marcia K. Cowan, RN, MSN, CPNP**
Pediatric Nurse Practitioner
The Pediatric Center of Tullahoma, PC
Tullahoma, Tennessee

**Cynthia E. Degazon, PhD, RN**
Associate Professor
Hunter Bellevue School of Nursing
Hunter College of the City University of New York
New York, New York

**Janna Dieckmann, PhD, RN**
Assistant Professor
School of Nursing
University of North Carolina at Chapel Hill
Chapel Hill, North Carolina

**Diane Downing, RN, MSN**
Public Health Program Specialist
Arlington County Department of Human Services
Clinical Instructor
Georgetown University
School of Nursing and Health Studies
Arlington, Virginia

**James J. Fletcher, PhD**
Associate Professor of Philosophy
Department of Philosophy and Religious Studies
George Mason University
Fairfax, Virginia

**Kathleen Ryan Fletcher, RN, MsN, APRN-BC, CNP**
Assistant Professor, School of Nursing
Administrator of Senior Services
University of Virginia Health Systems
Charlottesville, Virginia

**Beverly C. Flynn, PhD, RN, FAAN**
Emeritus Professor, Department of Environments
for Health
Director, Institute of Action Research for Community
Health
Head, World Health Organization Collaborating Center
in Healthy Cities
Indiana University School of Nursing
Indianapolis, Indiana

**Debra J. Giese, RN, MS**
Lecturer, PhD Candidate
College of Nursing
University of Kentucky
Lexington, Kentucky

**Doris F. Glick, RN, PhD**
Associate Professor and Director
Masters Program
School of Nursing
University of Virginia
Charlottesville, Virginia

**Jean Goeppinger, PhD, RN, FAAN**
Professor
Schools of Nursing and Public Health
University of North Carolina at Chapel Hill
Chapel Hill, North Carolina

**Patty J. Hale, RN, PhD, FNP**
Professor
Department of Nursing
Lynchburg College
Lynchburg, Virginia

**Shirley May Harmon Hanson, RN, PMHNP, PhD,
FAAN, CFLE, LMFT**
Professor
School of Nursing
Oregon Health and Science University
Portland, Oregon

**Susan B. Hassmiller, PhD, RN, FAAN**
Senior Program Officer
The Robert Wood Johnson Foundation
Chair, Disaster Services, American Red Cross
Princeton, New Jersey

**Diane C. Hatton, RN, CS, DNS, c**
Professor
Hahn School of Nursing and Health Sciences
University of San Diego
San Diego, California

**Kathleen Huttlinger, RN, PhD**
Director, Center for Nursing Research
College of Nursing
Kent State University
Kent, Ohio

**Janet T. Ihlenfeld, RN, PhD**
Professor
Department of Nursing
D'Youville College
Buffalo, New York

**L. Louise Ivanov, DNS, RN**
Associate Professor and Chair of
Community Practice Department
School of Nursing
University of North Carolina–Geensboro
Greensboro, North Carolina

**Alicia A. Jensen, RN, MSN**
Radford University
Radford, Virginia

**Kim Dupree Jones, PhD, RN, FNP**
Assistant Professor
Schools of Nursing and Medicine
Oregon Health and Science University
Portland, Oregon

**Joanna Rowe Kaakinen, PhD, RN**
Associate Professor
School of Nursing
University of Portland
Portland, Oregon

**Lisa M. Kaiser, RN, MSN, PhD, c**
Associate Faculty
National University
LaJolla, California

**Katherine K. Kinsey, PhD, RN, FAAN**
Associate Professor and Independence Foundation Chair
Director, Neighborhood Nursing Center
LaSalle University School of Nursing
Philadelphia, Pennsylvania

**Thomas Kippenbrock, MSN, EdD**
Department Chair and Professor
Department of Nursing
Arkansas State University
State University, Arkansas

**Sandra Caddell Kirkland, DNS, RN, CNA, BC**
Medical Information Specialist
Supportive Oncology Services, Inc.
Memphis, Tennessee

**Joyce Splann Krothe, DNS, RN**
Associate Professor
Indiana University School of Nursing
Director, Bloomington Campus
Bloomington, Indiana

**Pamela A. Kulbok, RN, DNSc**
Associate Professor
School of Nursing
University of Virginia
Charlottesville, Virginia

**Shirley Cloutier Laffrey, PhD, MPH, APRN, BC**
Associate Professor, Public Health Nursing
School of Nursing
The University of Texas–Austin
Austin, Texas

**Kären M. Landenburger, RN, PhD**
Associate Professor
Nursing Program
University of Washington–Tacoma
Tacoma, Washington

**Peggye Guess Lassiter, RN, MSN**
Adjunct Assistant Professor
College of Pharmacy, Nursing and Allied Health Sciences
Division of Nursing
Howard University
Washington, D.C.

**Susan C. Long-Marin, DVM, MPH**
Epidemiology Manager
Mecklenburg County Health Department
Charlotte, North Carolina

**Lois W. Lowry, RN, DNSc**
Professor
East Tennessee State University
Johnson City, Tennessee

**P. J. Maddox, MSN, EdD**
Professor
College of Nursing and Health Science
George Mason University
Fairfax, Virginia

**Karen S. Martin, RN, MSN, CARN, FAAN**
Health Care Consultant
Martin Associates
Omaha, Nebraska

**Mary Lynn Mathre, RN, MSN, CARN**
Nurse Consultant
Patients Out of Time
Charlottesville, Virginia

**Mary Ann McClellan, MN, CPNP, ARNP**
Assistant Professor
Coordinator–Pediatric Nurse Practitioner Track,
    Graduate Program
College of Nursing
University of Oklahoma
Oklahoma City, Oklahoma

**Robert E. McKeown, PhD, FACEP**
Graduate Director for Epidemiology
Department of Epidemiology and Biostatistics
Arnold School of Public Health
University of South Carolina
Columbia, South Carolina

**Kathleen M. McPhaul, RN, BSN, MPH**
Workplace Violence Project Director
Department of Community and Behavioral Health
University of Maryland
Baltimore, Maryland

**DeAnne K. Hilfinger Messias, RN, PhD**
Associate Professor
College of Nursing and Women's Studies
University of South Carolina
Columbia, South Carolina

**Lillian H. Mood, RN, MPH, FAAN**
Retired
State Director of Public Health Nursing, Assistant
    Commissioner, and Community Liaison
    for Environmental Quality Control
South Carolina Department of Health
    and Environmental Control
Columbia, South Carolina

**Marie Napolitano, RN, PhD, FNP**
Associate Professor
Coordinator for the Family Nurse Practitioner Program
Oregon Health and Science University
Portland, Oregon

**Lisa C. Onega, PhD, RN, FNP, GNP**
Associate Professor of Gerontological Nursing
Radford University
Radford, Virginia

**Bonnie Rogers, DrPH, COHN-S, LNCC, FAAN**
Director, North Carolina Occupational Safety
    and Health Education and Research Center
Director, Public Health/Occupational Health Nursing
    Programs
University of North Carolina
Chapel Hill, North Carolina

**Molly A. Rose, RN, PhD**
Associate Professor
Jefferson College of Health Professions
Department of Nursing
Thomas Jefferson University
Philadelphia, Pennsylvania

**Barbara Sattler, RN, DrPH, FAAN**
Associate Professor
School of Nursing
Director, Environmental Health Education Center
University of Maryland
Baltimore, Maryland

**Jennifer M. Schaller-Ayers, RN, PhD, BC**
Associate Professor
College of Nursing
East Tennessee State University
Johnson City, Tennessee

**Juliann G. Sebastian, ARNP, PhD, FAAN**
Professor and Assistant Dean for Advanced Practice
    Nursing
College of Nursing
University of Kentucky
Lexington, Kentucky

**George F. Shuster, RN, DNSc**
Associate Professor
College of Nursing
University of New Mexico
Albuquerque, New Mexico

**Mary Cipriano Silva, RN, PHD, FAAN**
Professor
College of Nursing and Health Science
George Mason University
Fairfax, Virginia

**Jeanne Merkle Sorrell, PhD, RN, FAAN**
Professor
Associate Dean, Academic Programs and Research
College of Nursing and Health Science
George Mason University
Fairfax, Virginia

**Francisco S. Sy, MD, DrPH**
Clinical Associate Professor
Department of Family and Preventive Medicine
School of Medicine
University of South Carolina
Columbia, South Carolina

**Anita Thompson-Heisterman, MSN, RN, CS, FNP**
Instructor
University of Virginia School of Nursing
Family Nurse Practitioner
Jefferson Area Board for Aging
Charlottesville, Virginia

**Heather Joy Ward, RN, MSN, ARNP**
College of Nursing
University of Kentucky
Lexington, Kentucky

**Cynthia J. Westley, RNC, MSN, ANPc**
Community Care Manager
University of Virginia Health System
Charlottesville, Virginia

**Carolyn A. Williams, RN, PhD, FAAN**
Dean and Professor
College of Nursing
University of Kentucky
Lexington, Kentucky

**Judith Lupo Wold, PhD, RN**
Associate Professor
School of Nursing
College of Health and Human Sciences
Georgia State University
Atlanta, Georgia

# Contributors to Canadian Boxes

**Jo-Ann Ackery, RN, BScN**
Manager, Communicable Disease, STD, HIV/AIDS
 Program
Toronto Public Health
Toronto, Ontario, Canada

**Betty Burcher, RN, BA, BScN, MSc**
Lecturer, Faculty of Nursing
University of Toronto
Toronto, Ontario, Canada

**Maureen Cava, BScN, MS**
Manager, Education and Research
Toronto Public Health
Toronto, Ontario, Canada

**Catherine Clarke, RN, BScN, MN**
Coordinating Manager, Tobacco Control
Toronto Public Health
Toronto, Ontario, Canada

**Karon Janine Foster, RN, BScN, MEd**
Lecturer, Faculty of Nursing
University of Toronto
Toronto, Ontario, Canada

**Jann Houston, BScN, MScN**
Manager
Toronto Public Health
Toronto, Ontario, Canada

**Lianne Patricia Jeffs, RN, MSc**
Faculty of Nursing
University of Toronto
Toronto, Ontario, Canada

**Barbara Mildon, RN, MN, CHE**
President, Community Health Nurses Association
 of Canada
Vice President, Nursing Leadership
Saint Elizabeth Health Care
Courtice, Ontario, Canada

**Pat Sanagan, RN, BScN, MEd**
Sanagan Consulting
Toronto, Ontario, Canada

**Karen Wade, RN, BN, MScN**
Clinical Nurse Specialist
Planning and Policy
Toronto Public Health
Toronto, Ontario, Canada

# Reviewers

**Michelle Ficca, DNSc, RN**
Assistant Professor, Department of Nursing
Bloomsburg University
Bloomsburg, Pennsylvania

**Olive Santavenere, RN, BS, MSOB, MSN, PhD, CNA**
Associate Professor, Department of Nursing
Southern Connecticut State University
New Haven, Connecticut

# Foreword

The national health agenda, Healthy People 2010, holds forth great hope and promise for the well-being of the people of this country. Nurses working in public and community health practice, research, and education are important factors in fulfilling this promise. However, protecting and preserving health in the face of our changing social, economic, political, and environmental realities requires heightened knowledge, skill, and sophistication. The sober realities of our times—the uncertainties that face us and the very tangible threats to health that surround all of us—have created an environment in which nurses bear more responsibility than ever for the well-being of those they serve. These are not easy times—nor are the roles of public and community health nurses easily fulfilled.

For educators, the challenge of preparing new generations of nurses who are effective in the community is increasingly more complex. The targets outlined in Healthy People 2010 require a knowledge and skill base that is truly rooted in the science of nursing and public health and interfaces meaningfully with disciplines that lie beyond both. The scope and depth of knowledge required by students and faculty alike demands educational resources that are authoritative, rigorous, timely, and interesting. Textbooks that meet this standard are rare and precious. Fortunately, this sixth edition of *Community &*
*Public Health Nursing* not only meets but surpasses the standard.

Students, faculty, and practicing public and community health nurses all stand to benefit from the views of the "star-studded" cast of nationally respected authors whose work is a part of this important text. Marcia Stanhope and Jeanette Lancaster have effectively woven a tapestry of topics and authors who impart crucial knowledge and insight to both the neophyte and the seasoned practitioner. This is a text that serves as both educational tool and ongoing reference—timely and timeless. It works well in both undergraduate and graduate contexts and can be used in survey and specialty courses.

The goals of Healthy People 2010 are attainable. Nursing does have the capacity to play critical roles in truly improving the health of the people of this nation. Marcia Stanhope and Jeanette Lancaster have provided us with an important resource that can only help to move the field forward and to build healthier communities in the process.

**Marla E. Salmon, ScD, RN, FAAN**
Dean, Nell Hodgson Woodruff School of Nursing
Professor, Rollins School of Public Health
Emory University
Atlanta, Georgia

# Preface

Since the fifth edition of this text was printed, many changes have occurred in society and also in health care. Indeed, many of society's changes are greatly influencing the amount and ways in which health care is delivered. The majority of people alive today have not lived in a time of global concerns about terrorism. In the past, limited funds have been available for disaster preparedness. The current shifting of funds to ensure greater safety to the public means that many of public health programs will be funded even less than they were in the past decade. If there is a bright spot to the concerns about terrorism, war, and limited financial resources, it is that far more people understand the importance and value of public health to individuals, families, communities, and nations.

It seems that some of the major issues at present relate to the quality of care, the cost of care, and access to care. The growing shortage of nurses and other health care providers will only increase the concerns about access to care and the fears of war and terrorism.

One of the ways in which quality of care could be improved would include new uses of technology to manage an information revolution. Great improvements in quality would require a restructuring of how care is delivered, a shift in how funds are spent, changing the workplace, and using more effective ways to manage chronic illness. There will be costs associated with quality improvements.

The United States continues to have a problem of increasing health care costs. At present these costs are consuming about $1.4 trillion or 15% of the Gross Domestic Product. These enormous costs are imposing heavy burdens on employers and consumers. Despite these costs, the number of uninsured continues to grow and is estimated to be around 41.2 million (U.S. Bureau of the Census, 2002*). This number of uninsured is larger than the population of either Canada or Australia. Despite spending more money per person in the United States for illness care than in any other country, Americans are not the healthiest of all people. The infant mortality and life expectancy rates—indexes of health care—while improving, are not close to what they should be given the amount spent on health care. Some of the most important factors leading to the high health care costs are diagnostic and treatment technologies, drugs, an aging population, more chronic illness, shortages in health care workers, and medical-legal costs.

Lifestyle continues to play a big role in morbidity and mortality. For example, half of all deaths are still caused by tobacco, alcohol, and illegal drug use; diet and activity patterns; microbial agents; toxic agents; firearms; sexual behavior; and motor vehicle accidents.

From 1990 to 1999 the biggest improvements in population health have come from public health achievements such as immunizations leading to eliminating and controlling infectious diseases; motor vehicle safety; safer workplaces; lifestyle improvements reducing the risk of heart disease and strokes; safer and healthier foods through improved sanitation; clean water and food fortification programs; better hygiene and nutrition to improve the health of mothers and babies; family planning; fluoride in drinking water; and recognizing tobacco as a health hazard. Continued changes in the public health system are essential if death, illness, and disability due to preventable problems are to continue to decline.

The need to focus attention on health promotion, lifestyle factors, and disease prevention led to the development of a major public policy about health for the nation. This policy was designed by a large number of people representing a wide range of groups interested in health. The policy has been updated and is reflected in the document Healthy People 2010, which identifies a comprehensive set of national health promotion and disease prevention objectives. Examples of these objectives are highlighted in chapters throughout the text.

The most effective disease prevention and health promotion strategies designed to change personal lifestyles are developed through partnerships between government, business, voluntary organizations, consumers, communities, and health care providers. According to Healthy People 2010, these partnerships aim to reduce health disparities among Americans by targeting care to children, minorities, elderly, and the uninsured, to increase the healthy life span of Americans and to achieve access to preventive services. The overall goals are to protect and promote health of populations, to prevent disease and injury, and to develop healthy communities. To develop healthy communities, individuals, families, and the communities must commit to those goals. Also, society, through the development of health policy, must support better health care, the design of improved health education, and new ways of financing strategies to alter health status.

What does this mean for the community-oriented nurse? Because people do not always know how to improve their health status, the challenge of nursing is to create change. Community-oriented nursing takes place in a variety of public and private settings and includes disease prevention, health promotion, health protection, education, maintenance, restoration, coordination, management, and evaluation of care of individuals, families, and populations, including communities.

---

*U.S. Bureau of the Census: Health insurance coverage 2001, available at www.census.gov/prod/2002puds/p60-220pdf,2002.

To meet the demands of a constantly changing health care system, nurses must have vision in designing new and changing current roles and identifying their practice areas. To do so effectively, the nurse must understand concepts and theories of public health, the changing health care system, the actual and potential roles and responsibilities of nurses and other health care providers, the importance of health promotion and disease orientation, and the necessity to involve consumers in the planning, implementing, and evaluating of health care efforts.

Since its initial publication 22 years ago, this text has been widely accepted and is popular among nursing students and nursing faculty in baccalaureate, BSN-completion, and graduate programs. The text was written to provide nursing students and practicing nurses with a comprehensive source book that provides a foundation for designing community-oriented nursing strategies for individuals, families, aggregates, populations, and communities. The unifying theme for the book is the integrating of health promotion and disease prevention concepts into the many roles of community-oriented nurses. The prevention focus emphasizes traditional public health practice with increased attention to the effects of the internal and external environment on health. The focus on interventions for the individual and family emphasizes community-oriented practice with attention to the effects of all of the determinants of health, including lifestyle, on personal health.

## CONCEPTUAL APPROACH TO THIS TEXT

The term *community-oriented* is now used to reflect the orientation of community and public health nursing. In 1998, the Quad Council of Public Health Nursing, comprised of members from the American Nurses Association Congress on Nursing Practice; the American Public Health Association Public Health Nursing section; the Association of Community Health Nursing Educators; and the Association of State and Territorial Directors of Public Health Nursing developed a statement on the *Scope of Public Health Nursing Practice*. Through this statement, the leaders in community-oriented nursing attempted to clarify the differences between public health nursing and the newest term introduced into nursing's vocabulary during health care reform of the 1990s, *community-based nursing*. The Quad Council recognized that the terms *public health nursing* and *community health nursing* have been used interchangeably since the 1980s to describe population-focused, community-oriented nursing practice and community-focused practice. They decided to make a clearer distinction between community-oriented and community-based nursing practice.

In this textbook, these same two but different levels of care in the community are acknowledged: community-oriented care and community-based care. Three role functions for nursing practice in the community are suggested: public health nursing, community health nursing, and community-based nursing. This text focuses only on public health nursing and community health nursing using the term *community-oriented nursing practice*.

For the fifth edition of this text, with consultation from C. A. Williams (author) and June Thompson (Mosby editor), Marcia Stanhope developed a conceptual model for community-oriented nursing practice. This model was influenced by a review of the history of community-oriented nursing practice from the 1800s to today. Marcia Stanhope studied Betty Neuman's model intensively while in school. This model is also influenced by the work of Neuman (see Chapter 9).

The model itself is presented as a caricature of reality—or an abstract, with a description of the characteristics and the philosophy upon which community-oriented nursing practice is built.

The *model* is shown as a flying balloon (see inside front cover of this book). The balloon represents community-oriented nursing practice and is filled with the knowledge, skills, and abilities needed in this practice to carry the world (the basket of the balloon) or the clients of the world who benefit from this practice. The *subconcepts* of public health nursing and community health nursing are the *boundaries* of the practice. The public health foundation pillars of assurance, assessment, and policy development hold up the world of communities, where people live, work, play, go to school, and worship. The ribbons flying from the balloon indicate the interventions used by community-oriented nurses. These ribbons (interventions) serve to provide lift and direction, tying the services together for the clients that are served. The intervention names and the services are listed on the inside cover of this book. The *propositions* (statements of relationship) for this model are found in the definitions of practice, public health functions, clients served, specific settings, interventions, and services. There are many *assumptions* that have served as the basis for the development of this model. Community-oriented nursing practice is a specialty within the nursing discipline. The practice has evolved over time, becoming more complex. The practice of nursing in public health is based on a philosophy of care rather than being setting specific. It is different from community-based nursing care delivery. The development of community-oriented nursing practice has been influenced by public health practice, preventive medicine, community medicine, and shifts in the health care delivery system. Community-oriented nursing practice requires nurses to have specific competencies to be effective providers of care.

The definition of community-oriented nursing practice appears on the inside front cover of this book. This practice includes both public health and community health nurses (see inside front cover). Community-based nurses differ from community-oriented nurses in many ways. These differences are described on the table in the inside back cover of this book. The differences are described as they relate to philosophy of care, goals, service, community, clients served, practice settings, ways of interacting with clients, type of services offered to clients, prevention levels used, goals, and priority of nurses' activities.

The four concepts of nursing, person (client), environment, and health are described for this model. These concepts appear in many works about nursing and in almost every educational curriculum for undergraduate students. Each of the four concepts may be defined differently in these works because of the beliefs of the persons writing the definitions. In this text nursing is defined as a community-oriented practice that focuses on providing "health care" through community diagnosis and investigation of major health and environmental problems. Health surveillance, monitoring, and evaluating community and population status are done to prevent disease and disability, and to promote, protect, preserve, and maintain health. This in turn creates conditions in which clients can be healthy. The person, or client, is the world, nation, state, community, population, aggregate, family, or individual.

The boundaries of the client *environment* may be limited only by the world, nation, state, locality, home, school, work, playground, religion, or individual self. *Health*, in this model, involves a continuum of health rather than wellness, with the best health state possible as the goal. The best possible level of health is achieved through measures of prevention as practiced by the nurse.

Community-oriented nursing practice is based on the belief that focus on the "health of all" clients is essential. The goals of this practice are to prevent disease and promote, preserve, protect, or maintain health. The client of the practice may be the world, nation, state, local community, population, group, family, or individual. The nurse engages in autonomous practice with the client, who is the primary decision maker about health issues. The nurse practices in a variety of environments, including, but not limited to, governments, organizations, homes, schools, churches, neighborhoods, industry, and community boards. The nurse interacts with diverse cultures, partners, other providers in teams, multiple clients and one-to-one or aggregate relationships. Clients at risk for the development of health problems are a major focus of nursing services. Primary prevention–level strategies are the key to reducing risk of health problems. Secondary prevention is done to maintain, promote, or protect health while tertiary prevention strategies are used to preserve, protect, or maintain health.

The community-oriented nurse has many roles related to community clients and roles that relate specifically to practice with populations (see inside back cover). Community-oriented nurses engage in activities specific to community development, assessment, monitoring, health policy, politics, health education, interdisciplinary practice, program management, community/population advocacy, case finding, and delivery of personal health services when these services are otherwise unavailable in the health care system. This conceptual model is the framework for this text.

## ORGANIZATION

The text is divided into seven sections:
- **Part 1, Perspectives on Health Care and Community-Oriented Nursing,** describes the historical and current status of the health care delivery system and community-oriented nursing practice, both domestically and internationally.
- **Part 2, Influences on Health Care Delivery and Community-Oriented Nursing,** addresses specific issues and societal concerns that affect public and community health nursing practice.
- **Part 3, Conceptual and Scientific Frameworks Applied to Community-Oriented Nursing Practice,** provides conceptual models for public and community health nursing practice, and selected models from nursing and related sciences are also discussed.
- **Part 4, Issues and Approaches in Community-Oriented Health Care,** examines the management of health care and select community environments, as well as issues related to managing cases, programs, disasters, and groups.
- **Part 5, Health Promotion With Target Populations Across the Life Span,** discusses risk factors and health problems for families and individuals throughout the life span.
- **Part 6, Vulnerability: Community-Oriented Nursing Issues for the Twenty-first Century,** covers specific health care needs and issues of populations at risk.
- **Part 7, Community-Oriented Nurses: Roles and Functions,** examines diversity in the role of community and public health nurses and describes the rapidly changing roles, functions, and practice settings.

## NEW TO THIS EDITION

New content has been included in the sixth edition of *Community & Public Health Nursing* to ensure that the text remains a complete and comprehensive resource:
- NEW! Chapter 12, Evidence-Based Practice, discusses the implementation of best practices based on scientific research and other evidence in community-oriented nursing.
- NEW! Healthy People 2010 boxes contain objectives and data from the most recent version of this federal government health promotion initiative. Each box contains objectives related to each chapter's topic that form the basis of community-oriented nursing practice.
- Expanded coverage of community-oriented nursing interventions at the primary, secondary, and tertiary levels of prevention illustrate their application to individuals, families, and communities.
- NEW! THE CUTTING EDGE boxes highlight significant issues and new approaches in community-oriented nursing practice.
- Increased coverage of the nurse's role in disaster management and infectious disease prevention highlight the challenges faced by today's community and public health nurse.
- NEW! Chapter openers contain a photograph and brief biography of the chapter author(s) to acknowledge the experts behind the content.
- NEW! Additional Resources boxes direct students to chapter-related tools and resources contained in the book's Appendixes or on its evolve website.

## PEDAGOGY

Other key features of this edition are detailed below.

Each chapter is organized for easy use by students and faculty. **Objectives** open each chapter to guide student learning and alert faculty to what students should gain from the content. **Key Terms** are identified at the beginning of the chapter and defined either within the chapter or in the glossary to assist students in understanding unfamiliar terminology. Finally, the **Chapter Outline** alerts students to the structure and content of the chapter.

**DID YOU KNOW?** boxes provide students with interesting facts that lend insight into the chapter content.

**WHAT DO YOU THINK?** boxes stimulate student debate and classroom discussion.

**HOW TO** boxes provide specific, application-oriented information.

**NURSING TIP** boxes emphasize special clinical considerations for nursing practice.

**Evidence-Based Practice** boxes in each chapter illustrate the use and application of the latest research findings in public health, community health, and community-oriented nursing.

Canadian boxes, written by practicing Canadian public health nurses, offer the Canadian perspective on community-oriented nursing issues and practice for Canadian readers and promote an international view of nursing care.

**Practice Application** At the end of each chapter a case situation helps students understand how to apply chapter content in the practice setting. Questions at the end of each case promote critical thinking while students analyze the case.

**Key Points** provide a summary listing of the most important points made in the chapter.

**Clinical Decision-Making Activities** promote student learning by suggesting a variety of activities that encourage both independent and collaborative effort.

The back of the book contains the following resources:
- The Appendixes provide additional content resources, key information, and clinical tools and references.
- Answers to Practice Application provide suggested solutions to the Practice Application case scenarios.

## evolve STUDENT LEARNING RESOURCES

Additional resources designed to supplement the student learning process are available on this book's website at http://evolve.elsevier.com/Stanhope, including:
- NEW! **Case Studies** with questions and answers
- **WebLinks** for direct access to websites keyed to specific chapter content
- NEW! **Content Resources** include chapter reference material such as screening tools, assessment questionnaires, and forms
- **Content Updates**
- **Answers to Practice Application questions**

- The **Glossary** offers complete definitions of all key terms and other important community and public health nursing concepts.

## INSTRUCTOR RESOURCES

Several supplemental ancillaries are available to assist instructors in the teaching process:

*Available on CD-ROM:*
- **Instructor's Manual,** with Lecture Outlines, Chapter Summaries, Critical Thinking Activities, and Additional Practice Application questions with answers
- **Computerized Testbank** with 1000 NCLEX-style questions and answers
- **Image Collection** with 70 illustrations from the text
- NEW! **Course Length** and **Integration Guides** help instructors use the textbook in community health nursing courses of varying lengths or when community health nursing is integrated within other nursing courses
- **Answers to Practice Application questions**
- **Glossary** of Key Terms
- **Content Resources** include chapter reference material such as screening tools, assessment questionnaires, and forms

*Available on evolve http://evolve.elsevier.com/Stanhope:*
All of the above **PLUS:**
- NEW! **Instructor's Community,** updated regularly with a variety of teaching strategies and other instructional resources
- NEW! **PowerPoint Lecture Slides** for each chapter
- **WebLinks** for direct access to websites keyed to specific chapter content
- **Content Updates**

## ACKNOWLEDGMENTS

Once again, for this the sixth edition of the text, we would like to thank our families, friends, and colleagues for their support and encouragement in this project. We particularly would like to thank our colleagues at the University of Kentucky College of Nursing and the University of Virginia School of Nursing for their support and assistance. Special thanks go to Linda Thomas and Nancy O'Brien at Elsevier and to Peg Teachey at the University of Kentucky, who have been steadfast and compassionate in their work with us on this edition.

We would also like to thank the contributors for the fifth edition. Their willingness to share their time, talent, and commitment to community-oriented nursing is greatly appreciated: Joyce Bonick, Mary Eure Fisher, Sara Fry, Patricia Howard, Cheryl Jones, Shirleen Lewis-Trabeaux, Carol Loveland-Cherry, Julie Novak, Demetrius Porche, Linda Sawyer, Cheryl Pandolf Shenk, Karen MacDonald Thompson, and Sally Weinrich.

**Marcia Stanhope**
**Jeanette Lancaster**

# Contents

## Part 1

### Perspectives in Health Care and Community-Oriented Nursing, 1

**1 Community-Oriented Population-Focused Practice: The Foundation of Specialization in Public Health Nursing . . . . . . . . . . . . . . . 2**

Public Health Practice: The Foundation for Healthy Populations and Communities, 3
Public Health Nursing as a Field of Practice: An Area of Specialization, 8
Public Health Nursing and Community Health Nursing Versus Community-Based Nursing, 13
Roles in Public Health Nursing, 15
Challenges for the Future, 18

**2 History of Public Health and Public and Community Health Nursing . . . . . . . . . . 22**

Change and Continuity, 22
Historical Measures to Provide for the Public's Health, 24
America's Colonial Period and the New Republic, 24
Nightingale and the Origins of Trained Nursing, 25
America Needs Trained Nurses, 26
School Nursing in America, 29
The Profession Comes of Age, 30
Public Health Nursing in Official Health Agencies, 30
World War I and the Importance of Public Health Nursing, 31
Paying the Bill for Community and Public Health Nurses, 31
Efforts to Shape Public Policy, 31
African-American Nurses in Public Health Nursing, 32
Between the Two World Wars: Economic Depression and the Rise of Hospitals, 33
Increasing Federal Action for the Public's Health, 34
World War II: Extension and Retrenchment in Community and Public Health Nursing, 35
The Rise of Chronic Illness, 36
Failure of Financing for Community-Oriented Nursing, 39
Consolidation of National Nursing Organizations, 39
Professional Nursing Education for Public Health Nursing, 39
New Forms of Payment for Community-Oriented Nursing, 41
Community Organization and Professional Change, 41
Community and Public Health Nursing from the 1970s to the Present, 41
Community and Public Health Nursing Today, 44

**3 Public Health and Primary Health Care Systems and Health Care Transformation . . . . . . . . . . . . . . . . . . . . . . 50**

Current Health Care System in the United States, 51
Trends Affecting the Health Care System, 53
Organization of the Health Care System, 55
Transformation of the Health Care System, 64
A Comprehensive Model: Integration of Public Health and Primary Care, 65

**4 Perspectives on International Health Care . . . . . . . . . . . . . . . . . . . . . . . . 72**

Overview of International Health, 72
The Role of Population Health, 76
Primary Health Care, 77
Nursing and International Health, 78
Major International Health Organizations, 78
International Health and Economic Development, 81
Health Care Systems, 83
Major World Health Problems and the Burden of Disease, 86

## Part 2

### Influences on Health Care Delivery and Community-Oriented Nursing, 96

**5 Economics of Health Care Delivery . . . . 98**

Principles of Economics, 99
The Context of the U.S. Health System, 103
Trends in Health Care Spending, 106
Factors Influencing Health Care Costs, 107
Financing of Health Care, 111
Health Care Payment Systems, 121
Other Factors Affecting Resource Allocation in Health Care, 122
Primary Prevention, 124
Economics and the Future of Community-Oriented Nursing Practice, 125

**6 Ethics in Community-Oriented Nursing Practice . . . . . . . . . . . . . . . . . . . . 130**

History, 131
Key Ethical Terms, 132
Ethical Decision Making, 132
Ethics, 134
Ethics and the Core Functions of Community-Oriented Nursing, 139
Nursing Code of Ethics, 140
Public Health Code of Ethics, 143
Advocacy and Ethics, 143

7 **Cultural Diversity and Community-Oriented Nursing Practice** .......................... 148

Immigrant Health Issues, 149
Culture, Race, and Ethnicity, 152
Cultural Competence, 153
Inhibitors to Developing Cultural Competence, 158
Cultural Nursing Assessment, 160
Variations Among Cultural Groups, 161
Culture and Nutrition, 166
Culture and Socioeconomic Status, 166

8 **Government, the Law, and Policy Activism** ............................. 170

Structure of Government in the United States, 171
Healthy People 2010: An Example of National Health Policy Guidance, 174
Organizations and Agencies That Influence Community Health, 175
Impact of Government Health Functions and Structures on Nursing, 178
The Law and Community-Oriented Nursing, 179
Nursing Practice and Law, 180
Special Community Health Practice Issues and the Law, 181
The Nurse's Role in the Policy Process, 184

**Part 3**

**Conceptual and Scientific Frameworks Applied to Community-Oriented Nursing Practice, 192**

9 **Organizing Frameworks Applied to Community-Oriented Nursing** ........ 194

Developing a Conceptual–Theoretical–Empirical Structure, 195
Using Conceptual Models, 196
Systems Models in Community-Oriented Nursing, 197
Neuman Systems Model, 198
Omaha System, 206
Merging of the Neuman Systems Model and the Omaha System, 212

10 **Environmental Health** ................ 220

Healthy People 2010 Objectives for Environmental Health, 222
Historical Context, 222
Environmental Health Sciences, 224
Assessment, 228
Precautionary Principle, 236
Reducing Environmental Health Risks, 237
Advocacy, 243
Referral Resources, 244
Roles for Nurses in Environmental Health, 244

11 **Epidemiology** ....................... 248

Definitions of Health, 249
Definitions and Descriptions of Epidemiology, 250

Historical Perspectives, 251
Basic Concepts in Epidemiology, 255
Screening, 265
Basic Methods in Epidemiology, 267
Descriptive Epidemiology, 269
Analytic Epidemiology, 271
Experimental Studies, 275
Causality, 276
Applications of Epidemiology in Community-Oriented Nursing, 278

12 **Evidence-Based Practice** .............. 284

History of Evidence-Based Practice, 284
Definitions, 285
Implementing Evidence-Based Practice in Nursing, 286
Barriers to Implementing Evidence-Based Practice in Nursing, 286
Current Perspectives, 287
Future Perspectives, 288
Year 2010 National Healthy People Objectives, 288
Evidence-Based Practice Nursing Application, 290
Nursing Interventions Related to the Core Public Health Functions, 291

13 **Community Health Education: Theories, Models, and Principles** .............. 294

Healthy People 2010 Educational Objectives, 296
Education and Learning, 298
Philosophical Perspectives of Learning, 298
Theories of Learning, 298
Educational Principles, 300
Educational Issues, 306
The Educational Process, 310
The Educational Product, 313

14 **Integrating Multilevel Approaches to Promote Community Health** ......... 318

Shifting the Emphasis From Illness and Disease Management to Wellness, 319
Historical Perspectives, Definitions, and Methods, 322
Application to Community-Oriented Nursing, 331

**Part 4**

**Issues and Approaches in Community-Oriented Health Care, 340**

15 **Community as Client: Assessment and Analysis** ........................ 342

Community Defined, 342
Community as Client, 344
Goals and Means of Community-Oriented Practice, 346
Community-Focused Nursing Process: An Overview of the Process From Assessment to Evaluation, 352
Personal Safety in Community Practice, 370

16  **Community and Public Health Nursing in Rural and Urban Environments ....374**

Historical Overview, 374
Definition of Terms, 375
Current Perspectives, 377
Rural Health Care Delivery Issues and Barriers to Care, 384
Nursing Care in Rural Environments, 385
Future Perspectives, 389
Building Professional–Community–Client Partnerships in Rural Settings, 391

17  **Health Promotion Through Healthy Communities and Cities ..............396**

History of the Healthy Communities and Cities Movement, 397
Definition of Terms, 398
Models of Community Practice, 399
Healthy Communities and Cities, 401
Future of the Healthy Communities and Cities Movement, 406
Implications for Community-Oriented Nursing, 407
Healthy People 2010, 408

18  **The Nursing Center: A Model for Community-Oriented Nursing Practice ...........................412**

What are Nursing Centers?  413
Types of Nursing Centers, 414
Foundations for Nursing Center Development, 419
The Nursing Center Team, 424
The Business Side of Nursing Centers, 430
Evidence-Based Practice: Outcome Data, 434
Education and Research, 436
Positioning Nursing Centers for the Future, 438

19  **Case Management ...................446**

Definitions, 447
Concepts of Case Management, 448
Public Health and Community-Based Examples of Case Management, 455
Essential Skills for Case Managers, 456
Issues in Case Management, 462

20  **Disaster Management ...............470**

Disasters, 470
Three Stages of Disaster Involvement: Preparedness, Response, and Recovery, 472

21  **Program Management ..............490**

Definitions and Goals, 491
Historical Overview of Health Care Planning and Evaluation, 492
Benefits of Program Planning, 493
Assessment of Need, 494
Planning Process, 495

Program Evaluation, 498
Advanced Planning Methods and Evaluation Models, 505
Cost Studies Applied to Program Management, 510
Program Funding, 512

22  **Quality Management .................516**

Definitions and Goals, 519
Historical Development, 520
Approaches to Quality Improvement, 521
TQM/CQI in Community and Public Health Settings, 524
Client Satisfaction, 530
Model QA/QI Program, 531
Records, 534

23  **Group Approaches to Practice ........540**

Group Concepts, 541
Promoting the Health of Individuals Through Group Work, 547
Community Groups and Their Contribution to Community Life, 554
Working With Groups Toward Community Health Goals, 555

**Part 5**

**Health Promotion With Target Populations Across the Life Span, 560**

24  **Family Development and Family Nursing Assessment ..........................562**

Challenges for Community-Oriented Nurses Working With Families, 563
Family Demographics, 565
Definition of Family, 568
Family Health, 569
Four Approaches to Family Nursing, 573
Theoretical Frameworks for Family Nursing, 573
Working With Families for Healthy Outcomes, 578
Barriers to Practicing Family Nursing, 582
Family Nursing Assessment, 583
Social and Family Policy Changes, 586

25  **Family Health Risks ..................594**

Early Approaches to Family Health Risks, 596
Concepts in Family Health Risk, 596
Major Family Health Risks and Nursing Interventions, 599
Community-Oriented Nursing Approaches to Family Health Risk Reduction, 607
Community Resources, 613

26  **Child and Adolescent Health .........616**

Status of Children, 616
Child Development, 617
Nutrition, 626

Immunizations, 630
Major Health Problems, 632
Current Issues, 641
Models for Delivery of Health Care to Vulnerable
    Populations, 644
Progress Toward Child Health: National Health
    Objectives, 645
Role of the Community-Oriented Nurse in Child
    and Adolescent Health, 645

## 27  Women's Health .....................652

Definitions, 652
Historical Perspectives on Women's Health, 653
Health Policy and Legislation, 654
Health, 655
Women's Health Concerns, 657
HIV, AIDS, 667
Health Disparities Among Special Groups
    of Women, 669
Complementary and Alternative Therapies, 672
U.S. Preventive Services Recommendations, 673

## 28  Men's Health ........................680

How Men Define Health, 680
The Health Status of Men in the United States, 681
Male Development, 682
Men's Health and Mortality, 683
Gender Differences, 686
Cultural Differences, 687
Leading Causes of Men's Deaths, 687
Men's Health Practices in Everyday Life, 694
The Community-Oriented Nurse's Role in Men's
    Health, 694

## 29  Health of Older Adults ..............700

Demographics, 700
Definitions, 703
Theories of Aging, 703
Multidimensional Influences on Aging, 704
Components of a Comprehensive Health
    Assessment, 706
Chronic Health Concerns of Older Adults
    in the Community, 707
Community-Based Models for Gerontological
    Nursing, 710
Role Opportunities for Nurses: Health Promotion,
    Disease Prevention, and Wellness, 714

## 30  The Physically Compromised .......720

Definitions and Concepts, 720
Scope of the Problem, 722
Effects of being Physically Compromised, 724
Special Populations, 729
Selected Issues, 730
Healthy People 2010 Objectives, 733
Healthy Cities/Healthy Communities, 734
Role of the Nurse, 735
Legislation, 736

# Part 6

# Vulnerability: Community-Oriented Nursing Issues for the Twenty-first Century, 744

## 31  Vulnerability and Vulnerable Populations: An Overview .........................746

Perspectives on Vulnerability, 746
Public Policies Affecting Vulnerable Populations, 751
Factors Contributing to Vulnerability, 753
Outcomes of Vulnerability, 760
Community-Oriented Nursing Approaches
    to Care, 760
Assessment Issues, 761
Planning and Implementing Care for Vulnerable
    Populations, 763
Evaluation of Nursing Interventions with Vulnerable
    Populations, 769

## 32  Poverty and Homelessness ...........774

Concept of Poverty, 775
Defining and Understanding Poverty, 776
Poverty and Health: Effects Across the Life Span, 778
Understanding the Concept of Homelessness, 783
Effects of Homelessness on Health, 785
Role of the Nurse, 789

## 33  Migrant Health Issues ...............794

Migrant Lifestyle, 795
Health and Health Care, 796
Occupational and Environmental Health Problems, 798
Children and Youths, 800
Cultural Considerations in Migrant Health Care, 801
Health Promotion and Illness Prevention, 802
Role of the Nurse, 802

## 34  Teen Pregnancy .....................808

Adolescent Health Care in the United States, 808
The Adolescent Client, 809
Trends in Adolescent Sexual Behavior and Pregnancy, 810
Background Factors, 811
Young Men and Paternity, 814
Early Identification of the Pregnant Teen, 815
Special Issues in Caring for the Pregnant Teen, 816
Teen Pregnancy and the Nurse, 822

## 35  Mental Health Issues .................826

Scope of Mental Illness in the United States, 827
Systems of Community Mental Health Care, 829
Evolution of Community Mental Health Care, 830
Deinstitutionalization, 832
Conceptual Frameworks for Community Mental
    Health, 833
Role of the Nurse in Community Mental Health, 835
Current and Future Perspectives in Mental Health
    Care, 837
National Objectives for Mental Health Services, 837

**36  Alcohol, Tobacco, and Other Drug
Problems in the Community** ......... 848

ATOD Problems in Perspective, 884
Psychoactive Drugs, 854
Predisposing/Contributing Factors, 859
Primary Prevention and the Role of the Nurse, 860
Secondary Prevention and the Role of the Nurse, 863
Tertiary Prevention and the Role of the Nurse, 866
Outcomes, 870

**37  Violence and Human Abuse** .......... 874

Social and Community Factors Influencing
      Violence, 876
Violence Against Individuals or Oneself, 878
Family Violence and Abuse, 881
Nursing Interventions, 889
Violence and the Prison Population, 895
Clinical Forensic Nursing, 896

**38  Infectious Disease Prevention
and Control** ......................... 902

Historical and Current Perspectives, 903
Transmission of Communicable Diseases, 905
Surveillance of Communicable Diseases, 907
Emerging Infectious Diseases, 908
Prevention and Control of Communicable Diseases, 910
Agents of Bioterrorism, 913
Vaccine-Preventable Diseases, 917
Food-Borne and Waterborne Diseases, 921
Vector-Borne Diseases, 924
Diseases of Travelers, 925
Zoonoses, 926
Parasitic Diseases, 926
Nosocomial Infections, 928
Universal Precautions, 928

**39  Communicable and Infectious Disease
Risks** ............................... 932

Human Immunodeficiency Virus Infection, 932
Sexually Transmitted Diseases, 938
Hepatitis, 944
Tuberculosis, 947
Nurse's Role in Providing Preventive Care
      for Communicable Diseases, 950

**Part 7**

**Community-Oriented Nurses: Roles and
Functions, 960**

**40  Community-Oriented Nurse in Home
Health and Hospice** ................. 962

Definition of Home Health Care, 963
History of Home Health Care, 964
Types of Home Health Care Agencies, 966
Scope of Practice, 968

Standards of Home Health Nursing Practice, 970
Hospice Care, 975
Interdisciplinary Approach to Home Health
      and Hospice Care, 976
Educational Requirements for Home Health
      Practice, 977
Accountability and Quality Management, 978
Financial Aspects of Home Health and Hospice
      Care, 979
Effects of Legislation on Home Health Care
      Services, 981
Legal and Ethical Issues, 982
Trends in Home Health Care, 983
Issues for the Twenty-First Century, 983

**41  The Advanced Practice Nurse
in the Community** ................... 990

Historical Perspective, 990
Educational Preparation, 992
Credentialing, 992
Advanced Practice Roles, 993
Arenas for Practice, 996
Issues and Concerns, 1001
Role Stress, 1002
Trends in Advanced Practice Nursing, 1003

**42  Community-Oriented Nurse Leader
and Consultant** .................... 1008

Major Trends and Issues, 1009
Definitions, 1012
Leadership and Management, 1012
Consultation, 1017
Competencies for Community-Oriented Nursing
      Leadership: Management, and Consultation, 1025

**43  Community-Oriented Nurse
in the Schools** .................... 1042

History of School Nursing, 1042
Standards of Practice for School Nurses, 1045
Educational Credentials of School Nurses, 1045
Roles and Functions of School Nurses, 1046
School Health Services, 1048
School Nurses and Healthy People 2010, 1049
The Levels of Prevention in the Schools, 1049
Controversies in School Nursing, 1061
Ethics in School Nursing, 1062
Future Trends in School Nursing, 1062

**44  Community-Oriented Nurse
in Occupational Health** ............. 1066

Definition and Scope of Occupational Health
      Nursing, 1067
History and Evolution of Occupational Health
      Nursing, 1067
Roles and Professionalism in Occupational Health
      Nursing, 1068
Workers as a Population Aggregate, 1070
Application of the Epidemiologic Model, 1074

Organizational and Public Efforts to Promote Worker Health and Safety, 1080
Nursing Care of Working Populations, 1081
Healthy People 2010 Related to Occupational Health, 1086
Legislation Related to Occupational Health, 1086
Disaster Planning and Management, 1087

## 45 Community-Oriented Nurse as Parish Nurse ................... 1092

Definitions in Parish Nursing, 1093
Heritage and Horizons, 1094
Parish Nursing Practice, 1099
Issues in Parish Nursing Practice, 1105
Healthy People 2010 Leading Health Indicators and Faith Communities, 1106
Population-Focused Parish Nursing: Faith Community and School, 1108

## 46 Public Health Nursing at the Local, State, and National Levels ........... 1114

Roles of Local, State, and Federal Public Health Agencies, 1114
History and Trends of Public Health, 1116
Scope, Standards, and Roles of Public Health Nursing, 1117
Issues and Trends in Public Health Nursing, 1119
Models of Public Health Nursing Practice, 1121
Education and Knowledge Requirements for Public Health Nurses, 1121
Certification for Public Health Nursing, 1122
National Health Objectives, 1122
Functions of Public Health Nurses, 1123

**Answers to Practice Application Questions .. P-1**


# Appendixes

## *A International/National Agendas for Health Care Delivery

A.1 Schedule of Clinical Preventive Services
A.2 Select Major Historical Events Depicting Financial Involvement of Federal Government in Health Care Delivery
A.3 Declaration of Alma Ata

## *B Community-Oriented Nursing Resources

## *C Contracts and Forms: Samples

C.1 Community-Oriented Health Record (COHR)
C.2 The Living Will Directive
C.3 OASIS: Start of Care Assessment

## *D Drug Immunization Information

D.1 Immunizing Agents and Immunization Schedules for Health Care Workers
D.2 Herbs and Supplements Used for Children and Adolescents

## *E Screening Tools

E.1 Vision and Hearing Screening Procedures
E.2 Screening for Common Orthopedic Problems

## F Health Risk Appraisal ................ A-3

F.1 Lifestyle Assessment Questionnaire, A-3
F.2 Healthier People Health Risk Appraisal, A-13
F.3 1999 Youth Risk Behavior Survey, A-21

## G Community Assessment Tools ....... A-27

G.1 Community-As-Partner Model, A-27

## H Family Assessment Tools ............ A-29

*H.1 Family Systems Stressor-Strength Inventory (FS3I)
H.2 Friedman Family Assessment Model (Short Form), A-29
*H.3 Case Example of Family Assessment

## I Individual Assessment Tools ........ A-31

I.1 Instrumental Activities of Daily Living (IADL) Scale, A-31
I.2 Comprehensive Older Persons' Evaluation, A-32
I.3 Comprehensive Occupational and Environmental Health History, A-35

## J Essential Elements of Public Health Nursing ........................... A-39

J.1 Examples of Public Health Nursing Roles and Implementing Public Health Functions, A-39
J.2 Public Health Guidelines for Practice, A-45
J.3 Core Competencies and Skill Levels for Public Health Nursing, A-47

---

*These appendixes can be found on the evolve website at http://evolve.elsevier.com/Stanhope*

---

*The Glossary can be found on the evolve website at http://evolve.elsevier.com/Stanhope*

# Part 1

Perspectives in
Health Care and
Community-Oriented
Nursing

Since the late 1800s, public health nurses have been leaders in making many improvements in the quality of health care for individuals, families, and aggregates including populations and communities. As nurses around the world meet and learn about one another, it is clear that, from one country to another, community-oriented nursing has more similarities than differences.

Important changes in health care occurred during the 1990s. The federal initiative to reform health care and initiate a national plan failed. This led to a shift of health care from the control of hospitals and health care professionals to control by insurers, investors, and venture capitalists. The positive aspects of the proposed health care reform plan were largely lost in the scramble for groups to carve out a market share and develop profitable systems of health care delivery.

The public health system, as a subset of the overall health care system, has been affected by the changes in health care organization, ownership, and financing. Specifically, public health is returning to its roots in the traditional core functions and moving away from providing primary care. If community-oriented nurses are to be effective in promoting the health of people, they must understand the history of public health nursing and the current status of the public health system.

Part 1 presents information about significant factors affecting health in the United States. Some contrasts and comparisons in health care are made to health care in Canada. Playing an instrumental role in changing the level and quality of services and the priorities for funding requires informed, courageous, and committed nurses. The chapters in Part 1 are designed to provide essential information so that community-oriented nurses can make a difference in health care by understanding their own roles and their functions in community-focused practice, and by understanding how the public health system differs from the primary care system.

Explanations are offered about exactly what it is that makes community and public health nursing unique. Often, community and public health nursing is confused with community-based nursing practice. There is a core of knowledge known as "public health" that forms the foundation for community and public health nursing. Working with people in the community is not necessarily community health or public health nursing. Community-oriented nursing practice involves more than the care of a person or family whose care has been moved from the hospital to the community.

# Chapter 1

*evolve* http://evolve.elsevier.com/Stanhope

# Community-Oriented Population-Focused Practice: The Foundation of Specialization in Public Health Nursing

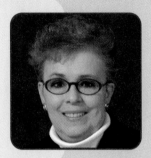

**Carolyn A. Williams, R.N., Ph.D., F.A.A.N.**

Dr. Carolyn A. Williams is Dean and Professor at the College of Nursing at the University of Kentucky, Lexington, Kentucky. Dr. Williams has held many leadership roles, including President of the American Academy of Nursing; membership on the U. S. Preventive Services Task Force, Department of Health and Human Services; and President of the American Association of Colleges of Nursing. She received the Distinguished Alumna Award from Texas Woman's University in 1983, and in 2001 she was the recipient of the Mary Tolle Wright Founder's Award for Excellence in Leadership from Sigma Theta Tau International.

## Objectives

After reading this chapter, the student should be able to do the following:

1. State the mission and core functions of public health and the essential public health services
2. Describe specialization in public health nursing and community health nursing, and the practice goals of each
3. Contrast clinical community health nursing practice with population-focused practice
4. Describe what is meant by population-focused practice
5. Name barriers to acceptance of population-focused practice
6. State key opportunities for population-focused practice

---

The twenty-first century has begun and the United States continues to grapple with ways to improve the health of the American people. The goal is to improve the functioning of the many public and private organizations involved in health care and health-related activities. Despite the failure of the efforts to make fundamental changes in health care through the twentieth century, private market forces and federal and state initiatives are bringing about changes in the health care system. With the changes have come new concerns about the growth of managed care, access to care, the ability to maintain affordable insurance coverage, quality of services, new warnings about possible increases in costs, and bioterrorism. Because of these factors, the goals of protecting health, promoting health, and preventing disease and disability, and the role of public health in achieving these goals, have gained new meaning. In short, there has been a renewed interest in public health and in population-focused thinking about health and health care in the United States.

Although populations have historically been the focus of public health practice, populations are also the focus of the "business" of **managed care.** Thus public health prac-

titioners and managed care executives are both population oriented. Increasingly, managed care executives and program managers are using the basic sciences and analytic tools of the field of public health. They focus particularly on epidemiology and statistics to develop databases and approaches to making decisions at the level of a defined population or subpopulation. Thus a population-focused approach to planning, delivering, and evaluating nursing care has never been more important.

This is a crucial time for public health nursing, a time of opportunity and challenge. The issue of growing costs together with the changing demography of the United States population, such as the aging of the population, is expected to put increased demands on resources available for health care. In addition, the threats of bioterrorism, highlighted by the events of September 11, 2001, and the anthrax scares, will divert health care funds and resources from other health care programs to be spent for public safety. Also important to the public health community is the emergence of modern-day epidemics and infectious diseases, such as the mosquito-borne West Nile virus and other causes of mortality, many of which affect the very

## Key Terms

**aggregate**, p. 10
**assessment**, p. 6
**assurance**, p. 6
**capitation**, p. 18
**community-based nursing**, p. 15
**Community Health Improvement Process**, p. 7

**community health nurse**, p. 14
**cottage industry**, p. 18
**integrated systems**, p. 18
**managed care**, p. 2
**policy development**, p. 6
**population**, p. 10
**population-focused practice**, p. 10

**public health**, p. 6
**public health core functions**, p. 6
**public health nursing**, p. 9
**Quad Council**, p. 7
**subpopulation**, p. 10
*See Glossary for definitions*

## Chapter Outline

Public Health Practice: The Foundation for Healthy Populations and Communities
*Definitions in Public Health*
*Public Health Core Functions*
*Core Competencies of Public Health Professionals*
Public Health Nursing as a Field of Practice: An Area of Specialization

*Educational Preparation for Public Health Nursing*
*Population-Focused Practice Versus Practice Focused on Individuals*
*Public Health Nursing Specialists and Core Public Health Functions: Selected Examples*
Public Health Nursing and Community Health Nursing Versus Community-Based Nursing

Roles in Public Health Nursing
Challenges for the Future
*Barriers to Specializing in Public Health Nursing*
*Establishing Population-Focused Nurse Leaders*

young. Most of the causes are preventable. What has all of this to do with nursing? Understanding the importance of community-oriented, population-focused nursing practice and developing the knowledge and skills to practice it will be critical to attaining a leadership role in health care regardless of the practice setting. Those who practice population-focused nursing in the context of community-based populations will be in a strong position to affect the health of populations and the decisions about how scarce resources will be used.

## PUBLIC HEALTH PRACTICE: THE FOUNDATION FOR HEALTHY POPULATIONS AND COMMUNITIES

In the last decade of the twentieth century, attention was focused on proposals to reform the American health care system. These proposals focused primarily on containing cost in medical care financing. They also focused on strategies for providing health insurance coverage to a higher portion of the population. Because medical treatment is estimated to account for up to 97% of all health expenses (U.S. Department of Health and Human Services [USDHHS],

2002), it is understandable that changes in health insurance would be the emphasis. However, many times the most benefit from the least cost is sought in the wrong place. As stated in the Public Health Services Steering Committee Report on the Core Functions of Public Health (1994), reform of the medical insurance system was thought to be necessary, but it was not adequate to improve the health of Americans.

Historically, gains in the health of populations have come largely from public health changes. Safety and adequacy of food supplies, the provision of safe water, sewage disposal, public safety from biological threats, and personal behavioral changes including reproductive behavior are a few examples of public health's influence. The dramatic increase in life expectancy for Americans during the 1900s, from less than 50 years in 1900 to more than 77 years in 2002, is credited primarily to improvements in sanitation, the control of infectious diseases through immunizations, and other public health activities (USDHHS, 2002). Population-based preventive programs launched in the 1970s are also largely responsible for the more recent changes in tobacco use, blood pressure control, dietary patterns (except obesity), automobile safety restraint, and injury control measures that have fostered declines in adult mortality rates up to 50% with declines in stroke and coronary heart disease deaths. Overall death rates for children have declined by 50% (USDHHS, 2002).

Another way of looking at the benefits of public health practice is to look at how early deaths can be prevented. The U.S. Public Health Service estimates that medical treatment can prevent only about 10% of all early deaths in the United States. However, population-wide public health approaches have the potential to help prevent some 70% of early deaths in America through measures targeted to the factors that contribute to those deaths. Many of these contributing factors are behavioral, such as tobacco use, diet, and sedentary lifestyle. Other factors that affect health are the environment, social conditions, culture, economics, working conditions, and housing (Institute of Medicine [IOM], 2003).

**DID YOU KNOW?**

The concept of using a population (or aggregate) approach in the practice of health nursing began to be seriously discussed in the 1970s.

Public health practice is of great value. The U.S. Public Health Service estimated in 2000 that only 3.4% (up from 1.5% in 1960) of all national health expenditures support population-focused public health functions, yet the impact is enormous. (Unfortunately, the public is largely unaware of the contributions of public health practice.) Federal and private monies were sought to support public health, so public health agencies began to provide personal care services for persons who could not receive care elsewhere. The health departments benefited

**Figure 1-1** Public health in America. *(From U.S. Public Health Service:* The core functions project, update 2000, *Washington, DC, 1994, Office of Disease Prevention and Health Promotion.)*

---

**PUBLIC HEALTH IN AMERICA**

**Vision:**
Healthy people in healthy communities

**Mission:**
Promote physical and mental health and prevent disease, injury, and disability

**Public health**
- Prevents epidemics and the spread of disease
- Protects against environmental hazards
- Prevents injuries
- Promotes and encourages healthy behaviors
- Responds to disasters and assists communities in recovery
- Ensures the quality and accessibility of health services

**Essential public health services by core function**
*Assessment*
1. Monitor health status to identify community health problems
2. Diagnose and investigate health problems and health hazards in the community

*Policy Development*
3. Inform, educate, and empower people about health issues
4. Mobilize community partnerships to identify and solve health problems
5. Develop policies and plans that support individual and community health efforts

*Assurance*
6. Enforce laws and regulations that protect health and ensure safety
7. Link people to needed personal health services and assure the provision of health care when otherwise unavailable.
8. Ensure a competent public health and personal health care workforce
9. Evaluate effectiveness, accessibility, and quality of personal and population-based health services

*Serving All Functions*
a. Research for new insights and innovative solutions to health problems

by getting Medicaid and Medicare funds. The result has been a shift of resources and energy away from public health's traditional and unique population-focused perspective (USDHHS, 2002).

Because of the importance of influencing a population's health and providing a strong foundation for the health care system, the U.S. Public Health Service and other groups strongly advocate a renewed emphasis on the population-focused essential public health functions and services, which have been most effective in improving the health of the entire population. As part

of this effort, a statement on public health in America was developed by a working group made up of representatives of federal agencies and organizations concerned about public health (Figure 1-1). The list of essential services presented in Figure 1-1 represents the obligations of the public health system to implement the core functions of assessment, assurance, and policy development. The How To box further explains these essential services and lists the ways public health nurses implement them (U.S. Public Health Service, 1994/ update 2000).

---

**HOW TO  Participate, as a Public Health Nurse, in the Essential Services of Public Health**

1. Monitor health status to identify community health problems.
   - Participate in community assessment.
   - Identify subpopulations at risk for disease or disability.
   - Collect information on interventions to special populations.
   - Define and evaluate effective strategies and programs.
   - Identify potential environmental hazards.
2. Diagnose and investigate health problems and hazards in the community.
   - Understand and identify determinants of health and disease.
   - Apply knowledge about environmental influences of health.
   - Recognize multiple causes or factors of health and illness.
   - Participate in case identification and treatment of persons with communicable disease.
3. Inform, educate, and empower people about health issues.
   - Develop health and educational plans for individuals and families in multiple settings.
   - Develop and implement community-based health education.
   - Provide regular reports on health status of special populations within clinic settings, community settings, and groups.
   - Advocate for and with underserved and disadvantaged populations.
   - Ensure health planning, which includes primary prevention and early intervention strategies.
   - Identify healthy population behaviors and maintain successful intervention strategies through reinforcement and continued funding.

4. Mobilize community partnerships to identify and solve health problems.
   - Interact regularly with many providers and services within each community.
   - Convene groups and providers who share common concerns and interests in special populations.
   - Provide leadership to prioritize community problems and development of interventions.
   - Explain the significance of health issues to the public and participate in developing plans of action.
5. Develop policies and plans that support individual and community health efforts.
   - Participate in community and family decision-making processes.
   - Provide information and advocacy for consideration of the interests of special groups in program development.
   - Develop programs and services to meet the needs of high-risk populations as well as broader community members.
   - Participate in disaster planning and mobilization of community resources in emergencies.
   - Advocate for appropriate funding for services.
6. Enforce laws and regulations that protect health and ensure safety.
   - Regulate and support safe care and treatment for dependent populations such as children and frail older adults.
   - Implement ordinances and laws that protect the environment.
   - Establish procedures and processes that ensure competent implementation of treatment schedules for diseases of public health importance.
   - Participate in development of local regulations that protect communities and the environment from potential hazards and pollution.

---

From the Association of State and Territorial Directors of Nursing: *Public health nursing: a partner for healthy populations,* Washington, DC, 2000, ASTDN.

*Continued*

**HOW TO** Participate, as a Public Health Nurse, in the Essential Services of Public Health—cont'd

7. Link people to needed personal health services and ensure the provision of health care that is otherwise unavailable.
   - Provide clinical preventive services to certain high-risk populations.
   - Establish programs and services to meet special needs.
   - Recommend clinical care and other services to clients and their families in clinics, homes, and the community.
   - Provide referrals through community links to needed care.
   - Participate in community provider coalitions and meetings to educate others and to identify service centers for community populations.
   - Provide clinical surveillance and identification of communicable disease.
8. Ensure a competent public health and personal health care workforce.
   - Participate in continuing education and preparation to ensure competence.
   - Define and support proper delegation to unlicensed assistive personnel in community settings.
   - Establish standards for performance.
   - Maintain client record systems and community documents.
   - Establish and maintain procedures and protocols for client care.
   - Participate in quality assurance activities such as record audits, agency evaluation, and clinical guidelines.
9. Evaluate effectiveness, accessibility, and quality of personal and population-based health services.
   - Collect data and information related to community interventions.
   - Identify unserved and underserved populations within the community.
   - Review and analyze data on health status of the community.
   - Participate with the community in assessment of services and outcomes of care.
   - Identify and define enhanced services required to manage health status of complex populations and special risk groups.
10. Research for new insights and innovative solutions to health problems.
    - Implement nontraditional interventions and approaches to effect change in special populations.
    - Participate in the collecting of information and data to improve the surveillance and understanding of special problems.
    - Develop collegial relationships with academic institutions to explore new interventions.
    - Participate in early identification of factors that are detrimental to the community's health.
    - Formulate and use investigative tools to identify and impact care delivery and program planning.

From the Association of State and Territorial Directors of Nursing: *Public health nursing: a partner for healthy populations,* Washington, DC, 2000, ASTDN.

## Definitions in Public Health

In 1988 the Institute of Medicine published a report on the future of public health. In the report, **public health** was defined as "what we, as a society, do collectively to assure the conditions in which people can be healthy" (IOM, 1988, p. 1). The committee stated that the mission of public health was "to generate organized community effort to address the public interest in health by applying scientific and technical knowledge to prevent disease and promote health" (IOM, 1988, p. 1; Williams, 1995).

It was clearly noted that the mission could be accomplished by many groups, public and private, and by individuals. However, the government has a special function "to see to it that vital elements are in place and that the mission is adequately addressed" (IOM, 1988, p. 7). To clarify the government's role in fulfilling the mission, the report stated that assessment, policy development, and assurance are the **public health core functions** at all levels of government.

- **Assessment** refers to systematic data collection on the population, monitoring of the population's health status, and making information available on the health of the community.
- **Policy development** refers to the need to provide leadership in developing policies that support the health of the population, including the use of the scientific knowledge base in making decisions about policy.
- **Assurance** refers to the role of public health in making sure that essential community-oriented health services are available, which may include providing essential personal health services for those who would otherwise not receive them. Assurance also refers to making sure that a competent public health and personal health care workforce is available.

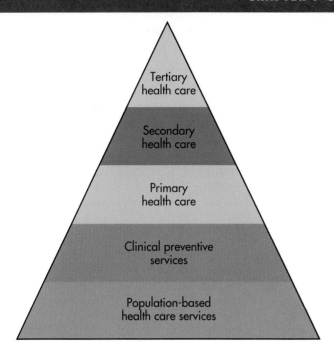

**Figure 1-2** Health services pyramid.

## Public Health Core Functions

The Core Functions Project (U.S. Public Health Service, 1994/2000) developed a useful illustration, the Health Services Pyramid (Figure 1-2), that shows that population-based public health programs support the goals of providing a foundation for clinical prevention services. These services focus on disease prevention, on health promotion and protection, and on primary, secondary, and tertiary health care services. All levels of services shown in the pyramid are important to the health of the population and thus must be part of a health care system with health as a goal. It has been said that "the greater the effectiveness of services in the lower tiers, the greater is the capability of higher tiers to contribute efficiently to health improvement" (U.S. Public Health Service, 1994/2000). Because of the importance of the basic public health programs, members of the Core Functions Project argued that all levels of health care, including the population-based public health care, must be funded or the goal of health of populations may never be reached.

Several new efforts to enable public health practitioners to be more effective in implementing the core functions of assessment, policy development, and assurance have been undertaken at the national level. In 1997 the Institute of Medicine published *Improving Health in the Community: A Role for Performance Monitoring* (Institute of Medicine, 1997). This monograph was the product of an interdisciplinary committee, co-chaired by a public health nursing specialist and a physician, whose purpose was to determine how a performance monitoring system could be developed and used to improve community health.

The major outcome of the committee's work was the **Community Health Improvement Process** (CHIP), a method for improving the health of the population on a community-wide basis. The method brings together key elements of the public health and personal health care systems in one framework. A second outcome of the project was the development of a set of 25 indicators that could be used in the community assessment process (see Chapter 15) to develop a community health profile (e.g., measures of health status, functional status, quality of life, health risk factors, and health resource use) (Box 1-1). A third product of the committee's work was a set of indicators for specific public health problems that could be used by public health specialists as they carry out their assurance function and monitor the performance of public health and other agencies.

The Centers for Disease Control and Prevention (CDC) established a Task Force on Community Preventive Services (CDC, 2000). The Task Force is working to collect evidence on the effectiveness of a variety of community interventions to prevent morbidity and mortality. This document will be a population-focused guide to providing services, much like the *Guide to Clinical Preventive Services* for personal care—the report of the U.S. Preventive Services Task Force (2000) (see Appendix A.1 for Schedule of Preventive Services). These efforts are important because they provide tools for public health practitioners, many of whom are public health nursing specialists, to enable them to be more effective in dealing with the core functions.

## Core Competencies of Public Health Professionals

To improve the public health workforce's abilities to implement the core functions of public health and to ensure that the workforce has the necessary skills to provide the 10 essential services listed in Figure 1-1, a group of academics and public health practitioners came together to form the *Council on Linkages*. This council, over a 10-year period, worked with the U.S. Public Health Service to develop a list of competencies for all public health practitioners, including nurses (Council on Linkages, 2001). The 34 competencies are divided among eight categories (Box 1-2). Furthermore, three levels of skill *(awareness, knowledge, proficiency)* are assigned to each competency on the basis of the public health job requirements. It is recommended that these categories of competencies be used for curriculum review and development, workforce needs assessment, competency development, performance evaluation, hiring, and refining of the personnel system job requirements (Council on Linkages, 2001).

A group of public health nursing organizations called the **Quad Council** has developed levels of skills to be attained by public health nurses for each of the competencies. Skill levels are specified for the generalist/staff nurse and the specialist in public health nursing (Quad Council, 1999). See Appendix I.3 for the Public Health Nursing Competencies and Skill Levels.

## THE CUTTING EDGE

The Council on Linkages (2001) developed a set of competencies for all public health professionals. The Quad Council developed skill levels for each of 34 competencies needed by public health nurses.

---

Council on Linkages Between Academia and Public Health Practice: *Core competencies for public health professional,* Washington, DC, 2001, Public Health Foundation/Health Resources and Services Administration; Quad Council of Public Health Nursing Organizations: *Scope and standards of public health nursing practice,* Washington, DC, 1999, American Nurses Association.

## PUBLIC HEALTH NURSING AS A FIELD OF PRACTICE: AN AREA OF SPECIALIZATION

What is public health nursing? Is it really a specialty, and if so, why? Public health nursing is a specialty because it has a distinct focus and scope of practice, and it requires a special knowledge base. The following characterizations distinguish public health nursing as a specialty:

- *It is population focused.* Primary emphasis is on populations whose members are free-living in the community as opposed to those who are institutionalized.
- *It is community oriented.* There is concern for the connection between the health status of the population and the environment in which the population lives (physical, biological, sociocultural). There is an imperative to work with members of the community to carry out core public health functions.

---

**BOX 1-1   Indicators Used to Develop a Community Health Profile**

### SOCIODEMOGRAPHIC CHARACTERISTICS

- Distribution of the population by age and race/ethnicity
- Number and proportion of persons in groups such as migrants, homeless, or the non-English speaking, for whom access to community services and resources may be a concern
- Number and proportion of persons aged 25 and older with less than a high school education
- Ratio of the number of students graduating from high school to the number of students who entered ninth grade 3 years previously
- Median household income
- Proportion of children less than 15 years of age living in families at or below the poverty level
- Unemployment rate
- Number and proportion of single-parent families
- Number and proportion of persons without health insurance

### HEALTH STATUS

- Infant mortality rate by race/ethnicity
- Numbers of deaths or age-adjusted death rates for motor vehicle crashes, work-related injuries, suicide, homicide, lung cancer, breast cancer, cardiovascular diseases, and all causes, by age, race, and sex as appropriate
- Reported incidence of AIDS, measles, tuberculosis, and primary and secondary syphilis, by age, race, and sex as appropriate
- Births to adolescents (ages 10 to 17) as a proportion of total live births
- Number and rate of confirmed abuse and neglect cases among children

### HEALTH RISK FACTORS

- Proportion of 2-year-old children who have received all age-appropriate vaccines, as recommended by the Advisory Committee on Immunization Practices
- Proportion of adults aged 65 and older who have ever been immunized for pneumococcal pneumonia; proportion who have been immunized in the past 12 months for influenza
- Proportion of the population who smoke, by age, race, and sex as appropriate
- Proportion of the population aged 18 and older who are obese
- Number and type of U.S. Environmental Protection Agency air quality standards not met
- Proportion of assessed rivers, lakes, and estuaries that support beneficial uses (e.g., approved fishing and swimming)

### HEALTH CARE RESOURCE CONSUMPTION

- Per capita health care spending for Medicare beneficiaries—the Medicare adjusted average per capita cost (AAPCC)

### FUNCTIONAL STATUS

- Proportion of adults reporting that their general health is good to excellent
- Average number of days (in the past 30 days) for which adults report that their physical or mental health was not good

### QUALITY OF LIFE

- Proportion of adults satisfied with the health care system in the community
- Proportion of persons satisfied with the quality of life in the community

- *There is a health and preventive focus.* The primary emphasis is on strategies for health promotion, health maintenance, and disease prevention, particularly primary and secondary prevention.
- *Interventions are made at the community or population level.* Political processes are used as a major intervention strategy to affect public policy and achieve goals.
- *There is concern for the health of all members of the population/community, particularly vulnerable subpopulations.*

---
( **NURSING TIP**
---

The primary features of the public health specialty are population focus, community orientation, emphasis on health promotion and disease prevention, and concern for and interventions at a population level.

---

In 1981 the public health nursing section of the American Public Health Association (APHA) developed the *Definition and Role of Public Health Nursing in the Delivery of Health Care* to describe the field of specialization. This statement was reaffirmed in 1996 (APHA, 1996). In 1999, The American Nurses Association, with input from three other nursing organizations—the Public Health Nursing Section of the American Public Health Association, the Association of State and Territorial Directors of Public Health Nursing, and the Association of Community Health Nurse Educators—published a statement on the *Scope and Standards of Public Health Nursing Practice* (Quad Council, 1999). In this document, the 1996 definition was supported. **Public health nursing** is defined as the practice of promoting and protecting the health of populations using knowledge from nursing, social, and public health sciences (APHA, 1996). Public health nursing is further described as population-focused, community-oriented nursing practice that emphasizes the prevention of disease and disability (Quad Council, 1999). Public health nursing practice takes place through assessment, policy development, and assurance activities of nurses working in partnerships with nations, states, communities, organizations, groups, and individuals. Nurses are expected to have organizational and political skills along with nursing and pub-

---

**BOX 1-2  Categories of Public Health Workforce Competencies**

- Analytic/assessment
- Policy development/program planning
- Communication
- Cultural competency
- Community dimensions of practice
- Basic public health services
- Financial planning and management
- Leadership and systems thinking

---

lic health knowledge to assess the needs and strengths of the population, design interventions to mobilize resources for action, and promote equity of opportunity for health (see Appendix I.1) (National Association of County and City Health Officials, 1994).

## Educational Preparation for Public Health Nursing

Targeted and specialized education for public health nursing practice has a long history. In the late 1950s and early 1960s, before the integration of public health concepts into the curriculum of baccalaureate nursing programs, special baccalaureate curricula were established in several schools of public health to prepare nurses to become public health nurses. (Today it is generally assumed that a graduate of any baccalaureate nursing program has the necessary basic preparation to function as a beginning staff public health nurse.)

Since the late 1960s, public health nursing leaders have agreed that a specialty in public health nursing requires a master's degree. Today, a master's degree in nursing is necessary to be eligible to sit for a certification examination. Perhaps because of the absence of a certification examination specifically for public health nursing, a master's degree for the specialty has not been widely recognized or required. The educational expectations for public health nursing were highlighted at the 1984 Consensus Conference on the Essentials of Public Health Nursing Practice and Education sponsored by the U.S. Department of Health and Human Services (USDHHS) Division of Nursing. The participants agreed "that the term 'public health nurse' should be used to describe a person who has received specific educational preparation and supervised clinical practice in public health nursing" (Consensus Conference, 1985, p. 4). At the basic or entry level, a public health nurse is one who "holds a baccalaureate degree in nursing that includes this educational preparation; this nurse may or may not practice in an official health agency but has the initial qualifications to do so" (Consensus Conference, 1985, p. 4). Specialists in public health nursing are defined as those who are prepared at the graduate level, with either a master's or a doctoral degree, "with a focus in the public health sciences" (Consensus Conference, 1985, p. 4) (Box 1-3). The consensus statement specifically pointed out that the public health nursing specialist "should be able to work with population groups and to assess and intervene successfully at the aggregate level" (Consensus Conference, 1985, p. 11).

Today, the Association of Community Health Nursing Educators reaffirms the results of the 1984 Consensus Conference (Association of Community Health Nursing Educators, 2000).

## Population-Focused Practice Versus Practice Focused on Individuals

The key factor that distinguishes public health nursing from other areas of nursing practice is the focus on populations, a focus historically consistent with public health philosophy. Although public health nursing is based on

---

> **BOX 1-3** Areas Considered Essential for the Preparation of Specialists in Public Health Nursing
>
> • Epidemiology
> • Biostatistics
> • Nursing theory
> • Management theory
> • Change theory
> • Economics
> • Politics
> • Public health administration
> • Community assessment
> • Program planning and evaluation
> • Interventions at the aggregate level
> • Research
> • History of public health
> • Issues in public health
>
> ---
>
> Consensus Conference on the Essentials of Public Health Nursing Practice and Education, Rockville, Md, 1985, U.S. Department of Health and Human Services, Bureau of Health Professions, Division of Nursing.

> **BOX 1-4** Prevention Levels, With Examples, in Public Health
>
> **PRIMARY PREVENTION**
> The public health nurse develops a health education program for a population of school-age children that teaches them about the effects of smoking on health.
>
> **SECONDARY PREVENTION**
> The public health nurse provides an influenza vaccination program in a community retirement village.
>
> **TERTIARY PREVENTION**
> The public health nurse provides a diabetes clinic for a defined population of adults in a low-income housing unit of the community.

clinical nursing practice, it is different. It may be helpful here to define the term *population.*

A **population** or **aggregate** is a collection of individuals who have one or more personal or environmental characteristics in common. Members of a community who can be defined in terms of geography (e.g., a county, a group of counties, a state) or in terms of a special interest (e.g., children attending a particular school) can be seen as constituting a population. Often there are **subpopulations** within the larger population—for example, high-risk infants under the age of 1 year, unmarried pregnant adolescents, or individuals exposed to a particular event such as a chemical spill. In **population-focused practice,** problems are defined (by assessments or diagnoses), and solutions (interventions), such as policy development or providing a particular preventive service, are implemented for or with a defined population or subpopulation (Box 1-4). In other nursing specialties, the diagnoses, interventions, and treatments are carried out at the individual client level.

Professional education in nursing, medicine, and other clinical disciplines focuses primarily on developing competence in decision making at the individual client level by assessing health status, making management decisions (ideally *with* the client), and evaluating the effects of care. Figure 1-3 illustrates three levels at which problems can be identified. For example, community-based nurse clinicians, nurse practitioners, and sometimes community-oriented nurses focus on individuals they see in either a home or a clinic setting. The focus is on an individual per-

son or an individual family in a subpopulation (the C arrows in Figure 1-3). The provider's emphasis is on defining and resolving a problem for the individual; the client is an individual.

In Figure 1-3, the individual clients are grouped into three separate subpopulations, each of which has a common characteristic (the B arrows). Public health nursing specialists often define problems at the population or aggregate level as opposed to an individual level. Population-level decision making is different from decision making in clinical care. For example, in a clinical, direct care situation, the community-oriented nurse may determine that a client is hypertensive and explore options for intervening. However, at the population level, the public health nursing specialist might explore the answers to the following set of questions:

1. What is the prevalence of hypertension among various age, race, and sex groups?
2. Which subpopulations have the highest rates of untreated hypertension?
3. What programs could reduce the problem of untreated hypertension and thereby lower the risk of further cardiovascular morbidity and mortality?

Public health nursing specialists are usually concerned with more than one subpopulation and frequently with the health of the entire community (in Figure 1-3, arrow A: the entire box containing all of the subgroups within the community). In reality, of course, there are many more subgroups than those in the figure. Professionals concerned with the health of a whole community must consider the total population, which is made up of multiple and often overlapping subpopulations. For example, the population of adolescents at risk for unplanned pregnancies would overlap with the female population 15 to 24 years of age. A population that would overlap with infants under 1 year of age would be children from 0 to 6 years of age. In addition, a population focus requires considering those who may need particular services but have not entered the health care system (e.g., children without immunizations or clients with untreated hypertension).

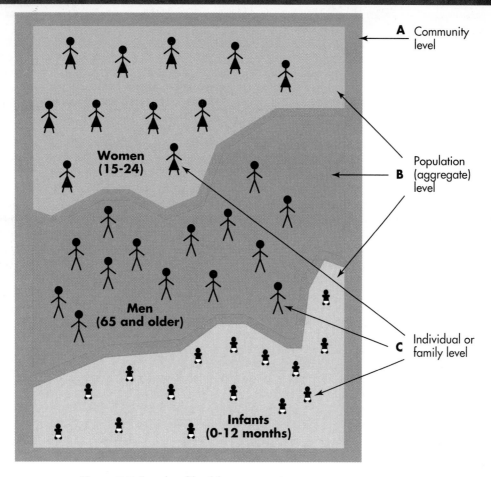

**Figure 1-3** Levels of health care practice.

## Public Health Nursing Specialists and Core Public Health Functions: Selected Examples

The core public health function of assessment includes activities that involve the collecting, analyzing, and disseminating of information on both the health and health-related aspects of a community or a specific population. Questions such as whether the health services of the community are available to the population and are adequate to address needs are considered. Assessment also includes an ongoing effort to monitor the health status of the community or population and the services provided. Excellent examples of assessment at the national level are the efforts of the USDHHS to organize the goal setting, data collecting and analysis, and monitoring necessary to develop the series of publications describing the health status and health-related aspects of the U.S. population. These efforts began with *Healthy People* in 1980 and continued with *Promoting Health, Preventing Disease: 1990 Health Objectives for the Nation* and *Healthy People 2000.* They are now moving into the future with *Healthy People 2010* (USDHHS, 2000).

Many states and other jurisdictions have developed publications describing the health status of a defined commu-

nity, a set of communities, or populations. Unfortunately, it is difficult to find published descriptions of health assessments on particular communities unless they demonstrate new methods or reveal unusual findings about a community. Such working documents and datasets should be available in specific settings, such as a county or state health department, and should be used by public health practitioners to develop services.

A survey was conducted to determine the extent to which local health departments were performing the core public health functions. The questions asked about *assessment* included (1) whether there was a needs assessment process in place that described the health status of the community and community needs, (2) whether there had been a survey of behavioral risk factors within the last 3 years, and (3) whether an analysis had been done of "the determinants and contributing factors of priority health needs, adequacy of existing health resources, and the population groups most affected" (Turnock, Handler, and Miller, 1998, p. 28). It should be part of the public health nurse specialist's role within a local health department to participate in and provide leadership for assessing community needs, health status of populations within the community, and environmental and behavioral risks;

## Healthy People 2010

In 1979, the surgeon general issued a report that began a 20-year focus on promoting health and preventing disease for all Americans. The report, entitled *Healthy People,* used morbidity rates to track the health of individuals through the five major life cycles of infancy, childhood, adolescence, adulthood, and older age.

In 1989, Healthy People 2000 became a national effort of representatives from government agencies, academia, and health organizations. Their goal was to present a strategy for improving the health of the American people. Their objectives are being used by public and community health organizations to assess current health trends, health programs, and disease prevention programs.

Throughout the 1990s, all states used Healthy People 2000 objectives to identify emerging public health issues. The success of the program on a national level was accomplished through state and local efforts. Early in the 1990s, surveys from public health departments

indicated that 8% of the national objectives had been met, and progress on an additional 40% of the objectives was noted. In the mid-course review published in 1995, it was noted that significant progress had been made toward meeting 50% of the objectives.

In light of the progress made in the past decade, the committee for Healthy People 2010 proposed two goals:
- To increase years of healthy life
- To eliminate health disparities among different populations

They hope to reach these goals by such measures as promoting healthy behaviors, increasing access to quality health care, and strengthening community prevention.

The major premise of Healthy People 2010 is that the health of the individual cannot be entirely separate from the health of the larger community. Therefore the vision for Healthy People 2010 is "Healthy People in Healthy Communities."

U.S. Department of Health and Human Services: *Healthy people 2000: national health promotion and disease prevention objectives,* DHHS Publication No. 91-50212, Washington, DC, 1991, U.S. Government Printing Office.

U.S. Department of Health and Human Services: *Healthy people 2010: understanding and improving health,* ed 2, Washington, DC, 2000, U.S. Government Printing Office.

U.S. Department of Health, Education, and Welfare: *Healthy people: the surgeon general's report on health promotion and disease prevention,* DHEW Publication No. 79-55071, Washington, DC, 1979, U.S. Government Printing Office.

## Evidence-Based Practice

This research used a participatory approach to explore environmental health (EH) concerns among Lac Courte Oreilles (LCO) Ojibwa Indians in Sawyer County, Wisconsin. The project focused on health promotion and community participation. Community participation was accomplished through a steering committee that consisted of the primary author and LCO College faculty and community members. The assessment method used was a self-administered survey mailed to LCO members in Sawyer County.

Concern for environmental issues was high in this tribal community, and what they would mean to future generations. Concern was higher among older members and tribal members living on rather than off the

reservation. Local issues of concern included environmental issues such as motorized water vehicles, effects from global warming, effects of aging septic systems on waterways, unsafe driving, and contaminated lakes/streams. Health concerns included diabetes, cancer, stress, obesity, and use of drugs and alcohol. The LCO community can use survey results to inform further data needs and program development.

**Nurse Use:** The community was most interested in developing a program on drug and alcohol use. The community participation in the assessment would promote a greater possibility that a drug and alcohol program would be successful.

Severtson C et al: A participatory assessment of environmental health concerns in an Ojibwa community, *Public Health Nurs* 19(1):47-58, 2002.

looking at trends in the health determinants; identifying priority health needs; and determining the adequacy of existing resources within the community (see the Evidence-Based Practice box on the Ojibwa Indians).

*Policy development* is both a core function of public health and a core intervention strategy used by public

health nursing specialists. Policy development in the public arena seeks to build constituencies that can help bring about change in public policy. In an interesting case study of her experience as director of public health for the state of Oregon, Gebbie (1999) describes her experiences in developing a constituency for public health. This enabled

### Evidence-Based Practice

The purpose of this study was to evaluate whether an 8-week support and education program could be beneficial for parents at high risk for parenting problems and at potential for child abuse. The participants were parents of infants and toddlers and the project was aimed at alleviating parental stress and improving parent–child interaction among parents who attended an inner-city clinic. Participants were 199 parents of children 1 through 36 months of age. Serious life stress including poverty, low social support, personal histories of childhood maltreatment, and substance abuse defined the parents at risk. Program effects were evaluated in terms of improvement in self-reported parenting stress and observed parent–child interaction. Positive effects were documented for the group as a whole and within each of three subgroups: two community samples and a group of mothers and children in a residential drug treatment program. Program attendance and the amount of gain in observed parenting skills were the factors related to a positive outcome.

**Nurse Use:** This program was offered in partnership with academic researchers and the public clinic. The nurses in this agency can assure better outcomes in parenting by providing a long-term program for high-risk parents.

Huebner C: Evaluation of a clinic-based parent education program to reduce the risk of infant and toddler maltreatment, *Public Health Nurs* 19(5):377-389, 2002.

her to mobilize efforts to develop statewide goals for Healthy People 2000 and also to update Oregon's disease reporting laws. Gebbie's experiences as a state director of public health illustrate how a public health nursing specialist can provide leadership at a very broad level. Gebbie left Oregon to go to Washington, D.C., to serve in the federal government as President Clinton's key official in the national effort to control acquired immunodeficiency syndrome (AIDS). Clearly, Gebbie is an example of an individual who has provided leadership in policy development at both state and national levels.

The third core public health function, *assurance,* focuses on the responsibility of public health agencies to make certain that activities have been appropriately carried out to meet public health goals and plans. This may result in public health agencies requiring others to engage in activities to meet goals, encouraging private groups to undertake certain activities, or sometimes actually offering services directly. Assurance also includes the development of partnerships between public and private agencies to make sure that needed services are available and that assessing the quality of the activities is carried out (see the Evidence-Based Practice box on parenting problems above).

## PUBLIC HEALTH NURSING AND COMMUNITY HEALTH NURSING VERSUS COMMUNITY-BASED NURSING

The concept of public health should include all populations within the community, both free-living and those living in institutions. Furthermore, the public health specialist should consider the match between the health needs of the population and the health care resources in the community, including those services offered in institutional settings. Although all direct care providers may contribute to the community's health in the broadest sense, not all are primarily concerned with the population focus—the big picture. All nurses in a given community, including those working in hospitals, physicians' offices, and health clinics, contribute positively to the health of the community. However, the special contributions of public health nursing specialists include looking at the community or population as a whole; raising questions about its overall health status and associated factors, including environmental factors (physical, biological, and sociocultural); and *working with the community* to improve the population's health status.

Figure 1-4 is a useful illustration of the arenas of practice. Because most community health nurses and many staff public health nurses, historically and at present, focus on providing direct personal care services, including health education, to persons or family units outside of institutional settings (either in the client's home or in a clinic environment), such practice falls into the upper right quadrant (section B) of Figure 1-4. However, specialization in public health nursing is community oriented and population focused and is represented by the box in the upper left quadrant (section A) (see the Nursing Tip, p. 9).

There are three reasons, in addition to the population focus, that the most important practice arena for public health nursing is represented by section A of Figure 1-4, the population of free-living clients:

1. Preventive strategies can have the greatest impact on free-living populations, which usually represent the majority of a community.
2. The major interface between health status and the environment (physical, biological, sociocultural) occurs in the free-living population.
3. For philosophical, historical, and economic reasons, population-focused practice is most likely to flourish in organizational structures that serve free-living populations (e.g., health departments, health maintenance organizations, health centers).

What roles in the health care system do public health nursing specialists (those in section A of Figure 1-4) have? Options include director of nursing for a health department, director of the health department, state commissioner for health, and director of maternal and child health services for a state or local health department. Nurses occupy all of these roles, but, with the exception of director of nursing for a health department, they are in the minority. Unfortunately, nurses who occupy these roles are often seen as administrators and not as public health nursing specialists.

Where does the staff public health nurse or community health nurse fit on the diagram? That depends on the focus of the nurse's practice. In many settings, most of the staff nurse's time is spent in community-based direct care activities, where the focus is on dealing with individual clients and individual families, which falls into section B (see Figure 1-4). However, although a staff public health nurse or a community health nurse may not be a public health nurse specialist, this nurse may spend some time carrying out core public health functions with a population focus, and thus that part of the role would be represented in section A of Figure 1-4. The field of public health nursing can be seen as primarily encompassing two groups of nurses:

- Public health nursing specialists, whose practice is community oriented and uses population-focused strategies for carrying out the core public health functions (section A).
- Staff public health nurses or community health nurses who are community based, who may be clinically oriented to the individual client, and who combine some population-focused, community-oriented strategies and direct care clinical strategies in programs serving specified populations (section B).

Figure 1-4 also shows that specialization in public health nursing, as it has been defined in this chapter, can be viewed as a specialized field of practice with certain characteristics within the broad arena of community health nursing and community-based nursing. This view is consistent with recommendations developed at the Consensus Conference on the Essentials of Public Health Nursing Practice and Education (1985). One of the outcomes of the conference was consensus on the use of the terms *community health nurse* and *public health nurse*. It was agreed that the term **community health nurse** could apply to all nurses who practice in the community, whether or not they have had preparation in public health nursing. Thus nurses providing secondary or tertiary care in a home setting, school nurses, and nurses in clinic settings (in fact, any nurse who does not practice in an institutional setting) may fall into the category of *community health nurse*. Nurses with a master's degree or a doctoral degree who practice in community settings could be referred to as *community health nurse specialists* regardless of the area of nursing in which the degree was earned. According to the conference statement,

"The degree may be in any area of nursing, such as maternal/child health, psychiatric/mental health, or medical–surgical nursing or some subspecialty of any clinical area"

(Consensus Conference, 1985, p. 4). The definitions of the three areas of practice have changed, however, over time.

In 1998, the Quad Council began to develop a statement on the scope of public health nursing practice (Quad Council, 1999). The council attempted to clarify the differences between the term *public health nursing* and the term introduced into nursing's vocabulary during health care reform of the 1990s, **community-based nursing.** The authors recognized that the terms *public health* and *community health nursing* had been used interchangeably since the 1980s to describe population-focused, community-oriented nursing practice and community-based practice. However, they decided to make a clearer distinction between community-oriented and community-based nursing practice. In contrast, community-based nursing care is the provision or assurance of personal illness care to individuals and families in the community whereas community-oriented nursing is the provision of disease prevention and health promotion to populations and communities. It is suggested that there be two terms for the two levels of care in the community: *community-oriented care* and *community-based care*. Three role functions are suggested for nursing practice: public health nursing and community health nursing (both of which are considered community-oriented) and community-based nursing (see front inside cover of the text).

In Figure 1-4, the words *Specialization in community health nursing* span boxes A and B. This suggests that there is a need and a place for a specialty in community health nursing; the nurse in this specialty is more than a clinical specialist with a master's degree who practices in a community-based setting, as was suggested by the Consensus Conference almost 20 years ago. Although in 1984 these nurses were referred to as community health nurses, today they are referred to as nurses in community-based practice. Those who provide community-oriented service to specific subpopulations in the community and who provide some clinical services to those populations may be seen as specialists in community health nursing. Although such practitioners may be community based, they are also community oriented as public health specialists but are usually focused on only one or two special subpopulations. Preparing for this specialty includes a master's degree in community health with emphasis in a direct care clinical area, such as school health or occupational health, and ideally some education in the public health sciences. Examples of roles such specialists might have in direct clinical care areas include case manager, supervisor in a home health agency, school nurse, occupational health nurse, parish nurse, and a nurse practitioner who also manages a nursing clinic.

## WHAT DO YOU THINK?

Are public health nursing, community health nursing, and community-based nursing practice all the same?

Sections C and D of Figure 1-4 represent institutionalized populations. Nurses who provide direct care to these clients in hospital settings fall into section D, and those who have administrative responsibility for nursing services in institutional settings fall into section C. Box 1-5 presents detailed definitions of the four key nursing areas in the community that are depicted in Figure 1-4.

BOX 1-5    Definitions of the Four Key Nursing Areas in the Community

**Community-oriented nursing practice** is a philosophy of nursing service delivery that involves the generalist or specialist public health and community health nurse. The nurse provides health care through community diagnosis and investigation of major health and environmental problems, health surveillance, and monitoring and evaluation of community and population health status for the purposes of preventing disease and disability and promoting, protecting, and maintaining health to create conditions in which people can be healthy.

**Public health nursing practice** is the synthesis of nursing theory and public health theory applied to promoting and preserving the health of populations. The focus of public health nursing practice is the community as a whole and the effect of the community's health status (including health care resources) on the health of individuals, families, and groups. Care is provided within the context of preventing disease and disability and promoting and protecting the health of the community as a whole.

**Community health nursing practice** is the synthesis of nursing theory and public health theory applied to promoting, preserving, and maintaining the health of populations through the delivery of personal health care services to individuals, families, and groups. The focus of community health nursing practice is the health of individuals, families, and groups and the effect of their health status on the health of the community as a whole.

**Community-based nursing practice** is a setting-specific practice whereby care is provided for clients and families where they live, work, and attend school. The emphasis of community-based nursing practice is acute and chronic care and the provision of comprehensive, coordinated, and continuous services. Nurses who deliver community-based care are generalists or specialists in maternal/infant, pediatric, adult, or psychiatric/mental health nursing.

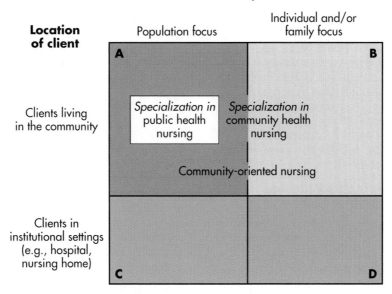

**Figure 1-4** Arenas for health care practice.

## ROLES IN PUBLIC HEALTH NURSING

In community-oriented nursing circles, there has been a tendency to talk about public health and community health nursing from the point of view of a role rather than the functions related to the role. This is limiting. In discussing such nursing roles, there is a preoccupation with the direct care provider orientation. Even in discussions about how a practice can become more population focused, the focus is frequently on how an individual practitioner, such as an agency staff nurse, can adopt a population-focused practice philosophy.

Rarely is attention given to how nurse administrators in public health (one role for public health nursing specialists) might reorient their practice toward a population focus, which is particularly important and easier for an administrator to do than for the staff nurse. This is because many agencys' nursing administrators, supervisors, or others (sometimes program directors who are not nurses) make the key decisions about how staff nurses will spend their time and what types of clients will be seen and under what circumstances. Public health nursing administrators who are prepared

## Community-Oriented, Population-Focused Practice: Foundation of Specialization in Nursing in Canada

Lianne Patricia Jeffs, R.N., M.Sc., Faculty of Nursing, University of Toronto

### MOVEMENT TOWARD COMMUNITY-ORIENTED, POPULATION-FOCUSED PRACTICE

The medical model focusing on treatment, cure, institutional care, and medical interventions dominated the Canadian health care arena until the mid 1970s. The Provincial Committee on the Costs of Health Services (Canada, 1969), the Hastings Report (Canada, 1973), and the Mustard Report (Ontario, 1974) all emphasized the need for less expensive community care, organizational and structural changes, and a focus on health promotion and disease prevention. Out of this emerged the lifestyle or behaviour approach decade (1974-1984). In 1974, LaLonde's *A New Perspective on the Health of Canadians* emphasized that the health care system was not the most important factor in determining health. In 1978, the World Health Organization's Alma Ata Declaration became the basis for primary health care (WHO, 1978). The last two decades of the twentieth century produced several reports on health care that highlighted the need to focus on the broader determinants of health in Canada, including *Achieving Health for All: A Framework for Health Promotion;* the *Ottawa Charter of Rights for Health Promotion,* and the *Population Health Promotion Model.* These reports provided the foundation for a more recent dialogue in Canada on the need for a population-based health promotion and disease prevention focus as part of the health care system reform (Romanow, 2002; Standing Senate Committee on Social Affairs, Science and Technology, 2002). The Canadian content box in Chapter 3 provides a more detailed discussion on the Canadian health care system reform.

### EVOLUTION OF COMMUNITY HEALTH NURSING AND PUBLIC HEALTH NURSING IN CANADA

In Canada, the terms *community health nursing* and *public health nursing* have been used interchangeably and debated in terms of the nature of the practice and the nature of the client. Definitions of *public health nurse* and *community health nurse* vary throughout the provinces and territories. The current discussion focuses on whether community health nursing refers to only registered nurses in traditional public health practice in health units, nurses in public health and home health services, or all nurses in community-based practice. Both public health nursing and community health nursing have evolved over the years as a result of the shift within the health care system from a medical model to a more population-focused health promotion. The role of public health nurse practice has diversified in the areas of health education, health promotion, illness and injury prevention, and primary health care for populations. Public health nurses have been defined as community health nurses who have sound knowledge of public health science, nursing science, and the social sciences, and who practice to promote, protect, and preserve the health of the population (Community Health Nurses Interest Group, 1998). Public health nurses provide services in the home, schools, workplaces, community centres, and other community agencies and institutions. Community health nursing emerged in the 1970s out of the growing industry of home care nursing in Canada.

Currently, Canada's public health care infrastructure is under considerable stress; it has deteriorated substantially as cuts in public spending have resulted in the downsizing and elimination of programs and services (Canadian Public Health Association, 2001). In addition, demand for home health care services continues to increase in Canada. In this context, a distinction between *public health nursing* and *community health nursing* is essential. It is recommended that *community health nursing* be used as the inclusive or umbrella term for community-based nursing practice, including public health nursing, home care nursing, community mental health nursing, and occupational health nursing. *Public health nursing* is defined as community-based nursing practice including population-focused health promotion and illness and injury prevention strategies working with individuals, families, groups, and communities (King, Harrison, and Reutter, 1995). Currently, national efforts are being undertaken to develop stan-

to practice in a population-focused manner will be more effective than those who are not prepared to do so.

Although their opportunities to make decisions at the population level are limited, staff nurses benefit from having a clear understanding of population-focused practice for three reasons. First, it gives them professional satisfaction to see how their individual client care contributes to health at the population level. Second, it helps them appreciate the practice of others who are population-focused specialists. Third, it gives them a better foundation from which to give clinical input into decision making at the program or agency level and thus to improve the effectiveness and efficiency of the population-focused practice.

A curriculum was proposed by representatives of key public health nursing organizations and other individuals that would prepare the staff public health nurse or generalist to function as a community-oriented practitioner (Association of State and Territorial Directors of Nursing, 2000). Box 1-6 lists the areas of study (which can be found in this book) that are essential to prepare the public health nurse generalist at the baccalaureate level.

Unfortunately, nursing roles as presently defined are often too limited to include population-focused practice, so it

dards of practice with corresponding competencies to reflect the uniqueness of each discipline.

## EDUCATIONAL PREPARATION

Educational preparation for community health nursing and public health nursing is predominately at the baccalaureate level, and in some cases an RN pursues further education and receives a diploma in public health. In some provinces, legislation exists that provides educational requirements for entry to practice and public health nursing (e.g., in Ontario, the Health Promotion and Protection Act of 1984 restricts the use of the title of public health nurse to those working in official programs who possess a baccalaureate or post-RN diploma in public health). Despite the need for educational preparation at the baccalaureate level for public health nursing, a discrepancy between educational preparation and the actual practice requirements emerging from the primary health care movement has been reported (Working Group, 1991). Epidemiologic surveillance, partnerships with groups and communities, population-based approaches, and community development were identified as areas that needed more emphasis within nursing curricula. Relatively few graduate programs that focus on community health and public health nursing are currently available in Canada (they can be found at Dalhousie University, University of Ottawa, University of Toronto, University of Calgary, and Memorial University). The discrepancy of educational preparation in community health nursing practice and the limited availability of graduate programs are barriers to recognizing and maximizing the unique scopes of practice of both public health nursing and community health nursing.

Continued efforts are needed to ensure that more graduate programs in community health nursing and public health nursing are developed in Canada, and that nursing curricula reflect the emerging primary health care principles and emphasis on epidemiology, population-based health promotion, and illness and injury prevention. In the current health care reform context, it is imperative to clearly articulate the roles of both the community health nurse and the public health nurse to ensure that primary health care, including population-based health promotion and illness/injury prevention strategies and programs, are at the core of public health and community health services.

## References

Canadian Public Health Association: *Creating conditions for health: submission to the future of health care commission,* Ottawa, 2001, Canadian Public Health Association, available at www.cpha.ca.

Community Health Nurses Interest Group of the Registered Nurses Association of Ontario: *Public health nursing position statement,* Toronto, 1998, Registered Nurses' Association of Ontario, available at www.chnig.org.

Epp J: Achieving health for all: a framework for health promotion. Ottawa, 1986, Health and Welfare Canada.

Information Canada: The community health centre in Canada. Report of the Community Health Centre Project to the Health Ministers. Ottawa, 1973, Information Canada.

King M, Harrison MJ, Reutter LI: Public health nursing or community health nursing: what's in a name? In Stewart MJ, editor: *Community nursing: promoting Canadians' health,* pp. 400-412, Toronto, 1995, Saunders Canada.

LaLonde M: *A new perspective on the health of Canadians,* Ottawa, 1974, Government of Canada.

Romanow R: *Building on values: the future of health care in Canada, final report,* Ottawa, 2002, Commission on the Future of Healthcare in Care in Canada, available at www.healthcarecommission.ca.

Standing Senate Committee on Social Affairs, Science and Technology: *The health of Canadians,* Vol. 6, *The Federal Role and Recommendations Report,* Ottawa, 2002, Standing Senate Committee, available at www.parl.gc.ca.

Toronto Ministry of Health. Report of the Health Planning Task Force. Toronto, 1974, Ministry of Health.

Working Group: *Report of the working group on the educational requirements of community health nurses,* Catalogue No. H39-235/1991E), Ottawa, 1991, Minister of Supply and Services.

World Health Organization: *Primary health care: report on the International Conference on Primary Health Care.* Alma Ata, USSR, 6-12 September, 1978, Geneva, WHO.

*Canadian spelling is used.*

is important not to think too narrowly. Furthermore, roles that entail population-focused decision making may not be defined as nursing roles—for example, directors of health departments, state or regional programs, and units of health planning and evaluation, and directors of programs such as preventive services within a managed care organization. If population-focused public health nursing is to be taken seriously, and if strategies for assessment, policy development, and assurance are to be implemented at the population level, more consideration must be given to organized systems for assessing population needs and managing care. Clearly, public health nurse specialists must move into po-

sitions where they can influence policy formation. This means, however, that some nurses will have to assume positions that are not traditionally considered nursing.

Redefining nursing roles so that population-focused decision making fits into the present structure of nursing services may not be possible just yet. It may be more useful to concentrate on identifying the skills and knowledge needed to make decisions in population-focused practice (see Appendix J.1), to define where in the health care system such decisions are made, and then to equip nurses with the knowledge, skills, and political understanding necessary for success in such positions. Although some of

---

### BOX 1-6 Areas of Study to Prepare the Public Health Staff Nurse

- Epidemiology
- Skills to effect organizational change
- Measurement of health status and organizational change
- How people connect to organizations
- Environmental health
- Policy
- Negotiation, collaboration, communication
- Advocacy
- Data analysis, statistics
- Health economics
- Interdisciplinary teams
- Program evaluation
- Coalition building
- Population-based principles, interventions
- Politics of health
- How to build on differences, diversity
- Quality-improvement approach

Association of State and Territorial Directors of Nursing: *Public health nursing: a partner for healthy populations,* Washington, DC, 2000, ASTDN.

---

these positions are in nursing settings (e.g., administrator of the nursing service and top level staff nurse supervisors), others are outside of the traditional nursing roles (e.g., commissioner of a health department).

## CHALLENGES FOR THE FUTURE
### Barriers to Specializing in Public Health Nursing

One of the most serious barriers to the development of specialists in public health nursing is the mindset of many nurses that the only role for a nurse is at the bedside or at the client's side (i.e., the direct care role), and indeed the heart of nursing is the direct care provided in personal contacts with clients. On the other hand, two things should be clear. First, whether a nurse is able to provide direct care services to a particular client depends on decisions made by individuals within and outside of the care system. Second, nurses need to be involved in those fundamental decisions. Perhaps the one-on-one focus of nursing and the historical expectations of the "proper" role of women have influenced nurses to view less positively other ways of contributing, such as administration, consultation, and research.

However, two things have changed. First, in all fields, within and outside of nursing, women have taken on every role imaginable. Second, the number of male nurses is steadily growing—nursing is no longer just a female occupation. These two changes have opened doors to new roles

that may not have been considered appropriate for nurses in the past.

A second barrier to population-focused public health nursing practice consists of the structures within which nurses work and the process of role socialization within those structures. For example, the absence of a particular role in a nursing unit may suggest that the role is undesirable or inaccessible to nurses. In another example, nurses interested in using political strategy to make changes in health-related policy, an activity clearly within the domain of public health nursing, may run into obstacles if their goals differ from those of other health care groups. Such groups may subtly but effectively lead nurses to conclude that involvement takes their attention away from the client and is not in their own, or in the client's, best interests.

A third barrier is that few nurses receive graduate level preparation in the concepts and strategies of the disciplines basic to public health (e.g., epidemiology, biostatistics, community development, service administration, and policy formation). As mentioned previously, master's level programs for public health nursing do not give the in-depth attention to population assessment and management skills that other parts of the curriculum, particularly the direct care aspects, receive. With few exceptions, graduate programs in public health and community health nursing do not aggressively develop the population-focused skills that are needed (Josten et al, 1995). For individuals who want to specialize in public health nursing, these skills are as essential as direct care skills, and they should be given more attention in graduate programs that prepare nurses for careers in public health. With the current revival in public health, there is a growing awareness among key decision makers that graduate preparation for nurses in community and public health requires a solid core of public health science.

### Establishing Population-Focused Nurse Leaders

The massive organizational changes occurring in the health delivery system present a unique opportunity to establish new roles for nurse leaders who are prepared to think in population terms. In the 1980s, Starr (1982) described the trend toward the use of private capital in financing health care, particularly institution-based care and other health-related businesses. The movement can be thought of as the "industrialization" of health care, which until recently operated very much like a **cottage industry.**

The implications and consequences of this movement are enormous. First, the goal is to provide investors a return on their investment. Other aspects include more attention to the delivery of primary and community-based care in a variety of settings; less emphasis on specialty care; the development of partnerships, alliances, and other linkages across settings in an effort to build **integrated systems,** which would provide a broad range of services for the population served; and an increasing adoption of **capitation,** a payment arrangement in which insurers agree to pay providers a fixed sum for each person per month or per year, independent of the costs actually incurred. With the spread of capitation, health professionals have become more interested in the concept of populations, sometimes referred to by financial officers and others as *covered lives* (i.e., individuals with insurance that pays on a capitated basis). For public health specialists, it is a new experience to see individuals involved in the business aspects of health care, and frequently employed by hospitals, thinking in population terms and taking a population approach to decision making.

This new focus on populations, coupled with the integrating of acute, chronic, and primary care that is occurring in some health care systems, is likely to create new roles for individuals, including nurses, who will span inpatient and community-based settings and focus on providing a wide range of services to the population served by the system. Such a role might be director of client care services for a health care system, who would have administrative responsibility for a large program area. There will also be a demand for individuals who can design programs of preventive and clinical services to be offered to targeted subpopulations. Who will decide what services will be given to which subpopulation and by which providers? How will nurses be prepared for leadership in the emerging and future structures for health care delivery and health maintenance?

Just as physician leaders are recognizing that other physicians need to be prepared to use population-focused methods, such as epidemiology and biostatistics, to make evidence-based decisions in the development of programs and protocols, the attention being given to preparing nurses for administrative decision making seems to be declining. This may be a result of (1) the recent lack of federal support for preparing nurse administrators and (2) the growing popularity of nurse practitioner programs. However, it is time that nurse leaders give more attention to preparing nurses for leadership in the area of population-focused practice. Perhaps it is time to combine the specialty in public health nursing and nursing administration, as suggested some time ago (Williams, 1985). Regardless of how the population is defined, there will be a growing need for nurses with population-level assessment, management, and evaluation skills. The primary focus of the health care system of the future will be on community-oriented strategies for health promotion and disease prevention, and on community-based strategies for primary and secondary care. Directing more attention to developing the specialty of public health nursing as a way to provide nursing leadership may be a good response to the health care system changes. Preparing nurses for population-focused decision making will require greater attention to developing programs at the master's and doctoral levels that have a stronger foundation in the public health sciences, while providing better preparation of baccalaureate-level nurses for community-oriented and community-based practice.

Some observers of public health have anticipated that if universal health insurance coverage for all Americans becomes a reality, public health practitioners can turn over the delivery of personal primary care services to other providers, such as health maintenance organizations and integrated health plans, and return to the core public health functions.

However, assurance (making sure that basic services are available to all) is a core function of public health. Thus even under the condition of universal coverage, there will still be a need to monitor subpopulations in the community to ensure that necessary care is available and that its quality is at an acceptable level. When these conditions are not met, public health practitioners will have to find a solution. Universal coverage, however, has not become a reality. Because of pressures in the health care system to cut costs, there is now a growing concern that the problem of access to basic primary care will get worse before it gets better, particularly for special, vulnerable populations (e.g., the homeless, the frail, older adults, and persons with AIDS).

The history of public health nursing shows that a common attribute of leaders is to move forward to deal with unresolved problems in a positive, proactive way. This is the legacy of Lillian Wald at the Henry Street Settlement, and many others who have met a need by being innovative. Within the context of the core public health function of assurance, public health nursing clearly has an opportunity to develop population-focused outreach programs that provide health care services to meet the needs of vulnerable populations. As a specialty, public health nursing can have a positive impact on the health status of populations, but to do so "it will be necessary to have broad vision; to prepare nurses for leadership roles in policy making and in the design, development, management, monitoring, and evaluation of population-focused health care systems and to develop strategies to support nurses in these roles" (Williams, 1992, p. 268).

## ■ Practice Application

Population-focused nursing practice is different from clinical nursing care delivered in the community. If one accepts that the specialist in public health nursing is population focused and has a unique body of knowledge, then it is useful to debate where and how public health nursing specialists practice. How does their practice compare with that of the specialist in community health nursing or community-based nursing?

A. In your public/community health class, debate with classmates which nurses in the following categories practice population-focused nursing:
- School nurse
- Staff nurse in home care
- Director of nursing for a home care agency
- Nurse practitioner in a health maintenance organization
- Vice president of nursing in a hospital
- Staff nurse in a public health clinic or community health center
- Director of nursing in a health department

B. Choose three categories in the list, and interview at least one nurse in each of the three. Determine what their scope of practice is. Are they carrying out population-focused practice? Could they? How?

**Answer is in the back of the book.**

## Key Points

- Public health is what we, as a society, do collectively to ensure the conditions in which people can be healthy.
- Assessment, policy development, and assurance are the core public health functions; they are employed at all levels of government.
- *Assessment* refers to systematic data collection on the population, monitoring of the population's health status, and making available information on the health of the community.
- *Policy development* refers to the need to provide leadership in developing policies that support the health of the population; it involves using scientific knowledge in making decisions about policy.
- *Assurance* refers to the role of public health in making sure that essential community-wide health services are available, which may include providing essential personal health services for those who would otherwise not receive them. Assurance also refers to making sure that a competent public health and personal health care workforce is available.
- Its setting is frequently viewed as the feature that distinguishes public health nursing from other specialties. A more useful approach is to use the following characteristics: a focus on populations that are free-living in the community, an emphasis on prevention, a concern for the interface between health status of the population and the living environment (physical, biological, sociocultural), and the use of political processes to affect public policy as a major intervention strategy for achieving goals.
- According to the 1984 Consensus Conference sponsored by the Nursing Division of the U.S. Department of Health and Human Services, *specialists in public health nursing* are defined as those who are prepared at the graduate level, either master's or doctoral, "with a focus in the public health sciences" (Consensus Conference, 1985).
- Specializing in public health nursing is a subset of community health nursing.
- Population-focused practice is the focus of specialists in public health nursing. This focus on populations and the emphasis on health protection, health promotion, and disease prevention are the fundamental factors that distinguish public health nursing from other nursing specialties.
- A *population* is defined as a collection of individuals who share one or more personal or environmental characteristics. The term *population* may be used interchangeably with the term *aggregate*.

## Clinical Decision-Making Activities

1. Define the following for your personal understanding, and suggest ways to check whether your understanding is correct.
   a. Essential functions of public health
   b. Specialist in public health nursing
   c. Specialist in community health nursing
2. State your opinion of the similarities and/or differences between a clinical nursing role and the population-focused role of the public health nursing specialist. What are some of the complex issues in distinguishing between these roles?
3. Review the model of public health nursing practice of the APHA as described in this chapter. Can you elaborate on the differences between the staff nurse and the specialist nurse?
4. With three or four of your classmates, identify some nurses in your community who are in an administrative role and discuss with them the following:
   a. How they define the populations they are serving
   b. Strategies they use to monitor the population's health status
   c. Strategies they use to ensure that the populations are receiving needed services
   d. What initiatives they are taking to address problems

   Do additional questions need to be asked to determine their views on population-focused practice and the responsibilities of the staff nurse? Elaborate.

## Additional Resources

Related resources are found either in the appendixes in the back of this book or on the book's website at **http://evolve.elsevier.com/Stanhope.**

### Appendix

Appendix J.1 Examples of Public Health Nursing Roles and Implementing Public Health Functions

Appendix J.2 Public Health Guidelines for Practice

### *evolve* Evolve Website

Appendix A.1 Schedule of Clinical Preventive Services

WebLinks: Healthy People 2010

# References

American Public Health Association: *The definition and role of public health nursing in the delivery of health care: a statement of the public health nursing section,* Washington, DC, 1981, APHA.

American Public Health Association: *The definition and role of public health nursing: a statement of the APHA public health nursing section, March 1996 update,* Washington, DC, 1996, APHA.

Association of Community Health Nursing Educators: *Graduate education for advanced practice in community public health nursing,* Lathrop, NY, 2000, ACHNE.

Association of State and Territorial Directors of Nursing: *Public health nursing: a partner for healthy populations,* Washington, DC, 2000, ASTDN.

Canadian Public Health Association: *Creating conditions for health: submission to the future of health care commission,* Ottawa, 2001, Canadian Public Health Association, available at www.cpha.ca.

Centers for Disease Control and Prevention: *Guide to community preventive services 2000,* retrieved 4/1/03 from http://www.cdc.gov/.

Community Health Nurses Interest Group of the Registered Nurses' Association of Ontario: *Public health nursing position statement,* Toronto, 1998, Registered Nurses Association of Ontario, available at www.chnig.org.

Consensus Conference on the Essentials of Public Health Nursing Practice and Education, Rockville, Md, 1985, U.S. Department of Health and Human Services, Bureau of Health Professions, Division of Nursing.

Council on Linkages Between Academia and Public Health Practice: *Core competencies for public health professional,* Washington, DC, 2001, Public Health Foundation/Health Resources and Services Administration.

Gebbie K: Building a constituency for public health, *J Public Health Manag Pract* 3:1, 1999.

Huebner C: Evaluation of a clinic-based parent education program to reduce the risk of infant and toddler maltreatment, *Public Health Nurs* 19(5):377-389, 2002.

Institute of Medicine: *The future of public health,* Washington, DC, 1988, National Academy Press.

Institute of Medicine: *Improving health in the community: a role for performance monitoring,* Washington, DC, 1997, National Academy Press.

Institute of Medicine: *The future of the public's health—the 21st century,* Washington, DC, 2003, National Academy Press.

Josten L et al: Public health nursing education: back to the future for public health sciences, *Fam Community Health* 18:36, 1995.

King M, Harrison MJ, Reutter LI: Public health nursing or community health nursing: what's in a name? In Stewart MJ, editor: *Community nursing: promoting Canadians' health,* pp. 400-412, Toronto, 1995, Saunders Canada.

LaLonde M: *A new perspective on the health of Canadians,* Ottawa, 1974, Government of Canada.

National Association of County and City Health Officials: Blueprint for a healthy community: a guide for local health departments, Washington, DC, 1994, NACCHO.

Public Health Futures Steering Committee: *Public health in America,* 1998, retrieved 4/1/03, from www.health.gov/phfunctions/public.htm.

Quad Council of Public Health Nursing Organizations: *Scope and standards of public health nursing practice,* Washington, DC, 1999, American Nurses' Association.

Romanow R: *Building on values: the future of health care in Canada, final report,* Ottawa, 2002, Author, available at www.healthcarecommission.ca.

Severtson C et al: A participatory assessment of environmental health concerns in an Ojibwa community, *Public Health Nurs* 19(1):47-58, 2002.

Standing Senate Committee on Social Affairs, Science, and Technology: *The health of Canadians,* Vol. 6, *The Federal Role and Recommendations Report,* Ottawa, 2002, Standing Senate Committee, available at www.parl.gc.ca.

Starr P: *The social transformation of American medicine,* New York, 1982, Basic Books.

Turnock B, Handler AS, Miller CA: Core function—related local public health practice effectiveness, *J Public Health Manag Pract* 4:26, 1998.

U.S. Department of Health and Human Services: *Healthy people 2000: national health promotion and disease prevention objectives,* DHHS Publication No. 91-50212, Washington, DC, 1991, U.S. Government Printing Office.

U.S. Department of Health and Human Services, Office of Public Health and Science: *Healthy people 2010 objectives: draft for public comment,* Washington, DC, 1998, U.S. Government Printing Office.

U.S. Department of Health and Human Services: *Healthy people 2010: understanding and improving health,* ed 2, Washington, DC, 2000, U.S. Government Printing Office.

U.S. Department of Health and Human Services: *Health US: 2000,* Washington, DC, 2002, National Center for Statistics.

U.S. Department of Health, Education, and Welfare: *Healthy people: the surgeon general's report on health promotion and disease prevention,* DHEW Publication No. 79-55071, Washington, DC, 1979, U.S. Government Printing Office.

U.S. Preventive Services Task Force: *Guide to clinical preventive services,* ed 3, Baltimore, 2000, Williams & Wilkins.

U.S. Public Health Service: *A time for partnership,* Prevention Report, Washington, DC, Dec 1994/Jan 1995, Office of Disease Prevention and Health Promotion.

U.S. Public Health Service: *The core functions project,* Washington, DC, 1994/update 2000, Office of Disease Prevention and Health Promotion.

Williams CA: Population-focused community health nursing and nursing administration: a new synthesis. In McCloskey JC, Grace HK, editors: *Current issues in nursing,* ed 2, Boston, 1985, Blackwell Scientific.

Williams CA: Public health nursing: does it have a future? In Aiken LH, Fagin CM, editors: *Charting nursing's future: agenda for the 1990s,* Philadelphia, 1992, Lippincott.

Williams CA: Beyond the Institute of Medicine report: a critical analysis and public health forecast, *Fam Community Health* 18:12, 1995.

Working Group: *Report of the working group on the educational requirements of community health nurses,* Catalogue No. H39-235/1991E, Ottawa, 1991, Minister of Supply and Services.

World Health Organization: *Primary health care: report on the International Conference on Primary Health Care.* Alma Ata, USSR, 6-12 September, 1978, Geneva, WHO.

evolve http://evolve.elsevier.com/Stanhope

# History of Public Health and Public and Community Health Nursing

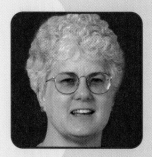

**Janna Dieckmann, Ph.D., R.N.**
Janna Dieckmann began her nursing practice in 1974 as a public health nurse with the Visiting Nurse Association of Cleveland, Ohio, and also practiced many years with the Visiting Nurse Association of Philadelphia. Today she is an assistant professor at The University of North Carolina at Chapel Hill, where she teaches public health nursing and health promotion. She uses written and oral historical materials to research the history of public health nursing and care of the chronically ill, and to comment on contemporary health policy.

## Objectives

After reading this chapter, the student should be able to do the following:
1. Interpret the focus and roles of community and public health nurses through a historical approach
2. Trace the ongoing interaction between the practice of public health and that of nursing
3. Identify the dynamic relationship between changes in social, political, and economic contexts and community-oriented nursing practice
4. Outline the professional and practice impact of individual leadership on community-oriented nursing, especially the leadership of Florence Nightingale and Lillian Wald
5. Identify structures for delivery of community-oriented nursing care such as settlement houses, visiting nurse associations, official health organizations, and schools
6. Recognize major organizations that contributed to the growth and development of community-oriented nursing
7. Relate the impact of legislative initiatives to changing opportunities for community-oriented nursing practice

Nurses use a historical approach to examine both the profession's present and its future. In doing so, several different questions might be asked: (1) Who are community and public health nurses? These nurses will be referred to in this text as community-oriented nurses; (2) How does the past contribute to who they are today? (3) What are the places and times in which community-oriented nurses have worked and continue to work? (4) When is a conscious process of critique and insight employed to look into past actions of the specialty, and what can be discovered from the process? (5) Can agreement with and endorsement of these past actions be achieved?

and (6) How might knowledge of community-oriented nursing history serve not only as a source of inspiration but also as a stimulus to solve creatively the emerging problems of the current period? This chapter serves as an introduction to consideration of these questions.

## CHANGE AND CONTINUITY

For over 100 years, public health nurses in the United States have worked to develop strategies to respond effectively to prevailing public health problems. The history of community-oriented nursing reflects changes in the specific focus of the profession while emphasizing continuity in approach and style. Community-oriented nurses have worked to improve the health status of individuals, families, and populations, especially those who belong to vulnerable groups. Part of the appeal of this nursing specialty

*The author acknowledges the important foundational work for this chapter developed by Dr. Jeanette Lancaster in previous editions of this book.*

## Key Terms

American Nurses Association, p. 39
American Public Health Association, p. 30
American Red Cross, p. 29
Mary Breckinridge, p. 31
district nursing, p. 25
district nursing association, p. 26
Frontier Nursing Service, p. 31

Metropolitan Life Insurance Company, p. 31
National League for Nursing, p. 39
National Organization for Public Health Nursing, p. 30
Florence Nightingale, p. 25
official (health) agencies, p. 34
William Rathbone, p. 26

settlement houses, p. 27
Sheppard-Towner Act, p. 31
Social Security Act of 1935, p. 34
Town and Country Nursing Service, p. 29
visiting nurse, p. 27
Lillian Wald, p. 27
*See Glossary for definitions*

## Chapter Outline

Change and Continuity
Historical Measures to Provide for the Public's Health
America's Colonial Period and the New Republic
Nightingale and the Origins of Trained Nursing
America Needs Trained Nurses
School Nursing in America
The Profession Comes of Age
Public Health Nursing in Official Health Agencies
World War I and the Importance of Public Health Nursing

Paying the Bill for Community and Public Health Nurses
Efforts to Shape Public Policy
African-American Nurses in Public Health Nursing
Between the Two World Wars: Economic Depression and the Rise of Hospitals
Increasing Federal Action for the Public's Health
World War II: Extension and Retrenchment in Community and Public Health Nursing
The Rise of Chronic Illnesses

Failure of Financing for Community-Oriented Nursing
Consolidation of National Nursing Organizations
Professional Nursing Education for Public Health Nursing
New Forms of Payment for Community-Oriented Nursing
Community Organization and Professional Change
Community and Public Health Nursing from the 1970s to the Present
Community and Public Health Nursing Today

has been its autonomy of practice and independence in problem solving and decision making, done in the context of a multidisciplinary practice. Many of the varied and challenging roles of community-oriented nurses can be traced to the late 1800s when public health efforts focused on environmental conditions such as sanitation, control of communicable diseases, education for health, prevention of disease and disability, and care of sick persons in their homes.

Although threats to health from communicable diseases, the environment, chronic illness, and the aging process have changed over time, the foundational principles and goals of community-oriented nursing have remained the same. Many communicable diseases, such as diphtheria, cholera, and typhoid fever, have been largely controlled in the United States, but others, including human immunodeficiency virus (HIV) and acquired im-

munodeficiency syndrome (AIDS), measles, tuberculosis, and hepatitis, continue to affect many lives. Emerging communicable diseases, such as West Nile virus, underscore the truth that health concerns are international. Even though environmental pollution in residential areas has been reduced, communities are now threatened by overcrowded garbage dumps and pollutants affecting the air, water, and soil. Periodic natural disasters continue to challenge public health systems, and the threat of human-made disasters and bioterrorism threatens to overwhelm existing resources. Research has identified means to avoid or postpone chronic disease, and nurses implement strategies to change individual and community risk factors and behaviors. Finally, with growth in the population of older adults in the United States and their preference to remain at home, additional nursing services are required to sustain the frail, the disabled, and the chronically ill in that community.

The roles of the community-oriented nurse in the United States developed from several sources and are a product of various social, economic, and political forces. This chapter describes the societal circumstances that influenced nurses to establish community-based and community-oriented practices. Community-oriented nurses rely heavily on public health science to complement their focus on nursing science and practice. The nation's need for community and public health nurses, the practice of community-oriented nursing, and the organizations influencing community and public health nursing in the United States during the nineteenth and twentieth centuries are outlined in this chapter.

## HISTORICAL MEASURES TO PROVIDE FOR THE PUBLIC'S HEALTH

Concern for the health and care of individuals in the community has characterized human existence. All people and all cultures have been concerned with the events surrounding birth, death, and illness. Human beings have sought to prevent, understand, and control disease. Their ability to preserve health and treat illness has depended on the contemporary level of science, use and availability of technologies, and degree of social organization.

## AMERICA'S COLONIAL PERIOD AND THE NEW REPUBLIC

In the early years of America's settlement, as in Europe, the care of the sick was usually informal and was provided by household members, almost always women. The female head of the household was responsible for caring for all household members, which meant more than nursing them in sickness and during childbirth. She was also responsible for growing or gathering healing herbs for use throughout the year. For the increasing numbers of urban residents in the early 1800s, this traditional system became insufficient.

American ideas of social welfare and the care of the sick were strongly influenced by the traditions of British settlers in the New World. Just as American jurisprudence is based on English common law, colonial Americans established systems of care for the sick, poor, aged, mentally ill, and dependents based on the model of the Elizabethan Poor Law of 1601. In the United States, as in England, the Poor Law guaranteed medical care for poor, blind, and "lame" individuals, even those without family. Early county or township government was responsible for the care of all dependent residents but provided almshouse charity carefully, economically, and only for their own. Those who were residents elsewhere were returned to their home counties for care. Few hospitals existed, and they were only in the larger cities. In 1751, Pennsylvania Hospital was founded in Philadelphia, the first hospital in what would become the United States.

Early colonial public health efforts included the collection of vital statistics, improved sanitation, and control of the communicable diseases that were introduced through seaports. The colonists lacked a continuing and organized mechanism for ensuring that public health efforts would be supported and enforced. Epidemics intermittently taxed the limited local organization for health during the seventeenth, eighteenth, and nineteenth centuries (Rosen, 1958). Early American efforts to provide for the public's health may be compared to early efforts in Canada by referring to the box titled A Historical Overview of Community and Public Health Nursing in Canada, later in this chapter.

After the American Revolution, the threat of disease, especially yellow fever, brought public support for establishing government-sponsored, or official, boards of health. With a population of 75,000 by 1800, New York City had established basic public health services, including a public health committee for monitoring water quality, sewer construction, drainage of marshes, planting of trees and vegetables, construction of a masonry wall along the waterfront, and burial of the dead (Rosen, 1958).

Increased urbanization and beginning industrialization contributed to increased incidence of disease, including epidemics of smallpox, yellow fever, cholera, typhoid, and typhus. Tuberculosis and malaria remained endemic with a high incidence rate, and infant mortality was about 200 per 1000 live births (Pickett and Hanlon, 1990). American hospitals in the early 1800s were generally unsanitary and staffed by poorly trained workers. Physicians received a limited education through proprietary schools or simple apprenticeship. Medical care was difficult to secure, although public dispensaries (similar to outpatient clinics) and private charitable efforts attempted to address gaps in the availability of sickness services, especially for the urban working class and poor. Environmental conditions in urban neighborhoods, including inadequate housing and sanitation, were additional risks to health.

Table 2-1 presents milestones of public health efforts that occurred during the seventeenth, eighteenth, and nineteenth centuries.

The federal government's early efforts for public health were targeted at securing its maritime trade and seacoast cities by providing health care for merchant seamen and by protecting seacoast cities from epidemics. The Public Health Service, still the most important federal public health agency today, was established in 1798 as the Marine Hospital Service. The first Marine Hospital was opened in Norfolk, Virginia, in 1800. Additional legislation to establish quarantine legislation for seamen and immigrants was passed in 1878.

During the early 1800s, experiments in providing nursing care at home usually focused more on moral elevation and less on illness intervention. The Ladies' Benevolent Society of Charleston, South Carolina, provided charitable assistance to the poor and sick beginning in 1813. In Philadelphia, lay nurses oriented in a brief training program cared for postpartum women and their newborns in

**Table 2-1   Milestones in History of Public Health and Community Health Nursing: 1600-1865**

| YEAR | MILESTONE |
|------|-----------|
| 1601 | Elizabethan Poor Law written |
| 1789 | Baltimore Health Department established |
| 1798 | Marine Hospital Service established; later became Public Health Service |
| 1812 | Sisters of Mercy established in Dublin where nuns visited the poor |
| 1813 | Ladies' Benevolent Society of Charleston, South Carolina, founded |
| 1836 | Lutheran deaconesses provide home visits in Kaiserwerth, Germany |
| 1851 | Florence Nightingale visits Kaiserwerth for 3 months of nurse training |
| 1855 | Quarantine Board established in New Orleans; beginning of tuberculosis campaign in the United States |
| 1859 | District nursing established in Liverpool, England, by William Rathbone |
| 1860 | Florence Nightingale Training School for Nurses established at St. Thomas Hospital in London, England |
| 1864 | Red Cross established in the United States |

their homes. In Cincinnati, Ohio, the Roman Catholic Sisters of Charity began a visiting nurse service in 1854 (Rodabaugh and Rodabaugh, 1951). Although these early programs provided services at the local level, they were not adopted elsewhere, and their influence on later community-oriented nursing is unclear.

During the middle of the nineteenth century, national interest grew to address public health problems and improve urban living conditions. The roles of urban boards of health reflected changing ideas of public health. Rather than addressing solely environmental hazards as they had in the past, attention was paid to communicable disease. Soon after it was founded in 1847, the American Medical Association (AMA) formed a hygiene committee to conduct sanitary surveys and to develop a system to collect vital statistics. The Shattuck Report, published in 1850 by the Massachusetts Sanitary Commission, called for major innovations: the establishment of a state health department and local health boards in every town; sanitary surveys and collection of vital statistics; environmental sanitation; food, drug, and communicable disease control; well-child care; health education; tobacco and alcohol control; town planning; and the teaching of preventive medicine in medical schools (Kalisch and Kalisch, 1995). However, these recommendations were not implemented in Massachusetts for 19 years, and in other states not until much later.

## NIGHTINGALE AND THE ORIGINS OF TRAINED NURSING

The origins of professional nursing are found in the work of Florence Nightingale in nineteenth-century Europe. With tremendous advances in transportation, communication, and other forms of technology, the Industrial Revolution led to deep social upheaval. Even with the growth of science, medicine, and technology in the two previous centuries, applied nineteenth-century public health measures continued to be very basic. Organization and management of cities improved slowly, and many areas lacked systems of sewage disposal and depended on private enterprise for water supply. Previous caregiving structures, which had depended on assistance of family, neighbors, and friends, became inadequate in the early nineteenth century because of migration, urbanization, and changing demand. During this period, a few Roman Catholic and Protestant women provided nursing care for the sick, poor, and neglected in institutions and sometimes in the home. For example, Mary Aikenhead, also known by her religious name, Sister Mary Augustine, organized the Irish Sisters of Charity in 1815 in Dublin. These sisters visited the poor at home and established hospitals and schools (Kalisch and Kalisch, 1995).

In nineteenth-century England, the Elizabethan Poor Law continued to guarantee medical care for all. This minimal care, provided most often in almshouses supported by local government, sought as much to regulate the poor as to provide care during illness. Many women who performed nursing functions in almshouses and early hospitals in Great Britain were poorly educated, untrained, and often undependable. With the increasingly complex practice of medicine in the mid 1800s, hospital work required skilled caregivers. Physicians and hospital administrators sought to advance the practice of nursing. Early experiments yielded some improvement in care, but the efforts of Florence Nightingale are credited with beginning a revolution.

**Florence Nightingale's** vision of trained nurses and her model of nursing education influenced the development of professional nursing and, indirectly, public health nursing in the United States. In 1850 and 1851, Nightingale had carefully studied nursing "system and method" by visiting Pastor Theodor Fliedner at his School for Deaconesses in Kaiserwerth, Germany. Pastor Fliedner had observed Mennonite deaconesses in Holland who were engaged in parish work for the poor and the sick, as well as Elizabeth Fry, the English prison reformer. Thus mid-nineteenth century efforts to reform the practice of nursing drew on a variety of interacting innovations across Europe.

The Kaiserwerth Lutheran deaconesses incorporated care of the sick at home with care in their hospital. Their system of **district nursing** (community-oriented nursing) had spread to other cities in Germany. American requests for the deaconesses to respond to epidemics of typhus and cholera in Pittsburgh provided only temporary assistance when local women proved uninterested in the work. The early efforts of the Lutheran deaconesses in the United States ultimately focused on developing systems of institutional care (Nutting and Dock, 1935).

Nightingale soon found a way to implement her ideas about nursing. During the Crimean War (1854 to 1856) between the alliance of England and France against Russia, the British military established hospitals for sick and wounded soldiers in Scutari, in Asia Minor. The care of soldiers was severely deficient, with cramped quarters, poor sanitation, lice and rats, insufficient food, and inadequate medical supplies (Kalisch and Kalisch, 1995; Palmer, 1983). When the British public demanded improved conditions, Nightingale sought and received an appointment to address the chaos. Because of her wealth, social and political connections, and knowledge of hospitals, the British government sent her to Asia Minor with 40 ladies, 117 hired nurses, and 15 paid servants.

In Scutari, Nightingale progressively improved the soldiers' health using a population-based approach that led to improvements in environmental conditions and nursing care. Using simple epidemiology measures, she documented a decreased mortality rate from 415 per 1000 at the beginning of the war to 11.5 per 1000 at the end (Cohen, 1984; Palmer, 1983). Paralleling Nightingale's efforts in Scutari, community-oriented nurses typically identify health care needs that affect the entire population, mobilize resources, and organize themselves and the community to meet these needs.

After the Crimean War and her return to England in 1856, with her fame established, Nightingale organized hospital nursing practice and nursing education in hospitals to replace untrained lay nurses with Nightingale nurses. Nightingale not only focused on establishing hospital nursing but also emphasized public health nursing. She said "The health of the unity is the health of the community. Unless you have the health of the unity, there is no community health" (Nightingale, 1894, p. 455). She differentiated "sick nursing" from "health nursing." The latter emphasized that nursing should strive to promote health and prevent illness. Nightingale (1946, p. v) found the task of nursing to be to "put the constitution in such a state as that it will have no disease, or that it can recover from disease." Proper nutrition, rest, sanitation, and hygiene were necessary for health. Community-oriented nurses continue to focus on the role of health promotion, disease prevention, and environment in their practice with individuals, families, and communities.

Nightingale's contemporary and friend, British philanthropist **William Rathbone,** founded the first **district nursing association** in Liverpool, England. Rathbone's wife had received outstanding nursing care from a Nightingale-trained nurse during her terminal illness at home. He wanted to offer similar care to relieve the suffering poor unable to afford private nurses. With Rathbone's verbal and economic support between 1859 and 1862, the Liverpool Relief Society divided the city into nursing districts and assigned a committee of

"friendly visitors" to each district to provide health care to needy people (Kalisch and Kalisch, 1995). On the basis of the Liverpool experience, Rathbone and Nightingale recommended steps to provide nursing in the home, and district nursing was organized throughout England. Florence Sarah Lees Craven shaped the profession through her "Guide to District Nurses," which recommended, for example, that the district nurse gain influence to improve the status of the whole family through the illness of one member of the family (Craven, 1889).

## AMERICA NEEDS TRAINED NURSES

As urbanization increased during the Industrial Revolution, the number of jobs for women rapidly increased. Educated women became elementary school teachers, secretaries, or saleswomen. Less educated women worked in factories of all kinds. The idea of becoming a trained nurse increased in popularity as Nightingale's successes became known across the United States. During the 1870s, the first nursing schools based on the Nightingale model opened in the United States.

Trained nurse graduates of the first Nightingale-style schools in the United States usually worked in private duty nursing or held the few positions of hospital administrators or instructors. Private duty nurses might live with families of patients receiving care. Although the trained nurse's role in improving American hospitals was clear, the cost of private duty nursing care for the sick at home was prohibitive for all but the wealthy.

The care of the sick poor at home was made economical by having home-visiting nurses attend several families in a day rather than attend only one patient as the private duty nurse did. In 1877 the Women's Board of the New York City Mission hired Frances Root, a graduate of Bellevue Hospital's first nursing class, to visit sick poor persons to provide nursing care and religious instruction (Bullough and Bullough, 1964). In 1878 the Ethical Culture Society of New York hired four nurses to work in dispensaries. In the next few years, visiting nurse associations were established in Buffalo, New York (1885), Philadelphia (1886), and Boston (1886). Wealthy people interested in charitable activities funded both settlement houses and visiting nurse associations. Upper-class women, freed of some of the social restrictions that had previously limited their public life, became interested in the charitable work of creating, supporting, and supervising the new visiting nurses. Community-oriented nursing in the United States began with organizing to meet urban health care needs, especially for the disadvantaged.

The public was interested in limiting disease among all classes of people both for religious reasons and as a form of charity, but also because the middle and upper classes feared the impact of diseases believed to originate in the large communities of new immigrants from Europe. In New York City in the 1890s, about 2.3 million people were packed into 90,000 tenement houses. The environmental conditions of immigrants in tenement houses and sweatshops were com-

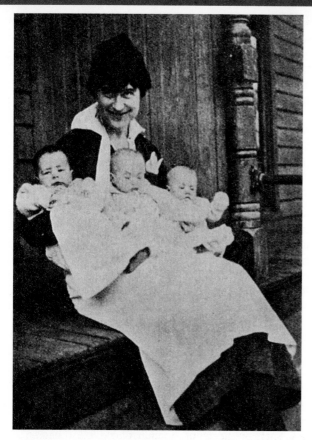

**Figure 2-1** Teaching well-child care was a significant public health nursing role. *(Courtesy Instructional Visiting Nurse Association of Richmond, Va.)*

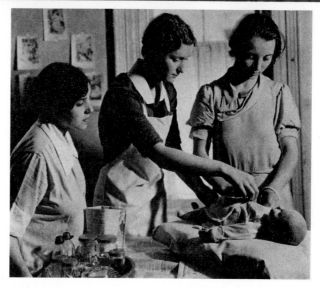

**Figure 2-2** Public health nurse demonstrating well-child care during a home visit. *(Courtesy the Visiting Nurse Service of New York.)*

mon to urban life across the northeastern United States and into the upper Midwest. "Slum dwellers were ravaged by epidemics of typhus, scarlet fever, smallpox, and typhoid fever, and many of them died or developed tuberculosis" (Kalisch and Kalisch, 1995, p. 172). From the beginning, community-oriented nursing practice included teaching and prevention (Figure 2-1). Community-oriented nursing interventions, improved sanitation, economic improvements, and better nutrition were credited with reducing the incidence of acute communicable disease by 1910.

New scientific explanations of communicable disease suggested that preventive education would reduce illness. The **visiting nurse** became the key to communicating the prevention campaign, through the home visit and well-baby clinics. These community health visiting nurses worked with physicians, gave selected treatments, and kept temperature and pulse records. The nurses emphasized education of family members in the care of the sick and in personal and environmental prevention measures, such as hygiene and good nutrition (Figure 2-2). Many early visiting nurse agencies employed only one nurse, who was supervised by members of the agency board, usually composed of wealthy or socially prominent ladies. These ladies were critically important to the success of visiting nursing through their efforts to open new agencies, financially sup-

port existing agencies, and render the services socially acceptable. The work of both visiting nurses and their lady supporters reflected changing societal roles for women as it became more acceptable for women to be active in public arenas than it had been earlier in the nineteenth century.

For example, in 1886, two Boston women approached the Women's Education Association to seek support for district nursing. To increase the likelihood of financial support, they used the term *instructive district nursing* to emphasize the relationship of nursing to health education. Support was also secured from the Boston Dispensary, which provided free medical care on an outpatient basis. In February of 1886, the first district nurse was hired, and in 1888 the Instructive District Nursing Association became incorporated as an independent voluntary agency. Sick poor persons, who paid no fees, were cared for under the direction of a trained physician (Brainard, 1922).

Other nurses established **settlement houses,** neighborhood centers that became hubs for health care and social welfare programs. For example, in 1893 Lillian Wald and Mary Brewster, both trained nurses, began visiting the poor on New York's Lower East Side. The nurses' settlement they established became the Henry Street Settlement and later the Visiting Nurse Service of New York City. By 1905, the public health nurses had provided almost 48,000 visits to over 5000 patients (Kalisch and Kalisch, 1995). **Lillian Wald** emerged as the established leader of public health nursing during its early decades (Box 2-1; Figure 2-3). Additional settlement houses influenced the growth of community-oriented nursing including the Richmond (Virginia) Nurses' Settlement, which became the Instructive Visiting Nurse Association. Others included the Nurses' Settlement in Orange, New Jersey, and the College Settlement in Los Angeles, California.

## BOX 2-1  Lillian Wald: First Public Health Nurse in the United States

Public health nursing developed in the United States in the late nineteenth and early twentieth centuries largely because of the pioneering work of Lillian Wald. Born on March 10, 1867, in Cincinnati, Ohio, Lillian Wald grew up in Rochester, New York, in a warm, nurturing family. When she was 16, Vassar College declined her application because of her youth. Wald found a life direction from discussions with a trained nurse who cared for a family member. At age 22 she entered, and in 1891 graduated from, the New York Hospital Training School for Nurses. The next year she spent working at the New York Juvenile Asylum, an orphanage, finding it institutional and impersonal. She enrolled for a year at Women's Medical College in New York, but she soon found an entirely new life.

During a severe economic depression of 1893, Wald led a class in home nursing for poor immigrant women on New York's Lower East Side. After one class, a young child asked Wald to visit her sick mother, who had given birth several days before. Wald found the mother in bed, isolated and alone, having hemorrhaged for 2 days. Doing what needed to be done, Wald cared for this family, finding a new purpose and direction for her life. Wald became determined "in a half-hour" to live in this neighborhood and work with its people (Wald, 1915).

Wald refused to tolerate poor people's lack of access to health care. With the financial support of two wealthy laypeople, Mrs. Solomon Loeb and Jacob Schiff, Wald and her friend Mary Brewster moved to the East Side and occupied the top floor of a tenement house on Jefferson Street. Wald and Brewster provided nursing care to their neighbors, leading to the establishment a year later of the Henry Street Settlement, whose health services later became the Visiting Nurse Service of New York. Wald invented the term *public health nursing* to describe this work. She believed that the nurse's visit "should be like that of a very interested friend rather than that of an impersonal, paid visitor" (Dolan, 1978). Ever political, Wald linked the Henry Street Settlement nurses to the New York City official health agency as her nurses wore the Board of Health insignia. During 1915 the Settlement's 100 nurses had cared for 26,575 patients and had made more than 227,000 home visits.

Beyond New York City, Wald took steps to increase access to public health nursing services through innovation. She persuaded the American Red Cross to sponsor rural health nursing services across the country, which stimulated local governments to sponsor public health nursing through county health departments. Beginning in 1909, Wald worked with Dr. Lee Frankel of the Metropolitan Life Insurance Company to implement the first insurance payment for nursing services. She argued that keeping working people and their families healthier would increase their productivity. Met Life found that nursing care for communicable diseases, injuries, and mothers and children reduced mortality and saved money for this life insurance company. Met Life nursing services continued for 44 years, yielding accomplishments in (1) providing home nursing services on a fee-for-service basis, (2) establishing an effective cost-accounting system for visiting nurses, and (3) reducing mortality from infectious diseases.

Convinced that environmental conditions as well as social conditions were the causes of ill health and poverty, Wald became actively involved in using epidemiologic methods to campaign for health-promoting social policies. She advocated for creation of the U.S. Children's Bureau as a basis for improving the health and education of children nationally. She fought for better tenement living conditions in New York City, city recreation centers, parks, pure food laws, graded classes for mentally handicapped children, and assistance to immigrants. She firmly believed in women's suffrage and considered its acceptance in 1917 in New York State to be a great victory. Wald supported efforts to improve race relations and championed solutions to racial injustice. She wrote *The House on Henry Street* (1915) and *Windows on Henry Street* (1934) to describe this public health nursing work.

Backer BA: Lillian Wald: connecting caring with action, *Nurs Health Care* 14:122, 1993.

Cristy TE: Lillian D. Wald: portrait of a leader. In Kelly LY: *Pages from nursing history,* pp. 84-88, New York, 1984, American Journal of Nursing Company.

Dock LL: The history of public health nursing, *Public Health Nurs* 14:522, 1922.

Dolan J: *History of nursing,* ed 14, Philadelphia, 1978, Saunders.

Duffus RL: *Lillian Wald: neighbor and crusader,* New York, 1938, Macmillan.

Frachel RR: A new profession: the evolution of public health nursing, *Public Health Nurs* 5(2):86, 1988.

Wald LD: *The house on Henry Street,* New York, 1915, Holt.

Wald LD: *Windows on Henry Street,* Boston, 1934, Little, Brown.

Williams B: *Lillian Wald: angel of Henry street,* New York, 1948, Julian Messner.

Zerwekh JV: Public health nursing legacy: historical practical wisdom, *Nurs Health Care* 13:84, 1992.

( NURSING TIP

Securing information about the organizational history of a practice agency, such as a visiting nurse association, may provide important perspectives on current agency values, decision-making structures, service areas, and clinical priorities.

In 1909, Yssabella Waters published her survey, *Visiting Nursing in the United States,* which found visiting nurse services concentrated in the northeastern quadrant of the nation. Emphasizing the rapid and divergent development of visiting nursing, New York City in 1909 had 58 different organizations with 372 trained nurses providing care in the community. However, nationally,

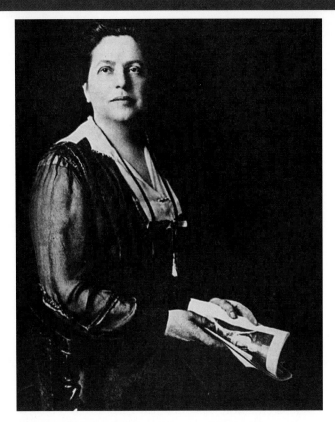

**Figure 2-3** Lillian Wald. *(Courtesy Visiting Nurse Service of New York.)*

68% of visiting nurses were employed in single-nurse agencies. In addition to visiting nurse associations and settlement houses, a variety of other organizations sponsored visiting nurse work, including boards of education, boards of health, mission boards, clubs, churches, social service agencies, and tuberculosis associations. With tuberculosis responsible for at least 10% of all mortality during this time, visiting nurses contributed to its control through gaining "the personal cooperation of patients and their families" to modify the environment and personal behavior (Buhler-Wilkerson, 1987, p. 45). Most visiting nurse agencies depended financially on the philanthropy and social networks of metropolitan areas. As today, service delivery in less densely populated (rural) areas was a challenge.

The **American Red Cross,** through its Rural Nursing Service (later the **Town and Country Nursing Service**), initiated home nursing care in areas outside larger cities. Lillian Wald secured initial donations to support this agency, which provided care of the sick and instruction in sanitation and hygiene in rural homes. The agency also improved living conditions in villages and isolated farms. The Town and Country nurse addressed diseases such as tuberculosis, pneumonia, and typhoid fever with a resourcefulness born of necessity. The rural nurse might use hot bricks, salt, or sandbags to substitute for hot water bottles; chairs as back-rests for the bedbound; and boards padded with quilts as stretchers (Kalisch and Kalisch,

1995). Immediately after World War I, the 100 existing Red Cross Town and Country Nursing Services expanded to 1800 in less than 2 years, eventually growing to almost 3000 programs in small towns and rural areas. This service demonstrated the importance and feasibility of public health nursing across the country at local and county levels. Once established by the Red Cross, these new agencies were passed on to be maintained by local voluntary agencies or local government.

Occupational health nursing began as industrial nursing and was a true outgrowth of early home visiting efforts. In 1895, Ada Mayo Stewart began work with employees and families of the Vermont Marble Company in Proctor, Vermont. As a free service for the employees, Stewart provided obstetric care, sickness care (e.g., for typhoid cases), and some postsurgical care in workers' homes. Unlike contemporary occupational health nurses, Stewart provided very few services for work-related injuries. A graduate of the Waltham (Massachusetts) Training School, Stewart continued to wear the Waltham school uniform and added a plain coat and hat. Although her employer provided a horse and buggy, she often made home visits on a bicycle. Before 1900, a few nurses were hired in industry, for example in department stores in Philadelphia and Brooklyn. Between 1914 and 1943, industrial nursing grew from 60 to 11,220 nurses, reflecting increased government and employee concerns for health and safety at work (American Association of Industrial Nurses, 1976; Kalisch and Kalisch, 1995).

## SCHOOL NURSING IN AMERICA

In New York City in 1902, more than 20% of children could be absent from school on a single day. The children suffered from the common conditions of pediculosis, ringworm, scabies, inflamed eyes, discharging ears, and infected wounds. Limited inspection of school students by physicians began in 1897 and focused on excluding infectious children from school rather than on providing or obtaining medical treatment to enable children to return to school. Familiar with this community-wide problem from her work with the Henry Street Nurses' Settlement, Lillian Wald sought to place nurses in the schools and gained consent from the city's health commissioner and the Board of Education for a 1-month demonstration project.

Lina Rogers, a Nurses' Settlement resident, became the first school nurse. She worked with the children in New York City schools and made home visits to instruct parents and to follow up on children excluded or otherwise absent from school. The school nurses found that "many children were absent for lack of shoes or clothing, because of malnourishment, or because they were serving their families as babysitters" (Hawkins, Hayes, and Corliss, 1994, p. 417). The school nurse experiment made such a significant and positive impact that it became permanent, with 12 more nurses appointed 1 month later. School nursing was soon implemented in Los Angeles, Philadelphia, Baltimore, Boston, Chicago, and San Francisco.

## THE PROFESSION COMES OF AGE

Established by the Cleveland Visiting Nurse Association, the publication of the *Visiting Nurse Quarterly* in 1909 initiated a professional medium of communication for clinical and organizational concerns. In 1911 a joint committee of existing nurse organizations convened, under the leadership of Lillian Wald and Mary Gardner, to standardize nursing services outside the hospital. Recommending formation of a new organization to address public health nursing concerns, 800 agencies involved in public health nursing activities were invited to send delegates to an organizational meeting in Chicago in June 1912. After a heated debate on its name and purpose, the delegates established the **National Organization for Public Health Nursing** (NOPHN) and chose Lillian Wald as its first president (Dock, 1922). Unlike other professional nursing organizations, the NOPHN membership included both nurses and their lay supporters. The NOPHN sought "to improve the educational and services standards of the public health nurse, and promote public understanding of and respect for her work" (Rosen, 1958, p. 381). With greater administrative resources than any of the other national nursing organizations existing at that time, the NOPHN was soon a dominant force in public health nursing (Roberts, 1955).

The NOPHN also sought to standardize public health nursing education. Visiting nurse agencies found that graduates of the hospital schools were unprepared for home visiting. It became apparent that the basic curriculum of many schools of nursing was insufficient. Because diploma schools of nursing emphasized hospital care of patients, public health nurses would require additional education to provide services to the sick at home and to design population-focused programs. In 1914, in affiliation with the Henry Street Settlement, Mary Adelaide Nutting began the first postgraduate nursing course in public health nursing at Teachers College in New York City (Deloughery, 1977). The American Red Cross provided scholarships for graduates of nursing schools to attend the public health nursing course. Its success encouraged development of other programs, whose curriculum might seem familiar to today's nurses. During the 1920s and 1930s, many newly hired public health nurses had to verify completion or promptly enroll in a certificate program in public health nursing. Others took leave for a year to travel to an urban center to obtain this further education. Correspondence courses were even acceptable to some agencies, for example, for public health nurses in upstate New York.

Public health nurses were also active in the **American Public Health Association** (APHA), which was established in 1872 to facilitate interdisciplinary efforts and promote the "practical application of public hygiene" (Scutchfield and Keck, 1997, p. 12). The APHA targeted reform efforts toward contemporary public health issues, including sewage and garbage disposal, occupational injuries, and sexually transmitted diseases. In 1923, the Public Health Nursing Section was formed within the APHA to provide an additional national forum for discussion of strategy for public health nurses within the context of the larger public health organization. The Section has continued to the present time as a focus of leadership and policy development for community/public health nursing.

> **◗ WHAT DO YOU THINK?**
>
> Lillian Wald demonstrated an exceptional ability to develop approaches and programs to solve the health care and social problems of her times. How would you apply this creativity to today's health care challenges? If Lillian Wald were looking over your shoulder, what would she recommend?

## PUBLIC HEALTH NURSING IN OFFICIAL HEALTH AGENCIES

Public health nursing in voluntary agencies and through the Red Cross grew more quickly than public health nursing in state, local, and national government. In the late 1800s, local health departments were formed in urban areas to target environmental hazards associated with crowded living conditions and dirty streets and to regulate public baths, slaughterhouses, and pigsties (Pickett and Hanlon, 1990). By 1900, 38 states had established state health departments, following the lead of Massachusetts in 1869, but the impact of these early state boards of health was limited. Only three states, Massachusetts, Rhode Island, and Florida, annually spent more than 2 cents per capita for public health services (Scutchfield and Keck, 1997). The federal role in public health gradually expanded. In 1912, the federal government redefined the role of the U.S. Public Health Service, empowering it to "investigate the causes and spread of diseases and the pollution and sanitation of navigable streams and lakes" (Scutchfield and Keck, 1997, p. 15).

During the 1910s, public health organizations began to target infectious and parasitic diseases in rural areas. The Rockefeller Sanitary Commission, active in hookworm control in the southeastern United States, concluded that concurrent efforts for all phases of public health were necessary to successfully address any individual public health problem (Pickett and Hanlon, 1990). For example, in 1911, efforts to control typhoid fever in Yakima County, Washington, and to improve health status in Guilford County, North Carolina, led to establishment of local health units to serve local populations. Public health nurses were the primary staff members of local health departments. These nurses assumed a leadership role on health care issues through collaboration with local residents, nurses, and other health care providers.

The experience of Orange County, California, during the 1920s and 1930s demonstrates the role of the public health nurse in these new local health departments. Following the efforts of a private physician, social welfare agencies, and a Red Cross nurse, the county board created the public health nurse's position, to begin in 1922. Presented with a shining new Model T car sporting the bright orange seal of the county, the nurse first addressed the serious communicable disease problems of diphtheria and scarlet fever. Typhoid became epidemic when a drainage pipe overflowed into a well, infecting those who drank the water and those who drank raw milk from an infected dairy. Almost 3000 residents were immunized against typhoid. Weekly baby conferences provided an opportunity for mothers to learn about care of their infants, and the infants were weighed and received communicable disease immunizations. Children with orthopedic and other disabilities were identified and referred for medical care in Los Angeles. At the end of this successful first year of public health nursing work, the Rockefeller Foundation and the California Health Department recognized the favorable outcomes and provided funding for more public health professionals.

## WORLD WAR I AND THE IMPORTANCE OF PUBLIC HEALTH NURSING

The personnel needs of World War I in Europe depleted the ranks of public health nurses, yet the NOPHN identified a need for second and third lines of defense at home. Jane Delano of the Red Cross, who was sending 100 nurses a day to the war, agreed that despite the sacrifice, the greatest patriotic duty of public health nurses was to stay at home. Soon after, a worldwide influenza epidemic swept from the Atlantic coast to the Pacific coast within 3 weeks and was met by a coalition of the NOPHN and the Red Cross. Houses, churches, and social halls were turned into hospitals. Some of the nurse volunteers lost their lives as well. The NOPHN also loaned a nurse to the U.S. Public Health Service to establish a public health nursing program for military outposts. This led to the first federal government sponsorship of nurses (Shyrock, 1959; Wilner, Walkey, and O'Neill, 1978).

## PAYING THE BILL FOR COMMUNITY AND PUBLIC HEALTH NURSES

Inadequate funding was the major obstacle to extending nursing services in the community. Most early visiting nurse associations sought charitable contributions from wealthy and middle-class supporters. Even poor families were encouraged to pay a small fee for nursing services, reflecting social welfare concerns against promoting economic dependency by providing charity. In 1909, as a result of Lillian Wald's collaboration with Dr. Lee Frankel, the **Metropolitan Life Insurance Company** began a cooperative program with visiting nurse organizations. The nurses assessed illness, taught health practices, and collected data from policyholders. By 1912, 589 Metropolitan Life nursing centers provided care through existing agencies or through visiting nurses hired directly by

the company. In 1918, Metropolitan Life calculated an average decline of 7% in the mortality rate of policyholders and almost a 20% decline in the mortality rate of children under age 3. The insurance company attributed this improvement and the reduced costs for the insurance company to the work of visiting nurses. Voluntary health insurance was still decades in the future; public and professional efforts to secure compulsory health insurance seemed promising in 1916 but had evaporated by the end of World War I.

## EFFORTS TO SHAPE PUBLIC POLICY

Nursing efforts to influence public policy bridged World War I and included advocacy for the Children's Bureau and the Sheppard-Towner Program. Responding to lengthy advocacy by Lillian Wald and other nurse leaders, the Children's Bureau was established in 1912 to address national problems of maternal and child welfare. Children's Bureau experts conducted extensive scientific research on the effects of income, housing, employment, and other factors on infant and maternal mortality, leading to federal child labor laws and the 1919 White House Conference on Child Health.

Problems of maternal and child morbidity and mortality spurred the Maternity and Infancy Act (often called the **Sheppard-Towner Act**) in 1921. This act provided federal matching funds to establish maternal and child health divisions in state health departments. Education during home visits by public health nurses stressed promoting the health of mother and child as well as seeking prompt medical care during pregnancy. Although credited with saving many lives, the Sheppard-Towner Program ended in 1929 in response to charges by the American Medical Association and others that the legislation gave too much power to the federal government and too closely resembled socialized medicine (Pickett and Hanlon, 1990).

In contrast to significant changes in public support for community-oriented nursing, some innovations were the result of individual commitment and private financial support. In 1925 the **Frontier Nursing Service** (FNS) was established by **Mary Breckinridge** on the basis of systems of care used in the Highlands and islands of Scotland (Box 2-2; Figure 2-4). Breckinridge introduced the first nurse-midwives into the United States. The unique pioneering spirit of the FNS influenced development of public health programs geared toward improving the health care of the rural and often inaccessible populations in the Appalachian sections of southeastern Kentucky (Browne, 1966; Tirpak, 1975) (Figure 2-5). FNS nurses were trained in nursing, public health, and midwifery. Their efforts led to reduced pregnancy complications and maternal mortality, and to one-third fewer stillbirths and infant deaths in an area of 700 square miles (Kalisch and Kalisch, 1995). Today the FNS continues to provide comprehensive health and nursing services to the people of that area and supports the Frontier School of Midwifery and Family Nursing.

---

**BOX 2-2   Mary Breckinridge and the Frontier Nursing Service**

Born in 1881 into the fifth generation of a Kentucky family, Mary Breckinridge devoted her life to the Frontier Nursing Service (FNS) and to promoting the health care of disadvantaged women and children. Educated by tutors and in private schools, Mary Breckinridge considered becoming a nurse only after her first husband died. In 1907 she entered St. Luke's Hospital School of Nursing in New York City. She later married for a second time, but her daughter died at birth and her son died at age 4 in 1918. In post–World War I France, Breckinridge administered maternal/child and public health programs, including a "goat crusade" in which Americans donated goats to provide milk for hungry European infants. In Great Britain, she became one of the first Americans to receive a nurse midwifery certificate. At this time, nurse midwifery training was not available in the United States. Breckinridge returned to the United States to take the 1-year public health nursing course at Teacher's College of Columbia University in New York.

Passionate about helping the children of rural America and prepared to begin her life's work, early in 1925 Breckinridge returned to Kentucky. She had determined that Kentucky's mountain region was an excellent place to demonstrate the value of public health nursing to improving the health of disadvantaged families living in remote areas. If it was possible to establish a nursing center in rural Kentucky, the program could be duplicated anywhere. Breckinridge applied her family inheritance to initiate her vision for the Frontier Nursing Service. Establishing the first FNS health center in a five-room cabin in Hyden, Kentucky, required not only nursing skills but also construction of the cabin, other buildings, and later the FNS hospital. Each step was difficult, including

securing a water supply, electric power, and sewage disposal, and stabilizing a mountain terrain prone to landslides. Despite these obstacles, six outpost nursing centers were built between 1927 and 1930. When the FNS hospital in Hyden was completed in 1928, physicians began providing service. Financial support for FNS nursing and medical care ranged from patient families' labor exchange and farm product donation to fundraising through annual family dues, philanthropy, and direct fundraising by Breckinridge herself.

Serving nearly 10,000 people spread out over 700 square miles, FNS provided nursing and midwifery services 24 hours a day and established medical, surgical, and dental clinics. Reduced mortality rates were especially remarkable considering the environmental conditions these rural Kentuckians faced. Many area homes lacked heat, electricity, and running water. During the 1930s, nurses lived in one of the six outposts. Transportation remained difficult, as nurse, midwives, and couriers climbed mountains by foot and rode horses great distances. Like her staff, Breckinridge traveled through the remote mountains of Kentucky on her horse, Babette, providing food, supplies, and health care to mountain families. Breckinridge documented her experiences in the book, *Wide Neighborhoods.*

Over the years, hundreds of nurses have worked with FNS. Since Mary Breckinridge died in 1965, FNS has continued to grow and provide needed services to people in the mountains of Kentucky. FNS remains a vital means to providing health services to rural families and as a creative model for nursing service delivery through its home health agency, outpost clinics, primary care, the Frontier School of Midwifery and Family Nursing, and the Mary Breckinridge Hospital.

---

Breckinridge M: *Wide neighborhoods, a story of the Frontier Nursing Service,* New York, 1952, Harper.

Browne H: A tribute to Mary Breckinridge, *Nurs Outlook* 14:54, 1966.

Frontier Nurse Service homepage, http://www.frontiernursing. org/fns.htm.

Holloway JB: Frontier Nursing Service 1925-1975, *J Ky Med Assoc* 13:491, 1975.

Tirpak H: The Frontier Nursing Service—fifty years in the mountains, *Nurs Outlook* 33:308, 1975.

## AFRICAN-AMERICAN NURSES IN PUBLIC HEALTH NURSING

African-American nurses seeking to work in public health nursing faced many challenges. Nursing education was absolutely segregated in the South until at least the 1960s, and it was also generally segregated elsewhere until this time. Even public health nursing certificate and graduate education were segregated in the South; study outside the South was difficult to afford and study leaves from the workplace were infrequently granted. The situation improved somewhat in 1936, when collaboration between the United States Public Health Service and the Medical College of Virginia (Richmond) established a certificate program in public health nursing for black nurses in which the federal government paid nurses' tuition. Although in

the North black and white visiting nurses received the same wage, in the South significantly lower pay rates were characteristic for black nurses. In 1925, just 435 black public health nurses were employed across the United States, and in 1930, just six black nurses held supervisory positions in public health nursing organizations. Jessie Sleet (Scales), a Canadian educated at Provident Hospital School of Nursing (Chicago), became the first black public health nurse when she was hired by the New York Charity Organization Society in 1900 (Buhler-Wilkerson, 2001; Hine, 1989; Thoms, 1929).

African-American public health nurses had a significant impact on the communities they served. The National Health Circle for Colored People was organized in 1919 to promote public health work in black communities in the

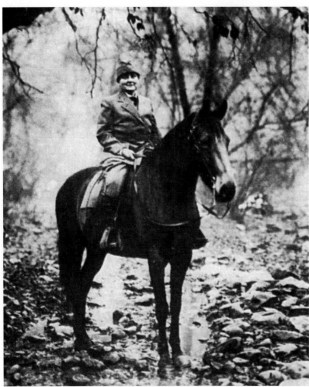

**Figure 2-4** Mary Breckinridge, founder of the Frontier Nursing Service. *(Courtesy Frontier Nursing Service of Wendover, Ky.)*

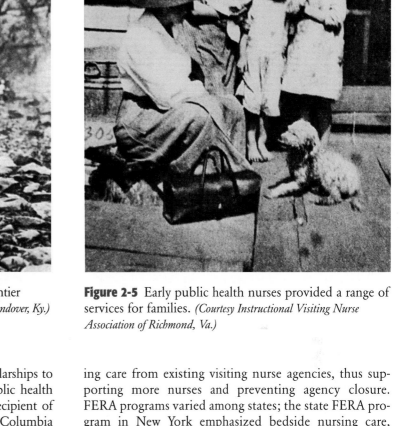

**Figure 2-5** Early public health nurses provided a range of services for families. *(Courtesy Instructional Visiting Nurse Association of Richmond, Va.)*

South. One strategy adopted was providing scholarships to assist black nurses to pursue university-level public health nursing education. Bessie M. Hawes, the first recipient of the scholarship, completed the program at Columbia University (New York) and was then sent by the Circle to Palatka, Florida. In this small, isolated lumber town, Hawes's first project was to recruit school-girls to promote health by dressing as nurses and marching in a parade while singing community songs. She conducted mass meetings, led Mother's Clubs, provided school health education, and visited the homes of the sick. Eventually she gained the community's trust, overcame opposition, and built a health center for nursing care and treatment (Thoms, 1929).

## BETWEEN THE TWO WORLD WARS: ECONOMIC DEPRESSION AND THE RISE OF HOSPITALS

The economic crisis during the Depression of the 1930s deeply influenced nursing. Not only were agencies and communities unprepared to address the increased needs and numbers of the impoverished but decreased funding for nursing services reduced the number of employed nurses in hospitals and in the community. The Federal Emergency Relief Administration (FERA) supported nurse employment through increased grants-in-aid for state programs of home medical care. FERA often purchased nurs-

ing care from existing visiting nurse agencies, thus supporting more nurses and preventing agency closure. FERA programs varied among states; the state FERA program in New York emphasized bedside nursing care, whereas in North Carolina, the state FERA prioritized maternal and child health and school nursing services. Some Depression-era federal programs built new services; public health nursing programs of the Works Progress Administration (WPA) were sometimes later incorporated into state health departments. In West Virginia, the Relief Nursing Service sought to assist unemployed nurses and provide nursing care for families on relief. Fundamental services included "(1) providing bedside care and health supervision for the family in the home; (2) arranging for medical and hospital care for emergency and obstetric cases; (3) supervising the health of children in emergency relief nursery schools; and (4) caring for patients with tuberculosis" (Kalisch and Kalisch, 1995, p. 306).

Over 10,000 nurses were employed by the Civil Works Administration (CWA) programs and assigned to official health agencies. "While this facilitated rapid program expansion by recipient agencies and gave the nurses a taste of public health, the nurses' lack of field experience created major problems of training and supervision for the regular staff" (Roberts and Heinrich, 1985, p. 1162). A 1932 survey of public health agencies found that only 7%

of nurses employed in public health were adequately prepared (Roberts and Heinrich, 1985). Basic nursing education focused heavily on the care of individuals, and students received limited information on groups and the community as a unit of service. Thus in the 1930s and early 1940s, new graduates continued to be inadequately prepared to work in public health and required considerable agency orientation and teaching (National Organization for Public Health Nursing, 1944).

Community-oriented nurses continued to evaluate the value of preventive care compared to bedside care of the sick. They also questioned whether nursing interventions should be directed toward groups and communities or toward individuals and their families. Although each nursing agency was unique and services varied from region to region, voluntary visiting nurse associations tended to emphasize care of the sick, whereas official public health agencies provided more preventive services. Not surprisingly, this splintering of services between "visiting," or community, and "public health" nurses further impeded development of comprehensive services (Roberts and Heinrich, 1985). In addition, some households received services from several community nurses representing several agencies (e.g., visits for a postpartum woman and new baby, for a child sick with scarlet fever, and for an older adult sick in bed). Nurses believed this confused families and duplicated scarce nursing resources. One solution was the "combination service," the merger of sick care services and preventive services into one comprehensive agency, most often ad-

ministered by a public agency. The downside was that, compared with visiting nurse organizations, nurses in **official agencies** might have less control over the program because physicians and politicians determined services and assignment of personnel in public health departments.

## INCREASING FEDERAL ACTION FOR THE PUBLIC'S HEALTH

Changes at the federal level affected the structure of community health resources. Credited as "the beginning of a new era in public nursing" (Roberts and Heinrich, 1985, p. 1162), Pearl McIver in 1933 became the first nurse employed by the U.S. Public Health Service to provide consultation services to state health departments. McIver was convinced that the strengths and ability of each state's director of public health nursing would determine the scope and quality of local health services. Together with Naomi Deutsch, director of nursing for the federal Children's Bureau, and with the support of nursing organizations, McIver and her staff of nurse consultants influenced the direction of public health nursing. Between 1931 and 1938, over 40% of the increase in public health nurse employment was in local health agencies. Even so, over one third of all counties nationally still lacked local public health nursing services.

The **Social Security Act of 1935** attempted to overcome the national setbacks of the Depression. Title VI of this act provided funding for expanded opportunities for health protection and promotion through education and

---

 **Evidence-Based Practice**

*No Place Like Home: A History of Nursing and Home Care in the United States* is a book-length analysis of the development of nursing care for those at home. Buhler-Wilkerson traces how the care of the sick moved from a domestic function to a charitable or public responsibility provided through visiting nurse associations and official health agencies. The central dilemma she raises is "why, despite its potential as a preferred, rational, and possibly cost-effective alternative to institutional care, home care remains a marginalized experiment in caregiving" (p. xi).

Buhler-Wilkerson follows the origins of home care from its beginnings in Charleston, South Carolina, to its expansion into northern cities at the end of the nineteenth century. She interprets the founding of public health nursing by Lillian Wald "as a new paradigm for community-based nursing practice within the context of social reform" (p. xii), and she particularly analyzes the effects of ethnicity, race, and social class. She traces the difficulties of organizing and financing care of the sick in the home, including the work of private duty nurses and the role of health insurance in shaping home ser-

vices. The concluding section of the book highlights contemporary themes of "chronic illness, hospital dominance, financial viability, and struggles to survive" (p. xii) and projects the future of home care.

Buhler-Wilkerson brings to bear the stories of patients' needs and nurses' work against the financial challenges that have characterized home care. While focusing on one element, this book raises important questions for nurses' work across elements of community/public health nursing. Clearly identified need does not by itself open the doors to adequate financing for nursing care of the sick, for public health nursing, or for population care for health promotion.

**Nurse Use:** This book points out the complex issues involved in trying to provide the most effective care to patients. The needs of patients and their families may not entirely correlate with what is financially available. A lesson for each of us to learn: identified need does not always influence the availability of funds to provide the desired care.

---

Buhler-Wilkerson K: *No place like home: a history of nursing and home care in the United States,* Baltimore, 2001, Johns Hopkins Press.

employment of public health nurses. Over 1000 nurses completed educational programs in public health in 1936. Title VI also provided $8 million to assist states, counties, and medical districts in the establishment and maintenance of adequate health services, as well as $2 million for research and investigation of disease (Buhler-Wilkerson, 1985, 1989; Kalisch and Kalisch, 1995).

A categorical approach to federal funding for public health services reflected the U.S. Congress's preference for funding specific diseases or specific groups. In categorical funding, funding is directed toward specific priorities rather than toward a comprehensive community health program. When funding is directed by established national preferences, it becomes more difficult to respond to local and emerging problems. Even so, local health departments shaped their programs according to the pattern of available funds (e.g., maternal and child health services and crippled children [1935], venereal disease control [1938], tuberculosis [1944], mental health [1947], industrial hygiene [1947], and dental health [1947]) (Scutchfield and Keck, 1997). This pattern of funding continues to be an element of the federal approach to health policy.

## WORLD WAR II: EXTENSION AND RETRENCHMENT IN COMMUNITY AND PUBLIC HEALTH NURSING

The U.S. involvement in World War II in 1941 accelerated the need for nurses, both for the war effort and at home. The Nursing Council on National Defense was a coalition of the national nursing organizations that sought to plan and coordinate activities for the war effort. National interest prioritized the health of military personnel and workers in essential industries. Many nurses joined the Army and Navy Nurse Corps. Through the influence and leadership of U.S. Representative Frances Payne Bolton of Ohio, substantial funding was provided by the Bolton Act of 1943 to establish the Cadet Nurses Corps, which increased enrollment in schools of nursing at undergraduate and graduate levels. Under management by the U.S. Public Health Service, the Nursing Council for National Defense received $1 million to expand facilities for nursing education. Training for Nurses for National Defense, the GI Bill, the Nurse Training Act of 1943, and Public Health and Professional Nurse Traineeships provided additional educational funds that expanded both the total number of nurses and the number of nurses with preparation in public health nursing (McNeil, 1967).

The war-related reduction in acute care services as a result of the depletion of nursing and medical personnel from civilian hospitals tended to shift responsibility for patient care to families and others. Nonnursing personnel assumed roles formerly held by registered nurses both at home and in hospitals. "By the end of 1942, over 500,000 women had completed the American Red Cross home nursing course, and nearly 17,000 nurse's aides had been certified" (Roberts and Heinrich, 1985, p. 1165). By the end of 1946, over 215,000 volunteer nurse's aides had received certificates.

In some cases, community-oriented nursing expanded its scope of practice during World War II. For example, nurses increased their presence in rural areas, and many official agencies began to provide bedside nursing care (Buhler-Wilkerson, 1985; Kalisch and Kalisch, 1995). The federal Emergency Maternity and Infant Care Act of 1943 (EMIC) provided funding for medical, hospital, and nursing care for the wives and babies of servicemen, but only when the services met the tough standards of the U.S. Children's Bureau. In other situations, community-oriented nursing roles were constrained by wartime and postwar nursing shortages. For example, the Visiting Nurse Society of Philadelphia ceased assisting with home births, drastically reduced industrial nursing care, and deferred care for the long-term chronically ill patient.

Reflecting the complex social changes of the war years, local health departments were faced immediately after the war with increased service needs, including sudden increases in client demand for care of emotional problems, accidents, alcoholism, and other responsibilities new to the domain of official health agencies. Changes in medical technology offered new possibilities for screening and treatment of infectious and communicable diseases, such as antibiotics to treat rheumatic fever and venereal diseases and photofluorography for mass case finding of pulmonary tuberculosis. Local health departments expanded, both to address underserved areas and to expand types of services, and they often fared better economically than the voluntary agencies.

Job opportunities for public health nurses grew because they constituted a large proportion of the staff in these health departments. Between 1950 and 1955, the proportion of U.S. counties with full-time local health services increased from 56% to 72% (Roberts and Heinrich, 1985). With more than 20,000 nurses employed in health departments, visiting nurse associations, industry, and schools, community and public health nurses at the middle of the twentieth century continued to be important in translating the advances of science and medicine into saving lives and improving health.

In 1946, representatives of agencies interested in community health met to improve coordination of various types of community nursing and to prevent overlap of services. The resulting guidelines proposed that a population of 50,000 be required to support a public health program and that there should be one nurse for every 2200 people. Community-oriented nursing functions should include health teaching, disease control, and care of the sick. Communities should adopt one of the following organizational patterns (Desirable organization, 1946):

- Administration of all community health nurse services by the local health department
- Provision of preventive health care by health departments, and provision of home visiting for the sick by a cooperating voluntary agency

## A Historical Overview of Community and Public Health Nursing in Canada

Karon Janine Foster, R.N., B.Sc.N., M.Ed., Lecturer, Faculty of Nursing, University of Toronto

### BEFORE CONFEDERATION

In Canada's early years as a French colony, residents of New France suffered from infectious diseases, malnutrition, injuries, and inadequate clothing and shelter. Physical, social, and spiritual care was provided by Christian religious orders. With the arrival of families, lay women in the community provided care to the community. One of the first lay healers was Marie Rollet Hébert of Quebec, who cared for the sick in settlers' homes. The first nurses in Canada were male attendants stationed at the sick bay in a French garrison in 1629.

The Duchess d'Aiguillon and three nuns from Hospitalières de la Misèricorde de Jèsus established a hospital in Quebec City in 1639. These nuns cared for the sick in the hospital and in residents' homes. Jeanne Mance was a co-founder of Hotel Dieu hospital on the Island of Montreal. At Hotel Dieu, care was provided to the sick, and shelter and education were provided to the poor, new immigrants, and the Aboriginals.

In 1738, Marguerite d'Youville founded the first community visiting nurses, the Grey Nuns of Montreal. The focus of their work was to provide direct care and education. They organized houses of refuge for older adults and the infirm, and they established hospitals. As Canada expanded, the Grey Nuns established health services in the 1840s in Red River Settlement (Manitoba) and Bytown (Ottawa) and in the 1860s in Saskatoon and the Northwest Territories.

In 1763, Canada came under British rule. There was a focus on controlling infectious diseases and building hospitals. Public health measures such as laws requiring meat inspection, building inspections, and quarantines were initiated. The cholera epidemics in the early 1800s prompted the establishments of boards of health. The Public Health Act of 1831 provided legal directives concerning personal and environmental cleanliness, quarantine, and the handling of contaminated objects or bodies.

### AFTER CONFEDERATION

On July 1, 1867, the provinces of Nova Scotia, New Brunswick, Quebec, and Ontario formed the Dominion of Canada. The British North America Act of 1867 outlined the responsibilities of the federal and provincial governments in relation to health care. The federal government was responsible for maintenance of marine hospitals and quarantines, and the provinces were responsible for the maintenance of hospitals, asylums, and welfare services. Regional variations in health care and public health services developed as a result of this decision.

From the 1870s to the early 1900s, the major threats to health were contagious diseases, maternal deaths, and deaths from childhood diseases. Economic expansion and immigration resulted in more settlers living in urban areas. The cities became overcrowded, and unsanitary conditions existed. Public support grew for comprehensive public health programs. In the 1880s, the first permanent boards of health were established in Ontario, and the appointed board was responsible for control of communicable diseases and the promotion of health. In 1874, the first school of nursing was established in St. Catherines, Ontario.

In 1890, the Countess of Aberdeen (wife of the governor general) was concerned about the health needs of women and the poor in cities and isolated settlements. She proposed the formation of a group of untrained workers to provide care to these populations; opposition came from doctors and nursing groups. She revised her plan, and graduate nurses with extra training in midwifery and home visiting were hired. The organization was called the Victorian Order of Nurses (VON). These nurses provided disease prevention and health promotion activities in the community. The first offices were set up in Halifax, Montreal, Ottawa, and Toronto. Charlotte MacLeod became the chief lady superintendent of the VON and was credited with establishing many branches and training schools during her tenure.

### TWENTIETH CENTURY

Public health services in the early 1900s were provided by both government and voluntary organizations, as federal department existed until 1919. The Canadian Red Cross became instrumental in promoting public health measures and training nurses to work in this

- A combination service jointly administered and financed by official and voluntary agencies with all services provided by one group of nurses

Table 2-2 highlights significant milestones in community and public health nursing from the mid 1800s to the mid 1900s.

## THE RISE OF CHRONIC ILLNESS

Between 1900 and 1955, the national crude mortality rate decreased by 47%. Many more Americans survived childhood and early adulthood to live into middle and older ages. Whereas in 1900 the leading causes of mortality were pneumonia, tuberculosis, and diarrhea/enteritis, by mid century the leading causes had become heart disease, cancer, and cerebrovascular disease. Nurses contributed to reductions in communicable diseases through immunization campaigns, improved nutrition, and better hygiene and sanitation. Additional factors included improved medications, better housing, and innovative emergency and critical care services. As the aged population grew from 4.1% of the total in 1900 to 9.2% in 1950, so did the prevalence of chronic illness. With extended life span and

area. They developed educational programs about public health, hygiene, and immunization. These types of programs eventually became the responsibility of the official public health agencies and resulted in the creation of the public health nurse (PHN) position. PHNs became the front-line workers in community health promotion and the maintenance of health providing programs such as maternal and child welfare, disease prevention, community education (e.g., first aid), health plays, and school health programs. Nursing divisions were developed within public health agencies in the early 1900s in Ontario, Manitoba, Alberta, and British Columbia and in the 1920s in Nova Scotia and New Brunswick.

In 1932, the Weir Report on Nursing Education evaluated the first nursing programs and made recommendations that influenced the preparation and practice of PHNs. Recommendations included requiring the completion of a 1-year public health nursing course after basic nursing training as the minimum requirement, doubling the number of practicing PHNs, increasing their salary, and a cost-sharing arrangement with provincial and municipal governments to fund the costs of public health services. The Red Cross provided grants to six Canadian universities to develop courses in public health. These programs eventually led to the development of baccalaureate programs in nursing.

Since the 1950s, the role of PHNs has continued to evolve. With the implementation of a publicly funded medical insurance plan in 1969, some of the health promotion activities done by PHNs (e.g., well-baby clinics, infant immunization clinics) were transferred to physicians. Today, the community health nurse role may include direct care to individuals and families as well as prevention efforts and promotion of health to individuals, families, groups, or communities. Community nurses continue to be concerned with social justice and the determinants of health, and they incorporate strategies of advocacy, education, and community organization and participation into their practice. They practice in a variety of venues including public health, visiting nurse agencies, home care, occupational health, community health centers, and agencies providing health promotion and care to the homeless.

## Bibliography

Allemang M: Development of community health nursing in Canada. In Stewart MJ, editor: *Community health nursing: promoting Canadians' health,* Toronto, 1995, Saunders.

Allemang M: Development of community health nursing in Canada. In Stewart MJ, editor: *Community health nursing: promoting Canadians' health,* ed 2, pp. 4-32, Toronto, 2000, Saunders.

Baumgart A: Evolution of the Canadian health care system. In Baumgart A, Larsen J, editors: *Canadian nursing faces the future,* ed 2, St Louis, Mo, 1992, Mosby.

Chalmers K, Kristjanson L: Community health nursing practice. In Baumgart A, Larsen J, editors: *Canadian nursing faces the future,* ed 2, St Louis, Mo, 1992, Mosby.

Duncan S, Leipert B, Mill J: "Nurses as health evangelists"? The evolution of public health nursing in Canada, 1918-1939, *ANS Adv Nursing Sci* 22(1):40-51, 1999.

Falk Rafael A: The politics of health promotion: influences on public health nursing practice in Ontario, Canada from Nightingale to the nineties. *ANS Adv Nurs Sci* 22(1):23-39, 1999.

Kerr Ross J: The growth of community health nursing in Canada. In Ross J, MacPhail J, editors: *An introduction to issues in community health nursing in Canada,* St Louis, Mo, 1996, Mosby.

Mill J, Leipert B, Duncan S: Frontiers and pioneers: a history of public health nursing in Alberta and British Columbia, 1918 to 1939, *Can Nurse* 98(1):18-23, 2002.

Pringle D, Roe D: Voluntary community agencies: VON Canada an example. In Baumgart A, Larsen J, editors: *Canadian nursing faces the future,* ed 2, St Louis, Mo, 1992, Mosby.

*Canadian spelling is used.*

increased duration of life after a diagnosis of chronic illness, community-oriented nurses faced new challenges related to chronic illness care, long-term illness and disability, and chronic disease prevention.

Studies such as the National Health Survey of 1935-1936 documented the national transition from communicable to chronic disease as the primary cause of significant illness and death. However, public policy and community-oriented nursing services were diverted from addressing the emerging problem, first by the 1930s Depression and then by World War II.

In official health agencies, categorical programs focusing on a single chronic disease emphasized narrowly defined services, which might be poorly coordinated with other agency programs. Screening for chronic illness was a popular method of both detecting undiagnosed disease and providing individual and community education. Some visiting nurse associations adopted coordinated home care programs to provide complex, long-term care to the chronically ill, often after long-term hospitalization. These home care programs established a multidisciplinary approach to complex patient care. For example, beginning

**Table 2-2   Milestones in History of Community Health and Public Health Nursing: 1866-1945**

| YEAR | MILESTONE | YEAR | MILESTONE |
|------|-----------|------|-----------|
| 1866 | New York Metropolitan Board of Health established | 1910 | Public health nursing program instituted at Teachers College, Columbia University, in New York |
| 1872 | American Public Health Association established | 1912 | National Organization for Public Health Nursing formed with Lillian Wald as first president |
| 1873 | New York Training School opens at Bellevue Hospital, New York City, as first Nightingale-model nursing school in United States | 1914 | First undergraduate nursing education course in public health offered by Adelaide Nutting at Teacher's College |
| 1877 | Women's Board of the New York Mission hires Frances Root to visit the sick poor | 1918 | Vassar Camp School for Nurses organized; U.S. Public Health Service (PHS) establishes division of public health nursing to work in the war effort; worldwide influenza epidemic begins |
| 1885 | Visiting Nurse Association established in Buffalo | | |
| 1886 | Visiting nurse agencies established in Philadelphia and Boston | 1919 | Textbook, *Public Health Nursing,* written by Mary S. Gardner |
| 1893 | Lillian Wald and Mary Brewster organized a visiting nursing service for the poor of New York, which later became the famous Henry Street Settlement; Society of Superintendents of Training Schools of Nurses in the United States and Canada was established (in 1912 became known as the National League for Nursing) | 1921 | Maternity and Infancy Act (Sheppard-Towner Act) |
| | | 1925 | Frontier Nursing Service using nurse-midwives established |
| | | 1934 | Pearl McIver becomes first nurse employed by PHS |
| | | 1935 | Passage of Social Security Act |
| 1895 | Associated Alumnae of Training Schools for Nurses established (in 1911 became the American Nurses Association) | 1941 | Beginning of World War II |
| 1902 | School nursing started in New York (Lina Rogers) | 1943 | Passage of Bolton-Bailey Act for nursing education and Cadet Nurse Program established; Division of Nursing begun at PHS; Lucille Petry appointed chief of Cadet Nurse Corps |
| 1903 | First nurse practice acts | | |
| 1909 | Metropolitan Life Insurance Company provides first insurance reimbursement for nursing care | 1944 | First basic program in nursing accredited as including sufficient public health content |

in 1949, the Visiting Nurse Society of Philadelphia provided care to patients with stroke, arthritis, cancer, and fractures using a wide range of services, including physical and occupational therapy, nutrition consultation, social services, laboratory and radiographic procedures, and transportation services. During the 1950s, often in reaction to family needs and the shortage of nurses, many visiting nurse agencies began experimenting with auxiliary nursing personnel, variously called housekeepers, homemakers, or home health aides. These innovative programs provided a

**THE CUTTING EDGE**

Nurse historians are increasingly using oral history methodology to uncover and preserve the history of public health nurses on audiotapes and in written transcripts.

substantial basis for an approach to sickness care that would be reimbursable by private health insurance and later by Medicare and Medicaid.

The increased prevalence of chronic illness encouraged growth in combination agencies—the joint operation of official (city or county) health departments and voluntary visiting nurse agencies using a unified staff. Nurses wanted services to be provided in a coordinated, cost-effective manner respectful to families served and to also avoid duplication of care. Where nursing services were specialized, one household might simultaneously receive care from three different agencies for postpartum and newborn care, tuberculosis follow-up, and stroke rehabilitation. In cities with combination agencies, a minimum number of nurses would provide improved services, assuring continuity of care at a cheaper price. No longer would an agency "pick up and drop a baby" but would follow the child through infancy, preschool, school, and into adulthood as part of one public health nursing program using one patient record. The "ideal program" of the combination agency proved difficult to administer, however, and many of the combination services implemented between 1930 and 1965 later retrenched into their former divided structures.

During the 1950s, public health nursing practice, like nursing generally, increased its focus on the psychological elements of patient, family, and community care. To be more effective as helping persons, nurses sought improved understanding of their own behavior, as well as the behavior of their patients and their co-workers. The nurse's responsibility for health and human needs now expanded to include stress and anxiety reduction associated with situational or developmental stressors, such as birth, adolescence, and parenting. Public health nurses sought a comprehensive approach to mental health that avoided dividing persons into physical components and emotional components (Abramovitz, 1961).

## FAILURE OF FINANCING FOR COMMUNITY-ORIENTED NURSING

Hospitals gradually became the preferred place for illness care and childbirth during the 1930s and 1940s. Improved technology and the concentration of physicians' work in the acute care hospital were influential, but the development of health insurance plans such as Blue Cross provided a way for the middle class to seek care outside the traditional arena of the home. Federal health policy after World War II supported the growth of institutional care in hospitals and nursing homes over community-based alternatives.

Financing for voluntary nursing agencies was greatly reduced in the early 1950s when both the Metropolitan and John Hancock Life Insurance Companies ceased to fund visiting nurse services for the care of their policyholders. The life insurance companies had found nursing services financially beneficial when communicable disease rates were high 30 years before, but reductions in communicable disease rates, improved infant and maternal health, and increased prevalence of chronic illness reduced financing and sponsor interest in home visiting. The American Red Cross also discontinued its programs of direct nursing service by mid 1950.

Beginning in the 1930s, the NOPHN collaborated with the American Nurses Association (ANA) through the Joint Committee on Prepayment. Voluntary nursing agencies developed a variety of initiatives to secure health insurance reimbursement for nursing services, including demonstration projects and educational campaigns directed toward nurses, physicians, and insurers. Blue Cross and other hospital insurance programs gradually adopted a formula that traded unused days of hospitalization coverage for postdischarge nursing care at home. Unlike organized medicine and hospital associations, the nursing profession contributed substantially to securing federal medical insurance for the aged, which was implemented as the Medicare program in 1966. The support of the ANA, so integral to the passage of Medicare legislation, was recognized by President Lyndon Baines Johnson at the ceremony to sign the bill.

## CONSOLIDATION OF NATIONAL NURSING ORGANIZATIONS

Despite the success and importance of the NOPHN, by the late 1940s its membership had declined and financial support was weak. At the same time, the vision of the nursing profession as a whole was to reorganize the national organizations to improve unity, administration, and financial stability. Three existing organizations—the NOPHN, the National League for Nursing Education, and the Association of Collegiate Schools of Nursing—were dissolved in 1952. Their functions were distributed primarily to the new **National League for Nursing,** and the **American Nurses Association,** which merged with the National Association of Colored Graduate Nurses, continued as the second national nursing organization. Occupational health nursing and nurse-midwifery declined to join the consolidation; both nursing specialties have continued to set their own course. Despite the optimism of the national reorganization and its success in some areas, the subsequent loss of public health nursing leadership and focus resulted in a weakened specialty.

### DID YOU KNOW?

Nurses, including public and community health nurses, interested in the history of nursing can join the American Association for the History of Nursing (AAHN), which holds annual research meetings. Look for the AAHN on the internet at www.aahn.org

## PROFESSIONAL NURSING EDUCATION FOR PUBLIC HEALTH NURSING

The National League for Nursing enthusiastically adopted the recommendations of Esther Lucile Brown's 1948 study of nursing education, reported as *Nursing for the Future.* Her recommendations to establish basic nursing preparation in colleges and universities was consistent with the NOPHN's goal of including public health nursing concepts in all basic baccalaureate programs. The NOPHN believed that this would remedy the problems of training found in nurses new to community-oriented nursing practice and would thus upgrade the profession. Unfortunately, the implementation of the plan fell short, and training programs in public health nursing concepts for college and university faculty were very brief. The population focus of public health nursing toward groups and the larger community was compromised and became less distinct in the hands of educators who themselves lacked education and practice in public health nursing.

During the 1950s, public health nursing educators carefully considered steps to enhance undergraduate and graduate education in the field. Education for public health nurses was actually divided between schools of nursing and schools of public health. Although both claimed legitimacy, collegiate education for nurses gradually moved completely into schools of nursing. The Haven Hill (1951) and Gull Lake (1956) Conferences clarified roles and definitions, built expectations for graduate education, and set standards for undergraduate field experiences. As public health nursing education drew closer to university schools of nursing, it adopted and applied broad principles char-acteristic of general nursing education. For example, rather than have the education director of the placement agency teach nursing students as done previously, collegiate programs themselves hired faculty who provided student supervision at community placements (NOPHN, 1951;

---

### BOX 2-3   Ruth Freeman: Public Health Educator, Administrator, Consultant, Author, and Leader of National Health Organizations

Public health nursing by the 1940s had emerged from its pioneer experiences and begun to develop into a professional discipline capable of functioning in an increasing complex health care system. To meet the challenges of providing health services to diverse communities, nursing needed leaders who possessed the necessary intellectual and political capabilities to keep the profession in the forefront of the national public health care movement. Ruth Freeman was one of these leaders.

Born in Methune, Massachusetts, on December 5, 1906, Ruth was the oldest of three children in a middle-class family. Encouraged by an aunt to become a nurse, Ruth entered the nursing program at Mount Sinai Hospital in New York City in 1923. As a student, she discovered that not only was nursing about caring for people but it was also intellectually challenging and offered many professional opportunities. After graduating in 1927, Ruth accepted a staff position at the Henry Street Visiting Nurse Service. This position profoundly influenced her career and her view of the power of nursing to help people deal with their illnesses and social problems. Recalling these formative years, Ruth noted that the families taught her an important nursing lesson: "that dying wasn't a calamity, that 'making do' was not demeaning, and helping was not controlling" (Safier, 1977, p. 68). Her Henry Street mentors, including Lillian Wald, reinforced her developing philosophy that the family was the principal decision-maker in their health activities, and that patience and optimism were essential characteristics of an effective nurse (Safier, 1977).

Recognized by faculty in her Columbia University baccalaureate program for her ability to lead, Ruth began her teaching career at the New York University Department of Nursing in 1937. She moved to the University of Minnesota School of Public Health to teach and to learn how health care was provided in rural communities. Ruth's insistence that she remain actively engaged in public health work allowed her opportunities to integrate the newly emerging social and biological knowledge into the direct care of clients. Her ability to use this information to alleviate health problems in the community enriched her students' education, and through her many articles and national presentations, she greatly influenced the practice of public health nurses and physicians in the nation.

Ruth's reputation as an innovative thinker and effective administrator led to positions as director of nursing at the American Red Cross and consultant to the National Security Board in Washington, DC (1946 to 1950). This experience solidified her belief in the interdisciplinary nature of community health services and the need for professional nurses to serve as administrators of health agencies and organizations. To ensure her own academic competency, she acquired an M.A. degree from Columbia University in 1939 and an Ed.D. from New York University in 1951 (Kaufman, 1988).

A new position at the Johns Hopkins University School of Hygiene and Public Health (1950 to 1971) led to Dr. Freeman's becoming a professor of public health administration and coordinator of the nursing program. During her tenure at Hopkins, her talents as teacher, author, consultant, and organizational leader flourished. Author of over 50 publications, several of her books, including *Public Health Nursing Practice, Administration in Public Health Services* (with E. M. Holmes), and *Community Health Practice*, became widely used texts in nursing programs. Her ability to provide insightful leadership led to her election and appointment to numerous national posts including president of the National League of Nursing (1955 to 1959), president of the National Health Council (1959 to 1960), and many of the major committees of the American Public Health Association. Dr. Freeman also served as a member of the 1958 White House Conference on Children and Youth and as a consultant to the World Health Organization and the Pan American Health Organization (Bullough, Church, and Stern, 1988).

The numerous national and international awards bestowed on her acknowledged Ruth Freeman's unique contributions to the professionalization of nursing and the improvement of public health services. These included the prestigious American Nurses Association's Pearl McIver Award, the American Public Health Association's Bronfman Prize, and the Florence Nightingale Medal given by the International Red Cross. She was named, in 1981, an honorary member of the American Academy of Nursing, and in 1984, 2 years after her death, she was awarded American nursing's highest honor, election to the American Nurses' Association's Nursing Hall of Fame (Bullough et al, 1988; Kaufman, 1988; Safier, 1977).

Contributed by Barbara Brodie, Ph.D., R.N., F.A.A.N., Director Emeritus of the Center for Nursing Historical Inquiry, University of Virginia, Charlottesville.

Bullough V, Church OM, Stern A: *American nursing: a biographic dictionary*, New York, 1988, Garland.

Kaufman M, editor: *Dictionary of American nursing biography*, New York, 1988, Greenwood Press.

Safier G: *Contemporary American leaders in nursing: an oral history*, New York, 1977, McGraw-Hill.

Robeson and McNeil, 1957). Ruth Freeman was an important nursing leader in this period (Box 2-3).

## NEW FORMS OF PAYMENT FOR COMMUNITY-ORIENTED NURSING

Beginning in earnest in the late 1940s but on the basis of advocacy begun in the late 1910s, policymakers and social welfare representatives sought to establish national health insurance. In 1965, Congress amended the Social Security Act to include health insurance benefits for older adults (Medicare) and increased care for the poor (Medicaid). Unfortunately, the revised Social Security Act did not include coverage for preventive services, and home health care was reimbursed only when ordered by the physician. Nevertheless, this latter coverage prompted the rapid proliferation of home health care agencies. Many local and state health departments rapidly changed their policies to allow the agencies to provide reimbursable home care as bedside nursing. This often resulted in reduced health promotion and disease prevention activities. From 1960 to 1968, the number of official agencies providing home care services grew from 250 to 1328, and the number of for-profit agencies continued to grow (Kalisch and Kalisch, 1995).

## COMMUNITY ORGANIZATION AND PROFESSIONAL CHANGE

The practice of public health and community-oriented nursing was influenced by social changes during the 1960s and 1970s. "The emerging civil rights movement shifted the paradigm from a charitable obligation to a political commitment to achieving equality and compensation for racial injustices of the past" (Scutchfield and Keck, 1997, p. 328). New programs addressed economic and racial differences in health care services and delivery. Funding was increased for maternal and child health, mental health, mental retardation, and community health training. Beginning in 1964, the Economic Opportunity Act provided funds for neighborhood health centers, Head Start, and other community action programs. Neighborhood health centers increased community access for health care especially for maternal and child care. The work of Nancy Milio in Detroit, Michigan, is an example of this commitment to action with the community. Milio built a dynamic decision-making process that included neighborhood residents, politicians, the Visiting Nurse Association and its board, civil rights activists, and church leaders. The Mom and Tots Center emerged as a neighborhood-centered service to provide maternal and child health services and a day-care center. Milio recorded this story in her book, *9226 Kercheval: The Storefront That Did Not Burn* (Milio, 1971).

New personnel also added to the flexibility of the community-oriented nurse to address the needs of communities. Beginning in 1965 at the University of Colorado, the nurse practitioner movement opened a new era for nursing's involvement in primary care, which had an impact on the delivery of services in community health clinics. Initially, the nurse practitioner was a public health

---

**HOW TO** Conduct an Oral History Interview

1. Identify an issue or event of interest.
2. Research the issue or event using written materials.
3. Locate a potential oral history interviewee or narrator.
4. Obtain the agreement of the narrator to be interviewed. Arrange an interview appointment.
5. Research the narrator's background and the time period of interest.
6. Write an outline of questions for the narrator. Open-ended questions are especially helpful.
7. Meet with the narrator. Bring a tape recorder and extra tapes to the interview.
8. Interview the narrator. Ask one brief question at a time. Give the narrator time to consider your question and answer it.
9. Ask clarifying questions. Ask for examples. Give encouragement. Allow the narrator to tell his or her story without interruption.
10. After the interview, transcribe the interview tape and prepare a written transcript.
11. Carefully compare the written transcript to the narrator's recorded interview. It may be appropriate to have the narrator review and edit the written transcript.
12. If you have made written arrangements with the narrator, place the oral history tape and transcripts in an appropriate archives or library (highly recommended).

Oral history is a type of nursing research. Please consider that oral history interviews may require formal consent by the interviewee or narrator before the interview, as well as prior approval of the research from an institutional review board.

---

nurse with additional skills in the diagnosis and treatment of common illnesses. Although some nurse practitioners chose to practice in other clinical areas, those who remained in practice made sustained contributions to improving access and providing primary care to people in rural areas, inner cities, and other medically underserved areas (Roberts and Heinrich, 1985). As evidence of the effectiveness of their services grew, nurse practitioners became increasingly accepted as cost-effective providers of a variety of primary care services.

## COMMUNITY AND PUBLIC HEALTH NURSING FROM THE 1970S TO THE PRESENT

During the 1970s, nursing was viewed as a powerful force for improving the health care of communities. Nurses made significant contributions to the hospice movement, the development of birthing centers, day care for older adult and disabled persons, drug abuse programs, and rehabilitation services in long-term care. Federal evaluation of the effectiveness of care was emphasized (Roberts and Heinrich, 1985).

By the 1980s, concern grew about the high costs of health care in the United States. Programs for health promotion and disease prevention received less priority as funding was shifted to meet the escalating costs of acute hospital care, medical procedures, and institutional long-term care. The use of ambulatory services including health maintenance organizations was encouraged, and the use of nurse practitioners increased. Home health care weathered several threats to adequate reimbursement and, by the end of the decade, had secured favorable legal decisions that increased its impact on the care of the sick at home. Individuals and families assumed more responsibility for their own health status because health education, always a part of community-oriented nursing, became increasingly popular. Advocacy groups representing both consumers and professionals urged the passage of laws to prohibit unhealthy practices in public such as smoking and driving under the influence of alcohol. Sophisticated media campaigns have contributed to improving health status. As federal and state funds grew scarce, the presence of nurses in official public health agencies diminished. Committed and determined to improve the health care of Americans, nurses continued to press for greater involvement in official and voluntary agencies (Kalisch and Kalisch, 1995; Roberts and Heinrich, 1985).

The National Center for Nursing Research (NCNR), established in 1985 within the National Institutes of Health in Washington, DC, has had a major impact on promoting the work of nurses. Through research, nurses analyze the scope and quality of care provided by examining the outcomes and cost effectiveness of nursing interventions. With the concerted efforts of many nurses, NCNR gained official institute status within the National Institutes of Health in 1993, becoming the National Institute of Nursing Research (NINR).

### WHAT DO YOU THINK?

The emphasis of community-oriented nursing has been varied and has changed over time. Given this chapter's review of the important issues that nursing can address, what priorities would you set for the work of the contemporary public and community health nurse?

By the latter part of the 1980s, public health as a whole had declined significantly in terms of effectiveness in implementing its mission and affecting the health of the public. The seriousness of reduced political support, financing, and impact was vividly described in the landmark report by the Institute of Medicine (IOM), *The Future of Public Health* (1988). The IOM study group found the state of public health in the United States to be in disarray and

concluded that, although there was widespread agreement about what the mission of public health should be, there was little consensus on how to translate that mission into action. Not surprisingly, the IOM reported that the mix and level of public health services varied extensively across the United States (Williams, 1995).

*The Future of Public Health* (IOM, 1988) found that "contemporary public health is defined less by what public health professionals know how to do than by what the political system in a given area decides is appropriate or feasible" (p. 4). Nurses working in health departments saw underfunding reduce the breadth and depth of their role. When local public health departments provided insufficient care, voluntary agencies such as visiting nurse associations stepped in to assist vulnerable groups. But without adequate funding for their care of the poor, visiting nurse associations faced hard economic choices, and some closed their doors.

The Healthy People initiative has influenced goals and priority setting in public health and in community-oriented nursing. In 1979, Healthy People proposed a national strategy to improve significantly the health of Americans by preventing or delaying the onset of major chronic illnesses, injuries, and infectious diseases. The initiative's specific goals and objectives provide a framework for periodic evaluation. Strategies recommended in *Healthy People 2010* are summarized on this book's website at http://evolve.elsevier.com/Stanhope/. Implementation of these strategies has influenced the work of community-oriented nurses through their employment in health agencies or through participation in state or local Healthy People coalitions. Many Healthy People 2010 objectives and intervention strategies are described in chapters throughout this text.

The 1990s debate about health care focused on the central issues of cost, quality, and access to direct care services. Despite considerable interest in health care reform and universal health insurance coverage, the core debate of the economics of health care—who will pay for what—emphasized reform of medical care rather than comprehensive changes in health care. The 1993 American Health Security Act received insufficient congressional support. Reflecting the weakness of public health, the aims of public health were never clearly considered in the proposed program. Proposals to reform existing services failed to apply the lesson learned from the Healthy People initiative—that health promotion and disease prevention appear to yield reductions in costs and illness/injury incidence while increasing years of healthy life.

In 1991 the ANA, the American Association of Colleges of Nursing, the National League for Nursing, and more than 60 other specialty nursing organizations joined to support health care reform. The coalition of nursing organizations emphasized key health care issues of access, quality, and cost, and proposed a range of interventions designed to build a healthy nation through improved primary care and public health efforts. Professional nursing's support contin-

## Healthy People 2010 | History of the Development of Healthy People 2010

In 1979, the groundbreaking *Healthy People: The Surgeon's General Report on Health Promotion and Disease Prevention* asserted that "the health of the American people has never been better" (p. 3). But this was only the prologue to deep criticism of the status of American health care delivery. Between 1960 and 1978, health care spending increased 700%—without striking improvements in mortality or morbidity. During the 1950s and 1960s, evidence accumulated about chronic disease risk factors, particularly cigarette smoking, alcohol and drugs, occupational risks, and injuries. Unfortunately, these new research findings were not systematically applied to planning and improving population health.

In 1974, the Government of Canada published *A New Perspective on the Health of Canadians* (Lalonde, 1974), which viewed death and disease to have four contributing factors: inadequacies in the existing health care system, behavioral factors, environmental hazards, and human biological factors. Applying the Canadian approach, in 1976 U.S. experts analyzed the 10 leading causes of U.S. mortality and found that 50% of American deaths were the result of unhealthy behaviors, and only 10% were the result of inadequacies in health care. Rather than just spending more to improve hospital care, clearly prevention was the key to saving lives, improving the quality of life, and saving health care dollars.

A multidisciplinary group of analysts conducted a comprehensive review of prevention activities. They verified that the health of Americans could be significantly improved through "actions individuals can take for themselves" and through actions that public and private

decision makers could take to "promote a safer and healthier environment" (p. 9). Like Canada's *New Perspectives, Healthy People* (1979) identified priorities and measurable goals. Healthy People grouped 15 key priorities into three categories: key preventive services that could be delivered to individuals by health providers, such as timely prenatal care; measures that could be used by governmental and other agencies, as well as industry, to protect people from harm, such as reduced exposure to toxic agents; and activities that individuals and communities could use to promote healthy lifestyles, such as improved nutrition.

In the late 1980s, success in addressing these priorities and goals was evaluated, new scientific findings were analyzed, and new goals and objectives were set for the period from 1990 to 2000 through *Healthy People 2000: National Health Promotion and Disease Prevention Objectives* (U.S. Public Health Service, 1990). This process was repeated 10 years later to develop goals and objectives for the period 2000 to 2010. Recognizing the continuing challenge to using emerging scientific research to encourage modification of health behaviors and practices, *Healthy People 2010* emphasizes reducing health disparities and increasing years of healthy life.

Like the nurse in the early twentieth century who spread the gospel of public health to reduce communicable diseases, today's community-oriented nurse uses Healthy People to reduce chronic and infectious diseases and injuries through health education, environmental modification, and policy development.

Lalonde M: *A new perspective on the health of Canadians,* Ottawa, Canada, 1974, Information Canada.

U.S. Department of Health and Human Services: *Healthy People 2010: understanding and improving health,* ed 2, Washington, DC, 2000, U.S. Government Printing Office.

U.S. Department of Health, Education, and Welfare: *Healthy people: the surgeon general's report on health promotion and disease prevention,* DHEW Publication No. 79-55071, Washington, DC, 1979, U.S. Government Printing Office.

U.S. Public Health Service: *Healthy people 2000: national health promotion and disease prevention objectives,* Washington, DC, 1991b, U.S. Government Printing Office.

ues for improved health care delivery and for extension of public health services to prevent illness, promote health, and protect the public (Table 2-3).

During the last decade, new and continuing challenges triggered growth and change in community-oriented health nursing. Nurse-managed centers provide a diversity of nursing services, including health promotion and disease/injury prevention, where existing organizations have been unable to meet community and neighborhood needs. New populations in communities continue to challenge schools of nursing, health departments, rural health clinics, and migrant health services to provide the range of services to meet specific needs. Transfer of official health services to private control has sometimes reduced professional flexi-

bility and service delivery. A nursing shortage reduces staffing in public health agencies when nurses seek institutional employment to increase their salaries. Nurse leadership in community-oriented nursing through the Association of Community Health Nurse Educators calls for increased graduate programs to educate community-oriented nurse leaders, educators, and researchers. Natural disasters (such as floods, hurricanes, and tornados) and human-made disasters (including explosions, building collapses, and airplane crashes) require innovative and time-consuming responses. Preparation for future disasters and potential bioterrorism demands the presence of community-oriented nurses. Some states hear new calls to deploy school nurses in every school; a new recognition of the

**Table 2-3   Milestones in History of Community Health and Public Health Nursing: 1946-2000**

| YEAR | MILESTONE | YEAR | MILESTONE |
|------|-----------|------|-----------|
| 1946 | Nurses classified as professionals by U.S. Civil Service Commission; Hill-Burton Act approved, providing funds for hospital construction in underserved areas and requiring these hospitals to provide care to poor people; passage of National Mental Health Act | 1990 | Association of Community Health Nursing Educators publishes *Essentials of Baccalaureate Nursing Education* |
| 1950 | 25,091 nurses employed in public health | 1991 | Over 60 nursing organizations joined forces to support health care reform and publish a document entitled *Nursing's Agenda for Health Care Reform* |
| 1951 | National organizations recommend that college-based nursing education programs include public health content | 1993 | American Health Security Act of 1993 published as a blueprint for national health care reform; the national effort, however, failed, leaving states and the private sector to design their own programs |
| 1952 | National Organization for Public Health Nursing merges into the new National League for Nursing; Metropolitan Life Insurance Nursing Program closes | 1994 | NCNR becomes the National Institute for Nursing Research, as part of the National Institutes of Health |
| 1964 | Passage of Economic Opportunity Act; public health nurse defined by the American Nurses Association (ANA) as a graduate of a BSN program; Congress amended Social Security Act to include Medicare and Medicaid | 1996 | Public health nursing section of American Public Health Association, *The Definition and Role of Public Health Nursing,* updated |
| 1965 | ANA position paper recommended that nursing education take place in institutions of higher learning | 1998 | *The Public Health Workforce: An Agenda for the 21st Century* published by the U.S. Public Health Service to look at the current workforce in public, health, and educational needs, and the use of distance learning strategies to prepare future public health workers |
| 1977 | Passage of Rural Health Clinic Services Act, which provided indirect reimbursement for nurse practitioners in rural health clinics | | |
| 1978 | Association of Graduate Faculty in Community Health Nursing/Public Health Nursing (later renamed as Association of Community Health Nursing Educators) | 1999 | The Public Health Nursing Quad Council through the American Nurses Association works on new scope and standards of a public health nursing document, which differentiates between community-oriented and community-based nursing practice |
| 1980 | Medicaid amendment to the Social Security Act to provide direct reimbursement for nurse practitioners in rural health clinics; ANA and APHA developed statements on the role and conceptual foundations of community and public health nursing, respectively | 2001 | Significant interest in public health because of threats of biological and other forms of terrorism after the destruction of buildings in New York City and Washington, D.C., by terrorists |
| 1983 | Beginning of Medicare prospective payments | 2002 | Establishment of the Office of Homeland Security to protect the public from threats to health |
| 1985 | National Center for Nursing Research established in National Institutes of Health (NIH) | | |
| 1988 | Institute of Medicine publishes *The Future of Public Health* | | |

link between school success and health is making the school nurse essential. Many of these stories are detailed in the chapters that follow.

**DID YOU KNOW?**

Many colleges and universities offer courses on the history of nursing, history of medicine, and the history of health care.

## COMMUNITY AND PUBLIC HEALTH NURSING TODAY

Today, community-oriented nurses look to their history for inspiration, explanation, and prediction. Information and advocacy are used to promote a comprehensive approach to address the multiple needs of the diverse populations served. Community-oriented nurses will seek to learn from the past and to avoid known pitfalls, even as they seek successful strategies to meet the complex needs of today's vulnerable populations. As plans for the future are made, as the public health challenges that remain unmet are acknowledged, it is the vision of what community-oriented nursing can accomplish that sustains these nurses.

## Practice Application

Mary Lipsky has worked for the county health department in a major urban area for almost 2 years. Her nursing responsibilities include a variety of services, including consultations at a senior center, maternal/newborn home visits, and well-child clinics. As she leaves work each evening and returns to her own home, she finds that she holds her clients in her thoughts. Why was it so difficult today to qualify a new mother and her baby to receive WIC (women, infants, and children) nutrition services? Why must she limit the number of children screened for high lead levels, when last year the health department screened twice as many children? Several children last month seemed asymptomatic, but the laboratory found lead levels that were high enough to cause damage. One mother she's gotten to know is having a very difficult time emotionally— Why is it so difficult to find a behavioral health provider for her? And the health department still cannot find a new staff dentist! And families on welfare cannot find a private dentist to care for their children.

  A. Why might it be difficult to solve these problems at the individual level, on a case-by-case basis?
  B. What information would you need to build an understanding of the policy background for each of these various populations?

Answers are in the back of the book.

## Key Points

- A historical approach can be used to increase understanding of public and community health nursing in the past, as well as its contemporary dilemmas and future challenges.
- The history of public and community health nursing can be characterized by change in specific focus of the specialty but continuity in approach and style of the practice.
- Public and community health nursing, referred to in this text as community-oriented nursing is a product of various social, economic, and political forces; it incorporates public health science in addition to nursing science and practice.
- Federal responsibility for health care was limited until the 1930s when the economic challenges of the Depression permitted reexamination of local responsibility for care.
- Florence Nightingale designed and implemented the first program of trained nursing, and her contemporary, William Rathbone, founded the first district nursing association in England.

- Urbanization, industrialization, and immigration in the United States increased the need for trained nurses, especially in community-oriented nursing.
- Increasing acceptance of public roles for women permitted public and community health nursing employment for nurses, as well as public leadership roles for their wealthy supporters.
- The first trained nurse in the United States, who was salaried as a visiting nurse, was Frances Root; she was hired in 1887 by the Women's Board of the New York City Mission to provide care to sick persons at home.
- The first visiting nurses' associations were founded in 1885 and 1886 in Buffalo, Philadelphia, and Boston.
- Lillian Wald established the Henry Street Settlement, which became the Visiting Nurse Service of New York City, in 1893. She played a key role in innovations that shaped public and community health nursing in its first decades, including school nursing, insurance payment for nursing, national organization for public health nurses, and the United States Children's Bureau.
- Founded in 1902 with the vision and support of Lillian Wald, school nursing sought to keep children in school so that they could learn.
- The Metropolitan Life Insurance Company established the first insurance-based program in 1909 to support community health nursing services.
- The National Organization for Public Health Nursing (founded in 1912) provided essential leadership and coordination of diverse public and community health nursing efforts; the organization merged into the National League for Nursing in 1952.
- Official health agencies slowly grew in numbers between 1900 and 1940, accompanied by a steady increase in public health nursing positions.
- The innovative Sheppard-Towner Act of 1921 expanded community health nursing roles for maternal and child health during the 1920s.
- Mary Breckinridge established the Frontier Nursing Service in 1925, which influenced provision of rural health care.
- Tension between the community health nursing role of caring for the sick and the role of providing preventive care, and the related tension between intervening for individuals and intervening for groups have characterized the specialty since at least the 1910s.
- As the Social Security Act attempted to remedy some of the setbacks of the Depression, it established a context in which community health nursing services expanded.
- The challenges of World War II sometimes resulted in extension of community health nursing care and sometimes in retrenchment and decreased public health nursing services.

- By mid-twentieth century, the reduced incidence of communicable diseases and the increased prevalence of chronic illness, accompanied by large increases in the population over 65 years of age, led to examination of the goals and organization of community health nursing services.
- Between the 1930s and 1965, organized nursing and community health nursing agencies sought to establish health insurance reimbursement for nursing care at home.
- Implementation of Medicare and Medicaid programs in 1966 established new possibilities for supporting community-based nursing care but encouraged agencies to focus on services provided after acute care rather than on prevention.
- Efforts to reform health care organization, pushed by increased health care costs during the last 40 years, have focused on reforming acute medical care rather than on designing a comprehensive preventive approach.
- The 1988 Institute of Medicine report documented the reduced political support, financing, and impact that increasingly limited public health services at national, state, and local levels.
- In the late 1990s, federal policy changes dangerously reduced financial support for home health care services, threatening the long-term survival of visiting nurse agencies.
- Healthy People 2000 and Healthy People 2010 have brought renewed emphasis on prevention to community-oriented nursing.

## Clinical Decision-Making Activities

1. Interview nurses at your clinical placement about the changes they have seen during their years in a community-oriented nursing practice. How do these changes relate to the changing needs of the community or the population?
2. Identify the visible record of community-oriented nursing agencies in your community. Note the buildings, plaques, display cases, and so on that are records of the past provision of nursing care in community settings. What forces have influenced these agencies over time? Which factors do they wish to make known publicly, and which factors are less apparent?
3. Secure a copy of your clinical agency's recent annual report. How is the history of the agency presented? How does this agency's history fit in with the points made in this chapter? What are your conclusions about how this agency's past influences its present?
4. Interview older relatives for their memories of community-oriented nursing care received by them, their families, and their friends. When they were younger, how was the public health nurse perceived in their community? What interventions were used by the public health nurse? How was the public health nurse dressed? How has the position of the public health or community health nurse changed?
5. What element or aspect of the history of public and community health nursing would you like to know more about? At your nursing library, review a period of 10 years of one journal from the past to identify trends in how this element or aspect was addressed. What conclusions do you reach?
6. The work and impact of several nursing leaders is reviewed or noted in this chapter. Of these leaders, which one strikes you as most interesting? Why? Locate and read further articles or books about this leader. What personal strengths do you note that supported this nurse's leadership?

## Additional Resources

These related resources are found either in the appendixes at the back of this book or on the book's website at **http://evolve.elsevier.com/Stanhope.**

**evolve Evolve Website**

WebLinks: Healthy People 2010

## References

Abramovitz AB, editor: *Emotional factors in public health nursing: a casebook,* Madison, Wisc, 1961, University of Wisconsin Press.

Allemang M: Development of community health nursing in Canada. In Stewart MJ, editor: *Community health nursing: promoting Canadians' health,* Toronto, 1995, Saunders.

Allemang M: Development of community health nursing in Canada. In Stewart MJ, editor: *Community health nursing: promoting Canadians' health,* ed 2, pp. 4-32, Toronto, 2000, Saunders.

American Association of Industrial Nurses: *The nurse in industry: a history of the American Association of Industrial Nurses, Inc.,* New York, 1976, AAIN.

Backer BA: Lillian Wald: connecting caring with action, *Nurs Health Care* 14:122, 1993.

Baumgart A: Evolution of the Canadian health care system. In Baumgart A, Larsen J, editors: *Canadian nursing faces the future,* ed 2, St Louis, Mo, 1992, Mosby.

Brainard A: *Evolution of public health nursing,* Philadelphia, 1922, Saunders.

Breckinridge M: Wi*de neighborhoods, a story of the Frontier Nursing Service,* New York, 1952, Harper.

Browne H: A tribute to Mary Breckinridge, *Nurs Outlook* 14:54, 1966.

Buhler-Wilkerson K: Public health nursing: in sickness or in health? *Am J Public Health* 75:1155, 1985.

Buhler-Wilkerson K: Left carrying the bag: experiments in visiting nursing, 1877-1909, *Nurs Res* 36:42, 45, 1987.

Buhler-Wilkerson K: *False dawn: the rise and decline of public health nursing, 1900-1930,* New York, 1989, Garland.

Buhler-Wilkerson K: *No place like home: a history of nursing and home care in the United States,* Baltimore, 2001, Johns Hopkins Press.

Bullough V, Bullough B: The *emergence of modern nursing,* New York, 1964, Macmillan.

Bullough V, Church OM, Stern A: *American nursing: a biographic dictionary,* New York, 1988, Garland.

Chalmers K, Kristjanson L: Community health nursing practice. In Baumgart A, Larsen J, editors: *Canadian nursing faces the future,* ed 2, St Louis, Mo, 1992, Mosby.

Cohen IB: Florence Nightingale, *Sci Am* 250(3):128, 1984.

Craven FSL: *A guide to district nursing,* New York, 1984, Garland (originally published in London, 1889, Macmillan).

Cristy TE: Lillian D. Wald: portrait of a leader. In Kelly LY: *Pages from nursing history,* pp. 84-88, New York, 1984, American Journal of Nursing Company.

Deloughery GL: *History and trends of professional nursing,* ed 8, St Louis, Mo, 1977, Mosby.

Denker EP, editor: *Healing at home: Visiting Nurse Service of New York, 1893-1993,* New York, 1994, The Carl and Lily Pforzheimer Foundation.

Desirable organization for public health nursing for family service, *Public Health Nurs* 38:387, 1946.

Dock LL: The history of public health nursing, *Public Health Nurs* 14:522, 1922.

Dolan J: *History of nursing,* ed 14, Philadelphia, 1978, Saunders.

Duffus RL: *Lillian Wald: neighbor and crusader,* New York, 1938, Macmillan.

Duncan S, Leipert B, Mill J: "Nurses as health evangelists"? the evolution of public health nursing in Canada, 1918-1939, *ANS Adv Nursing Sci* 22(1):40-51, 1999.

Falk Rafael A: The politics of health promotion: influences on public health nursing practice in Ontario, Canada from Nightingale to the nineties. *ANS Adv Nurs Sci* 22(1):23-39, 1999.

Frachel RR: A new profession: the evolution of public health nursing, *Public Health Nurs* 5(2):86, 1988.

Hawkins JW, Hayes ER, Corliss CP: School nursing in America—1902-1994: a return to public health nursing, *Public Health Nurs* 11(6):416, 1994.

Hine DC: *Black women in white: racial conflict and cooperation in the nursing profession, 1890-1950,* Bloomington, 1989, Indiana University Press.

Holloway JB: Frontier Nursing Service 1925-1975, *J Ky Med Assoc* 13:491, 1975.

Institute of Medicine: *The future of public health,* Washington, DC, 1988, National Academy of Science.

Kalisch PA, Kalisch BJ: *The advance of American nursing,* ed 3, Philadelphia, 1995, Lippincott.

Kaufman M, editor: *Dictionary of American nursing biography,* New York, 1988, Greenwood Press.

Kerr Ross J: The growth of community health nursing in Canada. In Ross J, MacPhail J, editors: *An introduction to issues in community health nursing in Canada,* St Louis, Mo, 1996, Mosby.

Lalonde M: *A new perspective on the health of Canadians,* Ottawa, Canada, 1974, Information Canada.

McNeil EE: *Transition in public health nursing,* John Sundwall Lecture, University of Michigan, Feb 27, 1967.

Milio N: *9226 Kercheval: the storefront that did not burn,* Ann Arbor, Mich, 1971, University of Michigan Press.

Mill J, Leipert B, Duncan S: Frontiers and pioneers: a history of public health nursing in Alberta and British Columbia, 1918 to 1939, *Can Nurse* 98(1):18-23, 2002.

National Organization for Public Health Nursing: Approval of Skidmore College of Nursing as preparing students for public health nursing, *Public Health Nurs* 36:371, 1944.

National Organization for Public Health Nursing: *Proceedings of work conference: Collegiate Council on Public Health Nursing Education,* New York, 1951, NOPHN.

Nightingale F: *Notes on nursing: what it is, and what it is not,* Philadelphia, 1946, Lippincott.

Nightingale F: Sick nursing and health nursing. In Billings JS, Hurd HM, editors: *Hospitals, dispensaries, and nursing,* New York, 1984, Garland (originally published in Baltimore, 1894, Johns Hopkins Press).

Nutting MA, Dock LL: *A history of nursing,* New York, 1935, Putnam.

Palmer IS: *Florence Nightingale and the first organized delivery of nursing services,* Washington, DC, 1983, American Association of Colleges of Nursing.

Pickett G, Hanlon JJ: Public health: administration and practice, St Louis, Mo, 1990, Mosby.

Pringle D, Roe D: Voluntary community agencies: VON Canada an example. In Baumgart A, Larsen J, editors: *Canadian nursing faces the future,* ed 2, St Louis, Mo, 1992, Mosby.

Roberts DE, Heinrich J: Public health nursing comes of age, *Am J Public Health* 75:1162, 1165, 1985.

Robeson KA, McNeil EE: *Report of conference on field instruction in public health nursing,* New York, 1957, National League for Nursing.

Roberts M: *American nursing: history and interpretation,* New York, 1955, Macmillan.

Rodabaugh JH, Rodabaugh MJ: *Nursing in Ohio: a history,* Columbus, Ohio, 1951, Ohio State Nurses' Association.

Rosen G: *A history of public health,* New York, 1958, MD Publications.

Safier G: *Contemporary American leaders in nursing: an oral history,* New York, 1977, McGraw-Hill.

Scutchfield FD, Keck CW: *Principles of public health practice,* Albany, NY, 1997, Delmar.

Shyrock H: *The history of nursing,* Philadelphia, 1959, Saunders.

Thoms AB: *Pathfinders: a history of the progress of colored graduate nurses,* New York, 1929, Kay Printing House.

Tirpak H: The Frontier Nursing Service—fifty years in the mountains, *Nurs Outlook* 33:308, 1975.

U.S. Department of Health and Human Services: *Healthy people 2010: understanding and improving health,* ed 2, Washington, DC, 2000, U.S. Government Printing Office.

U.S. Department of Health, Education, and Welfare: *Healthy people: the surgeon general's report on health promotion and disease prevention,* DHEW Publication No. 79-55071, Washington, DC, 1979, U.S. Government Printing Office.

U.S. Public Health Service: *Healthy communities 2000: model standards,* Washington, DC, 1991a, U.S. Government Printing Office.

U.S. Public Health Service: *Healthy people 2000: national health promotion and disease prevention objectives,* Washington, DC, 1991b, U.S. Government Printing Office.

Wald LD: *The house on Henry Street,* New York, 1915, Holt.

Wald LD: *Windows on Henry Street,* Boston, 1934, Little, Brown.

Waters Y: *Visiting nursing in the United States,* New York, 1909, Charities Publication Committee.

Williams B: *Lillian Wald: angel of Henry Street,* New York, 1948, Julian Messner.

Williams CA: Beyond the Institute of Medicine report: a critical analysis and public health forecast, *Fam Community Health* 18(1):12, 1995.

Wilner DM, Walkey RP, O'Neill EJ: *Introduction to public health,* ed 7, New York, 1978, Macmillan.

Zerwekh JV: Public health nursing legacy: historical practical wisdom, *Nurs Health Care* 13:84, 1992.

# Chapter 3

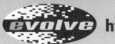 http://evolve.elsevier.com/Stanhope

# Public Health and Primary Health Care Systems and Health Care Transformation

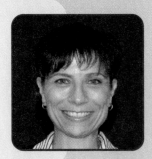

**Susan B. Hassmiller, Ph.D., R.N., F.A.A.N.**

Sue Hassmiller is a senior program officer at the Robert Wood Johnson Foundation in Princeton, New Jersey. The foundation provides support to improve the health and health care for all Americans. Dr. Hassmiller works in the areas of public health, primary care, and prevention, and on the health professions workforce on health and behavior, population health sciences, and priority populations program management teams. She comes to the foundation from the Health Resources and Services Administration, where she was the executive director of the U.S. Public Health Service Primary Care Policy Fellowship and other national and international primary care initiatives. She has also worked in public health settings at the local and state levels. Dr. Hassmiller has taught public health nursing at the University of Nebraska and at George Mason University in Fairfax, Virginia and has dedicated her career to the care of vulnerable populations and prevention. She is a fellow in the American Academy of Nursing and a member of the National Board of Governors for the American Red Cross.

## Objectives

After reading this chapter, the student should be able to do the following:

1. Analyze three trends in the United States that are affecting health care
2. Define public health, primary care, and primary health care
3. Differentiate between primary care and primary health care, including the workforce of each
4. Evaluate the significance of Alma Ata as the basis for primary health care
5. Analyze two of the most common health care systems that manage the personal care of Americans
6. Describe the current public health system in the United States
7. Compare and contrast the responsibilities of the federal, state, and local public health systems
8. Examine nursing roles in selected government agencies
9. Analyze the transformation of the U.S. health care system

The American health care system has done a remarkable job in many ways. It provides health care to the American people, particularly in technology development and skilled provider training. Today's health care facilities would defy the imagination of past health care providers.

This chapter describes the current primary care and public health systems in the United States and the trends that affect these systems. These systems are compared and contrasted both with one another and with the concept of primary health care. Box 3-1 presents a definition of terms used in this chapter.

Current concepts of health care transformation are described as the beginning of a discussion about what an emerging health care system might look like. This chapter describes a reformed health care system as one that weaves primary care and public health into a single integrated system. The role of the nurse is presented in all of the systems, current and future.

*The author wishes to thank Kathryn Hammes for her extensive and thoughtful assistance.*

## Key Terms

**advanced practice nurses**, p. 54
**certified nurse midwives**, p. 59
**community-based care**, p. 54
**community nursing centers**, p. 58
**community participation**, p. 56
**cost shifting**, p. 52
**Declaration of Alma Ata**, p. 56
**defined contribution**, p. 58

**digital divide**, p. 55
**health maintenance organizations**, p. 58
**managed care**, p. 52
**managed care organization**, p. 58
**National Health Service Corps**, p. 60
**nurse midwifery**, p. 59
**nurse practitioners**, p. 59
**physician assistants**, p. 59

**preferred provider organizations**, p. 58
**primary care**, p. 56
**primary care generalists**, p. 56
**primary health care**, p. 55
**report cards**, p. 64
**U.S. Department of Health and Human Services**, p. 54
*See Glossary for definitions*

## Chapter Outline

Current Health Care System in the United
   States
*Cost*
*Access*
*Quality*
Trends Affecting the Health Care System
*Demographic Trends*

*Social Trends*
*Economic Trends*
*Health Workforce Trends*
*Technological Trends*
Organization of the Health Care System
*Primary Health Care System*
*Primary Care System*

*Public Health System*
*Federal System*
*State System*
*Local System*
Transformation of the Health Care System
A Comprehensive Model: Integration of Public
   Health and Primary Care

## CURRENT HEALTH CARE SYSTEM IN THE UNITED STATES

Although the U.S. health care system can take credit for increasing the life span of most Americans through advances in medical technology, science, and medicines, the system is also plagued with problems related to cost, access, and quality. These problems are different for each person and affected by their health insurance. These issues are at the center of health care debates around the country.

## Cost

In 2002, Americans spent $1.4 trillion, nearly 15% of the gross domestic product (GDP), on health care, or 15 cents from every dollar (Health Care Financing Administration [HCFA], 2000a). The United States spends 40% more than Canada, the country that spends the next largest amount. Based on projections, by 2010, health care expenditures will account for nearly 16% of the U.S. GDP. The Centers for Medicare and Medicaid Services (CMS), projects that health care expenditures will increase by more than 7%

---

> ## BOX 3-1  Selected Health Care Definitions
>
> **Digital divide:** Gap in computer and internet access between population groups covered by income, educational level, race or ethnicity, age, disability, and ability
>
> **Disease prevention:** Activities that have as their goal the protection of people from becoming ill because of actual or potential health threats
>
> **Health:** A state of complete physical, mental, and social well-being; not merely the absence of disease or infirmity (WHO, 1986a, p. 1)
>
> **Health promotion:** Activities that have as their goal the development of human attitudes and behaviors that maintain or enhance well-being
>
> **Managed care organization:** An organization that provides or arranges by contract for specific health care services such as hospital care, outpatient visits, and prescription drugs
>
> **Primary care:** The providing of integrated, accessible health care services by clinicians who are accountable for addressing a large majority of personal health care needs, developing a sustained partnership with patients, and practicing in the context of family and community
>
> **Primary health care:** A combination of primary care and public health care made universally accessible to individuals and families in a community, with their full participation, and provided at a cost that the community and country can afford (WHO, 1978)
>
> **Primary prevention:** Active, health-promoting activities designed to reduce the likelihood of a specific illness occurring
>
> **Public health:** Organized community and multidisciplinary efforts, based on epidemiology, aimed at preventing disease and promoting health (Institute of Medicine, 1988, p. 4)
>
> **Secondary prevention:** Early diagnosis and prompt treatment of illness—for example, by screening for hypertension, breast cancer, blindness, deafness
>
> **Tertiary prevention:** Treatment, care, and rehabilitation to prevent further progression of disease (Pender, 1996)

Change (2002), nearly one in seven Americans reported some difficulty getting needed medical care in 2001—approximately the same number as in 1997. The American health care system is described as a two-class system: private and public. People with insurance or those who can personally pay for health care are viewed as receiving superior care, whereas people whose only source of care depends on public funds, or the working poor who do not qualify for public funds, either because they make too much money to qualify or because they are illegal immigrants, receive lower-quality care. In 2000, 42.6 million Americans (15% of the total population) were uninsured (U.S. Bureau of the Census, 2002). By 2003 the estimates are at 44 million. The number of uninsured people is currently rising at the rate of 500,000 people per year and will reach an estimated 47.9 million people by the year 2010 (Institute for the Future, 2000). Young adults 18 to 24 years of age, 27.3% of whom are uninsured, and minors under the age of 18 (21% of all uninsured) are more likely than other age groups to lack coverage, and older adults (0.63% of all uninsured) are the least likely to lack coverage (U.S. Bureau of the Census, 2002).

Finally, the gradual erosion of public health services has compounded the access problem in the United States. For example, funding to clinics in rural and heavily populated urban areas has been reduced, leading many uninsured people to seek care in the emergency department. To continue to care for the uninsured, hospitals automatically charge more for their services to those who have insurance. This process of making up for lost revenue by charging more to those who are able to pay is called **cost shifting.**

## Quality

Quality of care is the third major concern in the United States. Although **managed care** has succeeded in controlling some health care costs, many would say that it has been at the expense of quality. Consumer advocates believe that employers and managed care plans are more concerned with reducing costs than with offering needed services (Copeland, 1998). However, when care is delivered that is medically unneeded, the impact on quality of care is as significant as the impact of not providing enough care.

Federal and state health insurance plans (e.g., Medicare, Medicaid, and private managed care plans) have incorporated ways to improve the quality of care that they deliver. The best-known private group, the National Committee for Quality Assurance (NCQA), has developed a set of standard performance measurements that most managed care organizations are using. CMS, home to Medicare and Medicaid, has developed conditions of participation (CoPs) and conditions for coverage (CfCs) that health care organizations must meet to participate in the Medicare and Medicaid programs. CMS also ensures that the standards of the accrediting organizations it recognizes (through a process called "deeming") meet or exceed Medicare standards (HCFA, 2000b).

annually between 2004 and 2010, and health care expenditures in 2010, $2.638 trillion, will double those of 2000. Per-person health care expenditures, expected to increase every year over the next decade, are estimated to be $6186 in 2004 and almost $8708 in 2007 (HCFA, 1998). This means a choice between a down payment on a new car, for example, and health care. The efforts to contain costs that have been made since 1983 have attempted to curb the growth of costs, but they have not solved this tremendous problem. See Chapter 5 for details about the economics of health care.

## Access

Another significant problem is poor access to health care. According to the Center for Studying Health Systems

## THE CUTTING EDGE

As of March 2002, a patients' bill of rights had been passed in both the United States Senate and the House. The bills are identical on most issues. The major difference is that the Senate bill gives a patient more rights to sue a managed care organization that causes injury or death by wrongfully denying care. The House bill, on the other hand, focuses on increasing access to care and reducing the cost of premiums. The patients' bill of rights is expected to be passed and signed into law this year (Norwood, 2002).

## TRENDS AFFECTING THE HEALTH CARE SYSTEM

Because of the national concern about the cost, access, and quality of health care, significant change is expected in the next 10 years. Several trends, including demography, technology, and economics, will affect how these changes will occur.

## Demographic Trends

The population of the world is growing as a result of fertility and mortality rates. The most explosive growth is occurring in underdeveloped countries, and this is accompanied by a trend of decreased growth in the United States and other developed countries. The year 2000, however, marked the first time in over 30 years that the total fertility rate in the United States was above the replacement level. *Replacement* means that for every person who dies, another is born (Martin et al, 2002). Both the size and the characteristics of the population contribute to the changing demography.

### Size of the Population

The U.S. Bureau of the Census reported that the U.S. population increased by 33 million between 1990 and 2000, an increase of 13.2%. Immigration, both legal and illegal, also plays a major role in shaping the U.S. population. Roughly 350,000 to 500,000 legal immigrants enter the United States each year (Immigration and Naturalization Service, 2000).

The U.S. birthrate has fluctuated greatly in the last 55 to 60 years, going from the "baby boom" between 1946 and 1964 to the "baby bust" of the 1970s—when the population reached its lowest rate of growth in 1976. It was thought that the rise in birthrates experienced in the late 1970s would level out or decline as baby boom women passed through childbearing age. However, with women having children at more advanced ages, birthrates did not begin to decrease until 1991, and then they continued to decline until 1998 (Martin et al, 2002). From 1990 until 1997, birthrates declined a total of 7%. The year 2000 marked the third straight year of birthrate growth, with a 3% increase from 1999; this was the first time in over 30 years that the total fertility rate in the United States was above replacement level (Martin et al, 2002).

### Characteristics of the Population

The average age in the United States is increasing. In the 1990s, however, the older adult population grew more slowly than the total population (12% growth versus 13.2%) for the first time in census history. People who reached the age of 65 during the 1990s were born during the depression when the birthrate was extremely low (Administration on Aging, 2001). Between 2000 and 2010, the number of Americans aged 65 and older is expected to nearly double. From 2010 to 2030, the number of people 65 years of age and older will increase substantially, as the first baby boomers turn 65 in 2011. The number of people over 85 years of age is growing so rapidly that by 2050 they will make up approximately 24% of the older adult population.

The middle-aged population will also continue to increase, as nearly one third of Americans were born between 1945 and 1960. The entire baby boom generation was over 35 years of age by the turn of the century.

At the time of the 1990 census, African Americans were the largest minority group in the United States (U.S. Bureau of the Census, 1996). However, from 2000 until 2050, the African-American population is expected to see limited growth, whereas the Hispanic and Asian populations are projected to increase dramatically. If current trends continue, Hispanics will bypass African Americans to become the largest minority group by 2010. Whites are predicted to make up only 53% of the U.S. population in 2050 (Smelser, Wilson, and Mitchell, 2000).

The U.S. household composition is also changing. Families make up about 69% of all households, down from 81% in 1970 (U.S. Bureau of the Census, 2001). A single parent, usually the mother, heads 3 out of 10 families. Single-parent families constitute 19% of all white families, 32% of Hispanic families, and 52% of African-American families (U.S. Bureau of the Census, 2001).

In the last decade, mortality rates for both sexes in all age groups declined (U.S. Bureau of the Census, 2001). As a result of medical progress, the leading causes of death have changed from infectious diseases to chronic and degenerative diseases, such as osteoporosis. New treatments for infectious diseases have resulted in steady declines of mortality among children. The mortality rates for older Americans have also declined, especially during the 1970s and 1980s. However, people 50 years of age and older have higher rates of chronic illness, and they use a larger portion of health care services than other age groups.

## Social Trends

In addition to the size and changing age distribution of the population, other factors also affect the health care system.

Several social trends that influence health care include changing lifestyles, a growing appreciation of the quality of life, changing composition of families and living patterns, rising household incomes, and a revised definition of quality health care.

Historically, U.S. citizens have been driven by the "American dream," which emphasized hard work, getting a good education, and achieving a better life than the previous generation. However, the drive to achieve these goals has diminished, and there have been major shifts in American values and lifestyles. Replacing the work ethic is an increasing emphasis on an improved quality of life and the fulfilling of personal goals (Yin, 2001). This shift in values is changing the importance of financial success.

Americans spend more money on health care, nutrition, and fitness (U.S. Department of Labor, 2001). There is a growing belief that people are responsible for their own health. An awareness that health is a valued asset leads to efforts taken to improve it. Currently, it is estimated that 80% to 95% of all health problems are managed at home through self-care measures (Ory and DeFriese, 1998). In addition, centers for promoting all aspects of health and self-care are developing in response to this movement.

## Economic Trends

About 60 years ago, income was distributed in such a way that a relatively small portion of households earned high incomes; families in the middle-income range made up a somewhat larger proportion; and households at the lower end of the income scale made up the largest proportion. By the 1970s, household income had risen and income was more evenly distributed, largely as a result of dual-income families.

Since 1970, two trends in income distribution have been emerging. The first is that the average per person income in America is increasing. By 2010, 48 million households (52% of all households) will have an annual income of at least $50,000. The second and disturbing trend is that the gap between the richest 25% and the poorest 25% is widening because of the movement of middle-class families into higher income levels. Chapter 5 provides a detailed discussion of the economics of health care and how financial constraints influence decisions about public health services.

## Health Workforce Trends

In the 1990s there was a call for health care cost containment, which demanded a workforce that would help keep costs in line while maintaining quality and increasing access.

---

**❰ DID YOU KNOW?**

Research shows that overall health status of a population declines as income disparity widens in that population (Institute for the Future, 2000).

---

cess. Efforts by government agencies, such as the Bureau of Health Professions of the **U.S. Department of Health and Human Services** (USDHHS), and private foundations, such as the Robert Wood Johnson Foundation, provided money for programs to increase the primary care workforce. These strategies included increasing the number of both primary care physicians and **advanced practice nurses,** such as nurse practitioners and certified nurse midwives. Currently there are not enough primary care providers in the United States, especially in the most underserved areas such as the inner cities and very rural areas. Increasing the number of primary care providers and decreasing specialty physician salaries, in addition to the general cost-savings measures instituted by managed care, helped temporarily stabilize escalating health care costs in the 1990s. Costs, however, are on the rise again.

Historically, nursing care has been provided in a variety of settings, primarily in the hospital. Currently, 59% of all registered nurses (RNs) are employed in hospitals (USDHHS, 2000a); however, with a move to contain cost and a greater move to **community-based care,** hospitals are downsizing their acute care facilities. This will require a shift away from hospital settings to nursing homes, primary care settings, and skilled nursing facilities. With the current nursing shortage, however, the need for nurses in all areas is great. From 1998 to 2008, there are expected to be 450,864 new nursing positions. In this same time period, retired nurses, who will need to be replaced, are expected to number 331,000 (Braddock, 1999). By 2008, needs for RNs are expected to increase by a total of 21.7%. This total will include an increase of 7.9% in hospitals, of 41.9% in nursing homes, of 44.5% in physicians' offices, and of 82.2% in home health services. These numbers do not reflect the need to replace the large number of nurses who are expected to retire (Levine, 2001).

Increasing the number of minority nurses remains a priority and a strategy for addressing the current nursing shortage. It is also hoped this will help to decrease health disparities (Division of Nursing, 2000). For example, persons from minority groups, especially when language is a barrier, are more comfortable with and more likely to access care from a provider of their own minority group. Although minorities made up 30% of the U.S. population in 1996, minority nursing school enrollments accounted for only 12% (USDHHS, 2000a).

## Technologic Trends

Improved technology is rapidly changing the health care system and is having both positive and negative effects. On the positive side, technological advances promise improved health care services, reduced costs, and more convenience in terms of time and travel for consumers. Reduced costs come from a more efficient means of delivering care as well as from replacing people with machines. Contradictory as it may seem, cost is also the most significant negative aspect of advanced health care technology.

The more high-technology equipment and computer programs become available, the more they are used. High-technology equipment is expensive, quickly becomes outdated when newer developments occur, and often requires highly trained personnel. There are other drawbacks to new technology, particularly in the area of home health care. These include increased legal liability, the potential for decreased privacy, relying too much on technologic advances, and inconsistent quality of resources available on the internet and other places. For example, problems have been encountered when hand-held computers are used to monitor clients' blood pressure and cholesterol in the home and the results are sent to an agency base station for interpretation (Eng, 2001).

## THE CUTTING EDGE

Imagine a toothbrush with a biosensing chip that checks your blood sugar and bacteria levels while you're brushing your teeth. Optimally, the brush would come with a holder that would transmit information to a database containing your medical file (Lewis, 2001).

## DID YOU KNOW?

The same sensors that are being developed for automobiles, video cameras, and all other electronics will become cheap enough to be used in medical devices for the purpose of remote telemetry. Examples include monitoring vital signs with wireless heart monitors, respiratory meters, and blood pressure cuffs; blood glucose monitors; and alerts from pill dispensers that a needed pill has not been taken. Built into the sensors will be the software's capabilities to analyze, report, and react to abnormal results, which will ensure appropriate follow-up by a nurse (Institute for the Future, 1997; Lewis, 2001).

Advances in medical technology will continue. Medical technologies that are likely to have a large impact in the next decade include advances in radiology imaging, minimally invasive surgery, genetic mapping and testing, gene therapy, vaccines, and artificial blood (Institute for the Future, 2000). However, it is anticipated that the emphasis will shift away from using expensive diagnostic and therapeutic technologies. Efforts will focus on devising simpler, cheaper, and more mobile tests and procedures that are less oriented toward tertiary care and that can be used in nonhospital settings.

Products currently being developed include dramatically improved pacemakers, cochlear implants (for hearing), and medicine delivery systems. These devices no doubt will contain state-of-the-art technologies including microprocessors. In February of 2000, the U.S. Food and Drug Administration approved one of the latest telemedicine devices: it includes a blood pressure cuff, stethoscope, and thermometer, as well as a television monitor and camera, and the information gathered at home is transmitted directly to health professionals, including home-health nurses (Lewis, 2001).

People born between 1977 and 1995, known as generation Y, are largely driving the information era. Approximately 70 million strong, members of this generation are very comfortable with computers and technology. They have grown up with the internet and e-mail, using them as naturally as the telephone, and they would like to be able to contact their health providers by e-mail. They are likely to expect their health providers to be as attuned to technology as they are, to have websites, to use electronic medical records, and to have state-of-the-art equipment (Jacob, 2002).

The question of disparity of access is also raised as technology advances. The term **digital divide** is most often used to refer to the gap in computer and internet access between population groups because of income, educational level, race or ethnicity, age, disability, and other abilities. The people without access to computers and the internet are likely to be the same ones who already have limited access to health care resources. This new technology has the potential to increase disparity.

## ORGANIZATION OF THE HEALTH CARE SYSTEM

An enormous number and range of facilities and providers make up the health care system. These include physicians' and dentists' offices, hospitals, managed care organizations (MCOs), nursing homes, and other inpatient facilities. There are also mental health centers, ambulatory care centers, rehabilitation centers, and local, state, and federal official and voluntary agencies. In general, however, the American health care system is divided into two, somewhat distinct components: a private or personal care component and a public health component, with some overlap, as discussed in the following sections. Although the personal care component is composed of primary, secondary, and tertiary care, primary health care and primary care will be the focus of this chapter.

### Primary Health Care System

There is controversy over what the differences are between primary care and primary health care. Primary health care is different from primary care in several important ways. **Primary health care** (PHC) is generally defined more broadly than primary care. It includes a comprehensive range of services including public health, prevention, and diagnostic, therapeutic, and rehabilitative services. PHC is essential care made universally accessible to individuals and families in a community. Health care is made available to them with their full participation and is provided at a cost that the community and country can afford. Full participation means that individuals within the community help in defining health problems and in developing approaches to address the problems. The setting for primary health care is within all communities of a country and involves all aspects of society (World Health Organization, 1978).

PHC encourages self-care and self-management in health and the social welfare of daily life. People are educated to use their knowledge, attitudes, and skills in activities that improve health for themselves, their families, and their neighbors. A PHC strategy seeks to ensure individual, family, and community self-reliance and competence.

### Primary Health Care Workforce

The primary health care workforce consists of a multidisciplinary team of health care providers. Team members include **primary care generalists** and public health physicians, nurses, dentists, pharmacists, optometrists, nutritionists, community outreach workers, mental health counselors, translators, and other allied health professionals. Community members are also considered important to the team.

### Primary Health Care Movement

The primary health care movement officially began in 1977 when the 30th World Health Organization (WHO) Health Assembly adopted a resolution accepting the goal of attaining a level of health that permitted all citizens of the world to live socially and economically productive lives. At the international conference in 1978 in Alma Ata, in the former Soviet Union (Russia), it was determined that this goal was to be met through PHC. This resolution, the **Declaration of Alma Ata,** became known by the slogan "Health for All (HFA) by the Year 2000," which captured the official health target for all the member nations of the WHO. In 1998 the program was adapted to meet the needs of the new century and deemed "Health for All in the 21st Century."

In 1981 the WHO established global indicators for monitoring and evaluating the achievement of HFA. In the *World Health Statistics Annual* (WHO, 1986b), these indicators are grouped into four categories: health policies, social and economic development, provision of health care, and health status. An important part of the global indicators is the emphasis on health as an objective of socioeconomic development (Mahler, 1981). This means that health improvements are a result of efforts in many areas, including agriculture, industry, education, housing, communications, and health care. Because PHC is as much a political statement as a system of care, each United Nations member country interprets PHC according to its own culture, health needs, resources, and system of government.

Although the original definition of PHC has at times been misunderstood, it is important now to understand

the Alma Ata declaration as the basis for PHC, and to understand the global evolvement of this strategy over the past 10 to 15 years. For this reason the complete declaration is presented in Appendix A.3.

### Promoting Health/Preventing Disease: Year 2010 Objectives for the Nation

As a WHO member nation, the United States has endorsed primary health care as a strategy for achieving the goal of health for all in the twenty-first century. However, the PHC emphasis on broad strategies, **community participation,** self-reliance, and a multidisciplinary health care delivery team is not the primary strategy for improving the health of the American people. The national health plan for the United States focuses more on disease prevention and health promotion in the areas of most concern in the nation.

This focus is exemplified by the health objectives for the nation stated in *Healthy People 2010* (USDHHS, 2000c). Each decade since the 1980s has been measured and tracked according to health objectives set at the beginning of the decade. The U.S. Public Health Service of the USDHHS publishes the objectives after gathering data from health professionals and organizations throughout the country. Healthy People 2000 set 319 specific health objectives for the 1990s. During this time, progress was achieved on over 60% of the objectives, including surpassing the target for reducing deaths from coronary heart disease and cancer. The targets for the number of incidences of acquired immunodeficiency syndrome (AIDS), cases of syphilis, mammography exams, and violent deaths were also met. Healthy People 2000 also saw some failure, as backward movement was made for 15% of the objectives. Rather than a decrease there was an increase in the number of adults between the ages of 20 and 74 who were considered overweight, in the prevalence of diabetes, and in the prevalence of suicide attempts among adolescents (National Center for Health Statistics, 2001).

There is considerable overlap between the essential elements of PHC and the areas of concern stated in the year 2010 objectives. Table 3-1 relates the eight essential elements of PHC to the priority areas as defined by the Public Health Service.

## Primary Care System

**Primary care,** or what some refer to as primary medical care, is a combination of primary care and public health care made universally accessible to individuals and families within a community with full participation and provided at a cost that the community and country can afford (WHO, 1978).

Although primary care practitioners are encouraged to consider the client's social and environmental attributes in diagnosing, interventions are directed primarily toward the pathophysiological process (Institute of Medicine, 1996). Table 3-2 presents a comparison of primary health care and primary care.

## Healthy People 2010 | Objectives Relative to Health

In January of 2000, *Healthy People 2010* was released. The goals for this decade are even more ambitious than for previous decades. For example, instead of aiming to *reduce* health disparities, as was the goal for 2000, Healthy People 2010 aims to *eliminate* health disparities. The objectives focus on two overarching goals:

- Help Americans of all ages increase life expectancy and improve their quality of life.
- Eliminate the health disparities that exist between different segments of the U.S. population.
  Specific areas of concern for each of these goals are as follows:
- Health promotion: Nutrition; physical activity and fitness; consumption of tobacco, alcohol, and other drugs; family planning; violent and abusive behavior;

mental health; and educational and community-based programs
- Health protection: Environmental health, occupational safety and health, accidental injuries, food and drug safety, and oral health
- Preventive services priorities: Maternal and infant health; immunizations and infectious diseases; human immunodeficiency virus (HIV) infection; sexually transmitted diseases; heart disease and stroke; cancer, diabetes, and other chronic disabling disorders, and clinical preventive services for these; and mental and behavioral disorders
- System improvement priorities: Health education and preventive services, and surveillance and data systems (USDHHS, 2000c)

From U.S. Department of Health and Human Services: *Healthy people 2010: national health promotion and disease prevention objectives,* ed 2, Washington, DC, 2000, U.S. Government Printing Office.

### Table 3-1 Year 2010 Objectives and Elements of Primary Health Care (PHC)

| EIGHT ESSENTIAL ELEMENTS OF PHC | YEAR 2010 OBJECTIVES | OBJECTIVE NUMBER (FOCUS AREA) |
|---|---|---|
| Health education | Physical activity and fitness | 22 |
| | Tobacco, alcohol, and other drugs | 26, 27 |
| | Mental health | 18 |
| | Surveillance and data systems | 23 |
| | Violence and abusive behavior | 15 |
| Proper nutrition | Nutrition | 19 |
| Maternal and child health care; family planning | Maternal and infant health | 16 |
| | Family planning | 9 |
| Safe water and basic sanitation | Environmental health | 8 |
| Immunization | Immunization and infectious diseases | 14 |
| Prevention and control of locally endemic diseases | HIV infection | 13 |
| | Chronic disorders | 2, 4 |
| | Cancer | 3 |
| | Heart disease and stroke | 12 |
| | Sexually transmitted diseases | 25 |
| | Immunization and infectious diseases | 14 |
| | Clinical preventive services | 1 |
| Treatment of common diseases | HIV, STDs | 13, 25 |
| | Respiratory diseases, heart disease, stroke | 24, 12 |
| Provision of essential drugs | Medical product safety | 17 |

*HIV,* Human immunodeficiency virus; STDs, sexually transmitted diseases.

**Table 3-2** **Differentiating Between Primary Care and Primary Health Care**

| PRIMARY CARE | PRIMARY HEALTH CARE |
| --- | --- |
| Focused on individual | Focused on community |
| Preventive, rehabilitative, but with emphasis on cure | Curative, rehabilitative, but with emphasis on prevention |
| Care provided by generalist physicians, nurse practitioners, nurse midwives, and physician assistants with help of ancillary team members | Care provided by a wide variety of health care team members such as physicians, nurses, community outreach workers, nutritionists, sanitation experts |
| Professional dominance | Self-reliance |

## Primary Care Delivery System

Primary care is delivered in a variety of accessible community settings, such as physicians' offices, managed care organizations, community health centers, and **community nursing centers.** With the emphasis on containing costs toward the end of the last century, the health care delivery system focused its efforts on managed care as an increasingly large part of the primary care system. The two most common types of **managed care organizations** (MCOs) are **health maintenance organizations** (HMOs) and **preferred provider organizations** (PPOs). In 2000, more than 78 million Americans were enrolled in HMO plans (Interstudy Publications, 2002) and nearly 180 million Americans were enrolled in PPOs (InterStudy Publications, 2001).

MCOs in one form or another have existed for over 30 years. An HMO, the first common type of MCO, operates as an organized system of health care that, for a fixed fee, provides primary care services, emergency and preventive treatment, and hospital care to people who have agreed to obtain their medical care from the MCO for a specified period of time. An HMO can be a building in which all health care workers are direct employees (the staff model HMO), or the organization or plan can consist of a more loosely organized system whereby providers contract with the HMO on a fee-for-service basis (the network model HMO). Specialty care is received (and paid for) only as recommended by a primary care provider, sometimes referred to as the gatekeeper. However, because of "the hassle factor" of the gatekeeper system, some HMOs are allowing their patients to bypass the primary care provider when receiving certain aspects of specialty care, for which there is a general consumer demand. HMOs keep costs under control by encouraging prevention, keeping referrals to a minimum, and reducing unnecessary hospitalization.

A PPO, the second common type of MCO, is a health care arrangement between purchasers of care (employers, insurance companies) and providers that offers benefits at a reasonable cost by giving members incentives (such as lower deductibles and co-payments) to use providers within the network. Members who want to use nonpreferred physicians may do so but only at a higher cost (Our

> **WHAT DO YOU THINK?**
>
> A primary care provider in a managed care organization should refer patients to specialists only as outlined in the referral guidelines of their employing organization, whether they agree with the guidelines or not.

Health Plan, 2002). Physicians and other primary care providers can belong to several preferred provider plans. Other health care delivery organizations include community nursing centers and community health centers.

As consumers of health insurance continue to grow frustrated with MCOs, defined care may be the wave of the future. Defined care is based on the use of a **defined contribution** by employers rather than a defined health benefit. This type of plan enables employees to choose their own health plans on the basis of personal values, price, and insurance needs. The employers set aside a defined contribution each year for each employee to spend on benefits. Employees select from a wide range of health plan options, including MCOs, medical savings accounts (MSAs), or fee-for-service arrangements (Riddle, 2000). The employee, rather than the employer, has the burden of responsibility for being knowledgeable about different health plans. Currently, there are only a few defined care companies, but the market is expanding. Defined care is available in Portland, Chicago, and the Minneapolis/Twin Cities (Lutz and Henkind, 2000).

In the mid 1990s, Medicare managed care grew significantly. During this time the Centers for Medicare and Medicaid Services (CMS) made efforts to apply the same kind of cost-control methods to the Medicare and Medicaid programs that existed for the general population. Medicare managed care, part of the Medicare+Choice plan, works like other MCOs. The government contracts with MCOs, which market their plan to consumers. Medicare consumers select from the list of available plans, or they can elect to stay in a fee-for-service arrangement. The government pays each contracted plan the negotiated premium for every individual enrolled in that plan.

### Evidence-Based Practice

A study of the use of emergency department visits by children showed that a significant number of these visits were for needs that could be more appropriately met in primary care settings. The study found that the most likely users of the emergency department for nonurgent purposes were single-parent families and families on Medicaid. More than 20 million children seek medical care in emergency departments each year. Children are the patients in one in four emergency department visits. Previous studies showed that between a third and half of these are for nonurgent reasons. Use of the emergency department for nonurgent reasons greatly affects the cost and quality of health care. A visit to the emergency department for a nonurgent reason (otitis media) is approximately $170. This same visit in an office setting is likely to cost the patient only $55.

This study found that 65% of the emergency department visits made by children were nonurgent. The most common reasons given by the responsible adult for bringing a child to the emergency department were that the doctor's office was closed, that the child required immediate attention, that the emergency department was closer than the doctor's office, that the child is seen more quickly in the emergency department, and that the doctor could not be reached. These comments suggest that there is a perceived or true lack of primary care providers, and possibly that there is a lack of understanding of how to appropriately proceed when the provider is not available.

**Nurse Use:** Besides the financial costs, visits to the emergency department for nonurgent reasons are missed opportunities for preventive care and educational measures important to child health care. These measures are more likely to take place in an office or public health clinic setting than in an emergency department.

Phelps K et al: Factors associated with emergency department utilization for nonurgent pediatric problems, *Arch Fam Med* 9:1086, 2000.

Medicare members pay any additional premium and co-payments as necessary. The Balanced Budget Act of 1997 encouraged Medicare managed care by offering incentives for those choosing to join HMOs, such as reduced prescription co-payments (Managed Care Online, 2000). These efforts have not worked, and Medicare HMOs have complained of inadequate reimbursement and have begun closing. Enrollment in Medicare HMOs has declined from a peak of 6.1 million enrollees in 1999 to 5.6 million in May of 2001. Most Medicare beneficiaries remain in a fee-for-service plan (Sandy and Schroeder, 2001).

## Primary Care Workforce

Primary care developed in the 1960s as a need to reexamine the role of the general practitioner. The Millis Commission (Millis, 1966) expressed concern that a knowledge explosion, development of new technologies, and an increasing number of new specialties were threatening the role of the general practitioner. The specialty of family practice and the arrival of **nurse practitioners** (NPs) and **physician assistants** (PAs) emerged in response to the need to provide primary care.

Currently, primary care providers include generalists who possess skills in health promotion and disease prevention, assessment and evaluation of undiagnosed symptoms and physical signs, management of common acute and chronic medical conditions, and identification and appropriate referral for other needed health care services (USDHHS, 1992). The health care personnel trained as primary care generalists include family physicians, general internists, general pediatricians, NPs, PAs, and **certified nurse midwives** (CNMs). Some physicians with special training in preventive medicine, public health, or obstetrics/gynecology also deliver primary care (Institute of Medicine, 1996).

NPs and CNMs, both considered advanced practice nurses, are vital members of the primary care and primary health care teams. NPs receive advanced training, usually at the master's level, with most taking a certification examination in a specialty area, such as pediatrics, adult, gerontology, obstetrics/gynecology, or family. Training emphasizes clinical medical skills (history, physical, and diagnosis) and pharmacology, in addition to the traditional psychosocial- and prevention-focused skills that are normally thought of as nursing. Studies have shown that 60% to 80% of the primary care traditionally done by physicians can be delivered by an NP for less money and with equal or better quality (Office of Technology Assessment, 1986). An estimated 102,829 nurse practitioners are working today (USDHHS, 2000a). (See Chapter 41 for more information.)

**Nurse midwifery** is defined as "the independent management and care of essentially normal newborns and women antepartally, intrapartally, postpartally, and gynecologically, occurring within a health care system that provides for medical consultation, collaborative management, and referral" (Rooks and Haas, 1986, p. 9). The mother is the primary focus of care for CNMs, who spend the majority of their time on prenatal care, labor, delivery, and postpartum care, as well as family planning services. Nurse midwives receive training either at the master's level or by attending a school of nurse midwifery. All CNMs are certified by a national examination. Currently, an estimated 5800 CNMs practice in the United States (M. McCartney, American College of Nurse-Midwives, personal interview, 2002).

Physician assistants (PAs) operate under the license of the physician, unlike NPs and CNMs, who operate as independent practitioners. Most PAs receive their training at the baccalaureate level and are able to sit for their certification boards once they have graduated. PAs assist or substitute for physicians in the performance of specific medical tasks. Like NPs, PAs are skilled in history, physicals, and the diagnosing and treating of uncomplicated medical conditions. Both are trained in prescribing a limited number of medicines, but their ability to prescribe depends on the laws of the state in which they live. In the past, CNMs and NPs were pressured to limit their practice to avoid infringing on what physicians perceived as their role. However, many state practice laws have changed. With pressure from the federal government and consumers, NPs, and CNMs practice independently, prescribe, and receive third-party reimbursement. In the United States, there are currently 40,469 certified PAs in clinical practice (U.S. Department of Labor, 2002).

## Public Health System

Although the goal of the public health system is to ensure that the health of the community is protected, promoted, and ensured, there is overlap between this system and the primary care system. The overlap comes not only from the primary care system, which provides health promotion and disease prevention, but also through the public health system, which provides personal primary care services for those who cannot afford to receive their care elsewhere. For example, the USDHHS provides a commissioned corps of uniformed health personnel, the **National Health Service Corps,** to serve residents of medically underserved areas.

The public health system is mandated through laws that are developed at the national, state, or local level. Examples of public health laws instituted to protect the health of the community include a law mandating immunizations for all children entering kindergarten and a law requiring constant monitoring of the local water supply.

### Organization of the Public Health System

The public health system is organized into many levels in the federal, state, and local systems. Although not all local governmental units are involved in personal health care, most are. For example, school districts are responsible for health education and first aid, and many schools have on-site clinics that are responsible for a comprehensive array of the student's health, including mental health and family planning.

## Federal System

### U.S. Department of Health and Human Services

The U.S. Department of Health and Human Services (USDHHS) is the agency most heavily involved with the health and welfare concerns of U.S. citizens. The organizational chart of the USDHHS (Figure 3-1) shows the office of the secretary, 11 agencies, and a program support center. Although not shown on the chart, the position of U.S. surgeon general has been combined with that of the

---

**DID YOU KNOW?**

The U.S. Department of Health and Human Services is the largest health program in the world. Its mission is to enhance the health and well-being of the American people through the following (USDHHS, 2000b):
- Alcohol, drug abuse, and mental health programs
- Disease tracking and identification
- Health care access for all and integrity of the nation's health entitlement and safety net programs
- Identification and correction of health hazards
- Medical assistance after disasters
- Medical research
- Promotion of exercise and healthy habits
- Protection of the nation's food and drug supply

---

assistant secretary for health. The USDHHS is charged with regulating health care and overseeing the health status of Americans. Added to the USDHHS recently are the Office of Public Health Preparedness and the Center for Faith-Based and Community Initiatives. The Office of Public Health Preparedness was added to assist the nation and states to prepare for bioterrorism after September 11, 2001. The Faith-Based Initiative Center was developed by President Bush to allow faith communities to compete for federal money to support their community activities.

The USDHHS, directed by the secretary for health, is organized into 12 functional units (see Figure 3-1):
1. Administration for Children and Families (ACF)
2. Administration on Aging (AoA)
3. Centers for Medicare and Medicaid Services (CMS)
4. Agency for Healthcare Research and Quality (AHRQ)
5. Centers for Disease Control and Prevention (CDC)
6. Agency for Toxic Substances and Disease Registry (ATSDR)
7. Food and Drug Administration (FDA)
8. Health Resources and Services Administration (HRSA)
9. Indian Health Service (IHS)
10. National Institutes of Health (NIH)
11. Substance Abuse and Mental Health Services Administration (SAMHSA)
12. Program Support Center (PSC)

The PSC supports the secretary and all of the agencies listed. Ten regional offices are maintained to provide more direct assistance to the states. Their locations are shown in Table 3-3. The HRSA of the USDHHS contains the Bureau of Health Professions, which includes separate divisions for nursing, medicine, dentistry, public health, and allied health professions.

### Division of Nursing

The federal government looks to the Division of Nursing to provide the competence and expertise for administering nurse education legislation, interpreting trends and

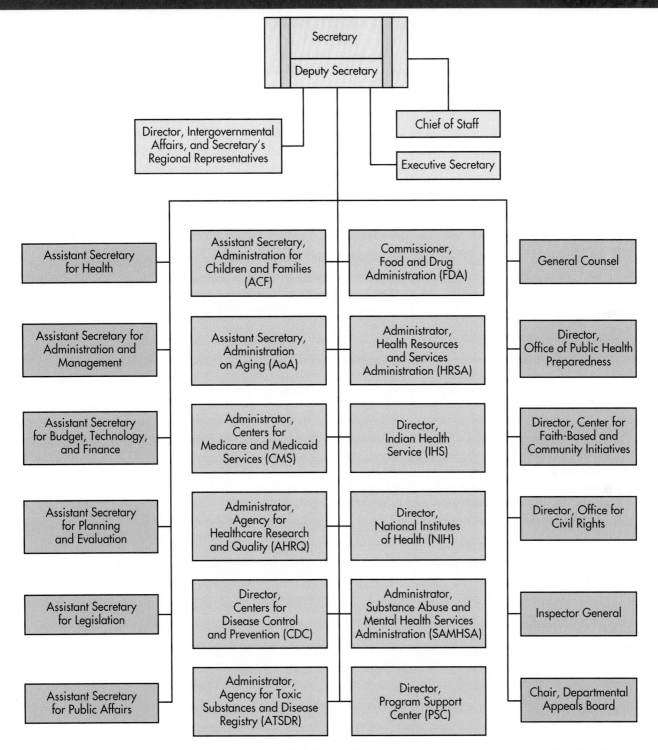

**Figure 3-1** Organization of the U.S. Department of Health and Human Services. *(From U.S. Department of Health and Human Services organization chart [www.hhs.gov/about/orgchart.html].)*

needs of the nursing component of the nation's health care delivery system, and maintaining a liaison with the nursing community and with international, state, regional, and local health interests. As the federal focus for nursing education and practice, the Division of Nursing identifies current and future nursing issues. Currently it is providing national leadership to ensure an adequate supply and distribution of qualified nursing personnel to meet the health needs of the nation. The division works collaboratively with other federal agencies and with national nursing organizations (U.S. Public Health Service, 1997).

*National Center for Nursing Research*

In late 1985, Congress overrode a presidential veto, allowing the creation of the National Center for Nursing Research within the National Institutes of Health. The research and research training activities previously supported by the Division of Nursing were transferred to this new center. In 1993 it was renamed the National Institute for Nursing Research (NINR), and it is the focal point of the nation's nursing research activities. It promotes the growth and quality of research in nursing and patient care, provides important leadership, expands the pool of experienced nurse researchers, and serves as a point of interaction with other bases of health care research.

*Agency for Health Care Research and Quality*

In 1999 President Clinton signed the Health Care Research and Quality Act changing the Agency for Health Care Policy and Research to the Agency for Health Care Research and Quality (AHRQ). This agency is charged with conducting research on effectiveness of medical services, interventions, and technologies, including research related to nursing interventions and outcomes that contribute to the improved health status of the nation. The name change reaffirms that it is a scientific research agency and not an agency that writes policy or regulations.

## Other Federal Government Agencies

The USDHHS has primary responsibility for federal health functions. The cabinet departments of the federal government carry out certain functions related to the health of the nation. Those departments include Commerce, Defense, Labor, Agriculture, and Justice.

*Department of Commerce*

Within the Department of Commerce, the Census Bureau provides health care information. Established in 1902, this bureau conducts a census of the population every 10 years.

Also a part of this department is the National Oceanic and Atmospheric Administration, which provides special services in support of controlling urban air quality, a major factor in community health today.

*Department of Defense*

The Department of Defense delivers health care to members of the military and their dependents. The assistant secretary of defense for health affairs administers the Civilian Health and Medical Program of the Uniformed Services (CHAMPUS). Each of the departments within Defense (Army, Navy, Air Force, and Marines) has a surgeon general. Health services, including community health services for members of the military, are delivered by a health services command in each department. In each command, nurses of high military rank are part of the administration of health services.

*Department of Labor*

The Department of Labor has two agencies with health functions: the Occupational Safety and Heath Administration (OSHA) and the Mine Safety and Health Administration. Both are charged with writing safety and health standards and ensuring compliance in the workplace. This includes conducting inspections, investigating complaints, and issuing citations if necessary. Each agency coordinates its activities with state departments of labor and health.

*Department of Agriculture*

The Department of Agriculture is involved in health care primarily through administering the Food and Nutrition Service. Although plant, product, and animal inspections by the Department of Agriculture are also related to health, the Food and Nutrition Service oversees a variety of food assistance activities. This service collaborates with state and local government welfare agencies to provide

| Table 3-3 | **Regional Offices of the U.S. Department of Health and Human Services** | |
|---|---|---|
| **REGION** | **LOCATION** | **TERRITORY** |
| 1 | Boston | Connecticut, Maine, Massachusetts, New Hampshire, Rhode Island, Vermont |
| 2 | New York | New Jersey, New York, Puerto Rico, Virgin Islands |
| 3 | Philadelphia | Delaware, District of Columbia, Maryland, Pennsylvania, Virginia, West Virginia |
| 4 | Atlanta | Alabama, Florida, Georgia, Kentucky, Mississippi, North Carolina, South Carolina, Tennessee |
| 5 | Chicago | Illinois, Indiana, Michigan, Minnesota, Ohio, Wisconsin |
| 6 | Dallas | Arkansas, Louisiana, New Mexico, Oklahoma, Texas |
| 7 | Kansas City | Iowa, Kansas, Missouri, Nebraska |
| 8 | Denver | Colorado, Montana, North Dakota, South Dakota, Utah, Wyoming |
| 9 | San Francisco | American Samoa, Arizona, California, Guam, Hawaii, Nevada, N. Mariana Islands, Trust Territories |
| 10 | Seattle | Alaska, Idaho, Oregon, Washington |

food stamps to needy persons to increase their food purchasing power. Other programs include school breakfast and lunch programs; the Supplemental Food Program for Women, Infants, and Children (WIC); and grants to states for nutrition education training.

### Department of Justice
Health services to federal prisoners are administered within the Department of Justice. The Medical and Services Division of the Bureau of Prisons includes medical, psychiatric, dental, and health support services. It also administers environmental health and safety, farm operations, and food service, along with commissary, laundry, and other personal services for inmates.

### Food and Drug Administration
The Food and Drug Administration (FDA) has the job of promoting and protecting public health by allowing safe and effective products to reach the marketplace in a timely way and monitoring products for continued safety after they are in use. Products that must have FDA approval before being sold in the United States include drugs, medical treatments, and food additives. Some products that do not require approval, including cosmetics and dietary aids, are closely monitored for safety. Besides the approval and monitoring of products, the FDA promotes food safety and tracks food-borne illnesses. It regulates consumer labels, creating the guidelines that are used to monitor the information on (and the truthfulness of) the label. It is also responsible for the safety of the nation's blood and plasma supply.

## State System
Although state health departments vary widely in their roles, they have an important role in health care financing (such as Medicaid), providing mental health and professional education, establishing health codes, licensing facilities and personnel, and regulating the insurance industry (Tulchinsky, 2000). State systems also have an important role in direct assistance to local health departments, including ongoing assessment of health needs. Box 3-2 provides a list of typical state health department programs.

As in international and federal agencies, nurses serve in many capacities in state health departments as consultants, direct services providers, researchers, teachers, and supervisors, as well as participating in program development, planning, and evaluation of health programs. Many health departments have a division or department of nursing.

Every state has a board of examiners of nurses. The board may be found either in the department of licensing boards of the health department or in an administrative agency of the governor's office. Created by legislation known as a state nurse practice act, the examiners' board is made up of nurses and consumers. A few states have other providers or administrators as members. The functions of this board are described in the practice act of each state and generally include licensing and examination of registered nurses and licensed practical nurses; approval of schools of nursing in the state; revocation, suspension, or denial of licenses; and writing of regulations about nursing practice and education.

## Local System
The local health department has direct responsibility to the citizens in its community or jurisdiction. Services and programs offered by local health departments vary greatly depending on the state and local health codes that must be followed, the needs of the community, and available funding and other resources. For example, one health department might be more involved with public health education programs and environmental issues, whereas another health department might emphasize direct client care.

Local health departments vary in providing sick care or even primary care. A list of health department programs, taken from an urban–suburban county health department in a mid-Atlantic state, is shown in Box 3-3. At the local level, as at the state level, coordinating health efforts between health departments and other county or city departments is essential. For example, local boards of education and departments of social services are an integral part of activities of local governments.

More often than at other levels of government, community health nurses at the local level provide direct services. Some community health nurses deliver special or selected services, such as follow-up of contacts in cases of tuberculosis or venereal disease, or providing child

---

**BOX 3-2   Typical Programs in a State Health Department**

Acquired immunodeficiency syndrome (AIDS) services
Bioterrorism/disaster management
Case management
Departmental licensing boards
Division of vital records
Environmental programs
Epidemiology
Health planning and development
Health services cost review
Juvenile services
Legal services
Media and public relations and educational information
Medical assistance: policy, compliance operations
Mental health and addictions
Mental retardation and developmental disabilities
Preventive medicine and medical affairs
Quality assurance
Referrals to resources
Service to the chronically ill and aging
Sexually transmitted diseases (screening and treatment)

---

**BOX 3-3    Examples of Programs Provided by Local Health Departments**

Addiction and alcoholism clinics
Adult health
Bioterrorism/disaster management
Birth and death records
Child day care and development
Child health clinics
Dental health clinic
Environmental health
Epidemiology and disease control
Family planning
Geriatric evaluation
Health education
Home health agency
Hospital discharge planning
Hypertension clinics
Immunization clinics
Information services
Maternal health
Medical social work
Mental health
Mental retardation and developmental disabilities
Nursing
Nursing home licensure
Nutrition
Occupational therapy
School health
Services for children with special needs
Speech and audiology

---

**BOX 3-4    Levels of Prevention in the Public Health Care System**

**PRIMARY PREVENTION**

Counsel clients in health behaviors related to lifestyle.

**SECONDARY PREVENTION**

Implement a family-planning program to prevent unintended pregnancies for young couples who attend the primary clinic.

**TERTIARY PREVENTION**

Provide a self-management asthma program for children with chronic asthma to reduce their need for hospitalization.

---

immunization clinics. Other community health nurses have a more generalized practice, delivering services to families in certain geographic areas. This method of delivery of nursing services involves broader needs and a wider variety of nursing interventions. The local level often provides an opportunity for nurses to take on significant leadership roles, with many nurses serving as directors or managers.

Box 3-4 gives examples of primary, secondary, and tertiary levels of prevention in the public health care system.

## TRANSFORMATION OF THE HEALTH CARE SYSTEM

The rising costs of health care in the United States, uneven access for consumers, and dissatisfied consumers and health care professionals have created an atmosphere of rapid change. Four important competing forces help to shape the health care system: consumers, employers (purchasers), managed care systems including HMOs and hospital systems, and state and federal legislation.

First, consumers want low-cost, high-quality health care without limits and with improved ability to access the providers of their choice. They are becoming more knowledgeable about appealing health care decisions that are being made for them and are joining and appealing to consumer groups to help them fight their battles in and outside of the court room. Consumer groups, especially those that are involved with creating managed care **report cards,** will continue to play a major role in helping to shape the future health care system.

Second, employers (purchasers of health care) want access to basic health care plans at reasonable costs. They put continual pressure on MCOs to decrease costs and are always threatening to change plans if their costs are not low enough or their benefits do not fit the needs of their employees. Employers are increasingly expecting their employees to pick up a greater share of this cost and employers continue to drop health care coverage for family members.

**◖ WHAT DO YOU THINK?**

Mandating small business owners to purchase health insurance for their employees (employer mandates) is a reasonable way to help ensure that the health needs of this nation, especially the working poor, will be taken care of.

Managed care organizations and other major health care systems continue to strive for a balance between consumer and purchaser demands, always keeping a close eye on their own budget and expenses. To maintain a profit while providing quality care, MCOs and other health care systems have had to downsize and create alliances, mergers, and other joint ventures.

Finally, legislation, especially concerning access and quality issues, continues to be debated and enacted, thus creating yet another force helping to shape a health care system based on changes. Legislators are pressured by a variety of groups, which include the following:

1. Constituents who seek changes because of an unsatisfactory experience with a health care system or provider
2. Consumer groups representing the uninsured
3. Employers who continually fight against mandated coverage for their employees

4. The managed care industry, which is trying to remain profitable in the face of rising costs

Other examples of a health care system in transformation include the following:

- Regionalizing managed health care in both the private and the public (Medicare and Medicaid) sectors on the basis of a competitive prepaid capitated (per person) system. Local communities will continue to be needed to address the needs of their homeless, underserved, and uninsured populations.
- Enormous growth in the home health care industry. Increased fraud within the last few years may cause Medicare to cut back on payments and has caused the growth rate of the industry to slow or even decrease.
- Consumers of health care will continue to feel empowered to make changes in the health care system. This will lead to healthier people in healthier communities. Consumers of health care will also become more informed and involved in their own health care.
- Advances in diagnostic and surgical technology may lead to higher survival rates and less time spent in sick care. However Americans still make health behavior choices such as smoking, not exercising, and excessive eating that keep them from living a long and healthful existence. In addition, leading-edge technology and surgical procedures will still benefit only those who can afford them.
- Experimenting in health personnel staffing will increase in an attempt to save costs and find new opportunities to substitute technology for human labor.
- The shortage of primary care providers for underserved populations such as those in rural and inner-city areas will continue.
- Efforts by health care personnel to bring back the "caring" side of health care as a revolt against the stringent cost-cutting efforts instituted by managed care in the 1990s will be seen.
- Increasing emphasis will be placed on population-based health care, not only as a cost-savings mechanism but also to promote disease prevention and to meet the health care needs of many people at one time.
- Emphasis will be placed on delivering care that leads to the best possible outcomes. This "evidence-based care" is done in an effort to ensure quality.
- Information systems, including the electronic medical record, will save time and effort and help ensure the delivery of appropriate care. Innovations in the field of information technology are also creating much debate and forthcoming legislation regarding the right to privacy.
- Major shifts of nurses from the acute care setting to the community will continue. Continuing education needs will expand to help nurses learn to transfer skills.

---

**◖ DID YOU KNOW?**

The Balanced Budget Act of 1997 provided $20 billion for children's health coverage to be distributed to the states and used over a 5-year period. Children to be covered by the State Children's Health Insurance Program (SCHIP) must be under age 19 in families with incomes of up to 200% of the federal poverty level, must not be covered by Medicaid, and must not be receiving coverage under a group or individual insurance plan (White House Press Office, 1999).

---

## A COMPREHENSIVE MODEL: INTEGRATION OF PUBLIC HEALTH AND PRIMARY CARE

The integration of public health and primary care for community-based health care is essential for improving the health of the nation (Lasker, 1997). The once-interrelated public health and primary care systems in this country have become separated over the last century. This separation has led to less effective health care with increasingly higher costs, less access, and poorer results (McKnight, 1995). Modern consumer societies, such as the United States, experience lower-quality health return for higher and higher medical investments. One of the reasons for the split of the two components has been the rapid advances in science in the last few decades. Preventing illnesses has become less important as the inventions of new technologies and procedures have provided treatments. As the importance of prevention has seemed to diminish, public health has also declined, and health professionals' "training has focused on preparing professionals to perform in specialized, acute care hospital environments" (Lasker, 1997, p. 18).

The overemphasis on technologies has led to a decrease in attention to the social, economic, behavioral, and environmental conditions that cause diseases to emerge in susceptible individuals. To achieve the specific health goals of programs such as Healthy People 2010 and the WHO's Health for All in the 21st Century, it will not be enough to be responsible for only the patients who seek care. It will become necessary to help those who do not actively seek care, to work towards higher patient compliance with care and to work within communities to establish health-seeking strategies. To achieve a true primary health care system, nurses must work not only with individual patients but with communities to evaluate the social, economic, behavioral, and environmental conditions that are causing disease in the community.

The interaction of the public health and primary care fields is necessary to achieve quality health, and many things have changed in the past 10 years that may make the process possible. The growing concern over the direction of the health care system in this country, along with the current strains on cost and access, have proven that neither of

## *Primary Health Care Systems and Health Care Transformation in Canada*

Lianne Patricia Jeffs, R.N., M.Sc., Faculty of Nursing, University of Toronto

### HEALTH STATUS AND OUTCOMES

In Canada, although wide variations exist depending on geography (e.g., underserviced and rural areas), ethnicity (e.g., First Nations populations), and socioeconomic status (e.g., low-income families), the overall health of Canadians is improving. Canada has a lower infant mortality rate (5.3 infant deaths per 1000 live births) than the United States (7.1 per 1000) (Organisation for Economic Co-Operation and Development [OECD], 2002). Life expectancy in Canada has been increasing continuously over the last 25 years. In 1999, life expectancy was 80.8 years for women and 74.4 years for men, compared to 79.4 years for women and 73.9 years for men in the U.S. population (OECD, 2002). Compared with other selected developed countries, Canada ranks second after the United States in percentage of the population reporting their health status as good, very good, or excellent. From 1979 to 1999, the potential years of life lost from causes such as unintentional injuries and acute myocardial infarction declined significantly (Statistics Canada, 2002). However, access to health care continues to be an issue: an estimated 4.3 million Canadians indicated that they had difficulties accessing first contact services for routine care, health information, and immediate care for a minor health problem (Health Canada, 2002).

### HEALTH CARE REFORM

Over the last three decades, several reports, studies, and strategies relating to improving the efficiency of the Canadian health care system have emerged at all levels of government. The Canadian content box in Chapter 1 provides a more detailed discussion of the reports. Recently, the Romanow commission (2002) and the Standing Senate on Social Affairs, Science and Technology (2002), released reports on how to improve the Canadian health care system. Both reports identified upward pressures in Canada's health care system resulting from increased pharmaceutical costs, new technologies, aging population, cost of health care human resources, growing public expectations around evidence-based quality health care, increased chronic illness and acuity of patients, health care restructuring, reemergence of communicable diseases, and environmental problems. These pressures are driving forces for a need for health care reform that involves a move from acute institutional care to community-based care and a more regionalized approach with emphasis on primary health care services and programs.

Part of the dialogue on health care reform is focused on ensuring that the supply of health care professionals involved in the provision of health care is adequate. Like the United States, Canada is faced with an actual shortage of nurses caused by the reduced number of educational seats in nursing programs in the past decade and an aging workforce; human management issues, which make it impossible to maximize the productivity of nurses; and insufficient funding for nursing positions (Canadian Nursing Advisory Committee, 2002). From 1997 to 2001, there was a small increase (from 6.9% to 9.2%) in community health nursing positions and a slight decrease (from 4.3% to 4.1%) in home care nurse positions (Canadian Institute of Health Information, 2001). This is a relatively small percentage of human resources growth compared to the magnitude of the shift from the hospital to the community health care sector. Mitigating strategies to address the nursing workforce and work environment issues have been developed and are in the process of implementation and evaluation at both the federal (National Nursing Strategy) and provincial/territorial (e.g., provincial nursing strategy based on the Nursing Task Force report in Ontario) levels. These efforts include the creation of senior bureaucratic positions for nursing at both the federal and the provincial/territorial governmental levels, with a mandate to provide policy advice and strategic direction for the current and future nursing services and health care needs in Canada.

### PRIMARY HEALTH CARE

Every major report on Canada's health care system released in recent years has recommended some version of primary health care reforms, and most outline models and approaches consistent with the Alma Ata Declaration (see Appendix A.3). Primary health care is the first level of care and the first point of contact of individuals and families to the health care system that emphasizes health promotion, illness prevention, management of chronic diseases, and links to other types of care including home care, palliative care (Cradduck, 1995). A variety of health professionals, working in collaborative teams of physicians, nurse practitioners, registered nurses, social workers, dieticians, physiotherapists, dentists, and health promoters, practise in a variety of settings such as public health units, community health centres, health service organizations, and family health networks (Ontario). The goal of these agencies is to provide an integrated and coordinated approach to meeting the complex needs of the populations they are providing care to.

A clear differentiation between primary care and primary health care continues to be needed in Canada, as does the operationalization of the principles of primary health care into the health care system. As part of the recent dialogue included in the Romanow report (2002), a common national platform for primary health care based on four essential building blocks (continuity of care, early detection and action, better information about needs and outcomes, and new and stronger incentives for health care professionals to participate in primary health care) is recommended. In addition, Romanow calls for a national immunization program. Primary health care reform was identified as a priority for the renewal of Canada's health care system at the First Ministers' meeting in September 2000. To support this goal, the government of Canada created the $800 million Primary Health Care Transition Fund, which provides financial support to provinces and territories for their efforts to improve the delivery of primary health care and its integration with other parts of the health care system.

## PUBLIC HEALTH SERVICES

Underlying public health practice in Canada is the legislative mandate designed to protect the public interest relative to communicable diseases and environmental risks. Public health services in Canada are administered primarily through governmental departments such as departments of health, Ministries of Health and Social Services, and departments of public health. Variations in structure occur across the provincial and territorial jurisdictions as well as in municipal/regional agencies (including health units and autonomous agencies). These agencies are responsible for providing basic public health services related to communicable disease control, regulation and enforcement of environmental standards and health promotion, and illness and injury prevention programs.

## THE ROLE OF THE REGISTERED NURSE IN THE PRIMARY HEALTH CARE SYSTEM

Registered nurses are key to the provision of comprehensive and effective primary health care services. The value of the registered nurse as a high-quality, cost-effective provider in the primary health care system is well documented (Registered Nurses Association of Ontario, 2002). The registered nurse has many roles in the primary health care system, depending on educational preparation and experience; these roles include community-oriented nurse, health promotion nurse, nursing administrator, and, in some jurisdictions, primary health care nurse practitioner. In each of these roles, the registered nurse can function as an educator, a consultant, a community developer, a facilitator, a leader, an enabler, an advocate, a communicator, a coordinator, a collaborator, a researcher, a social marketer, and a policy formulator.

For the health status of Canadians to improve, there needs to be a strong commitment to the principles of comprehensive and accessible primary health care. This commitment will strengthen the contribution of the multidisciplinary primary health care team, including the registered nurse, in the provision of care to individuals, families, and communities, which will ultimately lead to the overall effectiveness of the Canadian health care system.

### References

Canadian Institute of Health Information: *Supply and distribution of RNs in Canada in 2001,* 2001, available at www.cihi.ca.

Cradduck GR: Primary health care practice. In: Stewart MJ, editor: *Community nursing: promoting Canadians' health,* pp 454-474, Toronto, 1995, Saunders Canada.

Health Canada: *Healthy Canadians: a federal report on comparable health indicators,* Ottawa, 2002, available at www.healthcanada.ca.

Organisation for Economic Co-Operation and Development: *Health data,* 2002, available at www.oecd.org.

Registered Nurses Association of Ontario: *RN effectiveness project: clinical, financial and systems outcomes,* Toronto, 2002, available at www.rnao.org.

Romanow R: *Building on values: the future of health care in Canada: final report,* Ottawa, 2002, available at www.healthcarecommission.ca.

Standing Senate Committee on Social Affairs, Science and Technology: *Volume 6 of the health of Canadians: the federal role and recommendations report,* Ottawa, 2002, available at www.parl.gc.ca.

Statistics Canada: *Access to health care services in Canada,* 2001, available at www.statisticscanada.ca.

Statistics Canada, Vital Statistics Death and Demography Division: 2002, available at www.statisticscanada.ca.

*Canadian spelling is used.*

the two fields working alone will be able to accomplish its goals. It is no longer possible to make the health changes necessary in this country by simply putting more money into the current system. Fuchs (1998) said, "There is no reason to believe that the major health problems of the average American would be significantly alleviated by increases in the number of hospitals. . . . The greatest potential for improving the health of the American people is to be found in what they do and don't do for themselves . . . and collective decisions affecting pollution and other aspects of the environment are also relevant" (p. 54).

The W. K. Kellogg Foundation (1993), which financially supports efforts to improve the health of communities, states that a community-based practice must involve community members by allowing them to set their own priorities and solutions. Kellogg has found that when the right tools, such as power, information, and financial support, are shared with community members, they become more actively involved in the process. Building a consensus among the many community leaders who have a vested interest in the process will help to identify the community's health needs as well as a larger number of solutions to meet these needs. It must be remembered that health care cannot be separated from the broader scope of community development, such as housing and economic development. Consider the example of a young mother who has been scolded by a health professional for presenting her child with several infected insect bites without ever addressing the issue of the unavailability of window screens in the family's apartment.

### NURSING TIP

Many nurses in the United States are practicing illness-oriented care as a result of public need and the amount attached to these services (Miller et al, 1993). Salmon (1993) states that this has diverted community-oriented nurses away from their central roles in the activities of assessment, surveillance, policy development, health promotion, and disease and injury prevention.

A main focus in community-based health is to get the community to see that their actions, rather than the hospital's, determine their health. Community members on the west side of Chicago, for example, found that even though access to health care and hospitals had dramatically improved several years ago, their health had not. They analyzed the top reasons for hospitalizations and found that the most common reasons were not disease but rather social problems. Community members implemented programs to solve these problems, including dog catching, alternative traffic routes, and rooftop greenhouses (McKnight, 1995). Because nurses, like few other professionals, move in and are trusted in the community, they are ideally suited to work with the community for health change. They can be found in schools, homes, churches, and on street corners developing relationships, collecting data, assessing needs, and providing care.

### Practice Application

During a well-child clinic visit, Jenna Wells, R.N., met Sandra Farr and her 24-month-old daughter, Jessica. The Farrs had recently moved to the community. Mrs. Farr stated that she knew that Jessica needed the last in a series of immunizations, and because they did not have health insurance, she brought her daughter to the public health clinic. Upon initial assessment, Mrs. Farr told the nurse that her husband would soon be employed, but the family would not have any health care coverage for the next 30 days. The Farrs also need to decide which health care package they want. Mr. Farr's company offers a preferred provider option (PPO), a health maintenance organization (HMO), and a community nursing clinic plan to all employees. Neither Mr. nor Mrs. Farr has ever used an HMO or a community nursing clinic, and they are not sure what services are provided.

Mrs. Farr asks Nurse Wells what she should do. Nurse Wells should do which of the following?

A. Encourage Mrs. Farr to choose the HMO because it will pay more attention to the family's preventive needs, and direct Mrs. Farr to other sources of health care should the family need to see a provider while they are uninsured.

B. Encourage Mrs. Farr to choose the PPO because it will have a greater number of qualified providers to choose from, and direct Mrs. Farr to other sources of health care should the family need to see a provider while they are uninsured.

C. Encourage Mrs. Farr to choose the local community nursing center because it is staffed with nurse practitioners who are well qualified to provide comprehensive health care with an emphasis on health education, and direct Mrs. Farr to other sources of health care should the family need to see a provider while they are uninsured.

D. Explain the differences between a PPO, HMO, and community nursing clinic, and encourage Mrs. Farr to discuss the options with her husband, and direct Mrs. Farr to other sources of health care should the family need to see a provider while they are uninsured.

**Answers are in the back of the book.**

### Key Points

- Health care in the United States is composed of a personal care system and a public health system, with overlap between the two systems.
- Primary care is the providing of integrated, accessible health care services by clinicians who are accountable for addressing a large majority of personal health care needs, developing a sustained partnership with patients, and practicing in the context of family and community.
- Primary health care is essential care made universally accessible to individuals and families in a

community. Health care is made available to them through their full participation and is provided at a cost that the community and country can afford.

- Primary care is part of primary health care.
- Although primary care practitioners are encouraged to consider the client's biopsychosocial needs, interventions are directed primarily at the pathophysiologic process.
- Public health refers to organized community efforts designed to prevent disease and promote health.
- Important trends that affect the health care system are the demographic, social, economic, political, and technological trends.
- There are approximately 42.6 million uninsured people in the United States and many more who simply lack access to adequate health care.
- Many federal agencies are involved in government health care functions. The agency most directly involved with the health and welfare of Americans is the U.S. Department of Health and Human Services (USDHHS).
- Most state and local jurisdictions have government activities that affect the health care field.
- Health care reform measures seek to make changes in the cost, quality, and access of the present system.
- With an increasing emphasis on containing costs, the health care delivery system is focusing its efforts on developing managed care systems.
- The integration of primary care and public health is necessary for the future health of the nation. The disenfranchised systems have led to greater health care costs with less return.
- The development of scientific knowledge has made society more concerned about treatment than about prevention. Thus health professionals have become less dependent on public health.
- To achieve the specific health goals of programs such as Healthy People 2010, primary care and public health must work within the community for community-based care. It will not be enough to provide care to only those patients who seek it. Instead, increasing access for all, improving patient compliance, and promoting health-seeking strategies within the community will be necessary to accomplish these goals.
- The most sustainable individual and system changes come when there has been active participation from the people who live in the community.
- Building a consensus among the many diverse community leaders will help find the solutions to address the community's health needs.
- Nurses are more than able to fill the gap between personal care and public health because they have skills in assessment, health promotion, and disease and injury prevention; knowledge of community resources; and ability to develop relationships with community members and leaders.

## Clinical Decision-Making Activities

1. Compare the local and state services where you live with those that have been presented in this chapter. Give examples.
2. Debate the following: The major problem with the health care system is (choose one of the following topics):
   a. Escalating costs (including those from increased technology)
   b. Fragmentation
   c. Access to care
   d. Quality of care
   How does the answer help direct you to a solution to the problem?
3. Interview a nurse practitioner and a physician assistant to determine any philosophical differences in their scope of practice. What are some of the complex issues that have caused these differences?
4. If you were asked to plan a disease prevention program in your community, what would you do? Describe the plan you would implement. Give specific details.
5. If there is an MCO in your community, interview three providers and three consumers to determine what each sees as the advantages and disadvantages of this type of care delivery system. Do we need to consider their answers from another perspective? Why?
6. Visit your local health department and determine how its services fit into a primary care, public health, community-based health care system. Illustrate what you mean by your answer with examples.
7. Determine whether any agency in your community is promoting community-based care to deliver health care. Identify the principles the agency people *are* using and those they *could be* using. What are some of the difficulties they found in promoting community-based care?
8. Describe three factors that might discourage community-based care in your community or in the United States. Do these factors flow from the evidence you gathered in question 7? How do the factors relate to the problem?

## Additional Resources

These related resources are found either in the appendix at the back of this book or on the book's website at **http://evolve.elsevier.com/Stanhope**.

### evolve Evolve Website

Appendix A.3 Declaration of Alma Ata
WebLinks: Healthy People 2010

# References

Administration on Aging: *A profile of older Americans 2001,* available at www.aoa.gov/statistics/profile/2003/17.asp

Braddock D: Occupational employment projections to 2008, *Month Labor Rev* 122(11):51-57, 1999.

Canadian Institute of Health Information: *Supply and distribution of RNs in Canada in 2001,* 2001, available at www.cihi.ca.

Center for Studying Health Systems Change: *Data bulletin from the Community Tracking Study,* Washington, DC, 2002, Author.

Centers for Medicare and Medicaid Services, *Table 1: national health expenditures aggregate and per capita amounts, percent distribution, and average annual percent growth by source of funds: selected calendar years 1980-2000,* 2000a, available at www.cms.hhs.gov/media/press/release.asp?Counter=961

Centers for Medicare and Medicaid Services, *M+C Deeming glossary,* November 2000b, available at www.cms.hhs.gov/healthplans/deeming/deemingglossary.asp.

Copeland C: *Issues of quality and consumer rights in the health care market,* Employee Benefit Research Institute Issue Brief, April, 1998, p 196.

Cradduck GR: Primary health care practice. In: Stewart MJ, editor: *Community nursing: promoting Canadians' health,* pp 454-474, Toronto, 1995, Saunders Canada.

Division of Nursing: *A national agenda for the nursing workforce on racial/ethnic diversity,* Rockville, Md, 2000, USDHHS, available at ftp://ftp.hrsa.gov/bhpr/nursing/divreport/ DivFull.pdf.

Eng TR: *The eHealth landscape: a terrain map of emerging information and communication technologies in health and health care,* Princeton, NJ, 2001, Robert Wood Johnson Foundation.

Fuchs VR: *Who shall live? health, economics and social change* (expanded ed), Singapore, 1998, World Scientific.

Health Canada: *Healthy Canadians: a federal report on comparable health indicators,* Ottawa, 2002, available at www.healthcanada.ca.

Health Care Financing Administration: *Table 3: national health expenditure aggregate and per capita amounts, percent distribution and average annual percent change by source of funds: selected calendar years 1980-2010,* November 6, 1998, available at www.hcfa.gov/stats/NHE-Proj/proj2001/tables/ t3.htm.

Institute for the Future: *Piecing together the puzzle: the future of health and health care in America* (a commissioned report), Princeton, NJ, December 1997, Robert Wood Johnson Foundation.

Institute for the Future: *Health and health care 2010: the forecast, the challenge,* January 2000.

Institute of Medicine: *The future of public health,* Washington, DC, 1988, National Academy Press.

Institute of Medicine: *Primary care: America's health in a new era,* Washington, DC, 1996, National Academy Press.

InterStudy Publications: *InterStudy's PPO directory and performance report 2.0,* St Paul, Minn, 2001, Decision Resources.

InterStudy Publications: *HMO enrollment stabilizing, Medicaid continues to grow,* St Paul, Minn, 2002, Decision Resources.

Jacob JA: *The next patient wave: Y you should care, Am Med News* 45(16):21, 2002.

WK Kellogg Foundation: *Lessons learned in community-based health programming,* Battle Creek, Mich, 1993, The Foundation.

Lasker R: *Medicine and public health: the power of collaboration,* New York, 1997, New York Academy of Medicine.

Levine L: *A shortage of registered nurses: is it on the horizon or already here?* Washington, DC, 2001, Congressional Research Service.

Lewis C: Emerging trends in medical device technology: home is where the heart monitor is, *FDA Consumer Magazine,* May/June 2001.

Lutz S, Henkind J: The web fuels interest in defined contribution: the internet is facilitating an alternative model of health benefits financing as well as new types of health plans, *Health Plan Magazine,* Nov/Dec 2000.

Mahler H: The meaning of "health for all for the year 2000," *World Health Forum* 2(1):5, 1981.

Managed Care Online: *Managed care fact sheet,* Modesto, Calif, 2000, available at www.mcareol.com.

Martin JA et al: Births: final, *National Vital Statistics Report, Center for Health Statistics* 50(5), 2002.

McKnight J: *The careless society: community and its counterfeits,* New York, 1995, Basic Books.

Miller CA et al: Longitudinal observations on a selected group of local health departments: a preliminary report, *J Public Health Policy* 34(spring), 1993.

Millis JS: *The graduate education of physicians: report of the citizens' commission on graduate medical education,* Chicago, 1966, American Medical Association.

National Center for Health Statistics: *Healthy People 2000, final review,* Hyattsville, Md, 2001, Public Health Service.

Norwood C: *Break the patient's rights stalemate,* February 14, 2002, Roll Call, Inc.

Office of Technology Assessment (OTA): *Nurse practitioners, physicians' assistants, and certified nurse-midwives: a policy analysis* (Health Technology Case Study No. 37), Washington, DC, 1986, Government Printing Office.

Organisation for Economic Co-Operation and Development: *Health data,* 2002, available at www.oecd.org.

Ory MG, DeFriese GH: *Self care in later life: research, program and policy perspectives,* New York, 1998, Springer.

Pender NJ: *Health promotion in nursing practice,* ed 3, Norwalk, Conn, 1996, Appleton & Lange.

Phelps K et al: Factors associated with emergency department utilization for nonurgent pediatric problems, *Arch Fam Med* 9:1086, 2000.

Registered Nurses' Association of Ontario: *RN effectiveness project: clinical, financial and systems outcomes,* Toronto, 2002, available at www.rnao.org.

Riddle C: Is the market ready for defined care? *Managed Care Interfaces,* December 2000.

Romanow R: *Building on values: the future of health care in Canada: final report,* Ottawa, 2002, available at www.healthcarecommission.ca.

Rooks J, Haas JE, editors: *Nurse midwifery in America: a report of the American College of Nurse-Midwives Foundation,* Washington, DC, 1986, American College of Nurse-Midwives Foundation.

Salmon ME: Public health nursing: the opportunity of a century. *Am J Public Health* 83(12):1674, 1993.

Sandy L, Schroeder S: *Primary care in a new era: delusion and dissolution?* 2001, unpublished White Paper.

Smelser N, Wilson WJ, Mitchell F: *America becoming: racial trends and their consequences/commission on behavioral and social sciences and education,* National Research Council, Washington, DC, 2000, National Academy Press.

Standing Senate Committee on Social Affairs, Science and Technology: *Volume 6 of the health of Canadians: the federal role and recommendations report,* Ottawa, 2002, available at www.parl.gc.ca.

Statistics Canada: *Access to health care services in Canada,* 2001, available at www.statisticscanada.ca.

Statistics Canada, Vital Statistics Death and Demography Division: 2002, available at www.statisticscanada.ca.

Tulchinsky TH: *The new public health: an introduction to the 21st century,* San Diego, 2000, Academic Press.

U.S. Bureau of the Census: *Population projections of the United States by age, sex, race and Hispanic origin (1995-2050),* Washington, DC, 1996, Author.

U.S. Bureau of the Census: *Census 2000 summary file: DP-1 profile of general demographic characteristics,* 2000, available at http://factfinder.census.gov/bf/_lang=en_vt_name=DEC_2000_SF1_U_DPI_geo_id=01000US.html.

U.S. Bureau of the Census: *Statistical abstract of the United States: 2001,* ed 21, Washington, DC, 2001, Government Printing Office.

U.S. Bureau of the Census: *Health insurance coverage 2002, table A: people without health insurance coverage for the entire year by selected characteristics: 2001 and 2002,* 2003, available at www.census.gov/prod/2003pubs/p60-223.pdf.

U.S. Citizenship and Immigration Services: *2002 Yearbook, table 1: immigration to the United States: fiscal years 1820-2000,* available at http://uscis.gov/graphics/shared/aboutus/statistics/Yearbook2002.pdf.

U.S. Department of Health and Human Services: *Health personnel in the United States: eighth report to Congress 1991* [DHHS Publication No. HRS-P-OD-92-1], Washington, DC, 1992, U.S. Government Printing Office.

U.S. Department of Health and Human Services: *The registered nurse population,* Rockville, Md, 2000a, Health Resources and Services Administration.

U.S. Department of Health and Human Services: *Strategic plan FY 2001-2006,* September 2000b, available at http://aspe.hhs.gov/hhsplan.

U.S. Department of Health and Human Services: *Healthy people 2010,* November 2000c, Washington, DC: U.S. Government Printing Office.

U.S. Department of Labor, Bureau of Labor Statistics: *Consumer expenditures in 1999,* Washington, DC, May 2001, available at http://www.bls.gov/cex/csxann99.pdf.

U.S. Department of Labor, Bureau of Labor Statistics: *Occupational outlook handbook,* Washington, DC, 2002, available at http://stats.bls.gov/oco/oco2009.htm.

U.S. Public Health Service: *50 Years at the Division of Nursing,* Washington, DC, April 1997, available at ftp://ftp.hrsa.gov/bhpr/nursing/50years.pdf.

White House Press Office: *White House fact sheet on CHIP programs,* April 20, 1999, U.S. Government Printing Office.

World Health Organization: *Primary health care,* Geneva, 1978, WHO.

World Health Organization: *Basic documents,* ed 36, Geneva, 1986a, WHO.

World Health Organization: *World health statistics annual,* Geneva, 1986b, WHO.

Yin S: Shifting careers, *American Demographics* 23(12), 2001.

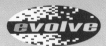

# Chapter 4

http://evolve.elsevier.com/Stanhope

# Perspectives on International Health Care

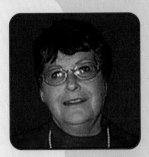

### Kathleen Huttlinger, Ph.D., F.N.P.

Kathleen Huttlinger began practicing population-based, community-oriented nursing in rural Alabama, where she became interested in how culture influences perceptions of health among individuals and families. This interest extended to population groups in Arizona, Mexico, Southeast Asia, and Africa. She is currently involved in a population-based research project that is investigating issues related to health care access in Appalachian communities.

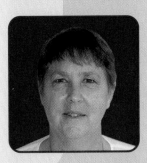

### Jennifer M. Schaller-Ayers, Ph.D., R.N., B.C.

Jennifer Schaller-Ayers began practicing population-based, community-oriented nursing in rural San Diego County, California, where she was first introduced to cultural influences on health and the perception of health. This interest was furthered by practice in Arkansas, Utah, and North Dakota, where she worked with African-American and Native American populations, and in El Paso, Texas, where she worked with people of Mexican heritage. She is currently involved in population-based research projects investigating issues related to health care access in Appalachian communities.

## Objectives

After reading this chapter, the student should be able to do the following:

1. Identify the major aims and goals for world health that were presented at the International Conference on Primary Health Care at Alma Ata

2. Identify the health priorities of Health for All in the 21st Century (HFA21)

3. Analyze the role of community-oriented nursing in international health care

4. Explain the role and focus of a population approach in international health care

5. Describe how world health is related to economic, industrial, and technological development

6. Compare and contrast the health care system in a developed country with one in a lesser-developed country

7. Define *burden of disease*

8. Discuss how countries can prepare for natural disasters and the role of nurses in these efforts

9. Describe at least five organizations that are involved in international health

10. Discuss some of the major international health concerns in developed and lesser-developed countries

---

This chapter presents an overview of the major public health problems of the world, along with a description of the role and involvement of nurses in international public and community health care settings. It discusses health care delivery from an international and population health perspective, illustrates how health systems operate in different countries, presents examples of organizations that address world health, and explains how economic development relates to health care throughout the world.

## OVERVIEW OF INTERNATIONAL HEALTH

In 1977, attendees at the annual meeting of the World Health Assembly maintained that a major social goal for member agencies should be "the attainment by all citizens of the world by the year 2000 a level of health that will permit them to lead a socially and economically productive life" (World Health Organization, 1986a, p. 65). The goals of **Health for All by the Year 2000** have been extended into the next century with **Health for All in the 21st Century** and have been promoted by numerous health-related conferences held around the world, including those sponsored by nursing. In fact, at the International Council of Nurses (ICN) in 1999, the director general of the World Health Organization (WHO) reaffirmed HFA21 and applauded the leadership role that nurses have played in promoting a healthy planet (Brundtland, 1999).

## Key Terms

bilateral organization, p. 79
bioterrorism, p. 91
developed country, p. 73
disability-adjusted life-years, p. 86
global burden of disease, p. 86
health commodification, p. 81
Health for All by the Year 2000, p. 72

Health for All in the 21st Century, p. 72
lesser-developed country, p. 74
multilateral organization, p. 79
nongovernmental organization, p. 79
Pan American Health Organization, p. 79
philanthropic organizations, p. 79
population health, p. 76

primary health care, p. 77
private voluntary organization, p. 79
religious organizations, p. 80
United Nations Children's Fund, p. 79
World Bank, p. 80
World Health Organization, p. 79
*See Glossary for definitions*

## Chapter Outline

Overview of International Health
The Role of Population Health
Primary Health Care
Nursing and International Health
Major International Health Organizations
*Multilateral Organizations*
*Bilateral Organizations*
*Nongovernmental or Private Voluntary
   Organizations*

International Health and Economic
   Development
Health Care Systems
*United Kingdom*
*Canada*
*Sweden*
*China*
*Mexico*

Major World Health Problems and the Burden
   of Disease
*Communicable Diseases*
*Maternal and Women's Health*
*Diarrheal Disease*
*Nutrition and World Health*
*Bioterrorism*

In 1978, concern for the health of the world's people was voiced at the International Conference on Primary Health Care that was held in Alma Ata, Kazakhstan, in what was then Soviet Central Asia. The conference was sponsored by WHO and the United Nations Children's Fund (UNICEF). The participants, who represented 143 countries and 67 organizations, adopted a resolution that proclaimed that the major key to attaining HFA2000 was the worldwide implementation of primary health care (Basch, 1990; Lucas, 1998).

Following the Alma Ata conference and as the twenty-first century has progressed, interest in world health and how best to attain it has grown. People around the world want to know and understand the issues and concerns that affect health on a global scale. This is important as many countries have not yet experienced the technological growth in health care systems that has been realized by more developmentally advanced countries such as the United States, Canada, and several in western Europe. Many terms are used to describe nations that have achieved a high level of industrial and technological advancement (along with a stable market economy) and those that have not. For the purposes of this chapter, the term **developed country** refers to those countries with a stable economy and a wide range of industrial and technological development—for example, the United States,

Canada, Japan, the United Kingdom, Sweden, France, and Australia. A country that is not yet stable with respect to its economy and technological development is referred to as a **lesser-developed country**—for example, Bangladesh, Zaire, Haiti, Guatemala, most countries in sub-Saharan Africa, and the island nation of Indonesia. Both developed and lesser-developed countries are found in all parts of the world and in all geographic and climatic zones (Evlo and Carrin, 1992).

Health problems exist throughout the world, but the lesser-developed countries are often faced with more exotic sounding health care problems such as buruli, leishmaniasis, schistosomiasis, pediculosis, typhus, yellow fever, and malaria (WHO, 2000b). Ongoing health problems in need of control in the lesser-developed countries include measles, mumps, rubella, and polio, whereas the current health concerns of the more developed countries reflect ongoing struggles with hepatitis, the appearance of new viral strains such as the hantavirus, and larger social yet health-related issues such as terrorism, warfare, violence, and substance abuse. Acquired immunodeficiency syndrome (AIDS) remains a major worldwide concern in both developed and lesser-developed countries (WHO, 2002a).

In addition to direct health problems, the effects of war and conflict can also have devastating effects on a country and the health of its population. For example, in the fall of 2002, conflict and warfare erupted in Afghanistan between the Taliban and the United States, which was allied with several European countries and Canada. The ruling Taliban government left the country with virtually no health care system. Continuing conflict there has taken a dramatic toll on its population, especially on older adults, women, and children. Serious nutritional problems have been reported throughout the country, along with outbreaks of influenza. Compounding the health risks are the increased incidence of violence against women and children, the hazards of unexploded weapons and land mines,

## WHAT DO YOU THINK?

The Taliban in Afghanistan has been ousted, but women who lived in an oppressive state under their rule are still tentative about reentering the workplace or going back to school and universities.

## DID YOU KNOW?

Mercy Corps International has initiated the Kosovo Women's Health Promotion Project (2001), in which nurse midwives actively participate in promoting midwifery care for positive reproductive outcomes. Kosovo is one of the countries where women's health care has suffered due to the ravages of war.

Heymann M: Reproductive health promotion in Kosovo, *J Midwifery Women's Health* 46(2):74-81, 2001.

and the not infrequent occurrence of earthquakes and other natural disasters (WHO, 2002b,c).

The escalation of conflicts in Afghanistan and other countries in the Middle East and the Balkans raises concerns about injuries, disabilities, and loss of life. Wherever conflict and open warfare take place, there is a disruption in health care services, with tragic consequences to vulnerable populations.

With the promotion of the objectives of HFA21, countries are realizing that they need to improve their economies and infrastructures and are therefore seeking monetary assistance and technological expertise from the wealthier and more developed countries (Lucas, 1998; World Bank, 2002). According to the WHO, HFA21 is not a single, finite goal but a strategic process that can lead to progressive improvement in the health of people (WHO, 2002a). It is a call for social justice and solidarity. As economic agreements between countries remove financial and political barriers, growth and development are stimulated. Simultaneously, global health problems that once seemed distant are brought closer to people all over the world, political and economic barriers between countries fall, and the movement of population groups increases, as does the risk of exposure to numerous kinds of diseases and other health risks (Basch, 1990; Howson, Fineberg, and Bloom, 1998). One such example that has potential worldwide health implications is the reappearance of the Ebola virus in central African countries (Cable News Network, 2000).

Not only do world travelers serve as hosts to various types of disease agents but they may expose themselves to diseases and environmental health hazards that are unknown or rare in their home country (Figure 4-1). Two examples of diseases from recent years that were once fairly isolated and rare but are now widespread throughout the world are AIDS and drug-resistant tuberculosis (TB) (Howson et al, 1998).

Despite efforts by individual governments and international health organizations to improve the general economy and welfare of all countries of the world, many health problems continue to exist, especially among poorer people. In many countries there is a lack of political commitment to health care, a lack of recognition of basic human rights issues, a failure to achieve equity in access to primary health care, inappropriate use of and allocation of resources for high-cost technology, and persistently low status of women (WHO, 2002a) (Figure 4-2). Currently, the lesser-developed countries experience high infant and child mortality rates, with diarrheal and respiratory diseases as major contributory factors (Lucas, 1998; WHO, 2002a; World Bank, 2002). Other major worldwide health problems include nutritional deficiencies in all age groups, women's health and fertility problems, sexually transmitted diseases (STDs), and illnesses related to the human immunodeficiency virus (HIV), malaria, drug-resistant TB, neonatal tetanus, leprosy, occupational and environmental health hazards, and abuses of tobacco, alcohol, and drugs.

Because of these continuing problems, the director general of the WHO has made a commitment to renew all

# THE CUTTING EDGE

The government of Thailand has initiated low-cost universal health coverage. This project is aimed at the poor and entitles people to visit a doctor for less than $1 per visit. The goal of this project is to reach millions of low-income people and especially those in the rural areas of Thailand.

British Broadcasting Company (BBC), World: *Health coverage for the poor in Thailand*, United Kingdom, October 20, 2001.

darity with an emphasis on the individual's, family's, and community's responsibility for health. HFA21 remains a priority for the WHO's executive board and the general assembly. Strategies for achieving the continuing goals of HFA21 include building on past accomplishments and the identification of global priorities and targets for the first 20 years of the new century (WHO, 2002a).

Being informed about world health is important, especially for nurses. Many of the world's health problems directly affect the health of individuals who live in the United States. For example, the 103rd U.S. Congress passed the North American Free Trade Agreement (NAFTA), which opened trade borders between the United States, Canada, and Mexico in 1994 and allowed an increased movement of products and people (Figure 4-3). Along the United States–Mexico border, an influx of undocumented immigrants in recent years has raised concerns for the health of people who live in this area. Many immigrants have settled

of the policies and actions of HFA21 (Brundtland, 1999). The WHO continues to develop new and holistic health policies that are based on the concepts of equity and soli-

## Healthy People 2010    An Example of Healthy People 2010 Goals Applied to Nigeria

Nigeria is a western African country that has large oil reserves that are extracted by foreign oil companies. In many instances, these foreign commercial interests have not paid much attention to the health and welfare of its locally employed Nigerian workers. Recently, the government of Nigeria has taken steps to protect and enhance the well-being of its native workforce.

The two interrelated goals of Healthy People 2010 are reflected in the general aims of Health for All by the 21st Century (HFA21). The first goal of Healthy People 2010 is to increase the quality and years of life and the second is to eliminate health disparities. There are 28 focal areas that include specific objectives. The WHO,

along with the country of Nigeria, has launched a workplace safety and protection program that incorporates the health promotional aspects of HFA21 and reflects seven of the focal areas of Healthy People 2010. These focal areas include the following:
- Arthritis, osteoporosis, and chronic back conditions
- Disability and secondary conditions
- Education and community-based programs
- Environmental health
- Health communication
- Injury and violence prevention
- Occupational safety and health

Ajo G: Workplace health promotion in Nigeria: a step towards health promotion and productivity, *Global Perspect* 4(2):6, 2001.
From U.S. Department of Health and Human Services: *Healthy people 2010: understanding and improving health*, ed 2, Washington, DC, 2000, U.S. Government Printing Office.

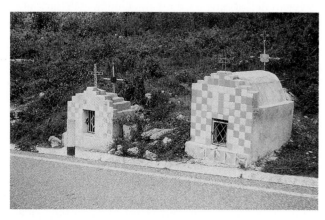

**Figure 4-1** A driver in rural Colombia may be confronted with many road hazards, as noted by these roadside shrines. *(Courtesy K. Huttlinger.)*

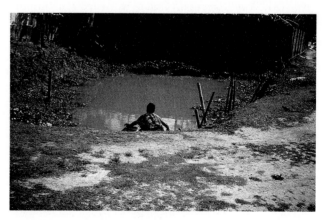

**Figure 4-2** Waterholes like this in rural Oman are used for drinking, bathing, and feeding livestock. *(Courtesy K. Huttlinger and L. Krefting.)*

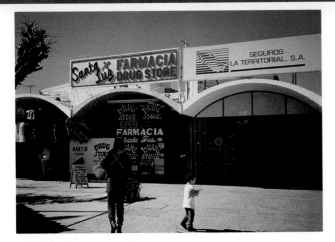

**Figure 4-3** The NAFTA encouraged trade between Mexico, Canada, and the United States. A local farmacia in Nogales, Mexico, supplies Americans with lower-cost prescription medicines. *(Courtesy K. Huttlinger.)*

> **HOW TO** **Stay Current About World Health**
>
> One of the ways that you can stay current with the world's health problems and advances is by reading the newspaper daily. Newspapers that cover international health include the *Wall Street Journal, USA Today,* and the *New York Times.*

> ## Evidence-Based Practice
>
> This binational study explored the migration patterns and health experiences of indigenous Mixtec and Zapotec women from the state of Oaxaca in southern Mexico. The researcher discovered a high degree of independent decision making among the women about migration and the various patterns of health-seeking behaviors for themselves and their families. Nearly always, their first recourse for treating health and illness conditions was the use of herbal and home remedies. They also used local public health departments and community clinics for children's well-care and immunizations, for acute episodes that were not responsive to treatment at home, and for themselves. They look for health care staff in the United States who are considerate of them as persons, who demonstrate affection and warmth to their children, and who are thorough and competent. Although some immigrant women have learned English, and all expressed a desire to learn, many work in the fields, in factories, and as domestics, lack the ability to speak English as a second language, are fully responsible for families, and have very complicated lives that present barriers to learning English. Some women speak their indigenous language and learned Spanish in northern Mexico before coming to the United States.
>
> **Nurse Use:** Spanish-speaking immigrants are very responsive to health care workers who speak some Spanish.
>
> Sharon McGuire, Ph.D., R.N.: "Migration patterns and health experiences of Mixtec and Zapotec women," unpublished research in progress at University of San Diego.

on unincorporated land, known as *colonias,* outside the major metropolitan areas in California, Arizona, New Mexico, and Texas, with no developed roads, transportation, or water or electrical services. The result has been an increase in numerous disease conditions including amebiasis, respiratory and diarrheal diseases, and environmental health hazards in the *colonias* that are associated with poverty, poor sanitation, and overcrowded conditions (Hernandez-Pena et al, 1993; VanderMeer, 1998).

Interestingly, Canadian worker groups are concerned that NAFTA will eventually lead to worsened working conditions as plants move to the lower-wage and largely nonunionized southern United States and Mexico (Hall, 1996). On a more positive note, NAFTA has provided an impetus and framework for the government of Mexico to modernize their medical system so that they can compete and respond to the demands of a more global competition. Although some improvements have been made, there is still an overriding concern that environmental and health regulations in Mexico have not kept up with the pace of increased border trade (Hall, 1996; Ortega-Cesena, Espinosa-Torres, and Lopez-Carillo, 1994). The Mexican National Academy of Medicine continues to make health and environmental recommendations to the government, which points out the beneficial interactions that are occurring between Mexico, Canada, and the United States as

part of this trade agreement (Gomez-Dantes, Frenk, and Cruz, 1997).

Nurses play an active role in the international border areas where political and economic boundaries mesh. For example, the geography along the United States–Mexican border is rugged, remote, and framed by inhospitable mountain ranges and deserts. Except in the larger metropolitan areas, health care for people who live along the border is scarce. Nurses supported by private foundations and by local and state public health departments often provide the only reliable health care in these areas, and they continue to serve as valuable resources for the residents.

## THE ROLE OF POPULATION HEALTH

**Population health** is an approach and perspective that focuses on the broad range of factors and conditions that have a strong influence on the health of populations. It is a holistic approach that considers the total health system, from prevention and promotion to diagnosis, treatment, and care. This approach emphasizes health for groups at the population rather than at the individual level and focuses on reducing inequities and improving health in these groups. In a public health sense, a population can be defined by a geographic boundary, by a group of people who share a common characteristic such as ethnicity or religion, or by the epidemiologic and social condition of a community that minimizes morbidity and mortality (Fox, 2001).

The factors and conditions that are important considerations in population health are called *determinants.* Population health determinants may include income and social factors, social support networks, education, employment, working and living conditions, physical environments, social environments, biology and genetic endowment, personal health practices, coping skills, healthy child development, health services, sex, and culture (Fox, 2001; Ibrahim et al, 2001). The determinants do not work independently of each other but form a complex system of interactions.

A leader in promoting the population health approach is Canada, which has been implementing programs using this framework since the mid 1990s and which builds on a tradition of public health and health promotion. A Canadian document, the Lalonde Report (1974), proposed that changes in lifestyles or social and physical environments lead to more improvements in health than would be achieved by spending more money on existing health care delivery systems. Following this report, in 1989 the Canadian Institute for Advanced Research (CIAR) introduced the population health concept, proposing that individual determinants of health do not act in isolation. The Canadian initiative was aimed at efforts and investments directed at root causes to increase potential benefits for health outcomes (Labonte, Jackson, and Chirrey, 1998; Zollner and Lessof, 1998). A key was the identification and definition of health issues and of the investment decisions within a population that were guided by evidence about what keeps people healthy. Therefore a population health approach directs investments that have the greatest potential to influence the health of that population in a positive manner. A significant factor is early intervention so that there can be greater potential for population health gains.

Canada has since implemented a broad range of projects across the country. Examples include a population division within the Calgary Regional Health Authority to reduce inequities in health status (Labonte et al, 1998) and policies in British Colombia directed at HIV/AIDS in aboriginal populations. Mexico has also integrated the health determinants into public policies. At the Fifth Global Conference on Health Promotion in Mexico City held on June 5-9, 2000, the theme of "Bridging the Equity Gap" addressed health determinants related to economically and socially disadvantaged populations. At this time, the Mexican government along with 87 other governments signed statements for the "Promotion of Health From Ideas to Action." This statement acknowledges that population-focused health promotion strategies contribute to the sus-

tainability of local, national, and international health activities (Levya-Flores, Kageyama, and Erviti-Erice, 2001).

## PRIMARY HEALTH CARE

The role of **primary health care** in international health is historically based on the worldwide conference that was held at Alma Ata (Levya-Flores et al, 2001; WHO, 1998a; WHO/UNICEF, 1978). WHO and UNICEF still actively promote primary health care. They maintain that all training needs to be based on current medical technology and practice methods. They also affirm that community members need to be involved in all aspects of the planning and implementation of health services.

Recognizing that there would be differences among countries with respect to the implementation of primary health care because of local customs and environments, it was anticipated that several major components should be included in each plan for health services (WHO/UNICEF, 1978):

- An organized approach to health education that involves professional health care providers and trained community representatives
- Aggressive attention to environmental sanitation, especially food and water sources
- Involvement and training of community and village health workers in all plans and intervention programs
- Development of maternal and child health programs that include immunization and family planning
- Initiation of preventive programs that are specifically aimed at local endemic problems such as malaria and schistosomiasis in tropical regions
- Accessibility and affordability of services for the treatment of common diseases and injuries
- Availability of chemotherapeutic agents for the treatment of acute, chronic, and communicable diseases
- Development of nutrition programs
- Promotion and acceptance of traditional medicine

The aim of the Alma Ata conference participants was to emphasize universal access and participation and to encourage a reallocation of resources, if needed, to reduce the inequality of health care that existed among the nations of the world. They encouraged community participation in all aspects of health care planning and implementation and the delivery of health care that was "scientifically sound, technically effective, socially relevant and acceptable" (WHO/UNICEF, 1978, p. 2). These aims continue to be reinforced, and they remain an integral part of the goals of the WHO to include essential health care that is accessible to all people of the world at a cost that the community and country can afford (Brundtland, 1999).

An example of a country that has made a particular effort to implement primary health care services is Mexico. Mexico has initiated a module program that is administered through the ministry of health. The program is characterized by village-based health posts, each of which is operated by a community volunteer and a health committee. The volunteer and committee are supervised by a community-oriented nurse who operates from a regional health center. It is believed that this module system can address community needs and will ultimately lead to better use of services and resources (Nigenda, Ruiz, and Montes, 2001).

## NURSING AND INTERNATIONAL HEALTH

Nurses have an important leadership role in health care throughout the world (Brundtland, 1999). In particular, nurses with community and public health experience provide much-needed knowledge and skill in countries where nursing is not an organized profession, and they give guidance not only to the nurses but also to the auxiliary personnel who are part of the primary health care team International Council of Nurses [ICN], 2001). In many settings throughout the world, nurses provide direct client care and facilitate the educational and health promotional needs of the community. Unfortunately, in the lesser-developed countries, the role of the nurse is defined poorly if at all (Figure 4-4), and care often depends on and is directed by physicians (Waller and Cammuso, 1997). In contrast, in developed countries, nursing is often seen as one of the strongest advocates for primary health care, through its social commitment to equality of health care and support of the concepts that are contained in the Alma Ata declaration (Andrews and Gottschalk, 1996; ICN, 2001). Examples of efforts led by nurses in international community health settings include a health promotion program in Japan (Murashima et al, 1999), a tuberculosis eradication program in India (Puri and John, 1997), an oral health promotion project in South Africa (Ogunbodede et al, 1999), and an assessment of training needs for district nurses in Uganda (Ziegler, Anyango, and Ziegler, 1997) (Figure 4-5).

One example of a changing role for nursing is in China. Nursing in China is undergoing a very dramatic change, largely because of an evolving political and economic environment. In the past, nursing was viewed as a trade, and the acquisition of nursing skills and knowledge took place in what is experienced as middle school or junior high in the United States. Increasing pressure on the health care system in China is providing an impetus for education at the university level. The Chinese government is sending many of its nurses to the United States, Europe, and Australia to receive university-level education in nursing at the undergraduate and graduate levels in hopes that these individuals will return to China to provide the nursing and nursing education needed there (Anders and Harrigan, 2002).

In some countries, such as Chile, the physician-to-population ratio is higher than the nurse-to-population ratio. In these cases, physicians influence nursing practice and place economic and political pressure on local, regional, and national governments to control the services that nurses offer. In Chile, nurses have set up successful and cost-effective clinics to deliver quality primary care services, but they are constantly being threatened by physicians who want to oust the nurses and replace them with physicians who will increase the cost for services (WHO, 2000a).

## MAJOR INTERNATIONAL HEALTH ORGANIZATIONS

A large number of international organizations have an ongoing interest in world health. Despite the presence of these well-meaning organizations, it is estimated that the lesser-developed countries still bear most of the cost for their own health care and that the major international organizations actually provide for less than 5% of those needed costs. Recent reports indicate that the majority of funds raised by international organizations are used for food relief, worker training, and disaster relief (International Medical Volunteer Association [IMVA], 2002). However, when considering the total effort, the poorer countries, such as those in sub-Saharan Africa, still receive the greatest amount of financial support from the more developed countries, often accounting for more

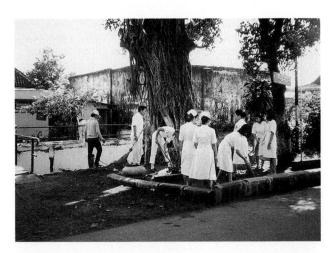

**Figure 4-4** When not providing direct client care, nurses in Indonesia must help keep the hospital grounds clean. *(Courtesy K. Huttlinger.)*

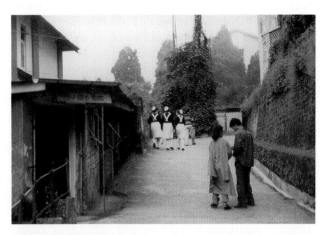

**Figure 4-5** Nursing students coming from a clinic in Nepal *(Courtesy J. Schaller-Ayers.)*

than 20% of the poorer country's health care expenditures (IMVA, 2002).

International health organizations may be classified as multilateral organizations, bilateral organizations, or nongovernmental organizations (NGOs) or private voluntary organizations (PVOs) (including philanthropic organizations). **Multilateral organizations** are those that receive funding from multiple government and nongovernment sources. The major ones are part of the United Nations (UN), and they include the World Health Organization (WHO), the United Nations Children's Fund (UNICEF), the Pan American Health Organization (PAHO), and the World Bank. A **bilateral organization** is a single government agency that provides aid to lesser-developed countries; an example is the U.S. Agency for International Development (USAID). **Nongovernmental organizations** (NGOs) or **private voluntary organizations** (PVOs), including the philanthropic organizations, are represented by such agencies as Oxfam, Project Hope, and the International Red Cross; various professional and trade organizations; Catholic Relief Services (CRS); church-sponsored health care missionaries; and many private groups.

## Multilateral Organizations

### World Health Organization

The **World Health Organization** (WHO) is a separate, autonomous organization that, by special agreement, works with the United Nations through its Economic and Social Council. The idea for a worldwide health organization developed from the First International Sanitary Conference in 1902, which is viewed as a precursor to the World Health Organization (Basch, 1990). Continued efforts by this and other worldwide agencies resulted in the formation of the WHO in 1946 as an outgrowth of the League of Nations and the UN charter. In this charter, the UN provided for the formation of a special health agency to address the wide scope and nature of the world's health problems.

The WHO, headed by a director general and five assistant generals, has three major divisions: the World Health Assembly approves the budget and makes decisions about health policies, the executive board serves as the liaison between the assembly and the secretariat, and the secretariat carries out the day-to-day activities of the WHO. The WHO headquarters is in Geneva, with six regional headquarters located in Copenhagen, Denmark; Alexandria, Egypt; Brazzaville, the Congo; New Delhi, India; Manila, Philippines; and Washington, D.C. The WHO's extremely broad scope includes more than 25 major functions with over 100 subfunctions; however, it is generally recognized that its principal work is to direct and coordinate international health activities and to provide technical medical assistance to countries in need.

More than 1000 health-related projects are ongoing within the WHO at any one time. Some projects may be operated and funded by the WHO itself or in collaboration with other governments, health care agencies, or private foundations and charities. The vast majority of projects involve technical services to individual governments. Requests for assistance may be made directly to the WHO by a country for a project, or they may be part of a larger collaborative endeavor involving many countries. Examples of current collaborative, multinational projects include comprehensive family planning programs in Indonesia, Malaysia, and Thailand; applied research on communicable disease and immunization in several East African nations; and projects that investigate the viability of administering AIDS vaccines to pregnant women in South Africa and Namibia.

In addition to multinational programs, there are projects that involve individual countries. In single-nation projects, the focus is generally placed on the training of medical personnel, the development of health services such as primary care, and specific disease control and intervention programs.

### United Nations Children's Fund

The **United Nations Children's Fund** (UNICEF) was formed shortly after World War II (WWII) to assist children in the war-ravaged countries of Europe, and it is a subsidiary agency to the UN Economic and Social Council. After the war, it became apparent to many social agencies that the world's children needed medical and other kinds of support. With financial assistance from the newly formed UN General Assembly, post-WWII programs were developed to control yaws, leprosy, and tuberculosis in children. Since then, UNICEF has worked closely with the WHO as an advocate for the health needs of women and children under the age of 5. In particular, there have been multinational programs aimed at the provision of safe drinking water, sanitation, education, and maternal and child health.

> **DID YOU KNOW?**
>
> Twenty-nine billion people lack access to adequate sanitation and safe water. In Nicaragua, Paraguay, Brazil, and Peru, less than 50% of the population have access to sanitation either in or near their homes.

### Pan American Health Organization

Founded in 1902, the **Pan American Health Organization** (PAHO) is one of the oldest continuously functioning international health organizations and predates the WHO. Presently, PAHO serves as a regional field office for the WHO in Latin America, with a focused effort to improve the health and living standards of the Latin American countries. It functions to distribute epidemiologic information, to provide technical assistance over a wide range of health and environmental issues, to support health care fellowships, and to promote health and environmentally related research along with professional education.

Focusing primarily on reaching people through their communities, PAHO works with a variety of governmental and nongovernmental entities to address the health issues of the peoples of the Americas. At present, a primary concern of PAHO is the prevention and control of AIDS and other sexually transmitted diseases. PAHO has developed some very special programs directed at the spread of AIDS in the most vulnerable groups in Latin America—mothers and children, workers, the poor, older adults, refugees, and displaced persons. Other focused efforts include public information, the control and eradication of tropical diseases, and the development of health system infrastructures in the poorer Latin American countries. PAHO collaborates with individual countries and actively promotes multinational efforts as well.

Of interest is a recent effort by PAHO to carefully examine the effects of health care reform on nurses and midwifery in the Latin American countries. Changes that countries in Latin America have made in their health care systems in recent years have affected nurses and midwives and their work environments in both positive and negative ways. Of special interest are the scope of practice for nursing and midwifery and the relationship of nurses with other health care workers and providers. So far, the countries of Belize, Colombia, and Mexico have published reports (available at http://www.paho.org).

### World Bank

The **World Bank** is another multilateral organization that is related to the UN. Although the major aim of the World Bank is to lend money to the lesser-developed countries so that they might use it to improve the health status of their people, it has collaborated with the field offices of the WHO for various health-related projects such as the control and eradication of the tropical disease onchocerciasis in West Africa. A poverty-reduction strategy in Yemen is significant because it involves many societal, community-based groups in Yemen including parliamentarians, academics, civic leaders, women's groups, and the media (see http://web.worldbank.org for additional information).

Other examples of World Bank projects in the lesser-developed countries include programs aimed at safe drinking water, affordable housing, developing sanitation systems, family planning, and childhood immunizations. The World Bank also sponsors programs that affect health indirectly. One such example is a $30 million project in Brazil to protect the Amazon ecosystem. The environmental effects, including health effects, of the decreasing rain forest in the Amazon are now just being realized. This project is important for Brazil and for the rest of the world in terms of effects on ozone and global climate.

The World Bank has provided financial assistance for people in lesser-developed countries to pursue careers in health care and has enabled these individuals to enroll in health care programs in the more developed nations. It has also lent money both to governments and to private foundations for economic initiatives that improve internal infrastructures, including communication systems, roads, and electricity, all of which ultimately impact health care delivery.

## Bilateral Organizations

Government agencies that operate within a single country and focus on providing direct aid to lesser-developed countries are known as bilateral organizations or agencies. The U.S. Agency for International Development (USAID) is the largest of these and operates totally out of the United States. Japan, France, Canada, Germany, Sweden, and Great Britain have similar organizations, although they are somewhat limited in their scope. All bilateral organizations are influenced by political and historical agendas that determine which countries receive aid. Incentives for engaging in formal arrangements may include economic enhancements for the benefit of both countries, national defense of one or both countries, or the enhancement and protection of private investments made by individuals in these nations.

Countries with advanced medical systems and technology may enter into a collaborative effort with a lesser-developed country to conduct medical research. For example, the Japanese government currently has an active collaborative arrangement with Indonesia to study ways to control the spread of yellow fever and malaria. France gives most of its aid to its former colonies.

## Nongovernmental or Private Voluntary Organizations

Nongovernmental (NGOs) or private voluntary organizations (PVOs) as well as the philanthropic organizations provide almost 20% of all external aid to lesser-developed countries. NGOs and PVOs are represented by many different kinds of religious and secular groups. **Religious organizations,** which reflect several denominations and religious interests, support many health care programs, including hospitals in rural and urban areas, refugee centers, orphanages, and leprosy treatment centers. For example, the Maryknoll Missionaries are sponsored by the Roman Catholic Church and carry out health service projects around the world. The missionaries comprise a large group of religious as well as lay people trained and educated in a variety of educational and health care professions.

Another religious group, Catholic Relief Services (CRS), specializes in providing food to starving people and those affected by war, famine, drought, and natural disasters. Thus it indirectly affects the health of the people it serves.

Many Protestant and Evangelical groups throughout the world function both as separate entities and as part of the Church World Service, which works jointly with secular organizations to improve health care, community development, and other needed projects. Other private and voluntary groups that assist with the worldwide health effort include CARE, Oxfam, and Third World First. Several of these organizations receive additional funding from developed countries including the United States, the United Kingdom, Sweden, Canada, and countries in western Europe.

Perhaps one of the best-known NGOs is the International Red Cross. Although the Red Cross is most often associated with disaster relief and emergency aid, it lays the groundwork for health intervention as a result of a country's emergency. It is a volunteer organization that consists of approximately 160 individual Red Cross societies around the world, and it prides itself on its neutrality and impartiality with respect to politics and history. Therefore it seeks permission from the country in which the disaster occurs before services are rendered.

Another NGO that provides health services and aid to countries experiencing warfare or disaster is Medicins San Frontieres (MSF). Unlike the Red Cross, MSF will provide services to victims without the permission of authorities and often speaks out against observed human rights abuses in the country it serves. MSF was the recipient of the Nobel Peace Prize in 1999 and the Conrad Hilton Prize in 1998.

Philanthropic organizations receive funding from private endowment funds. A few of the more active philanthropic organizations that are involved in world health care include the W. K. Kellogg Foundation, the Milbank Memorial Fund, the Pathfinder Fund, the Hewlett Foundation, the Ford Foundation, the Rockefeller Foundation, and the Carnegie Foundation. The purpose and programmatic goals of each organization differ widely with respect to funding, and their purposes often change as their governing boards change. Some of the worldwide health care activities that have been sponsored throughout past years include projects in public and preventive health; vital statistics; medical, nursing, and dental education; family planning programs; economic planning and development; and the formation of laboratories to investigate communicable diseases.

The professional and trade organizations are PVOs that are found mostly in the more developed and industrialized countries. One of the most famous of the professional and technical organizations is the Institut Pasteur, which has been in existence since the 1880s. In particular, its laboratories have facilitated the development of sera and vaccines for countries in need, have disseminated current health information, and have trained and provided fellowships for medical training and study in France.

Many private and commercial organizations such as Nestle and the Johnson & Johnson Company provide financial and technical backing for investment, employment, and access to market economies and to health care. Although these organizations have been present throughout the world for over 30 years, they have come under criticism for the promotion and marketing of infant formulas, pharmaceuticals, and medical supplies, especially to lesser-developed countries. The intense marketing that is done in these countries is known as *commodification*, and there is some controversy as to its legitimacy. For example, the **health commodification** of pharmaceuticals in southern India is a concern because

---

**DID YOU KNOW?**

Many NGOs and PVOs support internet web pages where you can get information about volunteering:
  WHO, www.who.int/home-page
  USAID, www.usaid.gov
  UNICEF, www.unicef.org
  OXFAM, www.oxfam.org.uk
  International Red Cross, www.icrc.org
  Catholic relief services, www.catholicrelief.org
  World Bank, www.worldbank.org

---

the companies give little consideration to the cultural and social structure of the country, thus interfering with the long-standing traditional Indian medical system. In southern India, good health and prosperity are related to certain social parameters bestowed to families and communities as a result of their conformity to the sociomoral order that was set down by their ancestors, gods, and patron spirits (Nichter, 1989). The taking of pharmaceutical agents thus disrupts the social and cultural order of things that have been traditionally addressed by cultural practices. Similar controversies in other countries have involved infant formulas and oral rehydration therapies.

## INTERNATIONAL HEALTH AND ECONOMIC DEVELOPMENT

The health of the world's people is related to economic, industrial, and technological development. Even though several studies of lesser-developed countries have indicated that the general demand for health care is related to health production technology, little evidence shows how and under what circumstances this technology affects the use of health care services (Wouters, 1992). Access to services and the removal of financial barriers alone do not account for use of health services. In fact, the introduction of health care technology from developed countries to lesser-developed countries has led to less-than-satisfactory results. For example, during the 1980s in an eastern Mediterranean country, two thirds of the high-output x-ray machines were not in use because of a lack of qualified and trained individuals to carry out routine maintenance and repairs (Perry and Marx, 1992). In another example, a hospital in a Latin American country was given a high-technology neonatal intensive care unit by a wealthier and more technologically advanced country. However, 70% of the infants died after discharge because there were no follow-up nutritional and prevention services and many of them experienced malnutrition and complications from dehydration on return to their home communities. These programs might have been more successful if they had focused on general public health and less complex kinds of health care technology (Perry and Marx, 1992). Quite simply, the most basic needs were not met, nor was recognition given to what resources and services the country could sustain.

Warfare presents another interesting challenge to delivering optimal health care. Afghanistan is a country that has been beset by more than 20 years of warfare, several years of severe drought, mass population displacement, abuses of basic human rights, and a health determinant index that is the worst in the world. In addition, internal state institutions, including those that direct health, have been virtually nonfunctional during the Taliban regime, economic performance in terms of production and financial services is defunct, and the tax and budget system is in ruin (WHO, 2002c). Even though over 200 international and national representatives of health organizations, governments, and NGOs are presently coming to the aid of Afghanistan, the question of restoration of the internal system to prewar functioning remains. It is hoped that this cooperative effort can chart a successful course for health recovery in Afghanistan (WHO, 2002b). Last, except for the demilitarized zone of Korea, Afghanistan is the most heavily land-mined region of the world. The presence of these land mines has serious consequences for the people, who risk losing limbs and dying as a result of contact with them.

On the basis of these examples, improvement in the overall health status of a population contributes to the economic growth of a country in several ways (Van der Gaag and Barham, 1998; World Bank, 1998b):

- By a reduction in production loss that was caused by workers who were absent from work because of illness
- By an increase in the use of natural resources that, because of the presence of disease entities, might have been inaccessible
- By an increase in the number of children who can attend school and eventually participate in their country's economic growth
- By monetary resources, formerly spent on treating disease and illness, now available for the economic development of the country

However, adequate health care coverage for individuals who reside in lesser-developed countries may be lacking if their governments reallocate financial resources from internal health needs and education and invest it instead in the country's market economy, or to develop technology, or to pay off the interest on their national debt. Many countries also divert resources to develop the underlying infrastructure that they believe is needed for technological and industrial improvement. Unfortunately, when governments experience an economic crisis, household expenditures are adversely affected. Most often, the provision of health services in lesser-developed countries depends on the importation of drugs, vaccines, and other health care products (Van der Gaag and Barham, 1998; World Bank, 1998a,b), which in turn depends on a network of foreign exchange that is influenced by economic and political factors. Often, lesser-developed countries have a difficult time maintaining a balance of payments, which leads to severe shortages of foreign exchange and subsequent reduction in the ability to import goods (Evlo and Carrin, 1992).

Because the economics of international development are complex, it is often difficult to convince governments to direct their resources away from perceived needs such as military and technology and instead place the resources in health and educational programs. Ideally, the role of the more developed countries is to assist lesser-developed countries in identifying internal needs and to support cost-efficient measures and share their technology and industrial expertise (Wouters, 1992).

It is important that nurses who work in international communities not only acknowledge the importance of technology and development but also recognize the political, economic, and cultural implications. Provision of health services alone will not ease a country's health care plight (Figure 4-6).

**NURSING TIP**

When conducting a health assessment interview, always ask if the client has recently traveled out of the United States or to one of the border areas along the United States–Mexico perimeter. Sometimes people bring back diseases that are hard to diagnose. Sometimes people cross into Mexico to fill a prescription for medicine, which is often less expensive there. Unfortunately, many times the medications brought back have been relabeled and are out of date.

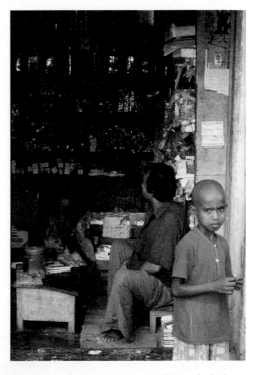

**Figure 4-6** A local pharmacy in rural Bangladesh. *(Courtesy K. Huttlinger and L. Krefting.)*

# HEALTH CARE SYSTEMS

The countries of the world present many different kinds of health care systems, but most consist of five fundamental elements (Basch, 1990):

- Usership, or who can use the system
- Benefits, or what kind of coverage a citizen might expect
- Providers who deliver health care
- Facilities, or where the provision of health care takes place
- Power, or who controls access and usability of the system

The roles of nursing in these countries are as diverse as the kinds of health care systems of which they are a part. A brief description of several health systems will help illustrate these concepts.

## United Kingdom

The United Kingdom has a tax-supported health system that is owned and operated by the government, and services are available to all of its citizens without cost or for a small fee. Administration of health services is conducted through a system of health authorities (Trusts). Each Trust plans and provides services for 250,000 to 1 million people. The services offered by each Trust are comprehensive, in that health care is available to all who want it and covers all aspects of general medicine, disability and rehabilitation, and surgery. Although physicians are the primary providers in this system, nurses and allied health professionals are also recognized and used. Services are made available through hospitals, private physicians and allied health professional clinics, health outreach programs such as hospice, boroughs, and environmental health services. Physicians are paid by the number of clients they serve and not by individual visits. Although the British system has come under criticism in past years, individual citizens still maintain a high level of support for government funding and control of their health services (Schoen et al, 2001).

District nursing (public or community health nursing) has been in Britain since the days of Florence Nightingale. In 1999, district nurses saw 2.75 million patients. As Britain faces a growing population of older adult citizens, the demand for district nursing is increasing. District nursing varies from Trust to Trust: some offer services 24 hours per day whereas others are more limited. District nursing faces many challenges—for example, over 50% of district nurses are near retirement age and fewer nurses at the entry level are selecting district nursing as a career choice (Audit Commission, 1999).

One of the hallmarks of the British system is a demonstrated reduction in infant mortality, from 14.3 deaths per 1000 births in 1975 to 5.6 in 2000. Overall life expectancy in Great Britain also improved during the same period (77.2 years in 2000). This has been done while holding down gross spending on health care. For comparison, in the United States, infant mortality was 6.9 in 2000 and life expectancy 76.9 years (Central Intelligence Agency, 2001). The United States spends "$4,090 per capita on health care annually (13.6% of GDP), Canada spends only $2,095 (9.3% of GDP) and the United Kingdom spends a mere $1,347 (6.7% of GDP)" (Health Care for All, 2001).

## Canada

The Canadian health care system is based on a national health insurance program that is operated by each provincial government. One notable feature of this system is that specialists are concentrated in centers, whereas primary care providers are evenly distributed throughout the Canadian provinces. Physicians are the primary providers, although nurses do play an active role in all aspects of health care delivery, including community and public health. Hospitals and other health care agencies have an annual budget that is set by the provincial government. Financing for the system is derived from provincial and federal governments, which receive monies through personal income taxes. Benefits are broad and cover every aspect of health care but limit certain kinds of elective surgeries as well as dental and eye care. As in Great Britain, infant mortality rates have decreased during the past 10 years, and overall life expectancy has increased.

Canada has had an organized system for health care for many years. The original plan for prepaid health care began during World War I when rural municipalities in Saskatchewan employed contract physicians to care for residents. The revenue to hire these general practice physicians came from local property taxes and "premiums" charged to non–property owners (Taylor, 1980, p. 184). The success of this early work in Saskatchewan supported the passage in 1947 of legislation to establish the first compulsory hospital insurance plan in North America by the cooperative Commonwealth Federation Party (Kerr and MacPhail, 1996). Several significant milestones in the development of a Canadian health plan included the following:

- *1949 National Health Grants Act:* Funded hospital construction (much like the Hill-Burton Act in the United States)
- *1957 Hospital Insurance and Diagnostic Services Act:* Prepaid universal coverage for all residents, for both inpatient and outpatient care, on a 50-50 cost-sharing basis between the province and federal funds
- *1966 Medical Care Insurance Act:* Expanded prepaid hospital coverage to include medical care (also began in Saskatchewan)
- *1977 Fiscal Arrangements and Established Programs Financing Act:* Replaced the increasingly expensive 50-50 cost sharing with block grants; the federal contribution was reduced to 25%; physicians became dissatisfied with their levels of reimbursement and began using co-payments and extra billing
- *1984 Canada Health Act:* Disallowed extra billing and co-payment fees and added a clause for federal reimbursement for "health practitioners," which

opened the door for nurse practitioners to provide primary care

Five basic principles of health care form the basis for the Canadian national health insurance system. These principles are similar to those proposed in the unsuccessful health reform plan in the 1990s in the United States:

- *Universality:* Coverage to the entire population
- *Comprehensiveness:* Coverage for all medically necessary services
- *Accessibility:* Because of the relatively sparsely populated, rural areas across Canada, accessibility has been a challenge. As in the United States, physicians prefer to work and live in urban, not rural, areas.
- *Portability:* Coverage for residents who require health services soon after they move to a different province or during a visit outside their home province
- *Public administration:* Nonprofit administration of services by an organization fiscally responsible to the provincial government

As can be seen from what is reimbursed, this system supports hospital and physician dominance. Health care services are provided through the private sector on a fee-for-service basis, and the vast majority of hospitals are owned and operated by nonprofit groups including municipalities, voluntary agencies, and religious groups. Although these institutions employ some physicians, most of the medical staff is composed of private physicians who are granted admittance privileges by each of the facilities (Health Canada, 2002). Hospitals and other health care agencies have an annual budget that is set by the provincial government. Financing for the system is derived from provincial and federal governments, which receive monies through personal income taxes. The federal government does provide block grants to help defray the cost. Most of the provinces have instituted some kind of expenditure target or limit to control the amount spent on physician services (Sokolovsky, 1993). Home and community care were not initially eligible for federal reimbursement.

As in the United States, in Canada there is a misdistribution of physicians, and nurses are underused. Nursing education entered the university after World War II, and Canada currently has excellent baccalaureate, masters, and doctoral programs in nursing. As their health care system continues to be examined, it is likely that nurses in Canada can carve out a greater role in a more cost-effective system. This will be especially true if the goal of HFA21 is achieved. For the last decade, Canadian provinces have examined the way they can incorporate principles of primary health care (PHC). There are unlimited opportunities for nurses to play key roles in a community-based primary health care system. Such a system is consistent with what nurses learn in baccalaureate education in both Canada and the United States. However, advances by nursing may be restricted by the severe nursing shortage that Canada has suffered from since the late 1990s.

In response to this nursing shortage, Canada held a summit to develop strategies for dealing with the shortage (Health Canada, 2002):

- Improvement in quality of work life
- Establishment of a nursing advisory committee in each province
- Effective planning and evaluation of nursing resources
- Identification of gaps in research
- Development of an education plan that promotes a positive image of nursing
- Increasing the number of educational allotments for students
- Examining means to have nurses reenter the workforce

A main component of Canada's health care system is health promotion and disease prevention. Several websites have been developed to make health education more available to citizens. One such site is Health Promotion On-Line, available at www.hc-sc.gc.ca/english/for_you/hpo/index.html. The use of the internet invites an opportunity for nurses to reach a wide base in health education efforts. In addition, nurses are playing an active role in the Commission on the Future of Health Care in Canada (CFHCC, 2001). The goal of this organization is "to ensure the sustainability of a universally accessible, publicly funded health system, that offers quality services to Canadians and strikes an appropriate balance between investments in prevention and health maintenance and those directed to care and treatment" (CHFCC, 2001).

## Sweden

Health care in Sweden is made available to all citizens. The system is based on a national health service that is operated almost completely by the Swedish government. The Board of Health and Welfare *(Socialstyrelsen)* has the responsibility for health care delivery in Sweden and has the goal of providing high-quality care on equal terms for all citizens (National Board of Health and Welfare, 2001). Local responsibility rests with 21 county councils that contain district medical centers that hire physicians. Several districts are in each council, and several councils are in a region. Each council has a hospital, and there are regional hospitals that provide specialty care in every region. The 1982 Health Care Act made it mandatory for all councils to plan for all health services (Health Care and Dental Care in Sweden, 2000). Also, private hospitals and physicians in private practice often have agreements with the Social Insurance Office. All children under 20 years receive health and medical care free if they are registered residents.

The role of nurses in the Swedish health care delivery system is not as pronounced as in the United States, Canada, or Great Britain, but there are indications that nurses are gaining in their professional role and autonomy. Sweden has hospital, clinic, and district (public) health nurses. District nurses have several roles, including triaging for referral, telephone information services, and direct care.

The financial basis for the Swedish health care delivery system is derived from a proportional wage tax of 13.5%. Federal revenues generate 35% of the total cost, and the last 4% is obtained through direct patient fees that vary by district (with a cap on the total amount a person pays per year for health care and prescriptions) (Health Care and Dental Care in Sweden, 2002). The services that are provided in this system are comprehensive and range from all hospital expenses to preventive services, physician and district nurses services, prescription drugs, dental and eye care, and psychiatric care. During the last 20 years, infant mortality has decreased and life expectancy has increased.

## China

Great advances in public health have been the hallmark of the People's Republic of China since it was founded in 1949. Examples of public health advances that were made in China include controlling contagious diseases such as cholera, typhoid, and scarlet fever and a reduction in infant mortality (Kennedy, 1999). These accomplishments in public health were credited to a political system that was and is largely socialistic and feature a health care system that is described in socialistic terms as collective. The Chinese collective system emphasized the common good for all people, not individuals or special groups. This system was financed through cooperative insurance plans. The collective health care system was owned and controlled by the state and was characterized by the use of barefoot doctors who were medical practitioners trained at the community level and who could provide a minimal level of health care throughout the country. Barefoot doctors combined Western medicine with traditional techniques such as acupuncture and herbal remedies. An emphasis was placed on improving the quality of water supplies and on disease prevention and massive public health campaigns against sanitation problems, such as flies, mosquitoes, and the snails that spread schistosomiasis. Recently, with the decrease in infectious diseases, there has been an increase in chronic diseases such as hypertension in the Chinese population (Dobie, 2002).

Today, health care in China is managed by the Ministry of Public Health, which sets national health policy. The current Chinese government continues to make health care a priority and has set goals to provide medical care to all of its citizens. However, with recent economic reforms, health care, especially in rural areas, has deteriorated because of lack of monetary support and the move toward the market economy (Qun, 2001). Health care costs are rising rapidly as more Western-style medicine is used, such as medical tests and prescription drugs. People tend to use health care episodically, and satisfaction has decreased as more people move from rural to urban settings (Dobie, 2001; Kennedy, 1999). China's health care system is being modified by the introduction of primary health care in community health clinics (CHC) based on the health care system in Canada. With this system, a family practice physician is assigned 500 or more individuals for whom to provide health care. CHCs work closely with other organizations, such as the Communist Party, to present health education programs (Dobie, 2002). In 2001 the cost for nursing services and health care in a hospital was about $3 (U.S.) and less than $3 (U.S.) for physician care and drugs (Loma Linda, 1998).

The ministry is also actively involved in medical and nursing education and sets standards for the curricula in schools and for placing graduates. Beijing Medical University established the first master's degree in nursing program in 1996. Currently there are 1.2 million nurses, 500 diploma schools, and 20 baccalaureate programs. In 2001, China started a distant learning project to educate baccalaureate-level nurses (International Council of Nurses, 1999). Since the 1980s, China's nurses have been visiting countries such as the United States, Canada, and Australia to seek baccalaureate and graduate nursing degrees. The W. K. Kellogg Foundation has sponsored exchange visits between China's nurse educators and Western nurse educators (University of Michigan, 2000). As a result of these visits, China has implemented home health nursing to reduce the prolonged stay (often a month or more) in hospitals to recuperate after surgery (University of Michigan, 2000). Mobile medical clinics staffed by physicians and nurses are making visits to isolated rural communities to deliver health care. In addition, faith-based health care delivery systems have recently been developed (Qun, 2001). China continues to try different avenues to bring health care to its citizens, and nursing is an important component of those efforts.

## Mexico

In 1995 Mexico initiated the Health Sector Reform Program to expand medical coverage, to provide efficient and quality services to the population, and to treat disorders arising from epidemiologic and demographic problems. The strategy to transform the public health care system, known as the social security system (IMSS), into a market-driven system has been a complex process that has not yet been completed (Laurell, 2001). The IMSS is the health sector that is the key to opening health care to private insurance companies, health maintenance organizations, and hospital enterprises, most of which represent foreign interests (Laurell, 2001). Basically, the IMSS is a fee-driven insurance that allows participants to choose a physician and may include total family insurance coverage for an additional cost. In theory, those who are able to pay may enroll voluntarily, but those who cannot pay (the uninsured) can receive services through the individual states in which they live.

Organization of health care is closely linked with employers, who provide part of the cost for health care services along with contributions from the government and from the employee. The system is coordinated by the secretariat of health, which oversees the integration and coordination of health services and encourages competition among service providers. In 1996 the secretariat of health implemented a program that expanded basic services for those with limited or no health care coverage to the most rural and remote areas of the country. People may also enroll for more expanded services by paying a fee that is met with a government contribution (Nigenda et al, 2001).

Mexico has strived to increase health services for all of its residents and has increased the number of outpatient clinics and hospitals each year. Health promotion, which is a major priority for the secretariat of health, focuses on programs for family health, comprehensive health of children and adolescents, healthy *municipios,* health care exercises, and development of educational content (Nigenda et al, 2001).

An additional 10 substantive program themes have a direct impact on health status: reproductive health, child health care, health care for adults and older adults, vector-borne diseases, *zoonoses, mycobacterioses,* epidemiologic emergencies and disasters, HIV/AIDS and other STDs, and addictions. Traditional healing is very important in all parts of the country but especially for indigenous people in rural and remote areas.

## MAJOR WORLD HEALTH PROBLEMS AND THE BURDEN OF DISEASE

As described, present population determinants of the world's health demonstrate that critical health care needs still exist despite ongoing attempts to attain good health. As world economies have lagged since the late 1970s and into the new century, the amount of debt incurred by lesser-developed countries has increased, and money that was once used for health care has been used to pay off debt. Therefore, even though attempts have been made by lesser-developed countries to address health care needs, major health problems still exist. Communicable diseases that are often preventable are still common throughout the world and are more common in lesser-developed countries. In addition, both developed and lesser-developed countries have to find ways to cope with the aging of their populations, which presents governments with the burden of providing care for people who become ill with more expensive noncommunicable and chronic forms of diseases and disabilities. Illnesses such as AIDS continue to raise concerns, and long-standing diseases such as TB and malaria still persist, adding to a growing burden of overextended health care delivery systems.

Mortality statistics do not adequately describe the outlook of health in the world. The WHO and the World Bank (1998a, 2002) have developed an indicator called the **global burden of disease** (GBD). The GBD combines losses from premature death and losses of healthy life that result from disability. Premature death is defined as the difference between the actual age at death and life expectancy at that age in a low-mortality population. People who have debilitating injuries or diseases must be cared for in some way, most often by family members, and thus they no longer can contribute to the family's or a community's economic growth (World Bank, 1998a, 2002). The GBD represents units of **disability-adjusted life-years** (DALYs) (Box 4-1) (World Bank, 1998a). In 2000, for example, 1.28

billion DALYs were lost worldwide, which equates to 39 million deaths of newborn children or to 80 million deaths of people who reach age 50. Approximately 13.7 million children under age 5 died during the same year in lesser-developed countries representing a tremendous loss of future

---

**BOX 4-1  Calculating Disability-Adjusted Life-Years**

There are five components of disability-adjusted life-years (DALYs).

1. *Duration of time lost due to a death at each age:* Measurement is based on the potential limit for life, which has been set at 82.5 years for women and 80 years for men.

2. *Disability weights:* The degree of incapacity associated with various health conditions. Values range from 0 (perfect health) to 1 (death). Four prescribed points between 0 and 1 represent a set of accepted disability classes.

3. *Age-weighting function, $Cxe^{-\beta x}$,*

   where $C = 0.16243$ (a constant), $\beta = 0.04$ (a constant), $e = 2.71$, a (constant), and $x = $ age; this function indicates the relative importance of a healthy life at different ages.

4. *Discounting function, $e^{-r(x-a)}$,*

   where $r = 0.03$ (the discount rate), $e = 2.71$ (a constant), $a = $ age at onset of disease, and $x = $ age; this function indicates the value of health gains today compared to the value of health gains in the future.

5. *Health is added across individuals:* Two people each losing 10 DALYs are treated as showing the same loss as one person losing 20 years.

   "In summary, the disability-adjusted life-year (DALY) is an indicator of the time lived with a disability and the time lost due to premature mortality. The duration of time lost due to premature mortality is calculated using standard expected years of life lost with model life-tables. The reduction in physical capacity due to morbidity is measured using disability weights. The value of time lived at different ages has been calculated using an exponential function which reflects the dependence of the young and older adults on the adults. Streams of time have been discounted at 3 percent. Accordingly the number of DALYs lost due to disability at age 'x' can be calculated using the following formula:" (Murray and Lopez, 1996, p. 15)

$$\text{DALY } (x) = (D)(Cxe^{-\beta x})(e^{-r(x-a)}),$$

   where $D = $ disability weight (ranging from 1 [death] to 0 [perfect health]).

---

Homedes N: 1995, available online at http://www.worldbank.org/htm./extrdr/hnp/hddflash/workp/wp-00068.html.

human potential. If these children could face the same risks as those in countries with developed market economies, the deaths would decrease by 90% to 1.1 million. This example demonstrates the importance of having accessible and affordable disease prevention programs for children around the world (World Bank, 1998c, 2002). Overall, premature deaths throughout the world during the 1990s accounted for 66% of all DALYs lost, with debilitating injuries and diseases accounting for 34%.

In lesser-developed countries, 67% of all DALY loss during the 1990s was attributed to premature death. In contrast, the developed countries reported only 55% from this same cause. Communicable diseases still account for the greatest proportion of calculated DALYs worldwide for both males and females, followed by noncommunicable diseases and injuries. Research studies have indicated that infections and parasitic diseases remain a threat to the health of many population groups. Results from these studies demonstrate the continuing need for intervention for infectious and other kinds of communicable diseases. Conditions that contribute to one quarter of the GBD throughout the world include diarrheal disease, respiratory infections, worm infestations, malaria, and childhood diseases such as measles. In 1992, sub-Saharan Africa demonstrated a GBD of 43% DALYs lost, largely because of preventable diseases among children, and 600,000 infants became infected with HIV (WHO/UNAIDS, 2002). Other countries and areas with comparable DALYs are India (29%) and the Middle Eastern crescent (29%). In adults, STDs and TB combine to account for 70% of the world's GBD (World Bank, 1998a, 2002).

Determining the total amount of loss, even using the GBD, is difficult because many consequences of disease and injury are hard to measure. For example, measuring the social and cultural impact of the disfigurements that result from accidents or debilitating diseases such as leprosy and river blindness is difficult. Likewise, it is problematic to measure social conditions such as familial and marital dysfunction, war, and familial violence.

The following sections describe selected communicable diseases that still contribute substantially to the worldwide disease burden: TB, AIDS, and malaria. Other health problems discussed include maternal and women's health, diarrheal disease in children, and nutrition.

## Communicable Diseases

One example of the long-term benefits of immunizing children against communicable diseases is the successful campaign against smallpox that was carried out during the 1960s and 1970s by the World Health Organization. Smallpox has been virtually eliminated throughout the world, with only occasional and incidental reportings from laboratory accidents and inoculation complications. The systematic and planned smallpox program formed the basis for a series of worldwide efforts that are now being implemented to control and eradicate other infectious and communicable diseases.

In 1974 the WHO formed the Expanded Programme on Immunization, which sought to reduce morbidity and mortality from diphtheria, pertussis, tetanus, TB, measles, and poliomyelitis throughout the world (WHO, 1986b, 2002a). At present, eight out of ten of the world's children are protected against these diseases, and the world's infant mortality rate has fallen by more than 37% since 1970 (WHO, 2000b). The major aim of immunization is to induce immunity to a disease without experiencing the actual disease (Thanassi, 1998).

### Tuberculosis

Predictions that 80 million new cases of TB would occur worldwide during the late 1990s and into the early years of the twenty-first century are being realized (Dye et al, 2002). Of these 80 million cases, it is estimated that close to 5 million are associated with HIV (Bleed, Dye, and Raviglione, 2000; Lienhardt and Rodrigues, 1997). In addition, it is estimated that 30 million people will die of TB during the same period (Dolin, Raviglione, and Kochi, 1994). At present, TB represents the largest cause of death from a single infectious agent, striking nearly 3 million people each year. This particular statistic represents 25% of premature adult deaths in lesser-developed countries that might have been prevented (WHO, 2000b, 2002e). The growth of the world's population, including an increase in the number of older adult individuals and the adverse effects of HIV, contributes to the large projected estimates for TB (Dolin et al, 1994).

A third of the world's population, or 1.7 billion people, harbor the TB pathogen *Mycobacterium tuberculosis*. Clinical manifestations of the disease include pulmonary TB, which is the most widespread form; TB meningitis, which is a leading cause of childhood mortality; and TB of a variety of other organs. The WHO (1992a) reported that of the 8 million new TB cases reported in 1992, 3.6 million were of the pulmonary form, and these numbers have remained constant during the late 1990s and into the twenty-first century (Lienhardt and Rodrigues, 1997; World Bank, 1998a; WHO, 2002d). Even though the disease affects all age groups, the heaviest toll is among young adults.

The presence of disease-causing bacilli in sputum examination is not evident in all forms of pulmonary TB. About half the cases are detectable by sputum smear examination, and these are of the infectious pulmonary type. Chemotherapy undoubtedly reduces the number of individuals who die from TB. However, many lesser-developed countries do not have organized treatment and prevention programs and therefore lose more people each year to TB than to either malaria or measles (Lienhardt and Rodrigues, 1997; WHO, 2002d).

Although TB is known worldwide, concern is greatest in certain areas: Southeast Asia (3 million new cases), sub-Saharan Africa (1.6 million cases), and eastern Europe, where there is a reoccurrence of TB and a quarter of a million cases (WHO, 2002b). This compares with 16,372 new cases in the United States (Centers for Disease Control, 2002). Interestingly, the incidence of TB in Russia has more than doubled since 1991, and a quarter of those cases are in Russian prisons (British Broadcasting Company, 1999). Worldwide, approximately 2.53 million deaths were attributable to TB in 1990, which exceeds the number of deaths that resulted from measles and malaria. The case fatality ratio for untreated TB is greater than 50%. Of these deaths, 1.1 million occurred in Southeast Asia and 0.6 million in the western Pacific. Also in 1990, 123,000 TB deaths could be attributed to HIV infection, with most of these deaths occurring in sub-Saharan Africa (Bleed et al, 2000). Additional estimates have indicated that one quarter of adult deaths that could be avoided in lesser-developed countries are caused by TB. This equates to a tremendous loss of social and economic potential for these countries.

Two factors are a threat to TB control and eradication. The first is the appearance of the HIV virus, which is one of the highest risk factors associated with the breakthrough of once-latent TB. HIV-associated TB infections most often progress to an active disease. Information currently available suggests that 5% to 10% of individuals infected with HIV and *M. tuberculosis* will develop TB each year. This can be compared with 2% of people infected with *M. tuberculosis* but not HIV who will develop TB (Maher and Raviglione, 1999). The appearance of HIV has added to the difficulty of treatment programs in both developed and lesser-developed countries. For example, in Africa, almost half of those individuals who are HIV seropositive are also infected with TB, and it is estimated that nearly 5% to 8% of these individuals will develop the clinical manifestations of TB. More importantly, HIV-positive individuals with infectious TB have an increased likelihood of transmitting TB to their families and to the community, further increasing the prevalence of this condition (Maher and Raviglione, 1999).

The second factor that poses a threat to the control and eradication of TB is the growing multidrug resistance of the TB bacillus to isoniazid and rifampin, the two drugs that are currently used to treat it. Resistance to these drugs is already evident around the world, including in the Mexico–Texas border communities. The WHO and other organizations maintain that a high priority should be given to TB control and eradication programs around the world. They advocate a short-term chemotherapy regimen for smear-positive patients as being one of the most cost-effective health interventions available.

Bacille Calmette-Guérin (BCG) consists of a series of vaccines that induce active immunity. These are used to prevent TB and have been available since the 1920s. Although the effectiveness of BCG is still questionable, research studies have demonstrated that it is effective in preventing the more lethal forms of TB, including meningitis and miliary disease in children (WHO, 1992a, 2002e). These same studies have demonstrated that more than 80% of the infants in lesser-developed countries have been vaccinated, with less coverage in sub-Saharan Africa. However, more studies are needed worldwide to determine the effect that BCG can have on the more infectious types of TB. Present indications are that BCG does not reduce the transmission of infectious types of TB.

The standard chemotherapeutic agents used in many countries for TB are isoniazid, thioacetazone, and streptomycin, and they are effective at converting sputum-positive cases to noninfectivity. The drug and the combinations that are used vary from country to country. To be effective, however, treatment must be carried out on a consistent basis, and many lesser-developed countries have difficulty getting patients to comply with any treatment regimen. Many of the TB intervention programs in these countries have been unable to carry out curative programs following standard treatment regimens (Pio, 1997; WHO, 1992a). In 1990, the WHO Global Tuberculosis Program (GTB) promoted the revision of national tuberculosis programs to focus on short-course chemotherapy (SCC), with directly observed treatment (DOT). The introduction of DOT programs has been successful in the United States and in several lesser-developed countries, including Malawi, Mozambique, Nicaragua, and Tanzania, producing a cure rate of approximately 80%. The SCC program involves aggressive administration of chemotherapeutic drugs combined with short-term hospitalization. The key to the program lies in a well-managed system with a regular supply of antituberculosis drugs to the treatment centers, follow-up care, and rigorous reporting and analysis of patient information (WHO, 2002d). Despite these efforts, little progress has been made, and little international support has been given to placing TB control programs as a number one priority worldwide.

## Acquired Immunodeficiency Syndrome

As discussed in Chapter 39, acquired immunodeficiency syndrome (AIDS) has rapidly become a major cause of morbidity and mortality throughout the world (WHO/UNAIDS, 2002). Since HIV/AIDS is discussed fully elsewhere, only a brief synopsis will be presented here.

Once infected with HIV, individuals harbor the virus for the remainder of their lives. The virus may produce no symptoms for years, but risk increases with the threat of a breakdown of the immune system and the subsequent infections that may occur. Worldwide prevention programs are important because failing to control this virulent disease will result in damaging and costly consequences for all countries in the future. Ideally, the goal is primary prevention of HIV. When prevention efforts fail at this level, the next goal is secondary prevention, or early diagnosis and treatment. In 2001, the director general of WHO appealed to the world's health professionals to set up targets for action to control and eradicate the spread of HIV/AIDS. In particular, WHO along with UNICEF, UNAIDS, women's health groups, and other international organizations, have promoted the use of nevirapine to prevent mother-to-child transmission of HIV. The regimen calls for a single dose of nevirapine to be given to the mother at delivery and a single dose to the newborn within

72 hours. WHO is recommending that nevirapine be included in the minimum standard package of care for HIV-positive women and their children (WHO/UNAIDS, 2002). Tertiary prevention with HIV includes both care of the patient and instructing, guiding, and teaching the family how to care for the person with HIV (Box 4-2).

## Malaria

Malaria continues to be one of the most important tropical parasitic disease, and it kills more people than any other communicable disease except tuberculosis (WHO, 1998b). Ninety countries and areas are considered malaria ridden (Thanassi, 1998; WHO, 1994). Countries where the disease is most endemic are those that lie in the tropical areas of Asia, Africa, and Latin America. It is estimated that 300 to 500 million people develop clinical cases of malaria each year, with more than 90% of these occurring in equatorial Africa (WHO, 1994). This current situation exists despite worldwide efforts to eradicate and control the spread of malaria over the last 50 years.

There are two primary modes of malarial control—vector reduction and chemotherapy (Basch, 1990). The methods of vector control vary widely, from using the larvae-eating fish tilapia to the use of insecticidal sprays and oils. Needless to say, the latter poses a potential threat to the environment in tropical areas where a delicate ecosystem is already threatened by other potential hazards such as lumbering and mining. Countries that do not have strict environmental laws continue to use DDT sprays to control mosquito populations despite the advent of DDT-resistant mosquitoes. The non-DDT insecticide sprays, such as malathion, generally cost more, presenting an extra financial burden to lesser-developed countries. Methods for control and eradication that are being considered by malaria-ridden countries are environmental management, reduction and control of the source, and elimination of the adult mosquito.

Chemotherapeutic agents can be used for both protection and treatment of the disease. Drugs for treatment and prophylaxis are expensive and often cause side effects. However, current evidence suggests that the *Plasmodium* sporozoites are becoming resistant to both treatment and preventive chemotherapeutic agents. Efforts are presently underway to develop an antimalarial vaccine, but so far the results have been unsuccessful. Individuals who live or travel to *Anopheles*-infested areas are urged to protect themselves with mosquito netting, clothing that protects vulnerable parts of the body, and repellents for both their bodies and their clothes.

## Maternal and Women's Health

The WHO and UNICEF have continued with worldwide initiatives to reform the health care received by women and children in lesser-developed countries (Heiby, 1998; WHO, 2000a). However, studies on women's health indicate that most deaths to women around the world are related to pregnancy and childbirth. Most of these deaths occur in lesser-developed countries (AbouZahr and Royston, 1992; Heiby, 1998; Tomlinson, 1996). Throughout the world, women between 15 and 44 years of age account for approximately one third of the world's disease burden, and women between 45 and 59 for one fifth of the burden. This burden comprises diseases and conditions that are either exclusively or predominantly found in women, including maternal mortality and morbidity, cervical cancer, anemia, STDs, osteoarthritis, and breast cancer (World Bank, 2002). Although most of these conditions can be dealt with by cost-effective prevention and screening programs, many lesser-developed countries have ignored women's health issues other than those directly related to pregnancy and childbirth. The health programs that are emphasized appear to be those that favor male children and men over women (Ganatra and Hirve, 1994).

Furthermore, lesser-developed countries presently account for 87% of the world's births. However, statistics from lesser-developed countries throughout the world indicate that prenatal services and safe birthing services are unavailable, inaccessible, and unaffordable to women, with the continent of Africa exhibiting the highest maternal mortality rates (Anderson, 1996). An African woman's risk of dying from pregnancy-related causes is 1 in 20 (AbouZahr and Royston, 1992; Andrews and Gottschalk, 1996). Africa is followed by the countries of Bangladesh, Pakistan, and India. These three countries account for nearly half of the world's maternal deaths but only 29% of the world's births. In fact, these three countries have more maternal deaths each week than Europe has in a single year (Basch, 1990). Still, an accurate reporting of maternal deaths is difficult to obtain because many of the women who die live in remote areas, they are poor, and their deaths are considered by many to be unimportant (Kestler, 1993).

The primary causes of maternal mortality, particularly in lesser-developed countries, vary. They include hemorrhage, infection, convulsions, and coma caused by eclampsia and obstructed labor, and infections from unsanitary conditions and nonsterile and poorly performed abortions. Risk factors for maternal mortality include poor nutritional status, disease conditions, high parity, and age below 20 and above 35 years.

To date, little attention has been paid to the problem of maternal mortality, even though the reported incidences are high throughout the world. There has been, however, a movement to address the issue by the WHO and by the UN Fund for Population Activities (UNFPA). These two organizations have called for government initiatives and actions to address direct obstetric deaths as well as those that arise from indirect causes. The WHO and UNFPA have argued that their initiatives and their call for action for programs addressing maternal health are associated with the health of infants and children.

In support of the recommendations of the WHO and UNFPA, the World Health Assembly's Technical Discussions on Women, Health, and Development in 1992 presented several suggestions to the WHO, including the following (WHO, 1992b):

- Assisting governments to initiate legislation that addresses women's health problems
- Supporting research that addresses socioeconomic implications of diseases in women
- Developing proactive strategies to intervene and reduce health problems among women

Even though these recommendations have been updated, safe motherhood initiatives are still needed throughout the world. These initiatives need to include accessible family planning services, access of prenatal and postnatal health care services, ensuring access to safe abortion, and improving the nutritional status of all women (Figure 4-7).

## Diarrheal Disease

Diarrhea, one of the leading causes of illness and death in children under 5 years of age throughout the world, is most prominent in the lesser-developed countries despite recent initiatives by the WHO to correct this problem (Heiby, 1998). For example, Guerrant (1986; Guerrant et al, 1992) indicates that diarrheal disease accounted for

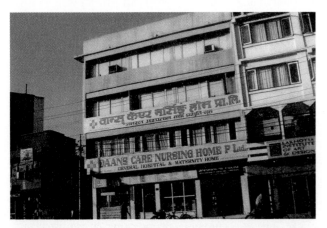

**Figure 4-7** General Hospital and Maternity Home in Katmandu, Nepal. *(Courtesy J. Schaller-Ayers.)*

more than half of all the causes of death among children in Brazil. The prevalence of diarrheal disease was so pervasive in 1978 that the World Health Assembly established a global program to reduce mortality and morbidity in infants and young children who suffered from all forms of the disease. This program continues today (Lucas, 1998).

Diarrhea is a symptom of a variety of different illnesses, and the definitions and perceptions of it vary greatly from country to country. For example, in Bangladesh, diarrhea is defined as more than two watery or loose stools in 24 hours, whereas Indonesians define it as four loose stools in 24 hours (Basch, 1990). Definitions are complicated by the observable presence of blood, mucus, or parasites. The age of the individual who is experiencing the diarrhea also complicates definitions.

Causes of diarrhea are just as varied and diverse as its definitions and perceptions. Some of the causes include (1) viruses such as the rotavirus and Norwalk-like agents; (2) bacteria, including *Campylobacter jejuni, Clostridium difficile, Escherichia coli, Salmonella,* and *Shigella;* (3) environmental toxins; (4) parasites such as *Giardia lamblia* and *Cryptosporidium;* and (5) worms. Nutritional deficiencies can also cause diarrhea and are most often secondary to infectious agents. Of these, the rotavirus has emerged as a major world concern, hospitalizing 55,000 American children and killing 1 million children in the world each year (Editor, 1998).

Dehydration is an immediate result of diarrhea and leads to a loss of fluid and electrolytes. The loss of up to 10% of the body's electrolytes can lead to shock, acidosis, stupor, and failure of the body's major organs (e.g., kidney, heart). Persistent diarrhea often leads to loss of body protein and increased susceptibility to infection. Prevention and control of diarrheal disease, especially in infants and children, should therefore be a major aim of countries around the world. In addition, many countries have developed diarrhea control programs that improve childhood nutrition. These programs focus on the promotion of breastfeeding, weaning practices, promotion of oral rehydration therapy, and supplementary feeding programs (Briscoe, 1984). However, all these programs must be considered in conjunction with improving the social and economic conditions that contribute to safe environmental, sanitary, and general living conditions of populations around the world (Basch, 1990).

## Nutrition and World Health

Good nutrition is an essential part of good health. Poor nutrition by itself or that associated with infectious disease accounts for a large portion of the world's disease burden (World Bank, 2002). Those environmental and economic conditions that are related to poverty contribute to underconsumption of nutrients, especially those nutrients that are needed for protein building, such as iodine, vitamin A, and iron. Worldwide, women and children suffer disproportionately from nutrition deficits, especially of the micronutrients just mentioned (Caballero and Rubinstein,

1997; Humphrey, West, and Sommer, 1992). For example, in war-torn Afghanistan, a critical shortage of fruits and vegetables led to an outbreak of scurvy that had devastating effects on the population, leaving them vulnerable to secondary diseases. In the same area, a vitamin A deficiency is evidenced by large numbers of people with night blindness (WHO, 2002b).

Another effect of poor nutrition is stunting, or low height and weight for a given age. Stunting is most frequently the result of eating foods that do not provide enough energy and do not contain enough protein (World Bank, 2002). Because protein foods are usually more expensive than nonprotein food sources, many households cut back on, or unconsciously eliminate, protein-rich foods to save money. Countries where populations are most affected by stunting are India (65%), Asia, not including India and China (50%), China (40%), and sub-Saharan Africa (40%) (World Bank, 2002).

## WHAT DO YOU THINK?

Nutritional support through promotion of continued breastfeeding and improved weaning practices using high-density, easily digestible, local foods is especially important during and after episodes of diarrhea.

Iron deficiencies are also common in lesser-developed countries and severely affect women and children. A deficiency of iron in the diet reduces physical productivity and affects the capacity of children to learn in school. Iron deficiency in the diet also affects appetite, causing many individuals, especially children, to experience a lessened desire to eat, which in turn affects overall food intake and growth over a prolonged time.

Women are most susceptible to iron deficiency as a result of menstruation and childbearing. Women who experience iron deficiency can develop a severe shortage of iron in their blood that results in anemia, which increases risk of hemorrhage during childbirth. A World Bank report (2002) indicates that 88% of all pregnant women in India are anemic, compared with 60% of the pregnant women in other parts of Asia. In developed, market-economy countries, only 15% of pregnant women experience iron deficiency anemia (Caballero and Rubinstein, 1997).

Other common dietary deficiencies observed throughout the world include iodine, vitamin A, folic acid, and calcium deficiencies. The total impact of malnutrition and dietary deficiencies cannot be underestimated. Any malnourished condition in a population can increase susceptibility to illness. For example, the principal causes of death among malnourished persons are measles, diarrheal and respiratory disease, TB, pertussis, and malaria. The loss of life from these diseases can be measured as 231 DALYs worldwide, with one fourth of the 231 being directly attributable to malnourishment and dietary deficiencies.

Worldwide initiatives that have been directed at overcoming nutritional deficits have included the following (World Bank, 2002):
- Control of infectious diseases
- Nutritional education
- Control of intestinal parasites
- Micronutrient fortification of food
- Food supplementation
- Food price subsidies

Contributions toward these initiatives have been made by individual governments, and organizations that have been most active in promoting them have included the International Red Cross, the WHO, and many international religious and private foundations.

## Bioterrorism

A new global health concern that has emerged in the twenty-first century is bioterrorism. **Bioterrorism** is a term that is used to describe terrorist activities in which biological substances are used to cause harm to other people (Federal Emergency Management Agency, 2002). Numerous diseases can be used by terrorists as weapons, including anthrax, plague, smallpox, cholera, botulism, salmonella, and tularemia. Terrorists can modify the disease-causing agents to be spread through the air and through water; those best transmitted through the air include anthrax and smallpox. Bacteria are easier to produce than the viruses and are the most dreaded of the biological weapons. Anthrax caused by *Bacillus anthracis*, plague caused by *Yersinia pestis*, and tularemia caused by *Francisella tularensis* are three of the most potent. Three el-

### Evidence-Based Practice

This research study examined the relationships among demographic characteristics, acculturation, psychological resilience, and symptoms of depression in midlife women from the former Soviet Union who immigrated to the United States. This cross-sectional study of 200 women revealed that the Russian immigrant women scored higher on the depression scales than those women native to the United States. Older women scored particularly high, but those younger women who learned English and held at least part-time jobs had lower scores.

**Nurse Use:** This study indicates that interventions that encourage the use of English may help decrease symptoms of depression in midlife immigrant Russian women.

Miller A, Chandler PJ: Acculturation, resilience, and depression in midlife women from the former Soviet Union. *Nurs Res*, 51(2):26-32, 2002.

ements are required to make disease agents effective air-borne weapons:

- The disease must be severe and have a short incubation time.
- The agent must be able to cause disease by inhalation.
- It must be possible to produce the causative agent in large amounts with minimal risk.

Another mode of transmission of biological agents is through drinking water and food. Diseases caused by swallowing organisms include cholera, botulism, and salmonella poisoning. Because food and water supplies could be contaminated, the threat of starvation, nutritional deprivations, and other food-related effects would be devastating (Sobel, Khan, and Swerdlow, 2002).

Nursing, through the International Congress of Nursing (ICN), has taken a strong position on terrorism and nursing preparedness. The ICN policy paper on disaster preparedness outlines actions, a risk assessment, and key management strategies essential to the delivery of an effective response to the health care needs of disaster-stricken populations (ICN, 2001).

## ■ Practice Application

The role of nurses in international health varies dramatically from country to country, as does the role of professional nursing. It is not surprising to learn that nursing plays a more active role in health care delivery in the more technologically advanced countries such as the United States, Canada, Australia, New Zealand, the United Kingdom, and other countries in western Europe. The more developed countries have a defined role for nurses, whereas the role is less well defined, if it is defined at all, in lesser-developed countries.

During the last decade, lesser-developed countries have implemented primary health care programs directed at prevention and management of important public health problems. With the increasing migration between and within countries because of war and famine, a greater need for nursing expertise to alleviate suffering of refugees and displaced persons has emerged. Starvation, disease, death, war, and migration underscore the need for support from the wealthier nations of the world.

More than 30 million refugees and internally displaced persons in lesser-developed countries currently depend on international relief assistance for survival. Mortality rates in these populations during the acute phase of displacement have been up to 60 times the expected rates. Displaced populations in Ethiopia and southern Sudan have suffered the highest mortality rates. In Afghanistan, infectious diseases accounted for one half of all admissions to the hospital—mostly malaria and typhoid fever. The greatest mortality rate has been in children 1 to 14 years old. The major causes of death have been measles, diarrheal diseases, acute respiratory infections, and malaria.

Nurses from abroad are often used to combat the major mortality in refugee camps—malnutrition, measles, diarrhea, pneumonia, and malaria. Nurses are following the principles of primary health care and are promoting adequate food intake, safe drinking water, shelter, environmental sanitation, and immunizations. These life-saving practices have been implemented in the following countries: Thailand (Myanmar refugees), Rwanda, Zaire, Angola, Afghanistan, the Sudan, and the former Yugoslavia.

You are sent to a country ravaged by war, in which many people are refugees. You are asked to work side by side with other nurses, both foreign and native to the country.

**A.** What would you do first to develop this group of nurses into a functioning team?

**B.** Which health and environmental problems would you attempt to handle early in your work?

**C.** Identify second-stage interventions and prevention once the initial crisis stage is relieved.

**Answers are in the back of the book.**

## ● Key Points

- Health for the world's people is a collective goal of its nations and is promoted by the major world health organizations.
- As the political and economic barriers between countries fall, the movement of people back and forth across international boundaries increases. This movement increases the spread of various disease entities throughout the world.
- Nurses can and do play an active role in the identification of potential health risks at U.S. borders, with immigrant populations throughout the nation, and as participants in international health care delivery.
- Understanding a population approach can be essential in understanding the health of specific populations
- Primary health care is one of the major keys in the provision of universal access to health care for the world's populations.
- The major organizations that are involved in world health include (1) multilateral, (2) bilateral and nongovernmental or private voluntary, and (3) philanthropic.
- The health status of a country is related to its economic and technical growth. More technologically and economically advanced countries are referred to as developed, whereas those that are striving for greater economic and technological growth are termed lesser developed. Many lesser-developed countries often divert financial resources from health and education to other internal needs, such as defense or economic development, that are not aimed at helping the poor.
- The global burden of disease (GBD) is a way to describe the world's health. The GBD combines losses from premature death and losses that result from disability. The GBD represents units of disability-adjusted life-years (DALYs).

- Critical world health problems still exist and include communicable diseases such as tuberculosis, measles, mumps, rubella, and polio; maternal and child health; diarrheal diseases; nutritional deficits; malaria; and AIDS.
- Bioterrorism is rapidly becoming a world health concern.

## Clinical Decision-Making Activities

1. In your class, divide into small groups and discuss how you might find out if there are immigrant communities in your area. You might want to contact your local health department, area social workers, or community social organizations and churches.
   a. Discuss how you might gain access to one of these immigrant groups. Upon gaining access, how would you go about determining what specific kinds of services the people might need? What are their beliefs about health and health care? What customs regarding health were followed in their country of origin? How does the American health care system differ from the health care system in their country?
   b. As a nurse, what kinds of interventions might you consider implementing with these immigrant populations? What special skills or knowledge might you need to provide care to these populations?
2. Write to one of the major international health organizations or go to their internet web page and obtain their mission and goal statements. What kinds of health-related activities do they focus on? Does the organization that you identified have a specific role defined for nurses? How can a nurse who is interested become involved in their programs and activities?
3. Pick a country or area of the world outside the United States that interests you. Go to the library or use the internet to obtain information about the following:
   a. Status of health care in that country
   b. Major health concerns
   c. GBD (global burden of disease)
   d. Whether this country is developed or lesser developed
   e. Which, if any, international health care organizations are involved with the delivery of health care in that country
4. Choose one or more of the following countries, and find out from your local or state health department the health risks that are involved in visiting that country: Indonesia, Zaire, Paraguay, Bangladesh, Kuwait, Kenya, Mexico, China, and Haiti.

### Additional Resources

These related resources are found either in the appendix at the back of this book or on the book's website at **http://evolve.elsevier.com/Stanhope.**

### *evolve* Evolve Website

Appendix A.3 Declaration of Alma Ata
WebLinks: Healthy People 2010

## References

AbouZahr C, Royston E: Excessive hazards of pregnancy and childbirth in the Third World, *World Health Forum* 13:343, 1992.

Ajo G: Workplace health promotion in Nigeria: a step towards health promotion and productivity, *Global Perspect* 4(2):6, 2001.

Anders R, Harrigan R: Nursing education in China: opportunities for international collaboration, *Nurs Educ Perspect* 23(3):137, 2002.

Anderson CM: Women for women's health: Uganda, *Nursing Outlook* 44:141, 1996.

Andrews CM, Gottschalk J: An international community-based nurse education program, *J Commun Health Nurs* 13(1):59, 1996.

Audit Commission: *District nursing services should modernise to manage growing patient demands,* retrieved 5/02 from http:// www.audit-commission.gov.uk/ news/prdnurse.shtml, 1999.

Basch PF: *Textbook of international health,* New York, 1990, Oxford University Press.

Bleed D, Dye C, Raviglione MC: Dynamics and control of the global tuberculosis epidemic, *Curr Opin Pulm Med* 6:174, 2000.

Briscoe J: Water supply and health in lesser developed countries, *Am J Public Health* 74:1009, 1984.

British Broadcasting Company (BBC), World: *Europe Russian TB threatens the world,* United Kingdom, September 17, 1999.

British Broadcasting Company (BBC), World: *Health coverage for the poor in Thailand,* United Kingdom, October 20, 2001.

Brundtland GH: *WHO's vision for health.* Presented at the International Council for Nurses Centennial Conference, June 30, 1999, London.

Caballero B, Rubinstein S: Environmental factors affecting nutritional status in urban areas of lesser developed countries, *Arch Latinoam Nutr* 47(2 Suppl 1):3, 1997.

Cable News Network (CNN): *Number of Ebola victims reaches 400: 160 dead in Uganda,* New York, 2000, Associated Press.

Centers for Disease Control: *TB, data and statistics,* Atlanta, 2002, CDC.

Central Intelligence Agency: *The world factbook, 2001,* retrieved 5/02 from http://www.cia.gov/cia/publications/factbook, 2001.

Commission on the Future of Health Care in Canada (CFHCC): *Home page,* retrieved 5/02 from http://www.healthcarecommission.ca, 2001.

Dobie M: *Why China's health needs fixing,* retrieved 5/02 from http://www.idrc.ca/books/reports/2001/04-02e.html, 2001.

Dobie M: *Strengthening community-based health in urban China,* retrieved 5/02 from Science from the developing world. http://www.idrc.ca/reports/read_article_english. cfm?article_num=857, 2002.

Dolin P, Raviglione M, Kochi A: Global tuberculosis incidence and mortality during 1990-2000, *Bull World Health Organ* 72(2):213, 1994.

Dye C et al: Erasing the world's slow staining strategies to beat drug resistant tuberculosis, *Science* 15:75, 2002.

Editor: Diarrhea vaccine OK'd, *San Francisco Chronicle* Sept 1, 1998.

Evlo K, Carrin G: Finance for health care: part of a broad canvas, *World Health Forum* 13:165, 1992.

Federal Emergency Management Agency (FEMA): *What is terrorism?* Washington DC, 2002, U.S. Government Printing Office.

Fox DM: The relevance of population health to academic medicine, *Acad Med* 76(1):6, 2001.

Ganatra B, Hirve S: Male bias in health care utilization for under-fives in a rural community in western India, *Bull World Health Organ* 72(1):101, 1994.

Gomez-Dantes O, Frenk J, Cruz C: Commence in health services in North America within the context of the North American Free Trade Agreement, *Rev Panam Salud Publica* 1(6):460, 1997.

Guerrant R: Unresolved problems and future considerations in diarrheal research, *Pediatr Infect Dis J* 5:S155, 1986.

Guerrant R et al: Diarrhea as a cause and effect of malnutrition: diarrhea prevents catch-up growth and malnutrition increases diarrhea frequency and duration, *Am J Trop Med Hyg* 47(1):28, 1992.

Hall CG: NAFTA and occupational health: an international perspective, *Mexican Labor News and Analysis* 12(1), 1996.

Health Canada: *Nursing strategy for Canada—executive summary,* retrieved 5/02 from http://www.hc-sc.gc.ca/english/for_you/nursing/index.htm, 2002.

*Health care and dental care in Sweden,* retrieved 5/02 from http://www.inv.se/svefa/sjukvard/engsjukvard/healthcarehome.html. 2002.

*Health Care for All,* retrieved 5/02 from http://www.ucsf.edu/shpsr/past_projects/hcfa.html 2001.

Heiby JR: Quality improvement and the integrated management of childhood illness: lessons from developed countries, *Qual Improv* 24(5):264, 1998.

Hernandez-Pena P et al: The free trade agreement and environmental health in Mexico, *Salud Publica Mex* 35(2):119, 1993.

Heymann M: Reproductive health promotion in Kosovo, *J Midwifery Women's Health* 46(2):74-81, 2001.

Homedes N: 1995, available online at http://www.worldbank. org/htm./extrdr/hnp/hddflash/workp/wp-00068.html.

Howson CP, Fineberg HV, Bloom BR: The pursuit of global health: the relevance of engagement for developed countries, *Lancet* 351(9102):586, 1998.

Humphrey J, West K, Sommer A: Vitamin A deficiency and attributable mortality among under-5-year-olds, *Bull World Health Organ* 70(2):225, 1992.

Ibrahim MA et al: Population-based health principles in medical and public health practice, *J Public Health Manag Pract* 7(3):75, 2001.

International Council of Nurses: *International nursing partnership project,* retrieved 5/02 from http://www.icn.ch/partnerpage40.htm, 1999.

International Council of Nurses: *ICN position statement on nurses and emergency preparedness,* Geneva, 2001, ICN.

International Medical Volunteer Association (IMVA): *The major international organizations,* Woodville, MA, 2002.

Kennedy B: *Serving the people: China's health care system may be headed for a crisis,* retrieved 5/02 from http://asia.cnn.com/SPECIALS/1999/china.50/dispatches/09.23.health/, 1999.

Kerr JR, MacPhail J: *An introduction to issues in community health nursing in Canada,* St Louis, Mo, 1996, Mosby.

Kestler E: Wanted: better care for pregnant women, *World Health Forum* 14:356, 1993.

Labonte R, Jackson S, Chirrey S: *Population health and health system restructuring: has our knowledge of social and environmental determinants of health made a difference?* A synthesis paper prepared for the Synthesis and Dissemination Unit, Health Promotion and Programs Branch, Health Canada, Ottawa, Ontario, 1998.

Lalonde M: *A new perspective on the health of Canadians: health and welfare Canada,* Ottawa, Ontario, 1974.

Laurell AC: Health reform in Mexico: the promotion of inequality, *Int J Health Serv* 31(2):291, 2001.

Levya-Flores R, Kageyama ML, Erviti-Erice J: How people respond to illness in Mexico: self-care or medical care? *Health Policy* 57(1):15, 2001.

Lienhardt C, Rodrigues LC: Estimation of the impact of the human immunodeficiency virus infection on tuberculosis: tuberculosis risks re-visited? *Int J Tuberc Lung Dis* 1(5):196, 1997.

Loma Linda School of Nursing News: *China Nurses' Association honorary president visits Medical Center, LLU School of Nursing,* retrieved 5/02 from http://www.llu.edu/ news/today/jan29/sn.htm, 1998.

Lucas A: WHO at country level, *Lancet* 351(9104):743, 1998.

Maher D, Raviglione MC: The global epidemic of tuberculosis. In Schlossberg D, editor: *Tuberculosis and non-tuberculosis mycobacterial infections,* pp 104-115, Philadelphia, 1999, Saunders.

Miller A, Chandler PJ: Acculturation, resilience, and depression in midlife women from the former Soviet Union, *Nurs Res* 51(1):26-32, 2002.

Murashima S et al: Public health nursing in Japan: new opportunities for health promotion, *Public Health Nurs* 16(2): 133, 1999.

Murray C, Lopez A: *Global burden of disease: 1996-2020—a World Bank and Harvard School of Public Health publication*, Cambridge, Mass, 1996, Oxford University Press.

National Board of Health and Welfare: Retrieved 5/02 from http://www.sos.se/fulltext/0000-043/0000-043.pdf, 2001.

Nichter M: Pharmaceuticals, health commodification, and social relations: ramifications for primary health care. In Nichter M, editor: *Anthropology and international health*, Boston, 1989, Kluwer Academic.

Nigenda G, Ruiz JA, Montes J: New trends in the regulation of medical practice in the context of health care reform: the Mexico case, *Rev Med Chil* 129(11):1343, 2001.

Ogunbodede EO et al: An oral health promotion module for the primary health care nursing course in Acornhoek, South Africa, *Public Health Nurs* 16(5):351, 1999.

Ortega-Cesena J, Espinosa-Torres F, Lopez-Carillo L: Health risk control for organophosphate pesticides in Mexico: challenges under the Free Trade Treaty, *Salud Publica Mex* 36(6):624, 1994.

Perry S, Marx ES: What technologies for health care in lesser developed countries? *World Health Forum* 13:356, 1992.

Pio C: National tuberculosis programme review: experience over the period 1990-1995, *Bull World Health Organ* 75(6):569, 1997.

Puri MM, John T: Nurses and fight against tuberculosis, *Nurs J India* 88(12):269, 1997.

Qun Y: Bridging the health care gap: Amity's response to health care reforms in China. *Quarterly Bulletin of the Amity Foundation*, retrieved 5/02 from http://www.amityfoundation.org/Amity/anl/Issue_56_1/gap.htm, 2001.

Schoen S et al: Equity in health care across five nations: summary findings from an international health policy survey, *Int Health Policy 2001*, retrieved 5/02 from www.cmwf. org/programs/international/schoen_snat_ib_388.asp.

Sobel J, Khan AS, Swerdlow DL: Threat of a biological terrorist attack on the US food supply: the CDC perspective, *Lancet* 359(9309):874, 2002.

Sokolovsky J: *CRS report for Congress:* Education and Public Welfare Division, Washington, DC, 1993, Library of Congress.

Taylor MG: The Canadian health insurance program. In Meilicke CA, Storch JL, editors: *Perspectives on Canadian health and social services policy: history and emerging trends.* Ann Arbor, Mich, 1980, Health Administration Press.

Thanassi WT: Immunizations for international travelers, *West J Med* 168(3): 197, 1998.

Tomlinson AJ: Maternal health in lesser developed countries, *Lancet* 347(9003): 769, 1996.

University of Michigan, College of Nursing: *Community-based international learning programs,* retrieved 5/02 from http:// www.nursing.umich.edu/usachina/introduction.html, 2000.

U.S. Department of Health and Human Services: *Healthy people 2010: understanding and improving health,* ed 2, Washington, DC, 2000, U.S. Government Printing Office.

Van der Gaag J, Barham T: Health and health expenditures in adjusting and non-adjusting countries, *Soc Sci Med* 46(8):995, 1998.

VanderMeer DC: *NAFTA prompts health concerns across the borders, September 11,* retrieved 5/02 from http://ehpnel.niehs.nih.gov/doc/1993/101-3/spheres.html, 1998.

Waller AJ, Cammuso BJ: Health care in the new Russia: a Western perspective, *Nurs Forum* 32(3):27, 1997.

World Bank: *World development indicators 1998,* New York, 1998a, Oxford University Press.

World Bank: *Annual review of development effectiveness,* New York, 1998b, Oxford University Press.

World Bank: *World development report 2002: building institutions for markets,* New York, 2002, Oxford University Press.

World Health Organization: *Twelve yardsticks for health,* New York, 1986a, WHO.

World Health Organization: *WHO-CDD: research on vaccine development* [WHO Document CDD/IMV/86.1], Geneva, 1986b, WHO.

World Health Organization: Tuberculosis control and research strategies for the 1990s: memorandum from a WHO meeting, *Bull World Health Organ* 70(1):17, 1992a.

World Health Organization: Women, health and development, *Int Nurs Rev* 40(1):29, 1992b.

World Health Organization: World malaria situation in 1991, *World Health Bull* 72:160, 1994.

World Health Organization: *Health for all: origins and mandate, special publication: the World Health Report: life in the 21st century—vision for all,* Geneva, Switzerland, 1998a, WHO.

World Health Organization: *Malaria: fact sheet #94,* Geneva, 1998b, WHO.

World Health Organization: *Global advisory group on nursing and midwifery,* Geneva, 2000a, WHO.

World Health Organization: *World health report 2000,* Geneva, 2000b, WHO.

World Health Organization: *Health for all* [press release], New York, 2002a, WHO.

World Health Organization: *Afghanistan health status update,* Geneva, 2002b, WHO.

World Health Organization: *WHO emergency and humanitarian action: Afghanistan,* Geneva, 2002c, WHO.

World Health Organization: *Global tuberculosis control: surveillance, planning and financing,* Geneva, 2002d, WHO.

World Health Organization: *Tuberculosis: fact sheet,* Geneva, 2002e, WHO.

World Health Organization/United Nations AIDS Program (WHO/UNAIDS): *WHO and UNAIDS continue to support use of nevirapine for prevention of mother-to-child HIV transmission* [press statement] (22 March), Geneva, 2002, WHO.

World Health Organization/United Nations Children's Fund: *Primary health care,* Geneva, 1978, WHO/UNICEF.

Wouters AV: Health care utilization in lesser developed countries: role of the technology environment in "deriving" the demand for health care, *Bull World Health Organ* 70(3):381, 1992.

Ziegler PB, Anyango H, Ziegler HD: The need for leadership and management for community nurses: results of a Ugandan district health nurse survey, *J Comm Health Nurs* 14(2):119, 1997.

Zollner H, Lessof S: *Population health: putting concepts into action: final report,* Geneva, 1998, WHO.

# Part 2

Influences on Health Care Delivery and Community-Oriented Nursing

In recent years, the U.S. health care system has been criticized for its rapidly rising health care costs, inequalities in the level and quality of services provided from one area of the country to another, and a general lack of accessibility to health services. With approximately 15% of all Americans uninsured, and with that percentage rapidly increasing, it has been recognized that equal access to health care services is not a right, as most Americans think it should be. The inconsistencies in health care are more significant when cost is considered. Health care costs in the United States increased from $24 million in 1960 to over $1 trillion in 2000. However, the budget for public health, the area of health care delivery that focuses on preventing disease and promoting and protecting health, has only about 3% of the total health care budget.

These factors have led to major public health care reform debates at the national and state levels. As a result of the debates, legal, economic, ethical, social, cultural, political, and health-policy issues have become extremely important. Now more than ever in the history of community-oriented nursing, nurses must understand how these issues affect their practice and the outcomes of care.

In the wake of bioterrorism, public health is redefining its role in improving and protecting the nation's health. Nurses, as the largest public health provider workforce, must be a force in redefining the renewed public health system. Understanding the issues that affect decisions about health care priorities is imperative. Knowledge is power.

The chapters in Part 2 provide the community-oriented nurse with an understanding of the economic, ethical, cultural, and policy issues that affect nurses in general and community-oriented nurses in particular.

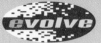
# Economics of Health Care Delivery

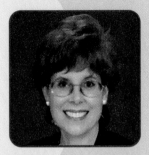

**P. J. Maddox, M.S.N., Ed.D.**
P. J. Maddox is dean of the College of Nursing and Health Science at George Mason University in Fairfax, Virginia. Prior to assuming the deanship, she was assistant dean for graduate health sciences and director of the Office of Research in the Center for Health Policy, Research, and Ethics. Her current research involves evaluation of state telehealth programs, development of federal program funding allocation methodologies, evaluation of state Medicaid program outcomes, and health workforce planning.

## Objectives

After reading this chapter, the student should be able to do the following:

1. Relate economics to nursing and health care
2. Describe the economic theories of microeconomics and macroeconomics
3. Identify major factors influencing national health care spending
4. Analyze the role of government and other third-party payers in health care financing
5. Identify mechanisms for financing health care services delivery
6. Discuss the implications of health care rationing from an economic perspective
7. Evaluate levels of prevention as they relate to health economics

The U.S. health care system is constantly changing, it is competitive, and its resources, available services, and access to technology are limited. The current system encourages health care providers to deliver care outside of traditional settings and discipline boundaries. The changing nature of health care has fostered competition in the health system between clinicians, administrators, providers, payers, consumers, and policy makers. Scarce resources must be managed and the rising costs of health care must be controlled. Policy makers and providers alike have struggled to balance access, quality of health care and services, and rising health care costs.

The United States spends more on health care than any other nation. The cost of health care has been rising more than the rate of inflation since the mid 1960s. Thus nurses are challenged to implement changes in practice and par-

ticipate in research and policy activities designed to provide the best return on investment of health care dollars (i.e., to design models of care, at a reasonable price, that improve access or quality of care). Meeting this challenge requires a basic understanding of the economics of the U.S. health care system. Nurses should be aware of the effects of nursing practice on the delivery of cost-effective care.

**Economics** is the science concerned with the use of resources; **health economics** is concerned with how scarce resources affect the health care industry (Jacobs, 2002). Economics provides the means to evaluate society's attaining its wants and needs in relation to limited resources. In addition to the day-to-day decision making about the use of resources, there is a focus on evaluating economics in health care. This presents challenges to public policy makers (legislators). The allocating of public money often causes conflict because the views and priorities of individuals and groups in our society may differ with those of the health care industry. If money is spent on health care, then money for other public needs, such as education, transportation, recreation, and defense, may be limited (Maddox, 1998).

*The author acknowledges the important foundational work for this chapter developed by Dr. Marcia Stanhope, Dr. Cheryl Bland Jones, and Dr. Karen Macdonald Thompson in previous editions of this book.*

## Key Terms

**budget limits**, p. 99
**business cycle**, p. 101
**capitation**, p. 122
**cost–benefit analysis**, p. 101
**cost–effectiveness analysis**, p. 101
**cost–utility analysis**, p. 101
**demand**, p. 100
**diagnosis-related groups**, p. 116
**economic growth**, p. 101
**economics**, p. 98
**effectiveness**, p. 101
**efficiency**, p. 100

**enabling**, p. 118
**fee-for-service**, p. 121
**gross domestic product**, p. 101
**gross national product**, p. 101
**health care rationing**, p. 123
**health economics**, p. 98
**inflation**, p. 101
**intensity**, p. 103
**macroeconomic theory**, p. 101
**managed care**, p. 119
**managed competition**, p. 120
**market**, p. 99

**means testing**, p. 111
**Medicaid**, p. 116
**medical technology**, p. 103
**Medicare**, p. 115
**microeconomic theory**, p. 99
**prospective payment system**, p. 116
**retrospective reimbursement**, p. 121
**safety net providers**, p. 123
**supply**, p. 100
**third-party payer**, p. 121
**utility**, p. 99
*See Glossary for definitions*

## Chapter Outline

Principles of Economics
*Supply and Demand*
*Efficiency and Effectiveness*
*Macroeconomics*
*Economic Analysis Tools*
The Context of the U.S. Health System
*First Phase*
*Second Phase*
*Third Phase*
*Fourth Phase*
Trends in Health Care Spending

Factors Influencing Health Care Costs
*Demographics Affecting Health Care*
*Technology and Intensity*
*Chronic Illness*
Financing of Health Care
*Public Support*
*Private Support*
Health Care Payment Systems
*Paying Health Care Organizations*
*Paying Health Care Practitioners*

Other Factors Affecting Resource Allocation
  in Health Care
*The Uninsured*
*The Poor*
*Access to Care*
*Rationing Health Care*
*Healthy People 2010*
Primary Prevention
Economics and the Future of Community-
  Oriented Nursing Practice

This chapter provides an overview of selected principles of health economics as a basis for understanding the development of the U.S. health care system and the complex relationships between consumers, providers, and payers of health care services. Knowledge about health economics is particularly important to community-oriented nurses because they are the ones who are often in a position to allocate resources to solve a problem or to design, plan, coordinate, and evaluate community-based health services and programs.

## PRINCIPLES OF ECONOMICS

Two branches of economics are important to understand for their application in health care: microeconomics and macroeconomics. **Microeconomic theory** deals with the behaviors of individuals and organizations and the effects of those behaviors on prices, costs, and the allocating and distributing of resources. Economic behaviors are based on (1) individual or organization choices and the consumer's level of satisfaction with a particular good (product) or service, or **utility,** and (2) the amount of money available to an individual or organization to spend on a particular good or service (its **budget limits**). Microeconomics applied to health care looks at the behaviors of individuals and organizations that result from tradeoffs in utility and budget limits.

A **market** is a network of buyers and sellers of a commodity, such as health care services (Jacobs, 2002). The competitive market explains how the resource allocating process works. However, not all market behavior is competitive. When and how suppliers and those demanding service in the health care market acquire power explains how the prices, quantity, and quality of health services are affected (health system output).

Because of the unique characteristics of health care, some economists believe that health care is special. There are debates about whether health care markets can ensure that health care is delivered efficiently to consumers. Cost–benefit and cost–effectiveness analyses are techniques used to judge the effect of interventions and policies on a particular outcome, such as health status (Jacobs, 2002).

## Supply and Demand

Two basic principles of microeconomic theory are **supply** and **demand,** both of which are affected by price. A simple illustration of the relationship between supply and demand is provided in Figure 5-1. The upward-sloping supply curve represents the seller's side of the market, and the downward-sloping demand curve reflects the buyer's desire for a given product. As shown here, suppliers are willing to offer increasing amounts of a good or service in the market for an increasing price (Jacobs, 2002). The demand curve represents the amount of a good or service the consumer is willing to purchase at a certain price. This curve illustrates that when few quantities of a good or service are available in the marketplace, the price tends to be higher than when larger quantities are available. The point on the curve where the supply and demand curves cross is the equilibrium, or the point where producer and consumer desires meet. Supply and demand curves can shift up or down as a result of the following factors (Jacobs, 2002):
- Competition for a good or service
- An increase in the costs of materials used to make a product
- Technological advances
- A change in consumer preferences
- Shortages of goods or services

Shifting of the supply and demand curve is, in reality, quite complex. For example, consider a specific utility that is available in the market but in low quantity, yet consumers want to purchase more of it. Its producers need time to make or bring to the market what is demanded. Consequently, price rises because of the costs of increased production and getting the product to market quickly. As more of the utility is offered in the marketplace, the consumer demand may fall for the item; then the supply increases, and the price goes down.

## Efficiency and Effectiveness

Two other terms are related to microeconomics: efficiency and effectiveness. **Efficiency** refers to producing maximal output, such as a good or service, using a given set of resources (or inputs), such as labor, time, and available money. Efficiency suggests that the inputs are combined and used in such a way that there is no better way to pro-

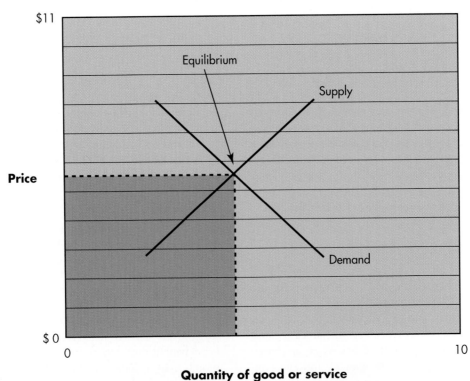

**Figure 5-1** Supply-and-demand curve.

duce the service, or output, and that no other improvements can be made. The word *efficiency* often focuses on time, or speed in performing tasks, and the minimizing of waste, or unused input, during production. Although these notions are true, efficiency depends on tasks as well as processes of producing a good or service, and the improvements made.

**Effectiveness,** on the other hand, refers to the extent to which a health care service meets a stated goal or objective, or how well a program or service achieves what is intended. For example, the effectiveness of a medication is related to how well that medication treats the clinical problem for which it is intended. Box 5-1 illustrates the differences between efficiency and effectiveness (Jacobs, 2002).

## Macroeconomics

Whereas microeconomics focuses on the individual or an organization, **macroeconomic theory** focuses on the "big picture"—the total, or aggregate, of all individuals and organizations (e.g., behaviors such as growth, expansion, or decline of an aggregate). In macroeconomics, the aggregate is usually a country or nation. Factors such as levels of income, employment, general price levels, and rate of economic growth are important. This aggregate approach reflects, for example, the contribution of all organizations and groups within health care, or all industry within the United States, including health care, on the nation's economic outlook.

### ( DID YOU KNOW?

When the media refer to "the economy," the phrase is typically used as a macroeconomic term to describe the wealth and financial performance of the nation in aggregate. Health care contributes to the economy through goods and services produced and employment opportunities.

The primary focuses of macroeconomics are the **business cycle** and economic growth. Business expands and contracts in cycles. These cycles are influenced by a number of factors, such as political changes (a new president is elected), policy changes (a new legislation is implemented), knowledge and technology advances (a new medication to treat depression is placed on the market), or simply the belief by a recognized business leader that the cycle is or should be shifting (e.g., when the head of the Federal Reserve Board changes interest rates).

**Economic growth** reflects an increase in the output of a nation. Two common measures of economic growth are the **gross national product** (GNP) and the **gross domestic product** (GDP). GNP is the total market value of all goods and services produced in an economy during a period of time (e.g., quarterly or annually). GDP is the total market value of the output of labor and property located in the United States (U.S. Department of Health and Human Services [USDHHS], 1998). GDP reflects only the na-

tional U.S. output, whereas GNP reflects national output plus income earned by U.S. businesses or citizens, whether within the United States or internationally. This discussion focuses on GDP, because U.S. health care spending reports are based on GDP (Jacobs, 2002).

Nurses face microeconomic and macroeconomic issues every day. For example, they are influenced by microeconomics when referring clients for services, informing clients and others of the cost of services, assessing community need for a particular service, evaluating client access to services, and determining health provider and agency response to client needs. Nurses who work with aggregates of individuals and communities are faced with macroeconomic issues, such as health policies that make the development of new programs possible; local, state, and federal budgets that support certain programs; and the total effect that services will have on improving the health of the community. In short, knowledge about health economics can enhance a nurse's ability to understand and argue a position for meeting society's needs.

## Economic Analysis Tools

The primary methods utilized to assess the economics of an intervention are **cost–benefit analysis** (CBA), **cost–effectiveness analysis** (CEA), and **cost–utility analysis** (CUA). CBA is considered the best of these methods. In simple form, CBA involves the listing of all costs and benefits that are expected to occur from an intervention during a prescribed time. Costs and benefits are adjusted for time and **inflation** (i.e., they are discounted). If the total discounted benefits are greater than the total discounted costs, the intervention has a *net positive value* (NPV). The top priority is given to the intervention with the highest

---

### BOX 5-1   Efficiency Versus Effectiveness

To illustrate the differences between efficiency and effectiveness, consider the case of a nurse who is designing a community outreach program to educate high-risk, first-time mothers about the importance of childhood immunizations. The most efficient method to disseminate the information to a large number of mothers might be to have the child health team from the public health department hold an evening educational session at the health department open to the public. The most effective means of offering the program might be to link public health nurses with new mothers for one-on-one, in-home counseling, demonstration, and follow-up. The goals of the program could be stated as follows:
- To change the behavior of the mothers regarding providing immunizations for their children
- To increase community mothers' knowledge and awareness of infectious diseases
- To reduce the incidence of preventable infections in the community
- To decrease the number of hospital admissions

## Evidence-Based Practice

Home care agencies, through the use of cost–effectiveness analysis, must explore alternative methods of care delivery if they are to remain competitive in the health care market of the future. The use of TeleHomecare can help agencies maintain a high level of quality while reducing costs. TeleHomecare can be defined as the provision of care, instruction, and education to patients in their place of residence using telecommunication technologies. When home care agencies use technology such as TeleHomecare to become more efficient, it is important that they be able to demonstrate favorable outcomes. The purpose of this article was to describe the strategies employed by an existing TeleHomecare program to document outcomes.

In May 1997, University Home Care (UHC) collaborated with an area health education center and a telemedicine program on a pilot project to evaluate the feasibility of using TeleHomecare to deliver home care services in a rural, underserved region. There are three general categories of outcome data that were collected for all clients receiving TeleHomecare: client health outcomes, agency outcomes, and system outcomes. The functional outcomes, such as bathing, ambulation, elimination, and pain control for TeleHomecare clients, were compared with outcomes for clients receiving traditional home care. The OASIS tool was used to evaluate functional status. Another important clinical indicator was patient satisfaction.

The second category of outcomes that were considered consisted of outcomes that were important for the agency providing the care. Most agencies want to compare the cost of a TeleHomecare visit with that of a traditional visit. Staff productivity was another important concern for the agency. The final agency outcome that was considered was the satisfaction of the nursing and medical staff with TeleHomecare.

Reliability and validity of the data were essential. Thus a systematic data collection procedure was put in place at the beginning of the TeleHomecare program. The TeleHomecare database included information from the UHC clinical record (demographics and OASIS); tools such as the quality-of-life and satisfaction surveys; and data from the parent organization, such as hospital admissions and emergency department visits.

To assess cost, clients with pregnancy-induced hypertension were studied. Those who received a combination of TeleHomecare and traditional home visits were compared with those treated with hospitalization. A significant cost savings was associated with the TeleHomecare approach to treating the clients. TeleHomecare represents how the use of technology can improve the care of clients while improving the financial bottom line of home care agencies.

**Nurse Use:** A nurse who provides only TeleHomecare visits can typically make 15 visits per day, whereas a nurse providing traditional home care typically makes six visits per day.

Britton B et al: Measuring costs and quality of TeleHomecare, *Home Health Care Manage Practice* 12(4):27-32, 2000.

NPV. This technique provides a way to estimate overall program and social benefits in terms of net costs.

CBA requires that all costs and benefits be known and be able to be quantified in dollars; herein lies the major problem with its use. Although it is fairly easy to estimate the direct dollar costs of a health care program, it is often very difficult to quantify the nondollar benefits and indirect costs. For example, benefits and costs could come in the form of increased income and expenses, which are fairly easy to measure. More difficult to measure are benefits such as improved community welfare resulting from a particular program, and the costs to the community that would result if the program did not exist. The value of potential lives lost because of lack of access to health care services is one example.

Cost–effectiveness analysis expresses the net direct and indirect costs and cost savings in terms of a defined health outcome. The total net costs are calculated and divided by the number of health outcomes. Although the data required for CEA are the same as for CBA, CEA does not require that a dollar value be put on the outcome (e.g., on an outcome such as quality of life). CEA is best used when comparing two or more strategies or interventions that have the same health outcome in the population. Both CEA and CBA are useful to nurses as they conduct community needs analyses and develop, propose, implement, and evaluate programs to meet community health needs. In both cases, the cost of a particular program or intervention is examined relative to the money spent and outcomes achieved. The Evidence-Based Practice box illustrates the use of a CEA in health care.

### DID YOU KNOW?

The value of money varies over time. Today's dollar is worth more than tomorrow's dollar. The causes include inflation and interest rates.

An objective commonly used when CEA is performed in health care is improvement in *quality of adjusted life-years* (QALYs) for clients. QALYs are the sum of years of life multiplied by the quality of life in each of those years. The QALY assigns a weight, ranging between 0 (death) and 1 (perfect health), to reflect quality of life during a given pe-

**HOW TO  Do a Cost–Effectiveness Analysis (CEA)**

In a CEA, the outcome of the service option is measured in a natural, nonmonetary unit such as length of stay, years of life gained, therapeutic successes, or lives saved. Results are expressed as the net cost required to produce an outcome. The cost to outcome is expressed as a ratio of cost per unit of outcome, where the numerator is a monetary value corresponding to the net expenditure of resources and the denominator is the net improvement in health expressed in nonmonetary terms. The steps for performing a CEA are as follows:

1. Establish program or service goals and objectives.
2. Consider all possible alternatives to achieve the goal or objectives.
3. Measure net effects to reflect a change in health status or health outcome.
4. Analyze costs for each alternative (adjusting costs for time and inflation) and conduct final cost–effectiveness analysis on marginal costs rather than on total costs.
5. Use multivariate sensitivity analysis and modeling to assess the effect of random error on the cost–effectiveness ratio.
6. Combine CEA results with other types of information, not included in the CEA, to make the most appropriate therapeutic or policy decision.

riod of years (Gold et al, 1996; Haddix et al, 1996). In conducting a CEA, the cost of a program or an intervention is compared with real or expected improvements in clients' quality of life. The How To box lists the steps involved in conducting a CEA. The QALY is often used in malpractice suits to award money to clients who have been injured by health care.

Depending on program or intervention goals, the most effective means of providing a service is not necessarily the least costly, particularly in the short run. This is particularly true in public health, when the cost effectiveness of a preventive service may not be known until some time in the future. For example, the total cost savings of a community no-smoking program might be difficult to project 10 years into the future. After 10 years, the number of lung cancer cases or deaths that have occurred can be compared to those in the 10 years before the program, and the cost effectiveness of the no-smoking program can be shown.

## THE CONTEXT OF THE U.S. HEALTH SYSTEM

The U.S. health care system is a diverse collection of industries that are involved directly or indirectly in providing health care services. The major players in the industry are the health professionals who provide health care services, pharmacy and equipment suppliers, insurers (public/

government and private), managed care plans (health maintenance organizations, preferred provider organizations), and other groups, such as educational institutions, consulting and research firms, professional associations, and trade unions. Today, the health care industry is large, and its characteristics and operations differ between rural and urban geographic areas.

In the twenty-first century, health policy and national politics reflect the importance of health care delivery in the general economy. Conflicts arise between competing special-interest groups who have different goals and objectives when it comes to the producing and consuming of health services. To some degree this is caused by federal and state policy changes about how health services are financed (public and private).

Figure 5-2 illustrates the four basic components that make up the framework of health services delivery: service needs and intensity, facilities, technology, and labor. **Intensity** is the extent of use of technologies, supplies, and health care services by or for the client. Intensity includes and is a partial measure of the use of technology (Banta, 1995a). **Medical technology** refers to "the set of techniques, drugs, equipment, and procedures used by health care professionals in delivering medical care to individuals. It also includes the system within which such care is delivered" (Banta, 1995a).

Health care systems have developed in four phases from the 1800s to today. These developmental stages correspond to different economic conditions. Developmentally, the four components of the health services delivery framework have changed over time, reflecting macro-level, or societal, changes in morbidity and mortality rates, national health policy, and economics (Figure 5-3).

### First Phase

The first developmental stage (1800 to 1900) was characterized by epidemics of infectious diseases, such as cholera, typhoid, smallpox, influenza, malaria, and yellow fever. Health concerns of the time related to social and public health issues, including contaminated food and water supplies, inadequate sewage disposal, and poor housing conditions (Banta, 1995b; Lee and Estes, 2001). Family and friends provided most health care in the home. Hospitals were few in number and suffered from overcrowding, disease, and unsanitary conditions. Sick persons who were cared for in hospitals often died as a result of these conditions. Most people avoided being cared for in a hospital unless there was no alternative. In this first developmental phase, health care was paid for by individuals who could afford it, through bartering with physicians, or through charity from individuals or organizations.

Technology to aid in disease control was very basic and practical but in keeping with the knowledge of the time. The physician's "black bag" contained the few medicines and tools available for treatment. The economics of health care is influenced by the types of health care providers and the number of practitioners, and the labor force then was

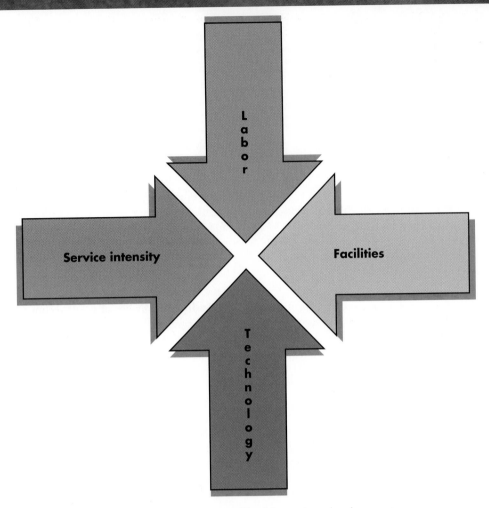

**Figure 5-2** Components of health services development.

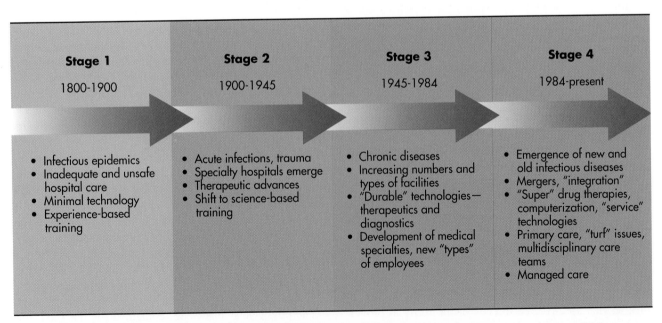

**Figure 5-3** Developmental framework for health service needs and intensity, facilities, technology, and labor.

composed mostly of physicians and nurses who attained their skills through apprenticeships, or on-the-job training. Nurses in the United States were predominantly female, and education was linked to religious orders that expected service, dedication, and charity (Kovner, 1999). The focus of nursing was primarily to support physicians and assist clients with activities of daily living.

## Second Phase

The second developmental stage (1900 to 1945) of U.S. health care delivery was focused on the control of acute infectious diseases. Environmental conditions influencing health began to improve, with major advances in water purity, sanitary sewage disposal, milk and water quality, and urban housing quality. The health problems of this era were no longer mass epidemics but individual acute infections or traumatic episodes (Pickett and Hanlon, 1990).

Hospitals and health departments experienced rapid growth during the late 1800s and early 1900s as technological advances in science were made (Kovner, 1999). In addition to private and charitable financing of health care, city, county, and state governments were beginning to contribute by providing services for poor persons, state mental institutions, and other specialty hospitals, such as tuberculosis hospitals. Public health departments were emphasizing case finding and quarantine. Although health care was paid for primarily by individuals, the Social Security Act of 1935 signaled the federal government's increasing interest in addressing social welfare problems.

Clinical medicine entered its golden age during this period. Major technological advances in surgery and childbirth and the identifying of disease processes, such as the cause of pernicious anemia, increased the ability to diagnose and treat diseases. The discovery and development of pharmacologic agents, such as insulin in 1922 for control of diabetes, sulfa drugs in 1932 for treatment of infectious diseases, and antibiotics such as penicillin in the 1940s, eradicated certain infectious diseases, increased treatment options, and decreased morbidity and mortality rates (Lee and Estes, 2001).

Advances in technology and knowledge shifted physician education away from apprenticeships to scientifically based college education, which occurred as a result of the Flexner Report in 1910. Nurses were trained primarily in hospital schools of nursing, with an emphasis on following and executing physicians' orders. Nurses in training were unmarried and under the age of 30. They provided the bulk of care in hospitals (Kovner, 1999). Public health nurses, who tracked infectious diseases and implemented quarantine procedures, worked more collegially with physicians (Kovner, 1999). In this period the university-based nursing programs were established to accommodate the expanding practice base of nursing. Client education became a nursing function early in the development of the health care delivery system.

## Third Phase

The third developmental stage (1945 to 1984) included a shift away from acute infectious health problems of previous stages toward chronic health problems such as heart disease, cancer, and stroke. These illnesses resulted from increasing wealth and lifestyle changes in the United States. To meet society's needs, the number and types of facilities expanded to include, for example, hospital clinics and long-term care facilities. The Joint Commission on Accreditation of Hospitals, established in 1951 and later renamed the Joint Commission on Accreditation of Health Care Organizations, focused on the safety and protection of the public and the delivery of quality care.

Changes in the overall health of American society also shifted the focus of technology, research, and development. Major technological advances included developments in the realms of chemotherapeutic agents; immunizations; anesthesia; electrolyte and cardiopulmonary physiology; diagnostic laboratories with complex modalities such as computerized tomography; organ and tissue transplants; radiation therapy; laser surgery; and specialty units for critical care, coronary care, and intensive care. The first "test tube baby" was born via in vitro fertilization, and other fertility advances soon emerged.

Health care providers constituted more than 5% of the total U.S. workforce during this period. The three largest health care employers were hospitals, convalescent institutions, and physicians' offices. Between 1970 and 1984 alone, the number of persons employed in the health care industry grew by 90%. The number of personnel employed in the community also increased. The expanding of care delivery into other sites, such as community-based clinics, increased not only the number but also the types of health care employees. For example, physician assistants were trained under the supervision of physicians and employed to assist physicians in delivering routine medical care.

Technologic advances brought about increased special training for physicians and nurses, and care was organized around these specialties. The ongoing shortage of nurses throughout the century was being seen in the 1970s and early 1980s. Nursing education expanded from hospital-based diploma and university-based baccalaureate education to include associate degree programs at the entry level. As the diploma schools of nursing began closing in the early-to-mid 1980s, the number of baccalaureate and associate degree programs began to increase. Graduate nursing education expanded to include the nurse practitioner (NP) and clinical nurse specialist (CNS) to meet increasing demands for the education of nurses in a specialty such as public health. The first doctoral programs in nursing were instituted to build the scientific base for nursing, and to increase the number of nurse faculty members.

The role of the commercial health insurance industry increased, and a strong link between employment and the providing of health care benefits emerged. Furthermore, the federal government's role expanded through landmark policy making that would affect health care delivery well into the twenty-first century. Specifically, the passage of Titles XVIII and XIX of the Social Security Act in 1965 created the Medicare and Medicaid programs, respectively.

The health care system appeared to have access to unlimited resources for growing and expanding.

Throughout the twentieth century, many public health advances were achieved. The life expectancy of U.S. citizens increased and has been related to public health activities. The most important achievements were in vaccinations, improved motor vehicle safety, safer workplaces, safer and healthier foods, healthier mothers and babies, family planning, fluoride in drinking water, and recognizing tobacco as a health hazard (Centers for Disease Control and Prevention, 2001).

## Fourth Phase

The fourth developmental stage (1984 to present) has been a period of limited resources, with an emphasis on containing costs, restricting growth in the health care industry, and reorganizing care delivery. For example, amendments were made to the Social Security Act in 1983 creating diagnostic-related groups and a prospective system of paying for health care provided to Medicare recipients. The 1997 Balanced Budget Act legislated additional federal changes in Medicare and Medicaid. Private-sector employer concerns about the rising costs of health care for employees and fear of profit losses spurred a major change in the delivery and financing of health care. Managed care systems were developed.

This period has included drastic change in the settings and organization of health care delivery. Transforming health care organizations became commonplace, and buzz words of the period were reorganization, reengineering, restructuring, and downsizing. Organization mergers occurred at an increased rate to consolidate care, to save money, and to coordinate care across the continuum (i.e., from "cradle to grave"). Merger discussions focused on *horizontal integration,* which indicated the union of similar agencies (e.g., a merger of hospitals), and *vertical integration* between different types of organizations (e.g., an acute care hospital, long-term care institution, and a home health facility).

These pressures brought about hospital closings and a shifting of care to other settings, such as ambulatory and community-based clinics and specialty diagnostic centers that offer technologies such as magnetic resonance imaging (MRI) and sonography. Rehabilitative, restorative, and palliative care, once delivered in the hospitals, was shifted to other settings, such as subacute care hospitals, specialty rehabilitation hospitals, long-term care institutions, and even individual homes. Although the basis of care delivery was no longer the traditional acute care hospital, the nature of the care delivered in hospitals changed remarkably, as evidenced by the following:
- Patients admitted to hospitals were more acutely ill.
- Length of stay for patients admitted to hospitals became shorter.
- Care delivery became more intense as a result of the first two items.

The widespread use of computers and the internet has enabled society to become increasingly sophisticated about health. The public's increasing knowledge about health care and awareness of health care advances has influenced the demand for health care, such as diagnostic and therapeutic services for treatment. Furthermore, pharmaceutical companies and other technological suppliers actively market their products through television, printed advertisements, the internet, and other sources, so clients rapidly become aware of the new technologies.

Health professionals are dependent on technology to care for clients. Distance, as a barrier to the diagnosis and treatment of disease, has been overcome through the use of telehealth. Health care professionals, along with payers, have become the principal buyers of technology for the client. They often make decisions about when and if a certain technology will be used for a client problem. Nurses have become dependent on technologies to monitor client progress, make decisions about care, and deliver care in innovative ways.

The shift away from traditional hospital-based care to the community, together with the need to consider new models of care, brought about an increased emphasis on primary care, on developing care delivery teams, and on collaborating in practice and education. The substituting of one type of health personnel for another was occurring to control care delivery costs. As examples, the NPs were replacing physicians as primary care providers, and unlicensed personnel were replacing staff nurses in hospitals and long-term care facilities. These replacements caused much debate, with territorial, or "turf," battles, for example, between physicians and nurses.

The increase in specialization by health professionals has led to changes in certification, qualifications, education, and standards of care in health professions. These factors, in turn, have caused an increase in the number and kinds of providers to meet the demands of the health care system. The Bureau of Labor Statistics predicts that health care employment will be among the top 10 industries, with significant employment growth through 2010 (Bureau of Labor Statistics, 1998).

## TRENDS IN HEALTH CARE SPENDING

Much has been written in the popular and scientific literature about the costs of U.S. health care and how society makes decisions about using available and scarce resources. Given that economics in general and health care economics in particular are concerned with resource use and decision making, any discussion of the economics of health care must consider past and current health care spending. The trends shown here reflect public and private decisions about health care and health care delivery in the past. Past spending reflects past decision making; likewise, past decisions reflect the values and beliefs held by society and policy makers that undergird policy making at any given point in time.

According to the Centers for Medicare and Medicaid Services (CMS), national health expenditures will reach $2.8 trillion in 2011 (Heffler et al, 2002). If these projections are accurate, health expenditures will grow at an average annual rate of 7.3%. Health spending will outpace increases in the gross domestic product by 2.5% per year, accounting for 17% of the GDP by 2011. This means that $17 of every $100 spent will be for health care. CMS relates the spending growth to new Medicare, Medicaid, and State Child Health Insurance Plans (SCHIP) (Balanced Budget Act, 1997). The effect of this economic growth represents a large increase in contrast to the approximately 13% GDP spent between 1992 and 2001.

## WHAT DO YOU THINK?

Projections indicate that health care spending will increase, perhaps even double, in less than 10 years, and that health care will represent approximately 17% of the GDP. If this happens, what impact will this increase have on the U.S. society and economy? Is spending 17% of the GDP on health care a concern? Provide rationales for your position.

Table 5-1 shows the growth in U.S. health care expenditures between 1970 and 2000. Spending for health care increased from approximately $24 million in 1960 to over $1.4 trillion in 2000. These numbers reflect per-person spending amounts of $124 in 1960 and $3759 in 1996, an increase of over 3000%. Note that the size of the U.S. population during this period increased by approximately 48% (Heffler et al, 2002; USDHHS, 1998).

## DID YOU KNOW?

The use of GNP versus GDP depends on whether labor and property used to produce a good or service are located in the United States. If labor and property are located in the United States, then output will be counted in the GDP; if labor and property are located outside of the United States, then output is not included in the GDP.

Figure 5-4 shows a breakdown of the distribution in health care expenses for 2000 (National Center for Health Statistics [NCHS], 2000). The largest portions of health care expenses were for hospital care and physician services, 32% and 22%, respectively. Although percentages for both of these categories have fluctuated over time, it is interesting to note that they have both changed since 1980, with hospital care declining from 41% and physician care increasing to 19.2% (USDHHS, 2002). Only a small fraction of total health care dollars was spent on home health (2.5%), public health (3.4%), and research and construction (2.0%) in 2000. For historical reference, these categories were funded at 1.0%, 2.7%, and 2.2% in 1980, suggesting that home health and public health have increased slightly in social value, and that research has declined slightly.

## FACTORS INFLUENCING HEALTH CARE COSTS

Health economists, providers, payers, and politicians have explored a variety of explanations for the rapid rate of increase in health expenses as compared to population growth. That individuals have, over time, consumed more health care is not an adequate explanation. The following factors are frequently cited as having caused the increases in total and per capita health care spending over the past 40 years (Levit, Lazenby, and Braden, 2002): inflation, changes in population demography, and technology and intensity of services. Predicted changes in health care costs are presented in Box 5-2.

## Demographics Affecting Health Care

A major demographic change underway in the United States is the aging of the population. Population changes are also affected by illnesses such as acquired immunodeficiency syndrome and by chemical dependency epidemics. These changes have implications for providers' health services, and they affect the overall costs of health care. Because the majority of older adults and other special

### Table 5-1  Health Care Expenditures 1980-2002

| CALENDAR YEAR | TOTAL HEALTH EXPENDITURES (IN BILLIONS) | TOTAL HEALTH EXPENDITURES PER CAPITA (PER PERSON) (IN BILLIONS) ($) | PERCENT (%) OF GROSS DOMESTIC PRODUCT |
|---|---|---|---|
| 1980 | $249.0 (actual) | $1067 (actual) | 8.8 (actual) |
| 1990 | $695.6 (actual) | $2737 (actual) | 12.0 (actual) |
| 2000 | $1311.1 (projected) | $4681 (projected) | 13.1 (projected) |
| 2001 | $1424.2 (projected) | $5043 (projected) | 13.4 (projected) |
| 2002 | $1541.9 (projected) | $5415 (projected) | 13.9 (projected) |

From Centers for Medicare and Medicaid Services: *National health expenditures,* Washington, DC, 2000, U.S. Government Printing Office.

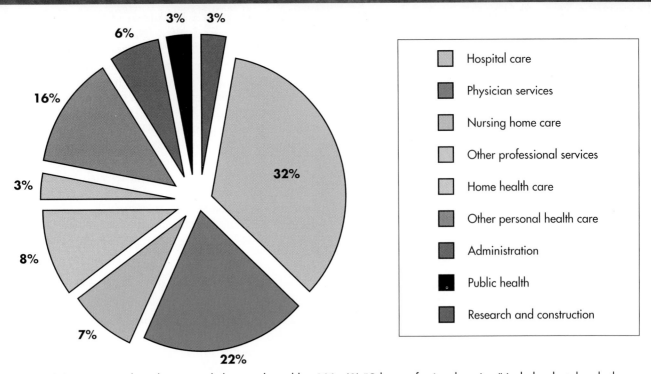

Notes: (1) Percentages have been rounded upward to add to 100. (2) "Other professional services" includes dental and other nonphysician health care services. (3) "Other personal services" includes drugs and other nondurable health care goods, vision products and other durable health care goods, and any other personal health care.

**Figure 5-4** Distribution of U.S. health care expenditures, 2000. *(Data from National Center for Health Statistics: Health: United States, 2000, Hyattsville, Md, 2002, U.S. Government Printing Office.)*

---

**BOX 5-2   Changes in Health Care Spending, 1997 to 2000**

All third-party payers pay the bill for health care. The bill is divided into categories. Health care bills have changed in the following ways:

- The hospital bill has declined from 33.7% of all dollars spent on health care, to 31.7%.
- Dollars for physician services remain about the same at 22% of the bill.
- The pharmaceutical bill has increased from 6.9% to 9.4% of all dollars spent on health care.
- The nursing home care bill has declined slightly from 7.8% to 7.1%.
- The home health care bill has changed from 3.2% to 2.5%.
- Specialists such as podiatrists, optometrists, and chiropractors were paid about 3.0% between 1977 and 2000.
- Although the overall cost of health care has increased faster than the growth in the health care bill, the number of uninsured has grown as individual employees increasingly become more responsible for their own insurance.

Centers for Medicare and Medicaid Services: *National health expenditures,* Washington, DC, 2000, U.S. Government Printing Office.

---

**Table 5-2   Projected Federal Spending for Social Security, Medicare, and Medicaid in 2001**

| | IN BILLIONS ($) | AS % OF TOTAL FEDERAL SPENDING |
|---|---|---|
| Social Security | 429 | 26.0 |
| Medicare | 238 | 14.4 |
| Medicaid | 131 | 7.9 |
| Subtotal | 796 | 48.3 |
| Rest of government | 882 | 52.6 |
| Total | 1651 | 100.0 |

From Congressional Budget Office: *The budget and economic outlook,* Washington, DC, August 2001, U.S. Government Printing Office.

### Table 5-3  Estimated Increases in Population by Age Cohort, Between 1995 and 2030

| AGE AND PERIOD | LOWEST ESTIMATE (%) | MIDDLE ESTIMATE (%) | HIGHEST ESTIMATE (%) |
|---|---|---|---|
| **65+** | | | |
| 1995-2010 | 10.8 | 17.5 | 24.2 |
| 1995-2030 | 75.6 | 106.8 | 136.4 |
| **75+** | | | |
| 1995-2010 | 14.5 | 24.1 | 35.0 |
| 1995-2030 | 71.8 | 116.2 | 164.0 |
| **85+** | | | |
| 1995-2010 | 37.9 | 56.0 | 79.1 |
| 1995-2030 | 59.1 | 132.7 | 235.1 |

From U.S. Bureau of the Census: National Aging Information Center, Washington, DC, 1999, U.S. Government Printing Office.

### Table 5-4  U.S. Health Spending for Older Adults, 1995

| SPENDING CATEGORY | AMOUNT $ (%) |
|---|---|
| Dollars (and percent) of total health spending on older adults | 4594 (38) |
| Estimated dollars (and percent) of gross domestic product (GDP) spent on health for older adults | 725 (5) |
| Dollars (and percent) of GDP spent on health | 1644 (13.6) |
| Dollars (and percent) of health spending per person | 12,090 (400) |

From Organization for Economic Cooperation and Development: *Health data 1999,* as presented in Andersen GF, Hussey PS: Population aging: a comparison among industrialized countries, *Health Aff* 19(3):195, 2000.

were 65 and older in 1990; 1 in 5 are projected to be 65 and older in 2030. In addition, the number of individuals 85 and older is expected to double between 1990 and 2030 (Maddox, 2001). Table 5-3 indicates projections for growth in older adult cohorts projected through 2030.

Although many older adults are independent and active, they are likely to experience multiple chronic conditions that may become disabling. They are admitted to hospitals three times more often than the general population, and their average length of stay is more than 3 days longer than the overall average. They visit physicians more often and make up a larger percentage of nursing home residents than the general population (Maddox, 2001). Table 5-4 shows the economic impact of funding health services for those over age 65, for the most recent year of available data.

Life expectancy and health status have been increasing in the United States. However, older adults continue to consume a large portion of financial resources. Health care providers are concerned about the growth in the older adult population because public funding sources, such as Medicare, have not been increasing their reimbursement rates sufficiently to cover inflation, and thus providers collect a smaller amount for visits by older adult clients each year.

## THE CUTTING EDGE

In 2003, the president suggested a 4% decrease in reimbursing visits for older adults to health care providers.

populations receive services through publicly funded programs, the growing health needs among these populations have great impact on costs, payments, and providers associated with Medicaid and Medicare programs (Table 5-2). As the population ages and the baby boom generation ages and retires, federal expenses for Social Security will increase from 4.2% of the GDP in 2001 to 6.5% of GDP in 2030 (Congressional Budget Office, 2001).

The aging population is expected to affect health services more than any other demographic factor. In 1950, more than half of the U.S. population was under 30 years of age; in 1994, half of the population was 34 years of age or older. In 1990, individuals 65 and older comprised 12% of the population; by 2030 they are estimated to comprise up to 21% of the population. That is, 1 in 8 Americans

The aging of the population also spurs concerns about funding their health care because of changes in the proportion of employed individuals to retired individuals. Persons in the workforce pay the majority of income taxes

**Table 5-5** **Federal Regulations Contributing to Technology/Cost Controls**

| YEAR | FEDERAL REGULATION |
|------|--------------------|
| 1906 | Prescription drug regulation: Food, Drug, and Cosmetic Act, now the U.S. Food and Drug Administration (FDA) |
| 1935 | Social Security Act (PL 74-271): Provides grants-in-aid to states for maternal and child care, aid to crippled children, the blind and aged |
| 1938 | Food, Drug, and Cosmetic Act PL 75-540: Establishes federal FDA protections for drug safety and protections for misbranded goods, drugs, cosmetics |
| 1946 | Hill-Burton Act (PL 79-725): Enacts Hospital Survey and Construction Act providing national direct support for community hospitals; establishes rudimentary standards for construction and planning; establishes community service obligation |
| 1954 | Hill-Burton Act amended (PL 83-482): Expands scope of program for nursing homes, rehabilitation facilities, chronic disease hospitals, and diagnostic or treatment centers |
| 1963 | Community Mental Health and Mental Retardation Centers Construction Act (PL 88-164) |
| 1965 | Medicare Title 18; Medicaid Title 19 (PL 89-97): Amendments to Social Security Act provide Medicare and Medicaid to support health care services for certain groups |
| 1966 | Comprehensive Health Planning Act (PL 89-749): For health services, personnel, and facilities in federal–state–local partnerships |
| 1971 | President Nixon introduces concept of HMOs as the cornerstone of his administration's national health insurance proposal |
| 1972 | Social Security Act amendments (PL 92-603): Extend coverage to include new treatment technologies for end-stage renal disease; provide for professional standards review organizations to review appropriateness of hospital care for Medicare/Medicaid recipients |
| 1973 | HMO Act (PL 93-222): Provides assistance and expansion for HMOs |
| 1975 | National Health Planning and Resources Development Act (PL 93-641): Designates local health system areas and establishes a national certificate-of-need (CON) program to limit major health care expansion at local and state levels |
| 1978 | Medicare End-Stage Renal Disease Amendment provides payment for home dialysis and kidney transplantation; Health Services Research, Health Statistics, and Health Care Technology Act establishes national council on health care technology to develop standards for use |
| 1981 | Omnibus Budget Reconciliation Act of 1981 (PL 97-351): Consolidates 26 health programs into four block grants (preventatives, health services, primary care, and maternal and child health) |
| 1982 | Tax Equity and Fiscal Responsibilities Act (PL 97-248): Seeks to control costs by limiting hospital costs per discharge adjusted to hospital case mix |
| 1983 | Amended Social Security Act (PL 98-21): Establishes new Medicare hospital prospective payment system based on diagnosis related groups (DRGs) |
| 1986 | 1974 Health Planning and Resource Development Act (PL 93-641): Moves CON program to states |
| 1989 | Omnibus Reconciliation Act of 1989 (PL 101-239): Creates physician resource-based fee schedule to be implemented by 1992, with emphasis on high-tech specialties of surgery; creates Agency for Health Care Policy and Research to research effectiveness of medical and nursing services, interventions, and technologies |
| 1990 | Ryan White Care Act (PL 101-381): Authorizes formula-based and competitive supplemental grants to cities and states for HIV-related outpatient medical services |
| 1990 | PL 101-629: Safe Medical Devices Act gives FDA authority to regulate medical devices and diagnostic products |
| 1993 | Omnibus Budget Reconciliation Act (OBRA 93) (PL 103-66): Cuts Medicare funding and ends ROE payments to skilled nursing facilities; provides support for immunizations for Medicaid children |
| 1996 | Health Insurance Portability and Accountability Act enacted to protect health insurance coverage for laid-off or displaced workers |
| 1997 | Balanced Budget Act of 1997 created a new program for states to offer health insurance to children in low-income and uninsured families |
| 1998 | PL 105-33: Authorizes third-party reimbursement for Medicare Part B services for NPs and CNSs |
| 2003 | HR 2295: The Medicaid Nursing Incentive Act expands direct reimbursement to all nurse practitioners and clinical nurse specialists and recognizes specialized services offered by advanced practice registered nurses such as primary care case management, pain management, and mental health services. |

## Table 5-6    Medical Expenditure Panel Survey (MEPS) Reported Health Conditions, 1996

| CONDITION | ESTIMATED NUMBER (MILLIONS) | NATIONAL COST ($, IN BILLIONS) | COST RANKING | ADL/IADL IMPAIRMENT (THOUSANDS) | ADL/IADL IMPAIRMENT (RANK) |
|---|---|---|---|---|---|
| Ischemic heart disease | 3.4 | 21.5 | 1 | 638.3 | 10 |
| Motor vehicle accidents | 7.3 | 21.2 | 2 | 808.6 | 8 |
| Acute respiratory infection | 44.5 | 17.9 | 3 | 1949.6 | 3 |
| Arthropathies | 16.8 | 15.9 | 4 | 3070.0 | 1 |
| Hypertension | 26.0 | 14.8 | 5 | 544.3 | 12 |
| Back problems | 13.2 | 12.2 | 6 | 1380.9 | 5 |
| Mood disorders | 9.0 | 10.2 | 7 | 1400.9 | 4 |
| Diabetes | 9.2 | 10.1 | 8 | 1954.0 | 2 |
| Cerebrovascular disease | 2.0 | 8.3 | 9 | 1084.1 | 6 |
| Cardiac dysrhythmias | 2.9 | 7.2 | 10 | 591.4 | 13 |
| Peripheral vascular disorders | 3.4 | 6.8 | 11 | 889.3 | 11 |
| Chronic obstructive pulmonary disease | 12.4 | 6.4 | 12 | 889.3 | 7 |
| Asthma | 8.6 | 5.7 | 13 | 690.4 | 9 |
| Congestive heart failure | 1.1 | 5.2 | 14 | 494.6 | 14 |
| Respiratory malignancies | 0.3 | 5.0 | 15 | 121.5 | 15 |

*ADL/IADL,* Activities of daily living/instrumental activities of daily living.
From Druss BG et al: The most expensive medical conditions in America, *Health Aff* 21(4):105-111, 2002.

and all Social Security payroll taxes. The funding base for Medicare decreases as the population ages, as retirement rates increase, and as the numbers in the workforce decrease. As a result, some policy makers believe that Medicare and system reforms are needed to ensure adequate financing and delivery of health care services to an aging population (Maddox, 2001).

Health policy reform options being considered include increased age limits to become eligible for Medicare, **means testing** (i.e., determining a lack of financial resources) for Medicare eligibility, increased coverage for long-term care insurance, increased incentives for prevention, and less expensive and more efficient delivery arrangements and care settings (e.g., managed care arrangements). Meanwhile, the debate continues over how to best handle the future funding of the growing Medicare program.

## Technology and Intensity

The introduction of new technology enhances the delivery of care, but it also has the potential to increase the costs of care. As new and more complex technology is introduced into the system, the cost is typically high. However, clients often demand access to the technology, and providers want to use it. In an effort to keep health care costs down, however, payers have attempted to restrict the use of certain technologies. For example, the drug Viagra, developed for the treatment of impotence by Pfizer Pharmaceuticals, is an example of a controversial technologic advance that,

as soon as it was available to the public, was in high demand and prescribed by providers. Use was restricted by payers because of cost.

The adopting of new technology demands investment in personnel, equipment, and facilities. Furthermore, new technology adds to administrative costs, especially if the federal government provides financial coverage for the service or is involved in regulating the technology. Table 5-5 outlines federal policy that has impacted technology and the cost of health care.

## Chronic Illness

Spending for the 15 highest-cost conditions (Table 5-6) accounted for 44.2% of total health care spending in 1996 (Druss et al, 2002). Using Medical Expenditure Panel Survey (MEPS) data, chronic medical conditions were identified by those costing the most, the number of bed days, work-loss days, and activity impairments. The most costly (ischemic heart disease) was ranked tenth in terms of impairment of activities of daily living/instrumental activities of daily living (ADL/IADL). These chronic illnesses account for a great portion of total health costs annually.

## FINANCING OF HEALTH CARE

Against the backdrop of today's chronic conditions, it must be appreciated that health care financing has evolved through the twentieth century from a system supported primarily by consumers, to a system financed by third-party

## *Economic Delivery of Health Care in Canada*

Lianne Patricia Jeffs, R.N., M.Sc., Faculty of Nursing, University of Toronto

### HEALTH EXPENDITURES

Health expenditures continue to rise in Canada, and it currently ranks fifth, with 9.1% of its gross domestic product (GDP) spent on health care, among Organization for Economic Cooperation and Development (OECD) countries in its total health care spending (OECD Statistics, 2002). Health expenditure expressed as a percentage of GDP is a measurement of the proportion of a country's wealth that is devoted to the health of its population. Despite its high ranking, Canada's level of public health expenditure is similar to that of other European countries.

### LEGISLATION GOVERNING CANADA'S FISCAL COMMITMENTS TO HEALTH CARE

Currently, Canada's national health care system is based on two statutes: the Canada Health and Social Transfer (CHST) and the Canadian Health Act (CHA). The CHST is the vehicle through which funds are transferred from the federal government to provinces in support of hospital and medical insurance programs defined by the CHA. The CHA (which operates under five principles—universality, comprehensiveness, accessibility, portability, and public administration) outlines the cost-sharing agreement between the federal and provincial governments. The major federal financial initiatives related to the Canadian health care system are listed (with their dates) in the following table. At first glance, the CHA appears to take a broad definition of health; however, it is restricted to care provided in hospitals and by physicians. Public health and home care are not formally a part of the CHA, which places health promotion and disease prevention programs in the community and public health services at the discretion of the provinces/territories and local municipalities.

| 1948 | Grants for hospital construction and some general services |
| 1953 | Child and Maternal Health Care: Social needs grants fixed amounts (per unit of activity—payment was contingent on provincial reporting to the federal government) |
| 1958 | Hospital Insurance and Diagnostic Services Act: Funding was based on 25% of national per capita costs in the specific province × provincial population. There were specified expenditures, |

no ceiling, and no conditions on provincial financing arrangements.

| 1968 | Medical Care Act (Medicare): Funding was based on 50% of national per capita cost × provincial population; provinces had to comply with four conditions: universality, comprehensiveness, public administration, portability. |
| 1976 | Ceilings were placed on growth of Medicare grant (ceiling limit = population growth + 13% in 1976, and 10.5% in 1977). |
| 1977 | Established Programs Financing (EPF) Act: Equal per capita payment, block funding. |
| 1984 | Canada Health Act: provinces receive full federal payments if they comply with the principles of the CHA—portability, public administration, accessibility, universality, and comprehensiveness. |
| 1996 | Canada Health and Social Transfer: Amalgamated EPF and Canada Assistance Plan into one cash transfer, fixed cash transfer for 1996-97 and 1997-98. |

A recent seminal report (Romanow, 2002) recommended the provision of stable, predictable, and long-term funding through a new, dedicated, cash-only transfer for Medicare (Canada Health Transfer—CHT—in place of the existing CHST) and modernizing the CHA by expanding (1) coverage to diagnostic services and priority home care services and (2) accountability as the sixth principle. Action, including policy direction and resource allocation, is now required at both the federal and provincial/territorial levels to operationalise these recommendations.

### FINANCING OF THE CANADIAN HEALTH CARE SYSTEM

Financing of health care in Canada shifted from the private to the public sector in 1957. For over 40 years, the publicly funded health care system has been financed mainly with taxes and premiums collected by federal and provincial governments. The shortage of resources in the health care system and pressures of globalization and trade liberalization have opened the door to private initiatives, which threatens the viability of a publicly funded health care system. Financing of the Canadian health care system has both public and private sources. The methods of funding in the public sector are the result of a redistribution of public funds to institutions.

payers (public and private). Table 5-7 shows changes in the percentage of financing according to the source. From 1980 to 2000, the percentage of third-party public insurance payments increased dramatically. Combined state and federal government payments are currently higher than those of private payers. In 2000, public sources paid the most.

## Public Support

The U.S. federal government became involved in health care financing for population groups early in its history. In 1798 the federal government created the Marine Hospital Service to provide medical care for sick and disabled sailors, and to protect the nation's borders against the im-

Public sources include consolidated revenue funds, earmarked taxes, intergovernmental transfers, employer-based taxes, and volunteer and federal expenditures. Private sources include private insurance, point-of-service charges, philanthropic donations, lotteries, and premiums (Deber et al, 1998; Maslove, 1998; Scott, 1998). The following chart outlines the financing of Canada's health care system (adapted from the Romanow Commission Interim Report, February 2002).

**Citizens**
- Payment of federal taxes
- Payment of provincial taxes
- Direct purchase of private insurance (often through employers)
- Direct purchase of medical and non-medical services

**Federal government**
- CHST (to provinces)
- Equalization support to less wealthy provinces
- Programs for medical and nonmedical research and public health
- Direct health services for selected First Nations populations, veterans, military personnel

**Provinces/territories**
- Program and service payments to providers, institutions, and health authorities for "medically necessary" doctor and hospital services under the CHA
- Supplementary programs not covered by the CHA (home care, long-term care, drug coverage for some residents)
- Programs for medical and nonmedical research and public health

In Canada, governments have five main methods of payment to finance activities of their institutions: payment by global budget, per capita payment, payment by episode of care, fee-for-service, and per diem payment (Deber et al, 1998). Funding is distributed from the provincial governments' central health budget directly to individual and institutional providers within the municipalities/regions in a single-payer funding mechanism. Community health centres (CHCs), health service organisations (HSOs), and Community Care Access Centres (CCACs) receive global funding from the provincial government, and the funds are allocated for salaries, services and operating costs according to the needs of the community they serve.

## FEDERAL, PROVINCIAL, AND MUNICIPAL ROLES IN THE ECONOMIC DELIVERY OF HEALTH CARE

Because health care is under provincial jurisdiction, the federal government has no direct power or influence to ensure that provincial insurance plans cover health care services of other health care providers outside hospitals and in the community and public health sectors. This has become problematic as technological advances have allowed more care to be provided in the community and in home settings, and it is delivered mainly by registered nurses and other nonphysician providers. Some of the provinces have made attempts to convert institution-based services to community-based services; however, resources have not always followed. With the current funding arrangements, it is difficult to shift funds from one organization to another. At the provincial level, health insurance acts and other legislation define what each health plan will pay for and under what conditions.

Several provinces have extended their funding umbrella to provide fairly inclusive and comprehensive public health and health promotion health systems; however, coverage varies among provinces and territories.

## References

Deber R et al: The public–private mix in health care. In *Striking a balance, vol 4: health care systems in Canada and elsewhere*, pp. 423-545, Quebec, 1998, Minister of Public Works and Government Services.

Maslove AM: National goals and the federal role in health care. In *Striking a balance, vol 4: health care systems in Canada and elsewhere*, pp. 413-414, Quebec, 1998, Minister of Public Works and Government Services.

Organization for Economic Cooperation and Development: *Health Data*, 2002: a comparative analysis of 30 countries. Pans, 2002, OECD. Available at www.oecd.org.

Romanow R: *Building on values: the future of health care in Canada: final report*, Ottawa, 2002, Commission on the Future of Healthcare in Canada, available at www.healthcarecommission.ca.

Romanow R: *Shape the future of health care: interim report*, Ottawa, 2002, Available at www.healthcarecommission.ca.

Scott G: International comparison of the hospital sector. In *Striking a balance, vol 4: health care systems in Canada and elsewhere*, pp. 3-31, Quebec, 1998, Minister of Public Works and Government Services.

*Canadian spelling is used.*

porting of disease through seaports. The Marine Hospital Service is considered the first national health insurance plan in the United States. The National Health Board was established in 1879 and was later renamed the United States Public Health Service (PHS). Within the PHS, the federal government developed a public health liaison with state and local health departments for the purpose of controlling communicable diseases and improving sanitation. Additional health programs were also developed to meet obligations to federal workers and their families within the PHS, the Department of Defense, and the Veterans Administration (see Chapters 3 and 8).

**Table 5-7   Health Services and Supplies, Expenditures in Aggregate Dollars by Source for Selected Years Between 1980 and 2010\***

| YEAR | TOTAL $ (BILLIONS/%) | OUT-OF-POCKET PAYMENTS ($/%) | TOTAL THIRD-PARTY PAYMENTS ($/%) | PRIVATE HEALTH INSURANCE ($/%) | OTHER PRIVATE ($/%) | PUBLIC TOTAL ($/%) | PUBLIC: FEDERAL ($/%) | PUBLIC: STATE/ LOCAL ($/%) | MEDICARE ($/%) | MEDICAID ($/%) |
|---|---|---|---|---|---|---|---|---|---|---|
| 1980 | $233.5 | $58.3 | $175.2 | $68.2 | $9.4 | $97.6 | $66.0 | $31.6 | $37.4 | $26.0 |
|  | 100.0 | 25 | 75 | 29.2 | 4.0 | 41.8 | 28.3 | 13.5% | 16.0 | 11.1 |
| 1990 | 669.2 | 137.8 | 531.5 | 232.6 | 31.2 | 267.6 | 181.7 | 85.9 | 110.2 | 73.6 |
|  | 100.0 | 20.6 | 79.4 | 34.8 | 4.7 | 40.0 | 27.2 | 12.8 | 16.5 | 11.0 |
| 2000* | 1268.2 | 202.5 | 1065.7 | 438.4 | 64.4 | 562.8 | 393.8 | 169.1 | 227.0 | 201.8 |
|  | 100.0 | 16.0 | 84.0 | 34.6 | 5.1 | 44.4 | 31.1 | 13.3 | 17.9 | 15.9 |
| 2002* | 1378.1 | 1492.8 | 239.5 | 1253.3 | 530.6 | 76.6 | 646.2 | 451.4 | 259.2 | 233.1 |
|  | 100.0 | 16.0 | 84.0 | 35.5 | 5.1 | 43.3 | 30.2 | 13.0 | 17.4 | 15.6 |
| 2010* | 2558.4 | 404.0 | 2154.4 | 902.6 | 122.8 | 1129.0 | 780.4 | 348.6 | 441.4 | 446.0 |
|  | 100.0 | 15.9 | 84.1 | 36.3 | 5.0 | 42.8 | 29.7 | 13.1 | 16.9 | 16.2 |

\*Projected.
From Centers for Medicare and Medicaid Services, Office of the Actuary, July 17, 2002.

**Table 5-8  Comparison of Medicare and Medicaid Program Features**

| FEATURE | MEDICARE | MEDICAID |
|---|---|---|
| Where to obtain information | Local Social Security Administration office | State welfare office |
| Recipients | Client is 65 years or older, disabled, or has permanent kidney failure | Specified low-income and needy, children, aged, blind, and/or disabled; those eligible to receive federally assisted income |
| Type of program | Insurance | Insurance |
| Government affiliation | Federal | Joint federal/state |
| Availability | All states | All states |
| Financing of hospital insurance | Medicare Trust Fund, mandatory payroll deduction, recipient deductibles, trust fund interest | Federal and state governments |
| Financing of medical insurance | Recipient premium payments; general revenue, U.S. Treasury | Federal and state governments |
| Types of coverage | Inpatient and outpatient hospital services, skilled nursing facilities (SNF), limited home health services | Inpatient and outpatient hospital services; prenatal care; vaccines for children; physician, dental, nurse practitioner, and nurse midwife services; SNF services for persons 21 or older; family services; rural health clinic |

From USDHHS, Centers for Medicare and Medicaid Services, 2002.

Medicare and Medicaid, two federal programs administered by the Centers for Medicare and Medicaid Services (formerly the Health Care Financing Administration), account for the majority of public health care spending. Table 5-8 compares these programs. CMS is the federal regulatory agency within the U.S. Department of Health and Human Services that is responsible for overseeing and monitoring Medicare and Medicaid spending. This agency routinely collects and reports actual health care use and spending and projects future spending trends. Through these programs, the federal government purchases health care services for population groups through independent health care systems, such as managed care organizations, private practice physicians, and hospitals.

## Medicare

The **Medicare** program, established in Title XVIII of the Social Security Act of 1965, provides hospital insurance and medical insurance to persons aged 65 and over, permanently disabled persons, and persons with end-stage renal disease—altogether approximately 39 million people. Medicare has two parts: Part A (hospital insurance) covers hospital care, home care, and skilled nursing care (limited); Part B (noninstitutional care insurance) covers medical care, diagnostic services, and physiotherapy.

Medicare Part A is primarily financed by a federal payroll tax that is paid by employers and employees. The proceeds from this tax go to the Hospital Insurance Trust Fund, which is managed by CMS. Part A coverage is available to all persons who are eligible to receive Medicare.

Older adults comprise the majority of individuals eligible. There is concern about the future of the Medicare Trust Fund, as projected expenses may be more than the trust fund resources. Payments to hospitals for covered services have been and continue to be higher than fund growth. Thus Medicare reimbursement policy has been changing in an attempt to control increasing hospital costs. As of 2002, Part A required a deductible from recipients of $812 for the first 60 days of services and $203 for 61 to 90 days of service, based on a rate equal to a 1-day stay in the hospital. The deductible has increased as daily hospital costs have increased (CMS, 2000). For skilled nursing facility care, persons pay nothing for the first 20 days and up to $101.50 per day for days 21 through 100.

The medical insurance package, Part B, is a supplemental (voluntary) program that is available to all Medicare eligible persons for a monthly premium. The vast majority of Medicare covered persons elect this coverage. The deductible is currently $100 per calendar year (CMS, 2000). Part B provides coverage for services (other than hospital, physician care, outpatient hospital care, outpatient physical therapy, and home health care) that are not covered by Part A, such as laboratory services, ambulance transportation, prostheses, equipment, and some supplies. After a deductible, up to 80% of reasonable charges are paid for these services. Part B resembles the major medical insurance coverage of private insurance carriers. Figure 5-5 shows the total expenses of the Medicare program from 1970 to 2000.

Since the passing of the Medicare amendments to the Social Security Act in 1965, the cost of Medicare has

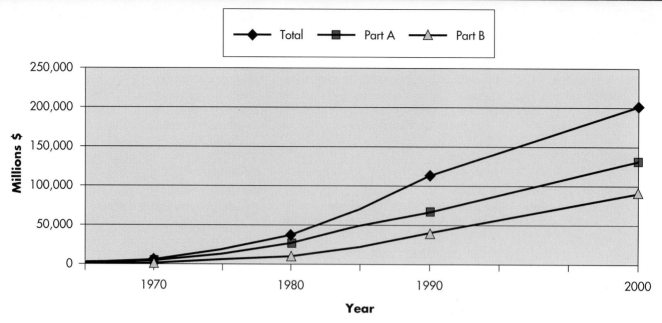

**Figure 5-5** Medicare expenditures for selected years from 1970 to 2000. Year 2000: *Total*, 222 million; *A*, 131 million; *B*, 91 million. *(Data from National Center for Health Statistics: Health: United States, 2000, Hyattsville, Md, 2002, U.S. Government Printing Office.)*

increased dramatically. Hospital care continues to be the major factor contributing to Medicare costs. However, because of the shorter hospital stays, home health and nursing home costs have increased dramatically. As a result of rising health costs, Congress passed a law in 1983 that radically changed Medicare's method of payment for hospital services. In 1983 federal legislation (PL98-21) mandated an end to cost-plus reimbursement by Medicare and instituted a 3-year transition to a **prospective payment system** (PPS) for inpatient hospital services. The purpose of the new hospital payment scheme was to shift the cost incentives away from the providing of more care and toward more efficient services. The basis for prospective reimbursement is the 468 **diagnosis-related groups** (DRGs). Also, the Balanced Budget Act of 1997 determined that payments to Medicare skilled nursing facilities (SNFs) would be made on the basis of the PPS, effective July 1, 1998. The PPS payment rates cover SNF services, including routine, ancillary, and capital-related costs (Health Care Financing Administration [HCFA], 1998b).

Older adults spend about 20% of their income on health care, and 66% of older adults who have Medicare purchase private supplemental health insurance (HCFA, 1998a). This is because of the limits in Medicare coverage, including certain preventive care, and the limited number of physicians and agencies who accept Medicare and Medicaid payment. Older adults who do not have supplemental insurance must cover the difference between the Medicare payment and the additional costs for services.

## Medicaid

The **Medicaid** program, Title XIX of the Social Security Act of 1965, provides financial assistance to states and counties to pay for medical services for poor older adults, the blind, the disabled, and families with dependent children. The Medicaid program is jointly sponsored and financed with matching funds from the federal and state governments. Currently, 23 million people are enrolled in Medicaid (NCHS, 2002). Medicaid expenditures from 1972 to 1998 are shown in Figure 5-6. Since the beginning of Medicaid, full payment has been provided for five types of services (USDHHS, 1998):

1. Inpatient and outpatient hospital care
2. Laboratory and radiology services
3. Physician services
4. Skilled nursing care at home or in a nursing home for people over 21 years of age
5. Early periodic screening, diagnosis, and treatment (EPSDT) for those under 21 years of age

The 1972 Social Security amendments added family planning to the list of full-pay services. States can choose to add prescriptions, dental services, eyeglasses, intermediate care facilities, and coverage for the medically indigent as program options. By law, the medically indigent are required to pay a monthly premium.

Any state participating in the Medicaid program is required to provide the six basic services to persons who are below state poverty income levels. Optional programs are provided at the discretion of each state. In 1989, changes in Medicaid required states to provide care for children less than 6 years of age and to pregnant women under 133% of the poverty level. For example, if the poverty level were $12,000, a pregnant woman could have a household income as high as $16,000 and still be eligible to receive care under Medicaid. These changes also provided for pediatric and family nurse practitioner reim-

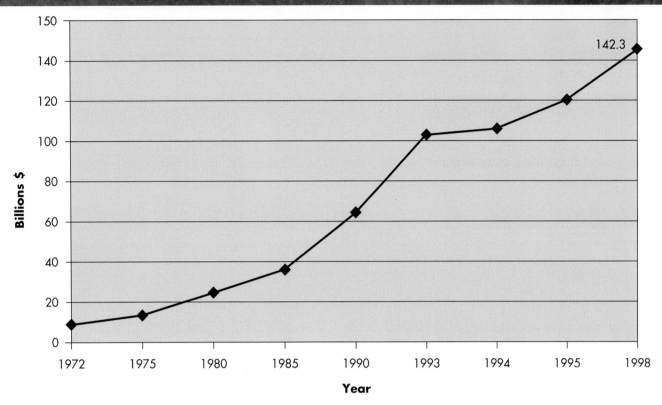

**Figure 5-6** Medicaid expenditures for selected years from 1972 to 1998. *(Data from National Center for Health Statistics: Health: United States, 2000, Hyattsville, Md, 2002, U.S. Government Printing Office.)*

bursement. In the 1990s, states were allowed to petition the federal government for a waiver. If the waiver was approved, the states could use their Medicaid monies for programs other than the six basic services. The first waiver to be approved was given to Oregon for their health care reform plan. Other states have received waivers to develop Medicaid managed care programs for special populations.

The major expense categories for the Medicaid program have historically been skilled and intermediate nursing home care and inpatient hospital care. When combined, these two categories account today for 37.5% of all costs to the program (NCHS, 2002).

## Public Health

Most public government agencies operate on an annual budget, and they plan for costs by estimating salaries, expenses, and costs of services for a year. Public health agencies, such as health departments and WIC programs (for women, infants, and children), receive primary funding from taxes, with additional money for select goods and services through private third-party payers. Selected public health programs receive reimbursement for services as follows: through grants given by the federal government to states for prenatal and child health; through Medicare and Medicaid for home health, nursing homes, WIC programs, and EPSDT; and through collecting of fees on a sliding scale for select client services, such as immunizations.

In 2000 only 3.4% of all health care–related federal funds were expended for federal health programs such as WIC, versus 96.6% for other types of health and illness care (such as hospital and physician services, for example). In addition to this 3.4% allotment, public health funds also come through states and territorial health agencies. State and local governments contributed 14.8% to public and general assistance, maternal and child health, public health activities, and other related services in 2000; the portion contributed to health care through state and local governments has remained the same since 1995 (NCHS, 2002).

## Other Public Support

The federal government finances health services for retired military persons and dependents through the Civilian Health and Medical Program of the Uniformed Services (CHAMPUS), the Veteran's Administration (VA), and the Indian Health Service (IHS). These programs are very important in providing needed health care services to these populations (see Chapters 3 and 8).

## Private Support

Private health care payer sources include insurance, employers, managed care, and individuals. Although insurance and consumers have been prominent health care payment sources for some time, the role of employers and managed care became increasingly prominent and powerful during the last two decades of the twentieth century, particularly as concerns grew about the use and changing nature of health insurance.

## Evolution of Health Insurance

Insurance for health care was first offered by the private sector in 1847 by a commercial insurance company. The purpose of the insurance was to provide security and protection when health care services were needed by individuals. The idea behind insurance was that it provided security, guaranteeing (within certain limits) monies to pay for health care services to offset potential financial losses from unexpected illness or injury related to accidents, catastrophic communicable diseases, such as smallpox and scarlet fever, and recurring (but unexpected) chronic illnesses.

A comprehensive study in the 1920s by the Committee on the Costs of Medical Care showed that a small portion of the population was paying most of the costs of medical care for the majority of the people. The Depression of the 1930s, rising medical costs, and the need to spread financial risk across communities spurred the development of the third-party payment system. The system began as a major industry in the 1930s with the Blue Cross system, which initially provided prepayment for hospital care. In 1939 Blue Shield created plans to provide physician payment. The Blue Cross plans began as tax-free, nonprofit organizations established under special **enabling** legislation in various states.

In the 1940s and 1950s, hospital and medical–surgical coverage increased. Employee group coverage appeared, and profit-making commercial insurance underwriters began offering health insurance packages with competitive premiums. The commercial insurance companies could offer lower premium rates because of the methods used to set rates. Insurance and premium setting, in general, are based on the notion of risk pooling (i.e., insurance companies were willing to risk the unlikely event that all or even a large portion of individuals covered under a plan would need payment for health services at any given time). Blue Cross used a *community rate*, establishing a similar premium rate for all subscribers regardless of illness potential. In contrast, the commercial companies used an *experience rate*, in which the premium was based on an estimate of the illness *risk* or the number of claims to be made by the subscriber (Jacob, 2001).

Premium competition, the offering of health insurance as a fringe benefit, and the use of health insurance as a negotiable collective bargaining item led to an increase in covered benefits, first-dollar coverage for medical care expenses, and increased employer-paid premiums. In turn, these factors pushed up insurance premium costs and health care costs and enabled insurance plans to cover high-cost segments of the population (the aged, poor, or disabled) because of the number of low-risk enrollees.

The health needs of high-risk populations led to the passage of Medicare and Medicaid legislation. These and other national health programs targeted health care coverage for specific population groups. Because these programs directed additional money into the health care system to subsidize care, there were financial incentives to encourage the providing of services (i.e., the more services that were ordered, the greater the amount of money that would be received). Other incentives were related to the use of services by clients (i.e., the more available the payment was for services that might otherwise have gone unused, the more services that were requested).

The Congressional Budget Office projected that private insurance premiums would on average increase about 5.1% per year between 1996 and 2007 (Congressional Budget Office, 2001). However, a greater increase in premiums may occur in the future as a result of pressure from employers, consumers, and policy makers. Driving forces behind this pressure are quality of care, clients' rights, and the concern that these areas are being compromised in the managed care system. Furthermore, the initial cost savings from managed care may have occurred already, and costs will have to be increased to simply maintain coverage, not to mention providing new services and technologies.

## Employers

Since the beginning of Blue Cross and Blue Shield, health insurance has been tied to employment and the business sector. This tie was strengthened during World War II to compensate, attract, and retain employees. Since that time, employers have played the major role in determining health insurance benefits.

Approximately 75% of private businesses provided for health insurance in 1997, compared with approximately 79% in 1965. Approximately 50% of the insurance premium was paid by employers (up from approximately 16% in 1965) and 50% by the employee (NCHS, 2002). This substantial contribution to health care by the private business sector gives the employer a lot of health care buying power in making policy about what services insurance will cover.

Before the growth of insurance (i.e., before 1930 and the beginning of Blue Cross), the health care consumer had more influence over health care costs because payment was out-of-pocket. Consumers made decisions about how they would spend their money, making certain tradeoffs—for

## THE CUTTING EDGE

Although employers originally offered health benefits to attract and retain employees, in the first 3 years of the twenty-first century employers were faced with increasing health insurance costs. Furthermore, the advantages of paying for employees' insurance were counterbalanced by reduced profits. With less money to pay for the programs, businesses began dropping the health insurance benefit or asking the employees to pay more of the cost.

example, about the type of health care they were willing to buy and how much they would pay. Entering the system was restricted in large part to those who could afford to pay for care, or to those few who could find care financed through charitable and philanthropic organizations. With the beginning of the insurance or third-party payer system, health care costs were set by payers, and they determined the type of care or service that would be offered and its price. This began to change somewhat in the 1980s with the increased use of managed care.

As the cost of health insurance has increased, some employers, in an effort to bypass the costs established by insurers, have found it less costly to self-insure. The employer does this by contracting directly with providers to obtain health care services for employees rather than going through health insurance companies. Some large businesses directly employ onsite providers for care delivery or offer onsite wellness programs. These programs within the private sector offer opportunities for nurses to provide wellness programs and health assessments to screen and monitor employees and their families. This move to self-insure has resulted in savings to companies and has reduced overall sick care costs (Knickman and Thorpe, 1999).

In a truly competitive market, the consumer buys goods and services at will, knowing the costs and expected value of services bought, and can choose the provider of those services. In the health system where a third party pays for the services, this transaction has less meaning. The third party makes decisions about the level and type of care that will be purchased for clients and determines how payment will be made. The service provider and client have no influence on how services will be reimbursed. However, the consumer may select the payer/plan and indeed may influence the system through political channels.

In 2000, individuals paid only approximately 17% of total health expenditures out-of-pocket (NCHS, 2002). However, these figures do not reflect the amount of money the consumer pays in taxes to finance government-supported programs such as Medicare and Medicaid, insurance premiums, and money paid for supplemental insurance to cover the gaps in a primary health insurance policy or Medicare.

The average monthly cost for private health insurance has increased greatly through the years. Premiums reflect a shift of the health care cost burden from employers to employees as the percent of employer contributions to health care declines. The decrease in employer contribution to health insurance premiums parallels the move away from traditional insurance plans and toward managed care plans by both small and large employers.

From an economic point of view, the shift in responsibility for the cost of health insurance is not bad. In theory, this shift makes consumers more knowledgeable about (sensitive to) the price of health services. This means that they have more information for health care decision making and consider price in making the decision to access types of health care services. Satisfaction with the quality

of service rests with the person buying the insurance and receiving health care. Two factors, then—the shifting of responsibility for health insurance premiums to employees and the changing demographics of the workforce in general—have resulted in a decline in employee enrollment in health insurance plans. Employees are choosing to use their resources in other ways and are willing to assume the risks of having an illness for which they may have to pay (Ginsberg, Gabel, and Hunt, 1998).

Given that access to health insurance is tied to employment, there was growing concern in the late 1980s and early 1990s about the employment layoffs and downsizing occurring in private business. Those who lost their jobs lost their ability to pay for health insurance and to qualify to purchase insurance privately. The Health Insurance Portability and Accountability Act of 1996 (HIPAA) was enacted to protect health insurance coverage for workers and families after a job change or loss (HCFA, 1999). Although this has increased the number of people who have access to health insurance and health care, there are claims that individual premiums are high, that insurance companies have lost their ability to pool risks, and that HIPAA is just one more federal control mechanism undermining competitive market influences (Nichols and Blumberg, 1998).

## Managed Care Arrangements

**Managed care** is the term for a variety of health care arrangements that integrate the financing and the delivery of health care. Managed care offers an array of services to purchasers, such as employers or Medicare, for a set fee. This fee, in turn, is used to pay providers through preset arrangements for services delivered to individuals who are covered (USDHHS, 1998). The concept of managed care is based on the notion that the use of costly care could be reduced if consumers had access to care and services that would prevent illness through consumer education and health maintenance. Therefore managed care uses disease prevention, health promotion, wellness, and consumer education. In addition to prevention and health promotion, managed care also makes use of *utilization review*—processes that determine how necessary and appropriate the care is. Utilization review often includes the use of second opinions to ensure that care was necessary, hospital admissions were preauthorized, and care was received as intended (Thorpe, 1995).

Two common types of managed care are health maintenance organizations (HMOs) and preferred provider organizations (PPOs). Box 5-3 provides an overview of HMOs and PPOs. Although they seem relatively new to many clients of care, HMOs have actually been around since the 1940s. The Health Maintenance Organization Act was enacted in 1972, and since that time, the number of individuals receiving care through HMOs and other types of managed care organizations has increased considerably: between 1976 and 2000, the number of individuals enrolled in an HMO increased from 6 million to almost

---

**BOX 5-3   Types of Managed Care**

1. A Health Maintenance Organization (HMO) is a provider arrangement whereby comprehensive care is provided to plan members for a fixed, "per member per month" fee. Common features include the following:
   a. Capitation
   b. Use of designated providers
   c. Point-of-service care, or receiving care from nondesignated plan providers
   d. One of the following models:
      (1) Staff model, whereby physicians are HMO employees
      (2) Group model, whereby a physician group practice contracts with the HMO to provide care
      (3) Individual practice association (IPA), whereby the HMO contracts with physicians in solo, small group practices, or physician networks to provide care
      (4) Mixed model, whereby the HMO uses a combination group/IPA arrangement
2. A Preferred Provider Organization (PPO) is a provider arrangement whereby predetermined rates are established for services to be delivered to members. Common features include the following:
   a. Hospital and physician providers
   b. Discounted rate setting
   c. Financial incentives to encourage plan members to select PPO providers
   d. Expedited claims payment to providers

From Folland S, Goodman AC, Stano M: The economics of health and health care, New York, 1993, Macmillan; U.S. Department of Health and Human Services: *Health: United States, 1998,* DHHS Publication No. (PHS) 98-1232, Washington, DC, 1998, U.S. Government Printing Office.

---

79 million; the percent of the population enrolled in an HMO increased from approximately 3% to 28% (NCHS, 2002).

Managed care is based, in part, on the principals of managed competition. **Managed competition** was introduced in health care in the late 1980s and early 1990s to address the increasing costs of health care and to introduce quality into the forefront of discussions. Managed competition simply means that clients make decisions, and choose the health care services they want, on the basis of the quality or reputation of the service. To make decisions, they use knowledge and information about health care problems, care, and providers, and they look at the costs of care.

Several basic issues, however, prevent the full implementation of managed competition in health care:

1. "Information asymmetry" exists in health care, whereby consumers do not have full knowledge of a health problem or health care delivery options, nor do they always want that knowledge. Although access to the internet and the readily accessible health care news in the media have increased awareness of certain health care problems, all information is not currently available to many individuals.
2. The costs of care are not openly shared. Providers are hesitant to give out cost information, and consumers do not know if the price is consistent with the level or quality of care received.
3. Information on outcomes and quality of care delivered by providers and health plans is not readily available, and even when related information *is* available, it is often overlooked in decision making. For example, a survey report of the Commonwealth Fund found that information is not frequently used by employers to make decisions about selection of managed care plans: accreditation data is required by only 9% of employers, and quality of care data is used by only 6% of employers. Furthermore, only 1% of surveyed employers pass information about health plan quality on to their employees (Commonwealth Fund, 1998).
4. Financial incentives for employees, employers, providers, and payers foster market resistance to change in the delivery and financing of health care. For example, labor unions want health benefits to remain a part of employment compensation, but employers are losing tax incentives to continue providing health benefits.
5. Adequate and sufficient data on which to base health care decisions are not available.

In short, health care is a complex market and not one wherein information about health care, health problems, and the costs of care is easy to get. Nonetheless, managed care represents a step toward managed competition, even if it does not fully embrace and realize all its issues.

## Medical Savings Accounts

Another insurance reform discussion at the political level concerns medical savings accounts (MSAs). MSAs are touted as a way of turning health care decision-making control over to the individuals receiving care. MSAs are tax-exempt accounts available to individuals who work for small companies, established usually through a bank or insurance company, that enable the individuals to save money for future medical needs and expenses (IRS, 1998). Money is contributed to an MSA by the employer, and the initial money put into an MSA does not come out of taxable income. Also, interest earned in MSAs is tax free, and unused MSA money can be held in the account from year to year until the money is used. MSAs, in theory, would allow individuals to make cost/quality tradeoffs and would require that individuals become knowledgeable about health care, become involved in health care decision making, and take responsibility for the decisions made. Providers, in turn, must be willing to provide and disclose information to individuals and give up control of health care decision making. The HIPAA and MSAs are examples of health insurance reform efforts, and these efforts will very likely remain in the forefront of political discussions for some time to come.

## HEALTH CARE PAYMENT SYSTEMS

Several methods have been used by public and private sources to pay health care providers for health care services. These include retrospective and prospective reimbursement for paying health care organizations, and fee-for-service and capitation for paying health care practitioners (Knickman and Thorpe, 1999).

## Paying Health Care Organizations

**Retrospective reimbursement** is the traditional reimbursement method, whereby fees for the delivery of health care services in an organization are set after services are delivered (Knickman and Thorpe, 1999). In this scenario, reimbursement is based on either organization costs or charges. The cost method reimburses organizations on the basis of cost per unit of service (e.g., home health visit, patient-day) for treatment and care. Costs include all or a percent of added, allowable costs. Allowable costs are negotiated between the payer and provider and include items such as depreciation of building, equipment, and administrative costs (e.g., administrative salaries, utilities, and office supplies) (Knickman and Thorpe, 1999). For example, the unit of service in home health is the visit, and the agreed-on price is a set amount of money that the home health agency will be paid for a home visit in the region of the United States in which the home care agency is located.

The *charge method* reimburses organizations on the basis of the price set by the organization for delivering a service (Knickman and Thorpe, 1999). In this case, the organization determines a charge for providing a particular service, provides the service to a client, and submits a bill to the payer, and the payer in turn provides payment for the bill. With this method, the charge may be greater than the actual cost to the agency to deliver the service. When the charge method is used, the client often has to pay the difference between what is paid and what is charged.

*Prospective reimbursement,* or payment, is a more recent method of paying an organization, whereby the **third-party payer** establishes the amount of money that will be paid for the delivery of a particular service before offering the services to the client (Knickman and Thorpe, 1999). Since the establishment of prospective payment in Medicare in 1983, private insurance has followed by requiring preapprovals before clients can receive certain services, such as hospital admission or mammograms more than once a year (Knickman and Thorpe, 1999). Under this payment scheme, the third-party payer reimburses an organization on the basis of the payer's prediction of the cost to deliver a particular service; these predictions vary by case mix (i.e., different types of clients, with different types, levels, and intensities of health problems), the

client's diagnosis, and geographic location. This process is used in the DRG system of the hospital (Knickman and Thorpe, 1999).

Similarly, ambulatory care services received by Medicare recipients are classified into ambulatory payment classes (APCs), which reflect the type of ambulatory clinical services received and resources required (HCFA, 1999). Prospective payment to skilled nursing facilities is also adjusted for case mix and geographic variations (HCFA, 1999).

Positive and negative incentives are built into these reimbursement schemes. The retrospective method of payment encourages organizations to inflate prices in one area to offset agency losses in another. These losses can result from providing service to nonpaying clients or from providing care to clients covered under plans that do not cover the total costs of delivering a service (Knickman and Thorpe, 1999). The major disadvantage of this system is that little regard is given to the costs involved. This practice of charging a payer at a higher rate to cover losses in providing care is referred to as *cost-shifting.*

Prospective cost reimbursement encourages agencies to stay within budget limits and adds an incentive for providing less service to contain or reduce costs. If an organization provides care to a particular patient or group of patients and keeps the costs of delivering the service lower than the amount of reimbursement, the provider keeps the difference; however, if the provider's costs exceed the reimbursement, the provider must assume the risk and pay the difference. The major disadvantage of this method is that organizations tend to overemphasize controlling costs and sometimes compromise quality of care.

A growth in contracting, or competitive bidding, for health care services, intended to create incentives for providers to compete on price, has occurred as managed care has increased in health care markets. For example, contracting has been used by states to provide Medicaid services to eligible persons. Hospitals and other health care providers who do not have a contract with the state to provide services are not eligible to receive Medicaid payments for client care. Managed care organizations also use this approach to negotiate with health care organizations, such as hospitals, for coverage of services to be provided to covered enrollees, often called *covered lives.*

## Paying Health Care Practitioners

The traditional method of paying health care practitioners is known as **fee-for-service** (Knickman and Thorpe, 1999) and is like the retrospective method just described. The practitioner determines the costs of providing a service, delivers the service to a client, and submits a bill for the delivered service to a third-party payer, and the payer pays the bill. This method is based on usual, customary, and reasonable (UCR) charges for specific services in a given geographic region, determined by periodic regional evaluations of physician charges across specialties (Knickman and Thorpe, 1999). Historically, Medicare, Medicaid, and private insurance companies have used this method of reimbursing physicians.

A major effort to regulate and control the costs of physician fees was introduced in 1990 in the Omnibus Reconciliation Act. After a study by the Physician Payment Review Commission established by Congress, the *resource-based relative value scale* (RBRVS) was established. The RBRVS method reimburses physicians for specific services provided and the amount of resources required to deliver the service (Knickman and Thorpe, 1999). Resources are defined broadly and include not only the costs of providing the service but also the training that is required to provide a particular service and the time required to perform certain procedures, including client diagnosis and treatment. The RBRVS method of reimbursement, adopted by Medicare in 1991, acknowledges the breadth and depth of knowledge required by primary care physicians in the community to provide services aimed at prevention, health promotion, teaching, and counseling.

( NURSING TIP

The Rural Health Clinic Services Act of 1977 provided indirect reimbursement for nurse practitioners (NPs) in rural health clinics, with payment going to clinics for nurses' salaries. The 1980 and 1989 Medicaid amendments to the Social Security Act provided direct reimbursement for nurse midwives, pediatric NPs, and family NPs. The 1989 amendments allow these nurses to provide services without physician supervision. In the 1990 Omnibus Budget Reconciliation Act, Medicare amendments included a provision for direct reimbursement of NPs and clinical nurse specialists (CNSs) working in collaboration with a physician for services provided in rural areas. Direct reimbursement is also available to these nurses.

**Capitation** is similar to prospective reimbursement for health care organizations. Specifically, third-party payers determine the amount that practitioners will be paid for a unit of care, such as a client visit, before the delivery of the service, thereby placing a limit on the amount of reimbursement received per patient (Knickman and Thorpe, 1999). In contrast to a fee-for-service arrangement, where the practitioner determines both the services that will be provided to clients and the charges for those services, practitioners being paid through capitation are given the rate they will be paid for a client's care, regardless of specific services provided. Therefore, for example, physicians and nurse practitioners are aware, in advance, of the payment they will receive to perform a routine, uncomplicated physical examination or a more complex, detailed physical examination, diagnosis, and treatment (Knickman and Thorpe, 1999).

In capitated arrangements, physicians and other practitioners are paid a set amount to provide care to a given client or group of clients for a set period of time and amount of money. This arrangement, typically used by managed care organizations, is one whereby the practitioner contracts with the managed care organization to provide health care services to plan members for a preset and negotiated fee. The agreed-on fee is negotiated between the practitioner and the managed care organization before the delivery of services and is set at a discounted rate, and the practitioner and managed care organization come to a legal agreement, or contract, for the delivery and payment of services. The managed care organization pays the predetermined fee to the practitioner, often before the delivery of services, to provide care to plan members for a set period of time (Knickman and Thorpe, 1999).

## Reimbursement for Nursing Services

Historically, practitioners eligible to receive reimbursement for health care services included physicians only. However, nurses who function in certain capacities, such as NPs, CNSs, and midwives, also provide primary care to clients and receive reimbursement for their services. Being recognized as primary care providers and eligible to receive reimbursement has not been an easy achievement.

Hospital nursing care costs have traditionally been included as part of the overall patient room charge and reimbursed as such. Other agencies, such as home health care agencies, include nursing care costs with administrative costs, supplies, and equipment costs. Nursing organizations, such as the American Nurses Association, have long advocated that nursing care should become a separate budget item in all organizations so that cost studies can show the efficiency and effectiveness of the nursing profession.

Spurred by efforts to control the costs of medical care, effective January 1, 1998, NPs and CNSs were granted third-party reimbursement for Medicare Part B services only, under Public Law 105-33 (American Nurses Association [ANA], 1999b). This new law sets reimbursement for NPs and CNSs at 85% of physician rates for the same service, an extension of previous legislation that allowed the same reimbursement rate to NPs and CNSs practicing in rural areas (Buppert, 1999). This law was passed after years of work in this area, including research documenting NP and CNS contributions to health care delivery and client outcomes, and after active lobbying efforts by professional nursing organizations.

Additionally, data about the cost–benefit ratio, efficiency, and effectiveness of nursing care in general have been collected. Today, nurse-managed clinics provide health care services to individuals in the United States who might not otherwise have access to health care, such as older adults, the homeless, and schoolchildren. All of these events have moved the discipline toward more autonomy in nursing practice and are serving as a means for evaluating and documenting nurses' contributions to health care delivery.

## OTHER FACTORS AFFECTING RESOURCE ALLOCATION IN HEALTH CARE

The distribution of health care is affected largely by the way in which health care is financed in the United States. Third-party coverage, whether public or private, greatly affects the distribution of health care. Also, socioeconomic status affects health care consumption, as it determines the ability to purchase insurance or to pay directly out-of-pocket. The effects of barriers to health care access and the effects of health care rationing on the distribution of health care follow.

## The Uninsured

In 1996, 68% of the total U.S. population had private health insurance. An additional 15% received insurance through public programs, and 17%, or 37 million, were uninsured. In 2003 the number of uninsured persons has increased to 44 million. The typical uninsured person is a member of the workforce or a dependent of this worker. Uninsured workers are likely to be in low-paying jobs, part-time or temporary jobs, or jobs at small businesses (Kaiser Commission on Medicaid and the Uninsured, 1998). These uninsured workers cannot afford to purchase health insurance, or their employers may not offer health insurance as a benefit. Others who are typically uninsured are young adults, especially young men, minorities, persons under 65 years of age in good or fair health, and the poor or near poor. These individuals may be unable to afford insurance, may lack access to job-based coverage, or, because of their age or good health status, may not perceive the need for insurance. Because of the eligibility requirements for Medicaid, the near poor are actually more likely to be uninsured than the poor.

## The Poor

Socioeconomic status is inversely related to mortality and morbidity for almost every disease. Poor Americans with an income below $10,000 a year have a mortality rate nearly three times that of Americans with incomes of $30,000 or more, even after accounting for age, sex, race, education, and risky health behaviors (smoking, drinking, overeating, and lack of exercise) (Lantz et al, 1998). Historically, the link between poor health and socioeconomic status resulted from poor housing, malnutrition, inadequate sanitation, and hazardous occupations. Today, explanations include the cumulative effects of a number of characteristics that explain the concept of poverty. These characteristics include low educational levels, unemployment or low occupational status (blue collar or unskilled laborer), and low wages.

## Access to Care

Medicaid is intended to improve access to health care for the poor. Although Medicaid persons have improved access (approximately twofold) when compared with the uninsured, Medicaid recipients are only about half as likely to obtain needed health services (medical/surgical care, dental care, prescription drugs, and eyeglasses) as the privately insured (Berk and Schur, 1998). Specifically, "the poorest Americans have Medicaid insurance, yet they also have the worst health" (Income and health, 1998).

Insurance coverage is often used as a ticket to access health care (i.e., insurance coverage provides an opportunity to get health services). In reality, access to care extends beyond insurance coverage. The poor and near poor are more likely to lack a usual source of care, more likely to postpone needed medical care, less likely to use preventive services, and, consequently, more likely to be hospitalized for avoidable conditions than those who are not poor (USDHHS, 1998).

The primary reasons for delay, difficulty, or failure to access care include inability to afford health care and insurance-related reasons, including insurer not approving, covering, or paying for care; having preexisting conditions; and doctors' refusing to accept the insurance plan. Other barriers include lack of transportation, physical barriers, communication problems, child care needs, lack of time or information, or refusal of services by providers (Weinick, Zuvekas, and Drilea, 1997). Additionally, lack of after-hours care, long office waits, and long travel distance are cited as access barriers (Forrest and Starfield, 1998). Community characteristics also contribute to individuals' ability to access care. For example, the prevalence of managed care and the number of **safety net providers,** as well as the wealth and size of the community, affect accessibility (Cunningham and Kemper, 1998).

Because reimbursement for services provided to Medicaid recipients is low, physicians are discouraged from serving this population. Thus people on Medicaid frequently have no primary care provider and may rely on the emergency department for primary care services. Although physicians can respond to monetary incentives in client selection, emergency departments are required by law to evaluate every client regardless of ability to pay. Emergency department co-payments are modest and are frequently waived if the client is unable to pay (Kellerman, 1994). Thus low out-of-pocket costs provide incentives for Medicaid clients and the uninsured to use emergency departments for primary care services.

## Rationing Health Care

Escalating health care spending has spurred renewed interest in **health care rationing.** With unsuccessful attempts at controlling and reducing costs, new plans are being considered to control the use of services and technologies.

Rationing health care in any form implies reduced access to care and potential decreases in acceptable quality of services offered. For example, a health provider's refusal to accept Medicare clients is a form of rationing. Rationing health care is a public health issue. Where care is not provided, the public health system and nurses must ensure that essential clinical services are available. Managed care was thought to offer the possibility of more appropriate health care access and better-organized care to meet basic health care needs of the total population. A shift in the general approach to health care from a reactionary, acute-care orientation toward a proactive, primary prevention orientation is necessary to achieve not only a more cost-effective but a more equitable health care system in the United States.

## Healthy People 2010

Healthy People 2010 goals are examples of strategies to provide better access for all people. Box 5-4 shows the levels of economic prevention strategies.

## PRIMARY PREVENTION

Society's investment in the health care system has been based on the premise that more health services will result in better health, but non–health care factors also have an effect. Of the four major factors that affect health—personal behavior (or lifestyle), environmental factors (including physical, social, and economic environments), human biology, and the health care system—medical services are said to have the least effect. Behavior and lifestyle have been shown to have the greatest effect, with the environment and biology accounting for 70% of all illnesses (USDHHS, 2000).

Despite the significant impact of behavior and environment on health, estimates indicate that 97% of health care dollars are spent on secondary and tertiary care. Such a reactionary, secondary-care system results in high-cost, high-technology, and disease-specific care and is consistent with the U.S. system's traditional emphasis on "sickness care." A more proactive investment in disease prevention and health promotion targeted at improving health behaviors,

lifestyle, and the environment has the potential to improve health status, thereby improving quality of life while reducing health care costs. The USDHHS has argued that a higher value should be placed on primary prevention. The goal of this approach is to preserve and maximize *human capital* by providing health promotion and social practices that result in less disease. An emphasis on primary prevention may reduce dollars spent and increase quality of life.

The return on investment in primary prevention through gains in human capital has, unfortunately, not been acknowledged. Consequently, large investments in primary prevention and public health care have not been made. Reasons given for this lack of emphasis on prevention in clinical practice and lack of financial investment in prevention include the following (Young, Griffith, and Kamerow, 1994):

- Provider uncertainty about which clients should receive services and at what intervals
- Lack of education about preventive services
- Negative attitudes about the importance of preventive care
- Lack of time for delivery of preventive services
- Delayed or absent feedback regarding success of preventive measures
- Lack of reimbursement for these services
- Lack of organization to deliver preventive services

A focus on prevention could mean reducing the need for and use of medical, dental, hospital, and health provider services. Under fee-for-service payment arrangements, this would mean that the health care system, the largest employer in the United States, would be reduced in size and would become less profitable. However, with the increasing costs of health care, consumer demand, and changes in financing mechanisms, there is a new trend toward financing more preventive care services.

Today, third-party payers are beginning to cover preventive services, recognizing that the growth of the health care system can no longer be supported. Under capitated health plans, health care providers stand to make money by keeping clients healthy and reducing health care use. Only through combining client interests with financial interests of the health care industry will primary prevention and public health be raised to the status and priority of acute care and chronic care.

---

**BOX 5-4   Economic Prevention Strategies**

**PRIMARY PREVENTION**

Work with legislators and insurance companies to provide coverage for health promotion to reduce the risk of diseases

**SECONDARY PREVENTION**

Encourage clients who are pregnant to participate in prenatal care and WIC to increase the number of healthy babies and reduce the costs related to preterm baby care

**TERTIARY PREVENTION**

Participate in home visits to mothers who are at risk for neglecting babies to reduce the costs related to abuse

---

**Healthy People 2010**   Objectives Related to Access to Care

**Goal 2:** Eliminate health disparities

**1-1** Increase the proportion of persons with health insurance.

**1-4.a** Increase the proportion of persons who have a specific source of ongoing care.

**16-6.a** Increase the proportion of pregnant women who begin prenatal care in the first trimester of pregnancy.

From U.S. Department of Health and Human Services: *Healthy people 2010: understanding and improving health,* ed 2, Washington, DC, 2000, U.S. Government Printing Office.

Despite difficulties, methods for determining prevention effectiveness, such as cost–effectiveness and cost–benefit analyses, are becoming standard and used more widely. Regardless of the method, prevention-effectiveness analyses are outcome oriented. This area of research seeks to link interventions with health outcomes and economic outcomes, and to reveal the tradeoffs between the two. In theory, support for increasing national investment in primary prevention is sound and long-standing. Since the public health movement of the mid-nineteenth century, public health officials, epidemiologists, and public health nurses have been working to advance the agenda of primary prevention to the forefront of the health care industry. Today, these efforts continue across a number of disciplines and in both the public and private sectors, as shown in Box 5-5.

## ECONOMICS AND THE FUTURE OF COMMUNITY-ORIENTED NURSING PRACTICE

The failure of sweeping health care reform during the 1990s opened the door to the growth of managed care. The American Nurses Association (ANA) notes that managed care offers the potential for bringing improvements in the health care delivery system, such as eliminating waste and redundancy, a greater focus on health promotion and disease prevention, more attention to chronic illness, and a focus on accountability of providers, practitioners, and payers. This potential has gone unrealized. An overt emphasis on profit-making, "bottom-line" approaches that often appear to come at the expense of quality and access has highlighted managed care as it exists today (ANA, 1999a).

---

### BOX 5-5  Promoting the Health and Well-Being of the American People

**PEW CHARITABLE TRUSTS**

**Pew's Health and Human Services Program (Public Voices, Public Choices) (Pew Health Professions Commission, 1993)**
- Public health
- Bioethics
- Health care delivery systems
- Welfare reform

**Pew Health Professions Commission**
- Access to care for all
- Cost-effective use of resources
- Market efficiency coupled with public compassion
- Orientation to health rather than medical care
- Participation by the public, both individually and collectively
- Evidence-based decision making

**FEDERAL RECOMMENDATIONS**

**Public Health Service: Healthy People (USDHEW, 1979)**
- Elimination of cigarette smoking
- Reduction of alcohol use
- Moderate dietary changes to reduce intake of excess calories, fat, salt, and sugar
- Moderate exercise
- Periodic screening for major causes of morbidity and mortality, such as cancer
- Adherence to speed laws and use of seat belts

**Public Health Service: Healthy People 2000 (USDHHS, 1990)**
- Health promotion
- Family planning
- Mental health
- Health protection

**Healthy People 2010 (USDHHS, 2000)**
- Reducing or eliminating illness, disability, and premature death among individuals and communities
- Improving access to quality health care
- Strengthening public health services
- Improving the availability and dissemination of health-related information

**NURSING'S AGENDA FOR HEALTH CARE REFORM (ANA, 1991)**
- Restructured health care system, emphasizing access, primary care, and community care
- Use of cost-effective providers
- Personal health and self-care
- A standard package of essential health care services for all citizens, phased in
- Planned health care services representing national demographics
- Steps to reduce health care costs based on managed care
- Case management
- Long-term care
- Insurance reforms
- No payment at point of care
- Establishing a public or private review to monitor the system

---

American Nurses Association: *Nursing's agenda for health care reform,* Washington, DC, 1991, American Nurses Publishing.
Pew Health Professions Commission: *Contemporary issues in health professions, education and workforce reform,* San Francisco, 1993, UCSF Center for the Health Professions.
U.S. Department of Health and Human Services: *Healthy people 2000: national health promotion and disease prevention objectives,* Washington, DC, 1990, USDHHS, Public Health Service.
U.S. Department of Health and Human Services: *Healthy people 2010,* Washington, DC, 2000, Public Health Service.
U.S. Department of Health, Education, and Welfare: *Healthy people: the surgeon general's report on health promotion and disease prevention,* DHEW Publication No. (PHS) 79-55071, Washington, DC, 1979, USDHEW.

| BOX 5-6 | Elements of the Patient Protection Act |

- *Guaranteeing a patient's right to know* will allow free and open communications between patients and doctors, enabling fully informed decisions about the best course of treatment. This is commonly referred to as lifting "gag rules" placed on medical providers.
- *Ensuring access to emergency care by applying prudent layperson standards* will guarantee that patients will be treated in emergency departments when they need care most by prohibiting health plans from arbitrarily refusing to pay for covered emergency benefits.
- *Providing direct access for obstetrics and gynecology services* will allow women the opportunity to bypass the insurance company's gatekeeper and go directly to their provider.
- *Disclosing plan information* will make it easier for patients to learn what their health plan specifically covers, including benefits, doctors, and facilities. It also enables patients to better compare coverage information between health plans.
- *Expediting internal review* will hold insurance companies accountable by giving patients access to immediate decisions from doctors about what is covered for emergency, urgent, and routine services without preventing legal options already provided under current law.
- *Providing independent medical expertise in external appeals* will guarantee unprecedented patient protection by requiring that an independent doctor decide if a requested service is medically necessary, if originally turned down by internal review.
- *Creating association health plans* will provide avenues for small businesses to pool together for their employees to enjoy the kinds of coverage afforded in big businesses.
- *Guaranteeing patient choice of doctors* will allow new avenues to health care coverage where quality and choice are unavailable by requiring health plans to offer point-of-service options.
- *Improving medical savings accounts* will make it easier for patients to increase access to health care services and have greater control over their health care dollars.
- *Creating health-marts* will increase consumer choice by providing a cooperative group marketplace where working families may choose from a menu of benefit options.
- *Creating community health organizations* will promote expansion of health coverage to all patients within their communities.
- *Reforming health care lawsuits* will hold down costs by ensuring that doctors are free to practice medicine responsibly without the fear of unnecessary litigation, excessive legal damages, or greedy trial lawyers.
- *Safeguarding medical record confidentiality* will protect personal and sensitive health care data from abuse.

From Patient Protection Act of 1998, HR 4250, 105th U.S. Congress, July 16, 1998.

Accounts of mistreatments in health care are frequently reported in the press. In response, numerous bills were introduced at the state and federal levels in 1996 and 1997 to regulate managed care and/or consumer protection. Notable enactments include the Patient Protection Act (Box 5-6) and the HIPAA. In 1998, the President's Advisory Commission on Consumer Protection and Quality in the Health Care Industry also developed a Consumer Bill of Rights and Responsibilities, and current efforts in Congress are underway to protect the public against unsafe service delivery practices and to ensure quality.

The balance of interest within society and health care will continue to shift toward a focus on quality. Health care system concerns of the twenty-first century are expected to focus on examining the quality of health care relative to the costs of care delivered. These changes will result from continued efforts of both the public and private sectors to reform the U.S. health care system. The current era of health care delivery will be noted as a time of vast changes in all sectors of health care delivery.

Nurses must plan for future changes in health care financing by becoming aware of the costs of nursing services, identifying aspects of care where cost savings can be safely achieved, and developing knowledge on how community-oriented nursing practice affects and is affected by the principles of economics. Nursing must continue to focus on improving the overall health of the nation, defining its contribution to the health of the nation, deriving the value of nursing care, and ensuring its economic viability within the health care marketplace. Nurses must effect changes in the health care system by providing leadership in developing new models of care delivery that provide effective, high-quality care and by assuming a greater role in evaluating client care and nurse performance. It is through their leadership that nurses will contribute to improved decision making about allocating scarce health care resources.

## Practice Application

Connie, a community health nursing student, has identified a caseload of five families in a home health nursing program offered by the local public health department. She is interested in assessing the costs of care to her clients and to the agency. Connie approaches the public health nurse administrator and asks the following questions:

**A.** How is the agency reimbursed for home health visits?
**B.** How is the payment for the visit determined?
**C.** Are nursing care costs known?
**D.** Are visits rationed to clients?

**Answers are in the back of the book.**

## Key Points

- From 1800 to the 1980s, the U.S. health care delivery system experienced three developmental stages, with different emphases on health care economics. In 1985, the health care delivery system entered a fourth developmental stage.
- Four basic components provide the framework for the development of health care services delivery: service needs and intensity, facilities, technology, and labor (workforce).
- Three major factors have been associated with the growth of the health care delivery system: price inflation, changes in population demographics, and technology and service intensity.
- Health care financing has evolved through the twentieth century from a system financed primarily by the consumer to a system financed primarily by third-party payers. In the twenty-first century, the consumer is being asked to pay more.
- To solve the problems of rising health care costs, a number of plans for future payment of health care are being considered; all include some form of rationing.
- Excessive and inefficient use of goods and services in health care delivery has been viewed as the major cause of rising health care costs.
- The goal of health economics is maximum benefits from services of health providers, leading to health and wellness of the population.
- Economics is concerned with use of resources, including money, to fulfill society's needs and wants.
- Health economics is concerned with the problems of producing services and programs and distributing them to clients.
- The goal of public health is providing the most good for the most people.
- Nurses need to understand basic economic principles to avoid contributing to rising health care costs.
- The GNP reflects the market value of goods and services produced by the United States.
- The GDP reflects the market value of the output of labor and property located in the United States.
- Microeconomic theory shows how supply and demand can be used in health care.
- Macroeconomic theory helps one look at national and community issues that affect health care.
- Social issues, economic issues, and communicable disease epidemics mark the problems of the twenty-first century.
- Medicare and Medicaid are two government-funded programs that help meet the needs of high-risk populations in the United States.
- A majority of the U.S. population has health insurance. The remaining uninsured segment represents millions of people, mostly the working poor, older adults, and children.
- Poverty has a detrimental effect on health.
- Health care rationing has always been a part of the U.S. health care system.
- Nurses are cost-effective providers and must be an integral part of health care delivery.
- Healthy People 2010 is a document that has established U.S. health objectives.
- Human life is valued in health economics, as is money. An emphasis on changing lifestyles and preventive care will reduce the unnecessary years of life lost to early and preventable death.

## Clinical Decision-Making Activities

1. Define the following terms in your own words: economics, health economics, gross national product, gross domestic product, consumer price index, and human capital. How do these terms relate to your work as a nurse?
2. Compare the advantages and disadvantages of applying economics to public health care issues. Be specific.
3. Compare and contrast efficiency and effectiveness of a community health program. What factors make these difficult to control?
4. Apply the concepts of supply and demand to an example from community health. Be exact in your answer.
5. Review Chapter 6. Debate in the class the ethical implications of the goal of rationing. Focus your debate on the implications for nursing practice. What are some of the complexities of this question?
6. Invite a public health nurse administrator to meet with your class or clinical conference group. Ask how inflation, changes in population, and technology have changed the public health care delivery system and nursing practice. How could we check for ourselves to find the answers?

## Additional Resources

These related resources are found either in the appendix at the back of this book or on the book's website at **http://evolve.elsevier.com/ Stanhope.**

### *evolve* Evolve Website

Appendix A.2: Select Major Historical Events Depicting Financial Involvement of Federal Government in Health Care Delivery

WebLinks: Healthy People 2010

# References

Agency for Health Care Policy and Research: *Medical Expenditure Panel Survey highlights: health insurance coverage in America 1996* (AHCPR Publication No. 98-0031), Rockville, Md, 1998, AHCPR.

American Nurses Association: *Nursing's agenda for health care reform*, Washington, DC, 1991, American Nurses Publishing.

American Nurses Association: *Managed care legislation—1997*, 1999a, available at www.nursingworld.org/gova/hod97/mgdcare.htm.

American Nurses Association: *Medicare reimbursement for NPs and CNSs*, 1999b, available at www.nursingworld.org/gova/medreimb.htm.

Andersen GF, Hussey PS: Population aging: a comparison among industrialized countries, *Health Aff* 19(3):195, 2000.

Balanced Budget Act: *State Children's Health Insurance Program*, Title XXI, Social Security Act, 1997, Section 210(a).

Banta HD: Technology assessment in health care. In Kovner A, editor: *Health care delivery in the United States*, New York, 1995a, Springer.

Banta HD: What is health care? In Kovner A, editor: *Health care delivery in the United States*, New York, 1995b, Springer.

Berk ML, Schur CL: Access to care: how much difference does Medicaid make? *Health Aff* 17(3):169, 1998.

Britton B et al: Measuring costs and quality of TeleHomecare, *Home Health Care Manage Practice* 12(4):27-32, 2000.

Buppert C: HEDIS for the primary care provider: getting an "A" on the managed care report card, *Nurse Pract* 24(1): 84-94, 1999.

Bureau of Labor Statistics, U.S. Department of Labor: *Occupational outlook handbook, 1998-99 edition* (Bulletin 2500), Washington, DC, 1998, Superintendent of Documents, U.S. Government Printing Office.

Centers for Disease Control: Ten great public health achievements—United States 1900-1999. In Lee P, Estes C, editors: *The national's health*, Boston, 2001, Jones and Bartlett.

Centers for Medicare and Medicaid Services: *National health expenditures*, Washington, DC, 2000, U.S. Government Printing Office.

Congressional Budget Office: *The budget and economic outlook*, Washington, DC, August 2001, U.S. Government Printing Office.

Cunningham PJ, Kemper P: Ability to obtain medical care for the uninsured: how much does it vary across communities? *JAMA* 280(10):921, 1998.

Deber R et al: The public–private mix in health care. In *Striking a balance, vol 4: health care systems in Canada and elsewhere*, pp. 423-545, Quebec, 1998, Minister of Public Works and Government Services.

Druss BG et al: The most expensive medical conditions in America, *Health Aff* 21(4):105-111, 2002.

Folland S, Goodman AC, Stano M: *The economics of health and health care*, New York, 1993, Macmillan.

Forrest CB, Starfield B: Entry into primary care and continuity: the effects of access, *Am J Public Health* 88(9):1330, 1998.

Ginsberg PB, Gabel JR, Hunt KA: Tracking small-firm coverage, 1989-1996, *Health Aff* 17(1):167, 1998.

Gold MR et al: *Cost-effectiveness in health and medicine*, New York, 1996, Oxford University Press.

Haddix AC et al: *Prevention effectiveness: a guide to decision analysis and economic evaluation*, New York, 1996, Oxford University Press.

Health Care Financing Administration: *1998 Medicare chartbook: a profile of Medicare*, 1998a, available at www.hcfa.gov/pubforms/chartbk.htm.

Health Care Financing Administration: *Case mix prospective payment for SNF's Balanced Budget Act of 1997*, retrieved June 24, 1998b, from www.hcfa.gov/medicare/overview.html.

Health Care Financing Administration: *HIPAA: the Health Insurance Portability and Accountability Act of 1996*, retrieved Feb 22, 1999 from www.hcfa.gov/HIPAA/HIPAAHm.htm.

Heffler S et al: Health spending projections for 2001-2001: the latest outlook, *Health Aff* 21(2):201-218, 2002.

Income and health: poor are left behind in health gains, *Am HealthLine*, July 30, 1998.

Internal Revenue Service: *Understanding MSAs*, retrieved Nov 19, 1998 from www.irs.gov/forms_pubs/pubs/p96901.htm.

Jacobs P: *The economics of health and medical care*, ed 5, Gaithersburg, Md, 2002, Aspen.

Kaiser Commission on Medicaid and the Uninsured: *Uninsured facts: the uninsured and their access to health care*, Washington, DC, 1998, Kaiser Commission.

Kellerman AL: Nonurgent emergency department visits: meeting an unmet need, *JAMA* 271(24):1953, 1994.

Knickman J, Thorpe K: Financing for health care. In Kovner A, editor: *Health care delivery in the United States*, New York, 1999, Springer.

Kovner C: The health care workforce in the United States. In Kovner A, editor: *Health care delivery in the United States*, New York, 1999, Springer.

Lantz PM et al: Socioeconomic factors, health behaviors, and mortality: results from a nationally representative prospective study of US adults, *JAMA* 279(21):1745, 1998.

Lee P, Estes C: *The nation's health*, Boston, 2001, Jones and Bartlett.

Levit KR, Lazenby HC, Braden BR: National health spending trends, *Health Aff* 21(1), 2002.

Maddox PJ: Administrative ethics and the allocation of scarce resources, *Online J Issues Nurs,* retrieved December 31, 1998, from www.nursisngworld.org/ojin/topic8/ topic8_5.htm.

Maddox PJ: Impact of financing arrangements and economics on nursing. In Doechterman G, editors: *Current Issues in Nursing,* ed 6, St Louis, Mo, Mosby, 2001.

Maslove AM: National goals and the federal role in health care. In *Striking a balance, vol 4: health care systems in Canada and elsewhere,* pp. 413-414, Quebec, 1998, Minister of Public Works and Government Services.

National Center for Health Statistics: *Health: United States: 2000,* Hyattsville, Md, 2002, U.S. Government Printing Office.

Nichols LM, Blumberg LJ: A different kind of "new federalism"? the Health Insurance Portability and Accountability Act of 1996, *Health Aff* 17(3):25-42, 1998.

Organization for Economic Cooperation and Development: *Health Data, 2002,* available at www.oecd.org.

Patient Protection Act of 1998, HR 4250, 105th U.S. Congress, July 16, 1998.

Pew Health Professions Commission: *Contemporary issues in health professions, education and workforce reform,* San Francisco, 1993, UCSF Center for the Health Professions.

Pickett G, Hanlon J: *Public health administration and practice,* St Louis, Mo, 1990, Mosby.

Romanow R: *Building on values: the future of health care in Canada: final report,* Ottawa, 2002, Author, available at www.healthcarecommission.ca.

Scott G: International comparison of the hospital sector. In *Striking a balance, vol 4: health care systems in Canada and elsewhere,* pp. 3-31, Quebec, 1998, Minister of Public Works and Government Services.

Smith S et al: The Health Expenditures Projection Team: the next ten years of health spending: what does the future hold? *Health Aff* 17(5):128, 1998.

Thorpe K: Health care cost containment. In Kovner A, editor: *Health care delivery in the United States,* New York, 1995, Springer.

U.S. Bureau of the Census: National Aging Information Center, Washington, DC, 1999, U.S. Government Printing Office

U.S. Department of Health and Human Services: *Healthy people 2000: national health promotion and disease prevention objectives,* Washington, DC, 1990, USDHHS, Public Health Service.

U.S. Department of Health and Human Services: *Health: United States,* 1998, DHHS Publication No. (PHS) 98-1232, Washington, DC, 1998, U.S. Government Printing Office.

U.S. Department of Health and Human Services: *Healthy people 2010: understanding and improving health,* Washington, DC, 2000, Public Health Service.

U.S. Department of Health, Education, and Welfare: *Healthy people: the surgeon general's report on health promotion and disease prevention,* DHEW Publication No. (PHS) 79-55071, Washington, DC, 1979, USDHEW.

Weinick RM, Zuvekas SH, Drilea SK: *Access to health care: sources and barriers, 1996,* MEPS Research Findings No. 3, AHCPR Publication No. 98-0001, Rockville, Md, 1997, Agency for Health Care Policy and Research.

Young S, Griffith H, Kamerow D: *Put prevention into practice: a program for community health centers, 1994,* available at www.hhs.gov/cgibin/waisgate? WAISdocID5870041254111010& WAISaction5retrieve.

# Chapter 6

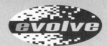 

# Ethics in Community-Oriented Nursing Practice

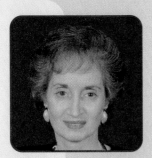

**Mary Cipriano Silva, R.N., Ph.D., F.A.A.N.**
Mary Cipriano Silva is currently professor of nursing and director of the Office of Health Care Ethics at George Mason University in Fairfax, Virginia. She undertook postdoctoral study in bioethics at the Hastings Center and at Georgetown University, where she was a Kennedy Fellow in Medical Ethics for Nursing Faculty. She is a prolific writer in the area of bioethics and won an *American Journal of Nursing* Book of the Year Award for her book on administrative ethics. She was a member of the American Nurses Association's Code of Ethics Project Task Force for the 2001 *Code of Ethics for Nurses with Interpretive Statements.*

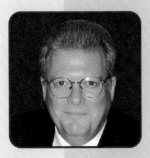

**James J. Fletcher, Ph.D.**
James J. Fletcher is an associate professor of philosophy in the Department of Philosophy and Religious Studies at George Mason University, where he specializes in bioethics and is the ethics collaborator in the Office of Health Care Ethics in the College of Nursing and Health Sciences. In addition to his research and teaching in bioethics, he is a member of the ethics committee and chair of the Human Research Review Committee of a community hospital. He sits on the Institutional Review Board of a local biotechnological company and serves as a member of Data and Safety Monitoring Boards for the National Institutes of Health.

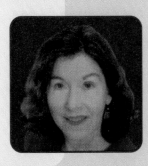

**Jeanne Merkle Sorrell, Ph.D., R.N., F.A.A.N.**
Jeanne Merkle Sorrell is currently professor of nursing and associate dean of academic programs and research at George Mason University in Fairfax. Her current research uses interpretive phenomenology to explore ethical concerns in the lived experience of patients and caregivers with Alzheimer's disease. She facilitated production of an educational video through the Office of Health Care Ethics at George Mason University. The video, "Quality Lives: Ethics in the Care of Persons with Alzheimer's," received the 2001 Sigma Theta Tau International Award for Nursing Electronic Media and a Bronze *Chris* Award, presented by the Columbus International Film & Video Festival.

## Objectives

After reading this chapter, the student should be able to do the following:

1. Describe a brief history of the ethics of community-oriented nursing
2. Analyze ethical decision-making processes
3. Compare and contrast ethical theories and principles, virtue ethics, the ethic of care, and feminist ethics
4. Comprehend the ethics inherent in the core functions of community-oriented nursing
5. Analyze codes of ethics for nursing and for public health
6. Apply the ethics of advocacy to community-oriented nursing

Both community health nursing and public health nursing are essentially ethical endeavors. Nurses who practice these two types of community-oriented nursing focus on protecting, promoting, preserving, and maintaining health while preventing disease. These goals reflect the ethical principles of promoting good and preventing harm. In addition, community health nurses struggle with the rights of individuals and families versus the rights of local groups within a community. On the other hand, public health nurses struggle with the rights of a community or population versus the rights of individuals, families, and local groups within a community. These two types of struggle reflect the tensions between respect for autonomy, rights-based ethical theory, and community-based ethical theory.

In addition, community health nurses and public health nurses deal with consequence-based ethical theory and obligation-based ethical theory. They also deal with the ethical components of advocacy, justice, health policy, caring, women's moral experiences, and the moral character of health care practitioners. Both community and public health nurses are guided by codes of ethics and ethical decision-making frameworks. The purpose of this chapter, then, is to make explicit the preceding content as it relates to the **ethics** inherent in community-oriented nursing.

## Key Terms

advocacy, p. 143
beneficence, p. 135
bioethics, p. 131
code of ethics, p. 140
communitarianism, p. 136
consequentialism, p. 134
deontology, p. 134
distributive justice, p. 135

ethical decision making, p. 132
ethical dilemmas, p. 132
ethical issues, p. 132
ethics, p. 130
feminine ethic, p. 138
feminist ethics, p. 138
feminists, p. 138
morality, p. 131

nonmaleficence, p. 135
principlism, p. 135
respect for autonomy, p. 135
utilitarianism, p. 134
values, p. 131
virtue ethics, p. 137
virtues, p. 137
*See Glossary for definitions*


## Chapter Outline

History
Key Ethical Terms
Ethical Decision Making
Ethics
*Definition, Theories, Principles*
*Virtue Ethics*
*Caring and the Ethic of Care*

*Feminist Ethics*
Ethics and the Core Functions of Community-
  Oriented Nursing
*Assessment*
*Policy Development*
*Assurance*
Nursing Code of Ethics

Public Health Code of Ethics
Advocacy and Ethics
*Definitions, Codes, Standards*
*Components of Advocacy*
*Conceptual Framework for Advocacy*
*Practical Framework for Advocacy*

# HISTORY

The history of public health and of public and community health nursing is discussed in detail in Chapter 2. The focus here is a brief history of nursing and public health ethics and the relationship between them and community-oriented nursing.

Modern nursing has a rich heritage of ethics and **morality**, beginning with Florence Nightingale (1820-1910). Her **values** and the moral significance she inculcated into the profession have endured. She saw nursing as a call to service. She viewed the moral character of persons entering nursing as important. She also viewed nursing within a broad social context, where poor people mattered and where soldiers harmed in the Crimean War (1854-1856) did not have to endure unhealthy environments. Because of her commitment to poor individuals in communities, as well as her stances on primary prevention and population-based evidence that healthy environments save soldiers' lives, she is seen as nursing's first enduring moral leader and community-oriented nurse.

In 1860, in London, Nightingale established the first nursing program. It was hospital based, but the curriculum contained not only care of the sick but also public health concepts with their inherent ethical tenets. Many of these programs were associated with religious institutions.

Students, therefore, often received ethics courses with a slant toward a particular religion's values. Soon thereafter in the United States, the notion of hospital-based nursing programs took hold, but community-oriented nursing practice was not a part of the curricula.

In the 1960s, two seminal events occurred. First, the American Nurses Association [ANA] recommended that all nursing education should occur in institutions of higher education. As this process slowly took place, ethics, as a course per se, was removed from many schools of nursing, although ethical values remained. Second, because of major advances in science and technology that affected health care, the field of **bioethics** began to emerge and was reflected in nursing curricula. Today, the vast majority of nursing programs integrate bioethical content into their courses or have separate courses on this topic; some do both. Although some of these courses relate bioethics to community-oriented nursing, more needs to be done as the emphasis has been primarily on acute care nursing.

Nurses' codes of ethics are important in the history of community-oriented nursing practice. The Nightingale Pledge is generally considered to be nursing's first code of ethics (ANA, 2001). After the Nightingale Pledge, a "suggested" code and a "tentative" code were published in the

**DID YOU KNOW?**

The Nightingale Pledge was written by Lystra Gretter in 1893.

*American Journal of Nursing* but were not formally adopted. In 1950, however, the *Code for Professional Nurses* was formally adopted by the ANA House of Delegates. In 1956, 1960, 1968, 1976, and 1985, the code was amended or revised. In 2001, after 5 years of work, the *Code of Ethics for Nurses with Interpretive Statements* was adopted by the ANA House of Delegates (ANA, 2001).

Community-oriented nurses should also be familiar with the first known international code of ethics, developed by the International Council of Nurses (ICN) in 1953. Like the ANA code, it has undergone various revisions and adoptions. The most recent version of the *ICN Code of Ethics for Nurses* was adopted in 2000.

In addition to codes of ethics, the nursing literature and nursing associations have consistently reflected a commitment to ethics, as well as an awareness of nursing's ethical obligations to society. From the 1980s to the present, the number of centers for nursing and health care ethics has increased steadily. The majority of these centers are located in academic settings; however, in 1991, the ANA founded its Center for Ethics and Human Rights. The historical contributions have affected the persistent ethicality of nursing and community-oriented nursing.

The bioethics movement of the late 1960s influenced not only nursing ethics but also public health ethics. However, until recently, the relationship between public health and ethics was implicit rather than explicit (American Public Health Association, 2001; Callahan and Jennings, 2002; Levin and Fleischman, 2002).

Finally, in 2000, public health professionals, individually and through their associations, initiated the writing of a code of ethics that was supported by the American Public Health Association (APHA). In 2001, the code was widely disseminated via the APHA website and critiqued. Its revisions were presented at the 2001 APHA annual meeting, and it is now being presented to relevant organizations for adoption (APHA, 2001).

## KEY ETHICAL TERMS

Before discussing ethics related to community-oriented nursing, some key ethical terms are defined in Box 6-1. Other ethical terms are defined within the context of the chapter.

## ETHICAL DECISION MAKING

**Ethical decision making** is that component of ethics that focuses on the process of how ethical decisions are made. The process is the thinking that occurs when health care professionals must make decisions about ethical issues

---

### BOX 6-1   Key Ethical Terms

**Ethics** is a branch of philosophy that includes both a body of knowledge about the moral life and a process of reflection for determining what persons ought to do or be, regarding this life.

**Bioethics** is a branch of ethics that applies the knowledge and processes of ethics to the examination of ethical problems in health care.

**Morality** is shared and generational societal norms about what constitutes right or wrong conduct.

**Values** are beliefs about the worth or importance of what is right or esteemed.

**Ethical dilemma** is a puzzling moral problem in which a person, group, or community can envision morally justified reasons for both taking and not taking a certain course of action.

**Codes of ethics** are moral standards that delineate a profession's values, goals, and obligations.

**Utilitarianism** is an ethical theory based on the weighing of morally significant outcomes or consequences regarding the overall maximizing of good and minimizing of harm for the greatest number of people.

**Deontology** is an ethical theory that bases moral obligation on duty and claims that actions are obligatory irrespective of the good or bad consequences that they produce. Because humans are rational, they have absolute value. Therefore persons should always be treated as ends in themselves and never as mere means.

**Principlism** is an approach to problem solving in bioethics that uses the principles of respect for autonomy, beneficence, nonmaleficence, and justice as the basis for organization and analysis.

**Advocacy** is the act of pleading for or supporting a course of action on behalf of a person, group, or community.

---

and ethical dilemmas. **Ethical issues** are moral challenges facing ourselves or our profession. In community-oriented nursing, one such challenge is how to prepare an adequate and competent workforce for the future. In contrast, **ethical dilemmas** are puzzling moral problems in which a person, group, or community can envision morally justified reasons for both taking and not taking a certain course of action. In community-oriented nursing, an example of an ethical dilemma is how to allocate resources to two equally needy populations when the resources are sufficient to serve only one of the populations. To facilitate the thinking processes needed to deal with ethical issues and dilemmas, ethical decision-making frameworks are helpful.

Ethical decision-making frameworks use problem-solving processes. They serve as guides to making sound ethical decisions that can be morally justified. Many such frameworks exist in the health care literature, and some are presented in this chapter. A caveat, however, is in order. According to

## Table 6-1  Rationale for Steps of Ethical Decision-Making Framework

| STEPS | RATIONALE |
| --- | --- |
| 1. Identify the ethical issues and dilemmas. | Persons cannot make sound ethical decisions if they cannot identify ethical issues and dilemmas. |
| 2. Place them within a meaningful context. | The historical, sociological, cultural, psychological, economic, political, communal, environmental, and demographic contexts affect the way ethical issues and dilemmas are formulated and justified. |
| 3. Obtain all relevant facts. | Facts affect the way ethical issues and dilemmas are formulated and justified. |
| 4. Reformulate ethical issues and dilemmas if needed. | The initial ethical issues and dilemmas may need to be modified or changed on the basis of context and facts. |
| 5. Consider appropriate approaches to actions or options. | The nature of the ethical issues and dilemmas determines the specific ethical approaches used. |
| 6. Make decisions and take action. | Professional persons cannot avoid choice and action in applied ethics. |
| 7. Evaluate decisions and action. | Evaluation determines whether or not the ethical decision-making framework used resulted in morally justified actions related to the ethical issues and dilemmas. |

Weston (2002), "Whether we admit it or not, we *do* make our own decisions. We cannot pretend that we are simply obeying some rules (or authorities) that settle matters—ours only to obey. Choosing is inescapable" (p. 28).

Keeping the preceding caveat in mind, the following generic ethical decision-making framework is presented:

1. Identify the ethical issues and dilemmas.
2. Place them within a meaningful context.
3. Obtain all relevant facts.
4. Reformulate ethical issues and dilemmas, if needed.
5. Consider appropriate *approaches* to actions or options (utilitarianism, deontology, principlism, virtue ethics, ethic of care, feminist ethics).
6. Make decision and take action.
7. Evaluate the decision and the action.

The steps of a generic ethics framework are often nonlinear, and, with one exception, they do not change substantially. Their rationales are presented in Table 6-1. Step 5 (the one exception) lists six approaches to the ethical decision-making process; these approaches are outlined throughout the chapter in the "How to" boxes.

One aspect of the preceding ethical decision-making framework needs additional discussion—the growing multiculturalism of American society. Community-oriented nurses often deal with ethical issues and dilemmas related to the diverse and at times conflicting values that result from ethnicity. From a moral perspective, what ought the nurse do when facing ethnicity conflicts?

Callahan (2000) offers useful insights into these conflicts. He describes four situations in which ethnic diversity can be judged in relationship to cultural standards:

1. Situations that place persons at direct risk of harm, whether psychological or physical

2. Situations where ethnic cultural standards conflict with professional standards
3. Situations where the greater community's values are jeopardized by specific ethnic values
4. Situations where specific ethnic community customs are annoying but not problematic for the greater community

### NURSING TIP

To create open-mindedness in ethics, when health care professionals or clients hold ethical positions with which you strongly disagree, do not interrupt or argue with them. First, let them state their position while you listen carefully. Then rephrase their position to them to ensure accuracy. Now ask the persons with the opposing positions to do the same for you. Once these steps are taken, try to find common ground between you, and make this the starting point for continued discussion.

Callahan (2000) then offers his perspectives on judging diversity in the four situations. Regarding situation one, he states that "we in America imposed some standards on ourselves for important moral reasons; and there is no good reason to exempt [ethnic] subgroups from those standards" (p. 43). Regarding situations two and three, he suggests a thoughtful tolerance but also some degree of moral persuasion (not coercion) for ethnic groups to alter values so that they are more in keeping with what is normative in the American culture. However, Callahan notes that "in the absence of grievous harm, there is no clear moral mandate to interfere with those values" (p. 43).

## Evidence-Based Practice

The purpose of this Canadian study was to identify recurring ethical problems in public health nursing practice. The design was an exploratory qualitative study in which 22 nurses who were deemed by supervisors to be reflective and articulate regarding ethical problems were interviewed. The nurses worked in public health nursing centers in both urban (*n* = 11) and rural (*n* = 11) settings. The interviews were tape recorded, were basically unstructured, and lasted from 30 minutes to 2 hours. The tape recordings were transcribed and then analyzed.

The analyses resulted in five interrelated themes: "relationships with health care professionals; systems issues; character of relationships; respect for persons; and putting self at risk" (p. 425). Each of the five themes had two or three subthemes related to ethical problems in public health nursing. Examples of subtheme ethical problems were perceived inequities in power, unacceptable practice, inequitable resource allocation, conflict between ethics and law, inadequate systems support for nursing, conflicts between individual and community rights, conflicts between nurses' and clients' values, and conflicts between service to clients and physical danger to self.

**Nurse Use:** This study concluded that ethics permeated every aspect of public health nursing.

Oberle K, Tenove S: Ethical issues in public health nursing, *Nurs Ethics* 7(5):425-438, 2000.

## HOW TO Apply the Utilitarian Ethics Decision Process

1. Determine moral rules that are important to society and that are derived from the principle of utility.*
2. Identify the communities or populations that are affected or most affected by the moral rules.
3. Analyze viable alternatives for each proposed action based on the moral rules.
4. Determine the consequences or outcomes of each viable alternative on the communities or populations most affected by the decision.
5. Select the actions on the basis of the rules that produce the greatest amount of good or the least amount of harm for the communities or populations that are affected by the action.

(Remember that the utilitarian ethics decision process is one of the approaches in step 5 of the generic ethical decision-making framework.)

*Moral rules of action that produce the greatest good for the greatest number of communities or populations affected by or most affected by the rules.

Finally, regarding situation four, he believes in moral tolerance of nonthreatening ethnic traditions, as there is no moral mandate to do otherwise.

## ETHICS

### Definition, Theories, Principles

Ethics is concerned with a body of knowledge that addresses such questions as How should I behave? What actions should I perform? What kind of person should I be? What are my obligations to myself and to fellow humans? There are general obligations that humans have as members of society. Among these general obligations are not to harm others, to respect others, to tell the truth, and to keep promises. Sometimes, however, a situation dictates that individuals tell a lie or break a promise because the consequences of telling the truth or keeping the promise may bring about more harm than good. For example, as a community-oriented nurse you have promised a family that you will visit them at a certain time, but your schedule has gone awry because of unexpected circumstances: One of the other families you visit is in a state of crisis—their adolescent child is suicidal—and your nursing inter-

vention is needed. Most community-oriented nurses would agree that this is not a good time to keep the original promise. You are morally justified in breaking your promise because you fear that more harm than good would be done if it were kept.

This example illustrates several things about ethical thinking. First, ethical judgments are concerned with values. The goal of an ethical judgment is to choose that action or state of affairs that is good or right in the circumstances. Second, ethical judgments generally do not have the certainty of scientific judgments. For example, in community-oriented nursing, nurses diagnose a situation on the basis of the best available information and then choose the course of action that seems to provide the best ethical resolution to the issue. In some situations, the decision is based on outcomes or consequences. That approach to ethical decision making is called **consequentialism.** It maintains that the right action is the one that produces the greatest amount of good or the least amount of evil in a given situation. **Utilitarianism** is a well known consequentialist theory that appeals exclusively to outcomes or consequences in determining which choice to make.

In other situations, community-oriented nurses touch upon options open to fundamental beliefs. In such circumstances, these nurses may conclude that the action is right or wrong in itself, regardless of the amount of good that might come from it. This is the position known as **deontology.** It is based on the premise that persons should always be treated as ends in themselves and never as mere means to the ends of others.

Members of the health professions have specific obligations that exist because of the practices and goals of the

**DID YOU KNOW?**

Deontology comes from the Greek roots *deon* meaning duty and *logos* meaning study of.

**HOW TO** Apply the Deontological Ethics Decision Process

1. Determine the moral rules (e.g., tell the truth) that serve as standards by which individuals can perform their moral obligations.

2. Examine personal motives for proposed actions to ensure that they are based on good intentions in accord with moral rules.

3. Determine whether the proposed actions can be generalized so that all persons in similar situations are treated similarly.

4. Select the action that treats persons as ends in themselves and never as mere means to the ends of others.

(Remember that the deontological ethics decision process is one of the approaches in step 5 of the generic ethical decision-making framework.)

---

**BOX 6-2** Ethical Principles

**Respect for autonomy.** Based on human dignity and respect for individuals, autonomy requires that individuals be permitted to choose those actions and goals that fulfill their life plans unless those choices result in harm to another.

**Nonmaleficence.** According to Hippocrates, nonmaleficence requires that we do no harm. It is impossible to avoid harm entirely, but this principle requires that health care professionals act according to the standards of due care, always seeking to produce the least amount of harm possible.

**Beneficence.** This principle is complementary to nonmaleficence and requires that we "do good." We are limited by time, place, and talents in the amount of good we can do. We have general obligations to perform those actions that maintain or enhance the dignity of other persons whenever those actions do not place an undue burden on health care providers. Health care professionals have special obligations of beneficence to clients.

**Distributive justice.** Distributive justice requires that there be a fair distribution of the benefits and burdens in society based on the needs and contributions of its members. This principle requires that, consistent with the dignity and worth of its members and within the limits imposed by its resources, a society must determine a minimal level of goods and services to be available to its members. For community and public health professionals, this principle takes on considerable importance.

---

profession. These health care obligations have been interpreted in terms of a set of principles in bioethics. *The primary principles are respect for autonomy, nonmaleficence, beneficence,* and *distributive justice,* as shown in Box 6-2. Because of their sociological grounding, these principles have dominated the development of the field of bioethics since its inception in the 1960s (Evans, 2000). This approach has been called **principlism,** and one of its best descriptions and fullest articulations is in the fifth edition of Beauchamp and Childress' *Principles of Biomedical Ethics* (2001). This approach to ethical decision making in health care arose in response to life-and-death decision making in acute care settings, where the question to be resolved tended to concern a single localized issue such as the withdrawing or withholding of treatment (Holstein, 2001). In these circumstances, preserving and respecting a patient's autonomy became the dominant issue.

Despite its success as a basis for analysis in bioethics, principlism has come under attack in recent years from a variety of quarters (e.g., Boylan, 2000; Callahan, 2000; Clouser and Gert, 1990), and there are grounds for the criticism. First, the principles are said to be too abstract to serve as guides for action. Second, the principles themselves can conflict in a given situation, and there is no independent basis for resolving the conflict. Third, some persons claim that effective ethical problem solving must be rooted in concrete, individual experiences. Fourth, ethical judgments are alleged to depend more on the judgment of sensitive persons than on the application of abstract principles.

**HOW TO** Apply the Principlism Ethics Decision Process

1. Determine the ethical principles (respect for autonomy, nonmaleficence, beneficence, justice) that are relevant to an ethical issue or dilemma.

2. Analyze the relevant principles within a meaningful context of accurate facts and other pertinent circumstances.

3. Act on the principle that provides, within the meaningful context, the strongest guide to action that can be morally justified by the tenets foundational to the principle.

(Remember that the principlism ethics decision process is one of the approaches in step 5 of the general ethical decision-making framework.)

---

The dominance of the principle of autonomy has also been challenged by critics concerned about decision-making in non–acute care settings, where the ethical decision is more likely to be about, for example, long-term care or access to health care (Callahan and Jennings, 2002). Thus,

> ┌─ WHAT DO YOU THINK? ─
> Should community-oriented nursing services be given to a smaller number of clients with greater needs or to a larger number of clients with fewer needs?

whereas autonomy may be stressed in acute care settings, an overemphasis on autonomy may inhibit ethical decisions in the arenas of community and public health. In community and public health, beneficence and distributed justice are frequently a greater issue than autonomy.

For this reason, many urge that we look to other models for ethical decision making. Utilitarianism and deontology were developed from the Enlightenment's focus on universals, rationality, and isolated individuals. Each theory maintains that there is a universal first principle, the principle of utility for utilitarianism and the categorical imperative for deontology, that serves as a rational norm for our behavior and allows us to calculate the rightness or wrongness of each individual action. Both utilitarianism and deontology also follow the lead of classic liberalism in asserting that the individual is the special center of moral concern (Arras and Steinbock, 1999). Giving priority to individual rights and needs means that the "rights and dignity of the individual should never (or rarely) be sacrificed to the interests of the larger society" (Arras and Steinbock, 1999, p. 26). The focus on individual rights leads to complications in the interpretation of distributive or social justice.

Distributive or social justice refers to the allocation of benefits and burdens to members of society. "Benefit" refers to basic needs, including material and social goods, liberties, rights, and entitlements. Among the benefits of society are wealth, education, and public services. Among the burdens to be shared are such things as taxes, military service, and the location of incinerators and power plants. Justice requires that the distribution of benefits and burdens in a society be fair or equal. There is wide agreement that the distribution should be based on what one needs and deserves, but there is considerable disagreement as to what these terms mean. Three primary theories of distributive justice are defended today. They are the egalitarian, libertarian, and liberal democratic theories.

Egalitarianism is the view that everyone is entitled to equal rights and equal treatment in society. Ideally, each individual has an equal share of the goods of society, and it is the role of government to ensure that this happens. The government has the authority to redistribute wealth if necessary to ensure equal treatment. Thus egalitarians are supportive of welfare rights—that is, the right to receive certain social goods necessary to satisfy basic needs. These include adequate food, housing, education, and police and fire protection (Boss, 1998). The weaknesses of egalitarianism are both practical and theoretical. It would be practically impossible to ensure the equal distribution of goods and services in any moderately complex society. Assuming that such a distribution could be accomplished,

it would require a coercive authority to maintain it (Hellsten, 1998). Further, egalitarianism is unable to provide any incentive for each of us to do our best, as there is no promise of our merit being rewarded.

The libertarian view of justice rests on the assertion that the right to private property is the most important right. Libertarians recognize only liberty rights, the right to be left alone to accomplish our goals. Hellsten (1998) notes, "The central feature of the libertarian view on distributive justice is that it is totally individualist. It rejects any idea that societies, states, or collectives of any form can be the bearers of rights or can owe duties" (p. 822). Libertarians see a very limited role for government, namely the protection of property rights of individual citizens through providing police and fire protection. While they also concede the need for jointly shared, publicly owned facilities such as roads, they reject the idea of welfare rights and view taxes to support the needs of others as coercive taking of their property. Given the libertarian rejection of the priority of the state, however, it is not clear where the right to property comes from (Hellsten, 1998).

The liberal democratic theory is well represented by the work of John Rawls (2001). Rawls attempts to develop a theory that values both liberty and equality. He acknowledges that inequities are inevitable in society, but he tries to justify them by establishing a system in which everyone benefits, especially the least advantaged. This is an attempt to address the inequalities that result from birth, natural endowments, and historic circumstances. Imagining what he calls a "veil of ignorance" to keep us unaware of our actual advantages and disadvantages, Rawls would have us choose the basic principles of justice (p. 15). Once impartiality is guaranteed, Rawls maintains that all rational people will choose a system of justice containing the following two basic principles:

Each person has the same indefeasible claim to a fully adequate scheme of equal basic liberties, which scheme is compatible with the same scheme of liberties for all; and social and economic inequalities are to satisfy two conditions: first, they are to be attached to offices and positions open to all under conditions of fair equality of opportunity; and second, they are to be to the greatest benefit of the least advantaged members of society (the difference principle). (Rawls, 2001, p. 42)

As the veil of ignorance device and the justice principles indicate, Rawls and other justice theorists all assume the Enlightenment concept of isolated, atomic selves in competition for scarce resources. The significance of justice, then, becomes the assurance of fairness to individuals. Violating the dictates of distributive justice is an offense to the dignity of the collective preferences of autonomous, rational moral agents. The interests of the community may be in conflict with the interests of individuals; yet, confined to the Enlightenment ideal, the needs of society are not directly addressed, nor is society given any priority. This Enlightenment assumption has been challenged recently by a number of ethical theories loosely grouped together under the heading *communitarianism*. **Communitarianism** maintains that abstract, universal principles are not an adequate basis for moral decision making; instead, these theorists argue, history, tradition, and concrete moral communities should be the basis of moral thinking and action (Solomon, 1993). Among the theories with a communitarian focus are virtue ethics, feminism, and care.

## Virtue Ethics

**Virtue ethics** is one of the oldest ethical theories; it belongs to a tradition dating back to the ancient Greek philosophers Plato and Aristotle. It is not concerned with actions, as utilitarianism and deontology are, but instead asks, What kind of person should I be? The goal of virtue ethics is to enable persons to flourish as human beings. According to Aristotle, **virtues** are acquired, excellent traits of character that dispose humans to act in accord with their natural good. During the seventeenth and eighteenth centuries, the Greek concept of the good as a principle of explanation went out of favor. Since virtue ethics was closely tied to the concept of the good, interest in virtues as an element of normative ethics also declined. Examples of virtues include benevolence, compassion, discernment, trustworthiness, integrity, and conscientiousness (Beauchamp and Childress, 2001, pp. 32-39).

Recently, there have been several attempts to revive virtue ethics (MacIntyre, 1984), including specific applications to the health care professions (Pellegrino, 1995). In a pluralistic society, there may be difficulty in reaching agreement about what it means to flourish as a human being, thus fulfilling the goal of virtue ethics. Although it may not be possible to agree on a single end for human beings, many persons believe it is possible to agree on what is meant by the good for more restricted aspects of our lives.

The appeal to virtues results in a significantly different approach to moral decision making in health care (Fletcher, 1999). In contrast to moral justification via theories or principles, the emphasis is on practical reasoning applied to character development.

## Caring and the Ethic of Care

Caring in nursing, the ethic of care, and feminist ethics are all interrelated and, historically, all converged between the mid 1980s and early 1990s. Regarding caring in nursing, seminal work was done by nurse–scholars (e.g., Leininger, 1984; Watson, 1985), who wrote about caring as the essence of or the moral ideal of nursing. This conceptualization occurred as a response to the technological advances in health care science and to the desire of nurses to differentiate nursing practice from medical practice. The discussion of the centrality of caring to nursing and to community-oriented nursing continues to the present. A current example is Eriksson's (2002) work on a caring science theory, which she sees as ethical in its essence. Proponents of caring support its premises; its distracters believe that nursing is not the only essentially caring profession and that caring, when placed within a broader societal context, represents the use of a disempowering concept to

---

> **HOW TO** **Apply the Virtue Ethics Decision Process**
>
> 1. Identify communities that are relevant to the ethical dilemmas or issues.
> 2. Identify moral considerations that arise from a communal perspective and apply the consideration to specific communities.
> 3. Identify and apply virtues that facilitate a communal perspective.
> 4. Modify moral considerations as needed to apply to the specific ethical dilemmas or issues.
> 5. Seek ethical community support to enhance character development.
> 6. Evaluate and modify the individuals or community character traits that impede communal living.
>
> ---
>
> (Remember that the virtue ethics decision process is one of the approaches in Step 5 of the generic ethical decision-making framework.)
> Modified from Volbrecht RM: *Nursing ethics: communities in dialogue*, p 138, Upper Saddle River, NJ, 2002, Prentice Hall.

---

identify the essence of nursing. However, most nurses, including community-oriented nurses, would agree that there is a relationship between caring and ethics or morality.

According to Volbrecht (2002), Carol Gilligan and Nel Noddings are considered to be the mothers of the *ethic of care*. For that reason, and because community-oriented nurses can identify with their writings, the seminal works of Gilligan (1982) and Noddings (1984) are briefly noted.

Gilligan (1982) speaks of a personal journey where, by listening and talking to people, she began to notice two distinct voices about morality and two ways of describing the interpersonal relationships between self and others. Contrary to what has been written about Gilligan and the two distinct voices (i.e., male and female) related to moral judgment, here is what she actually wrote: "The different voice I describe is characterized *not by gender* [italics added] but theme. Its association with women is an empirical observation, and it is primarily through women's voices that I trace its development. But this association is not absolute, and the contrasts between male and female voices are presented here to highlight a distinction between two modes of thought and to focus [on] a problem of interpretation rather than to represent a generalization about either sex" (Gilligan, 1982, p. 2). Her 1982 book is based on three qualitative studies about conceptions of morality and self and about experiences of conflict and choice. From these studies she formulated her basic premises about responsibility, care, and relationships. These premises, in Gilligan's (1982) own voice, are as follows:

1. "Sensitivity to the needs of others and the assumption of responsibility for taking care lead women to attend to voices other than their own" (p. 16).

2. "Women not only define themselves in a context of human relationships but also judge themselves in terms of their ability to care" (p. 17).
3. "The truths of relationship, however, return in the rediscovery of connection, in the realization that self and other are interdependent and that life, however valuable in itself, can only be sustained by care in relationships" (p. 127).

Noddings's (1984) personal journey started at a point different from that of Gilligan's. Noddings noticed that ethics was described in the literature primarily using principles and logic. The goal for Noddings's book, therefore, was to express a feminine view that could be accepted or rejected by women *or* men.

The basic premises of Noddings (1984), in her own voice, are as follows:

1. "The essential elements of caring are located in the relation between the one caring and the cared-for" (p. 9).
2. "Caring requires me to respond . . . with an act of commitment: I commit myself either to overt action on behalf of the cared-for or I commit myself to thinking about what I might do" (p. 81).
3. "We are not 'justified'–we are *obligated*–to do what is required to maintain and enhance caring" (p. 95).
4. "Caring itself and the ethical ideal that strives to maintain and enhance it guide us in moral decisions and conduct" (p. 105).

What both Gilligan and Noddings have in common has been called a **feminine ethic,** because they believe in the morality of responsibility in relationships that emphasize connection and caring. To them caring is not a mere nicety but a moral imperative. Nevertheless, a long-term healthy debate has surrounded their premises.

## Feminist Ethics

Although feminist ethics has begun to enter nursing, to date it has had limited impact on community-oriented nursing. Yet, according to Leipert (2001), the tenets of feminist ethics are highly relevant to community and public health nurses. According to her, "A feminist perspective facilitates critical thought and a focus on broad issues such as power, gender, and socioeconomic structures. Since these latter issues impact significantly on health, and since public health nurses work predominantly with power, gender, and socioeconomic determinants of health, feminist perspectives and approaches hold great import for public health nursing practice" (p. 54).

But what is meant by *feminists* and *feminist ethics?* **Feminists** are women *and* men who hold a worldview advocating economic, social, and political equality for women that is equivalent to that of men. Consequently, feminists reject the devaluing of women and their experiences through systematic oppression based on gender. According to Volbrecht (2002), "A feminist is also someone who works to bring about the social changes necessary to promote more just relationships among women and men" (p. 160). Feminists also can ascribe to the ethic of care.

**Feminist ethics** encompasses the tenets that women's thinking and moral experiences are important and should be taken into account in any fully developed moral theory, and that the oppression of women is morally wrong. Study of feminist ethics entails knowledge about and critique of classical ethical theories developed by men as well as ethical theories developed by women. Study of feminist ethics also entails knowledge about the social, cultural, political, economic, environmental, and professional contexts that insidiously and overtly oppress women as individuals, or within a family, group, community, or society.

Feminists and persons who ascribe to feminist ethics are not passive; they demand social justice and political action, preferably at the societal level and through legislation. Volbrecht (2002) has developed a feminist ethics decision-making process that readies women and men for such action.

---

**HOW TO** **Apply the Care Ethics Decision Process**

1. Recognize that caring is a moral imperative.
2. Identify personally lived caring experiences as a basis for relating to self and others.
3. Assume responsibility and obligation to promote and enhance caring in relationships.

---

(Remember that the care ethics decision process is one of the approaches in Step 5 of the generic ethical decision-making framework.)

---

**HOW TO** **Apply the Feminist Ethics Decision Process**

1. Identify the social, cultural, political, economic, environmental, and professional contexts that contribute to the identified problem (e.g., underrepresentation of women in clinical trials).
2. Evaluate how the preceding contexts contribute to the oppression of women.
3. Consider how women's lives are defined by their status in subordinate social groups.
4. Analyze how social practices marginalize women.
5. Plan ways to restructure those social practices that oppress women.
6. Implement the plan.
7. Evaluate the plan and restructure it as needed.

---

(Remember that the feminist ethics decision process is one of the approaches in Step 5 of the generic ethical decision-making framework.)

Modified from Volbrecht RM: *Nursing ethics: communities in dialogue,* p 219, Upper Saddle River, NJ, 2002, Prentice Hall.

## ETHICS AND THE CORE FUNCTIONS OF COMMUNITY-ORIENTED NURSING

In Chapter 1, the three foundational pillars or core functions of community-oriented nursing (i.e., assessment, policy development, and assurance) were identified and discussed. This discussion, however, did not include the basic assumption that community-oriented nursing is an ethical endeavor, with moral leadership at its core. Now the links of these three core functions to ethics are described.

### Assessment

To review, "*assessment* refers to systematic data collection on the population, monitoring of the population's health status, and making information available on the health of the community" (Williams, 2000, p. 4). Underlying this core function are at least three ethical tenets. The first relates to competency related to knowledge development, analysis, and dissemination. An ethical question related to competency is, Are the persons assigned to develop community knowledge adequately prepared to collect data on groups and populations? This question is important because the research, measurement, and analysis techniques used to gather information about groups and populations usually differ from the techniques used to assess individuals. Wrong research techniques can lead to wrong assessments, which in turn may hurt rather than help the intended group or population.

The second ethical tenet relates to virtue ethics or moral character. An ethical question related to moral character is, Do the persons selected to develop, assess, and disseminate community knowledge possess integrity? Beauchamp and Childress (2001) define *integrity* as "soundness, wholeness, and integration of moral character" (p. 36). The importance of this virtue is self-evident: without integrity, the core function of assessment is endangered. Persons with compromised integrity are easy prey for potential or real scientific misconduct.

The third ethical tenet relates to "do no harm." An ethical question related to "do no harm" is, Is disseminating appropriate information about groups and populations morally necessary and sufficient? The answer to "morally necessary" is yes, but to "morally sufficient" it is no. The fallacy with dissemination is that there is no built-in accountability that what is disseminated will be read or understood. If not read or understood, harm could come to groups and populations regarding their health status.

### Policy Development

To review, "*Policy development* refers to the need to provide leadership in developing policies that support the health of the population, including the use of the scientific knowledge base in making decisions about policy" (Williams, 2000, p. 4). Underlying this core function are at least three ethical tenets. The first purports that an important goal of both policy and ethics is to achieve the public good (Silva, 2002). According to several recent accounts, the concept of "the public good" is rooted in citizenship (e.g., Denhardt and Denhardt, 2000; Shapiro, 1999; Walters, Aydelotte, and Miller, 2000). For example, Denhardt and Denhardt (2000) view citizenship, or what they call "democratic citizenship" (p. 552), as a stance in which citizens play a more substantial role in policy development. For this to occur, however, citizens must be willing not only to be informed about policy but also to do what is in the best interests of the community. The approach is basically one in which the voice of the community is the foundation upon which policy is developed, rather than the voice of community *and* public health administrators.

The second ethical tenet purports that service to others over self is a necessary condition of what is "good" or "right" policy (Silva, 2002). Denhardt and Denhardt (2000) offer three perspectives on this matter:

- *Serve rather than steer.* An increasingly important role of the public servant (e.g., community health and public health nurses and administrators) is to help citizens articulate and meet their shared interests rather than to attempt to control or steer society in new directions (p. 553).
- *Serve citizens, not customers.* The public interest results from a dialogue about shared values rather than the aggregation of individual self-interests. Therefore public servants do not merely respond to the demands of "customers" but focus on building relationships of trust and collaboration with and among citizens (p. 555).
- *Value citizenship and public service above entrepreneurship.* The public interest is better advanced by public servants and citizens committed to making meaningful contributions to society rather than by entrepreneurial managers acting as if public money were their own (p. 556).

These three perspectives have at their core service, and service always has been one of the enduring values of nursing.

The third ethical tenet purports that what is ethical is also good policy (Silva, 2002). What is ethical should be the singular foundational pillar upon which community-oriented nursing is based. Moral leadership is critical to policy development because it is the highest human standard and therefore should result in ethical health care policies.

### Assurance

To review, "*assurance* refers to the role of public health in making sure that essential community-oriented health services are available, which may include providing essential personal health services for those who would otherwise not receive them. Assurance also refers to making sure that a competent public health and personal health care workforce is available" (Williams, 2000, p. 4). Underlying this core function are at least two ethical tenets.

The first purports that all persons should receive essential personal health services or, put in terms of justice, "to each person a fair share" or, reworded, "to all groups or populations a fair share." This is an egalitarian perspective

## *Ethics and Community Health Nursing in Canada*

Betty Burcher, R.N., B.A., B.Sc.N., M.Sc., Lecturer, Faculty of Nursing, University of Toronto

Nurses working in community health (public health, home health, primary care, community mental health, occupational health, and so on) are guided and directed by ethical principles, theories, policies, and legislation that encompass both individuals and populations. Professional nursing ethics tend to be more focused on individuals, whereas working in community health requires, in addition, ethical decision making based on the needs and rights of groups or all in society.

### CODE OF ETHICS FOR REGISTERED NURSES

The Canadian Nurses Association's code (CNA) of ethics (CNA, 2002) sets out ethical behaviour expected of registered nurses in Canada. Not only does the code give guidance for decision making concerning ethical behaviours and a process for self-evaluation and self-reflection but it also provides a basis for feedback, peer review, and advocacy for quality practice environments. The code is structured around eight primary values. These are safe, competent, and ethical care; health and well-being; choice; dignity; confidentiality; justice; accountability; and quality practice environments. Whereas the code of ethics is national in scope, health care is principally delivered and administered by the provinces, and nursing practice is regulated by each province or territory. Consequently, community health nurses need to understand not only the standards of practice and ethical guidelines set by their respective provincial regulatory body but also the applicable provincial, federal, and municipal legislation that provides the legal context for ethical decision making.

### RELATIONSHIPS WITH CLIENTS

Community health nurses need to be aware of their jurisdiction's legislation on the protection of privacy, the provision of informed consent, freedom of choice including the right to refuse treatment, determination of competency, cardiopulmonary resuscitation (CPR) and end-of-life treatment, and the legal status of advance directives. Advance directives are the "means used to document and communicate a person's preferences regarding life-sustaining treatment in the event they become incapable of expressing those wishes for themselves" (CNA, 1998). Advance directives are described as either an instruction directive in which the individual identifies what life-sustaining treatment he or she wishes in particular situations or a proxy directive in which the individual identifies who is to make the health care decisions if she or he becomes incompetent. Some provinces and territories recognize only proxy directives, and others recognize both proxy and instructional directives.

### ACCOUNTABILITY

Accountability includes providing an explanation of one's assigned responsibilities to oneself, the client, the employer, and the profession. In the last decade in Canada, there has been an increasing focus in the public sector on program, fiscal, and organizational accountability as politicians, taxpayers, and funders require performance outcomes and results. As a result, community health agencies must now provide evidence of improving health outcomes for targeted groups and popula-

---

of justice. This perspective does not mean that all persons in a society should share all of society's benefits equally, but that they should share at least those benefits that are essential. Few persons who see justice as fairness would disagree that basic health care for all is essential for social justice within a society.

The second ethical tenet purports that providers of public health services are competent and available. Although the *Public Health Code of Ethics* does not speak directly to workforce availability, it does speak directly to ensuring professional competency of public health employees. In addition to the *Public Health Code of Ethics, Healthy People 2010* not only addresses competencies but also notes workforce as depicted in the Healthy People 2010 box.

Goal 23-8 of Healthy People 2010 addresses the need for all public health workers not only to have knowledge of public health but also to have additional competencies as needed to fulfill their job responsibilities. Specific areas of knowledge noted in goal 23-8 include, among others, information technology, biostatistics, environmental health, and cultural and linguistic competence. Goals 23-9 and 23-10 address the present and future pub-

lic health workforce. This workforce represents future public health leaders, who must be educated to meet challenges in such areas as bioterrorism and technological disasters. Emphasis is also given to the availability and provision of life-long learning opportunities for public health employees.

## NURSING CODE OF ETHICS

As noted in the history section of this chapter, the *Code of Ethics for Nurses with Interpretive Statements* was adopted by the ANA House of Delegates in 2001. The three purposes of the 2001 code are the following:

- To be a succinct statement of the ethical obligations and duties of every individual who enters the nursing profession
- To be the profession's nonnegotiable ethical standard
- To be an expression of nursing's own understanding of its commitment to society (p. 5)

These purposes are reflected in the nine provisional statements of the code, as identified in Box 6-3. The **Code of Ethics** for nurses and its interpretive statements apply to community-oriented nurses, although the emphasis for

tions. Although this may assist in making decisions more explicit with regard to balancing harms and benefits for a population, it can also increase ethical dilemmas for community practitioners who must demonstrate program efficiency and balance the actual costs and benefits with providing for all who have health needs.

## CANADA HEALTH ACT

The Canada Health Act (1984) sets out the principles underlying the publicly funded health care system. They are comprehensiveness, universality, accessibility, portability, and public administration. For many Canadians, these principles articulate a social contract that defines health care as a basic right, that every person has an equal right to health care. Many also argue that the Canadian public health care system is equitable because the funding is derived from a progressive taxation system and is redistributed within the system on the basis of medical need, not the ability to pay. These two core ethical values, equality and equity, are fundamental to our health care system and lie beneath the current debate about the sustainability of the health care system. Although the content of the discourse focuses on provincial and federal responsibilities, decreased transfer payments, downloading, delisting of services, private versus public, health system restructuring, and so on, the debate is ultimately about these primary ethical values and their importance to Canadians. Accordingly, the Commission on the Future of Health Care in Canada has identified Canadian values as one of the four themes in its inquiry into ensuring the sustainability of a universally accessible publicly funded health system.

## Bibliography

Canada Health Act of 1984, Bill C–31: Ottawa, 1984, House of Commons, Government of Canada, available at http://www.hc-sc.gc.ca/medicare.

Canadian Nurses Association: Advance directives: the nurse's role. In Ethics for practice, Ottawa, 1998, CNA.

Canadian Nurses Association: Code of ethics for registered nurses, Ottawa, 2002, CNA.

Commission on the Future of Health Care in Canada: Shape the future of health care, Ottawa, 2002, Commission on the Future of Health Care in Canada, available at http://www.healthcarecommission.ca.

Community Health Nurses' Initiative Group of the Registered Nurses' Association of Ontario: Home health nursing position paper, Toronto, 2000, Registered Nurses Association of Ontario.

Community Health Nurses Interest Group of the Registered Nurses Association of Ontario: Public health nursing position statement, Toronto, 1998, Registered Nurses Association of Ontario.

Keatings M, Smith OB: Ethical and legal issues in Canadian nursing, Toronto, 2000, Saunders Canada.

Oberle K, Tenove S: Ethical issues in public health nursing, Nurs Ethics 7(5):425-438, 2000.

Storch JL, Meilicke CA: Political, social and economic forces shaping the health-care system. In Nursing management in Canada, Toronto, 1999, Saunders Canada.

Canadian spelling is used.

## Healthy People 2010 — Public Health Infrastructure and Workforce

The following are national goals (and their code numbers) for ensuring that all public agencies have the necessary infrastructure to provide essential and efficient public health services:

23-8 Increase the proportion of federal, tribal, state, and local agencies that incorporate specific competencies in the essential public health services into personnel systems.

23-9 Increase the proportion of schools for public health workers that integrate into their curricula specific content to develop competency in the essential public health services.

23-10 Increase the proportion of federal, tribal, state and local public health agencies that provide continuing education to develop competency in essential public health services for their employees.

From U.S. Department of Health and Human Services: Healthy people 2010: understanding and improving health and objectives for improving health, ed 2, Washington, DC, 2000, U.S. Government Printing Office.

each type of nursing sometimes varies. For example, provision 1 and its interpretive statement primarily address the individual but acknowledge that there are times when public health considerations override individual rights. Provisions 2 and 3 and their interpretive statements are pertinent to both community health nurses and to public health nurses. Keep in mind, however, that in provision 3, patient means the recipient of nursing care, whether a group, family, or community.

Whereas provisions 1 through 3 focus on the recipients of nursing care, provisions 4 through 6 focus on the nurse (in this case, the community-oriented nurse). This focus addresses nurses' accountability, competency, and contributions to their employment conditions.

## Evidence-Based Practice

The restructuring of health care has caused public health agencies to rethink how to educate competent public health nurses for the future. Two focus groups of knowledgeable participants were asked to synthesize published and unpublished materials related to the preceding goal. Knowledgeable participants included persons and organizations responsible for public health nursing education and practice at the local, state, and national levels. Staff public health nurses were also included, as well as persons recommended by their peers.

The first focus group identified knowledge and skills most needed by public health nurses, whereas the second focus group drafted content for a core curriculum in public health nursing continuing education. The focus groups identified epidemiology as the most needed knowledge, and bringing about organizational change as the most needed skill. Suggested content for the core continuing education curriculum included such topics as *ethics and values* [italics added], environmental health, health policy, partnership development, informatics, health economics, and conflict negotiation and resolution. An ideally proposed teaching method for the core curriculum was distance-based learning technology available 7 days a week around the clock.

**Nurse Use:** Apply this information to designing courses and programs to educate public health nurses.

Gebbie KM, Hwang I: Preparing currently employed public health nurses for changes in the health system, *Am J Public Health* 90(5):716, 2000.

## THE CUTTING EDGE

The American Nurses Association plans to have online continuing education modules of the *Code of Ethics for Nurses with Interpretative Statements* before 2004.

## BOX 6-3  Code of Ethics for Nurses

1. The nurse, in all professional relationships, practices with compassion and respect for the inherent dignity, worth, and uniqueness of every individual, unrestricted by considerations of social or economic status, personal attributes, or the nature of the health problems.
2. The nurse's primary commitment is to the patient, whether an individual, family, group, or community.
3. The nurse promotes, advocates for, and strives to protect the health, safety, and rights of the patient.
4. The nurse is responsible and accountable for individual nursing practice and determines the appropriate delegation of tasks consistent with the nurse's obligation to provide optimal patient care.
5. The nurse owes the same duties to self as to others, including the responsibility to preserve integrity and safety, to maintain competence, and to continue personal and professional growth.
6. The nurse participates in establishing, maintaining, and improving health care environments and conditions of employment conducive to the provision of quality health care and consistent with the values of the profession through individual and collective action.
7. The nurse participates in the advancement of the profession through contributions to practice, education, administration, and knowledge development.
8. The nurse collaborates with other health professionals and the public in promoting community, national, and international efforts to meet health needs.
9. The profession of nursing, as represented by associations and their members, is responsible for articulating nursing values, for maintaining the integrity of the profession and its practice, and for shaping social policy.

Reprinted with permission from the American Nurses Association, *Code of Ethics for Nurses with Interpretive Statements,* Washington, DC, 2001, American Nurses Foundation/American Nurses Association.

---

Provisions 7 through 9 focus on the bigger picture of both the nursing profession and national and global health concerns. Regarding the nursing profession, the emphasis is on professional standards, active involvement in nursing, and the integrity of the profession. All community-oriented nurses have a responsibility to meet these obligations. Regarding national and global health concerns, the emphasis is on social justice and reform. According to the ANA (2001), "The nurse has a responsibility to be aware not only of specific health needs of individual patients but also of broader health concerns such as world hunger, environmental pollution, lack of access to health care, violation of human rights, and inequitable distribution of nursing and health care resources" (p. 23). The ANA Code (2001) also stresses political action as the mechanism to effect social justice and reform regarding homelessness, violence, and stigmatization. All of the preceding responsibilities typically fall more in the domain of public health nursing than community health nursing, although all community-oriented nurses should be aware of the social activism embedded

> ### BOX 6-4  Levels of Prevention Related to Ethics
>
> **PRIMARY PREVENTION**
>
> Use the *Code of Ethics for Nurses* to guide your nursing practice.
>
> **SECONDARY PREVENTION**
>
> If you are unable to behave in accordance with the *Code of Ethics for Nurses* (for example, you speak in a way that does not communicate respect for a patient), take steps to correct your behavior. You could explain to the patient your error and apologize.
>
> **TERTIARY PREVENTION**
>
> If you have treated a patient or staff member in a way that is inconsistent with ethics practices, seek guidance on other choices you could have made.

in the 2001 code. Box 6-4 shows Levels of Prevention related to ethics.

## PUBLIC HEALTH CODE OF ETHICS

The *Public Health Code of Ethics* (Public Health Leadership Society, 2001) was noted in the history section of this chapter. This code consists of a preamble; 12 principles related to the ethical practice of public health (Box 6-5); 11 values and beliefs that focus on health, community, and action; and a commentary on each of the 12 principles. The preamble asserts the collective and societal nature of public health to keep people healthy. The 12 principles incorporate the ethical tenets of preventing harm; doing no harm; promoting good; respecting both individual and community rights; respecting autonomy, diversity, and confidentiality when possible; ensuring professional competency; trustworthiness; and promoting advocacy for disenfranchised persons within a community. Examples of values and beliefs include a right to health care resources, the interdependency of humans living in the community, and the importance of knowledge as a basis for action.

When the *Code of Ethics for Nursing* and the *Public Health Code of Ethics* are assessed, some commonalities emerge. These codes provide general ethical principles and approaches that are both enduring and dynamic. They force community-oriented nurses and public health personnel to think about the underlying ethics of their profession. Although the two codes do not specify (nor should they specify) details for every ethical issue, other mechanisms such as standards of practice, ethical decision-making frameworks, and ethics committees help work out the details. Nevertheless, the preceding two codes address most approaches to ethical justification, including traditional and emerging ethical theories and principles, humanist and feminist ethics, virtue ethics, professional–individual and/or community relationships, and advocacy.

## ADVOCACY AND ETHICS

### Definitions, Codes, Standards

**Advocacy** is a powerful ethical concept in community-oriented nursing. But what does *advocacy* mean? There are many definitions, but two definitions offered by Christoffel (2000) are useful in that they seem to differentiate between community health nursing and public health nursing. The following definition of community health nursing seems appropriate: "*Advocacy* is the application of information and resources (including finances, effort, and votes) to effect systemic changes that shape the way people in a community live" (p. 722). In contrast, "*Public health advocacy* is advocacy that is intended to reduce death or disability in groups of people . . . . Such advocacy involves the use of information and resources to reduce the occurrence or severity of public health problems" (pp. 722-723). The former definition is intended to address the quality of life of individuals in a community, whereas the latter definition is intended to address the quality of life for aggregates or populations. As such, both definitions have an ethical basis grounded in quality of life.

Several codes and standards of practice address advocacy. Three are noted here. Advocacy is addressed in the ANA and the Public Health Leadership Society's codes of ethics, as well as the ANA's (1999) *Scope and Standards of Public Health Nursing Practice*.

According to the ANA (2001) *Code of Ethics for Nurses with Interpretive Statements,* "The nurse promotes, advocates for, and strives to protect the health, safety, and rights of the patient" (p. 12). The focus of the interpretive statements regarding advocacy is the nurse's responsibility to take action when the patient's best interests are jeopardized by questionable practice on the part of any member of the health team, the health care system, or others.

According to the Public Health Leadership Society's (2001) *Public Health Code of Ethics,* "Public health should advocate and work for the empowerment of disenfranchised community members, aiming to ensure that the basic resources and conditions necessary for health are accessible to all" (p. 1). The Public Health Leadership Society's code elaborates on the preceding principle by addressing two issues: that the voice of the community should be heard and that the marginalized or underserved in a community should receive "a decent minimum" (p. 4) of health resources.

According to the ANA's (1999) *Scope and Standards of Public Health Nursing Practice,* public health nurses have a moral mandate to establish ethical standards when advocating for health care policy. The preceding standards extend the prior two concepts of advocacy by moving advocacy into the policy arena, particularly health and social policy as applied to populations.

### Components of Advocacy

According to Christoffel (2000), public health advocacy is composed of two components: products and processes. The

## BOX 6-5 Principles of the Ethical Practice of Public Health

1. Public health should address principally the fundamental causes of disease and requirements for health, aiming to prevent adverse health outcomes.

2. Public health should achieve community health in a way that respects the rights of individuals in the community.

3. Public health policies, programs, and priorities should be developed and evaluated through processes that ensure an opportunity for input from community members.

4. Public health should advocate and work for the empowerment of disenfranchised community members, aiming to ensure that the basic resources and conditions necessary for health are accessible to all.

5. Public health should seek the information needed to implement effective policies and programs that protect and promote health.

6. Public health institutions should provide communities with the information they have that is needed for decisions on policies or programs and should obtain the community's consent for their implementation.

7. Public health institutions should act in a timely manner on the information they have, within the resources and the mandate given to them by the public.

8. Public health programs and policies should incorporate a variety of approaches that anticipate and respect diverse values, beliefs, and cultures in the community.

9. Public health programs and policies should be implemented in a manner that most enhances the physical and social environment.

10. Public health institutions should protect the confidentiality of information that can bring harm to an individual or community if made public. Exceptions must be justified on the basis of the high likelihood of significant harm to the individual or others.

11. Public health institutions should ensure the professional competencies of their employees.

12. Public health institutions and their employees should engage in collaborations and affiliations in ways that build the public's trust and the institution's effectiveness.

Reprinted with permission from the Public Health Leadership Society (PHLS): *Code of Ethics for Public Health,* New Orleans, La, 2001, Louisiana Public Health Institute.

Members of the PHLS ethics work group who created the *Code of Ethics for Public Health* include Elizabeth Bancroft (Centers for Disease Control and Prevention, Los Angeles County), Kitty Hsu Dana (APHA), Jack Dillenberg (Arizona School of Health Sciences), Joxel Garcia (Connecticut Department of Health), Kathleen Gensheimer (Maine Department of Health), V. James Guillory (University of Health Sciences, Kansas City, MO), Teresa Long (Columbus, Ohio, Department of Health), Ann Peterson (Virginia Department of Health), Michael Sage (Centers for Disease Control and Prevention), Liz Schwarte (Public Health Leadership Society), James Thomas (University of North Carolina), Kathy Vincent (Alabama Health Department), Carol Woltring (Center for Health Leadership Development and Practice, Oakland, CA). The ethics project was funded in part by the Centers for Disease Control and Prevention.

end products are decreased morbidity and mortality. The intermediate products occur at the individual/family level (more community-health oriented) and at the extended family/community level (more public-health oriented). Examples of products at the individual/family level include healthy diet, stress reduction, and prenatal care. Examples of products at the extended family/community level include reduced dangers from the environment (e.g., pollution) and facilitation of community actions (e.g., school-based health services). To reduce public health problems effectively, multiple changes need to occur at both levels.

In addition, Christoffel (2000) views the processes involved in public health advocacy as follows: "(1) problem identification; (2) research and data gathering; (3) professional and clinical education, as well as education of those involved in the creation of public policy (including media coverage); (4) development and promotion of regulations and legislation; (5) endorsement of regulations and legislation via elections and government actions; (6) enforcement of effective policies; and (7) policy process and outcome evaluations" (p. 723). Community health nurses are more typically involved in one through three, and public health nurses are more typically involved in four through seven. In reality, however, all seven processes are interwoven within a context that best reduces morbidity and mortality. Two ethical principles underlying these products and processes are promoting good and preventing harm.

## Conceptual Framework for Advocacy

Christoffel (2000) goes on to identify three stages of her conceptual framework for advocacy: information stage, strategy stage, and action stage. The information stage focuses on gathering data about public health problems, including such factors as extent of the problem, patterns of frequency, and effectiveness of and barriers to public health programs. The strategy stage focuses on such tactics as disseminating the gathered information and policy statements to lay and professional audiences, identifying objectives, building and funding coalitions, and working with legislators. The action stage focuses on implementing the strategies through such tactics as lobbying, testifying, issuing press releases, passing laws, and voting. Several ethical tenets underlie the preceding conceptual framework for advocacy. These tenets include scientific integrity in data gathering and dissemination; respect for persons (i.e., lay and professional audiences); honesty regarding fundraising; truthfulness in lobbying and testifying; and justice in passing laws.

Modified from Bateman N: *Advocacy skills for health and social care professionals*, p 63, Philadelphia, 2000, Jessica Kingsley.

| BOX 6-6 Ethical Principles for Effective Advocacy |
|---|

1. Act in the client's (group's, community's) best interests.
2. Act in accordance with the client's (group's, community's) wishes and instructions.
3. Keep the client (group, community) properly informed.
4. Carry out instructions with diligence and competence.
5. Act impartially and offer frank, independent advice.
6. Maintain client confidentiality.

## Practical Framework for Advocacy

Bateman (2000) takes a practical approach to advocacy. He places the advocate's core skills (i.e., interviewing, assertiveness and force, negotiation, self-management, legal knowledge and research, and litigation) within the context of six ethical principles for effective advocacy, as shown in Box 6-6. His focus is on the individual client, although the focus could also apply to groups and communities as well.

Regarding the first ethical principle, Bateman (2000) is sensitive to the ethical conflict between clients' best interests and the best interests of groups, communities, or societies but does not elaborate on this conflict. The second ethical principle, which puts the client in charge, works in tandem with the first principle. It goes like this: "This is what I think we can do. What do you want me to do?" (Bateman, 2000, p. 51). Of course, the advocate can refuse the request if self or others may be harmed. By following the third ethical principle, the client is empowered to make knowledgeable decisions. The fourth ethical principal addresses standards of practice. The fifth ethical principle addresses fairness and respect for persons (community-oriented nursing is more collaborative in nature than independent.) The last ethical principle, confidentiality, ensures that information will be shared only on a need-to-know basis.

## Practice Application*

The retiring director of the Division of Primary Care in a state health department had recently hired Ann, a 34-year-old nurse with a master's degree in public health, to be director of the division. Ann's work involved the monitoring of millions of dollars of state and federal money as well as the supervising of the funded programs within her division.

Ann received many requests for funding from a particular state agency that served a poor, large district. The poor people of the district primarily consisted of young families with children and homebound older adults with chronic illnesses. Over the past 3 years, the federal government had allocated considerable money to the state agency to subsidize pediatric primary care programs, but no formal evaluation of these programs had occurred.

The director of the state agency was a physician who had been in this position for over 20 years. He was good at obtaining funding for primary care needs in his district, but the statistics related to the pediatric primary care program seemed implausible—that is, few physical exams were performed on the children, which had resulted in extra money in the budget. This unspent federal money was being used to supplement home health care services for the indigent homebound older adults in his district. The thinking of the physician was that he was doing good by providing some needed services to both indigent groups in his district. Ann felt moral discomfort because she did not have either the money or the personnel to provide both services. What should she do?

A. What facts are the most relevant in this scenario?
B. What are the ethical issues?
C. How can Ann resolve the issues?

*The preceding case and answers are adapted and paraphrased from a real practice application shared by J. L. Chapin in the inappropriate distribution of primary health care funds. In Silva M, editor: *Ethical decision making in nursing administration*, Norwalk, Conn, 1990, Appleton & Lange.

**Answers are in the back of the book.**

## Key Points

- Nursing has a rich heritage of ethics and morality, beginning with Florence Nightingale.
- During the late 1960s, the field of bioethics began to emerge and influence nursing.
- Ethical decision making is the component of ethics that focuses on the process of how ethical decisions are made.
- Many different ethical decision-making frameworks exist; however, underlying each of them is the problem-solving process.
- Ethical decision making applies to all approaches to ethics: utilitarianism, deontology, principlism, virtue ethics, the ethic of care, and feminist ethics.
- Cultural diversity makes ethical decision making more challenging.
- Classical ethical theories are utilitarianism and deontology.
- Principlism consists of respect for autonomy, nonmaleficence, beneficence, and justice.
- Other approaches to ethics include virtue ethics, the ethic of care, and feminist ethics.
- The core functions of community-oriented nursing (i.e., assessment, policy development, and assurance) are all grounded in ethics.
- Healthy People 2010, under public health infrastructure, addresses workforce competencies, training in essential public health services, and continuing education.

- The 2001 *Code of Ethics for Nurses* contains nine statements that address the moral standards that delineate nursing's values, goals, and obligations.
- The 2001 *Public Health Code of Ethics* contains 12 statements that address the moral standards that delineate public health's values, goals, and obligations.
- Advocacy is the act of pleading for or supporting a course of action on behalf of a person, group, or community.
- The *Code of Ethics for Nursing*, the *Public Health Code of Ethics*, and *The Scope and Standards of Public Health Nursing Practice* all address advocacy.
- Public health advocacy is composed of both products and processes.
- The products of advocacy are decreased morbidity and mortality.
- The processes of public health advocacy include, but are not limited to, identifying problems, collecting data, developing and endorsing regulations and legislation, enforcing policies, and assessing the policy process.

## Clinical Decision-Making Activities

1. Interview a long-retired community-oriented nurse about the most important ethical issues that this nurse faced when practicing. Next, interview an actively practicing community-oriented nurse about the most important ethical issues that this nurse is now facing. Compare and contrast the ethical issues in the two interviews and place each within a historical context.

2. In a local or national newspaper, read one or more articles that discuss health care public policy with which you agree or disagree. Compose a letter to the editor analyzing why you agree or disagree with the policy but only after you take into account any of your own biases or vested interests.

3. Analyze the 2001 *Code of Ethics for Nurses.* Critique it for clarity and relevance. Give specific examples to support your assessment.

4. Analyze the 2001 *Principles of the Ethical Practice of Public Health.* Critique it for clarity and relevance. Give specific examples to support your assessment. Compare and contrast the two codes.

5. Discuss why feminist ethics has not been well received in community-oriented nursing. Compose a logical position statement defending its merits for community-oriented nursing.

### Additional Resources

These related resources are found either in the appendix at the back of this book or on the book's website at **http://evolve.elsevier.com/Stanhope.**

**evolve** **Evolve Website**

WebLinks: Healthy People 2010

## References

American Nurses Association: *The scope and standards of public health nursing practice,* Washington, DC, 1999, ANA.

American Nurses Association: *Code of ethics for nurses with interpretive statements,* Washington, DC, 2001, ANA.

American Public Health Association: *Writing a public health code of ethics,* Washington, DC, 2001, APHA. Retrieved April 20, 2002, from http://www.apha.org/codeofethics/background.htm.

Arras J, Steinbock B, editors: *Ethical issues in modern medicine,* ed 5, Mountain View, Calif, 1999, Mayfield.

Bandman E, Bandman B: *Nursing ethics through the life span,* ed 4, Upper Saddle River, NJ, 2002, Prentice Hall.

Bateman N: *Advocacy skills for health and social care professionals,* Philadelphia, 2000, Jessica Kingsley.

Beauchamp TL, Childress JF: *Principles of biomedical ethics,* ed 5, New York, 2001, Oxford University Press.

Benjamin M: Between subway and spaceship: practical ethics at the outset of the twenty-first century, *Hastings Center Rep* 31(4):24, 2001.

Boss J: *Ethics for life.* Mountain View, Calif, 1998, Mayfield.

Boylan M: Interview with Edmund D. Pellegrino. In Boylan M, editor: *Medical ethics: basic ethics in action,* Upper Saddle River, NJ, 2000, Prentice Hall.

Boyle PJ et al: *Organizational ethics in health care: principles, cases, and practical solutions,* San Francisco, 2001, Jossey-Bass.

Brady GS et al: No care for the caregivers: declining health insurance coverage for health care personnel and their children, 1988-1998, *Am J Public Health* 92(3):404, 2002.

Callahan D: Universalism and particularism fighting to a draw, *Hastings Center Rep* 30(1):37, 2000.

Callahan D, Jennings B: Ethics and public health: forging a strong relationship, *Am J Public Health,* 92(2):169, 2002.

*Canada Health Act of 1984,* Bill C–31: Ottawa, 1984, House of Commons, Government of Canada, available at http://www. hc-sc.gc.ca/medicare.

Canadian Nurses Association: Advance directives: the nurse's role. In *Ethics for practice,* Ottawa, 1998, CNA.

Canadian Nurses Association: *Code of ethics for registered nurses,* Ottawa, 2002, CNA.

Centers for Disease Control and Prevention, and Health Resources and Services Administration: *Healthy people 2010,* 23: public health infrastructure, 2000, retrieved April 20, 2002 from http://web.health.gov/healthypeople/document/ HTML/Volume2/23PHI.htm.

Chapin JL: The inappropriate distribution of primary health care funds. In Silva M, editor: *Ethical decision making in nursing administration,* Norwalk, Conn, 1990, Appleton & Lange.

Christoffel KK: Public health advocacy: process and product, *Am J Public Health* 90(5):722-723, 2000.

Clouser KD, Gert B: A critique of principlism, *J Med Philos* 15:219, 1990.

Commission on the Future of Health Care in Canada: *Shape the future of health care,* Ottawa, 2002, Commission on the Future of Health Care in Canada, available at http://www.healthcarecommission.ca.

Community Health Nurses Interest Group of the Registered Nurses' Association of Ontario: *Public health nursing position statement,* Toronto, 1998, Registered Nurses' Association of Ontario.

Community Health Nurses Initiative Group of the Registered Nurses' Association of Ontario: *Home health nursing position paper,* Toronto, 2000, Registered Nurses' Association of Ontario.

Coughlin SS, Soskolne CL, Goodman KW: *Case studies in public health ethics,* Washington, DC, 1997, American Public Health Association.

Denhardt RB, Denhardt JV: The new public service: serving rather than steering, *Public Admin Rev* 60(6):549-552, 2000.

Elovainio M, Kivimaki M, Vahtera J: Organizational justice: evidence of a new psychosocial predictor of health, *Am J Public Health* 92(1):105, 2002.

Eriksson K: Caring science in a new way, *Nurs Sci Quarterly* 15(1):61, 2002.

Evans JH: A sociological account of the growth of principlism, *Hastings Center Rep* 30(5):31, 2000.

Fletcher JJ: Virtues, moral decisions, and healthcare, *Nurs Connections* 12(4):26, 1999.

Garrett TM, Baillie HW, Garrett RM: *Health care ethics: principles and problems,* ed 4, Upper Saddle River, NJ, 2001, Prentice Hall.

Gebbie KM, Hwang I: Preparing currently employed public health nurses for changes in the health system, *Am J Public Health* 90(5):716, 2000.

Gilligan C: In a different voice: women's conception of self and of morality, *Harvard Educ Rev* 47(4):481, 1977.

Gilligan C: *In a different voice: psychological theory and women's development,* Cambridge, 1982, Harvard University Press.

Governing Council of the American Public Health Association: Policy statements adopted by the Governing Council of the American Public Health Association, October 24, 2001, *Am J Public Health* 92(3):451, 2002.

Harman LB: *Ethical challenges in the management of health information,* Gaithersburg, Md, 2001, Aspen.

Hellsten S: Theories of distributive justice. In Chadwick R, editor: *Encyclopedia of applied ethics,* vol 1, pp. 815-827, New York, 1998, Academic Press.

Hinderer DE, Hinderer SR: *A multidisciplinary approach to health care ethics,* Mountain View, Calif, 2001, Mayfield.

Holstein MB: Bringing ethics home: a new look at ethics in the home and the community. In Holstein MB, Mitzen PB, editors: *Ethics in community based elder care,* New York, 2001, Springer.

International Council of Nurses: *ICN code of ethics for nurses,* Geneva, 1953, ICN.

International Council of Nurses: *ICN code of ethics for nurses,* Geneva, 2000, ICN.

Kass N: An ethics framework for public health, *Am J Public Health* 91(11):1776, 2001.

Keatings M, Smith OB: *Ethical and legal issues in Canadian nursing,* Toronto, 2000, Saunders Canada.

Leininger M, editor: *Care: the essence of nursing and health,* Thorofare, NJ, 1984, Slack.

Leipert BD: Feminism and public health nursing: partners for health. *Sch Inq Nurs Prac* 15(1):49, 2001.

Levin BW, Fleischman AR: Public health and bioethics: the benefits of collaboration, *Am J Public Health* 92(2):165, 2002.

MacIntyre A: *After virtue,* Notre Dame, Ind, 1984, University of Notre Dame Press.

Meslin EM: Some clues about the President's Council on Bioethics, *Hastings Center Rep* 32(1):8, 2002.

Noddings N: *Caring: a feminine approach to ethics & moral education,* Berkeley, Calif, 1984, University of California Press.

Oberle K, Tenove S: Ethical issues in public health nursing, *Nurs Ethics* 7(5):425-438, 2000.

Pellegrino ED: Toward a virtue-based normative ethics for the health professions, *Kennedy Inst Ethics J* 5(3):253, 1995.

Public Health Leadership Society: *Public health code of ethics,* New Orleans, La, 2001, Louisiana Public Health Institute. Retrieved April 5, 2002, from http://www.apha.org/codeofethics/ethics.htm.

Rawls J: *A theory of justice* (rev ed), Cambridge, Mass, 1971, 1999, Harvard University Press.

Rawls J: *Justice as fairness: a restatement,* Kelly E, editor, Cambridge, Mass, 2001, Harvard University Press.

Rosenstock L, Lee LJ: Attacks on science: the risks to evidence-based policy, *Am J Public Health* 92(1):14, 2002.

Shapiro HT: Reflections on the interface of bioethics, public policy, and science. *Kennedy Inst Ethics J* 9(3):209, 1999.

Silva MC: Ethical issues in health care, public policy, and politics. In Mason D, Leavitt J, Chaffee M, editors: *Policy and politics in nursing and health care,* ed 4, Philadelphia, 2002, Saunders.

Solomon RC: *Ethics: a short introduction,* Dubuque, Iowa, 1993, Brown & Benchmark.

Storch JL, Meilicke CA: Political, social and economic forces shaping the healthcare system. In *Nursing management in Canada,* Toronto, 1999, Saunders Canada.

U.S. Department of Health and Human Services: *Healthy people 2010: understanding and improving health,* ed 2, Washington, DC, 2000, U.S. Government Printing Office.

Veatch RM: *The basics of bioethics,* Upper Saddle River, NJ, 2000, Prentice Hall.

Volbrecht RM: *Nursing ethics: communities in dialogue,* Upper Saddle River, NJ, 2002, Prentice Hall.

Walters LC, Aydelotte J, Miller J: Putting more public in policy analysis, *Public Admin Rev* 60(4):349, 2000.

Watson J: *Nursing: human science and human care,* Norwalk, Conn, 1985, Appleton-Century-Crofts.

Weston A: *A practical companion to ethics,* ed 2, New York, 2002, Oxford University Press.

Williams CA: Community-oriented population-focused practice: the foundation of specialization in public health nursing. In Stanhope M, Lancaster J, editors: *Community & public health nursing,* ed 5, St Louis, Mo, 2000, Mosby.

Zoloth L: Heroic measures: just bioethics in an unjust world, *Hastings Center Rep* 31(6):34, 2001

# Chapter 7

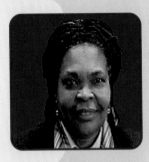

## Cultural Diversity and Community-Oriented Nursing Practice

**evolve** http://evolve.elsevier.com/Stanhope

### Cynthia E. Degazon, R.N., Ph.D.

Dr. Cynthia E. Degazon received a B.S. degree in nursing from Long Island University in New York. She received an M.A. degree in community health and a Ph.D. degree from the Division of Nursing, New York University. She is an associate professor at Hunter–Bellevue School of Nursing, City University of New York, and has been teaching courses on cultural diversity for 12 years. Dr. Degazon conducts research on that topic and has numerous publications. She has presented her findings throughout the United States, in the West Indies, and in Botswana, Africa.

### Objectives

After reading this chapter, the student should be able to do the following:

1. Analyze the effect of culture on nursing practice
2. Describe major barriers to developing cultural competence
3. Compare and contrast the effects of cultural organizational factors on health and illness among culturally diverse groups in a community
4. Examine issues related to minority access and use of cultural health practices
5. Conduct a cultural assessment of a person from a cultural group other than one's own
6. Develop culturally competent nursing interventions to promote positive health outcomes for clients
7. Analyze the role of the nurse as an advocate for culturally competent nursing care

---

Caring for culturally diverse groups has been a focus of nursing from its beginning. As early as 1893, nurses in New York City started public health nursing, and they provided home care to immigrants, particularly recent arrivals (Denker, 1994). Since nurses were not from the same cultural background as the immigrants, they had to deal with the cultural differences between themselves and the persons in their care.

Data from the 2000 census showed a greater shift than before in the population demographics (U.S. Census Bureau, 2001). In 1990, whites in 70 of the largest 100 cities in the United States represented more than 50% of the population; they are now a majority in 52 cities. This pattern of a decreasing white population is attributed to a rapidly growing Hispanic population, a strong increase in Asians, and a modest increase in Americans of African descent. These changes reflect a society that is becoming more diverse with regard to racial and ethnic groups. As a result, significant differences in beliefs about health and illness are becoming apparent between the various groups. Nurses who want to reflect their clients' beliefs of health and illness when intervening to promote and maintain wellness face many challenges.

Nurses need to know both the pathophysiology of the illness and the cultural views that affect its perception. According to Trossman (1998), the nursing workforce is overwhelmingly white (90%). African Americans account for 4.2%, Asian or Pacific Islanders make up 3.4%, Hispanics 1.6%, and Native Americans or Alaskan Natives 0.05% of the nursing workforce. Clearly, the number of racially and ethnically diverse nurses who are available to provide care is insufficient.

This chapter provides community-oriented nurses with strategies to provide culturally competent nursing care. A nurse who cares for clients (individuals; aggregates, including families; and communities) who are culturally different from the nurse will be able to apply strategies that are beneficial and appropriate. In this chapter, emphasis is on four groups: African Americans, Asians, Hispanics, and Native Americans. Not only is there much cultural and ethnic diversity present within and among these groups but also they are consistently identified in the literature as having more economic difficulties, less-accessible health care, and poorer health than other groups (Giger and Davidhizar, 1999; Spector, 2000; U.S. Department of Health and Human Services [USDHHS], 1998).

## Key Terms

**biological variations**, p. 165
**cultural accommodation**, p. 157
**cultural awareness**, p. 155
**cultural blindness**, p. 159
**cultural competence**, p. 153
**cultural conflict**, p. 159
**cultural desire**, p. 156
**cultural encounter**, p. 156
**cultural imposition**, p. 159
**cultural knowledge**, p. 155
**cultural nursing assessment**, p. 160

**cultural preservation**, p. 157
**cultural relativism**, p. 159
**cultural repatterning**, p. 157
**cultural skill**, p. 156
**culture**, p. 152
**culture brokering**, p. 158
**culture shock**, p. 160
**environmental control**, p. 165
**ethnicity**, p. 153
**ethnocentrism**, p. 159
**immigrants**, p. 149

**nonverbal communication**, p. 163
**prejudice**, p. 159
**race**, p. 152
**racism**, p. 159
**social organization**, p. 164
**space**, p. 163
**stereotyping**, p. 158
**time**, p. 164
**verbal communication**, p. 163
*See Glossary for definitions*

## Chapter Outline

Immigration Health Issues
Culture, Race, and Ethnicity
*Culture*
*Race*
*Ethnicity*
Cultural Competence
*Developing Cultural Competence*
*Dimensions of Cultural Competence*
Inhibitors to Developing Cultural Competence

*Stereotyping*
*Prejudice and Racism*
*Ethnocentrism*
*Cultural Imposition*
*Cultural Conflict*
*Culture Shock*
Cultural Nursing Assessment
Variations Among Cultural Groups
*Communication*

*Using an Interpreter*
*Space*
*Social Organization*
*Time*
*Environmental Control*
*Biological Variations*
Culture and Nutrition
Culture and Socioeconomic Status

## IMMIGRANT HEALTH ISSUES

Recent changes in immigration laws have increased migration to the United States (Battle, 1998). The 1965 amendment of the Immigration and Nationality Act changed the quota system that discriminated against individuals from southern and eastern Europe. The Refugee Act of 1980 provided a uniform procedure for refugees (based on the United Nations definition) to be admitted to the United States (U.S. Bureau of the Census, 2001). This included refugees from Cuba, Vietnam, Laos, and Cambodia, and Russian Jewish refugees. More recently, the 1986 Immigration Reform and Control Act permitted illegal aliens already living in the United States an opportunity to apply for legal status if they met certain requirements; this offer was extended to aliens employed in seasonal agricultural work. Table 7-1 summarizes the immigration patterns of selected immigrants by country of birth for the past 18 years.

However, people in the United States are ambivalent in their attitudes and policies about **immigrants,** and furthermore there is some misunderstanding about what distinguishes an immigrant. Also national debate about immigration policy has intensified since the events of September 11, 2001. The complex issues involved with im-

migrants and their health are beyond the scope of this discussion, but several issues will be discussed and suggestions made for nursing actions.

First, it is important to define *legal immigrant.* Also known as *lawful permanent residents,* these people are not citizens, but they are legally allowed to both live and work in the United States, often because they have useful job skills or family ties. There has been a trend toward more immigrants being "low skill" workers, and they compete with native low skill workers for jobs. The argument has been made that low skill workers take jobs that other Americans and "lawful residents" do not want. Since 1997, immigrants have needed to live in the United States for 10 years to be eligible for all entitlements, such as Aid to Families of Dependent Children, food stamps, Medicaid, and unemployment insurance (Riedel, 1998). About 85% of immigrants have entered the country legally (*Immigrant Policy Handbook,* 2000). The second category of immigrants consists of *unauthorized immigrants,* or undocumented or illegal aliens. These people may have crossed a border into the United States illegally, or their legal permission to stay may have expired. They are eligible only for emergency medical services (Riedel, 1998). A description of the immigrant populations and what benefits

**Table 7-1    Numbers of Selected Immigrants by Country of Birth: 1981 to 1998**

| CONTINENT/COUNTRY | 1981-1990 | 1991-1996 | 1997 | 1998 |
|---|---|---|---|---|
| All countries | 7338.1* | 6146.2 | 798.4 | 60.5 |
| Europe | 705.6 | 875.6 | 119.9 | 90.8 |
| Poland | 97.4 | 130.2 | 12.2 | 8.5 |
| Romania | 38.9 | 34.3 | 5.5 | 5.1 |
| Former Soviet Union | 84.0 | 339.9 | 49.1 | 30.2 |
| Russia | NA | 70.5† | 16.6 | 11.5 |
| Ukraine | NA | 92.2† | 15.7 | 7.4 |
| Yugoslavia | 19.2 | 31.7 | 10.8 | 8.0 |
| Asia | 2817.4 | 1941.9 | 265.8 | 219.7 |
| Bangladesh | 15.2 | 35.4 | 8.7 | 8.6 |
| Cambodia | 116.6 | 11.9 | 1.6 | 1.4 |
| China | 388.8 | 268.7 | 41.1 | 36.9 |
| Hong Kong | 63.0 | 52.9 | 5.6 | 5.3 |
| India | 261.9 | 236.5 | 38.1 | 36.5 |
| Iran | 154.8 | 79.4 | 9.6 | 7.9 |
| Korea | 338.8 | 114.1 | 14.2 | 14.3 |
| Laos | 145.6 | 37.8 | 1.9 | 1.6 |
| Pakistan | 61.3 | 70.5 | 13.0 | 13.1 |
| Philippines | 495.3 | 348.5 | 49.1 | 34.5 |
| Vietnam | 401.4 | 317.8 | 38.5 | 17.6 |
| North America | 3125.0 | 2740.7 | 307.5 | 253.0 |
| Mexico | 1653.3 | 1651.4 | 146.9 | 131.6 |
| Caribbean | 892.7 | 655.4 | 105.3 | 75.5 |
| Cuba | 159.2 | 94.9 | 33.6 | 17.4 |
| Dominican Republic | 251.8 | 258.1 | 27.1 | 20.4 |
| Haiti | 140.2 | 114.4 | 15.1 | 13.4 |
| Jamaica | 213.8 | 109.8 | 17.8 | 15.1 |
| Central America | 458.7 | 342.8 | 43.7 | 35.7 |
| El Salvador | 214.6 | 147.7 | 18.0 | 14.6 |
| Guatemala | 87.9 | 70.3 | 7.8 | 7.8 |
| South America | 455.9 | 344.0 | 52.9 | 45.4 |
| Argentina | 25.7 | 10.6 | 2.3 | 1.8 |
| Colombia | 124.4 | 81.7 | 13.0 | 11.8 |
| Peru | 64.4 | 66.7 | 10.9 | 10.2 |
| Africa | 192.3 | 213.1 | 47.8 | 40.7 |
| Egypt | 31.4 | 28.0 | 5.0 | 4.8 |
| Nigeria | 35.3 | 37.9 | 7.0 | 7.7 |

Data from U.S. Bureau of the Census: *Statistical abstract of the United States: 2001*, ed 121, Washington, DC, 2001, Government Printing Office.
*Multiply value by 1000 (e.g., 7338.1 represents 7,338,100).
*NA*, Not available.
†Covers years 1992-1996.

they are eligible for can be found in the *Handbook of Immigrant Health* (Loue, 1998, pp. 19-36).

Misperceptions abound about the economic value of allowing immigrants to enter, or to stay in, the United States. It is estimated that immigrants add about $10 billion to the economy annually, and that, in their lifetime in the United States, an immigrant family will pay $80,000 more in taxes than they consume in services *(Immigrants' Health Care Coverage and Access Fact Sheet*, 2001). The dilemma for communities, however, is that the taxes are typically paid to the federal government, whereas the services the immigrants use are paid for by the states and localities. Although federal matching funds for Medicaid are not available to the states for immigrants, some states have decided to use their own funds to cover new immigrant children, and other states cover pregnant women, the disabled, and older adults (Lillie-Blanton and Hudman, 2001). These states have found compelling public health reasons to provide some care to high-risk immigrant populations.

In addition to financial constraints on the provision of health care for immigrants, other serious factors need to be considered. Some of them are language barriers; differences in social, religious, and cultural backgrounds between the immigrant and the health care provider; providers' lack of knowledge about high-risk diseases in the specific immigrant groups for whom they care; and the fact that many immigrants rely on traditional healing or folk health care practices that may be unfamiliar to their U.S. health care providers.

## DID YOU KNOW?

Definitions for *immigrant* differ, and immigrants may be legal or illegal. They come from all parts of the world and bring with them unique cultural, health care, and religious backgrounds.
- Access to health care may be limited because of immigrants' lack of benefits, resources, language ability, and transportation.
- Nurses need to be astute in considering the cultural backgrounds of their immigrant clients and populations. Often, the family and community must be relied on to provide information, support, and other aid.
- Nurses need to know the major health problems and risk factors that are specific to immigrant populations.

When working with immigrant populations, nurses should take into account that their own background, beliefs, and knowledge may be significantly different from those of the people receiving their care. *Language barriers* may interfere with efforts to provide assistance. Community members may be excellent resources as translators, not only of the actual words but also of the cultural beliefs, expectations, and use of nontraditional health practices.

Nurses need to know if there are *specific risk factors* for a given immigrant population. For example, Southeast Asians are often at risk for hepatitis B (with its attendant effects on the liver), tuberculosis, intestinal parasites, and visual, hearing, and dental problems. Most of these conditions are either preventable or treatable if managed correctly (Riedel, 1998).

Nurses need to understand the *nontraditional healing practices* that their clients use. Many of these treatments have proven effective and can be blended with traditional Western medicine. The key is to know what practices are being used so the blending can be knowledgeably done. Community members are excellent sources of this information, and nurses working with immigrant populations should use the community assessment, group work, and family techniques described in other chapters.

Often children and adolescents adjust to the new culture more easily than their elders. This can lead to *family conflict* and, at times, violence. Be alert for warning signs of family stress and tension. On the other hand, family members can help translate their culture, religion, beliefs, practices, support systems, and risk factors for the health care provider. They also can assist with decision making and provide support to enable the person or group seeking care to change behaviors to become more health conscious. Nurses need to understand the role of the family in immigrant populations, and to treat individuals in the context of the families from which they come.

Similarly, the *role of the community* in the care of immigrants is important. Communities can help patients (and thus providers) with communication, explanation, crisis intervention, emotional and other forms of support, and housing. Nurses need to carefully assess the community and learn what strengths, resources, and talents are available. As noted, cultural and religious beliefs influence behaviors, and community groups can explain their value and meaning to the nurse.

Horowitz (1998) has identified six steps that clinicians can take to more effectively work with immigrant populations:
1. Know yourself: providers, like clients, are influenced by culture, values, language.
2. Get to know the families and their health-seeking behaviors. You might try using a simple genogram, which places family members on a diagram. Ask who the family members are, where they live, and who is missing or dead. You might also ask them to talk about holidays: who comes, who is missing, what do they do?
3. Get to know the communities common to your setting: read about them, take a course, get involved (e.g., volunteer to give talks), hold forums with free-flowing and two-way communication, learn who the formal and informal resources are.
4. Get to know some of the traditional practices and remedies used by families and communities, so you can work with, not against, them.
5. Learn how a community deals with common illnesses or events.
6. Try to see things from the viewpoint of the patient, family, or community.

## DID YOU KNOW?

As humans, we have more similarities with each other than we have differences.

## CULTURE, RACE, AND ETHNICITY

The concepts of culture, race, and ethnicity play a strong role in understanding human behavior. In everyday living, these three terms are often used incorrectly. Nurses are expected to understand the meaning of each when providing culturally competent health care to clients of diverse cultures.

### Culture

**Culture** is a set of beliefs, values, and assumptions about life that are widely held among a group of people and that are transmitted intergenerationally (Leininger, 2002a). Culture is a dynamic process that develops over time and is resistant to change. It takes many years for individuals to become familiar enough with a new value for it to become part of their culture. In response to the needs of its members and their environment, culture provides tested solutions to life's problems.

Individuals learn about their culture during the processes of learning language and becoming socialized, usually as children (Battle, 1998). Parents and family, the most important sources for the transfer of traditions, teach both explicit and implicit behaviors of the culture. The explicit behaviors, such as language, interpersonal distance, and kissing in public, can be observed and allow the individual to identify the self with other persons of the culture. In this way, people share traditions, customs, and lifestyles with others. The implicit behaviors are less visible and include the way individuals perceive health and illness, body language, difference in language expressions, and the use of titles. These behaviors are subtle and may be difficult for persons to articulate, yet they are very much a part of the culture. For example, deferring to older adults, standing when they enter the room, or offering them a seat suggests a cultural value related to older adults.

Another example of an implicit aspect of culture is the use of language to communicate. For example, in one culture a sign might read "No smoking is permitted." In another culture the sign might read "Thank you for not smoking." The former statement represents a culture that values directness, whereas the latter values indirectness. Each culture has an organizational structure that distinguishes it from others and provides the structure for what members of the cultural group determine as appropriate or inappropriate behavior. The organizational elements of cultures have been described by Andrews and Boyle (2003), Giger and Davidhizar (1999), Leininger (2002b), Purnell (2000), and Spector (2000). Such organizational elements include child-rearing practices, religious practices, family structure, space, and communication. In the case of language, there are idiomatic expressions unique to each language. It is important that nurses know these organizational elements to provide appropriate care to persons of diverse cultures. This does not mean, however, that one should overlook or fail to incorporate the individuality of any person within any culture when devel-

---

**BOX 7-1  Factors Influencing Individual Differences Within Cultural Groups**

- Age
- Religion
- Dialect and language spoken
- Gender identity roles
- Socioeconomic background
- Geographic location in the country of origin
- Geographic location in the current country
- History of the subcultural group with which clients identify in their current country of residence
- History of the subcultural group with which clients identify in their country of origin
- Amount of interaction between older and younger generations
- The degree of assimilation in the current country of residence
- Immigration status*
- Conditions under which migration occurred*

---

Except where noted with an asterisk (*), from Orque M: Orque's ethnic/cultural system: a framework for ethnic nursing care. In Orque MS, Bloch B, Monrroy LSA, editors: *Ethnic nursing care: a multi-cultural approach*, St Louis, Mo, 1983, Mosby.

---

oping a plan of care. Just as all cultures are not alike, all individuals within a culture are not alike. Each individual should be viewed as a unique human being with differences that are respected. Box 7-1 summarizes factors that may contribute to individual differences within cultures.

### Race

**Race** is primarily a social classification that relies on physical markers such as skin color to identify group membership (Bhopal and Donaldson, 1998). Individuals may be of the same race but of different cultures. For example, African Americans, who may have been born in Africa, the Caribbean, North America, or elsewhere, are a heterogeneous group, but they are often viewed as culturally and racially homogeneous. A frequent consequence of this is that the many cultural differences of these individuals from different countries are overlooked because of their similar racial characteristics (Snowden and Holschuh, 1992). This often blurs understanding of this culturally diverse group.

Another factor highlighting race's diminishing importance in comparison to ethnic identity is the interracial family. Physical changes in biracial and multiracial generations lead to changes in physical appearances of individuals and make race less important in ethnic identity. In the United States, children of biracial parents are assigned the race of the mother.

## Ethnicity

**Ethnicity** is the shared feeling of peoplehood among a group of individuals (Giger and Davidhizar, 1999). Ethnicity reflects cultural membership and is based on individuals sharing similar cultural patterns (such as beliefs, values, customs, behaviors, and traditions) that over time create a common history that is exceedingly resistant to change. Ethnicity represents the identifying characteristics of culture, such as race, religion, or national origin. It is influenced by education, income level, geographical location, and association with individuals from ethnic groups other than one's own. Therefore there is a reciprocal relationship between the individual and society. Members of an ethnic group give up aspects of their identity and society when they adopt characteristics of the group's identity. However, when there is a strong ethnic identity, the group maintains the values, beliefs, behaviors, practices, and ways of thinking.

## CULTURAL COMPETENCE

Many people are taught by and have knowledge of a dominant culture (Brislin, 1993). As long as the person is operating within that culture, responses occur without thought to a variety of situations and do not require examination of the cultural context. However, in today's climate of multiculturism, there is increasing emphasis from health care providers and organizations for nurses to provide quality and effective care. For example, a recent Mexican immigrant who speaks little English goes to a community health center because of urinary infection. The nurse understands that she must use strategies that would allow her to effectively communicate with the client; the client has the right to receive effective care, to judge whether she had received the care she wanted, and to follow up with appropriate action if she did not receive the expected care. Culturally competent care is provided not only to individuals of racial or ethnic minority groups but also to individuals belonging to groups held together by factors such as age, religion, sexual orientation, and socioeconomic status. Nurses must be culturally competent to provide nursing care that meets the needs of these persons.

**Cultural competence** in nurses is a combination of culturally congruent behaviors, practice attitudes, and policies that allows nurses to work effectively in cross-cultural situations. Culturally competent nurses function effectively when caring for clients of other cultures (Finch, Garcia-Calhoun, and Sockalingham, 1999). Cultural competence reflects a higher level of knowledge than cultural sensitivity, which was once thought to be all that was needed for nurses to effectively care for their clients.

Culturally competent nursing care is guided by four principles (AAN Expert Panel, 1992):

1. Care is designed for the specific client.
2. Care is based on the uniqueness of the person's culture and includes cultural norms and values.

# THE CUTTING EDGE

Standards for transcultural nursing have been developed to guide nurses in delivering culturally competent nursing care. The standards are available for all professional nurses to use as a basis for documenting, describing, teaching, and evaluating culturally competent care.

Leininger M: Part 1: the theory of culture care and the ethnonursing research method. In Leininger MM, McFarland M, editors: *Transcultural nursing: concepts, theories, research, and practices,* ed 3, pp. 71-98, New York, 2002b, McGraw-Hill.

3. Care includes self-empowerment strategies to facilitate client decision making in health behavior.
4. Care is provided with sensitivity and is based on the cultural uniqueness of clients.

Nurses must be culturally competent for a number of reasons. First, the nurse's culture often differs from that of the client. Nurses come from a variety of cultural backgrounds and have their own cultural traditions. Each nurse has a unique set of cultural experiences that gives meaning and understanding to his or her behavior. Because the nursing profession is a subsystem of the U.S. health care system, nurses also bring biomedical beliefs and values to the practice environment that may differ from client's beliefs and values. Because of these different beliefs and values, when the client and the nurse interact they may have different understandings about the meaning of the problem and different ideas about what to do to promote and protect health. In these circumstances, cultural competence helps nurses use strategies that respect client's values and expectations without diminishing the nurses' own values and expectations.

Second, care that is not culturally competent may further increase the cost of health care and decrease the opportunity for positive client outcomes. Failure to effectively respond to the health care needs and preferences of culturally and linguistically diverse individuals may (1) increase delays in clients seeking care, (2) create obstacles as nurses try to obtain information to make an appropriate diagnosis and develop effective treatment plans, and (3) inhibit effective communication between the client and the nurse. In the current climate of economic constraints, the health care industry is focused on cost effectiveness, which means balancing cost and quality (Irvine, Sidani, and Hall, 1998). Quality of care means that positive health outcomes are achieved. Care that is not focused on the clients' values and ideas is likely to increase cost and diminish quality. For example, when clients are using both folk medicine and traditional Western medicine and nurses fail to assess and use this information in teaching, the clients may not get the full benefits of the treatment

## Healthy People 2010 | Objective 5: National Goals for Reducing Diabetes

5-1  Increase the proportion of persons with diabetes who receive formal diabetes education.

5-2  Prevent diabetes.

5-3  Reduce the overall rate of diabetes that is clinically diagnosed.

5-4  Reduce the overall rate of persons with diabetes whose condition had been diagnosed.

5-5  Reduce diabetes related-death rate.

5-6  Reduce diabetes related-deaths among persons with diabetes.

5-7  Reduce deaths from cardiovascular disease in persons with diabetes.

5-8  (Developmental) Decrease the proportion of pregnant women with gestational diabetes.

5-9  (Developmental) Reduce the frequency of foot ulcers in persons with diabetes.

5-10 Reduce the rate of lower amputations in persons with diabetes.

5-11 (Developmental) Increase the proportion of persons with diabetes who obtain an annual urinary microalbumin measurement.

5-12 Increase the proportion of adults with diabetes who have a glycosylated hemoglobin measurement at least once a year.

5-13 Increase the proportion of adults with diabetes who have an annual dilated eye examination.

5-14 Increase the proportion of persons with diabetes who have at least an annual foot examination.

5-15 Increase the proportion of persons with diabetes who have at least an annual dental examination.

5-16 Increase the proportion of adults with diabetes who take aspirin at least 15 times per month.

5-17 Increase the proportion of adults with diabetes who perform self-blood-glucose monitoring at least once daily.

From U.S. Department of Health and Human Services: Healthy people 2010: *understanding and improving health and objectives for improving health,* ed 2, Washington, DC, 2000, U.S. Government Printing Office.

protocol. This suggests that positive outcomes, which are indicators of quality, may not be met. When quality is compromised, additional resources may be needed to achieve the health care outcomes. Increased use of resources means that cost is increased.

Third, specific objectives for persons of different cultures need to be met as outlined in Healthy People 2010 (USDHHS, 1998), but achievement of these objectives requires that clients' lifestyle and personal choices be considered. For example, the American health care system views excessive drinking as a sign of disease, and alcoholism as a mental illness. However, in the Native American culture, these signify a disharmony between the individual and the spirit world, and biomedical interventions alone may not be adequate to reduce alcoholism within this culture. In 1995, 19.2 per 100,000 Native Americans died of alcohol-related motor vehicle accidents, a rate that is three times higher than that in the general population (5.9 per 100,000) (USDHHS, 1998), and the national goal is to reduce this disparity. However, many Native Americans view the use of alcohol consumption as an acceptable way to participate in family celebrations and tribal ceremonies (Orlandi, 1992), and refusal to drink with family may be viewed as a sign of rejection. West (1993, p. 234) cautioned nurses that "if the government sends Indians to a health clinic where personnel do not understand the holistic health practices of Indians and where young white people serve as caregivers and authority figures, failure is likely to result." To have successful outcomes, nurses who develop population-based programs to reduce alcohol-related deaths must be willing to respect the cultural uniqueness of Native Americans and to explore individuals' life experiences to find the underlying causes of their behaviors.

## Developing Cultural Competence

Developing cultural competence is an ongoing life process that involves every aspect of client care. It is challenging and at times painful as the nurse struggles to break with the old and adopt new ways of thinking and performing. In developing cultural competence, nurses may be guided by the two principles suggested by Leininger (2002a): (1) maintain a broad objective and open attitude toward individuals and their cultures, and (2) avoid seeing all individuals as alike. Nurses develop cultural competence in different ways, but the key elements are experiences with clients of other cultures, an awareness of these experiences, and promotion of mutual respect for differences. As there are varying degrees of cultural competence, not all nurses may reach the same level of development.

Orlandi (1992) suggests that there are three stages in the development of cultural competence: culturally incompetent, culturally sensitive, and culturally competent (Table 7-2). Each stage has three dimensions—cognitive (thinking), affective (feeling), and psychomotor (doing)—that together have an overall effect on nursing care. Stop now and describe your cultural competence with persons of a culture different from your own by staging each of these three dimensions.

Campinha-Bacote (1998) offers a theoretical model to explain the process of developing cultural competence.

## Table 7-2 The Cultural Competence Framework: Stages of Competence Development

| | CULTURALLY INCOMPETENT | CULTURALLY SENSITIVE | CULTURALLY COMPETENT |
|---|---|---|---|
| Cognitive dimension | Oblivious | Aware | Knowledgeable |
| Affective dimension | Apathetic | Sympathetic | Committed to change |
| Skills dimension | Unskilled | Lacking some skills | Highly skilled |
| Overall effect | Destructive | Neutral | Constructive |

From Orlandi MA: Defining cultural competence: an organizing framework. In Orlandi MA, editor: *Cultural competence for evaluators*, Washington, DC, 1992, U.S. Department of Health and Human Services.

The five constructs of the model are (1) cultural awareness, (2) cultural knowledge, (3) cultural skill, (4) cultural encounter, and (5) cultural desire.

### Cultural Awareness

**Cultural awareness** involves the self-examination and in-depth exploration of one's own beliefs and values as they influence behavior (Campinha-Bacote, 2002; Misener et al, 1997). To be aware suggests that nurses are receptive to learning about the cultural dimensions of the client. Nurses who are culturally aware understand the basis for their own behavior and how it helps or hinders the delivery of competent care to persons from cultures other than their own (AAN Expert Panel, 1992). Culturally aware nurses recognize that health is expressed differently across cultures and that culture influences an individual's responses to health, illness, disease, and death. Culturally competent care can be delivered in a variety of modes consistent with the client's health values.

For example, at a community outreach program, a nurse was teaching a racially mixed group the screening protocol for breast and cervical cancer detection. An African-American woman in the group refused to give the return demonstration for breast self-examination. When encouraged to do so, she said, "My breasts are much larger than those on the model. Besides, the models are not like me. They are all white." After hearing the client's comments, the nurse realized that she had made no reference in her talk to the influence of culture or race on screening for breast and cervical cancer.

The nurse talked with the client, asked for her recommendations, and encouraged her to return the demonstration. The nurse coached the client through the self-examination process while pointing out that regardless of breast size, shape, and color, the technique is the same for feeling the tissue and squeezing the nipple to make certain that there is no discharge. Because this nurse was culturally aware, she neither became angry with herself or the client, nor did she impose her own values on the client. Rather, the client talked about her beliefs, attitudes, and feelings about screening for cancer that may be influ-

enced by her culture. Subsequently, the nurse purchased a model of an African-American woman's breast to be used in future health education programs with African-American women.

If the nurse had not been culturally aware, she might have misunderstood the client's concerns and acted in a defensive manner. Such an interaction would have failed in identifying client assets and barriers and appropriate intervention strategies. A confrontation might have ensued that would not have been helpful to the client or the nurse. McKenna (2001) urges nurses to champion the cause for clients to have their cultural traditions respected when they seek health care and interact with health care professionals. Box 7-2 identifies a number of factors on which nurses may focus as they try to know their own culture and the implications of their own cultural values.

### Cultural Knowledge

**Cultural knowledge** is information about organizational elements of diverse cultures and ethnic groups. Emphasis is on learning about the clients' worldview from an emic (native) perspective. An understanding of the client's culture decreases misinterpretations and misapplication of scientific knowledge and facilitates the client's cooperation with the health care regimen (Campinha-Bacote, 2002; Leininger, 2002a). Leininger points out that nurses who lack cultural knowledge may develop feelings of inadequacy and helplessness because they are often unable to effectively help their clients. On the basis of research findings, Eliason (1998) reports that there is a significant positive relationship between students' comfort level and the amount of experience they have had in caring for culturally diverse clients. This supports the need for nurses' education to include exposure to a variety of cultures. When knowledge of the client's culture is missing or inadequate, it can also lead to negative situations such as clients' lack of cooperation with the health care regimen and inadequate use of health services. Although it is unrealistic to expect that nurses will have knowledge of all cultures, they should be aware of and know how to obtain the knowledge of cultural influences that affect groups with

---

**BOX 7-2** **Early Cultural Awareness**

- Think about the first time you had contact with someone you realized was culturally different from you.
- Briefly describe the situation/event.
  How old were you?
  What were your feelings?
  What were your thoughts?
- What did your parents and other significant adults say about those who were culturally different from your family?
  What adjectives were used?
  What attitudes were conveyed?
- As you got older, what messages did you get about minority groups from the larger community or culture?
- As an adult, how do you see others in the community talk about culturally different people?
  What adjectives are used?
  What attitudes are conveyed?
  How does this reinforce or contradict your earlier experience?
- What parts of this cultural baggage make it difficult to work with clients from different cultural groups?
- What parts of this cultural baggage facilitate your work with clients?

---

From Randall-David E: *Culturally competent HIV counseling and education,* McLean, Va, 1994, Maternal and Child Health Clearinghouse.

---

whom they most frequently interact. Clients provide a rich source of information about their own cultures.

## Cultural Skill

The third construct in developing cultural competence is **cultural skill.** Cultural skill reflects the effective integration of cultural awareness and cultural knowledge to obtain relevant cultural data and meet needs of culturally diverse clients. Culturally skillful nurses use appropriate touch during conversation, modify the physical distance between themselves and others, and use strategies to avoid cultural misunderstandings while meeting mutually agreed-upon goals.

## Cultural Encounter

A **cultural encounter** is the fourth construct essential to becoming culturally competent. Nurses integrate at all levels of care the importance of culture as they work directly with clients from culturally diverse backgrounds (Campinha-Bacote, 2002). Cultural encounters involve all interactions and not only those that are health related (Jezewski, 1993). The most important ones are those in which nurses engage in effective communication, use appropriate language and

literacy level, and learn directly from clients about their life experiences and the significance of these experiences for health (Leininger, 2002a).

In some communities, nurses may have few opportunities to develop cultural competence by working directly with persons of other cultures. When nurses come into contact with persons who are culturally different from themselves, they should adapt general cultural concepts to the situation until they are able to learn directly from the clients about their culture (Figure 7-1). Developing cultural competence also comes from reading about, taking courses on, and discussing different cultures within multicultural settings.

Nurses should be aware that having cultural competence is not the same as being an expert on the culture of a group that is different from their own. A successful encounter may be judged on the basis of four aspects (Brislin, 1993):

1. The nurse feels successful about the relationship with the client.
2. The client feels that interactions are warm, cordial, respectful, and cooperative.
3. Tasks are done efficiently.
4. Nurse and client experience little or no stress.

## Cultural Desire

**Cultural desire** is the fifth construct needed in the process of developing cultural competence. It refers to the nurse's intrinsic motivation to provide culturally competent care (Campinha-Bacote, 2002). Nurses who have a desire to become culturally competent do so because they want to rather than because they are directed to do so. They demonstrate a sense of energy and enthusiasm, and they are goal directed in providing culturally competent nursing services. Unlike the other constructs, cultural desire cannot be directly taught in the classroom or other educational settings, but nurses are more likely to demonstrate cultural desire when their work environment reflects a philosophy that values cultural competence at all levels of the organization and for all its clients. Campinha-Bacote (1998) cautions nurses not to be fearful of making mistakes, and she provides a list of do's and don't's that could be helpful as they undertake the cultural competency journey.

## Dimensions of Cultural Competence

Nurses integrate their professional knowledge with the client's knowledge and practices to negotiate and promote culturally relevant care for a specific client. Leininger (2002a) suggests three modes of action, based on negotiation between the client and nurse, that guide the nurse to deliver culturally competent care: cultural preservation, cultural accommodation, and cultural repatterning. When these decisions and actions are used with cultural brokering, the nurse is able to fulfill the various roles vital to providing holistic care for culturally diverse clients.

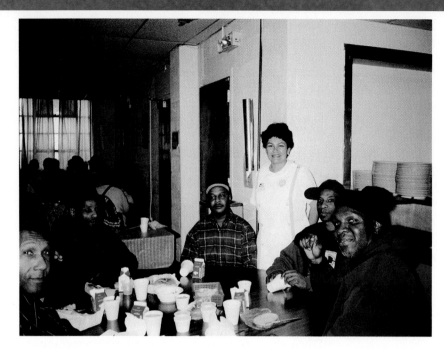

**Figure 7-1** A Hispanic nursing student interacting with African-American men at a nutritional center. To interact in a culturally competent manner, the student needs to have an awareness of and knowledge about the differences between her culture and the men's culture and the skill to portray this in her behavior toward them.

## Cultural Preservation

**Cultural preservation** means that the nurse supports and facilitates the use of scientifically supported cultural practices, such as acupuncture and acupressure, together with interventions from the biomedical health care system. For example, Ms. Lin, a 73-year-old Chinese woman, is discharged to home care after surgery for cancer of the large intestine. The nurse found her at home alone with her 76-year-old husband. After the physical assessment, the nurse discussed making a referral for Ms. Lin to have a home health aide to assist her with physical care and light housekeeping chores. The family was gracious but seemed hesitant to accept the referral. The nurse knew that the Chinese value the extended family network and family decision making. She asked the couple if they would like to discuss the situation with their daughters. Both the client and her husband seemed pleased with the idea, and the nurse promised to get back to them the next day. When the nurse returned for her visit, one of Ms. Lin's daughters was present and told the nurse that the family could manage without additional help. The three daughters had made a schedule to take turns caring for their parents. The nurse accepted and supported the family's decision and told them that if they decide at a later time to have the home health aide, they should call the agency, and she gave them the telephone number. She then scheduled the next follow-up visit with them.

## Cultural Accommodation

**Cultural accommodation** means that the nurse supports and facilitates the use of cultural practices, such as home burial of placenta (Helsel and Mochel, 2002), when such cultural practices have not been found to be harmful to clients. For example, the delivery nurse was very helpful when Ms. Sanchez asked her not to discard a piece of the amniotic sac that was present on her grandbaby's face immediately after birth. Ms. Sanchez asked the nurse to give it to her instead. The grandmother believed that being born with a piece of the amniotic sac on the face was a visible sign that something special was going to happen in the person's life. The grandmother explained that after she dried the piece of the amniotic sac, she would keep it in a safe place. She would also spend extra time protecting the baby to prevent her from being harmed. Although the delivery room nurse was not knowledgeable about this practice, she was assistive and gave the grandmother the piece of the sac as she requested. If, however, a particular cultural practice is found to be harmful, the nurse finds appropriate ways to modify the practice. Often, cultural practices can be successfully used alongside interventions from the biomedical health care system.

## Cultural Repatterning

**Cultural repatterning** means that the nurse works with clients to help them reorder, change, or modify their cultural practices when the practice is harmful to them. For example, a culturally competent nurse knows of the high incidence of obesity among Mexican-American women 20 years and older (USDHHS, 1998). A school nurse was invited to develop a health education program for Mexican teenagers in the local high school. While respecting their cultural traditions, the nurse discussed with the teenagers weight management strategies. The nurse understood the teenagers' cultural issues pertaining to food and knew how to negotiate with them. She discouraged the use of fried foods (such as tortillas), sour cream, and regular cheese and encouraged and demonstrated the use of baked tortillas and salsa as dip and topping.

In another example, a nurse who has been giving prenatal instructions to pregnant Haitian women discovered that many of them were visiting a herbalist to obtain teas to support their having a "strong baby." The nurse asked for the names of the herbs in the teas that they were drinking and scheduled a conference with the pharmacist to discuss the specific ingredients in the herbs and ways that they might help the client meet her cultural needs. The nurse found out that one of the herbs contributed to high blood pressure, a problem that many of the women were experiencing. She negotiated with the women not to take the tea with the specific herb. The nurse sought cooperation from the herbalist as she understood the importance of supernatural causes of illness in the Haitian culture (Miller, 2000).

### Culture Brokering

Culture brokering is another action used by culturally competent nurses to make certain that clients receive culturally competent care (Leininger, 2002a). **Culture brokering** is advocating, mediating, negotiating, and intervening

### Evidence-Based Practice

A study was conducted in South Carolina to determine differences in functional status, health status, and use of community services between older adult African Americans and whites diagnosed with diabetes. Data were collected over an 8-year period from the agency records for a four-county nonretirement and nonresort region. Results showed that there were no significant differences between the groups in functional status or health status. However, white older adults had significantly more difficulty in specific activities of daily living, such as house cleaning, food preparation, and transportation. Although both groups underused the community services, the use of services was significantly lower for the African-American older adults. Community services included case management, outreach, congregate meals, home-delivered meals, commodity distribution, recreation, and transportation.

Underuse of community services is a significant finding, particularly as it relates to older adults who live alone. Older adults who do not use community services are likely to be at an increased risk for developing diabetic complications, a poorer quality of life, and as a consequence, increased mortality.

**Nurse Usage:** When clients fail to use community resources, nurses should explore reasons for the inadequate use and take action to ensure the resources are available and accessible to all populations.

Witucki J, Wallace DC: Differences in functional status, health status, and community-based service use between black and white diabetic elders, *J Cult Divers* 6(3):94, 1998.

between the client's culture and the biomedical health care culture on behalf of clients. Culturally competent nurses are able to understand both cultures and to resolve or lessen problems that result from individuals in either culture not understanding the other person's values. To illustrate, migrant workers tend to have high occupational mobility; many are poor and have limited formal education. They may seek health care only when they are ill and cannot work. Whenever a nurse interacts with them, the opportunity should be taken to teach about prevention, health maintenance, environmental sanitation, and nutrition, because it may be the only opportunity that the nurse will ever have to treat a particular migrant worker. Nurses should also advocate for the rights of the migrant worker to receive quality health care. For example, the nurse may contact the migrant health services for follow-up or referral care for the migrant worker.

## INHIBITORS TO DEVELOPING CULTURAL COMPETENCE

When nurses fail to provide culturally competent nursing care, it may be because they have had minimal opportunity for learning about transcultural nursing, because their supervisors are encouraging them to increase productivity, or because they are pressured by colleagues who are not knowledgeable about cultural concepts and are offended when others use the concepts. These and similar issues would inhibit delivery of culturally competent care and may result in nurse behaviors such as stereotyping, prejudice and racism, ethnocentrism, cultural imposition, cultural conflict, and culture shock.

## Stereotyping

**Stereotyping** is ascribing certain beliefs and behaviors about a group to an individual without assessing for individual differences (Brislin, 1993). Stereotyping blocks the willingness of a person to be open and to learn about specific individuals or groups. When information is not immediately available, nurses may generalize about a group's behavioral pattern as a guide until they have had time to observe and assess the client's behavior. This can be a problem, and it may lead to a nurse's being unwilling to incorporate new and specific data about the client. New information may be distorted to fit with preconceived ideas. The generalizing that was a beginning point for understanding the individual becomes a final point, and the individual is thus stereotyped on the basis of the group's behavior (Galanti, 1997).

Stereotypes can be either positive or negative. For example, Asians are positively stereotyped as the "model" minority group, leading to an expectation that they will always behave in ways that reinforce the stereotypical notion. Other groups are stereotyped as "industrious and hard working." Nurses use negative stereotypes when they label a Native American who complains of abdominal pain as an alcoholic because they know that there is a high incidence of alcoholism in the group. Similarly, a nurse who believes that young African-American women tend to be sexually permissive may label a woman in this group who is complaining of abdominal pain as having a sexually transmitted disease. When clients perceive that they are being stereotyped, they may respond with anger and hostility. This in turn perpetuates the stereotype and creates barriers to health-seeking behavior. To minimize the use of stereotypes, nurses should be aware of their biases and recognize the effect of socialization on individual differences.

## Prejudice and Racism

**Prejudice** is the emotional manifestation of deeply held beliefs (stereotypes) about a group. These beliefs are directed toward a person who is a member of that group, and who is presumed to have the objectionable qualities ascribed to the group (Brislin, 1993). Prejudice usually refers to negative feelings, which are often the precursors for discriminatory acts based on prejudging, limited knowledge about, misinformation about, fear of, or limited contact with the individual. Those who are prejudiced wish to deny the individuals, on the basis of race, skin color, ethnicity, or social standing, the opportunity to benefit fully from society's offerings of education, good jobs, and community activities.

**Racism** is a form of prejudice that occurs through the exercise of power by individuals and institutions against people of other skin colors who are judged to be inferior— for example, in intelligence, morals, beauty, and self-worth (Brislin, 1993). The Tuskegee Syphilis Study is a well-known example of racism (Gamble, 1997). This study was conducted by the U.S. Public Health Service to observe the effects of syphilis on African-American men over a period of 40 years, beginning in 1932. African-American men with syphilis were recruited for the study, but instead of being told that they had syphilis, they were told that they were being treated for "bad blood," and treatment for syphilis was withheld. As a result, hundreds of men lost their lives because of the effects of syphilis. The consequence of such racism has contributed to the belief among some African Americans that research might be designed to harm them and that all care might be a part of a research study, especially government programs, designed to harm.

Prejudice and racism can be understood using a two-dimensional matrix: overt versus covert, and intentional versus unintentional. Locke and Hardaway (1992) depict four types of prejudice and racism that result from this matrix:

> ◖ WHAT DO YOU THINK?
>
> A 90-year-old South American woman refuses to have her nursing care provided by an African-American nurse. Should the community agency assign a nurse from another racial group to care for the client or should the client be transferred to another community health agency?

overt intentional, covert intentional, overt unintentional, and covert unintentional. Nurses too can exhibit prejudice and racism. Overt intentional prejudice or racism means that the behavior is both apparent and purposeful. The nurse is aware of personal biases and beliefs and integrates them into a plan of action to negatively manage client problems. With overt unintentional, the behavior is apparent but not purposeful, and no harm is intended. Covert intentional means that the behavior is subtle and purposeful but the person tries to avoid being viewed as prejudicial or racist. Covert unintentional means that the person's behavior is neither apparent nor is it purposeful. The person is unaware of the behavior. Regardless of the type of prejudice or racism, the behavior is harmful to the client (Box 7-3).

Nurses also may be recipients of prejudicial or racist acts. Nurses do not have to endure such behavior and should avoid internalizing the behavior, set limits with clients, and discuss the behavior with other colleagues (Miles and Awong, 1997).

## Ethnocentrism

**Ethnocentrism,** or cultural prejudice, is the belief that one's own cultural group determines the standards by which another group's behavior is judged. Ethnocentric nurses are unfamiliar and uncomfortable with that which is different from their culture (Sutherland, 2002). Their inability to accept different worldviews often leads them to devalue the experiences of others and judge them to be inferior, and to treat those who are different from them with suspicion or hostility (Andrews and Boyle, 2003).

This behavior is in contrast to **cultural blindness,** in which there is an inability to recognize the differences between one's own cultural beliefs, values, and practices and those of another culture. The tendency is to believe that the recognition of racial, ethnic, religious, or gender differences is itself prejudicial and discriminatory. Hence, nurses who state that they treat all clients the same, regardless of cultural orientation, are demonstrating cultural blindness.

## Cultural Imposition

The belief in one's own superiority, or ethnocentrism, may lead to cultural imposition. **Cultural imposition** is the act of imposing one's cultural beliefs, values, and practices on individuals from another culture. Nurses impose their values on clients when they forcefully promote biomedical traditions while ignoring the clients' value of non-Western treatments such as acupuncture, herbal therapy, or spiritualistic rituals. A goal for nurses is to develop an approach of **cultural relativism,** in which they recognize that clients have different approaches to health care, and that each culture should be judged on its own merit and not the nurse's personal beliefs.

## Cultural Conflict

**Cultural conflict** is a perceived threat that may arise from a misunderstanding of expectations when nurses are unable

---

**BOX 7-3    Types of Prejudice and Racist Behaviors**

### OVERT INTENTIONAL PREJUDICE/RACISM

Two homeless women, one African American and the other Irish, are clients at the neighborhood health care center. Both women are having financial difficulty. The African-American client's husband was laid off 4 years ago after his company merged with another company. The Irish client is undergoing radiation treatment for metastatic cancer and has lost her job as a result of her prolonged illness. Both women are without health insurance. A nurse referred the Irish client to social services but did not refer the African-American woman. The nurse believed that minority clients have direct experience with some local and national government programs. Therefore these clients know about available resources and can negotiate the social system for themselves and family. In contrast, the nurse believed that the Irish woman had a catastrophic illness, she had no prior experience negotiating government programs, and the nurse needs to advocate for her. The nurse, not knowing the health-seeking behaviors of either client, stereotyped both women and intentionally used her informational power to help one client while denying assistance to the other client.

### OVERT UNINTENTIONAL PREJUDICE/RACISM

A nurse was assigned to make an initial visit to two clients recently discharged from the hospital with a diagnosis of hypertension. The nurse performed physical assessments on both clients. He developed an extensive culturally relevant teaching plan with the Filipino client that included information on sodium restriction and the effect on kidney functioning, ways to integrate cultural foods into the diet, and support in lifestyle changes. With the Puerto Rican client, the nurse performed a routine physical assessment and did not discuss the client's culturally special dietary requirements. The nurse believed that the Puerto Rican client was not capable of understanding such complex information and was going to continue to seek help from her *cuarandera* (a folk practitioner) to manage the hypertension. At the end of his

visit, the nurse says to this client, "Take care of yourself. See you next time." This nurse did not realize that he had stereotyped the client and that his actions were hurtful. He believed that he was providing quality care on the basis of the client's needs.

### COVERT INTENTIONAL PREJUDICE/RACISM

A Native American nurse works in a home health agency that serves an ethnically diverse community. The nurse has observed that the clients are always among the poorest and live in the unsafe areas of the community, and she is very concerned about her client care assignment. Her nonminority colleagues are not assigned to those sections of the community. In a recent staff meeting, she raised the concerns with her nursing supervisors. On hearing her observations, the supervisors looked at her in a skeptical manner and asked what she was talking about. This is covert racism because the nursing supervisors were aware of the informal policy that they assign minority nurses to clients in a particular area of the community. They had discussed the practice among themselves but would never admit to it. The supervisors felt that the best way for minority clients to be the recipients of culturally competent care was to assign a minority nurse to care for them.

### COVERT UNINTENTIONAL PREJUDICE/RACISM

A lesbian middle-class couple legally adopted a physically challenged child. Their insurance refuses to pay for the child's medical care. The nurse, who has been working for the agency for many years, is aware but failed to tell the parents that the baby can qualify for Medicaid through the handicapped insurance program, even though both parents work and their income is above the Medicaid guidelines limit. This nurse was unaware that her dislike for the parent's sexual lifestyle influenced her thinking (she had in the past provided heterosexual couples with information on how to apply for Medicaid).

---

to respond appropriately to another individual's cultural practice because of unfamiliarity with the practice (Andrews and Boyle, 2003). Although cultural conflicts are unavoidable, the goal for nurses should be to manage conflicts so that they do not affect the delivery of culturally competent nursing care (Brislin, 1993).

## Culture Shock

**Culture shock** is the feeling of helplessness, discomfort, and disorientation experienced by an individual attempting to understand or effectively adapt to a cultural group whose beliefs and values are radically different from the individual's culture. Nurses may experience culture shock when they interact with a client whose culture is different from their own. It may be a normal reaction to a client's beliefs and practices that are not allowed, or are disapproved

of, in the nurse's own culture (Andrews and Boyle, 2003). Culture shock is brought on by anxiety that results from losing familiar signs and symbols of social interaction. As nurses change their practice environments and leave the safety of the hospital for community settings, they may experience heightened discomfort and feelings of powerlessness as they confront differences between themselves and clients. This is especially true when the nurse has little knowledge or exposure to the culture from which the client comes. Being aware of the clients' own cultural beliefs and having knowledge of other cultures may help nurses to be less judgmental and more accepting of cultural differences.

## CULTURAL NURSING ASSESSMENT

A **cultural nursing assessment** is "a systematic identification and documentation of the culture care beliefs, meanings, values, symbols, and practices of individuals or groups within a holistic perspective, which includes the worldview, life experiences, environmental context, ethnohistory, language, and divers social structure influences" (Leininger, 2002b, pp. 117-118). Cultural assessments should focus on those aspects relevant to the presenting problem, necessary intervention, and participatory education (Tripp-Reimer et al, 2001). Nurses use a component of data collection to help them identify and understand clients' beliefs about health and illness. By adopting a relativistic approach, nurses avoid judging or evaluating the client's beliefs and values in terms of their own culture.

A nonjudgmental approach toward the client's culture is helped through such skills as understanding, eliciting, listening, explaining, acknowledging, recommending, and negotiating. It is vital that nurses listen to clients' perceptions of their problems and, in turn, that nurses explain to clients their own perceptions of the problems. Nurses and clients should acknowledge and discuss similarities and differences between the two perceptions to develop suggestions for management of problems. Nurses also negotiate with clients the nursing care actions to be used.

A variety of tools are available to assist nurses in conducting cultural assessments (Andrews and Boyle, 2003; Leininger, 2002b; Ludwig-Beymer et al, 1998; Tripp-Reimer, Brink, and Saunders, 1997). The focus of such tools varies, and selection is determined by the dimensions of the culture to be assessed.

During initial contacts with clients, nurses should perform a general cultural assessment to obtain an overview of the clients' characteristics (Tripp-Reimer et al, 1997). Nurses ask clients about their ethnic background, religious preference, family patterns, cultural values, language, education, and politics. Such basic data help nurses to understand the clients from their own point of view and to recognize their uniqueness, thus avoiding stereotyping. Data from a general assessment help determine the need for an in-depth cultural assessment, which should be conducted over a period of time and should not be restricted to the first encounter with the client. This gives both the client and the nurse time to get to know each other and, especially beneficial for the client, time to see nurse in helping relationships. Tripp-Reimer and others (1997) suggest that an in-depth cultural assessment should be conducted in two phases: a data collection phase and an organization phase.

The data collection phase consists of three steps:
1. The nurse collects self-identifying data similar to those collected in the brief assessment.
2. The nurse raises a variety of questions that seek information on clients' perception of what brings them to the health care system, the illness, and previous and anticipated treatments.
3. After the nursing diagnosis is made, the nurse identifies cultural factors that may influence the effectiveness of nursing care actions.

In the organization phase, data related to the client's and family's views on optimal treatment choices are rou-

tinely examined, and areas of difference between the client's cultural needs and the goals of Western medicine are identified. Nurses may use Leininger's (2002a) three actions (discussed previously in this chapter) to guide them in selecting and discussing culturally appropriate interventions with clients.

Members of minority groups may distrust and fear the Western medical health care system of which nurses are a part. Persons from these cultures may initially have difficulty discussing their beliefs, values, and practices with nurses, especially when they do not know how nurses will receive the information.

**( DID YOU KNOW?**

Nurses can help clients meet people of other cultures who are recovering from similar illnesses. In these situations, clients may explore different approaches to handling their health issues.

The key to a successful cultural assessment lies in nurses being aware of their own culture. Randall-David (1989) developed a variety of principles that may be helpful as nurses conduct cultural assessments:
- Always be aware of the environment. Look around and listen to what is being said and understand nonverbal communications before taking action.
- Know about community social organizations such as schools, churches, hospitals, tribal councils, restaurants, taverns, and bars.
- Know the specific areas to focus on before beginning the cultural assessment.
- Select a strategy for gathering cultural data. Possible strategies include in-depth interviews, informal conversations, observations of the client's everyday activities or specific events, survey research, and a case method approach to study certain aspects of a client.
- Identify a confidante who will help "bridge the gap" between cultures.
- Know the appropriate questions to ask without offending the client.
- Interview other nurses or health care professionals who have worked with the specific client to get their input.
- Talk with formal and informal community leaders to gain a comprehensive understanding about significant aspects of community life.
- Be aware that all information has both subjective and objective aspects, and verify and cross-check the information that is collected before acting on it.
- Avoid pitfalls in making premature generalizations.
- Be sincere, open, and honest with yourselves and the clients.

## VARIATIONS AMONG CULTURAL GROUPS

Although all cultures are not the same, they do share basic organizational factors (Giger and Davidhizar, 1999). These

**Table 7-3   Cultural Variations Between Selected Groups**

| | AFRICAN AMERICANS | ASIANS | HISPANICS | NATIVE AMERICANS |
|---|---|---|---|---|
| Verbal communication | Asking personal questions of someone that you have met for the first time is seen as improper and intrusive | High level of respect for others, especially those in positions of authority | Expression of negative feelings is considered impolite | Speak in a low tone of voice and expect the listener to be attentive |
| Nonverbal communication | Direct eye contact in conversation is often considered rude | Direct eye contact among superiors may be considered disrespectful | Avoidance of eye contact is usually a sign of attentiveness and respect | Direct eye contact is often considered disrespectful |
| Touch | Touching someone else's hair is often considered offensive | It is not customary to shake hands with persons of the opposite sex | Touching is often observed between two persons in conversation | A light touch of the person's hand instead of a firm handshake is often used as a greeting |
| Family organization | Usually have close extended family networks; women play key roles in health care decisions | Usually have close extended family ties; emphasis may be on family needs rather than individual needs | Usually have close extended family ties; all members of the family may be involved in health care decisions | Usually have close extended family; emphasis tends to be on family rather than on individual needs |
| Time | Often present oriented | Often present oriented | Often present oriented | Often past oriented |
| Perception of health | Harmony of mind, health body, and spirit with nature | When the "yin" and "yang" energy forces are balanced | Balance and harmony between mind, body, spirit, and nature | Harmony of mind, body, spirit, and emotions with nature |
| Alternative healers | "Granny," "root doctor," voodoo priest, spiritualist | Acupuncturist, acupressurist, herbalist | Curandero, espiritualista, yerbero | Medicine man, shaman |
| Self-care practices | Poultices, herbs, oils, roots | Hot and cold foods, herbs, teas, soups, cupping, burning, rubbing, pinching | Hot and cold foods, herbs | Herbs, corn meal, medicine bundle |
| Biological variations | Sickle cell anemia, mongolian spots, keloid formation, inverted "T" waves, lactose intolerance, skin color | Thalassemia, drug interactions, mongolian spots, lactose intolerance, skin color | Mongolian spots, lactose intolerance, skin color | Cleft uvula, lactose intolerance, skin color |

**DID YOU KNOW?**

Some clients may view their illness as punishment for misdeeds and may have difficulty accepting care from nurses who do not share their belief.

---

**BOX 7-4 Levels of Prevention (of Hypertension, Stroke, and Heart Disease) Related to Cultural Differences**

**PRIMARY PREVENTION**

Provide health teaching about balanced diet and exercise.

**SECONDARY PREVENTION**

Teach clients and/or family to monitor blood pressure. Teach about diet, keeping in mind the client's cultural preferences. Talk about health beliefs and cultural implications, such as the use of alternative therapies; make sure alternative therapies are compatible with any medications that may be prescribed.

**TERTIARY PREVENTION**

If blood pressure cannot be controlled by diet, refer the client to a physician for medication; advise the client to engage in a cardiac program that will oversee diet and exercise.

---

factors—communication, space, social organization, time, environment control, and biological variations—should be explored in a cultural assessment because of their potential for highlighting differences between groups. Some of these factors and their variations are presented in Table 7-3. Box 7-4 gives examples of cultural strategies for primary, secondary, and tertiary levels of prevention.

## Communication

Understanding variations in patterns of **verbal** and **nonverbal communication** helps to achieve therapeutic goals. Verbal communication is the use of language in the form of words within a grammatical structure to express ideas and feelings and to describe objects. Variations in verbal communication among cultures are reflected in verbal styles, such as pronunciation, word meaning, voice quality, and humor. Nonverbal communication is the use of body language or gestures to send information that cannot or may not be said verbally. Nonverbal styles include eye contact, gestures, touch, interjection during conversation, body posture, facial expression, and silence. For example, when gathering data from a Hispanic woman, the nurse should be aware that the style may be low-keyed, and she may avoid eye contact and be hesitant to respond to questions. This behavior should not be interpreted as lack of interest or inability to relate to others (Randall-David, 1989).

Another example occurred when a nurse gave instructions to Asian clients about taking antituberculin drugs. The clients smilingly responded with "yes, yes." The nurse interpreted this response to mean that the clients understood the instructions and that they accepted the treatment protocol. A week later, when the clients returned for a follow-up visit, the nurse discovered that the medications had not been taken. The nurse knew that acceptance by and avoidance of confrontation or disagreement with those in authority are important behaviors in the Asian culture; interventions were adjusted accordingly. The nurse repeated the medication instructions and gave the clients an opportunity to raise questions and concerns and to repeat the instructions that were given. The nurse also discussed the cultural meaning and treatment of tuberculosis.

## Using an Interpreter

Effective communication with the client or family is required for all encounters, especially those involving a cultural assessment and teaching. When nurses do not speak or understand the client's language, they should make every effort to obtain assistance from an interpreter. Interpreters should be selected carefully, as all persons who speak the language may not be proficient in medical interpretation or in the cultural issues that are in play. Interpreters must also be able to understand what the clients are saying. Interpreters may emphasize their personal preferences by influencing both nurses' and clients' decisions to select and participate in treatment modalities. Nurses can minimize this by learning basic words and sentences of the most commonly spoken languages in the community. Additionally, nurses should provide written material in the client's primary language, so that family members can reinforce information when at home with the client. Strategies that nurses may use to select and effectively use an interpreter are listed in the How To Box.

**NURSING TIP**

Respect all information that a client shares with you, even when the information is in conflict with your own value system.

---

## Space

**Space** is the physical distance between individuals during an interaction (Giger and Davidhizar, 1999). When this space is violated, you or the client may experience discomfort. Findings from early research indicate that European-American nurses have specific spatial preferences related to an intimate zone (personal distance, social distance, or public distance) that may be observed when they care for clients.

Other cultural groups also have spatial preferences. To illustrate, Hispanics tend to be comfortable with less space because they like to touch persons with whom they are speaking. Filipinos may view touching strangers as inappropriate;

## HOW TO   Select and Use an Interpreter

1. When feasible, select an interpreter who has knowledge of health-related terminology.

2. Use family members with caution because of the client's need for privacy when discussing intimate matters, because family members may lack the ability to communicate effectively in both languages, and because family members may exhibit a bias that influences the client's decisions.

3. The sex of the interpreter may be of concern; in some cultures, women may prefer a female interpreter and men may prefer a male.

4. The age of the interpreter may also be of concern. For example, older clients may want a more mature interpreter. Children tend to have limited understanding and language skills, and when used as interpreters, they may have difficulty interpreting the information.

5. Differences in socioeconomic status, religious affiliation, and educational level between the client and the interpreter may lead to problems in translation of information.

6. Identify the client's origin of birth and language or dialect spoken before selecting the interpreter. For example, Chinese clients speak different dialects depending on the region in which they were born.

7. Avoid using an interpreter from the same community as the client to avoid a breach of confidentiality.

8. Avoid using professional jargon, colloquialisms, abstractions, idiomatic expressions, slang, similes, and metaphors (Randall-David, 1989). Speak slowly and use words that are common in the client's culture.

9. Clarify roles with the interpreter.

10. Introduce the interpreter to the client, and explain to the client what the interpreter will be doing

11. Observe the client for nonverbal messages, such as facial expressions, gestures, and other forms of body language (Giger and Davidhizar, 1999). If the client's responses do not fit with the question, the nurse should check to be sure that the interpreter understood the question.

12. Increase accuracy in transmission of information by asking the interpreter to translate the client's own words, and ask the client to repeat the information that was communicated.

13. At the end of the interview, review the material with the client to ensure that nothing has been missed or misunderstood.

Giger JN, Davidhizar R: *Transcultural nursing: assessment and intervention,* ed 3, St Louis, Mo, 1999, Mosby; Randall-David E: *Culturally competent HIV counseling and education,* McLean, Va, 1994, Maternal and Child Health Clearinghouse.

therefore nurses may stand farther away from Filipinos than from Hispanics. On the other hand, clients who are comfortable with closer distances may experience discomfort when nurses stand farther away, interpreting the behavior as rejecting. Nurses should take cues from clients to place themselves in the appropriate spatial zone and avoid misinterpretation of clients' behavior as they handle their spatial needs.

## Social Organization

**Social organization** refers to the way in which a cultural group structures itself around the family to carry out role functions. In African-American culture, for example, family may include individuals who are unrelated or remotely related. Members of families depend on the extended family and kinship networks for emotional and financial support in times of crises. Mothers and grandmothers play important roles in African-American culture and may need to be included in health care decisions. The significance of family also varies across cultures. Members of Hispanic and Asian cultures tend to believe that the needs of the family come before those of the individual. In the Native American family, members honor and respect their elders and look to them for leadership, believing that wisdom comes with increasing age (West, 1993). When working with clients from these cultures, nurses should be aware that it might be nonproductive to exclude family involve-

ment in decision making. At the same time, nurses should advocate for the individual, making sure that when families make decisions, the individual's needs are also being considered.

## Time

**Time,** in the sense used here, refers to past, present, and future time as well as to the duration of and period between events. Some cultures assign greater or lesser value to events that occurred in the past, occur in the present, or will occur in the future. The American middle-class culture tends to be future oriented, and individuals are willing to delay immediate gratification until future goals are accomplished. Clients valuing longevity may moderate their dietary intake and engage in exercise activities to minimize future health risks. In contrast, African-American and Hispanic families may place greater value on quality of life and view present time as being more important than future time. The future is unknown, but the present is known. When nurses discuss health promotion and disease prevention strategies with persons who have a present orientation, they should focus on the immediate benefits these clients would gain rather than emphasizing future outcomes. That is not to say that clients cannot or would not learn about preventing future problems, but the nurse needs to connect her teaching to the "here and now."

In cultures that focus on a past orientation (e.g., the Vietnamese culture), individuals may focus on wishes and memories of their ancestors and look to them to provide direction for current situations (Giger and Davidhizar, 1999). In a past-oriented culture, time is viewed as being more flexible than in a present-oriented culture. It has less of a fixed point, and individuals are not offended by being late or early for appointments. Nurses socialized in the Western culture may view time as money and equate punctuality with correctness and being responsible. Working with clients who have a different time perception than the nurse can be problematic. Nurses should clarify the clients' perceptions to avoid misunderstandings. It is not feasible to expect that clients will change their behavior and adopt the nurse's schedule. Nurses should explain the importance of keeping appointments from the Western perspective. For example, the nurse can communicate a willingness to be flexible in scheduling appointments and explain to the client that the time will be set aside specifically for that client. Along with culture, socioeconomic status and religion may influence perception of time.

## Environmental Control

**Environmental control** refers to the ability of individuals to control nature and to influence factors in the environment that affect them. Some cultural groups perceive individuals as having mastery over nature, being dominated by nature, or having a harmonious relationship with nature. Individuals who perceive mastery over nature believe that they can overcome the natural forces of nature. Such individuals would expect a cure for cancer through the use of medications, antibiotics, surgical interventions, radiation, and chemotherapy. They are willing to do whatever it takes to achieve health.

In contrast, those who view nature as dominant (e.g., African Americans and Hispanics) believe that they have little or no control over what happens to them. They may not adhere to a cancer treatment protocol because of the belief that nothing will change the outcome because it is their destiny. These individuals are less likely to engage in illness prevention activities than those who have other worldviews.

Persons who view a human harmony with nature (e.g., Asians and Native Americans) may perceive that illness is disharmony with other forces and that medicine can only relieve the symptoms rather than cure the disease. They would look to find the treatment for the malignancy from the mind, body, and spirit connection, where healing comes from within. These groups are likely to look to naturalistic solutions, such as herbs, acupuncture, and hot and cold treatments, to resolve or cure a cancerous condition (Figure 7-2).

## Biological Variations

**Biological variations** are the physical, biological, and physiological differences that exist between racial groups and distinguish one group from another. They occur in areas of growth and development, skin color, enzymatic dif-

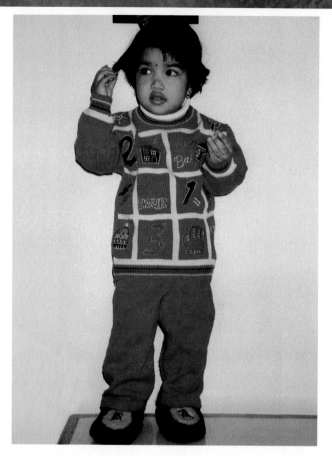

**Figure 7-2** A child from Nepal living in the United States. The child has a black dot on her forehead to protect her from the "evil eye."

ferences, susceptibility to disease, and laboratory tests (Andrews and Boyle, 2003; Giger and Davidhizar, 1999; Talbot and Curtis, 1996). For example, Western-born neonates are slightly heavier at birth than those born in non-Western cultures. Another variation is mongolian spots, which are present on the skin of African-American, Asian, Hispanic, and Native American babies. These are bluish discolorations that may be mistaken for bruises. When nurses are exposed to situations involving biological variations of which they are unfamiliar, they may create embarrassing situations. Consider the following scenario: The school nurse observes a bluish discoloration on the thigh of a Filipino child that she mistook for a bruise. The nurse reported her observation to the child protective agency in her state. When the child's mother arrived to pick her up at the end of the school day, she was accused of child abuse. The mother had to disprove the allegation before her child could be released into her care.

Other common and obvious variations include eye shape, hair texture, adipose tissue deposits, shape of earlobes, thickness of lips, and body configuration. Variations in growth and development may be influenced by environmental conditions such as nutrition, climate, and disease. Research findings suggest that sensitivity to codeine varies with ethnic background, and that Asian men experience significantly

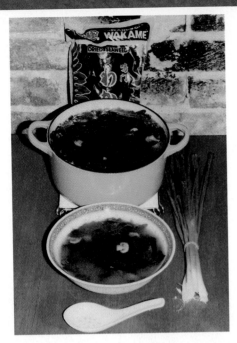

**Figure 7-3** Mi-yuk kook (seaweed soup) is a Korean dish eaten by postpartum women to stop bleeding and to cleanse body fluids. It is also eaten every birthday.

### BOX 7-5   Assessment of Dietary Practices and Food Consumption Patterns

- What is the social significance of food in the family?
- What foods are most frequently bought for family consumption? Who makes the decision to buy the food?
- What foods, if any, are taboo (prohibited) for the family?
- Does religion play a significant role in food selection?
- Who prepares the food? How is it prepared?
- How much food is eaten? When is it eaten and with whom?
- Where does the client live and what types of restaurants does he or she frequent?
- Has the family adopted foods of other cultural groups?
- What are the family's favorite recipes?

weaker effects from the drug than European men (Wu, 1997). Asian men are missing an enzyme called CYP2D6 that allows the body to metabolize codeine into morphine, which is responsible for the pain relief provided by codeine. When an individual is missing the enzyme, no amount of codeine will lessen the pain, and other pain-reducing medicines should be explored. A more common enzyme deficiency is glucose-6-phosphate dehydrogenase (G6PD), which is responsible for lactose intolerance in many ethnic groups (Giger and Davidhizar, 1999).

## CULTURE AND NUTRITION

Nutritional practices are an integral part of the assessment process for all families, especially because they play a prominent role in health problems of some groups (Greenberg et al, 1998). Efforts to understand dietary patterns of clients should go beyond relying on membership in a defined group. Knowing clients' nutrition practices makes it possible to develop treatment regimens that would not conflict with their cultural food practices (Figure 7-3). Box 7-5 identifies several questions that nurses should ask when conducting a nutritional assessment.

In mutual goal setting with the client and nutritionist to change harmful dietary practices, the nurse might need to consult culturally oriented magazines. A number of popular magazines, such as Essence, Ebony, and Latina, have created new dishes from old family recipes using healthier ingredients. These dishes are tasty and resemble old traditions, yet they are not as harmful.

Table 7-4 lists various dietary practices that are prevalent among some cultural groups in American society. Many of these practices may have their origin in religious as well as cultural traditions.

## CULTURE AND SOCIOECONOMIC STATUS

The relationship between socioeconomic status and health disparities is reflected in life expectancy, infant mortality rates, and many other health measures (Kington and Smith, 1997). Minority groups may not have the same opportunities for education, occupation, income earning, and property ownership that the dominant group has. According to the U.S. Census Bureau (2001), in 1999 there were more white families than minorities below the poverty level. However, the proportion of poor families in a minority group is greater. For example, white families represent 7.3% of those in poverty, whereas African Americans represent 21.9% and Hispanics represent 20.9%. Consequently, minority families are disproportionately represented on the lower tiers on the socioeconomic ladder. Poor economic achievement is also a common characteristic found among populations at risk, such as those in poverty, the homeless, migrant workers, and refugees. Nurses should be able to distinguish between culture and socioeconomic class issues and not misinterpret behavior as having a cultural origin, when in fact it should be attributed to socioeconomic class. Data suggest that when nurses and clients come from the same social class, it is more likely that they operate from the same health belief model, and consequently there is less opportunity for misinterpretation and communication problems.

There is also danger in believing that certain cultural behaviors, such as folk practices, are restricted to lower socioeconomic classes. Roberson (1987) found that health professionals, such as nurses and physicians, also used folk systems in conjunction with the biomedical system to promote their health and prevent disease. Therefore nurses

**Table 7-4   Food Preferences and Associated Risk Factors in Selected Cultural Groups**

| CULTURAL GROUP | FOOD PREFERENCES | NUTRITIONAL EXCESS | RISK FACTORS |
|---|---|---|---|
| African Americans | Fried foods, greens, bread, lard, pork, rice, foods with high sodium and starch content | Cholesterol, fat, sodium, carbohydrates, calories | Coronary artery disease, obesity |
| Asians | Soy sauce, rice, pickled dishes, raw fish, teas, balance between yin (cold) and yang (hot) concepts | Cholesterol, fat, sodium, carbohydrates, calories | Heart disease, liver disease, cancer of the stomach, ulcers |
| Hispanics | Fried foods, beans and rice, chili, carbonated beverages, high-fat and high-sodium foods | Cholesterol, fat, sodium, carbohydrates, calories | Heart disease, obesity |
| Native Americans | Blue corn meal, fruits, game and fish | Carbohydrates, calories | Diabetes, malnutrition, tuberculosis, infant and maternal mortality |

Data from Andrews MM, Boyle JS: *Transcultural concepts in nursing care,* ed 4, Philadelphia, 2003, Lippincott Williams & Wilkins; Giger JN, Davidhizar R: *Transcultural nursing: assessment and intervention,* ed 3, St Louis, Mo, 1999, Mosby.

must conduct a cultural assessment for all individuals when they first come in contact with them. Nurses should have guidance in integrating cultural concepts with other aspects of client care to meet their clients' total health care needs.

## Practice Application

Shu Ping was concerned about her father's deteriorating health and contacted her church friend, Jenny, a registered nurse, for advice. A public health nurse had been visiting the father since his recent discharge from the hospital, but the father had asked this nurse not to discuss his diagnosis with his family. After several weeks with the family, Jenny was able to establish a close enough relationship with the father so that she could engage him in a private discussion about his health. He confided in Jenny that he was diagnosed with cancer of the small intestine, and he feared he was dying. He did not want the family to know the "bad news." He refused treatment because his view was that people never got better after they were diagnosed with cancer; they always died.

Which of the following actions best characterizes the public health nurse's willingness to provide culturally competent care to the family?

**A.** Discussing the medical treatment and surgical intervention for cancer of the small intestine

**B.** Discussing with Shu Ping's father the prognosis for a person diagnosed with cancer of the small intestine in the United States

**C.** Requesting a conference involving the primary physician, the father, and the family to discuss the diagnosis and treatment options

**D.** Contacting the public health agency and discussing the problem with them

*Answers are in the back of the book.*

## Key Points

- The population of the United States is increasingly diverse. Changes in immigration laws and policies have increased migration, contributed to changes in community demographics, and heightened the need to recognize the impact of culture on health care and the need for nurses, particularly community-oriented nurses, to learn about the culture of the individuals to whom they give care.
- Culture is a learned set of behaviors that are widely shared among a group of people; a people's culture helps guide individuals in problem solving and decision making.
- Culturally competent nursing care is designed for a specific client, reflects the individual's beliefs and values, and is provided with sensitivity. Such nursing care helps to improve health outcomes and reduce health care costs.
- A culturally competent nurse uses cultural knowledge as well as specific skills, such as intracultural communication and cultural assessment, in selecting interventions to care for clients.
- There are four modes of action that nurses may use to negotiate with clients and give culturally competent care: cultural preservation, cultural accommodation, cultural repatterning, and culture brokering.

- Barriers to providing culturally competent care are stereotyping, prejudice and racism, ethnocentrism, cultural imposition, cultural conflict, and culture shock.
- Nurses should perform a cultural assessment on every client with whom they interact. Cultural assessments help nurses understand clients' perspectives of health and illness and thereby guide them in discussing culturally appropriate interventions. The needs of clients vary with their age, education, religion, and socioeconomic status.
- When nurses do not speak or understand the client's language, they should use an interpreter. In selecting an interpreter, nurses should consider the clients' cultural needs and respect their right to privacy.
- Dietary practices are an integral part of the assessment data. Efforts to understand dietary practices should go beyond relying on membership in a defined group and include individual nutritional practices and religious requirements.
- Members of minority groups are overrepresented on the lower tiers of the socioeconomic ladder. Poor economic achievement is also a common characteristic among populations at risk, such as those in poverty, the homeless, migrant workers, and refugees. Nurses should be able to distinguish between cultural and socioeconomic class issues and not interpret behavior as having a cultural origin when in fact it is based on socioeconomic class.

## Clinical Decision-Making Activities

1. Select a culture that you would like to learn more about. Go to an appropriate website and gather information about the cultural group. Identify the group's health-seeking behaviors. Validate this information with a member of the group. List differences between the two sources of data. How do you explain these findings? Explain how you can use this information in your clinical practice.
2. Recall a first meeting with a client whose culture differed from yours. Did you form an immediate impression about the reason for the individual's contact with the healthcare system? Discuss your assumptions about this client. What led you to make them? How did your assumptions influence your interaction with the client or family member? Give specific examples.
3. Interview an older person. What would you do to prepare for this interview? Discuss the individual's perspective of health and illness. Explore the use of Western and alternative health practices and determine the individual's decision-making process in seeking out these health services. Prepare a list of alternative health care specialists who practice in your community.
4. Explore with your community health agency the availability of culturally relevant policies and approaches for providing health care to the major cultural groups in the population it serves. On the basis of your findings, what gaps in services were evident? What input would you give the agency to augment services?
5. Which major ethnic and religious groups are represented in the community where you live? What resources are available to service their needs? What mechanisms are in place to facilitate access to these services by these groups?
6. On the basis of Healthy People 2010 objectives, identify an at-risk aggregate in your community. Develop a health education program that utilizes cultural interventions to promote positive health behaviors for the group.

### Additional Resources

These related resources are found either in the appendix at the back of this book or on the book's website at **http://evolve.elsevier.com/Stanhope.**

**evolve Evolve Website**

WebLinks: Healthy People 2010

## References

American Academy of Nursing Expert Panel on Culturally Competent Health Care: Culturally competent health care, *Nurs Outlook* 40:277, 1992.

Andrews MM, Boyle JS: *Transcultural concepts in nursing care,* ed 4, Philadelphia, 2003, Lippincott Williams & Wilkins.

Battle DE: *Community disorders in multicultural populations,* ed 2, Boston, 1998, Butterworth-Heinemann.

Bhopal R, Donaldson L: White, European, Western, Caucasian, or what? inappropriate labeling in research on race, ethnicity, and health, *Am J Public Health* 88(9):1303, 1998.

Brislin R: *Understanding culture's influence on behavior,* Fort Worth, Tex, 1993, Harcourt Brace.

Campinha-Bacote J: *The process of cultural competence in the delivery of healthcare services: a culturally competent model of care,* ed 3, Cincinnati, Ohio, 1998, Transcultural CARE Associates.

Campinha-Bacote J: The process of cultural competence in the delivery of healthcare services: a model of care, *J Transcultural Nurs* 13:181, 2002.

Denker EP, editor: *Healing at home: Visiting Nurse Service of New York, 1893-1993,* Dalton, Mass, 1994, Studley Press.

Eliason J: Correlates of prejudice in nursing students, *J Nurs Educ* 37(1):27, 1998.

Fielo S, Degazon CE: When cultures collide: decision making in a multicultural environment, *N&HC Perspectives on Community* 18:238, 1997.

Finch H, Garcia-Calhoun M, Sockalingham S: *Cultural competence: a tool to providing culturally competent family-based health care services for individuals and organizations,* Washington, DC, 1999, National Health Service Corps, Health Resources and Services Administration.

Galanti GA: *Caring for patients from different cultures,* ed 2, Philadelphia, 1997, University of Pennsylvania Press.

Gamble VN: Under the shadow of Tuskegee: African Americans and health care, *Am J Public Health* 87:1773, 1997.

Giger JN, Davidhizar R: *Transcultural nursing: assessment and intervention,* ed 3, St Louis, Mo, 1999, Mosby.

Greenberg MR et al: Region of birth and black diets: the Harlem household survey, *Am J Public Health* 88:1199, 1998.

Helsel DG, Mochel M: Afterbirth in the afterlife: cultural meaning of placental disposal in a Hmong American community, *J Transcultural Nurs* 13:282, 2002.

Hodges FS et al: Utilizing traditional storytelling to promote wellness in American Indian communities, *J Transcultural Nurs* 13:6, 2002.

Horowitz C: The role of the family and the community in the clinical setting. In Loue S: *Handbook of immigrant health,* pp. 163-182, New York, 1998, Plenum Press.

*Immigrants' Health Care Coverage and Access Fact Sheet:* Washington, DC, 2001, Kaiser Commission on Medicaid and the Uninsured.

*Immigrant Policy Handbook 2000:* Washington, DC, 2000, National Immigration Forum.

Irvine D, Sidani S, Hall LM: Finding value in nursing care: a framework for quality improvement and cultural evaluation, *Nurs Econ* 16(3):110, 1998.

Jezewski MA: Culture brokering as a model for advocacy, *Nurs Health Care* 14(2):78, 1993.

Kington RS, Smith JP: Socioeconomic status and racial ethnic differences in functional status associated with chronic diseases, *Am J Public Health* 8(5):805, 1997.

Leininger M: Essential transcultural nursing care concepts, principles, examples, and policy statements. In Leininger MM, McFarland M, editors: *Transcultural nursing: concepts, theories, research, and practices,* ed 3, pp. 45-69, New York, 2002a, McGraw-Hill.

Leininger M: Part 1: the theory of culture care and the ethnonursing research method. In Leininger MM, McFarland M, editors: *Transcultural nursing: concepts, theories, research, and practices,* ed 3, pp. 71-98, New York, 2002b, McGraw-Hill.

Leuning CL et al: Proposed standards for transcultural nursing, *J Cult Divers* 13(1):40-46, 2002

Lillie-Blanton M, Hudman J: Untangling the web: race/ethnicity, immigration and the nation's health [editorial], *Am J Public Health* 91(11):1736-1738, 2001.

Locke DC, Hardaway YV: Moral perspectives in interracial settings. In Cochrane D, Manley-Casimir M, editors: *Moral education: practical approaches,* New York, 1992, Praeger.

Loue S: *Handbook of immigrant health,* New York, 1998, Plenum Press.

Ludwig-Beymer P et al: Community assessment in a suburban Hispanic community: a description of method, *J Transcultural Nurs* 8(10):19, 1998.

McKenna M: A call for advocates for cultural awareness [editorial], *J Transcultural Nurs* 12(1):5, 2001.

Miles A, Awong L: When the patient is a racist, *Am J Nurs* 97(8):72, 1997.

Miller NK: Haitian ethnomedical systems and biomedical practitioners: directions for clinicians, *J Transcultural Nurs* 11:204, 2000.

Minnick A et al: Ethnic diversity and staff nurse employment in hospitals, *Nurs Outlook* 45:35, 1997.

Misener TR et al: Sexual orientation: a cultural diversity issue for nursing, *Nurs Outlook* 45:178, 1997.

Orlandi MA, editor: *Cultural competence for evaluators,* Washington, DC, 1992, U.S. Department of Health and Human Services.

Orque M: Orque's ethnic/cultural system: a framework for ethnic nursing care. In Orque MS, Bloch B, Monrroy LSA, editors: *Ethnic nursing care: a multi-cultural approach,* St Louis, Mo, 1983, Mosby.

Purnell LD: A description of the Purnell model for cultural competence, *J Transcultural Nurs* 11:40, 2000.

Randall-David E: *Strategies for working with culturally diverse communities and clients,* Bethesda, Md, 1989, Washington, DC, U.S. Department of Health and Human Services.

Randall-David E: *Culturally competent HIV counseling and education,* McLean, Va, 1994, Maternal and Child Health Clearinghouse.

Riedel RL: Access to health care. In Loue S: *Handbook of immigrant health,* pp. 101-123, New York, 1998, Plenum Press.

Roberson MHB: Folk health beliefs of health professionals, *West J Nurs Res* 9:257, 1987.

Snowden LR, Holschuh J: Ethnic differences in emergency psychiatric care and hospitalization is a program for the severely mentally ill, *Community Ment Health J* 28:281, 1992.

Spector RE: *Cultural diversity in health and illness,* ed 4, Norwalk, Conn, 2000, Appleton & Lange

Sutherland LL: Ethnocentrism in a pluralistic society, *J Transcult Nurs* 13:274, 2002.

Talbot L, Curtis L: The challenges of assessing skin indicators in people of color, *Home Healthcare Nurse* 14(3):167, 1996.

Tripp-Reimer T, Brink PJ, Saunders JM: Cultural assessment: content and process. In Spradley BW, Allender JA, editors: *Readings in community health,* ed 5, Philadelphia, 1997, Lippincott.

Tripp-Reimer T et al: Cultural barriers to care: inverting the problem, *Diab Spect* 14:13-22, 2001.

Trossman S: Diversity: a continuing challenge. *Am Nurse* 20(1):1, 24-25, 1998.

U.S. Department of Health and Human Services, Office of Public Health and Science: *Healthy people 2010 objectives: draft for public comment,* Washington, 1998, U.S. Government Printing Office.

U.S. Department of Health and Human Services: *Healthy people 2010: understanding and improving health,* ed 2, Washington, DC, 2000, U.S. Government Printing Office.

West EA: The cultural bridge model, *Nurs Outlook* 41:229-234, 1993.

Witucki J, Wallace DC: Differences in functional status, health status, and community-based service use between black and white diabetic elders, *J Cult Divers* 6(3):94, 1998.

Wu C: Drug sensitivity varies with ethnicity, *Science News* 152:165, 1997.

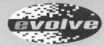

## Chapter 8

# Government, the Law, and Policy Activism

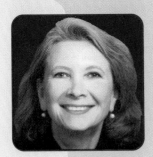

**Virginia Trotter Betts,**
**M.S.N., J.D., R.N., F.A.A.N.**

Virginia Trotter Betts served as the director for health policy at the University of Tennessee Health Sciences Center and was a professor of nursing from 2000 to January, 2003, when she was appointed by Governor Phil Bredesen to be commissioner of the Tennessee Department of Mental Health and Developmental Disabilities. Prior to this appointment, Ms. Betts served as the senior advisor on nursing and policy to the secretary and the assistant secretary of health of the U.S. Department of Health and Human Services (USDHHS). In this dual role, she advised the secretary and other USDHHS leaders on matters of federal legislation, regulation, and administrative processes that impact nursing and nurses in practice, such as scope of practice, professional autonomy, quality and safety of patient care, reimbursement, research, and education. Ms. Betts is the past president of the American Nurses Association (ANA), and she led the ANA and the nursing profession during the national debate on health care reform from 1992 to 1994. In 1995, she was appointed by President Clinton to serve on the Military Health Care Advisory Committee and shape the TriCare managed care health plan for military families and retirees. She also served as senior health advisor to the Clinton/Gore reelection campaign.

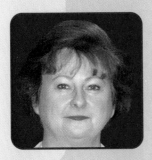

**Sandra Caddell Kirkland,**
**D.N.S., R.N., C.N.A., B.C.**

Sandra Kirkland was the primary designer of the graduate program in nursing administration at Union University in Tennessee, where she taught for 5 years. She attended the Health Policy Institute at George Mason University and taught numerous courses on health policy at the graduate level. Currently employed by Supportive Oncology Services, Dr. Kirkland is involved in the Community Oncology Alliance. This alliance grew out of a grassroots effort directed toward preventing Medicare cuts in reimbursement for community-based oncology services, where approximately 85% of all chemotherapy is administered.

## Objectives

After reading this chapter, the student should be able to do the following:

1. Discuss the structure of the United States government
2. List the functions of key governmental and quasi-governmental agencies that effect public health systems and nursing, both globally and in the United States
3. Identify the primary bodies of law that effect nursing and health care
4. Define health policy
5. Discuss the policy process
6. Define politics
7. Describe the relationships between nursing practice, health policy, and politics
8. Develop and implement a plan to communicate with policy makers on a chosen public health issue
9. Locate references related to nursing, public health, and health policy

urses are an important part of the health care system and are greatly affected by governmental and legal systems. Nurses who select community-oriented nursing as an area of practice must be especially aware of the impact of government, law, and health policy on nursing, health, and the communities in which they practice. Insight into how government, law, and political action have changed over time is necessary to understand how the health care system has been shaped by these factors. Also, understanding how these factors have influenced the current and future roles for nurses and the public health system is critical for better health policy for the nation. Nurses have historically viewed themselves as advocates for the health of the people of the nation. It is this heritage that has moved the discipline into the policy and political arenas. To secure a more positive health care system, nurse professionals must develop a working

*The authors acknowledge the contribution of Cynthia Northrup and Dr. Marcia Stanhope to the content of this chapter in previous editions.*

## Key Terms

advanced practice nurse, p. 184
Agency for Healthcare Research
    and Quality, p. 177
American Nurses Association, p. 184
block grants, p. 172
boards of nursing, p. 179
categorical funding, p. 178
categorical programs, p. 174
constitutional law, p. 179
devolution, p. 172

health policy, p. 189
judicial law, p. 180
legislation, p. 179
legislative staff, p. 184
licensure, p. 190
National Institute of Nursing Research,
    p. 173, 177
nurse practice act, p. 179
Occupational Safety and Health
    Administration, p. 176

Office of Homeland Security, p. 178
police power, p. 172
policy, p. 188
politics, p. 188
regulation, p. 179
U.S. Department of Health and Human
    Services, p. 172
World Health Organization, p. 175
*See Glossary for definitions*

## Chapter Outline

Structure of Government in the United States
*Trends and Shifts in Governmental Roles*
*Government Health Care Functions*
Healthy People 2010: An Example of National
    Health Policy Guidance
Organizations and Agencies That Influence
    Community Health
*International Organizations*
*Federal Health Agencies*
*Federal Non-Health Agencies*
*State and Local Health Departments*

Impact of Government Health Functions
    and Structures on Nursing
The Law and Community-Oriented Nursing
*Constitutional Law*
*Legislation and Regulation*
*Judicial and Common Law*
Nursing Practice and the Law
*Scope of Practice*
*Professional Negligence*
Special Community Health Practice Issues
    and the Law

*School and Family Health*
*Home Care and Hospice*
*Correctional Health*
The Nurse's Role in the Policy Process
*Legislative Action*
*Regulatory Action*
*The Process of Regulation*
*Nursing Advocacy*

knowledge of government, key governmental and quasi-governmental organizations and agencies, health care law, the policy process, and the political forces that are shaping the future of health care. This knowledge and the motivation to be an agent of change in the discipline and in the community are necessary ingredients for success as a community-oriented nurse.

## STRUCTURE OF GOVERNMENT IN THE UNITED STATES

In the United States, the federal and most state and local governments are composed of three branches, each of which has separate and important functions. The *executive branch* is composed of the president (or governor or mayor) and the staff and cabinet and various administrative and regulatory departments, and agencies such as the U.S. Department of Health and Human Services. The *legislative branch* (i.e., Congress at the federal level) is made up of two bodies: the Senate and the House of Representatives, whose members are elected by the citizens of particular ge-

> **DID YOU KNOW?**
>
> There is a federal Division of Nursing, a section within the Health Resources and Services Agency (HRSA) of the USDHHS, that refines criteria for nursing education programs as funded by Congress and affirmed by the president.

ographic areas. The *judicial branch* is composed of a system of federal, state, and local courts guided by the opinions of the Supreme Court. Each of these branches is established by the Constitution, and each plays an important role in the developing and implementing of health law and public policy.

The executive branch suggests, administers, and regulates policy. The role of the legislative branch is to identify problems and to propose, debate, pass, and modify laws to address those problems. The judicial branch interprets laws and their meaning, as in its ongoing interpretation of states' rights to define access to reproductive health services to citizens of the states.

One of the first constitutional challenges to a federal law passed by Congress was in the area of health and welfare in 1937, after the 74th Congress had established unemployment compensation and old-age benefits for U.S. citizens (U.S. Law, 1937b). Although Congress had created other health programs previously, its legal basis for doing so had never been challenged. In *Stewart Machine Co. v. Davis* (U.S. Law, 1937a), the Supreme Court (judicial branch) reviewed this legislation and determined, through interpreting the Constitution, that such federal governmental action was within Congress's powers to promote the general welfare.

Most legal bases for Congress's action in health care are found in Article I, Section 8 of the U.S. Constitution, including the following:

1. Provide for the general welfare.
2. Regulate commerce among the states.
3. Raise funds to support the military.
4. Provide spending power.

Through a continuing number and variety of cases and controversies, these Section 8 provisions have been interpreted by the courts to appropriately include a wide variety of federal powers and activities. State power concerning health care is called **police power.** This power allows states to act to protect the health, safety, and welfare of their citizens. Such police power must be used fairly, and the state must show that it has a compelling interest in taking actions, especially actions that might infringe on individual rights. Examples of a state using its police powers include requiring immunization of children before being admitted to school and requiring case finding, reporting, treating, and follow-up care of persons with tuberculosis. These activities protect the health, safety, and welfare of state citizens.

## Trends and Shifts in Governmental Roles

The government's role in health care at both the state and federal level began gradually. Wars, economic instability, and political differences between parties all shaped the government's role. The first major federal governmental action relating to health was the creation in 1798 of the Public Health Service (PHS). The Social Security Act of 1935 was passed to provide assistance to older adults and the unemployed, and it offered survivors' insurance for widows and children. It also provided for child welfare, health department grants, and maternal and child health projects. In 1948, Congress created the National Institutes of Health (NIH), and in 1965 it passed the most important health legislation to date—creating Medicare and Medicaid to provide health care service payments for older adults, the disabled, and the categorically poor. These legislative acts by Congress created programs that were implemented by the executive branch.

The **U.S. Department of Health and Human Services** (USDHHS) (known first as the Department of Health, Education, and Welfare [DHEW]) was created in 1953. The Health Care Financing Administration (HCFA) was created in 1977 as the key agency within the USDHHS to provide direction for Medicare and Medicaid. In 2002, HCFA was renamed the Center for Medicare and Medicaid Services (CMS). During the 1980s, a major effort of the Reagan administration was to shift federal government activities, including federal programs for health care, to the states. The process of shifting the responsibility for planning, delivering, and financing programs from the federal level to the states is called **devolution.** Throughout the 1980s and 1990s, Congress has increasingly funded health programs by giving **block grants** to the states. Devolution processes including block granting should alert professional nurses that state and local policy is growing in importance to the health care arena (USDHHS, 1998).

The role of government in health care is shaped both by the needs and demands of its citizens and by the citizens' beliefs and values about personal responsibility and self-sufficiency. These beliefs and values often clash with society's sense of responsibility and need for equality for all citizens. A recent federal example of this ideologic debate occurred in the 1990s over health care reform. The Democratic agenda called for a health care system that was universally accessible, with a focus on primary care and prevention. The Republican agenda supported more modest changes within the medical model of the delivery system. This agenda also supported the reducing of the federal government's role in health care delivery through cuts in Medicare and Medicaid benefits. The Democrats proposed the Health Security Act of 1993, which failed to gain Congress's approval. In an effort to make some incremental health care changes, both the Democrats and Republicans in Congress passed two new laws. The Health Insurance Portability and Accountability Act (HIPAA) allows working persons to keep their employee group health insurance for up to 16 months after they leave a job (U.S. Law, 1996). The State Child Health Improvement Act (SCHIP) of 1997 provides insurance for children and families who cannot otherwise afford health insurance (U.S. Law, 1997).

This discussion has focused primarily on trends in and shifts between different levels of government. An additional aspect of governmental action is the relationship between government and individuals. Freedom of individuals must be balanced with governmental powers. After the terrorist attacks on the United States in September (World Trade Center attack) and October (anthrax outbreak) of 2001, much government activity is being proposed in the name of protecting the safety of U.S. citizens. Yet it remains unclear just how much governmental intervention is necessary and effective and how much will be tolerated by citizens.

After the events of September 11, 2001, the Centers for Law and the Public's Health at Georgetown and Johns

> **WHAT DO YOU THINK?**
>
> Government has too much influence on the way health care services are delivered and on who receives care.

Hopkins University led a team in drafting the Model State Emergency Health Powers Act. The Model Act is designed to provide governors and public health officials with the power to act decisively in the event of a bioterror attack or an emerging infectious disease. The Model Act places a duty on states to plan for catastrophic events and build public health capacity to respond to bioterrorism. This legislation is on a fast track to be passed after input from the Centers for Disease Control (CDC), National Governors Association (NGA), the National Conference of State Legislatures (NCSL), National Association of Attorneys General (NAG), the Association of State and Territorial Health Officials (ASTHO), and the National Association of City and County Health Officers (NACCHO). The final law will then be ready to be enacted by the state legislatures and signed into law by governors for implementing by state public health authorities (Nicola, 2002).

## Government Health Care Functions

Federal, state, and local governments carry out four health care functions, which fall into the general categories of direct services, financing, information, and policy setting.

### Direct Services

Federal, state, and local governments provide direct health services to certain individuals and groups. For example, the federal government provides health care to members and dependents of the military, certain veterans, and federal prisoners. State and local governments employ nurses to deliver a variety of services to individuals and families, frequently on the basis of factors such as financial need or the need for a particular service, such as hypertension or tuberculosis screening, immunizations for children and older adults, and primary care for inmates in local jails or state prisons.

### Financing

Governments pay for some health care services; the current percent of the bill paid by the government is about 43.5%, and this is projected to increase to 44.7% by the year 2010. The government also pays for training some health personnel and for biomedical and health care research (U.S. Bureau of the Census, 2001). Support in these areas has greatly affected both consumers and health care providers. State and federal governments finance the direct care of clients through the Medicare, Medicaid, Social Security, and SCHIP programs. Many nurses have been educated with government funds through grants and loans, and schools of nursing, in the past, have been built and equipped using federal funds. Governments also have financially supported other health care providers, such as physicians, most significantly through the program of Graduate Medical Education funds. The federal government invests in research and new program demonstration projects, with the National Institute of Health (NIH) receiving a large portion of the monies. The **National Institute of Nursing Research** (NINR) is a part of the NIH and, as such, provides a substantial sum of money to the discipline of nursing for the purpose of developing the knowledge base of nursing and promoting nursing services in health care.

### Information

All branches and levels of government collect, analyze, and disseminate data about health care and health status of the citizens. An example is the annual report, *Health: United States*, compiled each year by the USDHHS (2001). Collecting vital statistics, including mortality and morbidity data, gathering of census data, and conducting health care status surveys are all government activities. Table 8-1 lists examples of available federal and international data sources on the health status of populations in the United States and around the world. These sources are available on the internet and in the governmental documents sections of most large libraries. This information is especially important because it can help nurses understand the major health problems in the United States and those in their own states and local communities.

### Policy Setting

Policy setting is a chief governmental function. Governments at all levels and within all branches make policy decisions about health care. These health policy decisions have broad implications for financial expenses, resource

### Evidence-Based Practice

The purpose of this study was to examine the changes in access to care, use of services, and quality of care among children enrolled in Child Health Plus (CHPlus), a state health insurance program for low-income children that became a model for the State Child Health Insurance Program (SCHIP). A before-and-after design was used to evaluate the health care experience of children the year before enrollment and the year after enrollment in the state health insurance program. The study consisted of 2126 children from New York State, ranging from birth to 12.99 years of age. Results indicated that the state health insurance program for low-income children was associated with improved access, use, and quality of care. The developing and implementing of SCHIP was an outcome of the soaring cost of health care and the fact that there are 11 million uninsured children in the United States. It was the largest public investment in child health in 30 years.

**Nurse Use:** This study supports the value of health policy and the need to evaluate the effectiveness of policy in accomplishing the purposes of the policy.

Szilagyi PG et al: Evaluation of a state health insurance program for low-income children: implications for state child health insurance programs. *Pediatrics* 105(2):363-371, 2000.

**Table 8-1  International and National Sources of Data on the Health Status of the U.S. Population**

| Organization Data Sources | |
| --- | --- |
| **International** | |
| United Nations | http://www.un.org/<br>*Demographic Yearbook* |
| World Health Organization | http://www.who.int/en/<br>*World Health Statistics Annual* |
| **Federal** | |
| Department of Health and Human Services | http://www.DHHS.gov<br>National Vital Statistics System<br>National Survey of Family Growth<br>National Health Interview Survey<br>National Health Examination Survey<br>National Health and Nutrition Examination Survey<br>National Master Facility Inventory<br>National Hospital Discharge Survey<br>National Nursing Home Survey<br>National Ambulatory Medical Care Survey<br>National Morbidity Reporting System<br>U.S. Immunization Survey<br>Surveys of Mental Health Facilities<br>Estimates of National Health Expenditures<br>AIDS Surveillance<br>Abortion Surveillance<br>Nurse Supply Estimates |
| Department of Commerce | http://www.commerce.gov<br>U.S. Census of Population<br>Current Population Survey<br>Population Estimates and Projections |
| Department of Labor | http://www.dol.gov<br>Consumer Price Index<br>Employment and Earnings |

use, delivery system change, and innovation in the health care field. One law that has played a very important role in the development of public health policy, public health nursing, and social welfare policy in the United States is the Sheppard-Towner Act of 1921 (USDHHS, 1992; USDHHS, HRSA, 2002).

The Sheppard-Towner Act made nurses available to provide health services for women and children, including well-child and child-development services; provided adequate hospital services and facilities for women and children; and provided grants-in-aid for establishing maternal and child welfare programs. The act helped set precedents and patterns for the growth of modern-day public health policy. It defined the role of the federal government in creating standards to be followed by states in conducting **categorical programs,** such as today's Women, Infants, and Children (WIC) and Early Periodic Screening and Developmental Testing (EPSDT) programs. Also defined was the position of the consumer in influencing, formulating, and shaping public policy; the gov-

ernment's role in research; a system for collecting national health statistics; and the integrating of health and social services. This act established the importance of prenatal care, anticipatory guidance, client education, and nurse-client conferences, all of which are viewed today as essential nursing responsibilities.

## HEALTHY PEOPLE 2010: AN EXAMPLE OF NATIONAL HEALTH POLICY GUIDANCE

In 1979, the surgeon general issued a report that began a 20-year focus on promoting health and preventing disease for all Americans (Department of Health, Education and Welfare, 1979). In 1989, Healthy People 2000 became a national effort with many stakeholders representing the perspectives of government, state and local agencies, advocacy groups, academia, and health organizations.

Throughout the 1990s, states used Healthy People 2000 objectives to identify emerging public health issues. The success of this national program was accomplished and measured through state and local efforts. The Healthy

**Healthy People 2010** | A Comparison of the Goals and Focus Areas of Healthy People 2000 and Healthy People 2010

**HEALTHY PEOPLE 2000**

**Goals**

- Increase the years of healthy life for Americans
- Reduce health disparities among Americans
- Achieve access to preventive services for all Americans

**Focus Areas**

- Cancer
- Clinical and preventive services
- Diabetes and chronic disabling conditions
- Educational and community-based programs
- Environmental health
- Family planning
- Food and drug safety
- Heart disease and stroke
- HIV infection
- Immunization and infectious diseases
- Maternal and infant health
- Mental health and mental disorders
- Nutrition
- Occupational safety and health
- Oral health
- Physical activity and fitness
- Sexually transmitted diseases
- Substance abuse: alcohol and other drugs
- Surveillance and data systems
- Tobacco
- Unintentional injuries
- Violent and abusive behavior

**HEALTHY PEOPLE 2010**

**Goals**

- Increase quality and years of healthy life
- Eliminate health disparities

**Focus Areas**

- Access to quality health services
- Arthritis, osteoporosis, and chronic back conditions
- Cancer
- Chronic kidney disease
- Diabetes
- Disability and secondary conditions
- Educational and community-based programs
- Environmental health
- Family planning
- Food safety
- Health communication
- Heart disease and stroke
- Human immunodeficiency virus
- Immunization and infectious diseases
- Injury and violence prevention
- Maternal, infant, and child health
- Medical product safety
- Mental health and mental disorders
- Nutrition and overweight
- Occupational safety and health
- Oral health
- Physical activity and fitness
- Public health infrastructure
- Respiratory diseases
- Sexually transmitted diseases
- Substance abuse
- Tobacco use
- Vision and hearing

From U.S. Department of Health and Human Services: *Healthy people 2010: understanding and improving health,* ed 2, Washington, DC, 2000, U.S. Government Printing Office.

People 2010 box shows the document's two overarching goals, with a vision of healthy people living in healthy communities. Box 8-1 shows an example of the goals for three of the 28 associated focus areas and objectives for 2010 (see Chapter 1 for more discussion).

## ORGANIZATIONS AND AGENCIES THAT INFLUENCE COMMUNITY HEALTH

### International Organizations

In June 1945, following World War II, many national governments joined together to create the United Nations (UN). By charter, the aims and goals of the UN deal with human rights, world peace, international security, and the promotion of economic and social advancement of all the world's peoples. The UN, headquartered in New York City, is made up of six principal divisions, several subgroups, and many specialized agencies and autonomous organizations. With the approval and support of the UN Commission on the Status of Women, four world conferences on women have been held. At these conferences, the health of women and children and their rights to personal, educational, and economic security, and initiatives to achieve these goals at the country level, are debated and explored, and policies are formulated (United Nations, 1975, 1980, 1985, 1995).

One of the special autonomous organizations growing out of the UN is the **World Health Organization** (WHO). Established in 1946, WHO relates to the UN through the Economic and Social Council to achieve its goal to attain the highest possible level of health for all persons. "Health for All" is the creed of the WHO. Headquartered in Geneva, Switzerland, the WHO has six regional offices. The office for the Americas is located in Washington, D.C., and is known as the Pan American Health Organization (PAHO). The WHO provides services worldwide to promote health, it cooperates with member countries in promoting their health efforts, and it coordinates the collaborating efforts between countries and the disseminating of biomedical research. Its services, which benefit all countries, include a day-to-day information service on the occurrence of internationally important diseases; the publishing of the international list of causes of disease, injury, and death; monitoring of adverse reactions to drugs; and establishing of world standards for antibiotics and vaccines. Assistance available to individual countries includes support for national programs to fight disease, to train health workers, and to strengthen the delivery of health services. The World Health Assembly (WHA) is the WHO's policy-making body, and it meets annually. The WHA's health policy work provides policy options for many countries of the world in their development of in-country initiatives and priorities, but, while important everywhere, WHA policy statements are guides and not law. The WHA's most recent policy statement on nursing and midwifery was released in 2001 as Resolution WHA.49.1, and the current worldwide shortage of professional nurses is now on the WHO agenda for further action in 2003 (WHA, 2001).

The presence of nursing in international health is increasing. Besides offering direct health services in every country in the world, nurses serve as consultants, educators, and program planners and evaluators. Nurses focus their work on a variety of public health issues, including the health care workforce and education, environment, sanitation, infectious diseases, wellness promotion, maternal and child health, and primary care. Dr. Naeema Al-Gasseer of Bahrain is the scientist for nursing and midwifery at the WHO; Marla Salmon, dean of nursing at Emory University chaired the Global Advisory Group on Nursing and Midwifery, and Linda Tarr Whelan served as the U.S. Ambassador to the UN Commission on the Status of Women. Virginia Trotter Betts, past president of the American Nurses Association (ANA), served as a U.S. delegate to both the WHA and the Fourth World Conference on Women in Beijing in 1995, where she participated on the negotiating team of the conference to develop a platform on the health of women across the life span. Many U.S. nurse leaders, such as Dr. Beverly Flynn and Dr. Carolyn Williams, authors in this book, have been WHO consultants.

## Federal Health Agencies

Laws passed by Congress may be assigned to any administrative agency within the executive branch of government for implementing, oversight, regulating, and enforcing. Congress decides which agency will monitor specific laws. For example, most health care legislation is delegated to the USDHHS. However, legislation concerning the environment would most likely be implemented and monitored by the Environmental Protection Agency (EPA), and that concerning occupational health by the **Occupational Safety and Health Administration** (OSHA) in the U.S. Department of Labor.

### U.S. Department of Health and Human Services

The USDHHS is the agency most heavily involved with the health and welfare of U.S. citizens. It touches more lives than any other federal agency. The organizational chart of the USDHHS (see Figure 3-1 in Chapter 3) shows and provides more discussion for the key agencies within the organization. The following agencies have been selected for their relevance to this chapter.

*Health Resources and Services Administration*

The Health Resources and Services Administration (HRSA) has been a long-standing contributor to the improved health status of Americans through the programs of services and health professions education that it funds. The HRSA contains the Bureau of Health Professions (BHPr), which includes the Division of Nursing, as well as the Divisions of Medicine, Dentistry, and Allied Health Professions.

The Division of Nursing has the following specific goals (USDHHS, 2000a):

- To enhance nursing's contribution to primary health care and public health
- To develop and promote innovative practice models for improved and expanded nursing services
- To enhance racial and ethnic diversity and cultural competency in the nursing workforce

- To promote improved and expanded linkages between education and practice
- To improve and expand nursing services to high-risk and underserved populations
- To enhance nursing's contributions to achieving the Healthy People 2010 objectives and health care reform
- To build capacity for meeting the nursing service needs of the nation

### Centers for Disease Control and Prevention

The Centers for Disease Control and Prevention (CDC) serve as the national focus for developing and applying disease prevention and control, environmental health, and health promotion and education activities designed to improve the health of the people of the United States. The mission of the CDC is to promote health and quality of life by preventing and controlling disease, injury, and disability. The CDC seeks to accomplish its mission by working with partners throughout the nation and the world in the following ways:

- To monitor health
- To detect and investigate health problems
- To conduct research that will enhance prevention
- To develop and advocate sound public health policies
- To implement prevention strategies
- To promote healthy behaviors
- To foster safe and healthful environments
- To provide leadership and training

### National Institutes of Health

Founded in 1887, the National Institutes of Health (NIH) today is one of the world's foremost biomedical research centers, and the federal focus point for biomedical research in the United States. The NIH is composed of 27 separate institutes and centers. The goal of NIH research is to acquire new knowledge to help prevent, detect, diagnose, and treat disease and disability, from the rarest genetic disorder to the common cold. The NIH mission is to uncover new knowledge that will lead to better health for everyone. The NIH works toward that mission by conducting research in its own laboratories; supporting the research of nonfederal scientists in universities, medical schools, hospitals, and research institutions throughout the country and abroad; helping in the training of research investigators; and fostering communication of medical and health sciences information. The National Institute of Nursing Research (NINR) is the focal point of the nation's nursing research activities. It promotes the growth and quality of research in nursing and client care, provides important research leadership, expands the pool of funded nurse researchers, and serves as a point of interaction with other health care researchers and projects.

### Agency for Healthcare Research and Quality

The mission of the **Agency for Healthcare Research and Quality** (AHRQ) is to support research designed to improve the outcomes and quality of health care, reduce its costs, address patient safety and medical errors, and broaden access to effective services. By examining what works and what does not work in health care, the AHRQ fulfills its missions of translating research findings into better patient care and providing consumers, policymakers, and other health care leaders with information needed to make critical health care decisions. In 1999, Congress, through legislation, specifically directed AHRQ to focus on measuring and improving health care quality; promoting patient safety and reducing medical errors; advancing the use of information technology for coordinating patient care and conducting quality and outcomes research; and seeking to eliminate disparities in health care delivery for the priority populations of low-income groups, minorities, women, children, older adults, and individuals with special health care needs.

### Centers for Medicare and Medicaid Services

One of the most powerful agencies within the USDHHS is the Centers for Medicare and Medicaid Services (CMS; formerly HCFA), which administers Medicare and Medicaid accounts and guides payment policy and delivery rules for services for 74 million people. In addition to providing health insurance, CMS also performs a number of quality-focused health care or health-related activities, including regulating of laboratory testing, developing coverage policies, and improving quality of care. CMS maintains oversight of the surveying and certifying of nursing homes and continuing care providers (including home health agencies, intermediate care facilities for the mentally retarded, and hospitals). It makes available to beneficiaries, providers, researchers, and state surveyors information about these activities and nursing home quality.

## Federal Non-Health Agencies

Although the USDHHS has primary responsibility for federal health functions, several other departments of the executive branch carry out important health functions for the nation. Among these are Defense, Labor, Agriculture, and Justice.

### Department of Defense

The Department of Defense delivers health care to members of the military, to their dependents and survivors, and to retired members and their families. The assistant secretary of defense for health affairs administers two health care plans for service personnel: TriCare Prime (a managed care arrangement) and an option for fee-for-service plans called TriCare Standard. In each branch of the uniformed services, nurses of high military rank are part of the administration of these health services.

### Department of Labor

The Department of Labor houses OSHA, which imposes workplace requirements on industries. These requirements shape the functions of nurses and the types of health services provided to workers in the workplace. A record-keeping system required by OSHA greatly affects health records in the workplace. Each state has an agency similar to OSHA that also monitors and inspects industries, as well as the health services delivered to them by nurses.

Needlestick injuries and other sharps-related injuries that result in occupational bloodborne pathogen exposure continue to be an important public health concern, especially to health care workers. In response to this serious situation, Congress passed the Needle Stick Safety and Prevention Act, which became law on November 6, 2000. To meet the requirements of this act, OSHA revised its Bloodborne Pathogen Standard to become effective on April 18, 2002. This act clarified the responsibility of employers to select safer needle devices as they become available and to involve employees in identifying and choosing the devices. The updated standard also required employers to maintain a log of injuries from contaminated sharps (Gerberding, 2003).

### Department of Agriculture

The Department of Agriculture houses the Food and Nutrition Service, which oversees a variety of food assistance activities. This service collaborates with state and local government welfare agencies to provide food stamps to needy persons to increase their food purchasing power. Other programs include school breakfast and lunch programs, WIC, and grants to states for nutrition education and training. While these programs have been successful, the increasing use of the process of giving federal block grants to states (rather than implementing national programs) may threaten the effectiveness of these programs because of differences in how decisions are made at the state level on how to spend money on nutrition.

### Department of Justice

Health services to federal prisoners are administered within the Department of Justice. The Federal Bureau of Prisons is responsible for the custody and care of approximately 160,000 federal offenders. The Medical and Services Division of the Bureau of Prisons includes medical, psychiatric, dental, and health support services with community standards in a correctional environment. Health promotion is emphasized through counseling during examinations, education about effects of medications, infectious disease prevention and education, and chronic care clinics for conditions such as cardiovascular disease, diabetes, and hypertension. The Bureau also provides forensic services to the courts, including a range of evaluative mental health studies outlined in federal statutes. Health care for prisoners is highly regulated due to a series of court decisions on inmates' rights.

## State and Local Health Departments

Depending on funding, public commitment and interest, and access to other resources, programs offered by state and local health departments vary greatly. Many state and local health officials report that employees in public health agencies lack skills in the core sciences of public health, and that this has hindered their effectiveness. The lack of specialized education and skill is a significant barrier to population-based preventive care and the delivery of quality health care to the public. Public health workforce specialists report that as many as 320,000 of the 400,000 people currently employed in state and local departments of public health have no formal education in public health. Additionally, it is estimated that less than 50% of the directors of local health departments have an education in public health. According to the HRSA, there is a shortage of properly educated public health nurses and physicians. More often than at other levels of government, nurses at the local level provide direct services. Some nurses deliver special or selected services, such as follow-up of contacts in cases of tuberculosis or venereal disease or providing child immunization clinics. Other nurses have a more generalized practice, delivering services to families in certain geographic areas (Nicola, 2002).

At the local and state levels, coordinating health efforts between health departments and other county or city departments is essential. Gaps in community coordination are showing up in glaring ways as states and communities scramble to address bioterrorism preparedness since September 11, 2001.

## IMPACT OF GOVERNMENT HEALTH FUNCTIONS AND STRUCTURES ON NURSING

The variety and range of functions of governmental agencies have had a major impact on the practice of nursing. Funding, in particular, has shaped roles and tasks of community-oriented nurses. The designation of money for specific needs, or **categorical funding,** has led to special and more narrowly focused nursing roles. Examples are in home health care, school nursing, and family planning. Funds assigned to communicable disease programs or family planning usually cannot be used to support other services such as home care.

The events of September 11, 2001, have the public and the profession of nursing concerned about the ability of the present public health system and its workforce to deal with bioterrorism, especially outbreaks of deadly and serious communicable diseases. For example, small pox vaccinations stopped in 1972, but immunity lasts for only 10 years, so although there have been no reported cases since the early 1970s, almost no one in the U.S. retains their immunity. Thus the population is vulnerable to a smallpox outbreak. Few public health professionals are knowledgeable of the symptoms, treatment, or mode of transmission of this disease. Most health professionals, including registered nurses (RNs), currently working in the United States have never seen a case of anthrax, smallpox, or plague, the three major biological weapons of concern in the world today. The USDHHS and the new federal **Office of Homeland Security** have plans and funding to address this serious threat to the people of the United States. One of the first things on their health agenda is to rebuild the crumbling public health infrastructures of each state to provide surveillance, intervention, and communication in the face of future bioterrorism events (Nicola, 2002).

## THE LAW AND COMMUNITY-ORIENTED NURSING

The United States is a nation of laws, which are subject to the U.S. Constitution. The law is a system of privileges and processes by which people solve problems on the basis of a set of established rules. It is intended to minimize the use of force. Laws govern the relationships of individuals and organizations to other individuals and to government. After a law is established, regulations further define the course of actions to be taken by the government, organizations, or individuals in reaching an agreed-on outcome. Government and its laws are the ultimate authority in society and are designed to enforce official policy whether it is related to health, education, economics, social welfare, or any other society issue. The number and types of laws influencing health care are ever increasing. Definitions of law (Catholic University of America, 2002) include the following:

- A rule established by authority, society, or custom
- The body of rules governing the affairs of people, communities, states, corporations, and nations
- A set of rules or customs governing a discrete field or activity (e.g., criminal law, contract law)

These definitions reflect the close relationship of law to the community and to society's customs and beliefs. The law has had a major impact on community-oriented nursing practice. Although community-oriented nursing emerged from individual voluntary activities, society passed laws to give formality to community health and, through legal mandates (i.e., laws), positions and functions for nurses in community settings were created. These functions in many instances carry the force of law. For example, if the nurse discovers a person with smallpox, the law directs the nurse and others in the public health community to take specific actions.

Three types of laws in the United States have particular importance to the community-oriented nurse. They are constitutional law, legislation and regulation, and judicial or common law.

### DID YOU KNOW?

Persons with communicable diseases such as tuberculosis may be confined to a prison hospital if they are considered a threat to their community by failing to follow their treatment regimen.

## Constitutional Law

**Constitutional law** derives from federal and state constitutions. It provides overall guidance for selected practice

situations. For example, on what basis can the state *require* quarantine or isolation of individuals with tuberculosis? The U.S. Constitution specifies the explicit and limited functions of the federal government. All other powers and functions are left to the individual states. The major constitutional power of the states relating to community-oriented nursing practice is the state's right to intervene in a reasonable manner to protect the health, safety, and welfare of its citizens. The state has *police power* to act through its public health system, but it has limits. First, it must be a "reasonable" exercise of power. Second, if the power interferes or infringes on individual rights, the state must demonstrate that there is a "compelling state interest" in exercising its power. Isolating an individual or separating someone from a community because that person has a communicable disease has been deemed an appropriate exercise of state powers. The state can isolate an individual even though it infringes on individual rights (freedom, autonomy) under the following conditions (Khan, Morse, and Lillibridge, 2000):

1. There is a compelling state interest in preventing an epidemic
2. The isolation is necessary to protect the health, safety, and welfare of individuals in the community or the public as a whole
3. The isolation is done in a reasonable manner

### WHAT DO YOU THINK?

The community's rights are more important than the individual's rights when there is a threat to the health of the public.

The legal and medical communities along with AIDS (acquired immunodeficiency syndrome) activists rejected (and made the case) that the social quarantine of individuals with AIDS was unnecessary. Thus individual freedom and autonomy of the individual come before "compelling state interest" unless science warrants another conclusion (Gerberding, 2003; Twitchell, 2003).

## Legislation and Regulation

**Legislation** is law that comes from the legislative branches of federal, state, or local government. Much legislation has an effect on nursing. **Regulations** are specific statements of law related to defining or implanting individual pieces of legislation. For example, state legislatures enact laws (statutes) establishing **boards of nursing** and defining terms such as *registered nurse* and *nursing practice*. Every state has a board of nursing. The board may be found either in the department of licensing boards of the health department or in an administrative agency of the governor's office. Created by legislation known as a state nurse practice act, the board of nursing is made up of nurses and consumers. The functions of this board are described in the **nurse practice act** of each state and generally include licensing and examination of registered nurses and licensed practical nurses; approval of schools of nursing in the state; revocation, suspension, or denying of licenses; and writing of regulations about nursing practice and education. The state boards of nursing operationalize, implement, and enforce the statutory law by writing explicit statements (called rules) on what it means to be a registered nurse, and on the nurse's rights and responsibilities in delegating work to others and in meeting continuing education requirements.

All nurses employed in community settings are subject to legislation and regulations. For example, home health care nurses employed by private agencies must deliver care according to federal Medicare or state Medicaid legislation and regulations, so the agency can be reimbursed for those services. Private and public health care services rendered by nurses are subject to many governmental regulations for quality of care, standards of documentation, and maintaining confidentiality of patient records and communications.

## Judicial and Common Law

Both judicial law and common law have great impact on nursing. **Judicial law** is based on court or jury decisions. The opinions of the courts are referred to as case law. The court uses other types of laws to make its decisions, including previous court decisions or cases. Precedent is one principle of common law. This means that judges are bound by previous decisions unless they are convinced that the older law is no longer relevant or valid. This process is called distinguishing, and it usually involves a demonstration of how the current situation in dispute differs from the previously decided situation. Other principles of common law such as justice, fairness, respect for individual's autonomy, and self-determination are part of a court's rationale and the basis upon which to make a decision.

## NURSING PRACTICE AND THE LAW

Despite the broad nature and varied roles of nurses in practice, two legal arenas are most applicable to nurse practice situations. The first is the statutory authority for the profession and its scope of practice, and the second is professional negligence or malpractice.

## Scope of Practice

The issue of scope of practice involves defining nursing, setting its credentials, and then distinguishing between the practices of nurses, physicians, and other health care providers. The issue is especially important to community-oriented nurses, who have traditionally practiced with much autonomy.

Health care practitioners are subject to the laws of the state in which they practice, and they can practice only with a license. The states' nurse practice acts differ somewhat, but they are the most important statutory law effecting nurses. The nurse practice act of each state accomplishes at least four functions: defining the practice of professional nursing, identifying the scope of nursing practice, setting educational qualifications and other requirements for **licensure,** and determining the legal titles nurses

may use to identify themselves. The usual and customary practice of nursing can be determined through a variety of sources, including the following:

1. Content of nursing educational programs, both general and special
2. Experience of other practicing nurses (peers)
3. Statements and standards of nursing professional organizations
4. Policies and procedures of agencies employing nurses
5. Needs and interests of the community
6. Updated literature, including research, books, texts, and journals

All of these sources can describe, determine, and refine the scope of practice of a professional nurse. Every nurse should know and follow closely any proposed changes in the practice acts of nursing, medicine, pharmacy, and other related professions. The nurse should always examine all legislation, rules, and regulations related to community-oriented nursing practice. For example, a review of the Pharmacy Act will let the nurse know whether to question the right to dispense medications in a family planning clinic in a local health department. Defining the scope of practice forces one to clarify independent, interdependent, and dependent nursing functions.

Just as practice acts vary by state, so do the evolving issues and tensions of scopes of practice among the health professions. In the last few years, several state legislatures (working closely with the National Council of State Boards of Nursing) have embarked on a legislative effort to develop the Interstate Nurse Licensure Compact. The compact allows mutual recognition of generalist nursing licensure across state lines in the compact states. To date, 19 states have adopted the compact (ANA, 2000).

## Professional Negligence

Professional negligence, or malpractice, is defined as an act (or a failure to act) that leads to injury of a client. To recover money damages in a malpractice action, the client must prove all of the following:

1. That the nurse owed a duty to the client or was responsible for the client's care
2. That the duty to act the way a reasonable, prudent nurse would act in the same circumstances was not fulfilled
3. That the failure to act reasonably under the circumstances led to the alleged injuries
4. That the injuries provided the basis for a monetary claim from the nurse as compensation for the injury

Reported cases involving negligence and community-oriented nurses are very few in number. However, the following is an example.

In *Williams v. Metro Home Health Care Agency, et al.* (U.S. Law, 2002), the patient brought a malpractice action against Edward Schiro, R.N., and his employer, a home health agency, alleging that the nurse's failure to visit and treat the patient (a paraplegic) in a manner that followed physician orders caused the progression of a decubitus ulcer on his hip to the extent that surgical intervention was required. The physician orders called for three visits per week, and the patient testified that the RN visited only once per week and had falsified the record as to the other visits.

The court determined that is was the nurse's duty to exercise the degree of skill employed by other nurses in the community, along with his best judgment on patient care to promote skin integrity. The failure of the nurse to both care for the patient's decubiti and to instruct the patient and his family concerning proper methods for self-care and assessment for decubitus ulcers contributed to the patient's deteriorating skin integrity and condition.

An integral part of all negligence actions is the question of who should be sued. When a nurse is employed and functioning within the scope of employment, the employer is responsible for the nurse's negligent actions. This is referred to as the doctrine of *respondeat superior.* By directing a nurse to carry out a particular function, the employer becomes responsible for negligence, along with the individual nurse. Because employers are usually better able to pay for the injuries suffered by clients, they are sued more often than the nurses themselves, although an increasing number of judgments include the professional nurse by name as a co-defendant.

Thus it is imperative that all nurses engaged in clinical practice carry their own professional liability insurance. Community-oriented nurses may have personal immunity for particular practice areas, such as giving immunizations. In some states, the legislature has granted personal immunity to nurses employed by public agencies to cover all aspects of their practice under the legal theory of *sovereign immunity* (Shinn, Gaffney, and Curtin, 2003).

Nursing students need to be aware that the same laws and rules that govern the professional nurse govern them. Students are expected to meet the same standard of care as that met by any licensed nurse practicing under the same or similar circumstances. Students are expected to be able to perform all tasks and make clinical decisions on the basis of the knowledge they have gained or been offered, according to their progress in their educational programs and along with adequate educational supervision.

## SPECIAL COMMUNITY HEALTH PRACTICE ISSUES AND THE LAW

Specific legal issues of nursing vary depending on the setting where care is delivered, the clinical arena, and the nurse's functional role. The law, including legislation and judicial opinions, significantly affects each of the following areas of special community-oriented nursing practice. Nurses responsible for setting and implementing program priorities need to identify and monitor laws related to each special area of practice.

## School and Family Health

Nurses employed by health departments or boards of education may deliver school and family health nursing. School health legislation establishes a minimum of services that must be provided to children in public and private schools. For example, most states require that children be immunized against certain communicable diseases before entering school. Children must have had a physical examination by that time, and most states require at least one physical at a later time in their schooling. Legislation also specifies when and what type of health screening will be conducted in schools (e.g., vision and hearing testing).

Statutes addressing child abuse and neglect make a large impact on nursing practice within schools and families. Most states require nurses to notify police and/or a social service agency of any situation in which they suspect a child is being abused or neglected. This is one instance in which the law mandates that a health professional breach patient confidentiality to protect someone who may be in a helpless or vulnerable position. There is *civil immunity* for such reporting, and the nurse may be called as a witness in a court hearing of the case.

Occupational health is another special area of practice that has specific legal requirements as a result of state and federal statutes. Of special concern are the state workers' compensation statutes, which provide the legal foundation for claims of workers injured on the job. Access to records, confidentiality, and the use of standing orders are legal issues that have great practice significance to nurses employed in industries.

## Home Care and Hospice

Home care and hospice services rendered by nurses are shaped through state statutes and have specific nursing requirements for licensure and certification. Compliance with these laws is directly linked to the method of payment for the services. For example, a service must be licensed and certified to obtain payment for services through Medicare. Federal regulations implementing Medicare/Medicaid have an enormous effect on much of nursing practice, including how nurses record details of their visits, record time spent in care activities, and document patient care and the patient's status and progress.

In addition, many states have passed laws requiring nurses to report elder abuse to the proper authorities, as is done with children and youths. Laws affecting home care and hospice services have focused on such issues as the right to death with dignity, rights of residents of long-term facilities and home health clients, definitions of death, and the use of living wills and advance directives. The legal and ethical dimensions of nursing practice are particularly im-

## *Policy, Politics, and the Law: Influences on Community Health Nursing Practice in Canada*

Lianne Patricia Jeffs, R.N., M.Sc., Faculty of Nursing, University of Toronto

### POLICY AND POLITICAL ACTION

Public policy in Canada is largely influenced by the prevailing dominant ideologies and societal values. Current ideologies include cost effectiveness and efficiency; individual freedom and responsibility; regional and geographic sensitivity; national identity, unity, and solidarity; responsiveness, accountability, and transparency; and evidence-based health care equity and fairness (Romanow, 2002). Public policy is commonly defined as what governments choose to do or not to do, as both decisions and indecisions represent policy action. Policy making is a process by which choices are made to allocate limited resources, and it usually is done by policy committees. These committees include representation from various levels of elected or appointed government officials and bureaucrats, representatives of organized societal groups, and influential individuals (Larsen and Baumgart, 1992).

### THE CANADIAN POLITICAL SYSTEM

Canada is made up of a confederation of 10 provinces and three territories that was established by the British North America (BNA) Act of 1867. This organizational structure divided power between the federal and provincial governments. Later in this box, there is a list of major federal initiatives related to the Canadian health care system. The Canadian government is grounded in British parliamentary roots. The power resides in the sovereignty of their representative (governor general at the federal level and lieutenant governor at the provincial/territorial level). The Canadian democratic electoral system is based on single-member constituencies in which the candidate with the most votes wins the electoral district. The leader of the party with the most votes becomes the prime minister (federal) or the premier (provincial/territorial). The prime minister selects an executive council, known as the *cabinet,* from the elected legislature, and each cabinet member is assigned a portfolio (department or ministry) of government.

### LEGISLATIVE PROCESS IN CANADA

The legislative process in Canada starts with a bill—a proposal to create a new law or change an existing one. Most bills considered by Parliament are public bills. There are two types of public bills: (1) government public bills introduced and sponsored by a minister, and (2) a bill sponsored by a private member. A bill can be introduced in the House of Commons (C-bills) or the Senate (S-bills); the majority of public bills start in the House of Commons. A bill can be passed, amended, delayed, or defeated. Once both houses have approved a bill, it is presented for royal assent and becomes law. The passing of a bill goes through several stages before becoming law. The process is described at the end of this box. Nurses have had experience in influencing federal legislation: strong lobbying efforts led by the Canadian Nurses Association resulted in an amendment to the Canada Health Act of 1984 that enabled provincial health plans to fund services of nurses and other health professionals on a direct reimbursement basis.

### ROLE OF GOVERNMENT IN HEALTH CARE IN CANADA

Health care is a shared responsibility between all levels of government in Canada. The federal government is responsible for setting and administering national principles or standards for the health care system (e.g., by the Canada Health Act); assisting in the financing of provincial health care services through fiscal transfers; delivering direct health services to specific groups; and fulfilling other health-related functions such as health protection, disease prevention, and health promotion. The provincial and territorial governments are responsible for managing and delivering health services; planning, financing, and evaluating the provision of hospital care and physician and allied health care services; and managing some aspects of prescription care and public health. Refer to the Canadian content box in Chapter 5 for further discussion of the roles of government in the economic delivery of health care in Canada.

### REGULATION OF NURSING PRACTICE IN CANADA

Registered nurses practice within an ethical and standards-of-practice framework (Keatings and Smith, 1995). The nursing profession is regulated at the provincial level. Each province and territory has passed statutes and regulations with respect to the governance of nursing, authority to establish educational requirements, prerequisites for entry to practice of nursing, fees, complaints, and disciplinary procedures. A fairly uniform system exists in most jurisdictions of Canada. In Ontario, however, both the Regulated Health Professions Act of 1991 (which has been recently reviewed and is responsible for the overall supervision of

---

portant. Individual rights, such as the right to refuse treatment, and nursing responsibilities, such as the legal duty to render reasonable and prudent care, may appear to be in conflict in delivering home and hospice services. Much case discussion (sometimes including outside ethics consultation) may be needed to resolve such conflicts.

## Correctional Health

Correctional health nursing practice is significantly shaped by federal and state laws and regulations and by recent Supreme Court decisions. The laws and decisions primarily relate to the type and amount of services that must be provided for incarcerated individuals. For exam-

health professions) and the Nursing Act of 1991 influence nursing practice.

The primary focus of the provincial and territorial regulatory body is protecting the welfare of the public relative to the nursing profession. All nursing regulatory bodies in Canada require applicants for membership to have graduated from an approved school of nursing and to have passed the requisite nursing registration examination before they are admitted as members of the association. The Canadian content box in Chapter 1 provides a more detailed discussion about educational preparation and standards of practice for community-oriented nursing.

To continue to have an influential role in the health care system, nurses need to have a more global view of health care, an understanding of political processes, and an understanding of the issues impacting the health of Canadians. Through political action, nurses can ensure that health care reform reflects the values of Canadians and provides a framework for the evolving health care system.

## IMPLICATIONS FOR COMMUNITY-ORIENTED NURSING PRACTICE

Community-oriented nurses require an understanding of the standards of practice that their particular provincial regulatory body requires, and of the federal, provincial, and municipal legislation that directly impacts their practice. The practice of public health is based on provincial public health acts. Other legislation includes mental health acts, communicable disease legislation, nursing acts, health unit acts, hospitals acts, medical professional acts, occupational health and safety acts (Miller, 1985), and pending personal health information privacy acts. Community-oriented nurses should also be aware of general legal principles, including consent to treatment, negligence, confidentiality, documentation of client care, criminal law, and family and child violence. Registered nurses who are employed by an official governmental health unit work with medical officers of health and public health inspectors to carry out the legislation and regulations by providing health services to community residents.

## FEDERAL GOVERNMENT INITIATIVES RELATED TO THE CANADIAN HEALTH CARE SYSTEM

1867   British North America Act (Provinces of Canada, Nova Scotia, and New Brunswick formed one dominion under the name of Canada)
1961   Hospital Insurance and Diagnostic Services Act (cost-sharing agreement of 50% between federal and provincial governments; provinces designed and operated their own health care services and federal government agreed to pay for specified services)
1968   Medical Care Act (emergence of Medicare: the federal government covers 50% of medical services provided by doctor and dental services in hospitals)
1977   Established Program Financing Act (reduced direct federal contribution for health care to 25% of the total 1975-1976 expenditures)
1984   Canada Health Act (merged Hospital Insurance and Diagnostic Services Act of 1961 and the Medical Care Act of 1968)

## HOW A BILL GETS PASSED IN THE CANADIAN GOVERNMENT

1. First reading in either House of Commons or Senate
2. Second reading (debate and vote on principle of the bill)
3. Parliamentary committee hearings and clause-by-clause examination
4. Report to the House of Commons or Senate
5. Report stage debate and vote on amendments from committee
6. Third reading (bill is debated for a final time and voted on)
7. Introduction of the bill into other house of Parliament (repetition of process)
8. Royal assent (the bill becomes law)

## References

Canadian Nurses Association: *Getting started: a political action guide for Canada's registered nurses,* Ottawa, CNA, available at www.cna-nurses.ca.

Keatings M, Smith O: *Ethical and legal issues in Canadian nursing,* Toronto, 1995, Saunders Canada.

Larsen J, Baumgart AJ: Overview: shaping of public policy. In Baumgart AJ, Larsen J, editors: *Canadian nursing faces the future,* ed 2, pp. 469-492, St Louis, Mo, 1992, Mosby.

Miller C: Legal issues. In Stewart M et al, editors: *Community health nursing in Canada,* pp. 70-90, Toronto, 1985, Gage.

Romanow R: *Building on values: the future of health care in Canada—final report,* Ottawa, 2002, Commission on the Future of Health Care in Canada, available at www.healthcarecommission.ca.

U.S. Department of Health and Human Services: *Leading indicators for healthy people 2010,* Washington, DC, 1998, USDHHS.

*Canadian spelling is used.*

ple, physical examinations are required for all prisoners after they are sentenced. Regulations specify basic levels of care that must be provided for prisoners, and access to care during illness is a particular focus. Court decisions requiring adequate health services are based on constitutional law. If minimal services are not provided, it is a violation of a prisoner's right to freedom from cruel and unusual punishment. Such decisions provide a framework that strongly influences the setting of nursing priorities. For example, providing care to the sick would take priority over wellness or health education classes.

# THE NURSE'S ROLE IN THE POLICY PROCESS

The number and types of laws influencing health care are increasing. Because of this, nurses need to be involved in the policy process and understand its effective touch points as important to nursing and to the clients they serve.

For nurses to effectively care for their client populations and their communities in the complex U.S. health care system, professional advocacy for logical health policy that considers equality is essential. Professional nurses working in the community know all too well about the health care problems they and their clients encounter daily, and it is through policy and political activism that both big-picture and long-term solutions can be developed.

Although the term *policy* may sound rather lofty, health policy is quite simply the process of turning health problems into workable action solutions. Health policy is developed on the three-legged stool of *access, cost,* and *quality.*

The policy process, which is very familiar to professional nurses, includes the following:

- Statement of a health care problem
- Statement of policy options to address the health problem
- Adoption of a particular policy option
- Implementation of the policy product
- Evaluation of the policy's intended and unintended consequences in solving the original health problem

Thus the policy process is very similar to the nursing process, but the focus is on the level of the larger society and the adoption strategies require political action. For most professional nurses, action in the policy arena comes most easily and naturally through participation in nursing organizations such as the **American Nurses Association** (ANA) at the state level and in certain specialty organizations.

### NURSING TIP

The nurse's basic understanding of the political process should include knowing who the lawmakers are, how bills become laws (see Figure 8-1), the process of writing regulations (see Figure 8-2), and methods of influencing the process and shaping health policy. With this knowledge, nurses can shape nursing practice.

## Legislative Action

The people within geographic jurisdictions elect their legislative representatives and senators. An important part of the legislative process is the work of the **legislative staffs.** These individuals do the legwork, research, paperwork, and other activities that move policy ideas into bills and then into law. In addition to the individual legislator's office, the congressional committee staffs are also important. They are usually experts in the content of the work of a committee,

### WHAT DO YOU THINK?

As a former Speaker of the House of Representatives noted, "all politics is local." Therefore should nurses focus their political activities only in the local community?

such as a health and welfare committee. Frequently, developing a working relationship with key legislative staffers can be as important to achieving a policy objective as the relationship with the policy maker (i.e., the legislator).

The legislative process begins with ideas (policy options) that are developed into bills. After a bill is drafted, it is introduced to the legislature, given a number, read, and assigned to a committee. Hearings, testimony, lobbying, education, research, and informal discussions follow. If the bill is passed from the legislative committee, the entire house hears the bill, amends it as necessary, and votes on it. A majority vote moves the bill to the other house, where it is read, amended, and voted on. Figure 8-1 shows the necessary formal process of the legislative pathway.

Nurses can be involved in the legislative process at any point. Many professional nursing associations have legislative committees made up of volunteers, governmental relations staff professionals, and sometimes political action committees (PACs), all engaged in efforts to monitor, analyze, and shape health policy.

Common methods of influencing health policy outcomes include face-to-face encounters, personal letters, mailgrams, electronic mail, telephone calls, testimony, petitions, reports, position papers, fact sheets, letters to the editor, news releases, speeches, coalition building, demonstrations, and law suits. Depending on the issue, any of these can be effective. Guidelines on communication are provided in the How To box. Tips on communication and visiting legislators and their staffs, as well as general tips on political action, are presented in Boxes 8-2, 8-3, and 8-4. Political activities in which nurses can and should be involved include a wide variety of activities such as informed voting (A MUST!), political party participation, registering others to vote, getting out the vote, fundraising for candidates, building networks or communication links for issues (e.g., a phone tree), and participating in organizations to ensure their effective involvement in health policy and politics.

The direct reimbursement of **advanced practice nurses** (APNs) in the Medicare program is one example of how nurses can use their influence. The inclusion of amendments to Medicare that authorized APN reimbursement regardless of specialty or client location in the Balanced Budget Act of 1997 required the sustained efforts of the ANA and other national nursing organizations over a long period (Nursing World, 2000). During that time, individual nurses provided testimony to Congress and to MEDPAC, the physicians' political action committee, on the importance of direct reimbursement to APNs. Many APNs worked closely and vigor-

**The Federal Level**

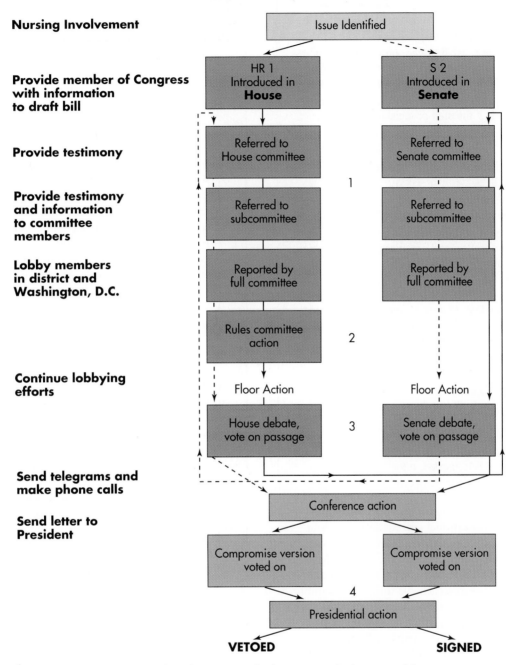

Nursing Involvement

Provide member of Congress
with information
to draft bill

Provide testimony

Provide testimony
and information
to committee
members

Lobby members
in district and
Washington, D.C.

Continue lobbying
efforts

Send telegrams and
make phone calls

Send letter to
President

[1] A bill goes to full committee first, then to special subcommittees for hearings, debate, revisions, and approval. The same process occurs when it goes to full committee. It either dies in committee or proceeds to the next step.

[2] Only the House has a Rules Committee to set the "rule" for floor action and conditions for debate and amendments. In the Senate, the leadership schedules action.

[3] The bill is debated, amended, and passed or defeated. If passed, it goes to the other chamber and follows the same path. If each chamber passes a similar bill, both versions go to conference.

[4] The President may sign the bill into law, allow it to become law without his signature, or veto it and return it to Congress. To override the veto, both houses must approve the bill by a two-third majority vote.

**Figure 8-1** How a bill becomes a law. *(From Mason DJ, Keavitt JK, Chaffee MW:* Policy and politics in nursing and health care, *ed 4, Philadelphia, 2002, Saunders.)*

## BOX 8-2  Tips for Visits With Legislators

- Call ahead and ask how much time the staff or legislator is able to give you.
- When you arrive, ask if the appointment time is the same or if a scheduled vote on the house/senate floor is going to need the legislator's attention.
- Engage in small talk at the beginning of the conversation only if the staff or legislator has time.
- Structure time so that the issue can be briefly presented.
- Allow an opportunity for the staff or Congress member to seek clarity or ask questions.
- Do not assume that the legislator or the legislator's staff is well informed on the issue.
- Numbers count. If the views you express are shared by a local nurses' organization or by nurses employed at a health care facility, let the legislator know.
- Invite Congress members and their staffs to conferences or meetings of nurses' organizations, or to tour nursing education facilities to meet others interested in the same policy issues.
- If appropriate, invite the media and let the legislator know.
- Send future invitations.
- Provide a one-page summary that gives key points at the conclusion of every meeting.

Modified from Milstead J: *Healthy policy and politics: a nurse's guide,* Gaithersburg, Md, 1999, Aspen.

## BOX 8-3  Tips for Written Communication With Legislators

- Communicate in writing to express opinions.
- Acknowledge the Congress member's work as positive or negative, but be courteous.
- Follow up on meetings or phone calls with a letter or e-mail.
- Share knowledge about a particular problem.
- Recommend policy solutions.
- The letter should be typed, a maximum of two pages, and focused on one or two issues at most.
- The purpose of the letter should be stated at the beginning.
- Present clear and compelling rationale for your concern or position on an issue.
- If the purpose of the letter is to express disappointment regarding a stance on an issue or a vote that has been cast, the letter should be as positive as possible.
- Write letters thanking a Congress member for taking a particular position on an issue.
- A letter to the editor of the local newspaper or a nursing newsletter praising a legislator's position (with a copy forwarded to the legislator) is welcome publicity, especially during an election year.
- Review the major points covered in person and answer any questions that were raised during conversation.
- Have business cards for yourself and include them with letters.
- Address written correspondence as follows (the same general format applies to state and local officials):

| U.S. Senator | U.S. Representative |
|---|---|
| Honorable Jane Doe | Honorable Jane Doe |
| United States Senate | House of Representatives |
| Washington, D.C. 20510 | Washington, D.C. 20515 |
| Dear Senator Doe: | Dear Representative Doe: |

Modified from Milstead J: *Healthy policy and politics: a nurse's guide,* Gaithersburg, Md, 1999, Aspen.

ously with their congressional representatives to lobby for this Medicare amendment. Even more wrote letters and provided position papers and fact sheets to help legislators understand the value of APNs. Although the process took more than 10 years to achieve fully, APN reimbursement in Medicare became a reality. Both the nursing profession and Medicare beneficiaries will benefit from the enhanced access of Medicare clients to APNs.

### WHAT DO YOU THINK?

What special interest group/groups has/have the most political influence in Washington, D.C., today? Why did you choose your answer?

The ANA was likewise a strong supporter for the Patient Safety Act of 1997 (ANA, 1997). This law requires health care agencies to make public some information on nurse staff levels, staff mix, and outcomes, and it requires the USDHHS to review and approve all health care acquisitions and mergers. All of these requirements are to determine any long-term effect on the health and safety of clients, communities, and staff.

On the state legislative level, all 50 states have passed title protection for APNs; this was achieved by individual nurses, state nurses associations, and various nursing specialty groups participating in the legislative process with the 50 state legislators. Title protection means that only certain nurses who meet state criteria can call themselves advanced practice nurses.

## Regulatory Action

The regulatory process, although it may not be as visible a process as legislation, can also be used to shape laws and dramatically affect health policy. This process should be

## BOX 8-4 Tips for Action

- Become involved in the state nurses' association.
- Build communication and leadership skills.
- Increase your knowledge about a range of professional issues.
- Expand and strengthen your professional network.
- Serve on committees and in elected positions.
- Build relationships within the profession and with representatives of public and private sector organizations with an interest in health care.
- Participate in political activities.
- Be aware of what is going on in health care beyond the environment and the practice in which you work.
- Be well informed across a range of health-related issues.
- Identify yourself as a nurse with associated education and expertise.
- Let people know that nurses are capable of functioning in many different roles and making substantial contributions.
- Be confident.
- Do not burn bridges behind you. On another occasion, they may provide the only route to your destination.
- Be friendly.
- Lend a hand to other nurses. It benefits all of us.
- If you are new to the policy arena, seek support from many people of diverse backgrounds. Accomplished people, whether nurses or not, often value mentoring others.

Modified from Milstead J: *Healthy policy and politics: a nurse's guide,* Gaithersburg, Md, 1999, Aspen.

## HOW TO Be an Effective Communicator

- Use simple communications that will be readily understood.
- Choose language that clearly conveys information to individuals of diverse cultures, different ages, and different educational backgrounds.
- Oral or written communication needs to be targeted to the issue and free of terminology unique to medicine and nursing (i.e., jargon).
- State your expertise on the issue first.
- Describe briefly your education and experience.
- Identify the relevance of the issue beyond nursing.
- Provide information regarding the impact of the issue on the legislator's constituents.
- Present accurate, credible data.
- Do not oversell or give inaccurate information about the problem.
- Present information in an organized, thorough, concise form that is based on factual data (when it is available).
- Give examples.

Modified from Milstead J: *Healthy policy and politics: a nurse's guide,* Gaithersburg, Md, 1999, Aspen.

on the radar screen of professional nurses who wish to successfully participate in policy activity. At each level of government, the executive branch can and, in most cases, must prepare regulations for implementing policy and new programs. These regulations are detailed, and they establish, fix, and control standards and criteria for carrying out certain laws. Figure 8-2 shows the steps in the typical process of writing regulations. When the legislature passes a law and delegates its oversight to an agency, it gives that agency the power to make regulations. Because regulations flow from legislation, they have the force of law.

## The Process of Regulation

After a law is passed, the appropriate executive department begins the process of regulation by studying the topic or issue. Advisory groups or special taskforces are sometimes formed to provide the content for the regulations. Nurses can influence these regulations by writing letters to the regulatory agency in charge or by speaking at open public hearings. After rewriting, the proposed regulations are put into final draft form and printed in the legally required publication (e.g., at the federal level, the *Federal Register*). Similar registers exist in most states, where regulations from state executive departments, including state health departments, are published. Public comment is called for in written form within a given period.

Revisions made to proposed regulations are based on public comment and public hearing. Depending on the amount and content of the public reaction, final regulations are prepared or more study of the area and issues is conducted. Final published regulations carry the force of law. When regulations become effective, health care practice is changed to conform to the new regulations. Monitoring administrative regulations is essential for the professional nurse, who can influence regulations by attending the hearings, providing comments, testifying, and engaging in lobbying aimed at individuals involved in the writing. Concrete written suggestions for revision submitted to these individuals are frequently persuasive and must be acknowledged by government in publishing the final rules. An excellent example of how nurses must continue to influence health policy outcomes, even after positive legislation has passed, occurred after the passage of the Balanced Budget Act of 1997 (BBA '97). The HCFA began to implement the BBA '97 through the publication of draft regulations seeking to define the how's of APN

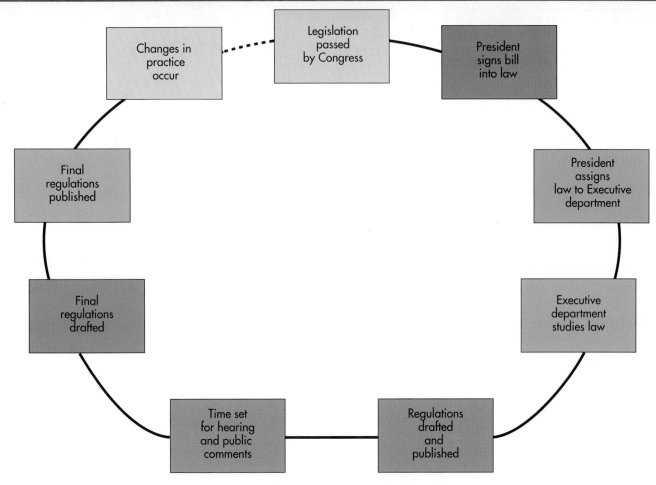

**Figure 8-2** The process of writing regulations.

practice and Medicare reimbursement. The nursing community responded vigorously with negative opinions about the initial restrictive definitions and requirement. Their reactions were effective and reshaped the final regulations to recognize the state definitions for APN practice autonomy.

Final regulations, published in a *Code of Regulations* (both federal and state), usually lead to changes in practice. For example, Medicare regulations setting standards for nursing homes and home health are incorporated into these agencies' manuals. In the case of APN reimbursement, some Medicare fiscal intermediaries have had difficulty in recognizing APNs as appropriate providers, but professional nursing organization advocates have forcefully addressed these implementation barriers.

## Nursing Advocacy

Advocacy begins with the art of influencing others **(politics)** to adopt a specific course of action **(policy)** to solve a societal problem. This is accomplished by building relationships with the appropriate policy makers—the individuals or groups that determine a specific course of action to be followed by a government or institution to achieve a desired end (policy outcome). Relationships for effective advocacy can be built in a number of ways.

### THE CUTTING EDGE

In January 2003, the Supreme Court heard a case presented by the managed care industry. This case challenged regulations requiring insurance companies to reimburse nonphysician health care providers, such as APNs, for care given outside the boundaries of health maintenance organizations. The lawyers suggested that paying providers such as APNs added to the cost of care.

Holland G: *High cost weighs state's HMO law,* Washington, DC, Jan 15, 2003, Associated Press.

A letter or visit to the district, state, or national office of a legislator to discuss a particular policy or health care issue can be interesting, educational, and effective. Contributions of money, labor, expertise, or influence may also be welcomed by the policy makers involved in setting a course of action to obtain a desired health outcome, either for an individual, a family, a group, a community, or society **(health policy).** Additionally one may develop a grassroots network of community and professional friends with a mutual interest in health policy advocacy. The network may be able to promote health policy initiatives for the community.

Many special-interest groups in health care have the potential, desire, and resources to influence the health policy process. A tremendous advantage that nursing has in advocating for issues and in influencing policy makers is the force of its numbers, as nursing is the largest of the health professions. However, nursing must organize its numbers in such a way that each nurse joins with others to speak with one voice. The greatest effect will be had when all nurses make similar demands for policy outcomes.

During 2002, nursing spoke clearly, distinctly, and together on a serious problem for the health arena and for the profession: the nursing shortage. Health care facilities and employers were having ever-increasing difficulty finding experienced nurses to employ. In addition, the need for RNs was predicted to balloon in the next 20 years because of the aging of the U.S. population, technologic advances, and economic factors. Demand for RNs is expected to increase by 22% by the year 2008. This increased demand for professional nurses, coupled with expected retirement of a rapidly aging nursing workforce, placed a tremendous stress on the health care system. A workforce supply study published recently estimated that by 2007, the number of nurses per capita (client) would begin to decline, and by 2020 supply will fall 20% short of demand. The workforce shortage results from a complex set of factors such as fewer young people entering the profession, declining nursing school enrollment, the aging of the current nurse work force, and uncomfortable working conditions in which nurses feel pressured to "do more with less" (Bloom, 2002).

The collective vision of the nursing community on the problems and solutions for nursing was developed through the ANA with the support of other nursing organizations at a national summit conference ("Call to the Nursing Profession") in 2001. *Nursing's Agenda for the Future* was put in motion (ANA, 2002). Many nursing organizations became involved, each one advocating for solutions in one of ten significant areas. One of the policy solutions that the summit attendees agreed was essential was the passage of the Nurse Reinvestment Act of 2002 (ANA, 2002). This act, passed by the 107th Congress in July 2002, provides nursing scholarships and loans, faculty development, public relations to attract new recruits into the profession, and financial incentives for health facilities to implement safe and satisfying work environments for professional practice.

Advocacy by expert and committed health professionals works; it can bring about positive change for the profession, the community, and the clients that nurses serve. Keeping up to date on issues within government, professional organizations, law, and public policy is vitally important. Informed activism directed toward a professional role, image, and value for professional nurses, and toward a health care system in the United States that provides universal access to health care that is of high quality and is affordable should be a lifelong commitment for all professional nurses.

## ■ Practice Application

Larry was in his final rotation in the Bachelor of Science in Nursing program at State University. He was anxious to complete his community-oriented nursing course, because upon graduation he would begin a position as a staff nurse specializing in school health at the local health department. His wife was expecting their first child, and she had been receiving prenatal care at the health department.

Larry was aware that a few years ago, the federal government had, by law, provided block grants to states for primary care, maternal child health programs, and other health care needs of states. He had read the *Federal Register* and knew that the regulations for these grants had been written through USDHHS departments. He was aware that these regulations did not require states to fund specific programs.

Larry read in the local paper that the health department was closing its prenatal clinic at the end of the month. When his state had received its block grant, they decided to spend the money for programs other than prenatal care. Larry found that a 3-year study in his own state showed improved pregnancy outcomes as a result of prenatal care. The results were further improved when the care was delivered by community-oriented nurses.

Larry was concerned that, as a student, he would have little influence. However, he decided to call his classmates together to plan a course of action.

What would such an action plan include?

**Answers are in the back of the book.**

## ▌ Key Points

- The legal basis for most congressional action in health care can be found in Article I, Section 8, of the U.S. Constitution.
- The four major health care functions of the federal government are direct service, financing, information, and policy setting.
- The goal of the World Health Organization is the attainment by all people of the highest possible level of health.
- Many federal agencies are involved in government health care functions. The agency most directly involved with the health and welfare of Americans is the U.S. Department of Health and Human Services (USDHHS).
- Most state and local governments have activities that affect nursing practice.
- The variety and range of functions of governmental agencies have had a major impact on nursing. Funding, in particular, has shaped the role and tasks of nurses.
- The private sector (of which nurses are a part) can influence legislation in many ways, especially through the process of writing regulations.

- The number and types of laws influencing health care are increasing. Because of this, involvement in the political process is important to nurses.
- Professional negligence and the scope of practice are two legal aspects particularly relevant to nursing practice.
- Nurses must consider the legal implications of their own practice in each clinical encounter.
- The federal and most state governments are composed of three branches: the executive, the legislative, and the judicial.
- Each branch of government plays a significant role in health policy.
- The U.S. Public Health Service was created in 1798.
- The first national health insurance legislation was challenged in the Supreme Court in 1937.
- *Health: United States* (USDHHS, 2001) is an important source of data about the nation's health care problems.
- In 1921, the Sheppard-Towner Act was passed, and it had an important influence on child health programs and community-oriented nursing practice.
- The Division of Nursing, the National Institute of Nursing Research, and the Agency for Health Care Policy and Research are governmental agencies important to nursing.
- Nurses, through state and local health departments, function as consultants, direct care providers, researchers, teachers, supervisors, and program managers.
- The state governments are responsible for regulating nursing practice within the state.
- Federal and state social welfare programs have been developed to provide monetary benefits to the poor, older adults, the disabled, and the unemployed.
- Social welfare programs affect nursing practice. These programs improve the quality of life for special populations, thus making the nurse's job easier in assisting the client with health needs.
- The nurse's scope of practice is defined by legislation and by standards of practice within a specialty.

## Clinical Decision-Making Activities

1. Conduct an interview with a local health officer. Ask for information from a 10-year period. Try to see trends in population size, health needs and corresponding roles, and activities of government that were implemented to meet these changes. What were some of the problems you identified?
2. Examine a current health department budget and compare it with a budget from previous years. Has there been any impact on health care because of changes in government spending (especially before and after September 11, 2001)? Give an example.
3. Locate your state register or other documents, such as newspapers, that publish proposed regulations. Select one set of proposed regulations and critique them. Submit your opinion in writing as public comment, or attend the hearing and testify on the regulations. Be sure to submit something in writing. Evaluate your participation by stating what you learned and whether the proposed regulations were changed in your favor.
4. Find and review your state nurse practice act and define your scope of practice. Give examples of your practice boundaries.
5. Contact your local public health agency to discuss the state's official powers in regulating epidemics, such as the recent West Nile virus outbreak and anthrax exposures related to bioterrorism. Explore the state's right to protect the health, safety, and welfare of its citizens. Ask about the conflict between the state's rights and individual rights and how such issues are resolved. Ask about the standards of care that apply to this issue and how it is decided which services offered to clients should be mandatory and which should be voluntary. Explore how the role of public health differs in these epidemics compared with the past epidemics of smallpox and tuberculosis. Be specific.

## Additional Resources

These related resources are found either in the appendix at the back of this book or on the book's website at **http://evolve.elsevier.com/Stanhope.**

**evolve** **Evolve Website**

WebLinks: Healthy People 2010

## References

American Nurses Association: *Code for nurses,* Kansas City, Mo, 1995a, ANA.

American Nurses Association: *Nursing's social policy statement,* ed 2, 1995b, ANA.

American Nurses Association: Press release, March 1997: *ANA applauds introduction of Patient Safety Act of 1997,* available at www.nursingworld.org.

American Nurses Association: *State legislative trends: interstate nurse licensure compact, Department of State,* Government Relations, May 2000, retrieved March 2003 from www.nursingworld.org.

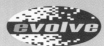
# Organizing Frameworks Applied to Community-Oriented Nursing

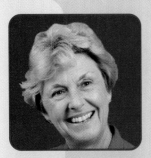

**Lois W. Lowry, R.N., D.N.Sc.**
Lois W. Lowry is a Professor in the College of Nursing at East Tennessee State University. She has been a trustee for the Neuman Systems Model since 1988, selected for this honor because of her expertise in using the model as a framework for educational programs. Lois consults with schools of nursing in the United States and internationally that wish to design model-based curricula.

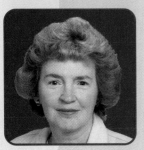

**Karen S. Martin, R.N., M.S.N., F.A.A.N.**
Karen S. Martin is a health care consultant who has been in private practice since 1993. She works with service and educational settings nationally and internationally as they evaluate and improve their practice, documentation, and information management systems. Karen has been employed as a staff nurse, director of a combined home care–public health agency, and, from 1978 to 1993, the director of research of the Visiting Nurse Association of Omaha, Nebraska, where she was the principal investigator of Omaha System research.

## Objectives

After reading this chapter, the student should be able to do the following:

1. Define the terms theory, model, concept, conceptual model, and paradigm
2. Differentiate between conceptual model and theory
3. Identify at least three uses of conceptual models for nursing
4. Describe key components of the Neuman Systems Model and the Omaha System
5. Apply the Neuman Systems Model to communities and aggregate populations
6. Apply the Omaha System to community-oriented practice
7. Describe how the Neuman Systems Model and Omaha System are complementary

All professional disciplines are based on a unique body of knowledge that is expressed through conceptual models and theories that guide practice. The hallmark of professional nursing is theory-based nursing (Fawcett, 1997). Before nurses can implement theory-based nursing in practice, they must understand the structure of nursing knowledge. The hierarchy of the structure differentiates the various components of nursing knowledge according to their abstract and concrete qualities (Fawcett, 2000). There are five components in the hierarchy, with the most abstract component at the top and the most concrete at the bottom. The components are metaparadigm, philosophies, conceptual models, theories, and empirical indicators (Fawcett, 2000). Each component of the hierarchy is made up of concepts. A **concept** is a word or phrase that provides a visual image of the phenomenon. A concept can represent a concrete image or an abstract image. For example, the concept "table" can be visualized as a four-legged object with a flat surface (concrete image) or as an underground water table or a table of contents; the latter two are more abstract images. Within the hierarchy of nursing knowledge, the concepts are words that convey abstract images. The statement that describes the concept is called a *nonrelational proposition,* or, simply stated, a definition. For example, the concept of person, or client, can be described as an individual, or a family, or a community. When this concept is linked to another concept in a statement, then it is called a *relational proposition.* An example of this could be how a client interacts with the environment.

Community-oriented nursing practice blends nursing and public health theory into a population-focused practice to promote and preserve the health of communities. This practice focuses on the care of individuals, families, and groups within the context of promoting and preserving the health of the community as a whole.

In 1988, the National Center for Nursing Research (NCNR) was established under the National Institutes of Health to facilitate nursing research. In 1993, the U.S. Congress expanded the scope and functions of the NCNR, making it one of the National Institutes of Health and renaming it the National Institute of Nursing Research (NINR). The NINR is crucial to the profession's movement to build a stronger knowledge base for practice. Although no conceptual or theoretical model will meet the needs of all community-oriented nurses, several nursing and public health models serve as frameworks for organizing educational programs and for making practice decisions.

In 1988, the Institute of Medicine report on the *Future of Public Health* identified the three primary or core functions of public health: (1) assessment through data collection and sharing of information, (2) policy development for family-, community-, and state-level health policies, and (3) assurance of available and necessary health services for clients. In 1993 the public health nursing directors of Washington State developed a model showing how public health/community health nurses perform the three core functions with all clients, whether individuals, families, or communities. In 2000, the Council on Linkages developed a list of competencies required of public health workers to provide quality care. In 2003, the Quad Council of Public Health Nursing Organizations applied the competencies to community-oriented nursing practice. These competencies help nurses recognize how they may implement the core functions of public health.

The scientific base provided by public health as a specialty remains the foundation for community-oriented nursing. In Part 3, chapters provide information about how to use conceptual models, epidemiology, and principles of education, and how to use evidence to organize community-oriented practice to meet the core functions of public health. Each chapter provides both theory and practical application of the specific topic to the clinical area. This section provides readers with tools that can be used to influence community-oriented nursing practice.

It has been estimated that the effect of the medical care system on usual indexes for measuring health is about 10%. The remaining 90% is determined by factors over which health care providers have little or no direct control, such as lifestyle, social, and environmental conditions. This text focuses on the processes and practices for promoting health, principally as used by the nurse, who is considered an ideal person to demonstrate and teach others how to promote health. To be effective, health promotion requires that people cease focusing on how to "fix" themselves and others only when they detect physical and emotional disequilibriums, and that they instead assume personal responsibility for health promotion. Such a change in emphasis requires that health care providers incorporate health promotion techniques into their practice.

Concern currently exists that the environment's effects on health and social conditions are causing an increase in the rate of infectious diseases. Community-oriented nurses are concerned with prevention, control, case-finding, reporting, and maintenance strategies as they relate to both communicable and infectious disease processes and to environment-related problems. Technological advances increasingly influence the environment and make it a potential threat to many aspects of health maintenance. Nurses must help others recognize how their actions as individuals, as well as in a composite group (aggregate) or community, are destroying vital parts of the environment.

# Part 3

## Conceptual and Scientific Frameworks Applied to Community-Oriented Nursing Practice

American Nurses Association: *Nursing profession unveils strategic plan to ensure safe, quality patient care and address root causes of growing shortage*, retrieved August 2002 from www.nursingworld.org.

Betts VT: Nurses and political action. In Chitty KK, editor: *Professional nursing concepts and challenges*, ed 3, pp. 529-549, Philadelphia, 2001, Saunders.

Bloom B: Crossing the quality chasm: a new health system for the 21st century, *JAMA* 287:646-647, 2002.

Canadian Nurses' Association: *Getting started: a political action guide for Canada's registered nurses*, Ottawa, CNA, available at www.cna-nurses.ca.

Catholic University of America: *Definitions of law*, retrieved March 2002, from www.faculty.cua.edu.

Department of Health, Education and Welfare: Improving health. In *Healthy people: the surgeon general's report on health promotion and disease prevention* (DHEW publication No. 79-55-71), Washington, DC, 1979, U.S. Government Printing Office, retrieved July 2002 from www.census.gov/ statab/www.

Gerberding J: Clinical practice: occupational exposure to HIV in health care settings, *N Engl J Med* 348(9):826-833, 2003.

Holland G: *High cost weighs state's HMO law*, Washington, DC, Jan. 15, 2003, Associated Press.

Keatings M, Smith O: *Ethical and legal issues in Canadian nursing*, Toronto, 1995, Saunders Canada.

Khan A, Morse S, Lillibridge S: Public-health preparedness for biological terrorism in the USA, *Lancet* 356(9236): 1179-1182, 2000.

Larsen J, Baumgart AJ: Overview: shaping of public policy. In Baumgart AJ, Larsen J, editors: *Canadian nursing faces the future*, ed 2, pp. 469-492, St Louis, Mo, 1992, Mosby.

Mason DJ, Talbott SW, Keavitt JK: *Policy and politics for nurses: action and change in the workplace, government, organizations, and community*, ed 2, Philadelphia, 1998, Saunders.

Miller C: Legal issues. In Stewart M et al, editors: *Community health nursing in Canada*, pp. 70-90, Toronto, 1995, Gage.

Milstead J: *Healthy policy and politics: a nurse's guide*, Gaithersburg, Md, 1999, Aspen.

Nicola B: The Model State Emergency Health Powers Act: turning point. In *Nursing concepts and challenges*, pp. 529-549, Philadelphia, 2002, Saunders.

Nursing World, Legislative Branch: *State government relations—advanced practice recognition with Medicaid reimbursement*, 2000, retrieved February 2003 from http://www.nuringworld.org.

Pearson L: Annual update of how each state stands on legislative issues affecting advanced nursing practice, *Nurse Pract* 24(1), 2002.

Romanow R: *Building on values: the future of health care in Canada—final report*, Ottawa, 2002, Commission on the Future of Health Care in Canada, available at www.healthcarecommission.ca.

Shinn L, Gaffney T, Curtin L: *An overview of risk management: an American Nurses Association educational program*, retrieved February 2003 from http://nursingworld.org/mods/working/rskmgt1/cerm1ful.htm.

Szilagyi PG et al: Evaluation of a state health insurance program for low-income children: implications for state child health insurance programs, *Pediatrics* 105(2):363-371, 2000.

Tennessee Nurses Association: *TNA legislative alert*, March 27, 2002.

Twitchell KT: Bloodborne pathogens. What you need to know: part I, *AAOHN J* 51(1):38-45; quiz 46-47, 2003.

United Nations: *Report of the World Conference of the International Women's Year*, Mexico City, 19 June-2 July, Chap. I, Sect. A.2, Publication No. E.76.IV.1, New York, 1975, UN.

United Nations: *Report of the World Conference of the United Nations Decade for Women*: equality, development and peace, Copenhagen, 24-30 July, Chap. I, Sect. A., Publication No. E.80.IV.3, New York, 1980, UN.

United Nations: *Report of the World Conference to Review and Appraise Achievements of the United Nations Decade for Women: Equality, Development and Peace*, Nairobi, 15-26 July, New York, 1985, UN.

United Nations: *Report of the Fourth World Conference on Women*, Beijing, 4-15 September, Chap. I, Resolution 1, Annex I, Publication No. E.96.IV.13, New York, 1995, UN.

United Nations: *Basic facts about the UN*, New York, 2002, UN.

U.S. Bureau of the Census: *Statistical abstract of the United States, health and nutrition table 119*, 2001, retrieved July 7, 2002, from http://www.census.gov/statab/www.

U.S. Bureau of the Census: *Access to quality health services, focus area 1—progress review*, June 4, 2002, retrieved July 2002 from http://factfinder.census.gov using the American factfinder tool.

U.S. Department of Health and Human Services: *Healthy people 2000: national health promotion and disease prevention objectives*, Washington, DC, 1991, U.S. Government Printing Office, available at http://www.health.gov/healthypeople.

U.S. Department of Health and Human Services: *Neonatal intensive care: a history of excellence*, NIH Publication No. 92-2786, October 1992, available at http://www.nichd.nih.gov/publications/pubs/neonatal/nic.htm.

U.S. Department of Health and Human Services: *The division of nursing resource and information guide*, Rockville, Md, 2000a, Division of Nursing.

U.S. Department of Health and Human Services: Leading indicators. In *Healthy People 2010: understanding and improving health*, ed 2, Washington, DC, 2000b, U.S. Government Printing Office.

U.S. Department of Health and Human Services: *Health: United States, 2000*, USDHHS Publication No. (PHS) 01-123(2), Hyattsville, Md, 2001, USDHHS.

U.S. Department of Health and Human Services, Health Resources and Services Administration (HRSA): *Community-based abstinence education program, Maternal and Child Health Bureau (MCHB) overview*, Special Projects of Regional and National Significance (SPRANS), December 2002, available at www.hrsa.gov.

U.S. Law: 42 SC 301, *Stewart Machine Co. v. Davis*, 1937a.

U.S. Law: 49 Stat 622, Title II, 1937b.

U.S. Law (Public Law 107-105): Health Insurance Portability and Accountability Act (HIPAA), 1996.

U.S. Law (Title XXI of the Social Security Act, BBA '97): State Child Health Improvement Act (SCHIP), 1997.

U.S. Law (wl 1044712 La. App. 4 Cir.): *Williams v. Metro Home Health Care Agency*, et al., 2002.

World Health Assembly: *Strengthening nursing and midwifery: progress and future*, Resolution 49.1, 2001, WHA, available at www.who.org.

World Health Organization: *The work of WHO, 1988-1990: biennial report of the director-general*, Geneva, 1990, WHO.

## Key Terms

**boundary**, p. 197
**client problem**, p. 207
**concept**, p. 194
**conceptual model**, p. 196
**documentation**, p. 208
**empirical indicator**, p. 196
**entropy**, p. 197
**environment**, p. 201
**equifinality**, p. 197
**evaluation**, p. 207
**feedback**, p. 198
**flexible line of defense**, p. 201

**general systems theory**, p. 197
**hypotheses**, p. 197
**information management**, p. 208
**intervention**, p. 207
**lines of resistance**, p. 201
**metaparadigm**, p. 196
**model**, p. 196
**negentropy**, p. 197
**Neuman Systems Model**, p. 199
**normal line of defense**, p. 201
**nursing diagnosis**, p. 207
**nursing intervention**, p. 207

**nursing practice**, p. 208
**nursing process**, p. 207
**Omaha System**, p. 208
**Omaha System Intervention Scheme**,
   p. 209
**Omaha System Problem Classification
   Scheme**, p. 209
**Omaha System Problem Rating Scale for
   Outcomes**, p. 208
**organization**, p. 197
**theory**, p. 196
*See Glossary for definitions*

## Chapter Outline

Developing a Conceptual–Theoretical–
   Empirical Structure
Using Conceptual Models
Systems Models in Community-Oriented
   Nursing
Neuman Systems Model
*Healthy People 2010*
*Application of the Neuman Systems Model
   to Communities*

*Use of the Neuman Systems Model
   for Community Outcomes*
Omaha System
*Definitions*
*Concepts of the Nursing Process*
*Description of the Omaha System*
*Application of the Omaha System in Practice
   and Education*

Merging of the Neuman Systems Model
   and the Omaha System
*Instrument Development*
*Using the Instrument*

This chapter provides an overview of the models and theories that are important and used most frequently in community-oriented nursing practice. First, the structural hierarchy of nursing knowledge is discussed, followed by a description of the competencies and essential functions of community and public health nursing. Next, two models for organizing data and guiding nursing practice are presented in detail: the Neuman Systems Model and the Omaha System. Over the last decade, these two models have demonstrated usefulness for nurses. This in no way implies that these are the only two models that effectively guide community-oriented nursing practice; however, there are data from practicing nurses to show that these models are frequently used with positive outcomes. Also, both models are used to guide curriculum design for courses in community and public health nursing and are guides for nursing practice in service agencies.

## DEVELOPING A CONCEPTUAL–THEORETICAL–EMPIRICAL STRUCTURE

The definitions of the components of the conceptual–theoretical–empirical (C-T-E) hierarchy follow. **Metaparadigm** refers to the major concepts that identify the phenomena (ideas or observations) of interest to a discipline. These concepts are agreed on by the members of the profession of nursing. They provide the boundaries for the subject matter of the discipline. The metaparadigm concepts for nursing are identified as *person, environment, health,* and *nursing.* When translated to community-oriented practice, *person* (or *client*) is usually an aggregate, a population, or an entire community. The *environment* is the physical, social, and political surroundings and settings for the aggregate populations and/or the entire community. *Health* is interpreted as the health state of the community or aggregate population, and the concept *nursing* includes the process or practice interventions that are used to care for this community or the aggregates within it. The second component in the C-T-E hierarchy is *philosophy,* which may be defined as a statement of beliefs and values (Kim, 1987) and what people assume to be true about the discipline of nursing. For example, nurses believe that clients are valuable human beings, and therefore nurses show them respect and dignity. The function of a philosophy is to inform those in the discipline and the community about the beliefs and values held by the discipline. **Conceptual models** are the third component in the C-T-E system. Conceptual models contain a set of abstract and general concepts that are of central interest to the profession of nursing. Usually, the **model** defines the four concepts in the metaparadigm according to the perspective of the theorist, and any unique concepts that help to explain the worldview of the theorist (Fawcett, 2000, p. 15).

There are several conceptual models in nursing, each based on a view of reality that stems from the philosophy and experience of the theorist. All conceptual models are abstract and must be linked with theories that help to explain the meaning of the concepts found in the models. A **theory** (the fourth level in the C-T-E hierarchy) has many definitions. For purposes of this chapter, it is defined as a set of concepts and relational propositions that state specific links between the concepts (Fawcett, 2000, p. 18). Theory provides a starting point to collect facts in a systematic way so that phenomena can be described, explained, or predicted (Fawcett, 1997). Theories vary in scope from grand theories that are very broad, to more concrete mid-range theories that can be tested through research. The final and most concrete component of the hierarchy is the **empirical indicator.** This term is defined as an actual instrument or procedure that can be used to

measure the mid-range theory concept (Fawcett, 2000, p. 20). For example, a sphygmomanometer is the empirical indicator for blood pressure measurement. Norbeck's social support instrument can be used to determine the means and strength of support networks for clients (Norbeck, Lindsey, and Carrierri, 1981). Nursing protocols can also be empirical indicators.

### WHAT DO YOU THINK?
Theoretical thinking is essential for community-oriented nurses to organize their actions.

Theoretical thinking is essential for nurses to integrate data into logical thinking and decision making to create order in their practices. Conceptual models and supporting theories identify the concepts that are essential for nursing and guide the actions that nurses should implement in their practices.

Table 9-1 defines several key terms useful in understanding the conceptual–theoretical–empirical structure of nursing knowledge.

## USING CONCEPTUAL MODELS
Conceptual models that are most useful to community-oriented nursing practice portray people as continually interacting with the environment. The environment is dynamic and can be either positive or negative. The unique feature of community-oriented nursing is the emphasis on assisting individuals, families, groups, and communities to maintain their highest possible level of health. To accomplish this, the community is viewed from a holistic perspective as a motivator or disrupter of health. The nursing

**Table 9-1 Key Terms to Understanding the Language of Theory**

| TERM | DEFINITION |
|---|---|
| Metaparadigm | The global concepts that identify the phenomena of central interest to a discipline |
| Philosophy | A statement encompassing ontologic claims about the phenomena of central interest to a discipline, epistemic claims about how the phenomena came to be known, and what members of the discipline value |
| Conceptual model | A set of concepts that provide a frame of reference for members of a discipline to guide their thinking, observations, and interpretations; propositions of a conceptual model are abstract and general. |
| Concepts | The building blocks of theory, which describe mental images of phenomena and can be concrete (chair) or abstract (fear) |
| Mid-range theory | One or more relatively concrete and specific concepts that are derived from a conceptual model, and the propositions that state relations among the concepts |
| Empirical indicators | Very concrete real-world proxies for a mid-range theory concept; an actual instrument, or clinical procedure, used to measure a mid-range theory concept |

Modified from Fawcett J: *Analysis and evaluation of contemporary nursing knowledge,* Philadelphia, 2000, Davis.

goal is to assess, plan, implement, and evaluate ways to make the community a healthier place to live.

To some extent, individuals have developed their own conceptual models because everyone has assumptions and beliefs about how the world operates. Everyone has a unique set of concepts guiding how ideas and information are categorized, how situations are viewed, and how responses are selected. A person's conceptual model influences behavior, and the person is influenced either consciously or subconsciously. In particular, a model directs one's worldview. *Worldview* refers to philosophical assumptions about the nature of interactions between a person and the environment. That is, a person's conceptual model determines what is considered relevant, what is eliminated, which concepts or constructs are identified, and how they are defined. For example, Neuman's worldview claims that environment is a source of stressors that can have positive and negative effects on the health of persons (Neuman and Fawcett, 2002). On the other hand, Rogers's (1980) worldview of person and environment regards them as wholes that cannot be reduced to parts, changing continuously, mutually, creatively, and inseparably. Each model states unique assumptions about the worldview that it represents.

Many nurses use one particular nursing model to guide practice; others merge more than one model into a unique guide for their practice. Sometimes nurses select nursing models that are supported by theories borrowed from other disciplines, such as psychology, sociology, and the biological sciences. Nurse educators use conceptual models to guide curriculum development and research studies. Later in this chapter, examples of the Neuman Systems Model are given as a guide for an undergraduate nursing course and nursing practice.

In nursing, mid-range theories are used to describe, explain, and predict client manifestations of actual or potential health problems (Neuman and Fawcett, 2002). A model, like a blueprint for building a house, describes the structure of how parts are related. A theory moves beyond description to explain relationships among the parts and to predict outcomes. By using models in practice, nurses can identify problems from which **hypotheses** can be generated. These hypotheses can then be tested in practice and education to validate them or prove the theory from which they are derived.

## SYSTEMS MODELS IN COMMUNITY-ORIENTED NURSING

As previously mentioned, a variety of conceptual models can be used to guide nursing actions. However, community and public health nursing as defined by both the American Nurses Association (ANA) and the American Public Health Association (APHA) can be logically understood from a systems perspective (see Chapter 1). Systems theory can be used to describe and explain the behaviors of individuals, groups, and communities. It emphasizes how each isolated part affects the whole and how the whole affects each part.

Conceptual models based on systems theory, known as systems models, are especially useful in community and public health nursing. Communities, made up of multiple subsystems and groups that interface with and influence each other, can be analyzed, interpreted, and understood from a systems theory perspective.

Systems models focus on the organizing, interacting, and integrating of parts and subparts and the interdependence of the parts on each other. Systems models are based on **general systems theory** as described by von Bertalanffy (1952, p. 11), who wrote, "Every organism represents a system, which is a complex of elements in mutual interaction." Concepts frequently discussed in relation to general systems theory are wholeness, **organization,** openness, boundary, entropy, negentropy, and equifinality. Using systems theory concepts, any community can be considered a whole made up of many parts. The parts are organized to function as a whole for the good of the community.

A community is an open system that exchanges materials such as energy, goods and services, values, and ideals with the environment inside and outside the community. The community as a system has boundaries, the most obvious being geographic lines such as mountains or rivers. The imaginary **boundary** is one that encompasses all the subsystems in the community and identifies what is inside and outside the subsystem-for example, where one community ends and the next one begins. **Entropy** is described as disordered energy, or energy that is bound and cannot be converted to work. In communities, an example of entropy is landfill garbage dumps, which disintegrate and may not be converted to something useful. **Negentropy,** on the other hand, is "free" energy that is converted into work and tends toward orderliness. In communities, negentropy can describe the resources, health, wealth, and altruistic values of the people. These are sources of energy that promote well-being and move the community to higher levels of wellness.

**Equifinality** means the end state of an open system, which is independent of the beginning state. For example, two communities may introduce new policies for health promotion at two different points in time, but in the long run both communities will have results from the policies. As another example, after a storm destroys part of a community, the members mobilize to restore stability by saving trees and planting new bushes in an attempt to attain or maintain balance and beauty, and thus they accomplish equifinality. All systems function through four processes: input, output, throughput, and **feedback.** These processes are continued through communication within the community so that subsystems relate to each other to provide effective functioning.

Each community is a social system made up of interrelated and interdependent subsystems. The subsystems are economics, education, religion, health care, politics, welfare, law enforcement, energy, and recreation. When any one of the subsystems is affected, the community as a whole is affected. One subsystem that immediately affects the whole community is the economic system. For example, if a major employer in the community lays off workers, the entire community, including its economic, social, educational, and health care institutions, is affected. The laid-off workers spend little or no money on movies or other paid recreational activities, buying only those clothes and groceries that are essential. Because they do not receive a paycheck, taxes are not paid to support the growth of the schools. When they must enter the health care system, they are unable to pay for care. Thus the whole community suffers.

Systems thinking, popularized in the 1960s, remains relevant in today's world. Several nurse theorists, including Johnson (2001), King (1981), Roy and Andrews (1999),

Neuman (Neuman and Fawcett, 2002), Rogers (1980), and Orem (2001), developed conceptual models of nursing based on systems theory. Table 9-2 summarizes the definitions of person (client), environment, health, and nursing according to these theorists. Although all these models are applicable to community-oriented nursing, the Neuman systems model is a particularly good fit and is discussed in detail in the next section.

## NEUMAN SYSTEMS MODEL

Betty Neuman developed the *Health Care Systems Model* as an organizing framework for graduate students to help in understanding client needs using a holistic viewpoint (Neuman and Young, 1972). Neuman defines, describes, and links together the four concepts of nursing's meta-paradigm (person, environment, health, nursing) within the model using the worldview of reciprocal interaction

---

### Table 9-2 Definitions of Person, Environment, Health, and Nursing

| PERSON (CLIENT) | ENVIRONMENT |
| --- | --- |
| "A whole being with parts that function as a unity for some purpose" (Roy and Andrews, 1999, p. 31). | "The world around and within persons that is the source of stimuli: focal, contextual, residual, or groups" (Roy and Andrews, 1999, p. 42). |
| "Unitary man—a four-dimensional, negentropic energy field identified by pattern and organization and manifesting characteristics and behaviors that are different from those of the parts and which cannot be predicted from knowledge of the parts" (Rogers, 1980, p. 332). | "A four-dimensional, negentropic energy field identified by pattern and organization and encompassing all that is outside and integral with any given human field" (Rogers, 1980, p. 332). |
| Behavioral system [made up of] all patterned, repetitive and purposeful ways of behaving that characterize each man's life (Johnson, 1990). | Encompasses internal and external environments from which malfunctions in behavioral systems may be caused (Johnson, 1990). |
| A patient is a receiver of care from health care professionals in some place (Orem, 2001). | "Encompasses physical, chemical, biological and socio/economic, cultural and community features" (Orem, 2001). |
| "A client system composed of the interrelationship of the five variables (physiologic, psychological, sociocultural, developmental, and spiritual), that are in varying degrees of development and interaction" (Neuman and Fawcett, 2002, p. 16). | "All internal and external forces surrounding the client system at any point in time. Created environment represents an open system exchanging energy with both the internal and external environments" (Neuman and Fawcett, 2002, p. 19). |
| "A social, sentient, rational, reacting, perceiving, controlling, purposeful, action-oriented, and time-oriented being" (King, 1981, p. 143). | Not explicitly defined, but it can be inferred that both internal and external environment are sources of stressors and energy (King, 1981). |

Johnson DE: The behavior system model for nursing. In Parker ME, editor: *Nursing theories in practice,* New York, 1990, National League for Nursing.
King I: *A theory for nursing: systems, concepts, process,* New York, 1981, Wiley.
Neuman B, Fawcett J, editors: *The Neuman Systems Model,* ed 4, Upper Saddle River, NJ, 2002, Prentice Hall.
Orem D: *Nursing: concepts of practice,* ed 6, St Louis, Mo, 2001, Mosby.
Rogers ME: Nursing: a science of unitary man. In Riehl JP, Roy CS, editors: *Conceptual models for nursing practice,* New York, 1980, Appleton-Century-Crofts.
Roy C, Andrews HA: *The Roy adaptation model,* ed 2, Stamford, Conn, 1999, Appleton-Lange.

(Fawcett, 2000). The intent of the Neuman Systems Model is to set forth a structure that shows the parts and subparts of the client, and their relationships to one another and the environment. The model provides the direction for nursing actions (Neuman and Fawcett, 2002, p. 11). Neuman believes that as nursing becomes more complex and comprehensive, a broad, flexible, expansive structure is required. Systems thinking enables nurses to focus on clients, themselves, and their surrounding environment in an interactive, creative way that is sensitive to change.

The Neuman Systems Model depicts an open system in which persons and their environments are in dynamic interaction (Neuman and Fawcett, 2002). The client system is composed of five interacting variables: physiological, psychological, sociocultural, developmental, and spiritual. These variables have a basic core structure unique to the individual but with a range of responses common to all human beings. Client systems may be individuals, families, groups, or communities.

The model, as seen in Figure 9-1, shows the client system as concentric rings surrounding the basic core. The outer ring is a broken circle, indicating an open system that exchanges energy with the environment. This ring, called the **flexible line of defense,** protects the system in a dynamic way, expanding when more protection is provided and contracting when less protection is available. The second ring, the **normal line of defense,** represents the usual wellness level of the client system. This line of defense represents what the client has become over time or the state to which the client has evolved (Neuman and Fawcett, 2002). Like the flexible line of defense, the normal line of defense is dynamic and may expand or contract when under the influence of stressors. This maintains system stability. A series of inner circles between the normal

## HEALTH

"A state and process of being and becoming integrated and whole that reflects person and environment mutuality" (Roy and Andrews, 1999, p. 13).

Health not specifically defined; however, disease and pathology are value terms (Rogers, 1980, p. 336) and since values change, phenomena perceived as disease (e.g., hyperactivity) may change over time and not be perceived as disease.

"It seems reasonable to assume that health would be considered behavior that is patterned, orderly, purposeful, predictable, and functionally efficient and effective" (Johnson, 1990, p. 25).

The state of wholeness and integrity of developed human structure and of bodily and mental functioning (Orem, 2001).

Health is equated with client system stability. The wellness–illness continuum implies energy flow is continuous between client system and environment (Neuman and Fawcett, 2002).

"Dynamic life experiences of a human being, which implies continuous adjustment to stressors in the internal and external environment through optimum use of one's resources to achieve maximum potential for daily living" (King, 1981, p. 5).

## NURSING GOALS

"Understanding how human systems cope with health and illness and what can be done to promote adaptive coping" (Roy and Andrews, 1999, p. 536).

"Goal of nursing is that individuals achieve their maximum health potential through maintenance and promotion of health, prevention of disease, nursing diagnosis, intervention, and rehabilitation" (Rogers, 1970, p. 86).

"Goal of nursing is to preserve the organization and integration of behavioral system balance and dynamic stability at the highest possible level for the individual" (Johnson, 1990, p. 29).

A helping service exercised by educated persons to bring about humanely desirable conditions in persons and their environments (Orem, 2001).

"Nursing's goal is to keep client system stability by assessing, and planning actions to assist individuals, families, and groups to attain, retain, and maintain optimal client health" (Neuman and Fawcett, 2002, p. 25).

"Nursing is a process of action, reaction and interaction whereby nurse and client share information about their perceptions of the situation; and through communication, they set goals, explore means, and agree on means to achieve goals" (King, 1981, p. 2).

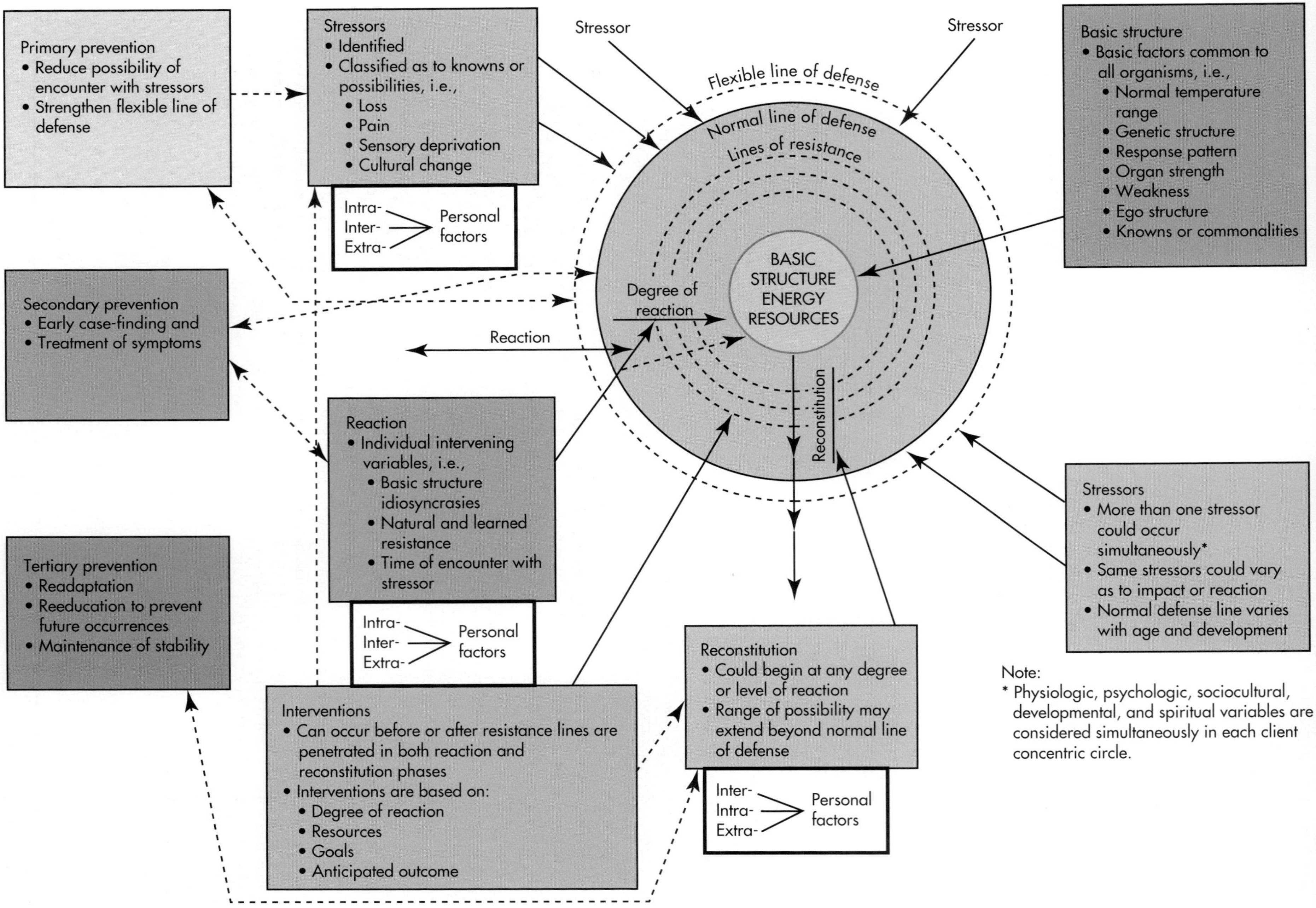

Basic structure
• Basic factors common to all organisms, i.e.,
  • Normal temperature range
  • Genetic structure
  • Response pattern
  • Organ strength
  • Weakness
  • Ego structure
  • Knowns or commonalities

Stressors
• More than one stressor could occur simultaneously*
• Same stressors could vary as to impact or reaction
• Normal defense line varies with age and development

Note:
* Physiologic, psychologic, sociocultural, developmental, and spiritual variables are considered simultaneously in each client concentric circle.

Stressor

Flexible line of defense

Normal line of defense

Lines of resistance

BASIC STRUCTURE ENERGY RESOURCES

Reconstitution

Degree of reaction

Reaction

Stressor

Stressor

Reconstitution
• Could begin at any degree or level of reaction
• Range of possibility may extend beyond normal line of defense

Inter-
Intra-
Extra-
Personal factors

Stressors
• Identified
• Classified as to knowns or possibilities, i.e.,
  • Loss
  • Pain
  • Sensory deprivation
  • Cultural change

Intra-
Inter-
Extra-
Personal factors

Reaction
• Individual intervening variables, i.e.,
  • Basic structure idiosyncrasies
  • Natural and learned resistance
  • Time of encounter with stressor

Intra-
Inter-
Extra-
Personal factors

Interventions
• Can occur before or after resistance lines are penetrated in both reaction and reconstitution phases
• Interventions are based on:
  • Degree of reaction
  • Resources
  • Goals
  • Anticipated outcome

Primary prevention
• Reduce possibility of encounter with stressors
• Strengthen flexible line of defense

Secondary prevention
• Early case-finding and
• Treatment of symptoms

Tertiary prevention
• Readaptation
• Reeducation to prevent future occurrences
• Maintenance of stability

**Figure 9-1** The Neuman Systems Model. (*Copyright 1970, Betty Neuman.*)

line of defense and the basic core, known as **lines of resistance,** contain factors that support the defense lines and protect the basic structure. The lines of resistance are activated when stressors invade the system. This assists the system in reconstituting to a higher wellness state. If lines of resistance are ineffective in their efforts, system energy is depleted and death of the system may occur (Neuman and Fawcett, 2002).

In the model, **environment** is defined as all internal and external influences surrounding and affecting the client system. The client may influence or be influenced by environmental forces, known as stressors, either positively or negatively, at any given point in time. Stressors occurring within and outside the client system can create instability. Thus the lines of resistance and defense are activated to defend the system in the presence of stressors. When system stability is attained, maintained, or retained, the result is a healthy system. In contrast, when stressors pile up and the lines of resistance are unable to handle these stressors, illness occurs. Figure 9-1 shows stressors invading the lines of defense and classifies stressors as intrapersonal, interpersonal, or extrapersonal factors. Neuman (Neuman and Fawcett, 2002) has identified another important environment called the *created environment.* Usually, clients are unaware of their created environment, which develops without their conscious input and serves as a protective buffer when stressors invade. Its purpose is to protect the system.

*Optimal system stability* is the best possible health state at any given time, occurring when all system variables are in balance and the lines of defense are functioning within the client system. Variance from wellness occurs when the system gets out of balance (Neuman and Fawcett, 2002). For example, client system energy levels are affected by actual or potential stressors that can increase energy with positive stress (eustress) or decrease energy with distress, or negative stress. When more energy is generated than used, the client system moves toward negentropy or health; conversely, when more energy is required than generated, movement is toward entropy or illness. Health is a manifestation of living energy available to the client system so that system integrity is enhanced (Neuman and Fawcett, 2002, p. 23).

The major goal of nursing in the Neuman Systems Model is to keep the client system stable through accurate assessment of actual and potential stressors, followed by implementing appropriate interventions. Three intervention strategies are suggested: (1) primary prevention strategies are implemented to strengthen the lines of defense by reducing risk factors and preventing stress, (2) secondary prevention begins after the occurrence of symptoms to strengthen the lines of resistance by establishing relevant goals and interventions to reduce the reaction, and (3) tertiary prevention can be initiated at any point after treatment when some degree of system stability has occurred. Reconstituting health at this point depends on the success of mobilizing client resources to prevent further stressor reaction or regression (Neuman and Fawcett, 2002, p. 29).

Figure 9-1 shows the three intervention strategies targeted toward the client system.

Three types of prevention as intervention can be used with communities. Primary prevention is appropriate to identify community risk factors and to plan mutually for health education programs with the community leaders. Health promotion and disease prevention activities are considered primary prevention or interventions. Secondary prevention interventions begin when one or more normal defenses of the community have been invaded, resulting in the development of specific health problems. At this point, nurses assist the community in identifying the stressors and begin intervention to correct the problem. Interventions are begun to strengthen the lines of resistance to prevent further dysfunction within the community system. For example a flu epidemic would require implementing secondary intervention strategies such as a mass flu vaccination clinic.

Tertiary prevention, the third intervention strategy, is most appropriate within a community that has become chronically dysfunctional over time. For example, a major disaster such as a hurricane or flood (external stressor) can create multiple health problems for the community and leave it severely compromised. A community that is isolated from other areas so that sufficient food is not available makes the community vulnerable to disease and malnutrition. Communities losing a major source of employment (e.g., coal mining, computer technology) or having a high incidence of heart disease are other examples. Over time, chronic health problems develop because of these stressors and lead to poor nutrition, postponement of medical care, and depression, and ultimately a chronically ill community results.

A perfect illustration for the twenty-first century is the epidemic of obesity throughout the United States. The nurse, partnering with the community, assists in identifying the stressors and then begins the process of reeducation that leads to readaptation to prevent further instability within the community. For example, in Sausalito, California, a community walking project was instituted to promote exercise to reduce obesity. The nurse also initiates health promotion strategies to reduce the possibility of further encounters with stressors and to strengthen community lines of defense.

The three prevention-as-intervention strategies can be used separately or together to direct nursing actions. Within the systems perspective, all strategies lead back toward primary prevention in a circular fashion. Health promotion, therefore, becomes a specific goal for nursing action in the Neuman Systems Model. For example, before or after stressor invasion, intervention goals include education and mobilizing of support resources to bolster lines of defense, reduce the effect of a stressor, and increase client resistance so illness will not occur. Health promotion efforts support secondary and tertiary goals to promote optimal wellness.

Health promotion within the Neuman Systems Model makes the model useful in meeting the objectives of

Healthy People 2010 (www.healthypeople.gov). Specifically, Healthy People 2010 defines the leading health indicators that reflect the major health concerns in the United States at the beginning of the twenty-first century. The Neuman Systems Model with its emphasis on primary prevention presents a theoretical framework through which strategies and approaches for achieving the objectives can be accomplished. Health promotion relates to activities conducted by nurses and clients that can optimize client wellness.

For more than 20 years, the Neuman systems model has been used by nurses in 14 countries. Its usefulness for community-oriented nurses in the United States and Canada is well documented (Neuman and Fawcett, 2002). The familiar vocabulary of the model, its systems perspective, and the integration of multiple psychosocial theories that support the model's propositions influence the usefulness of this model. Its comprehensive nature encourages other health care disciplines, such as physical therapy, social work, and public health, to use it as well. Using multidisciplinary approaches to health care, the Neuman Systems Model effectively directs quality care at an efficient cost.

## Healthy People 2010

The concepts and theories described in this chapter can be related to the goal of increasing the years and quality of healthy life. Selected examples of objectives related to this goal can be seen in the Healthy People 2010 box.

## Application of the Neuman Systems Model to Communities

The Neuman Systems Model is used frequently and successfully by nurses in the United States, Canada, and some European countries. Clients may be in their homes, at community clinics, or at other sites. Clients may be aggregates or entire populations. For example, Drew, Craig, and Beynon (1989) used the model as the theoretical basis for developing standards for the delivery of community-based preventive services for the populations in Manitoba and Ontario, Canada. Client assessments were accomplished by using a problem-oriented nursing assessment record based on Neuman terminology. Pierce and Fulmer (1995) used the Neuman Systems Model to plan care for an aggregate of older adults in the community to optimize their wellness.

Community-as-client goals often emphasize health promotion and health maintenance. When the community is the focus of service, the nurse and community must form a partnership to achieve mutual goals. In community partnerships, the members and professionals who have vested interests in the success of the effort actively participate in collaborative decision making (see Chapter 15). Assessment, diagnosis, planning, intervention, and evaluation focus on the entire community or aggregates within it. In the Neuman Systems Model, the community is seen as a whole system of interfacing subsystems. Optimal functioning within and between the subsystems results in optimal functioning of the whole system. Furthermore, dysfunction within or between any of the subsystems can compromise the function or health of the entire system. Stressors that affect any subsystem and create instability for the community must be assessed so that appropriate interventions can be designed to reduce the impact of these stressors and promote health. This process is interactive and collaborative between the nurses and the community. An example of community instability occurs when the government does not have enough money to support education programs and public health.

As seen in Figure 9-1, the core or basic structure of the community as client represents the energy, resources, and basic factors common to the infrastructure of the community. These can be classified as physiologic, psychosocial,

---

**Healthy People 2010** | **Health Objectives**

1-3  Increase the proportion of persons appropriately counseled about health behaviors

1-4  Increase the proportion of persons who have a specific source of ongoing care

1-15  Increase the proportion of persons with long-term care needs who have access to the continuum of long-term care services

6-10  Increase the proportion of health and wellness and treatment programs and facilities that provide full access for people with disabilities

6-12  Reduce the proportion of people with disabilities reporting environmental barriers to participation in home, school, work, or community activities

11-4  Increase the proportion of health-related World Wide Web sites that disclose information that can be used to assess the quality of the site

11-6  Increase the proportion of persons who report that their health care providers have satisfactory communication skills

17-2  Increase the use of linked, automated systems to share information

From U.S. Department of Health and Human Services: *Healthy People 2010: understanding and improving health*, ed 2, Washington, DC, 2000, U.S. Government Printing Office.

sociocultural, developmental, and spiritual variables (Neuman and Fawcett, 2002). Table 9-3 provides a definition and example of each variable; for example, physiologic community variables are the structure (e.g., geographic boundaries, rural or urban) and functions (e.g., local government, safety systems) of the community. Each of the five variables interfaces with the other variables; flexible boundaries exist between them. In fact, examples of some factors could be categorized under more than one variable, such as health beliefs (sociocultural and spiritual) or aging (developmental and physiologic). The purpose of categorizing within the variables is to provide a comprehensive framework for assessment. This eliminates the possibility of overlooking any community area. Understanding that the variables are interactive and interdependent supports the idea of a community gestalt (wholeness) as the Neuman Systems Model proposes.

Like people, however, communities do not function optimally all the time. Stressors, either positive or negative, affect one or more parts of the community, thus affecting the whole. As systems theory indicates, a change in one subsystem or part will affect the entire system. Stressors can be defined as intracommunity (originating from within one or more subsystems or the whole), intercommunity (originating from adjacent areas), or extracommunity, imposed from structures outside the community. For example, a hazardous waste dump adjacent to an elementary school would be an intracommunity stressor, whereas racial tension between in-town residents and out-of-town residents would be an intercommunity stressor. Examples of extracommunity stressors could be new industries encroaching on farm lands surrounding the community, an interstate highway system planned through town, or decreased federal funding for community health services. Table 9-4 provides further examples of stressors within each variable of community as client.

Nurses create partnerships between subgroups within the community and between communities to develop resources to help the community maintain health. Communication is the medium by which information is exchanged and plans are formulated to raise health standards. Sometimes the nurse must motivate the community to change and must provide the leadership for implementing change. The nurse begins the change process by becoming familiar with the basic structure of the community and developing a database of community variables. Assessment of the infrastructures that protect the community is paramount. For example, police and fire protection, health and illness services, and the penal system represent the lines of resistance within the community established to protect, stabilize, and maintain a steady state for the community. These are depicted as

## Table 9-3  Community Variables: Definitions and Examples

| VARIABLE | DEFINITION | EXAMPLE |
|---|---|---|
| Physiologic | Structures and functions of community | Urban, rural, suburban<br>Water, sewage systems<br>Geographic boundaries/location<br>Safety systems (police and fire)<br>Government<br>Transportation system |
| Psychological | Cognitive and affective characteristics | Happy/depressed town<br>Intelligence level<br>Isolation versus sensory overload |
| Sociocultural | Social, economic, demographic, political, recreational, and health characteristics, and communication patterns among subsets | Communication patterns<br>Liberal versus conservative<br>Poor/middle class/affluent<br>Race, ethnicity<br>Type of industry<br>Day care for older adults and children<br>Ambulance service<br>Clinics/hospitals |
| Spiritual | Moral, religious, and value systems of community | Churches<br>Health beliefs<br>Burial and birth practices<br>Adult bookstores |
| Developmental | History, stage, and evolution of subsystems and aggregates in community | National registry of homes<br>Aging/adolescent populations<br>Deteriorating/emerging city |

**Table 9-4  Stressors Affecting Community-as-Client Variables**

| PHYSICAL | PSYCHOLOGICAL | SOCIOCULTURAL | DEVELOPMENTAL | SPIRITUAL |
|---|---|---|---|---|
| **Intracommunity** | | | | |
| Increased infant mortality rate<br>Hazardous waste dump<br>Water supply contaminated | Insufficient health education about AIDS<br>Increased divorce rates<br>Potential for decreased emotional health in public housing areas | Homes crowded in downtown<br>Park land bought by developer<br>Decreased family income<br>Many ethnic groups in community | High teen pregnancy rate<br>Potential need for more child care centers<br>Deteriorating inner city community<br>High proportion of aging with no caregivers | Many religious sects<br>Health beliefs influenced by folk wisdom |
| **Intercommunity** | | | | |
| Poor roads connecting town or regional medical center<br>Distribution of physicians uneven | Anger between political parties<br>Potential for isolation of rural older adults<br>Inadequate communication system between rural and urban areas | Racial tension between migrants and townspeople | Historical significance of town<br>Young versus old communities | Diverse value systems between rural and urban sectors |
| **Extracommunity** | | | | |
| Interstate highway system planned through town<br>Nuclear power plant site outside town<br>Flu epidemic<br>Decreased state funding for services | Belief system of national political party in opposition to community's beliefs<br>Fear of environmental contamination | Failure of industry that employs people<br>Potential for unemployment related to industrial plant closing<br>Influx of ethnic groups | New industry encroaching on farmland<br>Potential for increase in young families to support new industry<br>Potential growth in schools | New morality in opposition to community values<br>Community selected as headquarters site for national denomination |

broken lines in concentric circles surrounding the core in the Neuman Systems Model (see Figure 9-1).

Neuman's normal line of defense represents the usual range of responses developed over time that mark the unique aspects of any community. These could include the type of politics and government structure, ways of doing business to maintain a stable economy, and communication lines within and among groups and organizations. The normal line of defense could also be viewed as the usual coping behaviors the community uses to maintain balance. The normal line of defense is protected by the flexible line of defense, which acts as a buffer zone so that the normal state of community wellness is maintained. If the community is stable, the flexible line of defense can expand to provide more services for citizens, greater economic opportunities for industry, or more recreation and parks within the community. On the other hand, if the community experiences a minor emergency, such as a fire or disease outbreak, the flexible line of defense contracts to protect the community. The lines of resistance then mobilize to protect the infrastructure of the community. In this example, the line of resistance could be mobilizing the health department to investigate and find where a food-borne illness (disease outbreak) came from. The source of the illness—perhaps a restaurant worker who does not wash his hands before preparing food—could be removed from the workplace and educated about personal hygiene before being returned to work. The restaurant could be reinspected by the health department on a more frequent basis.

Using the Neuman Systems Model perspective as just described, the nurse can develop a mental image of the community as client that includes variables that represent its structure and the lines of defense. A database can be established at this point that includes all the important aspects of the community. Each identified community subsystem becomes a part of one of the five variables (see Table 9-4).

The next step is to identify community stressors that affect each subsystem and to assess the degree of community or aggregate reaction to the stressors. Appropriate interventions are then targeted (Box 9-1). For example, primary prevention might include giving immunizations, supporting positive coping strategies of a group of clients with acquired immunodeficiency syndrome (AIDS), and providing health education seminars. Secondary interventions will include early case finding, followed by appropriate referrals and counseling about high-risk behaviors.

Common to all three models of intervention are client advocacy, coordinating health resources, and providing information to maintain or regain system stability. Community nurses are the appropriate professionals to lead these activities.

## Use of the Neuman Systems Model for Community Outcomes

An example of the use of the Neuman Systems Model in community health nursing education and practice follows. Nursing faculty members at Lander University in Greenwood, South Carolina, have used the model as the conceptual basis for the curriculum since 1985. One project (called TEAM MED) provides learning opportunities in a "real world" clinical laboratory that is shared by faculty members and students who work collaboratively under the guidance of an occupational health nurse to promote health for employees of the South Carolina Department of Transportation (SCDOT). TEAM MED provides a program of health promotion, early detection, and disease prevention for SCDOT employees and is a collaborative effort between the SCDOT and universities throughout the state.* Lander University assumes responsibility for the employees (about 425) in seven counties in upstate South Carolina (Freese, Natvig, and Douglas, 1997).

The TEAM MED project, based on the Neuman Systems Model, is used in several courses in the nursing curriculum. For example, in the wellness nursing course, students learn primary prevention as intervention by providing flu shot clinics for SCDOT employees. Likewise, in the public health nursing course, students learn how to assess a community as client by working with SCDOT employees as an aggregate client. Students of the nursing research course learn how to develop research proposals that are based on problems identified from TEAM MED and framed within the Neuman Systems Model. Senior and registered nurse students coordinate TEAM MED assessments and follow-up for junior students working with the project in the leadership and management course.

### Individual Client in Community

Through TEAM MED, students learn how to apply the Neuman Systems Model at both the individual and community-as-client levels. At the individual level, the

---

<table>
<tr><td>

**BOX 9-1 Prevention Strategies**

**PRIMARY PREVENTION**

Educate about the lack of seat belt use by adolescents as a major health risk in communities.

**SECONDARY PREVENTION**

Implement treatment for an epidemic outbreak.

**TERTIARY PREVENTION**

Help a community readapt after a major disaster or period of debilitation.

</td></tr>
</table>

*The information collected in this publication was accomplished through the efforts of TEAM MED, a collaborative program that provides a wellness program for the South Carolina Department of Transportation personnel with participation from Clemson University Joseph F. Sullivan Center, School of Nursing and the Department of Public Health; University of South Carolina, College of Nursing; University of South Carolina–Spartanburg, School of Nursing; University of South Carolina–Aiken, School of Nursing.*

client is the employee of the SCDOT. The normal line of defense is the state of health of the employee that evolved over time. Students collect data on the employee's normal line of defense by assessing wellness factors in the areas of general health status, exercise habits and preferences, eating habits, alcohol and drug patterns, stress and coping, safety habits, and health maintenance habits (such as dental care).

Follow-up health care for individual employees emphasizes health promotion through primary and secondary prevention; however, services are offered at all three levels of Neuman's typology as follows. Primary prevention as intervention includes a comprehensive risk assessment for each employee-client, with individual counseling based on his or her results. Secondary prevention as intervention includes treating symptoms (such as elevated cholesterol) appropriately and referring medical problems that require physician attention. Tertiary prevention as intervention is involved for the occasional employee who has required major medical intervention (such as coronary bypass surgery) followed by rehabilitation. Students assist with planning and implementing rehabilitation programs.

### Aggregate Client in Community

Students also learn how to view SCDOT employees as an aggregate client, defined by the policies and employment expectations that they share as employees of the SCDOT. On the basis of the work of Beddome (1989, p. 569), when the Neuman Systems Model is applied to an aggregate community client, the intrasystem is the group of people who share one or more characteristics. For the TEAM MED project, the intrasystem includes an "immediate caregiving system." For TEAM MED, the intersystem includes the SCDOT occupational health nurse working in a community-university partnership with nursing faculty and students. The aggregate extrasystem includes eight interdependent subsystems: communication, transportation and safety, economics, education, politics and government, health and social services, physical environment, and recreation (Anderson, McFarlane, and Helton, 1986). Interaction among these subsystems can affect the health of the aggregate community either positively or negatively. TEAM MED focuses on assessing and strengthening the health and safety subsystem, such as providing education on seat belt use and safe lifting techniques.

The community client's normal line of defense is the system's state of health developed over time. For SCDOT employees as an aggregate client, data from assessment of each employee's wellness factors are compiled into an aggregate form. Then each county is analyzed and wellness factors are listed by county. These reports are used to implement projects to improve employee health and safety.

The community client's flexible line of defense is composed of programs and activities that protect the client's normal state of wellness by serving as a buffer system. The TEAM MED program is one component of the flexible line of defense for the aggregate community of SCDOT

employees. Prevention-as-intervention strategies described previously (such as health assessment, teaching, and medical referrals) serve to promote client system stability as an occupational workforce.

This example illustrates a seamless process of education and practice. Students educated from a model perspective are prepared to practice in a community that is also familiar with the model's worldview. Thus the ultimate goal, positive health outcomes, can be achieved.

---

**DID YOU KNOW?**

The leading health indicators identified by Healthy People 2010 were selected on the basis of their ability to motivate action and provide data to measure progress toward a healthier nation.

---

## OMAHA SYSTEM

Nurses and administrators in community settings face urgent practice, documentation, and information management challenges (Handly et al, 2003; Monsen and Martin, 2002a, b). The scope of community and public health nursing practice has always been complex, diverse, and independent, as have been the individuals, families, and communities who are the clients of service. However, because of the magnitude and speed of current health care system changes, nurses and administrators have critical needs in three areas:

1. Timely, valid, and reliable data that describe clients' demographic characteristics, the severity and acuity of their needs, the type and location of services, and reimbursement methods
2. Timely, valid, and reliable data that quantify the clients receiving care, the services they receive, and the costs and outcomes of that care
3. Verbal and written methods for nurses to communicate with nurses and other professionals

According to Clark and Lang (1992, p. 27), "If we cannot name it, we cannot control it, finance it, teach it, research it or put it into public policy." Counting data must be added to naming data to address urgent practice, documentation, and data management challenges.

The ANA established a committee in 1991 to explore interrelated concerns involving changing nursing practice, standardizing nursing language, and automating it. Since then, the ANA committee (1) recognized 12 diverse classifications, data sets, and nomenclatures that met their research, practice, and information system criteria; (2) publicized the classifications and the related issues in publications and their website; and (3) collaborated with the National Library of Medicine to include the classifications in the *Metathesaurus*, a database that is available internationally (ANA, 2003; Coenen et al, 2001). The classifications most relevant to this chapter are the Omaha System, the North American Nursing

**Table 9-5    Comparison of Classification Systems**

| SYSTEMS AND ORIGINS | TAXONOMY STRUCTURE AND ORGANIZATION | SETTINGS WHERE ESPECIALLY APPLICABLE |
|---|---|---|
| North American Nursing Diagnosis Association (NANDA) | Nursing diagnoses with nine domains, 43 classes, and 149 diagnoses | Hospitals, ambulatory care, nursing homes (early 1970s) |
| Iowa Nursing Interventions classification (mid 1980s) | Nursing interventions with six domains | Hospitals, ambulatory care, nursing homes |
| Iowa Nursing Outcomes Classification (early 1990s) | Nursing outcomes with specific indicators and measurement scales | Hospitals, ambulatory care, nursing homes |
| Home Health Care Classification (1987) | Some NANDA nursing diagnoses; nursing interventions with four categories | Home care |
| Omaha System (early 1970s) | Nursing diagnoses/client problems with four domains; interventions with four categories; rating scale with three concepts and Likert-type scale | Community, including home care, public health, schools, nursing centers, emerging health delivery settings |

Diagnosis Association (NANDA) International nursing intervention and nursing outcomes classification, and the home health care classification. The Omaha System discussed here includes client problems, interventions, and an outcome rating scale and is used most frequently in community settings (Martin and Scheet, 1992a; Omaha System, 1999). NANDA International consists of nursing diagnoses that have been used most frequently in acute care settings (NANDA, 1999). The interventions and outcomes of the nursing interventions classification and nursing outcomes classification have been linked to NANDA and are also used in many acute care settings (Johnson, Maas, and Moorhead, 2000; Johnson et al, 2001; McCloskey and Bulechek, 2000). The home health care classification focuses on interventions generated by home health care agencies and includes some of the NANDA nursing diagnoses (Saba et al, 1991). Table 9-5 summarizes the five classifications.

## Definitions

Although the following concepts have been defined in various ways, their similarities involve evolving and interchangeable use as shown in this chapter. The concepts can be incorporated into community health programs as well as acute and long-term care programs. The concepts apply to the client as an individual, a family, or a community.

- **Nursing diagnosis** is a clinical judgment about individual, family, or community responses to actual and potential health problems and life processes. It provides the basis for selecting nursing interventions to achieve outcomes for which the nurse is accountable (NANDA, 1999).
- **Client problem** is a matter of difficulty or concern that historically, presently, or potentially affects adversely any aspect of the client's well-being; accu-

rately identifying the problem enables the professional to focus interventions (Martin and Scheet, 1992a).
- **Intervention** describes activity that follows a thought process or written exercise, usually referred to as planning. It is an action or activity implemented to address a specific client problem and to improve, maintain, or restore health or prevent illness (Martin and Scheet, 1992a).
- **Nursing intervention** is any treatment, based on clinical judgment and knowledge, that a nurse performs to enhance client outcomes. These treatments include direct and indirect care and nurse-initiated, physician-initiated, and other provider–initiated treatments (McCloskey and Bulechek, 2000).
- **Evaluation** is a process designed to determine a value or an amount, or to compare accomplishments with some standards. Donabedian's (1966) structure, process, and outcome framework is considered classic and has provided nurses with an evaluation model. Evaluation based on client outcomes assumes that changes in client health status and behavior result from or are consequences of care. Evaluation has been defined as measurement of client progress by comparing client knowledge, behavior, and status ratings at admission, regular intervals, and dismissal (Martin and Scheet, 1992a).

## Concepts of the Nursing Process

Nursing diagnosis or identifying the client problem follows the data collecting and assessing phases of the **nursing process.** Accurately identifying the nursing diagnosis or client problem is critical to the success of nursing care. Plans and interventions, the next phases of the nursing process, reflect the art and science of nursing. Interventions should be based on the best available evidence, and that should include research if it is available. The nurse's skill in selecting and implementing the best interventions is crucial to achieving the best possible outcomes. The final phase of the nursing process—evaluation—often receives little attention from clinicians or administrators in the practice setting. Without examining the results of care during and at the end of nursing service, accurate conclusions about the efficiency and effectiveness of care are not possible. Fortunately, heightened interest in evaluation and outcomes measurement is occurring because of new agency accrediting standards, federal regulations, legislation, escalating health care costs, and increasingly vocal consumers.

It is important for the nurse to recognize that the nursing process exists within a larger framework. In addition to nursing, other disciplines that require logical, scientific thinking and systematic nomenclature (naming) also employ a problem-solving approach. The problem-solving process includes generalized information gathering, problem identification, and analysis, as well as decision making based on fact, intuition, and experiences. Physicians employ a medical diagnostic process that is similar to the nursing process and the problem-solving approach. Table 9-6 illustrates the relationship of the nursing process to the medical diagnostic and problem-solving processes.

## Description of the Omaha System

As early as 1970, the staff and administrators of the Visiting Nurse Association (VNA) of Omaha, Nebraska, began addressing **nursing practice, documentation,** and **information management** concerns, and converting from their narrative method of documenting to a problem-oriented approach. At that time, no systematic nomenclature or classification of client problems existed that could be used with a problem-oriented record system. This reality provided incentive for beginning research on the topic.

With the assistance of people at seven different test sites, community-oriented nursing educators, other advisory committee members, and the VNA of Omaha staff conducted three research projects between 1975 and 1986 that were funded by contracts with the U.S. Department of Health and Human Services (USDHHS) Division of Nursing. The results of these projects were the problem classification scheme, the intervention scheme, and the problem rating scale for outcomes of care. A fourth research project was funded by a grant from the National Institute of Nursing Research, National Institutes of Health. That research was designed to examine reliability, validity, and usability of the Omaha System among different test agencies. Details about the research are included in other publications (Martin, Norris, and Leak, 1999; Martin and Scheet, 1992a; Omaha System, 1999).

> **( NURSING TIP**
>
> When using a data collection instrument, plan to collect data over several visits to avoid tiring the client. Always write down at least one nursing diagnosis goal and prevention strategy for each visit. This will keep your data accurate.

The theoretical framework for the **Omaha System** is based on the dynamic, interactive nature of the nursing or problem-solving process, the clinician-client relationship, and concepts of diagnostic reasoning, clinical judgment, and quality improvement. As shown in Figure 9-2, when the three Omaha System schemes are considered together, they make up the nursing process. The client as an individual, a family, or a community appears at the center of the model. This location shows the many ways the Omaha System can be used and the essential partnership between clients and clinicians.

The Omaha System is the only system developed inductively (initially) by and for practicing community-oriented nurses. Nurses who practice in different community settings need comprehensive tools to manage client data. Nurses, however, are not the only members of community-oriented health care delivery teams. The goals of the Omaha System research were (1) to develop a structured and comprehensive system that could be both understood and used by members of various disciplines and (2) to foster collaborative practice. Therefore the Omaha System was designed to guide practice decisions, sort and document pertinent client data uniformly, and provide a framework for an agency-wide, multidisciplinary

---

### Table 9-6  Relationship of Nursing Process to Problem-Solving and Medical Diagnostic Processes

| NURSING PROCESS | PROBLEM-SOLVING PROCESS | MEDICAL DIAGNOSTIC PROCESS |
| --- | --- | --- |
| Data collection | Information gathering | History and physical examination |
| Nursing diagnosis | Problem | Diagnosis |
| Plan | Plan | Plan |
| Intervention | Action | Treatment |
| Evaluation | Evaluation | Evaluation |

clinical information management system capable of meeting the needs of clinicians, managers, and administrators (Handly et al., 2003; Monsen and Martin, 2002b).

## Problem Classification Scheme

The **Omaha System Problem Classification Scheme** is a client-focused taxonomy of client problems or nursing diagnoses composed of simple and concrete terms. The language of the scheme is organized at four discrete levels. The vocabulary of each of the four levels is consistent and parallel. Because the scheme is not intended to be exhaustive, terms that are consistent with the scheme's classification rules can be added where the place-holder term *other* appears. The levels of the scheme are (1) domains, (2) problems, (3) modifiers, and (4) signs and symptoms. The content and relationship of the domain and problem levels are depicted in Box 9-2 and are further illustrated by the case example in the Practice Application at the end of this chapter.

The four domains define the scope of practice. These domains are (1) environmental, (2) psychosocial, (3) physiologic, and (4) health-related behaviors. Understanding the meaning of and relationships among the domains is a prerequisite to implementing the scheme accurately.

The 40 client problems are the second level of the problem classification scheme (excluding "other"; see Box 9-2). These client problems are the most critical portion of the scheme. Problems identified by the nurse are always documented in the client record.

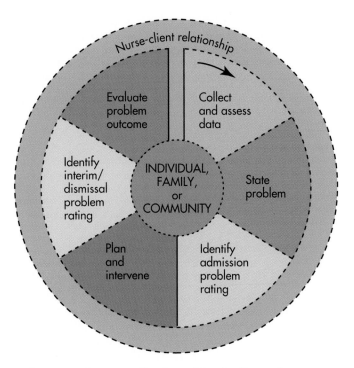

**Figure 9-2** Conceptualization of the family nursing process. *(Modified from Martin KS, Scheet NJ:* The Omaha System: applications for community health nursing, *Philadelphia, 1992a, Saunders.)*

Two sets of modifiers represent the third level of the scheme and are used in conjunction with each client problem. Modifiers selected by the nurse are (1) family or individual and (2) actual, potential, or health promotion. Using two modifiers with a problem enhances application across the health–illness continuum and adds an important degree of specificity and precision. Some nurses have expanded the "individual" and "family" modifiers to include groups and communities.

The fourth level of the problem classification scheme involves a cluster of signs and symptoms specific to each problem. Clues and cues are produced as the nurse gathers, sorts, and prioritizes data. These suggest signs and symptoms that, in turn, suggest the presence of actual client problems.

## Intervention Scheme

The **Omaha System Intervention Scheme** is a systematic arrangement of nursing actions or activities designed to help nurses and other health care professionals document both plans and interventions. The scheme is intended for use with client problems. Using the same principles as described for the problem classification scheme, the language is organized into three levels of specificity: (1) categories, (2) targets, and (3) client-specific information. The content and relationships of the category and target levels are shown in Box 9-3 and are further illustrated with the case example in the Practice Application.

The following four intervention categories represent the basis of community-oriented practice. When viewed together, they describe the clinician's primary functions in relation to importance and time. The categories are (1) health teaching, counseling, and guidance, (2) treatments and procedures, (3) case management, and (4) surveillance.

The second level of the intervention scheme is an alphabetical listing of 62 targets (excluding "other"; Box 9-4). Targets are the objects of nursing interventions. The targets are used to delineate a problem-specific intervention category by offering a more specific level of detail.

The third level of the intervention scheme is designed for client-specific information. Pertinent, concise words or short phrases are documented by clinicians as they develop plans or document care provided to a specific client. Although not part of the research projects, the VNA of Omaha staff organized care planning guides specific to each of the 40 problems of the problem classification scheme (Martin and Scheet, 1992b). Box 9-5 gives examples of problems and the signs and symptoms that help to identify the problem.

## Problem Rating Scale for Outcomes

The **Omaha System Problem Rating Scale for Outcomes** is a scale that offers a systematic, recurring way of measuring client progress throughout the time nursing service is given to the client. It was designed for use with any client problem in the problem classification scheme. In addition, the scale provides both a guide for practice and a method

## BOX 9-2  Domains and Problems of the Omaha System Problem Classification Scheme

I. Environmental Domain
  01. Income
  02. Sanitation
  03. Residence
  04. Neighborhood/workplace safety
  05. Other
II. Psychosocial Domain
  06. Communication with community resources
  07. Social contact
  08. Role change
  09. Interpersonal relationship
  10. Spirituality
  11. Grief
  12. Emotional stability
  13. Human sexuality
  14. Caretaking/parenting
  15. Neglected child/adult
  16. Abused child/adult
  17. Growth and development
  18. Other
III. Physiologic Domain
  19. Hearing
  20. Vision
  21. Speech and language

22. Dentition
23. Cognition
24. Pain
25. Consciousness
26. Integument
27. Neuromusculoskeletal function
28. Respiration
29. Circulation
30. Digestion, hydration
31. Bowel function
32. Genitourinary function
33. Antepartum/postpartum
34. Other
IV. Health-Related Behaviors Domain
  35. Nutrition
  36. Sleep and rest patterns
  37. Physical activity
  38. Personal hygiene
  39. Substance use
  40. Family planning
  41. Health care supervision
  42. Prescribed medication regimen
  43. Technical procedure
  44. Other

## BOX 9-3  Categories of the Omaha System Intervention Scheme

### I. HEALTH TEACHING, GUIDANCE, AND COUNSELING

Health teaching, guidance, and counseling are nursing activities that include giving information, anticipating client problems, encouraging client action and responsibility for self-care and coping, and assisting with decision making and problem solving. The overlapping concepts occur on a continuum, and variation results from the client's self-direction capabilities.

### II. TREATMENTS AND PROCEDURES

Treatments and procedures are technical nursing activities directed toward preventing signs and symptoms, identifying risk factors and early signs and symptoms, and decreasing or alleviating signs and symptoms.

### III. CASE MANAGEMENT

Case management includes nursing activities of coordination, advocacy, and referral. These activities involve facilitating service delivery on behalf of the client, communicating with health and human service providers, promoting assertive client communication, and guiding the client toward use of appropriate community resources.

### IV. SURVEILLANCE

Surveillance includes nursing activities of detection, measurement, critical analysis, and monitoring to indicate client status in relation to a given condition or phenomenon.

of documentation. When establishing the initial ratings for client problems, the nurse creates an independent data baseline. This captures the condition and circumstances of the client at a specific point in time. This admission baseline is used to compare client's ratings at later intervals and at dismissal. The content and relationship of the concepts and number ratings are shown in Table 9-7 and further illustrated by the case example in the Practice Application (Martin and Scheet, 1992b).

The problem rating scale for outcomes comprises three Likert-type ordinal scales, for knowledge, behavior, and sta-

tus. *Knowledge* involves what a client knows and understands about a specific health-related problem. *Behavior* involves the client's practices, performances, and skills. *Status* involves how a client is and how the client's conditions or circumstances improve, remain stable, or deteriorate. Although the three concepts are interrelated, they represent three distinct dimensions of client outcomes. The three dimensions of the scale are equal in importance, although they may not be equally important when used with a specific client.

The ratings have characteristics of ordinal scales: (1) mutually exclusive classes or categories, (2) each continuum

## BOX 9-4 Second Level of the Omaha System Intervention Scheme: Targets

01. Anatomy/physiology
02. Behavior modification
03. Bladder care
04. Bonding
05. Bowel care
06. Bronchial hygiene
07. Cardiac care
08. Caretaking/parenting skills
09. Cast care
10. Communication
11. Coping skills
12. Day care/respite
13. Discipline
14. Dressing change/wound care
15. Durable medical equipment
16. Education
17. Employment
18. Environment
19. Exercises
20. Family planning
21. Feeding procedures
22. Finances
23. Food
24. Gait training
25. Growth/development
26. Homemaking
27. Housing
28. Interaction
29. Laboratory findings
30. Legal system
31. Medical/dental care
32. Medication action/side effects

33. Medication administration
34. Medication setup
35. Mobility/transfers
36. Nursing care, supplementary
37. Nutrition
38. Nutritionist
39. Ostomy care
40. Other community resources
41. Personal care
42. Positioning
43. Rehabilitation
44. Relaxation/breathing techniques
45. Rest/sleep
46. Safety
47. Screening
48. Sickness/injury care
49. Signs/symptoms-mental/emotional
50. Signs/symptoms-physical
51. Skin care
52. Social work/counseling
53. Specimen collection
54. Spiritual care
55. Stimulation/nurturance
56. Stress management
57. Substance use
58. Supplies
59. Support group
60. Support system
61. Transportation
62. Wellness
63. Other

## BOX 9-5 Examples of Problems, Modifiers, and Signs/Symptoms from the Omaha System Problem Classification Scheme

01. Income
    Health promotion
    Potential deficit
    Deficit
        01. Low/no income
        02. Uninsured medical expenses
        03. Inadequate money management
        04. Able to buy only necessities
        05. Difficulty buying necessities
        06. Other
33. Antepartum/postpartum
    Health promotion
    Potential impairment
    Impairment
        01. Difficulty coping with pregnancy/body
           changes
        02. Inappropriate exercise/rest/diet/behaviors

        03. Discomfort
        04. Complications
        05. Fears delivery procedure
        06. Difficulty breastfeeding
        07. Other
39. Substance use
    Health promotion
    Potential
    Actual
        01. Abuses over-the-counter/street drugs
        02. Abuses alcohol
        03. Smokes
        04. Difficulty performing normal routines
        05. Reflex disturbances
        06. Behavior change
        07. Other

**Table 9-7  The Omaha System Problem Rating Scale for Outcomes**

| CONCEPT | 1 | 2 | 3 | 4 | 5 |
|---|---|---|---|---|---|
| Knowledge: The ability of the client to remember and interpret information | No knowledge | Minimal knowledge | Basic knowledge | Adequate knowledge | Superior knowledge |
| Behavior: The observable responses, actions, or activities of the client fitting the occasion or purpose | Not appropriate | Rarely appropriate | Inconsistently appropriate | Usually appropriate | Consistently appropriate |
| Status: The condition of the client in relation to objective and subjective defining characteristics | Extreme signs/ symptoms | Severe signs/ symptoms | Moderate signs/ symptoms | Minimal signs/ symptoms | No signs/ symptoms |

exhaustive, and (3) categories that fit into a specific order or sequence. Each scale has a continuum of five categories or degrees for response; very positive and negative categories are located at the ends of each continuum.

## Application of the Omaha System in Practice and Education

When results of the Omaha System surveys were published in 1992, approximately 250 sites in this country indicated that they used the system (Martin and Scheet, 1992a). Since then, the number and type of service and educational settings that use the Omaha System nationally and internationally have increased dramatically (Anderko and Kinion, 2001; Bowles, 2000; Clark et al, 2001; Marek and Rantz, 2000; Omaha System website, 2002; Schoneman, 2003). Approximately 400 service agencies and 50 nursing education programs have installed Omaha System software. Users include nurses and members of many disciplines: home care and public health agencies, nursing centers, clinics, schools, ambulatory care centers, parish programs, case management programs, correctional facilities, and nursing education programs.

Software offers numerous advantages to the nurses, managers, administrators, students, and faculty when they resolve their practice, documentation, and information management challenges mentioned earlier in this chapter. If clinicians or students enter standardized, comprehensive data accurately and consistently about the individual-, family-, and population-focused services they provide, they, their managers and administrators, and faculty members have access to equally standardized, comprehensive, accurate, and consistent aggregate data. The Evidence-Based Practice box describes a FITNE, Inc., study that was

## THE CUTTING EDGE

More community agencies are using computers and clinical information software, so nurses can document their care and client outcomes wherever they are in the community. In Minnesota, 85% of all counties now have one or more public health or home care agencies using Omaha System software.

designed to evaluate teaching strategies used when the Nightingale Tracker and Omaha System were introduced to students (Nightingale Tracker Clinical Field Test Nurse Team, 2000). The documentation and information experiences of the Washington County Department of Public Health and Environment, in Stillwater, Minnesota, are described (Monsen and Martin, 2002b). Their clinical experiences are described in the Practice Application. When nurses have a vision about the value of clinical data and they implement an appropriate action plan, they will generate information that becomes a powerful communication tool for themselves and their colleagues.

## MERGING OF THE NEUMAN SYSTEMS MODEL AND THE OMAHA SYSTEM

The following example illustrates how the Neuman Systems Model and the Omaha System Intervention Scheme are used together to plan and document care for senior citizens in southeastern Pennsylvania. The seniors who benefit from this project are frail elders from two sites—one a low-income

## Evidence-Based Practice

FITNE, Inc., conducted field test research to evaluate the teaching strategies used to introduce the Nightingale Tracker. The Tracker is a point-of-care information technology system that includes the Omaha System. Faculty members who represented baccalaureate, associate, and graduate degree nursing programs at five urban and rural sites were oriented to the Omaha System and the Tracker. In turn, they instructed their 44 students to use the Omaha System and the Tracker to document the services they provided in clinical settings. Data were collected from students using an attitudinal survey, a user profile questionnaire, journals, and videotapes. Students scored higher and felt more successful when they learned about the Omaha System prior to using the Tracker, practiced using the Omaha System and the Tracker with paper and pen simulations, and had more individualized hands-on practice time. Student frustration increased when network connections could not be maintained, technical support was not available, and they felt rushed. The findings from this field test have been incorporated into FITNE's orientation program and guidelines.

**Nurse Use:** As more computer technology is introduced into education and service settings, faculty and managers need to incorporate a complete orientation and practice opportunities.

Nightingale Tracker Clinical Field Test Nurse Team: A comparison of teaching strategies for integrating information technology into clinical nursing education, *J Nurs Educ* 25(3):136, 2000.

---

apartment complex and the other an ambulatory facility, the Community Nursing Center (CNC), established to provide health promotion and preventive services to independent seniors. The project originated in 1998 as a collaborative effort between two schools of nursing, a citizen's advisory committee, and the county office of aging. Several organizations provide funding so that cost-effective, safe, and accessible health care is available for this underserved population. Case managers employed by the Office of Aging in the county serve as coordinators of care for the elders. Baccalaureate and graduate nursing students from the two schools of nursing take part in the project by conducting the elder assessments and using the data to plan follow-up care and teaching projects for groups and individuals. The data become part of the elder's permanent health record. Referrals are made as necessary after the visits.

## Instrument Development

The data collection instrument was designed by Diana Newman, former Associate Professor at Neumann College, who was the first coordinator of the CNC. The instrument combines the breadth of the Neuman Systems Model (NSM) with the detail of the Omaha System Intervention Scheme. For example, the function of practice models is to specify the particular client (elders), the environment (housing project and senior center), health (aging issues), and nursing focus (wellness and health maintenance). The NSM indicated the variables for assessment, the focus on stressors of the elders, and the preventions as intervention. The NSM was then linked with the intervention scheme to provide the categories from which the nurse could select specific strategies for care.

The data collection instrument is divided into 11 sections with a total of 331 items. Each section includes specific questions appropriate to the Neuman variables and identified client stressors, strengths, and perceptions. After collecting these data, the nurse writes the nursing diagnoses and goals for the client and selects interventions from the Omaha System (Box 9-6).

Specific questions to elicit information about client health status and functional ability are shown in Table 9-8. The sample questions illustrate how the data collection instrument is organized according to NSM variables and the subsets of information under each variable. Note that some of the questions serve as triggers to jog the memory of the elders. For example, under the nutrition subset, elders are asked to recall what they had eaten in the last day. When they answer how they prepare their meals, memory is jogged about selection made during grocery shopping. Box 9-7 illustrates the integration of the three prevention-as-intervention categories of the NSM with the four subsets of the Omaha System Intervention Scheme that specify nursing actions.

## Using the Instrument

A request for client medical information is sent out to the client's primary care provider after the client is enrolled in the CNC. This form includes authorization by the client to obtain information such as medical diagnoses, medications, diet, and activity from the primary care provider, who signs and returns the form to the CNC. Client data are collected over several visits until the data collection instrument is complete. Nursing interventions are classified using the intervention scheme (Martin and Scheet, 1992a) and then placed in the appropriate intervention–primary, secondary, or tertiary–of the Neuman Systems Model (Neuman and Fawcett, 2002). The Neuman preventions are subsumed within the health teaching, guidance, and counseling section of the intervention scheme. The Omaha System is useful for coding primary, secondary, and tertiary preventions within the current physician terminology codes (Krischner et al, 1997) and the international classification of disease (Baierschmidt et al, 1996). All data are recorded in a format that is compatible with statistical computer programs.

Data are used to plan health teaching for individual elders and groups of elders with the same needs. For example, mobility issues, common among most elders, are addressed through passive (chair-bound) and active (line dancing)

## Evidence-Based Practice

The nurses, managers, and director at the Washington County Department of Public Health and Environment planned and implemented a comprehensive outcomes management program over a 5-year period. Critical components included the following:

1. Commitment of leaders and staff
2. Collaborative decision making related to clinical record software selection
3. Extensive staff orientation and support for documentation and automation
4. Ongoing evaluation

When the public health nurses in this program provided services to clients such as Tamika Brown (see Practice Application), they used the Omaha System and documented those services accurately and consistently on laptop computers. The data became the foundation of a successful program that provided reliable and valid quantitative, population-focused outcomes information.

**Nurse Use:** The information is now used by nurses and managers for the department's quality improvement program, by managers and the director for program planning and evaluation, and by the director to develop interim and annual reports that are shared with administrators and local government officials. Figure 9-3 is an example of aggregate data.

From Monsen KA, Martin KS: Developing an outcomes management program in a public health department, *Outcomes Manag* 6[2]:62-66, 2002a; Monsen KA, Martin KS: Using an outcomes management program in a public health department, *Outcomes Manag* 6[3]:120-124, 2002b.

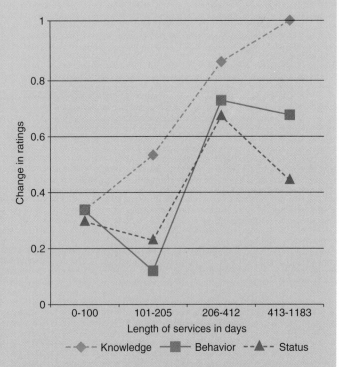

**Figure 9-3** Change in knowledge, behavior, and status ratings from the problem rating scale for outcomes for clients who had the problem, Caretaking/parenting (n = 83), by quartiles of time.

**BOX 9-6** NSM/OS Data Collection Instrument

A brief outline of the instrument follows:
- Background data (20 items): demographics, sources of health care
- Health history (24 items): diseases, surgeries, immunizations, and health behavior screening
- Variables:
  - Physiologic (200 items): divided into 11 subsections based on physiologic functions
  - Developmental (33 items): activities of daily living, functional status, safety, risk factors, housing
  - Psychological (9 items): mood, support systems, life transitions
  - Sociocultural (6 items): race, ethnicity, education, occupation, financial level
  - Spiritual (4 items): religion, beliefs
- Summary: client stressors, strengths, and perceptions
- Nursing diagnoses
- Nursing goals
- Intervention scheme
  - Health teaching, guidance, and counseling (6 items)
  - Treatments and procedures (5 items)
  - Case management (7 items)
  - Surveillance (6 items)
- Follow-up visits and signatures

**Table 9-8  Data Collection Instrument Sample Items**

| VARIABLE | DIMENSION | QUESTIONS | ANSWERS |
|---|---|---|---|
| Physiologic | Nutrition | a. I have an illness that made me change the kind or amount of food I eat. | a. YES/NO |
| | | b. I eat fewer than two meals a day. | b. YES/NO |
| | | c. I don't always have enough money to buy the food I eat. | c. YES/NO |
| | | d. I am not physically able to shop for myself. | d. YES/NO |
| | | e. I am drinking more than I used to. | e. YES/NO |
| | Mental Status | What is the (year) (date) (day) (month)? | |
| | Musculoskeletal status | Does client use aids for ambulation? | YES/NO |
| | Integumentary | Please indicate the presence or absence of skin characteristics<br>• Dry skin<br>• Pigmented spots<br>• Cyanosis<br>• Erythema | |
| Developmental | Housing | Please check the type of housing client lives in; add further information in the comments section.<br>1. Client lives in<br>a. An apartment ___<br>b. Own home ___<br>c. Lives with his or her family (please describe) ___<br>d. Other (please describe) ___<br>2. How many rooms does the client have? ___<br>3. Please check yes or no to the following statements:<br>a. Heat and ventilation are present.<br>b. Safety hazards are present.<br>c. Insect infestation is present.<br>d. Housing is clean.<br>e. Housing is well lit.<br>f. Elevator is present.<br>g. Walk-up<br>4. Comments: | <br><br><br><br><br><br><br><br>3a. YES/NO<br>3b. YES/NO<br>3c. YES/NO<br>3d. YES/NO<br>3e. YES/NO<br>3f. YES/NO<br>3g. YES/NO |
| Psychological | | 1. What is the client's mood?<br>2. Ask the client to describe his or her family structure.<br>3. Draw a genogram to document the family structure. | |
| Sociocultural | Education | What is the client's level of education (please circle): | 0 1 2 3 4 5 6 7<br>8 9 10 11 12<br>13 14 15 16 17<br>18 19 20<br>Grade school<br>High school<br>College<br>Graduate school |
| | Financial security | What is the client's source of financial security? (Check all that apply)<br>a. Employment ___<br>b. Retirement income ___<br>c. Public income ___<br>d. Savings ___<br>e. Family ___<br>f. Other ___ | |
| | Support system | With whom do you live?<br>What community support systems do you access? | |

*Continued*

**Table 9-8  Data Collection Instrument Sample Items—cont'd**

| VARIABLE | DIMENSION | QUESTIONS | ANSWERS |
|---|---|---|---|
| Spiritual | Religion | What is the client's religion?<br>a. Jewish ___<br>b. Protestant ___<br>c. Roman Catholic ___<br>d. Other ___ | |
| | Spiritual beliefs, support, and access | 1. What are the spiritual beliefs of the client?<br>2. What spiritual support is available to the client?<br>3. How does the client access spiritual support? | |

**BOX 9-7  Primary, Secondary, and Tertiary Prevention Examples Within the Omaha Scheme**

**PRIMARY PREVENTION**

1. Health teaching, guidance, and counseling:
   a. Information given ___
   b. Anticipatory guidance ___
   c. Encouraging self-care and coping ___
   d. Assistance with decision making and problem solving ___
Specific action taken:
Client response:

**SECONDARY PREVENTION**

2. Treatments and procedures:
   a. Prevention of signs and symptoms ___
   b. Identifying risk factors ___
   c. Decreasing and alleviating signs and symptoms ___
Specific action taken:
Client response:

**TERTIARY PREVENTION**

3. Case management:
   a. Coordination, advocacy, and referral ___
   b. Facilitate service delivery on behalf of the client by:
      1) Communicating with health and human service providers ___
      2) Promoting assertive client communication ___
      3) Guiding the client toward the use of appropriate community resources ___
Specific action taken:
Client response:
4. Surveillance: Please check which action(s) were taken to indicate client status in relation to a given condition or phenomenon.
      a. Detection ___
      b. Measurement ___
      c. Critical analysis ___
      d. Monitoring ___
Specific action taken:
Client response:

exercise classes. Adherence to medication protocols is another area requiring both individual and group teaching. Classes on proper diet that illustrate sources of hidden sodium and sugar have been very helpful to the clients. Not only are data used to design interventions for immediate use but also all data are entered into databases for future analyses.

This project has been ongoing for 4 years and has resulted in community-oriented, integrated, cost-effective, safe, and accessible health care for elders. Anecdotal evidence indicates that elders from the CNC and the housing area are more adherent to medication regimes and other health issues since they have received more regular care (K. Vito, personal communication, June 5, 2002). Word of the success of this project traveled to another housing authority in an adjacent geographic area. This housing authority decided to adopt the same assessment tool for use with its residents, rather than a competing tool, because it was more comprehensive and the taxonomy lent itself to computer tracking.

This real-world application of the development and use of a data collection instrument demonstrates the complementary nature of the Neuman Systems Model and the Omaha System Intervention Scheme. The systems approach of the Neuman Model provides the theoretical framework, whereas the Omaha System provides the specific classifications for coding reportable data. Used together, the structural hierarchy of nursing knowledge is illustrated. The conceptual Neuman Systems Model, supported by the mid-range Omaha System Theory, demonstrates a nursing structure applicable to quality practice and cost-effective outcomes.

| HOW TO | Apply the Omaha System in the Tamika Johnson Case | | | |
|---|---|---|---|---|

| Domain | Client data | Problems and signs/symptoms (see Boxes 9-2 and 9-5) | Ratings* (see Table 9-7) | Interventions (see Boxes 9-3 and 9-4) |
|---|---|---|---|---|
| Physiologic status | About 7 mo pregnant | Problem domain III<br>33. Antepartum/postpartum | K = 2 | I: 01, 25, 31 |
| Health-related behaviors | Weight before pregnancy: 120 lb<br>Gained 10 lb<br>Height: 5 feet 4 inches<br>Smokes ½ pack/day | Problem domain IV<br>35, 36, 39. Inappropriate exercise/rest/diet/behaviors | B = 2 | II: 57 |
| Potential deficits | No prenatal care<br>Nausea and vomiting for 5 mo<br>No medical insurance<br>Works part-time | 33. Antepartum/postpartum complications | S = 3 | III: 37<br>IV: 31<br>III: 52 |

*K, Knowledge; B, behavior; S, status.
See also Table 9-7 and Boxes 9-2 to 9-5 for the Omaha System. See Practice Application for the Tamika Johnson case.

## Practice Application

Tamika Johnson is a composite of many clients served by the nurses at the Washington County Public Health and Environment, Stillwater, Minnesota. She is a 19-year-old, single, African-American woman. She is living with a friend temporarily, although she would like to find her own apartment, and she works part-time at a convenience store for minimum wage. Tamika came to the Washington County WIC clinic seeking food and assistance. She is pregnant with her first baby. She is uncertain of her due date but believes she is about 7 months pregnant. She has not received medical care for her pregnancy and does not have medical insurance. Tamika experienced nausea and vomiting for about 5 months and lost weight during that time. She now weighs 10 pounds more than her reported pre-pregnancy weight. Her weight is appropriate for her height. Tamika reports that she smokes half a pack of cigarettes per day.

On the basis of her income, Tamika qualifies for the WIC program and agrees to schedule ongoing public health nursing visits. The nurse, Ellie Timm, observes and hears extensive data. On the basis of the data collected during the admission visit, the nurse identified three problems: Income, Antepartum/postpartum, and Substance use.

Which approach is most appropriate for Ellie to use as she gathers and documents pertinent pregnancy data for Tamika?

A. Use no guidelines for completing an assessment, but record all data that Tamika volunteers.
B. Base Tamika's prenatal assessment on Ellie's balanced diet and experience with her own problem-free pregnancy last year.
C. Use the Omaha System as a tool to explore Tamika's needs and strengths while focusing on her income, economic and insurance resources, pregnancy status, smoking patterns, and desire to have a healthy pregnancy and infant.
D. Focus on Tamika's smoking patterns, describe the dangers to her infant, and provide smoking cessation information and materials.

Answer is in the back of the book; see the How To box for an example of Omaha System use.

## Key Points

- Models can be physical, symbolic, or mental ways of viewing real phenomena.
- Conceptual models guide members of a discipline in their thinking, observing, and interpreting.
- Community-oriented health nursing is population focused, and the goal is to improve the health of the community.
- Community-oriented nursing practice is interdisciplinary and includes assessment, policy development, and a wide range of actions designed to provide assurance and promote healthy outcomes in a community.
- Systems models have particular usefulness for guiding education, practice, and research in nursing.
- The Neuman Systems Model can be effectively used to guide community and public health nursing education and practice.
- The Neuman Systems Model depicts an open system where people are in dynamic interaction with

the environment in regard to physiologic, psychological, sociocultural, developmental, and spiritual variables.

- The Neuman Systems Model includes primary, secondary, and tertiary intervention modes, which make it especially useful in community health.
- The Omaha System was developed and refined through a process of research. Reliability and validity were established for the entire system.
- The Omaha System is unique in that it is the only comprehensive vocabulary developed initially by and for practicing community-oriented nurses.
- The Omaha System was designed to follow specific principles. The system consists of a problem classification scheme, an intervention scheme, and a problem rating scale for outcomes.
- The Omaha System includes language and codes for nursing diagnoses, nursing interventions, and client outcomes.
- The Omaha System offers benefits in three principal areas: practice, documentation, and data management. These areas are of concern to community health educators and students as well as community health clinicians and administrators.
- The Neuman Systems Model and Omaha System are complementary systems that can be used in concert while retaining the integrity of each.

## Clinical Decision-Making Activities

1. Identify several concepts in nursing that you think are related and that guide actions. Using the concepts, try to construct a conceptual framework for your practice. Give an example of how it can be applied.
2. Debate one of these issues:
   a. Conceptual models should (should not) guide nursing practice. Be specific in your answer.
   b. Conceptual models help (hinder) community-oriented nursing practice. Illustrate what you mean.

3. Choose a clinical experience you had when you visited a family in their home, or create a fictitious family. Analyze their situation, including your nursing care plan, using the Neuman Systems Model. Does this approval make sense to you? Why?
4. Accompany an experienced home health, public health, or school health nurse on a home, clinic, or school visit. Observe and discuss whether that nurse uses a nursing diagnosis, intervention, or outcome measurement system or framework. Is it important to use a system or framework approach? Explain.
5. Work with a partner or in a small group. Select a community client whom you have visited, or invent a fictitious client. List typical referral and first-visit data. Independently apply the three parts of the Omaha System to the client data. Compare each portion of your selections with that of your partner or group members. Discuss and describe the levels of prevention that apply to the Omaha System in this case.
6. Use the Neuman Systems Model and Omaha System Intervention Scheme to prepare a data collection form. What are some of the complexities in developing such a form?

### Additional Resources

These related resources are found either in the appendix at the back of this book or on the book's website at **http://evolve.elsevier.com/Stanhope.**

**evolve** **Evolve Website**

WebLinks: Healthy People 2010

## References

American Nurses Association: *NIDSEC: recognized languages for nursing* [online], accessed Feb 2003, from http://www.nursingworld.org/nidsec/classlst.htm.

Anderko L, Kinion E: Speaking with a unified voice: recommendations for the collection of aggregated outcome data in nurse-managed centers, *Policy, Politics, Nurs Pract* 2(4):295, 2001.

Anderson E, McFarlane J, Helton A: Community-as-client: a model for practice, *Nurs Outlook* 34(5):220, 1986.

Baierschmidt C et al, editors: *International classification of diseases,* ed 5, Salt Lake City, Nev, 1996, Medicode.

Beddome G: Application of the Neuman systems model to the assessment of community-as-client. In Neuman B, editor: *The Neuman Systems Model,* ed 2, Norwalk, Conn, 1989, Appleton & Lange.

Bowles KH: Application of the Omaha system in acute care, *Res Nurs Health* 23(2):93, 2000.

Clark J, Lang N: An international classification for nursing practice, *Int Nurs Rev* 39(4):27, 109, 1992.

Clark J et al: New methods of documenting health visiting practice, *Community Practitioner* 74(3):108, 2001.

Coenen A et al: Toward comparable nursing data: American Nurses Association criteria for data sets, classification systems, and nomenclatures, *Comput Nurs* 19(6):240, 2001.

Donabedian A: Evaluating the quality of medical care, *Milbank Memorial Fund Q* 44(2):166, 1966.

Drew LJ, Craig DM, Beynon CE: The Neuman Systems Model for community health administration and practice: provinces of Manitoba and Ontario, Canada. In Neuman B, editor: *The Neuman systems model,* ed 2, Norwalk, Conn, 1989, Appleton-Lange.

Fawcett J: The structural hierarchy of nursing knowledge: components and their definitions. In King IM, Fawcett J, editors: *The language of theory and metatheory,* Indianapolis, Ind, 1997, Center Nursing Press.

Fawcett J: *Analysis and evaluation of contemporary nursing knowledge,* Philadelphia, 2000, Davis.

Freese BT, Natvig D, Douglas M: "TEAM MED," 1997 [unpublished manuscript].

Handly MJ et al: Essential activities for implementing a clinical information system in public health nursing. *J Nurs Adm* 33(1):14-16, 2003.

Johnson DE: The behavioral system model for nursing. In Parker ME, editor: *Nursing theories in practice,* New York, 2001, National League for Nursing.

Johnson M, Maas M, Moorhead S: *Nursing outcomes classification,* ed 2, St Louis, Mo, 2000, Mosby.

Johnson M et al: *Nursing diagnoses, outcomes, and interventions: NANDA, NIC, and NOC linkages,* St Louis, Mo, 2001, Mosby.

Kim HS: Theoretical thinking in nursing: problems and prospects, *Recent Adv Nurs* 2(4):106-122, 1987.

King I: *A theory for nursing: systems, concepts, process,* New York, 1981, Wiley.

Krischner CG et al, editors: *Physicians' current procedural terminology,* ed 4, Chicago, 1997, American Medical Association.

Marek KD, Rantz MJ: Aging in place: a new model for long-term care, *Nurs Adm Q* 24(3):1, 2000.

Martin KS, Norris J, Leak GK: Psychometric analysis of the problem rating scale for outcomes, *Outcomes Manag Nurs Pract* 3(1):20, 1999.

Martin KS, Scheet NJ: *The Omaha system: applications for community health nursing,* Philadelphia, 1992a, Saunders.

Martin KS, Scheet NJ: *The Omaha system: a pocket guide for community health nursing,* Philadelphia, 1992b, Saunders.

McCloskey JC, Bulechek GM, editors: *Nursing interventions classification,* ed 3, St Louis, Mo, 2000, Mosby.

Monsen KA, Martin KS: Developing an outcomes management program in a public health department. *Outcomes Manag* 6(2):62-66, 2002a.

Monsen KA, Martin KS: Using an outcomes management program in a public health department, *Outcomes Manag* 6(3):120-124, 2002b.

Neuman B, Fawcett J, editors: *The Neuman Systems Model,* ed 4, Upper Saddle River, NJ, 2002, Prentice Hall.

Neuman B, Young RJ: A model for teaching total person approach to patient problems, *Nurs Res* 21:264, 1972.

Nightingale Tracker Clinical Field Test Nurse Team: A comparison of teaching strategies for integrating information technology into clinical nursing education, *J Nurs Educ* 25(3):136, 2000.

Norbeck JS, Lindsey AM, Carrierri VL: The development of an instrument to measure social support, *Nurs Res* 30(5):264, 1981.

North American Nursing Diagnosis Association: *Nursing diagnoses: definitions, and classification 1999-2000,* Philadelphia, 1999, NANDA.

Omaha System: *On-line J Nurs Informatics,* 3(1), 1999, accessed Feb 2003, from http://www.eaa-knowledge.com/ojni.

Omaha System: Accessed Feb 2003 at http://www.omahasystem.org.

Orem D: *Nursing: concepts of practice,* ed 6, St Louis, Mo, 2001, Mosby.

Pierce AG, Fulmer TT: Application of the Neuman systems model to gerontological nursing. In Neuman B, editor: *The Neuman Systems Model,* ed 3, Stamford, Conn, 1995, Appleton-Lange.

Rogers ME: An introduction to the theoretical basis of nursing, Philadelphia, 1970, Davis.

Rogers ME: Nursing: a science of unitary man. In Riehl JP, Roy CS, editors: *Conceptual models for nursing practice,* New York, 1980, Appleton-Century-Crofts.

Roy C, Andrews HA: *The Roy adaptation model,* ed 2, Stamford, Conn, 1999, Appleton-Lange.

Saba VK et al: A nursing intervention taxonomy for home health care, *Nurs Health Care* 12(6):296, 1991.

Schoneman D: Surveillance as a nursing intervention: use in community nursing centers, *J Community Health Nurs* 19(1):33, 2002.

U.S. Department of Health and Human Services: *Healthy people 2010: understanding and improving health,* ed 2, Washington, DC, 2000, U.S. Government Printing Office.

von Bertalanffy L: *Problems of life: an evaluation of modern biological and scientific thought,* New York, 1952, Harper.

## Chapter 10

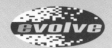
# Environmental Health

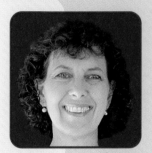

### Barbara Sattler, R.N., Dr.P.H., F.A.A.N.

Barbara Sattler is the Director of the Environmental Health Education Center at the University of Maryland School of Nursing, which houses a graduate program for nurses in environmental health and a post-master's certificate in environmental health. She is the principle investigator and co-investigator on several projects including a new Healthy Homes Initiative funded by the U.S. Department of Housing and Urban Development and, with the American Nurses Association, a continuing education initiative funded by the Environmental Protection Agency (EPA). Dr. Sattler is the principle investigator for a community outreach program for the EPA Hazardous Substance Research Center with the Johns Hopkins University Department of Geography and Environmental Engineering, in which she and staff are working with communities with concerns about hazardous waste sites. Her master's and doctorate degrees are in public health. She is a co-author of *Environmental Health and Nursing.*

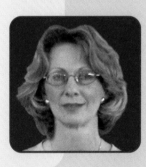

### Brenda Afzal, M.S.N., R.N.

Brenda M. Afzal has a master's degree in community/public health nursing from the University of Maryland School of Nursing. She is a project manager for the Environmental Health Education Center and is responsible for program development and outreach on issues related to environmental health advocacy, drinking water quality, the right to know, and community environmental health. Currently, using a geographic information system, she is piloting a project to investigate community environmental exposures and health outcomes experienced by clinic clients in an urban setting. She has authored a chapter about drinking water in *Environment and Health Nursing* (2002) and has co-authored continuing education materials for the American Nurses' Association on environmental health. She has been an advisory work group member of the Environmental Protection Agency's National Drinking Water Advisory Council and is an advisory member of Maryland's Governor's Commission on Environmental Justice and Sustainable Communities.

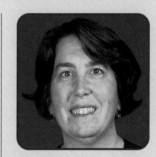

### Kathleen M. McPhaul, R.N., B.S.N., M.P.H.

Kate McPhaul, R.N., has a B.S.N. from the University of Virginia School of Nursing and an M.P.H. from the Johns Hopkins School of Public Health. She is currently a doctoral student at the University of Maryland School of Nursing. Ms. McPhaul has clinical experience directing mobile occupational health services and for 10 years (1991-2001) worked at the University of Maryland Occupational Health Project. There she directed asbestos, lead, and depleted uranium research studies, participated in teaching medical and nursing students, and coordinated outreach activities at the occupational health clinic. Ms. McPhaul has extensive experience teaching occupational/environmental health to a variety of audiences. She manages the University of Maryland School of Nursing website for environmental health and nursing, called EnviRN, and moderates the environmental health nursing list service (EH-Nurse).

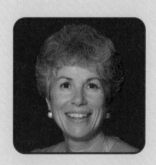

### Lillian H. Mood, R.N., M.P.H., F.A.A.N.

Lillian H. Mood is a retired public health nurse after a 30-year career with the South Carolina Department of Health & Environmental Control, where she was director of Risk Communication and Community Liaison, Environmental Quality Control, and, earlier, the assistant commissioner and state director of public health nursing. She serves as adjunct faculty for the University of South Carolina (USC) College of Nursing and the School of Public Health. She was a member of the Institute of Medicine committee that published *The Future of Public Health* (1988), chaired and co-edited an Institute of Medicine (IOM) study titled *Nursing, Health, & the Environment* (1995), and served on the IOM study to improve access to toxicology data bases (1998). She has been honored as a fellow by the American Academy of Nursing and the W. K. Kellogg Foundation, with the Order of the Palmetto from the Governor of South Carolina, the Lillian Wald Service Award from the Public Health Nursing Section of the American Public Health Association (1999), Outstanding Nurse Alumnus of the USC College of Nursing (2000), and the South Carolina Public Health Association's Outstanding Service Award (2002).

# Objectives

After reading this chapter, the student should be able to do the following:

1. Explain the relationship between the environment and human health and disease

2. Recognize the key disciplines that inform nurses work in environmental health

3. Apply the nursing process to the practice of environmental health

4. Describe legislative and regulatory policies that have influenced the impact of the environment on health and disease patterns in communities

5. Explain and compare the roles and skills for nurses practicing in the field of environmental health as well as those practicing in many other fields

6. Incorporate environmental principles in practice

# Key Terms

**agent**, p. 224
**compliance**, p. 242
**consumer confidence report**, p. 232
**enforcement**, p. 242
**environment**, p. 224
**environmental epidemiology**, p. 224
**environmental justice**, p. 242
**environmental standards**, p. 241
**epidemiologic triangle**, p. 224

**epidemiology**, p. 224
**host**, p. 224
**indoor air quality**, p. 228
**methyl mercury**, p. 243
**monitoring**, p. 241
**nonpoint sources**, p. 234
**permitting**, p. 239
**persistent bioaccumulative toxins**, p. 243

**persistent organic pollutants**, p. 243
**point sources**, p. 234
**precautionary principle**, p. 235
**right to know**, p. 232
**risk assessment**, p. 233
**risk communication**, p. 239
**toxicology**, p. 223
*See Glossary for definitions*

# Chapter Outline

Healthy People 2010 Objectives for Environmental Health
Historical context
Environmental Health Sciences
*Toxicology*
*Epidemiology*
*Multidisciplinary Approaches*
Assessment
*Environmental Exposure History*

*Environmental Health Assessment*
*The Right to Know*
*Risk Assessment*
*Assessing Risks in Vulnerable Populations: Children's Environmental Health*
**Precautionary Principle**
**Reducing Environmental Health Risks**
*Risk Communication*
*Ethics*

*Governmental Environmental Protection*
Advocacy
*Environmental Justice*
*Unique Environmental Health Threats in the Health Care Industry: New Opportunities for Advocacy*
Referral Resources
Roles for Nurses in Environmental Health

*Environmental health comprises those aspects of human health, including quality of life, that are determined by physical, chemical, biological, and social and psychological problems in the environment. It also refers to the theory and practice of assessing, correcting, controlling, and preventing those factors in the environment that can potentially affect adversely the health of present and future generations.*

From the World Health Organization draft definition, developed at WHO consultation in Sofia, Bulgaria in 1993.

Our homes, schools, workplaces, and communities are the environments in which most of us can be found at any given time. If you have children and regularly use insecticides in your home, you increase their risk of contracting leukemia. The more you use insecticides, the greater the risk of leukemia. The highest risk to the child occurs when the mother was exposed indoors to insecticides during pregnancy (Ma et al, 2002). Over 52 million homes in the United States have lead-based paint in them. Exposure to lead can cause premature births, learning disabilities in children, hypertension in adults, and other health problems. Of the top 20 environmental pollutants that were reported to the Environmental Protection Agency (EPA), nearly three quarters were known or suspected neurotoxics. This accounted for more than a billion pounds of neurotoxics being released into the air, water, and land (Goldman, 1998). Thirty million Americans drink water that exceeds one or more of the EPA's safe drinking water standards, and 50% of Americans live in an area that exceeds current national ambient air quality standards. Given such reported exposures, what is the role of community oriented nurses?

### DID YOU KNOW?

The number of waterborne outbreaks from infectious agents and chemical poisoning increased in the 1990s.

What exposures can you identify in your own home? Do you use pesticides? Does your home have lead-based paint? Is it chipping or peeling? Have you checked your home for radon, the second largest cause of lung cancer in the United States? How about our workplaces? Do we continue to use medical equipment that contains mercury, such as mercury thermometers and sphygmomanometers, which later contribute to the environmental mercury load that has contaminated fish in lakes and streams in 40 states?

*The authors wish to thank Robyn Gilden, R.N., B.S., and Laura Anderko, R.N., Ph.D., for their assistance with this chapter.*

### DID YOU KNOW?

There is a fish alert that warns pregnant women (or women who wish to become pregnant) to limit their fish consumption to one portion a week for certain fish, including tuna. Both the EPA and the Food and Drug Administration (FDA) have issued alerts because there are dangerously high amounts of mercury in these fish that create risks for the unborn child's developing nervous system. (See www.epa.gov/ost/fish or www.cfsan.fda.gov.)

Chemical, biological, and radiologic exposures contribute to health risks via the air we breathe, the water we drink, the food we eat, and the products we use. The media are alerting the public to health risks associated with food-borne illnesses, contaminated drinking water, triggers to asthma in indoor and outdoor air, and environmental threats from potential terrorists. Therefore it is critical that nurses understand how to assess the health risks posed by the environment and develop educational and other preventive interventions to help individual clients, their families, and communities understand and, when possible, decrease the risks. The National Academy of Science's Institute of Medicine (IOM) recommends that all nurses have a basic understanding of environmental health principles, and that these principles be integrated into all aspects of our practice, education, advocacy, policies, and research. This chapter explores the basic competencies recommended by the IOM (Box 10-1).

## HEALTHY PEOPLE 2010 OBJECTIVES FOR ENVIRONMENTAL HEALTH

Environmental health is one of the priority areas of the Healthy People 2010 objectives (as outlined in the Healthy People 2010 box). The federal government has long recognized the importance of the relationship between environmental risks and the underlying factors contributing to diseases.

## HISTORICAL CONTEXT

Nurses, like physicians, have been taught very little about the environment and environmental threats to health. This recognition led the IOM to evaluate the current state of environmental health knowledge and skills applied in nursing. The IOM study produced the report *Nursing, Health, and Environment* (Pope, Snyder, and Mood, 1995), which recognized early that the environment, as a determinant of health, is deeply rooted in nursing's heritage. Pictures of and quotes from Florence Nightingale are used throughout the report, not only because she is a recognized symbol of nursing but also because of the central focus of environment in her practice.

As mentioned in Chapter 2, Florence Nightingale, well known for her work in Crimea, is called by some "the mother of biostatistics" for her skilled use of data, both her

## BOX 10-1 General Environmental Health Competencies for Nurses

### BASIC KNOWLEDGE AND CONCEPTS

All nurses should understand the scientific principles and underpinnings of the relationship between individuals or populations and the environment (including the work environment). This understanding includes the basic mechanisms and pathways of exposure to environmental health hazards, basic prevention and control strategies, the interdisciplinary nature of effective interventions, and the role of research.

### ASSESSMENT AND REFERRAL

All nurses should be able to successfully complete an environmental health history, recognize potential environmental hazards and sentinel illnesses, and make appropriate referrals for conditions with probable environmental causes. An essential component is the ability to locate re-

ferral sources, access them, and provide information to clients and communities.

### ADVOCACY, ETHICS, AND RISK COMMUNICATION

All nurses should be able to demonstrate knowledge of the role of advocacy (case and class), ethics, and risk communication in client care and community intervention with respect to potential adverse effects of the environment on health.

### LEGISLATION AND REGULATION

All nurses should understand the policy framework and major pieces of legislation and regulations related to environmental health.

From Pope AM, Snyder MA, Mood LH, editors: *Nursing, health, and environment,* Washington, DC, 1995, Institute of Medicine, National Academy Press.

---

## Healthy People 2010 | Selected Objectives Related to Environmental Health

8-1 Reduce the proportion of persons exposed to air that does not meet the U.S. EPA health-based standards for harmful air pollutants

8-2 Increase use of alternative modes of transportation to reduce motor vehicle emissions and improve the nation's air quality

8-3 Improve the nation's air quality by increasing the use of cleaner alternative fuels

8-4 Reduce air toxic emissions to decrease the risk of adverse health effects caused by airborne toxicants

8-5 Increase the proportion of persons served by community water systems who receive a supply of drinking water that meets the regulations of the Safe Drinking Water Act

8-6 Reduce the waterborne disease outbreaks arising from water intended for drinking among persons served by community water systems

8-7 Reduce the per capita domestic water withdrawals

8-8 Increase the proportion of assessed rivers, lakes, and estuaries that are safe for fishing and recreational purposes

8-9 Reduce the number of beach closings that result from the presence of harmful bacteria

8-10 Reduce the potential human exposure to persistent chemicals by decreasing fish contaminant levels

8-11 Eliminate elevated blood levels of lead in children.

8-12 Minimize the risks to human health and the environment posed by hazardous sites

8-13 Reduce pesticide exposures that result in visits to a health care facility

8-14 Reduce the amount of toxic pollutants released, disposed of, treated, or used for energy recovery

8-15 Increase recycling of municipal solid waste

8-16 Reduce indoor allergen levels

From U.S. Department of Health and Human Services: *Healthy People 2010: understanding and improving health,* ed 2, Washington, DC, 2000, U.S. Government Printing Office.

---

own observations and the aggregate compilation of information, to compel action on conditions affecting health. Early in the twentieth century, Lillian Wald, who coined the term *public health nurses,* spent her life improving the environment of the Henry Street neighborhood and using her broad network of influential contacts to make changes in the physical environment and social conditions that had direct health impacts. As modern day nurses are rediscovering environmental health, they are reintegrating

many of the observations and skills that were practiced by our foremothers in nursing.

It is important to note how we began to understand the relationship between environmental chemical exposures and their potential for harm. There are several ways in which we have historically made such discoveries:

- When people present with signs and symptoms that can be connected to a specific chemical exposure. This has most commonly occurred when workers have been occupationally exposed. In such instances, the temporal and geographic relationships between the exposures and the health effects have helped to identify health hazards in the environment.

- When large, accidental releases of chemicals have occurred, contaminating the air or water in a community and resulting in health effects. When this has occurred, we have learned about the chemicals' toxicity to humans, as well as to other organisms in the environment.
- In rare instances, when human environmental (and occupational) epidemiologic studies have been performed. Through such studies, we have learned about the toxic effects of chemicals.

However, the most common way in which the relationships between chemical exposures and health risks are posited is when toxicologists study the effects of chemicals on animals and then estimate what the effects might be on humans. This estimation process is called *extrapolation*. More than 100,000 man-made (synthetic) chemical compounds have been developed and introduced to our environment since World War II, and we usually rely on the data emanating from animal studies to warn us about their potential toxicity to humans. For many of these chemicals, no toxicity data are available (Sattler and Lipscomb, 2002).

---

( NURSING TIP

"In watching diseases, both in private homes and in public hospitals, the thing which strikes the experienced observer most forcibly is this, that the symptoms or the sufferings generally considered to be inevitable and incident to the disease are very often not symptoms of the disease at all, but of something quite different—of the want of fresh air, or of light, or of warmth, or of quiet, or of cleanliness, or of punctuality and care in the administration of diet, of each or of all of these" (Nightingale, 1859, p. 8).

---

As a new millennium begins, it is important to note how radically different our environment is compared to a century ago. In addition to environmental contamination, many of the man-made chemicals can now also be found in our bodies (including breast milk) in measurable amounts. Understanding the health impacts that may be associated with these chemicals is an important part of a nurse's environmental practice.

## ENVIRONMENTAL HEALTH SCIENCES

### Toxicology

**Toxicology** is the basic science that studies the health effects associated with chemical exposures. Its corollary in health care is pharmacology, which studies the human health effects, both desirable and undesirable, associated with drugs. In toxicology, only the negative effects of chemical exposures are studied. However, the key principles of pharmacology and toxicology are the same. Just as

the dose of a drug makes the difference in its efficacy and its toxicity, the quantity of an air or water pollutant to which we may be exposed will determine whether or not we experience the risk of a health effect.

Both drugs and pollutants can enter the body by a variety of routes. Most drugs are given orally and absorbed via the gastrointestinal tract. Water- and food-associated pollutants, including pesticides and heavy metals, enter the body via the digestive tract. Some drugs are administered as inhalants, and some pollutants in the air (including indoor air) enter the body via the lungs. Some drugs are applied topically. In work settings, employees can receive dermal exposures from toxic chemicals when they immerse their unprotected hands in chemical solutions. Pollution can enter the body via the lungs (inhalation), gastrointestinal tract (ingestion), skin, and even the mucous membranes (dermal absorption). Some chemicals can cross the placental barrier and affect the fetus.

In the same way that we consider the age, weight, other drugs taken, and underlying health status of a client when we administer drugs, we must consider that these same factors may affect the way in which community members respond to environmental exposures. Because communities are composed of people of different ages and different health statuses, vulnerabilities to the effects of pollution vary. For example, children are much more vulnerable to virtually all pollutants. Similarly, immunocompromised community members are more vulnerable to food and waterborne pathogens. This includes people who are infected with the human immunodeficiency virus (HIV), who have acquired immunodeficiency syndrome (AIDS), who are taking chemotherapeutic drugs, or who are organ recipients. When assessing a community's environmental health status, it is important to review the general health status of the community to identify members who may have higher risk factors as well as to assess the environmental exposures.

The prospect of grasping and recalling all that is known about chemicals and incorporating that knowledge into practice is staggering. Fortunately, chemicals can be grouped into families, so that it is possible to understand the actions and risks associated within these groups. Examples are metals and metallic compounds (arsenic, cadmium, chromium, lead, mercury); hydrocarbons (benzene, toluene, ketones, formaldehyde, trichloroethylene); irritant gases (ammonia, hydrochloric acid, sulfur dioxide, chlorine); chemical asphyxiants (carbon monoxide, hydrogen sulfide, cyanides); and pesticides (organophosphates, carbamates, chlorinated hydrocarbons, bipyridyls).

With the ever-changing landscape of chemicals to consider, this is a time when technology is part of the solution.

---

( NURSING TIP

"Freedom from illness or injury is related to lack of exposure to toxic agents and other environmental conditions that are potentially detrimental to human health" (Pope, Snyder, and Mood, 1995, p. 3).

---

The National Library of Medicine (NLM) databases are now accessible on the internet and are increasingly user friendly. The NLM website provides access to medical databases (e.g., PubMed, GratefulMed) previously available only through professional Medline searches. The databases can be searched for possible environmental linkages to illnesses using illness and symptom search terms. The most recent public access point to the NLM toxicology databases is a website on the internet that can be accessed through the WebLinks component of this textbook's website at http://evolve.elsevier.com/Stanhope, or at www.nlm.nih.gov. Using chemical name search terms and display options of health effects, some potential environmental threats to health can be understood or ruled out.

## Epidemiology

Whereas toxicology is the science that studies the poisonous effects of chemicals, **epidemiology** is the science that helps us understand the strength of the association between exposures and health effects in human populations. Epidemiology is an applied science used in environmental health. It was through epidemiologic studies that we began to understand the association between learning disabilities and exposure to lead-based paint dust. Epidemiology has been widely employed for occupation-related illnesses.

The principles of epidemiology are covered in detail in Chapter 11 and should be reviewed and understood by community-oriented nurses. Epidemiology deals with patterns of the occurrence of diseases in people and the factors that affect the various patterns (Lilienfeld and Lilienfeld, 1980). Community-oriented nurses are well positioned to use this scientific tool to identify environmental hazards in communities, develop priorities based on dose-response data and level of risk, and evaluate hazard-control strategies.

**Environmental epidemiology** is the study of the effect on human health of physical, chemical, and biological factors in the external environment. By examining specific populations or communities exposed to different ambient environments, environmental epidemiology seeks to clarify the relationships between physical, chemical, and biological factors and human health. Environmental epidemiology explains the risk of lead poisoning, asthma exacerbation from air pollution, and waterborne outbreaks such as cryptosporidia (Goldman, 2000). Environmental surveillances, such as childhood lead registries, use epidemiologic methods to track and analyze incidences, prevalences, and health outcomes.

Three major concepts—**agent, host,** and **environment**—form the classic **epidemiologic triangle** (Figure 10-1). This simple model belies the often-complex relationships be-

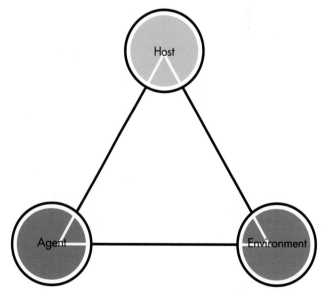

**Figure 10-1** The epidemiologic triangle. For a disease process to occur, there must be a unique combination of events (i.e., a harmful agent that comes into contact with a susceptible host in the proper environment). The occurrence of a disease can be blocked by intersecting the triangle on any of its three sides. A disease or outcome is never caused by one event but rather involves a chain of events that form a web (the epidemiologic web), which because of its complexity, may never be fully understood. *(From Cassens BJ:* Preventive medicine and public health, *ed 2, New York, 1992, John Wiley & Sons.)*

## Environmental Health in Canada

Catherine Clarke, R.N., B.Sc.N., M.N., Coordinating Manager, Toronto Public Health

### FEDERAL RESPONSIBILITIES

The two government agencies responsible for environmental health matters at the federal level are Health Canada and Environment Canada. Among other responsibilities, Human Resources Development Canada administers the Canada Labour Code, which regulates occupational health and safety requirements in areas of federal jurisdiction.

Health Canada provides national leadership in the development of health policy, the enforcement of federal health regulations, the prevention of disease and the promotion of healthy living. The Minister of Health is responsible to Parliament for administering approximately 20 health-related laws and associated regulations that govern the activities of the department. It works in collaboration with other federal departments to reduce health and safety risks to Canadians and participates in international knowledge development, surveillance, and regulatory activities. Through its administration of the Canada Health Act, Health Canada ensures that each provincial and territorial health care plan adheres to the five basic principles enshrined in the legislation:

- Universal availability to permanent residents
- Comprehensive services
- Accessibility without income barriers
- Portability within and outside the country
- Public administration

Several of Health Canada's agencies, branches, and programs deal with environmental health issues through research, technical and public education, and the development and enforcement of legislation.

- The Pest Management Regulatory Agency (www. hc-sc.gc.ca/pmra-arla) is responsible for protecting human health and the environment by minimizing risks associated with the use of pest control products through knowledge development, education, and the administration of the Pest Control Products Act.
- The Health Products and Food Branch (www. hc-sc.gc.ca/hpfb-dgpsa) is responsible for minimizing health risk factors associated with health products (medical devices and drugs, natural health products, biologics, and genetics), and food.

- The Healthy Environments and Consumer Safety Branch (www.hc-sc.gc.ca/hecs-sesc) reduces health risks posed by environmental factors such as radiation, air pollution (indoor and outdoor), and toxic substances. This branch regulates controlled substances, tobacco, and commercial and consumer chemicals, establishes workplace health and safety policies, and provides services to protect the health of the traveling public, including quarantine services.
- The Office of Children's Environmental Health (www.hc-sc.gc.ca/hecs-sesc/oceh/index.htm) has been established within this branch to act as the focal point for knowledge development about the special sensitivity of children to environmental factors and for action to reduce the risks posed by these exposures to children's health.
- The Population and Public Health Branch (www. hc-sc.gc.ca/pphb-dgspsp) has several programs that are important to environmental health, key among these being the Centre for Emergency Preparedness and Response (www.hc-sc.gc.ca/pphb-dgspsp/cepr-cmiu/index.html) and the National Microbiology Laboratory (www.nml.ca). The Centre for Emergency Preparedness and Response is a new program created to strengthen Health Canada's capacity to respond to global and public health threats including natural disasters, accidental and deliberate emergencies, and international public health risks. The National Microbiology Laboratory houses Canada's only Biological Safety Level (BSL 4) containment facility, which is one of only 15 such laboratories in the world.

Environment Canada, on the other hand, is concerned with protecting and conserving the natural environment, protecting water resources through the enforcement of International Joint Commission rules relating to boundary waters, forecasting weather, monitoring climate change, and promoting sustainable development. Climate change is acknowledged as a significant environmental problem with enormous implications for environmental and human health. Within the federal government, the Minister of the Environment and the Minister of Natural Resources co-

The views expressed in this box represent those of the writer and do not represent the views of the City of Toronto, Toronto Public Health.

---

tween *agent*, which may include chemical mixtures (i.e., more than one agent); *host*, which may refer to a community spanning different ages, genders, ethnicities, cultures, and disease states; and *environment*, which may include dynamic factors such as air, water, soil, and food as well as temperature, humidity, and wind. Limitations of environmental epidemiologic data include reliance on occupational health studies to characterize certain toxic exposures. Studies are usually per-

formed on healthy adults whose biological systems are quite different from those of neonates, pregnant women, children, the immunosuppressed, and older adults. Nevertheless, nurses need to review the epidemiologic studies of exposures of concern to their communities and use epidemiologic techniques to monitor environmental risks in communities.

Canada further explained the determinants of health in a document prepared in 1994 for the ministers of health

manage this important file. The government of Canada recently released its Climate Change Plan for Canada. In conjunction with this plan, the government of Canada has subsequently ratified the Kyoto Protocol, an international agreement developed in 1997 by more than 160 countries that established targets for reductions in the greenhouse gas emissions that contribute to global warming. Ratification of the Kyoto Protocol paves the way for the development and implementation of strategies that will produce the desired reductions of greenhouse gas emissions in Canada.

### PROVINCIAL AGENCIES

At the provincial level, Ministries of the Environment are responsible for establishing, monitoring, and enforcing requirements to protect the quality of the natural environment and encourage the efficient use and conservation of resources. Ministries of Health administer provincial health care systems that include community and public health as well as health promotion and disease prevention programs and services. They provide authority to local and regional boards of health and establish guidelines for the provision of programs and services that protect and promote health, including environmental health. Ministries of Labour set standards regarding environmental exposure levels in the workplace. All ministries administer relevant legislation, maintain databases, and publish technical and public education materials related to their areas of responsibility.

### LOCAL/REGIONAL BOARDS OF HEALTH

These agencies are responsible for enforcing local by-laws, conducting complaint investigations and risk assessments, and inspecting premises to ensure compliance with pertinent legislation. Staff are often first responders to community concerns, and liaise with, or refer to, provincial ministries responsible for monitoring and enforcement when appropriate. Their emphasis is on the provision of primary prevention strategies. The degree to which local and regional boards of health provide secondary prevention strategies, including screening and monitoring programs, varies considerably across regions and provinces.

### CANADIAN RESOURCES

There are Canadian equivalents to each of the categories listed in Box 10-14 of this chapter. The following

is a list of some specific sources of Canadian environmental health information.

**Federal**

Government of Canada (canada.gc.ca)
Government of Canada Climate Change website (climatechange.gc.ca)
Health Canada (www.hc-sc.gc.ca)
Environment Canada (www.ec.gc.ca)
Human Resources Development Canada (www.hrdc-drhc.gc.ca)

**Provincial**

Ministries of Health, Environment, Labour
Provincial public health associations

**Local/Regional**

Boards of health
Poison control centres

**Nongovernmental**

Canadian Cancer Society (www.cancer.ca)
Canadian Institute for Environmental Law and Policy (www.cielap.org)
Canadian Environmental Law Association (www.cela.ca)
Canadian Institute for Child Health (www.cich.ca)
Canadian Association of Physicians for the Environment (www.cape.ca)
Canadian Public Health Association (www.cpha.ca)
Children's Environmental Health Network (www.cehn.org)
Pollution Probe (www.pollutionprobe.org)
Learning Disabilities Association of Canada (www.ldac-taac.ca)
The Lung Association (www.lung.ca)
Toronto Cancer Prevention Coalition (www.city.toronto.on.ca/health/resources/tcpc)

**Bibliography**

Sutcliffe PA, Deber RB, Pasut G: Public health in Canada: a comparative study of six provinces, *Can J Public Health* 87(4):246, 1997.

*Canadian spelling is used.*

(Federal, Provincial, and Territorial Advisory Committee, 1994). The expanded list includes physical environments, and the report points out the necessary tools of research, information, and public policy for population health (Figure 10-2).

All of these perspectives from the past and present are reminders of the richness and necessity of the interdisciplinary nature of public health practice if a broad definition of health is the goal. To have a healthy population, we need a healthy planet. "Healing people and healing the planet are part of the same enterprise" (Roszak, 1992).

## Multidisciplinary Approaches

In addition to toxicology and epidemiology, a number of earth sciences help explain how pollutants travel in air, water, and soil. Geologists, meteorologists, and chemists

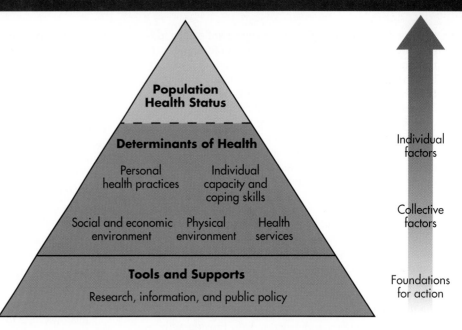

**Figure 10-2** Canadian model of determinants of health. *(From Federal, Provincial, and Territorial Advisory Committee on Population Health for Canadian Ministers of Health:* Strategies for population health: investing in the health of Canadians, *Ottawa, Ontario, 1994, Health Canada.)*

> **DID YOU KNOW?**
>
> Factors contributing to the reduction of lead levels in the United States include elimination of lead in paint, reduction of lead in gasoline, reduction in the number of manufactured food and drink cans and household plumbing components containing lead solder, lead screening laws, and lead paint abatement programs in communities.

> **DID YOU KNOW?**
>
> Dr. Claudia Smith, a community health nurse on the faculty at the University of Maryland in Baltimore, is a modern-day environmental health nursing pioneer. She is the director of a project in which community health nurses are working with community members to address a variety of health problems associated with poor housing conditions. For this project, which is funded by the U.S. Department of Housing and Urban Development, Dr. Smith has hired and trained community members to assess and reduce unhealthy conditions caused by lead-based paint, high levels of carbon monoxide, and asthma triggers (such as dust mites, pet dander, and pests), and she is teaching community members about safer choices for pest control using an integrated pest management approach.

all contribute information to help understand how and when humans may be exposed to hazardous chemicals, radiation (such as radon), and biological contaminants. The public health field also depends on food safety specialists, sanitarians, radiation specialists, and industrial hygienists.

The nature of environmental health requires a multidisciplinary approach to assess and decrease environmental health risks. For instance, to assess and address a lead-based paint poisoning case, the team might include a housing inspector with expertise in lead-based paint or a sanitarian to assess the lead-associated health risks in the home; clinical specialists to manage the clients' health needs; laboratory workers to assess lead levels in the clients' blood as well as in the paint, house dust, and drinking water; and lead-based paint remediation specialists to reduce the lead-based paint risk in the home. This approach could potentially involve the local health department, the state department of environmental protection, the housing department, a tertiary care setting, and public or private sector laboratories. A community-oriented nurse's role would be to understand the roles of each respective agency and organization, know the public health laws (particularly as they pertain to lead-based paint poisoning), and work with the community to coordinate services to address the community's needs. The nurse might also set up a blood-lead screening program through the local health department, educate local health providers to encourage them to systematically test children for lead poisoning, or work with local landlords to improve the condition of their housing stock.

## ASSESSMENT

When assessing environmental exposures, the environment can be divided into functional locations such as home, school, workplace, and community. In each of these locations, there may be unique environmental exposures as well as overlapping exposures. For instance, ethylene oxide, the toxic gas that is used in the sterilizing equipment in hospitals, would typically be found only in a workplace. However, pesticides might be found in all four areas. When assessing environments, determine whether an exposure is in the air, water, soil, or food (or a combination) and whether it is a chemical, biological, or radiologic exposure.

## HOW TO Apply the Nursing Process to Environmental Health

If you suspect that a client's health problem is being influenced by environmental factors, follow the nursing process and note the environmental aspects of the problem in every step of the process:

1. **Assessment.** Include inventories and history questions that cover environmental issues as a part of the general assessment.

2. **Diagnosis.** Relate the disease and the environmental factors in the diagnosis.

3. **Goal setting.** Include outcome measures that mitigate and eliminate the environmental factors.

4. **Planning.** Look at community policy and laws as methods to facilitate the care needs for the client; include environmental health personnel in planning.

5. **Intervention.** Coordinate medical, nursing, and public health actions to meet the client's needs.

6. **Evaluation.** Examine criteria that include the immediate and long-term responses of the client as well as the recidivism of the problem for the client.

## Environmental Exposure History

A helpful mneumonic was developed to help health professionals remember the questions to ask when taking an environmental history. Exposures may occur in any settings where people spend time; be sure to assess them all. The "I PREPARE" mneumonic can be used when interviewing an individual client or when assessing a family, or it can be adapted for use with a community (Box 10-2).

Figure 10-3 depicts various pathways by which toxic chemicals may be expressed in our environment.

## Environmental Health Assessment

A windshield survey is helpful as a first step to understanding the potential environmental health risks in a community. If the community is urban, the age and condition of the housing stock, and potential trash problems (and the associated pest problems) can be easily determined by driving around the neighborhood. Proximity to factories, dumpsites, major transportation routes, and other sources of pollution should be noted. In rural communities, the use of aerial and other types of pesticide and herbicide spraying should be noted.

To focus on the environmental health risks within a community, some specific tools are available in addition to the tools that you will use for a general community assessment. The Right to Know section (p. 233) describes the types of information that are available to the public regarding air and water emissions, drinking water quality, and other environmental sources. Additionally, Appendix I.3 is a community health assessment tool that provides an example of an environmental health assessment form with internet resources for each of the potential exposures being assessed.

## Air

The Clean Air Act regulates air pollution from both fixed sites (smokestacks) and nonpoint sources (automobiles, trucks, and buses). The EPA uses a set of pollutants ("criteria pollutants") to gauge overall air quality (Box 10-3). The greatest single source of air pollution in the United States is motor vehicles. The burning of fossil fuels (diesel, industrial boilers, and power plants) and waste incineration are two other major contributors. Health effects associated with air pollution include asthma and other respiratory diseases, cardiovascular diseases (including cardiac and hypertension), cancer, immunologic effects, reproductive health problems including birth defects, and neurologic problems.

**Indoor air quality** is a growing concern of the public, in office buildings, schools, and homes, especially because of an alarming rise in asthma incidence in the United States, particularly among children. Both the EPA and the American Lung Association provide excellent materials on indoor air quality (IAQ). The EPA has a free kit called *IAQ: Tools for Schools*, which includes a video and a number of materials helpful for people interested in improving the air quality in a school building. The major culprits contributing to poor indoor air are carbon monoxide, dusts, molds, dust mites, cockroaches, pests and pets, cleaning and personal care products (particularly aerosols), lead, and of course environmental tobacco smoke.

Because environmental health implies a relationship between the environment and health, it is important to assess both the environmental exposures and the human health status in a community. Health status is assessed using local, state, and national health data; by collecting our own data; or by a combination of the two. As we learn more about the exposures in our communities and their known or suspected health effects, health statistics can be targeted to review or collect. (Box 10-4 provides governmental, nongovernmental, and on-line resources.)

## DID YOU KNOW?

You can find out the major pollutants being released into your area (by zip code) by accessing www.scorecard.org, a website maintained by the Environmental Defense Fund, a national nonprofit organization. The data are provided by the Environmental Protection Agency.

## Water

Water is necessary for all life forms. Human bodies are 75% water. Only 2.5% of the water on this planet is freshwater, not salt water. Much of the freshwater is in the ice of the polar icecaps; groundwater makes up most of what remains, leaving only 0.01% in lakes, creeks, streams, rivers, and rainfall. Rudy Mancke, a noted naturalist, explains that because humans are not a chlorophyll-producing life form, we are simply consumers on this planet (Mancke, 1998). People's lives are inextricably tied to safe and adequate

*Text continued on p. 233*

## BOX 10-2 The "I PREPARE" Pneumonic

An exposure history should identify current and past exposures, have a preliminary goal of reducing or eliminating current exposures, and have a long-term goal of reducing adverse health effects. The "I PREPARE" mneumonic consigns the important questions to categories that can be easily remembered.

### I INVESTIGATE POTENTIAL EXPOSURES

Investigate potential exposures by asking,
- Have you ever felt sick after coming in contact with a chemical, pesticide, or other substance?
- Do you have any symptoms that improve when you are away from your home or work?

### P PRESENT WORK

At your present work,
- Are you exposed to solvents, dusts, fumes, radiation, loud noise, pesticides, or other chemicals?
- Do you know where to find material data safety sheets on the chemicals you work with?
- Do you wear personal protective equipment?
- Are work clothes worn home?
- Do co-workers have similar health problems?

### R RESIDENCE

At your place of residence,
- When was your residence built?
- What type of heating do you have?
- Have you recently remodeled your home?
- What chemicals are stored on your property?
- Where does your drinking water come from?

### E ENVIRONMENTAL CONCERNS

In your living environment,
- Are there environmental concerns in your neighborhood (i.e., air, water, soil)?
- What types of industries or farms are near your home?
- Do you live near a hazardous waste site or landfill?

### P PAST WORK

About your past work,
- What are your past work experiences?
- What is the longest job you held?
- Have you ever been in the military, worked on a farm, or done volunteer or seasonal work?

### A ACTIVITIES

About your activities,
- What activities and hobbies do you and your family engage in?
- Do you burn, solder, or melt any products?
- Do you garden, fish, or hunt?
- Do you eat what you catch or grow?
- Do you use pesticides?
- Do you engage in any alternative healing or cultural practices?

### R REFERRALS AND RESOURCES

Use these key referrals and resources:
- Environmental Protection Agency (www.epa.gov)
- National Library of Medicine, Toxnet programs (www.nlm.nih.gov)
- Agency for Toxic Substances & Disease Registry (www.atsdr.cdc.gov)
- Association of Occupational & Environmental Clinics (www.aoec.org)
- Material safety data sheets (www.hazard.com/msds)
- Occupational Safety & Health Administration (www.osha.gov)
- EnviRN website (www.enviRN.umaryland.edu)
- Local health department, environmental agency, poison control center

### E EDUCATE

Use this checklist of educational materials:
- Are materials available to educate the client?
- Are alternatives available to minimize the risk of exposure?
- Have prevention strategies been discussed?
- What is the plan for follow-up?

Prepared by Grace Paranzino, R.N., M.P.H., for the Agency for Toxic Substances and Disease Registry. For more information, contact ATSDR at 1-888-42-ATSDR, or visit ATSDR's website at ww.atsdr.cdc.gov.

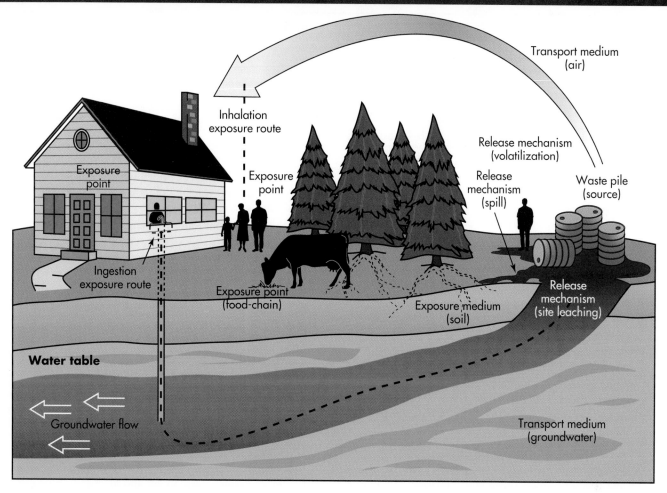

**Figure 10-3** Exposure pathways. *(From Agency for Toxic Substances and Disease Registry: Identifying and evaluating exposure pathways.* In Public health assessment guidance manual, *Atlanta, Ga, 1992, ATSDR.)*

### Evidence-Based Practice

This is a case study of childhood lead exposure in a family living at the poverty level. It is known that child lead exposure is endemic among those living in poverty and substandard housing. Children and families living along the U.S.-Mexican border experience multiple exposures to environmental hazards, especially lead. The impact of lead exposure on fetuses, infants, and children is dramatically compounded by poor nutrition, extreme poverty, inadequate access to health care, hazardous occupational exposures of other family members, social isolation, language and legal barriers,

high-risk home environments, lead-laden herbal home remedies, and medicinal and cultural practices.

In this case of Hispanic children and their families, the authors found evidence to support exposure to lead for many of the reasons listed here as well as likely exposure pathways, such as inhaling and ingesting lead-laden dust from auto repair, wire recycling, and paint chips.

**Nurse Use:** Community-oriented nurses play a key role in performing routine assessments of populations known to be at risk and providing community health services to reduce the long-term effects of lead exposure.

Amaya MA et al: Childhood lead poisoning on the US-Mexico border: a case study in environmental health nursing lead poisoning, *Public Health Nurse* 14(6):353, 1997.

## BOX 10-3  Criteria Air Pollutants (National Ambient Air Quality Standards)

- Ozone (ground level)
- Carbon monoxide
- Particulate matter
- Nitrogen dioxide
- Sulfur dioxide
- Lead

## BOX 10-4  Environmental Health Resources

### WEBSITES FOR ENVIRONMENTAL ASSESSMENTS

- The University of Maryland's School of Nursing (www.enviRN.umaryland.edu), a one-stop site for nurses interested in environmental health. All of the following linkages can be accessed from the enviRN portal.
- American Nurses' Association (www.nursingworld.org) for information on workplace health and safety and environmental health as it pertains to nursing
- *Nurses attack hidden dangers of health care* (www.nursingworld.org/tan/novdec001/pollutio.htm)
- Workplace issues, Occupational Safety and Health (www.nursingworld.org/DLWA/OSH)
- Children's environmental health (www.nursingworld. org/mods/mod250/CESAVERS.htm)
- Pollution prevention in health care (www.nursingworld. org/rnnoharm)
- U.S. Environmental Protection Agency (EPA) (www.epa.gov)
- IAQ Tool for Schools (www.epa.gov/iaq/schools); for a free copy of the EPA's IAQ Tools for Schools, call 1-800-438-4318
- Safe water (www.epa.gov/safewater); safe drinking water hotline, 1-800-426-4791
- "Surf Your Watershed" database (www.epa.gov/surf)
- Info on private wells (www.epa.gov/safewater/ pwells1.html)
- Office of Pesticides (www.epa.gov/pesticides); telephone: 703-305-5017
- National directory of IPM in schools (www.epa. gov/reg5foia/pest/matilla/ipm_dir.html)
- Children's page (www.epa.gov/children)
- EPA lead programs (www.epa.gov/lead)
- HUD lead programs (www.hud.gov/offices/lead)
- The National Lead Information Center: 1-800-424-LEAD
- National Pesticide Telecommunications Network: 1-800-858-7378
- Office of Pesticide Programs, Food Quality Protection ACT (FQPA) of 1996 (www.epa.gov/opppsps1/fqpa)
- Integrated pest management (IPM) in schools (www.epa.gov/pesticides/ipm/#fact)
- EPA software on mercury (www.epa.gov/seahome/mercury/Src/outmerc.htm)
- National Fish and Wildlife Contamination program (www.epa.gov/ost/fish)
- Heath Care Without Harm (www.noharm.org)

### RESOURCES ON ENVIRONMENTAL HEALTH RISKS ASSOCIATED WITH THE HEALTH CARE INDUSTRY

- Mercury elimination (www.noharm.org/library/docs/ SHEA_proceedings_Mercury_Elimination_White_Pap.pdf)
- Neonatal exposure to DEHP and opportunities for prevention in Europe (www.noharm.org/library/docs/ Neonatal_Exposure_to_DEHP-di-2-2ethylhexyl-phth. pdf)
- Children's Environmental Health Network (www.CEHN.org), a great on-line resource guide as well as a manual for health professionals on children's environmental health basics
- Healthy Schools Network (www.healthschools.org), great resources on school-based environmental health risk
- Center for Health, Environment and Justice (www.chej.org), excellent resources for communities that are experiencing environmental challenges
- Centers for Disease Control (CDC) National Center for Environmental Health (NCEH) (www.cdc.gov/nceh/ default.htm), provides expertise in environmental pesticide surveillance and disease outbreak investigations
- Agency for Toxic Substance Disease Registry (ATSDR) (http://atsdr1.atsdr.cdc.gov:8080/toxfaq.html), for hazardous chemical fact sheets and information on pesticides (Information Center toll-free at 1-888-422-8737 or e-mail ATSDRIC@cdc.gov)
- Preventing Harm (www.preventingharm.org), a resource and action center on children and the environment
- The American Lung Association (www.lungusa.org), good resources on reducing environmental triggers to asthma (1-800-LUNG-USA)
- Hospitals for a Healthy Environment (www.h2e-online. org); and h2e programs: Become a Partner (www. h2e-online.org/programs/partner/p_become.htm), Champion for Change Program (www.h2e-online/ programs/champion/c_desc.htm), Tools and Resources (www.h2e-online.org/tools/index.htm)
- Consumer Product Safety Council (www.cpsc.gov)

*Continued*

BOX 10-4 Environmental Health Resources—cont'd

**BOOKS AND PUBLICATIONS**

- Sattler B, Lipscomb L, editors: *Environmental health and nursing practice,* New York, 2002, Springer (http://www.springerpub.com)
- Schettler T et al: "In harm's way: toxic threats to development," a report by Greater Boston Physicians for Social Responsibility, prepared for a joint project with Clean Water, Cambridge, Mass, 2000, Physicians for Social Responsibility (http://www.igc.org/psr/pubs.htm and http://psr.igc.org)
- *An ounce of prevention: waste reduction strategies for health care facilities and guidebook for hospital waste reduction planning and program implementation,* call (800) AHA-2626
- *Preventable poisons: a prescription for reducing medical waste in Massachusetts,* call (617) 292-4821

- *The case against mercury: Rx for pollution prevention,* call (703) 548-5478
- *Guides to pollution prevention: selected hospital waste streams,* EPA publication # EPA/635/7-90/009
- *Protecting by degrees: what hospitals can do to reduce mercury pollution,* Environmental Working Group (www.ewg.org)
- Steingraber S: *Living downstream: a scientist's personal investigation of cancer and the environment,* New York, 1998, Vintage Books
- Steingraber S: *Having faith: an ecologist's journey to motherhood,* Cambridge, Mass, 2001, Perseus
- Schlosser E: *Fast food nation: the dark side of the all-American meal,* Boston, 2001, Houghton Mifflin

---

water. Water is necessary for the production of food—another essential to life. The quality of the soil is affected by its water supply, the chemicals that are intentionally added by man, and the deposition of pollutants from the air. Soil that is free from harmful contaminants and pathogens is basic to life and health.

Discharges into water bodies from industries and from wastewater treatment systems can contribute to degradation of water quality. Water quality is also affected by non-point sources of pollution, such as storm water run-off from paved roads and parking lots, erosion from clear-cut tracts of land (after timbering and mining), and run-off from chemicals added to soils such as fertilizers. The chain of potential damage continues with the additives to farm produce and to animal diets, such as antibiotics and growth hormones (which are then consumed by humans).

## THE CUTTING EDGE

Antibiotics, 17β-estradiol (an estrogen replacement hormone), and acetaminophen have been found in measurable quantities in U.S. streams.

### Food

Food and food production continue to be a source of concern. In recent years, food-borne illnesses have been associated with *Salmonella* and *Escherichia coli* H:057 in chicken, eggs, and hamburger. Good food preparation practices, such as washing and adequate cooking temperature and time, can prevent food-borne illnesses associated with most pathogens. Other food worries include the presence of pesticides in food, bovine growth hormones (given to dairy cows), low-level antibiotics (given to beef cattle, pigs, and chickens), irradiation of food, and the emerging use of genetically modified organisms and genetically engineered crops.

## The Right to Know

Several environmental statutes have been promulgated to give the public the right to know about hazardous chemicals in the environment. Under one of the **right to know** laws, health professionals and community members are permitted to access, by zip code, information regarding major sources of pollution being emitted into the air or water in their community. The EPA has an Envirofacts section on their website that provides data on sources of exposure.

When a community is provided drinking water by a water supplier (as opposed to individual wells), the water provider is responsible for testing the water according to EPA standards. The results of their testing are required to be reported to those who purchase the water, in the form of a **consumer confidence report.** Community-oriented nurses should review consumer confidence reports, sometimes referred to as right-to-know reports, to determine what pollutants have been found in the drinking water. If there is an immediate health threat posed by the drinking water, the water provider must send emergency warnings to the community via the local newspapers, radio, and television. The Freedom of Information Act is a federal law that allows citizens to request public documents.

### WHAT DO YOU THINK?

Access to information about the existence of toxic substances leaching into the water table of a community should be withheld from the public until the government completes negotiations with the party responsible for the toxic substance.

Robyn Gilden is a modern-day environmental health nursing pioneer. She is a community health nurse and manager for a new outreach program to work with communities who suspect or know that they are living near a hazardous waste site. She has become knowledgeable about the many laws and agencies that are involved in hazardous waste site assessments and cleanups. Hazardous wastes can impact our soil, water, and air. Sources of contamination may come from old, unlined landfills, uncontrolled dumpsites, spills or discharges from industry, or runoff from fields, just to name a few. The Agency for Toxic Substances and Disease Registry (ATSDR), a federal agency responsible for documenting the health hazards associated with environmental exposures, maintains a listing of the most serious contaminants found at polluted sites. They include arsenic, lead, mercury, vinyl chloride, benzene, polychlorinated biphenyls, cadmium, benzo[a]pyrene, polycyclic aromatic hydrocarbons, and benzo[b]fluoranthene. These toxicants top the list because they are the most commonly found contaminants and cause a significant threat to human health on the basis of routes of exposure and level of toxicity. Robyn has been busy learning about the resources that are available for her to access the best and most current toxicologic information. She relies heavily on the National Library of Medicine's Toxnet website and the web-site of the Agency for Toxic Substances and Disease Registry (www.atsdr.cdc.gov).

In working with communities, Robyn finds herself in meetings with government officials, including mayors of small towns, as well as with concerned parents, people from local governments, health departments, educational institutions, businesses, developers, bankers, realtors, and other community members. She has become knowledgeable about the many statutes that cover hazardous waste sites, such as the Superfund legislation (which covers our most polluted waste sites) and Brownfields legislation (which covers contaminated sites where economic development is involved). Both of these pieces of legislation mandate community involvement, which is where her skills come into play. Regardless of who is responsible for or in charge of a site, Robyn understands that the community must be an active and equal participant. It is the community who will be impacted by decisions and have to live with the results of cleanup and redevelopment.

As is true of most nurses, Robyn quickly became a trusted person to the community members. She has created an informational website for her new program (www.jhu.edu/hsrc), which includes an excellent set of frequently asked questions about waste sites and community involvement.

Employees have the right to know about hazardous chemicals with which they work through the federal Hazard Communication Standard. This standard requires employers (including hospitals) to maintain a list of all hazardous chemicals used on site. Each of these chemicals should have an associated chemical information sheet, known as a material safety data sheet, which is written by the chemical manufacturer. These safety sheets, available to any employee or their representative, should provide information about the chemical makeup, the health risks, and any special guidance on safe use and handling (such as requirements for protective gloves or respiratory protection). This standard is enforced by the Occupational Safety and Health Administration (OSHA) (see www.osha.org).

## Risk Assessment

Currently, the EPA uses a process called risk assessment when they develop health-based standards. The term **risk assessment** refers to a process to determine the probability of a health threat associated with an exposure. The following illustration describes the four phases of a risk assessment related to chemical exposures. First, access toxicologic and/or epidemiologic data to learn if a chemical is known to be associated with negative health effects (in animals or humans). Remember, the available toxicologic data will probably be based on animal studies (from which the potential effects on humans are estimated), whereas the results of the epidemiologic studies will be for human health effects.

Second, determine if the chemical has been released into the environment via the air, water, soil, or food. This is accomplished by testing for the presence of the suspected chemical in the various media (air, water, soil, food). Environmental professionals—for example, sanitarians, food inspectors, air and water pollution scientists, and environmental engineers—might be involved in this phase. When doing a risk assessment, it is important to note if there are multiple sources of the chemical in question. For example, is lead found in the drinking water, the ambient air, *and* in the paint within the houses of a given community?

The third phase is to estimate how much of the chemical might enter the human body, and by which route. This estimate can be based on a one-time exposure, a short-term exposure, or a projected lifetime exposure. Federal standards created for air, water, and other pollutants are based on an estimation of a lifetime exposure. However, in workplace settings, the chemical exposure standards are based on an average exposure during a typical work shift, or they are set for a maximum exposure at any given time.

Pollution sources are characterized as **point sources** or **nonpoint sources.** A point-source pollutant is released into the environment from a single site, such as a smoke stack, a hazardous waste site, or an effluent pipe into a waterway. A nonpoint source of pollution is more diffuse—for example, traffic, fertilizer, or pesticide runoff into waterways (whether from large-scale farming operations or from individual lawns and gardens). Another nonpoint source is animal waste, from wildlife or confined animal operations for food production (e.g., swine and poultry), that can get into nearby water bodies, resulting in coliform contamination and nutrient overload. The result can be illness from ingestion of contaminated water and the creation of conditions amenable to growth of toxic algae such as *Pfiesteria piscicida* (SC Task Group on Toxic Algae, 1998).

The final stage of the risk assessment process takes into account all three of the previous steps: Is the chemical toxic? What is the source and amount of the exposure? and What is the route and duration of the exposure for humans? The final synthesis attempts to predict the potential for harm on the basis of the estimated exposure. Like all science, risk assessment is subject to interpretation. In translating the risk assessment results for the purposes of policy development and recommendations for risk reduction activities, there are often several interpretations for each risk assessment step, and the result is different recommendations. Furthermore, areas of scientific uncertainty contribute to variations in assessment of risk. Also, environmental laws are often contentious because there are economic interests at stake and not just public or ecologic health concerns.

## Assessing Risks in Vulnerable Populations: Children's Environmental Health

A number of indicators show that problems in child development are on an upward trend. In the United States, 17% of our children suffer from one or more developmental disabilities (Boyle, Decoufle, and Yeargin-Allsopp, 1994). Learning disabilities alone may affect 5% to 10% of children in public schools (American Psychiatric Association, 1994). In the United States, 1.5 million children are taking Ritalin, 1% of all children are mentally retarded, and the increase in the prevalence of autism is up 200% in the last two decades. Although chemical pollutants probably do not account entirely for this trend, the scientific evidence that they make a contribution is strong.

In childhood cancer, the good news is that there are mounting successes in treatment; however, the very bad news is that childhood cancer rates appear to be increasing at a rate of 10% each year (Schmidt, 1998). Leukemia and tumors of the central nervous system, combined, account for approximately 50%. The list of possible causes of children's cancer includes genetic abnormalities, ultraviolet and ionizing radiation, electromagnetic fields, viral infections, certain medications, food additives, tobacco, alcohol, and industrial and agricultural chemicals (Schmidt, 1998). Clearly, the environment is playing an important role.

### WHAT DO YOU THINK?

When choosing a site for a school, should the government require the same environmental assessment of the land as it would if a commercial enterprise were being placed on the same site? (Currently, it requires less stringent environmental assessments.)

Children are not just little adults with regard to their responses to environmental exposures. As nurses, we know that infants and young children breathe more rapidly than adults. This increased respiratory rate translates to a proportionally greater exposure to air pollutants. While infants' lungs are developing, they are particularly susceptible to environmental toxicants. Because children are short, their breathing zones are lower than those of adults, so they have closer contact to the chemical and biological agents that accumulate on floors and carpeting.

### DID YOU KNOW?

Children's ability to readily absorb calcium and other nutrients is important for their growing bodies. But this mechanism also enhances the uptake of unwanted chemicals such as lead and other heavy metals.

Children's bodies also operate differently. Some protective mechanisms that are well developed in the adults, such as the blood–brain barrier, are immature in young children, making them more vulnerable to the effects of toxic chemicals. And finally, the kidneys of young children are less effective at filtering out undesirable, toxic chemicals, which then continue to circulate and accumulate.

Infants and young children drink more fluids per kilogram of body weight than adults, thus increasing their dose of contaminants found in their drinking water, milk (hormones and antibiotics), and juices (particularly pesticides). (To drink an amount equivalent to an infant's intake, an adult would have to drink about 50 glasses of water a day.) Children also eat more per kilogram of body weight than adults, and they eat different proportions of food and absorb it differently (Bucubalis and Balisitreri, 1997). How many adults could eat the same amount of raisins pound-for-pound as the average 2-year-old? Children consume more fruits and fruit juices than adults, once again adding exposure to pesticide residues. In proportion to body weight, the average infant consumes 15 to 17 times more apple juice than the national average (National Research Council, 1993).

Toxic chemicals can have different effects depending on the timing of exposure (Table 10-1). During fetal development, there are periods of exquisite sensitivity to the effects of toxic chemicals. During such times, even extraordinarily small exposures can prevent or change a process that may permanently affect normal development. The brain undergoes rapid structural and functional changes during late pregnancy and in the neonatal period.

### DID YOU KNOW?

Developmental toxicants such as lead, mercury, and pesticides (all found in hospitals and their waste streams) may directly interfere with processes required for normal brain development.

**TABLE 10-1  Environmental Agents Implicated in Adverse Reproductive Outcomes**

| EXPOSURE | KNOWN/SUSPECTED EFFECT |
|---|---|
| Anesthetic compounds | Infertility, spontaneous abortion, fetal malformations, low birthweight |
| Antineoplastics | Infertility, spontaneous abortion |
| Dibromochloropropane | Sperm abnormalities, infertility |
| Ionizing radiation | Infertility, microcephaly, chromosomal abnormalities, childhood malignancies |
| Lead | Infertility, spontaneous abortion, developmental disabilities |
| Manganese | Infertility |
| Organic mercury | Developmental disabilities, neurologic abnormalities |
| Organic solvents | Congenital malformations, childhood malignancies |
| CBs, PBBs | Fetal mortality, low birthweight, congenital abnormalities, developmental disabilities |

From Aldrich T, Griffith J: *Environmental epidemiology and risk assessment,* New York, 1993, Van Nostrand Reinhold.

Therefore, it is extremely important to safeguard women's environments when they are pregnant.

Alarmingly, 10 states have issued mercury contamination advisories for fish in *every* lake and river within their borders. According to the EPA, over 1 million women in the United States of childbearing age eat sufficient amounts of mercury-contaminated fish to risk damaging brain development of their children. Nurses in all settings need to understand the implications that the fish advisories have for their clients and communities, and the contribution that the health sector has made in creating these advisories, while counseling on the positive contribution of fish to a nutritionally balanced diet.

Of the tens of thousands of synthetic chemicals that are in air, water, food, workplaces, and products, 75% have undergone little or no toxicity testing. As of December 1998, only 12 chemicals had complete tests for developmental neurotoxicity at the EPA (Schettler et al, 2000). Companies are not required to divulge all the results of their private testing. A full battery of neurotoxicity tests is not required even for pesticides that may be sprayed in nurseries and labor and delivery areas of hospitals, not to mention in our homes. To make things even more complicated, risks from multiple chemical exposures are rarely considered when regulations are drafted. Such an omission ignores the reality that children (as well as adults) are exposed to many toxic chemicals, often concurrently. The only exception to this rule is in the case of regulations regarding pesticides that are used on food supplies. This new exception was created by the 1996 Food Quality Protection Act, in which Congress acknowledged that children eat foods that may be contaminated by more than one pesticide residue (Box 10-5).

## PRECAUTIONARY PRINCIPLE

With thousands of chemical compounds now creating a chemical soup in air and water (in our bodies, in our breast milk), it is increasingly difficult to prove a relationship between exposure to a single chemical and disease outcome in humans. It has been suggested that we adopt a precautionary approach when animal research or other indicators demonstrate a possible toxic relationship between a chemical and a health effect. The Wingspread statement on the **precautionary principle** (Box 10-6) calls for action to reduce potentially toxic exposure to humans in light of data or other indicators, rather than delaying until more conclusive studies are performed. Nurses are trained in disease prevention and can appreciate and should advocate for a precautionary approach when it may prevent injuries or illnesses.

The bottom line is that life depends on the environment, and what humans do collectively affects that vital resource for present and future generations. A central concept in Native American cultures is that humans are stewards, not proprietors, of the environment. Native Americans make the "Rule of Seven" central to all environmental decisions: What will be the effect on the seventh generation? A quote attributed to Chief Seattle, a nineteenth-century Native American, illustrates the need to think more holistically when we consider environmental impacts: "Whatever befalls the earth befalls the sons of the earth. Man did not weave the web of life; he is merely a strand in it. Whatever he does to the web, he does to himself."

Mary O'Brien, in her book *Making Better Environmental Decisions: Alternatives to Risk Assessments,* offers the observation that people are repeatedly given a short list of risk reduction choices, and that the public is not effectively engaged in the decision-making process. She suggests that a broader range of options would allow us to see the possibilities for further reducing (or even eliminating) risks, and that the process should be much more democratic in nature. O'Brien recommends that we "simultaneously employ information and emotion and a sense of relationship to others—other species, other cultures, and other generations" (O'Brien, 2000). Her method rings true for a nursing-based approach. But employing her approach will require that nurses more actively engage in

## BOX 10-5    Food Quality Protection Act of 1996

New provisions under the Food Quality Protection Act are related to protection of infants and children from pesticide exposure from multiple sources:

- **Health-based standard:** A new standard of a reasonable certainty of "no harm" that prohibits taking into account economic considerations when children are at risk
- **Additional margin of safety:** Requires that the EPA use an additional 10-fold margin of safety when there are adequate data to assess prenatal and postnatal developmental risks
- **Account for children's diet:** Requires the use of age-appropriate estimates of dietary consumption in establishing allowable levels of pesticides on food to account for children's unique dietary patterns
- **Account for all exposures:** In establishing acceptable levels of a pesticide on food, the EPA must ac-

count for exposures that may occur through other routes, such as drinking water and residential application of the pesticide

- **Cumulative impact:** The EPA must consider the cumulative impacts of all pesticides that may share a common mechanism of action
- **Tolerance reassessments:** All existing pesticide food standards must be reassessed over a 10-year period to ensure that they meet the new standards to protect children
- **Endocrine disruption testing:** The EPA must screen and test all pesticides and pesticide ingredients for estrogen effects and other endocrine disruptor activity
- **Registration renewal:** Establishes a 15-year renewal process for all pesticides to ensure that they have up-to-date scientific evaluations over time

From Environmental Protection Agency, Office of Pesticide Programs (http://www.epa.gov/oppfead1/fqpa).

## BOX 10-6    Wingspread Statement on the Precautionary Principle

In 1998, an international group of health and public health professionals, scientists, government officials, lawyers, grassroots activists, and labor activists met at a conference center called Wingspread in Wisconsin to define the "precautionary principle." The group issued the following consensus statement:

"The release and use of toxic substances, the exploitation of resources, and physical alterations of the environment have had substantial unintended consequences affecting human health and the environment. Some of these concerns are high rates of learning deficiencies, asthma, cancer, birth defects and species extinctions, along with global climate change, stratospheric ozone depletion and worldwide contamination with toxic substances and nuclear materials.

"We believe existing environmental regulations and other decisions, particularly those based on risk assessment, have failed to protect adequately human health and the environment the larger system of which humans are but a part.

"We believe there is compelling evidence that damage to humans and the worldwide environment is of such

magnitude and seriousness that new principles for conducting human activities are necessary.

"While we realize that human activities may involve hazards, people must proceed more carefully than has been the case in recent history. Corporations, government entities, organizations, communities, scientists and other individuals must adopt a precautionary approach to all human endeavors.

"Therefore, it is necessary to implement the Precautionary Principle: When an activity raises threats of harm to human health or the environment, precautionary measures should be taken even if some cause and effect relationships are not fully established scientifically. In this context the proponent of an activity, rather than the public, should bear the burden of proof.

"The process of applying the Precautionary Principle must be open, informed and democratic and must include potentially affected parties. It must also involve an examination of the full range of alternatives, including no action."

Available at http://www.gdrc.org/u-gov/precaution-3.html.

both assessing environmental health risks and developing risk-reduction strategies.

## REDUCING ENVIRONMENTAL HEALTH RISKS

As in every public health intervention, reducing risk with prevention strategies has significant value (Box 10-7). Preventing problems is less costly, whether the cost is mea-

sured in resources consumed or health effects. Education is a primary preventive strategy. When examining the sources of environmental health risks in communities and planning intervention strategies, it is important to apply the basic principles of disease prevention. For a home with lead-based paint, apply the primary prevention strategy of removing that specific source of lead (Box 10-8). Good surveillance, a secondary prevention strategy, will not prevent

## BOX 10-7    Risk Reduction: Everyone's Role in Protecting the Environment

Everyone has a role in protecting the environment. The decisions and choices that we make as individuals and as a society can have a profound effect on the health of our environment. Our individual choices to drive versus use public transportation and our societal choice to invest in public transportation can significantly affect our air quality, which can quickly affect our collective health status. In Atlanta, during the 1996 Olympics, residents of Atlanta and the surrounding area were encouraged to either work from home or take public transportation on the days that the Olympic Games were engaged. This resulted in a significant drop in emergency room visits for asthma, because there was less car-related pollution. There are many options for reducing car-related air pollution: we can take public transportation, choose cars that pollute less, add an additional tax to polluting cars (thus creating a disincentive for purchasing them), create a tax incentive to encourage car manufacturers to make cars that pollute less (and encourage consumers to buy them), encourage flexible work policies that allow people to work at home when possible, and build adequate sidewalks and paths in communities to encourage walking and biking. Each of these is a risk management choice. Similar options could be described for water protection or the promotion of healthy indoor environments in buildings such as schools.

## BOX 10-8    Levels of Prevention Related to the Environment

### PRIMARY PREVENTION

To prevent lead poisoning, instruct families to not use lead-based paint. If such paint has been used, instruct them in removing it and repainting with a non–lead-based paint.

### SECONDARY PREVENTION

Identify any household members who have a rising blood lead level.

### TERTIARY PREVENTION

Initiate treatment for lead poisoning that will reduce blood lead levels.

## BOX 10-9    Industrial Hygiene Controls

- Substitute less hazardous or nonhazardous substances for hazardous ones (e.g., use water-based products instead of solvent-based)
- Isolate the hazardous chemicals from human exposure (closed systems)
- Apply engineering controls (such as ventilation systems, including exhausts)
- Reduce the exposures through administrative controls (rotating employees)
- Utilize personal protective equipment (gloves, respirators, protective clothing)
- Educate employees about controls

Levy B, Wegman D: *Occupational health: recognizing and preventing work-related disease and injury,* ed 4, Philadelphia, 2000, Lippincott Williams & Wilkins.

## BOX 10-10    The Three R's for Reducing Environmental Pollution

The three R's adage of the environmentalist community—**reduce, reuse,** and **recycle**—helps us to consider ways to decrease our impact on the environment and thereby decrease environmental health risks. By *recycling,* we limit the need to extract more raw materials from the earth to manufacture new products. Choosing *reusable* products, instead of one-time-use products that are thrown away, limits the need to manufacture more products and decreases the waste stream. *Reducing* consumption reduces our waste stream as well as unnecessary packaging and other nonessentials.

lead exposure, but it may help with early identification of rising blood lead levels. For a symptomatic child brought to a health care provider, a system should be in place for immediate care provided by specialists familiar with lead poisoning; swift medical interventions to reduce blood levels of lead can reduce the risk of further harm. This might be a tertiary prevention response.

For workplace exposures, industrial hygienists have developed a list of precautions for avoiding or minimizing employee exposures to potentially hazardous chemicals. Industrial hygienists are public health professionals who specialize in workplace exposures to hazards-physical, chemical, and biological—that create conditions of health risk (Box 10-9). Once we have established that a human health threat exists, we must develop a plan of action to eliminate or manage (reduce) the risk. Risk management, which should be informed by the risk assessment process, involves the selection and implementation of a strategy to reduce risks, and this can take many forms (Box 10-10). For example, to reduce the risk from exposure to ultraviolet rays, people need to avoid being outside during peak sun hours, wear protective clothing, and/or wear sunblock. To reduce exposure to dangerous heavy metals, special processes can be employed at the water filtration plant that supplies the public water. In the home, running the cold water tap for 1 or 2 minutes each morning before collecting water for coffee or drinking will reduce the presence of lead that may have leached from old pipes (or the solder used on

---

**BOX 10-11   Definitions of Risk**

Risk has traditionally been defined by the following equation:

$$Risk = magnitude \times probability.$$

However, there is a growing body of literature from practitioners and researchers who have studied the human reaction to risk, real and perceived. Sandman, Chess, and Hane (1991) have written and spoken extensively on the factors related to risk that produce public "outrage." They propose a different formula for risk:

$$Risk = hazard + outrage.$$

Addressing only the hazard is doing only half of the necessary work; addressing the response (outrage) is equally important.

From Sandman PM, Chess C, Hane BJ: *Improving dialogue with communities,* New Brunswick, NJ, 1991, Rutgers University.

---

**BOX 10-12   Outrage Factors: Characteristics of Risk That Contribute to the Public's Feeling of Outrage**

**TWELVE PRINCIPAL OUTRAGE COMPONENTS**

| Safer (less outrage) | Less safe (more outrage) |
|---|---|
| Voluntary | Involuntary (coerced) |
| Natural | Industrial (artificial) |
| Familiar | Exotic |
| Not memorable | Memorable |
| Not dreaded | Dreaded |
| Chronic | Catastrophic |
| Knowable (detectable) | Unknowable (undetectable) |
| Controlled by the individual | Controlled by others |
| Fair | Unfair |
| Morally irrelevant | Morally relevant |
| Trustworthy sources | Untrustworthy sources |
| Responsive process | Unresponsive process |

**EIGHT SECONDARY OUTRAGE COMPONENTS**

| Safer (less outrage) | Less safe (more outrage) |
|---|---|
| Affects average populations | Affects vulnerable populations |
| Immediate effects | Delayed effects |
| No risk to future generations | Substantial risk to future generations |
| Victims statistical | Victims identifiable |
| Preventable | Not preventable (only reducible) |
| Substantial benefits | Few benefits (foolish risk) |
| Little media attention | Substantial media attention |
| Little opportunity for collective action | Much opportunity for collective action |

---

them) overnight. Reduction of risk can be accomplished not only by individuals and communities but also by nations. In recent years, there have been global agreements to reduce persistent pollutants and decrease global warming.

Nursing interventions to reduce environmental health risks can also take many forms. A prime mode of action is education. By working with an array of community members, nurses can further an understanding of the relationship between harmful environmental exposures and human health and guide the community toward risk reduction based on both individual behavior changes and community-wide approaches.

## Risk Communication

Risk is a familiar term in nursing practice. We counsel about risks of pregnancy, communicable disease (especially sexually transmitted disease), unintentional injury, and personal health-related choices (such as smoking, alcohol consumption, and diet). Risk assessment in environmental health has focused on characterizing the hazard (i.e., the source), its physical and chemical properties, its toxicity, and the presence of (or potential for) other elements in the exposure pathway—mode of transmission, route of exposure, receptor population, and dose. Risk has traditionally been formulated as magnitude (the size, severity, extent of area, or population affected) multiplied by the probability of occurrence (Sandman, Chess, and Hane, 1991) (Box 10-11). For example, an environmental risk assessment of a contaminated site includes a calculation of the dose that might be received through all routes of exposure, the toxicity of the chemical, the size and vulnerability (age, health) of the population potentially exposed (resident, future resident, transient), and the likelihood of exposure.

Sandman, Chess, and Hane (1991) noted that, in their experience, the reaction to things that scare people and the things that kill people are often not related to the actual hazard. They have gone further to probe what is behind those differences and identified a list of 20 "outrage" factors to explain people's responses to risk (Box 10-12). They maintain that the outrage is just as predictable and open to intervention as the science of addressing the hazard.

Communication of risk is both an area of practice and a skill. It involves understanding the outrage factors relevant to the risk being addressed so that both can be incorporated in the message, with the result that either action is taken to ensure safety or unnecessary fear is reduced. An example of raising outrage to produce action can be seen in the shift from emphasis on smokers (voluntary) to victims of passive smoking (involuntary) to stimulate public policy that limits or bans smoking in public places. When the emphasis on risk went from a voluntary choice of smokers to an involuntary exposure of nonsmokers, the outrage level of the nonsmoking public became high enough to result in legislation guaranteeing smoke-free public spaces (e.g., public buildings, airplanes, and restaurants) (see the Evidence-Based Practice box about smoking).

On the other hand, outrage diminishes when people get information about a situation from a trusted source, and doctors and nurses are often cited in surveys as trusted sources of information on environmental risks (University of South Carolina, 1990). The public trust is a compelling incentive to match professional knowledge and skills to a community's expectations. The outrage factor can also be a driving force for building credibility and trustworthiness in every person whose work involves interacting with the public.

**Risk communication** includes all the principles of good communication in general. It is a combination of the following:

- The right information: accurate, relevant, and in a language that audiences can understand. A good risk assessment is essential information for shaping the message.
- To the right people: those affected and those who may not be affected but are worried. Information about the community is essential: the geographic boundaries, who lives there (demographics), how they get information (flyers or newspapers, radio, television, word of mouth), where they get together (school, church, community center), and who within the community can help plan the communication.
- At the right time: for timely action or to allay fear.

## Ethics

Understanding ethics is essential for nurses making their own choices, in describing issues and options within groups, and in advocating for ethical choices. When the sticking points are around competing commodities, such as jobs versus environmental protection, or production versus conservation, the skillful nurse can change the discussion from "either/or" to "both" by opening new possibilities for ethical and mutually satisfactory outcomes. Ethical issues likely to arise in environmental health decisions are as follows:

- Who has access to information and when?
- How complete and accurate is the available information?
- Who is included in decision making and when?
- What and whose values and priorities are given weight in decisions?
- How are short- and long-term consequences considered?

## Governmental Environmental Protection

The federal government is involved with many major pieces of environmental legislation (Box 10-13). The government manages environmental exposures through the promulgation and enforcement of standards and regulations that limit a polluter's ability to put hazardous chemicals into our food, water, air, or soil. The government may

also be involved in educating the public about risks and risk reduction. Several federal agencies are involved in environmental health regulation, including the Environmental Protection Agency, the Food and Drug Administration, and the Department of Agriculture. In every state, an equivalent state agency exists as well. At the city or county level, environmental health issues are most often managed by the local health department. However, environmental protection issues are typically directed by the state using both federal and state laws. There is some variation among states in the organization and approach to environmental protection, but the common essential strategies of prevention and control via the permitting process, establishment of environmental standards, and monitoring, as well as compliance and enforcement, are found in every state.

Potentially harmful pollution that cannot be prevented must be controlled. The first step in the process of controlling pollution is **permitting,** a process by which the government places limits on the amount of pollution emitted into the air or water. Industries and businesses whose processes will result in releases (discharges, emissions) that have the potential for harm are required to obtain environmental permits to construct and operate. A range of permits may be required (e.g., storm water control, construction, operations for air and wastewater discharges, and waste management). It is in the permitting process that maximum opportunities to incorporate prevention strategies can be exercised. For example, waste minimization can be included as a permit condition, with the agreement of the industry, even if it is not required by a law or regulation. Once a condition exists in the permit, it has the force of law.

The permitting process includes submission of an application, which requires details on the proposed operation. Plans are studied, engineering processes are modeled and validated, and other technical requirements are reviewed by appropriate regulatory experts. Usually some form of public participation is required or included voluntarily. The public involvement can include public notice, public comment, and public meetings and hearings initiated by the regulatory agency. Public involvement can also take the form of voluntary agreements and dispute resolution between the industry and the community, which may or may not involve a government entity. Limits on what an industry or business can release or emit lawfully are based on environmental standards.

**Environmental standards** may be expressed as a permitted level of emissions, a maximum contaminant level (MCL) allowed, an action level for environmental cleanup, or a risk-based calculation. A standard often reflects the level of pollution that will limit a number of excess deaths at a given level of exposure over a specified period of time. For example, the MCL for a contaminant in drinking water may be the level of exposure that would produce one excess (over the expected rate) cancer death if a person drank 1 liter of the water a day for 70 years.

## BOX 10-13 Environmental Laws

### NATIONAL ENVIRONMENTAL POLICY ACT

The National Environmental Policy Act (NEPA) established the EPA and a national policy for the environment and provides for the establishment of a Council on Environmental Policy. All policies, regulations, and public laws shall be interpreted and administered in accordance with the policies set forth in this act.

### FEDERAL INSECTICIDE, FUNGICIDE, AND RODENTICIDE ACT

The Federal Insecticide, Fungicide, and Rodenticide Act (FIFRA) provides federal control of pesticide distribution, sale, and use. EPA was given the authority to study the consequences of pesticide usage and requires users such as farmers and utility companies to register when using pesticides. Later amendments to the law required applicators to take certification exams, registration of all pesticides used in the United States, and proper labeling of pesticides that, if in accordance with specifications, will cause no harm to the environment. (Summary from FIFRA 1972)

### CLEAN WATER ACT

The Clean Water Act (CWA) sets basic structure for regulating pollutants to U.S. waters. The law gave the EPA authority to set effluent standards on an industry basis and continued the requirements to set water quality standards for all contaminants in surface water. The 1977 amendments focused on toxic pollutants. In 1987 the CWA was reauthorized, and again focused on toxic pollutants, authorized citizen suit provisions, and funded sewage treatment plants.

### CLEAN AIR ACT

The Clean Air Act regulates air emissions from area, stationary, and mobile sources. The EPA was authorized to establish National Ambient Air Quality Standards (NAAQS) to protect public health and the environment. The goal was to set and achieve the NAAQS by 1975. The law was amended in 1977 when many areas of the country failed to meet the standards. The 1990 amendments to the Clean Air Act intended to meet unaddressed or insufficiently addressed problems, such as acid rain, ground-level ozone, stratospheric ozone depletion, and air toxics. Also in the 1990 reauthorization, a mandate for chemical risk management plans was included. This mandate requires industry to identify worst-case scenarios regarding the hazardous chemicals that they transport, use, or dispose of. (Summary from Clean Air Act 1970)

### OCCUPATIONAL SAFETY AND HEALTH ACT

The Occupational Safety and Health Act (OSHA) was passed to ensure worker and workplace safety. The goal was to make sure employers provide an employment place free of hazards to health and safety, such as chemicals, excessive noise, mechanical dangers, heat or cold extremes, and unsanitary conditions. To establish standards for the workplace, OSHA also created the National Institute for Occupational Safety and Health (NIOSH) as the research institution for OSHA.

### SAFE DRINKING WATER ACT

The Safe Water Drinking Act (SDWA) was established to protect the quality of drinking water in the United States. SDWA authorized the EPA to establish safe standards of purity and required all owners or operators of public water systems to comply with primary (health-related) standards.

### RESOURCE CONSERVATION AND RECOVERY ACT

The Resource Conservation and Recovery Act (RCRA) gave the EPA the authority to control the generation, transportation, treatment, storage, and disposal of hazardous waste. The RCRA also set forth a framework to manage nonhazardous waste. The 1984 Federal Hazardous and Solid Waste amendments to this Act required phasing out land disposal of hazardous waste. The 1986 amendments enabled the EPA to address problems of underground tanks storing petroleum and other hazardous substances.

### TOXIC SUBSTANCES CONTROL ACT

The Toxic Substances Control Act (TSCA) gives the EPA the ability to track the 75,000 industrial chemicals currently produced or imported into the United States. The EPA can require reporting or testing of chemicals that may pose environmental health risks and can ban the manufacture and import of those chemicals that pose an unreasonable risk. The TCSA supplements the Clean Air Act and the Toxic Release Inventory.

### COMPREHENSIVE ENVIRONMENTAL RESPONSE, COMPENSATION, AND LIABILITY ACT

The Comprehensive Environmental Response, Compensation, and Liability Act (CERCLA), known as the Superfund, created a tax on the chemical and petroleum industries and provided broad federal authority to respond directly to releases or threatened releases of hazardous substances that may endanger public health or the environment.

### SUPERFUND AMENDMENTS AND REAUTHORIZATION ACT (SARA)

The Superfund Amendments and Reauthorization Act (SARA) amended CERCLA. Changes included an increased size of the trust fund, encouragement of greater citizen participation in decision making about site cleanup, increased state involvement in every phase of the Superfund program, increased focus on human health problems related to hazardous waste sites, and new enforcement authorities and settlement tools stressing the importance of permanent remedies and innovative treatment technologies in cleanup of hazardous waste sites and Superfund actions to consider standards in other federal and state regulations. (Under Superfund legislation, the federal Agency for Toxic Substances and Disease Registry was established.)

*Continued*

---

**BOX 10-13    Environmental Laws—cont'd**

### EMERGENCY PLANNING AND COMMUNITY RIGHT-TO-KNOW ACT

The Emergency Planning and Community Right-to-Know Act (EPCRA), also known as Title III of SARA, was enacted to help local communities protect public health safety and the environment from chemical hazards. Each state was required to appoint a state Emergency Response Commission, and these were required to divide their states into emergency planning districts and to establish a local emergency planning committee for each district.

### NATIONAL ENVIRONMENTAL EDUCATION ACT

The National Environmental Education Act created the National Environmental Education and Training Foundation, which resulted in a new and better-coordinated environmental education emphasis at the EPA.

### POLLUTION PREVENTION ACT

The Pollution Prevention Act (PPA) focused industry, government, and public attention on reducing pollution through cost-effective changes in production, operation, and raw materials use. Other practices that increase efficient use of energy, water, and water resources include recycling, source reduction, and sustainable agriculture.

### FOOD QUALITY PROTECTION ACT

The Food Quality Protection Act (FQPA) amended FIFRA and the Federal Food, Drug, and Cosmetic Act. The FQPA changed the way the EPA regulates pesticides. The requirements include a new safety standard—reasonable certainty of no harm—to be applied to all pesticides used on foods.

### CHEMICAL SAFETY INFORMATION, SITE SECURITY AND FUELS REGULATORY ACT

The Chemical Safety Information, Site Security and Fuels Regulatory Act (an amendment to Section 112 of the Clean Air Act) removed from coverage by the Risk Management Plan (RMP) any flammable fuel when used as fuel or held for sale as fuel by a retail facility (flammable fuels held for sale at a wholesale facility are still covered). The law also limits access to off-site consequence analyses, which are reported in RMPs by covered facilities.

---

Cancer deaths have been the most frequently used outcome measure in environmental standards, but the risk calculations are now expanding to include birth defects, reproductive disorders, immune function disorders, and morbidity (kidney, liver, respiratory, neurotoxicity) (Pope et al, 1995). There is an urgency to conduct research that can facilitate the setting of protective environmental standards, but the cost for meaningful studies that explore the environmental determinants of health is high.

Once environmental standards are set, both as a basis for permitting and in individual facility permits, the next step in control is **monitoring.** Monitoring procedures, which must use methods approved by the EPA or scientific consensus, must follow accepted protocols (e.g., maintaining a documented chain of custody of samples to ensure accuracy and protection from contamination at the laboratory after sampling).

Environmental monitoring takes two main forms. One is actual inspections of permitted facilities to observe first-hand whether the plans submitted in the permit application are being implemented as approved. In addition to unannounced inspections, continuous monitoring of data and operating procedures required in permits is studied for any variations from what is allowed. Finally, periodic measurements of the facility outputs in air and water emissions are calculated or measured directly to ensure compliance with laws and regulations. An alternative or adjunct monitoring method is self-reported data from the regulated agency. Factors must be considered in deciding how much of the monitoring requirement can be met through self-reporting, such as costs, reliability, and public trust and acceptance.

Beyond the monitoring of individual permitted facilities, official regulatory agencies design sampling networks for measuring the quality of water and air throughout the geographic area for which they have responsibility. Routine samples of air and water are taken at designated monitoring sites and analyzed.

**Compliance** and **enforcement** are the next building blocks in controlling environmental damage. Compliance refers to the processes for ensuring that permitting requirements are met. When permit or other legally defined violations are found, the first effort is to get quick, voluntary compliance from the violator. Incentives in the form of reducing or eliminating fines and penalties may be negotiated in return for rapid and effective action to correct the problem. Formal enforcement actions are taken when voluntary compliance is not achieved. The range of enforcement tools that may be employed include fines or penalties, suspension of specific operations, or closure of the facility. If the violation is deemed to be willful and with full knowledge that it was unlawful, criminal law may provide for incarceration of the owners or operators, in addition to the other consequences.

Enforcement processes may also include provision for public involvement, although this is less common. The public often does not feel included at the level they desire in enforcement or permitting procedures. Rationales for excluding the public can range from a goal of early correction of the problem to a concern that time required for public comment or forums will delay a solution. Also, industry may guard information for fear of private party lawsuits. Another view, however, is that public involvement is essential to ensure aggressive enforcement.

Cleanup or remediation of environmental damage is the final step. The authority to direct and ensure adequate restoration of environmental quality may be entirely in the hands of state or federal government agencies, or it may be contracted out to private companies, with official oversight. Public information and involvement processes, such as citizen advisory panels or community forums, are integral to remediation where implications for future land use and remedies acceptable to the affected community are part of the decision process.

## ADVOCACY

One hundred years ago Isabel Hampton Robb was elected first president of the American Nurses Association (ANA). The 2.7 million nurses in the United States today can and should be a strong voice for change. As informed citizens, nurses can take a variety of actions to protect the environmental health of families, clients, and communities.

Nurses, who are perceived as trusted messengers and reliable sources of environmental health information (Carlson, 2000), have a responsibility to be informed and take action in the best interest of public health, and indeed they have used their abilities as educators, advocates, and communicators to affect public policy, laws, and regulations that protect public health. Nurses can serve as a resource for state and federal legislators and their staff. Often, legislators are called to vote on environmental legislation without a sound understanding of how the legislation may affect public health. Although every nurse cannot be an expert in all aspects of environmental health, every nurse does have a basic education in human health and can identify those who may be most vulnerable to environmental insult. Nurses' thoughts about the potential effects of new laws on the health of individuals and communities are valuable to legislators. As communicators and educators, nurses can write letters to local newspapers responding to environmental health issues affecting the community.

Grounded in science and using sound risk communication skills, nurses become extremely credible sources of information at community gatherings, formal governmental hearings, and professional nursing forums. Nurses, as trusted communicators, must not be silent when informed about environmental health issues. The nurse as an advocate works for environmental justice so that all members of the community have a right to live and work in an environment that is healthy and safe. The nurse can volunteer to serve on state, local, or federal commissions. It is important to be familiar with the zoning and permit laws that regulate the impacts of industry and land use on the community. Many nurse legislators began their careers by advocating for the rights of others. Nurses must read, listen, and ask questions. Then, as informed citizens, they will be leaders, fostering community action to address environmental health threats.

## Environmental Justice

Some diseases differentially affect different populations. Certain environmental health risks have notably disproportionately affected poor people and people of color in the United States. If you are a poor person of color, you are more likely to live near a hazardous waste site or an incinerator, and more likely to have children who are lead poisoned. Furthermore, you are more likely to have children with asthma, which has a strong association with environmental exposures. Campaigns in communities of color and poor communities to improve the unequal burden of environmental risks are striving to achieve **environmental justice** or environmental equity (Mood, 2002).

In 1993, the Environmental Justice Act was passed, and in 1994 Executive Order 12898, Federal Actions to Address Environmental Justice in Minority Populations, was signed. These created policies to more comprehensively reduce the incidence of environmental inequity by mandating that every federal agency act in a manner to address and prevent illnesses and injuries.

## Unique Environmental Health Threats in the Health Care Industry: New Opportunities for Advocacy

In the health care setting, many choices can be made that affect environmental health. The use of mercury-containing thermometers and sphygmomanometers (even though there are reliable, mercury-free alternatives) risks the possibility of breakage, which could result in the release of a highly toxic substance. Furthermore, if the facility disposes of waste by incineration, then the mercury will be released into the air. This airborne mercury will come down in raindrops, and when it lands in bodies of water (lakes, rivers, oceans), it is converted by microorganisms in the water to **methyl mercury,** which is highly toxic to humans. The methyl mercury is then bioaccumulated in fish: as larger fish eat smaller fish, the body burden of methyl mercury increases significantly.

Many synthetic chemicals that contaminate the environment are referred to as **persistent bioaccumulative toxins** (PBTs) or **persistent organic pollutants** (POPs). These are chemicals that do not break down, either in the air, water, or soil, or in the plant, animal, or human bodies to which they may be passed. Ultimately, as humans are at the top of the food chain, these chemicals may come to reside in our bodies. For instance, lead, which should not be found in the human body, can be found in the long bones of almost any human in the world because of its ubiquitous use and presence in the environment.

Dioxin is another pollutant that contaminates our communities. It is created, in part, by the health care industry. Dioxin is an unintentional byproduct of combusting chlorine compounds, and it is stored in fat cells as it works its way up the food chain. This phenomenon has resulted in dioxin deposition in breast tissue and then its expression in milk (both cow's milk and human milk). Virtually all women on earth now have dioxin in their breast tissue. Dioxin, which is an endocrine-disrupting chemical, a carcinogen, and associated with several neurodevelopmental problems including learning disabilities, is now in effect being expressed in all human milk. The solution to this concern is pollution prevention to remove the dioxin from our environment, not to stop breastfeeding, which is still the best nutritional choice for the baby.

An international campaign called Health Care Without Harm is working on the reduction and elimination of mercury and polyvinyl chloride (PVC) plastic in the health care industry, as well as the elimination of incineration of medical waste. When PVC plastic is incinerated, an unintentional byproduct of its combustion is dioxin, which is then released into the environment. The ANA was a founder of the Health Care Without Harm campaign, and nurses have taken many leadership roles in the activities in the United States and around the world. The Health Care Without Harm website (www. noharm.org) and the ANA's website (www.nursingworld. org/rnnoharm) provide outstanding information and resources about pollution prevention in the health care sector.

## REFERRAL RESOURCES

There is no single source of information about environmental health nor is there a single resource to which you can refer an individual or community should they suspect an environmental problem. Information is widely accessible on the worldwide web, but finding an actual person to assist you or the communities you serve may not be as easy. One starting point may be the environmental epidemiology unit or toxicology unit of your state health department or environmental agency. Another local or state resource may be environmental health experts in nursing or medical schools or schools of public health. The Association of Occupational and Environmental Clinics (www.AOEC.org) is a national network of specialty clinics and individual practitioners available for consultation and sometimes for provision of educational programs for health professionals.

Local resources include local health and environmental protection agencies, poison control centers, agricultural extension offices, and occupational and environmental departments in schools of medicine, nursing, and public health. Some local and state agencies have developed topical directories to assist in accessing the appropriate staff for specific questions. Many resources have websites that allow ready access through the internet and can be located by using any of the popular search methods (Box 10-14). (See also Box 10-4 and the WebLinks at http://evolve. elsevier.com/Stanhope.)

## ROLES FOR NURSES IN ENVIRONMENTAL HEALTH

Nurses can be involved in a number of roles in environmental health, in full-time work, as an adjunct to existing roles, and as informed citizens:

- *Community involvement and public participation.* Organizing, facilitating, and moderating. Making public notices effective, public forums accessible and welcoming of input, information exchange understandable, and problem solving acceptable to culturally diverse communities are valuable assets a nurse contributes. Skills in community organizing

---

> ### BOX 10-14  Information and Guidance Sources for Referrals
>
> **FEDERAL AGENCIES**
> - Agency for Toxic Substances and Disease Registry
> - Centers for Disease Control and Prevention
> - Consumer Product Safety Commission
> - Environmental Protection Agency
> - Office of Children's Environmental Health
> - Food and Drug Administration
> - National Institute for Occupational Safety and Health
> - National Institute of Environmental Health Sciences
> - National Institutes of Health
> - National Cancer Institute
> - National Institute of Nursing Research
> - Occupational Safety and Health Administration
>
> **STATE AGENCIES**
> - State Health Departments
> - State Environmental Protection Agencies
>
> **ASSOCIATIONS AND ORGANIZATIONS**
> - American Association of Poison Control Centers
> - American College of Occupational and Environmental Medicine
> - American Cancer Society
> - American Lung Association
> - Association of Occupational and Environmental Clinics
> - Center for Health and Environmental Justice
> - Children's Environmental Health Network
> - Children's Health and the Environment Coalition
> - National Environmental Education and Training Foundation
> - Pesticide Education Center
> - Society for Occupational and Environmental Health
> - Teratogen Exposure Registry and Surveillance

and mobilizing can be essential to a community's having a meaningful voice in decisions that affect it.
- *Individual and population risk assessment.* Using nursing assessment skills to detect potential and actual exposure pathways and outcomes for clients cared for in the acute, chronic, and healthy communities of practice.
- *Risk communication.* interpreting, and applying principles to practice. Nurses may serve as skilled risk communicators within agencies, working for industries, or working as independent practitioners. Amendments to the Clean Air Act require major industrial sources of air emissions to have risk management plans and to inform their neighbors of specifics of the risks and plans (Clean Air Act, 1996).

- *Epidemiologic investigations.* Nurses need to have the skills to respond in scientifically sound and humanly sensitive ways to community concerns about cancer, birth defects, and stillbirths that citizens fear may have environmental causes.
- *Policy development.* Proposing, informing, and monitoring action from agencies, communities, and organization perspectives.

The assimilation of the concepts of environmental health into a nurse's daily practice gives new life to the traditional public health values of prevention, building community, and social justice. There is great congruence with many personal, religious, and spiritual values of stewardship of creation, preserving the gifts of nature, and decision making that provides for quality of life for present and future generations. It is a context for practice where nurses are welcomed and valued for their contribution.

As nurses learn more about the environment, opportunities for integration into their practice, educational programs, research, advocacy, and policy work will become evident. Opportunities abound for those pioneering spirits within the nursing profession who are dedicated to creating healthier environments for their clients and communities.

## Practice Application

This Practice Application gives two case scenarios related to exposure pathways. The first involves lead poisoning and the second, gasoline contamination of groundwater.

At the county health department, a 3-year-old boy presents with gastric upset and behavior changes that have persisted for several weeks. Billy's parents report that they have been renovating their home to remove lead paint. They had been discouraged from routinely testing their child because their insurance does not cover testing and they could not find information on where to have the test done. Their concern has heightened with the persistent symptoms in their child.

You test level of lead in Billy's blood and find it to be 45 μg/dL. You research lead poisoning and discover that children are at great risk because of their inclination to absorb lead into their central nervous systems. You also find that chronic lead poisoning may have long-term effects, such as developmental delays and impaired learning ability. You refer Billy to his primary care physician. On further investigation, you find that Billy's home was built before 1950 and is still under renovation. The sanitarian tests the interior paint and finds a high lead content. Ample amounts of sawdust from sanding are noted in various rooms of the home. You determine that a completed exposure pathway exists.

A. What would you include in an assessment of this situation?
B. What prevention strategies would you use to resolve this issue?

- At the individual level?
- At the population level?

A citizen calls the local health department to report that his drinking water, from a private well, "smells like gasoline." A water sample is collected, and analysis reveals the presence of petroleum products. A nearby rural store with a service station has removed its old underground gasoline storage tanks and replaced them, as required by law. Contaminated soil from the old leaking tank has been removed, and a well to monitor groundwater contamination is scheduled for installation. However, sandy soil has allowed rapid movement of the contamination through the groundwater, and the plume has reached the neighbor's drinking-water well in levels that exceed the drinking-water standard. What are some possible responses?

**Answers are in the back of the book.**

## Key Points

- Nurses have responsibilities to be informed consumers and to be advocates for citizens in their community regarding environmental health issues.
- Models describing the determinants of health acknowledge the role of the environment in health and disease.
- For many chemical compounds, whether new or familiar, scientific evidence of possible health effects is lacking.
- Prevention activities include education, waste minimizing, and land use planning. Control activities include environmental permitting, environmental standards, monitoring, compliance and enforcement, and cleanup and remediation.
- Each nursing assessment should include questions and observations about intended and unintended environmental exposures.
- Environmental databases facilitate the easy and immediate access to environmental data useful in assessment, diagnosis, intervention, and evaluation.
- Both case advocacy and class advocacy are important skills for nurses in environmental health practice.
- Risk communication is an important skill and must acknowledge the outrage factor experienced by communities with environmental hazards.
- Federal, state, and local laws and regulations exist to protect the health of citizens from environmental hazards.
- Environmental health practice engages multiple disciplines, and nurses are important members of the environmental health team.
- Environmental health practice includes principles of health promotion, disease prevention, and health protection.

- Both Healthy People 2000 and Healthy People 2010 objectives address targets for the reduction of risk factors and diseases related to environmental causes.

## Clinical Decision-Making Activities

1. Explain why the source of drinking water is important to investigate in the assessment of an unusually high number of cancer cases in a community, in the assessment of increased lead levels in children from a certain school, and in the assessment of an outbreak of a gastrointestinal epidemic in an agricultural community.
2. Discuss the differences and similarities between the Canadian model and the epidemiologic triangle in explaining the determinants of health.
3. Discover if your jurisdiction has a law or regulation for the disclosure of radon levels on personal property as part of a real estate sale. If your community does not, investigate with the government officials of the community the reasons for the lack of disclosure requirement.

## Additional Resources

These related resources are found either in the appendix at the back of this book or on the book's website at **http://evolve.elsevier.com/Stanhope.**

### Appendix

Appendix I.3: Comprehensive Occupational and Environmental Health History

### *evolve* Evolve Website

WebLinks: Healthy People 2010

## References

Agency for Toxic Substances and Disease Registry: Identifying and evaluating exposure pathways. In *Public health assessment guidance manual,* Atlanta, Ga, 1992, ATSDR.

Aldrich T, Griffith J: *Environmental epidemiology and risk assessment,* New York, 1993, Van Nostrand Reinhold.

Amaya MA et al: Childhood lead poisoning on the US-Mexico border: a case study in environmental health nursing lead poisoning, *Public Health Nurs* 14(6):353, 1997.

American Psychiatric Association, *Diagnostic and statistical manual of mental disorders,* ed 4, 1994, New York, American Psychiatric Association.

Boyle CA, Decoufle P, Yeargin-Allsopp M: Prevalence and health impact of developmental disabilities in US children, *Pediatrics* 93(3):399-403, 1994.

Bucubalis JD, Balisitreri WF: The neonatal gastrointestinal tract. In Fanaroff AA, Marin RJ: *Neonatal-perinatal medicine: diseases of the fetus and infant,* ed 6, pp 1288-1344, St Louis, Mo, 1997, Mosby.

Carlson D: "Nurses remain at top of honesty and ethics poll," reported by the Gallup Organization for Gallop News Service, retrieved November 27, 2000, from www.gallup.com/ poll/ releases/pr00127iii.asp.

Children's Environmental Health Network: *Training manual on pediatric environmental health: putting it into practice,* 1998, available at www.cehn.org.

Clean Air Act, Risk Management Programs, Section 112 (7), Federal Register, Part III EPA, 40 CFR, Part 68, June 20, 1996.

Federal, Provincial, and Territorial Advisory Committee on Population Health for Canadian Ministers of Health: *Strategies for population health,* Halifax, Nova Scotia, 1994, the Committee.

Goldman LR: Chemicals and children's environment: what we don't know about risks. *Environ Health Perspect* 106:875-879, 1998.

Goldman LR: Environmental health and its relationship to occupational health. In Levy BS, Wegman DH, editors: *Occupational health recognizing and preventing work-related disease and injury,* Philadelphia, 2000, Lippincott Williams & Wilkins.

Levy B, Wegman D: *Occupational health: recognizing and preventing work-related disease and injury,* ed 4, Philadelphia, 2000, Lippincott Williams & Wilkins.

Lilienfeld AM, Lilienfeld DE: Laying the foundations: the epidemiologic approach to disease. In Lilienfeld AM, Lilienfeld DE, editors: *Foundations of epidemiology,* New York, 1980, Oxford University Press.

Ma X et al: Critical windows of exposure to household pesticides and risk of childhood leukemia, *Environ Health Perspect* 110:955-960, 2002.

Mancke R: Nature walk lecture, Congaree Swamp National Monument, South Carolina, April, 1998.

Mckeown RE, Weinrich SP: Epidemiologic applications. In Stanhope M, Lancaster J, editors: *Community and public health nursing,* St Louis, Mo, 2000, Mosby.

Mood LH: Environmental health policy: environmental justice. In Mason DJ, Leavitt JK, editors: *Policy and politics in nursing and health care,* ed 4, Philadelphia, 2002, Saunders.

National Research Council: *Environmental epidemiology, vol 1: public health and hazardous wastes.* Washington, DC, 1991, National Academy of Sciences.

National Research Council: *Pesticides in the diets of infants and children,* Washington, DC, 1993, National Academy Press.

National Research Council: *Environmental epidemiology, vol 2: use of the gray literature and other data in environmental epidemiology.* Washington, DC, 1997, National Academy of Science.

Nightingale F: *Notes on nursing: what it is and what it is not,* London, 1859, Harrison.

O'Brien M: *Making better environmental decisions: alternatives to risk assessment,* Cambridge, Mass, 2000, MIT Press.

Pope AM, Snyder MA, Mood LH, editors: *Nursing, health and environment,* Washington, DC, 1995, Institute of Medicine, National Academy Press.

Robinson JP, Switzer P, Ott W: Daily exposure to environmental tobacco smoke: smokers vs nonsmokers in California, *Am J Public Health* 86(9):1303, 1996.

Roszak T: *Voice of the earth: an exploration of ecopsychology,* New York, 1992, Simon & Schuster.

Sandman PM, Chess C, Hane BJ: *Improving dialogue with communities,* New Brunswick, NJ, 1991, Rutgers University.

Sattler B, Lipscomb L, editors: *Environmental health and nursing practice,* New York, 2002, Springer.

Schettler T et al: "In harm's way: toxic threats to development," a report by Greater Boston Physicians for Social Responsibility, prepared for a joint project with Clean Water, Cambridge, Mass, 2000, Physicians for Social Responsibility, available at http://www.igc.org/psr/pubs.htm.

Schmidt CW: Childhood cancer: a growing problem, *Environ Health Perspect* 106:18-23, 1998.

Sutcliffe PA, Deber RB, Pasut G: Public health in Canada: a comparative study of six provinces, *Can J Public Health* 87(4):246, 1997.

U.S. Department of Health and Human Services: *Healthy people 2010: understanding and improving health,* ed 2, Washington, DC, 2000, U.S. Government Printing Office.

University of South Carolina, College of Business Administration, Division of Research: USC report on the survey on environmental issues, Columbia, SC, 1990, University of South Carolina.

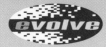

# Epidemiology

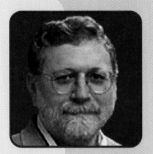

**Robert E. McKeown, Ph.D., F.A.C.E.**

Robert E. McKeown is an epidemiologist with doctoral degrees in epidemiology and theology. He is a fellow in the American College of Epidemiology (ACE) and active in national epidemiology professional organizations, serving as chair of the Epidemiology Section of the American Public Health Association and chair of the Ethics and Standards of Practice Committee of ACE. His research focuses on psychiatric epidemiology, especially in children and adolescents, perinatal epidemiology, women's health, public health ethics, and public health and the faith community. He is associate professor and graduate director for epidemiology and interim chair of the Department of Epidemiology and Biostatistics in the Norman J. Arnold School of Public Health, University of South Carolina.

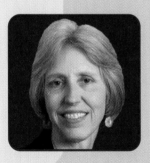

**DeAnne K. Hilfinger Messias, R.N., Ph.D.**

DeAnne Hilfinger Messias is an international community health nurse. She spent over two decades in Brazil, where she taught community health nursing and women's health, directed a primary health care project on the lower Amazon, and organized women's health initiatives among poor urban populations. Her research has focused on women's work and health, immigrant women, and community empowerment. Dr. Messias was recently selected as a Health Partners Fellow for 2002-2004 by the International Center for Health Leadership Development at the School of Public Health, University of Illinois at Chicago. She is an associate professor at the University of South Carolina, with a joint appointment in the College of Nursing and the Women's Studies Program.

## Objectives

After reading this chapter, the student should be able to do the following:

1. Define epidemiology and describe its essential elements and approach
2. Describe the history of epidemiology and how its scope and methods have evolved
3. Discuss the elements and interactions of the epidemiologic triangle
4. Explain the relationship of the natural history of disease to the various levels of prevention and to the design and implementation of community interventions
5. Interpret basic epidemiologic measures of morbidity and mortality
6. Discuss descriptive epidemiologic parameters of person, place, and time
7. Describe the features of common epidemiologic study designs
8. Describe essential characteristics and methods of evaluating a screening program
9. Explain the most common sources of bias in epidemiologic studies
10. Evaluate epidemiologic research and apply findings to community-oriented nursing practice
11. Discuss the role of the nurse in epidemiologic surveillance and primary, secondary, and tertiary prevention

What and who is an epidemiologist? The editors of the *American Journal of Public Health* raised that question in 1942 (Editorial, 1942) and received a wide range of responses from readers. More recent articles and editorials continue to address the nature, scope,

*The authors acknowledge the contributions of Carol Garrison and Sally Weinrich to this chapter in previous editions of this text.*

and direction of epidemiology (Koopman, 1996; Pearce, 1996; Susser and Susser, 1996a,b; Winkelstein, 1996). Although the question may not be settled, epidemiology has made major contributions to (1) understanding the factors that contribute to health and disease, (2) the development of health promotion and disease prevention measures, (3) the detection and characterization of emerging infectious agents, (4) the evaluation of health

## Key Terms

**agent**, p. 261
**analytic epidemiology**, p. 269
**attack rate**, p. 259
**bias**, p. 277
**case-control study**, p. 274
**cohort study**, p. 272
**confounding**, p. 277
**cross-sectional study**, p. 275
**descriptive epidemiology**, p. 269
**determinants**, p. 250
**distribution**, p. 250
**ecologic fallacy**, p. 275
**ecologic study**, p. 275

**environment**, p. 261
**epidemic**, p. 258
**epidemiology**, p. 250
**host**, p. 261
**incidence proportion**, p. 256
**incidence rate**, p. 256
**levels of prevention**, p. 262
**natural history of disease**, p. 262
**negative predictive value**, p. 266
**point epidemic**, p. 270
**popular epidemiology**, p. 278
**positive predictive value**, p. 266

**prevalence proportion**, p. 258
**rates**, p. 256
**reliability**, p. 265
**risk**, p. 256
**screening**, p. 265
**secular trends**, p. 270
**sensitivity**, p. 266
**specificity**, p. 266
**surveillance**, p. 267
**validity**, p. 266
**web of causality**, p. 261
*See Glossary for definitions*

## Chapter Outline

Definitions of Health
Definitions and Descriptions of Epidemiology
Historical Perspectives
Basic Concepts in Epidemiology
*Measures of Morbidity and Mortality*
  *Epidemiologic Triangle: Agent, Host,*
  *and Environment*
*Levels of Preventive Interventions*
Screening
*Reliability and Validity*
Basic Methods in Epidemiology
*Sources of Data*

*Rate Adjustment*
*Comparison Groups*
Descriptive Epidemiology
*Person*
*Place*
*Time*
Analytic Epidemiology
*Cohort Studies*
*Case-Control Studies*
*Cross-Sectional Studies*
*Ecologic Studies*

Experimental Studies
*Clinical Trials*
*Community Trials*
Causality
*Statistical Associations*
*Bias*
*Assessing for Causality*
Applications of Epidemiology in Community-
  Oriented Nursing
*Community-Oriented Epidemiology*
*Popular Epidemiology*

services and policies, and (5) the practice of community and public health nursing.

## DEFINITIONS OF HEALTH

The World Health Organization (WHO) defines health as "a state of complete well-being, physical, social, and mental, and not merely the absence of disease or infirmity" (Institute of Medicine [IOM], 1988, p. 39). The Institute of

Medicine's (IOM) 1988 study *The Future of Public Health* defined the mission of public health as "the fulfillment of society's interest in assuring conditions in which people can be healthy" and noted "the substance of public health [is] organized community efforts aimed at the prevention of disease and promotion of health" (IOM, 1988, p. 40). This definition implies establishment of public policies and programs and the delivery of specific services to individuals. It also suggests that the policies, programs, and services go beyond a narrow biomedical model of health. Public health activity is channeled in three directions: community prevention (proactive), disease control (reactive), and personal and community health (proactive and reactive) services. The IOM report notes that epidemiology is the core science of public health, and it is described as a constellation of disciplines with a common mission: optimal health for the whole community. The American Nurses Association's (ANA) definition of health as "the diagnosis and treatment of human responses to actual or potential health problems" coincides well with epidemiologic principles (ANA, 1995, p. 6). This holistic approach to health is particularly appropriate for community-oriented nurses. The concept of health employed clearly influences nursing practice. The IOM report cautions, however, that this broad understanding of health and the role of public health professionals and agencies forces "practitioners to make difficult choices about where to focus their energies and raises the possibility that public health could be so broadly defined so as to lose distinctive meaning" (IOM, 1988, p. 40). Nurses are especially well suited to address this concern because of their holistic view of health and broad, interdisciplinary approach to intervention. For that reason, nurses are critical to collaboration among health professionals, including epidemiologists, in order to ensure conditions to support health.

## DEFINITIONS AND DESCRIPTIONS OF EPIDEMIOLOGY

**Epidemiology** has been defined as "the study of the distribution and determinants of health-related states or events in specified populations, and the application of this study to control of health problems" (Last, 2001, p. 62). As the scope of epidemiology has broadened in the twentieth century,

the definition has changed. The term originally referred to epidemics that were primarily infectious in origin. However, now it includes chronic diseases, such as cancer and cardiovascular disease, and more recently, mental health and other health-related events, such as accidents, injuries and violence, occupational and environmental exposures and their effects, and positive health states. In addition, epidemiologic methods now are used to study health-related behaviors, such as diet and physical activity (Brownson, Remington, and Davis, 1998), and they are used in health services research (Brownson and Petitti, 1998) and to investigate such things as the association between poverty and poor living conditions with increased risk of infection, chronic diseases, and violence (National Center for Health Statistics [NCHS], 1998). Epidemiologic methods are used extensively to determine to what extent the goals of Healthy People 2000 (U.S. Department of Health and Human Services [USDHHS], 1991), the United States' health objectives, have been accomplished and to monitor progress toward the Healthy People 2010 objectives.

Epidemiology investigates the **distribution** or patterns of health events in populations and the determinants that influence those patterns. Epidemiologists characterize health outcomes in terms of what, who, where, when, and why: What is the outcome? Who is affected? Where are they? When do events occur? This focus of epidemiology is often called descriptive epidemiology, as it seeks to describe a disease entity according to person, place, and time. The **determinants** of health events are those factors, exposures, characteristics, behaviors, and contexts that determine (or influence) the patterns: How does it occur? Why are some affected more than others? Determinants may be individual, relational or social, communal, or environmental. This focus on investigation of causes and associations is called analytic epidemiology, as it is directed to-

---

## Healthy People 2010 — Categories Into Which Objectives Related to Epidemiology Fall

1. Access to quality health services
2. Arthritis, osteoporosis, and chronic back conditions
3. Cancer
4. Chronic kidney disease
5. Diabetes
6. Disability and secondary conditions
7. Educational and community-based programs
8. Environmental health
9. Family planning
10. Food safety
11. Health communication
12. Heart disease and stroke
13. Human immunodeficiency virus infection
14. Immunization and infectious diseases
15. Injury and violence prevention
16. Maternal, infant, and child health
17. Medical product safety
18. Mental health and mental disorders
19. Nutrition and overweight
20. Occupational safety and health
21. Oral health
22. Physical activity and fitness
23. Public health infrastructure
24. Respiratory disease
25. Sexually transmitted diseases
26. Substance abuse
27. Tobacco use
28. Vision and hearing

From U.S. Department of Health and Human Services: *Healthy people 2010: understanding and improving health,* ed 2, Washington, DC, 2000, U.S. Government Printing Office.

ward understanding the etiology (or origins and causal factors) of the disease. The results of these investigations are used to guide or evaluate policies and programs that improve the health of the community. The distinction between descriptive and analytic studies is inexact: analytic studies rely on descriptive comparisons, and descriptive comparisons shed light on determinants.

The first step in the epidemiologic process is to define a health outcome (the case definition, usually cases of disease but also of injuries, accidents, or even wellness). Epidemiology has played important roles in the refinement of the case definition for acquired immunodeficiency syndrome (AIDS) and in the development of precise diagnostic criteria for psychiatric disorders. Epidemiologic methods are then used to quantify the frequency of occurrence and characterize both the case group and the population from which they come (i.e., describing the distribution, or the who, where, and when) and to search for factors that explain the pattern or risk of occurrence (i.e., determinants, or the why and how).

Epidemiology builds on and draws from other disciplines and methods, including clinical medicine and laboratory sciences, social sciences, quantitative methods (especially biostatistics), and public health policy and goals, among others. Epidemiology differs from clinical medicine, which focuses on the diagnosis and treatment of disease in individuals. Epidemiology is the study of populations in order to (1) monitor the health of the population, (2) understand the determinants of health and disease in communities, and (3) investigate and evaluate interventions to prevent disease and maintain health. Effective community-oriented nursing bridges these disciplines in its focus on individual clients and services provided for them as well as on the broader context in which they live and the complex interplay of social and environmental factors that affect their well-being. This task involves using epidemiologic methods and findings in community health programs and preventive measures.

## HISTORICAL PERSPECTIVES

Some writers cite Hippocrates in the fourth century B.C. as an ancient precursor of epidemiology (Timmreck, 2002; Winkelstein and French, 1972). He maintained that to understand health and disease in a community, one should look to geographic and climatic factors, the seasons of the year, the food and water consumed, and the habits and behaviors of the people. His approach anticipates in a general way the major categories of descriptive epidemiology: namely, the distribution of health states by personal characteristics, place, and time. However, modern epidemiology emerged only within the last two centuries and developed as a discipline with a distinctive identity and method

### Table 11-1 Significant Milestones in the History of Epidemiology

| YEAR | RESPONSIBLE PERSON/ ORGANIZATION | SIGNIFICANT EVENT |
|---|---|---|
| 1662 | John Graunt | Used Bills of Mortality (forerunner of modern vital records) to study patterns of death in various populations in England. Published early form of life table analysis. |
| 1747 | James Lind | Studied scurvy using observation and comparison of responses to various dietary treatments (early precursor of clinical trial). |
| 1760 | Daniel Bernoulli | Used life table technique to demonstrate that smallpox inoculation conferred lifelong immunity. |
| 1775 | Percival Pott | First "cancer epidemiologist." Noted that a high proportion of patients presenting with cancer of the scrotum were chimney sweeps. Inferred that exposure to soot was the cause. (Lack of a comparison group would reduce validity of inference by today's standards.) |
| 1798 | Edward Jenner | Demonstrated effectiveness of smallpox vaccination. |
| 1798 | Marine Hospital Service | Forerunner of U.S. Public Health Service (1912) |
| 1836 | Pierre Charles-Alexandre Louis | Comparative observational studies to demonstrate ineffectiveness of bloodletting. Emphasized the importance of statistical methods ("la méthode numerique"). Influenced many of the pioneers in epidemiology in England and the United States. |
| 1836 | | Establishment of Registrar-General's Office in England as registry for births, deaths, and marriages. |

From Institute of Medicine: *The future of public health,* Washington, DC, 1988, National Academy Press; Learner M: A history of public health in South Carolina, accessed April 2003, from http://www.scdhec.net/co/elsa/publichealth; Lilienfeld DE, Stolley PD: *Foundations of epidemiology,* ed 3, New York, 1994, Oxford University Press; Susser M: Epidemiology in the United States after World War II: the evolution of technique, *Epidemiol Rev* 7:147, 1985; Timmreck TC: *An introduction to epidemiology,* ed 3, Boston, 2002, Jones & Bartlett; USDHHS: *Public health service fact sheet,* Washington, DC, 1984, USDHHS, Public Health Service.

*Continued*

**Table 11-1   Significant Milestones in the History of Epidemiology—cont'd**

| YEAR | RESPONSIBLE PERSON/ ORGANIZATION | SIGNIFICANT EVENT |
|---|---|---|
| 1840s | William Farr | Developed forerunner of modern vital records system in Registrar-General's Office. Study of mortality in Liverpool led to significant public health reform. Pioneered mortality surveillance and anticipated many of the basic concepts in epidemiology. His data provided much of the basis for Snow's work on cholera. |
| 1850 | | Founding of London Epidemiological Society. Known for influential reports on smallpox vaccination and studies of cholera. |
| 1850 | Lemuel Shattuck | Reported on sanitation and public health in Massachusetts. |
| 1850s | John Snow | Epidemiologic research on transmission of cholera. Used mapping and natural experiment, comparing rates in groups exposed to different water supplies. |
| 1870-1880s | Robert Koch | Discovered causal agents for anthrax, tuberculosis, and cholera; development of causal criteria. |
| 1887 | Joseph Kinyoun | Founded Laboratory of Hygiene, forerunner of the National Institute of Health (1930). |
| 1921 | Wade Hampton Frost | Founded first U.S. academic program in epidemiology at Johns Hopkins University. |
| 1942 | | Office of Malarial Control in War Areas established; became Communicable Disease Center (CDC) in 1946; then Centers for Disease Control (1973); now Centers for Disease Control and Prevention. |
| 1948 | | Framingham cohort study of cardiovascular disease begins. |
| 1950s | A. Bradford Hill and Richard Doll | Pioneering studies on smoking and lung cancer. |
| 1952 | Jonas Salk | Production of polio vaccine (Nationwide trial, 1954). |
| 1964 | U.S. Surgeon General | First surgeon general's report on smoking and health. |
| 1976 | Frank Speizer (with funding from National Institutes of Health) | Nurses' Health Study begins. |
| 1977 | World Health Organization | Organization's smallpox eradication campaign succeeds: last known case of smallpox in the world occurs. |
| 1983 | | HIV-I retrovirus is identified as the causal agent of AIDS. |
| 1980s | U.S. Department of Health and Human Services | Report of the Secretary's Task Force on Black and Minority Health, a landmark report documenting the health status disparities of minority populations in the United States. |
| 1991 | National Institutes of Health | Women's Health Initiative established. |
| 1990s | U.S. Department of Health and Human Services | Race and Health Initiative. |

From Institute of Medicine: *The future of public health,* Washington, DC, 1988, National Academy Press; Learner M: A history of public health in South Carolina, accessed April 2003, from http://www.scdhec.net/co/elsa/publichealth; Lilienfeld DE, Stolley PD: *Foundations of epidemiology,* ed 3, New York, 1994, Oxford University Press; Susser M: Epidemiology in the United States after World War II: the evolution of technique, *Epidemiol Rev* 7:147, 1985; Timmreck TC: *An introduction to epidemiology,* ed 3, Boston, 2002, Jones & Bartlett; USDHHS: *Public health service fact sheet,* Washington, DC, 1984, USDHHS, Public Health Service.

in the twentieth century (Susser, 1985). Notable events in the history of epidemiology are listed in Table 11-1. This section highlights a few major developments.

In the nineteenth century, germ theory developed with the isolation of organisms (including a number of infectious agents), induction of disease in susceptible hosts, and development of the idea of specificity in the relation of organism and outcome. These successes led to increased emphasis on the role of the agent in the genesis of disease. There is a parallel today in the emphasis on molecular and genetic studies in epidemiology. Pasteur also recognized the role of personal characteristics, such as immunity and host resistance, in explaining differential susceptibility to disease (Susser, 1973; Vandenbroucke, 1990). Furthermore, the accomplishments of the sanitary movement in reducing disease contributed to the acceptance of germ theory while emphasizing the importance of environmental influences for disease rates and variability by person, place, and time (IOM, 1988).

**Table 11-2** Household Cholera Death Rates by Source of Water Supply in John Snow's 1853 Investigation

| COMPANY | NUMBER OF HOUSES | DEATHS FROM CHOLERA | DEATHS PER 10,000 HOUSEHOLDS |
|---|---|---|---|
| Southwark and Vauxhall | 40,046 | 1263 | 315 |
| Lambeth | 26,107 | 98 | 37 |
| Rest of London | 256,423 | 1422 | 59 |

From Snow J: On the mode of communication of cholera. In *Snow on cholera,* New York, 1855, The Commonwealth Fund.

Two refinements in research methods in the eighteenth and nineteenth centuries were critical for the formation of epidemiologic methods: (1) use of a comparison group and (2) the development of quantitative techniques (numeric measurements, or counts). One of the most famous studies using a comparison group is the pivotal mid-nineteenth century investigation of cholera by John Snow, whom some call the "father of epidemiology" (Lilienfeld and Stolley, 1994; Timmreck, 2002). By mapping cases of cholera that clustered around a single public water pump in one outbreak, Snow demonstrated a connection between water supply and cholera. He later observed that cholera rates were higher among households supplied by water companies whose water intakes were downstream from the city than among households whose water came from further upstream, where it was subject to less contamination. Because in some areas households in close proximity to each other had different sources of water, differences observed in rates of cholera could not be attributed to location or economic status. Snow showed that households receiving water from the Lambeth Company, whose intake had been moved away from sewage contamination, had rates of cholera substantially lower than those supplied by Southwark and Vauxhall, a company whose intake was still in a contaminated section of the river (Table 11-2). Snow realized that his investigation was an example of what is called a "natural experiment," which added credibility to his argument that foul water was the vehicle for transmission of the agent that caused cholera (Rothman, 2002).

Another of what Lilienfeld called the "threads of epidemiology" (Lilienfeld and Lilienfeld, 1980) is found in the increased emphasis on a quantitative approach. Edwin Chadwick's 1842 *Report on the Sanitary Conditions of the Laboring Population of Great Britain* was an example of the use of quantitative methods to study large public health problems. This report looked at mortality (vital statistics) and morbidity data to demonstrate the association between mortality rate and environmental conditions: poor sanitation, overcrowding, and contaminated water (Chadwick, 1842). Chadwick recognized that the mortality rate was an indicator of a larger morbidity rate (i.e., the number who die from a disease is but "an indication of the much greater number" who suffer from the disease but survive)

(Lilienfeld, 1984). Even today, research indicates that income distribution is an important factor in variation of mortality rates (Lynch et al, 1998).

In the twentieth century, development and application of epidemiologic methods were stimulated by changes in society brought on by such factors as the Great Depression, World War II, a rising standard of living for many but horrible poverty for others, improved nutrition, new vaccines, better sanitation, the advent of antibiotics and chemotherapies, and declines in infant and child mortality and birth rates. These changes led to longevity and a shift in the age distribution of the population, which meant an increase in age-related diseases: coronary heart disease (CHD), stroke, cancer, and senile dementia (Susser, 1985). However, disparities remain among population subgroups in life expectancy and risk of many acute and chronic diseases. Figure 11-1 shows the 10 leading causes of death in the United States in 1900, 1950, and 2000, with the percentage of all deaths attributed to each. The top three causes of death have not changed since 1950, whereas the composition of the remaining seven leading causes *has* changed.

As chronic diseases increase, it is important to look beyond single agents, such as the infectious agent that causes cholera, toward a multifactorial etiology (i.e., many factors or combinations of factors contributing to disease, such as the complex of factors that cause cardiovascular disease). The possibility that behavioral and environmental causes existed for many conditions formerly thought to be degenerative diseases of aging raised the possibility of prevention or delay of onset (Susser, 1985). In addition, the development of genetic and molecular techniques (such as genetic markers for increased risk of breast cancer and sophisticated tests for antibodies to infectious agents or for other biological markers of exposures to environmental toxins, such as lead or pesticides) has increased the epidemiologist's ability to classify persons in terms of exposures or inherent susceptibility to disease. These two expansions of epidemiologic investigation—upward toward consideration of broader environmental contexts and community level factors (termed eco-epidemiology by some [Susser and Susser, 1996a,b]) and downward to the molecular and genetic levels—have prompted some to call

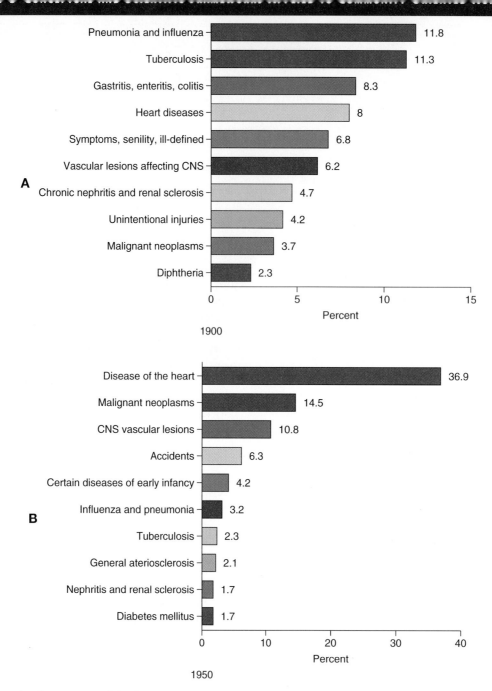

**Figure 11-1** Ten leading causes of death as a percentage of all deaths, United States. **A,** 1900. **B,** 1950. *(Data from Anderson RN: Deaths: leading causes for 2000,* Natl Vital Stat Rep *50(16), 2002; Brownson RC, Remington PL, Davis JR:* Chronic disease epidemiology and control, *ed 2, Washington, DC, 1998, American Public Health Association; U.S. Department of Health, Education, and Welfare:* Vital statistics of the United States: *1950, Vol 1, Washington, DC, 1954, USDHEW, Public Health Service.*

for a renewed look at both epidemiologic theory (Krieger, 1994; Krieger and Zierler, 1995) and methods incorporating multilevel analysis (Diez-Roux, 1998) in epidemiologic investigations. These developments are of particular interest to nurses who are in contact with people in their living and work environments and understand the role of those environments (even beyond chemical or biological expo-

sures) to their well-being. Furthermore, nurses in the community can assess a broad range of health outcomes as well as factors that contribute to wellness and illness.

In recent years, new infectious diseases, such as Lyme disease, legionnaires' disease, hantavirus, Ebola virus, human immunodeficiency virus (HIV), and AIDS; new forms of old diseases, such as resistant strains of tubercu-

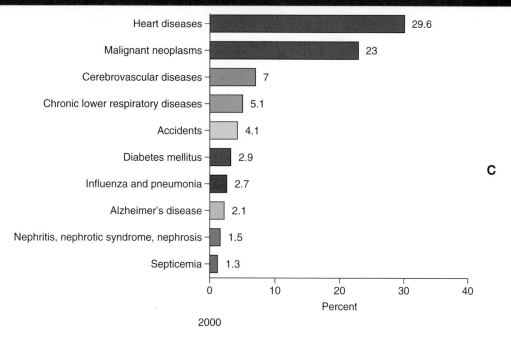

**Figure 11-1, cont'd** Ten leading causes of death as a percentage of all deaths, United States. **C,** 2000.

losis (TB), and new forms of *E. coli;* and potential threats from terrorist use of infectious agents, such as anthrax and smallpox, have emphasized the importance of infectious disease epidemiology. Epidemiologic methods are applied to a broader spectrum of health-related outcomes, including accidents, injuries and violence, occupational and environmental exposures, psychiatric and sociologic phenomena, health-related behaviors, and health services research. This demonstrates again the collaborative and multidisciplinary nature of epidemiologic investigations.

In the aftermath of the terrorist attacks of September 11, 2001, and the apparently unrelated anthrax letters that appeared, public health has taken on a broader mission, with heightened public awareness of its importance. Centers of public health preparedness are being funded by the federal government, and both researchers and practitioners are focusing on preparation, prevention, and response to attacks. There is renewed awareness of the importance of a sound public health infrastructure, especially with regard to surveillance and outbreak investigations, which can carry on critical day-to-day public health functions while also monitoring, alerting, and responding to events. Epidemiologists were among the first to respond to both the terrorist attacks of 9/11 and the anthrax letters. In the aftermath, numerous epidemiologic studies were designed and initiated to understand the impact of a range of exposures related to those events. Epidemiologic methods and epidemiologists are at the very center of public health planning and response to terrorist threats, another indication of the range and flexibility of the discipline and its central role in contributing to the health and well-being of the people.

## BASIC CONCEPTS IN EPIDEMIOLOGY
## Measures of Morbidity and Mortality
### Rates, Proportions, and Risk

Epidemiology focuses on the distribution of health states and events. Because people differ in their probability or risk of disease, the primary concern is how they differ. Mapping cases of a disease in an area, as John Snow mapped cases of cholera in one area of London and as many epidemiologists now map various health-related events, can be instructive, especially if other factors, such as industrial development, show similar patterns. However, mapping cases is limited in what it can reveal. A higher number of cases may simply be the result of a larger population with more people who are potential cases, or of a longer period of observation. Any description of disease patterns should take into account the size of the population at risk for the disease. That is, we should look not only at the numerator (the number of cases) but also at the denominator (the number of people in the population at risk) and at the amount of time each was observed. For example, 50 cases of influenza might be viewed as a serious epidemic in a population of 250 but would indicate a low rate in a population of 250,000. Using rates and proportions instead of simple counts of cases takes the size of the population at risk into account.

Epidemiologic studies rely on rates and proportions. A proportion is a type of ratio in which the denominator includes the numerator. For example, in 2000 there were 2,404,624 deaths recorded in the United States, of which

709,894 were reported as caused by diseases of the heart, so the proportion of deaths due to heart disease in 2000 was 709,894/2,404,624 = 0.295, or 29.5%. Because the numerator must be included in the denominator, proportions can range from 0 to 1. Proportions are often multiplied by 100 and expressed as a percent, literally meaning *per 100*. In public health statistics, however, if the proportion is very small, we use a larger multiplier to avoid small fractions, so the proportion may be expressed as a number per 1000 or per 100,000.

A **rate** is a measure of the frequency of a health event in "a defined population in a specified period of time" (Last, 2001, p. 151). A rate is a ratio, but it is not a proportion because the denominator is a function of both the population size and the dimension of time, whereas the numerator is the number of events. Furthermore, depending on the units of time and the frequency of events, a rate may exceed 1. As its name suggests, a rate is a measure of how rapidly something is happening: how rapidly a disease is developing in a population or how rapidly people are dying. Conceptually, a rate is the instantaneous change in a continuous process. Notice the use of the words *event* and *happening*. Rates deal with change: moving from one state of being to another, from well to ill, from alive to dead, or from ill to cure. Because they deal with events (moving from one state of being to another), time is involved. We must follow a population over time to observe the changes in state, and we typically exclude from the population being followed those persons who have already experienced the event.

By way of analogy, a common example of a rate is the rate of interest on money in a savings account (the true rate) and the accumulated return after some period of time (say, 5 years). If the rate were constant throughout the period, the total return on the investment would be a function of the amount of the initial investment, the interest rate, the frequency of compounding the interest, and the total length of time (in this case, 5 years). For disease processes, instead of adding to the population (parallel to the principal or initial investment) as interest is added to your investment, persons are taken away from the population (i.e., people are removed from the population at risk as they become ill). The incidence rate is analogous to the interest rate, but instead of assuming discrete periods for compounding, we assume that the rate is an instantaneous rate in a continuous process, equivalent to instantaneous and continuous compounding.

**Risk** refers to the probability that an event will occur within a specified time period. A population at risk is the population of persons for whom there is some finite probability (even if small) of that event. For example, although the risk of breast cancer in men is small, a few men do develop breast cancer and therefore could be considered part of the population at risk. There are some outcomes for which certain people would never be at risk (e.g., men cannot be at risk of ovarian cancer, nor can women be at risk of testicular cancer). A high-risk population, on the other hand, would include those persons who, because of exposure, lifestyle, family history, or other factors, are at greater risk for disease than the population at large. It seems that all persons are susceptible to HIV infection, although the degree of susceptibility may vary. Therefore everyone is in the population at risk for HIV and AIDS. Persons who have multiple sexual partners without adequate protection or who use intravenous drugs are in the high-risk population for HIV infection. However, others who do not fit these categories may unknowingly be at high risk. An example is women who consider themselves to be in monogamous relationships but are unaware that their partners have sexual relations with other women or men. As proportions, risk estimates have no dimensions, but they are a function of the length of time of observation. Given a continuous rate, increasing time will mean that a larger proportion of the population will eventually become ill, just as the longer an investment is left in an interest-paying account, the greater the total return will be even though the rate does not change.

Epidemiologists and other health professionals are interested in measures of morbidity, especially incidence proportions, incidence rates, and prevalence proportions. These measures provide information about the risk of disease, the rate of disease development, and the levels of existing disease in a population, respectively.

> **WHAT DO YOU THINK?**
>
> Genetic testing is becoming more common, but most tests for disease indicate only susceptibility to disease, not certainty. Similarly, screening tests are never perfect, so there is always some probability of misclassifying a person. How should these difficult concepts of probability and uncertainty be presented to clients when interpreting test results?

## Measures of Incidence

Measures of incidence reflect the number of *new* cases or events in a population at risk during a specified time. An **incidence rate** quantifies the rate of development of new cases in a population at risk, whereas an **incidence proportion** indicates the proportion of the population at risk who experience the event over some period of time (Rothman, 2002). The population at risk is considered to be persons without the event or outcome of interest but who are at risk of experiencing it. Note that existing (or prevalent) cases are excluded from the population at risk for this calculation, as they already have the condition and are no longer at risk of developing it. The incidence proportion is also referred to as the cumulative incidence rate (and erroneously simply as the incidence rate) because it reflects the cumulative effect of the incidence rate over the time period. An incidence proportion can be interpreted as an estimate of risk of disease in that population over that period—that is, as a probability with limits from 0 to 1. The risk of disease is a function of both the rate of new disease development and the length of time the population is at risk. The interpretation can be for an individual (i.e., the probability that the person will become ill) or for a population (i.e., the proportion of a population expected to become ill over that period). In epidemiology, we often calculate proportions on the basis of population frequencies. These frequencies are then translated into personal risk statements for people representative of the population on which the estimates are based.

For example, suppose a health department and community hospital jointly begin an intensive, broad-based screening program in an area characterized by overcrowded housing, limited access to services, and underuse of preventive health practices. Their program includes physical examinations; tuberculin skin tests with follow-up chest radiography where indicated; cardiovascular, glaucoma, and diabetes screening; and mammography for women and prostate screening for men over 45 years of age. Of the 8000 women screened, 35 were previously diagnosed with breast cancer, and 20 who have no history of breast cancer diagnosis are found by screening and follow-up to have cancer of the breast. One could follow the 7945 women in whom no breast cancer was detected and note the number of new cases of breast cancer detected over the following 5 years. Assuming no losses to follow-up (moved away or died from other causes), if 44 women were diagnosed over the 5-year period, then the 5-year incidence proportion of breast cancer in this population would be as follows:

$$\frac{44}{7945} = 0.005538, \text{ or } 553.8 \text{ per } 100,000.$$

Note the multiplication by 100,000, so that the number of cases is expressed as per 100,000 women. A cumulative incidence rate estimates the risk of developing the disease in that population during that time. Also, as a proportion, each event in the numerator much be represented in the denominator, and only those persons at risk of the event counted in the numerator may be included in the denominator.

We estimate incidence rates by counting events relative to the total amount of time persons in a population are observed, referred to as person-time. For many calculations it is generally assumed that rates are constant over the period of observation. A true incidence rate is an instantaneous rate of disease development, often approximated by incidence density. In calculating the person-time of observation for a denominator, we count the amount of time each person contributes from the time observation of that person begins until the person (1) experiences the event, (2) is lost to follow-up or dies from some other cause or otherwise is no longer at risk, or (3) reaches the end of observation. Incidence density is an estimate of the instantaneous rate (or *hazard*) of the event. It is an indication of how rapidly disease is developing in a population. Conceptually, a rate is the instantaneous change in a con-

tinuous process. Note that incidence density does have dimensions; it is not bounded by 1 (as a risk is); and its value depends on the units of time chosen. It may be interpreted as the reciprocal of the average time until disease onset (assuming no competing risks and fixed or steady state population with complete follow-up [Rothman, 2002; Rothman and Greenland, 1998]).

To continue the previous example, suppose the 7945 women we follow for 5 years accumulates a total of 39,615 person-years of observation. Remember, the assumption was there was no loss to follow-up or deaths from other causes. Note that the total person-time is not equivalent to $5 \times 7945$ (which is 39,725), because we stop counting time for the 44 women who developed breast cancer at the time of diagnosis. (You can imagine that determining the exact time of disease onset is often a problem in epidemiologic studies. Using time of diagnosis can be biased because diagnosis occurs at different stages of disease in populations.) So the incidence rate for breast cancer diagnosis in this population, after 5 years of observation, would be estimated as 44 newly diagnosed cases per 39,615 person-years of observation, or 0.0011107, which we could express as 11.1 cases per 10,000 person-years.

We often want to know about the risk—that is, the probability of disease occurring over some defined period of time, such as a year or several years. Earlier we estimated the risk directly as the number of new cases over a 5-year period in a population at risk. That was straightforward because we had no losses, and observation began at the same time for all the women. A more common situation is that people come under observation at different times and there are losses due to attrition or competing risks (i.e., other events or deaths). We can handle those easily by counting the amount of time that is observed and calculating the incidence density as an estimate of the incidence rate. The question is how the incidence density rate is related to an estimate of risk. We can say that the risk for individuals, accumulated over a population, gives rise to the rate observed in that population. In epidemiology, however, it is the observed rate in a population that allows us to estimate the risk of an event in that population, both in terms of the expected proportion of the population who would become ill and in terms of the risk to a representative member of the population. "A rate acts at an instant of time. As time moves across a time period, the cumulative action of the rate generates a risk across that time period" (Koopman, 1999). When certain assumptions are met, primarily a constant rate, the average incidence density over a period of time is related to the cumulative risk for that period by the following equation:

$$\textbf{Risk} = 1 - e^{[-I \times T]},$$

where $I$ is the mean per-person-time incidence rate, $T$ is the period of observation in the same units of time, and $e$ is the base of the natural logarithm. Again, to return to the example, suppose we observed the 44 new cases in 39,615 person-years of follow-up, but there were losses to follow-up, and women entered and left the population at different times. Assuming that the rate of new breast cancer is fairly constant over that 5-year period, the cumulative risk over 5 years is estimated as follows:

$$\text{Risk} = 1 - e^{[-0.0011107 \times 5]} = 0.005538,$$

which is the same as the risk we calculated for the simpler situation.

Note that the rate used is *not* the incidence proportion but the mean incidence densities for intervals of time comprising the total period, and the formula assumes that the rates do not vary over the period. Also, risk is a probability whose value depends on both the incidence rate and the period of observation, but not on the units of measurement for time, and whose range is restricted to between 0 and 1. The value of incidence density, on the other hand, does depend on the units of time and, because it is not a probability, is not restricted to the 0 to 1 range. Furthermore, when the incidence rate is low or the period of observation short—so that, relative to the size of the population, few people are removed from the population at risk by disease—the product of the per-person rate and the period of observation approximates the risk for the period. (Kelsey et al, 1996; Rothman and Greenland, 1998; Rothman, 2002; Szklo and Nieto, 2000).

A ratio can be used as an approximation of a risk. For example, the infant mortality "rate" is the number of infant deaths (i.e., infants here defined as being less than 1 year of age) in a given year divided by the number of live births in that same year. It approximates the risk of death in the first year of life for live-born infants in a specific year. Some of the infants who die that year were born in the previous year, and some of the infants born that year may die in the following year prior to their first birthday. However, because about two thirds of infant deaths occur within the first 28 days of life, the number of infants in the numerator (deaths in a given year) but not in the denominator (live births in that same year) will be small. It can be assumed that current year deaths from the previous year's cohort approximately equal the deaths from the current year's cohort occurring in the following year. Although technically a ratio, this is an approximation to the true proportion, and, therefore, an estimate of the risk. In NCHS publications, you may notice that the rate of infant death is not equivalent to the number of deaths divided by the number of live births. These rates take into account the changes in the rate of death over the first year of life—that is, they use a person-time denominator.

An **epidemic** occurs when the rate of disease, injury, or other condition exceeds the usual (endemic) level of that condition. There is no specific threshold of incidence that indicates an epidemic exists. Because smallpox has been eradicated, any occurrence of smallpox might be considered an epidemic by this definition. In contrast, given the high rates of ischemic heart disease in the United States, an increase of many cases would be needed before an epidemic was noted, although some might argue that the current high rates compared with earlier periods already indicate an epidemic.

## Prevalence Proportion

The **prevalence proportion** is a measure of existing disease in a population at a particular time (i.e., the number of existing cases divided by the current population). One also can calculate the prevalence of a specific risk factor or exposure. In the breast cancer example given earlier, the screening program discovered 35 of the 8000 women screened had previously been diagnosed with breast cancer, and 20 women with no history of breast cancer were diagnosed as a result of the screening. The prevalence proportion of current and past breast cancer events in this population of women would be as follows:

$$\frac{55}{8000} = 0.006875, \text{ or } 687.5 \text{ per } 100,000.$$

A prevalence proportion is not an estimate of the risk of developing disease, because it is a function of both the rate at which new cases of the disease develop and how long those cases remain in the population. In this example, the prevalence of breast cancer in this population of women is a function of how many new cases develop and how long women live after breast cancer diagnosis. One might see a fairly constant prevalence, for example, if improved survival after diagnosis were offset by an increasing incidence rate. The duration of a disease is affected by case fatality and cure. (For simplicity, in this example, women with a history of the disease are counted in the prevalence proportion even though they may have been cured.) A disease with a short duration (e.g., an intestinal virus) may not have a high prevalence proportion even if the rate of new cases is high, because cases do not accumulate (see Point Epidemic later in this chapter.) A disease with a long course will have a higher prevalence proportion than a rapidly fatal disease that has the same rate of new cases.

## Incidence and Prevalence Compared

The prevalence proportion measures existing cases of disease. The prevalence odds ($P/(1 - P)$) are roughly proportional to the incidence rate multiplied by the average duration of disease (Rothman, 2002). The prevalence proportion is, therefore, affected by factors that influence risk (incidence) and by factors that influence survival or recovery (duration). For that reason, prevalence measures are less useful when looking for factors related to disease etiology. Because prevalence proportions reflect duration in addition to the risk of getting the disease, it is difficult to sort out what factors are related to risk and what factors are related to survival or recovery. In mathematical notation,

$$P/(1 - P) \approx I \times D, \text{ or, when } P \text{ is small } (<0.1), \text{ the } P \approx I \times D,$$

where $P$ = prevalence, $I$ = incidence rate, and $D$ = average duration.

For example, the 5-year survival rate for breast cancer is about 85%, but the 5-year survival rate for lung cancer in women is only about 15%. Even if the incidence rates of breast and lung cancer were the same in women (and they are not), the prevalence proportions would differ because, on average, women live longer with breast cancer (i.e., it has a longer duration). Incidence rates and incidence proportions, on the other hand, are the measure of choice to study etiology because incidence is affected only by factors related to the risk of developing disease and not to survival or cure. Prevalence is useful in planning health care services because it is an indication of the level of disease existing in the population and therefore of the size of the population in need of services. In the previous example about screening, the health department would want to know both the existing level of TB in the area (the prevalence), to plan services and direct prevention and control measures, and the rate at which new cases are developing (the incidence), to study risk factors and evaluate the effectiveness of prevention and control programs.

> **HOW TO** **Quantify a Health Problem in the Community**
>
> Planning for resources and personnel often requires quantifying the level of a problem in a community. For example, to know how different districts compare in the rates of very-low-birthweight infants, one would calculate the prevalence of very-low-birthweight births in each district:
>
> 1. Determine the number of live births in each district from birth certificate data obtained from the vital records division of the health department.
> 2. Use the birthweight information from the birth certificate data to determine the number of infants born weighing less than 1500 grams in each district.
> 3. Calculate the prevalence of very-low-birthweight births by district as the number of infants weighing less than 1500 grams at birth divided by the total number of live births.
> 4. If the number of very-low-birthweight births in each district is small, use several recent years of data to obtain a more stable estimate.

## Attack Rate

One final measure of morbidity, often used in infectious disease investigations, is the **attack rate.** This form of incidence proportion is defined as the proportion of persons who are exposed to an agent and develop the disease. Attack rates are often specific to an exposure; food-specific attack rates, for example, are the proportion of persons becoming ill after eating a specific food item.

## Mortality Rates

Nurses need to understand a number of mortality rates (Table 11-3). Note that many commonly used mortality rates in Table 11-3 are not true rates but proportions (Gordis, 2000; Rothman, 2002), although the midyear population estimate for the denominator is intended to approximate the amount of person-time contributed by the population during a given year. Although measures of mortality reflect serious health problems and changing patterns of disease, they are limited in their usefulness. They are informative only for fatal diseases and do not provide direct information about either the level of existing disease in the population or the risk of getting any particular disease. Furthermore, it is not uncommon for a person who has one disease (e.g., prostate cancer) to die from a different cause (e.g., stroke).

Because the population changes during the course of a year, it is useful to take an estimate of the population at midyear as the denominator for annual rates. Using the approximation noted previously for small rates when the period of observation is a single unit of time, the annual mortality rate is an estimate of the risk of death in a given population for that year. These rates are multiplied by a scaling factor, usually 100,000, to avoid small fractions. The result is then expressed as the number of deaths per 100,000 persons. Although a crude mortality rate is calculated easily and represents the actual death rate for the total population, it has certain limitations. It does not reveal specific causes of death, which change in relative importance over time (see Figure 11-1). Also, it is affected by the age distribution of the population because older people are at much greater risk of death than younger people. For example, in 2000 the crude mortality rate for African Americans was 806.0 per 100,000 compared to a rate of 998.3 per 100,000 for non-Hispanic white Americans, even though the mortality rate was higher for African Americans than for whites in every age group up to age 85. This phenomenon will be discussed further.

Mortality rates also are calculated for specific groups (e.g., age-, sex-, or race-specific rates). In these instances, the number of deaths occurring in the specified group is divided by the population at risk, now restricted to the number of persons in that group. This rate may be interpreted as the risk of death for persons in the specified group during the period of observation.

The cause-specific mortality rate is an estimate of the risk of death from some specific disease in a population. It is the number of deaths from a specific cause divided by the total population at risk, usually multiplied by 100,000. Two related measures should be distinguished from the cause-specific mortality rate. The case fatality rate (CFR) is actually a proportion: the proportion of persons diagnosed with a particular disorder (i.e., cases) who die within a specified period of time. The CFR may be interpreted as an estimate of the risk of death within that period for a person newly diagnosed with the disease (e.g., the proportion of persons with breast cancer who die within 5 years). Because the CFR is the proportion of diagnosed persons who die within the period, 1 minus the CFR yields the survival rate. For example, if the 5-year CFR for lung cancer is 86%, then

## Table 11-3  Common Mortality Rates

| RATE/RATIO | DEFINITION AND EXAMPLE |
|---|---|
| Crude mortality rate | Usually an annual rate that represents the proportion of a population who die from any cause during the period, using the midyear population as the denominator<br>Example: In 2000 there were 2,403,351 deaths in a total population of 275,264,999, or 873.1 per 100,000. |
| Age-specific rate | Number of deaths among persons of given age-group per midyear population of that age-group<br>Example: 2000 age-specific mortality rate for 20- to 24-year-olds:<br>$$\frac{17,744}{18,484,615} = 96 \text{ per } 100,000 \text{ 20- to 24-year-olds}$$ |
| Cause-specific rate | Number of deaths from a specific cause per midyear population<br>Example: 2000 cause-specific rate for accidents:<br>$$\frac{97,900 \text{ accidental deaths}}{175,264,999 \text{ midyear population}} = 35.6 \text{ per } 100,000$$ |
| Case-fatality rate | Number of deaths from a specific disease in a given period/Number of persons diagnosed with that disease<br>Example: If 87 of every 100 persons diagnosed with lung cancer dies within 5 years, the 5-year case fatality rate is 87%. The 5-year survival rate is 13%. |
| Proportionate mortality ratio | Number of deaths from a specific disease per total number of deaths in the same period<br>Example: In 2000, there were 710,760 deaths from diseases of the heart, and 2,403,351 deaths from all causes.<br>$$\frac{710,760}{2,403,351} = 0.296 \text{ or } 29.6\% \text{ of all deaths were due to heart disease}$$ |
| Infant mortality rate | Number of infant deaths before 1 year of age in a year per number of live births in the same year<br>Example: In 2000, there were 28,035 infant deaths and 4,058,814 live births:<br>$$\frac{28,035}{4,058,814} = 0.0069 \text{ or } 6.9 \text{ deaths per } 1000 \text{ live births}$$ |
| Neonatal mortality rate | Number of infant deaths under 28 days of age in a year per number of live births in the same year<br>Example: In 2000, there were 18,776 neonatal deaths and 4,058,814 live births:<br>$$\frac{18,776}{4,058,814} = 4.63 \text{ per } 1000 \text{ live births}$$ |
| Postneonatal mortality rate | Number of infant deaths from 28 days to 1 year in a year per number of live births in the same year<br>Example: In 2000, there were 9,259 postneonatal deaths and 4,058,814 live births:<br>$$\frac{9,259}{4,058,814} = 2.28 \text{ deaths per } 1000 \text{ live births}$$ |

From Anderson RN: Deaths: leading causes for 2000, *Natl Vital Stat Rep* 50(16), 2002; Martin JA et al: Births: final data for 2000, *Natl Vital Stat Rep* 50(5), 2002; National Center for Health Statistics: *Health, United States, 1998,* Hyattsville, Md, 1998, Public Health Service.

the 5-year survival rate is only 14% (Brownson et al, 1998). Persons diagnosed with a particular disease often want to know the probability of surviving. These rates provide that information.

The second measure to be distinguished from the cause-specific mortality rate is the proportionate mortality ratio (PMR), the proportion of all deaths that are due to a specific cause. The denominator is not the population at risk of death but the total number of deaths in the population; therefore, the PMR is not a rate nor does it estimate the risk of death. The magnitude of the PMR is a function of both the number of deaths from the cause of interest and the number of deaths from other causes. If deaths from certain causes decline over time, deaths from other causes that remain fairly constant may have increasing PMRs. For example, motor vehicle accidents accounted for 4.3 deaths per 100,000 persons 5 to 14 years of age in the United States in 2000. This was 23.4% of all deaths in this age group (the PMR). By comparison, motor vehicle accidents caused 20.6 deaths per 100,000 persons 65 years of age and older in 2000, which was less than 0.4% of all deaths in the older age group (Minino and Smith, 2001). This demonstrates that, although the risk of death from a motor vehicle accident was almost five times as great in the older group (based on the rates), such accidents accounted for a far greater proportion of all deaths in the younger group (based on the PMR). The reason is that there is a much greater risk of death from other causes in the older group.

Health professionals also are interested in measures of infant mortality, which are used around the world as an indicator of overall health and availability of health care services. The most common measure, the infant mortality rate, is the number of deaths to infants in the first year of life divided by the total number of live births. Because the risk of death declines rather dramatically during the first year of life, neonatal and postneonatal mortality rates are also of interest (see Table 11-3).

> **HOW TO** **Epidemiologic Concepts in Community-Oriented Nursing**
>
> Epidemiologic concepts and data are used in ongoing assessments of both community and individual health problems. An initial component of a community health assessment is the collection of incidence, morbidity, and mortality rates for specific diseases. Health service data, such as immunization rates, causes of hospitalization, and emergency department visits, are also obtained. Additional areas for community assessment are outlined in the How To boxes on pp. 268 and 269. Individual health problems should incorporate evaluations of health risk based on lifestyle patterns along with the standard history and clinical examinations.

## Epidemiologic Triangle: Agent, Host, and Environment

Epidemiologists understand that disease results from complex relationships among causal agents, susceptible persons, and environmental factors. These three elements—**agent, host,** and **environment**—are called the epidemiologic triangle (Figure 11-2, *A*). Changes in one of the elements of the triangle can influence the occurrence of disease by increasing or decreasing a person's risk for disease. Risk is understood as the probability that an individual will experience an event (Last, 2001). Figure 11-2, *B*, suggests that both agent and host, as well as their interaction, are influenced by the environmental context in which they exist, and that they in turn may influence the environment. Some examples of these three components are listed in Box 11-1.

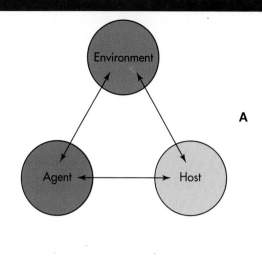

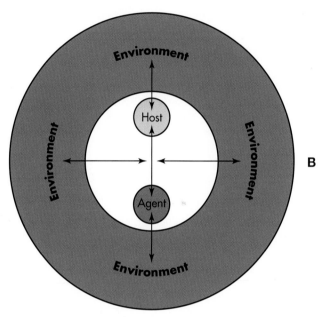

**Figure 11-2** Two models of the agent–host–environment interaction (the epidemiologic triangle).

Causal relationships are often more complex than the epidemiologic triangle conveys. It is common to speak of a **web of causality,** recognizing the complex interrelationships of numerous factors interacting, sometimes in subtle ways, to increase (or decrease) risk of disease. Furthermore, associations are sometimes mutual, with lines of causality going in both directions.

A common example of complex factors in a causal web is shown for cardiovascular disease in Figure 11-3. Fortunately, effective interventions to disrupt causal pathways and prevent disease are often possible even without a complete understanding of all causal elements and their interrelationships. Some authors use the term *black box epidemiology* to refer to research of associations without understanding how the factors and outcomes are related (Susser and Susser, 1996a,b). Recently, some researchers have advocated a new paradigm that goes beyond the two-dimensional causal web to consider multiple levels of factors that affect health and

> **BOX 11-1** **Examples of Agent, Host, and Environmental Factors in the Epidemiologic Triangle**
>
> **AGENT**
> - Infectious agents (bacteria, viruses, fungi, parasites)
> - Chemical agents (heavy metals, toxic chemicals, pesticides)
> - Physical agents (radiation, heat, cold, machinery)
>
> **HOST**
> - Genetic susceptibility
> - Immutable characteristics (age, sex)
> - Acquired characteristics (immunologic status)
> - Lifestyle factors (diet and exercise)
>
> **ENVIRONMENT**
> - Climate (temperature, rainfall)
> - Plant and animal life (agents or reservoirs or habitats for agents)
> - Human population distribution (crowding, social support)
> - Socioeconomic factors (education, resources, access to care)
> - Working conditions (levels of stress, noise, satisfaction)

disease (Diez-Roux, 1998; Krieger, 1994). This approach expands epidemiologic studies both upward to broader contexts (such as neighborhood characteristics and social context) and downward to the genetic and molecular level. This multilevel analytic approach should provide insight into the mysteries inside the "black box," even though public health practitioners continue to apply successful interventions in the absence of clear understanding of underlying processes and relationships. Epidemiologic studies often demonstrate what interventions are useful.

## Levels of Preventive Interventions

The goal of epidemiology is to identify and understand the causal factors and mechanisms of disease, disability, and injuries so that effective interventions can be implemented to prevent the occurrence of these adverse processes before they begin or before they progress. The **natural history of disease** is the course of the disease process from onset to resolution (Last, 2001). The three **levels of prevention** provide a framework commonly used in public health practice (Box 11-2). As practicing epidemiologists, community-oriented nurses are involved in primary, secondary, and tertiary prevention of communicable and noncommunicable diseases. At all three levels of prevention, nurses engage in the core public health functions of *assessment, policy development,* and *assurance* (IOM, 1988). Assessment involves

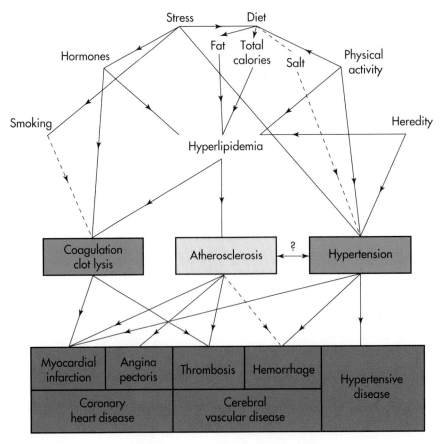

**Figure 11-3** An example of a web of causality for cardiovascular disease. *(From Stallones RA: Cerebrovascular disease epidemiology: a workshop,* Public Health Monogr *76:51-55, 1966.)*

## BOX 11-2  Levels of Prevention and Examples Related to Cardiovascular Disease

### PRIMARY PREVENTION
Counsel clients about low-fat diet and regular physical exercise.

### SECONDARY PREVENTION
Implement blood pressure and cholesterol screening, give treadmill stress test.

### TERTIARY PREVENTION
Provide cardiac rehabilitation, medication, surgery.

the regular and systematic collection, analysis, and dissemination of community health data in order to monitor health status and diagnose and investigate health problems and health hazards in the community. Policy development includes the incorporation of scientific knowledge and epidemiologic data in public health decision making and policy formulation within democratic processes. Information gathered through assessment processes provides the basis for policy development. The key processes of policy development are (1) to inform, educate, and empower people about health, (2) to mobilize community partnerships to identify and solve health problems, and (3) to develop policies and plans that support individual and community health efforts. The third core function of public health is to assure the members of the community that they will have access to needed health services; that laws and regulations that protect health and ensure safety will be enforced; that the heath care workforce is competent; that quality health services are effective and easily accessible; and that research is conducted and the resulting knowledge is applied in developing innovative solutions to health problems in the community (Turnock, 2001).

In their daily practice, nurses are often involved in activities related to all three levels of prevention. For example, community-oriented nurses use primary prevention in health promotion programs with both the general population and specific vulnerable groups (e.g., the homeless, HIV-positive persons, certain immigrant groups) to improve the general health status and to reduce the incidence of specific diseases such as TB. Secondary prevention activities include routine tuberculin testing of specific groups (e.g., health care providers, child care workers) and identification and screening of persons who have had contact with a known TB case. Diagnosis of individuals with active TB and using directly observed therapy fall within the realm of tertiary prevention. Given the emergence of new drug-resistant strains of TB, nurses are now facing the challenge of designing and implementing programs to increase long-term compliance and provide aftercare for clients in a variety of community settings.

## Primary Prevention

Primary prevention refers to interventions aimed at preventing the occurrence of disease, injury, or disability. Interventions at this level of prevention are aimed at individuals and groups who are susceptible to disease but have no discernible pathology (i.e., they are in a state of prepathogenesis). This first level of prevention includes broad efforts such as health promotion, environmental protection, and specific protection. Health promotion includes nutrition education and counseling and the promotion of physical activity. Environmental protection ranges from basic sanitation and food safety, to home and workplace safety plans, to air quality control. Examples of specific protection against disease or injury include immunizations, proper use of seat belts and infants' car seats, preconception folic acid supplementation to prevent neural tube defects, fluoridation of water supplies to prevent dental caries, and actions taken to reduce human exposure to agents that may cause cancer. Primary prevention occurs in homes, community settings, and at the primary level of health care (e.g., in public health clinics, physicians' offices, community health centers, and rural health clinics).

At the primary prevention level, nurses working in the community and in primary care settings are involved in general health promotion activities such as nutrition education and counseling, sex education, and family planning services. An example of a primary prevention intervention is providing health education and training for day-care workers regarding health and hygiene issues, such as proper hand hygiene, diapering, and food preparation and storage. Another example is teaching the asthmatic client to recognize and avoid exposure to asthma triggers and assisting the family in implementing specific protection strategies such as replacing carpets, keeping air systems clean and free of mold, and avoiding pets.

In terms of environmental protection, nurses work proactively to develop and advocate for policies and legislation that lead to prevention of environmental hazards. They can also provide consultation to industries, local governments, and groups of concerned citizens and public education for a wide range of preventable environmental health problems.

## Secondary Prevention

Secondary prevention encompasses interventions designed to increase the probability that a person with a disease will have that condition diagnosed at a stage when treatment is likely to result in cure. Health screenings are the mainstay of secondary prevention. Early and periodic screenings are critical for diseases for which there are few specific primary prevention strategies, such as breast cancer. Screening programs will be discussed later.

Interventions at the secondary level of prevention may occur in community settings as well as at primary and secondary levels of health care. Particularly in developing countries, when safe water can be made available, oral rehydration therapy (ORT) is a low-cost and effective way to treat infant diarrheal disease. The mother who is able to identify the early signs of infant dehydration and administer a homemade ORT solution of water, sugar, and salt is practicing secondary prevention. The nurse who asks about family history of cancer, heart disease, diabetes, and mental illness as part of a client's health history, and then follows up with education about appropriate screening procedures, is initiating the process of secondary prevention. Other examples of secondary prevention interventions include mammography to detect breast cancer, Papanicolaou (Pap) smears to detect cervical cancer, colonoscopy for early detection of colon cancer, and prenatal screening of pregnant women to screen for gestational diabetes.

## Tertiary Prevention

Tertiary prevention includes interventions aimed at disability limitation and rehabilitation from disease, injury, or disability. Tertiary prevention interventions occur most often at secondary and tertiary levels of care (e.g., specialized clinics, hospitals, rehabilitation centers) but may also occur in community and primary care settings. Medical treatment, physical and occupational therapy, and rehabilitation are interventions characterized as tertiary prevention.

## An Intervention Spectrum

The standard classification of preventive measures in public health is composed of the primary, secondary, and tertiary levels of prevention. However, this standard classification has been revised and refined for application to diverse settings and health issues. In the area of mental health, three generations of prevention have been identified, ranging from pre-intervention prevention to acute care (Figure 11-4). The IOM publication on prevention research in mental disorders (Mrazek and Haggerty, 1994) classified an intervention as *universal* when it is directed to the general population and provides general benefit with little risk at low cost; *selective* when it is directed toward persons or groups who are at increased risk for developing a problem, with risk and harms justified on the basis of the potential reduction in adverse outcomes; and *indicated* when more costly or higher-risk interventions target high-risk persons who already evidence a problem. This report reserved the term *prevention* for those interventions that occur before onset of disorder. The two components of *treatment interventions* include case identification and standard treatment for known disorders. Finally, the components of maintenance in an ongoing disorder are *compliance with long-term treatment* and *provision of aftercare services, including rehabilitation.* Although this classification system was designed from the perspective of mental health, it can

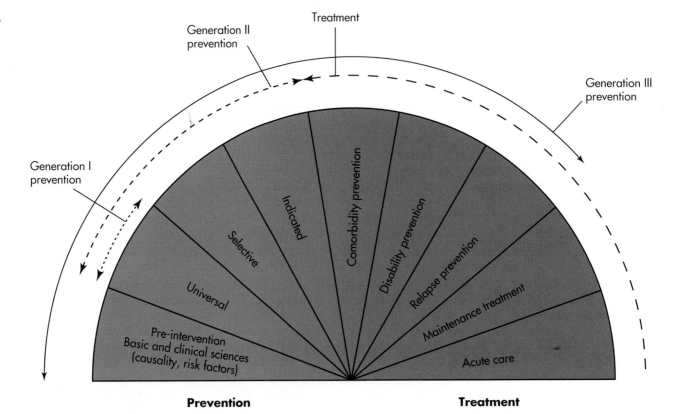

**Figure 11-4** Health intervention spectrum. *(From National Institute of Mental Health:* Priorities for prevention research at NIMH: a report by the National Advisory Health Council Workgroup on Mental Disorders Prevention Research, *Publication No. 98-4321, Washington, DC, 1998, NIH.)*

be applied to other public health issues, and community-oriented health nurses play critical roles at all points across the spectrum.

# SCREENING

**Screening,** a key component of many secondary prevention interventions, involves the testing of groups of individuals who are at risk for a certain condition but are as yet asymptomatic. The purpose is to classify these individuals with respect to the likelihood of having the disease. From a clinical perspective, the aim of screening is early detection and treatment when these result in a more favorable prognosis. From a public health perspective, the objective is to sort out efficiently and effectively those who probably have the disease from those who probably do not, again to detect early cases for treatment or begin public health prevention and control programs. A screening test is not a diagnostic test. Effective screening programs must have built-in referral mechanisms for subsequent diagnostic evaluation for those who screen positive, to determine if they actually have the disease and need treatment.

Nurses must keep abreast of screening guidelines, which are regularly reviewed and revised on the basis of epidemiologic research results. For example, the latest U.S. Preventive Services Task Force (USPSTF, 2002) strongly recommends routine screening for lipid disorders in men aged 35 years and older and women aged 45 years and older. Screening for younger adults (men aged 20 to 35 and women aged 20 to 45) is recommended when any of the following risk factors are present: diabetes, family history of cardiovascular disease before age 50 in men or age 60 in women relatives, family history suggestive of familial hyperlipidemia, or multiple coronary heart disease risk factors (e.g., tobacco use, hypertension). The Task Force also noted that all clients, regardless of lipid levels, should be offered counseling about the benefits of a diet low in saturated fat and high in fruits and vegetables, regular physical activity, avoidance of tobacco, and maintenance of healthy weight. The rationale for the current guidelines was explained as follows.

The clearest benefit of lipid screening is identifying individuals whose near-term risk of coronary heart disease is sufficiently high to justify drug therapy or other intensive lifestyle interventions to lower cholesterol. Screening men older than age 35 years and women older than age 45 years will identify nearly all individuals whose risk of coronary heart disease is as high as that of the subjects in the existing primary prevention trials. Younger people typically have a substantially lower risk, unless they have other important risk factors for coronary heart disease or familial hyperlipidemia. The primary goal of screening younger people is to promote lifestyle changes, which may provide long-term benefits later in life. The average effect of diet interventions is small, and screening is not needed to advise young adults about the benefits of a healthy diet and regular exercise since this advice is considered useful for all age groups. Although universal screening may detect some

clients with familial hyperlipidemia earlier than selective screening, it is not known whether this will lead to important reductions in coronary events (USPSTF, 2002, p. 95).

As community health advocates, nurses are responsible for planning and implementing screening and prevention programs targeted to the at-risk populations, such as prostate-screening programs among African-American men. Occupational and community-oriented nurses may work together to target at-risk populations on the basis of occupational risk. For example, worksites where there are occupational exposures associated with prostate cancer, such as sites that use or manufacture cadmium, batteries, and pesticides, could be targeted (S. Weinrich et al, 1998). However, in providing such programs, nurses need to be aware that research has demonstrated substantial race- and age-related differences in serum prostate-specific antigen (PSA) levels (M. Weinrich et al, 1998), which supports the use of population-specific reference ranges. Men with questionable PSAs need to be referred, especially if they have increased risk factors for prostate cancer, such as African-American race or family history of prostate cancer. Successful screening programs have several characteristics that depend on the tests and on population screened (Box 11-3). Desirable traits include the availability of reliable and valid screening tests (Gordis, 2000).

## Reliability and Validity

### Reliability

The precision, or **reliability,** of the measure (its consistency or repeatability) and the accuracy of the measure (whether it is really measuring what we think it is, and how exactly) are important considerations for any measurement. Suppose you want to do a blood pressure screening in a community. You will take blood pressures on a large

---

**BOX 11-3   Characteristics of a Successful Screening Program**

1. **Valid (accurate):** A high probability of correct classification of persons tested
2. **Reliable (precise):** Results consistent from place to place, time to time, and person to person
3. **Capable of large group administration:**
   a. Fast in both the administration of the test and the obtaining of results
   b. Inexpensive in both personnel required and in the materials and procedures used
4. **Innocuous:** Few if any side effects, and the test minimally invasive
5. **High yield:** Able to detect enough new cases to warrant the effort and expense (*yield* defined as the amount of previously unrecognized disease that is diagnosed and treated as a result of screening)

number of people, perhaps following up with repeated measures for individuals with higher pressures.

If the sphygmomanometer used for the screening varies in its readings so that it does not give the same reading for the same person twice in a row, then it lacks precision. The instrument would be unreliable even if the overall mean of repeated measurements were close to the true overall mean for the persons measured. The problem would be that the readings would not be reliable for any individual, which is what a screening program requires.

On the other hand, suppose the readings are reliably reproducible, but, unknown to you, they tend to be about 10 mm Hg too high. This instrument is producing precise readings, but the uncorrected (or uncalibrated) instrument lacks accuracy. In short, a measure can be consistent without producing valid results.

Three major sources of error can affect the reliability of tests:

- Variation inherent in the trait being measured (e.g., blood pressure changes with time of day, activity, level of stress, and other factors)
- Observer variation, which can be divided into intraobserver reliability (consistency by the same observer) and interobserver reliability (consistency from one observer to another)
- Inconsistency in the instrument, which includes the internal consistency of the instrument (e.g., whether all items in a questionnaire measure the same thing) and the stability (or test-retest reliability) of the instrument over time

## Validity: Sensitivity and Specificity

**Validity** in a screening test is measured by sensitivity and specificity. **Sensitivity** quantifies how accurately the test identifies those *with* the condition or trait. In other words, sensitivity represents the proportion of persons with the disease whom the test correctly identifies as positive (true positives). High sensitivity is needed when early treatment is important and when identification of every case is important.

**Specificity** indicates how accurately the test identifies those *without* the condition or trait (i.e., the proportion of persons whom the test correctly identifies as negative for the disease [true negatives]). High specificity is needed when rescreening is impractical and when reducing false positives is important. The sensitivity and specificity of a test are determined by comparing the results from the test with results from a definitive diagnostic procedure (sometimes called the gold standard). For example, the Pap smear is used frequently to screen for cervical dysplasia and carcinoma. The definitive diagnosis of cervical cancer requires a biopsy with histologic confirmation of malignant cells.

The ideal for a screening test is 100% sensitivity and 100% specificity. That is, the test is positive for 100% of those who actually have the disease, and it is negative for all those who do not have the disease. In practice, sensitivity and specificity are often inversely related. That is, if the test results are such that one can choose some point beyond which a person is considered positive (a "cutpoint"), as in a blood pressure reading to screen for hypertension or a serum glucose reading to screen for diabetes, then moving that critical point to improve the sensitivity of the test will result in a decrease in specificity, or an improvement in specificity can be made only at the expense of sensitivity.

Table 11-4 shows how to calculate sensitivity and specificity. Some writers refer to a false-positive rate, which is 1 minus the specificity, and a false-negative rate, or 1 minus the sensitivity. These "rates" are simply the proportions of subjects incorrectly labeled as nondiseased and diseased, respectively.

A third measure associated with sensitivity and specificity is the predictive value of the test. The **positive predictive value** (also called predictive value positive) is the proportion of persons with a positive test who actually have the disease, interpreted as the probability that an individual with a positive test has the disease. The **negative predictive value** (or predictive value negative) is the proportion of persons with a negative test who are actually disease free. Although sensitivity and specificity are relatively independent of the prevalence of disease, predictive values are affected by the level of disease in the screened

---

**Table 11-4  Classification of Subjects According to True Disease State and Screening Test Results for Calculation of Indices of Validity**

| RESULT OF SCREENING TEST | DISEASE | NO DISEASE |
|---|---|---|
| Positive | True positive (TP) | False positive (FP) |
| Negative | False negative (FN) | True negative (TN) |

Sensitivity = TP/(TP + FN)
Specificity = TN/(TN + FP)
False negative "rate" = 1 − sensitivity = FN/(FN + TP)
False positive "rate" = 1 − specificity = FP/(TN + FP)
Positive predictive value = TP/(TP + FP). Often multiplied by 100 and expressed as a percentage.

population and by the sensitivity and specificity of the test. When the prevalence is very low, the positive predictive value will be low, even with tests that are sensitive and specific. Additionally, lower specificity produces lower positive predictive values because of the increase in the proportion of false-positive results.

Consideration of the human and economic costs of missing true cases by lowering the sensitivity versus the cost of falsely classifying noncases by lowering the specificity is necessary in setting cutpoints. Factors to be considered include the importance of capturing all cases, the likelihood that the population will be rescreened, the interval between screenings relative to the rate of disease development, and the prevalence of the disease. A low prevalence typically requires a test with high specificity; otherwise, the screening will produce too many false positives in the large nondiseased population. On the other hand, a disease with a high prevalence usually requires high sensitivity; otherwise, too many of the real cases will be missed by the screening (false negatives).

Two or more tests can be combined, in series or in parallel, to enhance sensitivity or specificity. In series testing, the final result is considered positive only if all tests in the series were positive, and it is considered negative if any test was negative. For example, if a blood sample were screened for HIV, a positive enzyme-linked immunosorbent assay (ELISA) might be followed up with a Western blot, and the sample would be considered positive only if both tests were positive. Series testing enhances specificity, producing fewer false positives, but sensitivity will be lower. In series testing, sequence is important; a very sensitive test is often used first to pick up all cases including false positives, and then a second, very specific test is used to eliminate the false positives. In parallel testing, the final result is considered positive if *any* test was positive and negative only if all tests were negative. To return to the example of a blood sample being tested for HIV, a blood bank might consider a sample positive if a positive result was found on either the ELISA or the Western blot. Parallel testing enhances sensitivity, leaving fewer false negatives, but specificity will be lower.

# BASIC METHODS IN EPIDEMIOLOGY
## Sources of Data

One of the first issues to address in any epidemiologic study is how the data will be obtained (Kelsey et al, 1996). There are three major categories of data sources commonly used in epidemiologic investigations:
1. Routinely collected data, such as census data, vital records (birth and death certificates), and **surveillance** data (systematic collection of data concerning disease occurrence) as carried out by the Centers for Disease Control and Prevention (CDC)
2. Data collected for other purposes but useful for epidemiologic research, such as medical, health department, and insurance records

3. Original data collected for specific epidemiologic studies

### Routinely Collected Data

The United States census is conducted every 10 years and provides population data, including demographic distribution (age, race, sex), geographic distribution, and additional information about economic status, housing, and education. These data provide denominators for various rates.

Vital records are the primary source of birth and mortality statistics. Although registration of births and deaths is mandated in most countries, providing one of the most complete sources of health-related data, the quality of specific information varies. For example, on birth certificates, sex and date of birth are fairly reliable, whereas gestational age, level of prenatal care, and smoking habits of the mother during pregnancy are less reliable. On death certificates, the quality of the cause of death information varies over time and from place to place, depending on diagnostic capabilities and custom. Vital records are readily available in most areas; they are inexpensive, convenient, and allow study of long-term trends. Mortality data, however, are informative only for fatal diseases.

### Data Collected for Other Purposes

Hospital, physician, health department, and insurance records provide information on morbidity, as do surveillance systems, such as cancer registries and health department reporting systems, which solicit reports of all cases of a particular disease within a geographic region. Other information, such as occupational exposures, may be available from employer records.

### Epidemiologic Data

The National Center for Health Statistics sponsors periodic health surveys and examinations in carefully drawn samples of the U.S. population. Examples are the National Health and Nutrition Examination Survey (NHANES), the National Health Interview Survey (NHIS), and the National Hospital Discharge Survey (NHDS). The CDC also conducts or contracts for conduct of surveys such as the Youth Risk Behavior Survey (YRBS), Pregnancy Risk Assessment Monitoring System (PRAMS), and the Behavioral Risk Factor Surveillance System (BRFSS). These surveys provide information on the health status and behaviors of the population. For many studies, however, the only way to obtain the needed information is to collect the required data in a study specifically designed to investigate a particular question. The design of such studies is discussed later.

## Rate Adjustment

Rates, which are of central importance in epidemiologic studies, can be misleading when compared across different populations. For example, the risk of death increases rather dramatically after 40 years of age, so a higher crude death rate is expected in a population of older people compared with a population of younger people (Gordis, 2000; Rothman, 2002). Comparing the overall mortality rate in an area with a large population of older adults to the rate in a younger population would be misleading. Methods that adjust for differences in populations can be used to compare death rates. Age adjustment is based on the assumption that a population's overall mortality rate is a function of the age distribution of the population and the age-specific mortality rates.

Age adjustment can be performed by direct or indirect methods. Both methods require a *standard population*, which can be an external population, such as the U.S. population for a given year; a combined population of the groups under study; or some other standard chosen for relevance or convenience.

A direct adjusted rate applies the age-specific death rates from the study population to the age distribution of the standard population. The result is the (hypothetical) death rate of the study population if it had the same age distribution as the standard population.

The indirect method, as the name suggests, is more complicated. The age-specific death rates of the standard population applied to the study population's age distribution produce an index rate that is used with the crude rates of both the study and standard populations to produce the final indirect adjusted rate, which is also hypothetical. The indirect method may be required when the age-specific death rates for the study population are unknown or unstable (e.g., based on relatively small numbers).

Often, instead of an indirect adjusted rate, a standardized mortality ratio (or SMR) is calculated. This is the number of observed deaths in the study population divided by the number of deaths expected on the basis of the age-specific rates in the standard population and the age distribution of the study population (Gordis, 2000; Szklo and Nieto, 2000).

Although this discussion has focused on age adjustment, the process can be used to adjust for any factor that might vary from one population to another. For example, to compare infant mortality rates across populations with different birthweight distributions, these methods may be used to produce birthweight-adjusted infant mortality rates. Note that all adjusted rates are fictitious rates. They may resemble crude rates if the distribution of the study sample is similar to the distribution of the standard population. The magnitude of adjusted rates depends on the standard population used. The choice of a different standard would produce a different adjusted rate. The change from the 1940 U.S. population to the 2000 U.S. population as the standard for age-adjusted rates from the NCHS demonstrates the difference a change in standard population can make (Anderson and Rosenberg, 1998; Sorlie et al, 1999).

## Comparison Groups

The use of comparison groups is at the heart of the epidemiologic approach. Incidence or prevalence measures in

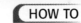

**HOW TO** Assess Health Problems in a Community

1. Examine local epidemiologic data (e.g., incidence, morbidity, and mortality rates) to identify major health problems.
2. Examine local health services data to identify major causes of hospitalizations and emergency department visits. Consult with key community leaders (e.g., political, religious, business, educational, health, and cultural leaders) about their perceptions of identified community health problems.
4. Mobilize community groups to elicit discussions and identify perceived health priorities within the community (e.g., focus groups, neighborhood or community-wide forums).
5. Analyze community environmental health hazards and pollutants (e.g., water, sewage, air, toxic waste).
6. Examine indicators of community knowledge and practices of preventive health behaviors (e.g., use of infant car seats, safe playgrounds, lighted streets, seat belt use, designated driver programs).
7. Identify cultural priorities and beliefs about health among different social, cultural, racial, or national origin groups.
8. Assess community members' interpretation of and degree of trust in federal, state, and local assistance programs.
9. Engage community members in conducting surveys to assess specific health problems.

groups that differ in some important characteristic must be compared to gain clues about which factors influence the distribution of disease (i.e., disease determinants or risk factors). Observing the rate of disease only among persons exposed to a suspected risk factor will not show clearly that the exposure is associated with increased risk until the rate observed in the exposed group is compared with the rate in a group of comparable unexposed persons. To illustrate, one might investigate the effect of smoking during pregnancy on the rate of low birthweight by calculating the rate of low-birthweight infants born to women who smoked during their pregnancy. However, the hypothesis that smoking during pregnancy is a risk factor for low birthweight is supported only when the low-birthweight rate among smoking women is compared with the (lower) rate of low-birthweight infants born to nonsmoking women.

The ideal approach would be to compare one group of people who all have a certain characteristic, exposure, or behavior, with a group of people *exactly* like them except they all *lack* that characteristic, exposure, or behavior. In the absence of that ideal, researchers either randomize people to exposure or treatment groups in experimental studies, or they select comparison groups that are comparable in observational studies. Advances in statistical techniques now make it possible to control for differences be-

**HOW TO** Assess Health Problems in an Individual

1. Obtain history of physical and mental health problems.
2. Ask the individual to identify major health problems. Always start interventions with what individual views as important.
3. Obtain family history of diseases. Identify possible genetic link based on early age of onset of disease or multiple family members with disease.
4. Perform clinical examination, including laboratory work.
5. Evaluate health risk based on lifestyle. Include smoking status, dietary patterns of fiber and fat, exercise patterns, stress factors, and risk-taking behaviors.
6. Identify immediate and long-range safety concerns.
7. Assess individual's cultural beliefs about health.
8. Assess social support.
9. Examine knowledge and practice of preventive health care.
10. Provide appropriate age-based screening (e.g., cancer screening, hypertension screening).

tween groups, but these advanced techniques are effective only in reducing the bias that results from confounding by variables we have measured.

## DESCRIPTIVE EPIDEMIOLOGY

**Descriptive epidemiology** describes the distribution of disease, death, and other health outcomes in the population according to person, place, and time, providing a picture of how things are or have been—the who, where, and when of disease patterns. **Analytic epidemiology,** on the other hand, searches for the determinants of the patterns observed—the how and why. That is, epidemiologic concepts and methods are used to identify what factors, characteristics, exposures, or behaviors might account for differences in the observed patterns of disease occurrence. Descriptive and analytic studies are observational, meaning the investigator observes events as they are or have been and does not intervene to change anything or to introduce a new factor. Experimental or intervention studies, however, include interventions to test preventive or treatment measures, techniques, materials, policies, or drugs.

### Person

Personal characteristics of interest in epidemiology include race, sex, age, education, occupation, income (and related socioeconomic status), and marital status. As noted previously, the most important predictor of overall mortality is age. The mortality curve by age drops sharply during and after the first year of life to a low point in childhood, then

it begins to increase through adolescence and young adulthood, and after that it increases sharply (exponentially) through middle and older ages (Gordis, 2000).

There are also substantial differences in mortality and morbidity rates by sex. Female infants have a lower mortality rate than comparable male infants, and the survival advantage continues throughout life (NCHS, 1998; Minino and Smith, 2001). However, patterns for specific diseases vary. For example, women have lower rates of CHD until menopause, after which the gap narrows. For rheumatoid arthritis, the prevalence among women is greater than among men (Brownson et al, 1998).

Although the concept of race as a variable for public health research has come under scrutiny (CDC, 1993; Fullilove, 1998), there are clear differences in morbidity and mortality rates by race in the United States (Peters, Kochanek, and Murphy, 1998; NCHS, 1998; USDHHS, 1985). According to the Office of Minority Health (OMH, 1999), although racial and ethnic minority groups are among the fastest-growing populations in the United States, they have poorer health and remain chronically underserved by the health care system. Data in the OMH report entitled *Elimination of Racial and Ethnic Disparities in Health* highlighted some of the significant health disparities within the leading categories of death in the United States. For example, in 1998, the overall U.S. infant mortality rate (IMR) was 7.2 deaths per 1000 live births, but the IMR among African Americans was 13.7 per 1000 live births. The incidence and prevalence of diabetes among ethnic and racial minorities is another example of current health disparities. African Americans experience diabetes at a rate that is 70% higher than white Americans, whereas Native Americans and Native Alaskans experience a diabetes death rate that is 3.5 times that of the rest of the U.S. population. The burden of HIV/AIDS is also greater among minority communities, which in official estimates account for 25% of the total U.S. population but 50% of all AIDS cases. An NCHS study of progress toward meeting the Healthy People 2000 goal of eliminating racial/ethnic disparities found that, although rates for most health status indicators did improve for all racial/ethnic groups, the improvements have not been uniform across groups and "substantial differences among racial/ethnic groups persist" (Keppel, Pearcy, and Wagener, 2002). Among Native Americans and Native Alaskans, several health indicators actually worsened from 1990 to 1998. The infant morality rate declined in all groups, but it remains 2.3 times higher for infants born to non-Hispanic African-American mothers than for those born to white non-Hispanic mothers. Similarly, the overall age-adjusted mortality rate was 30% higher in the African-American population than in the white population in 1998, and it was higher for 11 of the 15 leading causes of death (Hoyert et al, 2001). Reports from the NCHS provide further insight into health disparities across socioeconomic and racial/ethnic groups (Hoyert et al, 2001; Keppel et al, 2002; NCHS, 1998).

## Place

When considering the distribution of a disease, geographic patterns come to mind: Does the rate of disease differ from place to place (e.g., with local environment)? If geography had no effect on disease occurrence, random geographic patterns might be seen, but that is often not the case. For example, at high altitudes there is lower oxygen tension, which might result in smaller babies. Other diseases reflect distinctive geographic patterns. For example, Lyme disease is transmitted from animal reservoirs to humans by a tick vector. Disease is more likely to be found in areas where there are animals carrying the disease, a large tick population for transmission to humans, and contact between the human population and the tick vectors (Chin, 2000).

We might expect geographic variations to be caused by differences in the chemical, physical, or biological environment. However, variations by place also may result from differences in population densities, or in customary patterns of behavior and lifestyle, or in other personal characteristics. For example, geographic variations might occur because of high concentrations of a religious, cultural, or ethnic group who practice certain health-related behaviors. The high rates of stroke found in the southeastern United States are likely to be the result of a number of social and personal factors that have little to do with geographic features per se. Recent research has also focused on neighborhood-level variables, such as unemployment and crime rate, social cohesion, and access to important services (Caughy, O'Campo, and Patterson, 2001; Cohen et al, 2000; O'Campo et al, 1995; Sampson, Raudenbush, and Earls, 1997). These are factors that may be of particular interest to nurses, who are in a unique position to assess their effect on the health of communities.

## Time

### Secular Changes

Time is the third component of descriptive epidemiology. Is there an increase or decrease in the frequency of the disease over time, or are other temporal patterns evident? Long-term patterns of morbidity or mortality rates (i.e., over years or decades) are called secular trends. **Secular trends** may reflect changes in social behavior or practices. For example, increased lung cancer mortality rates in recent years reflect a delayed effect of the increased smoking in prior years. Also, the decline in cervical cancer deaths is

**◖ DID YOU KNOW?**

Lung cancer has now surpassed breast cancer as the leading cause of cancer mortality among women. The rapidly increasing rate of lung cancer deaths in women mirrors the patterns of increased rates of smoking among women and increased cigarette advertising directed toward women.

primarily due to widespread screening with the Pap test (Brownson et al, 1998).

Some secular trends may result from increased diagnostic capability or changes in survival (or case fatality) rather than in incidence. For example, case fatality from breast cancer has decreased in recent years although the incidence of breast cancer has increased. Some, though not all, of the increased incidence is due to improved diagnostic capability. These two trends result in a breast cancer mortality curve that is flatter than the incidence curve (Brownson et al, 1998; Holleb, Fink, and Murphy, 1991). Relying on the mortality data alone does not accurately reflect the true situation. Secular trends are affected by changes in case definition or revisions in the coding of a disease according to the International Classification of Diseases (ICD). Such changes can produce an artificial change in the rate (Peters et al, 1998).

### Point Epidemic

One temporal and spatial pattern of disease distribution is the **point epidemic.** This time-and-space-related pattern is particularly important in infectious disease investigations. It is also recognized as a significant indicator for toxic exposures in environmental epidemiology. A point epidemic is most clearly seen when the frequency of cases is plotted against time. The sharp peak characteristic of such graphs indicates a concentration of cases in some short interval of time. The peak often indicates the response of the population to a common source of infection or contamination to which they were all simultaneously exposed. Knowledge of the incubation or latency period (the time between exposure and development of signs and symptoms) for the specific disease entity can help to determine the probable time of exposure. A common example of a point epidemic is an outbreak of gastrointestinal illness from a food-borne pathogen. Nurses who are alert to a sudden increase in the number of cases of a disease can chart the outbreak, determine the probable time of exposure, and by careful investigation, isolate the probable source of the agent.

### Cyclical Patterns

In addition to secular trends and point epidemics, there are also cyclical time patterns of disease. One common type of cyclical variation is the seasonal fluctuation seen in a number of infectious illnesses. Seasonal changes may be influenced by changes in the agent itself, changes in population densities or behaviors of animal reservoirs or vectors, or changes in human behavior that result in changing exposures (e.g., being outdoors in warmer weather and indoors in colder months). There may also be artificial seasons created by calendar events, such as holidays and tax-filing deadlines, which may be associated with patterns of stress-related illness. Patterns of accidents and injuries also may be seasonal, reflecting differing employment and recreational patterns. Some disease cycles, such as influenza, have patterns of smaller epidemics every few years, depending on strain, with major pandemics occur-

## Evidence-Based Practice

### GEOGRAPHIC INFORMATION SYSTEM RESEARCH

The purpose of this study was to identify, map, and characterize geographic areas in New Jersey that have significantly high proportions of women diagnosed with breast cancer at the distant stage. The researchers used a geographic information system with spatial scan statistical software, U.S. Census data, New Jersey State Cancer Registry data, and mammography facility locations.

Included in the study were all reported cases of breast cancer that were histologically confirmed between 1995 and 1997 in women residing in New Jersey at the time of diagnosis. A spatial scan statistic was used to identify estimated geographic areas with significantly high proportions of women with breast cancer diagnosed in the distant stage. The identified areas were then mapped and characterized using data from the 1990 U.S. Census and locations of mammography facilities.

The results of the study included the identification of two separate geographic areas in northeastern New Jersey that accounted for nearly 10% of all the women diagnosed with breast cancer, and 14% of all the women diagnosed with breast cancer at the distant stage. The relative risks for women with breast cancer being diagnosed at the distant stage in the two geo-graphic areas compared to the state as a whole were 2.4 and 1.7 ($p < .01$). These areas' population characteristics included relatively high proportions of African-American or Hispanic women, foreign-born persons, linguistically isolated households, and adults without a high school diploma. The per capita income in these areas was lower than the population in the rest of the state, and the areas were also characterized by high unemployment (9%), high percentages of households on public assistance (10% to 12%), and low homeownership rates (30% to 45%). Of the 295 mammography facilities in New Jersey, 17 were located in the two estimated geographic areas.

The researchers noted that the results of this GIS research could be used by public health agencies, social service organizations, health care providers, local community groups, and other collaborators in developing breast cancer education and screening services to effectively target women in specific geographic areas.

**Nurse Use:** Geographic information is a useful way for nurses to identify priorities for their work in the community. By knowing which cohorts have the greatest risk of disease, nurses can focus their time and programs to most effectively fit the needs of their community.

Roche LS, Skinner R, Weinstein RB: Use of a geographic information system to identify and characterize areas with high proportions of distant stage breast cancer, *J Public Health Manag Pract* 3(2):26-32, 2002.

## THE CUTTING EDGE

A geographic information system (GIS) is a computer-based system of geographic, spatial, or location-based information. In public health, the advent of GIS has increased the ability of researchers to link demographic, epidemiologic, environmental, and health care system databases with spatial analysis to determine relationships between geographic patterns of disease distributions and social and physical environmental conditions. The result is that public health officials can more effectively allocate sparse public health resources in addressing health priorities.

From Roche LS, Skinner R, Weinstein RB: Use of a geographic information system to identify and characterize areas with high proportions of distant stage breast cancer, *J Public Health Manag Pract* 3(2):26-32, 2002; Rushton G, Elmes G, McMaster R: Considerations for improving geographic information system research in public health, *URISA Journal* 12(2):31-49, 2000; Taylor D, Chavez G: Small area analysis on a large scale: the California experience in mapping teenage birth "hot spots" for resource allocation, *J Public Health Manag Pract* 8(2)33-45, 2002.

ring at longer intervals (Chin, 2000). Workers in community health can prepare to meet increased demands on resources by careful attention to these cyclical patterns.

### Event-Related Clusters

A third type of temporal pattern is nonsimultaneous, event-related clusters. These are patterns in which time is not measured from fixed dates on the calendar but from the point of some exposure or event, presumably experienced in common by affected persons, although not occurring at the same time. An example would be vaccine reactions in an ongoing immunization program. If vaccinations are given on a regular basis, one might see nonspecific symptoms (e.g., fever, headaches, rashes) fairly consistently over, say, a year, making identification of a cluster related to the vaccinations difficult. If, however, the time of vaccination is artificially set as zero for each client, and the number of clients with symptoms is plotted against the time since time zero, the reactions are likely to show up as a peak at some period after the immunization.

## ANALYTIC EPIDEMIOLOGY

Descriptive epidemiology deals with the distribution of health outcomes, whereas analytic epidemiology seeks to discover the determinants of outcomes, the how and the why (i.e., the factors that influence observed patterns of health and disease and increase or decrease the risk of adverse outcomes). This section deals with analytic study designs and the related measures of association derived from them. Table 11-5 summarizes the advantages and disadvantages of each design.

## Cohort Studies

The **cohort study** is the standard for observational epidemiologic studies, coming closest to the ideal of a natural experiment (Rothman, 2002). In epidemiology, the term *cohort* is used to describe a group of persons who are born at

---

### Table 11-5  Comparison of Major Epidemiologic Study Designs

| STUDY DESIGN | ADVANTAGES | DISADVANTAGES |
|---|---|---|
| Ecologic | • Quick, easy, and inexpensive first study<br>• Uses readily available existing data<br>• May prompt further investigation or suggest other/new hypotheses<br>• May provide information about contextual factors not accounted for by individual characteristics | • Ecologic fallacy: the associations observed may not hold true for individuals<br>• Problems in interpreting temporal sequence (cause and effect)<br>• More difficult to control for confounding and "mixed" models (ecologic and individual data); more complex statistically |
| Cross-sectional (correlational) | • Gives general description of scope of problem; provides prevalence estimates<br>• Often based on population (or community) sample, not just those who sought care<br>• Useful in health service evaluation and planning<br>• Data obtained at once; less expense and quicker than cohort because no follow-up<br>• Baseline for prospective study or to identify cases and controls for case-control study | • No calculation of risk; prevalence, not incidence<br>• Temporal sequence unclear<br>• Not good for rare disease or rare exposure unless large sample size or stratified sampling<br>• Selective survival can be major source of selection bias; surviving subjects may differ from those who are not included (death, institutionalization, etc.)<br>• Selective recall or lack of past exposure information can create bias |
| Case-control (retrospective, case comparison) | • Less expensive than cohort; smaller sample required<br>• Quicker than cohort; no follow-up<br>• Can investigate more than one exposure<br>• Best design for rare diseases<br>• If well designed, can be important tool for etiologic investigation<br>• Best suited to disease with relatively clear onset (timing of onset can be established so that incident cases can be included) | • Greater susceptibility than cohort studies to various types of bias (selective survival, recall bias, selection bias in choice of both cases and controls)<br>• Information on other risk factors may not be available, resulting in confounding<br>• Antecedent–consequence (temporal sequence) not as certain as in cohort<br>• Not well suited to rare exposures<br>• Gives only an indirect estimate of risk<br>• Limited to a single outcome because of sampling on disease status |
| Prospective cohort (concurrent cohort, longitudinal, follow-up) | • Best estimate of disease incidence<br>• Best estimate of risk<br>• Fewer problems with selective survival and selective recall<br>• Temporal sequence more clearly established<br>• Broader range of options for exposure assessment | • Expensive in time and money<br>• More difficult organizationally<br>• Not good for rare diseases<br>• Attrition of participants can bias estimate<br>• Latency period may be very long; may miss cases<br>• May be difficult to examine several exposures |
| Retrospective cohort (nonconcurrent cohort) | • Combines advantages of both prospective cohort and case-control<br>• Shorter time (even if follow-up into future) than prospective cohort<br>• Less expensive than prospective cohort because relies on existing data<br>• Temporal sequence may be clearer than case-control | • Shares some disadvantages with both prospective cohort and case-control<br>• Subject to attrition (loss to follow-up)<br>• Relies on existing records that may result in misclassification of both exposure and outcome<br>• May have to rely on surrogate measure of exposure (such as job title) and vital records information on cause of death |

about the same time. In analytic studies, a cohort refers to a group of persons, generally sharing some characteristic of interest, who are enrolled in a study and followed over a period of time to observe some health outcome (Last, 2001). Because they enable us to observe the development of new cases of disease, cohort study designs allow calculation of incidence rates and therefore estimates of disease risk. Cohort studies may be prospective or retrospective (Gordis, 2000; Rothman, 2002; Szklo and Nieto, 2000).

---

**DID YOU KNOW?**

Epidemiologic studies conducted by nurse researchers have direct application to all areas of nursing?

---

## Prospective Cohort Studies

In a prospective cohort study (also called a longitudinal or follow-up study), subjects determined to be free of the outcome under investigation are classified on the basis of the exposure of interest at the beginning of the follow-up period. The different exposure groups constitute the comparison groups for the study. The subjects are then followed for some period of time to determine the occurrence of disease in each group. The question is, "Do persons with the factor (or exposure) of interest develop (or avoid) the outcome more frequently than those without the factor (or exposure)?"

For example, one might recruit a cohort of subjects classified as physically active ("exposed") or sedentary ("not exposed"). One might further quantify the amount of the "exposure" if there is sufficient information. These subjects would then be followed over time to determine the development of CHD. This study design avoids the problem of selective survival that sometimes affects other study designs. (See Figure 11-5, a cross-sectional study of physical activity and CHD later.) Because persons initially without the disease are followed over time, this design allows estimation of both incidence rates and incidence proportions. The cohort study can also estimate the relative risk of acquiring disease for those who are exposed compared with those who are unexposed (or less exposed). This ratio of incidence proportions is called the risk ratio (or relative risk), and a ratio incidence rate is called the rate ratio. For example, if the risk of CHD in smokers is twice as high as the risk among nonsmokers, the risk ratio would be 2. If a factor is unrelated to the risk of a disease, the risk ratio will be close to 1. A value less than 1 may suggest a protective association. For example, the risk of CHD is lower among those who are physically active than among sedentary persons, so the risk ratio for the association between physical activity and CHD should be less than 1.

Suppose 1000 physically active and 1000 sedentary middle-aged men and women enroll in a prospective cohort study. All are free of CHD at enrollment. Over a 5-year follow-up period, regular examinations detect CHD in 120 of the sedentary men and women, and in 48 of the active men and women. Assuming no other deaths or losses to follow-up, the data could be presented as shown in Figure 11-5.

The incidence proportion of CHD in the active group is a/(a + b), or 48/1000, and the incidence of CHD in the sedentary group is c/(c + d), or 120/1000. The risk ratio is as follows:

$$\left( \frac{48}{1000} \right) \div \left( \frac{120}{1000} \right) = 0.4.$$

Because physical activity is protective for CHD, the risk ratio is less than 1. The interpretation for this hypothetical example is that, over a 5-year period, the risk of CHD in persons who are physically active is about 0.4 as great as the risk among sedentary persons. If the risk were greater for those exposed, the risk ratio would be greater than 1. For example, if the risk ratio of CHD for overweight persons compared with normal weight is 3.5, it would be interpreted to mean that the risk of CHD among overweight persons is 3.5 times the risk of those with normal weight. The null value indicating no association is 1, because the incidence proportion and thus the risk would be equal in the two groups if there were no association.

Because subjects are enrolled before onset of disease, the cohort design can study more than one outcome, calculate incidence rates and proportions, estimate risk, establish the temporal sequence of exposure and outcome with greater clarity and certainty, and may avoid many of the problems of the other study designs with selective survival or exposure misclassification (discussed later). On the other hand, large samples are often necessary to ensure that enough cases are observed to provide enough statistical power to detect meaningful differences between groups. This is complicated by the long period required for some diseases to develop (the latency period). Also, the number of subjects required to observe sufficient cases makes longitudinal studies unsuitable for very rare diseases unless they are part of a larger study of a number of outcomes.

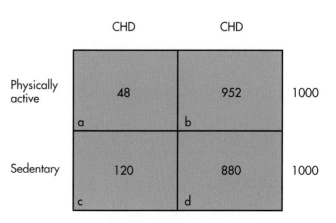

**Figure 11-5** Cohort study.

## Retrospective Cohort Studies

Retrospective cohort studies combine some of the advantages and some of the disadvantages of both case-control studies and prospective cohort studies. The epidemiologist relies on existing records, such as employment, insurance, or hospital records, to define a cohort, whose members are classified according to exposure status at some time in the past. The cohort is followed over time using the records to determine if the outcome occurred. Retrospective cohort (also called historical cohort) studies may be conducted entirely using past records or may include current assessment or additional follow-up time after study initiation. The obvious advantage of this approach is the time savings, because one does not have to wait for new cases of disease to develop. The disadvantages are largely related to the reliance on existing historical records. Retrospective cohort studies are frequently used in occupational epidemiology where industrial records are available to investigate work-related exposures and health outcomes.

## Case-Control Studies

The case-control design can be viewed against the background of an underlying cohort. The design uses a sample from the cohort rather than following the entire cohort over time. Because it uses only samples of cases and noncases, it is a more efficient design, although it is subject to certain types of bias (Rothman, 2002). In the **case-control study,** participants are enrolled because they are known to have the outcome of interest (cases) or they are known *not* to have the outcome of interest (controls). Case-control status is verified using a clear case definition and some previously determined method or protocol (e.g., by an examination, laboratory test, or medical chart review). Information is then collected on the exposures or characteristics of interest, frequently from existing sources, subject interview, or questionnaire (Armenian, 1994; Kelsey et al, 1996; Rothman, 2002; Schlesselman, 1982; Szklo and Nieto, 2000). The question in a case-control study is, "Do persons with the outcome of interest (cases) have the exposure characteristic (or a history of the exposure) more frequently than those without the outcome (controls)?"

Suppose a research group wanted to study risk factors for suicide attempts among adolescents. They were able to enroll 100 adolescents who had attempted suicide, and they selected 200 adolescents from the same community with no history of suicide attempt. One of the factors they want to investigate is a history of substance abuse (SA). Through a questionnaire and other medical records, they determine that 68 of the 100 adolescents who had attempted suicide had a history of substance abuse, whereas 36 of the 200 adolescents with no suicide attempt had such a history. The information could be presented as shown in Figure 11-6.

The odds of a history of substance abuse among suicide attempters is a/c, or 68/32, whereas the odds of substance

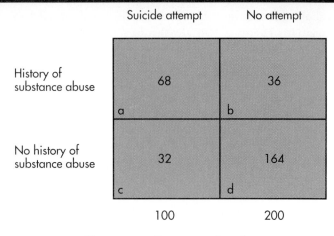

**Figure 11-6** Case-control study.

abuse among controls is b/d, or 36/164. The odds ratio (equivalent to ad/bc) is as follows:

$$\frac{(68 \times 164)}{(36 \times 32)} = 9.68.$$

This would be interpreted to mean that the odds of a history of substance abuse are about 10 times greater among adolescents who have attempted suicide than among adolescents who have not attempted suicide. Note that, as with the risk ratio, an odds ratio of 1 is indicative of no association (i.e., the odds of exposure are similar for cases and controls). An odds ratio less than 1 suggests a protective association (cases are less likely to have been exposed than controls).

Given the way subjects are selected for a case-control study, neither incidence nor prevalence can be calculated directly. However, if newly diagnosed cases are enrolled as they are ascertained, and if case ascertainment is fairly complete and the source population well defined, an estimate of incidence may be obtained. In a case-control study, an odds ratio tells how much more or less likely the exposure is to be found among cases than among controls. The odds of exposure among cases (a/c in Figure 11-6) are compared with the odds of exposure among controls (b/d in Figure 11-6). Under certain conditions, the ratio of these two odds provides an estimate of the risk ratio or rate ratio.

Because the number of cases is known or actively sought out, case-control studies do not demand large samples or the long follow-up time that is often required for prospective cohort studies. That is why many of the influential cancer studies have been of the case-control design.

Case-control studies are, however, prone to a number of biases (see further discussion under Bias, later in this chapter). Because these studies begin with existing cases, differential survival can produce biased results. The use of recently diagnosed, or "incident," cases may reduce this bias. Because exposure information is obtained from subject recall or past records, there may be errors in exposure assessment or misclassification. Because participants are selected precisely because they do or do not have a specific health outcome, case-control studies are limited to a single outcome, although they may investigate a number of potential risk factors.

## Cross-Sectional Studies

The **cross-sectional study** provides a snapshot, or cross section, of a population or group (Gordis, 2000). Information is collected on current health status, personal characteristics, and potential risk factors or exposures all at once. The cross-sectional study is characterized by the simultaneous collection of information necessary for the classification of exposure and outcome status, although there may be historical information collected (e.g., on past diet or history of radiation exposure).

Cross-sectional studies are sometimes called prevalence studies because they provide the frequency of existing cases of a disease in a population (Kelsey et al, 1996). One way cross-sectional studies evaluate the association of a factor with a health problem is by comparing the prevalence of the disease in those who have the factor (or exposure) with the prevalence in the unexposed. The ratio of the two prevalence rates indicates an association between the factor and the outcome. If the prevalence of CHD in smokers were twice as high as the prevalence among nonsmokers, the prevalence ratio would be 2. If a factor is unrelated to the prevalence of a disease, the prevalence ratio will be close to 1. A value less than 1 may suggest a protective association. For example, the prevalence of CHD is lower among those who are physically active than among sedentary persons, so the prevalence ratio for the association between physical activity and CHD should be less than 1. Prevalence ratios require caution in interpretation because the prevalence measure is affected by cure, survival, and migration and does not estimate the risk of getting the disease.

Cross-sectional studies are subject to bias resulting from selective survival (i.e., people who have survived to be in the study may be different from people diagnosed about the same time who have died and are not available for inclusion). Suppose that physical activity not only reduced the risk of CHD but also markedly improved survival among those with CHD. Sedentary persons with CHD would then have higher fatality rates than physically active persons who did develop CHD. One might observe higher rates of physical activity in a group of persons surviving with CHD than in a general population without CHD, both because of the survival advantage of those who previously were active and because of increased participation of other survivors in cardiac rehabilitation programs. It could erroneously appear that physical activity was a risk factor for CHD.

## Ecologic Studies

An epidemiologic study that is a bridge between descriptive epidemiology and analytic epidemiology is the **ecologic study.** The descriptive component involves examining variations in disease rates by person, place, or time. The ana-

lytic component lies in the effort to determine if there is a relationship between disease rates and variations in rates for possible risk (or protective) factors. The identifying characteristic of ecologic studies is that only aggregate data, such as population rates, are used rather than data on individuals' exposures, characteristics, and outcomes. For example, information on per capita cigarette consumption might be examined in relation to lung cancer mortality rates in several countries, in several groups of people, or in the same population at different times. Other examples include comparisons of rates of breastfeeding and of breast cancer, average dietary fat content and rates of CHD, or unemployment rates and level of psychiatric disorder.

Ecologic studies are attractive because they often make use of existing, readily available rates and are therefore quick and inexpensive to conduct. They are subject, however, to **ecologic fallacy** (i.e., associations observed at the group level may not hold true for the individuals that make up the groups, or associations that actually exist may be masked in the grouped data). This may be the result of other factors operating in these populations for which the ecologic correlations do not account. For that reason, ecologic studies may be suggestive but require confirmation in studies using individual data (Gordis, 2000; Lilienfeld and Stolley, 1994). However, recent studies have shown that ecologic data can add important information to analyses even when individual-level data are available (Lynch et al, 1998; O'Campo et al, 1995)

Uncertainty concerning the temporal sequence of events is a disadvantage that ecologic studies share with cross-sectional study designs. For example, in the study of unemployment rates and psychiatric disorder, it is unclear whether unemployed persons are at higher risk for psychiatric problems or persons with existing psychiatric problems are more likely to be unemployed. Although determining whether one event precedes or succeeds another may seem at first to be a simple matter, in practice it may be difficult to confirm.

## EXPERIMENTAL STUDIES

The study designs discussed so far are called observational studies because the investigator observes the association between exposures and outcomes as they exist but does not intervene to alter the presence or level of any exposure or behavior. Studies in which the investigator initiates some treatment or intervention that may influence the risk or course of disease are called intervention, or experimental, studies. Such studies test whether interventions are effective in preventing disease or improving health. Like observational studies, experimental studies generally use comparison (or control) groups, but unlike observational studies, they are subject to the consequences of randomly allocating persons to a particular intervention group and determining the type or level of the "exposure" (the treatment or intervention). Intervention studies are of two general types: clinical trials and community trials (Lilienfeld and Stolley, 1994; Meinert, 1986).

**WHAT DO YOU THINK?**

Epidemiologic studies are often inconclusive about causal associations. The same may be true for epidemiologically based evaluations of prevention programs. Should there be a difference in how we interpret results for purposes of designing future research as opposed to recommending guidelines? Should there be a difference in interpretation and application of epidemiologic results for individuals and for community or public policy?

## Clinical Trials

In clinical trials, the research issue is generally the efficacy of a medical treatment for disease, such as a new drug or an existing drug used in a new or different way, a surgical technique, or another treatment. The preferred method of subject allocation in clinical trials is randomization (i.e., assigning treatments to clients so that all possible treatment assignments have a predetermined probability but neither subject nor investigator determines the actual assignment of any participant). Randomization avoids the bias that may result if subjects self-select into one group or the other or if the investigator or clinician chooses subjects for each group.

A second aspect of treatment allocation is the use of masking, or "blinding," treatment assignments. The optimal design for most situations is the double-blind study in which neither the subject nor the investigator knows who is receiving which treatment. The aim of blinding is to reduce the bias from overestimating therapeutic benefit for the experimental treatment when it is known who is receiving it.

Clinical trials are generally thought to provide the best evidence of causality because of the assignment of treatment and the greater control over other factors that could influence outcome. Like cohort studies, clinical trials are prospective in direction and provide the clearest evidence of temporal sequence.

However, clinical trials are generally conducted in a contrived situation, under controlled conditions, and with select client populations. That means that the treatment may be less effective when it is applied under more realistic clinical or community conditions in a more diverse client population. There are also ethical considerations in experimental studies that go beyond those that apply to observational studies. Also, clinical trials tend to be costly in time, personnel, facilities, and other factors.

## Community Trials

Community trials are similar to clinical trials in that an investigator determines the exposure or intervention, but in this case the issue is often health promotion and disease prevention rather than treatment of existing disease. The intervention is usually undertaken on a large scale, with the unit of treatment allocation being a community, region, or group rather than individuals. Although a pharmaceutical product may be involved in a community trial (e.g., fluoridation of water or mass immunizations), community trials often involve educational, programmatic, or policy interventions. An example of community intervention is providing exercise programs and facilities and increasing the availability of healthy, fresh foods to study the effect on diabetes rates.

Although community trials provide the best means of testing whether changes in knowledge or behavior, policy, programs, or other mass interventions are effective, they are not without problems. For many interventions, it may take years for the effectiveness of the intervention to be evident. In the meantime, other factors also may influence the outcome, either positively (making the intervention look more effective than it really is) or negatively (making the intervention look less effective than it really is). Comparable community populations without similar interventions for comparative analysis are often difficult to determine. Even when comparable comparison communities are available, especially when the intervention is improved knowledge or changed behavior, it is difficult and unethical to prevent the control communities from making use of generally available information, effectively making them less different from the intervention communities. Also, because community trials are often undertaken on a large scale and over long periods of time, they can be expensive, requiring large staff, complicated logistics, and extensive communication resources.

## CAUSALITY

### Statistical Associations

One of the first steps in assessing the relationship of some factor with a health outcome is determining whether a statistical association exists. If the probability of disease seems unaffected by the presence or level of the factor, no association is apparent. If, on the other hand, the probability of disease does vary according to whether the factor is present, then there is a statistical association. The earlier discussion of null values is pertinent at this point. When an observed measure of association (such as a risk ratio) does not differ from the null value, it may not be assumed that there is an association between the factor and the outcome under investigation.

In many studies, a great deal of emphasis is placed on tests of statistical significance. This is a judgment that the observed results are or are not likely to be due to chance at some predetermined level of probability (usually 0.05). However, many epidemiologists contend that much more information is provided by an estimate of the association (the ratio or difference in rates or risks) and a confidence interval that indicates the precision of the estimate (Rothman, 2002). Note that statistical significance is determined by sample size, the amount of difference between groups, and the variance in the estimates.

## Bias

Although statistical testing and estimation are critical, it is important to remember that statistical testing and interval estimation generally assume that deviations from the true value are the result of chance. However, estimates may appear to be greater or less than they really are because of **bias,** a systematic error resulting from the study design, execution, or **confounding.** For example, if there were a gumball machine with colors randomly mixed and three red ones in a row came out, that would be due to chance. If, however, the person loading the gum ball machine had poured in a bag of red ones first, then green ones, then yellow, it would not be surprising to get three red ones in a row because of the way the machine was loaded. In epidemiologic studies, results are sometimes biased because of the way the study was "loaded" (i.e., the way the study was designed or subjects were selected or information collected and subjects classified). Although the types of bias are numerous, there are three general categories of bias (Rothman, 2002).

Bias attributable to the way subjects enter a study is called selection bias. It has to do with selection procedures and the population from which subjects are drawn. It may involve self-selection factors as well. For example, are teenagers who agree to complete a questionnaire on alcohol, tobacco, and other drug use representative of the total teenage population?

Bias attributable to misclassification of subjects once they are in the study is information, or classification (or misclassification), bias. It is related to how information is collected, including the information that subjects supply or how subjects are classified.

Bias resulting from the relationship of the outcome and study factor with some third factor not accounted for is called confounding. For example, there is a well-known association between maternal smoking during pregnancy and low-birthweight babies. There is also an association between alcohol consumption and smoking that is not due to chance nor is it causal (i.e., drinking alcohol does not cause a person to smoke, nor does smoking cause a person to drink alcohol). If one were to investigate the association of alcohol consumption and low birthweight, smoking would be a confounder because it is related to both alcohol consumption and low birthweight. Failure to account for smoking in the analysis would bias the observed association between alcohol use and low birthweight. In practice one can often identify potentially confounding variables and adjust for them in analysis.

## Assessing for Causality

The existence of a statistical association does not necessarily mean that there is a causal relationship or that causality is present. As the preceding paragraphs have shown, the observed association may be a random event (due to chance) or may be due to bias from confounding or from flaws in the study design or execution. Statistical associa-

---

### BOX 11-4    Criteria for Causality

1. **Strength of association:** A strong association between a potential risk factor and an outcome supports a causal hypothesis (i.e., a relative risk of 7 provides stronger evidence of a causal association than a relative risk of 1.5).

2. **Consistency of findings:** Repeated findings of an association with different study designs and in different populations strengthen causal inference.

3. **Biological plausibility:** Demonstration of a physiologic mechanism by which the risk factor acts to cause disease enhances the causal hypothesis. Conversely, an association that does not initially seem biologically defensible may later be discovered to be so.

4. **Demonstration of correct temporal sequence:** For a risk factor to cause an outcome, it must precede the onset of the outcome. (See under Prospective Cohort Studies and see Table 11-5.)

5. **Dose–response relationship:** The risk of developing an outcome should increase with increasing exposure (either in duration or quantity) to the risk factor of interest. For example, studies have shown that the more a woman smokes during pregnancy, the greater the risk of delivering a low-birthweight infant.

6. **Specificity of the association:** The presence of a one-to-one relationship between an agent and a disease (i.e., the idea that a disease is caused by only one agent and that agent results in only one disease lends support to a causal hypothesis, but its absence does not rule out causality). This criterion grows out of the infectious disease model, where it is more often, though not always, satisfied and is less applicable in chronic diseases.

7. **Experimental evidence:** Experimental designs provide the strongest epidemiologic evidence for causal associations, but they are not feasible or ethical to conduct for many risk factor–disease associations.

---

tions, although necessary to an argument for causality, are not sufficient proof. Some epidemiologists refer to *criteria for causality,* a term originally established to evaluate the link between an infectious agent and a disease but revised and elaborated to apply also to other outcomes. Although various lists of criteria have been proposed, the seven criteria listed in Box 11-4 are fairly commonly cited (Gordis, 2000; Lilienfeld and Stolley, 1994). Some have questioned the use of lists of criteria as misleading, especially because only temporal sequence is necessary, and none of the others really is a criterion (Rothman, 2002). Although no single epidemiologic study can satisfy all criteria, epidemiology relies on the accumulation of evidence and the strength of individual studies to provide a basis for effective public health interventions and policies.

## APPLICATIONS OF EPIDEMIOLOGY IN COMMUNITY-ORIENTED NURSING

Both knowledge and practical application of epidemiology are essential competencies for nurses (Gebbie and Hwang, 2000). Nurses incorporate epidemiology into their practices and function in epidemiologic roles in a variety of ways. In diverse settings, nurses are involved in the collection, reporting, analysis, interpretation, and communication of epidemiologic data as part of their daily practice. Nurses involved in the care of persons with communicable diseases use epidemiology daily as they identify, report, treat, and provide follow-up on cases and contacts of tuberculosis, gonorrhea, and gastroenteritis. School nurses also function as epidemiologists, collecting data on the incidence and prevalence of accidents, injuries, and illnesses in the school population. They are also key players in the detection and control of local epidemics, such as outbreaks of lice. As described earlier in this chapter, nurses across practice settings are actively involved in activities related to primary, secondary, and tertiary prevention (see Levels of Preventive Interventions, earlier, and Box 11-2).

Some nursing job descriptions are specifically based in epidemiologic practice. These include nurse epidemiologists and environmental risk communicators employed by local health departments, and hospital infection control nurses. Nurses are key members of local fetal and infant mortality review boards, which examine cases of newborn deaths for identifiable risk factors and quality of care measures. Members of these review boards may include public health and maternal child nurses as well as representatives from hospital labor and delivery and neonatal intensive care units.

Nursing documentation on patient charts and records is an important source of data for epidemiologic reviews. Patient demographics and health histories are often collected or verified by nurses. As nurses collect and document patient information, they might not be thinking about the epidemiologic connection. However, the reliability and validity of such data can be a key factor in the quality of future epidemiologic studies.

---

**❨ NURSING TIP**

Epidemiology uses a process similar to the nursing process.

---

## Community-Oriented Epidemiology

Nurses are often involved in environmental health issues, where they play important roles not only as epidemiologists but also as community liaisons (Mood, 2000). Community-oriented nurses serve as important professional contacts and liaisons for people in the community who are actively investigating or concerned about the health and illness issue, such as an increase in the number of cases of cancer, asthma, or traffic accidents. The role of community liaison involves observation, data collection, consultation, and interpretation. By talking and listening to community members around their kitchen tables, at local gathering places, or at community meetings, nurses gather information from the citizens' perspectives. They can also interpret scientific information for lay persons. The liaison role also involves consultation with public health and environmental professionals and participation in environmental inspections and investigations. Lillian Mood is a public health nurse with over 20 years' experience in South Carolina working with communities to detect and explain the causes of illness and disability. In describing her involvement with specific communities, Mood noted that the contact often began with a telephone call of concern about a planned or existing industrial facility or a first-hand observation of illness, expressed in lay terms as "too many cases of cancer," "several people have had miscarriages," or "more respiratory problems." The citizen's reasoning behind these observations is that "'If I am seeing more health problems in my community, I ask what they have in common? The common factor may be where we live. So it must be the air or the water.' This is basic epidemiologic thinking, not irrational fear. Citizens try to make sense of what they are seeing, and they want professional help to unravel the pattern of illness" (Mood, 2000, p. 24).

## Popular Epidemiology

In health departments and hospitals, nurses frequently work with other professionals who have training in epidemiology. However, in the community they may encounter citizens engaged in the practice of popular epidemiology (Brown and Ferguson, 1995; Brown and Masterson-Allen, 1994). **Popular epidemiology** is a form of epidemiology in which lay people gather scientific data as well as mobilize knowledge and resources of experts to understand the occurrence and distribution of a disease or injury. Popular epidemiology is more than just adding public participation to traditional epidemiology. Popular epidemiology also includes an emphasis on social structural factors as a component of disease etiology, as well as the involvement of social movements, political and judicial approaches to remedies, and challenges to basic assumptions of traditional epidemiology, risk assessment, and public health regulation (Brown and Ferguson, 1995, p. 149). Popular epidemiology considers the physiologic, psychological, and social effects of environmental hazards and attempts to show how racial, class, and gender differences are evident in the health effects of environmental toxic exposure. In contrast, many standard environmental health assessments are not designed to understand local cultures, traditions, or ethnic backgrounds and so are ineffective in identifying potential routes of toxic exposure (DiChiro, 1997).

Toxic waste activists are often women living in the community who have first-hand contact with toxic hazards and

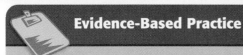
## Evidence-Based Practice

### The Epidemiologic Basis for Community Health Interventions

*Queso fresco,* a popular Latin American fresh cheese often made from raw milk, has been implicated as a source of *Salmonella typhimurium* definitive type (DT) 104 in the United States. From 1992 to 1996, the annual incidence of *S. typhimurium* DT104 infections in Yakima County, Washington, increased from 5.4 to 29.7 cases per 100,000 population, making it one of the highest rates in the country. Between January and May 1997, 89 cases of *S. typhimurium* were reported in the county, of which 54 were culture-confirmed as DT104, a strain that is resistant to five major antibiotics. The median age of infected persons was 4 years, and 90% of the clients had Spanish surnames. A case-control investigation conducted by the Centers for Disease Control and Prevention (CDC) indicated that the most probable source of the outbreak was raw-milk *queso fresco.* The CDC investigation also indicated that street vendors were the most frequent source (70%) of *queso fresco* among those who developed the illness.

In response to the outbreak, a multiagency intervention was initiated with the goal of reducing the incidence of *S. typhimurium* infections resulting from consumption of raw-milk *queso fresco,* while maintaining the traditional, nutritious food in the local Hispanic diet. A pasteurized-milk *queso fresco* recipe developed by a local Hispanic woman was modified by dairy scientists at Washington State University to inhibit undesirable microbial growth, increase shelf life, and improve ease of preparation. The new recipe was tested by local Hispanic persons and adjusted until flavor and texture were satisfactory.

A preintervention survey was conducted to gather background information for use in planning the multipronged intervention, which featured safe-cheese work-

shops introducing the new pasteurized-milk recipe, a mass media campaign about the risk of raw-milk cheese, and newsletter articles warning dairy farmers about the risks of selling or giving away raw milk. The safe-cheese workshops were conducted by older Hispanic women (*abuelas* means "grandmothers"), who were recruited from the community and trained to make the new *queso fresco* recipe from pasteurized milk. Following the training, each abuela educator signed a contract indicating her willingness to teach at least 15 additional members of the community how to safely make *queso fresco* with pasteurized milk. They followed through on their commitment, which included returning surveys completed by the women they taught.

The incidence of *S. typhimurium* infection in Yakima County decreased rapidly to below pre-1992 levels after the multilevel intervention was initiated. Between June and December 1997, only 16 cases were reported, of which two were associated with consumption of *queso fresco;* in 1998 there were 18 reported cases, none of which were associated with *queso fresco.* Postintervention surveys of Hispanic area residents who did not participate in the workshops indicated that consumption of *queso fresco* did not decrease as a result of the intervention.

**Nurse Use:** The *Abuela Project* is an example of a successful combination of applied epidemiology and community-based, culturally appropriate public health interventions. This activity clearly falls within the scope of good community-oriented nursing. To be successful in seeing correlations, nurses must be vigilant, have an inquiring mind, and be able to make associations between events and characteristics (e.g., in this example, the associations between how and by whom the cheese was being made, and by whom it was being eaten).

Bell RA, Hillers VN, Thomas TA: The Abuela project: safe cheese workshops to reduce the incidence of Salmonella typhimurium from consumption of raw-milk fresh cheese, *Am J Public Health* 89(9):1421-1424, 1999.

---

therefore have experiences and access to data that would otherwise be inaccessible to scientists (Brown and Ferguson, 1995). Community toxic waste activists engage in a process of linking traditional scientific practices with more narrative approaches. Their health surveys often make use of sampling techniques, laboratory testing, and mapping of suspected pollutants together with experiential narratives of the effects of toxic pollutants on the body and on their local environments (DiChiro, 1997). The information gathered can be used by community activists and health professionals to lobby for health services; advocate for policy development at local, state, and federal levels; establish preventive programs; educate medical professionals about environmental illness; and work with other agencies and community groups to reduce or eliminate toxic exposures.

## ■ Practice Application

You are a nurse at a local health department where Rob, a 46-year-old African American, comes for a routine blood pressure check. He mentions that his father recently died from prostate cancer and that he is worried about himself. Further assessment reveals that his father was diagnosed with prostate cancer when he was 52, and Rob's uncle, who is 56 years old, was recently diagnosed with prostate cancer. You know from Rob's health history that Rob smokes a pack of cigarettes a day and eats fried food frequently.

Which action would be your best choice?

**A.** Give Rob a digital rectal examination and prostate-specific antigen (PSA) test immediately to screen for prostate cancer.

**B.** Do not discuss or provide prostate cancer screening with Rob, because he is under 50 years old.

**C.** Advise Rob to be tested immediately for the prostate cancer gene because of his family history.

**D.** Inform Rob of the risks and benefits of prostate cancer testing, and of his increased personal risk of prostate cancer because of his family history, smoking, and dietary habits. Involve him in the decision-making process about prostate cancer screening.

---

**Answer is in the back of the book.**

## Key Points

- Epidemiology is the study of the distribution and determinants of health-related events in human populations and the application of this knowledge to improving the health of communities.
- Epidemiology is a multidisciplinary enterprise that recognizes the complex interrelationships of factors that influence disease and health at both the individual and the community level; it provides the basic tools for the study of health and disease in communities.
- Epidemiologic methods are used to describe health and disease phenomena and to investigate the factors that promote health or influence the risk or distribution of disease. This knowledge can be useful in planning and evaluating programs, policies, and services and in clinical decision making.
- Basic concepts important to epidemiology are the interrelationships between agent, host, and environment (the *epidemiologic triangle*); the interactions of factors, exposures, and characteristics in a causal web affecting risk of disease; and the levels of prevention corresponding to stages in the natural history of disease.
- Primary prevention involves interventions to reduce the incidence of disease by promoting health and preventing disease processes from developing.
- Secondary prevention includes programs (such as screening) designed to detect disease in the early stages, before signs and symptoms are clinically evident, to intervene with early diagnosis and treatment.
- Tertiary prevention provides treatments and other interventions directed toward persons with clinically apparent disease, with the aim of lessening the course of disease, reducing disability, or rehabilitating.
- Epidemiologic methods are also used in the planning and design of screening (secondary prevention) and community health intervention (primary prevention) strategies and in the evaluation of their effectiveness.
- Basic epidemiologic methods include the use of existing data sources to study health outcomes and related factors and the use of comparison groups to

assess the association between exposures or characteristics and health outcomes.

- Epidemiologists rely on rates and proportions to quantify levels of morbidity and mortality. Prevalence proportions give a picture of the level of existing cases in a population at a given time. Incidence rates and proportions measure the rate of new case development in a population and provide an estimate of the risk of disease.
- Descriptive epidemiologic studies provide information on the distribution of disease and health states according to personal characteristics, geographic region, and time. This knowledge enables practitioners to target programs and allocate resources more effectively and provides a basis for further study.
- Analytic epidemiologic studies investigate associations between exposures or characteristics and health or disease outcomes, with a goal of understanding the etiology of disease. Analytic studies provide the foundation for understanding disease causality and for developing effective intervention strategies aimed at primary, secondary, and tertiary prevention.

## Clinical Decision-Making Activities

1. Interview a local public health nurse or other public health professional from the local health department.
   a. Ask about the current public health priorities and how those priorities were determined.
   b. Describe the type of epidemiologic data utilized in determining local public health priorities.
2. Identify a current health issue in your local community (e.g., childhood lead poisoning, diabetes, HIV/AIDS).
   a. Describe primary, secondary, and tertiary prevention interventions related to this health issue.
   b. How could nurses improve the effectiveness of their prevention activities related to this health issues?
3. Look at a recent issue of the *Final Mortality Statistics* from the National Center for Health Statistics, or the most recent issue of *Health: United States.* Examine the trends in cause-specific mortality and choose one or two of the leading causes of death.
   a. On the basis of current epidemiologic evidence, what factors have contributed to the observed trend in mortality rates for this disease? Changes in survival? Changes in incidence?
   b. Are the changes the result of better (or worse) primary, secondary, or tertiary prevention? Are there modifiable factors, such as health behaviors, that lend themselves to better prevention efforts? What would they be?
4. Examine the leading causes of infant death in the United States.
   a. What differences in intervention approaches are suggested by the various causes of death?

b. How would you design an epidemiologic study to examine risk factors for specific causes of neonatal and postneonatal death? What types of epidemiologic measures would be useful? What study design(s) would be appropriate?

c. How would you use the information from your study to develop an intervention program and to define the target population for your intervention?

5. Find a report of an epidemiologic study in one of the major public health, nursing, or epidemiology journals. How do the findings of this study, if valid, affect your nursing practice? How do you incorporate the results of epidemiologic research into your nursing practice?

# References

American Nurses Association: *Nursing's social policy statement*, Washington, DC, 1995, American Nurses' Publishing.

Anderson RN: Deaths: leading causes for 2000, *Natl Vital Stat Rep* 50(16), 2002.

Anderson RN, Rosenberg HM: Age standardization of death rates: implementation of the year 2000 standard, *Natl Vital Stat Rep* 47(3), 1998.

Armenian HK: Applications of the case-control method, *Epidemiol Rev* 16(1):1, 1994.

Bell RA, Hillers VN, Thomas TA: The Abuela project: safe cheese workshops to reduce the incidence of *Salmonella typhimurium* from consumption of raw-milk fresh cheese, *Am J Public Health* 89(9):1421-1424, 1999.

Brown P, Ferguson FIT: "Making a big stink": women's work, women's relationships, and toxic waste activism, *Gender & Society* 9(2):145-172, 1995.

Brown P, Masterson-Allen S: Citizen action on toxic waste contamination: a new type of social movement, *Society and Natural Resources* 7:269-286, 1994.

Brownson RC, Petitti DB, editors: *Applied epidemiology: theory to practice*, New York, 1998, Oxford University Press.

Brownson RC, Remington PL, Davis JR: *Chronic disease epidemiology and control*, ed 2, Washington, DC, 1998, American Public Health Association.

Caughy MO, O'Campo PJ, Patterson J: A brief observational measure for urban neighborhoods, *Health & Place* 7:225-236, 2001

Centers for Disease Control and Prevention: Use of race and ethnicity in public health surveillance: summary of the CDC/ATSDR workshop, *MMWR Morb Mortal Wkly Rep* 42(RR-10), 1993.

Centers for Disease Control and Prevention: Addressing emerging infectious disease threats: a prevention strategy for the United States (executive summary), *MMWR Morb Mortal Wkly Rep* 43(RR-5):1, 1994.

Chadwick E: *Report on the sanitary conditions of the laboring population of Great Britain*, Edinburgh, 1842, University Press.

Chin J, editor: *Control of communicable diseases manual*, ed 17, Washington, DC, 2000, American Public Health Association.

Cohen D et al: "Broken windows" and the risk of gonorrhea, *Am J Public Health* 90(2):230-236, 2000.

DiChiro G: Local actions, global visions: remaking environmental expertise, *Frontiers* 18(2):203, 1997.

Diez-Roux AV: Bringing context back into epidemiology: variables and fallacies in multilevel analysis, *Am J Public Health* 88(2):216, 1998.

Editorial: *Am J Public Health* 32:414, 1942.

Fullilove MT: Comment: abandoning "race" as a variable in public health research: an idea whose time has come, *Am J Public Health* 88(9):1297, 1998.

Gebbie KM, Hwang I: Preparing currently employed public health nurses for changes in the health system, *Am J Public Health* 20:716-721, 2000.

Gordis L: *Epidemiology*, ed 2, Philadelphia, 2000, Saunders.

Holleb AI, Fink DJ, Murphy GP: *American Cancer Society textbook of clinical oncology*, Atlanta, Ga, 1991, American Cancer Society.

Hoyert DL et al: Deaths: final data for 1999, *Natl Vital Stat Rep* 49(8), 2001.

Institute of Medicine: *The future of public health*, Washington, DC, 1988, National Academy Press.

Kelsey JL et al: *Methods in observational epidemiology*, ed 2, New York, 1996, Oxford University Press.

Keppel KG, Pearcy JN, Wagener DK: Trends in racial and ethnic-specific rates for the health status indicators: United States, 1990-98, *Healthy People Statistical Notes*, No. 23, Hyattsville, Md, 2002, National Center for Health Statistics.

Koopman JS: Comment: emerging objectives and methods in epidemiology, *Am J Public Health* 86(5):630, 1996.

Koopman JS: Compartmental model analysis of epidemiologic processes, course at University of Michigan, accessed April 2003 from http://www.sph.umich.edu/jkoopman/802Web/Chap2/Chap2.htm (updated 1999).

Krieger N: Epidemiology and the web of causation: has anyone seen the spider? *Soc Sci Med* 39(7):887, 1994.

Krieger N, Zierler S: What explains the public's health? a call for epidemiologic theory, *Epidemiology* 7(1):107, 1995.

Last JM: *A dictionary of epidemiology,* ed 4, New York, 2001, Oxford University Press.

Learner M: *A history of public health in South Carolina,* accessed April 2003, from http://www.scdhec.net/co/elsa/publichealth.

Lilienfeld AM: Epidemiology and health policy: some historical highlights, *Public Health Rep* 99(3):237, 1984.

Lilienfeld AM, Lilienfeld DE: The 1979 Heath Clark lectures: the epidemiologic fabric—weaving the threads, *Int J Epidemiol* 9(3):199, 1980.

Lilienfeld DE, Stolley PD: *Foundations of epidemiology,* ed 3, New York, 1994, Oxford University Press.

Lynch JW et al: Income inequality and mortality in metropolitan areas of the United States, *Am J Public Health* 88(7):1074, 1998.

Martin JA et al: Births: final data for 2000, *Natl Vital Stat Rep* 50(5), 2002.

Meinert CL: *Clinical trials: design, conduct and analysis,* New York, 1986, Oxford University Press.

Minino AM, Smith BL: Deaths: preliminary data for 2000, *Natl Vital Stat Rep* 49(12), 2001.

Mood L: Toxic waste: deep in the roots of nursing comes a search for harmful sources, *Reflect Nurs Leadersh* 26(2):21-25, 2000.

Mrazek PJ, Haggerty RJ, editors: *Reducing risks for mental disorders: frontiers for preventive intervention research,* Committee on Prevention of Mental Disorders, Institute of Medicine, Washington, DC, 1994, National Academy Press.

National Center for Health Statistics: *Health: United States, 1998,* Hyattsville, Md, 1998, Public Health Service.

National Institute of Mental Health: *Priorities for prevention research at NIMH: a report by the National Advisory Health Council Workgroup on Mental Disorders Prevention Research,* Publication No. 98-4321, Washington, DC, 1998, NIH.

O'Campo P et al: Violence by male partners against women during the childbearing year: a contextual analysis, *Am J Public Health* 85(8):1092, 1995.

Office of Minority Health, United States Department of Health and Human Services: *Elimination of racial and ethnic disparities in health: report to Congress,* Washington, DC, 1999, Author.

Pearce N: Traditional epidemiology, modern epidemiology, and public health, *Am J Public Health* 86(5):678, 1996.

Peters KD, Kochanek KD, Murphy SL: Deaths: final data for 1996, *Natl Vital Stat Rep* 47(9):1-100, 1998.

Roche LS, Skinner R, Weinstein RB: Use of a geographic information system to identify and characterize areas with high proportions of distant stage breast cancer, *J Public Health Manag Pract* 3(2):26-32, 2002.

Rothman KJ: *Epidemiology: an introduction,* New York, 2002, Oxford University Press.

Rothman KJ, Greenland S: *Modern epidemiology,* ed 2, Philadelphia, 1998, Lippincott-Raven.

Rushton G, Elmes G, McMaster R: Considerations for improving geographic information system research in public health, *URISA Journal* 12(2):31-49, 2000.

Sampson RJ, Raudenbush SW, Earls F: Neighborhoods and violent crime: a multilevel study of collective efficacy, *Science* 277(15):918, 1997.

Schlesselman JJ: *Case-control studies: design, conduct, analysis,* New York, 1982, Oxford University Press.

Snow J: On the mode of communication of cholera. In *Snow on cholera,* New York, 1855, The Commonwealth Fund.

Sorlie PD et al: Age-adjusted death rates: consequences of the year 2000 standard, *Ann Epidemiol* 9:93-100, 1999.

Stallones RA: Cerebrovascular disease epidemiology: a workshop, *Public Health Monogr* 76:51-55, 1966.

Susser M: *Causal thinking in the health sciences,* New York, 1973, Oxford University Press.

Susser M: Epidemiology in the United States after World War II: the evolution of technique, *Epidemiol Rev* 7:147, 1985.

Susser M, Susser E: Choosing a future for epidemiology: I. eras and paradigms, *Am J Public Health* 86(5):668, 1996a.

Susser M, Susser E: Choosing a future for epidemiology: II. from black box to Chinese boxes and eco-epidemiology, *Am J Public Health* 86(5):674, 1996b.

Szklo M, Nieto FJ. *Epidemiology: beyond the basics,* Gaithersburg, Md, 2000, Aspen.

Taylor D, Chavez G: Small area analysis on a large scale: the California experience in mapping teenage birth "hot spots" for resource allocation, *J Public Health Manag Pract* 8(2)33-45, 2002.

Timmreck TC: *An introduction to epidemiology,* ed 3, Boston, 2002, Jones & Bartlett.

Turnock BJ: *Public health: what it is and how it works,* ed 2, Gaithersburg, Md, 2001, Aspen.

U.S. Department of Health and Human Services: *Healthy People 2010: understanding and improving health,* ed 2, Washington, DC, 2000, U.S. Government Printing Office.

U.S. Department of Health, Education, and Welfare: *Vital statistics of the United States: 1950,* Vol 1, Washington, DC, 1954, USDHEW, Public Health Service.

U.S. Department of Health and Human Services: *Public health service fact sheet,* Washington, DC, 1984, USDHHS, Public Health Service.

U.S. Department of Health and Human Services, Public Health Service: *Healthy people 2000: national health promotion and disease prevention objectives,* Washington, DC, 1991, U.S. Government Printing Office.

U.S. Department of Health and Human Services, Public Health Service, Health Resources and Services Administration, Bureau of Health Professions, Divisions of Disadvantaged Assistance: *Health status of minorities and low income groups,* Washington, DC, 1985, U.S. Government Printing Office.

U.S. Preventive Services Task Force: Screening for lipid disorders in adults: recommendations and rationale, *Am J Nursing* 102(6):91-95, 2002.

Vandenbroucke JP: Epidemiology in transition: a historical hypothesis, *Epidemiology* 1(2):164, 1990.

Weinrich M et al: Reference ranges for serum prostate-specific antigen in black and white men without cancer, *Urology* 52(6):967-973, 1998.

Weinrich S et al: Work sites: effective sites for recruitment of African American men into prostate cancer screening, *J Community Health Nurs* 15(2):113, 1998.

Winkelstein W: Editorial: eras, paradigms, and the future of epidemiology, *Am J Public Health* 86(5):621, 1996.

Winkelstein W, French FE, editors: *Basic readings in epidemiology,* ed 3, New York, 1972, MSS Educational.

# Evidence-Based Practice

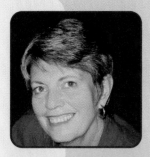

**Joyce Splann Krothe, D.N.S., R.N.**

Joyce Splann Krothe is an associate professor and director of the Bloomington campus of Indiana University School of Nursing. She has taught community health nursing since 1982. She has also served as the project director for the Brown County Health Support Clinic, a rural Indiana nurse-managed clinic, since 1996. The clinic utilizes a community development model to provide health care to underinsured and uninsured rural residents.

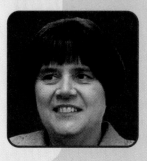

**Anne S. Belcher, D.N.S., R.N., P.N.P.**

Anne Schmidt Belcher is an associate professor and director of faculty affairs at the Indianapolis campus of Indiana University School of Nursing. She has taught community health nursing since 1983 and served as the project director for the Indiana Childhood Immunization Outreach Project. Most recently, Dr. Belcher has been involved in interprofessional collaboration with the Schools of Education and Social Work to develop community linkages for enhancing professional practice in school settings.

## Objectives

After reading this chapter, the student should be able to do the following:

1. Understand the history of evidence-based practice in health care
2. Analyze the relationship of evidence-based practice to community-oriented nursing
3. Provide examples of evidence-based practice in community-oriented nursing
4. Identify the barriers to evidence-based practice

Evidence-based practice (EBP) in nursing has its roots in international settings and has only recently expanded to nursing practice in the United States. The basic principles of EBP will be described as they apply to nursing in general and more specifically to the practice of community-oriented nursing. Dynamics of the practice setting will be described as they relate to implementing EBP in the current health care system.

## HISTORY OF EVIDENCE-BASED PRACTICE

Evidence-based medicine is at the foundation of the current EBP movement in the world. Physicians took the lead in the 1970s (Melnyk et al, 2000)—in particular, a British epidemiologist, Archie Cochrane, who criticized health professionals for their failure to evaluate the effects of their treatment methods. The first journal dedicated to advancing practice on the basis of scientific evidence soon followed (Melnyk et al, 2000).

The term *evidence-based practice* was coined in Canada in the 1980s to describe clinical learning strategies used at McMaster Medical School (Jennings and Loan, 2001). In nursing, EBP began in Great Britain, Canada, and Australia. It arrived in the United States in the 1990s and is currently moving to other health-related disciplines and to other fields as well, such as education. The underlying principle is that high-quality care is based on evidence rather than on tradition or intuition (Beyers, 1999). The current nursing literature on EBP is primarily associated with acute care settings and individual applications to nursing practice, and little is reported about its use in community-oriented nursing. However, the basic principles of EBP can be applied at the individual level or at the community level.

"Nursing practice based on scientific evidence is a rather recent phenomenon" (Melnyk et al, 2000, p. 78). A lack of understanding about the difference between research use, a focus in the 1970s in the United States, and EBP may be contributing to the "slow progress of evidence-based care in nursing" (Melnyk et al, 2000, p. 78). However, research use is a component of EBP, along with theories of practice,

## Key Terms

action research, p. 286
best practices, p. 285
community development model, p. 286
evidence-based practice, p. 285

gold standard, p. 285
knowledge manager, p. 288
randomized clinical trials, p. 285

situated perspective, p. 287
systematic review, p. 286
*See Glossary for definitions*


## Chapter Outline

History of Evidence-Based Practice
Definitions
Implementation of Evidence-Based Practice
Barriers to Implementing Evidence-Based
    Practice

Current Perspectives
Future Perspectives
Year 2010 National Healthy People Objectives
Evidence-Based Practice Nursing Application

Nursing Interventions Related to the Core
    Public Health Functions

expert opinions, clinical knowledge and judgment, and research studies of all type.

**Randomized clinical trials** are the **gold standard** of evidence gathering in evidence-based practice. Nursing has participated very little in randomized clinical trials, however, and all types of evidence, as mentioned earlier, may be equally applicable to nursing practice in communities.

## DEFINITIONS

**Evidence-based practice** is defined as those interventions in health care that are based on the best available (preferably scientific) evidence (Shorten and Wallace, 1997, p. 26). Rutledge (2002) defined EBP as both a process, requiring the evaluating of evidence, and a product, which requires that the evidence acquired is applied to practice. Although definitions of EBP vary widely in the literature, the common thread across disciplines is the application of the best available evidence to improve practice (Youngblut and Brooten, 2001). This is commonly referred to as **best practices.**

Pioneers in the use of evidence to guide practice decisions integrated individual clinical expertise with the best available evidence from systematic research (Closs and Cheater, 1999). Applied to community-oriented nursing, EBP includes the best available evidence from a variety of sources, including research studies, evidence from community-oriented nursing experience and expertise, and evidence from community leaders. Culturally and financially appropriate interventions need to be identified when working with communities.

EBP includes clients in decisions, presenting evidence to them in an understandable fashion, informing them of pros and cons of an intervention, and basing practice decisions on the values of the clients (Jennings and Loan, 2001). At the community level, this means that evidence would be applied with input from the community. For example, decisions related to the services to be offered in a nurse-managed clinic would be made with input from the clinic's advisory board. Advisory boards often include community leaders and consumers of the clinic's services.

A **systematic review** is a summary of the research evidence that relates to a specific question and to the effects of an intervention. Researchers follow rigorous methods to review the literature on a specific topic. Once the literature review is completed and summarized, conclusions are drawn and decisions are made about best practices (Ciliska, Cullum, and Marks, 2001). Nurses often have difficulty doing research because of lack of access and time to retrieve the volume of research reports available while in the work setting. Systematic reviews that include all types of evidence and have been performed by others can help solve this problem.

**Action research** is "a collaborative approach to inquiry that provides people with the means to take systematic action to resolve specific problems. Community-based action research focuses on methods and techniques of inquiry that ask questions about people's history, culture, international practices and emotional lives" (Springer, 1999, p. 17). Action research is responsive to community needs and consistent with the philosophy of a community development model. Qualitative methods, such as individual interviews and focus groups, are often more appropriate than quantitative methods for research involving community clients. The results of action research can benefit the community.

A **community development model** focuses on the achieving of community goals and describes a true partnership in which power and decision making are shared between community members and the academic community (Krothe et al, 2000). A community development model assumes that desired community change occurs through broad participation by community members. The model is an appropriate one to use as community-oriented nurses implement EBP.

## IMPLEMENTING EVIDENCE-BASED PRACTICE IN NURSING

The first step toward implementing EBP in nursing is recognizing the current status of one's own practice and believing that care based on the best evidence will lead to improved client outcomes (Melnyk et al, 2000). Implementation will be successful only when nurses practice in an environment that supports evidence-based care. Clinical performance evaluations should document nurses' use of EBP.

The evidence-based practice is the current catch phrase in health care. It is an approach to health care that assumes that practice grounded in research findings will ultimately provide a quality, cost-effective service (Hunter, 1999, p. 35). Nursing care, however, involves professional judgment gained through years of experience, which is frequently undervalued in EBP (Hunter, 1999).

Nurses in the United States view EBP as a process to improve practice and client outcomes, whereas nurses in other countries focus on its potential to influence policy and the use of limited resources (Jennings and Loan, 2001). Community-oriented nurses should consider EBP as a process to improve practice and outcomes, and they should use evidence to influence policies that will improve the health of communities.

Nurses should take an eclectic view of EBP, noting that "human beings require the benefits of science, but also need the benefits of humanism and personal experience" (Clarke, 1999, p. 89). A situation where evidence alone is the authority rather than the individual client is not appropriate in nursing care. This ignores the inherent differences found in communities. "Any evidence is only a tool, which ultimately requires human judgment" (Clarke, 1999, p. 92).

---

## THE CUTTING EDGE

The journal *Evidence-Based Nursing* started in 1998 as a collaborative effort between the United Kingdom and Canada to provide abstracts of quality nursing research in the international literature and to show clinical applications of the research.

---

Historically, nurses have used multiple sources of knowledge in their practice. Basing all practice on science, although desirable, is not possible. Nurses need to expand the rules of evidence to add intuition, observations of clients and communities, and how they are responding to intervention (Stetler et al, 1998). Important concerns for nurses beyond intervention include ethnicity, sex, age, cultural beliefs, and health status.

---

**HOW TO** **Perform a Systematic Review**

Systematic literature reviews help nurses who want to incorporate EBP principles into their practice but cannot find time to do the research. A quality review can be accomplished by doing the following:

- Reviewing several databases, including international sources
- Choosing and searching a reference list of relevant papers
- Searching key journals by hand
- Talking with key informants in the field to verify what was found in the literature

---

## BARRIERS TO IMPLEMENTING EVIDENCE-BASED PRACTICE IN NURSING

Barriers to the use of EBP "occur when time, access to journal articles, search skills, critical appraisal skills, and an understanding of the language used in research are lacking" (Ciliska, et al, 2001, p. 525). It is important for undergraduates to know how to review the literature to find best practice interventions to apply with clients. Graduate students will want to participate in developing best practice models through scientific analysis.

There are significant barriers that slow the merging of research and practice in an EBP environment. Common barriers to implementing EBP in nursing include misunderstood communication among nursing leaders about the process involved; inferior quality of available research evidence; inability to assess and use research evidence; unwillingness of organizations to fund research and make decisions based on evidence; and concern that EBP will lead to a cookbook approach to nursing while ignoring individual client needs and the nurse's ability to make clinical decisions (McCloughen, 2001; Melnyk et al, 2000).

Although a community-oriented agency may subscribe in theory to the use of EBP, actual implementation may be affected by the realities of the practice setting. Community-based nursing agencies may lack the resources needed for its implementation in the clinical setting, such as time, funding, computer resources, and knowledge. Nurses in the practice setting may lack the necessary skills to identify and evaluate the latest evidence. They may also be reluctant to accept the findings. Nurses may feel threatened when long-established practices are questioned. "The challenge for the clinician is how to access the evidence and integrate it into practice, thus moving beyond practice based solely on experience, tradition or ritual" (Barnsteiner and Prevost, 2002, p. 18).

### NURSING TIP

Systematic reviews of research evidence can potentially overcome barriers to putting evidence into practice. Systematic reviews, also known as evidence summaries and integrative reviews, have been called the heart of EBP (Stevens, 2001).

## CURRENT PERSPECTIVES

The following issues relate to the current status of EBP and nursing:

1. *Cost versus quality.* Much of the pressure to use EBP comes from third-party payers and is a response to the need to contain costs and reduce legal liability. Nurses must question whether the current agenda to contain health care costs creates pressure to focus on those research results that favor cost saving at the expense of quality outcomes for clients. Outcomes include client and community satisfaction, and the safety of care. Costs can be weighed against outcomes when EBP is used to show the best practices available to reduce possible harm to clients (Youngblut and Brooten, 2001).

2. *What is evidence?* The best practitioners "synthesize their clinical expertise and the best available external evidence, recognizing that neither is sufficient alone"

(Colyer and Kamath, 1999, p. 191). Research findings, knowledge from basic science, clinical knowledge, and expert opinion should all be considered sources of evidence for EBP (Youngblut and Brooten, 2001).

3. *Individual differences.* EBP cannot be applied as a universal remedy without attention to client differences. When EBP is applied at the community level, best evidence may point to a solution that is not sensitive to cultural issues and distinctions and thus may not be acceptable to the community. Ethical practice in communities requires attention to individual differences. Implementing EBP within the framework of a community development model should add community perspective in applying evidence to community issues (Shorten and Wallace, 1997).

4. *Appropriate EBP methods for community-oriented nursing practice.* Gaining a number of perspectives in a situated community is important for nurses using EBP. **Situated perspective** is defined as a view that begins in a specific environment and is developed in unique local circumstances (Zygouris-Coe et al, 2001, p. 400). Nursing has a legitimate role to play in interdisciplinary community health practice and can contribute to its evidence base. Nurses are obliged to ensure that the evidence applied to practice is acceptable to the community.

Establishing an EBP culture depends on the use of both qualitative and quantitative research approaches. For example, a quantitative research study of a community health center could provide information about patterns of client use, the cost of various services, and the use of different health care providers. However, when quantitative research is combined with an understanding of *why* clients use or do not use the services (i.e., qualitative information that can be obtained through action research), EBP can help the health center be both clinically and cost effective. Evidence from multiple research methods has the potential to enrich the application of evidence and improve nursing practice (Colyer and Kamath, 1999).

Nurses should cultivate the habit of using research evidence. To accomplish this goal, they must go beyond learning research in a formal course or reading research articles. New strategies will be required to develop the habit of regularly using research to guide practice (Fonteyn, 2002, p. 7).

EBP demands changes. It requires incorporating more practice-oriented research and more collaboration between clinicians and researchers. Emphasis should be on decision making using the varied sources of evidence including research studies and knowledge tailored to the needs of the individual community (Youngblut and Brooten, 2001).

Students should become involved in EBP: undergraduates should understand the research process and acquire the necessary tools for EBP; master's degree students should be highly skilled in accessing and evaluating evidence for practice and should be mentors to others in conducting EBP;

and doctoral students should use EBP to influence practice and health policy through conducting and disseminating research (Melnyk et al, 2000). There may be a lack of commitment to using EBP in the clinical setting, as some managers may tell students that the realities of limited resources and fiscal constraints do not allow for implementation of EBP.

Students are taught how to make practice decisions on the basis of the best available evidence rather than practicing in traditional ways. They learn to question long-standing nursing practice that is often based on intuition. Nurses in the practice setting may suggest that research is for the academic world, useful to satisfy course requirements but not used in the real world of nursing. Students can help resolve the disagreement between the mandate to use EBP and the realities of the clinical setting by exploring resource issues and suggesting creative strategies for overcoming the barriers that exist.

**WHAT DO YOU THINK?**

For EBP to be fully implemented, an organization must value EBP. What factors do you think support the development of an environment for nurses to implement EBP in the community?

## FUTURE PERSPECTIVES

Nurses need to acknowledge and understand EBP. They can participate by using it, or they can add to the research base for community health through active programs of research. Nurses should demonstrate leadership in supporting EBP. Using evidence in practice will demonstrate its value, but implementation can be difficult because of the sheer volume of evidence and the increasing client loads (Melnyk et al, 2000). Byers (2002) noted that despite the availability of quality research findings, it may take years for the evidence to be translated into practice.

**DID YOU KNOW?**

It is suggested that it takes 16 to 20 years for research to change practice.

Nurses have an important role to play in developing and using clinical guidelines for community practices. Use of a community development model will ensure that the community's perspective is included. Nurses active in the EBP movement should devote attention to understanding how best to incorporate the guidelines into practice (Kitson, 2001).

The rising cost of health care will demand a more critical look at the benefits and costs of EBP. Finding resources to implement EBP will continue to be a challenge requiring creative strategies (Cooke and Grant, 2002). An em-

phasis on quality care, equal distribution of health care resources, and cost control will continue. Implementing EBP can assist nurses in addressing these issues in the clinical setting.

As nurses implement EBP in an environment focused on cost savings, the potential for managed care organizations or other health care agencies to endorse reimbursement of treatment options solely on the basis of cost, without allowing for individual variation or considering environmental issues, will continue to be a concern (Stout, 2002). Nurses must use caution in adopting EBP in a prescriptive manner in different community environments.

In the future, the **knowledge manager** will be important in EBP. The knowledge manager will be responsible for collecting and disseminating the collective knowledge within an organization; gathering relevant knowledge and applying it to the community; and retrieving and evaluating the best evidence for clinical practice within a community, while staying informed about the community's politics and policy issues. Everyone within a community health organization would subscribe to the use of EBP, but one nurse would be designated the knowledge manager, responsible for ensuring that the practice is evidence based. This nurse would evaluate what is best practice and determine if it is effective for the given community considering community differences (Fennessy, 2001) (Box 12-1). Advanced practice nurses (APNs) are well prepared to integrate EBP into practice settings. The APN can provide information to support EBP at both an individual practitioner level and an organization level.

**DID YOU KNOW?**

Did you know that comprehensive EBP databases are available through various internet sites to assist nurses in applying the most recent best evidence to their clinical practice?

One source of evidence data is the internet (DeBourgh, 2001) (Box 12-2). However, there may be a lack of quality indicators to evaluate the myriad websites claiming to contain EBP information. For example, a recent survey published in the *Journal of the American Medical Association* noted that the majority of authors of an EBP clinical guideline had a vested interest in the company marketing the product recommended in the guideline, creating a potential conflict of interest (Stout, 2002).

## YEAR 2010 NATIONAL HEALTHY PEOPLE OBJECTIVES

Healthy People 2010 objectives offer a systematic approach to health improvement. These objectives cannot by themselves improve the health status of the nation, but they do provide general direction and focus for measuring progress within a specific amount of time. Healthy People 2010 is dedicated to the principle that every person in each com-

## BOX 12-1 Examples of Intervention Using Evidence-Based Practice at Three Levels of Prevention

### PRIMARY PREVENTION

According to the Centers for Disease Control (CDC) one out of every five Americans is obese, a 61% increase since 1991. One out of 16 Americans has diabetes, an increase of 49% since 1990. Lack of adequate physical activity is a significant risk factor for obesity and type II diabetes (McGinnis, 2002). Several community-level strategies have been suggested for increasing physical activity. At the primary prevention level, community-wide campaigns to support regular exercise, greater emphasis on school-based physical education programs, and environmental and policy initiatives to create or enhance places for physical activity in communities can make significant contributions to improving the lifestyle of sedentary people.

### SECONDARY PREVENTION

Low-income mothers of overweight children had personal and environmental challenges in preventing and managing obesity. Low-income mothers did not find pediatric growth charts useful or relevant in defining children's weight. They felt their children's weight was predestined by heredity, and they expressed difficulty in structuring their children's eating habits. The use of focus group interviews permitted clarification of maternal perceptions of obesity and provided information for community healthy nursing intervention (Jain et al, 2001).

### TERTIARY PREVENTION

The Task Force on Community Preventive Services published a report that demonstrated effective care strategies for managing people with diabetes. Nurses working in health care organizations can use case management to focus on the individual diabetic client. Population-focused strategies, such as implementing best practices for management of diabetic disease, contribute to an overall improvement in the health of all diabetics. McGinnis (2002) reports, "The potential for gain against the toll from diabetes is great, but only if we pair aggressive clinical interventions with equally aggressive community action fundamental to broad lifestyle changes" (p. 1). The responsibility to affect behavioral change lies not just with public health programs but also with community health nurses, primary care providers, local policy makers, health care systems, managed care organizations, and researchers. Use of proven strategies for behavioral and social change may result in achievement of a reduced number of obese Americans and fewer Americans diagnosed with type II diabetes. A population-focused strategy for diabetes disease management might be changing the foods found in vending machines. An individual-focused strategy might be managing the diet of the diabetic at the clinic.

---

Jain et al: Why don't low-income mothers worry about their preschoolers being overweight? *Pediatrics* 107(5):1138-1146, 2001; McGinnis JM: Report of independent task force on community preventive services, *Am J Prev Med* 22(4):330-331, 2002.

## BOX 12-2 Resources for Implementing Evidence-Based Practice

The following resources can assist nurses in developing an evidence-based nursing practice.

1. The Agency for Health Care Quality and Research (AHRQ) developed clinical guidelines based on the best available evidence for several clinical topics, such as pain management. The guidelines are accessible via the agency's website, http://www/ahcpr.gov, and serve as a resource to nurses involved in individual client care.

2. The Cochrane Database of Systematic Reviews is a collection of more than 1000 systematic reviews of effects of health care internationally. These reviews are accessible via the website http://www.cochrane.org. A nursing segment of this group, the Cochrane Collaboration Nursing Network, is being developed.

3. The Center for Evidence-Based Nursing established at the University of York, United Kingdom, identifies EBP through primary research and systematic literature reviews and can be accessed at the website www.york.ac.uk/inst/che.

4. The University of Sheffield, United Kingdom, developed a list of over 150 websites for EBP, which can be accessed at http://www.shef.ac.uk.

5. The University of Iowa Health Center, Department of Nursing, gained national recognition for its use of EBP to improve care. The success is attributed to an organization culture that supports EBP: clinicians consistently question what evidence can be used to improve care, and administrators support and value EBP (Titler et al, 2001). These resources can be accessed at www.nursing.uiowa.edu/ebp/index.htm.

6. The *Evidence-Based Nursing Journal* is in its fifth year of publication and is published quarterly. Its website, http://www.evidencebasednursing.com, was launched in 2001. The purpose of the journal is to select articles reporting studies and reviews from the health-related literature that warrant immediate attention by nurses attempting to keep pace with advances in their profession. Using predefined criteria, the best quantitative and qualitative original articles

*Continued*

---

**BOX 12-2    Resources for Implementing Evidence-Based Practice—cont'd**

are abstracted in a structured format, commented on by clinical experts, and shared in a timely fashion. The research question, methods, results, and evidence-based conclusions are reported.

7. Sigma Theta Tau International provides access to information resources globally through the society's website, http://www.nursingsociety.org. The online version of the journal contains direct links to the original published research report that is summarized in an abstract (Fonteyn, 2002).

8. The Task Force on Community Preventive Services is an independent, nonfederal task force appointed by the director of the Centers for Disease Control.

Information about the Task Force may be found at the website http://www.thecommunityguide.org. The Task Force has been charged with determining the topics to be addressed by the CDC's Community Guide and the most appropriate means to assess evidence regarding population-based interventions. The Task Force reviews and assesses the quality of available evidence on the effects of essential community preventive health services. The multidisciplinary Task Force determines the scope of the Community Guide that will be used by local health departments and agencies to determine best practices for preventive health in populations.

---

Fonteyn M: Implementation forum: print and online versions of evidence-based nursing: innovative teaching tools for nurse educators, *Evid Based Nurs* 5(1):6-7, 2002; Titler MG et al: The Iowa model of evidence-based practice to promote quality care, *Crit Care Nurs Clin North Am* 13(4):497-509, 2001.

---

## Healthy People 2010 | The Information Access Project

The Information Access Project is a resource for community-oriented nurses; it helps them identify research findings that have direct links to population-focused and community-based care. It has identified evidence-based strategies that assist with evaluation of progress toward achievement of Healthy People 2010 goals and objectives. The Information Access Project can be described as follows:

• It draws its citations from peer-reviewed literature available through PubMed.

• It is designed to yield more information about interventions and models than the extent or nature of the problems as addressed by a Healthy People Objective.

• All preformulated searches are reviewed by the staff of Public Health Foundation (a nonprofit organization in Washington, D.C.) or by external subject matter experts to ensure that searches adequately capture the largest amount of published research (available through PubMed) related to achieving the objective.

• It provides links to relevant guidelines related to the focus areas.

---

From U.S. Department of Health and Human Services: *Healthy people 2010: national health promotion and disease prevention objectives,* Washington, DC, 2000, U.S. Government Printing Office.

---

munity across the nation deserves equal access to comprehensive, culturally competent, community-based health care systems that are committed to serving the needs of individuals and promoting community health (U.S. Department of Health and Human Services [USDHHS], 2000). Nurses can implement and evaluate these objectives.

In preparing Healthy People 2010, the U.S. Department of Health and Human Services collaborated with other agencies and national organizations to address the need for information and data in meeting the goals. A group known as Partners in Information Access for Public Health Professionals formed to assist in meeting this goal. Their website (http://nnlm.gov/partners/hp/access.html) makes information and evidence-based strategies related to Healthy People 2010 available to health professionals. The National Library of Medicine, the Public Health Foundation, and the

National Network of Libraries of Medicine staff have worked together in a pilot project to develop preformulated search strategies for six focus areas of Healthy People 2010 objectives. These focus areas are access to quality health services, disability and secondary conditions, food safety, public health infrastructure, respiratory diseases, and environmental health.

## EVIDENCE-BASED PRACTICE NURSING APPLICATION

Evidence-based practice in community-oriented nursing challenges nurses to integrate outcomes of the best research into to their clinical practice. In community health, best-practice recommendations are translated from evidence that has broad application to communities and populations.

## Evidence-Based Practice

Family members find themselves largely responsible for provider care to persons with dementia. Being a family caregiver means not only providing direct care but paying out of pocket for some expenses. The caregiver may also experience physical and mental health effects, including stress and social isolation. This study tested an intervention that included classroom instruction, reading assignments, and exercises to help the caregiver learn to cope with the direct care role. The intervention through workshops was also designed to help caregivers understand the disease, their role, and their beliefs about caregiving. They were also given coaching to help them problem solve. The training occurred over 14 hours in seven 2-hour weekly sessions.

Family caregivers were referred by community health and social services agencies. Using random selection to assign participants to the intervention and initial groups, 94 caregiver/care receiver pairs were chosen over a 5-month period. The intervention group was given standard measures (tests) of beliefs about caregiving, burden, depression, and reaction to care. The results showed that the intervention provided benefits to the caregiver.

**Nurse Use:** The study indicated that the caregiver training would assist informal caregivers in understanding the disease process of dementia, in recognizing their own limits, and in reducing adverse outcomes.

Hepburn KW et al: Dementia family caregiver training: affecting beliefs about caregiving and caregiver outcomes, *J Am Geriatr Soc* 49:450-457, 2001.

## Evidence-Based Practice

This study focused on introducing a home-based strength and balance retraining program for persons 75 years and older. The clients were persons from a rehabilitation hospital in New Zealand. There were 240 participants, 88% of whom were followed for a 1-year period. The participants were randomly assigned to the intervention group or the control group. The 121 clients in the intervention group received exercise promotion interventions during home visits from a public health nurse. The intervention was done in five home visits that occurred over 6 months. Each participant agreed to exercise three times a week for 30 minutes, and to walk twice weekly for 1 year.

When comparing results between the exercise intervention group and the control group after 1 year, it was found that in the exercise group falls had been reduced and serious injuries from falls were reduced. The program showed a cost savings for fall treatment and hospital care.

**Nurse Use:** The nurse using a standard exercise protocol can be effective in reducing the risk of falls and serious injury in the older population.

Robertson MC, Devlin N, Gardner MM: A home-based, nurse delivered exercise program reduced falls and serious injuries in people >80 years of age, *Evid Based Nurs* 5(1):22, 2002.

## NURSING INTERVENTIONS RELATED TO THE CORE PUBLIC HEALTH FUNCTIONS

The public health functions that are considered to be core to all nursing practice in the community are assessment, policy development, and assurance. Nurses in official and nonofficial agencies focus their practice in these three areas (Conley and Dahl, 1993).

Nurses participate in the essential services of public health through a variety of interventions. The Association of State and Territorial Directors of Nursing have identified ways in which nurses can participate in interventions that contribute to the core functions of public health (see Chapter 1). Application of EBP to these interventions will support community-oriented nurses in assessment, policy development, and assurance activities as they work in collaboration with other disciplines to mobilize resources to promote the health of communities (Table 12-1).

## ■ Practice Application

The director of a part-time, nurse-managed clinic is in the process of analyzing how best to expand services to operate as a full-time clinic in the most cost-effective and clinically effective manner. The nurse who is the director gathers evidence on nurse-managed clinics in other rural settings to evaluate cost and clinical effectiveness of various models. The nurse also considers evidence from the following sources in the decision-making process: client satisfaction research data; knowledge of clinic staff; expert opinion of community advisory board members; evidence from community partners; and data on service needs in the state. Having examined the evidence, the nurse decides that incremental (step-by-step) growth toward full-time status is warranted. Evidence of needs in the community and analysis of statistical data indicate that addition of services for children is a priority, and a pediatric nurse practitioner is hired as a first step, while planning for full-time status continues.

**A.** Evaluation of the evidence gathered demonstrates which of the following?
- Effectiveness of the intervention in communities
- Application of the data to populations and communities

**Table 12-1    Core Public Health Functions and Related EBP Nursing Interventions**

| CORE FUNCTION | RELATED NURSING INTERVENTIONS |
|---|---|
| Assessment | • Diagnose and investigate health problems and hazards in the community.<br>• Mobilize community partnerships to identify and solve health problems.<br>• Link people to needed health services.<br>• Use EBP to research for new insights and innovative solutions to health problems. |
| Policy Development | • Inform, educate, and empower communities about health issues.<br>• Develop policies and plans using EBP that support individual and community health efforts. |
| Assurance | • Monitor health status to identify community health problems.<br>• Enforce laws and regulations that protect health and ensure safety.<br>• Ensure the provision of health care that is otherwise unavailable.<br>• Ensure a competent public health and personal health care workforce.<br>• Use EBP to evaluate effectiveness, accessibility, and quality of personal and population-based services. |

- Existence of positive or negative health outcomes
- Economic consequences of the intervention
- Barriers to implementation of the interventions in communities

**B.** Explain how this example applies principles of EBP.

**Answers are in the back of the book.**

## Key Points

- Evidence-based practice developed in other countries before coming to the United States.
- Application of evidence-based practice in relation to clinical decision making for nursing concentrates on interventions and strategies geared to communities and populations rather than to individuals.
- The goals, as evidenced through Healthy People 2010, are to increase the quality and years of healthy life and to eliminate health disparities in populations (USDHHS, 2000).
- Cost and quality of care are issues in evidence-based practice.
- Evidence-based practice includes intervention based on theory, expert opinions, provider knowledge, and research.
- Use of a community development model involves community leaders in making decisions about best practices in their community.
- Nurses need to recognize their current practice abilities.

## Clinical Decision-Making Activities

1. Give an example of how undergraduates can be involved in evidence-based practice.
2. The U.S. health care delivery system is thought to be one of the best in the world. Does it make sense that evidence-based practice came to the U.S. after being promoted in other countries? Explain your answer.
3. How does the nurse's knowledge of the community relate to evidence-based practice?
4. What are the barriers to implementing evidence-based practice?
5. Is the cost or quality of care more important in evidence-based practice? Debate this issue with classmates.
6. When working with a community to improve its health, is it more important to consider the perspectives of the community or those of the provider when defining the health problems? Elaborate.
7. Invite the director of nursing from the local health department to speak to your class. Ask if evidence is used to develop nursing policies and practice guidelines. If not, why not?
8. Explain the investment that you can make in applying evidence to your practice.

## Additional Resources

These related resources are found either in the appendix at the back of this book or on the book's website at **http://evolve.elsevier.com/Stanhope.**

**evolve** Evolve Website

WebLinks: Healthy People 2010

# References

Association of State and Territorial Directors of Nursing: *Public health nursing: a partner for progress,* Washington, DC, 1998, ASTDN.

Barnsteiner J, Prevost S: How to implement evidence-based practice: some tried and true pointers, *Reflect Nurs Leadersh* 28(2):18-21, 2002.

Beyers M: About evidence-based nursing practice, *Nurs Manag* 30(10):56, 1999.

Briss P et al: Developing an evidence-based guide to community preventive services: methods—The Task Force on Community Preventive Services, *Am J Prev Med* 18(suppl 1):35-43, 2000.

Byers JF: The relationship between continuous quality improvement and research, *J Healthcare Qual* 24(1):4-8, 2002.

Cameron G, Hayes V, Wren A: Using reflective processes in community-based participatory action research, *Reflect Pract* 1(2):215-231, 2000.

Carr C, Schott A: Differences in evidence-based care in midwifery practice and education, *J Nurs Scholarsh* 34(2):153-158, 2002.

Centers for Disease Control: Vaccine-preventable diseases: improving vaccination coverage in children, adolescents, and adults, 1999, *MMWR Morbid Mortal Wkly Rep* 48:1-15, 1999.

Ciliska D, Cullum N, Marks BA: Evaluation of systematic reviews of treatment or prevention interventions, *Evid Based Nurs* 4(4):100-103, 2001.

Ciliska DK et al: Resources to enhance evidence-based nursing practice, *AACN Clin Issues* 12(4):520-528, 2001.

Clarke JB: Evidence-based practice: a retrograde step? The importance of pluralism in evidence generation for the practice of health care, *J Clin Nurs* 8(1):89-94, 1999.

Closs SJ, Cheater FM: Evidence for nursing practice: a clarification of the issues, *J Adv Nurs* 30(1):10-18, 1999.

Colyer H, Kamath P: Evidence-based practice: a philosophical and political analysis: some matters for consideration by professional practitioners, *J Adv Nurs* 29(1):188-194, 1999.

Conley E, Dahl J: *Public health nursing with core public health functions: a progress report from the public health nursing directors of Washington,* Olympia, Wash, 1993, Washington State Department of Health.

Cooke L, Grant M: Support for evidence-based practice, *Oncol Nurs* 18(1):71-78, 2002.

DeBourgh GA: Champions for evidence-based practice: a critical role for advanced practice nurses, *AACN Clin Issues* 12(4):491-508, 2001.

Elliott J: Making evidence-based practice educational, *Br Educ Res J* 27(5): 555-575, 2001.

Fennessy G: Knowledge management in evidence-based healthcare: issues raised when specialist information services search for evidence, *Health Informat J* 7(1):4-8, 2001.

Fonteyn M: Implementation forum: print and online versions of evidence-based nursing: innovative teaching tools for nurse educators, *Evid Based Nurs* 5(1):6-7, 2002.

Hepburn KW et al: Dementia family caregiver training: affecting beliefs about caregiving and caregiver outcomes, *J Am Geriatr Soc* 49:450-457, 2001.

Higgs J, Burn A, Jones M: Integrating clinical reasoning and evidence-based practice, *AACN Clin Issues* 12(4):482-490, 2001.

Hunter S: Evidence-based nursing practice: a cautionary note, *Aust Nurs J* 6(6):35, 1999.

Jain et al: Why don't low-income mothers worry about their preschoolers being overweight? *Pediatrics* 107(5):1138-1146, 2001.

Jennings BM, Loan LA: Misconceptions among nurses about evidence-based practice, *J Nurs Scholarsh* 33(2):121-127, 2001.

Kitson AL: Approaches used to implement research findings into nursing practice: report of a study tour to Australia and New Zealand, *Int J Nurs Pract* 7(6):392-405, 2001.

Krothe JS et al: Community development through faculty practice in a rural nurse-managed clinic, *Public Health Nurs* 17(4):264-272, 2000.

McCloughen A: Identifying barriers to the application of evidence based practice in mental health nursing, *Contemp Nurse* 11(2-3):226-230, 2001.

McGinnis JM: Report of independent task force on community preventive services, *Am J Prev Med* 22(4):330-331, 2002.

Melnyk BM, Fineout-Overholt E: Putting research into practice, *Reflect Nurs Leadersh* 28(2):22-25, 2002.

Melnyk B et al: Evidence-based practice: the past, the present, and recommendations for the millennium, *Pediatr Nurs* 26(1):77-81, 2000.

Robertson MC, Devlin N, Gardner MM: A home-based, nurse delivered exercise program reduced falls and serious injuries in people >80 years of age, *Evid Based Nurs* 5(1):22, 2002.

Rutledge DN: Processes and outcomes of evidence-based practice, *Oncol Nurs* 28(2):3-10, 2002.

Shorten A, Wallace M: Evidence-based practice when quality counts, *Aust Nurs J* 4(11):26-28, 1997.

Springer ET: *Action research,* ed 2, Thousand Oaks, Calif, 1999, Sage.

Stetler CB et al: Utilization-focused integrative reviews in a nursing service, *Appl Nurs Res* 11(4):195-206, 1998.

Stevens KR: Systematic reviews: the heart of evidence-based practice, *AACN Clin Issues* 12(4):529-238, 2001.

Stout CE: Evidence-based practices: a clinical caveat, *Behav Health Accred Account Alert* 7(3):8-9, 2002.

Titler MG et al: The Iowa model of evidence-based practice to promote quality care, *Crit Care Nurs Clin North Am* 13(4):497-509, 2001.

U.S. Department of Health and Human Services: *Healthy people 2010: understanding and improving health,* ed 2, Washington, DC, 2000, U.S. Government Printing Office.

Youngblut JM, Brooten D: Evidence-based nursing practice: why is it important? *AACN Clin Issues* 12(4):468-476, 2001.

Zygouris-Coe V et al: Action research: a situated perspective, *Qual Stud Educ* 14(3):399-412, 2001.

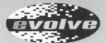
# Community Health Education: Theories, Models, and Principles

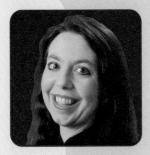

**Lisa C. Onega, Ph.D., R.N., F.N.P., G.N.P.**

Lisa L. Onega is an associate professor of gerontological nursing at Radford University, where she teaches in both the undergraduate and graduate programs. Her research and scholarship are related to depression in older adults. She is currently a Waldron Clinical Fellow and is in the process of establishing a gerontological clinical practice. She has participated in a number of community-based educational programs and health fairs for older adults.

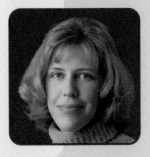

**Alicia A. Jensen, R.N., M.S.N.,**

Alicia A. Jensen began her nursing career in 1991 and has since practiced in home health care and in a number of acute care settings. She is currently working as a critical care nurse and as a graduate teaching fellow at Radford University.

## Objectives

After reading this chapter, the student should be able to do the following:

1. Identify the 12 educational objectives in Healthy People 2010 that may serve as a guide for community health education programs
2. Differentiate between the terms *education* and *learning*
3. Outline three philosophical perspectives of learning
4. Evaluate six theories of learning
5. Describe three domains of learning
6. Identify the nine events of instruction
7. Outline the six characteristics of effective educators
8. Discuss three educational issues
9. List the five steps of the educational process
10. Describe the importance of evaluating the educational product

Health education is a vital part of community-oriented nursing. The promotion, maintenance, and restoration of health require that community health clients receive a practical understanding of health-related information. Community health clients include individuals, families, communities, and populations (American Nurses Association [ANA], 1985, 2001). An individual is any person, regardless of age, sex, or other characteristic. Families are a group of individuals linked by ancestry, marriage, or household and may consist of nuclear, extended, biological, adoptive, or other alternative makeup. A community may be a small group, support system, club, church, school, neighborhood, or loosely tied and widely scattered group with a common interest or cause. A population is the complete set of individuals linked by a common char-

acteristic such as age, ethnicity, sex, or type of disease (Edelman and Fain, 1998). Because community-oriented nurses see clients with varying needs and abilities in a variety of settings, they are in key positions to deliver health education (ANA, 1985, 2001).

Community-oriented nurses may educate clients across three levels of illness prevention: primary, secondary, and tertiary (Edelman and Fain, 1998) (Box 13-1). The information that community-oriented nurses provide enables clients to attain optimal health, prevent health problems, identify and treat health problems early, and minimize disability. Education allows individuals to make knowledgeable health-related decisions, assume personal responsibility for their health, and cope effectively with alterations in their health and lifestyles.

Figure 13-1 identifies the sequence of actions that a community-oriented nurse follows when developing an educational program. The nurse educator identifies a population-specific learning need; decides which philo-

*The authors would like to thank Kevin Tapp for his guidance and assistance with the literature review and also Tanya Daniel and Tiffany Smith for their assistance with obtaining references for this chapter.*

## Key Terms

affective domain, p. 301
andragogy, p. 306
behavioral theory, p. 298
cognitive domain, p. 301
cognitive theory, p. 299
critical theory, p. 299
developmental theory, p. 300

education, p. 298
empiricism, p. 298
Healthy People 2010 educational objectives, p. 296
humanistic theory, p. 300
interpretivism, p. 298
learning, p. 298

long-term evaluation, p. 314
pedagogy, p. 306
pragmatism, p. 298
psychomotor domain, p. 301
short-term evaluation, p. 314
social learning theory, p. 300
*See Glossary for definitions*

## Chapter Outline

Healthy People 2010 Educational Objectives
Education and Learning
Philosophical Perspectives of Learning
Theories of Learning
*Behavioral Theory*
*Cognitive Theory*
*Critical Theory*
*Developmental Theory*
*Humanistic Theory*
*Social Learning Theory*

Educational Principles
*The Nature of Learning*
*The Events of Instruction*
*The Effective Educator*
Educational Issues
*Population Considerations*
*Populations Based on Culture*
*Barriers to Learning*
*Technological Issues*
The Educational Process

*Identify Educational Needs*
*Establish Educational Goals and Objectives*
*Select Appropriate Educational Methods*
*Implement the Educational Plan*
*Evaluate the Educational Process*
The Educational Product
*Evaluation of Health and Behavioral Changes*
*Short-Term Evaluation*
*Long-Term Evaluation*

---

### BOX 13-1  Levels of Prevention Related to Community Health Education

**PRIMARY PREVENTION**

Education at health fairs regarding immunizations for children, older adults, and people with chronic illnesses.

**SECONDARY PREVENTION**

Education at health fairs regarding early diagnosis and treatment of diabetes and hypercholesterolemia, along with providing health screenings, with the goal of shortening disease duration and severity.

**TERTIARY PREVENTION**

Education in rehabilitation centers to help individuals who have had a stroke maximize their functioning.

Modified from Edelman CL, Fain JA: Health defined: objectives for promotion and prevention. In Edelman CL, Mandle CL, editors: *Health promotion throughout the lifespan*, ed 4, pp 3-24, St Louis, Mo, 1998, Mosby.

---

sophical perspectives are appropriate to use in meeting that learning need; selects various aspects from the theories of learning to incorporate into the educational program; considers educational principles that will enhance learning; examines educational issues such as population-specific concerns, barriers to learning, and technological strategies to facilitate learning; designs and implements an educational program; and evaluates the effects of the educational program on learning and behavior.

The Sequence of Actions That a Community Health Nurse Follows When Developing an Educational Program

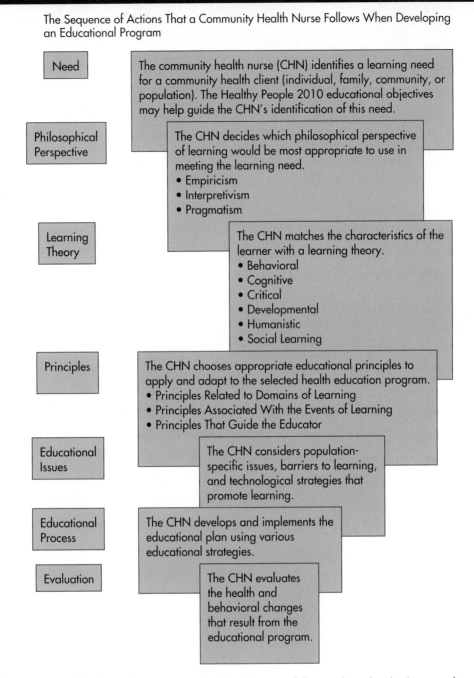

**Figure 13-1** The sequence of actions that a community health nurse follows when developing an educational program.

## HEALTHY PEOPLE 2010 EDUCATIONAL OBJECTIVES

Healthy People 2010 identifies national health needs and outlines goals and objectives designed to improve health. To meet and maintain many of the objectives of Healthy People 2010, community-based education programs across a variety of settings such as schools, worksites, and health care agencies are needed to promote healthy habits and lifestyles. The Healthy People 2010 box outlines the objectives that specifically address health education (Healthy People 2010 Online Documents, 2001).

The **Healthy People 2010 educational objectives** emphasize the importance of educating various populations (based on age and ethnicity) about health promotion activities such as avoiding cigarette smoking and illegal drug use, drinking alcohol in moderation, eating a well-balanced diet, exercising routinely, and making responsible sexual choices (Healthy People 2010 Online Documents, 2001). Nurses who use Healthy People 2010 as a guide in educating clients, strive to foster healthy communities mainly through primary and secondary prevention. One avenue for providing this primary and secondary preventative education is through developing and participating in health

**Goal:** To increase the quality, availability, and effectiveness of educational and community-based programs designed to prevent disease and improve health and quality of life

## SCHOOL SETTING

7-1 Increase completion of high school

7-2 Increase the proportion of middle, junior high, and senior high schools that provide comprehensive school health education to prevent health problems in the following areas: (1) unintentional injury, violence, and suicide; (2) tobacco use; (3) alcohol and other drug use; (4) unintended pregnancy and sexually transmitted infections; (5) unhealthy dietary patterns; and (6) inadequate physical activity

7-3 Increase the proportion of college and university students who receive information from their institution on each of the six priority health-risk behavior areas listed above

7-4 Increase the proportion of elementary, middle, junior high, and senior high schools that have a nurse-to-student ratio of at least 1:750

## WORKSITE SETTING

7-5 Increase the proportion of worksites that offer a comprehensive employee health promotion program to their employees

7-6 Increase the proportion of employees who participate in employer-sponsored health promotion activities

## HEALTH CARE SETTING

7-7 Increase the proportion of health care organizations that provide client and family education

7-8 Increase the proportion of clients who report that they are satisfied with the client education that they receive from their health organization

7-9 Increase the proportion of hospitals and managed care organizations that sponsor community disease prevention and health promotion activities that address the priority health needs identified by their community

## COMMUNITY SETTING AND SELECT POPULATIONS

7-10 Increase the proportion of tribal and local health service areas that establish community health promotion programs

7-11 Increase the proportion of local health departments that establish culturally appropriate and linguistically competent community health promotion and disease prevention programs

7-12 Increase the proportion of older adults who have participated during the preceding year in at least one organized health promotion activity

Modified from U.S. Department of Health and Human Services: *Healthy people 2010: national health promotion and disease prevention objectives,* Washington, DC, 2000, U.S. Government Printing Office.

---

**HOW TO**   **Set Up a Health Fair**

- Establish goals, outcomes, and screening activities in conjunction with desires of the population or community.
- Recruit a variety of health care professionals and sponsors to participate in the fair.
- Reserve the location and set the date and time of the fair approximately 1 year in advance.
- At least 6 months in advance, obtain a financial commitment from sponsors and develop a budget.
- About 4 months in advance, send letters to health care professionals and agencies verifying their participation and informing them of the location, date, and time of the fair.
- Approximately 2 months in advance, obtain tables, chairs, trash cans, decorations, and equipment needed for exhibits. Prepare program handouts and advertisements. Begin advertising for the fair. Verify that parking and security personnel are available.

- Approximately 1 week in advance, confirm that health care professionals and agency participants are planning to participate.
- The day before the health fair, set up tables, chairs, decorations, and equipment.
- On the day of the fair, greet health care professionals, agency representatives, sponsors, and members of the population being served. Solve problems as needed during the course of the day.
- Between 1 week and 1 month after the fair, send thank you letters to health care professionals, agencies, and sponsors. Pay bills associated with the fair.
- Work with the population of interest to evaluate the effectiveness of the health fair.

Modified from Kelemen A: Wellness promotion: how to plan a college health fair, *Am J Health Studies* 17(1):31-36, 2001; Lyman S, Benedik JR: Health fairs: timetable, pitfalls, & burnout, *College Student J* 33(4):534, 1999.

fairs designed for various populations. For example, nurses seeking to target primary prevention and improve the health of older adults in their communities may participate in health fairs that offer demonstrations, educational posters, and handouts related to healthy nutrition and age-appropriate exercises.

Typically, a nurse identifies a health need or problem in one particular population—for example, at the client, family, community, or population level. Then health education programs are designed to meet the health need or problem in that population. Generally these programs involve educating individual members of the population about health promotion, illness prevention, and treatment. For example, in a community where morbidity, mortality, and health care costs associated with childhood and adolescent asthma were problematic, a community-based asthma education and training program was established (Slutsky and Stephens, 2001). In another community, 60% of Hispanic/Latino women who delivered babies initiated breastfeeding; however, half of these women stopped breastfeeding in less than 2 months. To facilitate continued breastfeeding in this population, a community-based educational intervention was established (Stopka, Chapman, and Perez-Escamilla, 2002).

## EDUCATION AND LEARNING

A major reason that community-oriented nurses are concerned about learning is that learning enables individuals to improve their decision-making abilities and thereby change their behavior. There is a difference between **education** and **learning** (Knowles, Holton, and Swanson, 1998; Palazzo, 2001). Education is the establishment and arrangement of events to facilitate learning (Driscoll, 1994; Palazzo, 2001). Education emphasizes the provider of knowledge and skills. Learning emphasizes the recipient of knowledge and skills and results in behavioral changes. Learning is the process of gaining knowledge and expertise. Once an individual has learned or gained specified knowledge and expertise, the process is complete and behavioral change results (Driscoll, 1994; Knowles et al, 1998; Palazzo, 2001).

## PHILOSOPHICAL PERSPECTIVES OF LEARNING

Three philosophical perspectives frame the way that nurses view learning (Driscoll, 1994):

1. *Empiricism* is the objective and systematic method of observing and collecting information. Foundational information is assimilated to gain an understanding of complex issues.
2. *Interpretivism* is the use of reason and perception to structure and gain information. Knowledge is constructed so that it has personal meaning for the target audience, whether that is an individual or a particular group.
3. *Pragmatism* merges empiricism and interpretivism by acknowledging the existence of reality but accepting that it cannot be known completely.

Therefore pragmatism postulates that although knowledge is beneficial, the focus should be on what works in practical terms to yield positive behavioral changes (Table 13-1).

Nurses need to select the appropriate perspective when attempting to provide education. If the client is a group of adolescents, provision of empirical information regarding prevention of sexually transmitted infections and birth control options may be the first step in alerting the teens to their choices. The nurse may be the adolescents' only source of information about the consequences of sexually transmitted infections and the costs of teen pregnancy. Many adolescents will learn by empiricism and will subsequently make healthy behavioral choices. However, even when the information has been provided, some teens will need further learning to occur. The nurse may use interpretivism to help these adolescents to understand their individual perceptions about sexual decision making and to logically consider the implications of their choices. Ultimately, the nurse may use a variety of strategies including providing facts, having adolescents who have had an unwanted pregnancy or a sexually transmitted infection share their stories, having the teens write a personal paper about their sexual decision making, and offering counseling to adolescents who request it. This pragmatic view of learning enables the nurse educator to help adolescents with different learning styles and needs make healthy decisions.

## THEORIES OF LEARNING

A solid theoretical foundation of learning and health education enables nurses to educate clients successfully. Although many theories and principles related to learning are applicable to community-oriented nursing, samples of only the most useful and readily adaptable ones are included here. Theories of learning help nurses to understand how people learn and to design and implement client education. Table 13-2 provides an overview of six major theories of learning that are useful in community-oriented nursing. Theories of learning provide nurse educators with a choice of options as they apply the most appropriate theory to a specific health education situation. Often it is necessary to combine parts of a number of these theories in the education process (Driscoll, 1994).

### Behavioral Theory

**Behavioral theory** approaches the study of learning by concentrating on behaviors that can be observed and measured. The goal of these approaches to learning is behavioral change. A *target behavior,* which the nurse educator seeks to either increase or decrease, is identified. To increase a behavior, the nurse identifies and consistently uses a *reinforcer* to modify the target behavior. To decrease a behavior, the nurse identifies and consistently uses *withdrawal of a reinforcer (punishment)* to modify the target behavior (Dembo, 1994; Dobbins, 2001; Driscoll, 1994).

**Table 13-1   Philosophical Perspectives of Learning**

| EMPIRICISM | INTERPRETIVISM | PRAGMATISM |
|---|---|---|
| • Reality is objective, unique, and created by elemental parts. | • Reality is constructed, different for various individuals, and holistic. | • Reality is interpreted, negotiated, and consensual. |
| • Source of knowledge is experience. | • Source of knowledge is reason. | • Source of knowledge is experience and reason. |
| • Focus is on similarities. | • Focus is on differences. | • Focus is on both similarities and differences. |

Modified from Driscoll MP: *Psychology of learning for instruction,* Boston, 1994, Allyn and Bacon.

**Table 13-2   Theories of Learning**

| THEORY | FOCUS | METHOD |
|---|---|---|
| Behavioral | Change behavior | Reinforcement/punishment |
| Cognitive | Change thought patterns | Variety of sensory input and repetition |
| Critical | Increase depth of knowledge | Ongoing dialogue and open inquiry |
| Developmental | Consider human developmental stage | Educational opportunities match readiness to learn |
| Humanistic | Utilize feelings and relationships | Learners will do what is best for themselves (self-determination) |
| Social learning | Change expectations and beliefs | Link information, beliefs, and values |

Modified from Dembo MH: *Applying educational psychology,* ed 5, White Plains, NY, 1994, Longman; Driscoll MP: *Psychology of learning for instruction,* Boston, 1994, Allyn and Bacon; Knowles MS, Holton III EF, Swanson RA: *The adult learner: the definitive classic in adult education and human resource development,* ed 5, Houston, Tex, 1998, Gulf.

The behavioral approach is useful when the educator has full control over the rewards and consequences environment—that is, the feedback system. This approach is also useful when the learner has cognitive limitations, because the behavioral approach requires only the most rudimentary use of cognition (Dobbins, 2001; Driscoll, 1994).

For example, using Healthy People 2010 as a guide, a nurse working in a school system might want to decrease the number of adolescent deaths associated with alcohol use. The nurse identifies the target behavior as use of a designated driver. The nurse works to increase the use of designated drivers to transport students from school-related functions. Therefore after every school-related sporting or social event, four trained adults sit at the exit doors, evaluate the sobriety of designated drivers, and assign designated drivers to cars. Designated drivers each receive $10 for gasoline, have their names printed in the weekly school newspaper, and become eligible for a weekly prize drawing of $25.

## Cognitive Theory

**Cognitive theory** emphasizes that the way knowledge is organized, connected, and retrieved is important in learning. By *changing thought patterns* and *providing information,* learners' behavior will change. Cognitive theory posits that people's thought patterns undergo constant change as they interact with their environment. Thus the nurse educator provides information in a variety of ways that will change clients' thought patterns and ultimately lead to changes in behavior (Dembo, 1994; Dobbins, 2001; Driscoll, 1994).

For example, if a group of women do not do monthly breast self-examinations (BSEs), the nurse working with them instructs them to begin doing so. The nurse seeks to change their thought patterns by providing information about BSEs in a variety of ways. First, the nurse verbally teaches the women about the procedure and explains the reasons for doing BSEs and then shows them a video about them. Next, the nurse observes as each of the women practices breast examinations on a breast model. Finally, the nurse gives each woman a handout with the procedure written and diagrammed on it and instructs the women to hang the handout next to the bathroom mirror to remind them to do monthly BSEs. Thus, by using a variety of environmental cues and sensory input, the women's thought patterns can be changed, thereby influencing their behavior related to BSEs.

## Critical Theory

**Critical theory** approaches learning as an *ongoing dialogue.* An individual holds a belief about a health matter. Nurse educators attempt to change this belief by *questioning* the learner. As the learner answers the questions, the learner's beliefs begin to change, new questions arise, and the learner then asks the educator questions. The nurse educator responds to these questions. This process of *discourse* ultimately changes thinking and behavior (Driscoll, 1994).

For example, the nurse would like a newly diagnosed group of diabetic clients to assume responsibility for the management of their diabetes. The nurse asks the clients what they know about diabetes. The clients demonstrate that they can check their own blood sugar and prepare their own insulin injections. However, on further questioning, it is discovered that the clients are not familiar with the long-term complications of diabetes. The nurse then educates them about these complications. Next, the clients raise questions about what they can do to prevent long-term complications. As a result of this dialogue and exchange of information, the clients begin to go to an ophthalmologist every year and to check their feet daily for alterations in skin color or integrity.

## Developmental Theory

**Developmental theory** maintains that learning happens in concert with *developmental stages* that occur from infancy to old age. Each stage is a major transformation from the previous stage; therefore learning occurs quite differently in each developmental period. Knowledge acquisition is a process of continuous self-construction. Knowledge is invented and reinvented as individuals develop and interact with their world. *Readiness to learn* depends on each individual's developmental stage (Dembo, 1994; Driscoll, 1994).

For example, to help a family with a toddler prevent accidents in the home, nurses educate parents about safety practices. They also teach the parents how to educate the toddler simply and clearly about safety according to the toddler's developmental stage and readiness to understand concepts and to change behavioral patterns. The nurses recognize that the parents' and the toddler's levels of readiness to learn are quite different. Because the toddler cannot reach the stove top, teaching about the dangers of a hot stove at this stage of physical development is unnecessary. However, the toddler is at risk for accidental poisoning. Although the parents may teach the toddler not to open bottles and jars without their help, all poisons must be removed from the toddler's possible reach as a necessary precaution. The risk of poison ingestion is incomprehensible to the toddler because of the child's language and cognitive development. Thus the parents and the toddler receive different information depending on their developmental stages.

## Humanistic Theory

**Humanistic theory** describes the influence that *feelings, emotions,* and *personal relationships* have on behavior. Humanistic theorists think that learners should be encouraged to examine their feelings and engage in various forms of *self-expression.* Humanists also think that people need to be aware of and able to clarify their values. If people are given free choice, they will do what is best for themselves. Humanists encourage nurse educators not to be overly controlling and restrictive with learners but rather to help them grow and develop according to their natural inclinations (Dembo, 1994; Driscoll, 1994; Knowles et al, 1998).

For example, if members of a retirement community want to develop a health promotion program, they may invite the nurse to schedule meetings to assist them in furthering this goal. At the meetings, the nurse facilitates group discussion about the goals and strategies of the program and provides a variety of handouts related to health promotion. Finally, the nurse answers questions and offers encouragement to group members as they develop their own health promotion program.

## Social Learning Theory

**Social learning theory** builds on the principles of behavioral theory by stating that behavior is a function of an individual's *expectations* about the value of an outcome (Do I want the outcome?) or self-efficacy (Can I achieve the outcome?). If clients believe that an outcome is desired and attainable, they are more likely to change their behavior to achieve that goal. Thus nurse educators may use this theory to change behaviors by enabling clients to change either their expectations about the value of a certain outcome or their ability to achieve the desired outcome or both (Bandura, 1986; Dembo, 1994).

For example, if the nurse wants to help a group of obese women lose weight, the nurse instructs the women to eat less, select healthful foods, and exercise more. Through the presentation of scientific data describing balanced eating and the positive effects of exercise, the nurse helps the women develop the expectation that decreased food intake and increased exercise will result in weight loss. Through case study presentations and before-and-after photos, the nurse helps the women change their expectations about their power to achieve the goal of weight loss. Without the belief in their power to change, the women may be unable to remain motivated to change their target behaviors.

## EDUCATIONAL PRINCIPLES

A variety of educational principles can be used to guide the selection of health information for individuals, families, communities, and populations. Three of the most useful categories of educational principles include those associated with the nature of learning, the events of instruction, and guidelines for the effective educator.

## The Nature of Learning

One way to think about the nature of learning is to examine the cognitive (thinking), affective (feeling), and psychomotor (acting) domains of learning. Each domain has specific behavioral components that form a hierarchy of steps, or levels. Each level builds on the previous one. Understanding these three learning domains is crucial in providing effective health education (Bloom et al, 1956).

## Cognitive Domain

The **cognitive domain** includes memory, recognition, understanding, reasoning, application, and problem solving and is divided into a hierarchical classification of behaviors. Learners master each level of cognition in order of difficulty (Bloom et al, 1956; Dembo, 1994). For health education to be effective, the community-oriented nurse must first assess the cognitive abilities of the learner so that the instructor's expectations and plans are directed toward the correct level. Teaching above or below the client's level of understanding may lead to frustration and discouragement.

## Affective Domain

The **affective domain** includes changes in attitudes and the development of values. For affective learning, nurses consider and attempt to influence what individuals, families, communities, and populations feel, think, and value. Because the attitudes and values of nurses may differ from those of their clients, it is important to listen carefully to detect clues to feelings that learners have that may influence learning. It is difficult to change deeply rooted attitudes, beliefs, interests, and values. People need support and encouragement from those around them to make such changes and to reinforce new behaviors (Krathwohl, Bloom, and Masia, 1964). Like cognitive learning, affective learning consists of a series of steps. Steps in the affective domain are compared with those in the cognitive domain in Table 13-3.

## Psychomotor Domain

The **psychomotor domain** includes the performance of skills that require some degree of neuromuscular coordination and emphasize motor skills (Bloom et al, 1956).

Clients are taught a variety of psychomotor skills including bathing infants, changing dressings, giving injections, measuring blood sugars, taking blood pressures, and walking with crutches. The levels of psychomotor learning from the simplest to the most complex level of observable movements are outlined in Table 13-4.

To facilitate skill learning, the nurse should show learners the skill either in person, using pictures, or on a video. Then the educator should allow learners to practice and immediately correct any errors in performing the skill. Three conditions must be met before psychomotor learning occurs (Bloom et al, 1956; Dembo, 1994):

1. The learner must have the *necessary ability.* For example, the nurse may find that a client with Alzheimer's disease may be capable of following only one-step instructions. The nurse must adapt the education plan to fit the client's abilities.
2. The learner must have a *sensory image* of how to carry out the skill. For example, when educating a group of pregnant women about techniques to manage labor, the nurse asks the women to visualize themselves in calm control of their delivery.
3. The learner must have *opportunities to practice* the new skills being learned. Practice sessions should be provided during the program because many clients will not have the facilities, motivation, or time to practice what they have learned at home.

In assessing a client's ability to learn a skill, the educator should evaluate intellectual, emotional, and physical ability. Some clients do not have the intellectual ability to learn the steps that make up a complex procedure. Others may have cultural beliefs that conflict with healthy behaviors. Another may be a tremulous person with poor

---

**Table 13-3  Comparison of Learning Steps in the Cognitive and Affective Domains**

| LEARNING STEP | COGNITIVE DOMAIN | AFFECTIVE DOMAIN |
|---|---|---|
| Knowledge | Requires *recall* of information (dealing with specifics, universals, and abstractions in a field) | Learner *receives* the information. |
| Comprehension | *Combines* recall with understanding (translation, interpretation, and extrapolation) | Learner *responds* to what is being taught. |
| Application | New information taken in and *used* in a different way (problem solving) | Learner *values* the information. |
| Analysis | Breaks communication down into constituent parts to understand the parts and their *relationships* | Learner *makes sense* of the information. |
| Synthesis | Builds on the previous four levels by putting the parts back together into a *unified whole* | Learner *organizes* the information. |
| Evaluation | Judges the *value* of what has been learned (use of criteria for appraising learning) | Learner *adopts behaviors* consistent with the new value system. |

Modified from Bloom BS et al: *Taxonomy of educational objectives: the classification of educational goals—handbook 1: cognitive domain,* White Plains, NY, 1956, Longman; Krathwohl DR, Bloom BS, Masia BB: *Taxonomy of educational objectives: the classification of educational goals—handbook 2: affective domain,* New York, 1964, David McKay.

**Table 13-4    Levels of Psychomotor Learning**

| SKILL | DESCRIPTION OF SKILL | EXAMPLE |
|---|---|---|
| Reflex movements | Occur in response to a stimulus without conscious awareness | Blinking and tearing when a piece of dust gets in the eye |
| Basic movements | Develop from a combination of reflex movements | Moving your eyes to follow an object as an ophthalmologist moves it up, down, and from side to side |
| Perceptual abilities | Transfer visual stimuli into appropriate movements | Seeing an object on the floor and picking it up |
| Physical abilities | Combine basic body movements by incorporating agility, endurance, flexibility, and strength | Seeing a ball come toward you, catching it, and then throwing it to another person |
| Skilled movements | Are indicative of a degree of proficiency | Becoming skilled at inserting and removing contact lenses |
| Nondiscursive communication | Complex movements are used to communicate feelings, interests, or needs | Your eyes sparkle, you smile, and you say hello to someone else |

Developed from Dembo MH: *Applying educational psychology,* ed 5, White Plains, NY, 1994, Longman.

eyesight who is incapable of learning insulin self-injection. The nurse should teach at the level of the learner's ability.

## The Events of Instruction

To educate others effectively, one needs to understand the basic sequence of instruction. When nurses consider the following nine steps of instructing others, they can systematically plan health education so that learners gain as much as possible from the instruction (Driscoll, 1994; Knowles et al, 1998):

1. *Gain attention.* Before learning can take place, the educator must gain the learner's attention. One way to do this is by convincing the learner that the information about to be presented is important and beneficial to the learner.
2. *Inform the learner of the objectives of instruction.* Before teaching begins, the major goals and objectives of instruction should be outlined so that learners develop expectations about what they are supposed to learn.
3. *Stimulate recall of prior learning.* The educator should have learners recall previous knowledge related to the topic of interest. This assists learners in linking new knowledge with prior knowledge.
4. *Present the material.* The essential elements of a topic should be presented in as clear, organized, and simple a manner as possible. The material should be presented in a way that is congruent with the learner's strengths, needs, and limitations.
5. *Provide learning guidance.* For long-lasting behavioral changes to occur, the learner must store information in long-term memory. With guidance from the educator, the learner can transform general infor-

mation that has been presented into meaningful information that the learner can recall.
6. *Elicit performance.* Learners should be encouraged to demonstrate what they have learned. Educators should expect that during the educational process, learners will need to correct errors and improve skills.
7. *Provide feedback.* Educators should provide feedback to learners to assist them in improving their knowledge and skills. Learners can then modify their thinking patterns and behaviors on the basis of this feedback.
8. *Assess performance.* Learning should be evaluated. Knowledge and skills should be formally assessed with the expectation that new information has been understood.
9. *Enhance retention and transfer of knowledge.* Once a baseline level of knowledge and skills has been attained, educators should assist learners in applying this information to new situations.

By using these instructional principles, nurses may help clients to maximize learning experiences. If steps of this process are omitted, superficial and fragmented learning may occur.

## The Effective Educator

Nurse educators must be effective teachers. Six basic principles guide the effective educator (Box 13-2).

### Send a Clear Message

Regardless of the importance of the content or the interest level of learners, if the material is not presented in a clear and logical manner, learners will not receive or retain an optimum level of information. At various stages in the ed-

**BOX 13-2** Six Principles That Guide the Educator

**Message.** Sending a clear message to the learner
**Format.** Selecting the most appropriate learning format
**Environment.** Creating the best possible learning environment
**Experience.** Organizing positive and meaningful learning experiences
**Participation.** Engaging the learner in participatory learning
**Evaluation.** Evaluating and giving objective feedback to the learner

Modified from Knowles M: *The adult learner: a neglected species,* ed 4, Houston, Tex, 1990, Gulf.

**BOX 13-3** Guidelines for Clear Educational Programs

**Begin strongly.** People remember the first point.
**Use a clear, direct, succinct style.** This helps the learner remain focused.
**Use the active voice.** For example, the educator may say, "We will discuss relaxation techniques" instead of "Relaxation techniques will be discussed."
**Accentuate the positive.** For example, the educator may say, "The majority of individuals are able to lose weight with a well-balanced diet and exercise" instead of "A few people have not been able to lose weight with a well-balanced diet and exercise."
**Use vivid communication, not statistics or jargon.** Stories or examples are often more meaningful than dry statistics or general, nonspecific terms.
**Refer to trustworthy sources.** For example, "the surgeon general" is a more credible source than "some people."
**Base strategies on a knowledge of the audience.** Be aware of the perspectives and preferences of the audience.
**Use aids to highlight key points.** Provide a handout with learning objectives and an outline of the major points.
**Make points explicitly.** Be direct and give clear instructions.
**End strongly.** The last point made is likely to be remembered.

Modified from Babcock DE, Miller MA: *Client education: theory and practice.* St Louis, Mo, 1994, Mosby; Palazzo M: Teaching in crisis: patient and family education in critical care, *Crit Care Nurs Clin North Am* 13(1):83-92, 2001.

**HOW TO** Produce Videotapes for Health Education

Health education videos are a useful strategy for providing education in a low-cost, efficient manner. The following is a list of the steps needed to produce videotapes for health education.

- Determine the need for a health education video on a specific topic.
- Know the target audience and involve them in the planning and production process.
- Develop goals of the educational videotape and know how these goals are going to be measured.
- Identify stakeholders and key personnel who will be involved in the project.
- Develop a budget and find funding.
- Develop a timeline for production.
- Develop the script and information that will be included.
- Make sure that the content is appropriate for the target audience. Consider education levels, cultural background, and age of the target audience.
- Actively involve the production team.
- Plan for the filming of the video.
- Film the video.
- When editing, add narration, music, and graphics.

Modified from Meade CD: Producing videotapes for cancer education: methods and examples, *Patient Educ* 23(5):837-846, 1996.

ucational process, the educator must reassess learners' readiness and be aware of possible barriers to effective communication. Emotional stress and physical illness are only two factors that may limit the amount of information that learners are able to absorb. The nurse educator must be aware of various factors influencing learners and recognize that the needs and barriers influencing learners' receptivity may vary from session to session. Educational strategies and activities can be developed and adjusted to fit the dynamic needs of learners (Babcock and Miller, 1994; Palazzo, 2001).

The educator is responsible for providing information that is understandable (Box 13-3). Medical jargon and technical terms may interfere with the clarity of the intended message (Babcock and Miller, 1994; Palazzo, 2001). For example, in helping clients understand diet control for hypertension, the nurse might use the phrase *high blood pressure* rather than the term *hypertension* to tailor the message to learners' ability to understand.

### Select the Learning Format

The educator must decide how to teach. The educator selects an appropriate learning format, or strategy, for im-

## BOX 13-4  Examples of Learning Formats

**SMALL INFORMAL GROUP**

The client is a group of individuals from a shelter for victims of domestic violence. The format is a short poster session followed by an open discussion.

**HEALTH FAIR**

The client is a group of older adults in a community. The format is a health fair with posters, handouts, demonstrations, and various screenings, such as for cholesterol, osteoporosis, and vision.

**DEMONSTRATION**

The client is a classroom of preschoolers who are being taught various health promotion activities such as personal safety. The learning format is demonstration, return demonstration, and role playing, along with colorful handouts and posters.

**LECTURE**

The client is a large class of university students taking a personal health course that includes topics such as health promotion, exercise, nutrition, safety, sexuality, and substance use. The format is a lecture followed by a question-and-answer period.

**NONNATIVE LANGUAGE SESSIONS**

The client is a group of Hispanic migrant workers who do not speak English well. The learning format chosen for a community-based health promotion session is a brief presentation in Spanish along with handouts in Spanish, followed by individual and family health promotion sessions. After the brief presentation, 20 Spanish-speaking community health nurses are at stations where the migrant workers and their families go to receive family health promotion education that pertains to their specific needs and circumstances.

## BOX 13-5  Environmental Realms

**THE PHYSICAL REALM**

This realm includes setting up the program as well as positioning the presenter and the clients in physical relationship to one another. It includes bathroom facilities, decoration, equipment, furniture, lighting and temperature of the room, seating, ventilation, and volume of amplification equipment. The more subtle effects of the physical environment are those that create a stimulating setting, allow for few external distractions, assist the learner in concentration and attention, and are conducive to interaction.

**THE INTERPERSONAL REALM**

This realm consists of human relationships and should be therapeutic, supportive, and conducive to producing quality educational interactions. The interpersonal dynamic should be one in which learners experience a clear sense that the educator cares about their progress and needs. Learners can also contribute to the interpersonal environment by showing interest in the subject and remaining responsive both to peer and group interactions.

**THE ORGANIZATIONAL REALM**

This realm entails the administrative aspects of the educational program. Beginning with announcements, scheduling, and other preparations, this is the realm that makes the components of the program merge into an effective learning session. Arrangements for delivery of audiovisual materials, ensuring readability of printed or projected materials, ensuring parking, and being responsive to ongoing learner needs and requests are a few examples of organizational aspects of the environment.

Modified from Knowles M: *The adult learner: a neglected species,* ed 4, Houston, Tex, 1990, Gulf; Knowles MS, Holton III EF, Swanson RA: *The adult learner: the definitive classic in adult education and human resource development,* ed 5, Houston, Tex, 1998, Gulf.

plementing the learning program (Box 13-4). A format should be chosen that matches the goals and objectives of the program and should be adapted to meet the learning needs and abilities of the client. When selecting the learning format, consider factors such as the number of participants, their age, education, ethnicity, language, and literacy level. In addition, teaching tools such as printed materials or audiovisual aids that enhance learning should be selected (Babcock and Miller, 1994).

## Create the Best Learning Environment

The environment must be conductive to learning for educational programs to be effective. The nurse begins to establish an appropriate learning climate for an educational event when announcements of the program are made. The tone and appearance of letters, flyers, and media messages announcing the program draw a mental picture for participants of what the activity will be like.

By carefully considering both the program objectives and information about the culture, beliefs, and educational level of learners, the nurse can develop preparatory materials that appeal to the target population (Knowles, 1990). During the program, it is important to create a positive, supportive, and pleasant atmosphere for the client so that learning can be maximized. Three environmental realms that should be considered are described in Box 13-5.

## Organize the Learning Experience

Regardless of the nurse educator's level of knowledge or the quality of the interpersonal relationship that the educator has developed with the learner, sound organization of the material is essential for learning to occur. Materials should be presented in a logical and integrated manner, from simple foundational concepts to more complex ideas. Each concept and idea should represent building blocks in a well-designed structure with a clear and unambiguous blueprint. The educator should reduce difficult or confusing concepts to their component parts and show the learner how to reassemble them one at a time. The pace of the presentation should match the ability of the learner and leave adequate pause for the learner to absorb the material (Knowles, 1990; Palazzo, 2001).

The principles of continuity, sequence, and integration are important aids in the organization of educational programs (Knowles, 1990). A lack of *continuity* causes a break in the flow of logical thought and may confuse the learner. One valuable technique that helps maintain continuity for the learner is repeated emphasis of essential points.

*Sequencing* means that each learning experience builds on the previous one and requires a higher level of functioning. Learning activities should be sequenced so that participants start with simple, easy-to-master exercises or concepts and progress to more complex ones requiring greater skill, coordination, or understanding.

*Integration* of various aspects of the material demonstrates how each component fits into the whole. Without integration, the learner is left with a puzzle of disjointed facts that is difficult to assimilate in a productive way.

## Encourage Participatory Learning

People learn better when they are actively involved in the learning process. Participation increases motivation, flexibility, and learning rate. Participatory learning is not limited to the psychomotor domain. The cognitive and affective domains also call for a teaching strategy in which the nurse enlists the active involvement of the learner. Verbal response or feedback, as long as it engages the learner, is participatory. Merely sitting and listening is not as effective as discussion, even when the presentation is stimulating, interesting, and dynamic. Storytelling, role playing, hands-on training, acting out an experience, and similar activities are good examples of participatory learning. Immediate feedback, an important advantage of participatory learning, ensures that errors are corrected before problematic habits or misconceptions develop. Computer-assisted learning provides immediate feedback to learners (Knowles, 1990).

## THE CUTTING EDGE

Technologic advances in school systems have affected the community health education process. Some schools now have in-school CD-ROM interactive health education programs for children with disease processes such as asthma.

Modified from Yawn BP et al: An in-school CD-ROM asthma education program, *J School Health* 70(4):153-159, 2000.

In each educational situation, nurse educators need to decide whether they will be teachers or facilitators of learning (Table 13-5). According to Knowles et al (1998), teachers have (1) expertise about a topic that is important and can convey it well, (2) empathy for learners and an understanding of their needs and expectations, (3) enthusiasm about a topic (and energy), and (4) clarity; furthermore, they can be understood and followed by most learners, and they provide for learners who may not have comprehended the information being discussed during the initial presentation.

Facilitators of learning help learners identify and resolve the gap between their aspirations and their present level of knowledge and skills by (1) defining life problems that learners experience because of this gap, (2) respecting the worth of learners' feelings and ideas, (3) building relationships of mutual trust and helpfulness among learners, and (4) helping learners exploit their experiences as resources for learning by using strategies such as case analysis, discussion, and role play (Knowles et al, 1998). Facilitators of learning may also assist learners to develop learning contracts because a learning contract engenders more commitment to learning than being a recipient of a learning plan developed by the teacher (Knowles et al, 1998).

### HOW TO  Develop a Learning Contract

- Diagnose learning needs (include the knowledge, attitudes, and skills that the learner would like to obtain).
- Specify personal learning objectives.
- Identify learning resources and strategies.
- Specify evidence of accomplishment and how the evidence will be validated.
- Carry out the contract.
- Evaluate whether learning needs have been met.

Modified from Knowles MS, Holton III EF, Swanson RA: *The adult learner: the definitive classic in adult education and human resource development,* ed 5, Houston, Tex, 1998, Gulf.

The nurse educator can structure learning activities and the environment to facilitate participatory learning. Using proper teaching materials, learners can be provided with adequate prompting and modeling to ensure their ability to practice and to demonstrate mastery of the material. By using the principle of participatory learning, the material becomes more accessible and meaningful to learners and is more likely to be retained and used in the future (Knowles, 1990).

## Provide Evaluation and Feedback

It is essential to evaluate learning and provide constructive and helpful feedback to the learner throughout the educational process to avoid discouraging or offending the

**Table 13-5  Facilitator of Learning, or Teacher?**

| FACILITATOR OF LEARNING | TEACHER |
|---|---|
| Process designer and manager | Content planner and transmitter |
| Skills required include: | Skills required include: |
| • Relationship building | • Organization |
| • Needs assessment | • Excellent presentation abilities |
| • Involving students in planning | • Having a thorough knowledge of the content |
| • Linking students to learning resources | |
| • Encouraging student initiative | |

Modified from Knowles MS, Holton III EF, Swanson RA: *The adult learner: the definitive classic in adult education and human resource development,* ed 5, Houston, Tex, 1998, Gulf; Musinski B: The educator as facilitator: a new kind of leadership, *Nurs Forum* 34(1):23-29, 1999.

learner. Through clear and behaviorally focused feedback, clients can monitor their progress, level of knowledge, and learning needs. The educator may use tools such as quizzes, tests, study sheets, observation of skills, small-group tasks, and competency rating scales to evaluate learning outcomes (Knowles, 1990; Palazzo, 2001).

Not only should learners receive feedback but the educator should also elicit feedback from learners throughout the educational process. On the basis of the feedback that the educator receives from learners, modifications in the implementation and presentation of the educational program can be made (Babcock and Miller, 1994; Knowles, 1990; Palazzo, 2001). The components of the learning situation that the community-oriented nurse needs to evaluate before, during, and after the educational program include the following (Bandura, 1986; Knowles et al, 1998):
- Content
- Instructional objectives
- Principles of learning
- Learners' motivation
- Individual differences
- Educator behavior (beliefs, competency, and expectations)
- Method of instruction
- Teaching–learning process
- Evaluation of learners' behavior

## EDUCATIONAL ISSUES

As they are planning educational programs, nurse educators need to consider three important educational issues. First, different populations of learners require different teaching strategies. Second, nurse educators will need to be prepared to overcome barriers to learning. And third, they need to consider the appropriateness of technological advances in the educational programs that they design.

## Population Considerations

Education is a role of growing importance for the community-oriented nurse. The increase in populations of varying cultural and ethnic backgrounds and the aging of baby boomers requires that community health education cross age and cultural boundaries.

### Populations Based on Age

Children, adults, and older adults have different learning needs and respond to different educational strategies. In each age-group, nurses need to realize that learners vary in three ways (Knowles et al, 1998):
- By cognitive ability, having different innate intellectual abilities
- By personality, needing different amounts of encouragement and support
- By prior knowledge, having previously learned different amounts of information on a health topic

Learning strategies for children and individuals with little knowledge about a health-related topic are characterized as **pedagogy.** Learning strategies for adults, older adults, and individuals with some health-related knowledge about a topic are called **andragogy** (Table 13-6). Each

---

**NURSING TIP**

When planning community health education for children, the community-oriented nurse should address the following:
- What does the child need to learn?
- How can this information be presented so that it builds on existing knowledge and skills?
- What strategies can be used to convey the information?
- How should the new behavior be incorporated into the child's life?
- How can the child's learning be measured?

Modified from Whitener LM, Cox KR, Maglich SA: Use of theory to guide nurses in the design of health messages for children, *Adv Nurs Sci* 20(3):21-35, 1998.

**Table 13-6   Pedagogy Versus Andragogy**

| PEDAGOGY | ANDRAGOGY |
|---|---|
| Learners need to know that they must learn what the instructor teaches. | Learners need to know why they need to learn something before undertaking it. |
| Learners depend on teachers to teach them. | Learners seek self-direction. |
| Learners' experience is of little value as a resource for learning. | Learners have a variety of life experiences that need to be incorporated into learning experiences. |
| Learners need to be ready to learn when the teacher tells them that they are ready. | Learners become ready to learn the things that they need to know in order to cope effectively with real-life situations. |
| Learners have a subject-centered orientation to learning. | Learners have a life-centered or problem-centered orientation to learning. |
| Learners are motivated to learn by external motivators such as grades. | Learners are motivated to learn by intrinsic motivators such as a sense of satisfaction. |

Modified from Knowles MS, Holton III EF, Swanson RA: *The adult learner: the definitive classic in adult education and human resource development,* ed 5, Houston, Tex, 1998, Gulf; Palazzo M: Teaching in crisis: patient and family education in critical care, *Crit Care Nurs Clin North Am* 13(1):83-92, 2001.

model has useful elements (Knowles et al, 1998). For example, when learners are dependent and entering a totally new content area, they may require more pedagogical experiences. In addition to considering the age of the population to be educated, nurses think about the learning needs of the population and use the pedagogical and andragogical principles that will best meet these needs.

When educating children, it is important to provide educational programs that match their developmental abilities. The following age-specific strategies may help the nurse tailor educational programs for children (Whitener, Cox, and Maglich, 1998).

The younger the child, the more concrete the examples and word choices will need to be. For example, the nurse might tell a group of 3-year-old children that brushing their teeth twice a day is good to do. When discussing health promotion activities such as brushing teeth with children who are 10 years old, the nurse might explain to them the benefits of brushing their teeth and the risks of not brushing, and address issues such as the care of their teeth with braces.

When objects can be used, as opposed to discussion of ideas, attention will increase. Additionally, when children can interact with objects being incorporated into the educational experience, learning will be enhanced. For example, when teaching a group of children with asthma how to use inhalers, it is better to hand out inhalers to each participant and have them practice proper technique with the inhalers than it is to give them a handout with instructions or to demonstrate how to use an inhaler while they observe.

Incorporating repetitive health behaviors into games will help children retain knowledge and acquire skills. For example, singing songs while acting out healthy activities such as washing hands before eating helps children get in the habit of washing their hands and makes this health promotion behavior fun.

## Populations Based on Culture

By 2050, approximately 50% of the United States population will consist of ethnic minorities such as Asians, black Americans, Hispanic Americans, Native Americans, and Pacific Islanders. Culture influences family structure and interactions as well as views about health and illness. These demographic changes present new challenges to nurse educators. Nurses must understand the health belief systems of the ethnic populations they serve. They also need to be familiar with populations that are prone to develop certain health problems. Multilinguistic presentations of health education seminars and written materials need to be available to provide culturally competent health education (Go, 1998; Palazzo, 2001).

For example, in a rural area, nurse educators may have a large population of Mexican migrant crop workers in attendance. Knowing that this Spanish-speaking group is more likely to have tuberculosis than other segments of the community, nurses may visit the migrant worker camp to present information on tuberculosis, such as prevention, symptoms, early diagnosis, and treatment. An interpreter may accompany the nurses and provide oral content in Spanish. Written handouts may be in Spanish and designed to be read and understood on a second or third grade reading level.

## Barriers to Learning

Barriers to learning fall into two broad categories—one having to do with the educator and the other having to do with the learner.

### Educator-Related Barriers

Some common educator-related barriers to learning, together with strategies to minimize each barrier, follow (Knowles et al, 1998):

## Evidence-Based Practice

The purpose of this study was to determine whether a 34-minute video for self-instruction in cardiopulmonary resuscitation (CPR) was as effective or more effective than a 4-hour traditional CPR training program in an African-American community. Researchers found the following:

1. Knowledge test scores were comparable.
2. Performance as measured by observers and manikin recordings revealed that 40% of the individuals who used the video self-instruction were competent in their performance, compared to 16% of the individuals in the traditional training class.

**Nurse Use:** Community health nurses need to evaluate whether innovative educational strategies that target specific populations and are cost and time effective yield comparable or better educational results than traditional community-based educational programs.

Modified from Todd KH et al: Simple CPR: a randomized, controlled trial of video self-instructional cardiopulmonary resuscitation training in an African American church congregation, *Ann Emerg Med* 34(6):730-737, 1999.

- Educators may fear public speaking. Strategies to minimize fear include being well prepared, using icebreakers, and acknowledging the fear.
- Educators may think that they are not credible with respect to a certain topic. Strategies to increase confidence include not apologizing for not being an expert, having the attitude of an expert, and sharing personal and professional background.
- Educators may have a limited number of professional experiences related to a health topic. Strategies to deal with this obstacle are to share personal experiences, share experiences of others, and use analogies, illustrations, or examples from movies or famous people.
- Educators may need to deal with difficult people who need to learn health-related information. One strategy that may help with handling difficult learners is to confront the problem learner directly. Other strategies include using humor, using small groups to foster participation of timid people, asking disruptive people to leave, and circumventing dominating behavior, thereby enabling everyone to participate.
- Educators may feel unsure how to elicit participation. Strategies to foster participation include asking open-ended questions, inviting participation, and planning small group activities.
- Educators may be concerned about timing a presentation so that it is not too long and not too short. Strategies to be sure that the length of the presentation is appropriate include planning well and practicing the presentation.

- Educators may feel uncertain about how to adjust instruction. Strategies that can help the educator adjust instruction include knowing the participants' needs, requesting feedback, and redesigning during breaks.
- Educators may be uncomfortable when learners ask questions. Strategies to help include anticipating questions, concisely paraphrasing questions to be sure that the question is correctly understood, and recognizing that it is appropriate to admit when the educator does not know the answer to a question.
- Educators may want to obtain feedback from learners. Strategies to obtain feedback are to solicit informal feedback and to do program evaluations.
- Educators may be concerned about whether media, materials, and facilities will function properly. Strategies include having equipment ready and knowing how it works, having backup plans, obtaining assistance, being prepared, visiting the facility in advance, and arriving early.
- Educators may have difficulty with openings and closings. Strategies to foster successful openings and closings include developing a repertoire of openings and closings, memorizing the opening and closing, relaxing learners, concisely summarizing information, and thanking participants.
- Educators may be overly dependent on notes. Strategies to help include using note cards or visual aids as prompts, and practicing.

## Learner-Related Barriers

Two of the most important learner-related barriers are low literacy and lack of motivation to learn information and make needed behavioral changes.

### Low Literacy Levels

Nurses often deal with individuals and populations exhibiting illiteracy or low-literacy levels. People who are functionally illiterate are often embarrassed to admit this to health care providers and educators. They may not ask questions to clarify information and may have problems understanding health education materials (Baker et al, 1996).

The 1992 National Adult Literacy Survey, the largest literacy assessment study that has been done in the United States, showed that 23%, or 40 to 44 million adult Americans, are at the lowest literacy level (level 1), and that 27% were in the next literacy level (level 2). This means that 50% of Americans fell into the two lowest levels of literacy; the other 50% of Americans fell into the top three levels of literacy (levels 3, 4, and 5). Level 3 proficiency is the minimal standard needed to function in the workplace. This survey, now called the National Assessment of Adult Literacy, was repeated in 2002 and is expected to provide more current information (National Assessment of Adult Literacy, 2002; National Institute for Literacy, 2002; National Work Group on Literacy and Health, 1998).

It is currently recommended that health education materials be written at the eighth grade level or lower. Various

**Evidence-Based Practice**

The purpose of this study was to evaluate whether an interactive multimedia module for adults with limited literacy and without computer skills would be effective in assisting individuals with cancer to deal with fatigue. The module consisted of five units: using the computer; fatigue; saving, maintaining, and restoring energy; managing stress; and sleeping better. Findings revealed the following:

1. The individuals who used the interactive multimedia module had significantly greater improvement than individuals who did not use the module.
2. Of the individuals who used the interactive multimedia module, 94% liked the program very much, quite a lot, or some. The 6% who either did not like using the module at all or who liked using it a little had the greatest computer experience and the highest literacy and educational levels of the individuals in the study.
3. Of the individuals who used the interactive multimedia module, 92% found the program easy to use.

**Nurse Use:** Even when clients have limited literacy and little to no computer skills, nurses may successfully incorporate interactive multimedia methods in their population-based educational programs.

Modified from Wydra EW: The effectiveness of a self-care management interactive multimedia module, *Oncol Nurs Forum* 28(9):1399-1407, 2001.

screening devices such as the Rapid Estimate of Adult Literacy in Medicine, the Test of Functional Health Literacy, the Wide Range Achievement Test-3, and the Cloze procedure can be used to determine populations likely to have limited reading ability. When the nurse educates these populations, educational strategies such as videotapes can be selected (Davis et al, 1998; National Work Group on Literacy and Health, 1998).

Nurse educators may incorporate pictures, slide and video presentations, and models in educating clients with low literacy, but they still need to focus on individual learning capacity. It is important to understand the knowledge and beliefs of their clients with low literacy and tailor educational programs to the needs of these individuals. Often, a series of educational sessions are needed. At the first session, learning capacity is identified and a small amount of foundational information is provided. During subsequent sessions, new information that builds on existing knowledge and skills is provided and evaluated. Additional information is not provided until the nurse is sure that knowledge and skills are understood and are being incorporated into learners' lives (Davis et al, 2002; Marwick, 1997; Perdue, Degazon, and Lunney, 1999). This person-centered approach to community health education ultimately can decrease health care costs. It is estimated that the cost of health care for individuals with low literacy who do not receive health education that enables them to make behavioral changes is almost twice the cost of those who do (Marwick, 1997).

### Lack of Motivation

Often nurses find that their clients lack motivation to make behavioral changes; therefore they need to understand the importance of motivating clients whom they seek to educate. Motivation is influenced by three factors (Dembo, 1994):

- The value component (Why am I learning this?)
- The expectancy component (Can I do this?)
- The affective component (How do I feel about this?)

*Learned helplessness* occurs when individuals experience that over time they cannot control the outcome of events affecting their lives; there is no relation between effort and attainment of goals. *Self-efficacy* is individuals' evaluation of their performance capabilities related to a particular type of task (Driscoll, 1994). Motivation occurs when goal-directed behavior is initiated and sustained. Learners' beliefs about themselves in relation to task difficulty and outcome are important and influence self-efficacy. Strategies to increase motivation and self-efficacy include the following (Driscoll, 1994):

- *Enhance relevance.* The educator should explain how instruction relates to learners' goals and should build on learners' previous experiences.
- *Build confidence.* The educator should create positive expectations for success, provide opportunities for learners to successfully attain goals, and offer learners control over their learning.
- *Generate satisfaction.* The educator should provide learners with opportunities to use newly acquired skills and should provide them with positive feedback.

## Technological Issues

To facilitate health-related learning, nurses may use a variety of technologies, such as computer games and programs (de Vries and Brug, 1999; Dorman, 1997; Lewis, 1999; Lieberman, 2001; Yawn et al, 2000), the internet (Ferguson, 1997; Lewis, 1999), and videos (Dorman, 1997; Meade, 1996). These technologies may enable the learner to control the pace of instruction, offer flexibility in the time and

**DID YOU KNOW?**

Did you know that some physicians are now using e-mail as a primary means of client–provider contact?

Modified from Kane B, Sands DZ: Guidelines for the clinical use of electronic mail with patients, *J Am Med Inform Assoc* 5(1):104-111, 1998.

**WHAT DO YOU THINK?**

What do you think about the use of computer and video games to teach health education information to children?

**WHAT DO YOU THINK?**

What do you think about the quality of health-related information that clients may access from the internet?

location of learning, are engaging, and provide immediate feedback. Also, a computerized programmed instruction can be tailored to meet the needs of specific populations. Complex branching sequences and automatic record-keeping of learners' progress and responses can individualize learning (de Vries and Brug, 1999; Driscoll, 1994).

Many people have access to the internet and the World Wide Web, and this enables them to obtain a wealth of health education information (Ferguson, 1997). However, questions about the long-term behavioral effects that computer-based health education has on various populations have yet to be answered (Lewis, 1999). Clients may ask nurses to provide them with information regarding strategies to evaluate the quality and reliability of this information. The Agency for Health Care Research and Quality has suggested the following criteria for assessing the quality of internet health information (*Assessing the Quality of Internet Information,* 1999; Kotecki and Chamness, 1999; Silberg, Lundberg, and Musacchio, 1997):

* *Authorship.* Are the authors and contributors, as well as their credentials and affiliations, listed?
* *Caveats.* Does the site clarify whether its function is to provide information or to market products?
* *Content.* Is the information accurate and complete, and is an appropriate disclaimer provided?
* *Credibility.* Does the site include the source, currency, relevance, and editorial review process for the information?
* *Currency.* Are dates that the content was posted and updated listed?
* *Design.* Is the site accessible, capable of internal searches, easy to navigate, and logically organized?
* *Disclosure.* Is the user informed about the purpose of the site and about any profiling or collection of information associated with using the site?
* *Interactivity.* Does the site include feedback mechanisms and opportunities for users to exchange information?
* *Links.* Have the links been evaluated according to back linkages, content, and selection?

**DID YOU KNOW?**

Did you know that every year millions of Americans seek health information on the World Wide Web instead of contacting their health care provider?

Modified from Ferguson T: Health care in cyberspace: patients lead a revolution, *Futurist* Nov/Dec:29-33, 1997.

## THE EDUCATIONAL PROCESS

In addition to understanding philosophical perspectives of learning, theories of learning, the nature of learning, the events of instruction, strategies for effective education, and educational issues, knowledge of the educational process is essential for the community-oriented nurse. The five steps of the educational process (identify educational needs, establish educational goals and objectives, select appropriate educational methods, implement the educational plan, and evaluate the educational process) are discussed next.

### Identify Educational Needs

Nurses learn about the health education needs of their clients by performing a systematic and thorough needs assessment (Bartholomew et al, 2000), the steps of which are listed in Box 13-6. Once needs have been identified, they are prioritized so that the most critical educational needs are met first (Wolf, 2001).

A variety of factors influence clients' learning needs and their ability to learn. Demographic, physical, geographic, economic, psychological, social, and spiritual characteristics of learners should be considered when identifying learning needs (Babcock and Miller, 1994; Bartholomew et al, 2000). The educator must also understand how the learner's existing knowledge, skills, and motivation influence learning. Resources for and barriers to learning should be identified. Resources include printed materials, equipment, agencies, and other individuals. Barriers include lack of time, money, space, energy, confidence, and organizational support (Rankin and Stallings, 1996). Communication barriers may result from cultural and language differences between the nurse and the client or from printed materials that are inappropriate to the client's reading level (Babcock and Miller, 1994). Such adverse influences on the learning process can be minimized with a vigilant awareness of both initial and newly developing barriers during the educational process.

**NURSING TIP**

Consider the target audience carefully when developing a community health education project. Determine educational needs, educational and literacy levels, cultural backgrounds, and health beliefs.

### Establish Educational Goals and Objectives

Once learner needs are determined, goals and objectives to guide the educational program must be identified. Goals are broad, long-term expected outcomes such as, "Mr. Williams will become independently proficient in the care of his ostomy bag within 3 months." Goals of the program should directly address the client's overall learning needs (Knowles et al, 1998; Rankin and Stallings, 1996; Wolf, 2001).

Objectives are specific, short-term criteria that need to be met as steps toward achieving the long-term goal such as, "Within 2 weeks, Mr. Williams will properly reattach his own ostomy bag, after the nurse has cleaned the site, five consecutive times." Objectives are written statements of an intended outcome or expected change in behavior and should define the minimum degree of knowledge or ability needed by a client. Objectives must be stated clearly and defined in measurable terms (Bartholomew et al, 2000; Dembo, 1994; Knowles et al, 1998; Rankin and Stallings, 1996; Wolf, 2001). The four elements of an objective are listed in Table 13-7.

## Select Appropriate Educational Methods

Educational methods should be chosen to facilitate the efficient and successful accomplishment of program goals and objectives. The methods should also be appropriately matched to the client's strengths and needs. Caution should be used to avoid complex methodological designs. The educator should choose the simplest, clearest, and most succinct manner of presentation. The educator should be proficient in using a broad array of tools designed to convey information (Knowles, 1990). A few examples of strategies that may be used to enhance learning are listed in Box 13-7.

Educators need to implement various strategies for different learning orientations—for example, activity-oriented

learners enjoy participation, goal-oriented learners want to achieve a specific outcome, and learning-oriented learners enjoy learning new things (Knowles et al, 1998). Matching media and other tools to the needs of the learner is an important skill for educators to develop. Educators also need to be able to administer examinations, deliver presentations, lead group discussions, organize role plays, provide feedback to learners, share case studies, and use media and materials. Benefits of group teaching include cohesiveness among members, increased number of clients seen, clients' learning from each other, and cost effectiveness. Educational methods include structuring content, organizing instructional sequence, planning for the rate of delivery, identifying how much repetition is needed, practicing, evaluating the results, and providing reinforcement and rewards (Babcock and Miller, 1994; Knowles et al, 1998) (Box 13-8).

### NURSING TIP

When developing a health education presentation, use assorted methods and involve the audience.

When nurses select educational methods, they should consider age, developmental disabilities, educational level, knowledge of the subject, and size of the group. For example, clients with a visual impairment may need more verbal description. Clients with hearing impairments may need increased visual material, and speakers or translators who can use sign language may be necessary. Also, limitations in attention and concentration require creative methods and tools for keeping the learner focused. Such methods and tools include frequent breaks; austere, nondistractive surroundings; small-group interactions

## THE CUTTING EDGE

To individualize learning, the educator may opt to implement a personalized system of instruction in which material is broken up into units or modules, each with a set of behavioral objectives specifying what is to be learned in that unit. The emphases of this personalized system of instructions are on (1) individual study, (2) self-pacing, (3) unit mastery requirement, (4) use of proctors, and (5) supplementary instructional techniques.

Modified from de Vries H, Brug J: Computer-tailored interventions motivating people to adopt health promoting behaviours: introduction to a new approach, *Patient Educ Couns* 36:99-105, 1999; Knowles MS, Holton III EF, Swanson RA: *The adult learner: the definitive classic in adult education and human resource development,* ed 5, Houston, Tex, 1998, Gulf.

## Table 13-7   The Four Elements of an Objective*

| ELEMENT | EXAMPLE |
| --- | --- |
| Who is expected to exhibit the behavior? | (a) Ms. Smith<br>(b) Each member of the Jones family<br>(c) 80% of the target population |
| What behavior is expected? | (a) will do breast self-examinations<br>(b) will give an insulin injection to Billy<br>(c) will take their children to receive immunizations |
| Conditions and qualifiers of the behavior | (a) correctly on the same day each month<br>(b) with accuracy regarding the dosage and procedure<br>(c) within 1 month of the immunization due date |
| Standards of the behavior or performance | (a) 100% of the time for 1 year<br>(b) 100% of the time for 10 consecutive trials<br>(c) for 100% of the standard childhood disease immunizations |

Modified from Babcock DE, Miller MA: *Client education: theory and practice,* St Louis, Mo, 1994, Mosby; Bartholomew LK et al: Watch, discover, think, and act: a model for patient education program development, *Patient Educ Couns* 39:253-268, 2000.

*Instructions: String all "a" phrases together to make one sentence for the first example. String all "b" together for the second example, and all "c" phrases for the third.

### BOX 13-7   Strategies to Enhance Learning

- Audiovisual materials
- Brainstorming
- Case studies
- Computer-assisted learning
- Demonstrations
- Field trips
- Games
- Group participation
- Guest speakers
- Peer counseling and tutoring
- Peer presentations
- Printed materials
- Role plays
- Simulation

Modified from Dobbins KR: Applying learning theories to develop teaching strategies for the critical care nurse: don't limit yourself to the formal classroom lecture, *Crit Care Nurs Clin North Am* 13(1):1-11, 2001; Johnson PH, Kittleson MJ: A content analysis of health education teaching strategy/idea articles: 1970-1998, *J Health Educ* 31(5):282-298, 2000; Knowles M: *The adult learner: a neglected species,* ed 4, Houston, Tex, 1990, Gulf.

### BOX 13-8   How to Effectively TEACH Clients

Use the TEACH mneumonic:
**Tune in.** Listen before you start teaching. Client's needs should direct the content.
**Edit information.** Teach necessary information first. Be specific.
**Act on each teaching moment.** Teach whenever possible. Develop a good relationship.
**Clarify often.** Make sure your assumptions are correct. Seek feedback.
**Honor the client as a partner.** Build on the client's experience. Share responsibility with the client.

Modified from Hansen M, Fisher J: Patient-centered teaching from theory to practice, *Am J Nurs* 98(1):56-60, 1998.

that keep the learner involved and interested; and the use of hands-on equipment such as mannequins, models, and other materials that the learner can physically manipulate. Comprehension and retention are related to the depth or intensity of the learner's involvement (Knowles, 1990).

The educator tries to involve the learner appropriately and creatively in a variety of ways and as actively as possible. Educational programs that are interactive are more effective than those that are noninteractive. Interactive strategies include discussion, games, and role playing. Noninteractive strategies include demonstrations, films, and lectures (Knowles, 1990).

## Implement the Educational Plan

Once educational methods have been selected, they should be implemented through management of the educational process. Implementation entails the following (Knowles, 1990):

- Control over starting, sustaining, and stopping each method and strategy in the most effective and appropriate time and manner
- Coordination and control of environmental factors, the flow of the presentation, and other contributory facets of the program
- Keeping the materials logically related to the core theme and overall program goals

Additionally, administrative and political support is essential to successful program implementation (Edelman and Fain, 1998).

Educators must be flexible. They must modify educational methods and strategies to meet unexpected challenges that may confront both the educator and the learner. External influences such as time limitations, expense, administrative and political factors, and learner needs require an ongoing evaluation of their impact on the educational program (Babcock and Miller, 1994; Knowles, 1990). Thus implementation is a dynamic element in the educational process.

## Evaluate the Educational Process

Evaluation is as important in the educational process as it is in the nursing process. Evaluation provides a systematic and logical method for making decisions to improve the educational program (Babcock and Miller, 1994). Educational evaluation involves three areas:

- Educator evaluation
- Process evaluation
- Product evaluation

Educator and process evaluation are described next. Product evaluation is described later, under The Educational Product.

### Educator Evaluation

Feedback to the educator allows modifications in the teaching process and enables the nurse to better meet the learner's needs. The learner's evaluation of the educator occurs continuously throughout the educational program. The educator may receive feedback from the learner in written form, such as an evaluation sheet. The educator may also receive feedback verbally or nonverbally, as in return demonstrations and by facial expressions (Babcock and Miller, 1994; Knowles, 1990; Palazz, 2001).

The educator should assume that inadequate learner responses reflect an inadequate program, not an inadequate learner. If evaluation reveals that the learning objectives are not being met, the nurse must determine why the instruction is not effective. It is then that the educator must take the responsibility to present the material creatively and meaningfully in new ways that will increase learner re-

tention and the learner's ability to apply the new knowledge (Knowles, 1990). Ultimately, the educator must assume responsibility for the success or failure of the educational process and the development of learner knowledge, skills, and abilities.

### Process Evaluation

Process evaluation examines the dynamic components of the educational program. It follows and assesses the movements and management of information transfer and attempts to keep the objectives on track. Process evaluation is necessary *throughout* the educational program to determine whether goals and objectives are being met and the time required for their accomplishment. Ongoing evaluation also allows the teacher to correct misinformation, misinterpretation, or confusion (Babcock and Miller, 1994; Palazz, 2001).

Goals and objectives should also be periodically reconsidered. The nurse must ask if the desired health behavior change is really necessary. Such a question inevitably leads back to the original learning objectives and enables the nurse to rethink the practicality and merit of each of the objectives. Finally, factors that influence learner readiness and motivation should be reassessed if teaching seems to be ineffective. Process evaluation uses information gathered from the educator as well as from learner evaluations and assesses the dynamics of their interactions (Knowles, 1990).

## THE EDUCATIONAL PRODUCT

The educational product is the outcome of the educational process. The product is measured both qualitatively and quantitatively (Krathwohl et al, 1964). For example, a qualitative assessment should answer the question, "How well does the learner appear to understand the content?" A quantitative assessment should answer the question, "How much of the content does the learner retain?" Thus the quality of the product is measured by improvement and increase, or the lack thereof, in the learner's knowledge, skills, and abilities related to the content of the educational program. Selected outcomes for the population of interest need to be identified when the educational program is conceived. Measurement of changes in these outcomes determines the effectiveness of the program (Babcock and Miller, 1994). In community-oriented nursing, the educational product is assessed as a measurable change in the health or behavior of the client.

## Evaluation of Health and Behavioral Changes

A variety of approaches, methods, and tools can be used to evaluate health and behavioral changes. These include questionnaires, rating scales, surveys, checklists, skills demonstrations, testing, subjective client feedback, and direct observation of improvements in client mastery of materials (Babcock and Miller, 1994). Qualitative or quantitative strategies may be used, depending on the nature of the expected educational outcome. Evaluation of outcomes measured includes changes in knowledge, skills, abilities, attitudes, behavior, health status, and quality of life (Krathwohl et al, 1964). Approaches to evaluating health education effects will vary, depending on the situation (Babcock and Miller, 1994). For example, when considering a client's ability to perform a psychomotor skill, such as changing a dressing, viewing the actual performance of the skill is the most appropriate means of evaluation.

If evaluation of the educational product shows positive changes in health status and health-related behaviors, the educator can expect good results in similar health educational programs. If evaluation of the educational product shows that either no changes or negative changes in health status and health-related behaviors resulted, then various components of the educational process can be examined and modified to produce better results in the future (Babcock and Miller, 1994).

## Short-Term Evaluation

It is important to evaluate short-term health and behavioral effects of health education programs and to determine if they are really caused by the educational program. Short-term objectives are often easy to evaluate (Babcock and Miller, 1994). For example, a **short-term evaluation** of whether a client can perform a return demonstration of breast self-examination requires minimal energy, expense, or time; skill mastery can be determined within a matter of minutes. If the short-term objective is not met, the nurse determines why and identifies possible solutions so that successful learning can occur. If the short-term objective is met, the nurse can then focus on long-term evaluation designed to assess the lasting effects of the education program—in this case, that of ongoing monthly breast self-examinations performed by the learner independently at home.

## Long-Term Evaluation

The ultimate goal of health education is to help clients make lasting behavioral changes that will improve their overall health status (Babcock and Miller, 1994). Long-term follow-up with clients is a challenging task. When clients make positive behavioral changes and their health status improves, they may no longer require the health care services of the nurse. Other reasons long-term evaluation can be challenging are listed in Box 13-9.

**Long-term evaluation** is geared toward following and assessing the status of an individual, family, community, or population over time. The tools of evaluation are designed to assess whether specific goals and objectives were met. Also, the extent and direction of changes in health status and health behaviors that the client has experienced are monitored (Babcock and Miller, 1994; Kleinpell and Mick, 2001).

Often, for community-oriented nurse educators, the goal of long-term evaluation is an analysis of the effectiveness of the education program for the entire community, not the health status of a specific individual client. Nurses track the achievement of community objectives over time but not that of the individual community members. Thus,

---

**BOX 13-9 Long-Term Evaluation Is Challenging**

**COOPERATION**
Clients may show a lack of interest in their own health care.
Clients may think that it is too time consuming or expensive to follow up.
Clients may not keep scheduled appointments or return phone calls.

**TIME**
Follow-up requires the educator to keep track of clients and to locate those who have moved.
Follow-up requires making phone calls, evaluating clients, and reviewing and analyzing the results of the evaluation.

**ENERGY**
The nurse must obtain the cooperation of clients.
The nurse must balance long-term evaluation responsibilities with other demands.

**EXPENSE**
Mail, phone calls, staff time, and travel are expenses related to long-term evaluation.

Modified from Kleinpell RM, Mick DJ: Evaluating outcomes. In Fulmer TT, Foreman MD, Walker M, editors: *Critical care nursing of the elderly*, ed 2, pp 179-196, New York, 2001, Springer; Redman BK: Patient education at 25 years: where we have been and where we are going, *J Adv Nurs* 18(5):725, 1993.

---

in a changing population, long-term evaluation of the results of an education program is still possible. The percentage of objectives and goals met by sampling the target population gives valid statistics for program assessment, even though the population of individuals may have experienced a complete turnover (Kleinpell and Mick, 2001).

For example, a nurse notes that according to annual health department data, 60% of all pregnant women in the nurse's catchment area received some prenatal care. Wanting to increase this percentage to 100%, the nurse tries an educational intervention in which radio and television stations make public service announcements about the importance and availability of prenatal services.

After 1 year, the nurse discovers that 80% of all pregnant women now receive prenatal care. The nurse continues to use public service announcements the following year because good results are evident. However, the long-term goal of the education program to influence the behavior of 100% of the pregnant women in the community has not yet been met. Therefore the nurse also enlists volunteers to put informational posters in shopping malls, grocery stores, public transportation stops, laundries, and public transportation vehicles. The second year after implementing the revised educational program, again using the statistics from the health department, the nurse finds that 95% of all pregnant women in the target area now receive prenatal care. The nurse can thus evaluate and modify a community educational program over time to increase the rate, range, and consistency of progress made toward meeting the long-term goals of the project.

## Practice Application

Kristi is working toward her B.S.N. degree in a community health practicum at a local health department. The health department has been receiving numerous calls from people wanting information about anthrax, smallpox, and other potential weapons of biological warfare. For Kristi's community health intervention project, she decides to do a community educative piece on this topic. What is her best course of action?

A. Develop a poster presentation to have on display at the health department.

B. Put together an educative pamphlet to mail to anyone calling with questions.

C. Work with the health department staff to develop a community forum–style presentation and information brochures on biological warfare weapons.

D. Develop an inservice program for health department staff on potential weapons of biological warfare, so that they can provide accurate information to callers.

**Answer is in the back of the book.**

## Key Points

- Health education is a vital component of community-oriented nursing, because the promotion, maintenance, and restoration of health rely on clients' understanding of health care topics.
- The community-oriented nurse educator identifies a learning need, decides which philosophical perspectives are appropriate, selects aspects from the theories of learning, considers educational principles, examines educational issues, designs and implements an educational program, and evaluates the effects of the educational program on learning and behavior.
- The nurse often uses the Healthy People 2010 educational objectives as a guide to identifying community-based learning needs.
- Education and learning are different. Education is the establishment and arrangement of events to facilitate learning. Learning is the process of gaining knowledge and expertise and results in behavioral changes.
- The three philosophical perspectives that frame the way that community-oriented nurses view learning are empiricism, interpretivism, and pragmatism.
- Six important theories of learning are used to guide the practice of the nurse educator. They are behavioral, cognitive, critical, developmental, humanistic, and social learning.
- Three domains of learning are cognitive, affective, and psychomotor. Depending on the needs of the

learner, one or more of these domains may be important for the nurse educator to consider as learning programs are developed.

- Nine principles associated with instruction are gaining attention, informing the learner of the objectives of instruction, stimulating recall of prior learning, presenting the stimulus, providing learning guidance, eliciting performance, providing feedback, assessing performance, and enhancing retention and transfer of knowledge.
- Principles that guide the effective educator include message, format, environment, experience, participation, and evaluation.
- Educational issues include population considerations, barriers to learning, and technologic issues.
- The five phases of the educational process are identifying educational needs, establishing educational goals and objectives, selecting appropriate educational methods, implementing the educational plan, and evaluating the educational process and product.
- Evaluation of the product includes the measurement of short-term and long-term goals and objectives related to improving health and promoting behavioral changes.

## Clinical Decision-Making Activities

1. Review the theories of learning summarized in the chapter. Decide which one would most effectively fit the learning needs of a population of Hispanic Americans recently diagnosed with diabetes mellitus, a community in which adolescent cigarette smoking is on the rise, and families caring for an individual with Alzheimer's disease. What different choices would you use for each population?

2. Recall an educational interaction that you had with each type of client (individual, family, community, and population) that did not seem to go well. For each type of client, and on the basis of educational principles, identify what might have been the problem. Develop a plan for ways in which the interaction could have been improved, again on the basis of educational principles.

3. Recall a learning experience in which either the message, format, environment, experience, participation, or evaluation was unsatisfactory. Then develop a plan for how the problem could have been overcome and turned from a negative or neutral learning situation into a positive one.

4. Review the phases of the educational process. Apply this process to a population of individuals with hypertension, a community in which tuberculosis is on the rise, and families with a child who has attention deficit disorder.

5. Select one of the Healthy People 2010 educational objectives and design a population-specific education

program to meet that objective. Include the philosophical perspective, learning theory, educational principles, educational issues, educational process including teaching strategies, and evaluation procedures that you would use.

# References

American Nurses Association: *Code for nurses,* Kansas City, Mo, 1985, ANA.

American Nurses Association: *Code of ethics for nurses with interpretive statements,* Washington, DC, 2001, ANA.

*Assessing the Quality of Internet Information:* Retrieved 06/99 from http://www.ahcpr.gov/data/infoqual.htm.

Babcock DE, Miller MA: *Client education: theory and practice,* St Louis, Mo, 1994, Mosby.

Baker DW et al: The health care experience of patients with low literacy, *Arch Family Med* 5:329-334, 1996.

Bandura A: *Social foundations of thought and action: a social cognitive theory,* Englewood Cliffs, NJ, 1986, Prentice Hall.

Bartholomew LK et al: Watch, discover, think, and act: a model for patient education program development, *Patient Educ Couns* 39:253-268, 2000.

Bloom BS et al: *Taxonomy of educational objectives: the classification of educational goals—handbook 1: cognitive domain,* White Plains, NY, 1956, Longman.

Davis TC et al: Practical assessment of adult literacy in health care, *Health Educ Behav* 25(5):613-624, 1998.

Davis TC et al: Health literacy and cancer communication, *Cancer* 52(3):134-153, 2002.

Dembo MH: *Applying educational psychology,* ed 5, White Plains, NY, 1994, Longman.

de Vries H, Brug J: Computer-tailored interventions motivating people to adopt health promoting behaviours: introduction to a new approach, *Patient Educ Couns* 36:99-105, 1999.

Dobbins KR: Applying learning theories to develop teaching strategies for the critical care nurse: don't limit yourself to the formal classroom lecture, *Crit Care Nurs Clin North Am* 13(1):1-11, 2001.

Dorman SM: Video and computer games: effect on children and implications for health education, *J School Health* 67(4):133-138, 1997.

Driscoll MP: *Psychology of learning for instruction,* Boston, 1994, Allyn and Bacon.

Edelman CL, Fain JA: Health defined: objectives for promotion and prevention. In Edelman CL, Mandle CL, editors: *Health promotion throughout the lifespan,* ed 4, pp 3-24, St Louis, Mo, 1998, Mosby.

Ferguson T: Health care in cyberspace: patients lead a revolution, *Futurist* Nov/Dec:29-33, 1997.

Go GV: Changing populations and health. In Edelman CL, Mandle CL, editors: *Health promotion throughout the lifespan,* ed 4, pp 25-48, St Louis, Mo, 1998, Mosby.

Hansen M, Fisher J: Patient-centered teaching from theory to practice, *Am J Nurs* 98(1):56-60, 1998.

*Healthy people 2010:* Online documents retrieved 01-30-01 from http://www.health.gov/healthypeople/document/tableofcontents.htm.

Hooper JI: Health education. In Edelman CL, Mandle CL, editors: *Health promotion throughout the lifespan,* ed 4, pp 222-242, St Louis, Mo, 1998, Mosby.

Johnson PH, Kittleson MJ: A content analysis of health education teaching strategy/idea articles: 1970-1998, *J Health Educ* 31(5):282-298, 2000.

Kane B, Sands DZ: Guidelines for the clinical use of electronic mail with patients, *J Am Med Inform Assoc* 5(1):104-111, 1998.

Kelemen A: Wellness promotion: how to plan a college health fair, *Am J Health Studies* 17(1):31-36, 2001.

Kleinpell RM, Mick DJ: Evaluating outcomes. In Fulmer TT, Foreman MD, Walker M, editors: *Critical care nursing of the elderly,* ed 2, pp 179-196, New York, 2001, Springer.

Knowles M: *The adult learner: a neglected species,* ed 4, Houston, Tex, 1990, Gulf.

Knowles MS, Holton III EF, Swanson RA: *The adult learner: the definitive classic in adult education and human resource development,* ed 5, Houston, Tex, 1998, Gulf.

Kotecki JE, Chamness BE: A valid tool for evaluating health-related www sites, *J Health Educ* 30(1):56-59, 1999.

Krathwohl DR, Bloom BS, Masia BB: *Taxonomy of educational objectives: the classification of educational goals—handbook 2: affective domain,* New York, 1964, David McKay.

Lewis D: Computer-based approaches to patient education: a review of the literature, *J Am Med Inform Assoc* 6(4):272-282, 1999.

Lieberman DA: Management of chronic pediatric diseases with interactive health games: theory and research findings, *J Ambul Care Manage* 24(1):26-38, 2001.

Lyman S, Benedik JR: Health fairs: timetable, pitfalls, & burnout, *College Student J* 33(4):534, 1999.

Marwick C: Patients' lack of literacy may contribute to billions of dollars in higher hospital costs, *JAMA* 278(12):971-972, 1997.

Meade CD: Producing videotapes for cancer education: methods and examples, *Patient Educ* 23(5):837-846, 1996.

Musinski B: The educator as facilitator: a new kind of leadership, *Nurs Forum* 34(1):23-29, 1999.

*National Assessment of Adult Literacy:* Retrieved Nov 27, 2002 from http://www.negp. gov/NEGP/issues/publication/othpress/nalsdr.htm.

*National Institute for Literacy:* Retrieved Nov 27, 2002 from http://www.nifl.gov.

National Work Group on Literacy and Health: Communicating with patients who have limited literacy skills: report of the National Work Group on Literacy and Health, *J Family Pract* 46(2):168-175, 1998.

Palazzo M: Teaching in crisis: patient and family education in critical care, *Crit Care Nurs Clin North Am* 13(1): 83-92, 2001.

Perdue BJ, Degazon C, Lunney M: Case study: diagnoses and interventions with low literacy, *Nurs Diagn* 10(1):4, 1999.

Rankin SH, Stallings KD: *Patient education: issues, principles, and practices,* ed 3, New York, 1996, Lippincott.

Redman BK: Patient education at 25 years: where we have been and where we are going, *J Adv Nurs* 18(5):725, 1993.

Silberg WM, Lundberg GD, Musacchio RA: Assessing, controlling, and assuring the quality of medical information on the internet: let the reader and viewer beware, *JAMA* 277(15):1244-1245, 1997.

Slutsky P, Stephens TB: Developing a comprehensive, community-based asthma education and training program, *Pediatr Nurs* 27(5):449, 2001.

Stopka TJ, Chapman D, Perez-Escamilla R: An innovative community-based approach to encourage breastfeeding among Hispanic/Latino women, *J Am Diet Assoc* 102(6):766-767, 2002.

Todd KH et al: Simple CPR: a randomized, controlled trial of video self-instructional cardiopulmonary resuscitation training in an African American church congregation, *Ann Emerg Med* 34(6):730-737, 1999.

U.S. Department of Health and Human Services: *Healthy people 2010: understanding and improving health,* ed 2, Washington, DC, 2000, U.S. Government Printing Office.

Whitener LM, Cox KR, Maglich SA: Use of theory to guide nurses in the design of health messages for children, *Adv Nurs Sci* 20(3):21-35, 1998.

Wolf MS: Patient education. In Fulmer TT, Foreman MD, Walker M, editors: *Critical care nursing of the elderly,* ed 2, pp 162-178, New York, 2001, Springer.

Wydra EW: The effectiveness of a self-care management interactive multimedia module, *Oncol Nurs Forum* 28(9):1399-1407, 2001.

Yawn BP et al: An in-school CD-ROM asthma education program, *J School Health* 70(4):153-159, 2000.

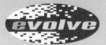
# Integrating Multilevel Approaches to Promote Community Health

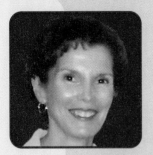

**Pamela A. Kulbok, R.N., D.N.Sc.**

Pamela A. Kulbok received her doctorate at Boston University and did postdoctoral work in psychiatric epidemiology at Washington University in St. Louis. She was a member of the U.S. Navy Nurse Corps, has worked in a visiting nurse service, and has been the director of a hospital-based home health agency. She is presently at the University of Virginia, where she is developing community-based participatory research to explore protective factors for youth nonsmoking. She has taught undergraduate and graduate courses in community/public health nursing, health promotion research, and nursing knowledge development. Dr. Kulbok has been active in the leadership of community and public health nursing professional organizations and is currently president-elect of the Association of Community Health Nursing Educators.

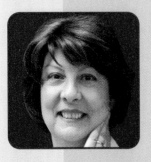

**Shirley Cloutier Laffrey, Ph.D., M.P.H., A.P.R.N., B.C.**

Shirley Cloutier Laffrey is an associate professor of public health nursing at the School of Nursing at the University of Texas at Austin. Dr. Laffrey's research has been in the area of how people visualize their health and what they do to be healthy. She has a particular interest in exercise and physical activity among older people. Her current research is an exercise intervention study with Mexican-American women.

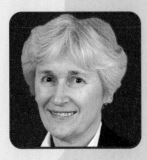

**Jean Goeppinger, Ph.D., R.N. F.A.A.N.**

Jean Goeppinger began her work in the community as a home-health nurse with the Visiting Nurse Association of Detroit. This work also provided an opportunity to work with an underserved and vulnerable inner-city African-American community. Since then, she has developed community-oriented nursing programs and courses and conducted research designed to improve the self-care abilities of community residents with chronic disease.

## Objectives

After reading this chapter, the student should be able to do the following:

1. Contrast the health paradigm and the pathogenic paradigm as the basis for health promotion, illness prevention, and illness care interventions.
2. Analyze the interrelationships of individual, family, aggregate, and community as the targets of health promotion strategies
3. Evaluate the methods used to assess the health risks of individuals, families, aggregates, and community groups
4. Analyze community-oriented nursing roles that are essential to health promotion, illness prevention, and illness care

Encouraging the pursuit of healthy **lifestyles** and participation in population-focused health programs is essential to achieve the national health objectives outlined in Healthy People 2010 (U.S. Department of Health and Human Services, 2000). Interest in healthy lifestyles is reflected in the scientific evidence linking lifestyle and health, as well as in the emphasis on public health programs for at-risk populations. People in many countries recognize the need to exercise regularly, maintain their weight at recommended levels, and manage stress in their lives. Despite increased interest in healthy lifestyles, more than 55% of adults in the United States are either overweight or obese (Jakicic et al, 2001), in excess of 60% of adults do not exercise regularly, and 25% of adults are sedentary (Seefeldt, Malina, and Clark, 2002). Nurses, other health professionals, and the public recognize that initiating and maintaining a healthy lifestyle is complex and requires different approaches directed toward individuals, families, and the environments in which they live.

In this chapter we describe how to integrate multilevel approaches to promote the health of the public and of communities. The integrative model of community health promotion (Laffrey and Kulbok, 1999) can help nurses plan care for clients (individuals, families, or groups in the community, or the **community** as a whole). The model

## Key Terms

**client system**, p. 321
**community**, p. 318
**community health**, p. 329
**disease management**, p. 320
**disease self-management**, p. 325
**focuses of care**, p. 321

**health**, p. 332
**health behavior**, p. 324
**health maintenance**, p. 325
**health promotion**, p. 325
**illness prevention**, p. 331
**lifestyle**, p. 318

**multilevel intervention**, p. 319
**risk appraisal**, p. 325
**self-care**, p. 322
*See Glossary for definitions*


## Chapter Outline

Shifting the Emphasis From Illness and Disease
    Management to Wellness
*Shifting the Emphasis From Individual to
    Population and Multilevel Interventions*
*An Integrative Model for Community Health
    Promotion*

Historical Perspectives, Definitions,
    and Methods
*Health and Health Promotion*
*Community*
**Application to Community-Oriented Nursing**

*Multilevel Community Health Projects*
*Application of the Integrative Model for
    Community Health Promotion*

synthesizes knowledge from public health, nursing, and the social sciences. In this chapter, we also define some of the basic concepts with which community-oriented nurses are concerned. We describe the historical roots of these concepts including how health and health promotion are defined for individuals, families, groups or aggregates, and communities. The concepts of community, illness care, illness prevention, risk reduction, self-care, and disease management are also discussed. These concepts and their linkages determine the direction and methods for community-oriented nursing practice. The chapter describes studies that illustrate **multilevel interventions.** The application of the integrative model of community and public health nursing (community-oriented nursing) shows that the way the concepts are viewed is important in the nurse's approach to practice.

## SHIFTING THE EMPHASIS FROM ILLNESS AND DISEASE MANAGEMENT TO WELLNESS

Community-oriented nurses recognize the need to shift the emphasis of health care from illness to wellness. In community-oriented nursing practice, it is abundantly clear that although illness and disease affect the health of individuals, families, groups, and communities, so do many other factors. The biomedical model, in which health is defined as absence of disease, does not explain why some individuals exposed to illness-producing stressors remain healthy, whereas others, who appear to be in health-enhancing situations, become ill. Nurses assist clients in identifying their health potential and in planning measures that enhance their health. However, viewing clients from the perspective of the biomedical model alone makes it difficult to identify health potential beyond the absence of disease. For example, most people over 65 years of age have at least one diagnosed chronic disease. Limiting the definition of health potential to the absence of disease or illness would result in these persons never being perceived as healthy. This is a pessimistic definition; nursing actions can help older and chronically ill persons become healthier if a broader definition of health is used.

Studies show that there is no better way to promote health and improve the quality of life of individuals than through basic health habits such as exercise, balanced nutrition, developing a positive and optimistic outlook, and not smoking (Hu et al, 2000; Rosenberg, 1994; Seefeldt, Malina, and Clark, 2002). The goal of health care must be directed toward helping individuals identify their health potential and providing nursing care that moves them toward their health potential.

Laffrey, Loveland-Cherry, and Winkler (1986) describe two paradigms from which the key concepts of nursing science (e.g., persons, health, environment) and nursing could be viewed:

1. The pathogenic, or disease paradigm, in which health is objectively defined as the absence of disease. The pathogenic paradigm assumes that humans are composed of organ systems and cells and that health care focuses on identifying what is not working properly with a given system and repairing it. Within this paradigm, health behavior is based on how the client complies with the recommendation of the health professional.

2. The health paradigm, in which health is subjectively defined and is a "fluid, flexible process" (Laffrey et al, 1986, p. 97). Within the health paradigm, humans are viewed as complex and interconnected with the environment. They are different from and greater than the sum of their parts. Health behavior within the health paradigm involves a holistic view of the person's total lifestyle and interaction with the environment and is therefore not judged simply by compliance with a prescribed regimen.

Both paradigms support the specific aims and processes of community-oriented nursing (Laffrey et al, 1986). The pathogenic approach directs nursing toward disease prevention, risk reduction, prompt treatment, and **disease management,** whereas the health approach directs community-oriented nursing practice toward promotion of greater levels of positive health. If health is defined broadly as the life process, taking into account the mutual and simultaneous interaction of humans and their environment, then disease and illness can be seen as potential manifestations of that interaction. Because the health paradigm does not exclude any part of the life process, it includes disease prevention and disease treatment, but it goes beyond these to positive and holistic health (Laffrey and Kulbok, 1999).

During the past decade, the growth of managed health care has encouraged an integrated focus on health promotion, disease prevention, and illness care. A related term, *disease management,* also implies integration of health promotion and disease prevention. Disease management refers to a clinical care process that is used with individuals who have chronic conditions. Disease management crosses the continuum from primary prevention to long-term health maintenance (Johnson, 1996, p. 54); it "shifts" the focus of managed care from treatment to prevention. During its early development, the first generation of managed care produced case management programs to manage high-cost, high-volume catastrophic diseases. The second generation expanded the focus of programs to include comprehensive analysis of resources and alternative settings for treatment for a broader range of chronic diseases. The third generation of managed care has been described as "proactive health management or preventive care—trying to keep people healthy" (Johnson, 1996, p. 54), which some see as a stage of maturity of the managed care movement. Many nurses acknowledge that case management has its roots in public health and district nursing (Issel, 1997; Utz and Kulbok, 1998). Regardless of whether one used the label *health management, disease management,* or *care management,* community-oriented nursing practice is based on meanings of health and actions taken by nurses and clients to optimize health potential.

## Shifting the Emphasis From Individual to Population and Multilevel Interventions

Because individuals ultimately make decisions to engage in healthy or risky behaviors, lifestyle improvement efforts typically focus on individuals as the target of care. Individuals generally focus on immediate personal rewards or threats when deciding whether or not to engage in specific behaviors, and within this perspective, they may convince themselves that their immediate personal risks from certain behaviors such as smoking are low, or that the immediate rewards outweigh the risks. However, from a public health perspective, 440,000 deaths annually were attributed to smoking in the United States during 1995 to 1999, and the annual health-related economic losses were estimated to total at least $157 billion (Centers for Disease Control and Prevention, 2002). Therefore it is clear that health behaviors have multilevel determinants both internal and external to the individual, to the family, to the community, and to the society. For instance, tobacco use by an adolescent is associated with personal attributes of the adolescent (e.g., self-esteem), family characteristics

---

**Healthy People 2010** | **Tobacco Use in Populations or Groups**

**Goal:** To reduce illness, disability, and death related to tobacco use and exposure to secondhand smoke

27-1 Reduce tobacco use by adults

27-2 Reduce tobacco use by adolescents

27-3 Reduce initiation of tobacco use among children and adolescents

27-4 Increase the average age of first use of tobacco products by adolescents and young adults

From U.S. Department of Health and Human Services: *Healthy people 2010: national health promotion and disease prevention objectives,* Washington, DC, 2000, U.S. Government Printing Office.

(e.g., parental attitudes toward smoking), aggregate characteristics (e.g., peer pressure to smoke), community factors (e.g., availability of cigarettes), and other social or environmental factors (e.g., taxation of cigarettes) (Tyas and Pederson, 1998). Therefore interventions to initiate or maintain healthy behaviors must be systematically directed toward the multiple targets of the individual, family, group or aggregate, community, and society.

Downie, Tannahill, and Tannahill (1996) argued that it is not realistic to emphasize individual responsibility for health behavior while excluding community. They cautioned against the danger of "victim blaming" by placing all of the responsibility for health behavior on the individual. Likewise, giving the community the sole responsibility for people's health behaviors is a patronizing, "top-down" attitude that leads people to feel as if they have no power or control. Both approaches result in people feeling helpless and victimized. Downie et al (1996) propose a "new sense of community responsibility" that empowers individuals to be informed "about their own health, and at the same time, empowers the community to provide needed leadership and professional assistance for community development—to work with and through the community to promote health. Health and well-being are, in the end, a set of relationships among citizens" (Downie, pp. 169-170).

## An Integrative Model for Community Health Promotion

Laffrey and Kulbok (1999) developed a model for community health promotion to guide community-oriented nursing. This model is based on two complementary paradigms for nursing: the health paradigm and the pathogenic (disease) paradigm described previously (Laffrey et al, 1986) (Figure 14-1). The health paradigm focuses on promoting health as a dynamic, creative, and positive quality of life and includes the promotion of physical, mental, emotional, functional, spiritual, and social well-

being. The pathogenic paradigm includes both the care and the prevention of illness, disease, and disability and focuses on reducing known risks and threats to health and preventing disease. Although some clinical strategies may be similar in the two paradigms, the ultimate goal of each is fundamentally different. This difference can be seen in the specific purpose of the nursing care and whether it is aimed at resolving a disease or illness or promoting greater health.

The integrative model includes two major dimensions: client system and focus of care. The **client system** is multidimensional and includes various levels of clients toward which community-oriented nursing care is targeted. The simplest level of the client system is its most delimited target, the individual. When the individual is the client, the environment includes the family, the population group, and the community of which the individual is a part. The nurse is concerned with how these environments affect the individual, and his or her health.

Each succeeding level of the client system is more complex, as the client can also be the family, an aggregate, or the community. The aggregate and community make up the environment for the family, and the community is the environment for the aggregate. Different kinds of assessments and nursing interventions appropriate at each level of client within the system are discussed later in this chapter. It is important to note that community-oriented nursing is holistic in nature and is population-focused in that it addresses multiple levels of clients and multiple levels of care within the total system.

The **focuses of care** in the model include health promotion, illness (disease or disability) prevention, and illness care. Each focus is appropriate for some aspects of nursing. Even more important is the awareness that the goal of community-oriented health care is a healthier community, and this is achieved through health promotion interventions. No matter where community-oriented nursing care

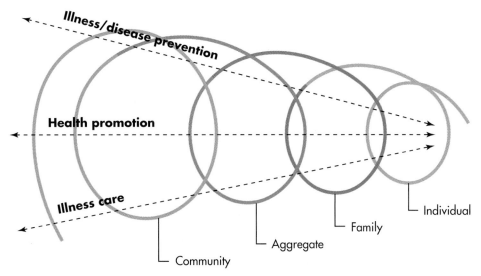

**Figure 14-1** An integrative model for community health promotion.

begins, it ultimately leads to health promotion of the community. This does not mean that one nurse provides all levels of care, but it does underscore the need for nurses to have a good understanding of care requirements at all of the client levels. The individual, family, aggregate, and community each has characteristics, strengths, and health needs that are unique and that differ from those at the other levels.

The integrative community health promotion model reflects the basic beliefs and values of community-oriented nursing. The model depicts continuity and expansiveness of the client systems and foci of care. The central axis, or core, of the model is health promotion. At its narrowest focus, illness care is provided to individuals. According to the model, at the broadest level of care, nurses work with community leaders and lay people to plan programs to promote optimal health of its citizens. The goals of nursing actions in the integrative model, at any client level from the individual to the community, are to achieve the maximal health potential through an active partnership between the nurse and the client system. When nurses facilitate an active partnership with the client system, whether the focus of care is health promotion, illness prevention, or illness care, they involve clients in every step of the process of managing health care from the assessment of their health needs and resources to implementation and evaluation of outcomes.

---

**⌈ NURSING TIP**

Facilitate active partnerships with clients by involving them in every step of the process of managing health care for individuals, families, aggregates, or communities, from assessment of their needs to planning, implementing, and evaluating outcomes.

---

# HISTORICAL PERSPECTIVES, DEFINITIONS, AND METHODS
## Health and Health Promotion
### Historical Perspectives on Health

**Health** is the key term in a model for community-oriented nursing practice. Beginning with Nightingale's efforts to discover and use the laws of nature to enhance humanity, nursing has always taken an active role in promoting the health of populations and the total community. How one defines health shapes the entire process of nursing, including making the decisions of what is to be assessed and with what level of client, and of how to evaluate the outcomes of care. When health is defined as alleviating illness symptoms, the assessment consists of the duration, intensity, and frequency of the specific symptoms. Intervention is aimed at symptom relief and perhaps treatment of the cause of the symptoms. Evaluation consists of a determination of whether the symptoms are alleviated. On the other hand, if health is defined as maximizing a commu-

nity's physical recreation opportunities, the assessment then focuses on existing recreation facilities, accessibility to the population, and beliefs and knowledge related to recreation and land use in the community.

The holistic view of health is not new. The ancient Greeks viewed health as the influence of environmental forces such as living habits; climate; and quality of air, water, and food on human well-being. Certain activities of daily living, such as exercise, were considered essential to the maintenance of health. Box 14-1 lists health perspectives over time. Scientific medicine emerged slowly and resistance to scientific discoveries, such as to the germ theory of disease, hindered the application of new medical science to medical practice. With the development of the scientific approach toward disease in the twentieth century, **self-care** was ignored in favor of professional care. During the last four decades, the idea of self-care as derived from a positive idea of health has reemerged and may compete with professional care. Some proponents of self-care emphasize lay diagnosis and self-treatment, whereas others focus on teaching people how to work with their health care providers. In both cases, the health care system is changing; roles are being renegotiated with an emphasis on collaboration between consumers and providers.

The self-care movement was accelerated by the political climate of the 1960s and 1970s and challenged profes-

---

**BOX 14-1   Health Perspectives Over Time**

**ANCIENT GREEK VIEW**
- Health was the totality of environmental forces influencing human well-being.
- Ways of living were essential to maintain health.

**1700s TO 1800s**
- Scientific discoveries were opposed (e.g., germ theory of disease and principle of antisepsis).
- An increasing emphasis on medical science was associated with a decreasing emphasis on self-care.

**EARLY TO MID 1900s**
- Holistic view of health was reintroduced as an antidote to the medical science model.
- Scientific and biological view of disease dominated.
- Self-care was deemphasized.

**LATE 1900s**
- Reemergence of the ideal of self-care was accelerated by the climate of political activism.
- Recognition that people produce health by what they do and do not do for themselves.
- Collaboration existed between consumers and providers, and renegotiation of professional roles in health care emerged.
- New chronic disease self-management models were developed under managed care.

sional health care. Racial minorities began to demand their rights in the 1960s, and women and older adults began to make their demands public in the 1970s. Illich wrote, "The medical establishment has become a major threat to health" (Illich, 1976, p. 3). He warned that politicians and legislators might promote self-care because of their interest in cost containment rather than a genuine belief in individuals' abilities to preserve health. More than 25 years later the same warning can be made about the cost-driven managed care movement.

Many health professionals contend that the individual is in a position to produce health. Fuchs (1974) suggests that the "greatest potential for improving health lies in what we do and don't do for and to ourselves" (p. 55). In the political arena, LaLonde introduced a similar conclusion in *A New Perspective on the Health of Canadians* (1974). LaLonde identified four major determinants of health: human biology, environment, lifestyle, and health care (Figure 14-2). In 1976 policymakers in the United States echoed these ideas. Efforts to improve health habits and the environment were viewed as the best hope of achieving any significant extension of life expectancy (U.S. Department of Health, Education, and Welfare [USDHEW], 1976, p. 69). Box 14-2 lists some landmark initiatives in health promotion and disease prevention.

The U.S. Public Health Service established the first national objectives involving disease prevention, health protection, and health promotion strategies in the surgeon general's Healthy People report (USDHEW, 1979). Disease prevention strategies focused on services such as family planning and immunizations delivered in clinical settings. Health protection strategies were directed to environmental measures to "significantly improve health and the quality of life for this and future generations of Americans"

(USDHEW, p. 101), including occupational health and accidental injury control. Health promotion strategies were designed to achieve well-being through community and individual lifestyle change measures. Healthy People (1979) also described inherited biological factors, the environment, and behavioral factors as the three categories of risks to health, which are identical to LaLonde's first three major determinants of health.

As described in Chapter 2, Healthy People 2010, the most recent set of health objectives for the nation, builds on initiatives pursued over the past two decades including *The 1979 Surgeon General's Report, Healthy People, and Healthy People 2000: National Health Promotion and Disease Prevention Objectives.* It is designed for use by individuals, states, communities, and professional organizations to help them develop programs to improve health. Nursing organizations, including the Association of Community Health Nursing Educators (ACHNE) and the Public Health Nursing (PHN) Section of the American Public Health Association, participated in the development of these new priorities and health directions.

## Definitions of Health

The World Health Organization (WHO, 1958) reflected a holistic perspective, in its classic definition of health as a state of complete physical, mental, and social well-being, and not merely the absence of disease and infirmity. In 1975 Terris noted that epidemiologists considered the WHO definition to be "vague and imprecise with a Utopian aura" (WHO, p. 1037). Terris expanded the definition: "Health is a state of physical, mental and social well-being and the ability to function and not merely the absence of illness and infirmity" (WHO, p. 1038). In deleting the word "complete" and adding "ability to function," the WHO definition was

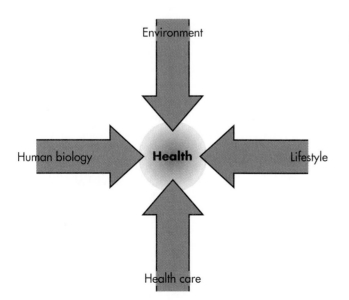

**Figure 14-2** Determinants of health. *(Modified from LaLonde M: A new perspective on the health of Canadians, Ottawa, 1974, Government of Canada.)*

> **BOX 14-2   Landmark Health Promotion/Disease Prevention Initiatives**
>
> - 1974    LaLonde's New Perspectives on the Health of Canadians
> - 1976    Forward Plan for Health, FY 1978-82
> - 1979    The surgeon general's report: Healthy People
> - 1989    Guide to Clinical Preventive Services (USPSTF, 1989)
> - 1990    Healthy People 2000
> - 1994    Put Prevention Into Practice (PPIP)
> - 2000    *Healthy People 2010* (second edition, *With Understanding and Improving Health and Objectives for Improving Health;* supercedes the January 2000 conference edition)
> - 2001    *Guide to Clinical Preventive Services,* second edition

placed in a more realistic context, providing a useful framework for health promotion.

Smith (1981) suggests that the "idea of health" directs nursing practice, education, and research. She clarifies the idea of health by observing that health was described as a comparative concept, allowing for "more" or "less" health along a health–illness continuum. Smith proposed four models of health, ordered from narrow and concrete to broad and abstract. These models were clinical health, or the absence of disease; role performance health, or the ability to perform one's social roles satisfactorily; adaptive health, or flexible adaptation to the environment; and eudaemonistic health, or self-actualization and the attainment of one's greatest human potential.

It is important for nurses to examine their own definition of health and recognize how the nursing care they provide is directed by their health definition. A nurse who views health as the absence of disease is likely to emphasize physical and biological signs and symptoms of disease, with minimal attention to the quality of social roles and evidence of subjective well-being. A nurse who broadly defines health as self-actualization is more likely to consider indicators of physical health, social health, and the potential for maximum well-being when planning nursing care. Community-oriented nurses emphasize health promotion while acknowledging the importance of illness and disease.

## Definitions of Health Promotion

Health promotion is an accepted aim of nursing practice, although it is rarely defined and is not often differentiated from disease prevention or health maintenance (Brubaker, 1983). Leavell and Clark (1965) strongly influenced the evolution of health promotion and disease prevention strategies through their classic definitions of primary, secondary, and tertiary levels of prevention that were rooted in the biomedical model of health and epidemiology. The application of preventive measures, according to Leavell and Clark, corresponds to the natural history or stages of disease (see Table 11-3 in Chapter 11). Primary preventive measures are directed toward "well" individuals in the prepathogenesis period to promote their health and to provide specific protection from disease. Secondary preventive measures are applied to diagnose or to treat individuals in the period of disease pathogenesis. Tertiary prevention addresses rehabilitation and the return of people with chronic illness to a maximal ability to function (Box 14-3).

Even though primary, secondary, and tertiary levels of prevention had their origins in the medical model, Leavell and Clark moved beyond the medical model. They conceptualized primary prevention as two distinct components: health promotion and specific protection. Health promotion focuses on positive measures such as education for healthy living and promotion of favorable environmental conditions as well as periodic selective examinations including, for example, well-child developmental as-

---

**BOX 14-3** **Levels of Prevention Related to Diabetes**

**PRIMARY PREVENTION**

For a person with identified risk factors for diabetes, the goal is to maintain a normal weight, to exercise regularly, and to reduce the intake of carbohydrates.

**SECONDARY PREVENTION**

Have regular blood sugar level testing done and be alert for any symptoms of the onset of diabetes.

**TERTIARY PREVENTION**

If the blood sugar level indicates that the client has diabetes, begin treatment, which might include a diabetic diet, regular exercise, and medication.

---

sessment and health education. Specific protection includes measures to reduce the threat of specific diseases such as hygiene and the elimination of workplace hazards.

When health promotion and specific protection are used as subconcepts of primary prevention, they appear to stem from a definition of health as the absence of disease. However, differences in health promotion and specific protection strategies suggest that they are not the same. Some terms used to describe health promotion are linked to a positive view of health (e.g., *health habits*), whereas other terms are linked to the negative view of the absence of disease (e.g., *disease prevention*). The confusion in terminology is increased when actions to promote health, protect health, and prevent disease are used interchangeably as indicators of preventive behavior (Kulbok and Baldwin, 1992; Kulbok et al, 1997).

The WHO described health promotion as "the process of enabling people to increase control over, and improve their health" (WHO, 1984, p. 3). According to the Ottawa Charter, health promotion combines both individual and community-level strategies including "building healthful public, creating supportive environments, strengthening community action, developing personal skills, and reorienting health services" (Bracht, 1990, p. 38). Health is a resource for daily living. For individuals or communities to realize physical, mental, and social well-being, they must become aware of and learn to use the social and personal resources available within their environment.

Kulbok (1985) proposed a resource model of health behavior, in which social and health resources were viewed as correlates of positive **health behaviors.** Two major findings were reported in studies to test this model (Kulbok, 1985; Kulbok et al, 1999). First, health behavior is multidimensional, and there are several categories of health behavior including positive behaviors (e.g., diet, exercise) and avoidance behaviors (e.g., substance use). Second, different health and social resources are associated with different health behaviors. Strategies to promote well-being often focus on helping clients practice new, healthy behaviors or to change unhealthy behaviors. Successful intervention is more likely when nurses understand how social and health resources are related to health behaviors of individuals and communities and how personal and community resources may affect behavior choices.

Laffrey (1990) differentiated between the terms *health promotion, illness prevention,* and *health maintenance.* **Health promotion** is behavior directed toward achieving a greater level of health. Illness prevention is behavior directed toward reducing the threat of illness or disease, and health maintenance is directed toward keeping a current state of health. Applying these definitions requires that one assess not only the behavior but also the basis on which one makes a choice to perform a given behavior. In a study of community-residing men and women with and without chronic diseases, Laffrey (1990) asked subjects to identify their five most important health behaviors. For each behavior reported, subjects were asked the major reason they usually performed that behavior. Responses indicated that behaviors were performed for each of the three reasons. For example, one individual reported that he exercises because he has several risk factors for coronary artery disease. Exercise, for him, is an illness-preventing behavior. Another person reported that he exercises because regular, vigorous exercise makes him feel more energetic and he functions at a higher level than he did when he was sedentary. For this individual, exercise is a health promotion behavior. A third individual who reported exercising regularly to maintain her weight used exercise as a **health maintenance** behavior.

Pender (1996) also differentiated between health-protecting and health-promoting behaviors. Health protection refers to behaviors that decrease one's probability of becoming ill, whereas health promotion refers to behaviors that increase well-being of either an individual or a group. Although health protection and health promotion are complementary, health promotion is a broader concept that encompasses both individuals and groups.

In 1997 Kulbok et al reported a content validity study of five national health promotion experts and found differences between the terms *health promotion* and *health promotion behavior.* The group of experts defined health promotion as activities undertaken by health professionals to promote health in their clients and the term includes health education and counseling. Health promotion behavior, on the other hand, was defined as behavior that an individual performs to promote his or her health and well-being.

In summary, there is considerable evidence of agreement regarding a positive view of health underlying health promotion directed toward individuals, families, and communities. For example, the WHO process of health promotion, the resource model of health behavior (Kulbok, 1985; Kulbok et al, 1999), Laffrey's (1990) notion of health behavior choices, and Pender's (1996) definition of health promotion are all conceptually grounded in the health paradigm. Clearly, health promotion and self-care are consistent with the goals of community-oriented nursing.

## Definitions of Self-Care and Disease Self-Management

The term *self-care* has influenced how nurses approach health promotion. Orem (1995) has developed a nursing model in which self-care describes activities that individuals initiate and perform on their own behalf to maintain life, health, and well-being. According to Orem, individuals are not always able to be completely self-sufficient in their self-care. Consequently, although self-care is a lay responsibility, professional care may be required to enhance an individual's capability for self-care. Within this model, nursing care depends on the capability of individuals and can range from total care to partial care to education and support of individuals to assist them in increasing their self-care capability. Orem's self-care focus is on the individual.

Goeppinger (1982) notes that self-care activities may be carried out by the individual, the community, or the society and are based on scientific, religious, philosophical, and cultural influences. The care provided by nurses and other primary care workers may be directed toward the individual by changing health beliefs and behaviors. From a public health perspective, it is important that self-care also emphasize community responsibility and social change. For example, the WHO definition of health promotion noted earlier includes one's use of personal and social resources within the environment to promote health and well-being. An important precursor to the use of resources by the population is to develop adequate resources within the environment to enhance the health of the entire population.

There is no question that self-care practices promote healthy lifestyles and prevent the onset of disease. However, it is also clear that individuals with chronic conditions can influence their comfort, ability to function, and other illness outcomes through self-care practices. Lorig (1996) argues that as chronic disease increases, a **disease self-management** model in which the professional and the client are partners in care, together learning to manage day-to-day living, is essential. Education to enhance a client's capacity for self-care practices and self-management of chronic conditions is an intervention that is consistent with the integrative model for community health promotion. Interventions are directed toward multiple client levels, supporting the individual's capacity for adopting self-care practices (e.g., knowledge and skills related to diabetes self-management) and maximizing environmental resources needed to sustain them (e.g., family support for dietary changes and affordable prescriptions, blood glucose testing equipment).

## Methods for Disease Prevention and Risk Reduction

Health providers use the disease prevention strategy of **risk appraisal** and risk reduction to help individuals and groups maximize their self-care activities. This strategy compares information supplied by individuals about their health-related practices, health habits, demographic characteristics, and personal and family medical history with data from epidemiologic studies and vital statistics. It uses these comparisons to predict individuals' risks of morbidity and mortality and to suggest areas in which disease risks may be reduced. The goal of risk appraisal and reduction is to prevent disease or detect disease in its earliest stages. The knowledge base for risk appraisal and reduction is the scientific evidence that relates risk factors and disease and the effectiveness of interventions in reducing both mortality and risks of mortality.

Risk appraisal and reduction are widely accepted strategies in population-focused health programming. This development was influenced by an emphasis on health promotion and disease prevention in the 1970s, epidemiologic studies that provided an empirical database for making predictions from risk appraisal methods, and a proliferation of risk appraisal tools for use in clinical practice. The health insurance industry recognized the potential of risk reduction for cost containment and promoted the approach in occupational and health care settings. Today, employers are documenting a decrease in health care costs as a result of participation in health risk appraisal programs (Anderson et al, 2000; Musich, Napier, and Edington, 2001).

In health risk appraisal (HRA), data about health risks experienced by an individual or group are collected and analyzed, and a health risk profile is generated. Health risk appraisal may be done at both individual and community levels. A clinical approach is used to identify risks in individuals, and an epidemiologic approach is frequently used to identify risks at the population level. Both of these approaches are important to community and public health nurses. In this section, the methods of individual and community health risk appraisal are discussed. Later in the chapter, some influential community and epidemiologic studies are reviewed.

Box 14-4 lists the three most common types of health risk appraisal approaches used to assess individuals. Each type of risk appraisal is complex, and only the basic concepts and selected procedures are described in this chapter. More complete explanations are found in the references cited at the end of the chapter. Clinical guidelines and an example of a risk appraisal tool are shown in Appendixes A.1 and F.

### Health Risk Appraisal

Robbins and Hall (1970) approached an individual's health from the perspective of what was likely to occur rather than what had already occurred. They recognized that most chronic diseases have a predictable sequence and that the characteristic precursors of many diseases can be monitored and controlled. Robbins and Hall put the concept of prospective medicine into practice by developing the health hazard appraisal to predict what diseases were likely to occur, given an individual's characteristics and lifestyle.

---

**BOX 14-4    Health-Risk Appraisal Approaches**

- The health hazard appraisal and its many versions
- Clinical guidelines and recommendations for preventive services
- Wellness appraisals or inventories

---

Risk appraisal instruments are convenient tools that determine individual health risks. One of the most comprehensive HRAs is the Healthier People Questionnaire (HPQ) developed by the Carter Center at Emory University and the Centers for Disease Control and Prevention (CDC). The CDC, along with a network of state health departments and universities, based the HPQ on a decade of development work and on the Risk Factor Update Project (Breslow et al, 1985). The HPQ is computer scored and is available

---

**HOW TO    Profile Client Risk**

1. Assess the total risks to a client's health on the basis of knowledge of the client.
2. Assess the history of certain diseases and major causes of mortality for aggregates of the client's age, sex, race, and family history.
3. Help the health provider to initiate lifestyle changes in the client to avoid health threats or to prevent complications.
4. Institute treatment or lifestyle changes early in the course of disease.
5. To accomplish these objectives, collect data with a self-administered questionnaire, basic laboratory tests, and clinical examination.
6. The questionnaire asks about personal characteristics and behaviors known to predict disease.
7. These data are compared with data compiled from the 10 major causes of death of an aggregate of the same age, sex, and race as the client.
8. On the basis of the comparison, the client's appraisal age and achievable age are calculated.
9. The appraisal age is the health age of the average person in the client's age, sex, and race aggregate with a similar risk profile. For example, a 20-year-old white woman might have an appraisal age of 15 years if she has good health habits and no family history of chronic disease. Another 20-year-old white woman might have an appraisal age of 26 years if she smokes, fails to wear a seat belt, does not perform regular breast self-examinations, and has a family history of hypertension. The second woman's achievable age could be lowered if she were to modify her behavior.
10. Achievable age is the health age the client could achieve by modifying health threats.

to the public. In 1991 the Healthier People Network (HPN) took responsibility for the ongoing scientific integrity of the health risk appraisal instrument. Version 6 (now called the HPN Health Risk Appraisal) was updated using 1990 mortality and census data. In addition, a new risk appraisal for older adults (55 to 90 years of age) predicts functional status and morbidity. Current program information is available from the HPN (see their website under Additional Resources, and see this book's website for information about how to contact them).

The Lifestyle Assessment Questionnaire (LAQ) from the National Wellness Institute (NWI, 1989) includes the HPQ, a wellness inventory, and a personal growth section. Users are provided with a personal wellness report, which summarizes their LAQ results and provides them with a sample action plan for increasing wellness behaviors. Also, the NWI offers age-specific risk appraisals and wellness inventories (see their website under Additional Resources, and see this book's website for information about how to contact them).

### Clinical Preventive Services Guidelines

Gradual acceptance of scientific evidence of the benefits associated with key preventive measures led to the development of clinical practice guidelines in the late 1970s. Breslow and Somers (1977) proposed the lifetime health-monitoring program to identify individuals' specific needs for health care. They provided a list of recommendations for preventive measures appropriate for each of 10 age groups. In 1989 the U.S. Preventive Services Task Force (USPSTF, 1989) published the first *Guide to Clinical Preventive Services* based on review of the scientific evidence on 169 clinical preventive services for 60 target conditions. The USPSTF was originally convened by the Public Health Service to evaluate clinical research and assess the merits of preventive measures, including screening tests, counseling, immunizations, and chemoprophylaxis. The second edition of the *Guide to Clinical Preventive Services* (USPSTF, 1996) provides the most recent recommendations for preventive interventions: screening tests, counseling, immunizations, and chemoprophylaxis regimens for more than 80 conditions. Many of these preventive measures are routine nursing interventions.

> ◖ **WHAT DO YOU THINK?**
>
> Many of the preventive measures in *A Guide to Clinical Preventive Services,* edition 2, are routine community-oriented nursing interventions and have individual-focused as well as population-focused applications.

To ensure implementation of the *Clinical Preventive Services Guidelines,* the Public Health Service of the U.S. Department of Health and Human Services (USDHHS), provider organizations, and major health-related groups collaborated to develop a program entitled Put Prevention into Practice (PPIP). The PPIP program uses materials designed to improve delivery of preventive services including the Child Health Guide and the Adult Personal Health Guide, which are passport-size, consumer-held mini-records (Griffith and Diguiseppi, 1994). The PPIP program is designed to influence the health promotion and disease prevention practices of health care professionals and consumers. PPIP materials are available in English and Spanish from the U.S. Government Printing Office.

### Wellness Inventories

Wellness inventories differ from health risk appraisal instruments and guidelines for preventive services by defining health risks more broadly and leading to health promotion as well as disease prevention and risk reduction. Typical wellness instruments include questions related to self-responsibility, nutrition awareness, physical fitness, stress management, and environmental sensitivity (Ardell, 1977). The wellness inventory of the LAQ (NWI, 1989) described previously covers six dimensions: physical, social, emotional, intellectual, occupational, and spiritual.

### Advantages and Disadvantages

There are both advantages and disadvantages to using health risk appraisals. These appraisals support individuals' self-care behaviors and provide direction for nurses to counsel and educate clients about healthy behaviors. Multilevel program participation, based on increased health risk awareness, has been shown to be associated with decreased health risk (Yen et al, 2001). Another advantage of HRAs is that they are used to measure the outcomes and economic costs of risk reduction interventions (Anderson et al, 2000; Musich et al, 2001). By completing HRAs, individuals and groups receive immediate feedback about how their behavioral changes can influence their health risks and life expectancy.

Despite these advantages, it is important to know the limitations of risk appraisal tools. Actual tool limitations are questionable validity and reliability of the instruments. Also, there is a concern that these instruments overemphasize lifestyle factors and do not address other important risks, such as environmental hazards and inadequate health care (Smith, McKinlay, and McKinlay, 1989). Furthermore, these instruments lack cultural sensitivity (Christopher, Christopher, and Dunnagan, 2000). When selecting an HRA tool, it is important to assess its overall strengths and limitations, and its relevance for specific populations.

For best results, it is wise to use health risk appraisals in conjunction with clinical observation, health assessment, and population-focused program planning. Although an educational message may have a great impact on some individuals, others may deny the message or avoid its implications (Becker and Janz, 1987). In general, knowledge is necessary but not sufficient to have a significant impact on behavior change. Even when individuals are motivated by health appraisal feedback, they may not have the behavioral skills or resources necessary to initiate and sustain changes in lifestyle (Clark and Becker, 1998). This is especially true regarding those behaviors that are difficult to change, such as smoking habits.

Another limitation of health risk appraisals is that they are probably more suitable for use with middle-aged people than for those younger than 35 or older than 65 years of age (Doerr and Hutchins, 1981). Some recent research indicates that age-specific HRA tools are effective in raising awareness of risk and motivating behavior change in older adult populations (Breslow et al, 1997). Health risk appraisals provide little incentive to the very young to change poor health habits, because the effects of lifestyle on health and illness are usually not detected until middle to late adulthood. In addition, because they were developed and tested with white, middle-class populations, existing appraisals are probably less useful with culturally diverse populations (Christopher et al, 2000). Their use with minorities is compromised by the inadequacy of epidemiologic data on risk factors, such as the lack of available and accessible health services for the poor. An individual's ability to change lifestyle is limited by living in a system that may restrict participation in decision making, by economic and educational opportunities, or by living in an environment that encourages risk taking and lifestyles that are not conducive to good health (Orlandi and Dalton, 1998).

## Community

### Historical Perspectives

After health and health promotion, the third major concept in an integrated model for nursing is community. The emphasis on community as the focus of practice has been gaining attention since the mid 1970s when the U.S. and Canadian governments and private health researchers attributed declining mortality and morbidity rates to better standards of living, such as sanitation, clean air and water, and availability of healthy foods. The Institute of Medicine's (IOM's) report on the future of public health also emphasized community by stating that the "mission of public health is to assure conditions in which people can be healthy by generating organized community effort to . . . prevent disease and promote health" (IOM, 1988, p. 7).

As discussed previously, the national health goals in the healthy people initiative (USDHHS, 1979, 2000, 2001) emphasized the environment and the community as central to achieving health. *Healthy People in Healthy Communities* (USDHHS, 2001) is a community-planning guide using Healthy People 2010 (Box 14-5). The objectives in Healthy People 2010 are included in the guide, along with a set of practical recommendations for coalition building, creating a vision, and measuring outcomes to improve the health of communities. Communities can tailor the recommendations to their own local needs, and health professionals

---

**BOX 14-5    Healthy People 2010: A Strategy for Creating a Healthy Community**

To achieve the goal of improving health, a community must develop a strategy supported by many individuals who are working together. The MAP-IT technique helps you to map out the path toward the change you want to see in your community. This guide recommends that you MAP-IT—that is, mobilize, assess, plan, implement, and track.

- Mobilize individuals and organizations that care about the health of your community into a coalition.
- Assess the areas of greatest need in your community, as well as the resources and other strengths that you can tap into to address those areas.
- Plan your approach: start with a vision of where you want to be as a community; then add strategies and action steps to help you achieve that vision.
- Implement your plan using concrete action steps that can be monitored and will make a difference.
- Track your progress over time.

Modified from U.S. Department of Health and Human Services: *Healthy people in healthy communities,* Washington, DC, 2001, U.S. Government Printing Office.

---

in public and private organizations can work together with community members to develop programs that fit the needs and resources of their own communities. Nurses participate in this process through community assessments, community development activities, and identification of key persons in the community with whom to build partnerships for health programs. The national health objectives and the healthy communities guide provide a logical link between the Healthy People 2010 and community-wide program planning.

In the first decade of the twenty-first century, community-oriented nurses have abundant opportunities to participate in community-wide health care. Edwards and Dees (1990) argued that the contribution of community-oriented nursing to problems of the environment lies in their ability to integrate concepts of health and disease, individual and aggregate, public health and nursing, and health promotion and disease prevention. This integration means that nurses must consider the complex relationship between the personal and environmental forces that affect health. Over 25 years ago, Milio (1976) offered a set of propositions for improving health behavior by considering personal choices in the context of available societal resources. These propositions (Box 14-6) constitute a fitting model for health promotion that addresses both personal and societal resources for this new millennium.

For community-oriented nurses, therefore, it is important to realize that individuals make choices about various

BOX 14-6 **Milio's Propositions for Improving Health Behavior**

- Health status of populations is a function of the lack or excess of health-sustaining resources.
- Behavior patterns of populations are related to habits of choice from actual or perceived limited resources and related attitudes.
- Organizational decisions determine the range of personal resources available.
- Individual health-related decisions are influenced by efforts to maximize valued resources in both the personal and societal domains.
- Social change is reflective of a change in population behavior patterns.
- Health education will impact behavior patterns minimally without new health-promoting options for investing personal resources.

Modified from Milio N: A framework for prevention: changing health-damaging to health-generating life patterns, *Am J Public Health* 66(5):435, 1976.

health practices. The degree of freedom in the personal choices of individuals is affected greatly by others in the family and peer group, options available within the immediate environment, and the norms and values within the community. Behavior change is based on interventions targeted to the person within the environment but must also include interventions targeted to the immediate and surrounding environment.

## Community Models and Frameworks

The theoretical frameworks developed within nursing are primarily oriented to individuals. There is an assumption in the nursing discipline that simply changing the word "man" or "human being" to "aggregate" or "community" is sufficient (Hanchett, 1988). Moe (1977) defined community as people and the relationships that emerge among them, developing and using common institutions and physical environment. Community-oriented nurses are aware that the community is more than the sum of the individuals, families, and aggregates within it and that interaction among the individuals, families, aggregates, and organizations must be considered for any real change to occur.

Despite a community-oriented ideal, the concept of the community as client is not easily integrated into practice. Consequently, nursing practice directed to the community has been neglected in favor of providing care to ill and disadvantaged individuals in the community. Chopoorian (1986) argues that a lack of consciousness of community may "contribute to the peripheral role of nurses in the larger arena of social, economic, and political affairs" (Chopoorian, 1986, p. 42). Nurses strengthen their position with the community by looking not at the profession

or to individual clients as objects of reform but rather at the environment, which can be reconceptualized as social, economic, and political structures; as human social relations; and as everyday life (Chopoorian, 1986). This dynamic perspective leads to interventions targeted to public health policy.

Several authors described community from a systems perspective (Anderson and McFarlane, 2000; Blum, 1981; Hanchett, 1988; Salmon-White, 1982) by viewing humans within a hierarchy of natural systems and health as a function of harmonious interrelationships among various levels of the hierarchy. Movement in one level of the hierarchy has a corresponding movement in all levels. If individual, family, aggregate, community, and society are different levels of the system's hierarchy, then any change in one level has a corresponding change in all other levels.

Anderson and McFarlane (2000) and Salmon-White (1982) developed models based on the assumption that assessing the various components of the system facilitates a healthy community. The community-as-partner model includes eight major community subsystems (Anderson and McFarlane, 2000). The basic core of the community, according to these authors, is its people and their values, beliefs, culture, religion, laws, and mores. Within a community system, the people interact with the other subsystems. A **community health** assessment must obtain information about the subsystems and the pattern of interactions among the subsystems and of the total community with the systems external to it.

The model created by Salmon-White (1982) is based on the public health mission of organized efforts to protect, promote, and restore health. It proposes that community-oriented nursing includes prevention, protection, and promotion strategies. The model embraces multiple health determinants and is consistent with the Canadian Framework for Health (LaLonde, 1974).

In these models, interventions are planned at the system level by participating with relevant subsystems. Although these models provide guidance for assessing community and aggregate systems, they cannot easily be used to direct interventions. Keller et al (1998) proposed a population-based model for pubic health nursing interventions. The model is based on the scope of public health nursing practice, which crosses multiple levels of care. It was designed to define more clearly the population-focused underpinning of public health nursing practice and to explain the work of public health nurses at the individual, community, and systems levels. The pubic health nursing interventions model is similar to the integrated model of community health promotion in that it delineates multiple levels of care or intervention.

These assessment and intervention models (Anderson and McFarlane, 2000; Salmon-White, 1982; Keller et al, 1998) focus on stability and equilibrium by protecting the community from specific disease risks; less attention is directed toward factors that promote an optimally healthy community. Nevertheless, several major community-wide studies have drawn on concepts such as those presented in these models. These community and epidemiologic studies are described next.

## Influential Multilevel Community Studies

Two significant community studies of health risks, morbidity, and mortality are the Framingham Heart study, initiated in 1949, and the Human Population Laboratory's longitudinal survey in Alameda County, California, initiated in the early 1970s. In the Framingham Heart study, 5209 adults agreed to be followed over their life span to identify factors contributing to coronary heart disease (CHD). Periodic health assessments were done, and morbidity and mortality data were collected. Major risk factors associated with CHD mortality rates were identified in the original cohort (e.g., elevated systolic blood pressure, elevated serum cholesterol level, and cigarette smoking) (Liao et al, 1999). The investigators proposed mathematical predictive models (e.g., health risk appraisal functions) that relate the risk factors identified among well individuals in the Framingham population to the probability of future cardiovascular disease. These complex statistical models have evolved since the 1960s and have been widely used to document the multifactorial nature of cardiovascular disease and the interrelationships among these major risk factors. This study is still in progress.

The Alameda County study was designed to follow a sample of 6928 individuals over a 4-year period. Social and behavioral factors were studied in relationship to mortality. The health behaviors studied included eating three meals daily, eating breakfast, sleeping 7 to 8 hours a night, using alcohol moderately, exercising regularly, not smoking, and maintaining a desirable weight-to-height ratio. Smoking and alcohol use were positively related to mortality (Berkman and Breslow, 1983). Physical exercise, 7 to 8 hours of sleep, optimal weight in relation to height, and social networks (e.g., contact with friends and relatives, church and group membership) were inversely related to mortality. These findings led to the inclusion of social and environmental variables, as well as personal behaviors, in health risk appraisal tools that are still in use today. Findings from these early large-scale surveys prompted a number of public health multilevel programs. Examples of community-oriented risk-reduction interventions were the Stanford Heart Disease Prevention program (Farquhar et al, 1990), the North Karelia study (Puska et al, 1983), the Pawtucket Heart Health program (Lasater et al, 1984), and the Minnesota Heart Health program (Luepker et al, 1994).

The Stanford Five-City project began in 1979 with a 6-year community health education program aimed at reducing cardiovascular (CV) risk factors. The program was delivered through multiple channels (Winkleby et al, 1996). Two treatment cities received a low-cost, comprehensive program based on social learning theory, communication theory, behavior change theory, community organization, and social marketing. Improvements in serum cholesterol levels, blood pressure, smoking rate, and resting heart rate were observed among the population of these cities after the program (Farquhar et al, 1990; Winkleby et al, 1996). A survey to evaluate the long-term effects of the intervention indicated that the changes after the intervention were sustained in the treatment cities. CV and all-cause mortality rates were maintained or improved in the treatment cities, whereas they leveled out or worsened in the comparison cities (Winkleby et al, 1996).

Positive changes were also found in the North Karelia Project (Puska et al, 1983). Citizens of North Karelia, a rural area in Finland, were selected for this program because they had had a high mortality rate from CV disease in the early 1970s. More than half of the North Karelia men smoked, consumed large amounts of animal fat, and had elevated serum cholesterol levels. In addition, many had untreated hypertension. The government directed the multilevel program at an individual and community level to help the citizens modify their high-risk behaviors. The North Karelia project involved retraining of health professionals, reorganization of public health services, production of low-fat and low-salt dairy products and meat, and community health education. Follow-up studies demonstrated that the three major risk factors for CV disease decreased much more in North Karelia than in a comparison county (Puska et al, 1983).

The Pawtucket Heart Health program (PHHP) is an ongoing project in a Rhode Island community that traditionally has had high rates of CV disease. The interventions are directed toward both individuals and the community to help individuals adopt new behaviors and to create a supportive environment (Carlton et al, 1995, p. 777). Churches, social groups, the business community, and volunteers provided the education intervention. The food industry offered "Heart Healthy" food items and menus, and media campaigns informed citizens about their cholesterol levels and other CV risk factors (Carlton et al, 1995). Although a follow-up survey, $8\frac{1}{2}$ years after the beginning of the program indicated lower obesity levels for the Pawtucket residents, as compared to the comparison city, there were no differences in blood pressure, cholesterol levels, or smoking prevalence. The authors concluded that possible national media exposure, high levels of unemployment, and stress during the time of the study might have contributed to the lack of difference between the two cities.

During the peak time of the PHHP intervention, a significant increase in heart-healthy behaviors, such as physical activity, was seen in the Pawtucket population, suggesting that community interventions can reach a large number of people. More recently, Levin et al (1998) reported on the success of a moderate-intensity physical activity campaign in Pawtucket, Rhode Island, that targeted inactive individuals in the community. The moderate physical activity program evolved from community research based on the original PHHP worksite fitness campaign, and it provides a model for other communities.

The Minnesota Heart Health program (Luepker et al, 1994) was initiated in 1980 with 400,000 persons in six

Midwestern communities. Three communities received the program and three served as controls. Risk factor improvements were seen in all six communities, but only modest differences were found between the treatment and control cities. Favorable health risk changes were found across age, education groups, and sex. Future programs must combine public policy initiatives and community-wide health education strategies with interventions directed to specific high-risk populations (Luepker et al, 1994).

These programs and others provided beginning scientific evidence for the implementation of community-level risk reduction programs. Although the outcomes of risk reduction interventions were in the expected direction, the relative effectiveness of specific interventions remains unclear. The results were modest and often not statistically significant (Winkleby, Feldman, and Murray, 1997). However, these studies have made major contributions to both theory and practice in community partnership, social marketing, behavior change, and evaluation. The programs make it clear that multiple levels of intervention are needed to reach the community in a meaningful way. Nurses have a close relationship with individuals, families, high-risk groups, and organizations such as schools and workplaces. They are positioned to contribute to risk reduction, disease and **illness prevention,** and health promotion by participating in community projects such as the ones described here. It is important that nurses develop health programs and document improved outcomes for high-risk groups with whom they interact.

### DID YOU KNOW?

Some community health promotion studies, such as the federally funded heart disease prevention trials, show only modest intervention effects. This may be due to the nature of the intervention (e.g., whether the intervention included a component for environmental change, or community members were involved in planning), to the target population, or to the way the intervention is evaluated.

Modified from Sellers DE et al: Understanding the variability in the effectiveness of community heart health programs: a meta-analysis, *Soc Sci Med* 44(9):1325, 1997.

## APPLICATION TO COMMUNITY-ORIENTED NURSING
### Multilevel Community Projects

The aim of community-oriented nursing is to create partnerships with individuals, families, groups, and communities to promote their health. Chapter 15 describes types of partnerships. In a passive partnership, nurses develop and direct interventions for the benefit of individuals or communities. As the partnership becomes more active, community members become more involved in assessing,

planning, implementing, and evaluating change. In an active partnership, both professionals and community residents determine health needs. As residents increase their awareness, they are better able to determine what they want for themselves, their families, and their community, and they are more likely to direct program development using the health professionals as consultants. Some examples from community studies, which address multiple levels of clients and foci of care, are described in the following paragraphs. These projects show expanded opportunities for assessment, planning, intervention, and evaluation.

### THE CUTTING EDGE

The use of community health workers (CHW) shows potential as a health promotion intervention strategy. However, high expectations, lack of a clear focus, inadequate supervision by professional nurses, and lack of documentation may decrease the effectiveness of the CHW role. Further research is required using stronger study designs, better documentation of CHW activities, and carefully defined target populations.

Modified from Swider S: Outcome effectiveness of community health workers: an integrative literature review, *Public Health Nurs* 19(1):11, 2002.

Glick et al (1996) used population-focused community development theory to assess the need for a nurse-managed clinic; citizen participation was paramount in the process. Faculty members provided clinical experiences over a 10-year period for undergraduate nursing students at a public housing facility for older adults and the disabled. A request by the local housing authority to expand services to a second site provided the impetus for obtaining grant funding for a community nursing center. Faculty and students conducted a community assessment that indicated that health problems of indigent residents far exceeded those of the state (e.g., an increased infant mortality rate among minorities). When residents and community leaders were asked what services were most needed from a nursing clinic, they listed well-child screening, parenting education, and medication management. Faculty, students, and community members collaborated in all project phases from planning to outcome evaluation.

Flick et al. (1994) and Van Hook (1997) describe other community partnerships. In the first, a partnership was developed by nurses with an urban neighborhood in St. Louis, Missouri, to enhance its capacity to improve its own health (Flick et al, 1994). This project, conducted over 7 years, was based on a community-organizing model; mobilization occurred through community participation and control, with health professionals serving as a resource to the community. The second partnership included East Tennessee State University and two counties in Tennessee

(Van Hook, 1997). It was designed to meet the service needs of underserved rural citizens and provide educational experience for health professional students. Faculty members, students, and community leaders served on advisory boards. On the basis of a community assessment, the School of Nursing opened a rural health clinic and provided a range of health services.

At the aggregate level of client systems, a smoking reduction program in San Francisco targeted Vietnamese men (Jenkins et al, 1997). A media campaign included articles in Vietnamese newspapers and magazines, television coverage, bumper stickers, posters, brochures, antitobacco billboards, and antitobacco presentations. Materials were distributed to Vietnamese physicians to give to clients, and antitobacco activities were developed in language schools. Smoking control ordinances and no-smoking signs were also provided to Vietnamese restaurants. Two years later, smoking rates were significantly lower, especially for young men and students, as compared with those of Vietnamese men in a comparison city.

Another program by Perry et al (1998) was directed to a healthy aggregate. This program was designed to increase fruit and vegetable consumption among fifth graders in 20 elementary schools in St. Paul, Minnesota. The program consisted of a school curriculum, parental education, school food services changes, education of food services staff, and involvement of the food industry in supplying nutritious foods. Eating habits were measured through diet recalls, observation of eating patterns during school lunch, and telephone surveys to the parents. After the intervention, fruit consumption and combined fruit and vegetable consumption increased for all of the children at lunch; vegetable consumption was increased only for girls. Total 24-hour recall indicated an increase in daily fruit and a decrease in fat consumption by both the girls and boys.

Amaya et al (1997) reported a project targeted to the individual and family levels of the client system. In this family living on the U.S.-Mexican border, two children were found to have elevated blood lead levels. The assessment of the family indicated that the exposure was probably related to the home and occupational environment. Risk factors included living near a waste dump, lack of sewage system and running water, peeling lead-based paint on the window sills, and auto parts and oil spills in the yard. In addition, the adults were employed in auto repair and recycling, and the family lacked access to health care and was socially isolated. The intervention included screening and education of individuals about hand washing, and family education about risk factors on the property and in the home. The authors recommended that a screening program be developed for the population living on the border and that programs be tailored to their needs.

Ruffing-Rahal and Wallace (2000) described a 7-year wellness intervention for urban-dwelling, culturally diverse older women with low levels of education and income. Despite their vulnerability, they exhibited indicators of successful aging. The small group intervention consisted of information-giving, dialogue, refreshments, musical accompaniment, and flexibility exercises. Six months after termination of the intervention, improved self-care and well-being indicated that the group of women sustained a "preventive-maintenance" benefit. The authors attributed the benefits to the social support the women derived from their group participation and concluded that social support is in itself an indicator of successful aging.

The projects described in the previous paragraph show the importance of multiple approaches to reaching the population. Cassano and Frongillo (1997) argue that a multilevel approach to community-oriented programs requires that one attend to all client levels. For example, in nutritional programs, it is important to address the individual, the household, grocery store accessibility and environment, the community, and the food environment. No one individual can address all of these levels, but there is increasing emphasis on working in teams and in developing partnerships consisting of health providers and residents. Nurses have an opportunity to work with and to lead these multidisciplinary teams to conduct assessments, develop strategies with the community and its populations, and facilitate the empowerment of community residents. It is increasingly important that nurses incorporate these strategies into their practice (see the Evidence-Based Practice box).

## Evidence-Based Practice

Investigators studied the 6-month impact of three cognitive–behavioral HIV risk-reduction programs on substance use and sexual risk behaviors and cognitive and psychological resources. The subjects included 325 women residing in emergency or sober-living shelters and their 308 intimate sexual partners. Participants were randomized by shelter into three groups: a peer-mentored, a nurse case-managed, or a standard care HIV risk-reduction program. Significant improvements were observed in all groups in risk behaviors and cognitive and psychological resources except for self-esteem. Participants in the peer-mentored and nurse case managed intervention groups did not differ significantly from the standard group in self-esteem, life satisfaction, psychological well-being, use of noninjection drugs, sex with multiple partners, and unprotected sex at 6 months.

**Nurse Use:** The authors concluded that the standard health care approach appears to effectively modify HIV risk behaviors for a majority of homeless participants and may have important economic and policy implications.

Nyamathi A et al: Evaluating the impact of peer, nurse case-managed, and standard HIV risk-reduction programs on psychosocial and health-promoting behavioral outcomes among homeless women, *Res Nurs Health* 24:410, 2001.

## Application of the Integrative Model for Community Health Promotion

In the previous sections, we described the importance of multiple levels of health care aimed at illness and disease prevention and health promotion of individuals, families, aggregates, and the total community. In the remainder of this chapter, we present some examples of the integrative model to assist the reader in applying these concepts. One example of community-oriented nursing care that reflects the four client systems and multiple foci of care is shown in Table 14-1. The health problem that comes to the nurse's attention in this example is a young child with a diagnosis of failure to thrive.

### Illness Care

The nurse initiates care at the individual level with a goal of resolving the failure to thrive. The child's health is assessed and monitored, and the mother is taught principles of nutrition, feeding, and care of her ill child. At the family level, the nurse assesses the presence of malnutrition within the family and refers other family members for care as needed. Also, the family is referred for counseling to relieve the stress related to the child's illness. At the aggregate level, the nurse assesses the community for the prevalence of failure-to-thrive children or teaches classes to raise awareness in the community about this condition and to educate groups about referral and emergency food sources. At the community level, the nurse works with key leaders and citizens to assess the prevalence of nutrition-related illnesses in the community. Community programs may also be instituted to enhance the identification of malnutrition among community members.

### Illness/Disease Prevention

At the individual level, well-balanced nutrition and childcare are taught to the mother to prevent recurrence of malnutrition in the child. A health risk appraisal and

### Table 14-1  Community Health Levels of Care: Malnutrition/Failure to Thrive

| | CLIENT SYSTEM | | | |
|---|---|---|---|---|
| FOCUS OF CARE | INDIVIDUAL | FAMILY | AGGREGATE | COMMUNITY |
| Illness care | • Weigh and measure the child<br>• Monitor the child's symptoms<br>• Teach mother basic nutrition and childcare for failure-to-thrive child | • Teach signs and symptoms of malnutrition to high-risk family members<br>• Refer family for care for nutrition-related problems | • Assess prevalence of failure-to-thrive children in the community<br>• Teach classes about emergency food sources and referral sources for aggregate of failure-to-thrive children | • Assess community for accessibility and adequacy of care providers to treat malnutrition and failure to thrive in the community |
| Illness/disease prevention | • Teach mother well-balanced nutrition and childcare to prevent recurrence of malnutrition and failure to thrive | • Teach nutrition to high-risk family members to prevent nutrition-related problems | • Assess community for prevalence of children at risk of malnutrition<br>• Develop classes about reducing risks of malnutrition in aggregate of high-risk children | • Participate in providing community-wide multimedia education for reduction of malnutrition<br>• Lobby for legislation to promote resources to ensure adequate nutrition to the community |
| Health promotion | • Support individual efforts to adopt health promotion lifestyle, including healthy nutrition | • Plan with family to adopt a healthy lifestyle and incorporate healthy foods into daily eating patterns | • Educate school personnel regarding healthy school lunches for aggregate of schoolchildren | • Work with community leaders and citizens to establish nutrition education programs in the community |

recommendations from the *Guide to Clinical Preventive Services* (USPSTF, 1996) provide direction for age-specific periodic health examination, assessment, and counseling interventions. In addition, the nurse selects an appropriate health risk appraisal tool for use with clinical observation and assessment. The high-risk family is taught nutrition principles and helped to incorporate healthy food into their diets to prevent nutrition-related problems. Using an aggregate approach, the nurse assesses the community for aggregates at risk for malnutrition (e.g., schoolchildren, poor persons, older adults, and the homeless), analyzes health-risk data, and works with others to institute programs to reduce their risk, thereby preventing malnutrition. Community multimedia education for malnutrition risk reduction and lobbying for legislation to promote resources for adequate nutrition within the community are examples of a community approach.

### Health Promotion

At the individual level, the nurse helps the individual adopt a healthy lifestyle as appropriate to age, culture, and resources. For the young child, this includes educating and supporting the parent to provide health-enhancing care. Using the perspective of the family as client, the approach includes the entire family and planning with the family on how to adopt healthy lifestyle activities. These activities range from balanced nutrition to planning for relaxation activities for the family. A wellness inventory helps the nurse design an intervention targeted to the family's awareness of personal self-care. At the aggregate level, the nurse educates school personnel about healthy lunches for the aggregate of students or teachers. Regardless of the level of health need or the client system at which care begins, the ultimate goal of the nurse is health promotion of the total community and its constituents. Participating with community leaders and citizens to establish nutrition education, and making nutritious foods available to all community members are examples of a community-level approach.

Although an important starting point is the care of the failure-to-thrive child, the nurse must recognize that solving the immediate problem is not sufficient. The child's health problem is viewed within a broader context of an optimally healthy child, family, aggregate of children, and community. This approach necessitates not that the nursing interventions be limited to solving the immediate problem of weight gain but rather that care be oriented toward interventions that promote optimal health for the child, family, aggregate of high-risk children, and the total community.

A second example (Table 14-2) concerns a referral of a middle-aged man with coronary heart disease (CHD). The

---

**Table 14-2  Community Health Levels of Care: Coronary Heart Disease (CHD)**

| | CLIENT SYSTEM | | | |
|---|---|---|---|---|
| **FOCUS OF CARE** | **INDIVIDUAL** | **FAMILY** | **AGGREGATE** | **COMMUNITY** |
| Illness care | • Administer medications<br>• Monitor heart rate of individual client in the home setting | • Teach signs/symptoms of CHD to high-risk family members | • Assess prevalence of CHD in the community<br>• Teach classes to high-risk groups about what to do in an emergency | • Assess community for accessibility and adequacy of care providers for clients with heart disease |
| Illness/disease | • Teach low-fat nutrition, progressive exercise, and relaxation to client to prevent recurrence of heart disease | • Teach low-fat nutrition and importance of regular exercise and relaxation to high-risk family members to prevent heart disease | • Develop classes for specific high-risk groups about cardiovascular risk reduction | • Community-wide multimedia education for cardiovascular risk reduction |
| Health | • Empower individual to adopt health promotion lifestyle | • Plan with family to incorporate health promotion activities into lifestyle | • Provide group education (classes) regarding benefits of regular exercise | • Work with community leaders and citizens to establish safe parks for community activities |

immediate goal of the nurse is to provide care that will help the individual client to resolve his illness. Therefore teaching him about the effects and side effects of his medications and how to monitor his condition at home are important interventions. Within the context of predisposing genetic, lifestyle, and environmental factors relative to CHD, the family members are also given information about this illness, including early recognition of signs and symptoms for themselves. Assessing the prevalence of CHD among high-risk aggregates in the community and developing media interventions and cardiopulmonary resuscitation (CPR) classes for high-risk aggregates is also an important aspect of illness care. An example is providing CPR classes in Spanish to monolingual Spanish-speaking persons in the community. At the community level, it is important to assess whether there are adequate providers and resources for identifying and treating heart disease in the community.

Prevention care is also addressed at the individual level by teaching measures, such as stress reduction, low-fat nutrition, and progressive exercise, to prevent recurrence of the disease. For high-risk family members, low-fat nutrition, smoking cessation, and regular moderate exercise are important preventive measures. Providing exercise programs to workers in high-stress and sedentary occupations is an example of an aggregate-level preventive intervention, and multimedia campaigns to provide intensive education to the community about prevention of heart disease during the month of February each year are an example of a community intervention.

Health promotion care similarly includes encouraging individuals to adopt a health-promoting lifestyle and helping them to become aware of their own power to do so. The nurse can also encourage families to incorporate health-promoting activities into their daily lives. This might include taking walks, swimming together, or joining an intergenerational baseball or bowling team in which families compete with other families. Aggregates can also benefit from heart-healthy classes or activities that are culturally specific to particular aggregates, such as older Hispanic women or African-American teenage girls. These activities can include stress management, well-balanced nutrition, exercise, or any other topic that can promote heart health. When looking at the total community, an example of a health promotion intervention is participating in a coalition to plan for parks and recreation areas within the community that are safe and accessible to the population.

In summary, the concepts of health, health promotion, and community are inextricably linked: it is difficult to discuss one without including the others. It is also important that nurses examine their definitions and beliefs about each concept as the basis for their practice. The essence of the community-oriented nursing perspective is the ability to see the totality of community while addressing its component parts and, at the same time, to see the total needs for health promotion, health protection, illness and disease prevention, and illness care and management. It is the integrative relationship among all these levels that distin-guishes community-oriented nursing from nursing in more circumscribed settings, such as hospitals and clinics.

## Practice Application

A rural health outreach program serves migrant workers, their families, and other vulnerable populations in the local community. The program's goals include increased knowledge about risk factors, services, and self-care; improved community health; increased access and affordability of individual- and community-level health promotion services; and reduced barriers to health services. The program offers health promotion and disease prevention educational materials and classes in English and Spanish throughout the region in churches, schools, community centers, fire departments, and migrant camps. In addition, clinics have been established in eight local sites across the county. Lay health promoters from the migrant community have been trained to deliver basic health education and resource information. Clinic services include health risk appraisal, disease screening, immunizations, health education, counseling, and referral. Funding from a variety of public and private sources supports the program. It is essential that the program show effective outcomes if it is to sustain funding.

Mary Ann, a nurse with a Bachelor of Science in Nursing degree, works for the outreach program. She is a member of a group asked to evaluate whether the outreach program (including the eight clinics) is effective in meeting the stated objectives.

A. Using the integrative model for community health promotion as a guide, how might you organize a comprehensive approach to assessment and data collection?
B. What are sources of data you might use for assessing individual, aggregate, and community health indicators?
C. What is the value of interviewing rural residents, migrant workers, and clinic participants about their perceptions of health and the value of health services?
D. Whom else can you interview to elicit important information about the usefulness of the outreach program?
E. How can you best use lay health promoters to increase participation and partnership among concerned health professionals, community residents, and migrant families and to ultimately sustain the program?

Be creative and comprehensive in your approach, and consider cultural factors associated with rural and migrant populations in the United States. Current spending limits on federal and state programs for health promotion and disease prevention require that nurses deal effectively with issues of outreach, sustainability, and success of community health programs.

**Answers are in the back of the book.**

## Key Points

- The idea of health shapes the process of community-oriented nursing practice, from assessment of health-related needs of individuals, families, aggregates, and communities to evaluation of behavioral outcomes.
- The greatest benefits in public health are likely to accrue from efforts to improve individual and family lifestyle, social conditions, and the physical environment.
- Community-oriented nurses have a history of commitment to primary health care and to enhancing levels of wellness in populations.
- When nurses examine their own definition of health, they recognize how nursing care is directed by this health definition.
- The goal of risk appraisal and reduction is the prevention or early detection of disease.
- The knowledge base for risk appraisal and risk reduction is the scientific evidence regarding the relationship between risk factors and mortality and the effectiveness of planned interventions in reducing both risks and mortality.
- Health risk appraisal is used to assess the total risks to an individual's health, and resulting knowledge of health risks may be used to initiate health-promoting and disease-preventing lifestyle changes.
- Clinical preventive guidelines use clinical and epidemiologic data to identify specific individual health risks, and they provide a detailed list of recommendations for preventive measures appropriate to different age-groups.
- Wellness inventories define health risks broadly and emphasize empowerment of individuals to achieve health.
- Clinical observation, assessment, and nursing interventions used in conjunction with health-risk appraisals are essential to obtain the best results.
- The Stanford Heart Disease Prevention program, the North Karelia Project, the Pawtucket Heart Health program, and the Minnesota Heart Health program contributed to the scientific knowledge base for the design, implementation, and evaluation of risk-appraisal and risk-reduction programs.
- Community-oriented nurses must function beyond resolving a specific illness to preventing the illness and promoting optimal health for the individual, the family, the aggregate, and the total community. All of these levels are important in population-focused care to promote the health of the community and its members.

## Clinical Decision-Making Activities

1. Elaborate on your own definition of health, and interview a nurse, client, and physician about their definitions of health. Use Smith's four models of health as a frame of reference to contrast different perspectives.
2. What are some difficulties encountered when you consider definitions of health promotion, disease prevention, and health maintenance? Illustrate these difficulties with examples of strategies that can be defined as health promoting, disease preventing, or health maintaining.
3. Define community health promotion, and provide examples of health promotion indicators for a specified community.
4. Develop a nursing care plan for adolescent substance abuse using Milio's (1976) propositions as a frame of reference.
5. Use the integrative model for community health promotion to identify the most important strategies in a community-wide plan for adolescent substance abuse.
6. Consider the role of partnership with the community from the perspectives of school health, public health, occupational health, and home health.
7. Illustrate community health levels of care including the client system and the focus of care:
   a. For teenage pregnancy, beginning with health promotion at the individual level
   b. For breast cancer, starting from the level of community illness/disease prevention

## Additional Resources

These related resources are found either in the appendix at the back of this book and on the book's website at **http://evolve.elsevier.com/Stanhope.**

### Appendixes

Appendix F Health Risk Appraisal

### evolve Evolve Website

Appendix A.1 Schedule of Clinical Preventive Services

Healthier People Network at http://www.mindspring.com/hpnhra/index.html

National Wellness Institute at http://www.nationalwellness.org/nwi_Home/nwi.asp

WebLinks: Healthy People 2010

# References

Amaya MA et al: Childhood lead poisoning on the US-Mexico border: a case study in environmental health nursing lead poisoning, *Public Health Nurs* 14(6):353, 1997.

Anderson DR et al: The relationship between modifiable health risks and group-level health care expenditures, *Am J Health Promot* 15(1):45, 2000.

Anderson ET, McFarlane J: *Community-as-partner: theory and practice in nursing,* Philadelphia, 2000, Lippincott, Williams & Wilkins.

Ardell DB: *High level wellness: an alternative to doctors, drugs, and disease,* Emmaus, Penn, 1977, Rodale.

Becker MH, Janz NK: Behavioral science perspectives on health hazard/health risk appraisal, *Health Serv Res* 22(4):537, 1987.

Berkman LF, Breslow L: *Health and ways of living, the Alameda County Study,* New York, 1983, Oxford University Press.

Blum HL: *Planning for health,* ed 2, New York, 1981, Human Sciences.

Bracht N, editor: *Health promotion at the community level,* Newbury Park, Calif, 1990, Sage.

Breslow L et al: *Risk Factor Update project: final report,* Atlanta, 1985, U.S. Department of Health and Human Services.

Breslow L et al: Development of a health risk appraisal for the elderly (HRA-E), *Am J Health Promot* 11(5):337-343, 1997.

Breslow L, Somers AR: The lifetime health-monitoring program: a practical approach to preventive medicine, *New Engl J Med* 296(11):601, 1977.

Brubaker BH: Health promotion: a linguistic analysis, *Adv Nurs Sci* 5(3):1, 1983.

Carlton RA et al: The Pawtucket heart health program: community changes in cardiovascular risk factors and projected disease risk, *Am J Public Health* 85(6):777, 1995.

Cassano PA, Frongillo EA: Annotation: developing and validating new methods for assessing community interventions, *Am J Public Health* 87(2):157, 1997.

Centers for Disease Control and Prevention: Smoking-attributable mortality and years of potential life lost, and economic costs: United States, 1995-1999, *MMWR Morb Mortal Wkly Rep* 51(14):300-303, 2002.

Chopoorian TL: Reconceptualizing the environment. In Moccia P, editor: *New approaches to theory development,* Publication No. 15-1992, New York, 1986, National League for Nursing.

Christopher S, Christopher JC, Dunnagan T: Culture's impact on health risk appraisal psychological well-being questions, *Am J Health Behav* 24(5):338, 2000.

Clark NM, Becker MH: Theoretical models and strategies for improving adherence and disease management. In Schuler SA et al, editors: *The handbook of health behavior change,* ed 2, New York, 1998, Springer.

Doerr BT, Hutchins EB: Health risk appraisal: process, problems, and prospects for nursing practice and research, *Nurs Res* 30(5):299, 1981.

Downie RS, Tannahill C, Tannahill A: *Health promotion models and values,* ed 2, New York, 1996, Oxford University Press.

Edwards LH, Dees RL: Environmental health: the effects of life style on the world around us. In Wold SJ, editor: *Community health nursing: issues and topics,* East Norwalk, Conn, 1990, Appleton & Lange.

Farquhar JW et al: Effects of community-wide education on cardiovascular disease risk factors: the Stanford five-city project, *JAMA* 264:359, 1990.

Flick LH et al: Building community for health: lessons from a seven-year-old neighborhood/university partnership, *Health Educ Q* 21(3):369, 1994.

Fuchs V: *Who shall live?* New York, 1974, Basic Books.

Glick DF et al: Community development theory: planning a community nursing center, *J Nurs Adm* 26(7/8):1, 1996.

Goeppinger J: Changing health behaviors and outcomes through self-care. In Lancaster J, Lancaster W, editors: *Concepts for advanced nursing practice: the nurse as a change agent,* St Louis, Mo, 1982, Mosby.

Griffith HM, Diguiseppi C: Guidelines for clinical preventive services: essential for nurse practitioners in practice, education, and research, *Nurse Pract* 19(9):25, 1994.

Hanchett ES: Nursing frameworks and community as client: bridging the gap, East Norwalk, Conn, 1988, Appleton & Lange.

Hu FB et al: Trends in the incidence of coronary heart disease and changes in diet and lifestyle in women, *New Engl J Med* 343(8):530, 2000.

Illich I: *Medical nemesis: the expropriation of health,* New York, 1976, Random House.

Institute of Medicine: *The future of public health,* Washington, DC, 1988, National Academy Press.

Issel LM: Measuring comprehensive case management interventions: development of a tool, *Nurs Case Manag* 2(4):132, 1997.

Jakicic JM et al: Appropriate intervention strategies for weight loss and prevention of weight regain for adults, *Med Sci Sports Exerc* 33(12):2145-2156, 2001.

Jenkins CNH et al: The effectiveness of a media-led intervention to reduce smoking among Vietnamese-American men, *Am J Public Health* 87(6):1031, 1997.

Johnson SK: The state of disease management, *Case Review* 2(4):53-54, 1996.

Keller LO et al: Population-based public health nursing interventions: a model for practice, *Public Health Nurs* 15(3):207, 1998.

Kulbok PA: Social resources, health resources, and preventive health behavior: patterns and predictors, *Public Health Nurs* 2(2):67, 1985.

Kulbok PA, Baldwin JH: From preventive health behavior to health promotion: advancing a positive construct of health, *Adv Nurs Sci* 14(4):50, 1992.

Kulbok PA et al: Advancing discourse on health promotion: beyond mainstream thinking, *Adv Nurs Sci* 20(1):12, 1997.

Kulbok PA et al: The multidimensional health behavior inventory, *J Nurs Measure* 7(2):177, 1999.

Laffrey SC: An exploration of adult health behaviors, *West J Nurs Res* 12(4):434, 1990.

Laffrey SC, Kulbok PA: The integrative model for community health nursing: a conceptual guide to education, practice, and research, *J Holist Nurs* 17(10):88, 1999.

Laffrey SC, Loveland-Cherry CJ, Winkler SJ: Health behavior: evolution of two paradigms, *Public Health Nurs* 3(2):92-97, 1986.

LaLonde M: *A new perspective on the health of Canadians,* Ottawa, 1974, Government of Canada.

Lasater T et al: Lay volunteer delivery of a community-based cardiovascular risk factor change program: the Pawtucket experiment. In Matarazzo JD et al, editors: *Behavioral health: a handbook of health enhancement and disease prevention,* Silver Spring, Md, 1984, Wiley.

Leavell HR, Clark EG: *Preventive medicine for the doctor in his community: an epidemiological approach,* ed 3, New York, 1965, McGraw-Hill.

Levin S et al: The evolution of a physical activity campaign, *Fam Community Health* 21(1):65-77, 1998.

Liao Y et al: How generalizable are coronary risk prediction models? Comparison of Framingham and two national cohorts, *Am Heart J* 137(5):837, 1999.

Lorig K: Chronic disease self-management: a model for tertiary prevention, *Am Behav Scientist* 39(6): 676, 1996.

Luepker RV et al: Community education for cardiovascular disease prevention: risk factor changes in the Minnesota Heart Health Program, *Am J Public Health* 84(9):1383, 1994.

McGinnis JM, Forge WH: Actual causes of death in the United States, *JAMA* 270(18):2207, 1993.

Milio N: A framework for prevention: changing health-damaging to health-generating life patterns, *Am J Public Health* 66(5):435, 1976.

Moe EV: Nature of today's community. In Reinhardt AM, Quinn MD, editors: *Current practice in community health nursing,* St Louis, Mo, 1977, Mosby.

Musich S, Napier D, Edington DW: The association of health risks with workers compensation costs, *J Occup Environ Med* 43(6):534-541, 2001.

National Wellness Institute: *Lifestyle assessment questionnaire,* Stevens Point, Wisc, 1989, National Wellness Institute.

Nyamathi A et al: Evaluating the impact of peer, nurse case-managed, and standard HIV risk-reduction programs on psychosocial and health-promoting behavioral outcomes among homeless women, *Res Nurs Health* 24:410-422, 2001.

Orem D: *Nursing: concepts of practice,* ed 5, St Louis, Mo, 1995, Mosby.

Orlandi MA, Dalton LT: Lifestyle interventions for the young. In Schuler SA et al, editors: *The handbook of health behavior change,* ed 2, New York, 1998, Springer.

Pender N: *Health promotion in nursing practice,* ed 3, East Norwalk, Conn, 1996, Appleton & Lange.

Perry CL et al: Changing fruit and vegetable consumption among children: the 5-a-Day Power Plus program in St. Paul, Minnesota, *Am J Public Health* 88(4):603, 1998.

Public Health Service: Healthy people: *Surgeon General's report on health promotion and disease prevention,* Washington, DC, 1979, U.S. Department of Health and Human Services.

Puska P et al: Change in risk factors for coronary heart disease during 10 years of a community intervention programme (North Karelia Project), *Br Med J* 287(6408):1840, 1983.

Robbins LC, Hall JN: *How to practice prospective medicine,* Indianapolis, 1970, Methodist Hospital of Indiana.

Rosenberg IH: Keys to a longer, healthier, more vital life, *Nutr Rev* 52(8 Pt 2): S50, 1994.

Ruffing-Rahal M, Wallace J: Successful aging in a wellness group for older women, *Health Care Women Int* 21:267, 2000.

Salmon-White M: Construct for public health nursing, *Nurs Outlook* 30(9):527, 1982.

Seefeldt V, Malina RM, Clark MA: Factors affecting levels of physical activity in adults, *Sports Med* 32(3):143, 2002.

Sellers DE et al: Understanding the variability in the effectiveness of community heart health programs: a meta-analysis, *Soc Sci Med* 44(9):1325, 1997.

Smith JA: The idea of health: a philosophical inquiry, *Adv Nurs Sci* 3(3):43, 1981.

Smith KW, McKinlay SM, McKinlay JB: The reliability of health risk appraisals: a field trial of four instruments, *Am J Public Health* 79(12):1603, 1989.

Swider S: Outcome effectiveness of community health workers: an integrative literature review, *Public Health Nurs* 19(1):11, 2002.

Terris M: Approaches to an epidemiology of health, *Am J Public Health* 65(10):1037-1038, 1975.

Tyas SL, Pederson LL: Psychosocial factors related to adolescent smoking: a critical review of the literature, *Tob Control* 7:409-420, 1998.

U.S. Department of Health, Education, and Welfare: *Forward plan for health,* FY 1978-82, DHEW PHS Publication No. (OS) 76-50046, Washington, DC, 1976, U.S. Government Printing Office.

U.S. Department of Health, Education, and Welfare: *Healthy people: the surgeon general's report on health promotion and disease prevention,* DHEW Publication No. 79-55071, Washington, DC, 1979, U.S. Government Printing Office.

U.S. Department of Health and Human Services: *Healthy people 2000: national health promotion and disease prevention objectives,* DHHS Publication No 91-50212, Washington, DC, 1991, U.S. Government Printing Office.

U.S. Department of Health and Human Services: *Healthy people 2010,* ed 2, *With understanding and improving health and objectives for improving health,* 2 vols, Washington, DC, 2000, U.S. Government Printing Office.

U.S. Department of Health and Human Services: *Healthy people in healthy communities,* Washington, DC, 2001, U.S. Government Printing Office.

U.S. Preventive Services Task Force: *Guide to clinical preventive services: report of the U.S. Preventive Services Task Force,* Baltimore, 1989, Williams and Wilkins.

U.S. Preventive Services Task Force: *A guide to clinical preventive services,* Alexandria, Va, 1996, USDHHS, available at http://www.hhs.gov/PPIP/handbook.html.

Utz S, Kulbok PA: Managing care through advanced nursing practice. In Lancaster JL, Lancaster W, editors: *Nursing issues in leading and managing change,* St Louis, Mo, 1998, Mosby.

Van Hook RY: East Tennessee State University: preparing health professionals for practice in Appalachia. In *USDHHS (HRSA): The third national primary care conference: community-based academic partnerships, case studies,* Washington, DC, 1997, USDHHS.

Winkleby MA et al: The long-term effects of a cardiovascular disease prevention trial: the Stanford five-city project, *Am J Public Health* 86(12):1773, 1996.

Winkleby MA, Feldman HA, Murray DM: Joint analysis of US three community intervention trials for reduction of cardiovascular disease risk, *J Clin Epidemiol* 50(6):645, 1997.

World Health Organization: *The first ten years of the World Health Organization,* New York, 1958, WHO.

World Health Organization: *Health promotion: a discussion document on the concept and principles,* Copenhagen, 1984, WHO Regional Office for Europe.

Yen L et al: Changes in health risks among the participants in the United Auto Workers-General Motors Life Steps Health Promotion Program, *Am J Health Promot* 16(1):7, 2001.

# Part 4

## Issues and Approaches in Community-Oriented Health Care

The primary orientation of health care delivery has been toward care and cure of the individual. There is increasing evidence that lifestyle and personal health habits influence the health of individuals, families, populations, aggregates, and communities.

Although it is necessary to identify health risk factors among individuals and groups in the community, it is of paramount importance that nurses learn to identify and work with health problems of the total community. This may be referred to as an aggregate approach or a population-focused approach to health care delivery. Healthy communities provide greater resources for growth and nurturing of individuals and families than do their unhealthy counterparts.

Certainly, community-oriented nurses use a public health approach to work with individuals and families in promoting health, intervening in disease onset or progression, and assisting with rehabilitation. Likewise, nurses often find that strategies used to introduce health behaviors directed at illness prevention and lifestyle changes are applicable to groups in the community and the community at large. Concepts for promoting health behaviors through groups, identifying community groups and their contributions to community life, and helping groups work toward community health goals are essential to community-oriented nursing practice.

Healthy Communities/Healthy Cities is an organized approach to helping communities organize and act to provide environments for healthful living for their populations. In this approach, health is described as encompassing the physical and mental health of individuals and families and of the social, political, economic, educational, cultural, and environmental settings of the total community.

The nurse will be able to help communities attain their health goals by understanding the organization of communities, the effects of rural versus urban settings on health issues, how and why programs are managed, and how to evaluate programs for quality and effectiveness. A community assessment provides the basis for helping communities establish their goals. The use of a nurse-managed clinic is one approach that community-oriented nurses have found to be successful in meeting the needs of aggregates, or vulnerable at-risk populations; these needs must be considered when trying to improve the health of a community. Case management is an approach that has been used by community-oriented nurses since its inception, to match the most appropriate services and health care delivery interventions to population needs.

Although all communities strive to protect their populations and provide a safe living environment, natural and human-made disasters may occur; community-oriented nurses can play a significant role in helping a community through crises such as the 9/11 crisis and other acts of terrorism. The chapters in this section of the text help the nurse learn how to work with aggregates and to develop healthy communities.

# Community as Client: Assessment and Analysis

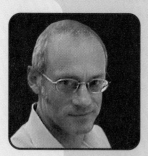

**George F. Shuster, R.N., D.N.Sc.**

George F. Shuster started community-oriented nursing as a volunteer nurse in one of the Seattle Neighborhood Free Clinics in 1981. Since that time, he has also practiced as a home-health nurse in San Francisco, California, and later in Charlottesville, Virginia. In Virginia he was involved with the American Lung Association in community-wide smoking cessation programs. In New Mexico he continues to teach community health at the undergraduate and graduate levels while also being involved in the development of a community-focused health promotion program for older Hispanic women.

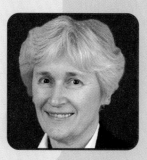

**Jean Goeppinger, Ph.D., R.N.**

Jean Goeppinger began her work in the community as a home-health nurse with the Visiting Nurse Association of Detroit. This work also provided an opportunity to work with an underserved and vulnerable inner-city African-American community. Since then she has developed community-oriented nursing programs and courses and conducted research designed to improve the self-care abilities of community residents with chronic disease.

## Objectives

After reading this chapter, the student should be able to do the following:

1. Decide whether nursing practice can be community oriented
2. Illustrate concepts basic to community-oriented nursing practice: community, community client, community health, and partnership for health
3. Understand the relevance of the nursing process to community-oriented nursing practice
4. Analyze the importance of community assessment in nursing practice
5. Decide which methods of assessment, intervention, and evaluation are most appropriate in given situations
6. Develop a community-oriented nursing care plan

---

Although in the past nurses have sometimes viewed the community as a client, many public and community health nurses have come to consider the community their most important client and, more recently, their partner (Anderson and McFarlane, 2000; Schwab and Syme, 1997; Westbrook and Schultz, 2000). This chapter clarifies community concepts and provides a guideline for nursing practice with the community client. The core functions of public health nursing include assessment, policy development, and assurance. A public and private group partnership called the Council on Linkages Between Academia and Public Health Practice has defined competencies for the core functions of public health practice (2001) (see Chapter 1 for more details). In the area of assessment, 11 competencies for the nurse and other health providers working in the community are listed (Box 15-1).

The nursing process from assessment through evaluation is used to promote community health. This process begins with **community assessment,** one of the core functions, which involves getting to know the community. It is a logical, systematic approach to identifying community needs, clarifying problems, and identifying community strengths and resources. This chapter provides the nurse with the knowledge necessary to develop the community assessment core competencies.

## COMMUNITY DEFINED

Definitions of the meaning of **community** vary widely. The Expert Committee Report on community health nursing of the World Health Organization includes this definition: "A community is a social group determined by geographic boundaries and/or common values and interests.

## Key Terms

aggregate, p. 344
APEXPH, p. 351
change agent, p. 367
change partner, p. 367
community, p. 342
community-as-partner model, p. 359
community assessment, p. 342
community competence, p. 347
community health, p. 346
community health problem, p. 356
community health strength, p. 356
community-oriented practice, p. 345
community partnership, p. 350
confidentiality, p. 359
database, p. 353
data collection, p. 353
data gathering, p. 353

data generation, p. 355
early adopters, p. 368
empowerment, p. 351
evaluation, p. 369
goals, p. 363
implementation, p. 366
informant interviews, p. 355
interacting groups, p. 368
interdependent, p. 344
intervention activities, p. 364
late adopters, p. 368
lay advisors, p. 368
MAPP, p. 351
mass media, p. 368
mediating structures, p. 368
nominal groups, p. 368
objectives, p. 363

participant observation, p. 355
partnership, p. 346
PATCH, p. 351
probability, p. 364
problem analysis, p. 356
problem correlates, p. 358
problem prioritizing, p. 362
program planning model, p. 358
role negotiation, p. 359
secondary analysis, p. 356
surveys, p. 353
target of practice, p. 344
typologies, p. 343
value, p. 364
windshield surveys, p. 355
*See Glossary for definitions*

## Chapter Outline

Community Defined
Community as Client
*Community Client and Nursing Practice*
Goals and Means of Community-Oriented
    Practice
*Community Health*

*Healthy People 2010*
*Community Partnerships*
*Strategies to Improve Community Health*
Community-Focused Nursing Process: An
    Overview of the Process From Assessment
    to Evaluation

*Community Assessment*
*Community-Oriented Nursing Diagnosis*
*Planning for Community Health*
*Implementing in the Community*
*Evaluating Community Health Intervention*
Personal Safety in Community Practice

Its members know and interact with one another. It functions within a particular social structure and exhibits and creates norms, values and social institutions" (World Health Organization [WHO], 1974, p. 7). Other theorists and writers present **typologies** (lists of types), which involve classifying communities by category rather than single definitions. One such typology of community was described by Blum in 1974. This typology is still used today. The categories, or types of communities, include communities defined by geopolitical boundaries, by their interactions (such as between schools, social services, and governmental agencies), and by their ability to solve problems. Some types of communities are listed in Box 15-2.

Nurses working in communities quickly learn that society consists of many different types of communities. Some of the communities listed in Box 15-2 are *communi-*

*ties of place*. In this type of community, interactions occur within a specific geographic area. Neighborhood and face-to-face communities are two examples of this type of community. Other communities, such as communities of special interest or resource communities, cut across geographic areas. Common concerns and interests, which can be long term or short term in nature, bring their members together—for example, a group to support a smoke-free environment. Another type of community is a *community of problem ecology*, which is created when environmental problems such as water pollution affect a widespread area. For example, a problem such as water pollution can bring people together from areas that would not otherwise share a common interest. Nurses also may work in partnership with *communities defined by geographic and political boundaries*, such as school districts, townships, or counties.

---

**BOX 15-1   Core Competencies for Public Health Professionals**

Public health professionals should be able to do the following:
- Define a problem
- Determine appropriate uses and limitations of both quantitative and qualitative data
- Select and define variables relevant to the defined public health problems
- Identify relevant and appropriate data and information sources
- Evaluate the integrity and comparability of data and identify gaps in data sources
- Apply ethical principles to the collection, maintenance, use, and dissemination of data and information
- Partner with communities to attach meaning to collected quantitative and qualitative data
- Make relevant inferences from quantitative and qualitative data
- Obtain and interpret information regarding risks and benefits to the community
- Apply data collection processes, information technology applications, and computer systems storage and retrieval strategies
- Recognize how the data illuminate ethical, political, scientific, economic, and overall public health issues

Council on Linkages Between Academia and Public Health Practice: *Core competencies for public health professionals,* Washington, DC, 2001, USDHHS and Public Health Foundation, available at www.phf.org/Link.htm.

---

**BOX 15-2   Types of Communities**

- Face-to-face community
- Neighborhood community
- Community of identifiable need
- Community of problem ecology
- Community of concern
- Community of special interest
- Community of viability
- Community of action capability
- Community of political jurisdiction
- Resource community
- Community of solution

From Blum HL: *Planning for health,* New York, 1974, Human Sciences Press.

---

Because the type of community varies, nurses planning community interventions must take into account each community's specific characteristics. Each community is unique, and its defining characteristics will affect the nature of the partnership.

In most definitions, the community includes three factors: people, place, and function. The people are the community members or residents. Place refers both to geographic and time dimensions, and function refers to the aims and activities of the community. Community-oriented nurses regularly need to examine how the person, place, and function dimensions of community shape their nursing practice. They can use both a definition and a set of measures for the community in their practice.

In this chapter, the following definition is used: Community is a locality-based entity, composed of systems of formal organizations reflecting society's institutions, informal groups, and aggregates. As defined in Chapter 1, an **aggregate** is a collection of individuals who have in common one or more personal or environmental characteristics. The parts of a community are **interdependent,** and their function is to meet a wide variety of collective needs. This definition of community includes person, place, and function dimensions and recognizes interaction among the systems within a community. Measures of the dimensions for this definition are listed in Table 15-1.

If the community is where community-oriented nurses practice and apply the nursing process, and the community is the client of that practice, then nurses will want to analyze and synthesize information about the boundaries, parts, and dynamic processes of the client community. The next section describes the community as client: it is both the setting for practice and the **target of practice** (i.e., the client) for the community-oriented health nurse.

## COMMUNITY AS CLIENT

Community-oriented nurses have often been considered unique because of their target of practice. The idea of health-related care being provided within the community is, however, not new. At the turn of the century, most persons stayed at home during illnesses. As a result, the practice environment for all nurses was the home rather than the hospital. As the range of community nursing services expanded, many different kinds of agencies were started, and their services often overlapped. For example, both privately owned voluntary agencies and official local health agencies worked to control tuberculosis. The nurses employed by these agencies were called community health nurses, public health nurses, and visiting nurses. They practiced in clients' homes and not in the hospital. *Today, these three types of nurses are called community-oriented nurses.*

Early public health nursing textbooks included lengthy descriptions of the home environment and tools for assessing the extent to which that environment promoted the health of family members. Health education about the

**Table 15-1    The Concept of Community Specified**

| DIMENSIONS | MEASURES | EXAMPLES OF DATA SOURCES |
|---|---|---|
| Place | Geopolitical boundaries | Maps |
| | Local or folk name for area | Local newspaper |
| | Size in square miles, acres, blocks, or census tracts | Census data |
| | Transportation avenues, such as rivers, highways, railroads, and sidewalks | Chamber of Commerce<br>City, county, or township government |
| | History | Library archives and local histories |
| | Physical environment such as land use patterns and condition of housing | Local housing office |
| People or person | Population: number and density | Census data |
| | Demographic structure of population, such as age, sex, socioeconomic, and racial distributions; rural and urban character, and dependency ratio | Census data<br>Churches, senior centers<br>Civic groups |
| | Informal groups such as block clubs, service clubs, and friendship networks | Local newspaper<br>Telephone directory<br>United Way<br>Social service agencies |
| | Formal groups such as schools, churches, businesses, industries, governmental bodies, unions, and health and welfare agencies | Chamber of Commerce<br>Tourist bureau<br>Local or state officials |
| | Linking structures (intercommunity and intracommunity contacts among organizations) | Chamber of Commerce |
| Function | Production, distribution, and consumption of goods and services | State departments<br>Business and labor<br>Local library |
| | Socialization of new members | Social and local research reports |
| | Maintenance of social control | Police station |
| | Adapting to ongoing and expected change | Social and local research reports |
| | Provision of mutual aid | United Way<br>Welfare agencies<br>Churches and religious organizations |

home environment was often a major part of home nursing care.

By the 1950s, schools, prisons, industries, and neighborhood health centers, as well as homes, had all become settings of practice for community-oriented nurses. Many of these new nurses did not consider the environments in which they practiced. Although their practices took place within the community, they focused on the individual client or family seeking care. The care provided was not community oriented; rather, it was oriented toward the individual or family who lived in the community, and this is now called community-*based* nursing practice. This commitment to direct, hands-on clinical nursing care delivered to individuals or families in community settings remains a more popular approach to community nursing practice than recognizing the whole community as the target of nursing practice. This remains true despite the American Public Health Association (APHA) (Public Health Nursing Section) definition of public health nursing as "the practice of promoting and protecting the health of populations us-

ing knowledge from nursing, social, and public health sciences" (American Nurses Association, 1999, p. 1; APHA, 1996, p. 1). When the location of the practice is the community and the focus of the practice is the individual or family, then the client remains the individual or family, and the nurse is practicing in the community as the setting.

The community is the client only when the nursing focus is on the collective or common good of the population instead of on individual health. **Community-oriented practice** seeks healthful change for the whole community's benefit (Shiell and Hawe, 1996). Although the nurse may work with individuals, families or other interacting groups, aggregates, or institutions, or within a population, the resulting changes are intended to affect the whole community. For example, an occupational health nurse's target might be preventing illness and injury and maintaining or promoting the health of an entire company workforce. Because of this focus, the nurse would help an individual disabled worker become independent in activities of daily living. The nurse would also become involved with promoting vocational rehabilitation services in the community and seek reasonable employment policies for all disabled workers through the community government.

## Community Client and Nursing Practice

Population-focused health care is experiencing a rebirth, and the community as client is important to nursing practice for several reasons. When focusing on the community as client, direct clinical care can be a part of population-focused community health practice (Abraham and Fallon, 1997a). For example, sometimes direct nursing care is provided to individuals and family members because their health needs are common community-related problems. Changes in their health will affect the health of their communities (Courtney et al, 1996).

---

**WHAT DO YOU THINK?**

Many nurses believe that home-health nursing is focused on the individual and it therefore should not be considered a part of community-oriented nursing. Other nurses argue that home-health nursing focuses on the family, takes place in the community, and should be considered a part of community-oriented nursing. Is home-health nursing focused on the individual, family, or community, or on all three? Is home-health nursing a part of community-oriented nursing? Why or why not?

---

In such cases, decisions are made at the individual level because the individual's health is related to the health of the population as a whole. Improved health of the community remains the overall goal of nursing intervention. Interventions to stop spousal or elder abuse are two examples of nursing interventions done primarily because of the effects of abuse on society and therefore on the population as a whole. Also, the treatment of a client for tuberculosis reduces the risk to other community members. This care reduces the risk of an epidemic in the community.

The community client also highlights the complexity of the change process. Change for the benefit of the community client must often occur at several levels, ranging from the individual to society as a whole. For example, health problems caused by lifestyle, such as smoking, overeating, and speeding, cannot be solved simply by asking individuals to choose health-promoting habits. Society also must provide healthy choices. Most individuals cannot change their habits alone; they require the support of family members, friends, community health care systems, and relevant social policies. Individuals who have lifestyle health problems are often blamed for their illness because of their choices (e.g., to smoke). In his classic work, Ryan (1976) points out that the "victim" cannot always be blamed and expected to correct the problem without changes also being made in the helping professions and public policy. Some communities have no-smoking areas

in restaurants to prevent secondhand smoke from harming others. This is an example of a community-level policy to change behavior.

Commitment to the health of the community client requires a process of change at each of these levels. One nursing role emphasizes individual and direct personal care skills. Another nursing role focuses on the family as the unit of service. A third focuses on the community as a unit of service. Collaborative practice models involving the community and nurses in joint decision making and specific nursing roles are required (Courtney et al, 1996). Clark and Mass (1998) note that nurses must remember that collaboration means a cooperative effort in which those participating want to do so. Participants must see themselves as part of a group effort and share in the process beginning with planning and including decision making. This means sharing not only the power but also the responsibility for the outcomes of the intervention. Viewing the community as client and thus as the target of service means a commitment to two key concepts: (1) community health and (2) partnership for community health. Together these form not only the goal **(community health)** but also the *means* of community-oriented practice **(partnership).**

## GOALS AND MEANS OF COMMUNITY-ORIENTED PRACTICE

In community-oriented practice, the nurse and the community seek healthy change together (Shiell and Hawe, 1996). Their common goal of community health involves an ongoing series of health-promoting changes rather than a fixed state. The most effective means of completing healthy changes in the community is through this same partnership. Specific examples of partnership between the nurse and the community (Jefferson County) are provided throughout this chapter.

## Community Health

Like the concept of community, community health has three common characteristics, or dimensions: status, structure, and process. Each dimension reflects a unique aspect of community health.

### Status

Community health in terms of status, or outcome, is the most well known and accepted approach; it involves biological, emotional, and social parts. The biological (or physical) part of community health is often measured by traditional morbidity and mortality rates, life expectancy indexes, and risk factor profiles. The question of exactly which risk factors are most important has been a matter of ongoing disagreement. In an effort to help resolve this question, *Morbidity and Mortality Weekly Report* published the work of a consensus committee involving representatives from a number of community-health-related organizations. This committee identified by consensus 18 community health status measures and risk factors (Box 15-3).

---

**BOX 15-3** **Consensus Set of Indicators for Assessing Community Health Status**

**INDICATORS OF HEALTH STATUS OUTCOME**

1. Race/ethnicity-specific infant mortality, as measured by the rate (per 1000 live births) of deaths among infants less than 1 year of age

**Death Rates (per 100,000 Population)\* for the Following:**

2. Motor vehicle crashes
3. Work-related injury
4. Suicide
5. Lung cancer
6. Breast cancer
7. Cardiovascular disease
8. Homicide
9. All causes

**Reported Incidence (per 100,000 Population) of the Following:**

10. Acquired immunodeficiency syndrome
11. Measles
12. Tuberculosis
13. Primary and secondary syphilis

**INDICATORS OF RISK FACTORS**

14. Incidence of low birth weight, as measured by percentage of total number of live-born infants weighing less than 2500 g at birth
15. Births to adolescents (girls 10 to 17 years of age) as a percentage of total live births
16. Prenatal care, as measured by percentage of mothers delivering live infants who did not receive prenatal care during first trimester
17. Childhood poverty, as measured by the proportion of children less than 15 years of age living in families at or below the poverty level
18. Proportion of persons living in counties exceeding U.S. Environmental Protection Agency standards for air quality during previous year

From Consensus set of health status indicators for the general assessment of community health status—United States, *MMWR Morb Mortal Wkly Rep* 40(27):449, 1991 (updated 8/01).
NOTE: Position of the indicator in the list does not imply priority.
\*Age-adjusted to the 1940 standard population.

---

The emotional part of health status can be measured by consumer satisfaction and mental health indices. Crime rates and functional levels reflect the social part of community health. Other status measures, such as worker absenteeism and infant mortality rates, reflect the effects of all three parts.

## Structure

Community health, when viewed as the structure of the community, is usually defined in terms of services and resources. Measures of community health services and resources include service use patterns, treatment data from various health agencies, and provider-to-client ratios. These data provide information, such as the number of available hospital beds or the number of emergency room visits to a particular hospital. The problems that can be found when structure measures are used are serious. For example, problems related to access to care and quality of care are well known through stories reported in local newspapers. Less well known, but of equal concern, is the false belief that simply *providing* health care improves health. Such problems require cautious use of health services and resources as measures of community health.

A structural viewpoint also defines the characteristics of the community structure itself. Characteristics of the community structure are commonly identified as social measures, or correlates, of health. Measures of community structure include demographics, such as socioeconomic and racial distributions, age, and educational level. Their relationships to health status have been thoroughly documented. For example, studies have repeatedly shown that health status decreases with age and improves with higher socioeconomic levels.

## Process

The view of community health as the process of effective community functioning or problem solving is well established. However, it is especially appropriate to community-oriented nursing because it directs the study of community health for community action.

**Community competence,** defined originally in a classic work by Cottrell (1976), provides a basic understanding of the process dimension of community health. Community competence is a process whereby the parts of a community—organizations, groups, and aggregates—"are able to collaborate effectively in identifying the problems and needs of the community; can achieve a working consensus on goals and priorities; can agree on ways and means to implement the agreed-on goals; and can collaborate effectively in the required actions" (Cottrell, 1976, p. 197). Cottrell also proposes eight essential conditions of competence. The conditions are listed and defined in Table 15-2.

The term *community health* as used in this chapter is the meeting of collective needs by identifying problems and managing behaviors within the community itself and between the community and the larger society. This definition emphasizes the process dimension but also includes the dimensions of status and structure. Measures for all

**Table 15-2  The Eight Essential Conditions of Community Competence**

| CONDITION | DEFINITION |
|---|---|
| Commitment | The affective and cognitive attachment to a community "that is worthy of substantial effort to sustain and enhance" (Cottrell, 1976, p. 198) |
| Awareness of self and others and clarity of situational definitions | The clear and realistic view of one's own and other persons' community components, identities, and positions on issues |
| Articulateness | The technical aspects of formulating and stating one's views in relation to other persons' views |
| Effective communication | The accurate transmission of information based on the development of common meaning among the communicators |
| Conflict containment and management of accommodation | The inventive and effective assimilation and management of true or realistically perceived differences |
| Participation | Active, community-oriented involvement |
| Management of relations with larger society | Adeptness at recognizing, obtaining, and using external resources and supports and, when necessary, stimulating the creation and use of alternative or supplementary resources |
| Machinery for facilitating participant interaction and decision making | Flexible and responsible procedures (formal and informal), participant interaction and facilities, interaction, and decision making |

From Cottrell LS: The competent community. In Kaplan BH, Wilson RN, Leighton AH, editors: *Further explorations in social psychiatry,* New York, 1976, Basic Books; Goeppinger J, Lassiter PG, Wilcox B: Community health is community competence, *Nurs Outlook* 30(8):464, 1982.

three dimensions are listed in Table 15-3. The use of status, structure, and process dimensions to define community health, as shown in Table 15-3, is an effort to develop a broad definition of community health, involving measures that are often not included when discussions focus only on risk factors as the basis for community health. Nevertheless, epidemiologic data related to health risks of aggregates and populations, commonly expressed as rates and confidence intervals, are vital measures of health status (Dever, 1997).

Considering health risks guides us to think upstream, to identify risks that could be prevented to make and keep people healthy. Most community- and population-oriented approaches to health are grounded in the notion that the earlier in the causal process (or more upstream) interventions occur, the greater the likelihood of improved health. Frequently, prevention or upstream action requires communitywide intervention directed toward social, economic, and environmental conditions that correlate with low health status (Health Canada, 2002). Examples of such interventions are presented under Implementing in the Community later in this chapter.

## Healthy People 2010

One important guideline that is available for nurses working to improve the health of the community is Healthy People 2010, a publication from the U.S. Department of Health and Human Services (USDHHS, 2000). It offers a vision of the future for public health and specific objectives to help attain that vision. The Healthy People 2010 vision recognizes the need to work collectively, in community partnerships, to bring about the changes that will be necessary to fulfill this vision. Healthy People 2010 provides the foundation for a national health promotion and disease-prevention strategy built on the two goals of increasing the "quality and years of healthy life" and eliminating "health disparities." The introduction to *Healthy People 2010* speaks directly to the relationship between individuals and their communities by stating, "Indeed, the underlying premise of Healthy People 2010 is that the health of the individual is almost inseparable from the health of the larger community." Furthermore, "community partnerships, particularly when they reach out to nontraditional partners, can be among the most effective tools for improving health in communities." Because Healthy People 2010 is dynamic rather than static, the Public Health Service (PHS) will continue to review progress.

## Community Partnerships

The introduction to Healthy People 2010 specifically refers to **community partnership** as a key to meeting program goals. Community partnership is necessary because community members and professionals who are active participants in a collaborative decision-making process have a

**Table 15-3  Concept of Community Health Specified**

| DIMENSION | MEASURES | EXAMPLES OF DATA SOURCES |
|---|---|---|
| Status | Vital statistics (live births, neonatal deaths, infant deaths, maternal deaths) | Census data<br>State health department annual vital statistics |
| | Incidence and prevalence of leading causes of mortality and morbidity | Census data<br>State health department |
| | Health risk profiles of selected aggregates | Local health department<br>Support groups<br>Local nonprofit organizations |
| | Functional ability levels | Census data<br>U.S. Department of Labor |
| Structure | Health facilities such as hospitals, nursing homes, industrial and school health services, health departments, voluntary health associations, categorical grant programs, and prepaid health plans | Local chamber of commerce<br>United Way |
| | Health-related planning groups | Local newspapers<br>Local magazines<br>Local government |
| | Health manpower, such as physicians, dentists, nurses, environmental sanitarians, social workers | Telephone directory<br>State and local labor statistics<br>Professional licensing boards |
| | Health resource use patterns, such as bed occupancy days and client/provider visits | Medicare and Medicaid databases (federal & state government)<br>Annual reports from hospitals, HMOs, nonprofit agencies |
| Process | Commitment to community health | Local government<br>Real estate agencies (turnover/ vacancy rates, for example) |
| | Awareness of self and others and clarity of situational definitions | Local history<br>Neighborhood help organizations |
| | Effective communication | Local/neighborhood newspapers and radio programs<br>Local government |
| | Conflict containment and accommodation | Social services department |
| | Participation | Existence of and participation in local organizations |
| | Management of relationships with society | Windshield survey—observation of interactions |
| | Machinery for facilitating participant interaction and decision making | Notices for community organizations and meetings in public places (supermarkets, newspapers, radio) |

vested interest in the success of efforts to improve the health of their community (Courtney et al, 1996). Therefore successful strategies for improving community health must include community partnership as the basic means, or key, for improvement (McClowry et al, 1996). Community partnership is a basic focus of such community-oriented approaches as Mobilizing for Action through Planning and Partnerships (MAPP; see p. 351).

Most changes must aim at improving community health through active partnerships between community residents and health workers from a variety of disciplines. Unfortunately, community residents are often viewed only as sources of information and receivers of intervention. This form of partnership is called passive participation. Passive participation is the opposite of the partnership approach in which all are involved in assessing, planning, and implementing needed community changes (Baker et al, 1997).

The community member–professional partnership approach specifically emphasizes active participation. Power

## Healthy People 2010 | Healthy People 2010 and Community as Partner

Healthy People 2010 promotes partnerships with communities, states, and national organizations and suggests the following:
- Taking a multidisciplinary approach to achieving health equity
- Using approaches to improving not only health but education, housing, labor, justice, transportation, agriculture, and the environment

- Empowering individuals to make informed health care decisions
- Promoting community-wide safety, education, and access to health care
- Tailoring approaches to prevention that are specific to the type of community and that ensure community participation in the process

From U.S. Department of Health and Human Services: *Healthy people 2010: understanding and improving health,* ed 2, Washington, DC, 2000, U.S. Government Printing Office.

### DID YOU KNOW?

The Healthy People 2010 website can be accessed through WebLinks on this book's website, http://evolve.elsevier.com/Stanhope. From the Healthy People 2010 website, at www.healthypeople.gov, information can be obtained about focus priority areas, the lead agencies, fact sheets, progress reviews, publications lists, and the Healthy People 2010 databases. Other valuable internet sites include the following:
- Behavior Risk Factor Surveillance System (BRFSS) developed and conducted to monitor state-level prevalence of the major behavioral risks among adults associated with premature morbidity and mortality and conducted by the National Center for Health Statistics (NCHS): http://www.cdc.gov/brfss/index.htm.
- Health Resources and Services Administration (HRSA) community health status indicators project provides data at the county level for all 50 states at htpp://www.communityhealth.hrsa.gov.

### BOX 15-4   Partnerships

The three main characteristics of a successful partnership are the following:
- **Being informed.** Community member and professional partners must be aware of their own and others' perceptions, rights, and responsibilities (Jackson and Parks, 1997).
- **Flexibility.** Community member and professional partners must recognize the unique and similar contributions that each can make to a given situation. For example, professionals often contribute important knowledge and skills that laypersons lack. On the other hand, laypersons' definitions of community health problems are often more accurate than those of professionals.
- **Negotiation.** Because contributions vary and each situation is different, the distribution of power must be negotiated at every stage of the change process.

Jackson EJ, Parks CP: Recruitment and training issues from selected lay health advisor programs among African Americans: a 20-year perspective [review], *Health Educ Behav* 24(4):418-431, 1997.

is shared among lay and professional persons throughout the assessment, planning, implementation, and evaluation processes. Partnership means the active participation and involvement of the community or its representatives in healthy change (Eng, Parker, and Harlan, 1997). For example, breast cancer is an issue for rural and Hispanic migrant and seasonal workers. Active community partnerships involving the Hispanic migrant and seasonal community helped develop and ensure an effective, ongoing program (Meade and Calvo, 2001) (Box 15-4).

Partnership, as defined here, is a concept that is as essential for nurses to know and use as are the concepts of community, community as client, and community health. Experienced nurses know that partnership is important because health is not a static reality. Rather, it is continuously generated through new and increasingly effective means of community member–professional collaboration.

However, such changes also require other active professional service providers, such as schoolteachers, public safety officers, and horticulturists. Partnership in identifying problems and setting goals is especially important because it brings commitment from all persons involved, which is essential to successful change (Flynn, 1998).

A growing body of literature supports the significance and effectiveness of partnership in improving community health. Studies document the use of partnership models involving urban areas and lay advisors (Baker et al, 1997; Parker et al, 1998; Schulz et al, 1997). The roles of these partners-in-health have included listening sympathetically, offering advice, making referrals, and starting programs among a wide range of communities. These include urban Hispanics, and rural and Hispanic migrant farmworkers

(Courtney et al, 1996; Meade and Calvo, 2001). They include partnerships with older adults in retirement communities as well as smaller, more rural communities (Clark and Mass, 1998; Lutz, Herrick, and Lehman, 2001). There are also examples of community partnerships for health promotion for at-risk students at the grade school or middle school level; for public educators at a museum; or for an adolescent pregnancy prevention program in a Midwestern military community (Kyba, Hathaway, and Okimi, 1997; Lewis et al, 1999; Lough, 1999; McMahon, Browning, and Rose-Colley, 2001; Miller et al, 2001).

Work by Hildebrandt et al (1996) and Kroeger et al (1997) shows the continuing use of partnership models for improving health in other countries. In international health, partnership models are generally viewed as empowering people, through their lay leaders, to control their own health destinies and lives. In the United States, partnership models have often involved informal community leaders, organizations such as churches, and communities.

Partnerships involving nurses working with community organizations offer one of the most effective means for interventions because they actively involve the community and build on existing community strengths. Nurses working with community groups and organizations fulfill many different roles. These roles include media advocacy, political action, "grass roots health communication and social marketing," and outreach facilitator to get more parents involved in a school health fair. Regardless of what roles nurses fulfill as their contribution to the partnership, they must remember to "start where the people are" (Courtney et al, 1996; Flynn, 1998; Lindsey, Stajduhar, and McGuinness, 2001; Maurana and Clark, 2000).

Courtney et al (1996, p. 179) sum up the characteristics of a community partnership as focusing on "fostering the skills and the capacity of the partner." Nurses do "with" rather than "to" the partner, and the partner's role throughout the process is active, not passive. Goal setting and the plan of action are mutually determined. Roles and responsibilities are negotiated and the partners become more effective at working independently to solve their own problems and make decisions for themselves, even if they do not solve the problems identified by the nursing diagnosis. In the language of community **empowerment** advocates, "Community participants have an active role in the change process. . . . The professional works hard to include members of a setting, neighborhood, or organization so they have a central role in the process" (Zimmerman, 2000, p. 45).

## Strategies to Improve Community Health

Healthy People 2010 has stimulated a number of joint efforts to develop strategies for achieving its goals. These efforts have involved such organizations as the Centers for Disease Control and Prevention (CDC), the American Public Health Association (APHA), the Association of State and Territorial Health Officials (ASTHO), and the National Association of County and City Health Officials (NACCHO). The results

### Evidence-Based Practice

The purpose of this intervention was to test the effectiveness of an interdisciplinary team's ability to build community partnerships and implement the core functions of public health nursing. This effort by the local public health department involved a wide variety of different community groups and organizations.
- The outcomes of the intervention supported a practice model built on core public health functions.
- The value of describing and measuring community capacity was apparent, as was the need for a "will to act" within the community—not just having knowledge and skills.
- The organizational climate of the health department shifted to a more participatory collegial model.

**Nurse Use:** Evaluation of the interventions indicated that both the agency and the community organizations were affected by this effort.

Westbrook L, Schultz P: From theory to practice: community health nursing in a public health neighborhood team, *Adv Nurs Sci* 23(2):50-61, 2000.

of these efforts are a number of publications and guidelines that provide detailed strategies for achieving the objectives in Healthy People 2010. These publications include Healthy People 2010 Took Kit: A Field Guide to Health Planning; Assessment Protocol for Excellence in Public Health **(APEXPH);** and Planned Approach to Community Health **(PATCH),** and more recently MAPP. Each of these four approaches offers step-by-step guidelines for community planning and interventions.

APEXPH and PATCH are two planning tools that can be used to help implement the Healthy People 2010 goals. APEXPH is a process that emphasizes local-level activity and focuses on improving the public health of communities by increasing the capacity of the local health care agencies to provide core functions, such as assessment and policy development. NACCHO, in collaboration with the CDC, produced Mobilizing for Action through Planning and Partnerships **(MAPP).** "MAPP is a community-wide strategic planning tool for improving community health." Finally, PATCH focuses more on the prevention of identified chronic disease and health promotion programs and their planning and implementation processes (APHA, 1993, 1994). Readers interested in contacting these organizations can refer to Box 15-5.

In addition to these approaches, there have been efforts to apply the evidence-based practice approach to community-level interventions. The *Community Guide*, located at http://www.thecommunityguide.org, provides recommendations for population-based interventions to promote health and to prevent disease, injury, disability,

---

**BOX 15-5  Website Information for Strategies to Improve Community Health**

**MODEL STANDARDS**

American Public Health Association
1015 15th Street, NW
Washington, DC, 20005
(202) 789-5618
www.apha.org/

**APEXPH AND MAPP**

National Association of County Health Officials
1100 17th Street, NW, 2nd Floor
Washington, DC 20036
(202) 783-5550
www.naccho.org/

**PATCH**

National Center for Chronic Disease Prevention and Health Promotion
Centers for Chronic Disease Control and Prevention
4770 Buford Hwy NE, Mailstop K-46
Atlanta, GA 30341-3717
(404) 488-5426
www.cdc.com

---

See also WebLinks on this book's website at http://evolve.elsevier.com/Stanhope.

---

and premature death, and it is appropriate for use by communities and health care systems. The *Community Guide* is a result of the work of the Task Force on Community Preventive Services, which systematically reviews published scientific studies, weighs the evidence, and determines the effectiveness of interventions in a particular area. They do not use the term *evidence-based practice*, but the *Community Guide* really is a guide to EBP for the community. Interventions are (1) strongly recommended, (2) recommended, or (3) labeled as having insufficient evidence to make a recommendation. For instance, in regard to physical activity promotion, the Task Force strongly recommends communitywide campaigns, individually adapted health behavior change programs, school-based physical education, social support interventions in community contexts, and creating or improving access to places for physical activity combined with informational outreach. The recommendations of the Task Force were published in a special supplement to the *American Journal of Preventive Medicine* in May 2002.

Another useful website is http://www.cdc.gov/nccdphp/dnpa/npa-proj.htm. This site includes links to CDC-supported public health programs found effective and links to guides and kits for the programs. The programs listed a year ago were 5-A-Day for Better Health (healthy eating); ACEs: Active Community Environments (activity); KidsWalk-to-School (activity); National Bone Health Campaign (healthy eating, activity); Well-Integrated

Screening and Evaluation for Women Across the Nation–WISEWOMAN (lifestyle intervention programs addressing cardiovascular and other chronic disease risk factors); and Ready, Set, It's Everywhere You Go (physical activity).

The World Health Organization's (WHO) Healthy Cities initiative offers yet another approach to community-oriented health promotion. First initiated in Europe during the middle 1980s, Healthy Cities has become a global movement with hundreds of Healthy Cities initiatives. Healthy Cities initiatives are based on the belief that the health of the community is affected by political, economic, environmental, and social factors. The Healthy Cities approach emphasizes community development through broad-based local citizen involvement to address local problems (Flynn, 1997). Healthy Cities efforts focus on social change, including developing supportive environments; developing personal skills; and reorienting health care services, health policy, and community action (Flynn, 1997). See Chapter 17 for more.

Several different community-oriented health promotion approaches have been noted here. Regardless of what approach is taken, specific strategies to improve community health often depend on whether the status, structure, or process dimension of community health is being emphasized (Courtney et al, 1996). If the emphasis is on the status dimension, the best strategy is usually at the level of primary or secondary prevention because the objective is either to prevent a disease or to treat it in its early stages. Immunization programs are an example of a nursing intervention at the primary prevention level. Laffrey and Kulbok's (1999) integrated model of holistic community health nursing provides an example of an approach emphasizing the health status dimension. See Chapter 14 for more.

Nursing intervention strategies focused on the structural dimension are directed to either health services or demographic characteristics. Interventions aimed at altering health services might include program planning. Interventions aimed at affecting demographic characteristics might include community development.

When the emphasis is on the process dimension, the best strategy is usually health promotion, also a primary prevention strategy. For example, if family-life education is lacking in a community because of ineffective communication among families, children, school board members, religious leaders, and health professionals, then the most effective strategy may be to open discussion among these groups and help community members develop education programs.

## COMMUNITY-FOCUSED NURSING PROCESS: AN OVERVIEW OF THE PROCESS FROM ASSESSMENT TO EVALUATION

Most nurses are familiar with the nursing process as it applies to individually focused nursing care. Using it to promote community health makes this same nursing process community focused (Flick, Reese, and Harris, 1996). The phases of the nursing process that directly involve the community as client begin at the start of the contract or partnership and include assessing, diagnosing, planning, implementing, and evaluating. Figure 15-1 provides an overview of the nursing process with the community as client.

The use of the nursing process with the community as client is presented in the following sections with a real case study taken from the practice of a nurse. For clarity, infant malnutrition is the only community health problem used to show how the nursing process is applied. In reality, several different community health problems were identified by the partnership. The relative importance of each was examined, and infant malnutrition was picked as the most important problem from among all of the identified problems before continuing with intervention.

## THE CUTTING EDGE

The assistant secretary for health of the U.S. Department of Health and Human Services has established an internet site with examples of best-practice programs in public health: http://www.osophs.dhhs.gov/ophs/BestPractice/default.htm.

## Community Assessment

Community assessment is one of three core functions of public health nursing and is the process of critically thinking about the community. This involves getting to know and understand the community as client. Community nurses start an assessment by clearly defining their client in terms of the three dimensions of place, people, and function presented in Table 15-1. Before data are collected in the assessment phase the nurse must be able to answer questions such as these: What are the geographic boundaries of this community? Which people are members of this community? What characteristics do they have in common? For example, homebound older adults in a particular city are a community of special interest with shared needs, who are defined by their age and homebound status. Once the nurse is clear about the boundaries of the community as client, the community assessment phase can be continued.

The community assessment phase itself involves a logical, systematic approach. Community assessment helps identify community needs, clarify problems, and identify strengths and resources. There are different types of community assessment. The longer and more complex process of a *comprehensive community assessment* is described here. This assessment process reflects the public health competencies essential for analysis and assessment in public health. Comprehensive community assessment is the necessary initial phase of the community nursing process with the community as client (Box 15-6).

Assessment data must be systematically collected, organized, and placed into assessment categories (Tables 15-1 and 15-3). The **database** form provided in Appendix C.1 is a useful means for entering and organizing these different types of data. Gathering the data and its initial interpretation are the first steps in the assessment phase of the nursing process (see Figure 15-1).

## DID YOU KNOW?

A complete set of blank forms for use in the different steps of the assessment process, including the database form, is available on this book's website at http://evolve.elsevier.com/Stanhope and in Appendix C.1. These blank data forms are identical to the forms completed throughout the chapter as part of the Jefferson County community assessment example. They can be used in steps of the community assessment presented in Figure 15-1 regardless of the type of community that is being assessed.

## Data Collection and Interpretation

The primary goal of **data collection** is to get usable information about the community and its health. The systematic collection of data about community health requires gathering or compiling existing data and generating missing data. These data are then interpreted, and community health problems and community abilities are identified.

### Data Gathering

**Data gathering** is the process of obtaining existing, readily available data. These data already exist. They usually describe the demography of a community: age, sex, socioeconomic, and racial distributions. They include vital statistics, such as selected mortality and morbidity data. Another source is **surveys,** such as the Behavior Risk Factor Surveillance System (BRFSS) developed and conducted to monitor state-level prevalence of the major behavioral risks associated with premature morbidity and mortality in adults (see the Did You Know? box in this chapter for the BRFSS website). Conducted by the National Center for Health Statistics (NCHS), these survey data, from sources such as the BRFSS, are important because they also provide data about trends. Other resources include data from community institutions, including health care organizations and the services they provide, and the characteristics of health care personnel. Often these data have been collected by others via structured interviews, questionnaires, or surveys and are available in published reports. State health departments gather extensive epidemiologic data in the form of rates, which are generally published at both county and state levels in the form of vital health statistics. Table 15-4 shows an example of existing epidemiologic data gathered as part of the Jefferson County assessment.

The USDHHS Health Resources and Services Administration has placed its Community Health Status Indicators

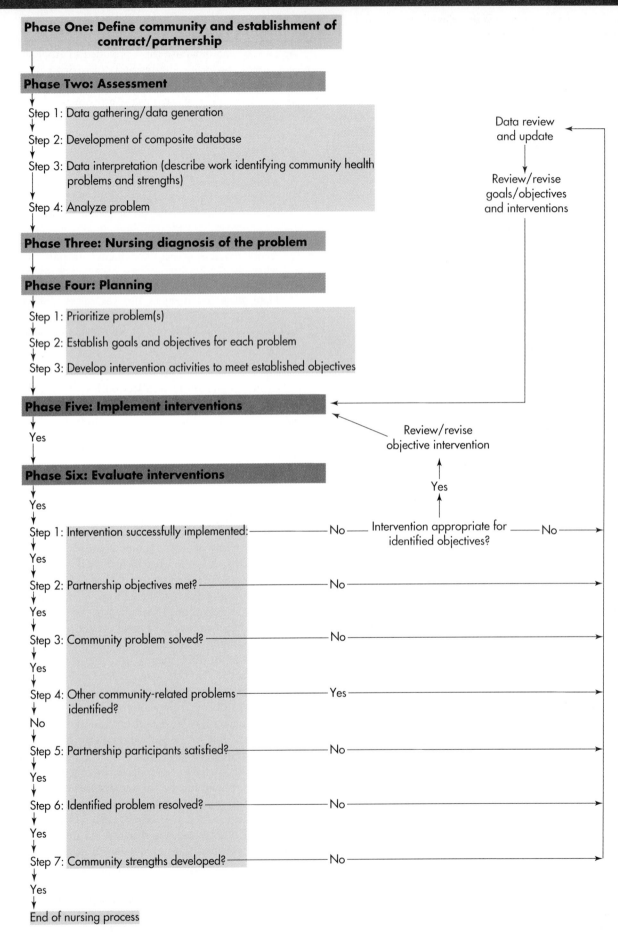

**Figure 15-1** Flowchart illustrating the nursing process with the community as client.

BOX 15-6 **Steps to Assessing Community Health**

**Step 1.** Gathering relevant existing data and generating missing data

**Step 2.** Developing a composite database

**Step 3.** Interpreting the composite database to identify community problems and strengths

**Step 4.** Analyzing the problem

---

Table 15-4 **Assessment Database**

Data Recording Sheet                    Page #____
Name of community: Jefferson County
Assessment category: Community health
Subcategory status: Vital statistics

| DATE | DATA SOURCE | DATA* |
|------|-------------|-------|
| 1/30/02 | National Center for Health Statistics Vital Statistics Reporting 2000 | Postneonatal infant mortality rate, 2.3 per 1000 live births (1-12 months) |
| | | Neonatal infant mortality, 6.4 per 1000 live births |
| | | 2.5% of births to teen mothers (less than 18 years old) |
| | | For 17.6% of births, the mothers had had no care in first trimester |

*Note with an asterisk the themes identified and meanings given.

---

project on the internet (access it through the WebLinks of this book's website [http://evolve.elsevier.com/Stanhope], or find the site in the Did You Know? box on p. 353). This site provides an excellent example of how data can be gathered to provide this part of the community assessment composite database. It also provides county-level data as well as a list of peer counties for almost every county in the United States.

### Data Generation

**Data generation** is the process of developing data that do not already exist through interaction with community members or groups. This type of information is harder to get and is generally not statistical in nature. Data that often must be generated include information about a community's knowledge and beliefs, values and sentiments,

goals and perceived needs, norms, problem-solving processes, power, leadership, and influence structures. These data, called qualitative data, are more likely to be collected by interviews and observation (Ludwig-Beymer et al, 1996).

Several methods to generate or collect data are needed. Methods that encourage the nurse to consider the community's perception of its health problems and abilities are as important as methods structured to identify knowledge that the nurse considers essential. Methods of collecting data rely either on what is directly observed *by* the data collector or on what is reported *to* the data collector.

**Generation of direct data.** Informant interviews, focus groups, participant observation, and **windshield surveys** are four methods of directly collecting data. All four methods require sensitivity, openness, curiosity, and the ability to listen, taste, touch, smell, and see life as it is lived in a community. Either informant interviews or focus groups, which consist of directed talks with selected members of a community about community members or groups and events, are basic to effective data generation (Parker, Barry, and King, 2000; Stevens, 1996). Also basic is **participant observation,** the deliberate sharing, to the extent that conditions permit, in the life of a community. **Informant interviews,** focus groups, and participant observation are good ways to generate information about community beliefs, norms, values, power and influence structures, and problem-solving processes. Such data can seldom be reported in numbers, so they are often not collected. Even worse, conclusions that are based on intuition and unchecked are sometimes used to replace these types of data. People providing information should confirm their conclusions from direct data-generation methods.

**HOW TO   Identify a Key Informant**

Talking to key informants is a critical part of the community assessment.

- Key informants are not always people who have a formal title or position.
- Key informants often have an informal role within the community.
- County health department nurses and church leaders are often key informants. They also know many community members and can identify other key informants.

In the example of the community with the infant malnutrition problem, informant interviews with social workers and religious leaders provided data indicating a community with well-defined clusters of persons with low incomes, concerns about adolescent pregnancy, and worries about the health of the community's babies. These data, which reflect the concerns and worries of the Jefferson County community, would have been difficult to acquire without personal interviews.

> ### HOW TO   Obtain a Quick Assessment of a Community
>
> - One way to get a quick, initial sense of the community is to do a windshield assessment using a format like the one provided as an example in Table 15-5.
> - Nurses interested in doing a windshield assessment need to either take public transportation, have someone else drive while they take notes, or plan to stop frequently to write down what they see.
> - The windshield survey example is organized into 15 elements with specific questions related to each element.
> - Nurses who use this approach will have an initial descriptive assessment of the community when they are done.
> - If interventions are planned, the more thorough and more comprehensive process described in this chapter will be necessary.

Windshield surveys are the motorized equivalent of simple observation (Table 15-5 shows an example). They involve the generation of data "which will help define the community, the trends, stability, and changes that will affect the health of the community" (Stanhope and Knollmueller, 2000). The nurse, driving a car or riding public transportation, can observe many dimensions of a community's life and environment through the windshield. Common characteristics of people on the street, neighborhood gathering places, the rhythm of community life, housing quality, and geographic boundaries can be observed readily. Again using the infant malnutrition example, the windshield survey suggested that the community had a large unemployed population because adults were observed "hanging out" at country crossroads during the day. A windshield survey can be used by itself for a short and simple assessment. However, it is used here as one part of the longer, more complex comprehensive community assessment.

**Collection of reported data.** Two methods of generating reported data are secondary analysis of data collected by someone else, and surveys. In **secondary analysis,** the nurse uses previously gathered data, such as minutes from community meetings. This type of analysis is extremely valuable because it saves time and effort. Many sources of data are readily available and useful for secondary analysis:

> ### NURSING TIP
>
> If you do a windshield survey as part of your community assessment, go twice: once during the day when people are at work and children are at school, and a second time in the evening after work is done and school is out.

public documents, health surveys, minutes from meetings, and statistical data (such as census and health records). In the Jefferson County infant malnutrition example, birth records noting low-birthweights and health department clinic records of low-weight-for-height children provided information that showed a higher-than-average rate of infant malnutrition.

Surveys report data from a sample of persons. They are equally useful, but they take more time and effort than observational methods and secondary analyses. They require time-consuming and costly data generation. Thus the survey method is not often used by the nurse. However, surveys are necessary for identifying certain community problems (Dever, 1997). For example, a lack of accessible personal health services cannot be documented readily and reliably in any other way.

### Composite Database
When new data that have just been collected or generated are combined with already-existing data (previously gathered by the nurse), the result is a composite database. Data analysis is used to make sense of the data in this composite database. First, data are analyzed and synthesized, and themes or trends are noted. For example, trends identified by comparing several years of epidemiologic data can identify certain kinds of problems. The analysis of data generated by interviews with key informants or focus groups can identify other kinds of problems. **Community health problems,** or needs for action, and **community health strengths,** or abilities, are determined. Problems are indicated by differences between (1) the community health goals of the nurse and community and (2) the themes or findings revealed by the data analysis. Strengths, on the other hand, are suggested by similarities between the nurse's and community's concepts of community health and the supporting data. The nurse and community, working in partnership, identify problems.

### Problem Analysis
**Problem analysis** seeks to clarify the nature of the problem. The nurse identifies the origins and effects of the problem, the points at which intervention might occur, and the parties that have an interest in the problem and its solution. Analysis often requires the development of a problem matrix, in which the direct and indirect factors that contribute to the problem and to the outcomes of the problem are identified and mapped. Relationships among the factors are noted. The map or matrix is important because the nurse can anticipate that several of the same factors that contribute to a problem and that affect the outcomes of a problem may also *cause* the problem. The problem of highest priority may share factors that also contribute to other problems and affect their outcomes as well.

Problem analysis should be done for each identified problem. This often requires organizing a special group composed of the nurse, persons whose areas of expertise relate to the problem, persons whose organizations are

**Table 15-5   Windshield Survey Components**

| ELEMENT | DESCRIPTION |
|---|---|
| Housing and zoning | What is the age of the houses, their architecture, of what materials are they constructed? Are all the neighborhood houses similar in age, architecture? How would you characterize the differences? Are they detached from or connected to others? Do they have space in front and behind? What is their general condition? Are there signs of disrepair—broken doors, windows, leaks, locks missing? Is there central heating, modern plumbing, air conditioning? |
| Open space | How much open space is there? What is the quality of the space—green parks or rubble-filled lots? What is the lot size of the houses? Are there lawns? Flower boxes? Do you see trees on the pavements, a green island in the center of the streets? Is the open space public or private? Used by whom? |
| Boundaries | What signs are there of where this neighborhood begins and ends? Are the boundaries natural (a river, a different terrain)? Physical (a highway, railroad)? Economic (real estate differences or presence of industrial, commercial units along with residential)? Does the neighborhood have an identity, a name? Do you see it displayed? Are there unofficial names? |
| "Commons" | What are the neighborhood hangouts (e.g., schoolyard, candy store, bar, restaurant, park, 24-hour drugstore)? For what groups, at what hours? Does the "commons" have a sense of "territoriality" or is it open to the stranger? |
| Transportation | How do people get in and out of the neighborhood? Car, bus, bike, walk? Are the streets and roads conducive to good transportation and also to community life? Is there a major highway near the neighborhood? Whom does it serve? How frequent is public transportation available? |
| Service centers | Do you see social agencies, clients, recreation centers, signs of activity at the schools? Are there offices of doctors, dentists? Palmists, spiritualists? Parks? Are they in use? |
| Stores | Where do residents shop? Shopping centers, neighborhood stores? How do they travel to shop? |
| Street people | If you are traveling during the day, who do you see on the street? An occasional housewife, a mother with a baby? Do you see anyone you would not expect? Teenagers, unemployed men? Can you spot a welfare worker, an insurance collector, a door-to-door salesman? Is the dress of those you see representative or unexpected? Along with people, what animals do you see? Stray cats, dogs, pedigreed pets, "watchdogs"? |
| Signs of decay | Is this neighborhood on the way up or down? Is it "alive"? How would you decide? Trash, abandoned cars, political posters, neighborhood meeting posters, real estate signs, abandoned houses, mixed-zoning usage? |
| Race | Which races are represented? Is the area integrated? |
| Ethnicity | Are there indexes of ethnicity—food stores, churches, private schools. What is the predominant language, and are other languages heard? |
| Religion | Of what religion are the residents? Do you see evidence of heterogeneity or homogeneity? What denomination are the houses of worship? Do you see evidence of their use other than on regular religious/holy days? |
| Health and morbidity | Do you see evidence of acute or chronic diseases or conditions? Of accidents, communicable diseases, alcoholism, drug addiction, mental illness? How far is it to the nearest hospital? Clinic? |
| Politics | Do you see any political campaign posters? Is there a local headquarters? Do you see any evidence of a predominant party affiliation? |
| Media | Do you see outdoor television antennas? What magazines, newspapers do residents read? Do you see *Forward Times, Hampton Post, Enquirer, Readers' Digest* in the stores? What media seem most important to the residents? Radio, TV? |

This example of a windshield survey is reprinted here with permission from Anderson ET, McFarlane J, editors: *Community as client: application of the nursing process,* Philadelphia, 1988, Lippincott.

capable of intervening, and representatives of the community experiencing the problem. Both content and process specialists must participate. Together they can identify the **problem correlates,** defined as factors contributing to the problem, and explain the relationships between each factor and the problem.

An example of problem analysis is shown in Table 15-6. Problem correlates (factors that contribute to or result from the problem) for infant malnutrition are listed in the first column. Correlates are from all areas of community life. Social or environmental correlates are as appropriate as those oriented to the individual. For example, teenage pregnancy is a social correlate of infant malnutrition, and high unemployment is an environmental correlate. In the second column, the relationships between each correlate and the problem are noted. The third column contains data from the community and the literature that support the relationship, using the suspected infant malnutrition example and a few of its correlates. Infant malnutrition is thought to be correlated with inadequate diet, community norms, poverty, disturbed mother–child relationships, and teenage pregnancy. Active community participation is critical for the data interpreting process, particularly in identifying problems.

The **program planning model,** first proposed by Delbecq and Van De Ven (1971), continues to be widely used to structure lay participation in defining problems. The model shows how to use active community participation in problem definition and program planning. It makes the most of the contributions by various groups with diverse interests, skills, and knowledge. This model depends heavily on **nominal groups,** "groups in which individuals work in the presence of one another but do not interact" (Delbecq and Van De Ven, 1971, p. 467); the separation of individual from collective (or group) problems; and a round-robin process for listing problems without evaluating or elaborating on them at the same time. This model is popularly known as the nominal group process.

Other consensus methods, such as the Delphi technique, are also used to define the extent of agreement among content experts, policy makers, and community members about the presence and importance of certain health problems. Experience shows that consensus methods produce useful results if the following conditions are met (MacLachlan, 1996; Redman et al, 1997):

1. Problems are carefully selected.
2. Participants in the process are deliberately selected and closely monitored.
3. Justified and reasonable levels of consensus are expected.
4. Findings are used as guides to decisions.

## Assessment Guides

Nursing assessment of community health—both data collecting and interpreting—must be focused. Focus, or perspective, can be provided by detailed assessment guides that are built on a conceptual framework of definitions of community and community health.

---

**Table 15-6  Problem Analysis: Infant Malnutrition**

Community: Jefferson County
Problem: Infant malnutrition

| PROBLEM CORRELATES* | RELATIONSHIP OF CORRELATE TO PROBLEM | DATA SUPPORTIVE TO RELATIONSHIPS† |
|---|---|---|
| 1. Inadequate diet | Diets lacking in required nutrients contribute to malnutrition. | All county infants and their mothers seen by PHNs in 2004 referred to nutritionist because of poor diets. |
| 2. Community norms | Bottle-fed babies are less apt to receive adequate amounts of safe milk containing necessary nutrients. | Area general practitioners and nurses agree that 90% of mothers in the county bottle-feed. |
| 3. Poverty | Infant formulas are expensive. | 60% of new mothers in county are receiving welfare. |
| 4. Disturbed mother–child relationship | Poor mother–child relationship may result in infant's failure to thrive. | Data from charts of 43 nursing mothers show infants diagnosed with failure to thrive. |
| 5. Teenage pregnancy | Teenage mothers are most apt to have inadequate diets prenatally, to bottle-feed, to be poor, and to lack parenting skills. | 90% of births in 2004 were to women 19 years of age or younger. |

*These are factors that contribute to problem and outcomes.
†Refer to appropriate sections of the database and relevant research of the findings in current literature.

Concepts that can be measured in behavioral or observable terms can serve as assessment guides. Community and community health have already been defined in such terms. The concept of community has been specified (see Table 15-1). The definition previously given includes three dimensions: person, place and time, and function. Several measures specify each of these dimensions.

A detailed description of community health—its status, structure, and process dimensions—is presented in Table 15-3. In the infant malnutrition example, status dimension data were gathered from morbidity and mortality data; structural dimension data were gathered from vital statistics and from informant interviews with social workers; and process dimension data were gathered from informant interviews with community religious leaders. In this way, the concepts of community and community health provide the framework for the assessment guide in Appendix C.1. Together, the concepts and assessment guide constitute the community health assessment model, the basis of the community-oriented health record (COHR) (Appendix C.1). Data, problems, and abilities are all organized by using the community health assessment model.

The **community-as-partner model** is another example of an assessment guide developed to show that nurses can work with communities as partners (Anderson and McFarlane, 2000). This model shows how communities change and grow best by full involvement and self-empowerment. The heart of this model is an assessment wheel that shows that the people actually are the community. Surrounding the people, and integral to the community, are eight identified subsystems: housing, education, fire and safety, politics and government, health, communication, economics, and recreation. These subsystems both affect and are affected by the people who make up the community. This model and additional information to understand it can be found in Appendix G.1.

## Assessment Issues

Gaining entry or acceptance into the community is perhaps the biggest challenge in assessment. The nurse is usually an outsider and often represents a health care agency that is neither known nor trusted by community members. Community members may therefore react with indifference or even active hostility to the nurse. In addition, nurses may feel insecure about their skills as a community worker, and

### HOW TO   Gain Community Trust

Often the nurse can gain entry to the community by doing the following:
- Taking part in community events
- Looking and listening with interest
- Visiting people in formal leadership positions
- Employing an assessment guide
- Using a peer group for support

the community may refuse to acknowledge its need for those skills. Because the nurse's success largely depends on the way he or she is viewed, entry into the community is critical.

Once the nurse gains entry at an initial level, **role negotiation** often becomes an issue. Role involves the values, behaviors, or goals that govern an individual's interactions with others. The nurse must decide how long to separate the roles of data collector and intervenor. Effective implementation of the nursing process requires an adequate database. The danger of a premature response to health needs and social injustice is great. Nurses can assist in negotiating roles by presenting thoughtful and consistent reasons for their presence in the community and by sincere demonstrations of their commitment to the community. Keeping appointments, clarifying community members' views of health needs, and respecting an individual's right to choose whether to work with the nurse are often useful approaches.

Maintaining **confidentiality** is also important. Nurses must be very careful to protect the identity of community members who provide sensitive or controversial data. In some cases, the nurse may consider withholding data; in other situations, the nurse may be legally required to disclose data. For example, nurses are required by law to report child abuse.

### WHAT DO YOU THINK?

In 1998 Howell and colleagues studied the Healthy Start initiative to reduce infant mortality rates and said that there can be problems when communities use a community empowerment model. Community involvement may interfere with the effectiveness of program operations, create goals that differ from the program's original goals, and slow the development of the program. Should Healthy Start sites use a different approach? Why or why not?

Howell EM, et al: Back to the future: community involvement in the healthy start program, *J Health Politics Policy Law* 23(2):291, 1998.

The difficulties raised in a small-area analysis are of a less personal nature (Dever, 1997). Potential problems of small-area analysis include the mistakes made when conclusions are based on data gathered from small areas. For example, calculations of mortality rates in a rural county may be skewed when the denominator is as small as 5000. This issue often raises questions about the validity of the identified health problems. It is useful to look at the same problem by comparing similar health problems at the state and national levels. Then the nurse can be more confident of the validity of the data.

Remember, a community assessment will identify multiple community health problems. Each of these problems must be analyzed and given a priority score to determine which are the most serious. Under the following headings, the infant malnutrition example is used to show how an identified problem generates a community-focused nursing diagnosis, which is analyzed and assigned a priority score.

## Community-Oriented Nursing Diagnosis

Creating a community assessment composite database will result in a list of community health problems. Each problem needs to be identified clearly and stated as a community health diagnosis. The statement of the problem in a community health diagnosis format is the third phase of the community-as-client process. Developing the community health diagnosis in this phase of the process helps clarify the problem and is an important first step to planning. In the planning phase, where each diagnosis is analyzed, priorities are established and community-focused interventions are identified. Community diagnoses clarify who gets the care (the community as opposed to an individual), provide a statement identifying problems faced by who is getting the care (i.e., the community), and identify the factors contributing to the identified problem.

Although the North American Nursing Diagnosis Association (NANDA) provides a taxonomy of nursing diagnoses familiar to most students, NANDA's focus has been on the individual rather than the community level. However, more recent NANDA work has also developed community-level diagnoses (Craft-Rosenberg, 1999; Parris et al, 1999). Furthermore, ongoing work with Nursing-sensitive Outcomes Classification (NOC) is an effort to produce a standard language across health care settings, including the community (Head, Maas, and Johnson, 1997). NANDA is only one accepted system of nursing diagnosis; for example, home-health nurses are familiar with the Omaha system of nursing diagnosis (Martin and Scheet, 1992). In this chapter, a version of a three-part nursing diagnosis format presented by Green and Slade (2001) is used:

1. Risk of
2. Among
3. Related to

"Risk of" identifies a specific problem or health risk faced by the community. "Among" identifies the specific community client with whom the nurse will be working in relation to the identified problem or risk (see Box 15-2). "Related to" describes characteristics of the community, including motivation, knowledge, and skills of the community and its environment. Environmental characteristics include physical, cultural, psychosocial, and political characteristics (Green and Slade, 2001). These data were identified in the composite database of the assessment phase and provide the basis for the community-level nursing diagnosis. Each community has its own unique characteristics. Some of these characteristics are strengths that the nurse can build on, but other characteristics contribute to the problem identified in the community health diagnosis. The characteristics, or factors, related to the identified problem are listed after the "related to" statement as the third part of the community health diagnosis.

Community nursing diagnosis language must describe at the aggregate level, and this means community level,

responses to actual and potential illnesses and life processes. This also means that the defining characteristics for community diagnoses must be observable and measurable at the aggregate level (Craft-Rosenberg, 1999, p. 127). To do this, community-level data must be used. Epidemiologic data or community survey data are two examples of community-level data. The comparison of local data with state, regional, or national data, as rates and across multiple years, is one key means of identifying community-level problems, as well as patterns and trends. Green and Slade (2001) provide a detailed example of how they developed community-level diagnoses involving "knowledge deficit" and "risk for adverse human health effects" that were related to the consumption of chemically contaminated fish by a local community. Their use of multiple sources of data also illustrates their development of a composite database to support their diagnosis. The example being used for illustration in this chapter is infant malnutrition. On the basis of assessment data, the community diagnosis for infant malnutrition using this format would be the following:

1. *Risk* of infant malnutrition
2. *Among* families in Jefferson County
3. *Related to* lack of regular developmental screening; lack of an outreach program to identify at-risk infants; knowledge deficit among families about infant-related nutrition and about WIC (Special Supplemental Nutrition Program for Women, Infants, and Children); and confusion among families about WIC program enrollment criteria.

Frequently, a number of community health diagnoses are made on the basis of the different problems identified during the assessment phase. The problems are stated in a community-focused nursing diagnosis format. In the next phase, planning for community health, weighting is done and priorities are established among these problems.

## Planning for Community Health

The planning phase includes analyzing the community health problems identified in the community nursing diagnoses and establishing priorities among them, establishing goals and objectives, and identifying intervention activities that will accomplish the objectives. Figure 15-2 shows the relationship between the prioritized problem, goals, objectives, and intervention activities in the fourth phase of the planning process.

### Problem Priorities

Infant malnutrition represents only one of several community health problems identified by the community assessment. The other community health problems included a mortality rate from cardiovascular disease that was higher than the national norm and, as expressed by many residents, a desire to quit smoking.

Each problem identified as part of the assessment process must be put through a ranking process to determine its importance. This ranking process, in which problems are

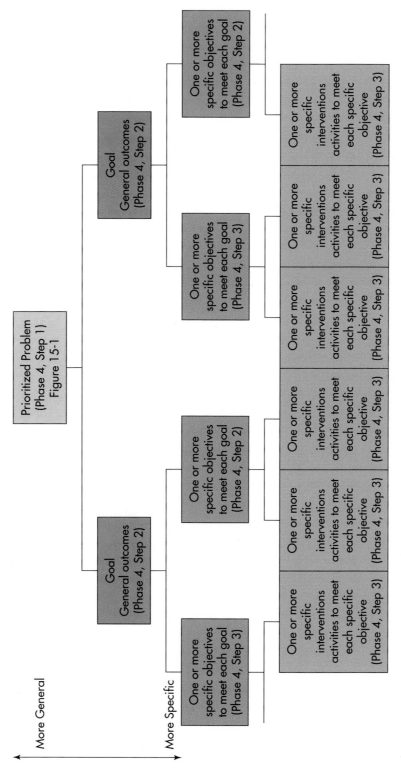

**Figure 15-2** Relationship between the prioritized problem, goals, objectives, and intervention activities in the phase four planning process.

evaluated and priorities established according to predetermined criteria, is termed **problem prioritizing.** It takes into account information provided by community members, content experts, administrators, and others who can provide resources (Box 15-7).

Using the example of infant malnutrition again, the six criteria in Box 15-7 are listed in the first column of Table 15-7.

---

### BOX 15-7  Problem Priority Criteria

Criteria that have been helpful in ranking identified problems include the following:
1. Community awareness of the problem
2. Community motivation to resolve or better manage the problem
3. Nurse's ability to influence problem solution
4. Availability of expertise to solve the problem
5. Severity of the outcomes if the problem is unresolved
6. Speed with which the problem can be solved

---

Given an acceptable and comprehensive set of criteria and a list of community health problems, the process of assigning priorities is rather simple. Each problem is considered independently, and an overall priority score is calculated. This calculation involves two separate but related weighted factors: the first factor involves criteria related to the problem itself, and the second factor involves the same criteria but is weighted on the basis of the partnership's ability to make a change in each of the criteria in the first factor.

Each of the six criteria listed in Table 15-7 is considered separately and independently and then assigned a weight. The criteria are weighted on a scale ranging from a low score of 1 to a high score of 10. Listed in the second column of Table 15-7, these criteria are weighted jointly by the members of the partnership on the basis of the perceived importance of each criterion to the identified community health problem. For example, when members of the partnership assigned a weight to the first criterion listed in Table 15-7, they had to ask each other, "How important is community awareness of infant malnutrition in Jefferson County so the problem can be solved?"

A second factor is related to the partnership's ability to resolve the problem. This factor, called the rating, is in the

---

### Table 15-7  Problem Prioritizing: Infant Malnutrition in Jefferson County

| CRITERION | CRITERION WEIGHT (1-10) | CRITERION RATING (1-10) | RATIONALE FOR RATING | PROBLEM RANKING (WEIGHT × RATE) |
|---|---|---|---|---|
| 1. Community awareness of the problem | 5 | 10 | Health service providers, teachers, and a variety of parents have mentioned problem. | 50 |
| 2. Community motivation to resolve the problem | 10 | 3 | Most believe that this problem is not solvable because most of those affected are indigent. | 30 |
| 3. Nurse's ability to influence problem resolution | 5 | 8 | Nurses are skilled at consciousness raising and mobilizing support. | 40 |
| 4. Ready availability of expertise relevant to problem resolution | 7 | 10 | WIC and nutritionists are available. A county extension agent is interested. | 70 |
| 5. Severity of outcomes if problem is left unresolved | 8 | 5 | Effects of marginal malnutrition are not well documented. | 40 |
| 6. Quickness with which problem resolution can be achieved | 3 | 3 | Time to mobilize rural community with no history of social action is lengthy. | 9 |

Note: Maximum possible problem ranking score = 600; total for Jefferson County = 239.

third column of Table 15-7. In deciding the rating to be given, the members of the partnership consider their ability to influence or change the situation. In the infant malnutrition example, they first ask each other to identify the extent of the community's awareness of the problem. After they talk about the criterion's importance and agree on its rating, the score is recorded. To understand the difference between the criterion weight and problem rating, consider that although a criterion might be weighted as extremely important, it might receive a low rating because the members of the community partnership believe that it would be difficult to influence or change things.

To understand the process of establishing a total score for a problem, or problem prioritizing, let us focus on the second criterion in Table 15-7, community motivation to resolve the problem of suspected infant malnutrition. The weighting of this criterion, 10, shows that it is considered very important to resolving the problem. However, most community residents believe that the problem cannot be solved because of the poverty of those affected. Partnership members do not believe they can actually have an impact on the poverty, so they give their ability to intervene the low rating of 3. The resultant problem ranking, obtained by multiplying the criterion weight by the criterion rating, was 30, a low score in comparison with the problem ranking scores of the other criteria in the table.

A similar process with the remaining five criteria listed in Table 15-7 yields a total ranking score of 239 for the infant malnutrition problem. This score is less than 50% of the total score possible. Other problems in the community would be ranked by the same procedure, and their ranking scores would be compared with the ranking of the infant malnutrition problem to reveal the partners' commitment to solving the problems. If 239 were found to be the highest-ranking score among the several identified community health problems, the problem of infant malnutrition would be the logical priority for intervention.

Arriving at a problem ranking score for each identified problem may appear complicated, but recall that the criteria were set up and weighted by the people taking part in the community partnership before prioritizing began. Also, the reasons for rating and each rating score are decided and set up with active input by all members in the community partnership. Although the number scores are subjective, the active involvement of the nurse and various community representatives helps to ensure that the data used to establish the rationale are real and accurate. Community participation also helps to ensure that the significance of the score for each problem reflects its importance relative to other community health problems.

Sometimes, the perceptions of the nurse and of community members differ. For example, if the issue is smoking in public buildings, the community nurse might identify smoking as a public health problem. Community members, on the other hand, might view smoking as an issue of individual choice and personal freedom.

Once infant nutrition has been established as the priority problem, what to do about infant nutrition becomes the focus of the second and third steps of phase four: step 2 is establishing goals and objectives, and step 3 is developing intervention activities to meet the established objectives.

> **HOW TO** Prioritize Community Health Problems
>
> List all community health problems defined and follow these steps for each problem:
>
> 1. Use nominal group technique to identify problem priorities.
> 2. The nurse and community partners answer the question "How important is community awareness to each problem so it can be solved?"
> 3. The nurse and community partners give a number score to the question, between 1 (low) and 10 (high).
> 4. The process is repeated to get a criterion score for each of the six criteria in Box 15-7.
> 5. For each problem and each criterion, ask the question "Can the partners influence or change the situation?"
> 6. By consensus, the nurse and partners agree on a criterion weight and a rating for each problem.
> 7. To find out the problem ranking, multiply the weight and rating for each criterion. Total the ranking score for the six criteria for each problem.
> 8. Compare the total scores for each problem to find the priority problem for the community.

## Establishing Goals and Objectives

Once high-priority problems are identified, **goals** and **objectives** are developed. Goals are generally broad statements of desired outcomes. Objectives are the precise statements of the desired outcomes.

Table 15-8 shows an example of one of the goals, and the specific objectives associated with it, for the infant malnutrition problem in Jefferson County. The goal is to reduce the incidence and prevalence of infant malnutrition. The objectives must be precise, behaviorally stated, incremental, and measurable. In this example, the specific objectives pertain to assessing infant developmental levels, determining WIC eligibility, implementing an outreach program, enrolling infants in WIC, and providing supplemental foods in existing diets.

Deciding on these goals and objectives involves collaboration between the nurse and representatives of the community groups affected by both the problem and the proposed intervention. This often requires a great deal of negotiating with everyone taking part in the planning process. One important advantage offered by the continuous active involvement of people affected by the outcomes is that they come to have a vested interest in those

## Table 15-8  Goals and Objectives: Infant Malnutrition

Community: Jefferson County
Problem/concern: Infant malnutrition
Goal statement: To reduce the incidence and prevalence of infant malnutrition

| PRESENT DATE | OBJECTIVE (NUMBER AND STATEMENT) | COMPLETION DATE |
|---|---|---|
| 1-03 | 1. 80% of infants seen by health department, neighborhood health center, and private physicians will have developmental levels assessed. | 8-05 |
| 1-03 | 2. WIC eligibility will be determined for 80% of infants seen by health department, neighborhood health center, and private physicians. | 5-05 |
| 1-03 | 3. An outreach program will be implemented to identify at-risk infants not now known to health care providers. | 8-05 |
| 1-03 | 4. WIC eligibility will be determined for 25% of at-risk infants. | 1-05 |
| 1-03 | 5. 75% of all infants eligible for WIC food supplements will be enrolled in the program. | 12-05 |
| 1-03 | 6. 50% of the mothers of infants enrolled in WIC will demonstrate three ways of incorporating WIC supplements into their infants' diets. | 5-05 |

outcomes and therefore are supportive of and committed to the success of the intervention. Once goals and objectives are chosen, intervention activities to accomplish the objectives can be identified.

### Identifying Intervention Activities

**Intervention activities** are the strategies used to meet the objectives, the ways change will be effected, and the ways the problem cycle will be broken. Usually, alternative intervention activities do exist, and they must be identified and evaluated. Sketching out possible interventions and selecting the best set of activities to achieve the goal of documenting and reducing infant malnutrition are shown in Tables 15-9 and 15-10.

To achieve the objective related to assessing infant developmental levels (objective 1 in Table 15-8), five intervention activities are listed in the second column of Table 15-9. Each is relevant to the first objective: 80% of infants seen by the health department, neighborhood health center, and private physicians will have their developmental levels assessed. The first two activities involve WIC personnel as the principal change agents. The last three involve the nurse, WIC personnel, and the staff of the health department, neighborhood health center, and private physicians' offices as the change partners (more about change agents and change partners later).

The expected effect of each activity is considered in the third and fifth columns of Table 15-9. The **value,** or the likelihood that the activity will help meet the objective and finally resolve the problem, is noted in the third column. Clearly, it is more valuable in the long term to educate others to assess infant development (activity 4) than to do it for them (activity 1). It is also valuable to analyze

the change process necessary to complete the objective (activity 5). As a result, activities 4 and 5 have higher value scores than activity 1, in which the professional staff alone carries out the intervention.

On the other hand, the **probability,** or the likelihood that the means can be implemented, is highest when only the nurse is involved, because the nurse has more control over self-behavior than over the behavior of others. Therefore activities 1 and 3 have higher probabilities than activities 2, 4, and 5, as recorded in the fifth column. Conditions explaining the numerical scores are noted briefly in the fourth column. A total score is computed by multiplying the value of the activity by the probability of implementation. These scores are listed in the last column. The activities with the highest total scores become the priority intervention activities, because it is important to be able to both achieve the objective (value) and carry out the means (probability). In this case, activities 4 and 5, with total scores of 64 and 80 respectively, would be selected.

Although the numbers assigned by the nurse to both value and probability are based on subjective judgment, their products are quite useful. When the scores in the two columns are multiplied, the products give the nurse a basis for judging which of the potential intervention activities will be most effective in meeting the objectives.

A second example of developing a plan is shown in Table 15-10. The activities relate to objective 3 of the goals and objectives (in Table 15-8), which involves starting up and carrying out an outreach program. These activities involve using lay advisors, hospital nurses, community and public health nurses, and WIC personnel. Activity 1 (with an activity ranking of 48) and activity 2 (with an activity ranking of 40) were selected. Activity 1 builds on existing

**Table 15-9  Plan: Intervention Activities to Assess Infants' Developmental Levels**

Community: Jefferson County
Objective number 1 and statement: 80% of infants seen by health department, neighborhood health center, and private physicians will have development levels assessed.

| DATE | INTERVENTION ACTIVITIES/MEANS | VALUE TO ACHIEVING OBJECTIVE (1-10) | ACTIVITY/MEANS FOR SELECTED IMPLEMENTATION | PROBABILITY OF IMPLEMENTING ACTIVITY (1-10) | ACTIVITY RANKING (VALUE × PROBABILITY) |
|---|---|---|---|---|---|
| 1-04 | 1. WIC supplies personnel to assess infant developmental levels. | 1 | Insufficient personnel and time; existing community resources (potential) are ignored. | 10 | 10 |
| 1-04 | 2. WIC provides inservice education to staff on assessment of infant development. | 5 | Antipathy between WIC personnel and other health workers is high. The need for education must be assessed first, and enthusiasm for objectives must be created. | 5 | 25 |
| 1-04 | 3. Community nurse (CN) provides inservice education to staff in assessment of infant development. | 3 | CN cannot do it alone. | 10 | 30 |
| 1-04 | 4. CN helps WIC personnel identify inservice educational needs of area health care providers related to assessment of infant development. | 8 | Most likely to build on existing community strengths; CN skilled in needs assessment, and interpersonal approaches are needed to increase interest. | 8 | 64 |
| 1-04 | 5. CN helps WIC personnel identify driving and restraining forces relative to implementation of objective. | 10 | Without this change, effort is likely to fail. | 8 | 80 |

## Table 15-10 Plan: Intervention Activities to Implement an Outreach Program

Community: Jefferson County

Objective number 3 and statement: An outreach program is implemented to identify at-risk infants not now known to health care providers.

| DATE | INTERVENTION ACTIVITIES/ MEANS | VALUE TO ACHIEVING OBJECTIVE (1-10) | ACTIVITY/ MEANS SELECTED FOR IMPLEMENTATION | PROBABILITY OF IMPLEMENTING ACTIVITY (1-10) | ACTIVITY RANKING (VALUE × PROBABILITY) |
|---|---|---|---|---|---|
| 1-04 | 1. Community nurse (CN) identifies and trains lay advisors in community as case finders. | 8 | Lay leaders already known, proven to be effective change agents; cannot, however, be paid. | 6 | 48 |
| 1-04 | 2. Local hospital administrators alter job descriptions of nurses in maternity and pediatrics to include case finding and referral. | 8 | Program to include all babies in Jefferson County born in hospital since 1994. Administrator interested in community. Administration powerful and can alter nurses' job descriptions. | 5 | 40 |
| 1-04 | 3. CN encourages public health nurses (PHNs) to do better job of case finding. | 8 | Public health nurses have historic role in case finding. CN not well known by PHNs. PHNs reported to be overworked. | 2 | 16 |
| 1-04 | 4. WIC personnel devote one evening per week to case finding. | 1 | One nurse (non-resident) eager to do this. Does not develop existing community resources. | 10 | 10 |

informal community leaders, and activity 2 addresses needed changes in the formal health care delivery system. See the How To box on p. 363 about prioritizing community health problems, and use a similar process for arriving at rankings. Note that in Tables 15-9 and 15-10, there is no total score.

Sufficient resources are not always available to implement all of the intervention activities, but the ranking process illustrated in Tables 15-9 and 15-10 will show which activities should be implemented first. To effectively implement each chosen activity, the health nurse must be clear about the availability of needed resources; who will be responsible for implementing the activity; how it will be evaluated; and when it will be completed. Table 15-11 provides a format for keeping track of these specific details.

## Implementing in the Community

**Implementation,** the fifth phase of the nursing process, involves the work and activities aimed at achieving the goals and objectives. Implementing efforts may be made by the person or group who established the goals and objectives, or they may be shared with, or even delegated to, others. Having a central authority to oversee the efforts to start up and carry out the plan is important, and the nurse's position on this issue can be affected by a variety of factors.

### Factors Influencing Implementation

Implementation is shaped by the nurse's chosen roles, the type of health problem selected as the focus for intervening, the community's readiness to take part in problem solving, and characteristics of the social change process.

**Table 15-11   Intervention Activity Implementation and Evaluation Details**

Community: Jefferson County

Objective number and statement: _____

| INTERVENTION ACTIVITY | RESPONSIBLE AGENCY/ INDIVIDUAL | HOW INTERVENTION ACTIVITY WILL BE EVALUATED (OBSERVABLE, MEASURABLE CRITERIA) | TARGET DATE FOR COMPLETION OF INTERVENTION ACTIVITY | RESULTS/ OUTCOMES OF INTERVENTION (COMPLETION DATE) |
|---|---|---|---|---|
| 1. Community nurse (CN) identifies and trains lay advisors in community as case finders (from Table 15-10, activity 1) | Community nurse | 1. Lay advisors will be able to verbally describe case-finding methods to the CN 2. Number of new WIC cases will be tracked by CN on monthly basis for 1 year. | Lay Advisor Training completed by 4-04. | |

The nurse taking part in community-oriented intervention has knowledge and skills that the partners do not have; the question is how the nurse uses the position, knowledge, and skills.

*Nurse's Role*

Nurses can act as content experts, helping communities select and attain task-related goals. In the example of infant malnutrition, the nurse used epidemiologic skills to find the incidence and prevalence of malnutrition. The nurse also serves as a process expert by fostering the community's ability to document the problem rather than by only providing help as an expert in the area.

Content-focused roles often are considered **change agent** roles, whereas process roles are called **change partner** roles. Change agent roles stress gathering and analyzing facts and implementing programs, whereas change partner roles include those of enabler-catalyst, teacher of problem-solving skills, and activist advocate.

*The Problem and the Nurse's Role*

The role the nurse chooses depends on the nature of the health problem, on the community's decision-making ability, and on professional and personal choices. Some health problems clearly require certain intervention roles. If a community lacks democratic problem-solving abilities, the nurse may select teacher, facilitator, and advocate roles. Problem-solving skills must be explained and modeled. A problem that involves determining the status of community health, on the other hand, usually requires fact-gatherer and analyst roles. Some problems, such as the example of infant malnutrition presented earlier, require multiple roles. In that case, managing conflict among the involved health care providers demands process

skills. Collecting and interpreting the data necessary to document the problem requires both interpersonal and analytical skills.

The community's history of taking part in decision making is a critical factor. In a community skilled in identifying and successfully managing its problems, the nurse may best serve as technical expert or advisor. Different roles may be required if the community lacks problem-solving skills or has a history of unsuccessful change efforts. The nurse may have to focus on developing problem-solving capabilities or on making one successful change so that the community becomes empowered to take on the job of promoting further change on its own behalf.

*Social Change Process and the Nurse's Role*

The nurse's role also depends on the social change process. Not all communities are open to innovation. Ability to change is often related to the extent to which a community adheres to traditional norms. The more traditional the community, the less likely it is to change. In 1995 Rogers wrote about the diffusion of innovation, and the book provides important information for nurses. Innovation is often directly related to high socioeconomic status; a perceived need for change; the presence of liberal, scientific, and democratic values; and a high level of social participation by community residents (Rogers, 1995). Innovations with the highest adoption rates are seen as better than the other available choices. They also fit with existing values, can be started as a limited trial, and are easily explained or demonstrated. They are also simple and convenient (Rogers, 1995). For example, people living in a community might go to an immunization clinic rather than a private physician if the clinic is nearby and less expensive and if the physician is not always available when needed.

Innovations also are easier to accept when the innovation is shared in ways that fit in with the community's norms, values, and customs and when information is spread by the best communication mode (mass media for early adopters and face-to-face for late adopters–more about these later). Other factors that positively influence acceptance include the support of other communities for the change efforts, identification and use of opinion leaders, and clear, straightforward communication about the innovation (Rogers, 1995).

Many complex factors combine to shape how the change process is started and maintained. Therefore the nurse must be adaptable. The roles required to begin change may differ from those used to maintain or stabilize it. Also, the roles required to initiate, maintain, and stabilize change may vary from community to community and from one intervention to another within the same community. Thus the nurse must be skilled in a variety of implementation mechanisms.

## Implementation Mechanisms

Implementation mechanisms are the vehicles, or modes, by which innovations are transferred from the planners to the community. The nurse alone is never considered an implementation mechanism. Change on behalf of the community client requires multiple implementation mechanisms. The nurse must identify and appropriately use all of them. Some important implementation mechanisms, or aids, include small **interacting groups, lay advisors,** the **mass media,** and health policies.

### Small Interacting Groups

Small interacting groups, formal and informal, are essential implementation mechanisms. *Formal* groups in the community include families, legislative bodies, health care clients, and service providers. *Informal* groups include neighborhoods and social action groups. The common tie among these diverse groups is that they are located between the community and individuals. Because of their intermediate position, they can and do act both to support and to prevent change efforts at the community and individual levels. They are potentially powerful precisely because they are **mediating structures.**

As a result, the nurse needs to identify which groups view the proposed change as beneficial and which do not. New small groups may need to be formed to encourage the change. Changes may be necessary in the innovation or in how the innovation is spread throughout the community to increase acceptance. At first the innovation may have to be directed to groups with a majority of **early adopters** (those with broad perspectives and abilities to adopt new ideas from mass media information sources) and to groups whose goals are reflected in the intervention plan (Eng et al, 1997). Using a small group to initiate community-oriented change is shown in Table 15-12.

### Lay Advisors

Lay advisors are people who are influential in approving or vetoing new ideas and from whom others seek advice and information about new ideas (Eng et al, 1997). They often perform a function similar to that of early adopters. Lay advisors, or opinion leaders, can be identified by their agreement with community norms, heavy involvement in formal social groups, specific areas of skill and knowledge, and a slightly higher social status than their followers (Rogers, 1995).

### Mass Media

Both small interacting groups and lay advisors are particularly useful in creating change among **late adopters,** those who are last to embrace change. However, groups dominated by early adopters and lay advisors can be reached through the mass media. Mass media, such as newspapers, television, and radio, represent an impersonal and formal type of communication and are useful in providing information quickly to a large number of people. Using the mass media is efficient because the ratio of money spent to population covered is low and populations can be targeted. For example, information about teenage pregnancy can be efficiently provided through rock music stations. In addition to being efficient, the mass media are effective aids in intervention.

### Health Policy

Health policy also can play a critical part in the adoption of healthful community-oriented change (Dever, 1997). The major intent of public policy in the health field is to address collective human needs, and it often limits individual choice in order to serve the public good. For example, drivers have been urged for several years to wear automobile seat belts. However, the incidence of automobile fatalities was not reduced until drivers were required to observe lowered speed limits and, in some states, to wear seat belts and use special restraining seats for children. Clearly, health policy can help encourage interventions that promote community health.

If public policy that will encourage or even simply allow health-generating choices is to become law, the nurse must actively lobby for it. See Chapter 8 for a more indepth discussion.

The nurse also must use small groups, lay advisors, and the mass media as aids to getting started. Working with naturally occurring small groups, such as the family, and with lay advisors is familiar to most community-oriented nurses. Working with legislators or the mass media is less familiar, yet all resources must be used to achieve healthful change in the community client. No matter what means are used, all efforts to start and maintain changes must be documented.

Evaluating, the sixth phase of this process, is also important to determine and improve the ability of community-oriented nursing practice to produce the desired results. Evaluating also increases the knowledge base and improves the rate of success in competing for funds for needed programs to solve community problems.

## Table 15-12 Progress Notes: Infant Malnutrition

Community: Jefferson County
Goal: To reduce the incidence and prevalence of infant malnutrition

| DATE | NARRATIVE, ASSESSMENT, PLAN* | BUDGET, TIME |
|---|---|---|
| 2-14-04 | Objective 1, means 4 | $200; 2 hours of meeting and 2 hours of preparation time |
|  | *Narrative:* Meeting to develop needs assessment was attended by community nurse (CN), two WIC personnel, and physicians from health department, neighborhood health center, and local medical society. Consensus rapidly achieved among 5 of 6 participants that goal, objectives, and means (especially objective 1, means 4) were appropriate. Physician representing medical society consistently objected, stating vehemently that private sector had long provided adequate medical care for area youngsters. Physician would not recommend that medical society support the effort. CN afraid that this would jeopardize entire effort. Eventually, however, physician left and plans were made to develop and conduct needs assessment and to continue seeking medical society's help. | |
|  | *Agenda:* CN to develop needs assessment tool with WIC personnel and health systems agency planner. Physicians to develop list of providers to be contacted. Neighborhood health center physician to get a place on medical society agenda and attempt to clarify plans. WIC personnel to contact nonphysician health workers to introduce plan and develop provider list. | |
|  | *Assessment:* Plans made to proceed with needs assessment and partner support essential to accomplishment of objective. Group process problematic, and CN ineffective because of discomfort with conflict between physician and WIC staff member. | |
|  | *Plans:* Meeting scheduled for 2-28-04 to deal with agreed-on agenda. | |
|  | Before 2-28 meeting, CN will discuss ways to better handle conflict with consultation group, collaborate on drafting needs assessment, and telephone others to determine their progress. J. Goeppinger, RN, CN | |

*Record both objective and subjective data. Interpret these data in terms of whether the objectives were achieved and whether the intervention activities were effective. The plan depends on the assessment and may include both new or revised objectives and activities.

## Evaluating Community Health Intervention

Simply defined, **evaluation** is the appraisal of the effects of some organized activity or program. Evaluating may involve the design and conduct of evaluation research, in which social science research methods are used to determine if the program is effective, efficient, adequate, and appropriate, and if there are unintended consequences (Dever, 1997). Evaluating may also involve the more elementary process of assessing progress by comparing the objectives and the results, as discussed here.

Evaluation begins in the planning phase, when goals and measurable objectives are established and goal-attaining activities are identified. After implementing the intervention, only the meeting of objectives and the effects of intervening activities have to be assessed. The progress notes direct the nurse to perform such appraisals during the implementing activities. In assessing the data recorded there, the nurse is requested to evaluate whether the objectives were met and whether the intervening activities used were effective.

The nurse also must decide whether the costs in money and time were worth the resulting benefits. This process is shown in the progress notes. In Table 15-12, the nurse has noted progress toward the needs assessed and the difficulties encountered in handling conflict among the group members.

Such an evaluating process is oriented to community health because the intervening goals and objectives come from the nurse's and the community's ideas about health. Simple as it appears, it is not without problems. The results must be compared to the baseline information collected on the nurse's community before the intervention, as well as to results obtained in other communities. Either of these comparisons will help reveal the success or failure of the intervention.

The lay role in evaluation is also important. Professionals have adopted partnerships in assessing and implementing more readily than in evaluating. The issue of who has the power to define, judge, and institute change in professional activities is an issue. With evaluation, the entire process is

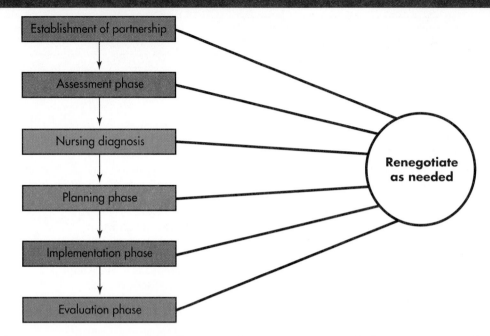

**Figure 15-3** Summary flow sheet illustrating the nursing process with the community as client.

open to renegotiation to achieve community health (Figure 15-3).

## Role of Outcomes in the Evaluation Phase

Students using the community-as-client process presented in this chapter must recognize that in a political climate where health resources are limited, the measurement of outcomes is a particularly important part of the evaluation process. This is one reason for emphasizing measurable objectives. Objectives must also be chosen with sensitivity to the changes that may result from the interventions. Dever (1997) recommends outcomes questions about appropriate and effective interventions—for example, Was the appropriate intervention done ineffectively or effectively? To answer these and other outcomes questions, Dever emphasizes the correct use of rates and numbers as one means of evaluating intervention outcomes in defined communities. Often, data collected over time can also provide important outcomes information about health trends within the community. As indicated previously, epidemiologic data and trends do not provide the only measures of success, but they do provide important information about the intervention. Nurses need to consider collecting this type of outcome data for use as part of the evaluation phase. Other types of evaluation questions focus on the intervention process itself—for example, Was the process of implementing the intervention efficient, and was it acceptable to the community?

## PERSONAL SAFETY IN COMMUNITY PRACTICE

Effective community-oriented nursing practice starts with personal safety, and this remains important throughout the process. An awareness of the community and common

sense are the two best guidelines for judgment. For example, common sense suggests not leaving anything valuable on a car seat and not leaving your car unlocked. Similar guidelines apply to the use of public transportation. Calling ahead to clients to schedule meetings will help prevent delays or confusion, and it gives the nurse an opportunity to lay the groundwork for the meeting. If there is no telephone and no access to a neighbor's telephone, plan to establish a time for any future meetings during the initial visit. Regardless of whether there has been telephone contact, there are rare situations when a meeting is postponed because the nurse arrives at a location where people are unexpectedly hanging out by the entrance and the nurse has concerns about personal safety.

For nurses who are either just beginning their careers in the community or who are just starting a new position, there are three clear sources of information that will help answer any questions about personal safety:

1. *Other nurses, social workers, or health care providers who are familiar with the dynamics of a given community.* They can provide valuable insights into when to visit, how to get there, and what to expect, because they function in the community themselves.

2. *Community members.* The best sources of information about the community are the community members themselves, and one benefit of developing an active partnership with community members is their willingness to share their insight about day-to-day community life.

3. *The nurse's own observations.* Knowledge gained during the data collection phase of the process should provide a solid base for an awareness of day-to-day

community activity. Nurses with experience practicing in the community generally agree that if they feel uncomfortable in a situation, they should trust their instincts and leave.

## Practice Application

Lily, a nurse in a small city, became aware of the increased incidence of respiratory diseases through contact with families in the community and the local chapter of the American Lung Association. During family visits, Lily noticed that many of the parents were smokers. Because most of the families Lily visited had small children, she became concerned about the effects of secondhand smoke on the health of the infants and children in her family caseload.

Further assessment of this community indicated that the community recognized several problems, including school safety and the risk of water pollution, in addition to the smoking problem that Lily had identified during her family visits. Talks with different community members revealed that they wanted each of these identified problems "fixed," although these same community members were uncertain about how to start. In deciding which of the three identified problems to address first, which criterion would be most important for Lily to consider?

**A.** The amount of money available
**B.** The level of community motivation to "fix" one of the three identified problems
**C.** The number of people in the community who expressed a concern about each of the three identified problems
**D.** How much control she would have in the process

**Answer is in the back of the book.**

## Key Points

- Most definitions of community include three dimensions: (1) networks of interpersonal relationships that provide friendship and support to members; (2) residence in a common locality; and (3) shared values, interests, or concerns.
- A community is defined as a locality-based entity, composed of systems of formal organizations reflecting societal institutions, informal groups, and aggregates that are interdependent and whose function or expressed intent is to meet a wide variety of collective needs.
- A community practice setting is insufficient reason for saying that practice is oriented toward the community client. When the location of the practice is in the community but the focus of the practice is the individual or family, then the nursing client remains the individual or family, not the whole community.

- Community-oriented practice is targeted to the community, the population group in which healthful change is sought.
- Community health as used in this chapter is defined as the meeting of collective needs through identifying problems and managing behaviors within the community itself and between the community and the larger society.
- Most changes aimed at improving community health involve, of necessity, partnerships among community residents and health workers from a variety of disciplines.
- Assessing community health requires gathering existing data, generating missing data, and interpreting the database.
- Five methods of collecting data useful to the nurse are informant interviews, participant observation, secondary analysis of existing data, surveys, and windshield surveys.
- Gaining entry or acceptance into the community is perhaps the biggest challenge in assessment.
- The nurse is usually an outsider and often represents an established health care system that is neither known nor trusted by community members, who may react with indifference or even active hostility.
- The planning phase includes analyzing and establishing priorities among community health problems already identified, establishing goals and objectives, and identifying intervention activities that will accomplish the objectives.
- Once high-priority problems are identified, broad relevant goals and objectives are developed.
- The goal (generally a broad statement of desired outcome) and objectives (the precise statements of the desired outcome) are carefully selected.
- Intervention activities, the means by which objectives are met, are the strategies that clarify what must be done to achieve the objectives, the ways change will be affected, and the way the problem will be interpreted.
- Implementation, the third phase of the nursing process, means transforming a plan for improved community health into achieving of goals and objectives.
- Simply defined, evaluation is the appraisal of the effects of some organized activity or program.

## Clinical Decision-Making Activities

1. Observe an occupational health nurse, community or public health nurse, school nurse, family nurse practitioner, or emergency department nurse for several hours. Determine which of the nurse's activities are community oriented, give specific examples, and present your reasons for considering them community oriented.

2. Using your own community as a frame of reference, develop examples illustrating the concepts of
community, community client, community health,
and partnership for health. What are some of the
complexities of this question?
3. Read your local newspaper and identify articles illustrating the concepts of community, community
client, community health, and partnership for
health. How does your article specifically relate to
the concept?
4. Using any two of the conditions of community
competence given in the chapter, briefly analyze
your own community. Give examples of each
condition.

**Additional Resources**

These related resources are found either in the appendix at the back of this book or on the book's
website at **http://evolve.elsevier.com/Stanhope.**

### Appendixes

Appendix G.1 Community-as-Partner Model

**evolve** Evolve Website

Appendix C.1 Community-Oriented Health Record
(COHR) and forms
WebLinks: Healthy People 2010

## References

Abraham T, Fallon PJ: Caring for the
community: development of the advanced practice nurse role, *Clin Nurse
Spec* 11(5):224-230, 1997a.

Abraham T, Fallon PJ: Community competence and empowerment: strategies
for rural change in women's health service planning and delivery, *Aust J Rural
Health* 5(1):26-30, 1997b.

American Nurses Association: Scope
and standards of public health nursing
practice, Washington, DC, 1999, ANA.

American Public Health Association:
*American public health association model
standards: the guide to implementing
model standards—eleven steps toward a
healthy community,* Washington, DC,
1993, APHA.

American Public Health Association:
*Community strategies for health: fitting
in the pieces,* Washington, DC, 1994,
APHA.

American Public Health Association,
Public Health Nursing Section: *The defi-
nition and role of public health nursing,*
Washington, DC, 1996, APHA.

Anderson ET, McFarlane J, editors:
*Community as client: application of the
nursing process,* Philadelphia, 1988,
Lippincott.

Anderson ET, McFarlane J, editors:
*Community as partner,* ed 3,
Philadelphia, 2000, Lippincott.

Baker EA et al: The Latino health advocacy program: a collaborative lay health
advisor approach, *Health Educ Behav*
24(4):495-509, 1997.

Blum HL: *Planning for health,* New York,
1974, Human Sciences Press.

Clark H, Mass H: Comox Valley nursing
centre: from collaboration to empowerment, *Public Health Nurs* 15(3):216-224,
1998.

Consensus set of health status indicators for the general assessment of community health status—United States,
*MMWR Morb Mortal Wkly Rep*
40(27):449-451, 1991 (updated 8/01).

Cottrell LS: The competent community.
In Kaplan BH, Wilson RN, Leighton AH,
editors: *Further explorations in social
psychiatry,* New York, 1976, Basic Books.

Council on Linkages Between Academia
and Public Health Practice: *Core competencies for public health professionals,*
Washington, DC, 2001, USDHHS and
Public Health Foundation, available at
www.phf.org/Link.htm.

Courtney R et al: The partnership
model: working with individuals, families, and communities toward a new vision of health, *Public Health Nurs*
13(3):177-186, 1996.

Craft-Rosenberg M: Diagnosis for community nursing, *Nurs Diagn* 10(3):127-
128, 1999.

Delbecq AL, Van De Ven AH: A group
process model for problem identification and program planning, *J Appl Behav
Sci* 62:467, 1971.

Dever GE: *Improving outcomes in public
health practice,* Gaithersburg, Md, 1997,
Aspen.

Eng E, Parker EA, Harlan C: Lay health
advisors: a critical link to community
capacity building, *Health Educ Behav*
24(4):413-522, 1997.

Flick LH, Reese C, Harris A:
Aggregate/community-centered undergraduate community health nursing
clinical experience, *Public Health Nurs*
13(1):36-41, 1996.

Flynn BC: Partnerships in healthy cities
and communities: a social commitment
for advanced practice nurses, *Adv Pract
Nurs Q* 2(4):1-6, 1997.

Flynn BC: Communicating with the public: community-based nursing research
and practice, *Public Health Nurs*
15(3):165-170, 1998.

Goeppinger J, Lassiter PG, Wilcox B:
Community health is community competence, *Nurs Outlook* 30(8):464, 1982.

Green PM, Slade DS: Environmental
nursing diagnoses for aggregates and
community, *Nurs Diagn* 12(1):5-13, 2001.

Head B, Maas M, Johnson M: Research
and development: outcomes for home
and community nursing in integrated delivery systems, *Caring* 16(1):50-56, 1997.

Health Canada: The population health
template: key elements and actions that
define a population health approach,
Ottawa, 2002, Health Canada, retrieved
June 2002 from http://www.hc-sc.ga.ca/
hppb/phdd/pdf/discussion_paper.pdf.

Hildebrandt E et al: Building community participation in health care: a
model and example from South Africa,
*J Nurs Scholarsh* 28(2):155-159, 1996.

Jackson EJ, Parks CP: Recruitment and
training issues from selected lay health
advisor programs among African Americans: a 20-year perspective [review],
*Health Educ Behav* 24(4):418-431, 1997.

Kroeger A et al: Operational aspects of bednet impregnation for community-based malaria control in Nicaragua, Ecuador, Peru and Colombia, *Trop Med Int Health* 2(6):589-602, 1997.

Kyba FN, Hathaway W, Okimi PH: Health promotion in a museum: a collaborative community partnership, *Nurse Educ* 22(4):32-35, 1997.

Laffrey SC, Kulbok PA: An integrative model for holistic community health nursing, *J Holist Nurs* 17(1):88-103, 1999.

Lewis RK et al: Reducing the risk for adolescent pregnancy: evaluation of a school/community partnership in a Midwestern military community, *Fam Community Health* 22(2):16-30, 1999.

Lindsey E, Stajduhar K, McGuinness L: Examining the process of community development, *J Adv Nurs* 33(6):828-835, 2001.

Lough MA: An academic-community partnership: a model of service and education, *J Community Health Nurs* 16(3):137-149, 1999.

Ludwig-Beymer P et al: Community assessment in a suburban Hispanic community: a description of method, *J Transcult Nurs* 8(1):19-27, 1996.

Lutz J, Herrick CA, Lehman BB: Community partnership: a school of nursing creates nursing centers for older adults, *Nurs Health Care Perspect* 22(1):26-29, 2001.

MacLachlan M: Identifying problems in community health promotion: an illustration of the nominal group technique in AIDS education, *J R Soc Health* 116(3):143-148, 1996.

Martin K, Scheet N: *The Omaha system: a pocket guide for community health nursing,* Philadelphia, 1992, Saunders.

Maurana CA, Clark MA: The health action fund: a community-based approach to enhancing health, *J Health Commun* 5(3):243-254, 2000.

McClowry SG et al: A comprehensive school-based clinic: university and community partnership, *J Soc Pediatr Nurses* 1(1):19-26, 1996.

McMahon B, Browning S, Rose-Colley M: A school-community partnership for at-risk students in Pennsylvania, *J Sch Health* 71(2):53-55, 2001.

Meade CD, Calvo A: Developing community-academic partnerships to enhance breast health among rural and Hispanic migrant and seasonal farmworker women, *Oncol Nurs Forum* 28(10):1577-1584, 2001.

Miller MP et al: Prevention of smoking behaviors in middle school students: student nurse interventions, *Public Health Nurs* 18(2):77-81, 2001.

Parker EA et al: Detroit's East Side Village health worker partnership: community-based lay health advisor intervention in an urban area, *Health Educ Behav* 25(1):24-45, 1998.

Parker M, Barry C, King B: Use of inquiry method for assessment and evaluation in a school-based community nursing project, *Fam Community Health* 23(2):54-61, 2000.

Parris KM et al: Integrating nursing diagnoses, interventions, and outcomes in public health nursing practice, *Nurs Diagn* 10(2):49-56, 1999.

Redman S et al: Consulting about priorities for the NHMRC National Breast Cancer Centre: how good is the nominal group technique? *Aust N Z J Public Health* 21(3):250-256, 1997.

Rogers E: *Diffusion of innovations,* ed 4, New York, 1995, Free Press.

Ryan W: *Blaming the victim,* New York, 1976, Free Press.

Schulz AJ et al: "It's a 24-hour thing . . . a living-for-each-other concept": identity, networks, and community in an urban village health worker project, *Health Educ Behav* 24(4):465-480, 1997.

Schwab M, Syme SL: On paradigms, community participation, and the future of public health, *Am J Public Health* 87(12):2049-2051, 1997.

Shiell A, Hawe P: Health promotion, community development and the tyranny of individualism, *Health Econ* 5(3):241-247, 1996.

Stanhope M, Knollmueller R: *Handbook of community-based and home health nursing practice,* ed 3, St Louis, Mo, 2000, Mosby.

Stevens P: Focus groups: collecting aggregate-level data to understand community health phenomena, *Public Health Nurs* 13(3):170-176, 1996.

U.S. Department of Health and Human Services: *Healthy people 2010: understanding and improving health,* ed 2, Washington, DC, 2000, U.S. Government Printing Office.

Westbrook L, Schultz P: From theory to practice: community health nursing in a public health neighborhood team, *Adv Nurs Sci* 23(2):50-61, 2000.

World Health Organization: *Community health nursing: report of a WHO expert committee,* Tech Rep Series No. 558, Geneva, 1974, WHO.

Zimmerman M: Empowerment theory: psychological, organizational and community levels of analysis. In Rappaport J, Seidman E, editors: *Handbook of community psychology,* pp 43-63, New York, 2000, Kluwer Academic/Plenum.

# Chapter 16

# Community and Public Health Nursing in Rural and Urban Environments

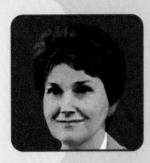

**Angeline Bushy, Ph.D., R.N., F.A.A.N.**

Angeline Bushy holds the Bert Fish Endowed Chair in community health nursing at the University of Central Florida, School of Nursing, Daytona campus. She holds a B.S.N. degree from the University of Mary in Bismarck, North Dakota; an M.N. degree in rural community health nursing from Montana State University in Bozeman; an M.Ed. in adult education from Northern Montana College in Havre; and a Ph.D. in nursing from the University of Texas at Austin. A clinical specialist in community health nursing, she has lived and worked for most of her life in rural facilities located in the north central and intermountain states. She has presented nationally and internationally on various rural nursing and rural health issues and has published six textbooks and numerous articles on that topic. She is actively involved in distributive education to off-campus sites and serves in the U.S. Army Reserve as a lieutenant colonel. She and Jack, her husband, have one daughter, Andrea.

## Objectives

After reading this chapter, the student should be able to do the following:

1. Compare and contrast definitions of rural and of urban

2. Describe residency as a continuum, ranging from farm residency to core inner city

3. Compare and contrast the health status of rural and urban populations on select health measures

4. Analyze barriers to care in health professional shortage areas and for underserved populations

5. Evaluate issues related to delivery of services for rural underserved populations

6. Describe characteristics of rural and small-town residency

7. Examine the role and scope of community and public health nursing practice in rural and underserved areas

8. Evaluate two professional–client–community partnership models that can effectively provide a continuum of care to residents living in an environment with sparse resources

---

Access to health care is a national priority, especially in regions with an insufficient number of health care providers. Recruiting and retaining qualified health professionals in underserved communities, particularly the inner city and rural areas of the United States, is difficult. Until recently, however, only limited research has been undertaken on the special challenges, problems, and opportunities of nursing practice—especially nursing in rural settings. This chapter presents major issues surrounding health care delivery in rural environments, which sometimes differs from that in urban or more populated settings. Common definitions for the term *rural* are discussed, as are its associated lifestyle, the health status of rural populations, barriers to obtaining a continuum of health care services, and nursing practice issues. Strategies are discussed to help nurses deliver more effective community-oriented health services to clients who live in isolated environments with sparse resources. This chapter describes rural nursing practice and can be used by students, nurses who practice in rural health departments, and those who work in agencies located in urban areas that offer outreach services to rural populations in their catchment area.

## HISTORICAL OVERVIEW

Formal rural nursing originated with the Red Cross Rural Nursing Service, which was organized in November 1912. The Committee on Rural Nursing was under the direction of Mabel Boardman (chair), Jane Delano (vice-chair), and Annie Goodrich along with other Red Cross leaders and philanthropists (Bigbee and Crowder, 1985). Before, care of the sick in a small community was provided by informal social support systems. When self-care and family care were not effective in bringing about healing, this task was assigned to healing women who lived in the community. Historically, the health needs of rural Americans have been numerous, and although not necessarily unique, they are different from those of urban populations. Consistent problems of maldistribution of health

## Key Terms

**farm residency**, p. 376
**frontier**, p. 381
**health professional shortage area**, p. 380
**medically underserved**, p. 391

**nonfarm residency**, p. 376
**rural**, p. 375
**rural–urban continuum**, p. 376
**suburbs**, p. 376

**urban**, p. 376
*See Glossary for definitions*


## Chapter Outline

Historical Overview
Definition of Terms
*Rurality: A Subjective Concept*
*Rural–Urban Continuum*
Current Perspectives
*Population Characteristics*
*Health Status of Rural Residents*
Rural Health Care Delivery Issues and Barriers
  to Care

Nursing Care in Rural Environments
*Theory, Research, and Practice*
*Community-Oriented Nursing*
*Research Needs*
*Preparing Nurses for Rural Practice Settings*
Future Perspectives
*Scarce Resources and a Comprehensive Health
  Care Continuum*

*Healthy People 2010 National Health Objectives
  Related to Rural Health*
Building Professional–Community–Client
  Partnerships in Rural Settings
*Case Management*
*Community-Oriented Primary Health Care*

professionals, poverty, limited access to services, ignorance, and social isolation have plagued many rural communities for generations.

Over the years, the history of the Red Cross Rural Nursing Service shows a consistent movement away from its initial rural focus, as demonstrated by its frequent name changes. Unfortunately, concern for rural health is similarly often temporary and replaced by other areas of greater need. It can be hoped that health care reform initiatives will soon focus on ensuring access to care for rural and urban residents.

## DEFINITION OF TERMS
### Rurality: A Subjective Concept

Everyone has an idea as to what constitutes rural as opposed to urban residence. However, the two cannot be viewed as two opposing entities. Moreover, with the increased degree of urban influence on rural communities, the differences are no longer as distinct as they may have been even a decade ago (Baer, Johnson, and Gessler, 1997; Cromartie and Swanson, 1995; U.S. Bureau of the Census, 2001). In general, **rural** is defined in terms of the geographic location and population density, or it may be described in terms of the distance from (e.g., 20 miles) or the time (e.g., 30 minutes) needed to commute to an urban center.

Nationally and regionally, many measures of health, health care use, and health care resources vary by urbanization level. In other words, communities at different urbanization levels differ in their demographic, environmental, economic, and social characteristics. In turn, these characteristics influence the magnitude and types of health problems that communities face. Additionally, urban counties tend to have a greater supply of health care providers in relation to population, and residents of more rural counties often live farther from health care resources (Centers for Disease Control and Prevention [CDC], 2001).

Other definitions equate rural with **farm residency** and **urban** with **nonfarm residency.** Some consider *rural* to be a state of mind. For the more affluent, rural may bring to mind a recreational, retirement, or resort community located in the mountains or in lake country where one can relax and participate in outdoor activities, such as skiing, fishing, hiking, or hunting. For the less affluent, the term can impose grim scenes. For example, some people may think of an impoverished Indian reservation as comparable to an underdeveloped country, or it may bring to mind images of a migrant labor camp with several families living in a one-room shanty with no access to safe drinking water or adequate sanitation.

Just as each city has its own unique features, it is also difficult to describe a "typical rural town" because of the wide population and geographic diversity. For example, rural towns in Florida, Oregon, Alaska, Hawaii, and Idaho are different from one another, and quite different from those in Vermont, Texas, Tennessee, Alabama, or California. Furthermore, there can be vast differences between rural areas within one state. Still, descriptions and definitions for *rural* tend to be more subjective and relative in nature than for urban.

For example, "small" communities with populations of more than 20,000 have some features that one may expect to find in a city. Then again, residents who live in a community with a population of less than 2000 may consider a community with a population of 5000 to 10,000 to be a city. Although some communities may seem geographically remote on a map, the residents who live there may not feel isolated. Those residents believe they are within easy reach of services through telecommunication and dependable transportation, although extensive shopping facilities may be 50 to 100 miles from the family home, obstetric care may be 150 miles away, or nursing services in the district health department in an adjacent county may be 75 or more miles away.

## Rural–Urban Continuum

Frequently used definitions to describe rural and urban and to differentiate between them are provided by several federal agencies (U.S. Bureau of the Census, 2001; U.S. Department of Agriculture [USDA], 1997) (Box 16-1). These definitions, which in many cases are dichotomous in nature, fail to take into account the relative nature of ruralness. Rural and urban residencies are not opposing lifestyles. Rather, they must be seen as a **rural–urban continuum** ranging from living on a remote farm, to a village or small town, to a larger town or city, to a large metropolitan area with a *core inner city* (Figure 16-1).

*United States, 2001: Urban and Rural Health Chartbook*, a publication by the CDC (2001), further classifies counties into five levels of urbanization, from the most urban to the most rural. Three subclassifications are listed for metropolitan (metro) counties and two subclassifications are listed for nonmetropolitan (nonmetro)

---

> ### BOX 16-1   Terms and Definitions
>
> **Farm residency:** Residency outside area zoned as "city limits"; usually infers involvement in agriculture
>
> **Frontier:** Regions having fewer than six persons per square mile
>
> **Large central:** Counties in large (1 million or more population) metro areas that contain all or part of the largest central city
>
> **Large fringe:** Remaining counties in large (1 million or more population) metro areas
>
> **Metropolitan county:** Densely populated county with more than 1 million inhabitants
>
> **Nonfarm residency:** Residence within area zoned as "city limits"
>
> **Nonmetropolitan statistical area (non-SMSA):** Counties that do not meet SMSA (see below) criteria
>
> **Rural:** Communities having less than 20,000 residents or fewer than 99 persons per square mile
>
> **Small:** Counties in metro areas with less than 1 million people
>
> **Standard metropolitan statistical area (SMSA):** Region with a central city of at least 50,000 residents
>
> **Suburban:** Area adjacent to a highly populated city
>
> **Urban:** Geographic areas described as nonrural and having a higher population density; more than 99 persons per square mile; cities with a population of at least 20,000 but less than 50,000

---

counties. Metropolitan subclassifications include the following:

- *Large central:* Counties in large (1 million or more population) metro areas that contain all or part of the largest central city
- *Large fringe:* Remaining counties in large (1 million or more population) metro areas
- *Small:* Counties in metro areas with less than 1 million population

Nonmetropolitan subclassifications include the following:

- Areas with a city of 10,000 or more population
- Areas without a city of 10,000 or more population

There has been a significant population shift from urban to less populated regions of the United States. The fastest growing rural counties are located in rural regions of the nation and along the edges of larger metropolitan counties. Demographers metaphorically refer to this demographic phenomenon as the "doughnut effect." That is to say, people are moving away from highly populated areas to far-flung **suburbs** of urban centers. Most of the population growth has been in counties with a booming economy, with room to grow, and in western and southern states. Of the 10 fastest growing counties with 10,000 persons or more, four were located in western states, five in southern states, and one in a midwestern state (Bowers and Cook, 1997; CDC, 2001; Johnson-Webb, Baer, and Gesler, 1997).

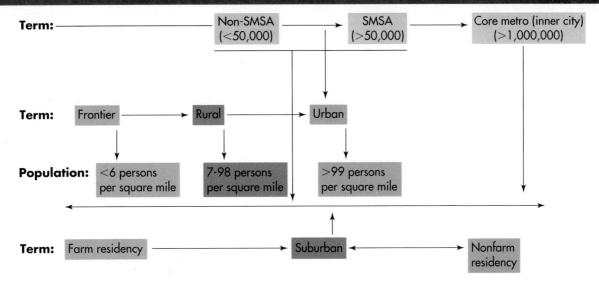

**Figure 16-1** The continuum of rural–urban residency.

Clearly, population shifts of this nature and size also affect the health status and lifestyle preferences of these communities. As beliefs and values change over time, urban–rural differences narrow in some aspects and enlarge in others. Depending on the definition that is used, the actual rural population might vary slightly. In general, about 25% of all U.S. residents live in rural settings. In this chapter, rural refers to areas having fewer than 99 persons per square mile and communities having 20,000 or fewer inhabitants.

## CURRENT PERSPECTIVES

### Population Characteristics

Adding to the confusion about what constitutes rural versus urban residency are the special needs of the numerous underrepresented groups (minorities, subgroups) who reside in the United States. In general, there is a higher proportion of whites in rural areas (about 82%) than in core metropolitan areas (about 62%). There are, however, regional variations, and some rural counties have a significant number of minorities. Of the total rural population, it is estimated that nearly 4 million are African American, almost 2 million are Native American, 34 million are Asian–Pacific Islanders, and 75 million are of other races. Little is documented on the needs and health status of special rural populations (National Rural Health Association, 1999, 2001a,b). Anthropologists are quick to report that, within a group, there often exists a wide range of lifestyles. Consequently, even in the smallest or most remote town or village, a subgroup may behave differently and have different values regarding health, illness, and patterns of accessing health care. Also, their lifestyle may be associated with health problems that are different from those of the predominant cultural group in a given community. Background infor-

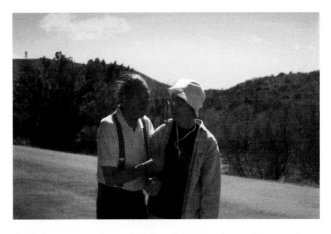

A higher proportion of older adults live in rural areas than in urban areas.

mation on selected populations can be found in Chapters 7 and 33. Table 16-1 presents demographic data comparing rural and urban populations.

Preliminary analysis of Census 2000 data reveals that rural communities are demographically bipolar. In respect to age distribution, there are higher-than-average numbers of younger and older residents in rural settings. One finds higher proportions of individuals between 6 and 17 years of age and over 65 years of age living in rural areas than in more populated settings. Persons 18 years of age and over living in rural areas are more likely to be, or to have been, married than are adults in the three urban categories. As a group, rural people also are more likely to be widowed. As for level of education, adults in rural areas have fewer years of formal schooling than do urban adults (U.S. Bureau of the Census, 2001).

Although there are regional variations, rural families in general tend to be poorer than their urban counterparts. Comparing annual incomes with the standardized index

### Table 16-1  Selected Population Characteristics by Place of Residence

| AGE (YR) | CORE METRO (%) | OTHER METRO (%) | URBAN NONMETRO (%) | RURAL (%) |
|---|---|---|---|---|
| 6-17 | 15.2 | 17.3 | — | 20 |
| 25-54 | 43.3 | 42.0 | 40.8 | 38.3 |
| 65+ | 12.0 | — | 10.0 | 17.3 |
| **Marital Status*** | | | | |
| Never married | 26.5 | 21.0 | 19.3 | 16.5 |
| Married/formerly married | 52.7 | 60.5 | 61.0 | 64.6 |
| **Education (yr)** | | | | |
| <12 | 25.0 | 25.0 | 40.0 | 36.0 |
| >12 | 40.0 | 40.0 | 30.0 | 24.0 |
| **Poverty Rate** | | | | |
| Below indices | 19.0 | 15.0 | 22.0 | 26.0 |

Data from Centers for Disease Control and Prevention: *United States, 2001—urban and rural chartbook*, Washington, DC, retrieved August 2001 from http://www.cdc.gov/nchs/data/hus/hus01.pdf; U.S. Department of Agriculture: *Agriculture fact book*, Washington, DC, 1997.
*Marital status determined in population over 17 years old.

established by the U.S. Bureau of the Census, more than one fourth of rural Americans live in or near poverty and nearly 40% of all rural children are impoverished (CDC, 2001; Packard Foundation, 1997a,b). Compared with those in metropolitan settings, a substantially smaller percentage of families living in nonmetropolitan areas are at the high end of the income scale. Accompanying the recent population shifts from urban to formerly rural areas, average income level may also be changing; however, no data are available at this time. Regardless, level of income is a critical factor in whether a family has health insurance or qualifies for public insurance. Thus rural families are less likely to have private insurance and more likely to have public insurance or to be uninsured.

The working poor in rural areas are particularly at risk for being underinsured or uninsured. In working poor families, one or more of the adults are employed but still cannot afford private health insurance. Furthermore, their annual income is such that it disqualifies the family from obtaining public insurance. A number of reasons are cited to explain why this phenomenon occurs more often in rural settings. For example, several individuals are self-employed in a family business, such as ranching or farming, or they work in small enterprises, such as a service station, restaurant, or grocery store. Also, an individual may be employed in part-time or in seasonal occupations, such as farm laborer and construction, in which health insurance is often not an employee benefit. In other situations, a family member may have a preexisting health condition that makes the cost of insurance prohibitive, if it is even available to them. A few rural families fall through the cracks and are unable to access any type of public assistance because of other deterrents, such as language barriers, being physically compromised, the

geographic location of an agency, lack of transportation, or having undocumented-worker status. Insurance, or the lack of it, has serious implications for the overall health status of rural residents and the nurses who provide services to them (CDC, 2001; National Rural Health Association, 1999, 2001a,b).

## Health Status of Rural Residents

Even though rural communities constitute about one fourth of the total population, the health problems and the health behaviors of the residents in them are not fully understood. This section summarizes what is known about the overall health status of rural adults and children. The health status measures that are addressed are perceived health status, diagnosed chronic conditions, physical limitations, frequency of seeking medical treatment, usual source of care, maternal–infant health, children's health,

### DID YOU KNOW?

Compared with urban Americans, rural residents have the following:
- Higher infant and maternal morbidity rates
- Higher rates of chronic illness, including heart disease, chronic obstructive pulmonary disease, unintentional motor vehicle traffic-related injuries, suicide, hypertension, cancer, and diabetes
- Unique health risks associated with occupations and the environment, such as machinery accidents, skin cancer from sun exposure, and respiratory problems associated with exposure to chemicals and pesticides
- Stress-related health problems and mental illness (although incidence not known)

mental health, minorities' health, and environmental and occupational health risks (CDC, 2001).

## Perceived Health Status

In general, people in rural areas have a poorer perception of their overall health and functional status than their urban counterparts. Rural residents over 18 years of age assess their health status less favorably than do urban residents. Studies show that rural adults are less likely to engage in preventive behavior, which increases their exposure to risk. Specifically, they are more likely to smoke and self-report higher rates of alcohol consumption and obesity; furthermore, they are less likely to engage in physical activity during leisure time, wear seat belts, have regular blood pressure checks, have Pap smears, and complete breast self-examinations. Ultimately, failure to participate in these healthy lifestyle behaviors affects the overall health status of rural residents, their level of function, physical limitations, degree of mobility, and level of self-care activities (CDC, 2001).

## Chronic Illness

Compared with their urban counterparts, rural adults are more likely to have one or more of the following chronic conditions: heart disease, chronic obstructive pulmonary disease, hypertension, arthritis and rheumatism, diabetes, cardiovascular disease, and cancer. Nearly half of all rural adults have been diagnosed with at least one of these chronic conditions, compared with about a quarter of nonrural adults. More specifically, the prevalence of diagnosed diabetes in rural adults is about 7 out of 100 as opposed to 5 out of 100 in nonrural environments. More rural adults have cancer (almost 7%) compared with urban adults (about 5%). Although most cases of acquired immunodeficiency (AIDS) are still found in urban areas, the rate is increasing in rural areas (CDC, 2001).

The percentage of rural adults who receive medical treatment for both life-threatening illness and degenerative or chronic conditions is higher than that of urban adults. Life-threatening conditions include malignant neoplasms, heart disease, cardiovascular problems, and liver disorders. Degenerative or chronic diseases include diabetes, kidney disease, arthritis and rheumatism, and chronic diseases of the circulatory, nervous, respiratory, and digestive systems. In essence, chronic health conditions, coupled with their poor health status, limit the physical activities of a larger proportion of rural residents than of their urban counterparts (Brooks, 1998; CDC, 2001; Edelman and Menz, 1996).

## Physical Limitations

Limitations in mobility and self-care are strong indicators of an individual's overall health status. Specific assessed measures on a national health survey included walking one block, walking uphill or climbing stairs, bending, lifting, stooping, feeding, dressing, bathing, and toileting. More rural adults (9%) experience at least three of these limita-

---

**DID YOU KNOW?**

- Americans who live in the suburbs are significantly better by many key health measures than those who live in the most rural and most urban areas of the nation.
- Death rates for working-age adults are higher in the most rural and the most highly populated urban areas. The highest death rates for children and young adults exist in the most rural counties.
- Residents of rural areas have the highest death rates for unintentional injuries in general, and for motor vehicle injuries in particular.
- Homicide rates are highest in the central counties of large metro areas. Suicide rates are highest in the most rural areas.
- Suburban residents are more likely to exercise during leisure time and more likely to have health insurance. Suburban women are the least likely to be obese.
- Both the most rural and the most urban areas have a high percentage of residents without health insurance. Residents in the most rural communities have the fewest dental visits.
- Teenagers and adults in rural counties are more likely to smoke.
- The AIDS rates are increasing more quickly in rural areas (30%) than in metropolitan areas (25.8%). Rural populations (fewer than 50,000) have the highest rates of increase in AIDS cases, representing 6.7% of all cases in the United States, with heterosexual contact accounting for most cases in many areas.
- In rural areas, gay men often are not openly gay and tend to engage in unprotected sex with strangers. Homophobia, racism, sexism, and AIDS stigma make HIV prevention efforts nearly impossible in some rural areas. Migration of people from urban to rural areas is cited as one possible contributor to the increased rates in rural areas. Among HIV-infected persons, more interstate than intrastate migration takes place from time of diagnosis until death.

From Centers for Disease Control and Prevention: *United States, 2001: urban and rural chartbook,* Washington, DC, retrieved August 2001 from http://www.cdc.gov/nchs/data/hus/hus01.pdf.

---

tions than metropolitan adults (6%). The increased prevalence of poor health status and impaired function is not necessarily due to the increased number of older adults found in rural areas. Similar patterns are evident in adults 18 to 64 years of age. Rural adults under 65 years of age are more likely than urban adults to assess their health status as fair to poor, and a greater percentage have been diagnosed with a chronic health condition (CDC, 2001).

On the basis of data from national health surveys, the overall health status of rural adults leaves much to be desired. This is attributed to a number of factors, including impaired access to health care providers and services, coupled with other rural factors. Thus nurses in rural practice settings play an important role in providing a continuum of care to clients living in these underserved areas. Specifically, nurses can help clients have healthier lives by teaching them how to prevent accidents, engage in more healthful lifestyle behaviors, and reduce the risk of chronic health problems. Once clients in rural environments have been diagnosed with a long-term problem, nurses can help them manage chronic conditions to achieve better health outcomes and functioning.

## Patterns of Health Service Use

When the use of health care services is measured, it is found that more than three fourths of adults in rural areas received medical care on at least one occasion during a year. Table 16-2 summarizes the frequency of visits to ambulatory care settings by rural and metropolitan residents. Despite their overall poorer health status and higher incidence of chronic health conditions, rural adults seek medical care less often than urban adults. In part, this discrepancy can be attributed to scarce resources and lack of providers in rural areas. Other reasons for this phenomenon are discussed later under Rural Health Care Delivery Issues and Barriers to Care (CDC, 2001).

NURSING TIP

Nurses must be especially thorough in their health assessment of rural clients who may not receive regular care for chronic health conditions.

### Table 16-2 Annual Number of Visits per Person to an Ambulatory Care Setting by Place of Residence

| PLACE OF RESIDENCE | VISITS PER YEAR |
|---|---|
| **Uninsured or Public Coverage** | |
| Rural/nonmetropolitan | 7.5 |
| All metropolitan | 7.5 |
| **Private Insurance** | |
| Rural/nonmetropolitan | 6.3 |
| All metropolitan | 7.4 |
| **Number of Visits by Place of Residence** | |
| Rural | 9.5 |
| Urban nonmetropolitan | 10.4 |
| Other metropolitan | 10.9 |
| Core metropolitan | 12.1 |

From Braden J, Beauregard K: National medical expenditure survey: health status and access to care of rural and urban populations, *Research Findings 18*, Rockville, Md, 1994, Agency for Health Care Policy and Research, Public Health Service (Publication No. 94-0031).

## Availability and Access of Health Care

The ability of a person to identify a usual source of care is considered a favorable indicator of access to health care and a person's overall health status. In essence, a person who has a usual source of care is more likely to seek care when ill and is more compliant with prescribed regimens. Having the same provider of care can enhance continuity of care, as well as a client's perceived perception of the quality of that care. Rural adults are more likely than urban adults to identify a particular medical provider as their usual source of care. As for the type of provider who delivers the care, general practitioners and advanced practice registered nurses (APRNs) usually are seen by rural adults, whereas urban adults are more likely to seek care from a medical specialist. However, this trend may be changing as managed care expands. Managed care advocates that primary care providers serve as gatekeepers, and it limits consumers' access to specialists (Health Resources Services Administration [HSRA], 1997, 2000; NRHA, 1999, 2001a,b; Schoenman, 1998).

Another measure of access to care is traveling time and/or distance to ambulatory care services. Rural persons who seek ambulatory care are more likely to travel more than 30 minutes to reach their usual source of care. Extended commuting time may also be a factor for residents in highly populated urban areas and those who must rely on public transportation. Upon arriving at the clinic or doctor's office, however, no differences between rural and urban residents have been found in the waiting time to see the provider.

Measures of usual place and usual provider suggests that rural residents are at least as well off as urban residents in regard to access to care. However, caution must be used when making this generalization, because 1 out of 17 rural counties is reported to have no physician. Among rural respondents on national surveys, the ability to identify a usual site of care or a particular provider often stems from a community or county having only one, perhaps two, health care providers. The limited number of health care facilities is reinforced by the finding that nearly all rural residents who seek health care use ambulatory services that are provided in a doctor's office as opposed to a clinic, community health center, hospital outpatient department, or emergency department (Bureau of Primary Health Care, 1997; CDC, 2001).

It is not unusual for rural professionals to live and practice in a particular community for decades. Moreover, in a **health professional shortage area** (HPSA), a physician, a nurse practitioner, or a nurse often provides services to residents who live in several counties. In the case of community and public health nursing, one or two nurses in a county health department usually offer a full range of services for all residents in a catchment area, which may span more than 100 miles from one end of a county to the other. Consequently, rural physicians and nurses frequently report, "I provide care to individuals and families with all kinds of conditions, in all stages of life, and across several generations." It should not come as a surprise that rural respondents who participate in national surveys are able to identify a usual source and a usual provider of health care (Bushy, 2000, 2001, 2002a).

## Maternal–Infant Health

Reports in the literature conflict regarding pregnancy outcomes in rural areas. Overall, rural populations have higher infant and maternal morbidity rates, especially counties designated as HPSAs, which often have a high proportion of racial minorities (Table 16-3). Here one also finds fewer specialists, such as pediatricians, obstetricians, and gynecologists, to provide care to at-risk populations.

There are extreme variations in pregnancy outcomes from one part of the country to another, and even within states. For example, in several counties located in the north central and intermountain states, the pregnancy outcome is among the finest in the United States. However, in several other counties within those same states, the pregnancy outcome is among the worst. Particularly at risk are women who live on or near Indian reservations, women who are migrant workers, and women who are of African-American descent and live in rural counties of states located in the Deep South (Bushy, 2002b; CDC, 2001; HRSA, 1997, 2000; NRHA, 1999, 2001a,b).

Most nurses understand the effects of socioeconomic factors, such as income level (poverty), education level, age, employment–unemployment patterns, and use of prenatal services, on pregnancy outcomes. There are other, less well known determinants, such as environmental hazards, occupational risks, and the cultural meaning placed on childbearing and child rearing practices by a community. The effects of these multifaceted factors vary.

## Health of Children

Reports on the health status of rural children show regional variations and conflicting data. Comparing rural with urban children less than 6 years of age on the measures of access to providers and use of services reveals the following (CDC, 2001; Packard Foundation, 1997a,b):

- Urban children are less likely to have a usual provider but are more likely to see a pediatrician when they are ill.
- Like rural adults, rural children are more likely to have care from a general practitioner who is identified as their usual caregiver.

School nurses play an important role in the overall health status of children in the United States. The availability of school nurses in rural communities also varies from region to region. More specifically, in **frontier** and rural areas of the United States, school nurses usually are scarce. In part, this deficit can be attributed to limited resources associated with low tax revenues and shortages of health personnel in those counties. In other words, there are fewer taxpayers living in those large geographic areas. Some frontier areas have fewer than four persons per square mile and a few have less than two persons per square mile. Consequently, rural county commissioners, like their urban counterparts, are forced to prioritize the allocation of scarce resources among such services as maintaining public utilities, roads, bridges, and schools; supporting a financially suffering county hospital; hiring a county health nurse; and offering school health services. In rural communities there are fewer resources overall, and certain public services must be provided to local residents.

Clearly, creativity is required by both community residents and local health care providers to resolve health care and school nursing needs. Partnership arrangements, for example, have been negotiated by two or more counties that agree to share the cost of a "district" health nurse. Other county commissioners have forged partnerships

| | NATIONAL AVERAGE | NON-HPSA | HPSA |
|---|---|---|---|
| Infant mortality rate | 10.4* | 9.1 | 12.6 |
| Low birth-weight | 6.8 | 5.8 | 8.3 |

**Table 16-3 Rates of Infant Mortality and Low Birth Weight Related to Residency in Health Professional Shortage Area (HPSA)**

From Braden J, Beauregard K: National medical expenditure survey: health status and access to care of rural and urban populations, *Research Findings 18,* Rockville, Md, 1994, Agency for Health Care Policy and Research, Public Health Service (Publication No. 94-0031).

*Number of cases per 1000 population.

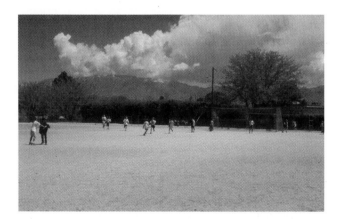

Schools in rural areas do not always have a full-time school nurse. Children living in rural areas do not usually have as much access to health care providers as children living in urban areas.

with an agency in an urban setting and contracted for specific health care services. In both of these situations, it is not unusual for the nurse to provide services to all children attending schools in the participating counties. In some frontier states, schools may be situated more than 100 miles apart and as many miles or more from the district health office. Because of the number of schools and distances between them, the county nurse may be able to visit each school only once, maybe twice, in a school term. Usually the nurse's visit is to update preschool immunizations and perhaps to teach maturation classes to students in the upper grades.

The health status of rural women, infants, and children is less than optimal. In part this can be attributed to inadequate preventive, primary, and emergency services to meet their particular health care needs. On one hand, scarce resources can pose a challenge to a nurse who provides care to rural residents, especially those in underserved areas. On the other hand, resource deficits encourage creativity, innovation, and they are an espoused characteristic of community-oriented nursing in general and of rural nurses in particular.

## Mental Health

As is true for other dimensions of the health of rural populations, the facts about their mental health status are also ambiguous and conflicting. Stress, stress-related conditions, and mental illness are prevalent among populations when severe economic difficulties persist. The depressed agriculture, lumber, and mining industries during the 1980s resulted in numerous job losses in rural communities, hence the term *farm stress*. Economic recession is also a contributing factor to a family's not having insurance or being underinsured. Interestingly, even if mental health services are available and accessible, rural residents delay seeking care when they have an emotional problem until there is an emergency or a crisis. This phenomenon is reflected in the lower number of annual visits for mental health services and chronic health problems by rural residents.

Mental health professionals who serve rural populations report a persistent, endemic level of depression among residents. They speculate that this condition is associated with the high rate of poverty, geographic isolation, and an insufficient number of mental health services. Depression may also contribute to the escalating incidence of accidents and suicides, especially among rural male adolescents and young men. The incidents have increased dramatically over the last decade and continue to rise in this group, to the point of being epidemic in some small communities (CDC, 2001; Substance Abuse and Mental Health Services Administration, 1997).

Reports on the incidence of domestic violence and alcohol and chemical substance use and abuse in rural populations are also conflicting. These behaviors are less likely to be reported in areas where residents are related or personally acquainted. After a period of time, in small, tight-knit communities destructive coping behaviors often come to be accepted as business as usual for a particular family. Family problems may also be ignored if formal social services and public health services are sparse or nonexistent and if the community does not trust the professionals who provide services within a local agency. In underserved rural areas, there are gaps in the continuum of mental health services, which, ideally, should include preventive education, anticipatory guidance, early intervention programs, crisis and acute care services, and follow-up care. As with other aspects of health care, nurses in rural areas play an important role in community education, case finding, advocacy, and case management of client systems experiencing emotional problems and chronic mental health problems (Bushy, 2000, 2002b).

## Health of Minorities

As mentioned previously, there is a significant number of at-risk minority groups in rural America who have some rather distinctive concerns (in particular, children, older adults, Native Americans, Native Alaskans, Native Hawaiians, migrant workers, African Americans, and the homeless) (Brooks, 1998; Brown et al, 2000; CDC, 2001; NRHA, 1999, 2001a,b; Office of Minority Health Resource Center, 1999; Sebastian and Bushy, 1999) (Table 16-4). The rural homeless, for example, may be seasonal farmworkers or families whose farm was foreclosed. Sometimes the family may be allowed by law to continue living in the house on the farm that once was theirs. The family no longer has a means of livelihood and often remains hidden in the community with insufficient income to purchase food or other necessary services. The particular health problems of these at-risk groups are discussed in Chapters 7 and 25 through 34. Nurses should be aware, however, that at-risk and underrepresented groups may experience some unique concerns related to rural lifestyle, isolation, and sparse resources.

## Environmental and Occupational Health Risks

A community's primary industry is an influencing factor in the local lifestyle, the health status of its residents, and the number and types of health care services it may need. For example, four high-risk industries identified by the Occupational Safety and Health Administration (OSHA) and found in predominantly rural environments are forestry, mining, fishing, and agriculture. Associated health risks of these industries are machinery and vehicular accidents, trauma, selected types of cancer, and respiratory disease stemming from repeated exposure to toxins, pesticides, and herbicides (CDC, 2001; USDA, 1997).

More specifically, agriculture-type businesses, such as farming and ranching, are often owned and operated by a family. Small enterprises do not fall under OSHA guidelines; therefore, safety standards are not enforceable on most farms and ranches. Moreover, small businesses, such as farms, are not covered under workman's compensation insurance. Additional concerns arise because family members participate in the farm or ranch work. This means that

**Table 16-4   Health Care Needs and Required Nursing Skills of Special Rural Populations**

| POPULATION/COMMUNITY | NEEDS/PROBLEMS |
| --- | --- |
| Farmers/ranchers | Advanced life support for cardiac emergencies<br>Emergency care for accident/trauma victims<br>Environmental hazards<br>Perinatal health care<br>Farmer's lung<br>Dermatitis<br>Farm stress/depression |
| Native Americans | Diabetes<br>Alcohol/substance abuse<br>Cirrhosis of the liver<br>Vehicular accidents<br>Hypothermic injuries<br>Trauma-related injuries<br>Tuberculosis (TB)<br>Sudden infant death syndrome (SIDS)<br>Perinatal health care |
| African Americans | Diabetes<br>Hypertension<br>Cardiovascular disease<br>Sickle cell anemia<br>Perinatal health care<br>HIV/AIDS prevention/diagnosis<br>Cancer screening and follow-up intervention |
| Migrant farmworkers | Field sanitation<br>Safe drinking water<br>Exposure to pesticides, herbicides<br>Infectious diseases (e.g., hepatitis, typhoid, TB, HIV/AIDS)<br>Maternal–child services |
| Native Alaskans | Exposure to petroleum byproducts<br>Toxic residue–contaminated seafood<br>Diabetes<br>Alcohol/substance abuse<br>Cirrhosis of the liver<br>Vehicular accidents<br>Hypothermic injuries<br>Trauma-related injuries<br>TB and other infectious diseases<br>SIDS<br>Perinatal health care |
| Coal miners | Occupational Safety and Health Administration standards<br>Respiratory diseases (black lung, chronic obstructive pulmonary disease)<br>Air/water quality standards<br>Substance abuse<br>Depression and associated mental health conditions<br>Trauma care |

some adults and children may operate dangerous farm machinery with minimal operating instructions on the hazards and on safety precautions. Consequently, agriculture-related accidents result in a significant number of deaths and long-term injuries, particularly among children and women. The morbidity and mortality rates associated with agriculture vary from state to state. The rising incidence of these injuries and deaths, however, has become a national concern. Nurses in rural settings can help address this problem by including farm safety content in school and community education programs.

In summary, it is risky to generalize about the health status of rural Americans because of their diversity coupled with conflicting definitions of what differentiates rural from urban residences. Many vulnerable individuals and families live in rural communities across the United

States, but little is known about many of them. This void is a potential research area for nurses who practice in rural environments.

## RURAL HEALTH CARE DELIVERY ISSUES AND BARRIERS TO CARE

Although each rural community is unique, the experience of living in a rural area has several common characteristics (Bushy, 2000; Office of Rural Health Policy [ORHP], 1994; Ramsbottom-Lucier et al, 1996; Schwartz, 2002) (Box 16-2). Concomitantly, barriers to health care may be associated with these characteristics (e.g., whether services and professionals are available, affordable, accessible, or acceptable to rural consumers).

Availability implies the existence of health services as well as the necessary personnel to provide essential services. Sparseness of population limits the number and array of health care services in a given geographic region. Therefore, the cost of providing special services to a few people often is prohibitive, particularly in frontier states where there is an insufficient number of physicians, nurses, and other types of health care providers. Consequently, where services and personnel are scarce, they must be allocated wisely. Accessibility implies that a person has logistical access to, as well as the ability to purchase, needed services. Affordability is associated with both availability and accessibility of care. It infers that services are of reasonable cost and that a family has sufficient resources to purchase them when they are needed. Acceptability of care means that a particular service is appropriate and offered in a manner that is congruent with the values of a target population. This can be hampered by both the client's cultural preference and the urban orientation of health professions (Box 16-3).

Providers' attitudes, insights, and knowledge about rural populations also are important. A demeaning attitude, lack of accurate knowledge about rural populations, or insensitivity about the rural lifestyle on the part of a nurse can perpetuate difficulties in relating to those clients. Moreover, insensitivity perpetuates mistrust, resulting in rural clients' perceiving professionals as outsiders to the community. On the other hand, some professionals in rural practice express feelings of professional isolation and community nonacceptance. To resolve these conflicting views, nursing faculty members should expose students to the rural environment. Clinical experiences should include opportunities to provide care to clients in their natural (e.g., rural) setting to gain accurate insight about that particular community.

To design community-oriented programs that are available, accessible, affordable, and appropriate, nurses must design strategies and implement interventions that mesh with a client's belief system. This implies that a family and a community are actively involved in planning and delivering care for a member who needs it. Nurses must have an accurate perspective of rural clients. Although the importance of forming partnerships and ensuring mutual exchange seems obvious, to date, most research about rural communities has been for policy or reimbursement purposes. There are minimal empirical data about rural family systems in terms of their health beliefs, values, perceptions of illness, health care–seeking behaviors, and what constitutes appropriate care. Therefore nurses must assume a more active role in implementing research on the community-oriented nursing needs of rural populations to expand the profession's theo-

---

### BOX 16-2 Characteristics of Rural Life

- More space; greater distances between residents and services
- Cyclic/seasonal work and leisure activities
- Informal social and professional interactions
- Access to extended kinship systems
- Residents who are related or acquainted
- Lack of anonymity
- Challenges in maintaining confidentiality stemming from familiarity among residents
- Small (often family) enterprises; fewer large industries
- Economic orientation to land and nature (e.g., agriculture, mining, lumbering, fishing)
- Higher prevalence of high-risk occupations
- Town as center of trade
- Churches and schools as socialization centers
- Preference for interacting with locals (insiders)
- Mistrust of newcomers to the community (outsiders)

---

### BOX 16-3 Barriers to Health Care in Rural Areas

- Great distances to obtain services
- Lack of personal transportation
- Unavailable public transportation
- Lack of telephone services
- Unavailable outreach services
- Inequitable reimbursement policies for providers
- Unpredictable weather and/or travel conditions
- Inability to pay for care
- Lack of "know-how" to procure entitlements and services
- Inadequate provider attitudes and understanding about rural populations
- Language barriers (caregivers not linguistically competent)
- Care and services not culturally appropriate

retical base and subsequently implement empirically based clinical interventions.

## NURSING CARE IN RURAL ENVIRONMENTS

### Theory, Research, and Practice

The body of literature on nursing practice in small towns and rural environments is growing, and several themes have emerged from it (Box 16-4). A nurse who practices in this setting can view each of these dimensions as an opportunity or a challenge.

Researchers from the University of Montana contend that existing theories do not fully explain rural nursing practice (Lee, 1998; Long and Weinert, 1999; Weinert and Long, 1990; Winstead-Fry, 1992). They examined the four concepts pertinent to a nursing theory (health, person, environment, and nursing/caring) and described relational statements that are relevant to clients and nurses in rural environments (see the Evidence-Based Practice box). Because the focus of their research was Anglo-Americans living in the Rocky Mountain area, care must be taken about generalizing those findings to other geographic regions and minorities. They propose that rural residents often judge their health by their ability to work. They con-

sider themselves healthy, even though they may suffer from several chronic illnesses, as long as they are able to continue working. For them, being healthy is the ability to be productive. Chronically ill people emphasize emotional and spiritual well-being rather than physical wellness.

Distance, isolation, and sparse resources characterize rural life and are seen in residents' independent and innovative coping strategies. Self-reliance and independence are demonstrated through their self-care practices and preference for family and community support. Community networks provide support but still allow for each person's and family's independence. Ruralites prefer and usually seek

---

### BOX 16-4 Characteristics of Nursing Practice in Rural Environments

- Variety/diversity in clinical experiences
- Broader/expanding scope of practice
- Generalist skills
- Flexibility/creativity in delivering care
- Sparse resources (materials, professionals, equipment, fiscal)
- Professional/personal isolation
- Greater independence/autonomy
- Role overlap with other disciplines
- Slower pace
- Lack of anonymity
- Increased opportunity for informal interactions with clients/co-workers
- Opportunity for client follow-up upon discharge in informal community settings
- Discharge planning allowing for integration of formal and informal resources
- Care for clients across the life span
- Exposure to clients with a full range of conditions/diagnoses
- Status in the community (viewed as prestigious)
- Viewed as a professional role model
- Opportunity for community involvement and informal health education

---

### Evidence-Based Practice

Nurse researchers at Montana State University proposed the following theoretical concepts and dimensions of rural nursing:

- **Health:** Defined by rural residents as the ability to work. Work and health beliefs are closely related for rural Montana sample.
- **Environment:** Distance and isolation are particularly important for rural dwellers. Those who live long distances neither perceive themselves as isolated nor perceive health care services as inaccessible.
- **Nursing:** Lack of anonymity, outsider versus insider, old-timer versus newcomer. Lack of anonymity is a common theme among rural nurses who report knowing most people for whom they care, not only in the nurse–client relationship but also in a variety of social roles, such as family member, friend, or neighbor. Acceptance as a health care provider in the community is closely linked to the outsider/insider and newcomer/old-timer phenomena. Gaining trust and acceptance of local people is identified as a unique challenge that must be successfully negotiated by nurses before they can begin to function as effective health care providers.
- **Person:** Self-reliance and independence in relationship to health care are strong characteristics of rural individuals. They prefer to have people they know care for them (informal services) as opposed to an outsider in a formal agency.

**Nurse Use:** In working with rural residents, it is important to know how they define their health and their environment, as their definitions may differ from yours. Understand that you may not find acceptance and trust immediately; rural residents often trust informal caregivers more than those in a formal organization.

Bushy A: *Orientation to nursing in the rural community,* Thousand Oaks, CA, 2000, Sage.

Bushy A: International perspectives on rural nursing: Australia, Canada, United States. *Aust J Rural Health* 10(2):104-111, 2002a.

Lee H, editor: *Conceptual basis for rural nursing,* New York, 1998, Springer.

## Rural Canada and Federal Government Commitment to Rural Health

Karon Janine Foster, R.N., B.Sc.N., M.Ed., Lecturer, Faculty of Nursing, University of Toronto

Almost 30% of Canadians live in rural or remote areas of this country (Health Canada, 2003). Health Canada has demonstrated their commitment to the health concerns of rural Canadians by establishing the Office of Rural Health in September 1998. This office ensures that the concerns of rural Canadians are considered in national health policies (Health Canada, 2001). Continued commitment was shown in June 2000 with the development of a Rural Health Strategy that identified major issues and offered ways for communities and the government of Canada to work together. Some of the issues identified were a need to improve the rural health infrastructure and to develop health information technology, a focus on primary health care, and the shortage of rural health practitioners (Health Canada, 2001). A review of this strategy occurred in 2001, and regional successes were identified. Examples of some successes are the obtaining of funding to develop a Telehealth network in Nunavut and Atlantic Canada, the establishment of a woman-focused primary health care facility in Nelson, British Columbia, and the development of a mobile diabetes screening service for Alberta First Nations communities.

### RURAL AND URBAN HEALTH

The Health of Canada's Communities is a report that compares the health indicators of life expectancy; disability-free life expectancy (DFLE); health behaviours such as smoking, drinking, and exercise; and psychosocial factors such as stress and depression, for 139 health regions. These regions have been grouped on the basis of similar sociodemographic characteristics, such as population size, level of education, percentage of minorities or aboriginal population, unemployment, and average income. The Canadian average life expectancy is 78.3 years and the DFLE is 68.6 years (Shields and Tremblay, 2002). National rates are as follows (Shields and Tremblay, 2002):

- For daily smoking, 22%
- For alcohol use (five drinks or more on one occasion), 16%
- For obesity (a body mass index over 30), 16%

- For infrequent exercise (less than three times in the past month), 22%

The results showed that residents of Richmond, B.C., were the healthiest, with a life expectancy of 81.2 years, a DFLE of 72.8 years, and the best lifestyle practices (Shields and Tremblay, 2002). People living in large metropolitan areas (e.g., Toronto, Montreal, Vancouver) or urban areas (e.g., Ottawa, Calgary, Peel, South Fraser Valley) were very healthy. These communities had life expectancies of 78.8 to 79.6 years and longer DFLEs. The rates for smoking, alcohol use, and obesity were the lowest in Canada.

People living in rural areas, in Canada's eastern and western provinces and the rural areas of Ontario and Quebec, were not as healthy as urbanites. They had average life expectancies of 77 to 77.8 years and DFLEs of 66.5 to 68.6 years (Shields and Tremblay, 2002). People living in these areas also had smoking, alcohol, and obesity rates that were above the national average. People in eastern and western rural communities did report lower rates of stress than the national average of 26% (Shields and Tremblay, 2002).

### CANADA'S FAR NORTH AND THE HEALTH OF NORTHERN RESIDENTS

One of the unique rural areas in Canada is the Far North, which extends from the Yukon in the west to Nunavut in the east and north to the Arctic Circle. The population is distributed among reserves, settlements, villages, towns, and cities and is composed of native groups such as the Metis, the Dene, the Inuit, and non-Aboriginal residents. Languages spoken in this area include English, French, Inuktitut, Slavey, Dogrib, Chipewyan, Cree, and Gwich'in.

Nurses have traditionally delivered health care in this remote area. From 1945 to 1988, the federal government was responsible for health care to the residents of the Far North until responsibility was transferred to the territorial governments. Health care is provided in health care facilities, which include hospitals, health centers, and health stations. Health centers include a treatment area, a few inpatient beds, a teaching area, and basic laboratory and x-ray equipment. Nursing stations are lo-

help through their informal networks, such as neighbors, extended family, church, and civic clubs, rather than seeking a professional's care in the formal system of health care, including services such as those provided by a mental health clinic, social service agency, or health department.

Although nursing is generally similar across settings and populations, there are some unique features associated with practice in a geographically remote area or in small towns where most people are familiar with one another. The following paragraphs highlight a few of the

variations that nurses in rural practice report (American Nurses Association [ANA], 1996; Barger, 1996; Dunkin et al, 1994; Pickard, 1996).

The work and home roles for professional nursing practice in rural areas may not be distinct. In many instances, a nurse may have more than one work role in the community; for example, a nurse may also be a Sears catalog store owner, may also work at the local hospital or doctor's office, or may also be actively involved in managing the family farm. For nurses, this means that many, if not all,

cated in small communities of 150 to 1500 people and may be staffed with one to five nurses. Often these health stations have access to larger centers only by air.

People living in Canada's most remote northern communities are the least healthy. The regions with the lowest life expectancy are the Yukon, Nunavut, northern regions of Quebec, Ontario, Manitoba, and Saskatchewan; these regions have a high Aboriginal population (Statistics Canada, 1999). Shields and Tremblay (2002) report that the Nunavut region has the lowest life expectancy at 65.4 years, whereas other regions have life expectancies that range from 71.8 to 76.7 years. The DFLE for these northern regions ranges from 62.7 to 66.7 years, lower than the national average (Shields and Tremblay, 2002). Mortality rates due to cancer, circulatory diseases, respiratory diseases, suicide, and infant mortality are also higher in regions with a high population of Aboriginals (Diverty and Perez, 1998). Obesity, smoking, alcohol, and infrequent exercise rates are the highest in the country (Shields and Tremblay, 2002). Rates of depression and stress were lower than the national average.

## DIVERSE NURSING ROLES AND CHALLENGES OF WORKING IN REMOTE AREAS

Like nurses working in other rural areas, nurses in the remote areas of Canada have diverse responsibilities and roles. They provide direct patient care that includes emergency care, monitoring of chronic health problems, prenatal and childcare clinics, and developing and implementing illness prevention and health promotion programs. Nonnursing roles may include pharmacist, environmental health officer, clerk, infection control officer, and social worker. To function effectively in this setting, nurses must have a broad knowledge base because they must function as both a generalist and a specialist in acute care and community health. Advanced assessment, diagnostic, prescribing, and clinical skills are needed to treat acute, chronic, and emergency health problems.

Nurses face many challenges when they work in these remote areas, such as isolation, a scarcity of community resources, a lack of anonymity, cultural and language barriers, and stress and burnout. Heavy workloads, understaffing, fatigue, culture shock, the challenges of weather, and lack of resources contribute

to the high turnover of staff. The community may be left without a nurse, or a pool of relief nurses may be used until the position is filled. It takes time for members of a community to trust the nurse, and high turnover rates can hamper the development of these relationships.

### References

Brumwell A, Janes C: Primary health care in Rae-Edzo, *Canadian Nurse* 90(3):38, 1994.

Diverty B, Perez C: The health of Northern residents: health reports, *Statistics Canada* 9(4):49-58, 1998.

Graham R: Inservice education for northern nurses, *Canadian Nurse* 90(3):33, 1994.

Gregory D: Nursing practice in native communities. In Baumgart A, Larsen J, editors: *Canadian nursing faces the future,* ed 2, St Louis, Mo, 1992, Mosby.

Health Canada: *Canada's rural health strategy: a one-year review,* Minister of Public Works and Government Services, 1-16, 2001.

Health Canada: *Rural health,* available at www.hc-sc.gc.ca/english/ruralhealth/index.html (updated 3/2003), and also through www.hc-sc.gc.ca (search for "rural").

Life expectancy (Health Reports): *Statistics Canada* 11(3):9-22, 1999.

Morewood-Northrop M: Nursing in the Northwest Territories, *Canadian Nurse* 90(3):26, 1994.

Roberts J: Outpost nurse responds to March column, *Canadian Nurse* 94(6):8, 1998.

Ross D: Nursing up north, *Canadian Nurse* 85(1):22, 1989.

Scott K: Northern nurses burnout, *Canadian Nurse* 87(10):18, 1991.

Shields M, Tremblay S: The health of Canada's communities, supplement to Health Reports, *Statistics Canada* 13:1-25, 2002.

The health of Canada's communities, 2000/01 (The Daily): *Statistics Canada,* July 4, 2002, available at www.statcan.ca/Daily/English/020704/d020704b.htm.

*Canadian spelling is used.*

clients are personally known as neighbors, as friends of an immediate family member, or perhaps part of one's extended family. Associated with the social informality is a corresponding lack of anonymity in a small town. Some rural nurses say, "I never really feel like I am off duty because everybody in the county knows me through my work." In part, this can be attributed to nurses' being highly regarded by the community and viewed by local people as experts on health and illness. It is not unusual for residents to informally ask a nurse's advice before see-

ing a doctor for a health problem. Moreover, health-related questions are asked by residents when they see the nurse (who may be a neighbor, friend, or relative) in a grocery store, at a service station, during a basketball game, or at church functions.

Nurses in rural practice must make decisions about individuals of all ages with a variety of health conditions. They assume many roles because of the range of services that must be provided in a rural health care facility. A nurse may assume several roles because of the scarcity of nursing and other health professionals. Stemming from rural residents' expectations of the health care delivery system, the skills needed by nurses in rural practice include technical and clinical competency, adaptability, flexibility, strong assessment skills, organizational abilities, independence, interest in continuing education, sound decision-making skills, leadership ability, self-confidence, skills in handling emergencies, teaching, and public relations. The nurse administrator is also expected to be a jack-of-all-trades (i.e., a generalist) and to demonstrate competence in several clinical specialties in addition to managing and organizing staff within the facility for which he or she is responsible.

There are challenges, opportunities, and rewards in rural community and public health nursing practice. The manner in which each factor is perceived depends on individual preferences and the situation in a given community. Challenges of rural practice include professional isolation, limited opportunities for continuing education, lack of other kinds of health personnel or professionals with whom one can interact, heavy work loads, the ability to function well in several clinical areas, lack of anonymity, and, for some, a restricted social life (Bushy, 2001, 2002b; Stratton, Dunkin, and Juhl, 1995; Stratton et al, 1995).

Of the many opportunities and rewards in rural nursing practice, those most commonly cited include close relationships with clients and co-workers, diverse clinical experiences that evolve from caring for clients of all ages who have a variety of health problems, caring for clients for long periods of time (in some cases, across several generations), opportunities for professional development, and greater autonomy. Many nurses value the solitude and quality of life found in a rural community personally and for their own family. Others thrive on the outdoor recreational activities. Still others thoroughly enjoy the informal, face-to-face interactions coupled with the public recognition and status associated with living and working as a nurse in a small community.

Prevention is important in rural communities. Box 16-5 shows the levels of prevention as they might be used by a community-oriented nurse in a rural locale.

### BOX 16-5 Levels of Prevention Related to Rural Health

**PRIMARY PREVENTION**
Using available community groups, teach women how to cook in a way that will offset the tendency to develop diabetes.

**SECONDARY PREVENTION**
Screen clients for the presence of diabetes.

**TERTIARY PREVENTION**
Teach clients with diabetes better eating and exercise habits, help them get medication if needed, and coach and encourage them.

## Community-Oriented Nursing

Although most of the publications about rural health care and nursing focus on hospital practice, much of that information is applicable to both community-oriented agencies and community-oriented nursing (Davis and Droes, 1993; Washington State Nursing Network, 1992). The work-related stressors of community-oriented nursing have received some attention in the literature. More than a decade ago, Case (1991) identified stressful experiences of nurses working in rural Oklahoma health departments including the following: political/bureaucratic problems and intraprofession and interpersonal conflicts associated with inadequate communication; unsatisfactory work environment and understaffing; difficult or unpleasant nurse-client encounters, such as with relatives who refuse to deliver needed care to clients, and with clients who are hostile, apathetic, dependent, or of low intelligence; fear for personal safety; difficulty locating clients, and clients falling through the cracks of the health care system. Even a decade later, similar stressors are cited by nurses who work in urban agencies. Anecdotal reports describe specific stressors associated with geographic distance, isolation, sparse resources, and other environmental factors that characterize rurality.

Nursing in rural practice settings is characterized by physical isolation that may lend itself to any one of the following: professional isolation; scarce financial, human, and health care resources; and a broad scope of practice. Because of personal familiarity with local residents, nurses often possess in-depth knowledge about clients and their families. Along with the acknowledged benefits, informal (face-to-face) interactions can significantly reduce a nurse's anonymity in the community and at times be a barrier to completing an objective assessment on a client. Like urban practice, rural community nursing takes place in a variety of locations, including homes, clinics, schools, occupational settings, and correctional facilities, and at community events, such as county fairs, rodeos, civic and church-sponsored functions, and school athletic events (Figure 16-2).

## Research Needs

Few empirical studies on rural nursing practice have been done. Much of what exists consists of anecdotal reports by nurses. Several specific areas for research are of particular importance to nursing practice in rural environments (Bushy, 2000).

1. Most nurses indicate that they enjoy practicing in rural areas and are proud of what they do. They believe, however, that their work deserves more recognition by professional nursing organizations. Furthermore, the retention rate of nurses in some practice settings is poor. The perspective of nurses who are dissatisfied with rural nursing is necessary to give a more complete picture of the rural experience. This information can be useful to a variety of people:

other nurses who are considering rural practice, nurse managers in need of better screening tools to assess the fit between the nurse and the environment when interviewing applicants, planners of continuing nursing education programs, and faculty members who teach community health to undergraduate and graduate students.

2. More information is needed about the stressors and rewards of rural practice. These data could lead to the development of stress management techniques to be used by nurses and their supervisors to retain nurses and to improve the quality of their workplace environment.

3. With the increasing number of rural residents in all regions of the United States, empirical data are needed on the particular community nursing needs of rural-client systems, especially underrepresented groups, minorities, and other at-risk populations that vary by region and state.

4. Because most of the reported research studies on rural nursing were performed on Anglo-Americans living in the intermountain and midwestern regions, data are needed from residents in other areas, especially the states east of the Mississippi River.

5. There also is a need for the international perspective on the health of rural populations, and on nursing practice within the rural community. Australian and Canadian nurse scholars have provided some insights into rural practice in their countries. Information is needed from less-developed countries as well as from other industrialized nations (Bushy, 2002a).

## Preparing Nurses for Rural Practice Settings

Nurses in rural practice must have broad knowledge about nursing theory. Topics important in this practice environment include health promotion, primary prevention, rehabilitation, obstetrics, medical–surgical specialties, pediatrics, planning and implementing community assessments, and

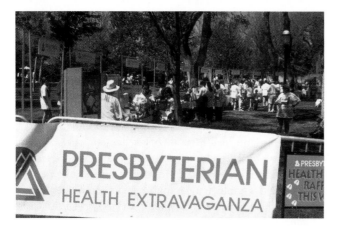

**Figure 16-2** A hospital-sponsored health fair is one example of a community event to provide health services to individuals in a rural area.

an awareness and understanding of the particular health concerns in a specific state. A community's demographic profile and its principal industry can present a snapshot of some of its social, political, and health risks. From this kind of information, a nurse can anticipate the particular skills that will be needed to care for clients in a catchment area (ANA, 1996; Pan and Straub, 1997; Pearson, 1997).

Because of their knowledge of resources and their ability to coordinate formal and informal services, nurses play an important role in offering a continuum of services for rural clients in spite of sparse resources and fragmentation in the health care delivery system. Preparing nurses to practice in rural environments demands creative and innovative nursing educational opportunities. Collaboration and partnerships must be established between educators, rural nurses, and administrators of health care facilities in rural settings. To meet the demands and expectations of practice in that setting, nursing faculty members must expose students to the rural environment, facilitate the development of generalist skills, and enhance the ability to function in several roles.

> **WHAT DO YOU THINK?**
>
> Within the nursing profession, there is disagreement as to whether rural nursing is a specialty practice. How could a nursing theory specific to rural practice settings be useful to nurse scholars?

## FUTURE PERSPECTIVES

Those concerned with rural health, including residents of rural communities, their elected representatives, and the administrators of public and private health care agencies, should be aware of the problems inherent in providing a continuum of care to underserved populations. Typically, media accounts focus exclusively on rural hospitals and the lack of primary care providers. Those reports generally neglect the public health perspective when discussing the continuum of health care in rural environments. Case management and community-oriented primary health care (COPHC), however, have proven to be effective models in helping to address some of those deficits and resolving rural health disparities (Box 16-6).

## Scarce Resources and a Comprehensive Health Care Continuum

The current health care system is fragmented, thereby creating even greater difficulty in providing a comprehensive continuum of care to populations living in areas having scarce resources, such as money, personnel, equipment, and ancillary services. In rural communities, the most critically needed services are usually preventive services, such as health screening clinics, nutrition counseling, and wellness education (CDC, 2001).

---

**BOX 16-6  Comparison of U.S. Urban (Metro) and Rural (Nonmetro) Residents' Health Status**

**RESIDENTS OF FRINGE COUNTIES OF LARGE METRO AREAS HAVE THE FOLLOWING:**

- Lowest levels of premature mortality, partly reflecting lower death rates for unintentional injuries, homicide, and suicide
- Lowest levels of smoking, alcohol consumption, and childbearing among adolescents
- Lowest prevalence of physical inactivity during leisure time among women
- Lowest levels of obesity among adults
- Greatest number of physician specialists and dentists per capita
- Lowest percentage of the population without health insurance
- Lowest percentage of the population who had no dental visits

**RESIDENTS IN THE MOST RURAL (NONMETRO) AREAS HAVE THE FOLLOWING:**

- Highest death rates for children and young adults
- Highest death rates for unintentional and motor vehicle traffic-related injuries
- Highest mortality rates among adults for ischemic heart disease and suicide
- Highest levels of smoking among adolescents
- Highest levels of physical activity during leisure time among men
- Highest levels of obesity among adults
- Highest percentage of adults with activity limitations caused by chronic health conditions
- Fewest physician specialists and dentists per capita
- Least likely to have seen a dentist
- Highest percentage of the population without health insurance

From Centers for Disease Control and Prevention: *United States, 2001–urban and rural chartbook,* Washington, DC, retrieved August 2001 from http://www.cdc.gov/nchs/data/hus/hus01.pdf.

---

Community-oriented nursing needs vary by community. However, there is a prevailing need in most rural areas, especially for the following:

- School nurses
- Family planning services
- Prenatal care
- Care for individuals with AIDS and their families
- Emergency care services
- Children with special needs, including those who are physically and mentally challenged
- Mental health services
- Services for older adults (especially frail older adults and those with Alzheimer's disease), such as adult day care, hospice, respite care, homemaker services, and meal deliveries to older adults who remain at home

Providing a continuum of care has been hindered by the closure of many small hospitals in the past two decades. Of those that remain, many report financial problems that could lead to closure (ORHP, 1994; Schoenman, 1998). A shortage or the absence of even one provider, most often a physician or nurse, could mean that a small hospital must close its doors. This event has a ripple effect on the health of local residents, other health care services, and the economic development efforts in many small communities.

The short supply and increasing demand for primary care providers in general, and nurses in particular, will continue for some time. To help solve this problem, elected officials and policy developers need nurses, especially those in advanced practice roles, to provide vital services in underserved areas. To respond to this opportunity, nurses need to be creative to ensure delivery of appropriate and acceptable services to at-risk and vulnerable populations who live in rural and underserved regions. Nurses must be sensitive to the health beliefs of clients, then plan and provide nursing interventions that mesh with communities' cultural values and preferences.

## Healthy People 2010 National Health Objectives Related to Rural Health

Because the demographic profile varies from community to community, each state has variations in the health status of its population. Healthy People 2010 has important implications for nurses in that a significant number of at-risk populations cited in that policy-guiding document live in rural areas across the United States (CDC, 2001; NRHA, 1999; 2001a,b; U.S. Department of Health and Human Services [USDHHS], 2002a,b,c). Consequently, priority objectives vary, depending on population mix, health risks, and health status of residents in the state.

At the local level, communities have used Healthy People 2000/2010 as a guide for action and to identify objectives and establish meaningful goals. *Healthy People in Healthy Communities: A Community Planning Guide Using Healthy People 2010* (known as *Healthy People in Healthy Communities 2010*) (USDHHS, 2002d) can be useful to local officials and health care planners to tailor the objectives to their community's needs. This document encourages the establishment of professional–community partnerships. Translating national objectives into achievable community health targets requires integration of the following components to ensure that services will be acceptable and appropriate for rural clients:

- Health statistics must be meaningful and understandable, and they must include appropriate process objectives that can be measured readily.
- Strategies must be designed that involve the public, private, and voluntary sectors of the community to achieve agreed-upon local objectives.
- Coordinated efforts are needed to ensure that the community works together to achieve the goals.

Consider, for example, these components in developing a health plan for a rural county having a large population of young people. Healthy People 2010 objectives for the county should target women of childbearing age, children, and adolescents. Priority objectives should include offering accessible prenatal care programs, improving immunization levels, providing preventive dental care instructions, implementing vehicular accident prevention and firearm safety programs, and educating teachers and health professionals for early identification of cases of do-

mestic violence. On the other hand, consider a rural county that has a higher number of individuals over 65 years of age than the national average. Priority objectives in the health plan should target the health risks and problems of older adults in that community. Specific objectives might include development of health-promoting programs to prevent chronic health problems and establishing community programs to meet the needs of those having chronic illness, specifically cardiovascular disease, diabetes, hypertension, and accident-related disabilities.

When implementing community-focused health plans that flow from Healthy People in Healthy Communities 2010, consideration must always be given to rural factors, such as sparse population, geographic remoteness, scarce resources, personnel shortages, and physical, emotional, and social isolation. In addition to being actively involved in empowering the community and planning and delivering care, nurses play an important role in representing their community's perspective to local, state, regional, and national health planners and to their elected officials.

## BUILDING PROFESSIONAL–COMMUNITY–CLIENT PARTNERSHIPS IN RURAL SETTINGS

Health care reform initiatives are focusing on cutting costs while improving access to care for all citizens, especially vulnerable and underserved populations. Active involvement by state and local groups is an essential element for any kind of reform to be successful, especially in rural areas. In other words, professional–client–community partnerships are important for reform to be meaningful at the local level. Two models have been found to be particularly useful in rural environments: case management and COPHC.

### Case Management

Case management is a client–professional partnership that can be used to arrange a continuum of care for rural clients, with the case manager tailoring and blending formal and informal resources. Collaborative efforts between a client and the case manager allow clients to participate in their plan of care in an acceptable and appropriate way, especially when local resources are few and far between. The Clinical Application at the end of this chapter demonstrates how nursing case management can allow an older adult resident to stay at home in a rural environment if adequate supports can be provided. Outcomes are often remarkably different when case management is used. Additional information on case management is found in Chapter 19.

### Community-Oriented Primary Health Care

COPHC is an effective model for delivering available, accessible, and acceptable services to vulnerable populations living in **medically underserved** areas. This model emphasizes flexibility, grassroots involvement, and professional–community partnerships. It blends primary care, public

---

## THE CUTTING EDGE

Community-based prevention programs need scientific evidence to demonstrate their effectiveness. Although rural public health departments implement many such programs, they are often not equipped to evaluate them. Rural public health agencies are often fettered by small budgets and small staffs, and they have less access to evaluation experts and information resources. Furthermore, community-based health promotion programs in rural areas may work differently from the way they work in more populated settings. Program evaluation can be hampered by lack of control groups and the instability that is associated with small populations. To help address rural concerns, the University of Kentucky has developed an innovative participatory model with the state Department of Public Health to facilitate program evaluations in rural parts of Kentucky. Essentially, a university-based evaluation expert trains staff in local public health departments in the technical skills, and serves as a mentor and technical consultant on an ongoing basis for program evaluation. This partnership between the university and the health department is expected to provide much-needed evidence-based outcomes on rural-based prevention programs. It could also serve as a model for other state health departments to learn about innovative prevention programs targeting rural populations.

Modified from Beaulieu J, Webb J: Challenges in evaluating rural health programs, *J Rural Health* 18(2):281-204, 2002.

**BOX 16-7  Community-Oriented Primary Health Care (COPHC): A Partnership Process**

The steps in the COPHC process include the following:
- Define and characterize the community
- Identify the community's health problems
- Develop or modify health care services in response to the community's identified needs
- Monitor and evaluate program process and client outcomes

**HOW TO  Build Professional–Community–Client Partnerships**

1. Gain the local perspective.
2. Assess the degree of public awareness and support for the cause.
3. Identify special interest groups.
4. List existing services to avoid duplication of programs.
5. Note real and potential barriers to existing resources and services.
6. Generate a list of potential community volunteers and professionals who are willing to assist with the project.
7. Create awareness among target groups of a particular program (e.g., individuals, families, seniors, church and recreation groups, health care professionals, law enforcement personnel, and members of other religious, service, and civic clubs).
8. Identify potential funding sources to implement the program.
9. Establish the community's health care priority list, and involve large numbers of community members in considering and selecting their health care options.
10. Incorporate business principles in marketing the program.
11. Measure the health system's local economic impact.
12. Educate residents about the important role the local health care system plays in the economic infrastructure of the community and the consequences of a system failure.
13. Develop local leadership and support for the community's health system through training and providing experience in decision making.

health, and prevention services, which are offered in a familiar and accessible setting. The COPHC model is interdisciplinary, uses a problem-oriented approach, and mandates community involvement in all phases of the process (Box 16-7).

Building professional–community partnerships is an ongoing process. At various times, nurses, other health professionals, and community leaders must assume the role of advocate, change agent, educator, expert, or group facilitator to gain both active and passive support from the community. Partnerships involve give-and-take by all participants in the negotiations to reach consensus. Essentially, the process begins with professionals gaining entrance into a community, establishing rapport and trust with local people, then working together to empower the community to resolve mutually defined problems and goals. As mentioned previously, Healthy People in Healthy Communities 2010 is an excellent guide for developing and defining those goals. Because of the central importance of churches and schools in a rural community, leaders from those institutions can be key players in building provider–community partnerships. The organizational phase should come first, as it lays the foundation for all other activities related to planning, implementing, and evaluating community services.

As was described for case management, professional–community partnerships allow more effective identification of existing informal social support systems that are accepted by rural residents. The goal is to integrate community preferences with new or existing formal services. Public input should be encouraged early in the planning process and must continue throughout the process to allow the community to feel that it has ownership in the project; this will help avoid having residents view it as an outsider bringing another bureaucratic program into town. Strategies that nurses can use to enhance the building of partnerships in rural environments are listed in the How To box.

Partnership models, such as case management and COPHC, have proven to be highly effective in areas with scarce resources and an insufficient number of health care providers. Individuals and communities who are informed, active participants in planning their health care are more likely to develop consensus about the most appropriate solution for local problems. Subsequently, they are more likely to use and support that system after it is

implemented. Partnership models enhance the ability of rural communities to do what they historically have done well (i.e., assume responsibility for the services and institutions that serve their residents). Knowledge about partnership models and the skills to effectively implement them are useful for nurses who coordinate services that are accessible, available, and acceptable for rural populations in their catchment area.

## Practice Application

Ethyl, a 73-year-old widow, was diagnosed more than 10 years ago with progressive Parkinson's disease. Her husband of more than 40 years died suddenly 3 years ago after a serious stroke. Her two married daughters live in California and Illinois. Her small midwestern town has 1000 residents, and the nearest health care is 100 miles away. Her 75-year-old widowed sister, Suzanna, also lives in town. Their brother Bill (age 71) has recently entered the county nursing home located in a town 20 miles away. Despite her physical rigidity and ataxia, Ethyl manages to live alone in her two-bedroom home with her dog and cat. Ethyl insists that she will not relinquish her private, independent lifestyle as her brother Bill has. Yet, within this past year she has been hospitalized three times: for a bad chest cold, for a bladder infection, and after a neighbor found her lying unconscious in the garden. Her doctor says that this last episode was related to "a heart problem."

After discharge, a home-health nurse, Liz, was assigned as her case manager. Liz's office is based at the County Senior Center near the nursing home where Bill is a resident. Bill is also one of the clients whom Liz checks on weekly. Liz provides outreach services to all the residents in the county who are referred by a large home health agency in the city. As a case manager, she works closely with the hospital's discharge planners to arrange a continuum of care for clients in the two-county area. Her activities include coordinating formal and informal services for clients, including nutrition, hydration, pharmacologic care, personal care, homemaker services, and routine activities, such as writing checks, home maintenance, and emergency backup services.

   A. Describe the nursing roles that Liz assumes in coordinating a continuum of care for Ethyl in terms of nutrition, transportation, and health care.
   B. Identify formal health care and support resources that can be accessed for Ethyl.
   C. Identify informal support resources that can be used to ensure that Ethyl is safe.
   D. Identify three outcomes that have been achieved by using nursing care management.
   E. Select a rural community in your geographic area. Create hypothetical situations, or select real clients with real health problems (e.g., an older adult with Alzheimer's disease, a middle-aged person with cancer requiring end-of-life care, a child who is dependent on technology as a result of a farm accident). Prepare a list of services and referral agencies in that community that could be used to develop a continuum of care for each of these cases. How are these the same as, or different from, the case described in this chapter?

**Answers are in the back of the book.**

## Key Points

- There is great diversity in rural environments across the United States.
- There are variations in the health status of rural populations, depending on genetic, social, environmental, economic, and political factors.
- There is a higher incidence of working poor in rural America than in more populated areas.
- Rural adults 18 years and older are in poorer health than their urban counterparts; nearly 50% have been diagnosed with at least one major chronic condition. However, they average one less physician visit each year than healthier urban counterparts.

- About 26% of rural families are below the poverty level; more than 40% of all rural children younger than 18 years of age live in poverty.
- General practitioners are the usual providers of care for rural adults and children.
- Rural residents must often travel more than 30 minutes to access a health care provider.
- Nurses must take into consideration the belief systems and lifestyles of a rural population when planning, implementing, and evaluating community services.
- Barriers to rural health care include the lack of availability, affordability, accessibility, and acceptability of services.
- Partnership models, in particular case management and community-oriented primary health care (COPHC), are effective models to provide a comprehensive continuum of care in environments with scarce resources.

## Clinical Decision-Making Activities

1. Compare and contrast the terms urban, suburban, rural, frontier, farm, nonfarm residency, metropolitan, and nonmetropolitan.
2. Describe residency as a continuum, ranging from farm residency to core metropolitan residency.
3. Discuss economic, social, and cultural factors that affect rural lifestyle and the health care–seeking behaviors of residents who live there.
4. Identify barriers that affect accessibility, affordability, availability, and acceptability of services in the health care delivery system.
5. Summarize key nursing concepts in terms of practice in rural environments.
6. Examine the characteristics of rural community nursing practice and how they differ from those of practice in more populated settings.
7. Identify challenges, opportunities, and benefits of living and practicing as a nurse in the rural environment.
8. Debate case management and community-oriented primary care as partnership models that can help nurses enhance the continuum of care for clients living in an environment with sparse resources.

## Additional Resources

These related resources are found either in the Appendix at the back of this book or on the book's website at **http://evolve.elsevier.com/Stanhope.**

**evolve** Evolve Website

WebLinks: Healthy People 2010

# References

American Nurses Association: *Rural/frontier health care task force: rural/frontier nursing: the challenge to grow,* Washington, DC, 1996, ANA.

American Public Health Association: *Healthy communities 2000: mid-course review,* Washington, DC, 1996, APHA.

Baer K, Johnson M, Gesler W: What is rural? a focus on urban influence codes, *J Rural Health* 13(4):329, 1997.

Barger S: Rural nurses: here today and gone tomorrow, *Rural Clin Q* 6(3):3, 1996.

Beaulieu J, Webb J: Challenges in evaluating rural health programs, *J Rural Health* 18(2):281-284, 2002.

Bigbee J, Crowder E: The Red Cross Rural Nursing Service: an innovation of public health nursing delivery, *Public Health Nurs* 2(2):109, 1985.

Bowers D, Cook P: Population: nonmetro population rebound continues: socioeconomic conditions issue, *Rural Conditions Trends* 7(3):6, 1997.

Braden J, Beauregard K: National medical expenditure survey: health status and access to care of rural and urban populations, *Research Findings 18,* Rockville, Md, 1994, Agency for Health Care Policy and Research, Public Health Service (Publication No. 94-0031).

Brown E et al: *Racial and ethnic disparities in access to health insurance and health care,* University of Southern California (UCLA) Research Center and the Henry J. Kaiser Family Foundation, 2000, available at http://www.healthpolicy.ucla.edu/pubs/publication.asp?pubID=31 and the Henry J. Kaiser Family Foundation website, www.kff.org.

Brooks J: Increasing AIDS rates in rural America deserve more attention, *Rural Clin Q* 8(1):1, 1998.

Brumwell A, Janes C: Primary health care in Rae-Edzo, *Canadian Nurse* 90(3):38, 1994.

Bureau of Primary Health Care: *Selected statistics of health professional shortage areas as of September 1996,* Washington, DC, 1997, Division of Shortage Designation, HRSA, USDHHS.

Bushy A: *Orientation to nursing in the rural community,* Thousand Oaks, CA, 2000, Sage.

Bushy A: International perspectives on rural nursing: Australia, Canada, United States. *Aust J Rural Health* 10(2):104-111, 2002a.

Bushy A: *Resource manual: rural minorities, their health issues and resources,* Kansas City, Mo, 2002b, National Rural Health Association.

Bushy A, Bushy A: Critical access hospitals: rural nursing issues, *J Nurs Adm* 31(6):301-310, 2001.

Case T: Work stresses of community health nurses in Oklahoma. In Bushy A, editor: *Rural nursing,* vol 2, Newbury Park, Calif, 1991, Sage.

Centers for Disease Control and Prevention: *United States, 2001—urban and rural chartbook,* Washington, DC, retrieved August 2001 from http://www.cdc.gov/nchs/data/hus/ hus01.pdf.

Cromartie J, Swanson L: *Defining metropolitan areas and the rural–urban continuum: a comparison of statistical areas based on county and sub-county geography,* Washington, DC, 1995, U.S. Department of Agriculture, Economic Research Division, Rural Economy Division, staff paper No. AGES-9603.

Davis D, Droes N: Community health nursing in rural and frontier counties, *Nurs Clin North Am* 28(1):159, 1993.

Diverty B, Perez C: The health of Northern residents: health reports, *Statistics Canada* 9(4):49-58, 1998.

Dunkin J et al: Characteristics of metropolitan and non metropolitan community health nurses, *Texas J Rural Health* 7(1):18, 1994.

Edelman M, Menz B: Selected comparisons and implications of a national rural and urban survey on health care access, demographics and policy issues, *J Rural Health* 11(3):197, 1996.

Graham R: Inservice education for northern nurses, *Canadian Nurse* 90(3):33, 1994.

Gregory D: Nursing practice in native communities. In Baumgart A, Larsen J, editors: *Canadian nursing faces the future,* ed 2, St Louis, Mo, 1992, Mosby.

Health Canada: *Canada's rural health strategy: a one year review,* Minister of Public Works and Government Services, 1-16, 2001.

Health Canada: *Rural health,* available at www.hc-sc.gc.ca/english/ruralhealth/index.html (updated 3/2003), and also through www.hc-sc.gc.ca (search for "rural").

Health Resources Services Administration: *Minorities and rural health, 1988 to 1997,* Rockville, Md, 1997, HRSA Information Center, available at www.ask.hrsa.gov.

Health Resources Services Administration: *A national agenda for nursing workforce: racial/ethnic diversity,* Rockville, Md, 2000, HRSA Information Center, available at ftp://ftp.hrsa.gov/bhpr/nursing/divreport/DivFull.pdf.

Johnson-Webb K, Baer I, Gesler W: What is rural? issues and considerations, *J Rural Health* 45(2):171, 1997.

Lee H, editor: *Conceptual basis for rural nursing,* New York, 1998, Springer.

Life expectancy (Health Reports): *Statistics Canada* 11(3):9-22, 1999.

Long K, Weinert C: Rural nursing: developing a theory base, 1989, *Sch Inq Nurs Pract* 3:113, 1999.

Morewood-Northrop M: Nursing in the Northwest Territories, *Canadian Nurse* 90(3):26, 1994.

National Rural Health Association, National Agenda for Rural Minority Health: *Issue paper,* Kansas City, Mo, retrieved May 1999 from www.NRHArural.org.

National Rural Health Association, National Agenda for Rural Minority Health: *The need for standardized data and information systems issue paper,* Kansas City, Mo, 2001a, available at www.NRHArural.org.

National Rural Health Association, National Agenda for Rural Minority Health: *The need for responsive rural health delivery systems issue paper,* Kansas City, Mo, 2001b, available at www.NRHArural.org.

Newbold KB: Problems in search of solutions: health and Canadian aboriginals, *J Community Health* 23(1):59, 1998.

Office of Minority Health Resource Center: *Closing the gap, the minority AIDS crises,* Washington, DC, 1999, available at http://www.omhrc.gov/ctg/aids1999.pdf.

Office of Rural Health Policy: *Seventh annual report on rural health: recommendations to the Secretary of Health and Human Services,* Washington, DC, 1994, ORHP.

Packard Foundation: *The future of children: welfare to work,* 7(1), 1997a.

Packard Foundation: *The future of children: children and poverty,* 7(2), 1997b.

Pan S, Straub L: Education for rural health professionals, *J Rural Health* 3(1):78, 1997.

Pearson L: Annual update of how each state stands on legislative issues affecting advanced nursing practice, *Nurse Pract* 22(1):18, 1997.

Pickard M: Rural nursing: a decade in review, *Rural Clin Q* 6(3):1, 1996.

Ramsbottom-Lucier M et al: Hills, ridges, mountains and roads: geographical factors and access to care in a rural state, *J Rural Health* 12(5):386, 1996.

Roberts J: Outpost nurse responds to March column, *Canadian Nurse* 94(6):8, 1998.

Ross D: Nursing up north, *Canadian Nurse* 85(1):22, 1989.

Schoenman J: *Impact of the Balanced Budget Act of 1997 on Medicare risk plan payment rates for rural areas,* Washington DC, 1998, Project Hope-Walsh Center for Rural Health Analysis.

Schwartz T: Making it safer down on the farm, *Am J Nurs* 102(3):114-115, 2002.

Scott K: Northern nurses burnout, *Canadian Nurse* 87(10):18, 1991.

Sebastian J, Bushy A, editors: *Special populations in the community: advances in reducing health disparities,* Gaithersburg, Md, 1999, Aspen.

Shields M, Tremblay S: The health of Canada's communities, supplement to Health Reports, *Statistics Canada* 13:1-25, 2002.

Stratton T, Dunkin J, Juhl N: Redefining the nursing shortage: a rural perspective, *Nurs Outlook* 43(2):71, 1995.

Stratton T et al: Retainment incentives in three rural practice settings: influence on the job satisfaction of registered nurses, *Appl Nurs Res* 8(2):73, 1995.

Substance Abuse and Mental Health Services Administration, Center for Substance Abuse Treatment: *Bringing excellence to substance abuse services in rural America: 1996 award for excellence papers,* Rockville, Md, 1997, US Government Printing Office, USDHHS Publication No. (SMA) 97-3134.

The health of Canada's communities, 2000/01 (The Daily): *Statistics Canada,* July 4, 2002, available at www.statcan.ca/Daily/English/020704/d020704b.htm.

The 1998 HHS Poverty Guidelines, *Federal Register* 63(36):9235, 1998.

U.S. Bureau of the Census: *Resident population of the United States by sex, race, and Hispanic origin: 2000,* retrieved April 2, 2001 from www.census.gov/population/estimates/nation.

U.S. Department of Agriculture: *Agriculture fact book,* Washington, DC, 1997, USDA.

U.S. Department of Health and Human Services: *Healthy people 2010: understanding and improving health,* ed 2, Washington, DC, 2000, U.S. Government Printing Office.

U.S. Department of Health and Human Services: *Selected statistics on health professional shortage areas,* Washington, DC, retrieved April 2002a from http://bphc.hrsa.gov/dsd/default.htm.

U.S. Department of Health and Human Services: *Healthy people 2000: final review,* Hyattsville, Md, 2002b, retrieved from http://www.cdc.gov/nchs/products/pubs/pubd/hp2k/review/highlightshp2000.htm.

U.S. Department of Health and Human Services: *Healthy people 2010,* vol I, vol II, and appendices, Washington, DC, 2002c, retrieved April 20 from http://www.health.gov/healthypeople/doc.

U.S. Department of Health and Human Services: *Healthy people in healthy communities: a community planning guide using Healthy People 2010,* Washington, DC, 2002d, retrieved April 20 from http://www.health.gov/healthypeople/Publications/HealthyCommunities2001/default.htm.

Washington State Nursing Network: Celebration of Public Health Nurse Committee: *opening doors: stories of public health nursing,* Olympia, Wash, 1992, Washington State Department of Health.

Weinert C, Long K: Rural families and health care: refining the knowledge base, *J Marriage Fam Rev* 15(1,2):57, 1990.

Winstead-Fry P, editor: *Rural health nursing: stories of creativity, commitment, and connectedness,* New York, 1992, NLN.

## Chapter 17

# Health Promotion Through Healthy Communities and Cities

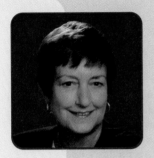

## Beverly C. Flynn, Ph.D., R.N., F.A.A.N.

Beverly C. Flynn recognizes that local communities hold the future of the world; yet, today they face some of the most complex health problems in human history. She is an emeritus professor at the Indiana University School of Nursing, the former director of the Institute of Action Research for Community Health (IARCH), and the head of the World Health Organization (WHO) Collaborating Center in Healthy Cities. In her work with Healthy Cities, she not only initiated the Healthy Cities Indiana project, one of the first Healthy Cities programs in the United States, but she also facilitated the development of the Healthy Cities and Communities program throughout the country and beyond. The basic tenets of her career in community health nursing include community-based nursing practice, community development, health promotion, and interdisciplinary action research, where the problems under investigation come from the community's need for information rather than questions generated from personal interests of researchers.

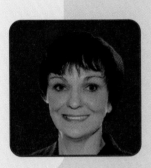

## L. Louise Ivanov, D.N.S., R.N.

Louise Ivanov started her community health practice as a public health nurse at the Tippecanoe County Health Department, Lafayette, Indiana. She became involved in the Healthy Cities movement in Indiana in 1990. Louise participated in an internship with the World Health Organization Healthy Cities project, working as an advisor to the St. Petersburg, Russia, Healthy City project, where she also conducted health systems research on delivery of prenatal care services. In 2000 she received a Fulbright Scholarship to teach public health nursing and health policy, not formerly taught in the nursing curriculum, to nurse educators at the St. Petersburg, Russia, Medical Academy of Postgraduate Studies. Currently, Louise is chair of the Community Practice Department at the University of North Carolina, Greensboro, School of Nursing.

## Objectives

After reading this chapter, the student should be able to do the following:

1. Trace the Healthy Communities and Cities movement
2. Examine the relationships between primary health care, health promotion, and the Healthy Communities and Cities movement
3. Describe the steps in working with communities in the Healthy Communities and Cities process
4. Apply the steps in working with Healthy Communities and Cities to the concepts of health promotion
5. Analyze the role for community-oriented nursing in Healthy Communities and Cities
6. Analyze the impact of the Healthy Communities and Cities process in health promotion at the community level

The development of the Healthy Cities movement began in Europe in 1986 and has spread to all regions of the world. Because in the United States many localities were not classified as cities, the movement was expanded to include Healthy Communities. The Healthy Communities and Cities movement shares common principles and concepts including support of a community problem-solving process for health promotion. Healthy Communities and Cities relies on a broad definition of health and a broad definition of community. It accepts a shared vision of the future that is based on community values. The goal is to address health and quality of life for all through a process that includes diverse citizen participation, mobilization of all sectors of the community, and community ownership. The focus is on "systems change," accomplished by placing health promotion on the political agenda of communities and cities. The emphases are on building capacity, using local assets and resources, and measuring progress and outcomes (Norris and Pittman, 2000; Tsouros, 1990). The Healthy Communities and Cities movement supports the strategy of primary care (World Health Organization [WHO] and United Nations

## Key Terms

**appropriate technology**, p. 399
**Community Health Promotion model**, p. 399
**community participation**, p. 399
**equity**, p. 399

**health promotion**, p. 399
**Healthy Communities and Cities**, p. 398
**healthy public policy**, p. 399
**Healthy People 2010 objectives**, p. 408
**international cooperation**, p. 398

**multisectoral cooperation**, p. 399
**primary health care**, p. 398
*See Glossary for definitions*

## Chapter Outline

History of the Healthy Communities and Cities
    Movement
Definition of Terms
Models of Community Practice
Healthy Communities and Cities
*United States*
*Canada*
*Russia*

*Denmark*
*Poland*
*Networks Link Cities in Europe*
*China*
*Nepal*
*El Salvador*
*Venezuela*
*Latin American Networks*

Future of the Healthy Communities and Cities
    Movement
*Facilitators and Barriers*
*Healthy Public Policy*
Implications for Community-Oriented Nursing
Healthy People 2010

Children's Fund [UNICEF], 1978), the principles of health promotion outlined in the Ottawa Charter for Health Promotion (WHO, 1986), and, in the United States, Healthy People 2010 (U.S. Department of Health and Human Services, 2000). Furthermore, Hancock (2000) indicates that healthy communities and cities must be both environmentally and socially sustainable. Communities and cities are challenged to do the following (Goldstein and Kickbusch, 1996; Tsouros, 1990):

- Develop projects that reduce inequalities in health status and access to services
- Develop healthy public policies at the local level
- Create physical and social environments that support health, strengthen community action for health, and help people develop new skills for health
- Reorient health services in a way that is consistent with the strategy of primary health care and the principles of health promotion

This chapter is an introduction to the history of the Healthy Communities and Cities movement and to the basic terminology related to the movement. It describes various models of community practice and indicates a com-

mon model that more clearly reflects the Healthy Communities and Cities process. To understand Healthy Communities and Cities as a worldwide movement, descriptive examples of Healthy Communities and Cities from a variety of regions of the world are included. The key facilitators and barriers to the Healthy Communities and Cities process emphasize the importance of healthy public policy in sustaining the health of communities and cities.

## HISTORY OF THE HEALTHY COMMUNITIES AND CITIES MOVEMENT

Although Healthy Communities and Cities can now be found in every region of the world, the European Healthy Cities Project was initiated by Dr. Ilona Kickbusch of the World Health Organization, Regional Office for Europe, in 1986. She recognized the potential for Healthy Cities to take action in health promotion at the local level (Hancock, 1993). There were 11 European cities that participated in the initial phase of the Healthy Cities project, and by 1991 there were 35 cities in the project. Today more than 1000 cities in 30 European countries participate. Some of these cities included Camden, England;

Horsens, Denmark; Rennes, France; Pecs, Hungary; Turku, Finland; and Athens, Greece.

Healthy Cities began with the recognition that about half of the world's population lives in urban areas, where the human and health-related problems are complex and coupled with increasingly fragmented policy and scarce resources. A key strategy of Healthy Cities is to mobilize the community by developing public, private, and not-for-profit partnerships to address the complex health and environmental problems in the city. The Healthy Cities process involves the following steps (Pan American Health Organization/WHO, 1999; WHO, 1992):

A. Start-up phase
    1. Develop a local task force.
    2. Build public awareness and support.
B. Organization phase
    3. Gain local government approval.
    4. Appoint broad-based partnership on the Healthy City committee.
    5. Establish priorities, goals, and city-wide action plans.
    6. Mobilize resources.
C. Implementation and evaluation phase
    7. Establish steering groups to carry out the action.
    8. Implement and evaluate progress.
    9. Review and modify local policies and programs.
    10. Network across Healthy Cities.

Healthy Communities and Cities was initiated in the United States in 1988, with Healthy Cities Indiana and the California Healthy Cities project. Healthy Cities Indiana adapted the European experiences to the American context. The concept of Healthy Communities was used to incorporate other localities that were not cities but rather smaller communities such as towns or counties. Since 1988, communities throughout the United States have initiated the Healthy Communities and Cities process with the result that thousands of communities have taken local action to promote health (Hospital Research and Educational Trust, 2002).

In 1994, the national network of Healthy Communities and Cities was initiated in the United States. The Coalition for Healthier Cities and Communities that evolved from this network not only helped to promote state networks of Healthy Communities and Cities but also assisted local communities through networking and information exchange. Since 1994, a number of documents have been published by the coalition, and in 1998 a web page (www.hospitalconnect.com) was initiated to help local communities through their various stages of developing the Healthy Communities and Cities process.

In other parts of the world, Healthy Communities and Cities has different names, including Healthy Islands, Healthy Villages, and, in Latin America, Healthy Municipalities and Healthy Cantons. In addition, national networks have also developed in Australia, Canada, Costa Rica, Iran, and Egypt. In Quebec, Canada, the Network of Healthy Towns and Villages has linked with Brazil, Colombia, Mexico, and Senegal (Kenzer, 1999). Other regional networks have been developed in Francophone Africa, Latin America, Southeast Asia, and the western Pacific.

Healthy Communities and Cities has become a movement and is labeled "the new public health" (Ashton and Seymour, 1988), although others claim that the concept of a healthy community or city is not new (Hancock, 1993). It is based on the belief that the health of the community is largely influenced by the environment in which people live and that health problems have multiple causes—social, economic, political, environmental, and behavioral. Healthy Communities and Cities is consistent with the definition of health promotion that promotes change in the broader environment to support health (*Declaration of Medellin*, 1999; *Mexico Ministerial Statement for the Promotion of Health*, 2000; WHO, 1986).

The Healthy Communities and Cities process has been applied to rural and metropolitan areas (Flynn, 1992; Focus on healthy communities, 2000). Healthy Communities and Cities engages local residents for action in health and is based on the premise that when people have the opportunity to work out their own locally defined health problems, they will find sustainable solutions to those problems (Chamberlin, 1996; Flynn, 1992; Focus on healthy communities, 2000).

## DEFINITION OF TERMS

Healthy Communities and Cities is an international movement that mobilizes local resources and political, professional, and community members to improve the health and quality of life of the community. A healthy city is one whose priority is to improve its environment and expand its resources so that community members can support each other in achieving their highest potential (Hancock and Duhl, 1988). **Healthy Communities and Cities** emphasizes partnerships and action and is based on guiding principles that include a broad definition of both health and community, a shared vision based on community values that addresses the health and quality of life for everyone, and diverse citizen participation and widespread community ownership. This movement focuses on "system change," by building the community's capacity to meet its needs and use its own local assets and resources, including building more capacity in the community to meet its needs. It also benchmarks against other programs or standards, and measures progress and outcomes (Norris and Pittman, 2000).

Instrumental in the development of the Healthy Cities movement were the principles of primary health care (WHO and UNICEF, 1978) and the Ottawa Charter for Health Promotion (WHO, 1986). **Primary health care,** the focus of health care system reform, refers to meeting the basic health needs of a community by providing readily accessible health services. Because health problems transcend international borders, **international cooperation** is important to ensure health. The principles of primary health care include equity, health promotion, community participation, multisectoral cooperation, appropriate technology, and international cooperation.

**Equity** implies providing accessible services to promote the health of populations most at risk for health problems (e.g., the poor, the young, older adults, minorities, the homeless, and refugees). **Health promotion** and disease prevention are focused on providing community members with a positive sense of health that strengthens their physical, mental, and emotional capacities. Individuals within communities become involved in health promotion through **community participation,** whereby well-informed and motivated community members participate in planning, implementing, and evaluating health programs. **Multisectoral cooperation** refers to coordinated action by all parts of a community, from local government officials to grassroots community members. **Appropriate technology** refers to affordable social, biomedical, and health services that are relevant and acceptable to individuals' health, needs, and concerns.

Health promotion had become a key strategy for the goal of health for all by the time the Ottawa Charter for Health Promotion was adopted in 1986. This charter provided a clear definition of health promotion and the framework for the Healthy Cities movement (Ashton, 1992; WHO, 1992). Health promotion was officially defined as the "process of enabling people to take control over and to improve their health" (WHO, 1986, p. 1). This is accomplished through enabling community members to increase control over and assume more responsibility for health; mediating among public, private, voluntary, and community sectors; and advocating on behalf of people who are powerless to make the necessary changes to promote health.

Five elements make up the strategic framework provided by the Ottawa Charter of Health Promotion (WHO, 1986). They are listed here in order of priority for health promotion action:

1. *Healthy public policy:* Policy based on an ecologic perspective and on multisectoral and participatory strategies, future oriented, and dealing with both local health problems and global health issues. (In contrast, medical policy is concerned mainly with the existing medical care system and use of technology and biomedical science to treat disease.)
2. *Creating supportive environments:* Physical, political, economic, and social systems that support the community's health
3. *Strengthening community action:* Promoting the community's capacity, ability, and opportunity to take appropriate action to protect and improve the health of the community
4. *Developing personal skills:* Helping people develop the lifestyle skills they need to be healthy
5. *Reorienting health services:* Changing the focus of health services toward primary health care, health promotion, disease prevention, and community-oriented care

At international conferences, health promotion has been reclaimed as the appropriate approach to reduce health gaps

(*Declaration of Medellin*, 1999; *Mexico Ministerial Statement for the Promotion of Health*, 2000). The Medellin Congress stated that health promotion would be the strategy of Healthy Municipalities (as Healthy Communities and Cities are called in Latin America). The Mexico Ministerial Statement concluded that health promotion must be a fundamental component of public policies and programs, and that national and international networks that promote health should be strengthened.

The **Community Health Promotion model,** developed at Indiana University School of Nursing, is a cyclical process and an adaptation of the European model of Healthy Cities in the United States (Figure 17-1). This nine-step process includes the following:

1. Orienting the community to community health promotion
2. Building the partnership for health
3. Development of the community structure for health promotion
4. Leadership development for health promotion
5. Assessing the community
6. Community-wide planning for health
7. Community action for health
8. Providing data-based information to policy makers
9. Monitoring and evaluating healthy progress

**DID YOU KNOW?**

Implementing the steps of the Community Health Promotion model will enable community-oriented nurses to gain an understanding of the linkages between health, community, and the policy process. Benefits to the community include increased access to services and improved health status, which promote equity in health.

## MODELS OF COMMUNITY PRACTICE

There are different models of community practice, and the assumptions that professionals have about communities shape the implementation of the Healthy Communities and Cities process. The classic work of Rothman and Tropman (1987) described these different models and continues to be relevant today (Fisher, 1998). These models include the following:

1. Locality development is a process-oriented model that emphasizes consensus, cooperation, and building group identity and a sense of community.
2. Social planning stresses rational–empirical problem solving, usually by outside professional experts. Social planning does not focus on building community capacity or fostering fundamental social change.
3. Social action, on the other hand, aims to increase the problem-solving ability of the community with concrete actions that attempt to correct the imbalance of power and privilege of an oppressed or disadvantaged group in the community.

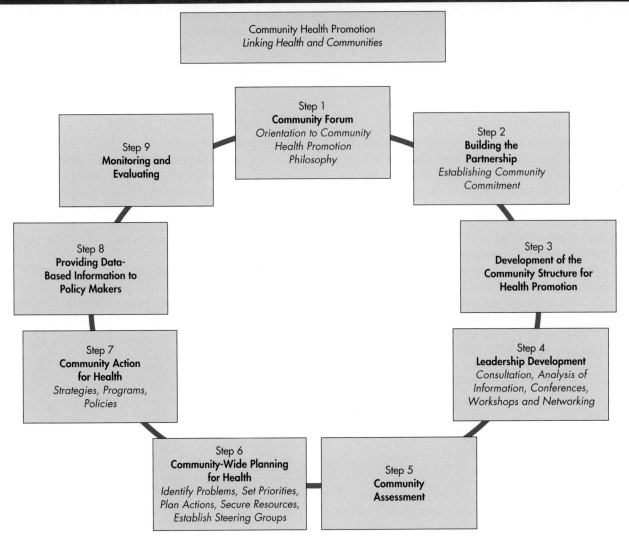

**Figure 17-1** Community Health Promotion model. *(Copyright 1994, Institute of Action Research for Community Health/Indiana University.)*

Although these models of community practice are not mutually exclusive, community efforts can generally be categorized within one model.

Arnstein (1969) depicts a ladder of citizen participation, with the lower levels of participation being manipulation, therapy, and informing; this can be equated with a top-down approach in which community practice and action are planned by professionals and experts. The higher levels of participation as described by Rothman and Tropman (1987) include partnership, delegated power, and citizen control; this represents a bottom-up approach, reflecting a multisectoral approach with community participation. However, Minkler and Pies (1998) note that much of current health promotion practice focuses on the lower rungs of the ladder and is not at a high level of community participation.

These models of community practice are summarized as top-down and bottom-up approaches. In a top-down approach, experts and health professionals take the lead in identifying community health problems and implement-

> **DID YOU KNOW?**
>
> Community participation can begin at town meetings, city council meetings, crime watch, and other settings where community members from different walks of life (including health professionals) identify the strengths and health needs of their community and plan appropriate action to address their needs. This is an example of social action—a bottom-up approach to community practice.

ing programs with little input from the individuals for whom these programs are being planned. The social planning model is an example that portrays a top-down approach where rational and empirical problem solving is usually conducted by outside experts.

A bottom-up approach uses broad-based community problem solving that includes health professionals, local officials, service providers, and other community members, in-

**WHAT DO YOU THINK?**

Community participation in health decisions is more effective in promoting healthy public policy than decision making by outside professional experts.

**Evidence-Based Practice**

The Healthy Cities process uses action research to empower communities to take action for health. Five concepts that link community empowerment and action research are focus on community, citizen participation, information and problem solving, sharing of power, and quality of life. Two case studies from Healthy Cities Indiana illustrate these concepts. The dynamics of community participation in action research and the successes and barriers to community participation are presented. Outcomes found to empower the community are the extent to which Healthy Cities projects are initiated, their progress is monitored, continued action in health is supported, resources are obtained, and policies are promoted that contribute to equity in health.

**Nurse Use:** The Healthy Cities process relies on a problem-solving approach to bring about community change. The goal is to encourage community members to take responsibility for the change they wish to see happen.

Flynn B, Ray D, Rider M: Empowering communities: action research through healthy cities, *Health Educ Q* 21(3):394, 1994.

cluding those at risk for health problems. The locality development and social action models are examples of a bottom-up approach, in which community participation is evident in all stages of community health planning and practice.

Healthy Communities and Cities emphasize a bottom-up approach, and at the same time it includes multisectoral planning and action for health (the top-down approach). The Community Health Promotion process aims at partnerships within the community and focuses on community leadership development for health that is consistent with the locality development model of Rothman and Tropman (1987).

## HEALTHY COMMUNITIES AND CITIES

In the following paragraphs, Healthy Communities and Cities initiatives in various regions of the world are discussed. These examples show the different models of community practice that are being implemented in the movement. The locality development and social planning models are used most frequently (Flynn, 1996).

### United States

Indiana and California have the longest history of Healthy Communities and Cities in the United States. Healthy Cities Indiana began as a pilot program in 1988 with a grant from the W. K. Kellogg Foundation as a collaborative effort among Indiana University School of Nursing, Indiana Public Health Association, and six Indiana cities. On the basis of this project's success, the W. K. Kellogg Foundation funded the dissemination phase, called CITYNET-Healthy Cities, in cooperation with the National League of Cities through their network of 19,000 local officials (Flynn, Rider, and Ray, 1991).

The Community Health Promotion process begins by holding a community forum to orient the community to health promotion. If those present desire to proceed with the process, a partnership begins and local leaders commit to the Healthy Communities and Cities process. Once the commitment is obtained, a Healthy Community or City committee is established that includes multisectoral representation of the community and citizen participation. Broad multisectoral involvement and citizen participation occur in all the remaining stages of the Community Health Promotion process (leadership development, community assessment, community-wide planning for health, community action, providing data-based information to policy makers, and monitoring and evaluation). The step-by-step process continues the cycle with feedback of progress to the broader community through the community forum. As the

healthy community or city develops, updates are made at each step of the process to ensure the relevant sustainability of Healthy Communities and Cities in health promotion. The Community Health Promotion process aims at partnerships within the community; health professionals need to recognize that, because of the city's complex nature, community problems cannot be solved by one sector alone, such as the health sector, but rather they need a multisectoral approach. "Professionalizing" community problems is working at the lowest level of participation—that is, providing therapy or treatment rather than community partnership (Arnstein, 1969).

Six cities were initially involved in Healthy Cities Indiana (Gary, Fort Wayne, New Castle, Indianapolis, Seymour, and Jeffersonville). Activities in these cities focused on problems of diverse populations. For example, actions were directed to local priorities that include problems of children, teen parents, the homeless, access to health care, crime and violence, and older adults. Action has also been taken on the broader environmental policy issues, including management of solid waste and promotion of air quality. For each of these projects, the Community Health Promotion process was followed, thereby providing a broad base of community participation at all stages of community planning (see Evidence-Based Practice box).

An early example of the use of the CITYNET process was the New Castle Healthy City community assessment. The committee questioned their community's high death rates caused by cancer, chronic obstructive pulmonary disease, and heart disease. The committee asked the following questions: Why were rates here higher than those of the state and the nation? What were the lifestyle choices of people in the community? What in the environment supported or inhibited healthy choices?

The committee decided to work with the staff at Indiana University School of Nursing, and they constructed a survey to obtain baseline data on health behaviors in the community. Indiana University staff trained local volunteers in survey data collection. One thousand surveys were distributed door-to-door using a system that ensured appropriate geographic coverage in the community. The response rate of 50% demonstrated the community's interest in health concerns. The committee used the national health objectives to compare their findings (U.S. Department of Health and Human Services [USDHHS], 1991). They found high levels of unhealthy behaviors, such as cigarette smoking and inadequate exercise, compared to the 2000 national objectives.

The committee then used the survey results to target their Healthy City initiatives. The data were used to testify before the county commissioners about the need for health education and to support the employment of a health educator in the local health department. The cigarette smoking results were used by the committee to testify before the city council in support of an ordinance banning smoking in city buildings. The committee also sponsored community health awareness programs. The 1994 program included a family fitness walk, safety checks of bicycles, and presentations on healthy food preparation emphasizing reduced fat and salt in meals.

New Castle has expanded its focus and is now known as Henry County Healthy Communities. Two 2002 initiatives are examples of a continuation of the earlier work of the committee. The first, which stemmed from the committee's concern with rising childhood obesity rates, was Walk-a-Child-to-School Day. This initiative identified opportunities for children to get exercise, and it also showed children a way to experience their community that many had missed by riding in cars or school buses. The second initiative was the planning of trails throughout Henry County that would promote walking and other exercise by community residents. Consultants worked with the committee in conducting a feasibility study and in writing a grant with the hope of obtaining funding.

Throughout the years, the committee obtained broad community support and cooperation, not only in defining their local problems but also in setting priorities and implementing their initiatives. Their interventions integrated individual lifestyle changes and policy changes aimed at promoting supportive environments for health.

The California Healthy Cities and Communities project has grown from a few initial cities to the California Network of Healthy Cities funded in part by the state Department of Health Service. It is built on the premise of shared responsibility among community members, local officials, and the private sector. Community participation is the cornerstone of the projects, and the mission is to re-

## THE CUTTING EDGE

Because of a local influx of a Latino population, Healthy Communities of Bartholomew County, Indiana, initiated nurse-managed services in a voluntary medical clinic to provide health care to low-income, uninsured Hispanic people. Nurses are beginning to evaluate the impact of the project on the Latino community, which will provide data for future evidenced-based nursing practice.

duce inequities in health status that exist among diverse populations in communities.

In 1989, Pasadena became a charter city of the California Healthy Cities project and produced a quality-of-life index with extensive input from residents, technical panels, and neighborhood groups. The index includes over 50 indicators affecting community life, such as safety, education, substance abuse, recreation, economy, and housing. The index guided policy development in tobacco control, alcohol availability, and infant health. In addition, it assisted city and community agencies in planning, priority setting, resource development, and budgeting. The quality of life index was revised in 1998, using the Healthy People 2000 targets or, in the absence of these targets, the 1992 index targets and the targets from the city's results-based budget were used.

Another example of California Healthy Cities and Communities is in Chico. A Healthy Chico Kids 2000 community-wide initiative was started, and it focused on nutrition and health promotion. Nutrition education was provided for students in kindergarten through sixth grade. A dietary assessment was conducted that led the school district to reduce calories from fat in school lunches. The initiative was expanded to increase awareness of cardiovascular risk factors among elementary school students.

There is a strong network of Healthy Communities and Cities in Massachusetts. Boston has at least 12 Healthy Communities and Cities initiatives. One example is the Chinatown Coalition, a community-based initiative involving community residents, community organizations, churches, businesses, and government agencies committed to improving the social, economic, environmental, and spiritual life of the Chinatown and Boston Asian community. The Chinatown Coalition facilitates and coordinates neighborhood-based efforts and resources to address community concerns. It also actively promotes advocacy and coordination with agencies that impact the Asian community.

Since the initial Healthy Cities efforts in the United States, there are thousands of Healthy Communities and Cities programs across the country that are seeking local solutions to complex problems. Statewide initiatives of Healthy Communities and Cities are in other states such as Maine, Colorado, New Mexico, and South Carolina. The national Coalition for Healthier Cities and Communities and other organizations that have supported networking among Healthy Communities and Cities include the Hospital Research and Educational Trust of the American Hospital Association, the Healthcare Forum, the Centers for Disease Control and Prevention, and the National Civic League.

## Canada

Toronto, Ontario, was one of the first cities to become involved in the Healthy Cities movement in North America. Toronto began with a strategic planning committee to develop an overall strategy for health promotion (Hancock, 1993). The committee conducted vision workshops in the community and a comprehensive environmental scan to help identify health needs in Toronto. The outcome was a final report outlining major issues, and it included a strategic mission, priorities, and recommendations for action. The Toronto Healthy City was involved in a number of projects. One of them, the Healthiest Babies Possible project, was an intensive antenatal education and nutritional supplement program for pregnant women who were identified by health and social agencies as being at high risk. The program included intensive contact and follow-up of women, along with food supplements. It has been successful in decreasing the incidence of low-birth-weight infants.

Another project, Parents Helping Parents, identified children at high risk for neglect or abuse. Parents of these children were linked with specially trained health workers from similar sociocultural backgrounds to help them cope with problems of parenting and learn new and more effective parenting skills. Community participation was especially evident in this program, in which community members, frequently from disadvantaged communities, were trained as health workers. The health workers were provided with new skills, a useful role in their communities, and a sense of self-esteem.

In 1998, the Toronto Healthy City office became part of the Chief Administrator's Office in the city of Toronto. More recent examples of initiatives include a neighborhood project, Caring and Sharing Across the Generations, in which senior citizens volunteer to share their life skills and build friendships with parents and young children. This outreach project includes cooking, reading, and arts and crafts activities. Another example is a city-wide initiative focused on community safety. The Toronto Task Force on Community Safety conducted a city-wide survey of safety concerns and resources and helped to develop the report "Toronto. My City. A Safe City" that was approved by the city council.

## Russia

In 1992, St. Petersburg was the largest city in the European Healthy Cities project and the first from the former Soviet Union. Government officials, health professionals, and consultants from the WHO European Region Healthy Cities project met to identify the major health problems in St. Petersburg. They decided to begin their health initiative by focusing on programs to decrease the city's high ma-

### Evidence-Based Practice

The St. Petersburg, Russia, Healthy Cities project began its health initiative by focusing on health care services for women, primarily because of a high maternal mortality rate and low attendance at prenatal care clinics. This study sought to explain and predict use and satisfaction with prenatal care services in St. Petersburg. A convenience sample of 397 women with uncomplicated pregnancies and normal deliveries was drawn, representing an 86% response rate. Survey data were collected retrospectively, after the women had delivered their infants but before they were discharged from the hospital, to answer the following questions:

1. Are there characteristics of pregnant women that predict the use of prenatal care services and satisfaction with the services?

2. To what extent do predisposing, enabling, and need characteristics contribute to explaining the use of prenatal care services and satisfaction with the services?

3. Is there a relationship between the use of prenatal care services and satisfaction with the services that explains the start of prenatal care?

Predictors of service use were attitude toward prenatal care, depression, marital status, and employment status. Russian women identified convenience of prenatal care clinics and doctors' behavior as measures of the quality of prenatal care received.

Predictors of satisfaction were a regular source of care and negative experiences with health care providers.

**Nurse Use:** Findings provide alternatives to improve the delivery of prenatal care services in St. Petersburg through a collaborative and multisectoral effort on the part of health policy makers, health care professionals, and educators to encourage an early start of prenatal care and provide quality prenatal services.

Ivanov LL, Flynn BC: Predictors of utilization and satisfaction with prenatal care services in St. Petersburg, Russia, *West J Nurs Res* 21(1):372, 1999.

ternal and infant mortality rates. Four projects were developed: a family planning center, a teen center, a maternity home with rooming-in and breastfeeding support (Baby Friendly Campaign), and a rehabilitation center for socially disadvantaged pregnant women (Flynn and Dennis, 1993). A consensus conference was held with international consultants to address how to improve the four projects. The local individuals who attended the conference were primarily health professionals, including physicians, nurses, and midwives. This was the first time many of these professionals had met together in an interdisciplinary approach to address health problems. The Evidence-Based Practice box details a study of prenatal services conducted in St. Petersburg. Currently, the family planning center continues to work with women and their partners, providing free brochures and consultation in methods of family planning that are individualized for each couple. The teen center has expanded to include exercise and sports facilities in an attempt to provide teens with a safe place to interact and learn about healthy lifestyles. The center also provides teens with weekly sessions on various topics, ranging from reproductive health to building self-esteem. Most recently, a 24-hour telephone line furnished with a psychologist is available for teens in crisis situations.

The city of Korolev, in the Moscow region of the Russian Federation, joined the Healthy Cities project in 1996 and focused on the effective use of energy resources. The city council accepted the energy savings program, which was projected to preserve natural resources, reduce environmental pollution, save budgetary funds, and provide improvement of working places and housing conditions. This comprehensive resource-saving program involves all aspects of city life, including economic, industrial, ecologic, and social areas. On the basis of experiences in Korolev, it appears that sustainable development of a city is impossible without efficient use of energy resources.

## Denmark

Horsens Healthy City in Denmark identified six steps necessary to transform a health promotion idea into action (Bragh-Matzon, 1992):

1. Political commitment and legitimacy
2. Building a small catalyst unit to secure the transformation process
3. Building an infrastructure to secure involvement and legitimization from essential powers in city life
4. Information, communication, visibility, and public debates on health issues
5. Combining short-term action and long-term planning
6. Promoting and securing the process over time

The first step involved obtaining a commitment from the city council to support the health-for-all strategy through the Healthy City model. In the second step, the catalyst unit was a small team that bridged the existing governmental and health structures with the multiple powers and resources within the city. The team included highly experienced professional community members from different disciplines. Nonprofessional community members, or grassroots people, were not directly involved in this team. However, their input was sought by professional team members. It was not until the third step that direct community participation occurred. Ordinary citizens were included on a steering committee that became the health committee for the city. The function of the health committee was to oversee projects and communicate with appropriate individuals and agencies in the city, thereby creating more effective links among politicians, health professionals, and citizens.

Horsens's first health initiative involved conducting a health survey to obtain a health profile for the city. This resulted in the Torsted West project. The goal of this project was to plan a new residential area along ecologic principles. This was accomplished through the six steps mentioned previously. Consultants from other Healthy Cities provided expertise to the project (Draper et al, 1993).

More recently, Horsens adopted an approach to community participation as a sustained feature of local governance and social, cultural, and environmental sustainability. The strategy was to turn the planning process around from a top-down to a bottom-up process. Methods included public meetings, mailings to all households, special meetings, study groups, and radio and press information bulletins. These methods resulted in about 1000 proposals, ideas, and requests. Working groups were formed and given specific topics to address, and new approaches to problem solving developed.

## Poland

In the 1990s, unemployment was an economic and a social problem in Poland. To combat this problem, the city of Tomaszow set their Healthy City objective as the improvement of local vocational training and the reduction of unemployment, which was above the national average. An employment forum was created to coordinate and reorganize local vocational training programs. The forum included representatives of training organizations, public officials from 10 counties, employers, and unemployed persons. A needs assessment was conducted that resulted in a database on local training needs, training capacity, and graduates of the training programs. On the basis of the needs assessment, the forum worked together to create a coalition of vocational training organizations, provide vocational training programs, and develop new training schemes for the unemployed. Currently, 65% of those trained in the vocational programs have found employment or are continuing in educational training.

## Networks Link Cities in Europe

Over the years, WHO has encouraged Healthy Cities in Europe to work together in seeking solutions to common problems. Multi-City Action Plans (MCAPs) and the European Healthy Cities Networks are two avenues that have promoted the Healthy Cities agenda. MCAPs provided platforms for international cooperation in health planning and sharing of professional experts in Europe. Groups of Healthy Cities in Europe worked together to address common health concerns. This enabled smaller cities and those new in the Healthy Cities movement to work together on common health problems, thereby expanding the number of partners and resources available to deal with problems. The goal of the MCAPs was to jointly develop, implement, and disseminate innovative models of health promotion. To achieve this goal, a partnership was developed between cities involved in the European Healthy Cities movement. These cities were committed to working together on one common health problem for at least 2 years. The result was open events that provided forums in which to present models of successful health promotion projects, exchange information, and monitor progress (Tsouros, 1995).

Examples of health concerns that MCAPs addressed include acquired immunodeficiency syndrome (AIDS) and human immunodeficiency virus (HIV), alcohol abuse, environment and health, diabetes, disability, health-promoting hospitals, nutrition, sports, tobacco-free cities, unemployment, and women's health (WHO, 1994). Specific MCAPs on AIDS activities included surveying users of services for their views on existing services and opinions on services needed; encouraging participation of gay, lesbian, and other community-based organizations in the HIV/AIDS work and policy development; exchanging educational material and expertise on prevention methods; and developing a guide on services available to travelers with HIV/AIDS. In addition, an MCAP newsletter on AIDS was published and distributed to member cities as a method of communicating and networking.

In 1993, the WHO encouraged the development of the European National Healthy Cities Networks to establish national and subnational networks. Since 1998, the WHO pledged to create stronger cooperation between the WHO and the national networks to further the Healthy Cities agenda and to form a powerful lobby for action at national, European, and international levels. In 2000, the European National Healthy Cities Networks adopted the Action Framework, which identified a common set of standards and a system of accreditation for national networks and their member cities in the WHO European region. Cities participating in these networks have developed and implemented a range of programs and policies that include city health profiles, city health plans, and community development initiatives addressing the needs of vulnerable populations, lifestyles, and environmental health issues.

## China

Chengdu, China, located on the upper parts of the Yangtze River and surrounded on four sides by the Fu and Nan Rivers, was one of the most polluted cities in southwestern China. The pollution created severe environmental problems as a result of industrial waste, raw sewage, and the intensive use of freshwater. The proliferation of slum and squatter settlements exacerbated the social, economic, and environmental problems of the city. The Fu and Nan Rivers Comprehensive Revitalization Plan was started in 1993 as a Healthy Community and City initiative to deal with the growing environmental problems. The principles of participatory planning and partnership were used to raise awareness of the problem among the general public and to mobilize major stakeholders to invest in a sustainable future for Chengdu and its inhabitants. The plan resulted in providing 30,000 households living in the slum and squatter settlements with decent and affordable housing, and with projects to deal with sewage and industrial waste. In addition, the plan was able to improve parks and

gardens, turning Chengdu into a clean and green city with the natural flow of its rivers.

## Nepal

Nepal is a small country where 70% of families live below the poverty level. Traditionally, Nepal is known as a male-dominated culture that discourages female education, restricts women's legal rights and participation in decision making, and allows women very little control over their lives. Only 20% of Nepalese women are literate. In 1998, the Women's Empowerment Program (WEP) was founded as a Healthy Community and City initiative to empower women through literacy, to finance training, and to further their understanding of their legal rights. Community participation was encouraged by having women develop the programs they desired, and by having them take ownership of the programs by creating group policies, providing facilities and supplies for the programs, and finding literacy volunteers. The WEP found that women were empowered when they participated and took ownership of the programs developed and by teaching themselves the skills needed to improve their lives.

## El Salvador

El Salvador, in Central America, is composed of 10 municipalities with a population of 2 million. A public–private Solid Waste Management and Environmental Sanitation project was started in El Salvador as a Healthy Municipalities initiative to deal with the critical environmental problems caused by inefficient and inadequate solid waste management. Using a community participation and democratic decision-making process, San Salvador took the lead in this project and joined efforts with the private sector, nongovernmental agencies, public organizations, and a university to develop and implement the Solid Waste Management program. The project included educational programs to improve health habits among community residents, and educational programs for waste collectors. The project resulted in innovative procedures to deal with solid waste management that included street cleaning, separation at source, composting, recycling, and the construction and operation of a sanitary landfill.

## Venezuela

In 1995, the Healthy Municipalities movement started in Venezuela. Today, the 28 municipalities involved in the movement make up the Venezuelan Network of Municipalities Toward Health. The network was established to support communication and coordination among municipalities and allow exchange and comparison of project experiences.

Zamora was the first Healthy Municipality in Venezuela. Community meetings were held and a needs assessment was conducted to identify areas of priority for health initiatives. These included the environment, adolescent pregnancy, basic sanitation, poor quality of education, and inadequate access to preventive services. Examples of creative projects to address the identified health problems include health-promoting murals painted by community youth, family gardens, and a children's orchestra that has even performed internationally. The family gardens project has been very popular, as it provides community members the opportunity to grow their own food and sell any extra produce to neighboring municipalities at a very low cost.

## Latin America Networks

The Pan American Health Organization (PAHO) is promoting Healthy Municipalities and Communities in Central and South America, and over 1000 Healthy Municipalities are now reported. Examples of Healthy Municipalities in Latin America are Cienfuegos, Cuba; Mexico City, Mexico; Manizales, Colombia; San Carlos, Costa Rica; Valdivia, Chile; San Salvador, El Salvador; and Zamora, Venezuela. The mission of the Healthy Municipalities and Communities movement is to strengthen the implementation of health promotion activities at the local level, placing health promotion at the highest priority of the political agenda and fostering the involvement of government authorities and active participation of the community. National networks of Healthy Municipalities and Communities exist to support the movement and the Latin American Network of Healthy Municipalities and Communities provides opportunities for cross-national collaboration and information exchange.

## FUTURE OF THE HEALTHY COMMUNITIES AND CITIES MOVEMENT

The future of Healthy Communities and Cities depends on a number of factors that can either facilitate or hinder the process. An important factor in the future of the movement is the extent to which Healthy Communities and Cities develops public policies that create healthier environments in which to live.

## Facilitators and Barriers

The continuance of the Healthy Communities and Cities movement is contingent on many factors that facilitate or impede the process (Flynn et al, 1991; Swartz, 2000; Wallerstein, 2000). The process can be influenced by the extent of the following:
- Political support
- Broad-based representation on the healthy community or city committee
- Leadership skills
- Program development
- Healthy public policy development
- Community participation
- Multisectoral collaboration
- Technical support
- Media support
- Resources
- Sustainability

The extent of official political support is important for the healthy community or city committee. Also, the level of political commitment can determine the action taken by the committee. Healthy Communities and Cities committees need to obtain broad-based representation to identify community problems, develop and implement appropriate solutions to the problems, and build consensus in the community for support of the solutions. The extent to which the Healthy Communities and Cities committee action is successful, in terms of program and policy development, enables the community to continue health promotion action. Such action requires a level of leadership skills, community participation, and multisectoral collaboration. Technical assistance to research the problems and solutions, as well as to evaluate existing programs, can influence the process. The extent of media support provides the image of the work conducted by the Healthy Communities and Cities committees to the broader community. Sustainability of efforts can be related to economic support and competition for scarce resources between other powerful organizations.

> **WHAT DO YOU THINK?**
>
> The support of local political officials in planning and implementing health and health-related programs in communities is critical to the development of the Healthy Communities and Cities program as well as to that of healthy public policies.

## Healthy Public Policy

As noted under Definition of Terms, healthy public policy is developed through a multisectoral and collaborative process with participation from those community members most affected by the policy (Pederson et al, 1988). Healthy public policy supports health in a broad ecologic sense that includes environmental, physical, social, and mental well-being. Although efforts to change individual behavior are important, the contributions of policies that affect the broader environment are thought to be more effective in social change (McKinlay, 1996). Healthy public policy transcends traditional departmental and governmental boundaries to include dialogue between policy makers and the public. The health effects of all public decisions can be considered. In this sense, healthy public policy proposes a new way of thinking about health and governmental policy, and it links policy makers, professionals, and common citizens through a concern for health. Examples of healthy public policies are seat belt legislation, no-smoking policies in public buildings, motorcycle helmet laws, handgun laws, and immunization policies for school-age children. Healthy public policies create supportive environments for health by "making the healthy choices the easy choices" for people to make (Ashton and Seymour, 1988, p. 22).

The Healthy Communities and Cities movement aims to support the promotion of healthy public policy at the local level through multisectoral action and community participation (see Figure 17-1). As the Healthy Communities and Cities movement continues to spread worldwide, healthy public policies may become the norm for providing healthier environments in which to live.

# IMPLICATIONS FOR COMMUNITY-ORIENTED NURSING

How can community-oriented nurses work with communities in the Healthy Communities and Cities process? They can use the nine steps of the Community Health Promotion model in their nursing practice. These steps will help them organize efforts around their particular community's problems and assets.

*Step 1:* Community forum. Community-oriented nurses can help organize a community forum to orient the community to health promotion and Healthy Communities and Cities and invite representatives of all sectors of the community, including local residents, to attend. They can also work with a task force of community people who are supportive of the concept and plan the agenda, invite speakers informed of community health promotion and the Healthy Communities and Cities process, and select a moderator for the session. Step 1 can be the first level of prevention by bringing together community members to begin developing a plan for better health (Box 17-1).

*Step 2:* Building the partnership for Healthy Communities and Cities. Community-oriented nurses can orient community leaders to the Healthy Communities and Cities process. They can identify key city leaders, politicians, and health providers and talk to them about the health benefits of becoming a healthy community or city. They can answer policy makers' questions about what political commitment means to the community's health. They also can meet with heads of community agencies to solicit their interest in the Healthy Communities and Cities process. Through this process, they help to establish community commitment to community health promotion using the Healthy Communities and Cities strategy.

*Step 3:* Development of the community structure for health promotion. On the basis of their knowledge of key community people and populations at risk for problems, the community-oriented nurses can contact community leaders and other citizens to serve on the Healthy Communities and Cities committee. Community-oriented nurses can ensure that the committee represents the various sectors of the community. They may also serve as a member of the committee, representing the public health sector.

*Step 4:* Leadership development in Healthy Communities and Cities. Community-oriented nurses recognize that although leaders exist in every community, they may not understand their potential in promoting health.

---

**BOX 17-1  Levels of Prevention Related to Healthy Communities and Healthy Cities**

**PRIMARY PREVENTION**
Develop a community forum to initiate communication regarding health promotion.

**SECONDARY PREVENTION**
Assess needs and strengths in the community to detect ways to address health problems.

**TERTIARY PREVENTION**
Initiate community action when problems have occurred and evaluate and monitor progress of programs and policies.

---

**DID YOU KNOW?**

Nurses can help community leaders apply the Community Health Promotion model in their communities. They should begin where the community is, no matter what step of the process the community begins with. Many communities begin with step 5, community assessment. Nurses often provide information that is used in a community assessment. They can use this as an opportunity to guide community leaders to report their findings back to the broader community. Communities may use the community assessment not only to identify needs and assets in the community but also to obtain community commitment for participation in the overall Healthy Communities and Cities process. Community leaders need to understand that all steps are necessary to sustain Healthy Communities and Cities as an ongoing process in their community.

---

Nurses can recommend relevant consultants, speakers, conferences, workshops, and network sessions that are related to local concerns.

*Step 5:* Community assessment. Community-oriented nurses can conduct community assessments, such as windshield surveys, and assessments of assets and needs. They can be a resource to the committee or work as a member of a team that conducts the community assessment. Step 5 can be the second level of prevention by assessing needs and strengths in the community to detect ways to address health problems.

*Step 6:* Community-wide planning for health. Community-oriented nurses can use group dynamics skills to help the Healthy Communities and Cities committee identify priorities and strategically plan for local health action.

*Step 7:* Community action for health. Community-oriented nurses can redirect community health services toward local priorities and plans. For example, they can expand a community health service, such as an exercise program for older adults or an immunization outreach program for Latino children.

*Step 8:* Providing data-based information to policy makers. Community-oriented nurses may be asked to testify or assist others in preparing testimony that will be given to the city council or county commissioners about issues identified by the Healthy Communities and Cities committee to promote the development of healthy public policy.

*Step 9:* Monitoring and evaluating progress. The Healthy Communities and Cities committee may ask the community-oriented nurse to provide the data relevant to community health services and to assist them in recommending policy changes. Nurses may also coordinate or be part of a research team conducting program evaluation research. Steps 7 through 9 can be the third level of prevention by initiating community action when problems have occurred and evaluating and monitoring progress of programs and policies.

The cycle then returns to the first step, community forum, whereby updated information about the healthy community or city is shared with the broader community. Community-oriented nurses can participate by organizing the community forum, by inviting speakers to present data and evaluation results, or by discussing projects that have been initiated. The cyclical process depicted in the Community Health Promotion model can help to sustain Healthy Communities and Cities.

---

( **NURSING TIP**

Because community-oriented nurses naturally work with community people from different walks of life and are respected health professionals in the community, they are well suited to promote Healthy Communities and Cities. Look for opportunities within existing community partnerships that you work with and that are also interested in promoting the community's health. Plan how to introduce them to the Healthy Communities and Cities process, and work together to find ways to initiate the Healthy Communities and Cities process with your combined network of contacts to develop activities that support improved health.

---

Although these examples demonstrate how the community-oriented nurse can participate in Healthy Communities and Cities, the ultimate goal is to promote the community's own leadership for health. In other words, the nurse must not do for the community what it can do for itself. The role of the nurse and of other health professionals in Healthy Communities and Cities is to work in partnership with community leaders (Flynn, 1997). John Ashton (1989), one of the founders of the European Healthy Cities project, summarizes the role of health professionals in Healthy Cities as being "on tap, not on top."

( **HOW TO**    **Organize a Community Meeting About Healthy Communities and Cities**

1. Identify who should be included in the community meeting. It is critical that all sectors and population groups in the community be involved.
2. How will they be invited to the meeting? Who will invite them? Allow at least 2 weeks so people can arrange their schedules.
3. Who will convene the meeting?
4. Set the date and time for the meeting and arrange for a neutral meeting place.
5. Plan the meeting agenda.
   a. Introduction of participants
   b. Introduction to Healthy Communities and Cities
   c. Identification of community people who should be there ("Whom did we miss?")
   d. Questions and discussion about Healthy Communities and Cities, and about community issues that are important
   e. Commitment to the Healthy Communities and Cities process
   f. Formation of the Healthy Communities and Cities committee (obtain names and addresses of those interested)
   g. Other suggestions

## HEALTHY PEOPLE 2010

The **Healthy People 2010 objectives** (USDHHS, 2000) are health objectives set through collaboration among government, voluntary and professional organizations, businesses, and individuals as the means of providing access to better health for all people and improving health outcomes for the nation. The 2010 objectives focus on prevention, surveillance and data systems, quality health care, changes in demographics that include an older and more culturally diverse population, and diseases new to the twenty-first century. In addition, there is a focus on implementation of community participation and intersectoral collaboration. The framework for the objectives is titled Healthy People in Healthy Communities. This framework incorporates mental, physical, and social well-being as dependent on health improvements at the individual, family, and community level. Within this framework, the overarching goals for the nation are as follows:

- Increase years of healthy life as well as quality of life
- Eliminate health disparities

These goals are accompanied by enabling goals that provide guidance to achieving the overarching goals:

- To promote healthy behaviors
- To protect health
- To ensure access to quality health care
- To strengthen community participation

**Healthy People 2010** | Educational and Community-Based Programs

**Goal:** To increase the quality, availability, and effectiveness of educational and community-based programs designed to prevent disease and improve health and quality of life

**NATIONAL GOALS FOR COMMUNITY SETTING AND SELECT POPULATIONS**

7-10 Increase the proportion of Tribal and local health service areas or jurisdictions that have established

a community health promotion program that addresses multiple Healthy People 2010 focus areas.

7-11 Increase the proportion of local health departments that have established culturally appropriate and linguistically competent community health promotion and disease prevention programs.

7-12 Increase the proportion of older adults who have participated during the preceding year in at least one organized health promotion activity.

From U.S. Department of Health and Human Services: *Healthy People 2010: understanding and improving health,* ed 2, Washington, DC, 2000, U.S. Government Printing Office.

The framework is further divided into 22 focus areas. Evaluating progress toward the objectives can be accomplished by measuring health outcomes and behavioral, health service, and community interventions that have been implemented (Poland, 1996).

The nurse who understands the Healthy Communities and Cities model of health promotion and can implement the steps of the Community Health Promotion model will be prepared to use the Healthy People in Healthy Communities 2010 objectives to improve the health of individuals, families, and communities through community participation and multisectoral cooperation. For example, the community may be working on educational and community-based programs and the community-oriented nurse could help the Healthy Communities and Cities committee by referring to the section of Healthy People 2010 that relates to those objectives (see the Healthy People 2010 box). Because communities vary in their needs and assets, other 2010 objectives could be applicable when working with communities in the Healthy Communities and Cities process. Community-oriented nurses can help the committee identify appropriate objectives because they are knowledgeable about the community, its needs and resources, and the particular issues that are being addressed. Nurses need to be familiar with all of the objectives and help communities to use them appropriately.

## Practice Application

Because the community-oriented nurse works in partnership with the community in Healthy Communities and Cities, the examples of outcomes of Healthy Communities and Cities initiatives reflect that partnership rather than a specific nursing intervention. An example of an outcome of a Healthy City initiative that used the Community Health Promotion process is Fort Wayne, Indiana, Healthy City.

Healthy City committee members of the Fort Wayne, Indiana, Healthy City project collaborated in a community-wide program to address the fact that only 65% of Fort Wayne preschool children were immunized. Access to

immunization services was expanded to five sites throughout the city at three different times in a program called Super-Shot Saturday.

A community health nurse, along with other members of the Fort Wayne, Indiana, Healthy City committee, would be using which of the following principles of health promotion to provide access to immunizations for preschool children?

**A.** Promoting healthy public policy
**B.** Creating supportive environments
**C.** Strengthening community action
**D.** Reorienting health services
**E.** Improving personal skills

**Answers are in the back of the book.**

## Key Points

- Although Healthy Cities began in 1986 in Europe, it is now an international movement of communities and cities focused on mobilizing local resources and political, professional, and community members to improve the health of the community.
- The principles of primary health care and health promotion guide the Healthy Communities and Cities movements.
- The models of community practice most frequently found in the Healthy Communities and Cities movement are locality development and social planning, with an emphasis on community partnerships.
- Examples of Healthy Communities and Cities initiatives indicate that a broad range of health problems and issues are being addressed at the local level.
- The continuance of Healthy Communities and Cities is contingent on the extent of facilitators and barriers to the process.
- As the Healthy Communities and Cities movement continues to spread worldwide, healthy public policies may become the norm for providing healthy environments in which to live.

- Implications of Healthy Communities and Cities for nursing can be organized by the steps of the Community Health Promotion model.
- Outcomes of Healthy Communities and Cities suggest the successes of multisectoral community partnerships formed.
- The Healthy People 2010 objectives incorporate community participation and intersectoral cooperation in their strategy for improving the health of individuals, families, and communities.

## Clinical Decision-Making Activities

1. In collaboration with a community group, conduct a community assessment. Identify the community's assets and problems.
2. Evaluate the effectiveness of a current approach to a health problem in your community (e.g., teen pregnancy). Describe how the approach would change with implementation of the Community Health Promotion process. Compare and contrast two approaches in addressing this problem.
3. Discuss the role of the community-oriented nurse in health promotion within a Healthy Communities and Cities model.
4. Identify city council members, the president of the Chamber of Commerce, the director of family services, the mayor, a religious leader, and other community leaders who are the "movers and shakers" in getting things done. Generate a list of questions that will help these leaders describe the major assets and problems of the community. Interview several local leaders and summarize their responses.
5. You are asked by the health commissioner to organize a community coalition for orientation to the Healthy Communities and Cities process. Outline the steps you would take.
6. Describe your philosophy of community leadership development for health promotion.
7. Debate the model that is most effective in health promotion: social planning, community develop-

ment, or social action. Present both the pro and con positions of the model you selected.
8. Discuss ways in which the Healthy People 2010 objectives can incorporate community participation and intersectoral cooperation. Examples of objectives are as follows:

27-7    Increase tobacco use cessation attempts by adolescent smokers (target, 84%; baseline, 76% of every-day smokers in grades 9 through 12 had tried to quit smoking in 1999).

19-5    Increase the proportion of persons aged 2 years and older who consume at least two daily servings of fruit (target, 75%; baseline, 28% of persons aged 2 years and older had consumed at least two daily servings of fruit in 1994-1996 (age-adjusted to the year 2000 standard population).

9. Access the internet to determine the extent of involvement of your community or another community elsewhere in the Healthy Communities and Healthy Cities movement. The following sites may be helpful:
   - www.hospitalconnect.com/healthycommunities/usa/index/html
   - www.who.int/hpr/archive/cities/index/html
   - www.paho.org/Project.asp?SEL=TP&LNG=ENG&CD=MUNIC
   - www.ulaval.ca/fsi/oms/p2En.html

### Additional Resources

These related resources are found either in the appendix at the back of this book or on the book's website at **http://evolve.elsevier.com/Stanhope.**

**evolve Evolve Website**

WebLinks: Healthy People 2010

## References

Arnstein S: A ladder of citizen participation, *J Am Institute Planners* 35:216, 1969.

Ashton J: *Creating healthy cities.* Paper presented at Healthy Cities Indiana Network Session, Seymour, Indiana, May, 1989.

Ashton J: *Healthy cities,* Milton Keynes, UK, 1992, Open University Press.

Ashton J, Seymour H: *The new public health,* Philadelphia, 1988, Open University Press.

Bragh-Matzon K: Horsens. In Ashton J, editor: *Healthy cities,* Milton Keynes, UK, 1992, Open University Press.

Chamberlin RW: World Health Organization healthy cities and the US family support movements: a marriage made in heaven or estranged bed fellows? *Health Promot Int* 11(2):137, 1996.

*Declaration of Medellin 1999:* Washington, DC, 1999, Pan American Health Organization.

Draper R et al: *WHO Healthy Cities project: review of the first five years (1987-1992),* Copenhagen, Denmark, 1993, WHO Regional Office for Europe.

Fisher R: Social action community organization: proliferation, persistence, roots, and prospects. In Minkler M, editor: *Community organizing & community building for health,* New Brunswick, NJ, 1998, Rutgers University Press.

Flynn BC: Healthy cities: a model of community change, *Fam Community Health* 15(1):13, 1992.

Flynn BC: Partners for healthy cities, *Health Forum J* 37(3):55, 1994.

Flynn BC: Healthy cities: toward worldwide health promotion. *Annu Rev Public Health* 17:299, 1996.

Flynn BC: Partnership is Healthy Cities and Communities: a social commitment for advanced practice nurses, *Adv Pract Nurs Q* 2(4):1, 1997.

Flynn BC, Dennis LI: Healthy families. In Altergott K, editor: *One world, many families,* Minneapolis, 1993, National Council on Family Relations.

Flynn BC, Ray DW, Rider MS: Empowering communities: action research through healthy cities, *Health Educ Q* 21(3):394, 1994.

Flynn BC, Rider MS, Ray DW: Healthy Cities: the Indiana model of community development in public health, *Health Educ Q* 18(3):331, 1991.

"Focus on healthy communities": *Public Health Rep* 115(2,3), 2000.

Goldstein G, Kickbusch I: A healthy city is a better city, *World Health* 49(1):4, 1996.

Hancock T: The evolution, impact, and significance of the Healthy Cities/Healthy Communities movement, *J Public Health Policy* 14(1):5, 1993.

Hancock T: Healthy communities must also be sustainable communities. *Public Health Rep* 115(2,3):151, 2000.

Hancock T, Duhl L: *Promoting health in urban context,* WHO Healthy Cities Paper No. 1, Copenhagen, 1988 FADL.

Hospital Research and Educational Trust, American Hospital Association: *Coalition for healthier cities and communities,* Chicago, Ill, retrieved September 24, 2002, from www.hospitalconnect.com.

Ivanov LL, Flynn BC: Predictors of utilization and satisfaction with prenatal care services in St. Petersburg, Russia, *West J Nurs Res* 21(1):372, 1999.

Kenzer M: Healthy Cities: a guide to the literature. *Environ Urbanization* 11(1): 201, 1999.

McKinlay JB: Health promotion through healthy public policy: the contributions of complementary research methods. In *Health promotion: an anthology,* Washington, DC, 1996, PAHO, WHO.

*Mexico Ministerial Statement for the Promotion of Health:* Fifth Global Conference on Health Promotion 2000, Mexico City, Mexico, June 5-9 2000, World Health Organization.

Minkler M, Pies C: Ethical issues in community organization and community participation. In Minkler M, editor: *Community organizing & community building for health,* New Brunswick, NJ, 1998, Rutgers University Press.

Norris T, Pittman M: The healthy communities movement and the coalition for healthier cities and communities. *Public Health Rep* 115(2,3): 118, 2000.

Pan American Health Organization/WHO: The healthy municipalities movement: a settings approach and strategy for health promotion in Latin America and the Caribbean. Washington, DC, 1999, PAHO.

Pederson AP et al: Coordinating healthy public policy: an analytic literature review and bibliography, Canada, 1988, Ministry of National Health and Welfare.

Poland BD: Knowledge development and evaluation in, of, and for healthy community initiatives, Part II: potential content foci, *Health Promot Int* 11(4):341, 1996.

Rothman J, Tropman JE: Models of community organization and macro practice: their mixing and phasing. In Cox FM et al, editors: *Strategies of community organization,* ed 4, Itasca, Ill, 1987, Peacock.

Swartz KJ: "Healthy cities/communities and healthy public policy: opportunities and challenges." Unpublished final paper for field research on issues in health promotion practice, 2000, Graduate Department of Public Health Sciences, University of Toronto.

Tsouros AD: *World Health Organization Healthy Cities Project: a project becomes a movement,* Copenhagen, Denmark, 1990, FADL.

Tsouros AD: World Health Organization Healthy Cities Project: state of the art and future plans, *Health Promot Int* 10(2):133, 1995.

U.S. Department of Health and Human Services: *Healthy people 2000: national health promotion and disease prevention objectives,* Washington, DC, 1991, USDHHS, Public Health Service.

U.S. Department of Health and Human Services: *Healthy people 2010: understanding and improving health,* ed 2, Washington, DC, 2000, U.S. Government Printing Office.

Wallerstein N: A participatory evaluation model for healthier communities: developing indicators for New Mexico. *Public Health Rep* 115(2,3):199, 2000.

World Health Organization: *Ottawa charter for health promotion,* Copenhagen, Denmark, 1986, WHO Regional Office for Europe.

World Health Organization: *Twenty steps for developing a healthy cities project,* Copenhagen, Denmark, 1992, WHO Regional Office for Europe.

World Health Organization: *Briefings on multi-city action plans: WHO Healthy Cities Project Phase II 1993-1997,* Copenhagen, Denmark, 1994, WHO Regional Office for Europe.

World Health Organization, United Nations Children's Fund: *Primary health care,* Geneva, Switzerland, 1978, WHO, UNICEF.

# Chapter 18

# The Nursing Center: A Model for Community-Oriented Nursing Practice

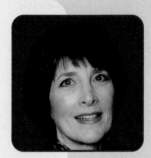

### Katherine K. Kinsey, Ph.D., R.N., F.A.A.N.

Katherine K. Kinsey is the director of a nationally recognized nurse-managed health center. The center is an essential safety net provider targeting the needs of underserved, vulnerable urban populations. Dr. Kinsey has an extensive background in maternal child health, home care, hospice, school health, nursing education, and program evaluation. She serves as consultant to other nurse-managed health centers, and to public health and community-based social service organizations. Dr. Kinsey serves on several nonprofit boards and is the president of the Kingsley Foundation, which is committed to improving the health of vulnerable populations who reside in southeastern Pennsylvania and southern New Jersey. She has a particular interest in advancing public health nurses and nurse-managed health centers as mainstream health care providers in the twenty-first century.

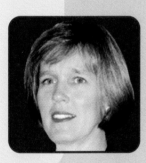

### Marjorie Buchanan, R.N., M.S.

Marjorie Buchanan, Consultant, Program Development, Center on Aging, University of Maryland, works with national, regional, and local public health organizations, foundations, professional associations, academic institutions, and nonprofit agencies. Her services include community health assessment, strategic planning, program development, project management, funding and other resource development, and evaluation. She has a particular commitment to nursing centers, having spent the past 25 years helping to develop centers and support systems to ensure their place in health care and human service systems.

Dr. Kinsey and Ms. Buchanan have collaborated on numerous public health and nurse-managed health center projects for more than 15 years. They have discovered that the art, science, and business of nursing in community settings can make genuine differences in the lives of people served.

## Objectives

After reading this chapter, the student should be able to do the following:

1. Describe key characteristics of community nursing center models
2. List population groups served by nursing centers
3. Discuss essential roles and responsibilities for community collaboration
4. Identify interventions that address Healthy People 2010 goals, leading health indicators, and disease prevention and health promotion focus areas
5. Describe roles for advanced practice nurses in nursing centers
6. Determine the feasibility of establishing and sustaining a nursing center
7. Identify key quality improvement indicators for evidence-based practice
8. Describe opportunities for education, practice, and research in nursing centers
9. Discuss the future of nursing in the twenty-first century

A growing body of evidence documents that **nursing centers** improve health outcomes. The nurse-managed health center model increases access to care; provides a more comprehensive approach to health and illness; decreases racial, ethnic, and geographic disparities in health status; and has the potential to reduce the overall costs of health care. This chapter describes nursing centers—their origins, evolution, and future potential. It describes nursing roles and responsibilities in delivering community-based services, managing center operations, and implementing education, service, and research programs. Emphasis is placed on the Healthy People 2010 framework, community collaboration, and multilevel interventions to improve access and reduce health disparities. Emerging health, economic, social, and political factors influencing nursing center operations, community health nursing practice, and the future of nursing are highlighted.

**advanced practice nurse**, p. 415
**business plan**, p. 430
**community collaboration**, p. 419
**community health worker**, p. 441
**community-oriented nurse**, p. 416
**comprehensive primary health care**,
    p. 416
**contracts**, p. 433

**cost effectiveness**, p. 433
**evidence-based practice**, p. 434
**feasibility study**, p. 432
**grants**, p. 433
**health and wellness centers**, p. 415
**multilevel interventions**, p. 414
**nursing centers**, p. 412
**nursing models of care**, p. 413

**organizational framework**, p. 426
**program evaluation**, p. 437
**reimbursement systems**, p. 414
**special care center**, p. 416
**stakeholders**, p. 420
**strategic planning**, p. 420
**sustainability**, p. 424
*See Glossary for definitions*

## Chapter Outline

What Are Nursing Centers?
*Definition*
*Nursing Models of Care*
Types of Nursing Centers
*Health and Wellness Centers*
*Comprehensive Primary Health Care Centers*
*Special Care Centers*
*Other Designations*
Foundations for Nursing Center Development
*World Health Organization*
*Healthy People 2010*
*Community Collaboration*
*Community Assessment*

*Multilevel Interventions*
*History Has Paved the Way*
The Nursing Center Team
*Other Providers and Community Members*
*Students*
*Educators and Researchers*
*Others on the Nursing Center Team*
The Business Side of Nursing Centers
*Start-up and Sustainability*
Evidence-Based Practice: Outcome Data
*Health Insurance Portability*
    *and Accountability Act*
*Quality Indications*

*Quality Improvement*
*Essential Technology and Information Systems*
Education and Research
*Community-Based Education*
*Research Opportunities in Nursing Centers*
*Program Evaluation*
Positioning Nursing Centers for the Future
*Emerging Health Care Systems*
*National and Regional Organizations*
*Nursing Workforce*
*Policy Development and Health Advocacy*

# WHAT ARE NURSING CENTERS?

## Definition

The most frequently cited and referenced definition of nursing centers continues to be the one developed in the mid 1980s by the Nursing Centers Task Force of the American Nurses Association (ANA) (Box 18-1).

Nursing centers provide unique opportunities to improve the health status of individuals, families, and communities through direct access to nurses and **nursing models of care** (Lancaster, 1999). Over the past 25 years, various definitions and operational terms have been used to describe nurse-managed health centers. Some centers provide health and wellness services for general or particular population groups. Others offer full primary health care services, and still others provide select services that address special health care needs. Regardless of the specific focus or scope of practice, all nursing centers possess char-

acteristics that reflect the values, beliefs, and scientific knowledge and skills inherent in nursing models of care. Furthermore, each is guided, managed, and primarily staffed by nurses, thus ensuring that decision making and ultimate accountability for this model of care rests with professional nurses.

The nurse-managed health center is supported by the ANA position paper, *Health Promotion and Disease Prevention* (1995). The paper recognizes health promotion strategies as the pivotal points of any health care system designed to control costs and reduce human suffering. The statement acknowledges nursing's scope of practice, incorporates prevention, and underscores that nursing's efforts should focus on the health promotion and disease prevention interventions.

Nursing center models combine human caring; scientific knowledge about health and illness; an understanding of family and community characteristics, interests, assets,

---

**BOX 18-1    American Nurses Association Nursing Centers Task Force Definition of *Nursing Center***

"Nursing centers—sometimes referred to as community nursing organizations, nurse-managed centers, nursing clinics and community nursing centers—are organizations that give the client direct access to professional nursing services. Using nursing models of care professional nurses in these centers diagnose and treat human responses to actual and potential health problems, and promote health and optimal functioning among target populations and communities. The services provided in these centers are holistic and client-centered and are reimbursed at the reasonable fee level. Accountability and responsibility for client care and professional practice remain with the professional nurse. Overall accountability and responsibility remain with the nurse executive. Nursing centers are not limited to any particular organizational configuration. Nursing centers can be freestanding businesses or may be affiliated with universities or other service institutions like home health agencies and hospitals. The primary characteristic of the organization is responsiveness to the health needs of the population."

Aydelotte et al: *The nursing center: concept and design,* p. 1, Kansas City, Mo, 1987, American Nurses Association.

---

needs, and goals for health promotion; disease prevention; and disease management. They deemphasize the illness-oriented and institutional care that has dominated the health care landscape since World War II. Figure 18-1 shows the perspective and philosophical approach of nursing center services.

## Nursing Models of Care

Nursing centers are strategically positioned to improve the health and well-being of vulnerable populations (Kinsey, 1999) and build on the core values and beliefs of the profession (Matherlee, 1999). Trust, health, caring, personal respect, equity, and social justice serve as the foundation from which health is viewed as a resource for everyday life (Buchanan, 1997). Efforts focus on enhancing people's capacity to meet their personal, family, and community responsibilities and interests and typically include the following:

- *Community-based, culturally competent care* that is accessible, acceptable, and responsive to the populations being served
- *A holistic approach* to care based on complex and interrelated biopsychosocial factors
- *Interorganizational and interdisciplinary collaboration* that crosses health and human service systems and increases opportunities for comprehensive and seamless services among care providers, agencies, and payers

- *Multilevel interventions* that acknowledge organizational, environmental, and health and social policy contributions to health, health problems, and issues of access to care
- *Multisector community partnerships* that establish and support the center's health efforts
- *Relationship-based practice* with individuals, families, organizations, and communities that fosters understanding of context, interests, and needs for health care

Nursing center models combine people, place, approach, and strategy in everyday life to develop appropriate health interventions. Nurses work in close partnership with the communities they serve in providing public health programs, communitywide health education, and primary health care services (National Health Policy Forum, 1998). They establish relationships with families, community representatives, policymakers, and others in designing, implementing, and evaluating appropriate health intervention strategies, services, and programs.

Each center's population is unique and complex. Client needs can rarely be met by working only with the individuals or families who seek care. Absent or limited personal resources, family support needs, and community dynamics require skilled nurses to develop interventions at the individual and family levels as well as at the community and system levels. Multilevel interventions foster and sustain positive change for clients and the community.

A nursing center's health and community orientation builds strong connections to the community served. These strong relationships with community leaders, residents, and clients foster a deep awareness of local factors that influence everyday life. The Lundeen model reflects this important interconnection with the community. The Lundeen community nursing center model (Lundeen, 1999) guides the work of the Silver Spring Community Health Center in Milwaukee, Wisconsin. This center has served the community for more than two decades, earning a respected place in the local health care system. The Lundeen model places the nursing center at the hub, and the spokes are the reciprocal relationships with the community, its residents, nursing, medicine, related organizations, other human service providers, policymakers, payers, and funders.

## TYPES OF NURSING CENTERS

There are many types of nursing centers, and each has a personality of its own that reflects the particular community in which it is located and the services it provides (Gerrity and Kinsey, 1999). A center's mission, values, goals, and strategies as well as its commitment to community well-being contribute to its profile.

A center is typically defined by its particular array of health services and programs (Clear, Starbecker, and Kelly, 1999). Organizational structure, federal tax status, and **reimbursement systems** also define centers. The nursing center category (Box 18-2) frames its specific

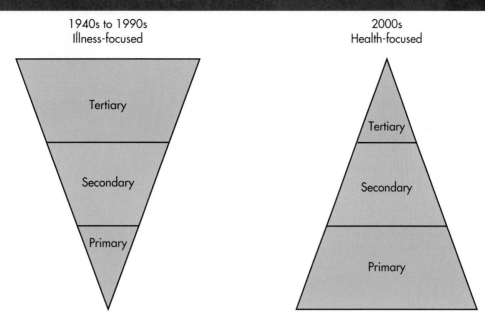

1940s to 1990s
Illness-focused

2000s
Health-focused

**Figure 18-1** The paradigm shift from illness-focused care between 1940 and 1990, to health-focused care in the twenty-first century.

---

**BOX 18-2  Nursing Center Categories**

**SERVICE MODEL**
- **Health and wellness centers:** Provide health promotion and disease prevention programs
- **Comprehensive primary care centers:** Provide health-oriented primary care and public health programs
- **Special care centers:** Provide programs that target specific health conditions, such as diabetes, or population groups, such as frail older adults

**ORGANIZATIONAL STRUCTURE**
- **Academic nursing center:** Housed within a school of nursing
- **Free standing center:** Independent center with its own governing board
- **Subsidiary:** Part of larger health care systems, such as home health agencies, community centers, senior centers, schools, and others
- **Affiliated center:** Legal partnership association with health organization, human services organization, or other

**INTERNAL REVENUE SERVICE DESIGNATION**
- **501(c)3:** Not-for-profit business
- **Proprietary:** Incorporated as a for-profit business

**REIMBURSEMENT MECHANISM**
- **Fee-for-service:** Payment at time of service; may include sliding-fee scale
- **Health maintenance organization (HMO) provider:** Payment at contracted rates by health maintenance organization
- **Federally qualified health center (FQHC):** Federal designation that allows cost-based reimbursement per encounter
- **Third party reimbursement:** Client billing to public program or commercial/private insurance
- **Contributions:** Individuals, donations, philanthropic gifts, fund-raising activities to support a program

---

health care focus, its reimbursement sources, and its program offerings.

## Health and Wellness Centers

**Health and wellness centers,** designed in partnership with community leaders and residents, focus on health promotion, disease prevention, and management programs. In health and wellness centers, **advanced practice nurses** and community workers provide outreach and public awareness services, health education, immunizations, family assessment and screening services, home visiting, and social support efforts (Evans et al, 1997). Public health education and support programs may include smoking cessation, weight management counseling, parenting classes, violence prevention, and many others. Enabling services help people access and appropriately use health care services. Enabling services include language translation, cultural interpretation, childcare, advocacy, policy development, program evaluation, registration for entitlement programs, and providing transportation vouchers.

Health and wellness centers are designed to complement existing primary care services in the community. Typically, a center's staff has a strong relationship with local health care providers in community health centers, clinics, private practices, emergency departments, long-term care facilities, and other organizations. Staff members link people to community resources and work collaboratively with housing organizations, schools, senior centers, and others to address issues of shared concern (Hurst and Osban, 2000). In general, financial support for center programs comes from public health department and other service contracts, foundation grants, fee for services, voluntary contributions, and shared resources from affiliated organizations (Oros et al, 2001).

## Comprehensive Primary Health Care Centers

In many communities, nursing centers offer **comprehensive primary health care**. In addition to the health and wellness programs just described, these centers also serve as the primary care home for families in the communities where they are located. Both physical and mental/behavioral health care services are provided by nurse practitioners and other advanced practice nurses. These centers address the needs of individuals and families across the life span, ensuring access to specialized health care as needed. **Community-oriented nurses** and community workers provide outreach, social support, and an array of public health programs. The public health programs include health education, screening, immunizations, home visiting, and enabling services (Figure 18-2).

Comprehensive primary health care centers are challenged to establish systems for documentation of clinical care; utilization patterns; demographic profiles; accounting, billing, and reimbursement documentation; quality improvement; and client satisfaction. Nursing centers must meet standards established by government, insurers, health maintenance organizations, and other payers.

Some centers are designated as federally qualified health centers (FQHCs) by the Bureau of Primary Health Care (BPHC) of the U.S. Department of Health and Human Services (USDHHS). The purposes of FQHCs are (1) to provide population-based comprehensive care in medically underserved areas, and (2) to possess the appropriate mission and organizational and governance structure. The FQHC designation is important from a number of perspectives, but primarily it helps support a primary care center's efforts to serve low-income and uninsured populations and remain fiscally solvent. There is great interest in achieving this status; many nursing centers need to overcome internal and external organizational hurdles to initiate the FQHC application process.

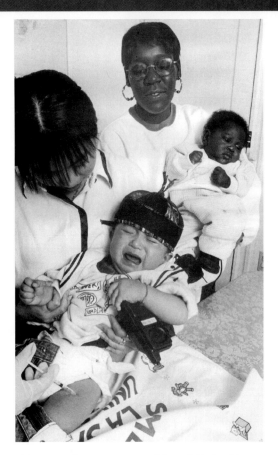

**Figure 18-2** Nursing centers provide public health programs such as immunizations.

## Special Care Centers

Some nursing centers focus on a particular demographic group or on those with special health care needs. Services are designed to respond to the characteristics and needs of a particular aggregate, and to provide specialized health knowledge and skills to this population. These models are limited in number and are often attached to comprehensive primary health care models. Examples of **special care centers** are those that focus on the needs of people with diabetes, human immunodeficiency virus (HIV), or acquired immunodeficiency syndrome (AIDS); adolescent mothers; and frail older adults. Special care centers may also provide continence programs for women, and emotional and psychological support services for people with cancer.

## Other Designations

Many nurse-managed health centers are in academic settings. Known as *academic nursing centers*, they are housed within, or closely affiliated with, schools of nursing. They actively integrate service, education, and research in their model. They build on public health and primary care nurse practitioner educational programs; draw on the knowledge and skills of their faculty; and provide rich learning experiences for nursing students at all levels. Furthermore, they utilize the knowledge, skills, and resources of other schools of health professions, business, communications, and law to expand the center's service capacity (Shiber and D'Lugoff, 2002).

Other centers may be freestanding organizations, subsidiaries of health care or other human service organizations, or formal affiliates of such entities. Each of these organizational arrangements requires carefully established legal agreements. To conduct business, these organizations must become incorporated, apply to the Internal Revenue Service (IRS) for a tax status designation, and receive a statement of tax status determination. Organizations are generally categorized as a not-for-profit (501[C]3) entity or some form of proprietary (for-profit) organization. Most community nursing centers are not-for-profit organizations; others select the proprietary business model, and others operate as subsidiaries of established organizations. In all cases, staff must be familiar with the particular laws and regulations associated with the IRS tax status under which they operate.

Another way to describe nursing centers involves the health care system's financial reimbursement methods that support services and programs. These include fee-for-service, designated health maintenance organization (HMO) provider, Medicaid provider, Medicare provider, and FQHC (described previously). Each designation requires a center to possess certain characteristics, meet a set of standards, and possess identification numbers that allow participation in particular billing and reimbursement systems.

Regardless of the type of nursing center, the many personal, social, educational, economic, and environmental concerns indicate the need for and continued interest in nursing centers. Increasing population density and diversity, challenging community conditions, and long-standing and emerging health problems indicate the role such models of care can play (Kinsey, 2002). Population groups that use a nursing center include the following:

- Older adults and their caregivers
- Culturally and linguistically diverse groups, such as immigrants, refugees, or religious sects
- Homeless persons and families
- Migrant and other workers
- Children and youths in public and independent schools
- Underimmunized children and adults
- HIV-positive individuals and those with AIDS
- Incarcerated persons
- Childbearing adolescents and adult women
- Minority men with a history of hypertension
- Working adults
- Frail older adults
- Isolated rural families

### DID YOU KNOW?

Nursing centers can trace their origins back to Lillian Wald's public health nursing work and the establishment of the Henry Street Settlement (in New York City) in 1893.

Each center's vision, mission, purpose, and goals are designed to address the interests and needs of particular populations. The mission and scope of the center determines the extent to which the center engages in primary, secondary, and/or tertiary interventions. For example, (1) health and wellness centers would focus on primary prevention to teach clients how to care for themselves and prevent health disruption; (2) special care centers might do secondary and tertiary prevention for a special population to help them manage their condition and prevent complications. Examples of specific nursing center designs and models are displayed in Boxes 18-3 and 18-4.

### BOX 18-3 Overview of the Guiding Framework of the La Salle Neighborhood Nursing Center (Philadelphia)

**Mission:** The La Salle Neighborhood Nursing Center supports and enhances the teaching, learning, and service mission of La Salle University and the School of Nursing through the development and implementation of exemplary health care and educational programs.

**Vision:** The School of Nursing and its Neighborhood Nursing Center will be positioned as a nationally recognized provider of quality health care services in urban settings.

**Purpose:** To provide access to public health, educational, counseling, and primary care services to underserved populations residing in a multicultural, diverse, urban community. Emphasis is placed on health promotion, disease and injury prevention, screening, detection, early intervention, and rehabilitation.

**Goals**

- To exemplify Lasallian values in everyday life
- To provide optimal community-based educational experiences for students and clients
- To improve the health of individuals, families, and communities
- To provide direct access to primary health care services to underserved individuals, families, and groups
- To emphasize disease prevention and health promotion initiatives
- To incorporate Healthy People 2010 goals and objectives in individual, group, and community programs through outreach and case finding
- To promote 100% access, 0% disparity for all
- To provide community consultation
- To evaluate program services and population outcomes
- To promote organizational, environmental, and public policy change
- To share evidence-based practice and program outcomes in regional and national forums

---

**BOX 18-4** Other Examples of Frameworks That Guide Nurse-Managed Health Centers

### ABBOTTSFORD & SCHUYLKILL FALLS FAMILY PRACTICE AND COUNSELING CENTERS, PHILADELPHIA, PENNSYLVANIA

**Mission Statement:** The Health Centers exist to improve the health status of all the people we serve, with special attention to vulnerable people and residents of public housing communities.

**Beliefs That Guide the Work of Health Centers' Staff:**

- The Health Center is a partnership between residents and the staff
- The Center must provide health education to empower residents to make choices about their health
- Staff members must ensure the confidentiality of every client's contact with the Center
- Health care is a right, not a privilege
- No one will be turned away because of an inability to pay
- Health care must be delivered in a sensitive and compassionate manner by caring for the whole person—body, mind, and spirit
- The Health Center must also nurture the staff and encourage each individual to be creative
- The Center is a model of community-based health care and must work to encourage others to follow its example

### UNIVERSITY OF AKRON, CENTER FOR NURSING, AKRON, OHIO

**Mission Statement:** To provide service to the University community as well as underserved and vulnerable populations in the local community, to offer graduate and undergraduate nursing education in community health and primary care, to provide nursing and interdisciplinary practice opportunities for faculty, and to generate and share clinical research.

**Objectives Derived From the Mission Statement:**

- To fully integrate the clinical practice opportunities in the Center for Nursing into the undergraduate and graduate programs
- To provide primary care and special programs that target the Healthy People 2000-2010 objectives for minorities, medically underserved, and vulnerable persons
- To serve as a leader and advocate for community partnerships that will address access to care for minorities, medically underserved, and vulnerable persons

### UNIVERSITY OF MARYLAND, SCHOOL OF NURSING'S CLINICAL ENTERPRISE, BALTIMORE

**Mission Statement:** University of Maryland School of Nursing's Clinical Enterprise reinvents nursing practice and education through the development, implementation, and evaluation of new models of clinical learning and practice that emphasize hands-on, community-based experiences for both students and faculty nursing mentors. The framework is an evidence-based clinical practice model, which uses systems theory to define the set of relationships between community and student needs, the clinical practice program, and student and community outcomes. The evidence-based clinical practice model ensures that every component of the clinical enterprise rests on a solid foundation of research in striving to promote improved health status and the elimination of racial and ethnic health disparities in the target communities served.

**Goals**

- To provide increased access to health care services in target communities around the state of Maryland, with a focus on medically underserved communities suffering from significant barriers to health care services
- To improve through measurable outcomes the health status of patients served by the clinical enterprise
- To expand the clinical education of graduate and undergraduate nursing students in community-based practice
- To expand faculty practice through the clinical enterprise
- To promote interdisciplinary and collaborative practice and education opportunities through the clinical enterprise
- To expand faculty research in community-based health care delivery

### UNIVERSITY OF MICHIGAN, ANN ARBOR

**Mission and Vision:** The Community Family Health Center and North Campus Family Health Services provides primary care services by advanced practice nurses working collaboratively with physicians and other health care providers, along with the community, to do the following:

- Provide a community-based service with a full range of primary health care services
- Increase access to health care for the neighboring residents and their families
- Improve the health behaviors of individuals and families
- Provide an educational experience for both graduate and undergraduate students in the School of Nursing
- Provide opportunities for faculty practice

---

**BOX 18-5**    **Integration of Primary Health Care Into the Nursing Center Model**

**ELEMENTS OF PRIMARY HEALTH CARE**
- It is essential health care.
- It is based on practical, scientifically sound, and socially acceptable methods and technology.
- It is universally accessible to all in the community through their full participation.
- Its cost is affordable.
- It is directed toward self-reliance and self-determination.

**WAYS IN WHICH PRIMARY HEALTH CARE IS INTEGRATED INTO THE COMMUNITY**
- It forms an integral part of both the health system and the overall social and economic development of the community.
- It is the main focus and central function of the health system.
- It is the first level of contact of people with the health system.
- It is as close as possible to where people live and work.
- It constitutes the first element of a continuing health process.

**ESSENTIAL CONCEPTS IN ENSURING HEALTH CARE FOR ALL**
- Maximum involvement of people in their own health care and the development of self-reliance

- Involvement and cooperation of persons and agencies from many sectors (safety and transportation, communications, and so forth)
- Use of scientifically sound technologies that are appropriate, acceptable, and affordable
- Availability of essential medicines

**PRIORITIES FOR ACTION**
- To teach people about identification and prevention/control of prevailing health problems
- To make available proper food supplies and nutrition
- To ensure adequate supply of safe water and basic sanitation
- To provide maternal and childcare, including family planning
- To immunize against the major infectious diseases, and to prevent and control locally endemic diseases
- To provide appropriate treatment of common diseases using appropriate technology
- To promote mental health
- To provide essential drugs

From Anderson E, McFarlane J: *Community as a partner,* Philadelphia, 1996, Lippincott-Raven.

---

## FOUNDATIONS FOR NURSING CENTER DEVELOPMENT

The foundations for integrating primary care and public health services through the nurse-managed health center model include the perspective of the World Health Organization (WHO) and the Healthy People 2010 systematic approach to improving individual and community health.

### World Health Organization

The World Health Organization's (1978) definition of health and its framework to address global health needs supports the nurse-managed health center's integration of primary care and public health services in community settings. Nursing center services reflect the nursing focus on prevention and promotion, and the shift in focus from sickness to wellness interventions. Box 18-5 outlines the integration of primary health care in the nursing center model.

### Healthy People 2010

The Healthy People initiative has guided the nation's health promotion and disease prevention agenda since 1980. Healthy People 2010 goals are to increase quality and years of healthy life and to eliminate health disparities. Healthy

People 2010 accounts for demographic changes (as the nation's population has become older and more racially and culturally diverse); it recognizes the escalating global influences on personal and national health status; and it factors in anticipated changes in the health care system (USDHHS, 2000b). The Healthy People box focuses on the Healthy People 2010 agenda that pertains to nursing centers.

The concept of Healthy People 2010 is based on shared responsibility to improve the nation's health. It is based on the belief that communities have the potential for change, but that no one person or organization can do this alone. Achieving Healthy People 2010 goals requires a long-term commitment to community collaboration, and powerful, productive partnerships among many diverse people and groups. Nursing centers are well positioned to guide and facilitate interventions directed at meeting Healthy People 2010 goals.

### Community Collaboration

**Community collaboration** is needed to achieve the goals of Healthy People 2010 and to develop new services, share resources, and have cost efficiency (Keefe, Leuner, and Laken, 2000). Productive collaboration

## Healthy People 2010 | Leading Health Indicators

**Overarching Goals:** To increase quality and years of healthy life and to eliminate health disparities

### PHYSICAL ACTIVITY

22-2 Increase the proportion of adults who engage regularly, preferably daily, in moderate physical activity for at least 30 minutes per day

22-7 Increase the proportion of adolescents who engage in vigorous physical activity that promotes cardiorespiratory fitness 3 or more days per week for 20 or more weeks per occasion

### OVERWEIGHT AND OBESITY

19-2 Reduce the proportion of adults who are obese

19-3c Reduce the proportion of children and adolescents who are overweight or obese

### TOBACCO USE

27-1a Reduce cigarette smoking by adults

27-2b Reduce cigarette smoking by adolescents

### SUBSTANCE ABUSE

26-10a Increase the proportion of adolescents not using alcohol or any illicit drugs during the past 30 days

26-11c Reduce the proportion of adults engaging in binge drinking of alcoholic beverages during the past month

### RESPONSIBLE SEXUAL BEHAVIOR

25-11 Increase the proportion of adolescents who abstain from sexual intercourse, or who use condoms if currently sexually active

### MENTAL HEALTH

18-9b Increase the proportion of adults with recognized depression who receive treatment

### INJURY AND VIOLENCE

15-15a Reduce deaths caused by motor vehicle crashes

### ENVIRONMENTAL QUALITY

27-10 Reduce the proportion of nonsmokers exposed to environmental tobacco smoke

### IMMUNIZATION

14-29a,b Increase the proportion of noninstitutionalized adults who are vaccinated annually against influenza, and who have ever been vaccinated against pneumococcal disease

### ACCESS TO HEALTH CARE

1-4a Increase the proportion of persons who have a specific source of ongoing care

From U.S. Department of Health and Human Services: *Healthy People 2010: national health promotion and disease prevention objectives,* ed 2, Washington, DC, 2000, U.S. Government Printing Office.

---

requires staff expertise and commitment from many to change communication patterns and professional agendas, and to speak in a common voice to generate positive community transformation (Cross and Prusak, 2002). The community transformation will occur through policy, legislative, and funding changes that improve the health status of many (Figure 18-3).

Collaborators include individuals, families, groups and organizations, policymakers, and staff. Referred to as **stakeholders,** each entity has diversity in perspective and particular knowledge and skills to aid the community's efforts to address critical needs and solve problems. Stakeholders facilitate or undermine strategic efforts to improve health. It is impossible to fully know and address issues and concerns in a community without hearing all perspectives. Each stakeholder should be respectful of different opinions and experiences (Hansen-Turton and Kinsey, 2001).

### NURSING TIP

Take the time to carefully listen to others' perspectives and experiences before taking action.

Collaboration takes time, effort, and resources. It requires nurturing and support to make it work. Relationships among people and organizations serve as the foundation for the collaborative process and for community change. Relationships begin with introductions and open discussion times to listen to and learn from one another. From this, relationships will grow toward a collective willingness to work together toward a common purpose, sharing *risks, responsibilities, resources,* and *rewards* along the way. The working definition of *collaboration* developed by Mattessich and Monsey (1992) guides the work of stakeholders (Box 18-6).

Nursing centers are typically established on a foundation of community collaboration. Each center develops its philosophy, goals, and activities through a process of community collaboration, community assessment, and **strategic planning.** This process addresses the many levels of intervention needed to bring about and sustain change. Partnership relationships and agreements are established with diverse sectors, such as housing organizations, schools, religious groups, childcare programs, and advocacy coalitions, to address their shared commitment to improving health in the community. Box 18-7 presents an

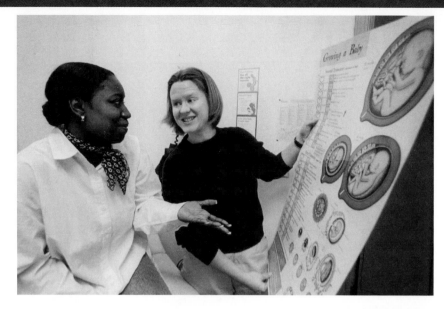

**Figure 18-3** Nursing centers guide and facilitate interventions directed at meeting Healthy People 2010 goals.

---

**BOX 18-6  Working Definition of Collaboration**

Collaboration can be defined as "a mutually beneficial and well-defined relationship entered into by two or more organizations to achieve common goals. The relationship includes a commitment to: a definition of mutual relationships and goals; a jointly developed structure and shared responsibility; mutual authority and accountability for success: and a sharing of resources and rewards" (Mattessich and Monsey, 1992, p. 7).

From Mattessich P, Monsey B: *Collaboration: what makes it work,* St Paul, Minn, 1992, Amherst H. Wilder Foundation.

---

**BOX 18-7  Potential Stakeholders in Community Collaboration**

- Educational systems: public and independent
- Home care agencies/Visiting Nurse Associations
- Homeless shelters/soup kitchens
- Industries with full- and part-time employees
- Juvenile/family court
- Local hospitals
- Local police district
- Parish nurses
- Public housing for low-income families and seniors
- Recreation centers
- Religious organizations
- School nurses
- Senior centers
- Small businesses

---

array of potential partners. Many others could also be involved.

Center staff members need skills in networking, coordination, and cooperation to collaborate (Floyd, 2001). A few basic premises help set the stage for a long-term process of discussion, decision making, and action. Once established, they are reviewed and rigorously adhered to throughout the life of the collaboration:

- Regular meetings, in which diverse perspectives are heard and respected
- A mutually agreed on decision-making process
- Consistent and accurate communications, so all participants have the necessary information to make decisions
- Agreement by all participants to support collaborative decisions once they are made—both within the groups or organizations they represent and publicly in the community

Perhaps the most important feature in community collaboration is the capacity of those involved to enhance the capacity of *another* person, group, or organization to serve the common purpose. For example, rather than the nursing center serving as the lead organization every time, different participating organizations will serve from time to time in the leadership role, or hold greater responsibility, or perhaps receive additional funds to support their common purpose. In this way, mutual benefit is realized by all who are involved (Goffee and Jones, 2001).

Mattessich and Monsey (1992) have identified six critical elements in the overall success of a given collaborative endeavor: the environment, membership characteristics, process and structure of the group, communication patterns, purpose of the collaboration, and resources within and outside the group. In Table 18-1, influencing factors for each element are listed.

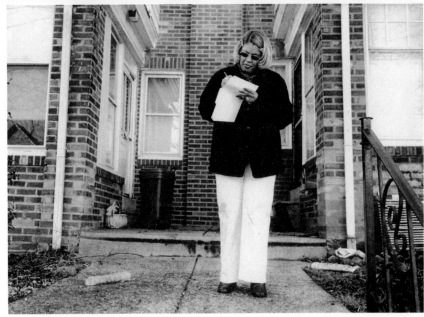

**Figure 18-4** Neighborhood walks provide insight into the community's health.

| Table 18-1 | Factors Influencing the Success of Collaboration |
|---|---|
| **CATEGORY OF FACTOR** | **FACTORS HAVING A POSITIVE EFFECT** |
| Factors related to the environment | • History of collaboration or cooperation in the community<br>• Collaborative group seen as a leader in the community<br>• Favorable political/social climate |
| Factors related to membership characteristics | • Mutual respect, understanding, and trust<br>• Appropriate cross section of members<br>• Collaboration seen as being in members' self-interest<br>• Ability to compromise |
| Factors related to process/structure | • Members share a stake in both processes and outcome<br>• Multiple layers of decision making (participative)<br>• Flexibility<br>• Development of clear roles and policy guidelines<br>• Adaptability |
| Factors related to communication | • Open and frequent communication<br>• Established informal and formal communication links |
| Factors related to purpose | • Concrete, attainable goals and objectives<br>• Shared vision<br>• Unique purpose |
| Factors related to resources | • Sufficient funds<br>• Skilled convener |

From Mattessich P, Monsey B: *Collaboration: what makes it work,* St Paul, Minn, 1992, Amherst H. Wilder Foundation.

## Community Assessment

Nurse-managed centers must conduct community assessments. Essential elements in community assessment, including data collection processes and needs analyses, are described in detail in other chapters. This chapter reemphasizes the importance of data about and analysis of community needs and assets in determining the type of nursing center established.

Through the assessment process, nurses learn both the community's formal and informal infrastructure and communication networks (Baker, White, and Lichtveld, 2001). Neighborhood walks, bus rides, car trips, and discussions with elected officials, administrators of health care systems, and public health department staff provide insight into the community's health and the many other influencing factors (Figure 18-4).

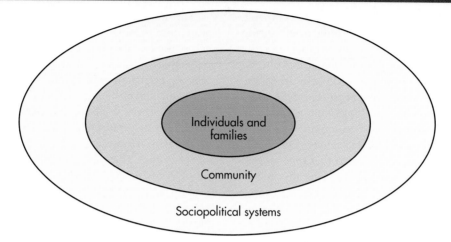

**Figure 18-5** Multilevel intervention.

Assessment activities identify community assets and health problems. For example, there may be a rich network of block captains who serve as leaders and communication liaisons with the community. There may be a local community college that can provide space and support for meetings. If high rates of childhood asthma are discovered, there may be human service organizations well positioned to help in disease prevention and management efforts.

As nurses conduct individual interviews and focus groups, hold larger community meetings, develop surveys, review health care data, and examine various indices (social, educational, employment), they gather detailed information about the health status of the community. These sources of information build the center's understanding of the community and its traditions, strengths, interests, concerns, problems, needs, and preferences.

The assessment process includes sharing current health data, historical trends, and future projections with the community. Center staff can discuss the findings, share perspectives and ideas, and encourage involvement in the collaborative process. From this, the nursing center's overall direction, services, and programs emerge (Anderko, 2000). Over time, the community and the nursing center together guide the services provided and advance the center's future.

## Multilevel Interventions

As the community and the center work together for health, a multilevel approach is needed (Figure 18-5). Some impact occurs through individual and family health behavior change. However, for comprehensive community health improvement, changes are needed at organizational, community, and sociopolitical levels. Nursing center staff may focus their efforts on system issues, community capacity, and family and individual health care access concurrently. Alternatively, the staff may concentrate program efforts solely at the individual or family level and later address system and community issues. There is no one approach, but most interventions take place in community rather than institutional settings.

> **NURSING TIP**
>
> In nurse-managed health centers:
> - People can be understood within the context of everyday life.
> - Community residents can be encouraged and educated about health lifestyles and health care practices through public health education programs.
> - Common barriers to care, such as transportation, childcare, language, and cultural differences, can be overcome with an array of enabling and supportive services.
> - People can enter earlier, with greater ease and confidence, and continue in care long enough to realize positive outcomes.
> - A multilevel intervention approach is essential.

The implementation of multilevel interventions requires nursing center staff to be committed to working with diverse groups and to have advanced skills in this area. The staff must have the administrative support and expertise to make constructive contributions to communal well-being. If applied appropriately, the multilevel intervention approach helps people enter the health care system earlier, with greater ease and confidence, and continue in care long enough to realize positive outcomes (Berkman and Lochner, 2002).

> **WHAT DO YOU THINK?**
>
> Using the multilevel approach, how might one address increasing childhood obesity in the community served by your nursing center?

## History Has Paved the Way

The foundations of nursing center development are rooted in public health nursing history and the evolution of the nursing profession (Reverby, 1993). Other chapters provide historical details and factors that have influenced nursing education, practice, service, and research throughout the twentieth century. The current nursing center model was a new and untested dimension of the health care landscape in the 1970s and 1980s. In the twenty-first century, nursing centers have achieved national recognition as essential safety net providers in underserved communities.

Most current nursing center models emerged from academic nursing programs in the 1970s. At that time, opportunities did not exist within the traditional health care system for faculty or their nurse practitioner students to apply their knowledge and skills in a framework of nursing care. Bold ideas in the schools of nursing at the University of Wisconsin at Milwaukee, Arizona State University, and others established practice settings in partnership with nearby communities that simultaneously provided health care to the community and learning experiences for students.

( DID YOU KNOW?

Nursing centers can be found in every region of the nation.

The success of these early efforts has generated other academic nursing centers in colleges and universities across the country. Interest in this practice model is growing rapidly among community service organizations, schools, churches, public housing facilities, and organizations that serve the homeless (Bellack and O'Neil, 2000). Although there is no central databank that shows how many nursing centers have been developed and where they are located, it appears that there are or have been centers in every state, and in urban, suburban, and rural communities. Most are viewed as safety net providers that provide care for vulnerable populations who face significant barriers to accessible and affordable health care (National Health Policy Forum, 1998). Many centers are expanding and providing services in satellite sites.

Table 18-2 highlights the evolution of nursing centers over the past century. It lists educational, political, legislative, and funding factors that have influenced the development and **sustainability** of nursing centers.

## THE NURSING CENTER TEAM

Nursing center models support the skill development of advanced practice nurses, allied health professionals, and support staff. Nurses, the community at large, other

---

### Table 18-2   The Evolution of Nursing Centers

**Where We Are Now**

2000s
- National Nursing Centers Consortium emerges in 2001 from the Regional Nursing Centers Consortium of Pennsylvania, New Jersey, and Delaware.
- Midwest Regional Consortium established and housed at the University of Wisconsin.
- Michigan Academic Nursing Centers Consortium established with support from the W. K. Kellogg Foundation.
- USDHHS, HRSA, Bureau of Health Professions publishes *Fact Sheet* about nursing centers' unique solutions to filling health care gaps.
- Applications to become federally qualified health center (FQHC) models submitted to USDHHS, Bureau of Primary Health Care, by academic nursing centers, freestanding centers, and public entities nursing centers.

**The Start-Up Years**

1990s
- Senator Daniel Inouye speaks on the Senate floor urging support of nursing school–administered primary care centers.
- National Health Policy Forum site visits to nursing centers in Pennsylvania and Utah in 1998 conducted for congressional and government staff.
- USDHHS, HRSA Bureau of Health Professions *Models That Work* awards presented to nursing centers.
- Data collection and management systems tested for continuous quality improvement, documentation of nursing efforts/outcomes, and center operations.
- Medicare reimbursement for nurse practitioner practice throughout the nation in place.
- Regional Nursing Centers Consortium established in 1996 in Philadelphia, as similar organizational associations are launched in the Midwest.
- National League for Nursing returns to a nursing education mission, phasing out its practice councils in 1997, including the Council for Nursing Centers.
- Independence Foundation supports critical mass of nursing centers serving vulnerable populations in metropolitan Philadelphia to document impact, outcomes, and visibility of community nursing.

| Table 18-2 | The Evolution of Nursing Centers—cont'd |
|---|---|

**The Start-Up Years—cont'd**

**1990s—cont'd**
- Abbottsford Family Practice and Counseling Center located in Philadelphia public housing complexes is awarded FQHC status by USDHHS, Bureau of Primary Care.
- New nursing center organizational models emerge, including business ventures, freestanding entities, and those affiliated with an array of human service entities.

**1980s**
- Academic nursing centers emerge across the country, serving urban, suburban, rural and special needs populations in the course of educating students.
- W. K. Kellogg and Robert Wood Johnson Foundations provide significant national philanthropic support for nursing centers.
- Centers affiliate with the National League for Nursing in 1988, forming the Council for Nursing Centers, a formal communication and leadership hub.
- American Nurses Association Nursing Centers Task Force establishes first definition of *nursing center.*
- Nursing Centers Conference Group, an informal association, holds conferences in 1982, 1984, and 1986, reaching consensus on nursing center model and affiliation plans with a national nursing organization to further promote nursing centers.
- Model of grouping by diagnosis/treatment with reimbursement criteria introduced in New Jersey: diagnosis related groups (DRGs).

**1970s**
- First special project grants made in 1973 to nursing centers by the USDHHS, Bureau of Health Professions, Division of Nursing to improve public access to nurses in noninstitutional community settings.
- First academic nursing centers established at Arizona State University, University of Wisconsin, and elsewhere to provide primary health care services, student learning experiences, and sites for faculty practice and research.
- First independent nursing practice established in 1971 by Lucille Kinlein.
- Nurses challenged to develop new means for providing nursing and primary health services in community settings.
- Introduction of managed care models supported by federal planning grants.

**Our Foundation in Nursing and Public Health**

**1980s**
- States begin extending direct reimbursement privileges to nurse practitioners for publicly funded programs (Medicaid).
- Paradigm shift from post–World War II (WWII) illness-focused care to health-oriented care.
- USDHEW establishes 1990 Objectives for the Nation.

**1970s**
- Nations commit to *primary health care for all* by the year 2000.
- WHO expands definition of *health* in 1978 . . . *to allow the person to live a productive life in the community.*
- Public health nurse positions eliminated from many health departments across the nation because of fiscal constraints.

**1960s**
- Nurse practitioner role created in 1965 to provide primary health care to clients.
- Expansion of nursing homes.
- Title XVIII (Medicare) and Title XIX (Medicaid) became part of the Social Security Act.

**1940s-1950s**
- Post-WWII creation of institutional facilities and biomedical model, dominating health care landscape and diminishing community care.
- WHO provides definition of health in 1948 as biopsychosocial well-being.

**1890s-1920s**
- Frontier Nursing Service established by Mary Breckenridge in 1925 in rural Kentucky.
- First birth control clinic established in New York City by Margaret Sanger in 1916.
- Henry Street Settlement established in NYC by Lillian Wald in 1893.

health professionals, and support staff make up the team. The type of nursing center and its services determine staff patterns and roles, responsibilities, and reporting lines. A fundamental premise to any nursing center is that the *community* in which the model is placed has the most power and influence on model development and team composition. A rural nursing center may have staff needs that are different from those of a nursing center in a distressed urban community (Jacobson, 2002). A center's success relates to how well the team works together to ensure the delivery of high-quality health care to target populations. Positive collegial and professional relationships set the tone for the work.

Like any successful social enterprise, the interview and hiring process for any member of the team should be conducted carefully and thoughtfully with the nursing center model and its mission in mind. Each team member should be familiar with the organizational structure and collective contributions to the success of the model. In some centers, the staff may consist of only one provider and the support staff. In other centers where there is extensive program funding and community need, the staff may be substantial.

The organizational chart of the nursing center should clearly depict reporting relationships in the organization, as well as staffing patterns and responsibilities. Depending on funding streams, the **organizational framework** may be relatively fixed, or it may be dynamic and adaptive to newly funded programs. The roles held by team members are critical to the overall functioning of the center and are considered the glue that holds the center together (Figure 18-6). Table 18-3 further details staff positions, responsibilities, and key characteristics critical to nursing center operations.

## Other Providers and Community Members

Nursing centers may engage a variety of providers such as physicians, students, faculty, administrators, and clinical social work and outreach staff of various community organizations. Representation is diverse and variable. The staff of local churches, synagogues, and mosques, independent and public schools, Headstart programs, day-care centers, hospitals, and county health departments may work with nursing center staff, clients, and their families. As the reputation of the nursing center expands, other disciplines

A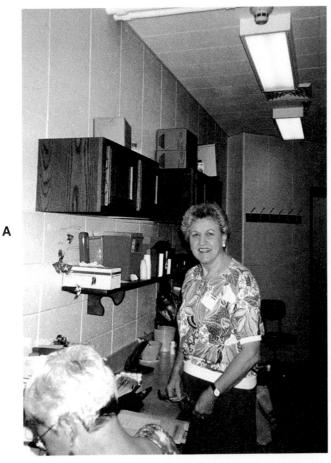

B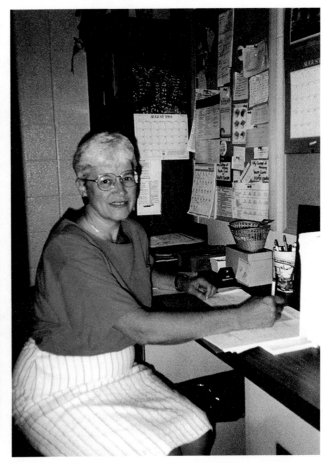

**Figure 18-6** Two staff members at a university nursing center. **A,** Nurse volunteer Agnes Black assists nursing staff in delivery of care at the nurse-managed Center for the Homeless at the University of Kentucky College of Nursing. **B,** Public Health Clinical Nurse Specialist Ruth Berry serves as director at the University of Kentucky College of Nursing's nurse-managed center for the homeless.

## Table 18-3   Nursing Center Positions

| POSITION | ROLES AND RESPONSIBILITIES | KEY CHARACTERISTICS |
|---|---|---|
| Executive director | • Administrative and fiscal oversight<br>• Development of community board<br>• Grants and contracts management<br>• Personnel<br>• Data analyses<br>• Quality improvement<br>• Liaison responsibilities<br>• Policy development<br>• Annual reports<br>• Community advocate<br>• Contributing member to community boards | • Commitment to model<br>• Background in community development and program planning<br>• Refined communication skills<br>• Knowledge of target community<br>• Vision<br>• Pragmatism<br>• Collaborative philosophy<br>• Interest in education, practice, and program evaluation |
| Advanced practice nurses | • Expanded level of health services<br>• Oversight of clinical staff<br>• Specific clinical program development | • Additional training and education beyond basic nursing program<br>• Preparation in specific area (e.g., diabetes education) |
| Public health nurses | • Assessment of community needs and interests<br>• Health education<br>• Case management<br>• Health screenings<br>• Oversight of clinical staff<br>• Specific clinical program administration and development<br>• Community building<br>• Advocacy<br>• Promotion of social justice | • Advanced preparation in public health or community health<br>• Collaborative skills |
| Nurse practitioners | • Administrative and clinical responsibilities in specific practice area (e.g., children's, geriatric, or women's health) or generalized practice as family nurse practitioner<br>• Flexible practice skills (on site, in home, institutional)<br>• Program and practice development and management<br>• Liaison with medical providers<br>• Referrals to other providers and organizations<br>• Data analysis | • Advanced education<br>• Certification<br>• State licensure<br>• National accreditation<br>• Current insurance credentials<br>• Eligible for Medicaid and Medicare reimbursement<br>• Knowledge of key support groups and organizations<br>• Established relationships with other health care providers and like models of care |
| Nurse midwives | • Advanced skills in comprehensive women's health with specialty training in midwifery<br>• Oversight of clinical staff<br>• Home visits<br>• On site and in hospital services<br>• Referrals to other providers and organizations<br>• Data analysis | • Advanced education<br>• Certification<br>• State licensure<br>• National accreditation<br>• Current insurance credentials<br>• Eligible for Medicaid and Medicare reimbursement<br>• Knowledge of key support groups and organizations |
| Clinical specialists | • Advanced skills in specialty area: mental health, substance abuse, family therapy<br>• Oversight of clinical staff<br>• Individual and group work<br>• On-site and in-home visits<br>• Program management<br>• Data analysis | • Advanced education and certification as clinical specialist or therapist<br>• Eligible for third-party reimbursement |

*Continued*

**Table 18-3  Nursing Center Positions—cont'd**

| POSITION | ROLES AND RESPONSIBILITIES | KEY CHARACTERISTICS |
|---|---|---|
| Ambulatory care nurses | • Practice management on-site for continuity of care<br>• Individual and small group health education<br>• Counseling and direct care services under the supervision of advanced practice nurse<br>• Outreach to community<br>• Appointment follow-up<br>• Marketing of services to community<br>• Data entry | • Basic nursing education<br>• Professional licensure<br>• Interest in working in nurse-managed model and primary care services with the underserved<br>• Public health perspective |
| Social worker | • Services to individuals, families, and groups with social service needs including housing, finances, family dynamics<br>• Liaison with all center providers<br>• Referrals and linkages to supporting agencies<br>• On-site and in-home visits<br>• Community group work<br>• Data entry and analysis | • Basic and advanced education in practice area<br>• Certification or licensure<br>• Interest in working in nurse-managed model with underserved populations<br>• Knowledge of community resources |
| Medical assistants | • Provision of routine health care functions in primary care under supervision of nurse practitioners and office manager<br>• Routine office responsibilities: telephone triage, appointments, insurance and billing forms<br>• Community liaison<br>• Client follow-up<br>• Data entry | • Completion of formal education program<br>• Interest in working in nurse-managed model<br>• Interest in working with diverse populations |
| Community health workers | • Community outreach<br>• Supervised family case management<br>• Specific program work with health education focus<br>• Community liaison<br>• Health fairs<br>• Data entry | • Completion of high school<br>• Preferably two years of college<br>• Local resident familiar with community needs and resources<br>• Interest in helping others |
| Support staff | • Business and office management<br>• Information systems<br>• Public relations and marketing<br>• Communications | • Completion of college; advanced education preferred in specific area<br>• Interest in working in nurse-managed center<br>• Public speaking skills |

such as law, nutrition, education, and public policy may affiliate or provide direct services.

## Students

Staffing patterns and roles in many nursing center programs are student oriented (Box 18-8). Nursing students can participate in different programs or projects and learn about the overall center functions and how health care is related to economics, service, education, and research (Hamner et al, 2002). Students can experience varied and challenging work with community members, learning communication strategies that engage community members in determining health practices for themselves and their families (Hemphill, 2001). If the nursing center is part of an academic health center or a school of nursing, faculty roles include clinical oversight of graduate and undergraduate students assigned to the nursing center or involved in related community projects, such as influenza inoculation campaigns.

## Educators and Researchers

The education and research roles held by faculty, staff, and consultants are essential if the nursing center model is to advance in today's changing and uncertain health care system (American Association of Colleges of Nursing, 2002). If the nursing center model is located in an educational institution with a nursing program, faculty members with community and primary health background and the com-

---

**BOX 18-8  Student Roles**

- Advocate
- Collaborator
- Data collector
- Educator
- Evaluator
- Facilitator
- Learner
- Partner
- Planner
- Provider

---

mitment to improve the health of those who live in the catchment area are key (Aydelotte and Gregory, 1989). The opportunity for faculty involvement through clinical training of students as well as community-focused research programs is evident. These centers can attract faculty and students interested in advancing the nursing center model and documenting nursing contributions that improve the health status of the vulnerable and increase primary care access to all.

The nursing center model offers academic and service challenges to nurses who have education and research roles. Such challenges include time management, research protocols in primary care settings, and community expectations. Faculty and students involved in education and research must possess the communication skills and commitment to fully engage the community in the work at hand, be it student education, research models, or program development and evaluation. Collaboration is the key at all levels.

## Others on the Nursing Center Team

As discussed, collaboration with the others on the team is a key part of a successful nursing center. A nursing center may not last long if collaboration is fragmented or nonexistent. Working together through honest communication is essential, with value placed on each team member's contributions and opinions. The extended team members include community advocates, board of directors/advisory board members, multidisciplinary health professionals, and organizational partners.

### Community Advocates

Community advocates want to improve the health and well-being of people. They have a genuine commitment to participating in activities that are productive, that are proactive, and that directly invest in the people who live or work in the target area. Frequently, community advocates are already active in their community. Advocates hold in common the idea that life can be better for people, and that the nursing center model contributes to the overall well-being of people. Nursing center staff, faculty, and students should reach out to community members who want to contribute to the life of their community and enlist their support. Community voices are often the most influential and most listened to by elected officials and bureaucrats.

### Board of Directors/Advisory Board Members

The organizational structure of a nursing center (whether part of a larger institution or a freestanding entity) dictates the type of board members that govern or advise staff on the direction of the center. A *board of directors* has oversight responsibilities, including fiscal management, for the nursing center model. An *advisory board* guides the work of a nursing center but holds no fiduciary or voting responsibilities. Regardless of the type of board, members are part of the team and each has particular expertise. They should represent diverse professions and occupations and be knowledgeable about the target community and its residents. Board members are guided by center bylaws and generally serve for 3 years, with another 3-year reappointment. When board members rotate off the board, nominations from the community are sought for new board members.

It is important to know the governance structure and the persons responsible for daily decision-making processes as well as for overall administrative and fiscal oversight. For example, if the parent organization is a university, its board of trustees is the overall governing body. In this example, a nursing center will have input by an advisory board or committee. This committee does not have fiduciary responsibilities; the board of trustees does. The advisory board is responsible for clinical oversight of the programs, professional development, fund-raising, and community networking. It is composed of community members, professionals, and representatives of other groups. Members commit to periodic meetings and workgroups that support the development and growth of the nursing center.

The composition of either type of board should reflect the community's demographic profile. The nomination and selection of members is critical for the future of the nursing center. The members represent diverse work, educational, and professional backgrounds. Quarterly (or more frequent) meetings are held. Students and staff should have opportunities to attend scheduled meetings and workgroups.

### Multidisciplinary Health Professionals

The nursing center model is in the unique position to engage diverse health professionals and to utilize their skills and expertise in many ways. Primary care physicians, pediatricians, and other medical providers in the community are resources to the staff. Nutritionists, dentists, sanitation officers, communicable disease officials, social workers, educators, and attorneys involved in health care insurance for low-income people can make significant contributions to the well-being of clients served by the nursing center. Other professionals include podiatrists, lactation specialists, and clinicians with interests in holistic health. Nursing center staff should have on hand an up-to-date index of health professionals in other disciplines who can be resources for clients and supporters of the nursing center model (Lutz, Herrick, and Lehman, 2001).

## Organizational Partners

Similarly, representatives of local, regional, and national organizations make contributions to the collaborative team effort. Local and state health department administrators and clinical staff are frequently involved in one or more of the nursing center programs. The American Cancer Society, the Girl Scouts of America, the Boys and Girls Clubs, the local coalition on aging, the Lion's Club, the Rotary Club, the local hospitals, the public housing administrators, and the Salvation Army are examples of key organizational partners. Nursing centers that develop and maintain organizational relationships through collaboration benefit from service agreements and contracts with one or more of the partners. For example, the local chapter of the American Cancer Society may have an outreach program in the nursing center's target area and offer specific training in cancer prevention and early intervention services for the staff. Salvation Army staff may identify a critical health issue for children in day care and engage a nursing center in providing immunizations to children and education to parents on childhood communicable diseases (Figure 18-7).

## THE BUSINESS SIDE OF NURSING CENTERS

Nurses who enjoy working in nursing centers are committed to working with diverse people in noninstitutional settings. They use community characteristics, population profiles, health indices, epidemiologic findings, and positive working relationships with professionals and the public to develop the model (Gerrity and Kinsey, 1999). The model requires careful planning and structure to be a successful education, service, and business enterprise. During the planning and implementation phases, interrelated elements must be considered. An outline of essential services (Box 18-9) is useful when developing a center and as an annual checklist to measure growth and maturity of a nursing center as well as to guide sound decisions regarding sustainability and future planning.

## Start-up and Sustainability

In planning and establishing a nursing center (Schultz, Krieger, and Galea, 2002), nurses need to seek expert advice and support throughout the exploratory phases. This includes having financial advisors. A nursing center is a business enterprise in which the art and science of nursing is practiced. Before deciding to establish a nursing center, consider these essential areas:

- Organizational goals, commitments, and resources
- Community interests, assets and needs
- Feasibility studies, internal and external to the parent organization
- A strategic plan
- A business plan
- An information management plan and resources
- Existing social policy and health care financing
- Legal and regulatory considerations
- Mission, vision, and commitment of lead organization

### Assessment Phase

Efforts to assess the interests, resources, and capacity of an organization to begin a nursing center are separate but interrelated. For example, a feasibility study may be undertaken prior to the development of a **business plan.** Elements of the feasibility study are incorporated into the business plan. Similarly, a strategic plan builds on feasibility data as well as on economic principles and practices. Other considerations include workforce needs, personnel management plan, public information and outreach campaigns, community capacity, and the health care environment relative to funding streams (Shortell et al, 2002).

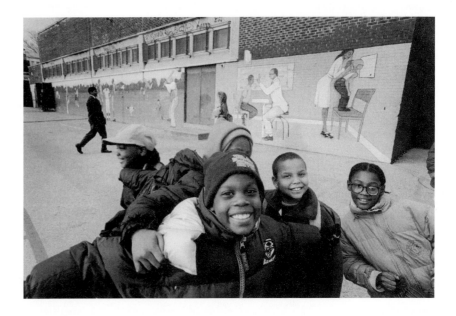

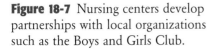

**Figure 18-7** Nursing centers develop partnerships with local organizations such as the Boys and Girls Club.

## BOX 18-9 Outline of Essential Elements in Nursing Center Development

I. Organizational development
  A. Governance structure and process guidelines
    • Governance structure and process (board member composition, roles and responsibilities, subgroups/committees, leadership positions, decision-making process, voting privileges, linkages to program administration and staff)
    • Meeting schedule for all groups, committees
    • Mechanisms for communicating information, project progress, meetings
    • Mechanisms for follow-up action on governing board decisions/actions
  B. Administrative activities
    • Role and responsibilities of project directors, administrators and site managers
    • Fiscal management system and personnel
    • Information management system and personnel
    • Oversight of overall project progress, process, outcomes, cost
    • Personnel policies, hiring and staff supervision
  C. Board or advisory committee(s)
    • Structure (connections to governing board, project administration, program services)
    • Membership composition, appointment process, terms of membership
    • Leadership positions and process for elections
    • Roles and responsibilities
    • Working groups or committees
    • Meeting schedule

II. Program development
  A. Needs assessment (project director, collaborating partners, and community)
    • Overview of community
    • Target populations for each program
    • Specific community assessments of target populations
  B. Plan for community collaboration and project governance
    • Model for multisector collaboration (health, education, business, law, community residents) in project governance
    • System for community communication about the project (public forums, public information campaigns)
    • Structures for community advisement on program services (advisory committees, community workers as staff)
  C. Program plan (advanced practice nurse responsibility)
    • Program goals for improvements in community health status, client services, student education, faculty practice and research, objectives (stated as measurable outcomes)

    • Program activities to meet objectives and timeline for implementation
    • Communication plan with multidisciplinary professional resources (physician, nutritionist)
    • Communication plan with referral agencies
    • Monitoring and coordination of program service delivery (quality management)
    • Program staff supervision
    • Reporting mechanisms
    • Fiscal reports
  D. Administrative/business plan (nurse administrator/business manager)
    • Follow-up action to governing board decisions
    • Overall project oversight (ensuring adherence to policies and procedures, achievement of goals and objectives)
    • Systems oversight (fiscal management, information management, program management, collaboration process management, service contracts/linkages with other systems—education or other)
    • Personnel management
  E. Information management plan (data systems analyst)
    • Preparation of summarized program records
    • Generation of cost reports relative to services and expected outcomes
    • Summarized health status indicators/project benchmark data
    • Oversight of technology support
    • Shared information with funders and community
  F. Evaluation plan (nurse evaluator)
    • Formative (monitoring ongoing collaborative process, progress in meeting project goals and objectives, making midcourse corrections)
    • Summative (measuring degree to which overall goals and objectives were met, their impact on health status or other elements of project), and analysis of outcomes with regard to balance in quality of care, access to care and cost of care/project
  G. Sustainability plan (project directors and collaborating partners)
    • Balance between quality of care, access to care, and cost of care
    • Expansion of reimbursement options for services
    • Development of long-term strategic plan
    • Identification of sources of other support (federal grants, private foundation grants, volunteer development, miscellaneous fund-raising activities)
    • Ensure fiscal stability

## Feasibility Study

A **feasibility study** depicts the strengths, limitations, and capacity of an organization and the community to support the establishment–in other words, the viability of a nursing center. It requires interviews with key individuals, surveys and data collection, focus groups, and community forums. Epidemiologic and environmental community assessment data from local public health agencies should be examined and interpreted. Local government, social service agencies, and tertiary care institutions can provide data about health needs and gaps in care for targeted groups. Legal and regulatory policies must be examined. States vary in their regulations for advanced practice nurses, particularly nurse practitioners. The planners must also investigate required professional credentialing, site accreditation, state Medicaid waivers, physician collaborative agreements, and any local or state requirements (Stacy, 2000). Planners will participate in all review processes and support community collaboration. The overall process supports the emergence of business plans, strategic plans, and timelines. Feasibility studies and assessment phases are often concurrent activities.

## Business Plan

A sound business plan considers all aspects of establishing a nursing center and describes the development and direction of the nursing center and how goals will be met (see the How To box about developing a business plan). In today's uncertain health care environment, a business plan is essential; however, flexibility is required to be able to modify the plan to take advantage of opportunities that may present at a moment's notice.

A business plan is built on the known or predictable sources of funding at the time the plan is developed. However, new funding sources can emerge that could not have been anticipated by the staff (Swan and Catroneo, 1999). Legislative changes and reimbursement regulations can significantly alter the business plan. In addition, no grant allocation should ever be included in the business plan until the grant is awarded. A strategic plan is critical for any nursing center under development or in operation.

## Strategic Plan

The strategic plan complements the business plan. It looks into the future and guides the work of the nursing center in a chosen direction. Strategic plans have a regular timeline and change as required by local events and community input. Strategic planning meetings are periodically scheduled to review and refine the plan. The plan includes goals, objectives, and target dates for implementation and evaluation of projected and ongoing services. Questions to be addressed in a strategic plan include (1) Where will the center be after start-up? (2) Where should the center be in 5, 7, 9 years? (3) How can the staff move the center in the appropriate direction? (4) What resources will be needed?

---

**HOW TO Develop a Business Plan**

1. Cover page includes date, name, address, and phone number of the person(s) responsible for the nursing center, and of any consultants to the business plan.
2. Executive summary: a one- or two-page overview of the center and the plan.
3. Table of contents.
4. Description of the business plan. This details what the center is and what services it will provide.
5. Survey of the industry. This summarizes the past, present, and future of the local and regional health care market.
6. Market research and analysis. This description outlines existing competition and the potential market share, and it identifies target groups.
7. Marketing plan. This details how the center will reach its targeted clients.
8. Organizational chart with a description of the management team.
9. List of supporting professional staff, such as accountants.
10. Operations plan. This describes how and where services will be provided.
11. Research and development. This projects program improvement and opportunities for new initiatives.
12. Overall schedule. The timeline establishes the start date and development phase of the nursing center.
13. Critical risks and problems. This examines the internal and external threats to the center and how these will be addressed.
14. Financial plan. The fiscal projections for the first 3 to 5 years are presented. A budget, cash flow forecast, and break-even point are included.
15. Proposed funding. Specific sources are listed that can provide funding.
16. Legal structure of the center. This describes the status of the center, such as freestanding, corporation, or part of a larger organization.
17. Appendixes and supporting documents.

---

Feasibility studies and business and strategic plans lay the foundation for strong nursing centers. The plans are crucial to the day-to-day functioning of a newly opened nursing center and reflect the abilities of the management team to build community coalitions and collaboratives. Shared resources and interests across groups and organizations demonstrate a nursing center's (1) credibility in the community, (2) commitment to use community recommendations, (3) flexibility and creativity in working with particular population groups, and (4) functional linkages with organizations and institutions.

**WHAT DO YOU THINK?**

What might happen if the organization drives the desire to establish a nursing center model?

Once community assessment, feasibility studies, business and strategic plans, and organizational networking have been done, key people need to ask these questions:

- Why would the organization want to do this?
- What will the immediate and long-term outcomes be for the organization and the community?
- Can the investment (staff, money, time, space) be made?
- Does the community truly want and need a nursing center?

The organization cannot drive the desire for the nursing center. If a nursing center is established solely from the organization's vantage point, long-term sustainability may be jeopardized. Thus the final question is the most critical one: Does the community truly want and need a nursing center? No assessment, study, or plan can ignore this question. If the answer is not clear, more time must be invested to find out if there is a match in need, interest, and a center's potential capacity.

For example, if the community is focused on helping young women move from public assistance into jobs, and the immediate need is day care, a nursing center that offers linkages with day-care providers and on-site physical examinations and childhood immunizations will be an essential community resource. If the nursing center moves ahead with a plan to offer only senior citizen services, the immediate and expressed need of the community has been ignored.

**NURSING TIP**

There must be a match between the services wanted and needed and those that are offered by the center.

The establishment of a nursing center is warranted if there are documented rationales regarding the match of the model with the target population or geographic area, the economic feasibility, and the long-term commitment of the planners and, if necessary, the parent organization. Careful planning builds the foundation that supports research and program evaluation, and that promotes opportunities to secure the nursing center's future. The parent organization's mission, vision, and commitment to this model will influence the viability of the nursing center model. Planners must determine the support of the parent organization before investing the time, effort, and collaborative work necessary to develop the model. If there is uncertainty at the administrative level about the long-term support of the model, it is foolhardy to move forward until there is strong and documented commitment from the organization that matches the community commitment.

## Funding: Finance and Operations

It is challenging for those involved in the planning process to forecast programs, determine service patterns, integrate outcome measures, and project costs. The planning process can be daunting, and planners may not devote sufficient time to the matter of nursing center revenue sources. If money matters are not thoroughly considered, any nursing center's future will be compromised and may not withstand the stresses of changing funding streams, political decisions, and policies. Consequently, planners must scrutinize funding needs and sources (Kinsey and Gerrity, 1997). These sources are variable and include private, public, and corporate funding.

The business plan provides information that forecasts the minimum funding necessary to start up a nursing center and to project income over 1 to 3 years from inception. A break-even analysis is essential. Other needed components include existing local fiscal resources, such as the health department; anticipated changes in health and social service funding streams; potential client characteristics; and commercial and public reimbursement structures for advanced nurse clinicians, including practitioners and public health nurses. Examine carefully the managed care reimbursement criteria in a particular state and the state's reimbursement parameters for nurse practitioners.

Potential income includes fee for service, commercial reimbursement, self-pay, and fund-raising. Depending on the nursing center model developed and the anticipated client users, fee for service may be the most viable economic strategy. Commercial reimbursement includes private company health care insurers with an established fee schedule. Clients without a source of health insurance would be self-pay. Costs and charges for services must be established. Nursing centers located in medically underserved areas, or working with medically underserved populations, may use a sliding fee schedule based on yearly published federal poverty guidelines. Managed care contracts with particular insurance companies are another source of income; however, the monthly reimbursements do not cover the cost of providing health care to the most vulnerable and underserved populations (Carlson et al, 2001). **Cost effectiveness** is a key concern as providers deal with managed care reimbursement issues and the cost of delivering health care services to those in need.

Support may also come from foundations, charitable contributions, private pledges, and fund-raising. Fund-raising can take the form of direct mailings, pledges, and events that raise money.

Start-up funds may include personal or borrowed funds; **grants** or **contracts** from local, state, or federal agencies or foundations; and private contributions. The Division of Nursing of the Public Health Service (USDHHS) has been a principal source of start-up funding for nursing centers operated by schools of nursing. The U.S. Bureau of Primary Care has been a source of funding for nursing centers located in public housing complexes. Other centers have obtained funding from the Robert Wood Johnson and W. K. Kellogg Foundations.

Grants are a source of initial and ongoing funding. Funding organizations generally release guidelines of what they will fund. The guidelines are frequently released as a request for proposals (RFP). A proposal developed in response to an RFP specifies how the nursing center would meet the goals of the granting organization in the given timeline. The description of services and client outcomes must be presented in relation to the RFP guidelines.

Ongoing agreements and contracts are necessary to open and sustain the nursing center model. Nursing staff must know about potential funding opportunities and seek to develop consultation and service agreements as well as specific contracts.

## Agreements and Contracts

Nursing centers have agreements and contracts in place for specific services. Agreements and contracts may have different language as well as reporting and fiscal management requirements; however, their basic premises are similar. The nursing center enters into a written agreement to provide services to a select population group or to develop a program that targets a specific area. For example, a nursing center has an agreement with the American Cancer Society to develop a cancer education program for minority seniors in a low-income senior housing complex. The agreement is time limited, has target goals and objectives, and outlines staff assignments and expectations, but there is no budget related to the program.

A contract is a legal document that lists the purchase of services, reporting requirements, invoicing, and expected client outcomes. An example would be a city health department that issues a contract to a nursing center to immunize 100 adults against influenza for a specified sum per vaccine. Comprehensive primary care nursing centers have contracts with managed care insurers and commercial insurers to provide primary care that adheres to core standards. Each nursing center may have one or many contracts and agreements; however, a nursing center should enter into each arrangement with a clear understanding of the business side of the model. All contracts and agreements should be fiscally sound and should not deplete center resources.

## EVIDENCE-BASED PRACTICE: OUTCOME DATA

**Evidence-based practice** represents the clinical application of particular nursing interventions and documented client and population outcome data. The necessity of measuring client needs and the application of various strategies to improve health and stay in business is evident (Deaton, 2002). Trends in health care services, client responses, and changes in community features must be documented and summarized periodically. Sources of ill health, including noncommunicable conditions, are to be assessed as well as social and community influences on economic, environmental, behavioral, and physical health, and they are to be reported. The findings (evidence) need to have collection and analysis mechanisms in place and timelines to share the evidence in appropriate forums. The challenges are to define the criteria, develop measurements and collection modalities, compare the evidence with broader community findings, interpret the data to funders, and disseminate findings to the wider health care community. Nursing center staff must seek a variety of forums to share findings, including professional publications, popular press, multimedia venues, and public hearings. Figure 18-8 shows an evidence-based practice model.

Evidence-based practice is relevant when nursing center administrators and managers review program costs in light of outcome data and quality improvement measures (Forrest and Whelan, 2000). Client-oriented outcome data must relate to the projected and then the actual cost expenditures and include meaningful quality-of-care measures, such as client satisfaction. The information is particularly important when prevention strategies have eliminated or reduced the need for expensive tertiary care and cost savings are quantifiable.

Directors should use measurement tools to learn what their consumers and the public in general want the health care system and providers to do. Surveys indicate that the American public has five concerns: (1) access and communication (e.g., being treated respectfully, understanding what is said, and having access to services and providers); (2) being healthy (i.e., through prevention and education); (3) getting better (e.g., returning to normal functioning

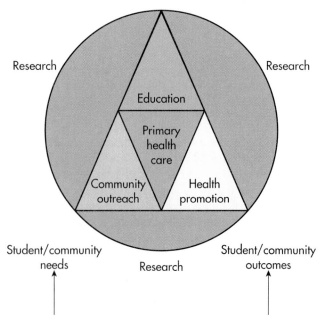

**Figure 18-8** The University of Maryland School of Nursing Evidence-Based Practice Model. *(Modified from Oros M et al: Community-based nursing centers: challenges and opportunities in implementation and sustainability, Policy Polit Nurs Pract 2(4):277-287, 2001.)*

through early intervention); (4) living with a chronic condition (i.e., being as functional and as independent as possible); and (5) coping with changes resulting from disability and death (e.g., having sources of comfort and support) (Eddy, 1998).

Outcome measurements can include client access and use of on-site services, childhood and adult immunization patterns, pregnancy outcomes, emergency department and hospital use, and other health indices as well as client satisfaction and quality-of-life measures. Measurement instruments require technologic support and staff expertise (Garrett and Yasnoff, 2002), and these are essential for center success.

## Health Insurance Portability and Accountability Act

The federal regulations relative to the Health Insurance Portability and Accountability Act (HIPAA) increase the nursing center's financial investment in administrative and oversight services. HIPAA is Public Law 104-191, passed by the 104th Congress. The regulations regarding this law pertain to new practices regarding patient confidentiality. Specifically, staff must monitor client records and keep them secure, have mechanisms to transfer client information securely and appropriately, and strictly adhere to client confidentiality. HIPAA and its evolving regulations and the concurrent need to collect, summarize, and report client data must be priorities in any nursing center. Another priority is the quality health indicators and attached performance measures that can be evaluated and reported (Stryer, Clancy, and Simpson, 2002). These indicators and measurements, which show the nursing center's contributions to the health and welfare of the community, are presented to the nursing center's board, funders, and the community.

Outcome measures and quality indicators may be the same, or the staff may decide at the time of review that some outcome measures that were not predetermined appear to be meaningful. For example, the nurse practitioners may have put in place a call-back system that improves timely utilization of primary care services. This can now be documented through client satisfaction, adherence to advised health practices, and changes in health behaviors. This outcome may now be included as a quality indicator that emerged from the day-to-day practices and policies of the nurse practitioners as contributing to changed client behaviors.

## Quality Indications

Nursing center staff must carefully consider which outcome measures and quality indicators are worthy of their investment and are meaningful to the community and the health care system. Although the staff might want to measure everything, it is prudent to begin with particular indicators and measures and incrementally add more. To do otherwise is to tax the staff and the system, and valid measurements may not emerge.

The Quality Care Task Force of the National Nursing Centers Consortium has developed *Guidelines for Quality Management for Nursing Centers with Standards for Community Nursing Centers*. The guidelines incorporate elements presented in earlier sections and will be a vital tool to the staff. The guidelines can be accessed on the internet (www.nationalnursingcenters.org). The standards will enable any nursing center to assess growth and development and areas that need improvement. The standards also include quality indicators, population groups, and performance targets and measures. The indicators are grouped into the areas of prevention, utilization, client satisfaction, functional status, symptom severity, and other primary care and prevention indicators.

Utilization of the standards and select indicators and associated processes will enable a nursing center to document evidence-based practice (see the Evidence-Based Practice box and Table 18-4). Sources for developing the standards include the National Committee for Quality Assurance (NCQA) (2000), which can be accessed at their website, http://www.Ncqa.org/Docs/Policies/2001BENCH.pdf.

## Quality Improvement

The evidence-based practice box together with Table 18-4 shows what nurses can do to measure outcomes, strive to improve those outcomes given particular standards, and make meaningful contributions to the public's health. Accurate data collection, measurements, summary statistics, and preparation of evidence practice reports are fundamental standards in any nurse-managed health center. As the nursing center model continues to grow throughout the nation, the potential for collectively summarizing data and outcomes will further strengthen the movement. Through collaboration and the pooling of data, this model will advance further into the mainstream health care system (Christensen, Bohmer, and Kenagy, 2000). However, the staff must be as committed to data collection as to the provision of services. Inservice conferences must be periodically held to reinforce the responsibilities of all staff to improve services. The data will enable the staff to clearly understand what goals are in place and, if areas need improvement, to develop action plans to improve services and client outcomes (Campbell, 2000). However, the emphases on service and on data collection can stress the capacity of a nursing center to manage both effectively (Goetzel, 2001).

## Essential Technology and Information Systems

It is essential to utilize available technology to collect, collate, and analyze data and to support the provision of quality health care services. Technology and information systems will continue to change given HIPAA, Health Plan Employer Data and Information Set (HEDIS) measures, and Healthy People 2010 objectives (Partridge, 2001). Computer software programs enable nurses to collect, store,

**Table 18-4 Examples of Quality Health Indicators for Nursing Center Application**

| INDICATOR | POPULATION | PERFORMANCE TARGETS | MEASURE |
|---|---|---|---|
| **Prevention** | | | |
| Annual influenza vaccine | High risk groups: age 65+ or those with heart or lung disease and other chronic conditions | HP 2010 = 90% age 65+ HP 2010 = 60% high risk, age 18-64 years | Client self-report and/or clinical records/audit |
| **Utilization** | | | |
| Mammogram within past 2 years | HEDIS: women age 52-69 years HP 2010: women 40 years and over | HEDIS 2001 = 81% HP 2010 = 70% | Client self-report and/or clinical records/audit |
| **Client Satisfaction** | | | |
| Patient satisfaction, annual | 100 consecutive clients per quarter | Performance targets to be determined by individual nursing center and/or health care plan | Survey |
| **Functional Status** | | | |
| Quality-of-life indicator | Adults age 18 years and older | Determined by individual nursing center and relate to baseline indicators and improvement goals | Screen utilizing Short Form 12 or 36 |

*HEDIS,* Health Plan Employer Data Information Set; *HP,* Healthy People.

retrieve, and analyze client and population characteristics and outcomes, and nurses must be current in that technology. Furthermore, nurses in nurse-managed health centers must know HIPAA regulations and guide the staff to effectively implement them with the concurrent expectation to maintain data inputs and outputs. Confidentiality of client records is key (Callahan and Jennings, 2002). Transferal of information must be carefully monitored. The use of computers by staff for entering and retrieving data will be governed by role, responsibility, and passwords.

## EDUCATION AND RESEARCH
### Community-Based Education

Student education in nursing centers must be thoughtfully coordinated, supervised, and evaluated. A faculty liaison enables students to have a resource within the educational system as well as a link with the center. Student and nursing center schedules must be coordinated. A year-round nursing center that provides 24-hour coverage of services must accommodate academic schedules and students moving in and out of clinical assignments. Center staff and faculty should maintain communication with clients and community agencies about student rotations, program assignments, and student projects. Students should be encouraged to share their work and clinical projects with the community, because learning is a mutual exchange. And, in the nursing center model, nothing is done in isolation.

## Research Opportunities in Nursing Centers

Research in nursing centers provides the opportunity to gain answers to questions and to share the findings with colleagues and the public (Gaus and Fraser, 1996). Critical questions involve individual and population health status, client outcomes, roles and capacities to address health promotion within the existing health system, and the value and affordability of care. In addition, many nursing centers serve as clinical laboratories for nursing and other health professional students. Centers offer many opportunities for educational research.

Each center needs a research agenda. The WHO's priorities for a common nursing research agenda offer a reference framework (Box 18-10). The research focus must include identification and clarification of client needs, particularly those not engaged in an existing health system; description of nursing interventions and linkages with consumer needs and resources; demonstration of effective interventions that produce appropriate outcomes; and cost analysis and documented cost-effectiveness of services.

Over the past two decades, nursing center research has principally focused on the development and characteristics of nursing centers (Glick, Thompson, and Ridge, 1999). Descriptive data have been collected about clients, types of services, financial supports, and community relationships. Currently, more than descriptive clinical studies are needed. Efforts are under way to capture and name the unique features of nursing models of care and to link them with health outcomes. For example, the significance

## Evidence-Based Practice

In 1997, the La Salle Neighborhood Nursing Center staff noted an increasing number of uninsured infants and children presenting for primary health care. The parents or caregivers of the children did not have health insurance for themselves, or if they did have health insurance, the children were not included on their policies. Parents or caregivers found that the cost of adding their children to their policies was prohibitive, so they took the risk that their children would remain healthy. However, when their young children were seen by a primary nurse practitioner, expenses were incurred because they needed immunizations, school physicals, and other health needs that required immediate attention and specialty referrals.

In 1998, the La Salle Neighborhood Nursing Center wrote a grant to the Patricia Kind Family Foundation to support the identification of uninsured children through community outreach and the provision of primary care to children while the parents/caregivers applied for the appropriate health care insurance. The insurance coverage for low-income families in the Commonwealth of Pennsylvania is Medicaid or the Children's Health Insurance Plan (CHIP). Eligibility for one or the other plan is based on income, family size, the child's age, and yearly renewal of the plan. During the first year of the grant, the La Salle Neighborhood Nursing Center identified more than 300 children who did not have health insurance and had documented health needs. The needs included inadequate immunizations, lack of well-child screenings, lack of lead screening for age-appropriate children, acute illnesses including ear infections, and chronic health problems such as scoliosis.

The first year showed that there were more families who applied for Medicaid coverage than for CHIP and that there was significant lag time between identification of the uninsured child, the completed application process, and health insurance coverage issued. During the second year of the grant award, other processes were put into place to hasten the completed application process and to monitor the numbers of families who received Medicaid or CHIP for their children and their ongoing use of primary health care services. Approximately 50% of the families selected the La Salle Neighborhood Nursing Center as a primary care provider; others (after they had received health care coverage) returned to community providers that they had used in the past.

Data (evidence of the practice) document that the La Salle Neighborhood Nursing Center has been effective in community outreach, family enrollment in the appropriate health care plan, and provision of primary care to high-risk children during the enrollment process. Families are now connected with primary health care homes. The grant support has enabled the nursing center to document interventions that have improved the well-being of children. The grant with meaningful data enabled the nursing center to apply for and successfully receive a Commonwealth of Pennsylvania Department of Insurance contract to extend community outreach to locate and enroll more uninsured children into the appropriate health care insurance plan.

**Nurse Use:** Data indicate that families do not know community resources, how to access those resources, or how to advocate on behalf of themselves or their children. Given the data and the current community status of more unemployed adults, the nursing center staff will use related evidence-based outcomes to seek other sources of funding to continue the services. Work with uninsured children and the acquisition of appropriate family health care coverage is an atypical quality health indicator and one that evolved from the direct experience and documentation of the nursing center staff.

---

of psychosocial interventions such as listening, support, and interpretation of information is being examined. Client satisfaction studies document the perceived value by those who use nursing centers. Factors associated with access to services are being examined. These include availability, timeliness, acceptability, and affordability of services. Environmental conditions, housing, transportation, criminal activities, and welfare-to-work transitions that influence health care access and use patterns are being examined. Box 18-11 presents a template for research in nursing centers.

## Program Evaluation

**Program evaluation** is essential in nursing centers, and research questions emerge from it. The evaluation process is a systematic approach to improve and account for public health and primary care actions. Evaluation is integrated in routine program operations. It is an expected component of all programs offered through the nursing center model and is a driving force when planning community-focused strategies, measuring resource allocations, improving existing programs, and identifying the need for additional services. Program evaluation separates what is working from what is not and enables clinicians, faculty, and students to ask difficult questions and deal with pressing challenges (Richards et al, 2002). Resources are available to help staff understand and apply program evaluation in their particular setting. Resources include courses offered through the Centers for Disease Control and Prevention (CDC) Public Health Training Network, the Community Toolbox, available through the internet and updated by the CDC Evaluation Working Group (www.cdc.gov/eval/index/htm). These resources will enable center staff to implement the six essential program evaluation steps in their particular model and community. The essential steps are outlined in Box 18-12.

Program evaluation, research focuses, and clinical outcomes contribute to quality management plans for nursing

---

**BOX 18-10   WHO Priorities for a Common Nursing Research Agenda**

- Evaluation of the effects of health care reform on equity, sustainability, and quality care, as well as on the workforce, particularly nursing personnel
- Comparative analysis of supply and demand of the health workforce
- Evaluation of the effects of health care organization, work conditions, technology, and supervision on the motivation and productivity of nursing personnel
- Analyses of the feasibility, effectiveness, and quality of education and practice:
  (1) where nurses have the responsibility for the entire range of care in a given community—promotive, preventive, curative, rehabilitative, long-term, and palliative care (including mental health/illness); and
  (2) where the focus of care is on individual as opposed to community/public health as opposed to environment/intersectoral
- Under which conditions are there feasible options, providing sound models of quality service delivery
- Comparative analysis of the effectiveness of education and quality of services provided by nurses as opposed

to the effectiveness of education and quality of services based on different options of skill mix (within nursing and with other professions)
- Action research on delivery modes and necessary context for quality nursing care to vulnerable populations (e.g., homeless, chronically mentally ill, urban slum dwellers, nomads, refugees)
- Quality of care at different levels of the health care system and to different population groups (e.g., what are the educational and legal requirements for appropriate care to women, minorities, and so on?)
- Ethics research related to different population groups, and ethical considerations in research
- Culturally appropriate models of care and culturally appropriate human resource recruitment, retention, and deployment strategies
- Specific focus on home care, occupational health, and infection control in light of emerging trends

---

center models. The costs of care are linked to various outcome measures. Analysis of care costs is crucial to long-term sustainability of nursing centers. The effects of nursing models of care must be considered within society's continuing efforts to contain health care costs while improving health status. More refined studies are needed in this area, and more studies across nursing centers are needed to document common client outcomes.

The stronger the research agenda and the program evaluation capacity, the greater is the potential for nursing centers to survive and thrive in the emerging health care environment. Centers must integrate research efforts into all aspects of their operations and must reach out to similar models, share common goals and data, and commit to working with each other. One example of working together is the National Nursing Centers Consortium and other regional consortiums situated in the Midwest.

## POSITIONING NURSING CENTERS FOR THE FUTURE

### Emerging Health Care Systems

Nationally, nursing is strategically placed to make significant contributions to the health of people and achieve the Healthy People 2010 goals of reducing health disparities and increasing years of productive life (Buhler Wilkerson, 1993). Nursing centers offer unique opportunities to develop preventive services to improve the well-being of individuals, families, and communities. Nurses can continue to build the community trust, support, and capacity nec-

essary to move the nursing center model into the mainstream of health care by 2010 and beyond. Challenges and opportunities exist to advance this model. The traditionalist health care system is changing, particularly since the September 11, 2001, terrorist attack on the nation and the threat of widespread bioterrorism in this nation and the world. The public health system and community models of care will be in the forefront of prevention, early intervention, and communitywide education should further attacks occur. Nurse-managed health centers and their community counterparts must be prepared to meet the everyday needs of people as well as the sudden, catastrophic events that threaten our society's future.

Other threats, such as the escalating numbers of uninsured adults and children who seek (or fail to seek) care, will continue to vex health care providers and legislators (Agency for Healthcare Research and Quality, 2002). Any extended economic downswings will increase the number of people without health care coverage, and more public dollars will be consumed to support those in need. One threat to community and personal well-being is social isolation, particularly for older adults or those who are disenfranchised because of geography or a community's social anomie (Case and Paxson, 2002). Nursing center staff grapple with the complex health, social, and environmental issues presented by their clients and the community. Membership in professional organizations, including nursing center consortiums, will enable people to organize around one or more critical health threats and strategize about what interventions work locally, regionally, and nationally. In addition, lessons learned and programmatic

## BOX 18-11   Template for Research in Nursing Centers

### PRINCIPLES FOR NURSING CENTER RESEARCH

- Responsibility and accountability for research projects conducted in or through the center
- Community participation in research endeavors
- Staff collaboration in operational and relevant aspects of research endeavors
- Public dissemination of information about findings of all research projects conducted in or through the center

### DOMAINS OF NURSING CENTER RESEARCH

- The community's health
- Individual and family primary care
- Public health programs
- Nursing education
- Education of students and practitioners in other health professions and related fields
- Quality, methods, and cost of nursing center operations
- Emerging research questions in nursing, community health, primary care, and education of health professions

### EXAMPLES OF RESEARCH PRIORITIES FOR NURSING CENTERS

- Nursing approaches to the delivery of community and primary health care services
  - Population-focused and primary health care practice
  - Community, family, and health-oriented care
  - Multisector, multidisciplinary, and interorganizational collaboration
  - Nurses as health advocates on community, non-profit, governmental, and corporate boards and advisory groups
- Strategies for working with and in the community
  - Community collaboration and partnership
  - Working with community health workers/advocates
  - Links between health and the environment
  - Dissemination of public health information
- Integrating with a complex and shifting health care system
  - Managing health care quality and costs
  - Fiscal and health care data management systems
  - Associations, partnerships, and mergers
  - Achieving federally qualified health centers (FQHC) status
- Responding to emerging community and personal health challenges
  - Changing demographic, geographic, and economic indicators
  - Bioterrorism response competencies and capacity
  - Health promotion and disease prevention for such conditions as obesity, heart disease, cancer, violence, and HIV/AIDS
  - Chronic and communicable disease management

### CONDUCTING CENTER-BASED NEEDS

- Staff research project liaison
  - Senior member of nursing center staff liaison for each research project (selected tasks may be delegated to other staff, as appropriate)
  - Responsible for guiding and facilitating individual or teams of investigators through research principles, procedures, operational systems, internal problem-solving
  - Responsible for tracking progress and issues, overseeing any fiscal matters related to project, internal and external communications, reporting to internal and community groups as indicated by project
- Community collaboration
  - Guided/facilitated by staff liaison or designee
  - To occur through center's community advisors
  - To also include other appropriate community leaders, involved or related community organizational leaders, and involved or related health providers
  - Written description of purpose, research team members, nursing center liaison, research methods, community impact, participation, confidentiality/anonymity procedures and signature forms, and procedures for review of public information materials
  - Letters of approval/recommendation from each of above
- Staff collaboration
  - Guided/facilitated by staff liaison or designee
  - To include communications with all involved or relevant clinical, program, and administrative staff (informational, educational, and evaluative, as indicated by project)
  - To include communications with all involved or relevant administrative staff (informational, educational, and evaluative, as indicated by project)
  - Approval signatures from divisional heads of all involved or otherwise relevant center department/divisions
- Nursing center research committee
  - Members to include (a) appointed/elected staff, (b) appointed/elected community representatives, (c) relevant research experts
  - Written application submitted by primary investigator and center staff liaison (copy of research proposal, research team members/credentials, nursing center liaison, methods for community collaboration, ensuring/protecting anonymity, confidentiality, reporting process, impact and outcomes of research to community, acknowledgment and appreciation for community involvement)

| | | |
| --- | --- | --- |

**BOX 18-12   Essential Program Evaluation Steps**

- Engaging stakeholders
- Describing the program
- Focusing the evaluation design
- Gathering credible evidence
- Justifying conclusions
- Ensuring use and sharing lessons learned

successes can be shared, compared, and utilized to build legislative support for nurse-managed health centers.

## National and Regional Organizations

Professional organizations abound for nurses to join and contribute their skills to advance the future of nursing. Nurses choose membership in organizations on the basis of clinical interest, academic preparation, and employment. Nurses involved in the nurse-managed health centers across the nation have several consortiums available to advance their administrative and clinical skill base.

An example of these consortiums is the Regional Nursing Centers Consortium (RNCC), founded in 1996 to meet the needs of nursing centers in Pennsylvania, New Jersey, and Delaware. Since 1996, membership has expanded beyond the tri-state area. In 2001, the RNCC board voted to change the name to the National Nursing Centers Consortium (NNCC) to better represent members throughout the nation. NNCC headquarters are located in Philadelphia. The NNCC membership services include nursing center development, marketing, public relations, data warehouse and information systems technical assistance, public policy development, and health care advocacy (Box 18-13).

The potential for far-reaching change has been created through the consortiums. Time will tell the effectiveness and long-lasting community value of nursing centers at the national level. Much will depend on nurses uniting for common causes and a shared vision of what nursing is and can be in this century.

## Nursing Workforce

Over the past two decades, fewer people have entered the nursing workforce. Legislators, health care systems, the nursing profession, educational institutions, and the public are now examining the interrelated factors that have contributed to the decline in the number of new nursing graduates and the increasing number of nurses who leave the profession (Bingham, 2002). The need for skilled nurses with the commitment and passion for nursing work regardless of the clinical setting is dramatic. People are living longer and advances in technology and drug therapies require that nurses possess current knowledge

**BOX 18-13   Overview of National Nursing Centers Consortium (NNCC)**

**Vision:** To improve community health through neighborhood-based primary health care services that are accessible, acceptable, and affordable.

**Mission:** To serve its neighborhood-based health center members by enhancing their potential for sustainability and growth.

**The NNCC was established for the following purposes:**
- To foster understanding, recognition, and use of nursing centers, as essential primary health care providers through health promotion, disease prevention, health education, and primary care services
- To provide a forum for communication and collaboration among consortium members
- To offer services that enhance members' management capabilities and health care programs

**The values to which the NNCC ascribes include the following:**
- Nursing models of care
- Individual, family, and community health
- Community collaboration
- Interorganization and multidisciplinary alliances for health care

**Goals**
- NNCC is a catalyst in health care policy development and legislative change.
- Nursing centers are positioned as a recognized mainstream health care model.
- NNCC and member centers are able to receive optimal multisource funding.
- NNCC fosters partnerships with people and groups who share common goals.
- NNCC ensures the collection and sharing of pertinent health outcome data from its member centers to demonstrate the impact of the nursing center model.
- NNCC ensures continued work on defining quality care for nursing centers.
- NNCC enhances the growth of nursing centers.

and skills to care for acutely ill people in hospitals, homes, and extended care facilities. The increasing demand for nurses coupled with the decline in workforce numbers and the aging of the nursing workforce have placed institutional and community premiums on working nurses. Salaries, benefits, and working hours have changed for the better; however, working conditions for nurses have not improved dramatically. Mandatory overtime and client mix (number of clients and acuity levels) are challenges nurses confront daily. Sometimes they make other career choices because they want more control over their work and personal lives, and often they gravitate toward the nursing center model. Their work hours and salaries may not change, but the opportunity to use their expertise to make meaningful differences and to shape the nursing model is both appealing and fulfilling. Nurses attracted to this model often discover their professional need to be an advocate for people in need and become involved in public policy development at the local and national levels (Drevdahl, 2002). Through the nursing center model, the voices of nurses are heard, and lasting changes are made in public policy because of their work with legislators and bureaucrats.

## Policy Development and Health Advocacy

Policy development and health advocacy are essential roles in nursing centers. Nurses focus on health disparities and access to care for all as principal agendas. They also promote the nursing center model as a system of public health and primary care services that reduces health disparities and improves ongoing access to healthy care. The roles of advocate can be diverse, from working with a community group to reduce the exposure of children to lead-based paint to testifying in the House of Representatives about the contributions of nurse-managed health centers as safety net providers. Advocates often integrate policy development work as they learn more about community needs, document clinical outcomes, and conduct program evaluations. In addition, nurses who work closely with local and state health departments, state nursing organizations, and state departments of public welfare are in unique positions to contribute to the processes that change laws and regulations.

Nursing centers represent an innovative and therefore disruptive approach to the delivery of health care services. Pressing issues are legislative and insurance barriers that reduce access to appropriate funding resources; the public's increasing disenchantment with managed care programs; the increasing double-digit percentage of the gross national product spent on health care; the necessity for nurse-managed health centers to be fiscally sustainable despite the numbers of uninsured adults and children who seek health care services; and the national emphasis on achieving Healthy People 2010 goals and objectives despite the absence of universal health insurance.

There is no better time to be a nurse and to advance the profession. The profession is undergoing change and more nurses are needed to meet health needs in many settings. Nurses in nurse-managed health centers are uniquely positioned to introduce nursing to community members, to speak on behalf of the profession, and to educate those seeking a career with a social mandate to improve health and provide care. Nurses involved in the nurse-managed health centers are advocates for social justice and equality for all and their work is a lasting legacy for those who follow. The Practice Application box gives an example of the contributions of nurses and a nursing center to the life of one urban community.

## Practice Application

The William Penn Foundation has funded a Youth Opportunities Initiative (YOI) in certain areas of Philadelphia. La Salle Neighborhood Nursing Center is one of the funded entities. The 3-year grant supports the work of one public health nurse and ancillary staff, **community health workers** and nursing students to work with minority children and youths in organized youth programs. The youth programs are offered in public housing complexes, local schools, and recreation centers. The program focuses on self-esteem, responsible decision making, recognizing personal assets, and goal setting.

The YOI students in the La Salle program are introduced to La Salle University. They have coordinated campus visits, meet faculty, and participate in educational, recreational, and multimedia events. Prior to this program, youths in this neighborhood had never been on the La Salle campus and did not know what the university had to offer to the community. Students also participate in sports events including football, basketball, and track. The university cosponsors the youth activities and the youths begin to bond with the university within their neighborhood. The youths also participate in the development of public service announcements regarding public health topics that are aired on the university's cable television channel.

Throughout the program, goal setting by the youths is emphasized, particularly because the graduation rate from high school in the target neighborhoods hovers around 50%. Goal setting includes school attendance, improving grades, staying in school, graduating on time, and considering higher education. As the nurses work with the youths, careers in the health professions are discussed. Nurses, social workers, nutritionists, physicians, and others speak to the youths about their health career choices and the paths taken to accomplish their goals. It is too soon to tell what choices the youths will make; however, an intermediate goal is to monitor their progress and performance in school and keep in contact with them after the YOI grant ends.

A. What do you think the short-term outcomes will be in terms of student participation?
B. What might be intermediate outcomes?
C. Identify a possible long-term outcome.

**Answers are in the back of the book.**

## Key Points

- Nursing centers provide unique opportunities to improve the health status of individuals, families, and communities through direct access to nursing care.
- Nursing center models combine people, place, approach, and strategy in everyday life to develop appropriate health care interventions.
- A nursing center's health and community orientation builds strong connections to the community served.

- A center is defined by its particular array of services and programs; examples are comprehensive primary health care centers and special care centers.
- The foundations for the nursing center model include the perspective of the World Health Organization and the Healthy People 2010 systematic approach to improving individual and community health.
- Each center develops its philosophy, goals, and activities through a process of community collaboration, assessment, and strategic planning.
- As the community and the center work together for health, a multilevel approach is used that includes individuals and expands to legislators.
- Nursing center development is rooted in public health nursing history and the evolution of the nursing profession.
- Most current nursing center models emerged from academic nursing centers in the 1970s.
- Nursing center models support the skill development of advanced practice nurses, allied health professionals, and paraprofessionals.
- Any nursing center must have a board of directors or an advisory board to guide program development, fund-raising, community networking, and other work.
- The nursing center requires careful planning and structure to be a successful education, service, and business enterprise.
- Start-up and sustainability are based on a community-focused feasibility study, a sound business and financial plan, operational support, and resource management.
- Evidence-based practice in nursing centers is essential and represents the clinical application of particular nursing interventions and documented client outcomes.
- The Health Insurance Portability and Accountability Act (HIPAA) will increase the center's investment in administrative and oversight services.
- Available technology and systems management must be used to collect, collate, and analyze center data.
- Education and research opportunities abound in this model.
- Program evaluation is an organizational practice in nursing centers; research questions are developed from program evaluation.
- Threats to the viability of nursing centers include the uninsured or underinsured, erratic funding resources, community decline, and disenfranchised populations at high risk.
- Nurses attracted to the nursing center model discover professional fulfillment in advocating for people in need and becoming involved in public policy change.
- Nursing centers represent a disruptive and innovative approach to the delivery of health care services.
- Nurses involved in the nursing center model are advocates for social justice and equality for all.

## Clinical Decision-Making Activities

1. Interview one nursing center staff member about the organization. How does the nurse-managed health center fit into the current health care system? Give one or more illustrations using community and client data.
2. Investigate your state certification requirements for nurse practitioners, and the criteria for independent practice. What factors support or limit the certification of nurse practitioners to function as independent primary health care providers? How do the factors influence the operation of a nursing center?
3. Examine a nursing center's annual budget and report. Compare to a previous year and to projections for a future year. Describe any impact on the past, current, or projected budget given the current political and legislative climate in your region, the nation, and the world. Cite two examples and what might happen to the provision of high-quality health care to vulnerable groups.
4. Identify one public policy that has influenced the health care access of adults and/or children in need of ongoing primary health care. Investigate the history of the public policy and make recommendations to support, change, or abolish the policy.
5. Select a health care position that you wish to learn more about. Interview two or more staff members in those positions. Ask about roles and responsibilities, review the job descriptions, and determine their contributions to the community and the nursing center. Learn about career mobility, salary ranges, and future aspirations. Determine if the nursing center model supports staff growth and development.
6. Contact a local elected official or staff member and determine if this person is familiar with the nurse-managed health center model and the essential services it provides. Determine if more information and detail is needed by the official and staff, and suggest effective strategies to educate the staff.

## Additional Resources

These related resources are found either in the appendix at the back of this book or on the book's website at **http://evolve.elsevier.com/Stanhope.**

### *evolve* Evolve Website

WebLinks: Healthy People 2010

# References

Agency for Healthcare Research and Quality: Medicaid program expansions to cover otherwise uninsured poor children appear to be relatively inexpensive, *AHRQ Research Activities,* February 2002, AHRQ, available at http://www.ahrq.gov/.

American Association of Colleges of Nursing: *Hallmarks of the professional nursing practice movement,* Washington, DC, January 2002, AACN, available at www.aacn.nche.edu.

American Nurses Association: *Health promotion and disease prevention: a position statement,* Kansas City, Mo, 1995, ANA.

Anderko L: The effectiveness of a rural nursing center in improving health care access in a three-county area, *J Rural Health* 16(2):177-184, 2000.

Anderson E, McFarlane J: *Community as a partner,* Philadelphia, 1996, Lippincott-Raven.

Aydelotte MK, Gregory MS: Nursing practice: innovative models, *NLN Publ* (21-2311):1-20, 1989.

Aydelotte et al: *The nursing center: concept and design,* Kansas City, Mo, 1987, ANA.

Baker EL, White LE, Lichtveld MY: Reducing health disparities through community-based research, *Public Health Rep* 116(6):517-519, 2001.

Bellack JP, O'Neil EH: Recreating nursing practice for a new century: recommendations and implications of the Pew Health Professions Commission's final report, *Nurs Health Care Perspect* 21(1):14-21, 2000.

Berkman LF, Lochner KA: Social determinants of health: meeting at the crossroads, *Health Aff* 21(2):291-293, 2002.

Bingham R: Leaving nursing, *Health Aff* 21(1):211-217, 2002.

Buchanan M: The new system of care. In *Teaching in the community: preparing nurses for the 21ˢᵗ century,* New York, 1997, National League for Nursing.

Buhler Wilkerson K: Bring care to the people: Lillian Wald's legacy to public health nursing, *Am J Public Health* 83(12):1778-1786, 1993.

Callahan D, Jennings B: Ethics and public health: forging a strong relationship, *Am J Public Health* 92(2):169-176, 2002.

Campbell BS: Preventive health service outcomes in three government funded health centers, *Fam Community Health* 23(1):18-28, 2000.

Carlson BL et al: Primary care of patients without insurance by community health centers, *J Ambul Care Manage* 24(3):47-59, 2001.

Case A, Paxson C: Parental behavior and child health, *Health Aff* 21(2):164-178, 2002.

Christensen CM, Bohmer R, Kenagy J: Will disruptive innovations cure health care? *Harv Bus Rev* 78(5):102-112, 2000.

Clear JB, Starbecker M, Kelly DW: Nursing centers and health promotion: a federal vantage point, *Fam Community Health* 21(4):1-14, 1999.

Cross R, Prusak L: The people who make organizations go—or stop, *Harv Bus Rev* 80(6):104-112, 2002.

Deaton A: Policy implications of the gradient of health and wealth, *Health Aff* 21(2):13-30, 2002.

Drevdahl D: Social justice or market justice? the paradoxes of public health partnerships with managed care, *Public Health Nurs* 19(3):161-169, 2002.

Eddy DM: Performance measurement: problems and solutions, *Health Aff* 17(4):7-25, 1998.

Evans LK et al: *Health care for the 21ˢᵗ century—greater Philadelphia style,* paper prepared for the Independence Foundation, March 28, 1997.

Floyd JM: Envisioning new nursing roles and scopes of practice, *Reflect Nurs Leadersh* 27(2):52-53, 2001.

Forrest CB, Whelan EM: Primary care safety-net delivery sites in the United States: a comparison of community health centers, hospital outpatient departments, and physicians' offices, *JAMA* 284(16):2077-2083, 2000.

Garrett NY, Yasnoff WA: Disseminating public health practice guidelines in electronic medical record systems, *J Public Health Manag Pract* 8(3), 2002.

Gaus CR, Fraser I: Shifting paradigms and the role of research, *Health Aff* 15(2):235-242, 1996.

Gerrity P, Kinsey KK: An urban nurse-managed primary health care center: health promotion in action, *Fam Community Health* 21(4):29-40, 1999.

Glick DF, Thompson KM, Ridge RA: Population-based research: the foundation for development, management, and evaluation of a community nursing center, *Fam Community Health* 21(4):41-50, 1999.

Goetzel R: The financial impact of health promotion, *Am J Health Promot* 15(5):277-280, 2001.

Goffee R, Jones G: Followership: it's personal, too, *Harv Bus Rev* 79(11):147, 2001.

Hamner JB et al: Community-based service learning in the engaged university, *Nurs Outlook* 50(2):67-71, 2002.

Hansen-Turton T, Kinsey K: The quest for self-sustainability: nurse-managed health centers meeting the policy challenge, *Policy Polit Nurs Pract* 2(4):304-309, 2001.

Hemphill JC: Integration of research, education, and practice, *Nurs Leadersh Forum* 6(2):47-54, 2001.

Hurst CP, Osban LB: Service learning on wheels: the Nightingale mobile clinic, *Nurs Health Care Perspect* 21(4):184-187, 2000.

Jacobson PD: Form versus function in public health, *J Public Health Manag Pract* 8(1):92-94, 2002.

Keefe MF, Leuner JD, Laken MA: Caring for the community initiative integrating research, practice, and education, *Nurs Health Care Perspect* 21(6):287-292, 2000.

Kinlein ML: Independent nurse practitioner, *Nurs Outlook* 21(1):22-24, 1972.

Kinsey KK: Models that work: an interview with Dorothy Harrell, Philadelphia community activist, *Fam Community Health* 21(4):74-79, 1999.

Kinsey KK: *La Salle Neighborhood Nursing Center annual report,* Philadelphia, 2002, The Center.

Kinsey KK, Gerrity P: Planning, implementing, and managing a community-based nursing center: current challenges and future opportunities, *Handbook Home Health Care Admin* 77:903-912, 1997.

Lancaster J: From the editor, *Fam Community Health* 21(4), 1999.

Lundeen SP: An alternative paradigm for promoting health in communities: the Lundeen Community nursing center model, *Fam Community Health* 21(4): 15-28, 1999.

Lutz J, Herrick CA, Lehman BB: Community partnership: a school of nursing creates nursing centers for older adults, *Nurs Health Care Perspect* 22(1):26-29, 2001.

Matherlee K: The nursing center in concept and practice: delivery and financing issues in serving vulnerable people, *Issue Brief Natl Health Policy Forum* 746:1-10, 1999.

Mattessich P, Monsey B: *Collaboration: what makes it work?* St Paul, Minn, 1992, Amherst H. Wilder Foundation.

National Health Policy Forum: *Providing community-based primary care: nursing centers, CHC's, and other initiatives:* a site visit report, George Washington University, July 1998.

National Health Policy Forum: *Essential community health services on the frontier:* a site visit report, George Washington University, January 1999.

Oros M et al: Community-based nursing centers: challenges and opportunities in implementation and sustainability, *Policy Polit Nurs Pract* 2(4):277-287, 2001.

Partridge L: *The APHSA Medicaid HEDIS database project,* Report for the Third Project Year, December 2001.

Reverby S: From Lillian Wald to Hilary Rodham Clinton: what will happen to public health nursing? *Am J Public Health* 83(12):1662-1663, 1993.

Richards L et al: Achieving success in poor urban minority community-based research: strategies for implementing community-based research within an urban minority population, *Health Promot Pract* 3(3):410-420, 2002.

Schultz AJ, Krieger J, Galea S: Addressing social determinants of health: community-based participatory approaches to research and practices, *Health Educ Behav* 29(3):287-295, 2002.

U.S. Department of Health and Human Services: *Healthy people 2010: understanding and improving health,* ed 2, Washington DC, 2000, U.S. Government Printing Office.

Shiber S, D'Lugoff M: A win-win model for an academic nursing center: community partnership faculty practice, *Public Health Nurs* 19(2):81-85, 2002.

Shortell SM et al: Evaluating partnerships for community health improvement: tracking the footprints, *J Health Polit Policy Law* 27(1):49-91, 2002.

Stacy NL: The experience and performance of community health centers under managed care, *Am J Managed Care* 6(11):1229-1239, 2000.

Stryer D, Clancy C, Simpson L: Minority health disparities: AHRQ efforts to address inequities in care, *Health Promot Pract* 3(2):125-129, 2002.

Swan BA, Catroneo M: Financing strategies for a community nursing center, *Nurs Econ* 17(1):44-48, 1999.

U.S. Department of Health and Human Services: *Fact sheet—health care access: it all starts with quality professionals,* Washington, DC, Oct 2000, U.S. Government Printing Office.

U.S. Department of Health and Human Services: *Healthy People 2010: Understanding and Improving Health,* Washington, DC, Nov 2000, U.S. Government Printing Office.

World Health Organization: *Primary health care: report of the International Conference on Primary Health Care,* Alma-Ata, USSR, 6-12 September, 1978.

# Chapter 19

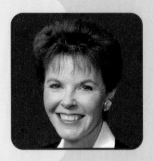

# Case Management

**Ann H. Cary, Ph.D., M.P.H., R.N., A.-C.C.C.**

Ann H. Cary began practicing public health nursing in the 1970s as a home-health nurse in New Orleans, Louisiana, where she executed case management functions daily. She has served on national workgroups that established the standards of practice for case managers; created certification exams for case managers; authored numerous articles on case management issues; taught baccalaureate and graduate-level courses in case management; and directed graduate programs in case management and continuity of care. She was the first director of the Institute for Research, Education and Consultation at the American Nurses Credentialing Center in Washington, D.C.

## Objectives

After reading this chapter, the student should be able to do the following:

1. Define continuity of care, care management, case management, and advocacy
2. Describe the scope of practice, roles, and functions of a case manager
3. Compare and contrast the nursing process with processes of case management and advocacy
4. Identify methods to manage conflict, as well as the process of achieving collaboration
5. Define and explain the legal and ethical issues confronting case managers

---

The health care industry has created delivery systems that integrate financing, management, and delivery of services. Care may be financed and paid through insurance using fee-for-service or capitation plans, or by self-pay. Delivery of care may come through a network of providers, such as negotiated contracts with hospitals, physicians and nurse practitioners, pharmacies, ancillary health services, and outpatient centers. Managing the health of populations served by the integrated systems is essential. Population management includes wellness and health promotion, illness prevention, acute and subacute care, rehabilitation, end-of-life care, and care coordination. The use of integrated systems has had important consequences in the focus of care (Qudah and Brannon, 1996):

- Emphasis is on population health management across the continuum, rather than on episodes of illness for an individual.
- Management has shifted from inpatient care as the point of management to primary care providers as points of entry.
- Care management services and programs provide access and accountability for the continuum of health.

- Successful outcomes are measured by systems performance (rather than limited to individual provider performance) to meet the needs of populations.

The contemporary focus of the integrated health systems defines the nature of the client as a population rather than as an individual. In these systems, **population management** entails the following activities:

- Assessing the needs of the client population through health histories (and, in the future, genotypes), claims, use of service patterns, and risk factors
- Creating benefits and network designs to address these needs
- Prioritizing actions to produce a desired outcome with available resources
- Selecting programs related to wellness, prevention, health promotion, and demand management, and educating the population about them
- Instituting a care management process that coordinates care across the health continuum for a population aggregate
- Assigning case managers to clients and to primary care providers

## Key Terms

**advocacy**, p. 456
**affirming**, p. 458
**allocation**, p. 460
**amplifying**, p. 457
**assertiveness**, p. 461
**autonomy**, p. 465
**beneficence**, p. 465
**brainstorming**, p. 459
**care management**, p. 447
**CareMaps tool**, p. 453
**case management**, p. 448
**case management plans**, p. 453
**case manager**, p. 448
**clarifying**, p. 458
**collaboration**, p. 461

**constituency**, p. 457
**cooperation**, p. 461
**coordinate**, p. 449
**critical path**, p. 453
**demand management**, p. 448
**disease management**, p. 448
**distributive outcomes**, p. 460
**information exchange process**, p. 457
**informing**, p. 457
**integrative outcomes**, p. 460
**intermediate criteria**, p. 454
**justice**, p. 465
**life care planning**, p. 455
**negotiating**, p. 460
**nonmaleficence**, p. 465

**outcome criteria**, p. 454
**population management**, p. 446
**problem–purpose–expansion method**,
  p. 459
**problem solving**, p. 459
**risk sharing**, p. 454
**social mandate**, p. 447
**supporting**, p. 458
**timelines**, p. 454
**utilization management**, p. 447
**variance**, p. 454
**veracity**, p. 465
**verifying**, p. 458
*See Glossary for definitions*

## Chapter Outline

Definitions
Concepts of Case Management
*Case Management and the Nursing Process*
*Characteristics and Roles*
*Knowledge and Skill Requisites*
*Tools of Case Managers*

Public Health and Community-Based Examples
  of Case Management
Essential Skills for Case Managers
*Advocacy*
*Conflict Management*

*Collaboration*
Issues in Case Management
*Legal Issues*
*Ethical Issues*

Establishing a relationship between financing, managing, delivering, and coordinating services is critical to reach the goal of population management: that is, achieving healthy outcomes at the population level. The Healthy People 2010 goals to increase both quality of life and years of healthy life, and to eliminate health disparities, frame the **social mandate** for health care. In the first decade of the twenty-first century, case management will be an intervention of choice to positively influence the leading health indicators and focus areas of Healthy People 2010.

Establishing evidence-based strategies is critical to the success of case management for individuals and populations. In their practice, nurse case managers have the following core values: increasing the span of healthy life, reducing disparities in health among Americans, and promoting access to care and to preventive services. Many of the interventions nurses use with clients and health care systems help to further the progress toward the Healthy People objectives.

## DEFINITIONS

**Care management** is an enduring process in which a population manager establishes systems and processes to monitor the health status, resources, and outcomes for a targeted aggregate of the population. The population manager is the tactical architect for a population's health in the delivery system. Building blocks that are used by the manager include risk analysis; data mapping; monitoring for health processes, indicators, and unexpected illnesses; epidemiologic investigation of unexpected illnesses; development of multidisciplinary action plans and programs for the population; and identifying case management triggers or events (e.g., when dramatic results are obtained by prevention or early intervention) that indicate the need for early referrals of high-risk clients (Qudah and Brannon, 1996).

Care management strategies were initially developed by health maintenance organizations (HMOs) in the late 1970s to manage the care of different populations. The purpose was to promote quality and ensure appropriate use and costs of services. Care management strategies include utilization management, critical pathways, case management, disease management, and demand management. **Utilization management** attempts to promote optimal use of services to redirect care and monitor the appropriate use of provider care/treatment services for both acute and community/ambulatory services. Providers are offered

**Healthy People 2010** | **Case Management Strategies Offer Opportunities for Nurses to Help Meet the Following Healthy People 2010 Objectives for Target Populations**

1-2 Increase the proportion of insured persons with coverage for clinical preventive services

1-3 Increase the proportion of persons appropriately counseled about health behaviors

1-5 Increase the proportion of persons with a usual primary care provider

1-6 Reduce the proportion of families that experience difficulties or delays in obtaining health care, or who do not receive needed care for one or more family members

1-7 Increase the proportion of schools of medicine, schools of nursing, and other health professional training schools whose basic curriculum for health care providers includes the core competencies in health promotion and disease prevention

1-15 Increase the proportion of persons with long-term care needs who have access to the continuum of long-term care services

From U.S. Department of Health and Human Services: *Healthy People 2010: national health promotion and disease prevention objectives,* ed 2, Washington, DC, 2000, U.S. Government Printing Office.

multiple options for care with different economic implications. Through the use of utilization management, clients who have repetitive readmissions (i.e., they fail to respond to care) are often referred to care management programs (Llewellyn and Moreo, 2001).

Critical pathways are tools that specify activities providers may use in a timely sequence to achieve desired outcomes for care. The outcomes are measurable, and the pathway tools strive to reduce differences in client care. Case management services are used for clients with specific diagnoses who may have high use patterns, noncompliance issues, cost caps (e.g., no more than $10,000 or $20,000 can be spent on their case), or threshold expenses.

**Disease management** activities target chronic and costly disease conditions that require long-term care interventions (e.g., diabetes, asthma, depression). These strategies are an acceptable approach to organizing services for a specific population across a continuum of primary, secondary, and tertiary prevention interventions and self-care management activities (McClatchey, 2001). Disease management information systems use treatment guidelines to streamline the process, avoid unnecessary care, and act proactively to slow or reduce the effects or complications of the disease process for populations (Llewellyn and Moreo, 2001).

**Demand management** seeks to control use by providing clients with correct information and education strategies to make healthy choices, to use healthy and health-seeking behaviors to improve their health status, and to make fewer demands on the health care system (Coleman and Zagor, 1998).

**Case management** comprises the activities implemented with individual clients in the system. The **case manager** builds on the basic functions of the traditional nurse's role and adapts new competencies for managing transition from hospital to home—for example, wellness and prevention, and multidisciplinary teams. Additionally, case managers in care-managed programs are expanding

their clinical expertise to embrace the process of disease management, a successful strategy for population outcomes. Specialty case management by master's-prepared advanced practice nurses (APNs) is an emerging role in this field. In implementing case management, APNs work with client or community aggregates, systems of disease, and outcomes management processes, whereas nurses with bachelor's degrees focus on care at the individual level (Stanton and Dunkin, 2002).

This chapter will describe the nature and process of case management for individual and family clients. Case management has a rich tradition in public health nursing. More recently, it is becoming important in the acute care setting (Llewellyn and Moreo, 2001). Nursing has maintained the leadership among health care providers in coordinating resources to achieve health care outcomes based on quality, access, and cost. As health care delivery embraces capitation, the most efficient management of client outcomes can be done with case management.

## CONCEPTS OF CASE MANAGEMENT

Reviewing multiple or historical definitions of case management helps to demonstrate the complex process. Weil and Karls (1985) describe case management as a "set of logical steps and process of interacting within a service network which ensures that a client receives needed services in a supportive, effective, efficient and cost-effective manner" (p. 4). Case management is defined by the American Hospital Association (AHA, 1986) as the process of planning, organizing, coordinating, and monitoring services and resources needed by clients, while supporting the effective use of health and social services. Bower (1992) describes the continuity, quality, and cost-containment aspects of case management as a health care delivery process whose goals are to provide quality health care, decrease fragmentation, enhance the client's quality of life, and contain costs. Secord (1987) defines case management as a systematic process of assessing, planning, and coordinating the service, referrals, and monitoring that meets the multiple needs of clients. A focus on collaboration is important in the National Case Management Task Force definition: "a collaborative process which assesses, plans, implements, coordinates, monitors and evaluates the options and services to meet an individual's health needs, using communication and available resources to promote quality, cost effective outcomes" (Mullahy, 1998a).

As a competency, case management is defined in the public health nursing literature as the "ability to establish an appropriate plan of care based on assessing the client/family and coordinating the necessary resources and services for the client's benefit" (Kenyon et al., 1990, p. 36). Knowledge and skills required to achieve this competency include the following:

- Knowledge of community resources and financing mechanisms
- Written and oral communication and documentation
- Proficient negotiating and conflict-resolving practices
- Critical-thinking processes to identify and prioritize problems from the provider and client viewpoints
- Identifying the best resources for the desired outcomes

The American Nurses Credentialing Center (ANCC) indicates that nursing case management is a dynamic and systematic collaborative approach to providing and coordinating health care services to a defined population (Llewellyn and Moreo, 2001). In the latest *Standards of Practice for Case Management,* case management is defined as "involving the timely coordination of quality health care services to meet an individual's specific health care needs in a cost effective manner" (Case Management Society of America [CMSA], 2002, p. 7). CMSA further describes the spectrum of case management activities as four: assessment, planning, facilitating, and advocacy (Aliotta, 2003; CMSA, 2002)

That case management practice is complex is further seen by the need to **coordinate** activities of multiple providers, payers, and settings throughout a client's continuum of care. Care provided must be assessed, planned, implemented, adjusted, and evaluated on the basis of goals designed by many disciplines, and goals of the client, the family, significant others, and community organizations. Although the community-oriented nurse may be employed and located in one setting, the nurse will be influencing the selecting and monitoring of care provided in other settings by formal and informal care providers. With the increased use of electronic care delivery through telehealth activities, case management activities are now handled via telephone, e-mail, and fax, and through video visits and electronic monitoring in a client's residence. They may also be delivered to a global network of clients located in different countries. A particularly challenging problem is the fragmenting of services, which can result in overuse, underuse, gaps in care, and miscommunication. This can result in costly client outcomes.

Case management differs between urban and rural settings. In the rural setting, where the population is more spread out, there are fewer organized community-based systems and the distance to the delivery site is often greater. Furthermore, the economics, pace and style of life, values, and social organization all differ. In a recent study by Stanton and Dunkin (2002), rural residents identified four barriers to access to care that confront case managers in rural areas: lack of proximity to providers, limited services, scarcity of providers, and reduced available emergency and acute care services. Transportation, both for nurses and for clients, and lack of health insurance and benefits were documented challenges to rural clients of case managers. These were also identified by Waitzkin, Williams, and Bock (2002) as problems for rural clients in managed care systems.

**DID YOU KNOW?**

Although the activities in case management may differ among providers and clients, the following four goals are shared.
- To promote quality in the services provided to populations
- To reduce institutional care while maintaining quality processes and satisfactory outcomes
- To manage resource utilization through the use of protocols, evidence-based decision making, guidelines utilization, and disease management programs
- To control expenses by managing care processes and outcomes

Modified from Flarey DL, Blancett SS: Case management: delivering care in the age of managed care. In Flarey DL, Blancett SS, editors: *Handbook of nursing case management: health care delivery in a world of managed care,* Gaithersburg, Md, 1996, Aspen.

## Case Management and the Nursing Process

The community-oriented nurse views the process of case management through the broader health status of the community. Clients and families receiving service represent the microcosm of health needs within the larger community. Through a nurse's case management activities, general community deficiencies in quality and quantity of health services are often discovered. For example, the management of a severely disabled child by a nurse case manager may uncover the absence of respite services or parenting support and education resources in a community. While managing the disability and injury claims within a corporation, the nurse may discover that alternative care referrals for home health visits and physical therapy are generally underused by the acute care providers in the community. Through a nurse's case management of brain-injured young adults, the absence of community standards

**Table 19-1   The Nursing Process and Case Management**

| NURSING PROCESS | CASE MANAGEMENT PROCESS | ACTIVITIES |
|---|---|---|
| Assessment | • Case finding<br>• Identification of incentives for the target population<br>• Screening and intake<br>• Determination of eligibility<br>• Assessment | • Develop networks with target population<br>• Disseminate written materials<br>• Seek referrals<br>• Apply screening tools according to program goals and objectives<br>• Use written and on-site screens<br>• Apply comprehensive assessment methods (physical, social, emotional, cognitive, economic, and self-care capacity) |
| Diagnosis | • Identification of the problem | • Hold interdisciplinary, family, and client conferences<br>• Determine conclusion on basis of assessment<br>• Use interdisciplinary team |
| Planning/outcome | • Problem prioritizing<br>• Planning to address care needs | • Validate and prioritize problems with all participants<br>• Develop activities, time frames, and options<br>• Gain client's consent to implement<br>• Have client choose options |
| Implementation | • Advocating of clients' interests | • Contact providers<br>• Negotiate services and price |
| Evaluation | • Arrangement of delivery of service<br>• Monitoring of clients during service<br>• Reassessment | • Coordinate service delivery<br>• Monitor for changes in client or service status<br>• Examine outcomes against goals<br>• Examine needs against service<br>• Examine costs<br>• Examine satisfaction of client, providers, and case manager |

and legislative policy for helmet use by bicyclists and motorcyclists may be revealed, stimulating advocacy efforts for changing community policy. Case management activities with individual clients and families will reveal the broader picture of health services and health status of the community. Community *assessment, policy development,* and *assurance* activities that frame core functions of public health actions are often the logical next steps for a community-oriented nurse's practice. When observing lack of care or services at the individual and family intervention levels, the nurse can, through case management, intervene at the community level to make changes. Clearly, the core components of case management and the nursing process are complementary (Table 19-1).

**NURSING TIP**

Use the components of the nursing process when executing the functions of a case manager with clients.

Secord's (1987) classic illustration of case management remains an appropriate picture of the process that nurses use (Figure 19-1). The CMSA model is also illustrative of the case manager's process (Figure 19-2).

## Characteristics and Roles

Case management can be labor intensive, time consuming, and costly. Because of the increasing number of clients with complex problems in nurses' caseloads, the intensity and duration of activities required to support the case management function may soon exceed the demands of direct caregiving. Managers and clinicians in community health are exploring methods to make case management more efficient. In an earlier effort to achieve efficiency (Weil and Karls, 1985), the characteristics desired for case manager effectiveness were described. These characteristics, which incorporated the four CMSA activities (previously noted under the heading Concepts of Case Management), are used today (CMSA, 2002):

1. The technical qualifications to understand and evaluate specific diagnoses, generally requiring clinical credentials (and experience) and financial analyses
2. Capability in language and terminology (able to understand and then to explain to others in simple terms)
3. Assertiveness and diplomacy with people at all levels
4. The ability to *assess* situations objectively and to *plan* appropriate case management services

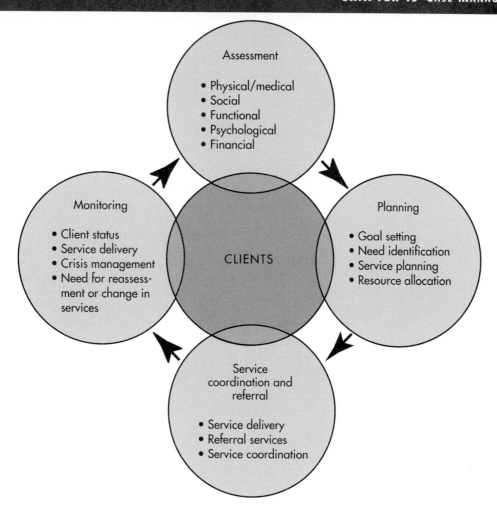

**Figure 19-1** Core components of case management. *(From Secord LJ: Private case management for older persons and their families, Excelsior, Minn, 1987, Interstudy.)*

5. Knowledge of available resources and of the strengths and weaknesses of each
6. The ability to act as *advocate* for the client and payer in models relying on third-party payment
7. The ability to act as a counselor or *facilitator* to clients in providing support, understanding, information, and intervention

Cary (1998) and Llewellyn and Moreo (2001) have described the roles that case managers assume in the practice setting (Box 19-1). The roles demanded of the community-oriented nurse as case manager are greatly influenced by the forces that support or detract from the role. Figure 19-3 presents factors that demand the attention of both the nurse and the client during the case management process.

## Knowledge and Skill Requisites

Community-oriented nurses do not automatically adopt the role of case manager. First, they develop and refine the knowledge and skills that are essential to implementing the role successfully. Stanton and Dunkin (2002), Llewellyn and Moreo (2001), and Cary (1998) suggest

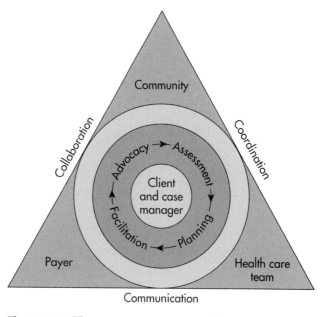

**Figure 19-2** The case management model. *(Permission to reprint granted by the Case Management Society of America, Standards of Practice for Case Management, Little Rock, Ark, p. 6, 2002 CMSA. All rights reserved.)*

**BOX 19-1** **Case Manager Roles**

**Broker:** Acts as an agent for provider services that are needed by clients to stay within coverage according to budget and cost limits of health care plan

**Consultant:** Case managers who work with providers, suppliers, the community, and other case managers to provide case management expertise in programmatic and individual applications

**Coordinator:** Arranges, regulates, and coordinates needed health care services for clients at all necessary points of services

**Educator:** Educates client, family, and providers about case management process, delivery system, community health resources, and benefit coverage so that informed decisions can be made by all parties

**Facilitator:** Supports all parties in work toward mutual goals

**Liaison:** Provides a formal communication link among all parties concerning the plan of care management

**Mentor:** Case managers who counsel and guide the development of the practice of new case managers

**Monitor/reporter:** Provides information to parties on status of member and situations affecting patient safety, care quality, and patient outcome, and on factors that alter costs and liability

**Negotiator:** Negotiates the plan of care, services, and payment arrangements with providers; uses effective collaboration and team strategies

**Patient advocate:** Acts as advocate, provides information, and supports benefit changes that assist member, family, primary care provider, and capitated systems

**Researcher:** Case managers who utilize and apply evidence-based practices for programmatic and individual interventions with clients and communities, participate in protection of clients in research studies, and initiate/collaborate in research programs and studies

**Standardization monitor:** Formulates and monitors specific, time-sequenced critical path and care map plans (see text) and disease management protocols that guide the type and timing of care to comply with predicted treatment outcomes for the specific client and conditions; attempts to reduce variation in resource use; targets deviations from standards so adjustments can occur in a timely manner

**Systems allocator:** Distributes limited health care resources according to a plan or rationale

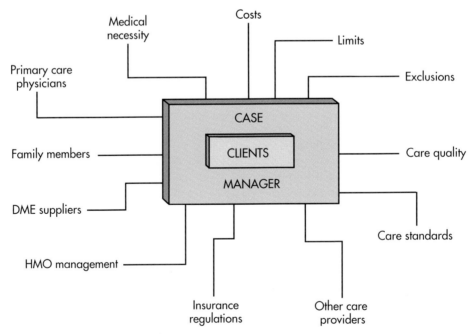

**Figure 19-3** Forces affecting solutions in the case management process. *(Hicks LL, Stallmeyer JM, Coleman JR:* The role of the nurse in managed care, *Washington, DC, 1993, American Nurses Publishing.)*

## BOX 19-2 Knowledge Domains for Case Management

- Knowledge of health care financial environment and the financial dimension of client populations managed by nurses
- Clinical knowledge, skill, and maturity to direct quality-induced timing and sequencing of care activities
- Care resources for clients within institutions and communities: facilitating the development of new resources and systems to meet clients' needs
- Transition planning for ideal timing and sequencing of care
- Management skills: communication, delegation, persuasion, use of power, consultation, problem solving, conflict management, confrontation, negotiation, management of change, marketing, group development, accountability, authority, advocacy, ethical decision making, and profit management
- Teaching, counseling, and education skills
- Program evaluation and research
- Performance improvement techniques
- Peer consultation and evaluation
- Requirements of eligibility and benefit parameters by third-party payers
- Legal issues
- Information systems: clinical and management
- Health care legislation/policy
- Technical information skills
- Outcomes management and applied research

## HOW TO Learn About Telehealth Interventions for Clients

To learn more about telehealth interventions for clients, case managers can do the following:

- Make it a point to learn how telehealth works in your community.
- Consider telehealth as an option when considering available resources.
- Seek continuing education courses that will educate you on the art and science of telehealth application.
- Seek networking opportunities with professional organizations and other case managers about the uses of telehealth.
- Improve your personal interaction skills to better assist in decision making about the use of telehealth services.

From Wrinn MM: The emerging role of telehealth in health care, *Continuing Care* 17(8):18-22, 40, 1998.

knowledge domains useful for nurses in systems desiring to implement quality case management roles (Box 19-2).

When a community health nurse seeks a case manager position, some of the skills and knowledge will need to be acquired through academic and continuing education programs, literature reviews, and orientation and mentoring experiences. Basic nursing education may need to be updated, and practical experiences in case management may be required.

## Tools of Case Managers

The five "rights" of case management are right care, time, provider, setting, and price. How does the nurse judge the effectiveness of case management? Three tools are useful for case management practice: case management plans, disease management, and life care planning tools.

**Case management plans** have evolved through various terms and methods (e.g., critical paths, critical pathways, care maps, multidisciplinary action plans, nursing care plans). Regardless of the title given, standards of client care, standards of nursing practice, standards of practice, and clinical guidelines using evidence-based practices for

case management serve as core foundations of case management plans. Likewise, in multidisciplinary action plans, core professional standards of each discipline guide the developing of the standard process.

As early as 1985, the New England Medical Center in Boston instituted a system of critical path development to guide the case management process in the acute care setting. A **critical path** is a case management tool composed of abbreviated versions of discipline-specific processes; it is used to achieve a measurable outcome for a specific client "case" (Zander, Etheredge, and Bower, 1987). The critical path details the essential and sequential activities in care, so that the expected progress of the client is known at a point in time. Outcomes from critical paths can include satisfaction, client competency, continuity of care, continuity of information, and costs and quality of care. However, a criticism is that critical paths are rarely evidence based (Renholm, Leino-Kilpi, and Suominen, 2002). The prevailing method of establishing critical paths is by internal, "expert knowledge" from a specific institution, the result being that they cannot be applied generally or tested under systematic, scientific methods (Baily, Litaker, and Mion, 1998). In the New England model, key incidents included consults, tests, activities, treatments, medication, diet, discharge planning, and teaching. The paths showed the differences between clients' progress. However, the paths are not revised unless a body of evidence is found to adjust the expected actions.

Care maps became the second generation of critical pathways of care. As described by Zander and McGill (1994), a **CareMaps tool** is a "cause-and-effect grid which identifies expected patient/family and staff behaviors against a timeline for a case-type or otherwise defined

## Evidence-Based Practice

Info-Santé Local Community Service Center (CLSC), the Québec telenursing service, is a telephone health-line nursing service that was implemented in 1995 in 141 community service centers. It operates in continuity with the other resources in the health and social service system. Info-Santé CLSC operates 24 hours a day, 7 days a week, and it received more than 2,260,000 calls in 1997. This report describes the findings from the first province-wide survey of the service, based on a stratified random sample of 4696 callers.

Info-Santé CLSC provides the population of Québec with a first-line response to their physical, psychosocial, and mental health needs. The telenursing protocols used by Info-Santé CLSC are based on a holistic approach to health and have various functions: once nurses have greeted callers and assessed their situation, they provide the relevant information about health, social, and community services; they give professional advice when there is no need for specialized or immediate intervention; and finally, they refer callers to the most appropriate resources when needed.

The descriptive survey evaluation was performed to assess, among other factors, the capacity of the service to develop self-care abilities among users. The services were perceived as useful and effective for solving problems, and as helping respondents develop a feeling of self-reliance. It would seem that telenursing leads to two factors that predispose the adoption of health care behaviors: perceived self-efficacy and perceived behavior effectiveness.

**Nurse Use:** The findings revealed that most respondents were highly satisfied with the service; they followed the nurses' advice and carried out self-care measures as recommended. Nursing interventions helped respondents feel self-reliant, and that they could solve the same or similar problems should they occur in the future.

Hagan L, Morin D, Lepine R: Evaluation of telenursing outcomes: satisfaction, self-care practices, and cost savings, *Public Health Nurs* 17(4):305-313, 2000.

---

The timeline plan can be in hours, days, weeks, or months. **Variance** is the difference between what is expected and what is occurring with the client. Cohen and Cesta (1993) describe variances as *operational* (broken equipment, staffing mix, delays, lost documentation), health care *provider* (variance in provider practice, level of expertise/experience), client (client refusal to accept care, lack of availability, change in status), and *unmet clinical quality indicators*. Variance data are useful in understanding why expected client outcomes and indicators have not been met, and they allow early correction of the care process.

The adapting of the case management care plan to each client's characteristics is a crucial skill for standardizing the process and outcome of care. It links multiple provider interventions to client responses and offers reasonable predictions to clients about health outcomes. Institutions report that sharing case management plans with clients empowers the clients to assume responsibility for monitoring and adhering to the plan of care. Self-responsibility by clients incorporates autonomy and self-determination as the core of case management. For the community-oriented nurse employed to function as a case manager, ample opportunity exists to develop, test, and revise critical path prototypes for a target population experiencing acute health problems.

Disease management is an organized program of services for all clients with specific conditions such as cancer, depression, asthma, or diabetes. For clients with conditions such as these, disease management programs may contain the following (LaPensee, 1997; McClatchey, 2001):

- Case management and **risk sharing** arrangements between payers and providers
- Programs for monitoring the use of prescriptions and treatment interventions, to assess outcomes and costs
- Protocols for clinical and administrative processes
- Education initiatives to meet the learning needs of both clients and providers about knowledge of cost-effective treatments
- Interventions to modify health behaviors and increase compliance with treatment regimens

Clients with chronic diseases benefit from a disease management approach, as the goals are to interrupt continued development of a disease and prevent future disease and complications through secondary and tertiary prevention interventions. Promotion of wellness is necessary for success (McClinton, 1998a). Research has shown that disease management programs promote greater control of signs and symptoms in clients (Solberg et al, 1997). Disease management programs also reduce emergency department visits and school absences (McClatchey, 2001). As the science of disease management evolves to predict direct relationships between outcomes and protocols of care, case managers will be able to ensure cost-effective, optimal clinical care across the continuum—a goal of care management for populations. In fact, disease management is viewed as a top strategy by employers; compared

homogeneous population" (p. 4). The four components of the care maps tool are (1) index of problems with intermediate and outcome criteria, (2) timeline, (3) critical path, and (4) variance record (client differences). **Outcome criteria** are the measurable health goals to be achieved on the basis of the problems presented by the client's condition of health or illness. **Intermediate criteria** are incremental (step-by-step), measurable incidents that serve to monitor progress toward outcomes. **Timelines** are landmarks of an episode of health or illness care from initial encounter to client self-care. Timelines with standard nursing (and other discipline) diagnoses and outcomes constitute the map.

to traditional wellness programs, a disease management industry program produces a higher level of wellness among employees in a shorter time (AHA, 2002). For case managers, disease management strategies, which are part of the care management programs, shift the client interventions from specific, episodic care to holistic care functions that are proactive and population based (Rieve, 1998; Ward and Rieve, 1995). The Joint Commission on the Accreditation of Healthcare Organizations (JCAHO) certifies and the American Accreditation HealthCare Commission accredits disease management organizations and programs on the basis of their respective standards (see websites www.jcaho.org, www.urac.org). This may influence the choice of programs a case manager selects to use with clients.

**Life care planning** is another tool used in case management. It assesses the current and future needs of a client for catastrophic or chronic disease over a life span. The life care plan is a customized, medically based document that provides assessment of all present and future needs (medical, financial, psychological, vocational, spiritual, physical, and social), including services, equipment, supplies, and living arrangements for a client (Llewellyn and Moreo, 2001). These plans may be used by either plaintiff or defense lawyer to analyze damages. They are also used to set financial rewards, which can be used to pay for care in the future and create a lifetime care plan. Life care plans are typically used for clients experiencing catastrophic illness or adverse events resulting from professional malpractice. A systematic process is used and multidisciplinary input is required. The first phase of the plan is crafted to include a thorough assessment of the client, financial/billing agreements, an information release signed by the client, and a targeted date for report completion. Development of the plan is the second phase. Case management plans are based on a number of factors: social situation, leisure activities, educational and employment status, medical history, physical abilities, current status, and assistance required for daily living. The plan includes projected costs and resources needed for the frequency and duration of treatments, equipment, and supplies. It also includes plans for future evaluations. The life care plan seeks to portray the needs of a client that are consistent with the changes in a client's life over the predicted life span, taking into account the injury or diagnosis (McKinley and Zasler, 1998).

## PUBLIC HEALTH AND COMMUNITY-BASED EXAMPLES OF CASE MANAGEMENT

Carondelet Health at St. Mary's Hospital in Tucson, Arizona, has developed a community nursing network in which enrollees are distributed among a number of community health centers. Professional nurse case managers assist older clients to attain healthier lifestyles and maintain themselves in the community. Nurses have been successful in delivering economical services per month for Medicare enrollees. Through nurse case management services, this nursing HMO was reported to have reduced the number of inpatient days per 1000 enrollees by one third, at an average cost of $900 per day, for a savings of $300,000 for every 1000 enrollees (ANA, 1993; American Nurses Foundation, 1993).

Community-based statewide programs in New Jersey use case management methods to promote early identification, selection, evaluation, diagnosis, and treatment of children who are potentially physically compromised. Local case management units provide coordinated and comprehensive care. Collaboration with existing local and regional agencies serving children supports this process. The nurse case manager (1) provides counseling and education to parents and children about identifying problems and increasing their knowledge, (2) develops individual plans incorporating multidisciplinary services (education, social issues, medical development, rehabilitation), (3) obtains appropriate community services, (4) acts as a family resource in crises and service concerns, (5) facilitates communication between child and family, and (6) monitors services for outcomes. Interdisciplinary teams include public health nurses and social workers (with master's degrees) for larger caseloads. A recommended caseload is 300 to 350 children per case manager (Bower, 1992).

The case management program for persons with acquired immunodeficiency syndrome (AIDS) pioneered at San Francisco General Hospital focused on the support of community-based outpatient services. These services were developed to reduce dependency on unnecessary hospital admission and length of stay, using community-based services and brokering with a strong network of community services: housing, home, hospice delivery, and respite care. The San Francisco Department of Public Health used its positive reputation with the gay community to plan, develop, and evaluate care (Bower, 1992; Foster and Hall, 1986).

A national study of 2437 people who tested positive for human immunodeficiency virus (HIV) and who have case managers demonstrated that, regardless of the model, these patients were more likely to be using life-prolonging HIV medications and meeting the needs for income, health insurance, home care, and supportive emotional counseling than those without case management. Having contact with a case manager was not significantly related to use of outpatient care, hospital admission, or emergency department visits. Case managers in this study example included social workers, nurses, and AIDS service organization staff (Katz et al, 2001).

Liberty Mutual Insurance Company has used case management principles for more than 30 years in workers' compensation cases and has expanded services for employees whose conditions were noted as chronic or catastrophic (Box 19-3). Case managers coordinate all clients, providers, and services to reduce expenses caused by lack of coordination, failure to use beneficial alternatives, duplicating, and fragmenting of services (Bower, 1992).

## BOX 19-3 Examples of Case-Managed Conditions

- Acquired immunodeficiency syndrome (AIDS)
- Amputations
- Cerebrovascular accident (CVA)
- Chronic diseases and disabilities
- Coma
- High-risk neonates
- Multiple fractures
- Severe burns
- Severe head trauma
- Spinal cord injury
- Substance abuse
- Terminal illness
- Transplantation
- Ventilator dependency
- Work-related injuries

Important guidance in developing a community-based case management program can be found in the United States. Case management is a key component of federally financed and many state-financed health delivery options. The experiences of states over the past two decades provide testimony to the importance of case management for populations at risk. For older clients, state-derived case management provides objective advice and assistance with care needs. It also provides access to multidisciplinary providers and services. For payers (federal, state, clients), case management serves as a way to ensure that funds are allocated appropriately to those in greatest need. Case management serves a policy assurance and accountability function for communities.

Within the states, the types of agencies designated to conduct case management are often district offices of state government, area agencies on aging, county social services departments, and private contractors. States maintain the oversight responsibilities for case management agencies to (1) ensure they are complying with program standards, contracts, reporting, and fiscal controls; (2) identify emerging problems and issues to be resolved by additional state policies; and (3) provide on-site technical assistance and consulting to improve performance. States' payment methods for case management include daily/monthly rates, hourly/quarterly rates, capped rates for services, and capped aggregate rates to cover both case management and provider costs (Congressional Research Service, 1993).

The models of case management delivery vary. Taylor (1999) describes three models by their focus: client, system, and social service. *Client-focused models* are concerned with the relationship between case manager and client to support continuity of care and to access providers of care, as in the case of the Carle Clinic's Association Community Nursing Organization (Schroeder and Britt, 1997). Another example is the case of the public health nurse working with the chronically ill and families with young children needing age-specific health maintenance (Kaiser et al, 1997).

*System-focused models,* in contrast, address the structure and processes of using the population-based tools of disease management and critical pathways to offer care for client populations. The *social service models* provide services to clients to assist them in living independently in the community and in maintaining their health by eliminating or reducing the need for hospital admissions or long-term care.

These models offer a solution to unnecessary health care expenses by reducing costs and accessing appropriate health care services. Imagine the impact on health status if these saved resources were shifted to primary prevention and health promotion activities.

## HOW TO Ensure High-Quality Care

According to the president's Advisory Commission on Consumer Protection and Quality (1997), the following actions can ensure high-quality care for clients and should be used by case managers in their practice:

- Provide access to easily understood information for each client
- Provide access to appropriate specialists
- Ensure continuity of care for those with chronic and disabling conditions
- Provide access to emergency services when and where needed
- Disclose financial incentives that could influence medical decisions and outcomes
- Prohibit "gag clauses" (which mean that providers cannot inform clients of all possible treatment options)
- Provide antidiscrimination protections
- Provide internal and external appeal processes to solve grievances of clients

Modified from McClinton DH: Protecting patients, *Continuing Care* 17(7):6, 1998b.

## ESSENTIAL SKILLS FOR CASE MANAGERS

Three skills are essential to the role performance of the case manager: advocacy, conflict management, and collaboration.

### Advocacy

For community-oriented nurses, **advocacy** involves a number of activities, ranging from exploring self-awareness to lobbying for health policy. Advocacy is essential for practice with clients and their families, communities, organizations, and colleagues on an interdisciplinary team. The functions of advocacy require scientific knowledge, expert communication, facilitating skills, and problem-solving and affirming techniques. As the *Code of Ethics for Nurses* (ANA, 2001) states, "The nurse establishes relationships and delivers nursing services with respect. . . . Such consideration does not suggest that the nurse necessarily agrees with or condones certain individual choices, but rather that the nurse respects the client as a person" (p. 7). However, this goal is a contemporary one. The perspective regarding the advocacy function has shifted through time. The nurse advocate has been described in earlier writings as one who acted on behalf of or interceded for the client (Nelson, 1988). An example of the nurse interacting on behalf of the client is the community-oriented nurse who calls for a well-child appointment for a mother visiting the family planning clinic when the mother is capable of making an appointment on her own.

The advocate role evolved to that of mediator and is described as a response to the complex configuration of social change, reimbursers, and providers in the health care system (Winslow, 1984). Mediating is an activity in which a third party attempts to provide assistance to those who may be experiencing a conflict in obtaining what they desire. The goal of the nurse advocate as mediator is to assist parties to understand each other on many levels so that agreement on an action is possible. In the example of a nurse as case manager for an HMO, mediating activities between an older adult client and the payer (the HMO) could accomplish the following results: the client may understand the options for community-based skilled nursing care, and the payer may understand the client's desires for a less restrictive environment for care, such as the home. The case manager as mediator does not decide the plan of action but facilitates the decision-making processes between the client and the payee so that the desired care can be reimbursed within the options available.

In contemporary practice, the nurse advocate places the client's rights as the focus of highest priority. The goal of promoter for the client's autonomy and self-determination may result in an optimal degree of independence in decision making. For example, when a group of young pregnant women is the collective "client" (the aggregate), the nurse advocate's role may be to inform the group of the benefits and consequences of breastfeeding their infants. However, if the new mothers decide on formula feeding, the nurse advocate should support the group and continue to provide parenting, infant, and well-child services. This example shows a different perspective of the nurse as advocate. It holds that the nurse's role as advocate may demand a variety of functions that are influenced by the client's physical, psychological, social, and environmental abilities.

The nurse adapts the advocacy function to the client's dynamic capabilities as the client moves from one health state to another. Even clients who desire access to more substantial health promotion activities can benefit from a partnership with the nurse advocate. As Yarmo (1998) indicates, case managers will be called on to mediate between client needs and payer requirements/economic constraints without becoming a barrier to quality care. Examples of advocacy in such cases might include promoting a client group's access to on-site physical fitness programs in the occupational setting, or supporting parents' and students' concerns about the high-fat content of vending machine food in the school system. With the cost of health care exceeding a trillion dollars annually and consumers assuming a larger financial portion of the care they choose, the promoter role of advocacy for those clients capable of autonomy is expected to increase.

## THE CUTTING EDGE

Pharmaceutical companies may have a program of free supplies of drugs for clients who have no health coverage or who do not qualify for other programs. Call a pharmaceutical company for information about clients' eligibility.

## Process of Advocacy

The goal of advocacy is to promote self-determination in a **constituency.** The constituency may be a client, family, peer, group, or community. The classic process of advocacy was defined by Kohnke (1982) to include informing, supporting, and affirming. All three activities are more complex than they may initially seem, and they require self-reflection by the nurse as well as skill development. It is often easier for the nurse to inform, support, and affirm another person's decision when it is consistent with the nurse's values. When clients make decisions within their value systems that are different from the nurse's values, the advocate may feel conflict about contributing to the process of informing, supporting, and affirming those decisions. Promoting self-determination in others demands that the nurse have a philosophy of free choice once the information necessary for decision making has been discussed.

### Informing

Knowledge is essential, but it is not enough to make decisions that affect outcomes. Interpreting knowledge is affected by the client's values and the meanings assigned to the knowledge. Interpreting facts is the result of both objective and subjective processing of information. Subjective processes greatly influence client decisions.

**Informing** clients about the nature of their choices, the content of those choices, and the consequences to the client is not a one-way activity. The **information exchange process** is composed of interactions that reflect three subprocesses: amplifying, clarifying, and verifying. **Amplifying** occurs between the nurse and the client to assess the needs and demands that will eventually frame the client's decision. Information is exchanged from both viewpoints. Although the exchange may be initiated at the objective, factual level, it is likely to proceed to incorporate the subjective perspectives of both parties.

---

**HOW TO** **Provide for Information Exchange Between Nurse and Client**

1. Assess the client's present understanding of the situation.
2. Provide correct information.
3. Communicate with the client's literacy level in mind, making the information as understandable as possible.
4. Use a variety of media and sources to increase the client's comprehension.
5. Discuss other factors that affect the decision, such as financial, legal, and ethical issues.
6. Discuss the possible consequences of a decision.

---

The tone of the amplifying process can direct the remainder of the information exchange. It is important to relate with clients in a manner that reflects the advocate's endorsement of their self-determination. Setting aside the time necessary to listen to clients is critical. Clients will sense they are part of a mutual process if the nurse can engage them during the information exchange with a message that says, "I respect your needs and desires as I share my knowledge with you." Nonverbal behaviors, including using direct eye contact, sitting at the client's level, arriving and concluding at a prescribed time, and employing verbal patterns that foster exchange (e.g., open-ended statements, questions, probes, reflections of feelings, paraphrasing), convey the nurse's desire to promote the client's ability to self-determine.

A client may not desire to exchange information because of lack of self-esteem, fear of the information, or inability to comprehend the content of the communication. In such a case, the focus is to understand the client's desire to be given no information and to express to the client the consequences of such inaction. The nurse may invite the client to ask for the information exchange at a later time, when the client is ready, and can periodically check with the client whether information exchange and amplifying is desired. In these cases, the nurse should document the implemented nursing actions to reflect the guidelines just discussed. This can reduce the basis for lawsuits and misunderstanding by other parties.

**Clarifying** is a process in which the nurse and client strive to understand meanings in a common way. Clarifying builds on the breadth and depth of the exchange developed in amplifying to determine if the nurse and client understand each other. During this process, misunderstandings and confusions are examined. The goal of clarifying is to avoid confusion between the nurse and the client. To foster clarifying, nurses can use certain verbal prompts:

- "What do you understand about . . . ?"
- "Please tell me more about how you . . . ."
- "I don't think I am clear. Let me explain the situation in another way."
- "As an example, . . ."
- "What other information would be helpful so that we both understand?"

**Verifying** is the process used by the nurse advocate to establish accuracy and reality in the informing process. If the nurse discovers that a client is misinformed, the nurse may return to the clarifying or amplifying stage and begin the process again. Verifying produces the chance for the advocate and client to examine "truth" from their points of view, which may include knowledge, intuition, previous experiences, and anticipated consequences.

Promoting a client's self-determination may take the advocate and client through the information exchange process several times, as new dimensions, or obstacles, to an issue develop. Information exchange is a critical process for advocacy and is applicable to all advocacy clients: individuals, families, groups, and communities.

### Supporting

The second major process, **supporting,** involves upholding a client's right to make a choice and to act on it. People who are aware of clients' decisions fall into three general groups: supporters, dissenters, and obstructers. Supporters approve and support clients' actions. Dissenters do not approve and do not support clients. Obstructers cause difficulties when clients try to implement their decisions.

The nurse advocate needs to implement several actions that fulfill the supporting role. Important interventions are assuring clients that they have the right and responsibility to make decisions, and reassuring them that they do not have to change their decisions because of others' objections (Cary, 1998).

### Affirming

The third process in the advocacy role is **affirming.** It is based on an advocate's belief that a client's decision is consistent with the client's values and goals. The advocate validates that the client's behavior is purposeful and consistent with the choice that was made. The advocate expresses a dedication to the client's mission, and a purposeful exchange of new information may occur so that the client's choice remains possible. Recognizing that a client's needs may fluctuate with changing resources, the affirming activity must encourage a process of reevaluation and rededication to promote client self-determination.

The importance of affirming activities cannot be emphasized strongly enough. Many advocacy activities stop with assuring and reassuring, but affirming is often critical in promoting a client's self-determination. Table 19-2 compares the nursing process with the advocacy process.

**Table 19-2  Comparison of Nursing Process and Advocacy Process**

| NURSING PROCESS | ADVOCACY PROCESS |
| --- | --- |
| Assessment/diagnosis | • Information exchange<br>• Gather data<br>• Illuminate values |
| Planning/outcome | • Generate alternatives and consequences<br>• Prioritize actions |
| Implementation | • Decision making<br>• Support of client<br>• Assure<br>• Reassure |
| Evaluation | • Affirmation<br>• Evaluation<br>• Reformulation |

The advocate's role in the decision-making process is *not* to tell the client that an option is correct or right. The advocate's role is to provide the opportunity for information exchange, and to arm clients with tools that can empower them in making the best decision from their point of view. Enabling clients to make an informed decision is a powerful tool for building self-confidence. It gives clients the responsibility for selecting the options and experiencing the success and consequences of their decisions. Clients are empowered in their decision making when they recognize that although some events are beyond their control, other events are predictable and can be affected by decisions they can make.

Nurses can promote client decision making by using the information exchange process, promoting the use of the nursing process, incorporating written techniques (contracts, lists), using reflecting and prioritizing techniques, and using role playing and sculpturing to "try on" and determine the "fit" of different options and consequences for the client. By engaging clients in the information-sharing process and assisting them to recognize the progression of activities they experience as they build their informed decision-making base, the nurse advocate is empowering clients with skills that can strengthen their autonomy and confidence in the future.

Advocacy is a complex process. There is a delicate balance between doing for and promoting autonomy. The process is influenced by the client's physical, emotional, and social capabilities. The goal of advocacy is to promote the maximum degree of client self-determination, given the client's current and potential status; for most clients, this goal can be realized. When clients are comatose, unborn, or legally incompetent, nurse advocates have unique functions. The advocate's role is usually determined by the legal system; however, in some cases, nurses must decide what roles they will play. These are areas requiring inten-

sive self-exploration, research, and collaboration with professionals, family members, and significant others.

## Skill Development

Skills needed by the nurse advocate are not unique to their profession. Nursing demands technical, relationship, and problem-solving skills. Advocacy applies nursing skills of communication and competency to promote client self-determination.

Knowledge of nursing and other disciplines as well as of human behavior is essential for the advocacy role in establishing authority, authenticity, and developing skills. The capacity to be assertive for personal rights and the rights of others is essential.

## Systematic Problem Solving

The nursing process—assessment, diagnosis, planning, implementing, and evaluating—is an example of a method of **problem solving** that can be used in the advocacy role. Advocates can be particularly helpful with clients in identifying values and generating alternatives.

### Illuminating Values
People's values affect their behavior, feelings, and goals. In the process of amplifying, clarifying, and validating, the advocate understands a client's values. Through the process of self-revelation, an emerging value (environment, people, cost, quality) may become more apparent to a client. This can have an effect in two ways. The client may be able to focus on actions on the basis of the value, or the value may confuse the decision process. The nurse can assist the client in prioritizing action and clarifying the value. Values can also change as new or relevant data are processed. The advocate's role is to assist clients in discovering their values. This process can be particularly demanding in the information exchange and affirming process.

### Generating Alternatives
Clients and advocates may feel limited in their options if they generate solutions before completely analyzing the problems, needs, desires, and consequences. Several techniques can be used to generate alternatives, including brainstorming and a technique known as the problem-purpose–expansion method. In **brainstorming,** the nurse, client, professionals, or significant others generate as many alternatives as possible, without placing a value on them. Brainstorming creates a list that can then be examined for the critical elements the client seeks to preserve (e.g., environmental preferences, degree of control). The list can be analyzed according to the consequences and the effect of the alternatives on self and others.

The **problem–purpose–expansion method,** as described by Volkema (1983), is a way to broaden limited thinking. It involves restating the problem and expanding the problem statement so that different solutions can be generated. For example, if the problem statement is to convince the insurance company to approve a longer hospital stay, the nurse and client have narrowed their options. However, if the problem statement is to improve the client's convalescence and safety, several solutions and options are available, such as the following:

- Obtaining skilled nursing facility placement
- Obtaining home health skilled services
- Arranging physician home visits
- Paying for custodial care
- Paying for private skilled care
- Obtaining informal caregiving

## Impact of Advocacy

Advocacy empowers clients to participate in problem-solving processes and decisions about health care. Clients try to understand changing opportunities in the health care system for access, use, and obtaining continuity of care. Nurse advocates promote client self-determination and management of behavior as it relates to health and the adhering to therapeutic regimens. Clients are part of larger systems: the family, the work environment, and the community. Each system interacts with the client to shape the available options through resources, needs, and desires. Each system also exhibits both confirming and conflicting goals and processes that need to be understood for client self-determination to be successful. For example, the practice of advocacy among minority groups may involve the ability to focus attention on the magnitude of problems caused by diseases affecting minority clients. Whether the client is an individual, family, group, or community, the advocacy function can promote the interest of self-determination, which influences the progress of societies.

Advocacy is not without opposition. Clients and advocates may find barriers to services, vendors, providers, and resources. A community may experience a shortage in nursing home beds, a childcare facility may experience staffing shortages, a family may not have the money to keep a child at home, and a client may find that the school system cannot fund a full-time nurse for its clinic. The reality of scarce resources creates a difficult barrier for advocates. However, it is often events such as these that stimulate a community's self-determination and lead to innovative actions to correct gaps in service (Box 19-4).

## Allocation and Advocacy: Complements or Conundrum?

Whereas advocacy holds a traditional role in the nursing profession, **allocation** is a staple of market competition. Nurses perform allocation roles when they triage clients or perform the gatekeeping and rationing functions. The field of medicine has struggled with the allocation debate, as Mechanic (1997) notes. Nurses often reflect that clinical judgments are influenced by their values and ethics as well as technology and science (American Association of Colleges of Nursing, 1997). When working in organizations, nurses experience allocation demands at the systems level through budgetary decisions and staffing assign-

---

> ### BOX 19-4  Levels of Prevention Applied to Case Management
>
> **PRIMARY PREVENTION**
> Use the information exchange process to increase the client's understanding of how to use the health care system.
> **SECONDARY PREVENTION**
> Use case finding to identify existing health problems.
> **TERTIARY PREVENTION**
> Monitor the use of prescription medications and adherence to treatment to reduce risk of illness complications.

---

ments. At the clinical level, demands relate to implementing treatment protocols. When nurses act as client advocates by clarifying a client's desires or needs, they can conflict with systems procedures for allocation of limited resources within these systems. Case managers need to balance efficient use of resources by comparing costs of alternative options to care, calculating private and public costs of provider services recommended, and monitoring service expenses over time (Geron and Chassler, 1994).

Nurses who shoulder both advocacy and allocation responsibilities may benefit from a clear understanding of their personal and professional values. A systematic procedure for mediating conflict between the two competing responsibilities is also helpful (Cary, 1998).

## Conflict Management

Case managers help clients manage conflicting needs and scarce resources. Techniques for managing conflict include a range of active communication skills. These skills are directed toward learning all parties' needs and desires, detecting their areas of agreement and disagreement, determining their abilities to collaborate, and assisting in discovering alternatives and activities for reaching a goal. Mutual benefit with limited loss is a goal of conflict management.

Conflict and its management vary in intensity and energy in a number of ways. The effort needed to manage a conflict depends on different factors: the existing evidence to support facts, and the objective and subjective perceptions of the parties involved.

**Negotiating** is a strategic process used to move conflicting parties toward an outcome. The outcome can vary from one in which one party gains benefit at the other's expense **(distributive outcomes)**. The outcome may be one in which mutual advantages override individual gains **(integrative outcomes)**. Integrative outcomes are usually based on problem-solving and solution-generating techniques (Bisno, 1988).

The process of negotiating can be characterized in three stages: prenegotiating, negotiating, and aftermath. Prenegotiating activities are designed to have parties agree to collaborate. Parties must see the possibility of agreeing and

BOX 19-5    Categories of Behaviors Used in Conflict Management

**Accommodating:** An individual neglects personal concerns to satisfy the concerns of another.
**Avoiding:** An individual pursues neither his or her concerns nor another's concerns.
**Collaborating:** An individual attempts to work with others toward solutions that satisfy the work of both parties.
**Competing:** An individual pursues personal concerns at another's expense.
**Compromising:** An individual attempts to find a mutually acceptable solution that partially satisfies both parties.

Modified from Thomas KW, Kilmann RH: Thomas-Kilmann conflict mode instrument, New York, 1974, Xicom.

the costs of not agreeing. Preparations must be made as to time, place, and ground rules concerning participants, procedures, and confidentiality.

The negotiation stage consists of phases in which parties must develop trust, credibility, distance from the issue (to limit the feeling of "one best way"), and the ability to retain personal dignity. Bisno (1988) characterizes the phases as the following:

*Phase 1:* Establishing the issues and agenda. This is accomplished by identifying, clarifying, presenting, and prioritizing the issues.
*Phase 2:* Advancing demands and uncovering interests. Negotiations center on presenting parties' interests and differentiating parties' demands and positions on the conflict.
*Phase 3:* Bargaining and discovering new options. Debates include gathering facts based on reasoning that will generate understanding and promote re-learning. Bargaining reduces differences on issues by giving or removing rewards or desired objects. Creating new solutions or options through brainstorming, reflective thinking, and problem–purpose–expansion techniques is important in achieving options that provide mutual benefits.
*Phase 4:* Working out an agreement. This may involve settling on some but not all points. Parties can agree to reexamine the issues later, and steps for implementing and follow-up must be clarified.

The aftermath is the period following an agreement in which parties are experiencing the consequences of their decisions. The reality of their decisions may lead to reevaluating their values. In a conflict situation, parties engage in behaviors that reflect the dimensions of assertiveness and cooperation. **Assertiveness** is the ability to present one's own needs. **Cooperation** is the ability to understand and meet the needs of others. Each person uses a primary and secondary orientation to engage in conflict (Box 19-5). Depending on the situation, each of the behaviors described in Box 19-5 can be used as a primary or secondary behavior, as described by Thomas and Kilmann in 1974.

Clearly, flexibility in conflict management behavior can facilitate an outcome that meets the client's goals. Helping parties navigate the process of attaining a goal requires effective personal relations, knowledge of the situation and alternatives, and a commitment to the process.

## Collaboration

In case management, the activities of many disciplines are needed for success. Clients, the family, significant others, payers, and community organizations contribute to achieving the goal. **Collaboration** is achieved through a developmental process. It occurs in a sequence and is reciprocal (Cary and Androwich, 1989) and can be characterized by seven stages and activities (Figure 19-4).

The goal of communication in the collaborative development process is to amplify, clarify, and verify all team members' points of view. Although communication is essential in collaboration, it is not sufficient to result in or maintain collaboration. Although the collaboration model recognizes the contributions of joint decision making, one member of the team should be accountable to the system and to the client. This team member should be responsible for monitoring the entire process.

Case managers encounter conflict on a daily basis. Competing needs, resources, organizational demands, and professional role boundaries present opportunities and pitfalls for conflict management and collaboration (Box 19-6). Barriers to collaborating effectively include: time restraints, lack of information, and failure to communicate essential, complete information in a timely manner (Birmingham, 2002).

Teamwork and collaborating clearly demand knowledge and skills about clients, health status, resources, treatments, and community providers. The ability to assess clients' and families' complex needs involves knowledge of intrapersonal, interpersonal, medical, nursing, and social dimensions. Demonstrating team member and leadership skills in facilitating a goal-directed group process is essential. It is unlikely that any single professional possesses the

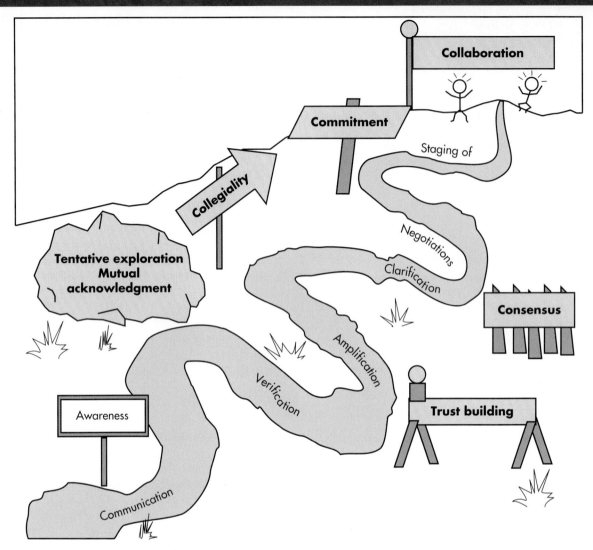

**Figure 19-4** Collaboration is a sequential yet reciprocal process. *(From Cary A, Androwich I: A collaboration model: a synthesis of literature and a research survey, paper presented at the Association of Community Health Nursing Educators Spring Institute, Seattle, June, 1989.*

expertise required in all dimensions. It is likely, however, that the synergy produced by all can result in successful outcomes.

## ISSUES IN CASE MANAGEMENT

### Legal Issues

Liability concerns of case managers exist when three conditions are met: (1) the provider had a duty to provide reasonable care, (2) a breach of contract occurred through an act or an omission to act, and (3) the act or omission caused injury or damage to the client. Case managers must strive to reduce risks, practice wisely within acceptable standards, and limit legal defense costs through professional insurance coverage. Five general areas of risk are reviewed:

1. *Liability for managing care* (Hinden et al, 1994; Llewellyn and Moreo, 2001)
   a. Inappropriate design or implementation of the case management system

   b. Failure to obtain all pertinent records on which case management actions are based
   c. Failure to have cases evaluated by appropriately experienced and credentialed clinicians
   d. Failure to confer directly with the treating provider (physician or nurse practitioner) at the onset and throughout the client's care
   e. Substituting a case manager's clinical judgment for that of the medical provider
   f. Requiring the client or his or her provider to accept case management recommendation instead of any other treatment
   g. Harassment of clinicians, clients, and family in seeking information, and setting unreasonable deadlines for decisions or information
   h. Claiming orally or in writing that the case management treatment plan is better than the provider's plan
   i. Restricting access to otherwise necessary or appropriate care because of cost

BOX 19-6 Stages of Collaboration

1. Awareness
   - Make a conscious entry into a group process; focus on goals of convening together; generate a definition of collaborative process and what it means to team members.
2. Tentative exploration and mutual acknowledgment
   - Exploration: Disclose professional skills for the desired process; disclose areas where contributions cannot be made; disclose values reflecting priorities; identify roles and disclose personal values, including time, energy, interest, and resources.
   - Mutual acknowledgment: Clarify each member's potential contributions; verify the group's strengths and areas needing consultation; clarify member's work style, organizational supports, and barriers to collaborative efforts.
3. Trust building
   - Determine the degree to which reliance on others can be achieved; examine congruence between words and behaviors; set interdependent goals; develop tolerance for ambiguity.
4. Collegiality
   - Define the relationships of members with each other; define the responsibilities and tasks of each; define entrance and exit conditions.
5. Consensus
   - Determine the issues for which consensus is required; determine the processes used for clarifying and decision making to reach consensus; determine the process for reevaluating consensus outcomes.
6. Commitment
   - Realize the physical, emotional, and material actions directed toward the goal; clarify procedures for reevaluating commitments in light of goal demands and group standards for deviance.
7. Collaboration
   - Initiate a process of joint decision making reflecting the synergy that results from combining knowledge and skills.

Modified from Cary A, Androwich I: *A collaboration model: a synthesis of literature and a research survey,* paper presented at the Association of Community Health Nursing Educators Spring Institute, Seattle, June 1989; Mueller WJ, Kell B: *Coping with conflict,* Englewood Cliffs, NJ, 1972, Prentice Hall.

j. Referring clients to treatment furnished by providers related to the case management agency without proper disclosure
k. Connecting case managers' compensation to reduced use and access of services
l. Inappropriate delegation of care
2. *Negligent referrals* (Hyatt, 1994; Llewellyn and Moreo, 2001)
   a. Referral to a practitioner known to be incompetent
   b. Substituting inadequate treatment for an adequate but more costly option
   c. Curtailing treatment inappropriately when treatment was actually needed
   d. Referral to a facility or practitioner inappropriate for the client's needs
   e. Transfer to another facility that lacks care requirements
3. *Experimental treatment and technology* (Saue, 1994)
   a. Failure to apply the contractual definition of "experimental" treatment found in the client's insurance policy
   b. Failure to review sources of information referenced in the applicable insurance policy (e.g., Food and Drug Administration, or published medical literature)
   c. Failure to review the client's complete medical record
   d. Failure to make a timely determination of benefits in light of timeliness of treatment
   e. Failure to communicate coverage determined to be needed, to the insured client or participant
   f. Improper economic considerations determining the coverage
4. *Confidentiality/security* (Llewellyn and Moreo, 2001; Scheutzow, 1994)
   a. Failure to deny access to sensitive information that is awarded special protection by federal or state law
   b. Failure to protect access to computerized medical records
   c. Failure to adhere to regulatory provisions (e.g., Health Insurance Portability and Accountability Act provisions [http://hipaa.cms.gov]; Americans With Disabilities Act)
5. *Fraud and abuse* (Llewellyn and Moreo, 2001; Sollins, 1994)
   a. Making false statements of claims or causing incorrect claims to be filed
   b. Falsifying the adhering to conditions of participation of Medicare and Medicaid
   c. Submitting claims for excessive, unnecessary, or poor-quality services
   d. Engaging in remuneration, bribes, kickbacks, or rebates in exchange for referral
   e. Upcoding intensity of care or intervention requirements

Legal citations relevant to case management and managed care include negligent referrals, provider liability, payer liability, breach of contract, and bad faith. As in any scope of nursing practice, proactive risk management strategies can lower the provider's exposure to legal liability.

Saue (1994) notes that court cases influence the legal considerations of case managers. When courts find that cost considerations affect medical care decisions, all parties to the decision will be liable for resulting damages. Guidelines to reduce risk exposure include the following:

1. Clear documentation of the extent of client participation in decision making and reasons for decisions

---

**BOX 19-7** **Credentialing Resources for Case Managers (Individual Certification Options)**

| Organization | Phone number/website | Credential/initials |
|---|---|---|
| American Nurses Credentialing Center | 1-800-284-2378 | Nurses, RNC or RN, BC for Case Management |
| Case Management Administrators | 212-356-0660, www.ptcny.com | CMA for Case Management Administrators |
| Certification of Disability Management Specialists Commission | 1-847-394-2106 | Multidisciplinary, CDMS for Certified Disability Management Specialist |
| Commission for Case Manager Certification | www.ccmcertification.org | Multidisciplinary, CCM for Certified Case Manager |
| Commission on Disability Examiner Certification (CDEC) | | CDEC for specialty certification for life care planners |
| National Academy of Certified Care Managers | 1-800-962-2260 | Multidisciplinary, CMC for Care Manager Certified |
| National Board for Certification in Continuity of Care | www.ptcny.com | Multidisciplinary, A-CCC for Continuity of Care Certification—Advanced |
| Rehabilitation Nursing Certification Board | 1-800-229-7530 | CRRN for Certified Rehabilitation Registered Nurse |

---

**BOX 19-8** **Websites for Case Management Resources**

| | | |
|---|---|---|
| Advocacy | www.infonet.welch.jhu.edu/advocacy.html | 1-800 numbers for patient organizations |
| AIDS Global Information System | www.aegis.com | Contains largest AIDS library |
| American Accreditation Healthcare Commission (URAC) | www.urac.org | Accredits disease management programs and other services |
| American Association of Health Plans | www.aahp.org | Provides information relevant to managed care organizations |
| American Nurses Credentialing Center | www.nursecredentialing.org | Offers review course materials for case managers preparing for certification exams by any certifying body |
| American Medical Association | www.ama-assn.org | Includes CEU programs |
| Case Management Society of America | www.cmsa.org | Specialty organization for case managers |
| Center for Medicare and Medicaid Services | www.cms.gov | Formerly the Health Care Financing Administration, HCFA. Oversees execution of rules and regulations for clients of state and federally funded services |
| Center Watch Clinical Trial Listing Service | www.centerwatch.com | Reviews all clinical trials in the United States |
| Centers for Disease Control and Prevention | www.cdc.gov | Provides education, training, research for infectious diseases, and on appropriate strategies to prevent disease (e.g., asthma, obesity) |
| Joint Commission on Accreditation of Healthcare Organizations | www.jcaho.org | Accredits delivery organizations |
| Medscape | www.medscape.com | Features clinical updates for professionals |
| National Action Plan on Breast Cancer | www.napbc.org | Provides information on breast cancer |
| National Committee for Quality Assurance | www.ncqa.org | Publishes HEDIS performance indicators for provider systems and accredits managed care organizations |
| National Library of Medicine | www.nlm.nih.gov | |
| Nurseweek | www.nurseweek.com | Provides information links to other sites |
| Oncology | www.oncolink.upenn.edu | Oncology links |
| Online Journal | www.nursingworld.org | Issues in nursing |
| Rehabilitation Accreditation Commission | www.carf.org | Accredits globally the services that may be used by case management clients such as adult day care, assisted living, behavioral health, employment and community services and medical rehabilitation |
| Webster's Death, Dying and Grief | www.katsden.com | Includes link for advance directives, wills, CEU programs, and resource material |

Modified from Cary AH: Managed care. In Lundy K, James S, Hartman S, editors: *Nursing in the community: continuity of care of individuals, families and populations,* Sudbury, Mass, 1999, Jones and Bartlett; Wrinn MM: The emerging role of telehealth in health care, *Continuing Care* 17(8):18-22, 40, 1998.

2. Records demonstrating accurate and complete information on interactions and outcomes
3. Use of reasonable care in selecting referral sources, which may include verifying of licensure of providers
4. Written agreements when arrangements are made to modify benefits other than those in the contract
5. Good communication with clients
6. Informing clients of their rights of appeal

## Ethical Issues

Case managers as nursing professionals are guided in ethical practice by the *Code of Ethics for Nursing* (ANA, 2001), by performance indicator for ethics in the *Standards of Practice for Case Management* (CMSA, 2002), and by the contract expressed in *Nursing's Social Policy Statement* (ANA, 1995, p. 4):

> *Nursing is a caring-based practice in which processes of diagnosis and treatment are applied to the human experiences of health and illness. Nurses are guided by a philosophy of caring and advocacy. Nurses have a high regard for patient self-determination, independence and informed choice in decision making. Recognizing that responses to illness and disability may limit independence and self-determination, nurses focus on the rights of individuals, families and communities to define their own health-related goals and seek out health care that reflects their values.*

This philosophy of nursing practice is ideally suited to preserving the principles of autonomy, beneficence, justice, nonmaleficence and veracity in case management processes. Banja (1994a) and Llewellyn and Moreo (2001) describe how case managers may confront dilemmas in each of these areas.

Case management may hamper a client's **autonomy,** meaning the individual's right to choose a provider, if a particular provider is not approved by the case management system. If a new provider must be found who can be approved for coverage, continuity of care may be disrupted.

**Beneficence,** or doing good, can be impaired when excessive attention to containing costs supersedes the nurse's duty to improve health or relieve suffering. "If cost containment goals are accomplished by diminishing services, at what point do health providers' behaviors subordinate the good of their (clients) to the interests of restraining expenditures?" (Banja, 1994a, p. 39).

**Justice** as an ethical principle for case managers considers equal distribution of health care with reasonable quality. Tiers of quality and expertise among provider groups can be created when quality providers refuse to accept reimbursement allowances from the managed system, leaving less experienced or lower-quality providers as the caregiver of choice for clients being managed.

**Nonmaleficence** is doing no harm. When case managers incorporate outcomes measures, evidence-based practice, and monitoring processes in their plans of care, this principle is addressed.

**Veracity,** or truth telling, is absolutely necessary to the practice of advocacy and building a trusting relationship with clients. Clients particularly complain that in the changing health care system, payers do not seem to be able to provide comprehensive yet inexpensive options for care.

Standards of practice and care, codes of ethics, licensure laws, credentialing through certification, and organizational policies and procedures (e.g., ethics committees, risk management units) offer the case manager information and support in managing ethical conflicts and dilemmas in the case management system. Maintaining familiarity with ethical issues published in the case management literature can offer specific assistance for practicing case managers (Boxes 19-7 and 19-8).

## ▪ Practice Application

During her regularly scheduled blood pressure clinic in a local apartment cluster, Mrs. B., 45 years old, complained of feeling dizzy and forgetful. She could not remember which of her six medications she had taken during the last few days. Her blood pressure readings on reclining, sitting, and standing revealed gross elevation. The nurse and Mrs. B. discussed the danger of her present status and the need to seek medical attention. Mrs. B. called her physician from her apartment and agreed to be transported to the emergency room.

In the emergency room, Mrs. B. manifested the progressive signs and symptoms of a cerebrovascular accident (a CVA, or stroke). During hospitalization, she lost her capacity for expressive language and demonstrated hemiparesis and loss of bladder control. Her cognitive function became intermittently confused, and she was slow to recognize her physician and neighbors who came to visit. The utilization review nurse contacted the case manager from the health department to screen and assess for the continuum of care needs as early as possible, as she lived alone and family members resided out of town.

It became apparent that family caregiving in the community could be only intermittent because family members lived too far away. Mrs. B. had residual functional and cognitive deficits that would demand longer-term care.

As the case manager contracted by the plan, place the following actions in the correct sequence to construct a case management plan:

**A.** Discuss with the family their schedule of availability to offer care in the client's home.
**B.** Call the client and introduce yourself, as a prelude to working with her.
**C.** Obtain information on the scope of services covered by the benefit plan for your client.
**D.** Arrange a skilled nursing facility site visit for the patient and family.

**Answer is in the back of the book.**

## Key Points

- An important role of the community-oriented nurse is that of client advocate.

- The goal of advocacy is to promote the client's self-determination.

- When performing in the advocacy role, conflicts may emerge about the full disclosure of information, territoriality, accountability to multiple parties, legal challenges to clients' decisions, and competition for scarce resources.

- The functions of advocacy and allocation can pose dilemmas in practice.

- Amplification, clarification, and verification are three communication skills necessary in the advocacy process.

- Additional skills important to fulfilling the role of client advocate include the helping relationship, assertiveness, and problem solving.

- Problem solving is a systematic approach that includes understanding the values of each party and generating alternative solutions.

- Brainstorming and the problem–purpose–expansion method are two techniques to enhance the effectiveness of problem-solving skills.

- During conflict, negotiations can move conflicting parties toward an outcome.

- Prenegotiation, negotiation, and aftermath are three phases of managing a conflict.

- Each individual has a predominant orientation when engaging in conflict: competing, accommodating, avoiding, collaborating, or compromising.

- Collaboration may result by moving through seven stages: awareness, tentative exploration and mutual acknowledgment, trust building, collegiality, consensus, commitment, and collaboration.

- Care management is a strategic program to maintain the health of a population enrolled in a delivery system.

- Continuity of care is a goal of community-oriented nursing practice. It requires making linkages with services to improve the client's health status.

- As the structure of the health care system moves toward delivering more services in the community, the achievement of continuity of care will present a greater challenge.

- Case management is typically an interdisciplinary process in which the client is the focus of the plan.

- Documentation of case management activities and outcomes are essential to community-oriented nursing practice.

- Case management is a systematic process of assessment, planning, service coordination, referral, monitoring, and evaluation that meets the multiple service needs of clients.

- Community-oriented nurses have within their scope of practice advocacy, allocation, and case management functions.

- Nurses functioning as advocates and case managers need to be aware of the ethical and legal issues confronting these components of their practice.

- Standardization of care for predictable outcomes can be achieved through critical paths, disease management protocols, and multidisciplinary action plans.

- Telehealth application provides new alternatives within resource delivery options but must be customized for clients.

## Clinical Decision-Making Activities

1. Observe a typical workday of a community health nurse, noting the types of activities that are done in coordination and case management, as well as the amount of time spent in these areas. Interview several staff members to determine whether they perceive that their time spent in case management is changing. To what degree are the staff members involved in care management activities?

2. Initiating, monitoring, and evaluating resources are essential components of community health nursing practice. Describe a client situation and the case management process that might occur in the following practices:
   a. A school nurse in an elementary school and one in a high school
   b. An occupational health nurse in a hospital and one in a manufacturing plant
   c. A nurse working in a well-child clinic
   d. A case manager employed by a managed care organization
   e. A care manager employed in a health benefits corporation

3. The values and beliefs held by a community health nurse influence the nurse's ability to be an advocate for clients. Discuss your values and beliefs about rationing health care and how they may affect your ability to be a client advocate.

4. Read the following article: Cary A: Advocacy or allocation, *Nursingconnections* 11(1):35-40, 1998. Discuss your reactions to the statement, "Allocation always works within the mixed interests of the individual and society" (p. 39).
   a. What are the mixed values of individuals?
   b. What are the mixed values of delivery systems?
   c. What are the mixed values of society in the United States? In underdeveloped nations?

**Additional Resources**

These related resources are found either in the appendix at the back of this book or on the book's website at **http://evolve.elsevier.com/Stanhope.**

**evolve** **Evolve Website**

WebLinks: Healthy People 2010

# References

Advisory Commission on Consumer Protection and Quality in the Health Care Industry: *Consumer bill of rights and responsibilities—report to the president of the United States,* Washington, DC, 1997, U.S. Government Printing Office.

Aliotta S: Coordination of care, *Case Manager* 14(2):49-52, 2003.

American Association of Colleges of Nursing: T*he essentials of baccalaureate education for professional nursing practice,* Washington, D.C., 1997, AACN.

American Hospital Association: *Glossary of terms and phrases for health care coalitions,* Chicago, 1986, AHA Office of Health Coalitions and Private Sector Initiatives.

American Hospital Association: URAC announces new disease management standards, retrieved from www.ahanews.com, July 15, 2002.

American Nurses Association: *Managed care: cornerstone for health care reform—a fact sheet,* Washington, DC, 1993, ANA.

American Nurses Association: *Nursing's social policy statement,* Washington, DC, 1995, ANA.

American Nurses Association: *Code of ethics for nurses,* Washington, DC, 2001, ANA.

American Nurses Foundation: *America's nurses: an untapped natural resource,* Washington, DC, 1993, ANF.

Baily D, Litaker D, Mion L: Developing better critical paths in health care: combining "best practice" and the quantitative approach, *J Nurs Adm* 8(7/8):21-26, 1998.

Banja JD: Ethical challenges of managed care, *Case Manager* 5(3):37-40, 1994a.

Banja JD: Ethical dimensions of cultural diversity in case management, *Case Manager* 5(4):27-29, 1994b.

Birmingham J: Managing the dynamics of collaboration, *Case Manager* 13(3):73-77, 2002.

Bisno H: *Managing conflict,* Beverly Hills, Calif, 1988, Sage.

Bower KA: Case management by nurses, Washington, DC, 1992, American Nurses' Association.

Cary AH: Advocacy or allocation, *Nursingconnections* 11(1):1-7, 1998.

Cary AH: Managed care. In Lundy K, James S, Hartman S, editors: *Nursing in the community: continuity of care of individuals, families and populations,* Sudbury, Mass, 1999, Jones and Bartlett.

Cary A, Androwich I: *A collaboration model: a synthesis of literature and a research survey,* paper presented at the Association of Community Health Nursing Educators Spring Institute, Seattle, June 1989.

Case Management Society of America: *Standards of practice for case management,* Little Rock, Ark, 2002, CMSA.

Cohen EL, Cesta TG: *Nursing case management: from concept to evaluation,* St Louis, Mo, 1993, Mosby.

Coleman JR, Zagor KB: Effective care management, *Contin Care* 17(7):64, 1991.

Congressional Research Service: *Case management standards in state community-based long-term care programs for older persons with disabilities,* CRS-91-55, Washington, DC, 1993, CRS, Library of Congress.

Flarey DL, Blancett SS: Case management: delivering care in the age of managed care. In Flarey DL, Blancett SS, editors: *Handbook of nursing case management: health care delivery in a world of managed care,* Gaithersburg, Md, 1996, Aspen.

Foster J, Hall H: Public health and AIDS, *Caring* 5(6):4-11, 73-78, 1986.

Geron S, Chassler D: *Guidelines for case management practice across the longterm care continuum,* Boston, 1994, Boston University School of Social Work.

Hagan L, Morin D, Lepine R: Evaluation of telenursing outcomes: satisfaction, self-care practices, and cost savings, *Public Health Nurs* 17(4):305-313, 2000.

Hicks LL, Stallmeyer JM, Coleman JR: *The role of the nurse in managed care,* Washington, DC, 1993, American Nurses' Publishing.

Hinden RA et al: Legal hazards on the case management highway, *Case Manager* 5(3):97-111, 1994.

Hyatt TK: Negligent referral, *Case Manager* 5(3):102-106, 1994.

James M: At the heart of the disease management revolution, *Case Manager* 9(2):47-50, 1998.

Kaiser KL et al: Patterns of health resource utilization, costs, and intensity of need for primary care clients receiving public health nursing case management, *Nurs Case Manag* 4(2):53-62, 1997.

Katz MH et al: The effects of case management on unmet needs and utilization of medical care and medications among HIV-infected persons, *Ann Intern Med* 135(8):557-565, 2001.

Kenyon V et al: Clinical competencies for community health nursing, *Public Health Nurs* 7(1):33-39, 1990.

Kohnke MF: *Advocacy risk and reality,* St Louis, Mo, 1982, Mosby.

LaPensee KT: Pricing specialty carve-outs and disease management programs under managed care, *Manag Care Q* 5(2):10-19, 1997.

Llewellyn A, Moreo K: *The essence of case management,* Washington, DC, 2001, American Nurses Credentialing Center.

May CA, Schraeder C, Britt T: Managed care and case management: roles for professional nursing, Washington, DC, 1997, American Nurses Publishing.

McClatchey S: Disease management as a performance improvement strategy, *Top Health Inform Manag* 22(2):15-23, 2001.

McClinton DH: Promoting wellness, *Continuing Care* 17(4):6, 1998a.

McClinton DH: Protecting patients, *Continuing Care* 17(7):6, 1998b.

McKinley LL, Zasler CP: Weaving a plan of care, *Continuing Care* 17(7):19-22, 1998.

Mechanic D: Muddling through elegantly: finding the proper balance in rationing, *Health Aff* 16(5):83-92, 1997.

Mueller WJ, Kell B: *Coping with conflict,* Englewood Cliffs, NJ, 1972, Prentice Hall.

Mullahy C: *The case managers handbook,* ed 2, Gaithersburg, Md, 1998a, Aspen.

Mullahy CM: *Essential readings in case management,* Gaithersburg, Md, 1998b, Aspen.

Nelson ML: Advocacy in nursing, *Nurs Outlook* 36(3):136-141, 1988.

Qudah FJ, Brannon M: Population-based case management, *Qual Manag Health Care* 5(1):29-41, 1996.

Renholm M, Leino-Kilpi H, Suominen T: Critical pathways: a systematic review, *J Nurs Adm* 32(4):196-202, 2002.

Rieve J: Disease management concerns, *Case manag* 9(2): 34-36, 1998.

Saue JM: Legal issues related to case management. In Fisher K, Weisman E, editors: *Case management: guiding patients through the health care maze,* Chicago, 1994, Joint Commission on the Accreditation of Healthcare Organizations.

Scheutzow SO: Confidentiality, *Case Manger* 5(3):108-109, 1994.

Schroeder C, Britt T: The Carle clinic. *Nurs Manag* 28(3):32-34, 1997.

Secord LJ: *Private case management for older persons and their families,* Excelsior, Minn, 1987, Interstudy.

Solberg LI et al: Using continuous quality improvement to improve diabetes care in populations: the ideal model, *Jt Comm J Qual Improv* 23(11):581-592, 1997.

Sollins HI: Fraud and abuse, *Case Manager* 5(3):109-110, 1994.

Stanton MP, Dunkin J: Rural case management: nursing role variations, *Case Manag* 7(2):48-58, 2002.

Taylor P: Comprehensive nursing case management: an advanced practice model, *Nursing Case Manag* 4(1):2-10, 1999.

Thomas KW, Kilmann RH: *Thomas–Kilmann conflict mode instrument,* New York, 1974, Xicom.

U.S. Department of Health and Human Services: *Healthy People 2010: understanding and improving health,* ed 2, Washington, DC, 2000, U.S. Government Printing Office.

Volkema RJ: *Problem–purpose–expansion: a technique for reformulating problems* [unpublished manuscript], 1983, University of Wisconsin.

Waitzkin H, Williams RL, Bock JA: Safety net institutions buffer the impact of Medicaid managed care, *Am J Public Health* 92(4):598-610, 2002.

Ward MD, Rieve J: Disease management: case management's return to patient-centered care, *J Care Manag* 1(4):7-12, 1995.

Weil M, Karls JM: Historical origins and recent developments. In Weils M et al, editors: *Case management in human service practice,* San Francisco, 1985, Jossey-Bass.

Winslow GR: From loyalty to advocacy: a new metaphor for nursing, *Hastings Cent Rep* 14:32-40, 1984.

Wrinn MM: The emerging role of tele-health in health care, *Continuing Care* 17(8):18-22, 40, 1998.

Yarmo D: Research directions for case management, *J Case Manag* 7(2):84-89, 1998.

Zander K, Etheredge ML, Bower KA: *Nursing case management: blueprints for transformation,* Waban, Mass, 1987, Winslow Printing Systems.

Zander K, McGill R: Critical and anticipated recovery paths: only the beginning, *Nurs Manag* 25(8):34-40, 1994.

# Chapter 20

# Disaster Management

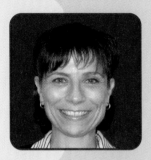

**Susan B. Hassmiller, Ph.D., R.N., F.A.A.N.**

Sue Hassmiller is a senior program officer at The Robert Wood Johnson Foundation in Princeton, New Jersey. The Foundation provides support to improve the health and health care for all Americans. Dr. Hassmiller works in the areas of public health, primary care, prevention, and the health professions workforce, including the nursing shortage. Dr. Hassmiller has taught public health nursing at the University level and has dedicated her career to the care of vulnerable populations and prevention. She is a member of the National Board of Governors for the American Red Cross. She is a 2002 recipient of both the national American Red Cross Ann Magnussen Award and regional American Red Cross Clara Barton Award, both recognizing her outstanding leadership in the field of nursing.

## Objectives

After reading this chapter, the student should be able to do the following:

1. Discuss types of disasters, including natural, human-made, and epidemics
2. Evaluate how disasters affect people and their communities
3. Discuss disaster management, including preparedness, response, and recovery
4. Examine the nurse's role in the preparedness, response, and recovery phases of disaster management
5. Describe the priorities in a triage situation
6. Identify how the community (including voluntary, governmental, and community organizations; business; and labor) works together to prepare for, respond to, and recover from disasters
7. Analyze the role of the American Red Cross in disaster management

---

*Wherever disaster calls there I shall go. I ask not for whom, but only where I am needed.*

From the Creed of the Red Cross Nurse
(American Red Cross, 1981)

"We do not expect disasters, but they happen. With living come natural calamities; with industry and technologic advances come accidents; with socioeconomic and political stagnation or change come dissatisfaction, terrorism, and war" (Waeckerle, 1991, p. 820). Although disasters, man-made or natural, are inevitable, there are ways to prevent or manage how people and their communities respond to disasters. This chapter describes management techniques throughout the preparedness, response, and recovery phases of disaster. The nurse's role in these phases is highlighted.

The author wishes to thank the following individuals for their thoughtful review and critique of this chapter: Jane Morgan, R.N., manager, External Relations and Direct Services for Disaster Services at the American Red Cross; Victoria Child, R.N., B.S.N., senior associate, Disaster Services at the American Red Cross; and Johanna Tracy, M.S.N., A.P.R.N., B.C., Red Cross nurse liaison. The author also wishes to thank Kathryn Hammes for her extensive and thoughtful assistance.

## DISASTERS

Children often first hear about a natural disaster through the story of Noah and the flood in the Book of Genesis in the King James Bible. The fairy tale fashion in which the story is often told is inadequate preparation for the destruction and devastation that disasters truly leave behind. Disasters can affect one family at a time, as in a house fire, or they can kill thousands and have economic losses in the millions, as with floods, earthquakes, tornadoes, hurricanes, and bioterrorism. From 1991 until 2000, major natural disasters cost an estimated $78.7 billion dollars per year (International Federation of Red Cross [IFRC], 2001). The loss of life was also dramatic. Just over 3 million lives have been lost in the past decade as a result of conflict (including terrorism) and both natural and technologic disasters. In addition to the mortality, 5 billion more people each year have had to deal with the injuries, disease, and homelessness that follow disasters (IFRC, 2001).

The burden of natural disasters throughout the world falls mostly on developing countries. A person living in a developing country is 12 times more likely to perish in a natural disaster than a person living in the United States. This fact is supported by projections suggesting that by 2050, 80% of the world's population will live in develop-

## Key Terms

**bioterrorism**, p. 477
**delayed stress reaction**, p. 484
**disaster**, p. 471
**disaster medical assistance teams**, p. 479
**emergency support functions**, p. 479
**Federal Emergency Management Agency**, p. 473
**Federal Response Plan**, p. 479

**human-made disasters**, p. 471
**level I disaster**, p. 478
**level II disaster**, p. 478
**level III disaster**, p. 478
**mitigation**, p. 472
**natural disasters**, p. 471
**Office of Emergency Management**, p. 474
**preparedness**, p. 473

**recovery**, p. 473
**response**, p. 473
**triage**, p. 482
**Volunteer Organizations Active in Disasters**, p. 476

*See Glossary for definitions*

## Chapter Outline

Disasters
*Defining Disasters*
*Disaster Mitigation*

*Healthy People 2010 Objectives*
Three Stages of Disaster Involvement:
    Preparedness, Response, and Recovery

*Preparedness*
*Response*
*Recovery*

ing countries (United Nations Office for the Coordination of Humanitarian Affairs, 1998).

### DID YOU KNOW?

Disasters create the most devastation in developing countries, where the death rate is up to 12 times higher than in developed countries. The poor suffer the most because their houses are less sturdy and they have fewer resources and less means of social security.

The urbanizing and the overcrowding of cities have increased the danger of **natural disasters** because communities have been built in areas that are vulnerable to disasters, such as in known tornado zones or near rivers. Increases in population and the investing of money in areas vulnerable to natural disasters have led to major increases in insurance payouts in the United States in every decade. Projections suggest that by 2050, at least 46% of the world's population will live in areas vulnerable to natural floods, earthquakes, and severe storms.

Overcrowding and urban development have also increased **human-made disasters.** The stress caused by overcrowding has caused civil unrest and riots. In some parts of the world, modern wars waged over land rights and space have markedly increased the risk of injury and death from disaster. In the United States and other countries, school violence, such as the 1999 Columbine High School incident, has been increasing in intensity and magnitude. This is considered a human-made disaster.

The cost of disaster recovery efforts has also risen sharply because of the number of people involved and the amount of technology that must be restored. People in industrialized countries are becoming less self-sufficient because they rely heavily on technology and social and economic systems within their community. People who live on the brink of disaster every day, physically, emotionally, or economically, are among the first to be affected when disaster strikes.

## Defining Disasters

A **disaster** is any human-made or natural event that causes destruction and devastation that cannot be relieved without assistance. The event need not cause injury or death to be considered a disaster. For example, a hurricane may cause millions of dollars in damage without causing a single death or injury. Box 20-1 lists examples of human-made and natural disasters.

Although natural disasters will always occur, much can be done to prevent further increases in accidents, death, and destruction after impact. A concise, realistic, and well-rehearsed disaster plan, as well as sustained and open communication among involved organizations and workers, can prevent further damage. Also, many of the human-made disasters listed in Box 20-1 can be prevented (e.g., major transportation accidents and fires resulting from substance abuse).

**WHAT DO YOU THINK?**

Much of the destruction caused by natural disasters in the 1990s could have been avoided. In many documented cases, building codes were ignored, warnings were not issued or followed, communities were located in dangerous areas, and plans were forgotten. An "ounce of prevention," or preparedness, would have made a real difference.

Modified from Gerrity ET, Flynn BW: Mental health consequences of disasters. In Noji EK, editor: *The public health consequences of disasters,* New York, 1997, Oxford University Press.

## Disaster Mitigation

As the life and economic losses caused by natural disasters increased, the United Nations (UN) declared the 1990s to be the International Decade for National Disaster Reduction resulting in heightened public–private partnering emphasizing **mitigation** (i.e., actions or measures that can either prevent the occurrence of a disaster or reduce the severity of its effects [American Red Cross, 1998a]). Mitigation activities include:

1. Awareness and education, such as holding community meetings on disaster preparedness
2. Disaster prevention, such as building a retaining wall to divert flood water away from a residence
3. Advocacy, such as supporting actions and efforts for effective building codes and proper land use

Dozens of national, state, and local agencies, such as the Institute for Business and Home Safety, American Red Cross, Centers for Disease Control and Prevention (CDC), and local communities of faith, came together during this internationally declared decade for disaster reduction to work proactively to save lives and property.

## Healthy People 2010 Objectives

Because disasters affect the health of people in many ways, they have an effect on almost every Healthy People 2010 objective. For example, although nutrition and exercise are two important Healthy People 2010 objectives, they become less significant when the more pressing need for people to be housed in temporary shelter arises. There are, however, some objectives that are more directly affected. Disasters do play a direct role in the objectives related to unintentional injuries, occupational safety and health, environmental health, and food and drug safety. Professionals, such as those who work at the CDC, study the effects that disasters have on objectives such as these and are constantly developing new prevention strategies. Other organizations, such as the American Psychological Association and the American Red Cross, work with communities in the immediate recovery phase of a disaster and sometimes for years thereafter to effect the Healthy People 2010 objectives related to mental health. International groups also work to reduce the psychological effects that follow a disaster.

The Pan American Health Organization has an educational program set up for emergency response personnel including nurses. The Stress Management in Disaster program is designed to prevent and lessen the psychological dysfunction that occurs in disaster situations (Bryce, 2001).

## THREE STAGES OF DISASTER INVOLVEMENT: PREPAREDNESS, RESPONSE, AND RECOVERY

Disaster management includes the three stages of a disaster: preparation, response, and recovery. Figure 20-1 shows the disaster management cycle. A key to disaster preparedness is that the plan must be kept both realistic and sim-

**Healthy People 2010** | Examples of Objectives Developed to Avoid Disasters

8-12 Minimize the risks to human health and the environment posed by hazardous sites
10-1 Reduce infections caused by food-borne pathogens

15-39 Reduce weapon carrying by adolescents on school property
20-5 Reduce deaths by work-related homicides

From U.S. Department of Health and Human Services: *Healthy People 2010: national health promotion and disease prevention objectives,* ed 2, Washington, DC, 2000, U.S. Government Printing Office.

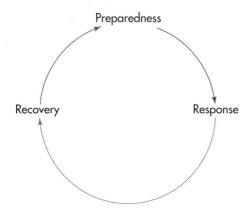

**Figure 20-1** Disaster management cycle *(Modified from American Red Cross:* Disasters happen, *Washington, DC, 1994, ARC.)*

ple. The reasons for this are that (1) plans will never exactly fit the disaster as it occurs, and (2) all plans must be able to be implemented no matter what key members of the disaster team are there at the time (CDC, 2002; U.S. Department of Health and Human Services, 2001). The following discussion elaborates on all three stages, including what the role of the nurse should be.

## Preparedness

### Personal Preparedness

Nurses with client responsibilities can also become disaster victims (Gebbie and Qureshi, 2002). Conflicts arise between family-related and work-related responsibilities. For example, a mother whose childcare needs go unmet will not be able to participate fully, if at all, in disaster relief efforts. Personal and family preparation can help ease some of the conflicts that arise and will allow nurses to attend to client needs sooner. In addition, the nurse assisting in disaster relief efforts must be as healthy as possible, both physically and mentally. A disaster worker who is not well is of little service to his or her family, clients, and other disaster victims.

The American Red Cross and the **Federal Emergency Management Agency** (FEMA), two well-known authorities on disaster **preparedness, response,** and **recovery,** have devised a personal checklist to help individuals and families prepare for disasters before they strike (FEMA, 1997). The

How To box shows an adapted version of the FEMA's recommendations entitled Four Steps to Safety. Also, the Nursing Tip lists emergency supplies that should be prepared and stored in a sturdy, easy-to-carry container. Important documents should always be kept in a waterproof container.

### Professional Preparedness

Professional preparedness requires that nurses become aware of and understand the disaster plans at their workplace and community. Nurses who take disaster preparation seriously will take the time to read and understand workplace and community disaster plans and will participate in disaster drills and community mock disasters. Adequately prepared nurses can function in a leadership capacity and assist others toward a smoother recovery phase. Personal items that are recommended for nurses preparing to help in a disaster include the following (American Red Cross, 1995):

- Copy of professional license
- Personal equipment, such as a stethoscope
- Flashlight and extra batteries
- Cellular phone
- Cash and traveler's checks
- Warm clothing and a heavy jacket (or weather-appropriate clothing)
- Change of protective shoes
- Change of clothing
- Record-keeping materials
- Pocket-sized reference books
- Watch

Disaster work is not high tech. Fieldwork, including shelter management, requires that nurses be creative and willing to improvise in delivering care. All workers should be certified in first aid and cardiopulmonary resuscitation (CPR). In addition, the American Red Cross provides a comprehensive program of disaster training for health professionals, to enable them to provide assistance within their own communities and to other stricken communities and countries. The courses teach nurses how to adapt their existing nursing skills to a disaster setting and to the scope of the Red Cross disaster nursing.

### Community Preparedness

The level of community preparedness for a disaster is only as high as the people and organizations in the community

**HOW TO** Prepare for Safety in a Disaster: Four Steps

1. Find out what could happen to you.
   a. Determine what types of disasters are most likely to happen.
   b. Learn about warning signals in your community.
   c. Ask about postdisaster pet care (shelters usually will not accept pets).
   d. Review the disaster plans at your workplace, school, and other places where your family spends time.
   e. Determine how to help older adult or disabled family members or neighbors.

2. Create a disaster plan.
   a. Discuss types of disasters that are most likely to happen, and review what to do in each case.
   b. Pick two places to meet, including outside your home and outside your neighborhood.
   c. Choose an out-of-state friend to be your family contact; this person will verify the location of each family member. After a disaster, it may be easier to call long distance than to make local calls.
   d. Review evacuation plans, including care of pets. Identify ahead of time where to go if evacuation is necessary.

3. Complete this checklist.
   a. Post emergency phone numbers by telephones.
   b. Teach everyone how and when to call 911.

   c. Determine when and how to turn off water, gas, and electricity at the main switches.
   d. Check adequacy of insurance coverage for self and home.
   e. Locate and review use of fire extinguisher.
   f. Install and maintain smoke detectors.
   g. Conduct a home hazard hunt and fix potential hazards.
   h. Stock emergency supplies and assemble a disaster supplies kit.
   i. Acquire first aid and CPR certification.
   j. Locate all escape routes from your home. Find two ways out of each room.
   k. Find the safe spots in your home for each type of disaster.

4. Practice and maintain your plan.
   a. Review the plan every 6 months.
   b. Conduct fire and emergency evacuation drills.
   c. Replace stored water every 3 months and stored food every 6 months.
   d. Test and recharge fire extinguisher according to manufacturer's instructions.
   e. Test your smoke detectors monthly and change the batteries at least once a year.

make it. Some communities stay prepared for a possible disaster by having a written disaster plan and by participating in yearly disaster drills. Other communities are less vigilant and depend on luck and the fact that they have never been hit before to see them through. Some organizations within the community may be more prepared than others. For example, most health care facilities have written disaster plans and require employees to perform annual mock drills, but many businesses do not have these requirements.

Most states and counties have an **Office of Emergency Management** (OEM) that is responsible for developing and coordinating emergency response plans within their defined area. The state office supports local OEMs and other state agencies that participate in disaster response. The office helps in all three phases of emergency management. It provides planning and training services to local governments, including financial and technical assistance. During an actual emergency or disaster, the state OEM coordinates a state response and recovery program if necessary. County OEMs are in charge of creating a comprehensive, all-hazard plan that should address realistic dangers to the community and list available resources (Alson, Leonard, and Stringer, 1997).

Nurses need to review the disaster history of the community, including how past disasters have affected the health care delivery system and how their particular organization fits into the plan. Understandings of past disasters

influence planning for future disasters. For example, disaster history may reveal that the local disaster services committee has not appropriately used the county's nurses because of a lack of education about their roles. It might be beneficial for this committee to receive an educational program on what nurses do and what role they can play in a disaster. A solid disaster plan requires the talents, coordination, and cooperation of many different people and organizations, both in and outside the health profession (Box 20-2).

Working together cooperatively and with clear role definitions *before* a disaster gives greater assurance that assistance will be delivered smoothly once disaster hits. Communication is the key in setting up and implementing a disaster plan. Knowing in advance exactly what is expected of each organization during an emergency or disaster gives the staff the opportunity to acquire necessary knowledge and to practice necessary skills beforehand (Gebbie and Qureshi, 2002).

## THE CUTTING EDGE

In the United States, 100 cities are listed as potential targets for terrorism.

## BOX 20-2 Key Organizations and Professionals in Disaster Management

### HEALTH CARE COMMUNITY

- Hospitals
- Mental health professionals
- Pharmacies
- Public health departments
- Rescue personnel

### NON-HEALTH CARE COMMUNITY

- Clergy
- Firefighters
- Funeral directors
- The mayor and other municipal or government officials
- Media
- Medical examiners
- Medical supply manufacturers
- Morticians
- Police

Finally, the community must have an adequate warning system and a backup evacuation plan to remove those individuals from areas of danger who hesitate to leave. Some people refuse to leave their homes because they are afraid that their possessions will be lost or destroyed by the disaster or from looting after the disaster. It may take a face-to-face encounter with law enforcement personnel or others in authority to convince them to leave their homes and retreat to safer quarters. Also, some people mistakenly believe that experience with a particular type of disaster is enough preparation for the next one. People must be convinced that pre-disaster warnings are official, serious, and personally important before they are motivated to take action. A template for a community/health care facilities readiness plan has been developed to help prepare for bioterrorism. The template includes the recognized bioterrorism potential of four diseases: anthrax, botulism, plague, and smallpox (English and Malone, 1999).

### Role of the Nurse in Disaster Preparedness

Nurses in disaster preparedness facilitate preparation within the community and place of employment (Figure 20-2). Nurses employed in emergency departments generally know their role in citywide disaster plans for the community. Nurses working in other settings, such as home health, may not have the same preparation (Gebbie and Qureshi, 2002).

Within the employing organization, the nurse can help initiate or update the disaster plan, provide educational programs and materials regarding disasters specific to the area, and organize disaster drills. The nurse is also in a unique position to provide an updated record of vulnerable populations within the community. When calamity strikes, disaster workers must know what kinds of populations they are attempting to assist. For example, after a tornado strikes a retirement village, the needs are quite different from those seen after the tornado hits a church filled with families or a center for the physically challenged. In addition to knowing where special populations exist, the nurse should be involved in educating these special populations about what impact the disaster might have on them. Individual strategies should be reviewed, including available specific resources, in the event of an emergency.

The nurse who leads a preparedness effort can help recruit others within the organization who will help if and when a response is required. Although there is no psychological profile of a disaster leader, it is wise to involve persons in this effort who are flexible, decisive, and emotionally stable, and who have physical endurance (Bryce, 2001). The nurse leader should also possess an intimate knowledge of the institution and be familiar with the individuals who work there. Persons with disaster management training, and especially those who have served during real disasters, also make valuable members of any preparedness team.

Within the community, the nurse may be involved in many roles. As community advocates, nurses help keep a safe environment. Recalling that disasters are not only natural but may be human-made as well, the nurse in the community needs to assess for and report environmental health hazards. For example, the nurse should be aware of and report unsafe equipment, faulty structures, and the beginning of disease epidemics such as measles or flu.

Nurses should also understand what the available community resources will be after a disaster strikes, and, most important, how the community will work together.

### NURSING TIP

Emergency supplies needed in case of disaster:
- A 3-day supply of water (1 gallon per person per day) and food that will not spoil
- One change of clothing and protective footwear per person, and one blanket or sleeping bag per person
- A first-aid kit that includes your family's prescription medications
- Emergency tools including a battery-powered radio, flashlight, and plenty of extra batteries
- Candles and matches
- An extra set of car keys and a credit card, cash, or traveler's checks, picture identification, proof of address
- Sanitation supplies, including toilet paper, soap, feminine hygiene items, and plastic garbage bags
- Special items for infant, older adult, or disabled family members
- An extra pair of eyeglasses

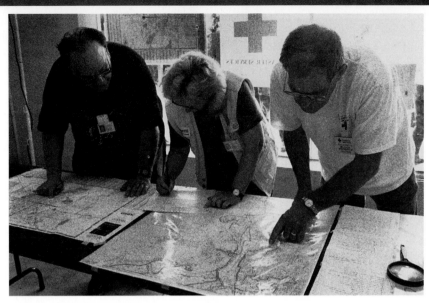

**Figure 20-2** Understanding the community's disaster plan is a key role for nurses who seek greater involvement in disaster management. *(Courtesy American Red Cross. All rights reserved in all countries.)*

A communitywide disaster plan will help nurses understand what "should" occur before, during, and after the response and their role within the plan. Nurses who seek to be more involved or who seek an in-depth understanding of disaster management can become involved in any number of community organizations that are part of the official response team, such as the American Red Cross or Emergency Medical System/Ambulance Corps. It is also possible to become involved in **Volunteer Organizations Active in Disasters** (VOAD) such as the Salvation Army. The American Red Cross offers classes on disaster health services and disaster mental health services to help participants identify disaster health services preparedness measures that should take place on the local unit level and to become familiar with Red Cross disaster health services procedures and protocols in local disaster operations (American Red Cross, 2000). The Red Cross requires workers to complete the disaster health services or a disaster mental health services course work before assigning an individual to a disaster site as a Red Cross representative. For nurses who choose to volunteer with agencies such as the Red Cross, there are many ways to become involved. After several hours of disaster training, nurses may wish to take the following steps to get actively involved:

- Join a local disaster action team (DAT).
- Act as a liaison with local hospitals.
- Determine health-related appropriateness for shelter sites.
- Plan with pharmacies, opticians, morticians, and other health personnel to facilitate services for disaster victims.
- Plan for needed supplies and keep them available.
- Teach disaster nursing in the community.

It is important to keep the nursing and medical protocols and intervention standards, whether they are with the Red Cross or employing institution, up to date and consistent with local public health standards (American Red Cross, 2000). Nurses are needed for national and international disaster assignments as well.

## Mass Casualty Drills or Mock Disasters

Mass casualty drills or mock disasters are valuable components of preparedness. Whether the drills are carried forth in a desktop manner or through realistic scenarios, the objectives are as follows (Gebbie and Qureshi, 2002):

- To promote confidence
- To develop skills
- To coordinate activities
- To coordinate participants

It is critical for those who will be involved in an actual disaster to be involved in a drill (Waeckerle, 2000). Also, the drill leader needs special skills in disaster management, including the ability to coordinate many organizations at one time. Although a successful disaster drill can allow participants to evaluate the rescue plan and make further recommendations, it should not create a misplaced sense of security (Alson et al, 1997).

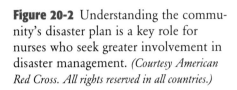

## THE CUTTING EDGE

In 2002, the federal government gave states money to prepare for disasters, including bioterrorism.

## Agencies Involved in Disaster Preparedness

Many community agencies contribute to disaster preparedness. Table 20-1 describes the preparedness responsibilities assumed by the American Red Cross, other voluntary organizations, business and labor organizations, and local government.

## Table 20-1 Disaster Preparedness Responsibilities by Agency

| AMERICAN RED CROSS | OTHER VOLUNTARY ORGANIZATIONS | BUSINESS AND LABOR ORGANIZATIONS | LOCAL GOVERNMENT |
|---|---|---|---|
| • Participates with government in developing and testing community disaster plan<br>• Designates persons to serve as representatives at government emergency operations centers and command posts<br>• Develops and tests local Red Cross disaster plans<br>• Identifies and trains personnel for disaster response<br>• Collaborates with other voluntary agencies to develop and maintain local Voluntary Organizations Active in Disaster groups to promote cooperation and coordinate resources and people for disaster work<br>• Works with business and labor organizations to identify resources and people for disaster work<br>• Educates the public about hazards and ways to avoid, prepare for, and cope with their effects<br>• Acquires material resources needed to ensure effective response | • Collaborate in developing and maintaining local Voluntary Organizations Active in Disaster groups to identify roles, resources, and plans for disasters<br>• Identify and train personnel for disaster response<br>• Identify community issues and special populations for consideration in disaster preparedness<br>• Make plans to continue to serve regular clients after a disaster<br>• Identify facilities, resources, and people to serve in time of disaster<br>• Educate specific client groups on disaster preparedness | • Develop disaster plans for business locations and integrate their plans with the community disaster plan<br>• Develop procedures to facilitate continuity of operations in times of disaster<br>• Develop plans for assisting business employees after a disaster<br>• Identify union and business facilities, resources, and people who may be able to support community disaster plans<br>• Provide volunteers, financial contributions, and in-kind gifts to Red Cross and other voluntary organizations to support disaster preparedness<br>• Educate employees and union members about disaster preparedness | • Coordinates the development of the community plan and conducts evaluation exercises<br>• Trains staff to carry out the plan<br>• Passes legislation to mitigate the effects of potential disasters<br>• Designs measures to warn the population of disaster threats<br>• Conducts building safety inspections<br>• Develops procedures to facilitate continuity of public safety operations in times of disaster<br>• Identifies public facilities, resources, and public employees for disaster work<br>• Educates the public about disaster threats in the community and safety procedures |

From American Red Cross: *Disasters happen* (ARC publication No. 1570), Washington, DC, 1994, ARC.

## The Future of Disaster Preparation

The terrorist events of September 11, 2001, and the later anthrax cases have increased the awareness of the need to plan for disaster. Since then there has been a growing amount of information compiled on how to specifically plan for human-made disasters, which often occur with no forewarning. Part of planning for a **bioterrorism** attack is learning the symptoms of illnesses that are likely to be caused by infectious agents. For both natural and human-made disasters, there are often early warning signs. For example, signs of a tornado include hail, strong rain, and a green sky. Signs for a human-made disaster may not be as clear, but being aware of suspicious activities is still important (Box 20-3).

### BOX 20-3 Precautions for a Terrorist Attack

• Be aware of the surrounding area and unusual activity.
• Take extra precautions when traveling, such as watching luggage carefully.
• Locate emergency exits wherever you go.

Federal Emergency Management Agency: *National situation updates,* Washington, DC, 2001, FEMA, available at www.fema.gov/emanagers/nat091201.htm.

## Office of Homeland Security

On October 8, 2001, President Bush signed an Executive Order that established the Office of Homeland Security. The mission of the office is to develop and coordinate the implementing of a comprehensive national strategy to secure the United States from terrorist threats or attacks. The office will work with executive departments and agencies, state and local governments, and private agencies to ensure adequate strategies for detecting, preparing for, preventing, protecting against, responding to, and recovering from terrorist threats or attacks.

## Response

### Levels of Disaster and Agency Involvement

Many small disasters, such as single-family home fires, and even many extensive disasters do not require the assistance of FEMA. In these cases, the American Red Cross and other organizations such as the Salvation Army work to assist disaster victims. When the president of the United States declares a disaster, the Red Cross works with FEMA to assist with recovery efforts. Table 20-2 describes disaster response responsibilities of the American Red Cross, other voluntary organizations, business and labor organizations, and local government.

According to the American Red Cross (2003), there are three ways of classifying a disaster:

1. Disaster type: The agent that produced the event, such as a hurricane, a hazardous material accident, or a transportation accident.

2. The Level: The anticipated or actual Red Cross disaster response and relief cost required by the event.
   - Level I—costs less than $10,000
   - Level II—costs $10,000 or more, but less than $50,000
   - Level III—costs $50,000 or more, but less than $250,000
   - Level IV—costs $250,000 or more, but less than $2.5 million
   - Level V—costs $2.5 million or more

3. The Scope: The basic characteristics of the event's magnitude, and the Red Cross unit or units affected and responding to the event.
   - Single Family Disaster—A disaster that affects an individual or a single family unit, occurs within the jurisdiction of a single Red Cross chapter, and may require the short-term application of limited human and material resources from that chapter.
   - Local Disaster—A disaster that affects more than one family, occurs within the jurisdiction of a single Red Cross chapter, and generally requires the application of limited human and material resources from the Red Cross chapter.
   - State Disaster—A disaster that affects multiple families, occurs within the jurisdiction of one or more Red Cross chapters within a single state, generally requires the focused commitment of human and material resources from the affected chapter(s), and may require support and assistance from other Red Cross units.
   - Major Disaster—A disaster that generally has one or more of the following characteristics: requires the

---

**Table 20-2    Disaster Response Responsibilities by Agency**

| AMERICAN RED CROSS | OTHER VOLUNTARY ORGANIZATIONS | BUSINESS AND LABOR ORGANIZATIONS | LOCAL GOVERNMENT |
|---|---|---|---|
| • Operates shelters<br>• Provides feeding services<br>• Provides individual and family assistance to meet immediate emergency needs (including purchase of groceries, clothing, and household items)<br>• Provides disaster health services, including mental health support<br>• Handles inquiries from concerned family members outside the area<br>• Coordinates relief activities with other agencies, business, labor, and government<br>• Informs the public of services available<br>• Seeks and accepts contributions from those wanting to help | • Provide services that are identified in pre-disaster planning<br>• Provide regular services to ongoing client groups<br>• Identify unanticipated needs and provide resources to meet those needs<br>• Act as advocates for their client groups<br>• Coordinate services with all other groups involved with the disaster response<br>• Seek and accept donations from those wanting to help | • Take action to protect employees and to ensure the safety of the facility<br>• Advise public safety forces of hazardous conditions<br>• Identify resources such as union halls, generators, and heavy equipment that are available to support the disaster response<br>• Provide volunteers, financial contributions, and gifts of goods and services to the relief effort | • Provides for coordination of the overall relief effort<br>• Advises the public on safety measures such as evacuation<br>• Provides public health services<br>• Provides fire and police protection to the affected area<br>• Inspects facilities for safety and health codes<br>• Provides ongoing social services for the community<br>• Repairs public buildings, sewage and water systems, streets, and highways |

From American Red Cross: *Disasters happen* (ARC publication No. 1570), Washington, DC, 1994, ARC.

coordinated response and/or resources of multiple Red Cross units; affects more than a single state; creates national news media attention; is expected to result in an emergency or major disaster declaration by the President of the United States or the mobilization and application of federal government human and/or material resources; involves nuclear power plants, nuclear, chemical, or biological weapons; involves impact of material from space; requires international involvement; has the potential for similar extraordinary or unusual effect; or is expected to require types and/or quantities of services and/or assistance that exceed the combined capacity of the affected Red Cross chapter.

- Presidentially Declared Disaster—A disaster that requires full or partial implementation of the Federal Response Plan (FRP). Such a disaster generally has one or more of the following characteristics: exceeds the capabilities of a state and its local governments to provide a timely and effective response to meet the needs of the situation; causes or has the potential to cause a substantial number of deaths or injuries; causes or has the potential to cause substantial health and medical problems; or causes or has the potential to cause significant damage, particularly to the economic and physical infrastructure of the state or political subdivisions.

In any large-scale or major national disaster, not only do official agencies respond but many other concerned citizens, including health professionals, come on their own to help as well. At times, so many people come "out of the woodwork" to help that role conflict, anger, frustration, and helplessness occur. The World Trade Center attacks of September 11, 2001 like many other disasters, brought many qualified but unassociated citizens to the site, "many well-intentioned local physicians, in shirt sleeves and light footwear, proceeded to the area and attempted to find victims, risking further injuries to themselves and getting in the way of structured rescue protocols. In fact unauthorized would-be rescuers are legally prohibited from participating in rescue operations within any area designated as a disaster by the Fire Department of New York" (Crippen, 2002). After the bombing of the Alfred P. Murrah building in Oklahoma City in 1995, one nurse rushed in to rescue people. During her heroic efforts, she was killed by a fall. Thus it is best that nurses attach themselves to an official agency with assigned disaster management responsibilities (Alson et al, 1993; Switzer, 1985).

## The Federal Response Plan

Once a federal emergency has been declared, the **Federal Response Plan** (FRP), also known as Public Law 93-288, may take effect depending on the specific needs of the disaster. The FRP is implemented "to assist state and local governments when a major disaster or emergency overwhelms their ability to respond effectively to save lives; protect public health, safety, and property; and restore their communities" (FEMA, 1999, p. iii). Box 20-4 lists the purpose of the FRP.

Within the FRP there are 12 **emergency support functions** (ESFs), each one headed by a primary agency. Each primary agency is responsible for coordinating efforts in a particular area with all of its designated support agencies. In all, 26 federal agencies and the American Red Cross must respond if called on. For example, in a presidentially declared disaster, all ongoing health and medical services fall under the auspices of the U.S. Public Health Service. The U.S. Public Health Service divides its responsibilities among its own agencies as needed (see Chapter 3). The CDC, for example, under ESF numbers 8 to 10, may "assist in establishing surveillance systems to monitor the general population and special high-risk population groups; carry out field studies and investigations; monitor injury and disease patterns and injury control measures and precautions" (FEMA, 1999). Sheltering, feeding, emergency first aid, providing a disaster welfare information system, and coordinating bulk distribution of emergency relief supplies is the mass care emergency support function number 6. For this, the American Red Cross is the primary agency. It is conceivable that the nurse could be involved with any of these response efforts within the local community or, with appropriate training, on a national basis.

The National Disaster Medical System (NDMS) is part of the ESF of Health and Medical Services. In a presidentially declared disaster, including overseas war, the U.S. Public Health Service can activate **disaster medical assistance teams** (DMATs) to an area to supplement local and state medical care needs. DMATs can also be activated by the Assistant Secretary for Health on the request of a state health officer. Teams of specially trained civilian physicians, nurses, and other health care personnel can be sent to a disaster site within hours of activation. DMATs can provide triage and continuing medical care to victims until they can be evacuated to a national network of hospitals prearranged by the NDMS (FEMA, 1999).

Within hours of the September 11 terrorist attacks, five DMAT teams were on site in the New York City area. Three

---

### BOX 20-4 Purpose of the Federal Response Plan

- Establishes fundamental assumptions and policies
- Establishes a concept of operations that provides an interagency coordination mechanism to facilitate the immediate delivery of federal response assistance
- Incorporates the coordination mechanisms and structures of other appropriate federal plans and responsibilities into the overall response
- Assigns specific functional responsibilities to appropriate federal departments and agencies
- Identifies actions that participating federal departments and agencies will take in the overall federal response in coordination with the affected state

From Federal Emergency Management Agency: *The federal response plan (FRP)*, Washington, DC, 1999, FEMA.

additional teams were sent to assist at the site of the Pentagon attack. In total, 190 DMAT personnel were working in New York City after the attack. As of October 1, 2001, they had treated 5574 patients, most of whom where police officers, firefighters, and construction workers who had sustained injuries at the site (FEMA, 2001). Because of the nature of this country's disasters since the initiation of DMATs, these teams have been used primarily to staff community health outpatient clinics in the affected areas.

### Response to Bioterrorism

Biological or chemical terrorist attacks require a very different response. An unannounced dissemination of a biological agent may easily go unnoticed, and the victims may have left the area of exposure long before the act of terrorism is recognized. The first signs that a biological agent has been released probably would not be apparent until days to weeks later, when the victims become ill and go to health care professionals for evaluation. In this case, it is the health care professionals, including nurses, who are considered the "first on the scene." There are five components to a comprehensive public health response to outbreaks of illness. These include detecting the outbreak, determining the cause, identifying factors that place people at risk, implementing measures to control the outbreak, and informing the medical and public communities about treatments, health consequences, and preventive measures (Rotz et al, 2000).

### How Disasters Affect Communities

People in a community can be affected physically and emotionally, depending on the type, cause, and location of the disaster; on its magnitude and extent of damage; on its duration; and on the amount of warning that was provided. For example, an earthquake may not cause any deaths; however, the structural damage to buildings and the continuous aftershocks that may last for weeks can cause intense psychological stress. In addition, the longer it takes for structural repairs and other cleanup, the longer the psychological effects can last.

The terrorist attacks of September 11, 2001, created extreme anger and grief but also led to a huge increase in compassion and patriotism. Thousands of people helped, from donating blood and money to rescuing victims from the buildings. Four days after the attack, buying an American Flag was nearly impossible, as most stores had sold out (Associated Press, 2001). Within 1 month of the attack, an estimated $757 million in cash contributions and hundreds of truckloads of goods had been donated to help the families of victims and rescue workers (Yates, 2001). Although this was the worst man-made disaster in American history, killing over 230 firefighters, policemen, and medical personnel in the heroic rescue mission, the terrorist attacks of September 11 will also be remembered for how they unified the country (Fire Department of New York, 2002).

Individuals react to the same disaster in different ways depending on their age, cultural background, health status,

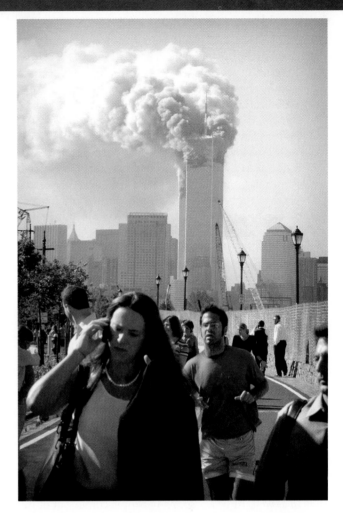

**Figure 20-3** New York residents in the immediate aftermath of the September 11 World Trade Center terrorist attacks. *(Copyright 2001 Thomas A. Ferrara/Corbis Sygma.)*

**WHAT DO YOU THINK?**

Is it reasonable for people to drop off chronically ill family members, especially those suffering from Alzheimer's disease, at Red Cross shelters for extended periods of time during the preparedness, response, and recovery phases of disaster?

social support structure, and their general ability to adapt to crisis (Figure 20-3). The sequencing of reactions and level of intensity depend to some extent on the characteristics of the disaster, such as the suddenness of the impact, the duration of the event, and the probability of recurrence (Gerrity and Flynn, 1997).

Box 20-5 describes common reactions of adults and children to disasters. In adults, the typical first reaction to a disaster is an extreme sense of urgency (Bryce, 2001). Victims become obsessed with personal losses. Other initial reactions include fear, panic, disbelief, reluctance to abandon property, feeling disoriented and numb, difficulty in

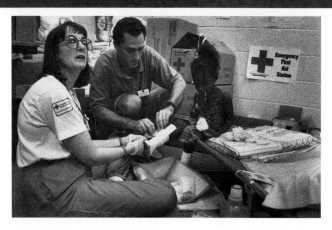

**Figure 20-4** The effects of a disaster on young children can be especially disruptive. *(Courtesy American Red Cross. All rights reserved in all countries.)*

---

### BOX 20-5  Common Reactions to Disasters

**ADULTS**
- Extreme sense of urgency
- Panic and fear
- Disbelief
- Disorientation and numbing
- Reluctance to abandon property
- Difficulty in making decisions
- Need to help others
- Anger and blaming
- Blaming and scapegoating
- Delayed reactions
- Insomnia
- Headaches
- Apathy and depression
- Sense of powerlessness
- Guilt
- Moody and irritable
- Jealousy and resentment
- Domestic violence

**CHILDREN**
- Regressive behaviors (bedwetting, thumb sucking, crying, clinging to parents)
- Fantasies that disaster never occurred
- Nightmares
- School-related problems, including an inability to concentrate and refusal to go back to school

---

making decisions, need for information, seeking help for self and family, and offering help to other disaster victims (American Red Cross, 2002). Disturbances in bodily functions, such as gastrointestinal upsets, diarrhea, and nausea and vomiting, are also common (Gerrity and Flynn, 1997).

Anger, especially blaming and scapegoating, is common among victims soon after a disaster (Gerrity and Flynn, 1997). Anger and blaming stem from an increasing awareness of what has been lost, physical fatigue, emotional stress, and a continuing change in personal comfort. Victims being interviewed on television after a disaster often say that FEMA, the American Red Cross, and other response organizations simply did not do all that was possible. Later, victims have difficulty sleeping, headaches, apathy and depression, moodiness and irritability, anxiety about the future, domestic violence, feelings of being overwhelmed, feelings of frustration and powerlessness over one's own future, and guilt over not being able to prevent the disaster or do more to help resolve it (American Red Cross, 2002).

The psychological effects of September 11 were slightly different from those of more contained, single-event disasters. What makes these attacks different is that they were totally unexpected and of great magnitude. There was much uncertainty and the fear about what might happen next (American Red Cross, 2002). Never knowing when or if the next attack is going to occur prevents individuals from moving beyond their fear and anger. One doctor compared the attacks with being diagnosed with cancer, "the attacks seem to have evoked the identical feelings that I felt upon diagnosis. It is as if we, as a nation, were diagnosed with cancer on September 11. From diagnosis, to treatment, to living with the fear of recurrence" (Raji, 2002, p. 286). The treatment for terrorism, including military, economic, and other ways to contain the enemy, is all guesswork. As with cancer, there is no sure method. Unlike for other disasters that just seem to pass, treatment for terrorism is necessary and long term. This event, like cancer, is a chronic disease. Raji goes on to state, "The next attack could happen anytime, anywhere, without warning. This is the invisible stalking, continuously lurking fear of cancer—and so it seems with terrorism" (p. 286). The fear of recurrence has slowed the recovery process because it has not allowed us to feel comfortable about letting down our guard.

An exacerbation of an existing chronic disease is also common. For example, the emotional stress of being a disaster victim may make it difficult for people with diabetes to control their blood sugar levels. Grief results in harmful effects on the immune system. It reduces the function of cells that protect against viral infections and tumors. As a result of these immunologic deficits, studies indicate that grief is associated with a rise in the frequency of health care visits (Goodkin, 2002). Hormones that are produced by the body's flight-or-fight mechanism also play a role in mediating the effects of grief.

The effects on young children can be especially disruptive (Figure 20-4). Regressive behaviors such as thumb sucking, bedwetting, crying, and clinging to parents can

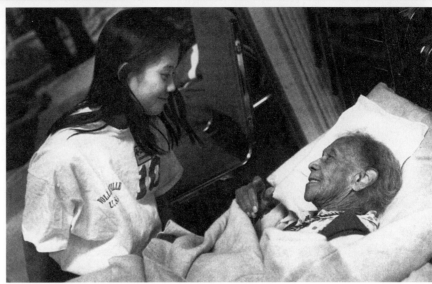

**Figure 20-5** Elderly persons' reactions to a disaster depend greatly on their physical health, strength, mobility, self-sufficiency, and income source and amount. *(Courtesy American Red Cross. All rights reserved in all countries.)*

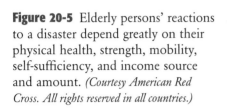

**BOX 20-6** **Populations at Greatest Risk for Disruption After a Disaster**

• Persons with disabilities
• Persons living on a low income, including the homeless
• Non–English speaking persons and refugees
• Persons living alone
• Single-parent families
• Persons new to the area
• Institutionalized persons or those with chronic mental illness
• Previous disaster victims or victims of traumatic events
• Undocumented individuals
• Substance abusers

occur (American Red Cross, 2001). Fantasies that the disaster never occurred and nightmares are common as well. School-related problems may also occur, including an inability to concentrate and even refusal to go back to school (Gerrity and Flynn, 1997).

Older adults' reactions to disaster depend a great deal on their physical health, strength, mobility, self-sufficiency, and income source and amount (Ellen, 2001) (Figure 20-5). They react deeply to the loss of personal possessions because of the high sentimental value attached to the items and the limited time left to replace them (Gerrity and Flynn, 1997). Anticipatory guidance may help older adults who have to move into a nursing home, either temporarily or permanently, or who must adjust to moving in with an adult child. The need for relocation depends on the extent

of damage to their home or their compromised health. Older adults may hide the seriousness of their losses because of a fear of loss of independence (Oriol, 1999). Box 20-6 lists other populations at risk for severe disruption from a disaster.

## Role of the Nurse in Disaster Response

The role of the nurse during a disaster depends a great deal on the nurse's experience, professional role in a community disaster plan, specialty training, and special interest. The most important attribute for anyone working in a disaster, however, is flexibility (American Red Cross, 2002). If there is one thing certain about disaster, it is that there is continuing change.

Although valued for their expertise in community assessment, case finding and referring, prevention, health education, surveillance, and working with aggregates, there may be times when the nurse is the first to arrive on the scene. In this situation, it is important to remember that all life-threatening problems take priority. Once rescue workers begin to arrive at the scene, plans for triage should begin immediately.

**Triage** is the process of separating casualties and allocating treatment on the basis of the victims' potentials for survival. Highest priority is always given to victims who have life-threatening injuries but who have a high probability of survival once stabilized (Ciancamerla and Debacker, 2000). Second priority is given to victims with injuries that have systemic complications that are not yet life threatening and could wait 45 to 60 minutes for treatment. Last priority is given to those victims with local injuries without immediate complications and who can wait several hours for medical attention.

Nurses working as members of an assessment team need to feed back accurate information to relief managers to facilitate rapid rescue and recovery. Often nurses make home visits to gather needed information. Types of information in initial assessment reports include the following (Noji, 1996):

- Geographic extent of the disaster's impact
- Population at risk or affected
- Presence of continuing hazards
- Injuries and deaths
- Availability of shelter
- Current level of sanitation
- Status of health care infrastructure

These assessments help match available resources to a population's emergency needs. Noji (1996) also points out that disaster assessment priorities are related to the type of disaster that has occurred. For example, sudden-impact disasters, such as tornadoes and earthquakes, are more concerned with ongoing hazards, injuries and deaths, shelter requirements, and clean water. Gradual-onset disasters, such as famines, are most concerned with mortality rates, nutritional status, immunization status, and environmental health.

Lack of or inaccurate information regarding the scope of the disaster and its initial effects contributes to the misuse of resources. For example, after hurricane Andrew, a well-meaning public continued to ship thousands of pounds of clothing to South Florida, well beyond what it could ever hope to use. Much of the clothing eventually had to be burned because there were inadequate onsite personnel to sort and distribute the clothing, and the piles eventually became a public health nuisance. The tragedy of September 11 produced a similar outpouring of goods, much of which never reached the intended recipients. Pan American Health Organization (PAHO) officials caution "that despite good intentions, aid that does not answer real needs can became a burden" (Voelker, 1998). Local and regional emergency management and public health resources can be readjusted as assessment reports continue to come in. Prioritizing needs that benefit the largest aggregate of affected individuals with the most correctable problems is consistent with the most basic tenets of triage (PAHO, 2000).

Ongoing assessments or surveillance reports are just as important as initial assessments. Surveillance reports indicate the continuing status of the affected population and the effectiveness of ongoing relief efforts. They continue

---

## HOW TO  Gather Disaster Information

1. Interview
2. Observation
3. Individual physical examinations
4. Health and illness screening
5. Surveys (sample and special health)
6. Records (census, school, vital statistics, disease reporting)

From Landesman L: Public health management of disasters: the practice guide, Washington, DC, 2001, APHA.

---

to inform relief managers of needed resources. Nurses involved in ongoing surveillance can use the methods listed in the How To box to gather information. Surveillance continues into the recovery phase of a disaster.

## Shelter Management

Shelters are generally the responsibility of the local Red Cross chapter, although in massive disasters the military may be used to set up "tent cities" for the masses who need temporary shelter. Nurses, because of their comfort with delivering aggregate health promotion, disease prevention, and emotional support, make ideal shelter managers and team members. Although initially physical health needs are the priority, especially among older adults and the chronically ill, many of the predominant problems in shelters revolve around stress. The shock of the disaster itself, the loss of personal possessions, fear of the unknown, living in close proximity to total strangers, and even boredom can cause stress.

Common-sense approaches work best in working with victims dealing with stress. Basic measures that can be taken by the shelter nurse include the following (American Red Cross, 2002):

- Listen to victims tell and retell their feelings related to the disaster and their current situation.
- Encourage victims to share their feelings with one another if it seems appropriate to do so.
- Help victims make decisions.
- Delegate tasks (reading, crafts, and playing games with children) to teenagers and others to help combat boredom.
- Provide the basic necessities (food, clothing, rest).
- Attempt to recover or gain needed items (prescription glasses, medication).
- Provide basic compassion and dignity (e.g., privacy when appropriate and if possible).
- Refer to a mental health counselor if the situation warrants.

The American Red Cross provides specialized training in disaster mental health services. Its objective is "assisting the worker or client to understand disaster-related stress and grief reactions, develop adaptive coping and problem-solving skills, and return to a pre-disaster state of equilibrium or seek recommended further treatment" (American Red Cross, 1991, p. 5. Highly trained mental health counselors, such as psychologists, psychiatrists, clinical social workers, and nurses, are always available in large-scale disasters. They are important members of any disaster team, no matter what the level of disaster, and their services should be used as often as necessary.

Nurses in shelter functions are involved in assessment and referral, including medical needs (prescription glasses, medications), first aid, meal serving, keeping client records, ensuring emergency communications and transportation, and providing a safe environment (American Red Cross, 1998a). The Red Cross provides training for shelter support and using appropriate protocols.

## International Relief Efforts

Clearly, disasters do not occur just in industrialized countries. Other countries, especially those involved with political upheavals, suffer not only from natural disasters but from human-made disasters as well. Civil strife leads to war, famine, and communicable disease outbreaks. Sometimes disaster or relief workers are sent to these international disasters at the request of the affected country's government. At other times, workers are not welcomed but instead may go with the support of the UN. When workers are not welcomed, their lives may be in danger, even though they go as peacekeeping agents of the Federation of Red Cross and Red Crescent Societies and the International Committee of Red Cross or as health representatives from the World Health Organization. International disaster or relief workers generally have intense training and preparation before embarking on a mission.

## Psychological Stress of Disaster Workers

Psychological stress among victims and workers during disasters is well documented (Gerrity and Flynn, 1997). The degree of workers' stress depends on the nature of the disaster, their role in the disaster, individual stamina, and other environmental factors. Environmental factors include noise, inadequate workspace, physical danger, and stimulus overload, especially exposure to death and trauma. Other sources of stress may emerge when workers do not think that they are doing enough to help, from the burden of making life-and-death decisions, and from the overall change in living patterns (Bryce, 2001).

Disaster nurses who live in the community where disaster has struck and who are also victims of the disaster may experience additional stress. Anger and resentment may occur as the job demands time away from their own situation.

Symptoms of early stress and burnout include minor tremors, nausea, loss of concentration, difficulty thinking, and problems with memory (Bryce, 2001). Suppressing feelings of guilt, powerlessness, anger, and other signs of stress will eventually lead to symptoms such as irritability, fatigue, headaches, and distortions of bodily functions. It is normal to experience stress, but it must be dealt with. The worst thing anyone can do is to deny that it exists.

The American Red Cross (2002) and the PAHO (2000) recommend the following strategies for dealing with stress while working at the disaster:

- Get enough sleep.
- Take time away from the disaster (i.e., take breaks).
- Avoid alcohol.
- Eat frequently in small amounts.
- Use humor to break the tension and provide relief.
- Use positive self-talk.
- Take time to defuse or debrief.
- Stay in touch with people at home.
- Keep a journal.
- Provide mutual support.

**Delayed stress reactions,** or those that occur once the disaster is over, include exhaustion and an inability to adjust to the slower pace of work or home (Bryce, 2001). Other emotions out of the ordinary may occur but are normal for someone who has been involved with a disaster. Disappointment may be felt if family members and friends do not seem as interested in what the worker has been through and because coming back home, in general, does not live up to expectations.

Frustration and conflict may occur as the worker's needs seem totally inconsistent with those of the family and co-workers. Frustration and conflict also occur as a result of having left the disaster site, when there remains a real or perceived belief that much more could have been done (Bryce, 2001). Issues or problems that once seemed pressing may now seem trivial. Anger may emerge as others present problems that seem trivial compared with those faced by the victims who were left behind. Disaster workers may fantasize about returning to the disaster site if they think that their actions are appreciated more than at home or the office. Mood swings are common and serve to resolve conflicting feelings. Feelings or actions that persist or that the worker perceives are interfering with daily life should be dealt with by a trained mental health professional (American Red Cross, 2002).

## Recovery

The stage of disaster known as recovery occurs as all involved agencies pull together to restore the economic and civic life of the community (American Red Cross, 1993). For example, the government takes the lead in rebuilding efforts, whereas the business community attempts to provide economic support. Many religious organizations help with rebuilding efforts as well. The Internal Revenue Service educates victims as to how to write off losses and the Housing and Urban Development Department provides grants for temporary housing. The CDC provides continuing surveillance and epidemiologic services. Voluntary agencies continue to assess individual and community needs and meet those needs as they are able.

**DID YOU KNOW?**

The best time to start thinking about the lessons learned from a recent disaster is during the recovery phase of the disaster cycle.

Gerrity ET, Flynn BW: Mental health consequences of disasters. In Noji EK, editor: *The public health consequences of disasters,* New York, 1997, Oxford University Press.

## Role of the Nurse in Disaster Recovery

The role of the nurse in the recovery phase of a disaster is as varied as in the preparedness and response phases (Box 20-7). Flexibility remains important for a successful recovery operation. Community cleanup efforts can cause a

## Evidence-Based Practice

The aftermath of a natural disaster presents many challenges to health care workers. Most epidemiologic investigations after natural disasters have focused on physiological problems and containing infectious disease outbreaks. However, these investigations tend to neglect the long-term effects of disasters on affected populations, specifically the long-term mental health effects. Two years after hurricane Iniki struck the island of Kauai (one of the Hawaiian Islands), the Department of Psychiatry and Pediatrics of Mount Sinai School of Medicine and the National Center for Posttraumatic Stress Disorder studied the effectiveness of public health–inspired, school-based screening and treatment of mental distress following a natural disaster. There were two main objectives of the study. The first objective was to see if it is possible to identify symptomatic cases in a large population of children, given that few children may be symptomatic and not all symptomatic children outwardly display disordered behavior. The second goal was to determine the efficiency of providing treatment to relatively large numbers of affected children.

The study found that certain children were more likely to experience symptoms of mental health distress. These children included those of the female sex, younger age, and lower socioeconomic status. These children reacted with panic to the attack and feared for the physical safety of family and self during the disaster.

After being screened, children who were assessed to have high levels of trauma-related symptoms were provided school-based treatment. Children were randomly assigned to group or to individual treatment. Treatment consisted of four weekly sessions. The children were assessed again after treatment was complete, and then again a full year later.

The study found that the levels of mental health distress were significantly lower after treatment and remained at that level a year later without additional treatment. Group and individual treatments did not differ in their effectiveness, but group treatment was associated with higher levels of completion rates. The similarity of clinical ratings and self-report findings, as well as control for the passage of time and for the effects of assessment, suggest that these results did not merely reflect an immediate response but showed a long-term response to disaster.

**Nurse Use:** This study suggests that using schools as a natural means to screen and treat children affected by natural disasters is cost effective and valid. This public health inspired strategy may be useful in other posttraumatic environments. For example, children's psychological recovery in the aftermath of human-made disasters, including community violence and terrorism, may be facilitated in this way.

Chemtob CM, Nakashima JP, Hamada RS: Psychosocial intervention for postdisaster trauma symptoms in elementary school children, *Arch Pediatr Adolesc Med* 156:211-216, 2002.

---

### BOX 20-7  Prevention Levels in Disaster Management

**PRIMARY PREVENTION**

Participate in developing a disaster management plan for the community.

**SECONDARY PREVENTION**

Assess disaster victims and triage for care.

**TERTIARY PREVENTION**

Participate in home visits to uncover dangers that may cause additional injury to victims or cause other problems (e.g., house fires from faulty wiring).

---

host of physical and psychological problems. For example, the physical stress of moving heavy objects can cause back injury, severe fatigue, and even death from heart attacks. An additional burden that is often present is the continuing threat of communicable disease due to an inadequate water supply and crowded living conditions (Noji, 1996).

Nurses must remain vigilant in teaching proper hygiene and making sure immunization records are up to date.

Acute and chronic illnesses can become worse by the prolonged effects of disaster. The psychological stress of cleanup and/or moving can cause feelings of severe hopelessness, depression, and grief (Figure 20-6). Recovery can be impeded by short-term psychological effects that eventually merge with the long-term results of living in adverse circumstances (Bryce, 2001). In some cases, stress can lead to depression and suicide (Vastag, 2002). Although the majority of people eventually recover from disasters, mental distress may persist in members of vulnerable populations who continue to live in chronic adversity (Stephenson, 2001). Referrals to mental health professionals should continue as long as the need exists.

Nurses need to be alert for environmental health hazards during the recovery phase of a disaster. During home visits, they may uncover situations such as a faulty housing structure or lack of water or electricity. Objects that have been blown into the yard by a tornado or that floated in from a flood may be dangerous and must be removed. Also, the nurse should assess the dangers of live or dead animals and

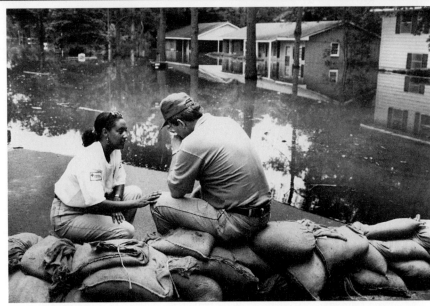

**Figure 20-6** The psychological stress of cleanup and moving can bring about feelings of severe hopelessness, depression, and grief. *(Courtesy American Red Cross. All rights reserved in all countries.)*

rodents that are harmful to a person's health. An example of this would be finding poisonous snakes in and around homes once the waters from a flood start to recede. The role of case finding and referral remains critical during the recovery phase and will continue, in some cases, for a long time. For example, for a full 2 years after the Oklahoma City bombing of the Alfred P. Murrah Federal Building, the American Red Cross supported the Bombing Recovery Project (American Red Cross, 1998b). Follow-up home visits were made for all those in need, although the recovery process for some will last for years. In the end, all of the nurses and organizations in the world can only provide partnerships with the victims of a disaster. Ultimately, it is up to individuals to recover on their own.

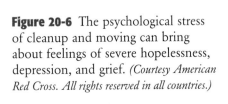

## Practice Application

Paula, a nurse in a medium-size public health department in Lincoln, Nebraska, was called to serve on her first national disaster assignment. Her disaster skills were tested when a level I hurricane hit Miami and its surrounding areas. Paula left Lincoln to help manage a shelter in an elementary school cafeteria in Homestead, Florida, near Miami.

The devastation that Paula saw en route to the school had a negative effect on her. She was assigned to help with client intake. She patiently listened to the disaster victims, referred many of her most distraught clients to the mental health counselor, and set priorities for other needs as they arose. For example, she found that many of her clients had left their medications behind and needed therapy. Other needs included diapers and formulas for infants, prescription eyeglasses, and clothing. By identifying their needs, Paula helped to ensure that the master "needs list" was complete.

As the days went on, the stress level in Paula's shelter began to intensify. The crowded living conditions and lack of privacy began to take its toll on the residents. Around the tenth day of Paula's assignment, she began to experience pounding headaches and was finding it difficult to concentrate. Paula believed she would be fine, but the mental health counselor told her that she was experiencing a stress reaction.

Which of the following actions would probably be the most useful for Paula to take?

**A.** Share her feelings with the on-site mental health counselor on a regular basis

**B.** Call home to share her feelings with family members

**C.** Meet the needs of her clients to the best of her ability, and accept the fact that stress is a part of the job

**Answer is in the back of the book.**

## Key Points

- The number of disasters, both human-made and natural, continue to increase, as do the number of people affected by them.
- The cost to recover from a disaster has risen sharply because of the amount of technology that must be restored.
- The director-general of the World Health Organization designated the decade of the 1990s the International Decade for Natural Disaster Reduction on the basis of a worldwide need for disaster education and a need to curtail the fatalistic approach to disasters that so many people take.
- Professional preparedness involves an awareness and understanding of the disaster plan at work and in the community.

- To counteract a historical lack of use or misuse of nurses in disaster planning, response, and recovery, nurses must get involved in their community's planning efforts, through their local health department or local government.
- Disaster health and disaster mental health training from an official agency such as the American Red Cross will help prepare nurses for the many opportunities that await them in disaster preparedness, response, and recovery.
- The response to a disaster is determined by its assigned level. Levels are not determined by the number of casualties but by the amount of resources needed.
- Helping clients maintain a safe environment and advocating for environmental safety measures in the community are key roles for the nurse during all phases of disaster management.
- Becoming knowledgeable about available community resources, especially for vulnerable populations, during the preparedness stage of disaster management will ensure smoother response and recovery stages.
- The Federal Response Plan may be activated if a disaster is so significant in its effect that it will overwhelm the capability of state and local governments to carry out the extensive emergency operations needed for community restoration.
- In all, 26 federal agencies and the Red Cross have specific functions to carry out in such an event.
- People in a community react differently to a disaster depending on the type, cause, and location of the disaster; its magnitude and extent of damage; its duration; and the amount of warning that was provided.
- Individual variables that cause people to react differently include their age, cultural background, health status, social support structure, and general adaptability to crisis.
- A great deal of stress is exhibited by nurses who are not only caring for clients but are also disaster victims themselves.
- Disaster shelter nurses are exposed to a variety of physical and emotional complaints, including stress. Stress may be instigated by the shock of the disaster, the loss of personal possessions, fear of the unknown, living in close proximity to strangers, and boredom.
- The degree of worker stress during disasters depends on the nature of the disaster, role in the disaster, individual stamina, noise level, adequacy of workspace, potential for physical danger, stimulus overload, and, especially, being exposed to death and trauma.

- Symptoms of worker stress during disasters include minor tremors, nausea, loss of concentration, difficulty thinking and remembering, irritability, fatigue, and other somatic disorders.
- A key attribute in aiding disaster victims is flexibility.
- The stage of disaster known as recovery occurs as all involved agencies pull together to restore the economic and civic life of the community.

## Clinical Decision-Making Activities

1. Select a vulnerable population within your community and determine what special needs the group would have in time of disaster. What community resources are currently available to help this group?
2. Describe the role of the nurse in the preparedness, response, and recovery stages of disaster. Does all of this make sense to you?
3. Interview a nurse who has participated in a disaster to determine what role was played and the nurse's reaction to that role. Ask the nurse to give you specific examples.
4. Conduct an interview with an official from the fire department, civil defense department, American Red Cross, or other agencies involved with disaster preparation and response to determine what your community's plan is. How can you find out if your community has a disaster plan?
5. Discuss the advantages and disadvantages of serving on a disaster team, in either your own community or another community. Decide whether you would be a good candidate to serve on a disaster team. Have you examined your ability to be flexible?
6. Contact your local public health department to determine its role in a local disaster, including the role of the nurses who work there. How could you check out a specific nurse's role in disaster management?
7. Find out what the disaster plan is for your place of employment. Give specific details.

## Additional Resources

These related resources are found either in the appendix at the back of this book or on the book's website at **http://evolve.elsevier.com/Stanhope**.

**evolve** Evolve Website

WebLinks: Healthy People 2010

# References

Alson RL, Leonard RB, Stringer LW: Disaster response in North Carolina, *N C Med J* 58(4):248-252, 1997.

Alson R et al: Analysis of medical treatment at a field hospital following hurricane Andrew, 1992, *Ann Emerg Med* 22(11):1721-1728, 1993.

American Red Cross: *The creed of a Red Cross nurse,* Washington, DC, 1981, ARC.

American Red Cross: *Disaster mental health services* (ARC publication No. 3050M), Washington, DC, 1991, ARC.

American Red Cross: *Disaster mental health services I* (ARC publication No. 3077-1A), Washington, DC, 1993, ARC.

American Red Cross: *Disasters happen* (ARC publication No. 1570), Washington, DC, 1994, ARC.

American Red Cross: The American Red Cross and mitigation, *Disaster Services News Sheet* Feb 3, 1998a.

American Red Cross: Oklahoma City bombing recovery project: answering the call: Roberta Flynn offers encouragement to victims, *Disaster Services News Sheet* Feb 27, 1998b.

American Red Cross: *Disaster health services simulation: instructor manual* (ARC publication No. 3076-2), Washington, DC, 2000, ARC.

American Red Cross: *How do I deal with my feelings?* Washington, DC, 2001, ARC.

American Red Cross: *Disaster mental health services: an overview* (ARC publication No. 3077-2A), Washington, DC, 2002, ARC.

American Red Cross: *Foundations of the disaster services program* (ARC publication No. 3000, pg. 12), Washington, DC, 2003, ARC.

Associated Press: As patriotism soars, flags are hard to come by, *USA Today* Sept 16, 2001, retrieved from www.usatoday.com/news/nation/2001/09/16/flag-shortage.htm.

Bryce CP: *Stress management in disasters,* Washington, DC, 2001, Pan American Health Organization.

Center for Disease Control and Prevention: *Local emergency preparedness and response inventory,* Atlanta, Ga, 2002, Public Health Program Office, available at www.bt.cdc.gov.

Chemtob CM, Nakashima JP, Hamada RS: Psychosocial intervention for post-disaster trauma symptoms in elementary school children, *Arch Pediatr Adolesc Med* 156:211-216, 2002.

Ciancamerla G, Debacker M: Triage. In de Boer J et al, editors: *Handbook of disaster medicine,* Zeist, The Netherlands, 2000, International Society of Disaster Medicine.

Crippen DW: *Disaster management: lessons from September 11, 2001,* presented at 8th World Congress of Intensive and Critical Care Medicine, Sydney, Australia, 2002.

Ellen EF: The elderly may have advantage in natural disasters, *Psychiatric Times* 18(1), 2001.

English J, Malone J: *Bioterrorism readiness plan: a template for healthcare facilities,* Atlanta, Ga, 1999, Centers for Disease Control and Prevention, available at www. cdc.gov.

Federal Emergency Management Agency, American Red Cross: *Your family disaster plan,* Washington, DC, 1997, FEMA, ARC.

Federal Emergency Management Agency: *The federal response plan (FRP),* Washington, DC, 1999, FEMA.

Federal Emergency Management Agency: *National situation updates,* Washington, DC, 2001, FEMA, available at www.fema.gov/emanagers/nat091201.htm.

Fire Department of New York: *Daily World Trade Center update,* 2002, available at www.ci.nyc.us.

Gebbie KM, Qureshi K: Emergency and disaster preparedness: core competencies for nurses—what every nurse should but may not know, *Am J Nurs* 102(1):46-51, 2002.

Gerrity ET, Flynn BW: Mental health consequences of disasters. In Noji EK, editor: *The public health consequences of disasters,* New York, 1997, Oxford University Press.

Goodkin K: Effective new treatments for grief: Facts of Life Issue Briefing for Health Reporters, Center for the Advancement of Health, 7(3), 2002, available at www.cfah.org/pdfs/ grief_march_2002.pdf.

International Federation of Red Cross and Red Cross Societies: *World disaster report 2001,* Washington DC, 2001, available at www.ifrc.org.

Landesman L: Public health management of disasters: the practice guide, Washington, DC, 2001, APHA.

Noji EK: Disaster epidemiology, *Emerg Med Clin North Am* 14(2):289, 1996.

Oriol W: Pyschosocial issues for older adults in disasters, Washington, DC, Emergency Services and Disaster Relief Branch, Center for Mental Health Services, Substance and Abuse Mental Health Services Administration, 1999, available at http://www.mentalhealth. org/publications/allpubs/SMA99-3323/ 99-821.pdf.

Pan American Health Organization: *A quick guide to effective donations,* Washington, DC, 2000, PAHO, available at www.paho.org/english/ped/ humanitarianassistnce.htm.

Raji A: A piece of my mind: the body politic, *JAMA* 287(3):286, 2002.

Rotz LD et al: Bioterrorism preparedness: planning for the future, *J Public Health Manag Pract* 6(4):45, 2000.

Stephenson J: Medical, mental health communities mobilize to cope with terror's psychological aftermath, *JAMA* 286(15):1823, 2001.

Switzer KH: Functioning in a community health setting. In Garcia LM, editor: *Disaster nursing: planning, assessment, and intervention,* Rockville, Md, 1985, Aspen.

United Nations Office for the Coordination of Humanitarian Affairs: Natural disasters and sustainable development: linkages and policy options, *OCHA-Online,* Nov 6, 1998, available at http:// 156.106.192.130/dha_ol/programs/ idndr/presskit/options.html.

U.S. Department of Health and Human Services: *The public health response to biological and chemical terrorism,* Washington, DC, 2001, available at www.bt. cdc.gov/documents/planning/ planningguidance.pdf.

Vastag B: PTSD and depression in NYC, *JAMA* 287(15):1930, 2002.

Voelker R: The world in medicine: pinpointing disaster needs, *JAMA* 280(22): 1898, 1998.

Waeckerle JF: Disaster planning and response, *N Engl J Med* 324(12):815-821, 1991.

Waeckerle JF: Domestic preparedness for events involving weapons of mass destruction, *JAMA* 283(2):252, 2000.

Yates J: Gifts, letters piling up at N.Y. relief centers, *Chicago Tribune* Oct 6, A1, 2001.

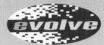
# Program Management

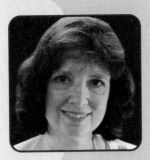

**Doris F. Glick, R.N., Ph.D.**
Doris F. Glick is currently an associate professor and director of the master's program at the School of Nursing of the University of Virginia in Charlottesville. Her work has focused on teaching, research, and scholarship in community and public health nursing. She has taught courses in community and public health nursing, epidemiology, management, and global women's health. She has developed a community nurse-managed center, has served as a public health nursing consultant for the state of Florida, and has served on numerous community health boards. Her research and publications focus on access to care for vulnerable populations and on management of community-focused services. She has presented widely at national and international meetings.

## Objectives

After reading this chapter, the student should be able to do the following:

1. Compare and contrast the program management process and the nursing process
2. Analyze the application of the program planning process to community-oriented nursing
3. Critique a program planning method to use in community-oriented nursing practice
4. Analyze the components of program evaluation methods, techniques, and sources
5. Compare different types of cost studies applied to program management

**P**rogram management consists of assessing, planning, implementing, and evaluating a program. This chapter focuses primarily on planning and evaluation. Although presented in separate discussions, these factors are related and interdependent processes that work together to bring about a successful program. This chapter does not deal with implementing programs, because most other chapters in this text focus on implementation.

The program management process is parallel to the nursing process. One is applied to a program that addresses the needs of a specific population, whereas the other is applied to individuals or families. The process of program management, like the nursing process, consists of a rational decision-making system designed to help nurses know when to make a decision to develop a program (assessment and identifiable problem), where they want to be at the end of the program (goal setting), how to decide what to do to have a successful program (planning), how to develop a plan to go from where they are to where they want to be (implementing), how to know that they are getting there (formative evaluation), and what to measure to know that the program has successful outcomes (summative evaluation).

Today, there is a greater need for the nurse to be accountable for nursing actions and client outcomes. Introducing prospective payment systems, health care reform, and managed care has changed the focus of nursing. Planning for nursing services is necessary today if the nurse is to survive in the field of health care delivery.

Community-oriented nurses are expected to demonstrate leadership in addressing community health problems. This chapter examines how nurses can act, instead of reacting, by planning programs that can be evaluated for their effectiveness. This discussion focuses on the historical development of health planning and evaluation, a generic program planning and evaluation method, the benefits of planning and evaluation, the elements of planning and evaluation, how cost studies are applied to program evaluation, and how programs may be funded. Some sections of this chapter can be used by undergraduate students, whereas other sections are more appropriately used by graduate students.

*The author acknowledges the important foundational work for this chapter developed by Dr. Marcia Stanhope in previous editions of this book.*

## Key Terms

**case registers**, p. 509
**community assessment**, p. 494
**community health planning**, p. 494
**cost accounting**, p. 510
**cost benefit**, p. 510
**cost effectiveness**, p. 510
**cost efficiency**, p. 511
**cost studies**, p. 510
**evaluation**, p. 491

**formative evaluation**, p. 505
**grant writing**, p. 512
**health program planning**, p. 495
**outcome**, p. 508
**planning**, p. 491
**planning process**, p. 495
**population needs assessment**, p. 494
**process**, p. 508
**program**, p. 491

**program effectiveness**, p. 505
**program evaluation**, p. 498
**program management**, p. 490
**project**, p. 491
**strategic planning**, p. 493
**structure**, p. 508
**summative evaluation**, p. 505
**tracer**, p. 509
*See Glossary for definitions*

## Chapter Outline

Definitions and Goals
Historical Overview of Health Care Planning
   and Evaluation
Benefits of Program Planning
Assessment of Need
*Community Assessment*
*Population Needs Assessment*
Planning Process
*Basic Program Planning Model Using a*
   *Population-Level Example*
Program Evaluation

*Benefits of Program Evaluation*
*Planning for the Evaluation Process*
*Evaluation Process*
*Formulating Objectives*
*Sources of Program Evaluation*
*Aspects of Evaluation*
Advanced Planning Methods and Evaluation
   Models
*Planning, Programming, and Budgeting System*
*Program Planning Method*
*Program Evaluation Review Technique*

*Critical Path Method*
*Multi-Attribute Utility Technique*
*Evaluation Models and Techniques*
Cost Studies Applied to Program Management
*Cost Accounting*
*Cost Benefit*
*Cost Effectiveness*
*Cost Efficiency*
Program Funding

# DEFINITIONS AND GOALS

**Community health planning** is population focused, and it puts the well-being of the public above private interests (Rohrer, 1996). A **program** is an organized approach to meet the assessed needs of individuals, families, groups, populations, or communities by reducing the effect of or eliminating one or more health problems. Community health programs are planned to meet the needs of designated populations or subpopulations in a community. Examples of specific programs in public health nursing are home health programs, immunization programs, health-risk screening programs for industrial workers, and family planning programs. These programs are usually conducted under the direction of the total program plan of a local health department or a managed care agency. More broadly based group and community programs are the community school health program, the occupational health and safety program, the environmental health program, and community programs directed at preventing specific illnesses through special-interest groups (e.g., American Heart Association, American Cancer Society, March of Dimes). Programs are ongoing organized activities that become part of the continuing health services of a community, whereas **projects** are smaller, organized activities with a limited time frame. A health fair and a blood pressure screening day at the mall are examples of projects that nurses may implement.

**Planning** is defined as the selecting and carrying out of a series of actions to achieve stated goals (Kropf, 1995). The *goal* of planning is to ensure that health care services are acceptable, equal, efficient, and effective. **Evaluation** is determining whether a service is needed and can be used, whether it is conducted as planned, and whether the service actually helps people in need (Posavac and Carey, 2000). Evaluation for the purpose of assessing whether objectives are met or planned activities are completed is referred to as *formative* or *process evaluation*. This type of evaluation begins with an assessment of the need for a program. Evaluation to assess program outcomes or as a follow-up of the results of the program activities is called *summative* or *impact evaluation*.

Program evaluation is an ongoing process from the beginning of the planning phase until the program ends. It is used to make judgments about improving, managing, and continuing programs. The major goals of program evaluation are to determine the relevance, adequacy, progress, efficiency, effectiveness, impact, and sustainability of program activities (Kaluzny and Veney, 1999).

## HISTORICAL OVERVIEW OF HEALTH CARE PLANNING AND EVALUATION

As the health care delivery system has grown in the past century, emphasis on health planning and evaluation has increased. Factors that have increased interest in planning and evaluation are advances in health care technology and consumer education, increased consumer expectations, third-party payers, budget pressures, increased professional conflicts, focus on preventive care, new focus on health care as a business, unionizing of health care workers, urbanization, increased health risks, personnel shortages, and increased health care costs. From the 1920s to the 1940s, specific actions were taken that related to health planning. Table 21-1 outlines the development of health planning.

The post–World War II era after 1944 brought an interest in evaluating program effectiveness. As government and third-party payers began to finance health care services and money became more plentiful, public demand for health services grew. As a result, numbers and kinds of health care agencies increased; laws were passed to increase the scope of and control over health care, and the health

---

### Table 21-1 Historical Development of Health Planning and Evaluation

| YEAR | ACTOR | ACTION |
|------|-------|--------|
| 1920 | Committees on administrative practice and evaluation of American Public Health Association | Called for public health officers to engage in better program planning<br>Reduced haphazard methods used to develop public health programs |
| 1920s | Committee on costs of medical care | Studied social and economic aspects of health services<br>Cited the need for comprehensive health care planning because of rising costs and unequal health care services to target populations |
| 1944 | American Hospital Association | Established committee on postwar planning<br>Began regional planning for nationwide health services |
| 1946 | Federal government, Congress | Passed the Hospital Survey and Construction Act (Hill-Burton Act) to legislate health planning, which resulted in increase in number of hospitals |
| 1963 | Federal government, Congress | Emphasis on Great Society programs<br>Community Mental Health Centers Act (Public Law 88-464) was passed to provide mental health programs in the states; defined the role of consumers in making decisions and of professionals as advisors in the planning process |
| 1965 | Federal government, Congress | Passed Regional Medical program legislation (Public Law 89-239); upgraded quality of tertiary health care services for the leading causes of death<br>Coined the term *Partnership for Health* |
| 1965 | U.S. Department of Health and Human Services | Office of Health Planning opened<br>No direct authority for health planning given |
| 1966 | Federal government, Congress | Passed the Comprehensive Health Planning (CHP) and Public Health Services amendments (Public Law 89-749)<br>Developed a national health planning system |
| 1974 | Federal government, Congress | Passed National Health Planning and Resources Development Act (Public Law 93-641), which provided specific directions for developing the structure, process, and functions of a national health planning system |
| 1993 | President Clinton | Introduced the Health Security Act to provide for health care reform and planning based on population needs |
| 1994-1999 | States | Introduced legislation for health care based on planning and evaluating state reform population needs (Kentucky, Hawaii, Minnesota, Oregon, Florida, California, Washington, New York) |
| 2001-2003 | Federal government | New focus on need to protect the health of the public; focus on planning for community response to disasters |

care delivery system began to be held accountable for its actions. During this time, legislation was passed to require health care providers and consumers to work together in groups to address issues in health care.

Through the 1970s, laws were passed that gradually changed to provide a more comprehensive structure and more power over federal program funds. In 1974 Congress enacted the National Health Planning and Resources Development Act. This legislation had the goal of reducing the growth of health care costs by ensuring that only needed services and facilities would be added to the health care system. Under this legislation, health care providers were required to obtain a certificate of public need (COPN) in order to add services or facilities. However, there was very little authority to carry out some of the more critical tasks of improving the health of clients, increasing access and quality of services, restraining costs, and preventing the duplication of unnecessary services. Power over the private health care sector continued to be absent.

As "the new federalism" became the catch phrase of the 1980s and emphasis was placed on cost shifting, reducing costs, and more competition within the health care system, President Ronald Reagan proposed doing away with the federal government's role in health planning. In 1981, with cutbacks in federal spending, states began the takeover or dismantling of their own health planning systems. The national health planning system came to a halt. The federal, state, and consumer partnership for health care was ended.

In 1993, with President Bill Clinton's emphasis on health care reform, the decision was made that the government would continue to be not involved in health planning. It would use its power to set limits on health insurance costs and limit overall health care spending. In this way, it would influence health planning decisions made by the private health care agencies and providers (Kropf, 1995). Although national health care reform did not occur, many states are engaged in reforming their systems.

Today, at the beginning of the twenty-first century, the process of health planning is not coordinated but is largely in the control of different interests in the health care industry. The health care system is largely shaped by decisions of hospitals, physicians, pharmaceutical companies, equipment companies, insurance companies, and managed care organizations, which determine where, how, and for whom health care will be delivered. Although the Federal Health Planning legislation is no longer in effect, some states continue to have health systems agencies (HSAs), although these organizations have much less authority than when they were established in the 1970s. In some states, the health systems agency must approve the planned expanding of agencies or services, and a COPN must be issued by the state before these plans may proceed. The primary purpose of such health planning is to improve the health of local communities by increasing available and accessible services, preventing the duplicating of services, and controlling health care costs.

The political party in power often influences the outcome of the national and state health planning efforts. Nurses must be involved in aspects of health planning for the community in which they live in order to influence the direction of health care reform.

In addition to health planning in the external environment, internal health care agency planning is necessary to meet the goals and objectives of providing efficient, effective health care services to clients at a reasonable cost. Community health personnel have a responsibility to participate in internal planning and evaluation to solve the problems of a client population and to ensure the delivery of health services that are accessible, acceptable, and affordable. Both health care planning within the community and national health care planning affect health care planning within an agency. For example, today there is much emphasis on developing national and community health plans to prevent bioterrorism. The federal government is developing a plan, and states and communities have been given federal monies to develop their own plans. Agencies within communities have been asked to develop bioterrorism prevention plans and to be a part of the community plans.

## BENEFITS OF PROGRAM PLANNING

Systematic planning for meeting the health needs of populations in a community has benefits for clients, nurses, the employing agencies, and the community. Planning ensures that available resources are used to address the actual needs of people in the community, and it focuses attention on what the organization and health provider are attempting to do for clients. Planning assists in identifying the resources and activities that are needed to meet the objectives of client services. Planning reduces role ambiguity (uncertainty) by giving responsibility to specific providers to meet program objectives.

Planning also reduces uncertainty within the program environment and increases the abilities of the provider and the agency to cope with the external environment. Everyone involved with the program can anticipate what will be needed to implement the program, what will occur during the implementing process, and what the program outcomes will be. Planning helps the provider and the agency anticipate events. Also, planning allows for quality decision making and better control over the actual program results. Today, this type of planning is referred to as **strategic planning,** and it involves the successful matching of client needs with specific provider strengths and competencies and agency

## THE CUTTING EDGE

A major national program to assist communities to plan, organize, and develop programs specific to their needs is called Turning Point. See the website, www.turningpointprogram.org.

resources. The planning process reflects the desires to implement a reality-based program that can be readily evaluated and can reduce the number of unexpected events that occur.

## ASSESSMENT OF NEED

Planning for effective and efficient programs must be based on identifying the needs of populations within a community. Identifying at-risk groups and documenting the health needs of the targeted population are the reasons and rationale for the program plan. Such documenting of need is essential if funding will be sought to implement the plan. An assessment of health needs may be approached as either a community assessment or a population needs assessment.

## Community Assessment

A thorough assessment of a community is necessary to provide a clear understanding of the overall health status of a community and to identify populations at risk. Public health agencies, health planners, and nurses and agencies wishing to address the true needs of a community benefit from accurate and thorough community assessment data.

A **community assessment** is comprehensive. It is a community-oriented approach that views the entire community as the client. Community assessment considers all of the people in a community for the purpose of identifying the most vulnerable populations and determining unmet health needs. All of the services of a community are examined to assess their effect on the health of the population, and the environment is assessed for its impact on the health of the people. For example, some vulnerable groups may lack access to existing services because of lack of transportation, or there may be a high prevalence of asthma because of air pollution from a particular industrial source.

Community assessment begins with the collection of existing data (secondary data). Variables related to the characteristics of the population in the community include demographic data such as age, sex, ethnic group/race, income, occupation, education, health status, norms, and values. Such data, which for most communities are readily available on the internet, are derived from census data and morbidity and mortality statistics. Data about communities may be found in local libraries, courthouse records, service agencies, newspapers, the phonebook, and other local resources.

New data about the community may be collected through surveys or interviews with community members and key informants. When community members have a voice in identifying needs and in program planning, community acceptance and use of that program are likely to be increased.

Variables related to people, resources, and the environment of a community be determined by using existing models that provide an organizing framework for the collecting and analyzing of data (Box 21-1). (For more information about community assessment and the community-

### BOX 21-1 Example of a Real-Time Community Assessment

Community assessment data will help social groups and government understand residents' needs. LexLinc and the University Research Center for Families and Children released results yesterday of the first County Self-Assessment, a demographic study of the community. Those involved with the study hope the findings will help local groups more accurately address the needs of the county.

The results are a tool to help community organizations, government, businesses, faith-based organizations and neighborhood groups make more informed decisions. The survey has data about households, finances, health, crime and other topics from more than 1,500 families. The data show geographic areas with high-service and low-income characteristics.

In the county the average reported income is between $40,000 and $49,000, while the same figure for the targeted areas is $25,000 and $29,000. In nontargeted areas, 97% of those surveyed consider their neighborhood safe, compared with 79% in target sectors.

The findings are helpful for agencies applying for grants to develop needed programs.

Excerpted from Meredith Kesner, staff writer: Lexington (Kentucky) *Herald-Leader,* March 7, 2003, p. B3

as-partner model, see Chapter 15.) Also, check out this textbook's website at http://evolve.elsevier.com/Stanhope to find assessment tools for the vulnerable population group: the physically compromised.

## Population Needs Assessment

Agencies or health care providers are frequently interested in providing a specific service in a community and want to assess the need for that service in the target population. In this case, an assessment may be focused on determining the needs of a specific population in a community. The *assessment of need* is defined as a systematic appraisal of type, depth, and scope of problems as perceived by clients, health providers, or both.

A **population needs assessment** focuses on the characteristics of a specific population, their health needs, and the resources available to address those needs. For example, a nurse may want to initiate a health education program for older adult diabetics, or to establish an immunization program for children of a certain age or health services for migrant workers. In each case, assessment would focus on the characteristics and health status of the target population and the resources available to address the identified need for that group. When assessing a population, the same types of data collected for community assessment are collected and entered for the population—such as demographic data.

## Table 21-2  Summary of Needs Assessment Tools

| NAME | DEFINITION | ADVANTAGES | DISADVANTAGES |
|---|---|---|---|
| Community forum | Community, group, organization, open meeting | • Low cost<br>• Learn perspectives of large number of persons | • Limited data<br>• Limited expression of views<br>• Discourages less powerful<br>• Becomes arena to discuss political issues |
| Focus groups | Open discussion with small representative groups | • Low cost<br>• Clients participate in identification of need<br>• Initiates community support for the program | • Time consuming<br>• Allows focus on irrelevant or political issues |
| Key informant | Identify, select, and question knowledgeable leaders | • Provides picture of services needed | • Bias of leaders<br>• Community<br>• Characteristics may be incorrectly perceived by informants |
| Indicators approach | Existing data used to determine problem | • Excellent data on problems and characteristics of client groups | • Growth and change in population may make data outdated |
| Survey of existing agencies | Estimates of client populations via services used at similar community agencies | • Easy method to estimate size of client group<br>• Know extent of services offered in existing programs | • Records and data may be unreliable<br>• All cases of need may not be reported<br>• Exaggeration of services may occur |
| Surveys | Measurement of total or sample client population by interview or questionnaire | • Direct and accurate data on client population and their problems | • Expensive<br>• Technically demanding<br>• Need many interviews or observations<br>• Interviews may be biased |

It is important to avoid planning services that do not target the health needs of a community and services already provided by other agencies. A needs assessment determines gaps in or duplication of needed services (i.e., their availability), examines the quality of existing resources to meet the identified needs (i.e., their adequacy), and identifies barriers to the use of existing resources (i.e., their acceptability).

A number of needs assessment tools exist to assist the nurse in the needs assessment process. The major sources of information used for needs assessment, summarized in Table 21-2, are census data, key informants, community forums, surveys of existing community agencies with similar programs, surveys of residents of the community to be served (client population), and statistical indicators (Rossi and Freeman, 1999).

## PLANNING PROCESS

**Health program planning** is affected by government control over licensure and funding, by society, and by the culture and belief system of the population in which the program must function. Program planning is required by federal, state, and local governments; by philanthropic organizations; and by the employing agency. Planning programs and planning for the evaluation of programs are two very important activities, whether the program being planned is a national health insurance program such as Medicare, a state health care program such as an early childhood development screening program, or a local program such as vision screening for elementary schoolchildren. Regardless of the type of program, the planning process is the same.

Nutt (1984) describes a basic **planning process** that is reflected in the steps of most planning methods. The process includes five planning stages: formulating, conceptualizing, detailing, evaluating, and implementing (Table 21-3).

---

**( DID YOU KNOW?**

Nurses working in community-oriented agencies who identify unmet needs among vulnerable populations can initiate program development and find funding to provide needed services.

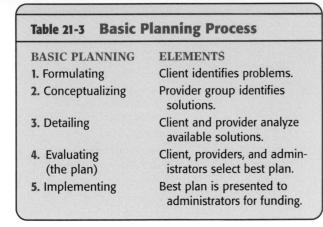

**Table 21-3   Basic Planning Process**

| BASIC PLANNING | ELEMENTS |
|---|---|
| 1. Formulating | Client identifies problems. |
| 2. Conceptualizing | Provider group identifies solutions. |
| 3. Detailing | Client and provider analyze available solutions. |
| 4. Evaluating (the plan) | Client, providers, and administrators select best plan. |
| 5. Implementing | Best plan is presented to administrators for funding. |

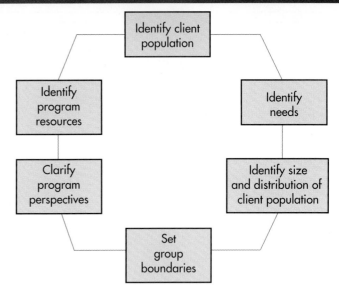

**Figure 21-1** Steps in the needs assessment process.

## Basic Program Planning Model Using a Population-Level Example

### Formulating

The initial and most critical step in planning a health program is defining the problem and assessing client need. This stage in the planning process can be *preactive*, projecting a future need; *reactive*, defining the problem based on past needs; *inactive*, defining the problem on the basis of the existing health state of the population to be served; or *interactive*, describing the problem using past and present data to project future population needs.

Needs assessment is a key ingredient in the planning process. The target population or client to be served by any program must be identified and involved in designing the program. Program planners must verify that a current health problem exists and is being either ignored or unsuccessfully treated in a client group. Data provide the rationale to establish a new program or revise existing programs to meet the needs of the client group. The client population should be defined specifically by its demographic and psychosocial characteristics, by geographic location, and by the problems to be addressed. For example, in a community with a large number of preschool children who require immunizations to enter school, the client population may be described as all children between 4 and 6 years of age residing in Central County who have not had up-to-date immunizations (Figure 21-1).

A health education program may be necessary to alert the population to the existing need. In the example of the need for immunizing preschool children, public service announcements on television and radio and in newspapers may be used to alert parents to laws requiring immunizations, to the continuing problems with communicable diseases, and to the outcomes of successful immunizing programs, such as vaccination programs that have been successful in eliminating smallpox worldwide. A good example of the use of media was seen when an outbreak of rubella occurred in Los Angeles. Local and national television was used to bring attention to the problem, to encourage parents to have children immunized, and to en-

courage other communities to launch campaigns to prevent additional outbreaks.

*Specifying the size and distribution of a client population* for a program involves more than counting the number of persons in the community who may be eligible for the program. It involves determining the number of persons with the problem who are unserved by existing programs and the numbers of eligible persons who have and who have not taken advantage of existing services. For example, consider again the community need for a preschool immunization program. In planning the program, the size of the population of preschool children in the county may be obtained from census data or birth certificates. The nurse then must determine the number of children unserved and the number of children who have not used services for which they are eligible.

*Boundaries* for the client population are primarily established by defining the size and distribution of the client population. The boundaries will stipulate who is included in and who is excluded from the health program. If the fictional immunization program were designed to serve only preschool children of low-income families, all other preschool children would be excluded.

*Perspectives on the program,* or what people think about the need for a program, might differ between health providers, agency administrators, policy makers, and potential clients. These groups are considered the stakeholders in the program. Collecting data on the opinions and attitudes of all persons, whether directly or indirectly involved with the program's success, is necessary to determine if the program is feasible, the need to redefine the problems, or the decision to develop a new program or expand or modify an existing program. For example, policy makers in the 1970s decided that neighborhood health clinics were the answer to providing services for low-income residents. They discov-

| Solution | Alternatives | Uncertain risks | Consequences |

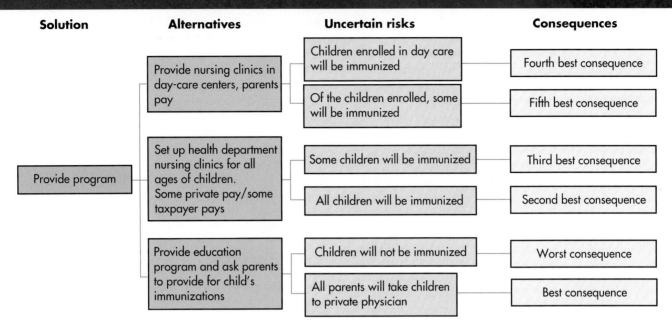

**Figure 21-2** Ranking of solutions to problem: providing a preschool immunization program to low-income children using a decision tree.

ered that their perspective was not the same as those of most health providers or of the clients, who were not supportive of developing neighborhood clinics. The neighborhood health clinics failed because the clients would not use them. If the policymakers had explored the perspectives of the clients when planning the program, they might have chosen another type of service to offer.

Before implementing a health program, the nurse must also identify available resources. *Program resources* include personnel, facilities, equipment, and financing. The number and kinds of personnel available to implement a program must be determined. Available supplies and up-to-date equipment are as essential for implementing a program as the source and amount of funds. If any one of the four categories of resources is unavailable, the program is likely to be inadequate to meet the needs of the client population. If planners consider the problem to be a critical one, funding may be sought by seeking donations or by writing a proposal for grant funds to support the program. A well-done assessment provides direction and suggests strategies for appropriate interventions.

## Conceptualizing

The need and demand for a program are determined through the formulating process. The conceptualizing stage of planning creates options for solving the problem and considers several solutions. Each option for program solution is examined for its uncertainties (risks) and consequences, leading to a set of *outcomes*.

Some alternative solutions to the problem will have more risk or uncertainties than others. The nurse must decide between a solution that involves more risk and a solution that is free of risk. A "do nothing" decision is always the decision with the least risk to the provider. When choosing a solution, the nurse looks at whether the desired outcome can be achieved. After careful thought about each possible solution to the problem, the nurse rethinks the solutions. The assessment data compiled during the formulation stage should be used to develop alternative solutions.

Decision trees are useful graphic aids that give a picture of the solutions and the risks of each solution. Such a picture graph of the process of identifying a solution helps clients and administrators rank the consequences of a decision. Figure 21-2 shows an example of a decision tree.

As shown in Figure 21-2, the best consequence would be for each family to provide immunizations for its children. One must consider the value of this action to the parents, the odds that immunizations will be given if a formal clinic is not available, the cost to the parents as opposed to the taxpayer, and the cost to the community. Costs to the community include the possibility of increased incidence of communicable disease or mortality and increased need for more expensive services to treat the diseases if children are not immunized. If the parents provide the immunizations for their own children, costs to the taxpayer and to the community are low.

## Detailing

In this phase, the provider, with client input, considers the possibilities of solving a problem using one of the solutions identified. The provider details (or is specific about) the costs, resources, and program activities needed to choose one of the solutions from the conceptualizing phase. For each of the three proposed alternatives shown in the immunization scenario in Figure 21-2, the program planner lists the activities that would need to be implemented. Using the proposed solution of encouraging the parents to provide the immunizations (the best consequence), examples of activities include developing a script for a health education program and implementing a television program to encourage parents to take children to the physician. If an alternative that produced the second, third, fourth, or fifth best consequence was chosen, offering a clinic 8 hours per day at the health department and providing a mobile clinic to each day-care center for 4 hours each day to provide the immunizations would be possible activities.

For each alternative, the nurse lists the resources needed to implement each activity. The resources to be considered include all costs of personnel, supplies, equipment, and facilities, and the potential acceptance by the clients and the administrators of the program. In the example, personnel could include nurses, volunteers, and clerks; supplies might include handouts, Band-Aids, vaccine, records, and consent forms; equipment might include syringes, needles, stethoscopes, and blood pressure cuffs; and facilities might include a television studio for a media blitz on the education program and a room with examination tables, chairs, and emergency carts. The total costs of each solution must be considered. As indicated, clients should review each solution for acceptance.

## Evaluating

In the evaluation phase of the plan, each alternative is weighed to judge the costs, benefits, and acceptance of the idea to the client population, community, and provider. The information outlined in the detailing phase would be used to rank the solutions for choice by the client population and provider on the basis of cost, benefit, and acceptance. Consideration must be given to the solution that will provide the desired outcomes. Looking at available information through literature reviews or interviews might suggest whether someone else had previously tried each of the options in another place. The experience of others may be helpful in deciding whether a chosen solution would be useful.

## Implementing

In the implementing phase of the planning process, the clients, providers, and administrators select the best plan to solve the original problem. Change theory is useful to help create an environment in which the best solution may be supported. Providing reasons why a particular solution was chosen will help the provider get the approval of the agency administration for the plan. On approval, the plan is implemented.

Community members may participate in implementing the program either as volunteers or as paid staff. Program success will be increased if community residents are included in the work of the program and on advisory boards and if they participate in program evaluation. The greater the participation of community members in developing a program, the greater will be the sense of ownership of that program by members of the target population, and therefore the greater will be the probability that the program will achieve its objectives and result in positive changes in health (Glick et al, 1996).

## PROGRAM EVALUATION

### Benefits of Program Evaluation

**Program evaluation** is a method of ensuring that a program has met its goals. The major benefit of program evaluation is that it shows whether the program is fulfilling its purpose. It should answer the following questions:

1. Are the needs for which the program was designed being met?
2. Are the problems it was designed to solve being solved?

This is critical information for program managers, funding agencies, top-level decision makers, program accreditation reviewers, health providers, and the community. Evaluation data are used to make judgments about a program and may be used to justify making adjustments in the program, expanding or reducing the program, or even closing it.

Hale, Arnold, and Travis (1994) describe process evaluation, also referred to as formative evaluation, as examining, documenting, and analyzing the progress of a program. Changes are required when there is unacceptable difference between what was observed and what was anticipated. Corrective action may then be taken to get the program back on track. This description of process evaluation is consistent with what Rossi and Freeman (1999) and Veney and Kaluzny (1998) refer to as program monitoring. Three critical questions are addressed when monitoring a program (Glick and Kulbok, 2001): (1) Does the program reach the target population? (2) Were activities to reach the goals carried out as planned? (3) What was the resource use in implementing the program?

Quality assurance programs are prime examples of program evaluation in health care delivery. Evaluation data are used to justify continuing programs in community health. Program evaluation focuses on whether goals were met and the efficiency and effectiveness of program activities. Many methods of program evaluation are described in the literature. The primary method of evaluation used in health care today is Donabedian's (1982) evaluative framework, which examines the structure, process, and outcomes of a program. Other models and frameworks

## HOW TO   Develop a Program Plan

A. Define the problem
B. Formulate the plan
  1. Assess population need
     a. Who is the program population?
     b. What is the need to be met?
     c. How large is the client population to be served?
     d. Where are they located?
     e. How does the target population define the need?
     f. Are there other programs addressing the same need? (Describe.)
     g. Why is the need not being met?
  2. Establish program boundaries
     a. Who will be included in the program?
     b. Who will not be included? Why?
     c. What is the program goal?
  3. Program feasibility
     a. Who agrees that the program is needed (stakeholders: administrators, providers, clients, funders)?
     b. Who does not agree?
  4. Resources (general)
     a. What personnel are needed? What personnel are available?
     b. What facilities are needed? What facilities are available?
     c. What equipment is needed? What equipment is available?
     d. Is funding available to support the project? Is additional funding needed?
     e. Are resources being donated (space, printing, paper, medical supplies)?
        (1) Type
        (2) Amount
  5. Tools used to assess need
     a. Census data
     b. Key informants
     c. Focus groups
     d. Community forums
     e. Existing program surveys
     f. Surveys of client population
     g. Statistical indicators (e.g., demographic and morbidity/mortality data)
C. Conceptualize the problem
  1. List the potential solutions to the problem
  2. What are the risks of each solution?
  3. What are the consequences?
  4. What are the outcomes to be gained from the solutions?
  5. Draw a decision tree to show the problem-solving process used.
D. Detail the plan
  1. What are the objectives for each solution to meet the program goal?
  2. What activities will be done to conduct each of the alternative solutions listed under C1 and based on objectives.
  3. What are the differences in the resources needed for each of the alternative solutions?
  4. Which of the alternative solutions would be chosen if the resources described under B4 were the only resources available?
  5. Who would be responsible or accountable for implementing the plan?
E. Evaluate the plan
  1. Which of the alternative solutions is most acceptable to the following:
     a. The client population
     b. The agency administrator
     c. You
     d. The community
  2. Which of the alternative solutions appears to have the most benefits to the following:
     a. The client population
     b. The agency administrator
     c. You
     d. The community
  3. On the basis of cost, which alternative solution would be chosen by the following:
     a. The client population
     b. The agency administrator
     c. You
     d. The community
F. Implement the program plan
  1. On the basis of data collected, which of the solutions has been chosen?
  2. Why should the agency administrator approve your request? Give a rationale.
  3. Will additional funding be sought?
  4. When can the program begin? Give date.

Developed by Marcia Stanhope and based on the Basic Program Planning Model (Nutt, 1984).

have been developed using this approach. The tracer method and case register are examples of other methods applied to program evaluation.

Program records and community indices serve as the major source of information for program evaluation. Surveys, interviews, observations, and diagnostic tests are ways to assess client and community responses to health programs. *Cost studies* help identify program benefits and effectiveness.

As financial resources become scarce, nursing and the health care system must be able to justify their existence, prove that their services are responsive to client needs, and show their professional concern for being accountable. Planning and evaluation will assist in meeting these objectives.

## Planning for the Evaluation Process

Planning for the evaluation process is an important part of program planning. When the planning process begins, the plan for evaluating the program should also be developed. All persons to be involved in implementing a program should be a part of the plan for program evaluation. Assessment of need is one component of evaluation. The basic questions to be answered, after carefully considering the data collected from a census, key informants, community forums, surveys, or health statistics indicators, are as follows:

1. Will the objectives and resources of this program meet the identified needs of the client population?
2. Is the program relevant?

Once need has been established and the program is designed, the nurse must continue plans for program evaluation (see the Evidence-Based Practice box).

As a part of the planning process, Posavac and Carey (2000) describe six steps to use for continuing program evaluation (Figure 21-3):

---

### Evidence-Based Practice

The purpose of the project was twofold: (1) to develop a program to prevent diabetes and hypertension in the Chinese population in Chinatown, Hawaii, and (2) to develop a relationship with the Chinese community association. This article provides evaluation of the program, which was a collaborative effort between the community, the public health nurse, and diabetes nurse educators. The authors used several approaches to developing the program: volunteers helped them access the community, the community association identified participants for the program, and surveys of participants were conducted to determine interest. The authors used techniques of community education and health promotion to implement this self-care management program with 200 Chinese residents of the community. Case studies, laboratory diagnostic tests, blood pressure monitoring, and surveys were used to evaluate the outcomes of the program. The evaluation showed the effectiveness of the education, counseling, support, and outreach approaches used in the program to improve blood glucose and blood pressure levels in the population.

**Nurse Use:** The nurse can use this study to find appropriate ways to work with culturally diverse groups and ways to provide culturally sensitive health care programs.

Wang C, Abbott L: Development of a community based diabetes and hypertension prevention program, *Public Health Nurs* 15(6):406, 1998.

---

1. Identify the key people for evaluation. Program personnel, program funders, and the clients of the program should be included in planning for evaluation.
2. Arrange preliminary meetings to discuss the question of how the group wants to evaluate the program and where to start. If the program planners and others agree on an evaluation, the resources needed to do the evaluation must be identified. Evaluation is necessary even though some may not be interested in it. Community-oriented nurses can help others see that without evaluation, money to support programs will not be available, or the need for a new nurse to help with the work cannot be justified. In health care today, there is great emphasis on outcomes of care. The only way to see outcomes is through evaluation.
3. After the key people have met and considered the questions in the previous steps, they are ready to begin the evaluation process. Even though evaluation may be desired, the decision to conduct the evaluation may be an administrative one, based on available resources and existing circumstances. For example, if a program evaluation were attempted in a situation in which program personnel wanted it and clients chose to be uncooperative, evaluation efforts would fail.
4. Examine the literature for suggestions about the appropriate methods and techniques for evaluation

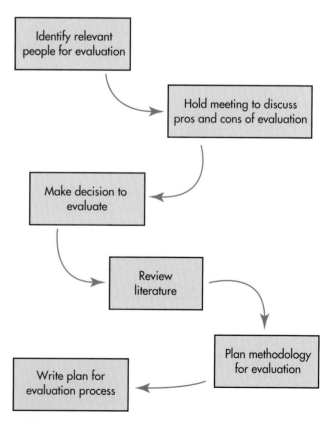

**Figure 21-3** Six steps in planning for program evaluation.

and their usefulness in program evaluation. If an agency has chosen to use an external evaluator, this person may make suggestions about the questions to be answered in the evaluation process. These questions are based on the program goals. Nurses who have reviewed the literature and talked with others affected by the evaluation can determine whether the evaluation suggestions are appropriate for the situation.

5. Plan the method to be used, including decisions about what goals and objectives will be measured, how they will be measured, and for what population.

6. Write a plan that outlines the purpose and goals of the overall program, the type of evaluation to be done, the operational measures to be used to evaluate the program goals, the choice of who will do the evaluation, internal or external personnel, the available resources for conducting the evaluation, and the readiness of the organization, personnel, and clients for program evaluation.

> ( **WHAT DO YOU THINK?**
> Nurses at all levels of education and preparation can participate in program planning and evaluation.

## Evaluation Process

The evaluation process presented by Rossi and Freeman (1999) is explained in this section. Its steps are very similar to the steps in the planning process (Figure 21-4):

1. *Goal setting.* The values and beliefs of the agency, the providers, and the clients provide the basis for goal setting and should be considered at every step of the evaluation process. In the preschool immunization example, the fact that children should not be exposed to early childhood diseases would lead to a program goal to decrease the incidence of early childhood diseases in the county where the program is planned.

2. *Determining goal measurement.* In the case of the previous goal, reduced disease incidence would be an appropriate goal measurement.

3. *Identifying goal-attaining activities.* These activities include, for example, media presentations urging parents to have their children immunized.

4. *Making the activities operational.* This involves the actual administrating of the immunizations through the health department clinics.

5. *Measuring the goal effect.* This consists of reviewing the records and summarizing the incidence of early childhood disease before and after the program.

6. *Evaluating the program.* This involves determining whether the program goal was achieved. Keep in mind that only one program goal is used in this example. Most programs have multiple goals.

## Formulating Objectives

The most important step in the planning and evaluation process is the writing of program objectives. The objectives provide direction for conducting the program, and they provide the mechanism for evaluating specific activities and the total program. The following discussion addresses the development of well-written objectives. Development of program objectives begins with the initial phases of program planning.

### Specifying of Goals and Objectives

Clear, concise, and measurable objectives help with evaluating the program. If the objectives are too general, program evaluation becomes impossible. The objectives must be specific and stated so that anyone reading them could conduct the program without further instruction. To be truly effective, objectives should begin with a general program goal and move on to specific objectives that will help meet the program goal.

The document Healthy People 2010 (USDHHS, 2000a) may be used as a template to guide the development of more specific objectives that are tailored to address the needs of a given community.

Useful program objectives include a statement of the specific behaviors that the program will accomplish, and success criteria, or expected results, for the program. Each

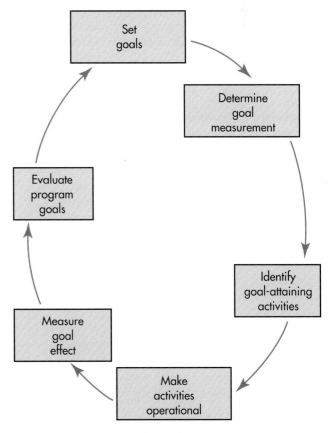

**Figure 21-4** The evaluation process.

**Healthy People 2010** | **Examples of Healthy People 2010 Goals for Program Planning**

The following two objectives are examples from Healthy People 2010; they relate to immunization as a health indicator.

14-24 Increase the proportion of young children who receive all vaccines that have been recommended for universal administration for at least 5 years

14-29 Increase the proportion of noninstitutionalized adults who are vaccinated annually against influenza and ever vaccinated against pneumococcal disease.

From U.S. Department of Health and Human Services: *Healthy people 2010: understanding and improving health,* ed 2, Washington, DC, 2000, U.S. Government Printing Office.

program objective requires a *strong, action-oriented verb* to specify the behavior, a *statement of a single purpose,* a *statement of a single result,* and a *time frame for achieving the expected result.* In this continuing example, a program objective that meets these criteria may be to decrease (action verb) the incidence of early childhood disease in Center County (result) by providing immunization clinics in all schools (purpose) between August and December of 2007 (time frame).

As objectives are developed, an *operational indicator* for each objective should be considered so the evaluator knows when and if the objective has been met. For instance, an operational indicator for the previous objective would be a 10% to 25% decrease in the incidence rates of the most frequently occurring childhood vaccine-preventable illnesses in Center County. Such indicators provide a target for persons involved with implementing programs. A review of Healthy People 2010 health indicators and objectives will give the reader examples of objectives that include all the elements just listed.

### Levels of Program Objectives

It is customary for objectives to be stated in levels from general to specific. The first level consists of general and broad statements that are sometimes called goals. Their purpose is to focus on the major reason for the program.

A general program goal may be to reduce the incidence of low-birth-weight babies in Center County by 2010 by improving access to prenatal care. Several specific objectives are required to meet a general program goal. A specific objective for this program may be to open (action verb) a prenatal clinic in each health department within the county by January 2005 (time frame) to serve the population within each census tract of the county (purpose) to improve pregnancy outcomes (result).

Specific program activities are then planned to meet each specific objective. These activities address resources, such as number of nurses, equipment, supplies, and location. A time frame is planned for each activity. It is assumed that as each specific objective is met, progress toward achieving the general program objective (or goal) is made.

## Sources of Program Evaluation

Major sources of information for program evaluation are the program clients, program records, and community indices. The program participants, or clients of the service, have a unique and valuable role in program evaluation. Whether the clients, for whom the program was designed, accept the services will determine to a large extent whether the program achieves its goal. Thus their reactions, feelings, and judgments about the program are very important to the evaluation.

To assess the response of participants in a program, the evaluator may use a written survey in the form of a questionnaire or an attitude scale. Interviews and observations are other ways of obtaining feedback about a program. Attitude scales are probably used most often, and they are usually phrased in terms of whether the program met its objectives. The client satisfaction survey is an example of an attitude scale often used in the health care delivery system to evaluate the program objectives.

The second major source of information for program evaluation is program records, especially clinical records. Clinical records provide the evaluator with information about the care given to the client and the results of that care. To determine whether a program goal has been met, one might summarize the data from a group of records. For example, if one overall goal were to reduce the incidence of low-birth-weight babies through prenatal care, records would be reviewed to obtain the number of mothers who received prenatal care and the number of low-birth-weight babies born to them. Records would be reviewed from the beginning of the program and at the end of a specific time frame—for example, at the end of each year.

The third major source of evaluation is epidemiologic data. Mortality and morbidity data measuring health and illness are probably cited more frequently than any other single index for program evaluation. These health and illness indicators are useful in evaluating the effects of health care programs on the total community. Incidence and prevalence data are valuable indices for measuring program effectiveness and impact (see Chapter 11 for further discussion of rates and ratios).

## Healthy People 2010 — Focus Areas

1. Access to quality health services
2. Arthritis, osteoporosis, and chronic back conditions
3. Cancer
4. Chronic kidney disease
5. Diabetes
6. Disability and secondary conditions
7. Educational and community-based programs
8. Environmental health
9. Family planning
10. Food safety
11. Health communication
12. Heart disease and stroke
13. Human immunodeficiency virus
14. Immunization and infectious diseases
15. Injury and violence prevention
16. Maternal, infant, and child health
17. Medical product safety
18. Mental health and mental disorders
19. Nutrition and overweight
20. Occupational safety and health
21. Oral health
22. Physical activity and fitness
23. Public health infrastructure
24. Respiratory diseases
25. Sexually transmitted diseases
26. Substance abuse
27. Tobacco use
28. Vision and hearing

From U.S. Department of Health and Human Services: *Healthy people 2010: understanding and improving health,* ed 2, Washington, DC, 2000, U.S. Government Printing Office.

## Healthy People 2010 — Example of a Measurable National Health Objective

In the Healthy People focus area of injury and violence prevention, the general goal is to reduce injuries, disabilities, and deaths due to unintentional injuries and violence.

15-13 Reduce *(action verb)* deaths caused by unintentional injuries *(result)* to no more than 20.8 per 100,000 people *(operational indicator)* by the year 2010 *(time frame)*

From U.S. Department of Health and Human Services: *Healthy people 2010: understanding and improving health,* ed 2, Washington, DC, 2000, U.S. Government Printing Office.

An example of a national program based on a needs assessment of the U.S. population is the national health objectives program, Healthy People 2010 (USDHHS, 2000a). Healthy People 2010 is designed to achieve two overarching goals: to increase quality and years of healthy life, and to eliminate health disparities. These two goals are supported by specific objectives in 28 focus areas, shown in the Healthy People 2010 box titled Focus Areas.

The Healthy Communities program (USDHHS, 2000b) suggests activities to evaluate national health objectives related to communities. The example shown in the next Healthy People 2010 box highlights injury and violence prevention. This box shows that objectives include an action verb, a result, an operational indicator, and a time frame (10 years, beginning in 2000).

Box 21-2 provides examples of applying levels of prevention to program planning and evaluation.

## Aspects of Evaluation

The aspects of program evaluation include the following (Kaluzny and Veney, 1999):

1. *Relevance.* Need for the program
2. *Adequacy.* Program addresses the extent of the need
3. *Progress.* Tracking of program activities to meet program objectives
4. *Efficiency.* Relationship between program outcomes and the resources spent
5. *Effectiveness.* Ability to meet program objectives and the results of program efforts
6. *Impact.* Long-term changes in the client population
7. *Sustainability.* Enough resources to continue the program

The How To box suggests questions that may be asked to achieve program evaluation using this process.

**Relevance.** Evaluation of relevance is an important component of the initial planning phase. As money, providers, facilities, and supplies for delivering health care services are more closely monitored, the needs assessment done by the nurse will determine whether the program is needed.

**Adequacy.** Evaluation of adequacy looks at the extent to which the program addresses the entire problem defined in the needs assessment. The magnitude of the problem is determined by vital statistics, incidence, prevalence, and expert opinion.

**HOW TO    Do a Program Evaluation**

To do a program evaluation, first choose the type of evaluation you wish to do. Second, identify the goal and objectives for evaluation. Third, decide who will be involved in the evaluation. Fourth, answer the questions related to the type of evaluation as follows:

A. Program relevance: needs assessment (formative)
  1. Use answers to all questions listed in section B of How To Develop a Program Plan (p. 499).
  2. On the basis of the needs assessment, was the program necessary?

B. Adequacy
  1. Is the program large enough to make a positive difference in the problem/need?
  2. Are the boundaries of the services defined so that the problem/need can be addressed for the target population?

C. Program progress (formative)
  1. Monitor activities (circle which this reflects: daily, weekly, monthly, annually)
    a. Name the activities provided.
    b. How many hours of service were provided?
    c. How many clients have been served?
    d. How many providers?
    e. What types of clients have been served?
    f. What types of providers were needed?
    g. Where have services been offered (home, clinic, organization)?
    h. How many referrals have been made to community sources?
    i. Which sources have been used to provide support services?
  2. Budget
    a. How much money has been spent to carry out activities?
    b. Will more/less money be needed to conduct activities as outlined?
    c. Will changes to objectives and activities be needed to keep the program going?
    d. What changes do you recommend and why?

D. Program efficiency (formative and summative)
  1. Costs
    a. How do costs of the program compare with those of a similar program to meet the same goal?
    b. Do the activities outlined in C1 compare with the activities in a similar program?
    c. Although this program costs more/less than expected, is it needed? Why?
  2. Productivity (may use national or state averages for comparison)
    a. How many clients does each type of staff see per day (public health nurses, community health nurses, nurse practitioners)?

  b. How does this compare with similar programs?
  c. Although the productivity level of this program is low/high, is the program needed? Why?
  3. Benefits
    a. What are the benefits of the program to the clients served?
    b. What are the benefits to the community?
    c. Are the benefits important enough to continue the program? Why? (Look at cost, productivity, and outcomes of care.)

E. Program effectiveness (summative)
  1. Satisfaction
    a. Is the client satisfied with the program as designed?
    b. Are the providers satisfied with the program outcomes?
    c. Is the community satisfied with the program outcomes?
  2. Goals
    a. Did the program meet its stated goal?
    b. Are the client needs being met?
    c. Was the problem solved for which the program was designed?

F. Impact (summative)
  1. Long-term changes in health status (1 year or more)
    a. Have there been changes in the communities' health?
    b. What are the changes seen (e.g., in morbidity or mortality rates, teen pregnancy rates, pregnancy outcomes)?
    c. Have there been changes in individuals' health status?
    d. What are the changes seen?
    e. Has the initial problem been solved or has it returned?
    f. Is new or revised programming needed? Why?
    g. Should the program be discontinued? Why?

G. Sustainability
  1. Was the program funded as a demonstration or by an external agency?
  2. Can money and resources be found to continue the program after the initial funding is gone?

Depending on the answers to the questions, the program can be found to be successful or not.

Developed by Marcia Stanhope using the framework in Veney A, Kaluzny J: *Evaluation and decision making for health services,* 1998, Chicago, Health Administration Press.

BOX 21-2 Levels of Prevention Applied to Program Planning and Evaluation

**PRIMARY PREVENTION**

Plan a communitywide program with the local government and health department to make all public businesses smoke free to prevent exposure to secondhand smoke.

**SECONDARY PREVENTION**

Develop screening programs for all workers in businesses to determine the incidence/prevalence of respiratory illness, cardiovascular diseases, and lung cancer before implementing the program.

**TERTIARY PREVENTION**

Evaluate the incidence/prevalence of respiratory illness, cardiovascular disease, and lung cancer among nonsmoking workers after the implementation of the program and provide programs to reduce complications from the diseases.

**WHAT DO YOU THINK?**

The combination of prenatal care programs delivered by nurses and the supplemental nutritional program for women, infants, and children (WIC) produces better pregnancy and postnatal outcomes for mothers and babies than traditional medical care.

**Progress.** The monitoring of program activities, such as hours of services, number of providers used, number of referrals made, and amount of money spent to meet program objectives, provides an evaluation of the progress of the program. This type of evaluation is an example of formative or process evaluation, which occurs on an ongoing basis while the program exists. This provides an opportunity to make effective day-to-day management decisions about the operations of the program. Progress evaluation occurs primarily while implementing the program. The nurse who completes a daily or weekly log of clinical activities (e.g., number of clients seen in clinic or visited at home, number of phone contacts, number of referrals made, number of community health promotion activities) is contributing to progress evaluation of the nursing service.

**Efficiency.** If the reason for evaluation is to examine the efficiency of a program, it may occur on an ongoing basis as **formative evaluation** or at the end of the program as a **summative evaluation.** The evaluator may be able to determine whether the program provides better benefits at a lower cost than a similar program, or whether the benefits to the clients, or number of clients served, justify the costs of the program.

**Effectiveness and impact.** An evaluation of **program effectiveness** may help the nurse evaluator determine both client and provider satisfaction with the program activities, as well as whether the program met its stated objectives. However, if evaluation of impact is the goal, long-term effects such as changes in morbidity and mortality must be investigated. Both effectiveness and impact evaluations are usually *summative evaluation* functions primarily performed as end-of-program activities.

**Sustainability.** A program can be continued if there are resources for the program. Ongoing evaluation of sustainability is important!

## ADVANCED PLANNING METHODS AND EVALUATION MODELS

After a need and a client demand for a program have been determined through the needs assessment process, the next step in the development of the program is to choose a procedural method that will assist the nurse in planning the program to be offered. The following is offered for students who are more advanced in their career and need to consider several methods of program planning plus more extensive evaluation models for program management.

Five planning methods are discussed in this section:
1. Planning, programming, and budgeting system (PPBS)
2. Program planning method (PPM)
3. Program evaluation review technique (PERT)
4. Critical path method (CPM)
5. Multi-attribute utility technique (MAUT)

PPM and PPBS are more general approaches to program planning, whereas PERT, CPM, and MAUT offer guidelines for identifying and tracking specific program activities essential to program success. All of these approaches establish the basis for program evaluation.

## Planning, Programming, and Budgeting System

PPBS is a procedural tool initially developed for use by the Department of Defense and other government agencies. PPBS is an outcome-oriented accounting system, the effect of which is to determine the most efficient method of resource allocation to attain measurable objectives.

PPBS is an economic method of describing a program plan and is compared with the Nutt model of program planning. Steps of PPBS are listed in Box 21-3. In PPBS, planning represents the formulating of objectives and conceptualizing or identifying of alternatives and methods for accomplishing the objectives; programming represents detailing of resources (personnel, facilities, equipment, and financing) for each identified alternative; and budgeting represents the assignment of dollar values to resources required for implementing the program or the evaluating of program costs and benefits (Figure 21-5).

PPBS is widely used for planning broad-scale government programs. It is a system that can also be used to plan programs for an agency or for client groups. For example, PPBS could be used to develop the annual program plan

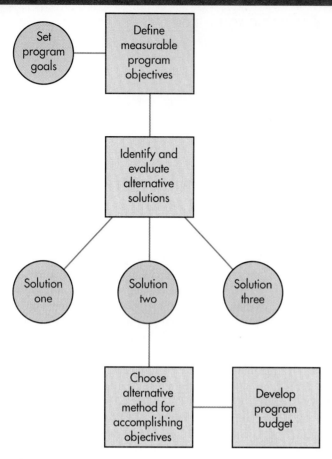

**Figure 21-5** Planning, programming, and budgeting system.

---

**BOX 21-3    Steps Involved in PPBS**

1. Setting program goals
2. Defining measurable program objectives
3. Identifying and evaluating alternatives to accomplish program objectives
4. Choosing the method for accomplishing the objectives
5. Developing a program budget with justification for minimizing costs while maximizing program benefits

---

for the health department or a prenatal program for the local community. A nurse could also use this method to develop a health education program for the school population on sexually transmitted diseases. Because PPBS uses objectives that can be operationally defined by nursing standards, or performance criteria, it is a system that lends itself to effective program evaluation.

## Program Planning Method

PPM is a technique employing the nominal group technique described by Delbecq and Van de Ven in 1971. The nurse can use this method to involve clients more directly in the planning process. PPM is a five-stage process to identify program needs. It focuses on three levels of planning groups composed of clients, providers, and administrators. The client or consumer group relays a list of problems to the provider group, who in turn aids the client group in presenting the solutions to the problems to the administrative group (Nutt, 1984).

The stages of PPM are compared with Nutt's planning process in Table 21-4. The five stages are as follows:

1. *Problem diagnosis.* Each client in the group works with all other members of the group to develop a written problem list, one problem at a time. After all problems have been shared and recorded, they are discussed by the total client group. After the discussion, clients select the problems with the highest priority by voting on the ranking of each problem.
2. *Expert provider group identifies solutions for each of the problems identified by the clients.*
3. *Client and provider groups present their problems and suggested solutions* to the administrative group to determine the possibilities of developing a program to resolve one or more of the problems using one or more of the solutions. In this phase, clients and providers are seeking acceptance from the administrators who control the program resources.
4. *Alternative solutions to the problem are identified,* and the pros and cons of each are analyzed.
5. *Client, providers, and administrators select the best plan* for program implementation. In this phase, the link between the planned solutions and the problem are evaluated, pointing out strengths and limitations of the proposed program plan.

A nurse might use this technique for developing school health services within the total community or in one school. A nurse working with a senior citizens group might use this method to identify the priority needs for nursing clinic services at the health department. It is important to note that this method is used to get consensus among all persons involved in the program: clients, providers, and administrators. Consensus is most helpful in having a successful program. The process may also be used in a community decision-making activity in which community representatives come together to decide health care service needs for the entire community.

## Program Evaluation Review Technique

PERT is a network programming method developed in the 1950s through a joint effort of the United States Navy, Lockheed Aircraft Corporation, and Booz-Allen and Hamilton, Incorporated. The method was developed for planning and controlling the program activities involved in developing the Polaris missile.

The PERT method is primarily useful for large-scale projects that require planning, scheduling, and controlling a large number of activities. PERT is mentioned here to in-

## Table 21-4  Planning Methods Compared With Basic Planning Process

| BASIC PLANNING | PPBS | PPM | PERT/CPM | MAUT |
|---|---|---|---|---|
| Formulating | Identify the goals and define in measurable terms | Problems identified by client | Identify program activities | Identify target population and program objectives |
| Conceptualizing | Identify alternatives | Provider group identifies solution | Explore time and events required to meet program activities | Identify alternative problem solutions |
| Detailing | Evaluate alternatives for use of resources | Analyze available solutions | Determine sequencing of events and resources to meet activities | Identify criteria for choice; rank and weight; calculate value |
| Evaluating | Choose method for accomplishing objectives and develop budget to evaluate costs and compare with benefits | Clients, providers, and administrators select best plan | Select appropriate events | Choose best alternatives |
| Implementing | | Best plan presented to administrators for funding | | |

---

### BOX 21-4  Major Objectives of PERT

- To focus attention on the key developmental parts of a program
- To identify potential program problems that could interfere with movement toward program goals
- To evaluate program progress toward goal attainment
- To provide a prompt reporting method
- To facilitate decision making

troduce the reader to the concept of network, or systems, planning. Its objectives are listed in Box 21-4. PERT as a planning method has been used successfully in hospitals to plan for the development of nursing services such as primary care services and for designing projects such as the installation and use of computers for organizing and providing nursing services.

PERT involves the concepts of time and events. The basic tool used in the technique is the network or flow plan, which is a series of circles, ovals, or squares representing the program events, or goals, and their relationships with the activities of the program. The program activities are the time-consuming events of the program and are represented by arrows that connect the program accomplishments or goals (Figure 21-6). Note in the flow plan that it may take several activities to attain a program event (goal), and that some events (goals) must be accomplished before

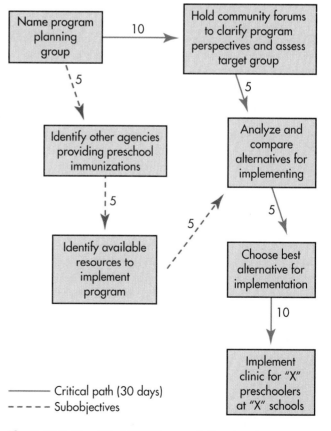

**Figure 21-6** Simplified PERT network for planning a preschool immunization program. Numbers represent days required for completion of activities.

other events may be attained. The relationship of several program events (subgoals) may be essential to attain the ultimate program event (goal).

Another element in PERT is the estimate of the time it will take to implement activities leading to program goals. In PERT, three estimates of activity time are given: the optimistic time it will take to complete activities, given minimal difficulties; the most likely time it will take to complete activities, given experiences with normal development of such activities; and the pessimistic time it will take to complete activities, given maximal difficulties. From the time estimates, a simple formula can be applied to indicate the probability of completing a project in a given time. The numbers next to the arrows in Figure 21-6 are the estimated number of days (after calculation) required for completion of activities leading to a particular event.

## Critical Path Method

CPM is a network program planning method that is described by some authors as a technique and by others as an element of PERT (Longest, Rakich, and Darr, 2000). CPM is a technique that focuses the program planner's attention on the program activities, the sequencing of activities for the best use of time and resources, and the estimated time it will take to complete the project from beginning to end. Using this method, the planner can determine the amount of time it will take to accomplish each activity and can identify those activities that may take longer. The planner can then determine the amount of resources needed (personnel, money, facilities, and supplies) to accomplish tasks at given points in time along the program's critical path.

CPM allows for frequent review of progress by program planners. Problems can be identified early in the program implementation, and corrective action can be taken or alternative activities can be substituted for activities that are not meeting program requirements. The amount of time and resources being used during program implementation can be assessed, and time and resources can be increased or decreased as necessary and can be compared with initial estimates of program need.

Hospital nursing services and home health agencies are using CPM to develop protocols for caring for clients with specific health problems (e.g., breast cancer, hypertension, or total hip replacement). These are called critical paths, or CareMaps. The CPM protocols identify the estimated number of days the client will be in the hospital, and the estimated nursing care activities for each day the client is hospitalized, from admission to discharge. The CPM extends to the home, estimating nursing care activities and rehabilitation in the home (see Chapter 19). Nurses must document reasons why activities may not have been accomplished. These notes are used to change nursing care plans and set new goals for clients. CPM as a program model and CPM as an individual client evaluation approach are two different processes.

PERT and CPM use the five generic stages of planning described by Nutt. However, these two methods focus on specific activities, times, and events essential to program success. The emphasis in these two models is on detailing and evaluating (see Table 21-4).

## Multi-Attribute Utility Technique

MAUT is a planning method based on decision theory (Edwards, Guttentag, and Snapper, 1975). This method can be adapted for making decisions about the care of a single client or about national health care programs. The purpose of MAUT is to separate all elements of a decision and to evaluate each element separately for its effects on the overall decision, considering available options.

If money is no object, then the option with the highest use value is the best decision. However, if this option exceeds the budget, the next best option may be the alternative to choose. The steps of MAUT (listed in Box 21-5) relate closely to the basic planning process described by Nutt (1984) as shown in Table 21-3.

Steps 1 and 2 of MAUT relate to problem formulating. Step 3 involves conceptualizing the program alternatives, and steps 4 through 9 focus on detailing and the implications of each option. Step 10 involves the evaluating phase of planning or the choice of the best solution as identified in steps 4 through 9. Placing quantitative values on solutions to meet program needs is most helpful in the implementing phase of planning (e.g., convincing administrators of the need for such a program). However, caution must be taken in using all planning methods, because the best solution reflects the bias of the planner.

## Evaluation Models and Techniques

### Structure–Process–Outcome Evaluation

The method for evaluation of programs by Donabedian (1982) was initially directed primarily toward medical care but is applicable to the broader area of health care. He describes three approaches to assessment of health care: structure, process, and outcome.

- **Structure** refers to settings in which care occurs. It includes materials, equipment, qualification of the staff, and organizational structure (Donabedian, 1982). This approach to evaluation is based on the assumption that, given a proper setting with good equipment, good care will follow. However, this assumption is not strongly supported.
- **Process** refers to whether the care that was given was "good" (Donabedian, 1982), competent, or preferred. Use of process in program evaluation may consist of observing practice but more likely consists of review of records. The review could focus on whether documentation of preventive teaching was on the clinical record. Audits using specific criteria are examples of the use of process.
- **Outcome** refers to results of client care and restoration of function and survival (Donabedian, 1982), but it is also used in the sense of changes in health status or changes in health-related knowledge, atti-

## BOX 21-5 Ten Basic Steps of the MAUT Method

1. Identify the person or aggregate for whom a problem is to be solved. Who is the client for whom the program is being planned?

2. Identify the issue(s) or decision(s) that are relevant. This step involves the identification of the program objectives.

3. Identify the options to be evaluated. The program planner identifies the available options or action alternatives to accomplish the program goals.

4. Identify the relevant criteria related to the value of each option. The program planner places a value on competing options or alternatives or identifies criteria to be considered in making a choice between them.

5. Rank the criteria in order of importance. The program planner decides which of the criteria are most important and which are least important for meeting program goals.

6. Rate criteria in importance. In this step the program planner assigns an arbitrary rating of 10 to the least important criterion. In considering the next least important criterion, the planner decides how many times more important it is than the least important criterion. If it is considered twice as important, the dimension will be assigned a 20. If it is only considered half as important, it will be assigned a 15. If it

is considered four times as important, it will be assigned a 40. The process is continued until all criteria have been rated.

7. Add the importance rate, divide each by the sum, and multiply by 100. This process is called *normalizing* the weights. It is recommended that the number of criteria be kept between 6 and 15. Therefore, in this initial process, the planner can be concerned with only general criteria for choosing action alternatives.

8. Measure the location of the option being evaluated by each criterion. The planner may ask a colleague or expert to estimate on a scale of 0 to 100 the probability that a given option from step 3 will maximize the value of the criterion from step 4.

9. Calculate the use of options. The program planner will obtain the usefulness of each identified action alternative by multiplying the weight for each criterion (step 7) by the rating of an option for each criterion (step 8) and adding the products. The sum of the products for each action is termed the *aggregate utility*.

10. Decide on the best alternative to meet the program objective. The action alternative with the highest aggregate use is considered the best decision for meeting the program objectives.

---

tude, and behavior. Thus program outcomes may be expressed in terms of mortality, morbidity, and disability for given populations, such as infants, but they could be expressed in a broader sense through health promotion behaviors such as weight control, exercise, and abstinence from tobacco and alcohol.

Donabedian's model of evaluating program quality is a popular model and is widely used for evaluation in the health care field. It can be useful in evaluating program effectiveness. The Center for Medicare and Medicaid Service and other third-party payers are currently placing more emphasis on outcome evaluation. It is essential that nurses begin to develop outcome criteria for client interventions.

### Tracer Method

The Board of Medicine of the National Academy of Sciences developed a program to evaluate health service delivery called the tracer method (Veney and Kaluzny, 1998). The **tracer** method of evaluation of programs is based on the premise that health status and care can be evaluated by viewing specific health problems called tracers. Just as radioactive tracers are used to study the thyroid gland, specific health problems are selected to evaluate the delivery of health and nursing services. Examples of conditions selected as tracers are middle ear infection and associated hearing loss, vision disorders, iron deficiency anemia, hy-

pertension, urinary tract infections, and cervical cancer. This approach can be used to compare the following:

- Health status among different population groups
- Health status in relation to social, economic, medical care, nursing care, and behavioral variables
- Various arrangements for health care delivery

The tracer method is a useful technique for looking at efficiency, effectiveness, and effect of a program.

### Case Register

Systematic registration of contagious disease has been a practice for many years. Denmark began a national register of tuberculosis in 1921 (Friis and Sellers, 1999). Its contribution to the reduction in the incidence of contagious diseases has been widely recognized. **Case registers** are also used for acute and chronic diseases (e.g., cancer and myocardial infarction).

Registers collect information from defined groups, and the information may be used for evaluating and planning services, preventing disease, providing care, and monitoring changes in patterns and care. The method is described here because of its use in evaluation of services. The answers to the questions listed in Box 21-6, asked before and after implementing a program, give information about the effects of the program. A tuberculosis register indicates the degree to which infection is being controlled. Cancer registers make state, regional, national, and international

BOX 21-6    Examples of Questions Asked
About Cases for Case Register

1. What is the incidence of disease? What is the prevalence? What differences in incidence and prevalence are there between one community and another?

2. What percentage of clients recover? What percentage die?

3. Where does death occur?

4. How long do clients wait before contacting a health care provider?

5. How long is it before they are seen by a health care provider?

6. How many cases are associated with other major risk factors?

7. How many cases are associated with environmental factors such as water hardness or air pollution?

8. What happens after clients leave the hospital and when they return to work? Are there rehabilitation programs?

9. How many had been seen by a health care provider shortly before the problem occurred?

10. What prevention measures are taken for persons considered susceptible?

comparisons possible, and they provide clues to causes of disease. They are also used to direct the development of programs specific to population needs.

## COST STUDIES APPLIED TO PROGRAM MANAGEMENT

Although cost must be considered in planning and evaluating, it is particularly significant in programs involving nursing services. The major types of **cost studies** primarily applied to health care industry are cost accounting, cost benefit, cost efficiency, and cost effectiveness. A discussion of the types of cost studies is presented to give the reader an idea of the kinds of questions that can be answered with such studies. Nurses must be willing to answer these questions to help show the actual costs of nursing programs and the relevance of the programs to the clients they have served. Note that regardless of the type of method used, all methods require a comparison to another program (see Box 21-6).

### Cost Accounting

**Cost accounting** studies are performed to find the actual cost of a program. A question answered by this method could be, "What is the cost of providing a family planning program in Anytown, USA?" To answer the question, the total costs of equipment, facilities (rental), personnel (salaries and benefits), and supplies used over a period are

calculated. The total program costs are divided by the number of clients participating in the program during that time. The total program cost per client is the end product. Thus a cost accounting study can provide data about total program costs and about total cost per client, which makes program management easier. A simple example of cost accounting is the monthly balancing of a personal checkbook. One looks at the costs of providing food, shelter, and clothing for a family and relates these costs to the family income.

### Cost Benefit

**Cost benefit** studies are a way of assessing the desirability of a program by placing a specific dollar amount on all costs and benefits. If benefits outweigh the costs, the program is said to have a *net positive impact*. The major problem with cost benefit analysis is placing a quantifiable value on all benefits of the program. Can a dollar value be placed on human life, on safety, on the relief of pain and suffering, or on prevention of illness? These are all program benefits. If an attempt is made to perform cost benefit analysis of a hospice program, can a dollar amount be placed on the family and client support and comfort provided or on the relief of pain of the terminally ill client? Can such benefits be weighed against costs to justify continuing the program? Should the program be continued despite costs?

It is recognized that public health programs have net positive impacts because preventing morbidity with illness prevention programs such as hypertension screening reduces the future cost of chronic long-term illnesses such as cerebrovascular accident (stroke) or cardiovascular disease. To do a cost benefit study for a program, it must be decided which costs and which benefits are to be included, how the costs and benefits are to be valued, and what constraints are to be considered legal, ethical, social, and economic. For example, in a home health care program funded by the state health department to offer care to clients with acquired immunodeficiency syndrome (AIDS), the mortality rate would continue to be high because a cure is not available. Would the program be considered to have a low cost-to-benefit ratio *(a negative impact)* because clients cannot be cured? The program would be considered to have a high cost-to-benefit ratio *(a positive net impact)* if the cost of home health care services was less expensive than providing similar care in the hospital. The benefits of the program would include reducing the costs to the client and reducing the hospital services (Rossi and Freeman, 1999). The cost per client to use the intervention is considered a negative net impact because the nation has had to spend money on illness that could be prevented and there have been lost work productivity and lost lives (increased mortality rate) as a result of the preventable illness.

### Cost Effectiveness

**Cost effectiveness** analysis, which measures the quality of a program as it relates to cost, is the most frequently

## BOX 21-7  Steps in Cost Effectiveness Analysis

1. Identify the program goals or client outcome to be achieved.
2. Identify at least two alternative means of achieving the desired outcomes.
3. Collect baseline data on clients.
4. Determine the costs associated with each program activity.
5. Determine the activities each group of clients will receive.
6. Determine the client changes after the activities are completed.
7. Combine the costs (step 4), the amount of activity (step 5), and outcome information (step 6) to express costs relative to outcomes of program goals.
8. Compare cost outcome information for each goal to that in a similar program to present cost effectiveness analysis.

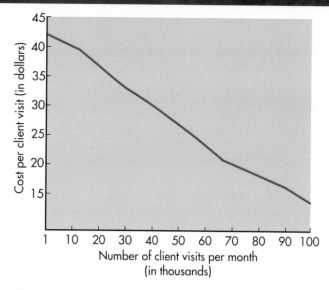

**Figure 21-7** Cost per client visit at a home health agency.

used analysis in nursing. Cost effectiveness is a subset of cost benefit analysis and is designed to provide an estimate of costs to achieve an outcome. A cost effectiveness study can answer several questions: Did the program meet its objectives? Were the clients and nurses satisfied with the effects of the interventions? Are things better as a result of the interventions? (Kaluzny and Veney, 1999). In cost benefit analysis, both costs and outcomes are quantitative, whereas in cost effectiveness analysis, the outcomes are qualitative and quantitative. Outcome measures addressed by cost effectiveness might identify the increase in client knowledge after health teaching, a change in the client's condition after treatment, the difference in graduates of two nursing programs with similar goals, and the ability of two screening programs to detect hearing loss.

A cost effectiveness study requires collecting baseline data on clients before the program is implemented and evaluated. This occurs after the program is completed. Box 21-7 shows the procedure for completing such a study. There are several potential outcomes of a cost effectiveness study. For example, a nurse is interested in comparing two methods for implementing a program to teach diabetic clients self-care techniques. The nurse chooses self-teaching modules and a group instruction program for comparison. There are several potential outcomes of comparing the two teaching methods. Of the potential outcomes in a cost effectiveness study, the program of choice would be the more effective teaching method for the lesser cost. However, if the more costly program demonstrates superior outcomes, it may be chosen. If the less costly program is of poor quality, the more costly program would be appropriate.

## Cost Efficiency

**Cost efficiency** analysis is the actual cost of performing a number of program services. To determine the cost efficiency of a program, its productivity must be analyzed. Productivity is the relationship between what the nurse does and how much it costs to do it.

To determine the nurse's activities with a group of clients, a nurse's workload is of primary concern. This includes direct client care and indirect care activities such as charting, phone calls, client care conferences, and travel. The functions are then related to the client load, client need, and the number of nurses available to meet the needs of all clients served by a program.

Figure 21-7 shows an example of the cost efficiency of a home health agency. The graph indicates that as the number of client visits per year increases, the cost per client visit decreases. The graph assumes that the number of nurses from the beginning to the end of the period is the same, that the nurses' workloads were necessary to provide home health services, that caseloads were assigned on the basis of staff mix and client need, and that the organizational structure helped nurses be highly productive.

All cost studies have three major tasks: financial, research, and statistical. The financial tasks involve identifying total program costs and breaking them down into smaller parts. To identify the costs of a nurse's participation in a teaching program, the costs for facilities, equipment, supplies, and salaries would have to be examined. All costs associated with the program, such as the nurse's time and use of facilities, equipment, and supplies, should be compared with the total program costs. The statistical tasks involve the identifying of appropriate quantifiable measures for analyzing data, and the research tasks involve setting up an appropriate study design to answer the questions of benefit, efficiency, or effectiveness.

Nurses with various educational backgrounds may be involved in cost studies with the assistance of people knowledgeable in research statistics and accounting techniques. Nurses with undergraduate degrees may be involved in the actual implementing of a cost study, whereas nurses with graduate degrees may be involved in planning, designing, implementing, analyzing, and evaluating study results as they relate to program management.

Cost studies are essential to show the worth of nursing in the marketplace of the future, and nurses should be familiar with the results of cost studies so that sound decisions can be made about future program management. Nurses must be ready to identify appropriate program outcomes, client outcomes, the roles that graduates have in health care delivery, and the requirements to perform nursing procedures so that appropriate decisions about program management will be made on the basis of adequate information.

## PROGRAM FUNDING

Providing adequate funding for programs to meet the needs of populations can be a challenge to nurse managers in communities. When money is not available to support endeavors that serve the public good, nonprofit organizations may seek funding from outside the organization. Such funding may be in the form of gifts, grants, or contracts.

Gifts are philanthropic contributions from individuals, foundations, businesses, religious or civic organizations, or voluntary associations. Many organizations engage in extensive development efforts to solicit monetary gifts that support the agency's goals. Contracts are awarded for the performance of a specific task or service, usually to meet guidelines specified by the organization making the award. Contracts are frequently used by government to purchase services of others to perform certain services. Grants are awards to nonprofit organizations to allow recipients to implement activities of their own design that address the interests of the funding agency. Grants are given by government and by foundations and corporations (Lauffer, 1997).

Nurse leaders working in nonprofit agencies may write grants to fund community programs that meet the needs of at-risk populations. Successful **grant writing** meshes the plan for the envisioned program of the applying organization with the criteria set forth by the funding agency. Grant writing uses planning and evaluation concepts and approaches described in this chapter into a written document. Funding agencies provide guidelines for grant applications, and it is essential to follow those specific guidelines if grant funding is to be acquired. In general, however, most grant proposals include certain essential components.

First, it is important to identify the target population and define the problem(s) that the project intends to address. Specific data, conditions, or circumstances that illustrate the problem and that document the need, such as environmental characteristics, economic conditions, population characteristics, and health status indicators,

should be included and discussed. Health services should be discussed in relationship to availability, accessibility, and acceptability to the target population within both the public and private sectors. Identification of duplication or gaps in services that result in unmet needs should be addressed.

The second component is the description of the program that is being proposed. The program description should provide details about what is planned, how it will be done, where it will be done, and by whom. This section should present the reviewer with a clear understanding of the details of the program structure and function. It should be apparent that the program is realistic and can be done. This section includes goals, objectives, action steps, and anticipated outcomes that describe how, when, and by whom each activity will be accomplished to achieve the outcome of objective for which it was written.

Plans for evaluation address the method that will be used to ensure ongoing and timely review of the specific action steps and objectives involved in achieving the stated goal (formative) and to assess program outcomes (summative).

Applicants for grant funds should develop a realistic operating budget that is commensurate with the requirements of the project. The budget represents the plan for how the program will be implemented and reflects the project's proposed spending plan.

## Practice Application

The following is a real-life example of the application of the program management process by an undergraduate community health nursing student. This activity resulted in the development and implementation of a nurse-managed clinic for the homeless. This example shows how students as well as providers can make a difference in health care delivery. It also shows that no mystery surrounds the program management process.

Eva was listening to the radio one Sunday afternoon and heard an announcement about the opening of a soup kitchen within the community for the growing homeless population. She was beginning her community health nursing course and wanted to find a creative clinical experience that would benefit herself as well as others. The announcement gave her an idea. Although it mentioned food, clothing, shelter, and social services, nothing was said about health care.

Eva was interested in finding a way to provide nursing and health care services at the soup kitchen. Which of the following should she do?

A. Talk with key leaders to determine their interest in her idea.
B. Review the literature to find out the magnitude of the problem.
C. Survey the community to find out if others were providing services.
D. Discuss the idea with members of the homeless population.

E. Consider potential solutions to the health care problems.

F. Consider where she would get the resources to open a clinic.

G. Talk with church leaders and community health nursing faculty members to seek acceptance for her idea.

---

**Answers are in the back of the book.**

## Key Points

- Planning and evaluation are essential elements of program management and vital to the survival of the nursing discipline in health care delivery.
- The program management process is population focused and is parallel to the nursing process. Both are rational decision-making processes.
- The health care delivery system has grown in the past century, making health planning and evaluation very important.
- Comprehensive health planning grew out of a need to control costs.
- A program is an organized approach to meet the assessed needs of individuals, families, groups, populations, or communities by reducing or eliminating one or more health problems.
- Planning is defined as selecting and carrying out a series of actions to achieve a stated goal.
- Evaluation is defined as the methods used to determine if a service is needed and will be used, whether a program to meet that need is carried out as planned, and whether the service actually helps the people it intended to help.
- To develop quality programs, planning should include four essential elements: problem diagnosis and assessment of need, identification of problem solutions, analysis and comparison of alternative methods, and selection of the best plan and planning methods.
- The initial and most critical step in planning a health program is assessment of need. Assessment focuses on the needs of the population who will use the services planned.
- Some of the major tools used in needs assessment are census data, community forums, surveys of existing community agencies, surveys of community residents, and statistical indicators about demographics, morbidity, and mortality of the population.
- The major benefit of program evaluation is to determine whether a program is fulfilling its stated goals. Quality assurance programs are prime examples of program evaluation.
- Plans for implementing and evaluating programs should be developed at the same time.
- Program records and community indices serve as major sources of information for program evaluation.

- Planning programs and planning for their evaluation are two of the most important ways in which nurses can ensure successful program implementation.
- Cost studies help identify program benefits, effectiveness, and efficiency.
- Program planning helps nurses and agencies focus attention on services that clients need.
- Planning helps everyone involved understand their role in providing services to clients.
- The assessment of need process provides an evaluation of the relevance that a new service may have to clients.
- A decision tree is a useful tool to choose the best alternative for solving a problem.
- Setting goals and writing objectives to meet the goals are necessary to evaluate program outcomes.
- Healthy People 2010 is an example of a national program based on needs assessment that has stated goals and objectives on which the program can be evaluated.
- Cost accounting studies (which are similar to balancing a checkbook) help to determine the actual cost of a program.
- Cost benefit studies are used to assess the desirability of a program by examining costs and benefits, such as the value of human life.
- Cost effectiveness studies measure the quality of a program as it relates to cost.
- Cost efficiency studies examine the actual cost of performing program services and focus on productivity versus cost.
- Program planning models include PPBS, PERT, CPM, and MAUT.
- Program evaluation includes assessing structure, process, and outcomes of care.
- The critical path method of evaluating care is a popular model.
- Grant writing is a tool used by nurse managers to provide resources for needed services.
- Grant proposals are documents that incorporate principles of program planning and evaluation.

## Clinical Decision-Making Activities

1. Choose the definitions that best describe your concept of a program, of planning, and of evaluation. Explain how each of these definitions can help you in accomplishing planning and evaluation.

2. Apply the program planning process to an identified clinical problem for a client group with whom you are working in the community. Give specific examples.

   a. Assess the client need.

   b. Choose tools appropriate to the assessment of needs.

   c. Analyze the overall planning process of arriving at decisions about implementing a program.

    **d.** Summarize the benefits for program planning that apply to your situation.

**3.** Given the situation just described, choose three or four of your classmates to work with you on the following projects:

    **a.** Plan for evaluation of the program in activity 2.

    **b.** Apply the evaluation process to the situation.

    **c.** Name the measures you will use to gather data for evaluating your program.

    **d.** Name the sources you will tap to gain information for program evaluation.

    **e.** Analyze the benefits of program evaluation that apply to your situation.

    **f.** Talk with a community-oriented nurse or administrator about the application of program planning and evaluation processes at the local agency. Compare their answers to your readings. What are some of the difficulties that your group and the agency had in evaluating a program?

## Additional Resources

These related resources are found either in the appendix at the back of this book or on the book's website at **http://evolve.elsevier.com/Stanhope.**

### Appendix

Appendix G.1 Community-As-Partner Model

### evolve Evolve Website

Assessment Tools: Communities With Physically Compromised Members

Assessment Tools: Families With Physically Compromised Members

WebLinks: Healthy People 2010

# References

Delbecq A, Van de Ven A: A group process model for problem identification and program planning, *J Appl Behav Sci* 7(4):466, 1971.

Donabedian A: *Explorations in quality assessment and monitoring,* vol 2, Ann Arbor, Mich, 1982, Health Administration Press.

Edwards W, Guttentag M, Snapper K: A decision-theoretic approach to evaluation research. In Struening E, Guttentag M, editors: *Handbook of evaluation research,* Beverly Hills, Calif, 1975, Sage.

Friis R, Sellers T: *Epidemiology for public health practice,* Gaithersburg, Md, 1999, Aspen.

Glick DF, Kulbok PK: Program revision: a dynamic outcome of evaluation, *Qual Manag Health Care* 10(1):37, 2001.

Glick DF et al: Community development theory: planning a community nursing center, *J Nurs Adm* 26(7/8):1, 1996.

Hale CD, Arnold F, Travis MT: *Planning and evaluating health programs: a primer,* Albany, NY, 1994, Delmar.

Kaluzny A, Veney J: Evaluating health care programs and services. In Williams S, Torrens P, editors: *Introduction to health services,* New York, 1999, Wiley.

Kropf R: Planning for health services. In Kovner A, editor: *Health care delivery in the United States,* New York, 1995, Springer.

Lauffer A: *Grants, etc.,* ed 2, Thousand Oaks, Calif, 1997, Sage.

Longest B, Rakich J, Darr K: *Managing health services organizations and systems,* Baltimore, 2000, Health Professions Press.

Nutt P: *Planning methods for health and related organizations,* New York, 1984, Wiley.

Posavac EJ, Carey RG: *Program evaluation: methods and case studies,* Englewood Cliffs, NJ, 2000, Prentice Hall.

Rohrer JE: *Planning for community-oriented health systems,* Baltimore, 1996, American Public Health Association, United Book Press.

Rossi P, Freeman H: *Evaluation: a systematic approach,* Beverly Hills, Calif, 1999, Sage.

U.S. Department of Health and Human Services: *Healthy people 2010: understanding and improving health,* ed 2, Washington, DC, 2000a, U.S. Government Printing Office.

U.S. Department of Health and Human Services: *Healthy people in healthy communities: a community planning guide using Healthy People 2010,* Washington, DC, 2000b, U.S. Government Printing Office.

Veney J, Kaluzny A: *Evaluation and decision making for health service programs,* Englewood Cliffs, NJ, 1998, Prentice Hall.

Wang C, Abbott L: Development of a community based diabetes and hypertension prevention program, *Public Health Nurs* 15(6):406, 1998.

# Chapter 22

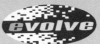 http://evolve.elsevier.com/Stanhope

# Quality Management

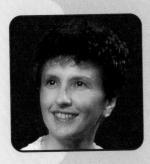

**Judith Lupo Wold, Ph.D., R.N.**

Judith Wold is a visiting scholar at the Nell Hodgson Woodruff School of Nursing and interim director of the International Health MSN/MPH Program and the Office of Service Learning. Dr. Wold was formerly the director of the School of Nursing at Georgia State University, where she is presently a tenured associate professor of nursing. She holds a B.S. and a Ph.D. from Georgia State University and a master's of nursing in family and community health from Emory University in Atlanta. Dr. Wold's primary research focus has been in health promotion and prevention of cardiovascular disease in rural occupational sites. She has extended this project into former Soviet Georgia, where she compared health risks of physicians and nurses. She is negotiating the first university-based school of nursing in Tbilisi, Georgia. She has led two trips to Cuba with Emory nursing students to study Cuba's primary health care system. Additionally, Dr. Wold been instrumental in the successful implementation of the Farm Worker Family Health Program to deliver health care to migrant farm workers in Georgia and in developing inner-city community partnerships to promote the health and well-being of Atlanta's children.

## Objectives

After reading this chapter, the student should be able to do the following:

1. Explain total quality management/continuous quality improvement (TQM/CQI)
2. State the goals of TQM/CQI in a health care system
3. Define quality assurance/quality improvement (QA/QI)
4. Evaluate the role of QA/QI in continuous quality improvement
5. Analyze the historical development of the quality process in nursing and the changes developing under managed care
6. Evaluate approaches and techniques for implementing continuous quality improvement
7. Examine how managed care is changing the way quality is ensured in health care
8. Plan a model QA/QI program
9. Identify the purposes for the types of records kept in community and public health agencies
10. Evaluate a method for documentation of client care in community-oriented nursing

Although the concept of quality assurance has been a part of the health care arena for a number of years, it is only in the last few years that major movement to improve health care quality has begun in the United States. The Institute of Medicine (IOM) (2001), not confident of the current health care systems' ability to deliver the quality of care expected, has set forth a series of recommendations to transform current systems to meet American's expectations. Very little is known about quality of care in this country for two reasons: (1) a variety of definitions of *quality* are used, and (2) it is difficult to get comparable data from all providers and health care agencies.

In a changing health care market, the demand for quality has become a rallying point for health care consumers. All consumers, including private citizens, insurance companies, industry, and the federal government, are concerned with the highest quality outcomes at the lowest cost (Young, 1998). In addition to the demand for higher quality and lower cost, the public wants health care delivered with greater access, and health care that is accountable, efficient, and effective. Moreover, consumers want information about quality. Information is empowering to the consumer. With the expanded use of the internet, access to information on quality in health care is readily available on topics ranging from talking to consumers about quality health care (www.talkingquality.gov) to clinical practice guidelines that promise to improve care for all (www.guideline.gov). **Total quality management/continuous quality improvement** (TQM/CQI), a management style that includes quality assurance, or quality control, is one method used to ensure that the client is getting high-quality care at top value for the

## Key Terms

accountability, p. 519
accreditation, p. 522
audit process, p. 527
certification, p. 522
charter, p. 522
concurrent audit, p. 527
credentialing, p. 521
evaluative studies, p. 529
licensure, p. 522
malpractice litigation, p. 530
managed care, p. 518

outcome, p. 529
partnerships, p. 518
practice guidelines, p. 526
process, p. 529
Professional Review Organization, p. 529
Professional Standards Review
    Organization, p. 529
quality assurance/quality improvement,
    p. 519
recognition, p. 522
records, p. 535

report cards, p. 526
retrospective audit, p. 528
risk management, p. 528
staff review committees, p. 527
structure, p. 529
total quality management/continuous
    quality improvement, p. 516
utilization review, p. 528
*See Glossary for definitions*

## Chapter Outline

Definitions and Goals
Historical Development
Approaches to Quality Improvement
*General Approaches*
*Specific Approaches*
TQM/CQI in Community and Public Health
    Settings

*Using QA/QI in TQM/CQI*
*Traditional Quality Assurance*
Client Satisfaction
*Malpractice Litigation*
Model QA/QI Program
*Structure*
*Process*

*Outcome*
*Evaluation, Interpretation, and Action*
Records
*Community and Public Health Agency Records*

money spent. Although relatively new in health care, the concept of TQM/CQI has been tried and proven in industry. The terms total *quality management, continuous quality improvement, total quality,* and *organization-wide quality improvement* are often used interchangeably. These terms refer to a management philosophy that focuses on the processes by which work is done with the goal of continuously improving those processes. CQI should be implemented not only to address system problems but to maintain and enhance good performance (Durch, Bailey, and Stoto, 1997). By obtaining facts about work processes (e.g., all the steps in certifying a child for the women, infants, and children nutritional program [WIC]), it is possible to discover which steps are unnecessary (i.e., non–value adding) and to eliminate those steps to produce better health outcomes for individuals

and communities (Verhey, 1996). Box 22-1 presents several abbreviations that are commonly used in health care and quality management.

Both consumers and providers have a vested interest in the quality of the health care system. According to Jonas (2002), the health care provider has three basic reasons to be concerned about health care quality:

1. The principle of nonmaleficence (above all, do no harm) has been a basic ethical principle of the health care system since the writing of the Hippocratic oath.
2. The principle of beneficence (do good work) is a basic ethical principle of professionalism.
3. The strong social work ethic in the culture places a high value on "doing a good job" (see Chapter 6 for more discussion about ethics).

---

**BOX 22-1  Commonly Used Abbreviations**

| | |
|---|---|
| AACN | American Association of Colleges of Nursing |
| ACHNE | Association of Community Health Nursing Educators |
| AHRQ | Agency for Healthcare Research and Quality (formerly AHCPR) |
| ANA | American Nurses Association |
| APHA | American Public Health Association |
| CCNE | Commission on Collegiate Nursing Education |
| CHAP | Community Health Accreditation Program |
| CMS | Centers for Medicare and Medicaid Services (formerly HCFA) |
| CQI | Continuous Quality Improvement |
| HEDIS | Health Plan Employer Data and Information Set |
| IOM | Institute of Medicine |
| JCAHO | Joint Commission on Accreditation of Healthcare Organizations |
| MCO | Managed Care Organization |
| NCQA | National Committee for Quality Assurance |
| NLN | National League for Nursing |
| PRO | Professional Review Organization |
| QA | Quality Assurance |
| QI | Quality Improvement |
| TQI | Total Quality Improvement |
| TQM | Total Quality Management |

---

Kovner and Jonas say that in health care there is a direct link between doing a good job and individual and professional survival. Health care providers pride themselves on individual achievement and responsibility for good client outcomes (Kovner and Jonas, 1998). Health care organizations are natural extensions of health care providers and thus can demonstrate their responsibility for optimal outcomes through a rigorous quality improvement process. Leatherman and McCarthy (2002) state that application of quality improvement strategies to six areas of performance could affect both process and outcomes of health care (p. 12):

1. Consistently providing appropriate and effective care
2. Reducing unjustified geographic variation in care
3. Eliminating avoidable mistakes
4. Lowering access barriers
5. Improving responsiveness to patients
6. Eliminating racial/ethnic, gender, socioeconomic, and other disparities and inequalities in access and treatment

The United States has entered a new era of community-oriented, community-controlled delivery of care in which **managed care** organizations (MCOs) play an integral role (Weiss, 1997). MCOs are agencies designed to monitor and deliver health care services within a specific budget (Halverson, Kaluzny, and McLaughlin, 1998). Weiss (1997)

states that "in the future, quality will be measured based on the health status of both MCO-enrolled populations and the community or population served as well as individual perceptions of health status" (p. 29). Although the Health Plan Employer Data and Information Set (HEDIS), a data collection arm of the National Committee for Quality Assurance (NCQA), provides performance information, or report cards, for managed care organizations, no such single report card exists for public health agencies. As a part of a movement to provide quality health care in communities, health departments are examining their place in promoting this quality (Joint Council Committee on Quality in Public Health, 1996). Mays et al (1999) say that public health and CQI are connected because of the use of systems approaches that public health takes in identifying problems and developing interventions. Aspects of planning, implementing, and evaluating by TQM/CQI fall under each of the core public health functions of assessment, assurance, and policy development. It is, however, with the assurance core function related to ensuring available access to the health care services that are essential to sustain and improve the health of the population, that TQM/CQI programs must be undertaken. Public health cannot ensure services that improve health if those services lack quality. Public health must maintain quality in its workforce and continually evaluate the effectiveness of its services whether service is delivered to the individual, the community, or the population.

---

**DID YOU KNOW?**

Although managed care was expected to save money and improve the quality of health care in this country, neither expectation has resulted. In fact, for all the money spent on quality improvement, little is known about the quality of health care in America.

---

Community-oriented nurses are in a perfect position to implement strategies to improve community-oriented health care. Community assessments, identifying high-risk individuals, targeting interventions, case management, and managing illnesses across a continuum of care are strategies suggested as part of the focus on improving the health of communities (Weiss, 1997). These strategies have long been used by community-oriented nurses.

The growth of the managed care industry has changed the face of health care in the United States, both in how health care is delivered and in how it is received by consumers. Consumers are forming **partnerships** in communities to counteract the power of MCOs by holding them accountable for health outcomes in relation to costs. Partnerships are using data-based community assessments to improve health and to ensure that communities receive quality services (Al-Assaf, 1998; Bushy, 1997; Lasker et al, 1997).

Because of managed care agencies and consumer demands for quality nursing, objective and systematic evalu-

---

### BOX 22-2    The Areas of Public Health Nursing Interventions for Quality Community-Oriented Health Care

| Interventions | Chapter |
|---|---|
| Advocacy | 5, 6, 10, 19, 28, 30, 32, 35, 46 |
| Case finding | 19, 30, 31, 43 |
| Case management | 16, 19, 28, 30, 31, 43, 46 |
| Coalition building | 8, 15, 17 |
| Collaborating | 18, 19, 23, 30, 40, 42, 45 |
| Community organizing | 15, 17 |
| Consulting | 41, 42 |
| Counseling | 9, 27, 30, 34, 38, 39, 43, 45, 46 |
| Delegated functions | 42 |
| Disease and health event investigation | 11, 38, 39 |
| Health teaching | 9, 13, 14, 17, 22, 34, 36-39, 41, 43-46 |
| Outreach | 31, 33, 46 |
| Policy development and enforcement | 1, 8, 10, 15, 24, 27, 31 |
| Referral and follow-up | 10, 19, 24, 25, 30, 46 |
| Social marketing | 15, 32, 36, 37 |
| Survey | 15, 21 |

Minnesota Department of Health, Division of Community Health Services: *Public health interventions: applications for Public health nursing practice,* p 1, Public Health Nursing Section, St Paul, March 2001.

---

## THE CUTTING EDGE

In Minnesota, interventions for public health nursing that have been developed to document outcomes of care are adding to the means for evaluating total quality of care.

---

ation of nursing care is a priority for the nursing profession. Since organized nursing is committed to direct individual **accountability,** is evolving as a scientific discipline, and is concerned about how costs of health services limit access, it demands delivery and valuating of quality service aimed at superior client outcomes (Lindsey, Henly, and Tyree, 1997; Stevens-Barnum and Kerfoot, 1995). In the public health arena in Minnesota, researchers identifying competencies for public health nursing to document outcomes attributable to nursing interventions are adding methods for evaluating total quality (Lia-Hoagberg, Schaffer, and Strohschein, 1999; Strohschein, Schaffer, and Lia-Hoagberg, 1999). Box 22-2 is a list of the areas of nursing interventions that community-oriented nurses must be able to use. The chapters that discuss the interventions are noted.

Additionally competencies for public health leadership have been developed to ensure quality and performance of the public health workforce (Wright et al, 2000). (See Appendix J.3 for a list of the competencies.)

Records are maintained on all health care system clients to provide complete information about the client and to show the quality of care being given to the client within the system. Records are a necessary part of a CQI process, as are the tools and methods for evaluating quality.

## DEFINITIONS AND GOALS

Quality is defined as a continual striving for excellence and a conforming to specific approaches or guidelines (Davis, 1994). However, a definition of quality rests largely on the perception of the client, the provider, the care manager, the purchaser, the payer, or the public health official. Whereas the physician views quality in a more technical sense, the client may look at the personal outcome; the manager, purchaser, or payer may consider the cost effectiveness; and the public health official will look at the appropriate use of health care resources to improve population health (Leatherman and McCarthy, 2002). The Institute of Medicine (IOM) (2001) defines quality as "the degree to which health services for individuals and populations increase the likelihood of desired health outcomes and are consistent with current professional knowledge" (p. 1000). Problems with quality of health care are divided into three groups: overuse, underuse, and misuse (Chassin and Galvin, 1998). The category of misuse is the focus of the IOM's push toward greater client safety. The category of underuse focuses on health disparities as defined in Healthy People 2010. The term *health services* applies to a wide range of health delivery institutions. Of particular interest to public health is the question of access to appropriate and needed services, a well-prepared workforce, and improvement in the status of the population's health. Client satisfaction and well-being, and the processes of client–provider interaction, should be considered.

TQM/CQI (the terms TQM and CQI are used here interchangeably) is a process-driven, customer-oriented management philosophy that includes leadership, teamwork, employee empowerment, individual responsibility, and continuous improvement of system processes to yield improved outcomes (Berwick, 1989). Under TQM/CQI, quality is defined as customer satisfaction. **Quality assurance/ quality improvement** (QA/QI) is the promise or guarantee that certain standards of excellence are being met in the delivery of care. The quality assurance, or quality control, process does three things (Kinney, Freedman, and Cook, 1994):

1. It sets standards for care.
2. It evaluates care provided on the basis of the standards.
3. It takes action to bring about change when care does not meet standards.

## Healthy People 2010
### Goal of Improving Access to Comprehensive, High-Quality Health Care, and Examples of Objectives to Eliminate Health Disparities

**1-1**  Increase the proportion of persons with health insurance

**1-4**  Increase the proportion of persons who have a specific source of ongoing care

**1-6**  Reduce the proportion of families that experience difficulties or delays in obtaining health care or do not receive needed care for one or more family members

**1-7**  Increase the proportion of schools of medicine, schools of nursing, and other health professional training schools whose basic curriculum for health care providers includes the core competencies in health promotion and disease prevention

**1-8**  In the health professions, allied and associated health profession fields, and the nursing field, increase the proportion of all degrees awarded to members of underrepresented racial and ethnic groups

From U.S. Department of Health and Human Services: *Healthy people 2010: understanding and improving health,* ed 2, Washington, DC, 2000, U.S. Government Printing Office.

*Quality assurance* is concerned with the accountability of the provider and is only one tool in achieving the best client outcomes (Davis, 1994). Accountability means being responsible for care and answerable to the client (McLaughlin and Kaluzny, 1999). Under QA/QI, quality may have a variety of definitions.

Quality traditionally has been an important issue in the delivery of health care. Quality assurance programs historically have ensured this accountability. According to Jonas (2002), the goals of quality assurance and improvement are (1) to ensure the delivery of quality client care, and (2) to demonstrate the efforts of the health care provider to provide the best possible results. However, standards are a static measurement and do not provide incentive for improvement beyond that standard. Under a CQI philosophy, quality assurance and improvement is but one of the many tools used to ensure that the health care agency fulfills what the client thinks are the requirements for the service. Quality assurance focuses on finding what providers have done wrong in the past (e.g., deviations from a standard of care found through a chart audit). Sprague (2001) says that CQI operates at a higher level on the quality continuum but requires the commitment of more organization resources to move in a positive direction. CQI focuses on the sources of differences in the ongoing process of health care delivery and seeks to improve the process (Sprague, 2001).

The process of health care includes two major components: technical interventions (e.g., how well procedures are accomplished, accurate diagnosis, and effective treatment) and interpersonal relationships between practitioner and client. Both contribute to quality care, and both can be evaluated (Donabedian, 1990). Several approaches and techniques are used in quality programs. *Approaches* are methods used to ensure quality, and *techniques* are tools for measuring differences in quality (Kovner and Jonas, 1998).

The term *quality assurance/quality improvement,* or (QA/QI), is used in place of *quality assurance* in this chapter to more accurately reflect the current thinking about health care quality. Traditional approaches to quality focus on assessing or measuring performance, ensuring that performance conforms to standards, and providing remedial work to providers if those standards are not met. Such a definition of quality is too narrow in health care systems that try to meet the needs of many clients, both internal and external to the agency (Donabedian, 1990). Bellin and Dubler (2001) state that CQI requires constant attention and should involve surveillance of all records while there is still the opportunity to intervene in both the client's care and the practitioner's actions. Comprehensive data analysis is necessary to detect process failure. Many agencies use some of the TQM/CQI concepts, such as client satisfaction questionnaires, but have not adopted the entire management philosophy. However, because QA/QI methods have traditionally been used and are still in use in many agencies, the QA/QI concept will be covered.

## HISTORICAL DEVELOPMENT

Improving the quality of care has been a part of nursing since the days of Florence Nightingale. In 1860, Nightingale called for the development of a uniform method to collect and present hospital statistics to improve hospital treatment. Nightingale was a pioneer in setting standards for nursing care. The movement to establish nursing schools in the United States came in the late 1800s from a desire to set standards that would upgrade nursing care. In the early 1900s, efforts were begun to set similar standards for all nursing schools. From 1912 to 1930, interest in quality nursing education led to the development of nursing organizations involved in accrediting nursing programs. Licensure has been a major issue in nursing since 1892. By 1923, all states had permissive or mandatory laws directing nursing practice.

After World War II, the attention of the emerging nursing profession focused on establishing a scientific method

of practice. The nursing process was the chosen method and included evaluation of how nursing activities helped clients (Maibusch, 1984). QA/QI is the evaluative step in the nursing process.

The 1950s brought the development of tools to measure quality assurance. One of the first tools was Phaneuf's nursing audit method (1965), which has been used extensively in community-oriented nursing practice.

In 1966 the American Nurses Association (ANA) created the Divisions on Practice. As a result, in 1972 the Congress for Nursing Practice was charged with developing standards to institute quality assurance programs. The Standards for Community Health Nursing Practice were distributed to ANA Community Health Nursing Division members in 1973. In 1986 and 1999, the standards were revised.

In 1972, the Joint Commission on Accreditation of Hospitals (JCAH) clearly stated the responsibilities of nursing in its description of standards for nursing services. The JCAH called on the nursing industry to clearly plan, document, and evaluate nursing care provided. In the mid 1980s, JCAH became the Joint Commission on Accreditation of Healthcare Organizations (JCAHO) and began developing quality control standards for hospital and home health nursing. JCAHO presently incorporates continuous quality improvement principles in its standards.

Also in 1972, the Social Security Act (Public Law [PL] 92-603) was amended to establish the Professional Standards Review Organization (PSRO) and to mandate the process review of the delivery of health care to clients of Medicare, Medicaid, and maternal and child health programs. The PSRO program later became the Professional Review Organization (PRO) under the 1983 Social Security amendments. The purpose of the PROs was to monitor the implementing of the prospective reimbursement system for Medicare clients (the diagnosis-related groups [DRGs]). Although PSROs were intended for physicians, PROs have made quality improvement a primary issue for all health care professionals.

In response to increasing charges of malpractice, the government passed the National Health Quality Improvement Act of 1986. Although it was not funded until 1989, its two major goals were to encourage consumers to become informed about their practitioner's practice record and to create a national clearinghouse of information on the malpractice records of providers. The emphasis of this act continued to be on the structure of care rather than the process or outcomes of care (National Association for Healthcare Quality, 1993). (See Chapter 21 for discussion of structure, process, and outcome.)

Efforts to strengthen community-oriented nursing practice have been carried out by several nursing organizations. These include the ANA, the Public Health Nursing Section of the American Public Health Association (APHA), the Association of State and Territorial Directors of Nursing (ASTDN), and the Association of Community Health Nursing Educators (ACHNE). These organizations

are now called the QUAD Council. The quality of nursing education is a major concern of the ACHNE, which was established in 1978. In 1993 and 2000, three reports published by this organization identified the curriculum content required to prepare community nursing students for practice (ACHNE, 1993, 2000a,b). In 1997, the Quad Council reviewed scopes and standards of population-focused (public health) and community-based nursing practice and developed new standards to guide the profession in obtaining the best health outcomes for the populations they serve (ANA, 1999). QA/QI programs remain the enforcers of standards of care for many agencies that have not elected to engage in a program of CQI. These activities are called *assurance activities* because they make certain that those policies and procedures are followed so that appropriate quality services are delivered.

## APPROACHES TO QUALITY IMPROVEMENT

Two basic approaches exist in quality improvement: *general* and *specific*. The general approach involves a large governing or official body's evaluation of a person's or an agency's ability to meet criteria or standards. Specific approaches to quality improvement are methods used to manage a specific health care delivery system in an attempt to deliver care with outcomes that are acceptable to the consumer. QA/QI programs that evaluate provider and client interaction through compliance with standards historically have been used alone to monitor quality care. In a TQM/CQI management approach, QA/QI methods are an integral, but not the only, tool for ensuring quality or customer satisfaction.

### General Approaches

General approaches to protect the public by ensuring a level of competency among health care professionals are *credentialing, licensure, accreditation, certification, charter, recognition,* and *academic degrees*. Although there has been a long history of public oversight of quality in the United States, this public oversight increasingly involves the private sector. Jost (1995) says that public oversight for quality emerged when the private market failed to focus on health care quality. Diminishing public involvement in quality could leave gaps in external quality assurance mechanisms in the United States (Young, 1998).

**Credentialing** is generally defined as the formal recognition of a person as a professional with technical competence, or of an agency that has met minimum standards of performance (Kamajian et al, 1999). These mechanisms are used to evaluate the agency structure through which care is provided and the outcomes of care given by the provider. Credentialing can be mandatory or voluntary. Mandatory credentialing requires laws. State nurse practice acts are examples of mandatory credentialing.

Voluntary credentialing is performed by an agency or an institution. The certification examinations offered by the ANA through the American Nurses Credentialing Center are examples of voluntary credentialing. Licensing, certification, and accreditation are all examples of credentialing.

**Licensure** is one of the oldest general quality assurance approaches in the United States and Canada. Individual licensure is a contract between the profession and the state. Under this contract, the profession is granted control over entry into, and exit from, the profession and over quality of professional practice.

The licensing process requires that written regulations define the scope and limits of the professional's practice. Job descriptions based on these regulations set minimum and maximum limits on the functions and responsibilities of the practitioner. Licensure of nurses has been mandated by law since 1903. Today all 50 states have mandatory nurse licensure, which requires all individuals who practice nursing, whether it be for money or as a volunteer, be licensed. Some critics cite licensure as a barrier to quality practice (Gragnola and Stone, 1999). A new approach to interstate practice requires a pact between states so that nurses can practice across state borders. Although reciprocity (which means nurses can have their license accepted through an application process if there is agreement between the states requiring application) exists among states for nursing licensure, interstate practice without approval is an issue for state boards of nursing.

---

### WHAT DO YOU THINK?

Historically, licensure has protected the public by ensuring at least a beginning level of competence. Nurses are licensed by state government, even though all nurses take the same licensing examination. What do you think about allowing nurses to practice across state lines without registering in each state?

---

**Accreditation,** a voluntary approach to quality control, is used for institutions. Since 1954, the National League for Nursing (NLN), a voluntary organization, has established standards for inspecting nursing education programs. In 1997, the NLN board established an accrediting body as an independent organization, the NLN Accrediting Commission (NLNAC). In 1997, the American Association of Colleges of Nursing (AACN), also a voluntary organization supporting baccalaureate and higher degree programs, established an affiliate, the Collegiate Commission on Nursing Education (CCNE), to accredit baccalaureate and higher degree nursing programs. In 1966, community health/home health program standards were established by the NLN for the purpose of accrediting these programs through their Community Health Accreditation Program (CHAP). In addition, state boards of nursing accredit basic nursing programs so that their graduates are eligible for the licensing examination.

The accreditation function is quasi-voluntary. Although accreditation appears to be a voluntary program, it is often linked to government regulation that encourages programs to participate in the accrediting process. Examples include the federal Medicare regulations restricting payments only to accredited public health and home health care agencies.

Accreditation, whether voluntary or required, provides a means for effective peer review and an opportunity for an in-depth review of program strengths and limitations. Accreditation applies external pressure and places demands on institutions to improve quality of care (Bodenheimer, 1999). In the past, the accreditation process primarily evaluated an agency's physical structure, organizational structure, and personnel qualifications. However, beginning in 1990, more emphasis was placed on evaluation of the outcomes of care and on the educational qualifications of the person providing the care.

**Certification,** another general approach to quality, combines features of licensure and accreditation. Certification is usually a voluntary process within professions. Educational achievements, experience, and performance on an examination determine a person's qualifications for functioning in an identified specialty area. The American Nurses Credentialing Center provides certification in several areas. For example, to become a certified community health nurse, one must have a baccalaureate degree in nursing and 2 years of practice as a community health nurse immediately before application.

Although usually a voluntary process, certification also can be a quasi-voluntary process. For example, to function as a nurse practitioner in some states, one must show proof of educational credentials and take an examination to be certified to practice within the boundaries of the state.

Major concerns exist about certification as a quality assurance mechanism. Data are lacking about the clinical competence of the practitioner at the time of certification because clinical competency is usually not measured by a written test. Although better data exist about the quality of the practitioner's work after the certification process, the American Nurses Credentialing Center has a research program to look at how certification is related to the work of the certified nurse (Cary, 2000). Except for occupational health nurses and nurse anesthetists, certification has not been recognized by employers as an achievement beyond basic preparation, so financial rewards are few. Although the nursing profession has accepted the certification process as a mechanism for recognizing competence and excellence, certifying bodies must help nurses communicate the importance of certified nurses to the public.

Charter, recognition, and academic degrees are other general approaches to quality assurance. **Charter** is the mechanism by which a state government agency, under state laws, grants corporate status to institutions with or without rights to award degrees (e.g., university-based nursing programs).

**Recognition** is a process whereby one agency accepts the credentialing status of and the credentials conferred by another. For example, some state boards of nursing accept nurse practitioner credentials that are awarded by the

American Nurses Credentialing Center or by one of the specialty credentialing agencies. Academic degrees are titles awarded to individuals recognized by degree-granting institutions as having completed a predetermined plan of study in a branch of learning. There are four academic degrees awarded in nursing, with some variety at each degree level: associate of arts/science; bachelor of science in nursing; master's degrees, such as master of science in nursing and master of nursing; and doctoral degrees such as doctor of philosophy, doctor of nursing science, doctor of science in nursing, doctor of nursing, and doctor of nursing practice.

Although these general quality management methods are important and should continue, newer and better approaches must be devised. If performance in the area of quality health care is to advance, better diagnosis of problems and corrective strategies that are effective will be necessary (Leatherman and McCarthy, 2002).

A recent approach to reorganization is the Magnet nursing services recognition given by the American Credentialing Center to agency nursing services that, after an extensive review, are considered excellent. This program began with reorganizations of excellent hospital nursing services. It is being expanded to include nursing home and home health agencies.

## Specific Approaches

Historically, quality assurance programs conducted by health care agencies have measured or assessed the performance of individuals and how they conformed to standards set forth by accrediting agencies. TQM/CQI is a management philosophy and method that incorporates many tools, including quality assurance, to increase customer satisfaction with quality care. Quality care has four components: *professional performance, efficient use of resources, minimal risk to the client of illness or injury associated with care,* and *client satisfaction* (Davis, 1994, p. 6). TQM/CQI seeks to eliminate errors in a process before negative outcomes can occur rather than waiting until after the fact to correct individual performance.

Health care agencies have only recently paid heed to the tenets of TQM/CQI, although Donabedian's early concepts of quality bear a striking similarity to writings of the industry's TQM leaders. This management philosophy has been used in Japanese industry since the post–World War II era when W. Edwards Deming was invited to Japan to help rebuild its broken economy. In addition to Deming, people associated with the total quality concept are Walter Stewart, who first published in this area, Joseph M. Juran, Armand F. Feigenbaum, Phillip B. Crosby, Genichi Taguchi, and Kaoru Ishikawa. Unlike traditional quality assurance programs, the focus of CQI is the *process* of delivering health care. This focus on process avoids placing personal blame for less-than-perfect outcomes. Applying TQM in health care allows management to look at the contribution of all systems to outcomes of the organization.

Deming's guidelines are summarized by his 14-point program (Deming, 1986, p. 23):

1. Create, publish, and give to all employees a statement of the aims and purposes of the company or other organization. The management must demonstrate constantly their commitment to this statement.
2. Learn the new philosophy, top management and everybody.
3. Understand the purpose of inspection, for improvement of processes and reduction of costs.
4. End the practice of awarding business on the basis of price tag alone.
5. Improve constantly and forever the system of production and service.
6. Institute training.
7. Teach and institute leadership.
8. Drive out fear. Create trust. Create a climate for innovation.
9. Optimize toward the aims and purposes of the company the efforts of teams, groups, staff areas.
10. Eliminate exhortations for the work force.
11a. Eliminate numerical quotes for production. Instead, learn and institute methods for improvement.
11b. Eliminate management by objective. Instead, learn the capabilities of processes and how to improve them.
12. Remove barriers that rob people of pride of workmanship.
13. Encourage education and self-improvement for everyone.
14. Take action to accomplish the transformation.

Deming's first point emphasizes that an organization must have purpose and values. Health care providers have a clear idea of their values and have been committed to quality in the past, as demonstrated by codes of ethics and standards of care. However, successful TQM/CQI processes rely on a cultural change within an organization and the full support of management. With respect to providing quality health care, a paradigm shift from individual provider responsibility to team responsibility must occur (McLaughlin and Kaluzny, 1999). A guiding principle is a customer orientation focused on positive health outcomes and perceived satisfaction. Customer (client) satisfaction surveys must be done for both internal and external users of services.

Personnel policies that are motivating and continuous training/learning opportunities are crucial to any quality improvement program. Deming's eighth point addresses driving out fear. Fear in this context means the fear of being fired for being innovative or taking risks. In the CQI process, individuals are not blamed for failures in the system and therefore are motivated through the group to continually look for problems and improve system performance.

TQM/CQI exists best in a flat organizational structure. This means there are very few supervisors between the staff and the director. This organization operates with a multi-disciplinary team approach and a separate but parallel management quality council that monitors strategy and implementation. Teams are empowered to solve problems and locate opportunities for system improvement. Shewhart's plan/do/check/act cycle serves as a guideline for the team approach to problem solving. Steps include the following (Deming, 1986, p. 88):

1. What could be the most important accomplishments of this team? What changes might be desirable? What data are available? Are new observations needed? If yes, plan a change or implement a test. Decide how to use the observations.
2. Carry out the change or test decided upon.
3. Observe the effects of the change.
4. Study the results. What did we learn? What can we predict?
5. Repeat cycle.

A suggested way to start the problem-solving process with a team in step 1 is *brainstorming* (Al-Assaf, 1993). Brainstorming is getting everyone's input about a possible process situation with no team member criticizing the suggestion. Because TQI/CQI organizations are data driven, moving to step 2 requires that ongoing statistics be collected. Differences from the mean or norm are detected through consistent use of tools, such as the flow chart, the Pareto chart (used to compare the importance of differences between groups of data), cause-and-effect diagrams, check sheets, histograms, control charts, regression, and other statistical analyses (e.g., quality assurance data and techniques, risk management data, risk-adjusted outcome measures, and cost effectiveness analysis) (McLaughlin and Kaluzny, 1999). Steps 3, 4, and 5 are self-explanatory.

Joseph Juran built on Deming's initial quality work and became a supporter of building quality into all processes. The Juran trilogy provides an effective way to compare the tasks of quality planning, quality control, and quality improvement. Quality planning involves determining who the clients are, the needs of those clients, the service that fulfills the need, and the process to produce that service. Quality control evaluates the performance of that service, compares it with the service goals, and then makes corrections if necessary. Quality improvement makes sure the infrastructure exists to enable individuals to identify improvement projects. Management of quality improvement establishes project teams and provides those teams with the resources needed to carry out improvement projects (Juran, 1998).

## TQM/CQI IN COMMUNITY AND PUBLIC HEALTH SETTINGS

Guidelines provided by the 1991 APHA Model Standards linked standards to meeting the health goals for the nation in the year 2000 (Mays et al, 1999). Healthy People 2000 and APHA Model Standards (1991) provided not only lists of priority health objectives for the nation and a way for public health to implement TQM/CQI but also the most

current statistics and scientific knowledge about health promotion and disease prevention (Durch et al, 1997). Now Healthy People in Healthy Communities (U.S. Department of Health and Human Services [USDHHS], 2000a) provides the objectives with their stated targets, measurement tools, and reflected intended performance expectations.

Healthy People 2010 builds on Healthy People 2000 and contains modified and additional objectives for promoting health and preventing disease (USDHHS, 2000b). An important part of the framework of Healthy People 2010 is eliminating health disparities and ensuring access to quality health care for all. Additionally, the Planned Approach to Community Health (PATCH) (Centers for Disease Control and Prevention [CDC], 1995), and the Assessment Protocol for Excellence in Public Health (APEXPH) and APEXPH in Practice (National Association of City and County Health Officials, 1995) provide methods of assessing community needs and how well health departments are operating to meet existing standards.

As health care reform continues, public health agencies face competition and are trying to reform themselves. A promising outcome of reform is the Community Health Improvement Process (CHIP) described by the Institute of Medicine (Durch et al, 1997) in their report *Improving Health in the Community: A Role for Performance Monitoring.* This report describes how private health care and public health can come together in a community-level effort to monitor performance and improve health.

Recognizing the many factors that cause health problems and the fragmenting that continues to exist in the health care system, this public–private collaborative framework involves many stakeholders, including public health, in monitoring the health of entire communities. Performance monitoring is defined as "a continuing community-based process of selecting indicators that can be used to measure the process and outcomes of an intervention strategy for health improvement . . . making the results available to the community as a whole . . . to inform assessments of an effective intervention and the contributions of accountable agencies to this" (Durch et al, 1997, p. 418). The performance indicators developed by a CHIP (Figure 22-1) relate to TQM/CQI. These indicators would measure processes or states that contribute to health and thus the processes are potentially alterable.

Home health care agencies have increasingly adopted quality improvement programs because of the competition that exists. Congruent with the TQM/CQI philosophy, meeting customer expectations is essential for home health care agencies. Davis (1994) presents a systems quality productivity model for home health care based on Deming's work. Under the first step, labeled *specifier,* Davis states that straightforward definitions of requirements and processes are necessary before embarking on a CQI process. This reinforces the need for the continuing learning process called for under Deming's 14 points. The model then proceeds with quality control, quality assurance, and quality continuation processes that should result

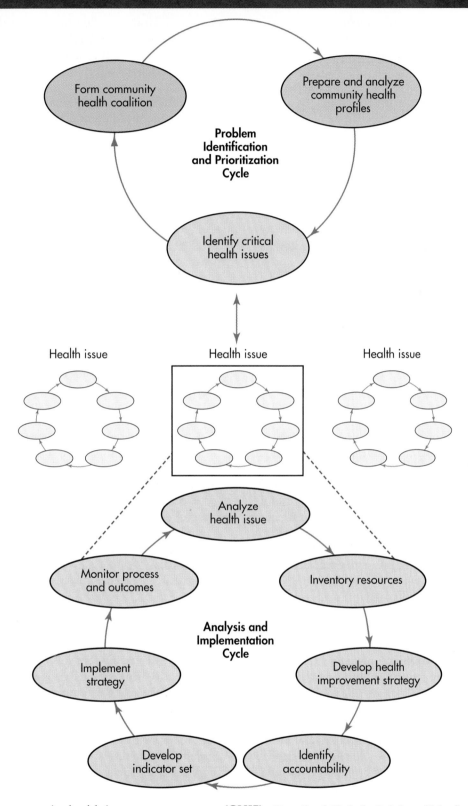

**Figure 22-1**  The community health improvement process (CHIP). *(From Durch JS, Bailey LA, Stoto MA, editors:* Improving health in the community: a role for performance monitoring, *Washington, DC, 1997, National Academy Press.)*

in quality improvement. *Quality control* is a proactive process and flows from specifiers being written in measurable terms and taught to all employees. *Quality assurance* activities are implemented through a proactive continuing quality sequence (or series of steps). Quality assurance retrospectively validates measures of policies, procedures, and standards set forth under quality control. In addition to the quality assurance function, it is important to eliminate errors before they happen. Quality assurance can alert organizations to unwanted trends. The *quality continuation sequence* is an "alignment of quality policy, procedure, practice, hiring criteria, training, rewards, and recognition" (Davis, 1994, p. 11). Quality improvement results from all preceding activities and is an ongoing process with continuing higher standards for achievement reintroduced into the system.

Other models for QA/QI in home health care have been developed to improve the quality of care in TQM/CQI frameworks emphasizing processes, empowerment, collaboration, consumers, data and measurement, and standards and outcomes (Verhey, 1996). One model is a provider partnership that emphasizes processes and systems developed by Care Home Health Services (CHH–Northern California Region). CHH evaluated eight system and process categories, which included condition, available and courteous service, timely responses, accuracy of paperwork, promise keeping, cost, and overall satisfaction. Implementing this model led to increased satisfaction of the provider partners and increased revenue (Smith, 1993).The Home Care Client Satisfaction instrument is a consumer-focused quality management tool designed to measure overall satisfaction with care through a 15-question Likert scale instrument (Westra et al, 1995). Another consumer model yielding positive results using focus group feedback from clients and caregivers was developed by the Visiting Nurses' Association (VNA) of Cleveland (Stricklin, 1995). Datasets of clinical information, such as those developed through the Omaha System and the National Association of Home Care (NAHC) (Clark et al, 2001; NAHC, 1994) are useful in measuring quality of care. **Report cards** of outcomes of health care agencies are becoming more readily available to consumers of health care.

Finally, in the area of standards and guidelines, Leatherman and McCarthy (2002) address six areas of performance that need improvement. One of these areas is consistently providing appropriate and effective care. This area is applicable to all health care practitioners including community-oriented nurses. Evidence-based **practice guidelines** are one way to deliver consistent, up-to-date care and to improve outcomes for individuals, communities, and populations. In 2001, five Minnesota health plans, covering most of the state's insured population, endorsed standard treatment and prevention guidelines for 50 common diseases (Sprague, 2001). The use of guidelines helps gather data on the effectiveness and outcomes of nurse interventions (Strohschein et al, 1999). The

Agency for Healthcare Research and Quality (AHRQ), formerly the Agency for Health Care Policy and Research (AHCPR), has played a major role in developing clinical practice guidelines.

*Guidelines* are protocols or statements of recommended practice developed by professional organizations; they are based on the distilling of scientific evidence and expert opinion that guide a clinician in decision making (Sprague, 2001). "Framing research findings as guidelines can provide a user friendly approach that increases nurses' awareness of existing research and ways to apply research to practice. Such evidence-based guidelines than can be used to document effective outcomes of nurse's interventions at the community and systems levels" (Strohschein et al, 1999, p. 84). Guidelines provide research-based evidence for interventions and promote improved health outcomes. An example of criteria for clinical practice guidelines are those set forth by AHRQ and available on the internet at the National Guideline Clearinghouse (NGC) website (www.guideline.gov/index.asp) (NGC, 2000):

- The guideline must contain systematically developed recommendations, strategies, or other information to assist health care decision making in specific clinical circumstances
- The guideline must have been produced under the auspices of a relevant professional organization (e.g., medical specialty society, government agency, health care organization, or health plan)
- The guideline development process must have included a verifiable, systematic literature search and review of existing evidence published in peer-reviewed journals
- The guideline must be current and the most recent version (developed, reviewed, or revised in the last 5 years)

Primary care practice guidelines already available are the *Guide to Clinical Preventive Services* (U.S. Preventive Services Task Force, 2000) and the population–based *Guide to Community Preventive Services* available on the website of the CDC. This guide is an ongoing process of the Taskforce on Community Preventive Services that offers information on changing risk behaviors, reducing specific disease, injuries and impairments, environmental concerns, and crosscutting public health activities. Community-oriented nurses need guidelines to reduce differences in care practices, to improve outcomes on the basis of the best research available, and to deliver effective care to individuals, communities, and populations.

## Using QA/QI in TQM/CQI

Although the methods differ, the objective of both TQM/CQI and QA/QI programs is quality outcomes for clients. QA/QI methods and tools help agencies conform to standards required by external accrediting agencies. QA/QI provides a way to identify examples of substandard care and to improve that care when standards are not met. QA is focused on problem detection, whereas

TQM/CQI is focused on problem prevention and continuous improvement. The total quality philosophy states that quality cannot be "inspected in"; it must be "built in." In QA/QI, little attention is paid to preventing errors or problems and finding out who owns the quality issues. Furthermore, the QA process may stop unless another problem is found. McLaughlin and Kaluzny (1999) point out differences in traditional management models that use performance standards versus those that use TQM/CQI (Table 22-1).

Because common ground exists between TQM/CQI and QA/QI, positive steps of a known quality assurance program can be integrated into a total quality approach. Strengths of quality assurance include a history of expertise in developing evaluation of structure, identifying high-priority problems, and developing knowledge in quality assessment and information systems. These strengths can be used to advantage in a CQI effort.

## Traditional Quality Assurance

Traditional quality assurance programs can fit well with the CQI process. Because organizations may implement only parts of the TQM process, it is important to understand existing traditional quality assurance programs. The overall goal of specific quality assurance approaches is to monitor the process and outcomes of client care. The goals are as follows:

1. To identify problems between provider and client
2. To intervene in problem cases
3. To provide feedback regarding interactions between client and provider
4. To provide documentation of interactions between client and provider

The specific approaches are often implemented voluntarily by agencies and provider groups interested in the quality of interactions in their setting. However, state and federal governments require mandatory programs within public health agencies. For example, periodic utilization review, peer reviews (audits), and other quality control measures are required in public health agencies that receive funds from state taxes, Medicaid, Medicare, and other public funding sources. Examples of specific approaches to quality control are agency **staff review committees** (peer review), utilization review committees, research studies, PRO monitoring, client satisfaction surveys (see the Evidence-Based Practice box on p. 530), risk management, and malpractice lawsuits.

### Staff Review Committee

Staff review committees are the most common specific approach to quality assurance in the United States. Staff committees are designed to monitor client-specific aspects of certain levels of care. The audit is the major tool used to evaluate quality of care.

The **audit process** (Figure 22-2) consists of six steps:

1. Select a topic for study.
2. Select explicit criteria for quality care.
3. Review records to determine whether criteria are met.
4. Do a peer review for all cases that do not meet criteria.
5. Make specific recommendations to correct problems.
6. Follow up to determine whether problems have been eliminated.

Two types of audits are used in nursing peer review: concurrent and retrospective. The concurrent audit is a process audit that evaluates the quality of ongoing care by looking at the nursing process. **Concurrent audit** is used

| Table 22-1 Traditional Management Compared With TQM Model | |
|---|---|
| **TRADITIONAL MODEL** | **TQM MODEL** |
| Legal or professional authority | Collective or managerial responsibility |
| Specialized accountability | Process accountability |
| Administrative authority | Participation |
| Meeting standards | Meeting process and performance expectations |
| Longer planning horizon | Shorter planning horizon |
| Quality assurance | Continuous improvement |

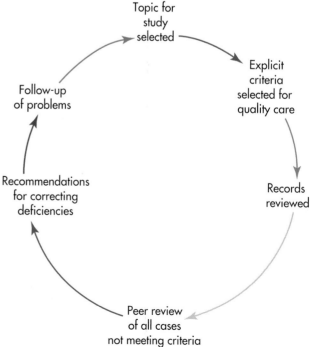

**Figure 22-2** The audit process.

by Medicare and Medicaid to evaluate care being received by public health/home health clients. The advantages of this method are as follows:

- Identification of problems at the time care is given
- Provision of a mechanism for identifying and meeting client needs during care
- Implementation of measures to fulfill professional responsibilities
- Provision of a mechanism for communicating on behalf of the client

The disadvantages of the concurrent audit are as follows:

- It is time consuming.
- It is more costly to implement than the retrospective audit.
- Because care is ongoing, it does not present the total picture of care that the client ultimately will receive.

The **retrospective audit,** or outcome audit, evaluates quality of care through evaluating the nursing process after the client's discharge from the health care system. The advantages of the retrospective audit are that it provides the following:

- Comparison of actual practice to standards of care
- Analysis of actual practice findings
- A total picture of care given
- More accurate data for planning corrective action

Disadvantages of the retrospective audit method are as follows:

- The focus of evaluation is directed away from ongoing care.
- Client problems are identified after discharge.

Thus corrective action can be used only to improve the care of future clients.

## Utilization Review

The purpose of **utilization review** is to ensure that care is needed and that the cost is appropriate (Davis, 1994). There are three types of utilization review:

1. *Prospective:* An assessment of the necessity of care before giving service
2. *Concurrent:* A review of the necessity of services while care is being given
3. *Retrospective:* An analysis of the necessity of the services received by the client after the care has been given

Each of these reviews assesses the appropriate cost of care. Prospectively, care can be denied and money saved. Concurrently, services can be cut if they are not found to be essential. Retrospectively, payment can be denied to the provider if the care was not necessary.

Utilization review began in the middle part of the twentieth century out of concern for increasing health care costs. The first committees were developed by insurance companies and professional groups. Utilization review committees became mandatory under the 1965 Medicare law as a way to control hospital costs (Davis, 1994).

The utilization review process includes development of explicit criteria regarding the need for services and the length of service. Utilization review has been used primarily in hospitals to establish the need for client admission and to determine the length of hospital stay. In community and public health, especially home health care, utilization review establishes criteria for admission to agency service, the number of visits a client may receive, the eligibility for client services, such as a nursing aide or physical therapist, and discharge.

Utilization review has several advantages:

- It helps clients avoid unnecessary care.
- It may encourage clients to consider alternative care options, such as home health care rather than hospital care.
- It can provide guidelines for staff and program development.
- It provides for agency accountability to the consumer.

The major disadvantage of utilization review is that not all clients fit the classic picture presented by the explicit criteria used to determine approval or denial of care. For example, an older adult client was admitted to a home health care agency for management after hospital discharge. The client was paraplegic as a result of a cerebrovascular accident. After several weeks of physical and speech therapy, the client showed little sign of progress. The utilization review committee considered the client's condition to be stable and did not recognize the continued need for management to prevent future complications; therefore Medicare payment was denied.

Appeal mechanisms have been built into the utilization review process used by Medicare and Medicaid. The appeal allows providers and clients to present additional data that may help to reverse the original decision to deny payment.

## Risk Management

**Risk management** committees often are a part of the QA/QI program of a community agency. Risk management seeks to reduce the agency's liability because of grievances brought against them. The risk management committee reviews all risks to which an agency is exposed. It reviews client and personnel safety policies and procedures and determines whether personnel are following the rules. Examples of problems reviewed by a risk management committee include administering incorrect vaccination dosage, pediatric client injury caused by a fall from an examining table, or injury to the nurse as a result of an accident while making a home visit. Incident reports are reviewed by the risk management committee for appropriate, accurate, and thorough documentation of any problem that occurs relating to clients or personnel. In addition, patterns are identified that may require changes in policy or staff development to correct the problem. As a part of risk management, grievance procedures are established for both clients and personnel.

## Professional Review Organizations

The **Professional Standards Review Organization** (PSRO) was established in 1972 in an amendment to the Social Security Act (PL 92-603) as a publicly-mandated utilization and peer review program. This law provided that medical, hospital, and nursing home care under Medicare, Medicaid, and Title V Maternal and Child Health Programs would be reviewed for appropriateness and necessary care to be reimbursed.

In 1983 Congress passed the Peer Review Improvement Act (PL 97-248), creating **Professional Review Organizations** (PROs). PROs replaced PSROs and are directed by the federal government to reduce hospital admissions for procedures that can be performed safely and effectively in an ambulatory surgical setting on an outpatient basis. The goal was to reduce inappropriate or unnecessary admissions or invasive procedures by specific practitioners or hospitals. Quality measures include reducing unnecessary admissions caused by previous substandard care, avoidable complications and deaths, and unnecessary surgery or invasive procedures (Sprague, 2001).

Institutions contract with PROs for quality reviews. PROs are local (usually state) organizations that establish criteria for care on the basis of local patterns of practice. They can be for-profit or not-for-profit organizations. They have access to physicians or may include physicians in their membership. PROs must define their operational objectives and are required to consult with nurses and other nonphysician health care providers when reviewing the activities of those professionals. PROs monitor access to care and cost of care. Professionals working under the regulation of PROs should develop accurate and complete documenting procedures to ensure compliance with the criteria of the PRO.

Debate has occurred over the limits and benefits of the federally mandated quality review process. Limits include jeopardizing professional autonomy because decision making regarding care includes professionals, consumers, and government representatives. Another limitation of this process is the development of a costly control mechanism whereby client care activities may be determined by cost rather than by professional criteria. The benefit of the PSRO/PRO system has been the development of standards and the peer review mechanisms to increase accountability for care provided (Greenberg and Lezzoni, 1995). In 1985, PRO authority was expanded to include review of services offered by health maintenance organizations (HMOs) and competitive medical plans. In addition, the Medicare Quality Assurance Act was passed to strengthen quality assurance programs and to improve access to care after hospitalization. This act required hospitals receiving Medicare payments to provide to Medicare beneficiaries written forms of discharge planning supervised by registered nurses and social workers.

## Evaluative Studies

**Evaluative studies** for quality health care increased during the twentieth century. Studies demonstrate the effect of nursing and health care interventions on client populations. Three key models have been used to evaluate quality: Donabedian's structure–process–outcome, the tracer, and the sentinel.

Donabedian's (1981, 1985, 1990) model introduced three major methods for evaluating quality care:

1. *Structure.* Evaluating the setting and instruments used to provide care. Examples of structure are facilities, equipment, characteristics of the administrative organization, client mix, and the qualifications of health providers.
2. *Process.* Evaluating activities as they relate to standards and expectations of health providers in the management of client care
3. *Outcome.* The net change that occurs as a result of health care or the net result of health care

The three methods may be used separately to evaluate a part of care. However, to get an overall picture of quality of care, they should be used together.

The tracer method described by Kessner and Kalk (1973) is a measure of both process and outcome of care. This method is more effective in evaluating health care of groups than of individual clients. It is also more effective in evaluating care delivered by an institution than by an individual provider. Kessner and Kalk (1973) described the following essential characteristics for implementing the tracer method:

1. A tracer, or a problem, that has a definite impact on the client's level of functioning
2. Well-defined and easily diagnosed characteristics
3. Population prevalence high enough to permit adequate data collection
4. A known variation resulting from use of effective health care
5. Well-defined management techniques in prevention, diagnosis, treatment, or rehabilitation
6. Understood (documented) effects of nonmedical factors on the tracer

Stevens-Barnum and Kerfoot (1995) provided a classification system for selecting client groups for tracer outcome studies in nursing. The client groups would have the following:

1. A particular disease
2. Similar treatment
3. Similar needs

---

**DID YOU KNOW?**

TQM/CQI gives direction for managing a system of care, whereas QA/QI focuses on the care a client receives within the system.

4. Similar community
5. Similar lifestyle
6. Similar illness stage

The tracer method provides nurses with data to show the differences in outcomes as a result of nursing care standards.

The sentinel method of quality evaluation is based on epidemiologic principles. This method is an outcome measure for examining specific instances of client care. Changes in the sentinel indicate potential problems for others. For example, increases in encephalitis in certain communities may result from increases in mosquito populations. New information technologies available improve surveillance of process and outcome and can eliminate the need for sentinel events to trigger a QA review (Bellin and Dubler, 2001).

---

**HOW TO   Conduct a Sentinel Evaluation**

- Identify cases of unnecessary disease, disability, complications. Example: tuberculosis (TB).
- Count the deaths from these causes.
- Examine the circumstances surrounding the unnecessary event (or sentinel), in detail.
- Review morbidity and mortality rates as an index for comparison; determine the critical increase in the untimely event, which may reflect changes in quality of care. Example: compare the incidence and prevalence of TB cases before the increased population occurred.
- Explore health status indicators, such as changes in social, economic, political, and environmental factors that may have an effect on health outcomes. Example: Overcrowding in the shelter where migrant workers stay (environmental) and the inability to follow up on testing because of the transient nature of the population (social).

---

## CLIENT SATISFACTION

Client satisfaction is another approach to measuring quality of care. Client satisfaction can be assessed using in-person or telephone interviews and mailed questionnaires. Satisfaction surveys are used to assess care received during an admission to a specific agency; to assess a client's personal nursing care; or to assess the total care that the client received from all services (see the Evidence-Based Practice box).

Satisfaction surveys may measure the interventions used for client care, attitudes about the care received and the providers of care, and perceptions of the situation (environment) in which the care was received. Clients are often more critical of interpersonal and situational components of care than of the interventions of care.

Satisfaction surveys are an essential aspect of quality assessment. Survey data provide clues to reasons for client compliance or noncompliance with plans of care. Although consumers may not view quality in the same

---

**Evidence-Based Practice**

Client satisfaction remains an important outcome measure in determining quality in health care organizations, but there are weaknesses in the methods used to measure it. This study sought to investigate the reliability of the client satisfaction tool (CST) and looked at client satisfaction in a nurse-managed senior health clinic. The Cox interactional model of client satisfaction consists of 12 questions with scores ranging from 12 (worst) to 60 (best). It has five Likert-type questions, ranging from 1 (worst) to 5 (best), that represent elements of client–professional interaction thought to influence health outcomes. A convenience sample of 38 clients completed the CST. A descriptive correlational research design was used, and data were collected through an interview format twice at 1-week intervals to look at test–retest reliability.

Data revealed that client satisfaction with the clinic was high, with a mean score of 52.06 (range, 31 to 60). Answers to individual questions also produced a high score, with mean responses ranging from 4.13 to 4.50. Reliability analysis yielded a high overall internal consistency. Stepwise regression identified that elements of care were the best predictors of overall satisfaction with care. "Care decisions are of high quality" and "helped me to take care of myself at home" were found to explain 90% of the reasons for overall client satisfaction.

**Nurse Use:** The CST provides a comprehensive indicator of client satisfaction with the nurse practitioner model.

Bear M, Bowers C: Using a nursing framework to measure client satisfaction at a nurse managed clinic, *Public Health Nurs* 15(1):50, 1998.

---

light as the health professional, surveys provide data about health-seeking behaviors, the probability of malpractice litigation, and the likelihood of continuing client–provider–agency relationships, always an important measure for HMOs (Bodenheimer, 1999) (Figure 22-3).

## Malpractice Litigation

**Malpractice litigation** (i.e., a lawsuit) is a specific approach to quality assurance imposed on the health care delivery system by the legal system. Malpractice litigation typically results from client dissatisfaction with the provider and with the content of the care received. Nursing is not immune from malpractice litigation. Nursing must continue to have a sound quality assurance program that ensures quality care. This will reduce the risk of quality control measures being imposed by an external source, such as the legal system.

Please mark the following questions using the scale.

| Domain | Example | Strongly Agree | Somewhat Agree | Agree | Somewhat Disagree | Strongly Disagree |
|---|---|---|---|---|---|---|
| Affective support | 1. The clinic staff were understanding of my health concerns. | | | | | |
| | 2. The clinical staff gave me encouragement in regard to my health problems. | | | | | |
| Health information | 3. I got my questions answered in an individual way. | | | | | |
| | 4. The information I received at the clinic helped me to take care of myself at home. | | | | | |
| Decision control | 5. I was included in decision making. | | | | | |
| | 6. I was included in the planning of my care. | | | | | |
| Technical competencies | 7. The treatments I received were of high quality. | | | | | |
| | 8. Decisions regarding my health care were of high quality. | | | | | |
| Accessibility | 9. The clinic staff was available when I needed them. | | | | | |
| | 10. The appointment time at the clinic was when I needed it. | | | | | |
| Overall satisfaction | 11. Overall, I was satisfied with my health care. | | | | | |
| | 12. The care I received at the clinic was of high quality. | | | | | |

**Figure 22-3** Client satisfaction tool domains and examples.

## MODEL QA/QI PROGRAM

The primary purpose of a QA/QI program is to ensure that the results of an organized activity are consistent with the expectations. All personnel affected by a quality assurance program should be involved in its development and implementation. Although administration and management are responsible for the quality of services, the key to that quality is in the personnel who deliver the service: their knowledge, skills, and attitudes.

Figure 22-4 shows a model, which identifies the basic components of a quality assurance program. Quality as-surance programs answer the following questions about health care services and nursing care:

1. What is being done now?
2. Why is it being done?
3. Is it being done well?
4. Can it be done better?
5. Should it be done at all?
6. Are there improved ways to deliver the service?
7. How much does it cost?
8. Should certain activities be abandoned or replaced?

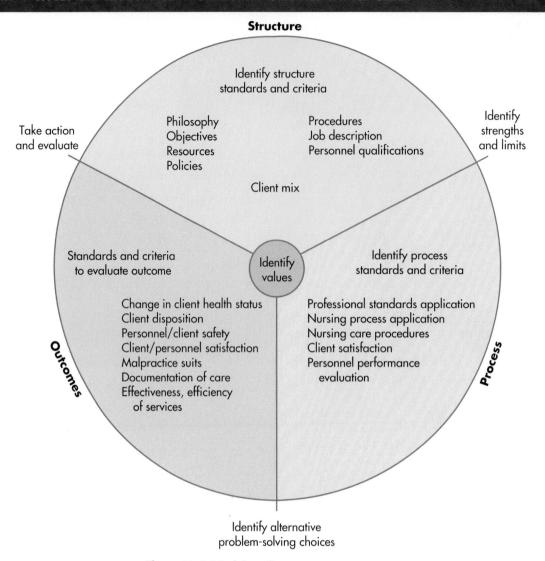

**Figure 22-4**  Model quality assurance programs.

Donabedian's framework for evaluating health care programs using the components of structure, process, and outcome can be used in developing a quality assurance program. *Outcome* is the most important ingredient of a program because it is the key to evaluating providers and agencies by accrediting bodies, by insurance companies, and by Medicare and Medicaid through PROs and other accrediting agencies.

## Structure

The vision, values, philosophy, and objectives of an agency serve to define the structural standards of the agency. Evaluation of structure is a specific approach to looking at quality. In evaluating the structure of an organization, the evaluator determines whether the agency is adhering to the stated philosophy and objectives and to its vision and stated values. Is the agency providing services to populations across the life span? Are primary, secondary, and/or tertiary preventive services offered? Standards of structure are defined by the licensing or accrediting agency (e.g., the NLN standards for accrediting

home health agencies) (Council of Home Health Agencies, Community Health Services, 1986).

Identifying values, the first step in a quality assurance program, serves to define the beliefs of the agency about humanity, nursing, the community, and health. The beliefs of the community, the population to be served, and the providers of care are equally important to the agency, and all need to be considered to provide quality service.

Identifying standards and criteria for quality assurance begins with writing the philosophy and objectives of the organization. Program objectives define the intended results of nursing care, descriptions of client behaviors, and/or change in health status to be demonstrated on discharge.

Once objectives are formulated, the resources needed to accomplish the objectives should be identified. The personnel, supplies and equipment, facilities, and financial resources that are needed should be described. Once resources are determined, policies, procedures, and job descriptions should be formed to serve as behavioral guides to the employees of the agency. These documents should reflect the essential nursing and other health provider qualifications needed to implement the services of the agency.

Standards of structure are evaluated internally by a committee composed of administrative, management, and staff members for the purpose of doing a self-study. Standards of structure are also evaluated by a utilization review committee, often composed of an external advisory group with community representatives for all services offered through an agency, such as a nurse, a physical therapist, a speech pathologist, a physician, a board member, and an administrator from a similar agency. The data from these committees identify the strengths and weaknesses of the agency structure.

## Process

The evaluation of process standards is a specific look at the quality of care being given by agency providers, such as nurses. Agencies use a variety of methods to determine criteria for evaluating provider activities: conceptual models, such as a developmental model or Neuman Systems Model (see Chapter 9); the standards of care of the provider's professional organization, such as the ANA's *Scope and Standards of Public Health Nursing Practice* (1999) (see Chapter 1); or the nursing process. The activities of the nurse are evaluated to see whether they are the same as the nursing care procedures defined by the agency.

The primary approaches used for process evaluation include the peer review committee and the client satisfaction survey. The techniques used for process evaluation are direct observation, questionnaire, interview, written audit, and videotape of client and provider encounters.

---

**◖ NURSING TIP**

Know the standards of care for your agency and for your practice area (e.g., ANA *Scope and Standards of Practice for Public Health Nursing*). Keep your eyes open for recurring practices that are not up to the quality standards of your agency. (For example, your clients complain daily about long waits for service.) Chances are that these same practices may be occurring in other areas of the agency, and knowing this helps the agency improve quality.

---

Once data are collected to evaluate nursing process standards, the peer review committee reviews the data to identify strengths and weaknesses in the quality of care delivered. The peer review committee is usually an internal committee composed of representatives of the nursing staff who are trained to administer audit instruments and conduct client interviews.

## Outcome

The evaluation of outcome standards, or the result of nursing care, is one of the more difficult tasks facing nursing today. Identifying changes in the client's health status that result from nursing care provides nursing data that demonstrate the contribution of nursing to the health care deliv-

ery system. Research studies using the tracer or sentinel method to identify client outcomes and client satisfaction surveys can be used to measure outcome standards. Measures of outcome standards include client admission data about the level of dependence or the acuity of problems and discharge data that may show changes in levels of dependence and activity.

From these data, strengths and weaknesses in nursing care delivery can be determined. The most common measurement methods are direct physical observations and interviews. Instruments also have been developed to measure general health status indicators in home health. The Omaha Visiting Nurse Association problem classification system (see Chapter 9) includes nursing diagnosis, protocols of care, and a problem rating scale to measure nursing care outcomes (Clark et al, 2001; O'Brien-Pallas et al, 2001, 2002). Additionally, the ANA has developed 10 areas for data collection of outcome criteria in community-based, non–acute care settings, including pain management, consistency of communication, staff mix, client satisfaction, prevention of tobacco use, cardiovascular disease prevention, caregiver activity, identification of primary caregiver, activities of daily living, and psychosocial interactions (Rowell, 2001). Nursing has been involved primarily in evaluating program outcomes to justify program expenses rather than in evaluating client outcomes.

Outcome evaluation assumes that health care has a positive effect on client status. The major problem with outcome evaluation is determining which nursing care activities are primarily responsible for causing changes in client status. In nursing, many uncontrolled factors in the field, such as environment and family relationships, have an effect on client status. Often it is difficult to determine whether these factors are the cause of changes in client status or whether nursing interventions have the most effect.

Types of problems studied in a quality assurance program include reasons for the following:

- Client death
- Client injury
- Personnel and client safety
- Agency liability
- Increased costs
- Denied reimbursement by third-party payers
- Client complaints
- Inefficient service
- Staff noncompliance with standards of structure
- Lack of resources
- Unnecessary staff work and overtime
- Documenting of care
- Client health status

Table 22-2 summarizes quality assurance measures.

## Evaluation, Interpretation, and Action

Interpreting the findings of a quality care evaluation is an important part of the process. It allows differences between the quality care standards of the agency and the

**Table 22-2　Quality Assurance Measures**

| STRUCTURE | PROCESS | OUTCOME |
|---|---|---|
| **Internal Agency** | **Peer Review Committees** | **Internal Agency Committees** |
| Self-study | Prospective audit | Evaluative studies |
| Review agency documents | Concurrent audit | Survey health status |
| | Retrospective audit | |
| **External Agency** | **Client** | **Client** |
| Regulatory audit | Satisfaction survey | Malpractice suits |
| | Utilization review | Satisfaction survey |

actual practice of the nurse or other health providers to be identified. These patterns reflect the total agency's functioning over time and generate information for decisions to be made about the strengths and limits of the agency. Regular intervals for evaluation should be established within the agency, and periodic reports should be written so that the combined results of structure, process, and outcome efforts can be analyzed and health care delivery patterns and problems can be identified. These reports should be used to establish an ongoing picture of changes that occur within an agency to justify nursing services.

Identifying choices of possible courses of action to correct the weaknesses within the agency should involve both the administration and the staff. The courses of action chosen should be based on their importance, cost, and timeliness. For example, if there is a nursing problem in the recording of client health education, the agency administration and staff may analyze the problem to see why it is occurring. Reasons for lack of record keeping given by the nurses include a lack of time to do paperwork properly, case overloads that reduce the amount of time spent with clients, and lack of available resources for health education. If such reasons are given, it would not be appropriate for management to deal with the problem by providing a staff development program on the importance of doing and recording health education. It would be more important to assess how to provide the time and resources necessary for the nurses to offer health education to the clients. Economically, it may be more beneficial to provide handheld or laptop computers and clerical assistance so that nurses can make notes at the point of care, thereby providing more client contact time, or it may be more beneficial economically to employ an additional nurse and reduce caseloads.

Taking action is the final step in the QA/QI model. Once the alternative courses of action are chosen to correct problems, actions must be implemented for change to occur in the overall operation of the agency. Follow-up and evaluating of actions taken must occur to improve quality of care. Although health provider evaluation will continue to be included in a quality improvement effort, the focus of a CQI effort emphasizes the process and not the person. The assumption here is that health care professionals and other employees customarily want to do the best job possible for the client, and problems or differences in a process should not be automatically attributed to their behavior. Although frequent feedback should be given to all employees, the hallmark of quality improvement is continuous learning. Staff development must be ongoing for all employees (see Box 22-3 for prevention levels related to quality management).

Documentation is essential to evaluating quality care in any organization. The following paragraphs focus on the kinds of documentation that normally occur in a community agency.

## RECORDS

**Records** are an important part of the communication structure of the health care organization. Accurate and complete records are required by law and must be kept by all government and nongovernment agencies. In most states, the state departments of health stipulate the kinds of records to be kept and their content requirements for community agencies.

Records provide complete information about the client, indicate the extent and quality of services being given, resolve legal issues in malpractice suits, and provide information for education and research.

### Community and Public Health Agency Records

Within the community or public health agency, many types of records are kept and used to predict population trends in a community, to identify health needs and problems, to prepare and justify budgets, and to make administrative decisions. The kinds of records kept by the agency may include reports of accidents, births, census, chronic disease, communicable disease, mortality rates, life expectancy, morbidity rates, child and spouse abuse, occupational illness and injury, and environmental health.

Other types of records kept within the agency are those used to maintain administrative contact and control of the organization. Three types of records make up this category:

---

**BOX 22-3** **Levels of Prevention Applied to Quality Management**

**PRIMARY PREVENTION**

Staff development program to teach nurses and other providers how to reduce risk by properly documenting interventions.

**SECONDARY PREVENTION**

Agency evaluation of individual nurse competencies in completing a community assessment on which program decisions will be made.

**TERTIARY PREVENTION**

Staff development program to teach nurses skills in community assessment when the nurse's competency evaluation indicated that he or she did not have the proper skills.

---

clinical, service, and financial. The *clinical record* is the client health record. The *provider service records* include information about the number of clinic clients seen daily, the immunizations given, home visits made daily, transportation and mileage, the provider's time spent with the client, and the amount and kinds of supplies used. The service record is completed on a daily basis by each provider and is summarized monthly and annually to indicate trends in health care activities and costs related to personnel time, transportation, maintenance, and supplies. The provider service records are used to compare with the agency's *financial records* of salaries, overhead, and transportation costs, and they serve as the basis for the cost accounting system (see Chapter 21). These records are basic to peer review and audit.

Three additional kinds of service records seen in the community agency are the central index system, the annual implementation plan, and the annual summary of agency activities. The *central index system* is a data-filing system that indicates the services requested, services offered, active and inactive clients of the agency, and a profile of the agency's clients.

The *annual implementation plan* is developed at the beginning of each fiscal year to define the short-term and long-term goals of the agency. The annual implementation plan serves as the basis for the agency's annual summary. The *annual summary* reflects the success of the agency in meeting the annual objectives, changes in population trends and health status during the year, the actual versus the projected budget requirements, the number of services offered, the number of clients served, and the plans and changes recommended for the future. This plan serves as the basis for the evaluation of agency structure.

As an outgrowth of quality assurance efforts in the health care system, comprehensive methods are being designed to document and measure client progress and client outcome from agency admission through discharge. An example of such a method is the client classification system developed at the Visiting Nurses Association of Omaha, Nebraska (Martin and Norris, 1996). This comprehensive method for evaluating client care has several components: a classification system for assessing and categorizing client problems, a database, a nursing problem list, and anticipated outcome criteria for the classified problem. Such

schemes are viewed as having the potential to improve the delivery of nursing care, documentation, and the descriptions of client care. Briefly, implementing a comprehensive documentation method improves nursing assessment, planning, implementing, and evaluating of client care, and it allows the organization of important client information for more effective and efficient nurse productivity and communication (see Figure 22-3 and Chapter 9).

## Practice Application

Menaka, a community health nursing student, has been working in the clinic area and has noted that each practitioner uses a different educational method for teaching parenting skills to new mothers and fathers. Menaka knows that practice guidelines for teaching parenting skills exist in her clinical facility and that charts have an area to note parenting skills information. She also knows that for nurses to be most effective and ensure quality client outcomes, research-based practice guidelines should be used by all nurses in the health department.

As part of the community health course, Menaka must prepare a teaching plan and conduct a class on a health care problem. She obtains permission from her instructor and the director of the clinic to conduct an inservice program on teaching parenting skills to the nursing staff. She obtains and studies the guidelines about teaching parenting skills, and she researches the methodologic background for development of the guidelines.

As part of her inservice program, Menaka keeps demographic records on attendees and conducts before-and-after tests of knowledge, adding questions about the present use of the guidelines. She plans to follow up with the nurses in 6 months with a further test and questions about use of the guidelines. The director will help her determine an outcome measure that can be used with the client population to show effective use of the guidelines.

**A.** What outcome measure would be useful in this project?

**B.** How will this help in the overall assessment of quality in the community nursing service?

---

**Answers are in the back of the book.**

## Key Points

- The health care delivery system is the largest employing industry in the United States; society is demanding increased efficiency and effectiveness from the system. Little is known about the actual quality of care in this country because of varying definitions, logistics, and data collection methods.
- Quality control is the tool used to ensure effective and efficient care.
- The managed care industry is changing the face of the American health care delivery system and how quality is defined and measured.
- Objective and systematic evaluation of nursing care has become a priority within the profession for several reasons, including the effects of cost on health care access, consumer demands for better quality care, and increasing involvement of nurses in formulating public and health agency policy.
- Total quality management/continuous quality improvement (TQM/CQI) is a management philosophy new to the health care arena. It is prevention oriented and process focused. Its primary focus is to deliver quality health care. One measure of quality is customer satisfaction.
- Public and private sectors are forming partnerships to monitor performance of all players in health care delivery to improve the health of communities. The different players in the health care system have different perceptions of quality.
- Quality assurance/quality improvement (QA/QI) is the monitoring of client care activities to determine the degree of excellence attained in implementing activities.
- Quality assurance has been a concern of the profession since the 1860s, when Florence Nightingale called for a uniform format to gather and disseminate hospital statistics.
- Licensure has been a major issue in nursing since 1892.
- Two major categories of approaches exist in QA/QI today: general and specific.
- Accreditation is an approach to quality control used for institutions, whereas licensure is used primarily for individuals.
- Certification combines features of both licensing and accreditation.
- Three major models have been used to evaluate quality: Donabedian's structure–process–outcome model, the sentinel model, and the tracer model.
- Seven basic components of a quality assurance program are (1) identifying values; (2) identifying structure, process, and outcome standards and criteria; (3) selecting measurement techniques; (4) interpreting the strengths and weaknesses of the care given; (5) identifying alternative courses of action; (6) choosing specific courses of action; and (7) taking action.
- Records are an integral part of the communication structure of a health care organization. Accurate and complete records are by law required of all agencies, whether governmental or nongovernmental.
- QA/QI mechanisms in health care delivery are the mechanisms for controlling the system and requesting accountability from individual providers within the system. Records help establish a total picture of the contribution of the agency to the client community.
- Delivering quality care to individuals, communities and populations falls under the 10 essential services of public health.
- Evidence-based practice guidelines can help community-oriented nurses document the outcomes and effectiveness of their interventions.

## Clinical Decision-Making Activities

1. Write your own definition of TQM/CQI; compare your definition with the one given in the text. Are they the same or different? Give justification for your answer.
2. How does traditional QA/QI fit into the TQM/CQI effort? Explain the relative importance of a continuing QA/QI effort.
3. Interview a nurse who is a coordinator of or is responsible for QA/QI in a local health agency. Ask the following questions and add your own. Do the answers to the questions relate to what you have learned about QA/QI? Explain!
   a. Does the agency subscribe to the TQM/CQI approach to management?
   b. If not, is the agency incorporating elements of the TQM/CQI process as outlined by Deming (1986) in his 14 points?
   c. Is a traditional method of quality assurance used to ensure quality?
   d. Describe the components of the QA/QI program.
   e. How are records used in your QA/QI effort?
   f. Discuss the approaches and techniques that are used to implement the QA/QI program.
   g. How has the QA/QI program changed in the health agency over the past 20 years?
   h. What influence has the QA/QI program had on decreasing problems attributable to process? To provider accountability?
   i. List and describe the types of records usually kept in a community health agency. Explain the purpose of each type of record.
4. Identify partnerships necessary to ensure quality health outcomes for your community from data gathered in a community assessment. Explain why these partners are necessary.

5. Find the *Guide to Community Preventive Services* on the CDC website, and look for the segments on smoking cessation or tuberculosis control. How could you use this information in your practice in community health?

## References

Al-Assaf AF: Data management for total quality. In Al-Assaf AF, Schmele JA, editors: *The textbook of total quality in healthcare,* Delray Beach, Fla, 1993, St Lucie Press.

Al-Assaf AF: Historical evolution of managed care quality. In Al-Assaf AF, editor: *Managed care quality: a practical guide,* New York, 1998, CRC Press.

American Nurses Association: *The scope and standards of public health nursing practice,* Washington, DC, 1999, ANA.

American Public Health Association: Healthy communities 2000: model standards, guidelines for community attainment of the year 2000 national health objectives, ed 3, Washington, DC, 1991, APHA.

Association of Community Health Nursing Educators: Perspectives on doctoral education in community health nursing, Lexington, Ky, 1993, ACHNE.

Association of Community Health Nursing Educators: *Graduate education for advanced practice education in community/public health nursing,* Chapel Hill, NC, 2000a, ACHNE.

Association of Community Health Nursing Educators: *Essentials of baccalaureate nursing education for entry level community health nursing practice,* Chapel Hill, NC, 2000b, ACHNE.

Bear M, Bowers C: Using a nursing framework to measure client satisfaction at a nurse managed clinic, *Public Health Nurs* 15(1):50, 1998.

Bellin E, Dubler NN: The quality improvement–research divide and the need for external oversight, *Am J Public Health* 91(9):1512, 2001.

Berwick DM: Continuous improvement as an ideal in healthcare, *N Engl J Med* 320:52, 1989.

Bodenheimer T: The American health care system: the movement for improved quality in health care, *N Engl J Med* 340(6):488-492, 1999.

Bushy A: Empowering initiatives to improve a community's health status, *J Nurs Care Qual* 11(4):32, 1997.

Cary AH: Data drives policy: the case for certification research, *Pol Polit Nurs Pract* 1(3):165-171, 2000.

Centers for Disease Control and Prevention: *Planned approach to community health: guide for local coordinators,* Atlanta, Ga, 1995, CDC, National Center for Chronic Disease Prevention and Health Promotion.

Chassin MR, Galvin RW: The urgent need to improve health care quality, *JAMA* 280:1000, 1998.

Clark J et al: New methods of documenting health visiting practice, *Community Practitioner* 74(3):108, 2001.

Council of Home Health Agencies, Community Health Services: *Accreditation of home health agencies and community nursing services: criteria and guide for preparing reports,* New York, 1986, National League for Nursing.

Davis ER: *Total quality management for homecare,* Gaithersburg, Md, 1994, Aspen.

Deming WE: *Out of the crisis,* Cambridge, Mass, 1986, Massachusetts Institute of Technology, Center for Advanced Engineering Study.

Donabedian A: *Exploration in quality assessment and monitoring,* vol 2, Ann Arbor, Mich, 1981, Health Administration Press.

Donabedian A: *Explorations in quality assessment and monitoring,* vol 3, Ann Arbor, Mich, 1985, Health Administration Press.

Donabedian A: The seven pillars of quality, *Arch Pathol Lab Med* 114:1115, 1990.

Durch JS, Bailey LA, Stoto MA, editors: *Improving health in the community: a role for performance monitoring,* Washington, DC, 1997, National Academy Press.

Gragnola CM, Stone E: Considering the future workforce regulation, San Francisco, 1997, Pew Health Profession Commission.

Greenberg LG, Lezzoni LI: Quality. In Calkins D, Fernandopulle RJ, Marino BS, editors: *Health care policy,* Cambridge, Mass, 1995, Blackwell Science.

Halverson PK, Kaluzny AD, McLaughlin CP: *Managed care and public health,* Gaithersburg, Md, 1998, Aspen.

Institute of Medicine: *Crossing the quality chasm,* Washington, DC, 2001, National Academy Press.

Joint Council Committee on Quality in Public Health: *Promoting quality care for communities: the role of health departments in an era of managed care,* Washington, DC, 1996, National Association of City and County Health Officials.

Jonas S: Measurement and control of the quality of health care. In Kovner AR, editor: *Health care delivery in the United States,* New York, 2002, Springer.

Jost TS: Oversight of the quality of medical care: regulation, management or the market? *Arizona Law Rev* 37:825, 1995.

Juran JM: *Juran's quality handbook,* New York, 1998, McGraw-Hill.

Kamajian MF et al: Credentialing and privileging of advanced practice nurses, *AACN Clin Iss* 10(3):316, 1999.

Kessner DM, Kalk CE: Assessing health quality—the case for tracers, *N Engl J Med* 288:189, 1973.

Kinney ED, Freedman JA, Cook CA: Quality improvement in community-based, long-term care: theory and reality, *Am J Law Med* 20(1-2):59, 1994.

Kovner A, Jonas S, editors: *Jonas and Kovner's health care delivery in the United States,* New York, 1998, Springer.

Lasker RD et al: *Medicine and public health: the power of collaboration,* New York, 1997, New York Academy of Medicine.

Leatherman S, McCarthy D: *Quality of health care in the United States: a chartbook,* New York, 2002, Commonwealth Fund.

Lia-Hoagberg B, Schaffer M, Strohschein S: Public health nursing practice guidelines: an evaluation of dissemination and use, *Public Health Nurs* 16(6):397, 1999.

Lindsey DL, Henly SJ, Tyree EA: Outcomes in an academic nursing center: client satisfaction with student services, *J Nurs Care Qual* 11(5):30, 1997.

Maibusch RM: Evolution of quality assurance for nursing in hospitals. In Schroder PS, Maibusch RM, editors: *Nursing quality assurance,* Rockville, Md, 1984, Aspen.

Martin KS, Norris J: The Omaha System: a model for describing practice, *Holist Nurs Pract* 11(1):75, 1996.

Mays GP et al: CQI in public health organizations. In McLaughlin CP, Kaluzny AD, editors: *Continuous quality improvement in healthcare: theory, implementation and applications,* Gaithersburg, Md, 1999, Aspen.

McLaughlin CP, Kaluzny AD: Defining quality improvement: past, present and future. In McLaughlin CP, Kaluzny AD, editors: *Continuous quality improvement in healthcare: theory, implementation and applications,* Gaithersburg, Md, 1999, Aspen.

Minnesota Department of Health, Division of Community Health Services: *Public health interventions: applications for public health nursing practice,* Public Health Nursing Section, St Paul, March 2001.

National Association of City and County Health Officials: *APEXPH in practice,* Washington, DC, 1995, NACCHO.

National Association for Healthcare Quality: *Risk management: NAHQ guide to quality management,* Skokie, Ill, 1993, NAHQ Press.

National Association of Home Care: Draft uniform data set for home care and hospice, *Caring* 12(6):10, 1994.

National Guideline Clearinghouse: *Fact sheet,* AHRQ publication No. 00-0047, Rockville, Md, 2000, Agency for Healthcare Research and Quality.

O'Brien-Pallas LL et al: Evaluation of a client care delivery model, part 1: variability in nursing utilization in community home nursing, *Nurs Econ* 19(6):267, 2001.

O'Brien-Pallas LL et al: Evaluation of a client care delivery model, part 2: variability in nursing utilization in community home nursing, *Nurs Econ* 20(1):13, 2002.

Phaneuf M: A nursing audit method, *Nurs Outlook* 5:42, 1965.

Rowell PA: Beyond the acute care setting: community-based nonacute care nursing-sensitive indicators, *Outcomes Manag Nurs Pract* 5(1):24, 2001.

Smith BA: A TQM model for home care coordination and provider partnering, *Caring* 12(9):54, 1993.

Sprague L: Quality in the making, *Am J Med* 111(5):422, 2001.

Stevens-Barnum B, Kerfoot K: *The nurse as executive,* Gaithersburg, Md, 1995, Aspen.

Stricklin MLV: Home care consumers speak out on quality, *Home Healthcare Nurse* 11(6):10, 1995.

Strohschein S, Schaffer M, Lia-Hoagberg B: Evidenced-based guidelines for public health nursing practice, *Nurs Outlook* 47(2):84, 1999.

U.S. Department of Health and Human Services: *Healthy People in healthy communities: a community planning guide using Healthy People 2010,* Washington, DC, 2000a, U.S. Government Printing Office.

U.S. Department of Health and Human Services: *Healthy people 2010: understanding and improving health,* ed 2, Washington, DC, 2000b, U.S. Government Printing Office.

U.S. Preventive Services Task Force: *Guide to clinical preventive services,* Baltimore, 2000, Williams & Wilkins.

Verhey M: Quality management in home care: models for today's practice, *Home Care Provid* 1(4):180, 1996.

Weiss M: The quality evolution in managed care organizations: shifting the focus to community health, *J Nurs Care Qual* 11(4):27, 1997.

Westra BL et al: Development of the home care client satisfaction instrument, *Public Health Nurs* 12:393, 1995.

Wright K et al: Competency development in public health leadership, *Am J Public Health* 90(8):1202-1207, 2000.

Young G: The privatization of quality assurance in health care. In Halverson PK, Kaluzny AD, McLaughlin CP: *Managed care and public health,* Gaithersburg, Md, 1998, Aspen.

# Chapter 23

# Group Approaches to Practice

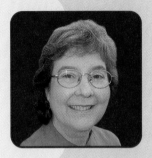

**Peggye Guess Lassiter, R.N., M.S.N.**

Peggye Guess Lassiter is currently an adjunct assistant professor at Howard University's Division of Nursing, Washington, D.C. Her career has centered on nursing with community clients and the teaching of community health nursing. Her areas of subspecialization include group work with families and communities, rural nursing, and community health assessment, intervention, and evaluation. From 1996 through 1999 she was project coordinator for the Mississippi Delta Project: Education and Preparation of Nurses, a project initiative awarded to Howard University through the Minority Health Professions Foundation and the Agency for Toxic Substances and Disease Registry. Through this environmental health nursing initiative, a modular curriculum, *Environmental Health and Nursing: The Mississippi Delta Project* (Powell, 1999), was published and distributed to faculty and students throughout the southeastern United States.

## Objectives

After reading this chapter, the student should be able to do the following:

1. Describe member interaction and group purpose as the major elements of a group
2. Analyze the effect of cohesion on group effectiveness
3. Identify the influence of group norms on group members
4. Explain the usefulness of groups in promoting individual health
5. Evaluate nursing behaviors that assist groups in promoting health for individuals
6. Identify the groups that constitute a community and illustrate links between them
7. Describe the role of the nurse working with established groups toward community health goals

---

Working with groups is an important community nursing skill. Groups are an effective and powerful way to initiate and implement changes for individuals, families, organizations, and the community. People naturally form groups in the home setting, and groups in the community dramatically influence the community's health. Nurses who work with groups understand group concepts and group process. Groups form for various reasons. They may form for a clearly stated purpose or goal, or they may form naturally as shared values, interests, activities, or personal characteristics attract individuals to each other.

Community groups represent the collective interests, needs, and values of individuals; they provide a link between the individual and the larger social system. Individual attitudes are developed in families and friendships. Throughout life, membership in other groups influences thoughts, choices, behaviors, and values as people socialize and interact. Through groups, people may express personal views and relate them to the views of others. Groups serve as communication networks and may be viewed as an organization of community parts.

Groups can bring about changes to improve the health and well-being of individuals and communities. Some individual changes for health are difficult or impossible to achieve without group support and encouragement.

All nurses have group experience. In daily practice, nurses routinely plan and use health-focused action with clients, other nurses, and other health care workers. Nurses often participate in groups in which they observe their own responses to members and leaders. Such study and experience aid nurses in applying group concepts in a variety of settings.

As discussed in Chapter 13, groups can be used to communicate health information in a cost-effective way to a number of clients who meet together, rather than having to repeat the information several times to individuals. During a time of decreasing resources, groups are an increasingly popular format for nursing intervention.

Understanding the community and assessing its health begin by identifying groups and their goals, member characteristics, and their place in the community structure. Through community groups, nurses help people identify priority health needs and capabilities and make valuable community changes.

## Key Terms

cohesion, p. 542
communication structure, p. 546
conflict, p. 550
established groups, p. 548
formal groups, p. 554
group, p. 541
group culture, p. 544

group purpose, p. 541
group structure, p. 546
informal groups, p. 554
leadership, p. 545
maintenance functions, p. 542
maintenance norms, p. 544
member interaction, p. 541

norms, p. 544
reality norms, p. 544
role structure, p. 546
selected membership groups, p. 548
task function, p. 542
task norm, p. 544
*See Glossary for definitions*

## Chapter Outline

Group Concepts
*Definitions*
*Group Purpose*
*Cohesion*
*Norms*
*Leadership*
*Group Structure*

Promoting the Health of Individuals Through Group Work
*Choosing Groups for Health Change*
*Beginning Interactions*
*Conflict*
*Strategies for Change*
*Evaluation of Group Progress*

*Building Effective Work Teams*
Community Groups and Their Contribution to Community Life
Working With Groups Toward Community Health Goals

# GROUP CONCEPTS

The basic group concepts described in this section may be used in nursing practice to identify community groups and their contributions to community life and to assist groups in working toward community and individual health goals.

## Definitions

A **group** is a collection of interacting individuals who have a common purpose or common purposes. Each member influences and is in turn influenced by every other member to some extent. Key elements in this definition of group are **member interaction** and **group purpose.** Families are a unique and familiar example of a community group. Family purposes are numerous, including providing psychological support and socialization for their members. Usually, families share kinship bonds, living space, and economic resources. Interactions are diverse and frequent.

A second example is groups formed in response to particular community needs, problems, or opportunities. For example, in one community, residents banded together to form a neighborhood association to protect their health and welfare. This neighborhood of upper-middle-class homes was located in an unincorporated area. For 3 years the residents were threatened with multiple environmental hazards, including a forest fire (fire hydrants had been overlooked in developing part of the area), establishment of a small airport near the homes, and construction of an interstate highway adjacent to the homes. To protect their interests, residents formed a neighborhood association and elected officers to represent their interests in a constructive manner.

Other groups in the community occur spontaneously because of mutual attraction between individuals and obvious and keenly felt personal needs. Young and single adults sharing similar desires for socialization and recreation may form loosely structured groups. Through parties and other social meetings, the young adults establish new ways of behaving and relating. They select partners, test ideas and attitudes, and establish their identity within a group of people with similar developmental needs. Their unstated purpose is to test and become familiar with adult roles.

A fourth example is health-promoting groups, which are formed as people meet in the community and health care settings and discover common challenges to their physical and emotional well-being. The purposes of health-promoting groups are to improve members' health and to deal with specific threats to health. Chapters of Alcoholics Anonymous, Parents without Partners, and La Leche League illustrate health-promoting groups. Members both give and receive personal support and participate in group problem solving and education. These groups may be one of two types: established groups or selected membership groups. Both types of groups are discussed later in this chapter.

> ### NURSING TIP
>
> When the purpose for a group is clearly stated and agreed on, the group becomes increasingly attractive to members.

How do purpose and interaction vary in these four examples? Some groups, such as the neighborhood association and La Leche League, have an obvious purpose that can be easily stated by members. For families, social groupings, and many spontaneously formed groups, the purposes are unstated. However, the purpose can be determined by studying their activities as a group over time. Purpose and member interaction are important components of all groups.

## Group Purpose

When the need for a particular health change is identified and group work is selected as the most effective way to make it happen, a clear statement and presentation of the proposed group's purpose are essential. A clear purpose helps in establishing criteria for member selection.

A clear statement of purpose proved valuable in forming a new group in one city's housing development. The local department of social services had received numerous reports of child abuse and neglect. Routine home visits for well-child care documented high stress between parents and their offspring, and some parents requested guidance from the nurse in child discipline. The nurse proposed that a parent group address this community need. Nurses selected the following purpose for the group: dealing with kids for child and parent satisfaction. The purpose indicated both the process (to help parents deal with children) and the desired outcome (satisfaction for parents and children). As potential members were approached, this statement of purpose for the group helped the individuals decide whether they wanted to join.

When a group makes a public appeal for members and accepts everyone who wants to join, the membership is self-selected on the basis of the group's stated purpose. In this type of recruitment, publicity must reach those in need of particular health changes. Prospective members often want to discuss the purpose with leaders or clarify questions concerning the purpose at the first group meeting. Their commitment to group health is partly based on

individual goals and how well the group goal satisfies personal objectives.

## Cohesion

**Cohesion** is the attraction between individual members and between each member and the group. Individuals in a highly cohesive group identify themselves as a unit, work toward common goals, endure frustration for the sake of the group, and defend the group against outside criticism. Attraction increases when members feel accepted and liked by others, see similar qualities in one another, and share similar attitudes and values (Figure 23-1). Group effectiveness also improves as members work together toward group goals while still satisfying the needs of individual members (Brandler, 1999).

Members' traits that increase group cohesion and productivity include the following:

- Compatible personal and group goals
- Attraction to group goals
- Attraction to other selected members
- Appropriate mix of leading and following skills
- Good problem-solving skills

A **task function** is anything a member does that deliberately contributes to the group's purpose. Members with task-directed abilities become more attractive to the group. These traits include strong problem-solving skills, access to material resources, and skills in directing. Of equal importance are abilities to affirm and support individuals in the group. These functions are called **maintenance functions** because they help other members stay with the group and feel accepted. The ability to help people resolve conflicts and ensure social and environmental comfort is also a maintenance function. Both task and maintenance func-

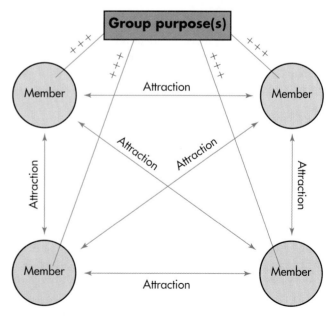

**Figure 23-1** Cohesion is the measure of attraction between members, and of member attraction to group purpose(s).

tions are necessary for group progress. Naturally, those members who supply such group requirements are attractive, and an abundance of such traits within the membership tends to increase group cohesion.

Other group members' traits may decrease cohesion and productivity. These include the following:

- Conflicts between personal and group goals
- Lack of interest in group goals and activities
- Poor problem-solving and communication abilities
- Lack of both leadership and supporter skills
- Disagreement about types of leadership
- Aversion to other members
- Behaviors and attributes that are poorly understood by others

Usually, the more alike group members are, the stronger a group's attraction, whereas differences tend to decrease attractiveness. Members' perceptions of differences can create marked competition and jealousy. At the same time, personal differences can increase group cohesion if they support complementary functioning or provide contrasting viewpoints necessary for decision making. This only reinforces the idea that cohesion factors are complex; many factors influence member attraction to each other and to the group's goal. In either case, group productivity and member satisfaction are positively affected by high group cohesion. Two examples illustrate factors that influence group cohesion.

A nurse initiated, and provided beginning leadership for, a group of clients who had been treated for burns. Ten residents, all from one town, had been discharged after a month in the local burn unit. The stated purpose for the group was to assist members in the difficult transition from hospital to home. Each individual had been treated for extensive burns in an intensive care treatment center; each had relied heavily on health workers for physical, social, and emotional rehabilitation; and each had faced the challenge of resuming work and family roles. Individuals shared some similar experiences and hopes for the future

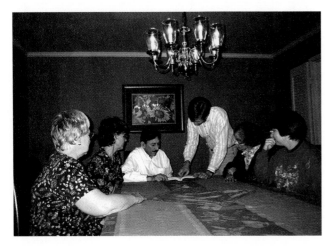

Cohesive community groups can support and help one another.

but varied in the amount of trauma and stress experienced. They also differed widely in psychological readiness for return to ordinary daily routines. One woman in the group was able to return quickly to her job as cashier in a large supermarket. The strength of her determination to overcome public reaction to her scars, coupled with an ability to "use the right words" and an empathy for others, distinguished her from others in the group. These differences proved attractive to other members, inspiring them to work toward a return to their own roles in life. These members saw her differences as attainable.

The cohesion for this group was provided by the members' attraction to the common purpose of returning to successful life patterns and managing relationships with others. Each member also believed that interaction with others with similar burn experiences could help them reach that goal. This example shows that certain member experiences, such as crises or traumas, may help individuals identify with each other and may increase member attraction.

Being different from the general population and similar to the other group members is, for some, a compelling force for membership in the group. Others are repelled by the group because they do not want to be identified by an aversive characteristic, such as disfigurement. Empathy for another's pain, learned only through mutual experience, may provide each individual with a required perspective for problem solving or affirming another's view. The nurse in this example helped members use common experiences and learn from their differences. The group was effective.

Differences created tension in one self-help group for victims of spouse abuse; in this group, nurses met a severe challenge stemming from the differences they presented as nonvictims. The nurses had been invited by professional staff to assist the group in its process toward the goal of "learning to manage: safety, health, and independence." Victim members of the group believed that the nurses could not truly understand the intensely personal and devastating injury each had experienced and told the nurses so. They isolated the nurses from membership but tolerated their presence. Attraction of the group diminished, and attendance at meetings fell. Discussion of superficial issues occupied group time as the victim members avoided topics of member safety and violence in general. Differences between the nurses and victims hampered group cohesion; the group was not effectively addressing its goal, and members felt isolated.

In response to this deterioration, the nurses encouraged all members to describe experiences seen as threatening to self-respect in their family and work roles. The nurses revealed some of their own struggles for responsible self-direction and control. Revealing their vulnerability made the nurses more attractive to the group. The members were able to accept the nurses, whom they now saw as more similar to themselves. They promptly refocused their efforts on the purpose of the group.

Group members supported one another to assert individual rights for safety, to locate employment, to make necessary living arrangements for independence from the abuser, and to identify needs for personal interactional changes. The clear purpose of maintaining member safety combined with the new, broader common goal of asserting one's self-respect, contributed to successful group work.

Members' attraction to the group also depends on the nature of the group. Factors include the group programs, size, type of organization, and position in the community. When individuals perceive goals clearly and group activities are believed to be effective, attraction to the group is increased.

The concept of cohesion helps to explain group productivity. Some cohesion is necessary for people to remain with a group and accomplish the set goals. Attractiveness positively influences members' motivation and commitment to work on the group task. Cohesion for groups may be increased as members better understand the experiences of others and are able to identify common ideas and reactions to various issues. Nurses facilitate this process by pointing out similarities, contrasting supportive differences, or helping members redefine differences in ways that make those dissimilarities compatible.

## Norms

**Norms** are standards that guide, control, and regulate individuals and communities. Group norms set the standards for group members' behaviors, attitudes, and perceptions. Group norms suggest what a group sees as important, what it accepts, objects to, or is indifferent about. This commonly held view of what ought to be provides motivation for the members to use the group for their mutual benefit (Northen and Kurland, 2001). All groups have norms and mechanisms whereby conformity is accomplished. Group norms serve three functions:

1. They ensure movement toward the group's purpose or tasks.
2. They maintain the group through various supports to members.
3. They influence members' perceptions and interpretations of reality.

Even though certain norms keep the group focused on its task, a certain amount of diversion is permitted as long as members respect central goals and feel committed to return to them. This commitment to return to the central goals is the **task norm;** its strength determines the group's keeping to its work.

**Maintenance norms** create group pressures to affirm members and maintain their comfort. Individuals in groups seem most productive and at ease when psychological and social well-being is nurtured. Maintenance behaviors include identifying the social and psychological tensions of members and taking steps to support those members at high-stress times. Health supportive maintenance norms may direct the group's attention to conditions such as temperature, space, and seating to ensure the physical comfort of the group during meeting times. This attention to arrangements may include meeting in places

that are easily accessible and comfortable to the participants, providing refreshments, and scheduling meetings at convenient times.

A third and equally important function of group norms relates to members' perceptions of reality. Daily behavior is largely based on the way each aspect of life is understood. Through socialization, individuals learn how to gather information, assign meaning, and react to situations in a way that satisfies needs. Decision-making and action-taking processes are influenced by the meanings ascribed by a group's **reality norms.** Individuals look to others to reinforce or to challenge and correct their ideas of what is real. Groups serve to examine the life situations confronting individuals. As individuals gather information, attempt to understand that information, make decisions, and consider the facts and their implications, they can take responsible action, not only in relation to themselves and their group but also for the community. Group (task, maintenance, and reality) norms combine to form a **group culture.** Although working with a group does not mean dictating its norms, the nurse can support helpful rules, attitudes, and behaviors. Norms form when these rules, attitudes, and behaviors become part of the life of the group, independent of the nurse.

Figure 23-2 shows that reality norms influence each member to see relevant situations in the same way the

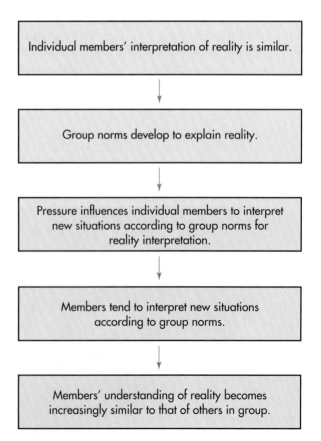

**Figure 23-2** Influence of group reality norms on individual members.

other members see them. They may feel strong normative pressures to support members who are considering change. Benne (1976), describing how small groups contribute to planned changes, points out that people develop their values by internalizing their particular small groups' norms, especially their families' norms. "Changes in value orientations of individuals may be accomplished by seeking and finding significant membership in a small group with norms that are different in some respects from the normative orientation these individuals bring to a group" (Benne, 1976, p. 76).

To illustrate, suppose a group of individuals with diabetes defines an uncontrolled diet as harmful; members may try to influence one another to maintain diet control. The role of the nurse in this group is to provide accurate information about diet and the disease process, including cause and effect between food intake and disease. The nurse also continually displays a belief that health through diet control is attainable and desirable.

When members of any group have similar backgrounds, their scope of knowledge may be limited. For example, female members in a spouse abuse group may believe that men are exploitive and harmful on the basis of common childhood and marriage experiences. Such a stereotypical view of men could be reinforced by similar perceptions in other members; this might lead to continuing anger, fear of interactions with men, and a hostile or helpless approach to family affairs. Nurses or group members who have known men in loving, helpful, and collaborative ways can describe their different and positive perceptions of men, thereby adding information and challenging beliefs. Thus the group functions to influence members' perceptions and interpretations of reality. The health and condition of the individual improves as members' perceptions of reality become based on a full range of data and as cause-and-effect factors are understood. Nurses bring an important perspective to groups in which similar backgrounds limit the understanding and interpretation of personal concerns.

## Leadership

**Leadership** is a complex concept. It consists of behaviors that guide or direct members and determine and influence group action. Positive leadership defines or negotiates the group's purpose, selects and helps implement tasks that accomplish the purpose, maintains an environment that affirms and supports members, and balances efforts between task and maintenance. An effective leader attends to member communications and interactions as they unfold in the here and now. Attention to both spoken words and body language provides leaders and members continuous feedback, alerting members to changing group needs and encouraging them to take responsibility and pride in their own involvement.

Leadership is essential for effective groups. Leading may be concentrated in one or a few persons, or it may be shared by many. Generally, shared leadership increases

productivity, cohesion, and satisfying interactions among members.

After initiating or establishing a group, nurses may facilitate leadership within and among members, frequently relinquishing central control and encouraging members to determine the ultimate leadership pattern for their group. Of course, nurses differ widely in their leadership style preferences. In some settings and circumstances, a single authority seems necessary (e.g., when members have limited skills or limited time, or when groups claim discomfort with shared responsibility for leading). A leadership style that shares leading functions with other group members is effective when there are many alternatives and issues of values and ethics are involved in the group's action

Experiences with committees, work teams, and client groups promote self-confidence and increase appreciation of the leading capabilities of others. Practice teaches that getting selected tasks done is only one group outcome. A second, equally valuable result is watching members become more competent and able to share more responsibility. Shared leadership limits power seekers and supports group wholeness, flexibility, and freedom.

Leadership behaviors and definitions are listed in Box 23-1. Sources of leader influence are knowledge, ability,

---

**BOX 23-1   Examples of Leadership Behaviors**

- **Advising:** Introducing direction on the basis of knowledgeable opinion
- **Analyzing:** Reviewing what has occurred as encouragement to examine behavior and its meaning
- **Clarifying:** Checking out meanings of interaction and communication through questions and restatement
- **Confronting:** Presenting behavior and its effects to the individual and group to challenge existing perceptions
- **Evaluating:** Analyzing the effect or outcome of action or the worth of an idea according to some standard
- **Initiating:** Introducing topics, beginning work, or changing the focus of a group
- **Questioning:** Bringing about analysis of a view or views by questions that support examination
- **Reflecting behavior:** Giving feedback on how behavior appears to others
- **Reflecting feelings:** Naming the feelings that may be behind what is said or done
- **Suggesting:** Proposing or bringing an idea to a group
- **Summarizing:** Restating discussion or group action in brief form, highlighting important points
- **Supporting:** Giving the kind of emotionally comforting feedback that helps a person or group continue ongoing actions

access to needed resources, personal attractiveness, status or position in the community or organization, and ability to control sanctions for others.

Leadership is typically described as patriarchal, paternal, or democratic; each of these styles has a particular effect on members' interaction, satisfaction, and productivity. Groups may reflect one or a combination of styles.

When one person has the final authority for group direction and movement, the leadership style is patriarchal or paternal. Patriarchal leadership may control members through rewards and threats, often keeping them in the dark about the goals and rationale behind prescribed actions. Paternal leadership wins the respect and dependence of its followers by parent-like devotion to members' needs. The leader controls group movement and progress through interpersonal power. Patriarchal and paternal styles of leadership are authoritarian. These styles are effective for groups such as a disaster team, in which the immediate task accomplishment or high productivity is the goal. Group morale and cohesiveness are typically low under authoritarian styles of leadership, and members may fail to learn how to function independently. In addition, issues of authority and control may disrupt productivity if the group members challenge the power of the leader.

Paternal leadership was effective in the following situation. Mary Jones, a nurse, called her neighbors together to alert them to the threat of drug traffic in the neighborhood. The residents agreed with Mary that several recent drug-related arrests in the area signaled a need for community concern. No one knew what to do, but all believed that quick action was necessary. Mary had experience in organizing people, knew of local resources, and thought that information, education, and residents' collaboration with police could substantially control the local drug traffic problem. She organized the neighborhood group, assigned and monitored their tasks, and praised them as they made progress toward the goal of keeping the area free of drug sales.

Democratic leadership is cooperative in nature and promotes and supports members' involvement in all aspects of decision making and planning. Members influence each other as they explore goals, plan steps toward the goals, implement those steps, and evaluate progress.

A more common experience for nurses is illustrated in the following example. A committee of nurses for a small community health organization met weekly to improve nursing services. Tom initiated a revision of the written standards. Several members of the group felt threatened by Tom's idea. They feared that their daily work would change and that a resulting evaluation using new standards would find them inferior or necessitate that they alter familiar procedures. Jane supported updating the standards. She also recognized the necessity of continuing support and affirmation of each nurse's worth on the committee. While Tom pushed the committee toward revising the standards, she often interrupted to ask members to respond and to make suggestions, noting to the group the

---

> ### BOX 23-2   Levels of Prevention Related to Working With Groups
>
> **PRIMARY PREVENTION**
> Teach residents ways to avoid getting involved in the use of illegal drugs.
>
> **SECONDARY PREVENTION**
> Screen for the early signs of drug use.
>
> **TERTIARY PREVENTION**
> Mobilize resources to intervene in drug use in the community. Refer any identified clients to treatment programs.

excellent contributions that were made. Sara provided a touch of humor whenever group tension became high. Amber provided a critical, questioning support to the decision-making process and encouraged the members to evaluate each step. In these and other ways, group members shared leadership tasks. Some served predominantly to push the group toward its objective, whereas others facilitated that movement by maintaining member involvement through support. For this group, the chairperson served as convener but did not dominate. The members were able to write and implement an audit for new nursing standards in a democratic leadership style. Levels of prevention as they relate to groups are shown in Box 23-2.

## Group Structure

Structure describes the particular arrangement of group parts as they combine to make up the group as a whole. A **communication structure** identifies message pathways and member participation in sending and receiving messages. People who are active in receiving and sending messages and who serve as channels for messages are important in the structure. These "central" individuals influence the group because of their access to and interpretive control over communication flow. Communication and role structures are interrelated.

**Role structure** describes the expected behaviors of members in relation to each other as the group interacts. The role assumed by each member serves a purpose in the life of that group. Examples of roles are leader, follower, task specialist, maintenance specialist, evaluator, peacemaker, and gatekeeper (Box 23-3). Members' roles in the group may be described by their predominant actions. Identification of communication patterns helps to determine roles because people occupying particular roles characteristically use certain kinds of communication.

**Group structure** emerges from various member influences, including the members' understanding and support of the group purpose. Nurses assess the group structure as it relates to goal accomplishment. Many groups also consider their own structure, assess its usefulness in relation to member comfort and productivity, and then plan for a different division of tasks that is agreeable to the whole.

In the earlier example of nurses working on standards of nursing service, Tom served as task specialist, Jane as maintenance specialist, and Amber as evaluator. They consistently occupied particular roles and were expected by others to maintain their behavior to serve the group purposes.

A person occupying a gatekeeper's role controls outsiders' access to the group. Gatekeepers either facilitate or block communication between outsiders and group members. Identification of those in gatekeeper roles is crucial when established groups are used for community health. The gatekeeper usually confronts the nurse after beginning contacts are attempted. An invitation to communicate further with group members is extended only after the nurse and gatekeeper determine mutual benefits and possible risks from continued contact between the nurse and the group.

## PROMOTING THE HEALTH OF INDIVIDUALS THROUGH GROUP WORK

Health behavior is influenced greatly by the groups to which people belong. Individuals live within a social structure of significant others such as family members, friends, co-workers, and acquaintances. The patterns and directions of everyday activities are learned in a family, and these are later reinforced or challenged by new groups. These groups constitute the context in which values, beliefs, and attitudes are formed; individuals usually consider the responses of others in all types of decisions regarding personal welfare.

The following example illustrates the effects of a person's social network on health behavior. Mary Berton was worried about a lump she had recently discovered in her breast. She first asked her husband, Lew, to confirm its presence, which he did. He agreed that she should arrange for a diagnostic evaluation, and an appointment was arranged. Mary talked with Lew about the possible consequences of malignancy, and she noted Lew's concern for her safety. She was fearful of radical surgery and its effects on her relationship with Lew, but she did not discuss that with him. Mary telephoned two close friends from her workplace and asked them to meet her for coffee. Although they thought it was premature to fret about the lump being malignant, they discussed all they knew about treatment for breast cancer, including the trials, defeats, and successes of three mutual friends who had had surgery for breast cancer. Each of the friends had reacted differently to her own situation, and Mary's friends retold familiar details. The retelling seemed important to understanding the current situation and helped Mary sort out her feelings. The outcome for Mary of retelling was her improved understanding of the situation and of her own response to it. She was assisted in facing the reality of risk, in recognizing the need to follow through with diagnostic procedures, in selecting able medical sources, and in managing her emotional stress.

Mary's friends' and her husband's responses to her situation influenced her assessment, decision making, and subsequent behavior. The work done by Mary and her social network in response to her health need was important. It illustrates a common mechanism among individuals and the groups to which they belong. The groups described in this example are Mary's family group, which includes Mary and Lew, and Mary's friendship group, of which those who met for coffee are a subset.

Groups who will support an individual's health changes are unavailable to some people because of their social or emotional isolation. Isolated individuals may have low self-esteem, be mentally ill, or occupy positions of low status in their family or community. They may be disadvantaged, gifted, or deviant, or they may simply live in a rural area or be engaged in solitary work. These individuals benefit greatly from newly organized groups established for specific purposes.

Although social support is basic to health, the absence of negative social interactions is of equal importance to well-being. Groups sometimes oppose health. Friends who use addictive drugs are a clear example of such a group. It may be impossible for an individual to quit drug use while associating with such friends. To effect a lasting behavior change, an addicted individual needs support and new friends who do not abuse drugs. In such circumstances the individual must leave his or her group of associates, even if he or she must move from the neighborhood where they gather. Through participation with others, meaning is confirmed, confounded, contradicted, or compromised. This is how social reality is created. Within groups, people believe or are encouraged to believe in their created, shared realities (Goldberg and Middleman, 1997).

As nurses increase their knowledge of group concepts, develop skills in working with varied groups, and learn to employ the power in groups for individual changes, they will become available, visible, and sought for group work.

## Choosing Groups for Health Change

Nurses frequently use groups to help individuals within a community after studying the overall needs of the community and its people. Such a study is based on client contacts, expressed concerns from various community spokespersons, health statistics for the area, available health resources, and the community's general well-being. These data point to the community's strengths and critical needs. Just as other nursing interventions are based on the assessment of needs and knowledge of effective treatment, group formation is determined by the assessment of priority community needs for individual health change.

At times nurses work with existing groups, and at other times they form new groups. Initiation of change and recruitment of a nurse may come not just from the nurse but from individuals, the affected groups, or a related organization. A decision about whether to work in established groups or to begin new ones is based on the clients' needs, the purpose of existing groups, and the membership ties in existing groups.

### Established Groups

There are advantages to using **established groups** for individual health change. Membership ties already exist, and the structure already in place can be used. It is not necessary to find new members because compatible individuals already form a working group. Established groups usually have operating methods that have already proved successful; an approach for a new goal is built on this history. Members are aware of each other's strengths, limitations, and preferred styles of interaction. Members' comfort levels, stemming from their experience together, facilitate their focus on the new goal.

Established groups have a strong potential for influencing members. Ties between members have been enhanced through successful group endeavors. Their bonds are usually multidimensional because of the length of time they have spent together. Such rich ties support group change efforts for individuals' health.

Before deciding to work with particular established groups, the nurse must judge whether introducing a new focus is compatible with existing group purposes. In some cases, individual health goals will enhance existing group purposes, and the nurse is an important resource for bringing information for health, behavior, and group process.

How can the nurse enter existing groups and direct their attention to individual health needs? One nurse employed by an industrial firm noted the harmful effect of managerial stress on several individuals. They had elevated blood pressure, stomach pain, and emotional tension. The nurse learned that the employees with stress were all members of a jogging team that met weekly for conversation in addition to regular workouts. The other joggers readily accepted the offer to work together on individual stress management, recognizing that their fellow members were facing high-stress circumstances and the accompanying danger to health. High-level health had been a value shared by all team members, but although jogging was seen as an enjoyable and health-promoting activity, they had never talked about a shared purpose for improved health. In this circumstance the nurse saw a need for stress reduction, thought that the individuals at risk could achieve stress reduction if supported through a group process from valued friends, and proposed that a new purpose be added to the jogging team's activities.

### Selected Membership Groups

In some situations, using existing groups is undesirable or impossible. The nurse then begins a selection process and brings a new group into existence. Nurses are familiar with group work in which members are selected because of their health. For instance, individuals with diabetes are brought together to consider diet management and physical care and to share in problem-solving remedies; community residents are brought together for social support and rehabilitation after treatment for mental illness; or isolated older adults are brought together for socialization and hot meals.

Members' attributes are an important consideration in composing a new group. Members are attracted to others from similar backgrounds, with similar experiences, and with common interests and abilities. It is important to select members so that common ties or interests balance out dissimilar traits.

> **WHAT DO YOU THINK?**
> Will a group of similar individuals work together better than a group of dissimilar individuals? List similarities among individuals that increase their attraction to each other.

Membership ties are influential; even in newly formed groups, people bring emotional and social ties from previous and parallel group memberships. People are influenced by the interaction in the newly formed group and by their alliance with other important groups to which they belong. Memory serves to keep the norms and role expectations from one group present as a person moves from one group to another. Individual behavior is then influenced not only by the membership, purpose, attraction, norms, leadership, and structure of the group, but also by those processes remembered from other valued group memberships. Consideration of the multiple influences on members helps to determine an appropriate grouping for each situation and its particular dimensions.

When the nurse is able to arrange it, the membership for **selected membership groups** should contain one or more individuals with expressive and problem-solving skills and others who are comfortable in supportive roles. Many people demonstrate abilities in task and maintenance functions, and others have undeveloped potential for such functions. Support and training for group effectiveness within the unit build cohesion. As members perform increasingly valuable functions for the group, they become more attracted to it and more attractive to others.

The size of the group influences effectiveness; generally, a good number for group work focused on individual health changes is 8 to 12 people. Groups of up to 25 members may be effective when their focus is on community needs, such as the group discussed previously that formed a neighborhood association. Large groups often divide and assign tasks to the smaller subgroups, with the original large groups meeting less frequently for reporting and evaluation.

Setting member criteria can facilitate recruitment and selection of the most appropriate members for any group. The criteria usually suggest a mixture of member traits, allowing for balance for the processes of decision making and growth.

## Beginning Interactions

Once a group forms, work begins on the stated purpose. Early meetings require further clarification of both individual and group goals. Members with varying degrees of openness present themselves and their backgrounds. They begin to interact with each other by seeking and giving information about themselves and their circumstances and simultaneously demonstrating their capabilities in problem solving and group participation. The nurse assists by supporting ideas and feelings, inviting participation, giving information, seeking and providing clarification, and suggesting structure. Subsequent steps are then planned not only according to the nurse's skill and preference but also according to the group composition and the skills brought by members.

Nurses in the beginning groups should place the priority on helping members interact with a degree of satisfaction. This requires close attention to maintenance tasks of attending, eliciting information, clarifying, and recognizing contributions of members. Attending includes simple responses to people, such as listening carefully to their speech and noting their mood, dress, and informal conversation as they enter the meeting. Attending behavior communicates recognition and acceptance of the person and his or her presentations to the group.

A beginning format that focuses on whatever brought each member to the group provides recognition and helps the individual acknowledge similar and different perspectives. Members may be asked to describe what each hopes to accomplish in the group and what experiences each has previously had in groups. Member-to-member exchanges are encouraged; individuals are recognized and supported as they take on leadership functions. Even in these beginning sessions, roles and a structure for the new group begin to take shape. Members try out familiar roles and test their individual abilities. Those approaches to member support, leadership, and decision making that are comfortable and productive become normative ways for the group to work. The nurse helps by creatively evaluating the appropriateness of style and productivity of roles. The work of the group is

begun even as the goals for health change are examined carefully and are realistically accepted. During this early period, members' attractions to one another and to the group begin to develop. How to initiate and conduct group work in the community setting, using the example of addressing disease prevention through a community agency, is presented in the How To box. The core competency skills for communication recommended by the Public Health Foundation are useful to nurses engaged in group work in the community. Box 23-4 lists these competencies.

## Conflict

Although conflict occurs normally in all human relations, people generally see conflict as the opposite of harmony, a state of interference to guard against. This view is an unfortunate one because the tensions of difference and potential

---

**HOW TO** | **Initiate and Conduct Group Work in the Community Setting**

**Example:** Group work to address disease prevention through a community agency

**PURPOSES FOR GROUP MEMBERS**

1. To increase awareness of common risks to health
2. To improve health through problem solving
3. To foster health promotion behaviors

**PLANNING AND IMPLEMENTATION STEPS**

1. Seek consultation from community agency staff about priority health concerns and interests of the population that the agency serves.
2. Determine times when members can meet, when meetings can be held, and standards and procedures related to working within the agency.
3. Select a health-focused topic of interest. Develop a teaching plan; submit the plan to a designated agency contact for information and approval.
4. Market group teaching through a variety of strategies. Make the purpose, benefits to members, length of meeting, place, and time clear in the recruitment. Group members may volunteer, be referred, or be selected through leaders' interviews. Number should be limited to 10 to 15 per group.
5. Meet with group at designated times. Stick to teaching plan; submit needed revision to agency contact.
6. Record and evaluate process and outcome of group teaching. Keep a meeting journal.
7. Keep agency staff up to date on progress throughout the group meeting block of time.
8. Meet with agency staff for a summary report of the group project; make recommendations for continued teaching or other health-focused follow-up for members.
9. Write a summary report.

**BOX 23-4   Core Competencies for Communication Skills**

**COMMUNICATION SKILLS**

- Communicates effectively both in writing and orally, or in other ways
- Solicits input from individuals and organizations
- Advocates for public health programs and resources
- Leads and participates in groups to address specific issues
- Uses the media, advanced technologies, and community networks to communicate information
- Effectively presents accurate demographic, statistical, programmatic, and scientific information for professional and lay audiences

**ATTITUDES**

- Listens to others in an unbiased manner, respects points of view of others, and promotes the expression of diverse opinions and perspectives

From Council on Linkages Between Academia and Public Health Practice: *Core competencies for public health professionals,* Washington, DC, Public Health Foundation, retrieved April 2001 from www.trainingfinder.org/competencies/list_nolevels.htm.

ness and also hold the potential to satisfy the frustrated parties include confrontation, competition, compromise, reconciliation, and collaboration.

Resolving conflict within groups depends on open communication among all parties, diffusion of negative feelings and perceptions, focusing on the issues, fair procedures, and a structured approach to process. The How To box on conflict resolution shows a sequence of behaviors that support and encourage participants to acknowledge and resolve conflicts.

**HOW TO   Resolve Conflict in Groups**

1. Give a full description of concerns and divergent views.
2. Clarify assumptions on the conflict issue.
3. Specify underlying factors, including beliefs, individual desires, and expectations.
4. Identify the real issue or issues.
5. Jointly search for a collaborative resolution through a problem-solving approach.
6. Finalize resolution agreement (either a full agreement or a compromise in which each party is satisfied on important points).

conflict actually help groups work toward their purposes. Understanding common causes of conflict, conflict management approaches, and conflict resolution models is especially important in this decade of challenges to health and health care systems and increasingly violent expressions of community conflict.

**Conflict** occurs when group members feel obstructed or irritated by one or more others (Northen and Kurland, 2001). Conflict signals that antagonistic points of view must be considered and that one must reexamine beliefs and assumptions underlying relationships. Some sources of concern for people are security, control of self and others, respect between parties, and access to limited resources; in groups, members express frustrations about trust, closeness and separation, and dependence and independence. These themes of interpersonal conflict operate to some extent in all interactions; they are not unique to groups. Within a group, because of members' regular and committed associations toward a common purpose, such issues are key; responding to them appropriately encourages personal growth and the facing of frustrations in the group.

Avoidance, forcing with power, capitulation, and excluding a member are conflict responses that fail to satisfy the concerns of frustrated parties. Two potentially positive dimensions of response to conflict are assertiveness (attempting to satisfy one's own concerns) and cooperativeness (attempting to satisfy the concerns of others). Behaviors that reflect either assertiveness or cooperative-

Conflict can be overwhelming, especially when members believe that the expression of controversy is unacceptable or unremitting. Conflict suppressed over time tends to build up and finally explode out of proportion to the current frustration. A group that repeatedly avoids expressing conflict becomes fragile, unable to adapt to growth within the group, and helpless to face challenges. Conflict may be destructive if contentious parties fail to respect the rights and beliefs of others.

Conflict-acknowledging and problem-solving approaches that respect others and represent self-concerns are first learned in families and other small groups. These lessons teach people to embrace conflict as a natural occurrence that supports growth and change. Other individuals learn to avoid conflict or to disregard others in the promotion of self. Teams that embrace a united desire for harmony to the extent of avoiding conflict in interactions may hinder collaboration and personal growth (Gerow, 2001). However, individuals may evaluate conflict management styles and refine skills in collaborative groups that support expression and resolution of conflict. Examination of conflict and resolution in supportive groups results in enhanced working relationships, stress reduction, and better coping.

The following example illustrates conflict resolution through collaboration. A small church in a rural town initiated a project for youth recreation because fast driving around the countryside was the primary form of recreation for the teens. A roadway was frequently used as a speedway by the restless youth. The church enlisted the high school principal and the nurse to work with a project group. All supported the development of a local youth center and worked energetically toward the goal.

After 2 months of steady cooperation, arguments began to erupt at meetings. Conflict about the supervision of the proposed center, the site for the physical plant, and numerous smaller concerns dominated planning time. The group consisted of active, aggressive members; four individuals dominated the discussions and resisted argument resolution. After several frustrating meetings, the nurse asked the group to explore each person's concerns and individual views on the direction and interaction of their work together. Welcoming an opportunity to relieve tension, members described their hopes, misgivings, and frustrated expectations related to the project. Each person elaborated on his or her assumptions about who would do what and how work should proceed. From this full discussion, the real issue became clear to all: disagreement related to members' functions in the project. The four dominant individuals expressed personal wishes to direct the planning and displayed aggravation when these attempts were thwarted. Other members described supportive and task functions but did not seek dominance in leadership functions. The open analysis of role structure made it clear to the members that arguments grew out of competition for directing roles rather than from true disagreements about the recreation project. Members searched for a collaborative resolution to the issue. They reached an agreement to divide the work into several task areas to be led by separate area directors. Members expressed relief that basic agreement about the purpose remained intact, and they were able to modify their role expectations to accommodate all members. They joked together about being a collection of bosses and renewed their productive work.

## Strategies for Change

Nurses can help groups meet established health goals through their knowledge of health and health risks for individuals, groups, and communities. Skill in problem solving for change is essential for accomplishing health goals.

Change, whether welcome or not, is disruptive to the client. Even though moving from a familiar way of being and interacting with others is uncomfortable (and resisted), all human systems do change over time because of development within the system and adaptation to outside stimuli. A change for one person in a group has effects on every other member. The disruption of growth, new opportunities, and threats to security trigger a fertile period for reevaluating, selecting new directions, improving, and maturing. Change creates opportunity for learning that is more than mastery of new information and identification of appropriate adjustment resources.

As discussed throughout this chapter, healthful change requires knowledge, practice of new skills, examination of attitudes and values about the change, and adjustment of roles in one's personal group or network. Helping people accomplish needed changes is ideally done in the small group context.

Basic teaching helps members understand the known associations between environment, body response, wellness, and pathological states that are pertinent to desired changes. Together, group members focus on the reality of the problems and ways to understand them. A group reaches its full potential for effecting individual change when members work actively and directly through discussion and other approaches to problem solving. Such group work produces individual outcomes for healthful change.

Expectant-parent groups illustrate a type of community group in which teaching is an appropriate method. Participants need to understand facts concerning pregnancy, labor and delivery, self-care, infant care, parenting, and adjusting to change. They also need to practice the skills required in anticipated tasks and to explore their attitudes and emotional responses to the anticipated family changes. Specific learning activities in the group might include demonstration and practice for baby baths and situation enactment of family activity after the baby comes home. Such experiential learning activities, which require interaction among members and involve topics highly relevant to the goal of change, are useful.

One approach for improved health involves analyzing both supportive and interfering forces that affect movement toward the particular change proposed for improved health, including sources such as important individuals within the family, work, and community groups. These forces are identified during group meetings when group members learn from one another and the nurse how to help overcome interferences and promote facilitative factors.

With the support of a group, people often make needed changes for health that they are unable to accomplish on their own or with the help of just one individual. Skillful use of group methods can help the client analyze the problem, help sustain motivation for change, support the client during vulnerable periods, and provide quick interpersonal feedback for success and failure. The discomfort associated with change is greatly mitigated through the relationships with others in beneficial groups. Most of the Healthy People 2010 priorities may be effectively addressed in health promotion and disease prevention groups where individuals may learn healthier behaviors and gain support from others in changing from risky to healthy lifestyle choices. For example, groups may support physical activity and fitness, sound nutrition, and safe sexual practices. Through group support, individuals may conquer smoking, drug abuse, or abusive relationships. They may identify and reduce exposure to environmental hazards and promote safer physical settings for all.

## Evaluation of Group Progress

Evaluation of individual and group progress toward health goals is important. Action steps toward the goal are identified early in the planning stage. These small steps may be responses to learning objectives (listed action steps designed to support facilitative forces and deal with resistive forces), or they may reflect the group's problem-solving plan. The action steps and the indicators of achievement are discussed and written in a group record. Celebration is built into the group's evaluation system to help individuals recognize and reinforce each step toward the health goal. Celebration may include concrete rewards such as special foods and drinks, or it may be the personal expression of joy and member-to-member approval. Celebration for group accomplishments marks progress, rewards members, and motivates each person to continue.

---

**HOW TO   Evaluate Group Effectiveness**

The following questions focus evaluation on group task accomplishment, member satisfaction, conflict management, and group purpose. Answer each question for the group and write a descriptive summary of group effectiveness.

1. Describe the group's task goal. List the steps proposed or acted on by members relative to the goal. How well do members achieve these steps?
2. Describe leadership behavior for the group. How well do members carry out other group roles?
3. Describe the comfort level for group members. Do members support each other? Is the level of tension conducive to productive behavior?
4. Is disagreement expressed clearly and openly? How do members manage and resolve conflict?
5. By what bonds are members attracted to each other and to the group?
6. Are there implicit goals for the group, and do these goals interfere with the group's work toward the explicit goal?

---

## Building Effective Work Teams

Teamwork is essential for nursing in all health care settings (see the Healthy People 2010 box). In community work, the team often includes workers from other health care disciplines and community residents. Team members' satisfaction and work team effectiveness depends on several key factors, including behavioral traits of team members, their expertise for producing the work product, and the leader's and members' skill at team building, coordination of work, and knowledge of group process. Group process concepts such as cohesion, purpose, task function, maintenance function, leadership, and conflict resolution guide nurses in effective team functioning.

---

**NURSING TIP**

Help-group members recognize traits and interests that they have in common and how some differences in skills among individuals help to complement the main group purpose.

---

Effective teams begin with selection of members who have the specialized knowledge and skill to produce the desired product. Nurses who want effective teams become part of the hiring and personnel selection process. Training for skills can occur after hiring for some, if most members come with relevant education and experience for the work. Good teams need a balance of member behavior types, including people who are self-reliant and task oriented, those who are enthusiastic and people oriented, those who are loyal and close in interpersonal relationships, and those who are factual and evaluative in style. Once a core team is selected, the leader and team members should evaluate

---

## Healthy People 2010 | Working With Groups

Healthy People 2010 recommends that community health promotion programs include the following:
- Community participation with representation from at least three of the following community sectors: government, education, business, faith organizations, health care, media, voluntary agencies, and the public
- Community assessment to determine community health problems, resources, and perceptions and priorities for action
- Measurable objectives that address at least one of the following: health outcomes, risk factors, public awareness, or services and protection

- Monitoring and evaluation processes to determine whether the objectives are reached
- Comprehensive, multifaceted, culturally relevant interventions that have multiple targets for change—individuals (e.g., racial, ethnic, age, socioeconomic groups), organizations (e.g., worksites, schools, faith), and environments (e.g., local policies and regulations)—and multiple approaches to change, including education, community organization, and regulatory and environmental reforms

From U.S. Department of Health and Human Services: *Healthy people 2010: national health promotion and disease prevention objectives,* ed 2, Washington, DC, 2000, U.S. Government Printing Office.

the mix of member behavior types and target recruitment for persons exhibiting personal styles needed by the team. A periodic change in membership as new members are added or some members are replaced may benefit the productivity; older members pass on their knowledge, and new members' ideas challenge old ways of doing business.

Cohesiveness in the team, as in other groups, is increased by the connections among members. Cohesion and member attraction is built through regular contacts and interactions that strengthen team identity. For example, identity is enhanced by pointing out cooperation and success in meeting goals. Members are asked to share their experiences and expertise. They are encouraged to work together on parts of the work assignments.

Some tension among team members energizes work. Differences challenge set patterns of working toward task and may contribute to improved procedures. Dissent within the group contributes to team innovation whenever there is a high degree of member participation in decision making (De Dreu and West, 2001). (See the Evidence-Based Practice box on minority dissent in working teams.) In groups where differences are welcomed, devil's advocacy or espousing an opposition view is not defined as conflict.

Antagonistic conflict is addressed quickly by a successful team. Often the issue that divides team co-workers is the purpose or perceived reason for conducting work. The purpose of teamwork must be understood. If there is a disagreement about the guiding goal and secondary objectives, members will function at cross-purposes and find tension in interaction. As in other groups, team leaders must clearly define and negotiate purposes, objectives, and member roles. Coordination, an essential component of successful team performance, is the way in which group members synchronize their actions.

## WHAT DO YOU THINK?

Under what circumstances will a member of a group taking a devil's advocate position improve group creativity?

Work projects are divided into the tasks that must be undertaken. Responsibilities of each team member should relate directly to the purpose of the unit's function. The most important criteria in assigning and delegating responsibility are the ability of the team member to carry out the task and the fairness of the assignment. Coordination may occur before work begins or during the process of work. The coordination may be tacit, based on unspoken expectations and intentions, or explicit, based on verbal agreements or formally adopted plans that fully and clearly designate who is to do what and when. Tacit coordination may be sufficient when member abilities are easily identified, and when work is under considerable time pressure for a task that is simple, stable, and requires low to moderate interdependence among members. When the group task is uncertain or variable, or when membership changes, the need for explicit coordination planning increases (Wittenbaum et al, 1998). As tasks are assigned or negotiated among members, differences in interpretation of work purpose will be identified. Sometimes the guiding purpose is rightfully redefined; more often team members refine their understanding of the work goal and adjust role expectations accordingly.

A successful team attends to the maintenance needs of members by observing for physical, social, and emotional comfort. Members' comfort includes satisfaction with progress and others' affirmation of individuals' parts in accomplishing the work. Support from others and the leader leads to strong team identification with the work unit. Clear leadership in work teams is essential, as it is for all groups. Leader directiveness in group process improves group satisfaction and group performance (Peterson, 1997) (see the Evidence-Based Practice box on directiveness).

## Evidence-Based Practice

Two Netherlands research studies show that minority dissent in working teams increases group innovation whenever the degree of decision-making participation is high. Participants in study 1 included 109 respondents from 21 work teams, a homogeneous sample of self-managing teams employed by an international postal service. Participants in study 2 worked in management and (cross-functioning) project teams from several different organizations.

Minority dissent (defined as instances when a minority of a group publicly opposes the beliefs, ideas, procedures, or policies assumed by the majority of the group) appears to prevent premature movement to consensus, promotes cognitive complexity, and prevents defective group decision making. The unique contribution of minority dissent is that it stimulates divergent thinking and creativity. These reported studies support the notion that organizational culture that values the process of continuous learning fosters dissent as a necessary and desirable part of organizational life. Groups that want to benefit from minority dissent not only need to foster dissent but also need to ensure high degrees of participation in decision making.

**Nurse Use:** When working with groups, appreciate the usefulness of dissent and disagreement by a minority of the participants. This dissent may help the group think through the work more carefully and evaluate more options.

De Dreu CK, West MA: Minority dissent and team innovation: the importance of participation in decision making, *J Appl Psychol* 86(6):1191-1201, 2001.

### Evidence-Based Practice

Leader directiveness in the group decision-making process was shown to improve group performance in three studies reported in 1997. Leader directiveness, as specified in these studies, has two components: (1) outcome directiveness (the degree to which the leader advocates a favored solution) and (2) process directiveness (the degree to which the leader regulates the process by which a group reaches a decision). One of the reported studies was an experimental control design; one was observational, a study of decision making in city councils in the San Francisco Bay area; and the third was a study of a selected set of groups. Findings showed that process directiveness of group leaders predicts improved group process and outcome. This was not so, however, when the group leaders were directive to advocate a favored solution or outcome. When leaders advocated a favored outcome, there was no predictable improvement in group process or in group outcome.

**Nurse Use:** In a working group, typically the outcome is more productive when the leader uses the process to arrive at the outcome rather than directing the members toward a preferred solution.

Peterson RS: A directive leadership style in decision making can be both virtue and vice: evidence from elite and experimental groups, *J Personality Soc Psych* 72:1107, 1997.

Although leadership and decision making may be concentrated in one person or more equally shared among all, the pattern and legitimacy of leading should be firmly established and agreed on by the team. Leading patterns may change over the life of the group; at each pattern change, the team adjusts expectations on lines of direction, responsibility, and evaluation. Clear communication holds top priority among effective team members. Messages are quickly clarified when they seem vague or contradictory.

Members are alert to the factors within and from outside that facilitate their performance. Barriers to accomplishing purpose are acknowledged, and the group makes decisions about how to deal with such barriers. Work is monitored by evaluating the group process in attaining purposes and by evaluating outcomes as they relate to the stated team purpose. From time to time, the team reassesses its purposes, effectiveness in working together, and levels of member satisfaction.

## COMMUNITY GROUPS AND THEIR CONTRIBUTION TO COMMUNITY LIFE

Locality communities consist of related and integrated parts. These components fit within the community according to residents' beliefs and definitions of who belong there, who are included within an organization or group, and how they relate to each other. Community organizations include service sectors, neighborhood sectors, and professional, social, employment, worship, and cultural associations. Community components reflect the major social institutions of society: economy, government, family, education, religion and medicine (Renzetti and Curran, 1998).

### DID YOU KNOW?

Voluntary associations are formal organizations that individuals join simply for the personal satisfaction of participating in them or because they believe it is morally right. In the United States, membership in voluntary associations has declined, especially for young people.

Modified from Renzetti CM, Curran DJ: *Living sociology,* Boston, 1998, Allyn & Bacon.

An understanding of group concepts provides a starting point for identifying community groups and how they function as components of the community. Because individuals develop, refine, and change their ideas within the context of the groups to which they belong, groups are vital to community well-being. Groups help identify community problems and are important in the management of interactions within the community and between the community and the larger society.

Community groups may be informal or formal. **Formal groups** have a defined membership and a specific purpose. They may or may not have an official place in the community's organization. In **informal groups,** the ties between members are multiple, and the purposes are unwritten yet understood by members. Informal groups can be identified through interviews with key spokespersons. Information about when and why they gather is learned through interviews or by observing gatherings to which the nurse is invited. Informal groups are often featured in the news when they are distinguished for community action or service. Formal groups can usually be identified in a variety of community media with meetings announced and business reported publicly. Membership lists, goals, and mission statements are usually written and available to interested persons. Typically, residents willingly describe the informal and formal groups in their communities after they learn the nurse's purpose for entering and studying their community. Public health nurses have traditionally facilitated linkages or initiated new ones between community groups (Schulte, 2000).

Community residents' interactions across groups influence the overall harmony and free exchange in the community. Natural links occur among groups through family, friendships, and other relationships. Many communities encourage cooperation among groups through interagency councils.

When citizens experience threats to community well-being, they seek others with similar concerns to collectively explore the problem and consider relevant action. Citizens utilize focal concern groups to address perceived threats to community well-being. Focal concern groups provide a context through which persons influence and are influenced by the community.

As communities become increasingly aware of specific needs for residents and particular populations, they may support development of local leadership to address these needs. In California, for example, the Woman's Health Leadership (WHL) recruits and trains individuals in leadership skills to lead efforts in community health and social justice.

## THE CUTTING EDGE

The Women's Health Leadership (WHL) program is building leadership capacity of diverse community leaders committed to promoting health and social justice in the community. The WHL Alumnae Network consists of 383 women representing 45 of 58 California counties and 22 ethnic and cultural groups. The program builds on the capacity of women who already make a difference in their communities and have the desire to strengthen and build on their current work.

Modified from Littlefield D et al: Mobilizing women for minority health and social justice in California, *Am J Public Health* 92(4):576, 2002.

Nurses have a historical role and acceptance in communities, especially low-income and underserved communities. Nurses are in a privileged position to work with and assist community groups as they respond to actual and potential threats to their health (Powell, 1999). For example when populations are exposed to environmental toxins, nurses provide information and links to information; they support community groups to organize and address such threats.

The nurse discerns goals for the community and for various groups through media reports, from community informants, and from local archives. These goals tell of resources and visions for change as perceived by the people living and working in the local community. Data may be organized according to the opinions and behaviors of the groups identified. Such information about community groups and assessment data are used with community representatives to plan desired interventions. Community working alliances or coalitions bring together diverse interest groups who share a common interest in perceived threats to community health. Nurses and other professionals are active in groups formed to address community issues. Groups are both units of community analysis and vehicles for change.

Small groups can influence and change the larger social community of which they are a part. The social system depends on groups for governing, making policy, determining community needs, taking steps to alleviate those needs, and evaluating program outcomes. The small group is a mechanism for interrelatedness between community subsystems, certain subsystems and their counterparts in the larger social structure, and factions within subsystems. Change in the composition and function of strategic small groups may produce change for the wider social system that depends on small groups for direction and guidance (Benne, 1976).

## WORKING WITH GROUPS TOWARD COMMUNITY HEALTH GOALS

Nurses use their understanding of group principles to work with community groups to make needed health changes. The groupings appropriate for this work include both established, community-sanctioned groups and groups for which nurses select members representing diverse community sectors.

Existing community groups formed for community-wide purposes such as elected executive groups, health-planning groups, better business clubs, women's action groups, school boards, and neighborhood councils are excellent resources for community health assessment, because part of their ongoing purpose is to determine and respond to community needs. In addition, they are already established as part of the community structure. When a group representing one community sector is selected for community health intervention, the total community structure is studied. Groups reflect existing community values, strengths, and normative forces.

How might nurses help established groups to work toward community goals? The same interventions recommended for groups formed for individual health change are beneficial to groups focused on community health. Such interventions include the following:

- Building cohesion through clarifying goals and individual attraction to groups
- Building member commitment and participation
- Keeping the group focused on the goal

- Maintaining members through recognition and encouragement
- Maintaining member self-esteem during conflict and confrontation
- Analyzing forces affecting movement toward the goal
- Evaluating progress

When nurses enter established groups, they need to assess the leadership, communications, and normative structures. This facilitates group planning, problem solving, intervention, and evaluation. The steps for community health changes parallel those of decision making and problem solving in other methodologies.

One nurse, Mrs. Winter, was asked to meet with a neighborhood council to help them study and "do something about" the number of homeless living on the streets. Mrs. Winter was known to residents from a local clinic, and they knew she also consulted at a shelter for the homeless in an adjacent community. When the council invited her, they stated that "our intent is to be part of the solution rather than part of the problem." Mrs. Winter accepted the invitation to visit. She learned that the neighborhood council had addressed concerns of the neighborhood for 20 years—protecting zoning guidelines, setting up a recreational program for teens, organizing an after-school program for latchkey children, and generally representing the homeowners of the area. The neighborhood was composed of low-income families who took great pride in their homes. After meeting with the council and listening to their description of the situation, Mrs. Winter agreed to help, and she joined the council.

As the first step in addressing the problem, the council conducted a comprehensive problem analysis on the homeless situation. All known causes and outcomes of homeless persons on the street were identified, and the relationships between each factor and the problem were documented from literature and from the local history. Mrs. Winter lent her expertise in health planning and her knowledge of the homeless and health risks. She suggested negotiation between the council and the local coalition for the homeless, recognizing that planning would be most relevant if homeless individuals participated. The council was cohesive and committed to the purpose, had developed working operations, and did not need help with group process. They made adjustments in their usual group operation to use the knowledge and health-planning skills of Mrs. Winter.

Interventions for the homeless included establishment of temporary shelters at homes on a rotating basis, provision of daily meals through the city council or churches, and joining the area coalition for the homeless. This example shows how an established, competent group addressed a new goal successfully by building on existing strengths in partnership with the nurse. Community groupings, because of their interactive roles, seem to be logical and natural ways for people who work together for community health change. As the decision-making and problem-solving capa-

bilities of community groups are strengthened, the groups become more able representatives for the whole community. Nurses improve the community's health by working with groups toward that goal.

## Practice Application

Two case scenarios are listed in this Practice Application. The first explores a situation in which conflict within a group is ignored. The second presents effective group work.

Four nursing students in Chicago decided to work with parents at a drop-in family resource center as part of their undergraduate field experience. Parents at the center wanted to learn how to provide nutritious low-cost meals at home. The four students recruited three of the center parents who used the drop-in center's programs regularly. The group of students and parents decided to teach economical food planning and preparation through cooking and serving simple meals and explaining how to plan, select, and prepare them. The meals were planned for three consecutive Mondays at the center.

On the first scheduled Monday, everyone in the group worked together successfully. Eight parents attended the class, enjoyed a good economical meal, and were interested in learning how to plan and prepare it. At the close of the evening, three of the students announced that they would be unable to come the following Monday. The parents and remaining student on the teaching team felt abandoned and resentful but carried on planning for the next session. They did not talk about their resentment to the offending students even though they were left unfairly "holding the bag."

**A.** What went wrong in this example?

Two nurses worked with a group of 12 high school juniors as part of a health education course in an inner-city neighborhood. The class met weekly in 90-minute sessions for 6 weeks. Faculty members for the class from the high school selected participants, shared their existing curriculum, and supported the purpose of the group. That purpose was to address issues that students identified as the most troublesome in their lives through group process.

As the class began, students asked for a review of sexually transmitted diseases, how to identify symptoms, and how to avoid risky behaviors. The leaders responded to requests with complete descriptions of prevention approaches and treatment. Discussion moved to teen relationships and communication. It became clear that verbal and physical violence were of even more importance to the teens than their concern about STDs.

The teens said that they were comfortable with the nurses, who identified themselves as helpers who cared about students and their daily challenges. Students described how violence played an important part in everyday interactions. They described a culture in which a person must fight to be honorable, one in which fighting often occurred before irritations and provocations were carefully considered. One would fight first, in this culture, and ask questions later. Some felt safe in the neighborhood only when armed with a gun or knife. Both girls and boys were expected to fight for self and friends. The norm for fighting was clearly named. The teens were at risk for harm and death related to beliefs that problems are best solved through violent means.

With this knowledge, the group members refocused on conflict resolution through means other than violence. The group lent support as members described recent deaths of friends from fierce acts. Because of their fears, students were willing to consider peaceful ways to solve problems in spite of the norms that were held about fighting. Students questioned their own attitudes and beliefs. They realized that friends greatly influenced how they thought they should behave. They began to change some of their ideas. Initiated by the class group, a nonviolent support club was established with the full sponsorship of the high school. It was one means to encourage continuing change for nonviolent resolution of conflict.

B. Can individuals develop healthy attitudes and change risk behaviors even when their peer culture values run counter to these changes?

---

**Answers are in the back of the book.**

## Key Points

- Working with groups is an important skill for nurses. Groups are an effective and powerful vehicle for initiating and implementing healthful changes.
- A group is a collection of interacting individuals with a common purpose. Each member influences and is influenced by other group members to varying degrees.
- Group cohesion is enhanced by commonly shared characteristics among members and diminished by differences among members.
- Cohesion is the measure of attraction between members and the group. Cohesion or the lack of it affects the group's function.
- Norms are standards that guide and regulate individuals and communities. These norms are unwritten and often unspoken and serve to ensure group movement to a goal, to maintain the group, and to influence group members' perceptions and interpretations of reality.
- Some diversity of member backgrounds is usually a positive influence on a group.
- Leadership is an important and complex group concept. Leadership is described as patriarchal, paternal, or democratic.
- Group structure emerges from various member influences, including members' understanding and support of the group purpose.

- Conflicts in groups may develop from competition for roles or member disagreement about the roles ascribed to them.
- Health behavior is greatly influenced by the groups to which people belong and for which they value membership.
- An understanding of group concepts provides a basis for identifying community groups and their goals, characteristics, and norms. Nurses use their understanding of group principles to work with community groups toward needed health changes.

## Clinical Decision-Making Activities

1. Consider three groups of which you are a member. What is the stated purpose of each one? Are you aware of unstated but clearly understood purposes? What is the nature of member interaction in each group? How do purpose and interaction differ in the three groups?
2. Observe two working groups in session, from the community, a health care agency, or a school. Notice the attractiveness of each group through the eyes of its members.
3. List actions that nurses may take to assist groups in various aspects of their work, such as member selection, purpose clarification, arrangements for comfort in participation, and group problem solving.
4. Observe a nurse working with a health promotion group. Does the nurse function in the way you anticipated? What nursing behavior facilitates the group process? List the areas of skill and knowledge most likely to be expected of the nurse by the community residents' groups.
5. Identify areas of conflict in a work group to which you belong. Describe how one of these expressed or potential conflicts could be managed. Use the steps for conflict resolution outlined in the How To box on resolving conflicts in groups. What role would you take? Practice conflict-acknowledging and problem-solving behaviors in the next conflict you encounter.

## Additional Resources

These related resources are found either in the appendix at the back of this book or on the book's website at **http://evolve.elsevier.com/Stanhope.**

**evolve** **Evolve Website**

WebLinks: Healthy People 2010

## References

Benne KD: The current state of planned changing in persons, groups, communities, and societies. In Bennis WG et al, editors: *The planning of change,* New York, 1976, Holt, Rinehart, & Winston.

Brandler S: *Group work: skills and strategies for effective intervention,* ed 2, New York, 1999, Haworth Press.

Council on Linkages Between Academia and Public Health Practice: *Core competencies for public health professionals,* Washington, DC, Public Health Foundation, retrieved April 2001 from www.trainingfinder.org/competencies/list_nolevels.htm.

De Dreu CK, West MA: Minority dissent and team innovation: the importance of participation in decision making, *J Appl Psychol* 86(6):1191-1201, 2001.

Gerow SJ: Teachers in school-based teams: contesting isolation in schools. In Sockett HT et al, editors: *Transforming teacher education: lessons in professional development,* Westport, Conn, 2001, Bergin & Garvey.

Goldberg G, Middleman RR: Constructivism, power, and social work with groups. In Parry JK, editor: *From prevention to wellness through group work,* New York, 1997, Haworth Press.

Littlefield D et al: Mobilizing women for minority health and social justice in California, *Am J Public Health* 92(4):576, 2002.

Northen H, Kurland R: *Social work with groups,* ed 3, New York, 2001, Columbia University Press.

Peterson RS: A directive leadership style in decision making can be both virtue and vice: evidence from elite and experimental groups, *J Personality Soc Psych* 72:1107, 1997.

Powell DL: Environmental Justice. In Howard University Division of Nursing: *Environmental health and nursing: the Mississippi Delta project, a modular curriculum,* Atlanta, Ga, 1999, Agency for Toxic Substances and Disease Registry.

Renzetti CM, Curran DJ: *Living sociology,* Boston, 1998, Allyn & Bacon.

Schulte JA: Finding ways to create connections among communities: partial results of an ethnography of urban public health nurses, *Public Health Nurs* 17(1):3, 2000.

U.S. Department of Health and Human Services: *Healthy people 2010: understanding and improving health,* ed 2, Washington, DC, 2000, U.S. Government Printing Office.

U.S. Department of Health and Human Services: *Healthy people 2010: national health promotion and disease prevention objectives,* ed 2, Washington, DC, 2000, U.S. Government Printing Office.

Wittenbaum GM et al: Coordination in task-performing groups. In Tindale RS et al, editors: *Theory and research on small groups,* New York, 1998, Plenum Press.

# Part 5

## Health Promotion With Target Populations Across the Life Span

The family is a major influence on the individual's concept of health and illness. It is within the family that a person's sense of self-esteem and personal competence is developed. The action taken by or for the person with a health problem depends on this sense of self-worth and the family's definition of illness. Environmental, social, cultural, and economic factors, as well as the resources of the community to meet health needs, influence the family's health risks and reaction to health. The goals of the nation for the year 2010 focus on changing the overall health of the nation, with the community as the primary target. Through family support, the individual may develop the responsibility to participate in activities that will lead to a healthier lifestyle.

Major health problems of individuals can be identified and related to their developmental phase. This factor becomes evident when age-specific morbidity data are reviewed. Nurses can influence the actions and reactions to health of all individuals in the community from birth through senescence. The nurse can influence the health of children by introducing healthy parenting behaviors, risk factor appraisal, and age-appropriate interventions.

Women and men are faced with many life changes and challenges, some of which are gender specific. Previous lifestyles and increases in stress from social, environmental, and economic constraints often result in risk for major health problems during adulthood.

The nurse's primary function with persons of all ages should be to promote quality and length of life. As the older adult segment of the population continues to grow, the health care delivery system and nurses must address and plan strategies to cope with increasing longevity, and chronic health problems.

Attention is also focused on the needs of a special population, the physically compromised. Nursing interventions must be refined to assist this group in meeting their health care needs. The nurse who studies and gathers evidence about the health issues of a population (such as children, women, men, the older adults) can better understand how to assess and plan for care of individuals who make up these populations. Community-oriented nurses assess the risk of age-related issues in populations, promote the development of programs and policies that will support initiatives to enhance population health status, and ensure that such programs are available to address the health risks of these target populations.

## Chapter 24

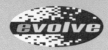
# Family Development and Family Nursing Assessment

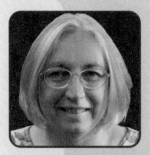

**Joanna Rowe Kaakinen, Ph.D., R.N.**

Joanna Rowe Kaakinen has been a family nurse scholar for the last 13 years. She has written extensively about family nursing theory. She is a reviewer for the *Journal of Family Nursing* and has presented nationally and internationally on family nursing. Currently, Dr. Kaakinen teaches at the School of Nursing at the University of Portland in Portland, Oregon.

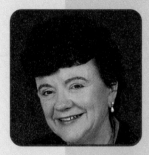

**Shirley May Harmon Hanson, R.N., P.M.H.N.P., Ph.D., F.A.A.N., C.F.L.E., L.M.F.T.**

Shirley M. H. Hanson is a professor in the School of Nursing at Oregon Health Sciences in Portland, Oregon. Her teaching and research interests include families and health, single-parent families, parenthood, and fatherhood, and child/adolescent/family mental health and therapy. She is a member of the American Nurses Association, Sigma Theta Tau. She is also a certified family life education (CFLE) nurse with the National Council on Family Relations and an approved supervisor for the American Association of Marriage and Family Therapy. In addition to her academic work, Dr. Hanson has an independent practice in child, couple, and family therapy. She has written many articles and book chapters and has co-authored or edited seven books. She is on the editorial boards and is a reviewer for *Family Relations, Western Journal of Nursing Research, Journal of Family Nursing, Advances in Nursing Science,* and *Marriage and Family Review.* Dr. Hanson is a fellow of the American Academy of Nursing and a fellow of the National Council on Family Relations.

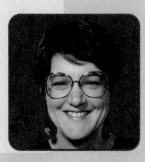

**Linda K. Birenbaum, R.N., Ph.D.**

Linda K. Birenbaum began practicing family nursing as a mental health clinical nurse specialist in 1976 at Morrison Center Children and Family Services. Her public health experience was with the Oregon Health Division as a nursing consultant to county health departments. Today she teaches graduate students community nursing at the School of Nursing at the University of Portland and consults for the Department of Human Services, Oregon Health Division.

## Objectives

After reading this chapter, the student should be able to do the following:

1. Explain the challenges of family nursing in the community setting
2. Describe family demographic trends
3. Predict how demographic changes affect health of families
4. Define family, family nursing, family health, and healthy/nonhealthy/resilient families
5. Analyze changes in family function and structure
6. Compare and contrast four social science theoretical frameworks for the family
7. Explain the various steps of the Outcomes Present–State Testing nursing process as it relates to family
8. Compare and contrast the four ways to view family nursing
9. Compare and contrast two different models and approaches that can be used for family assessment and intervention
10. Summarize how the genogram and ecomap assist family assessment
11. Describe barriers to family nursing
12. Discuss implications for social and family policy

Family nursing is practiced in all settings. The trend in the delivery of health care has been to move health care to community settings; thus family nursing is related to community-oriented nursing practice. **Family nursing** is a specialty area that has a strong theory base; it is more than just common sense or viewing the family as the context for individual health care. Family nursing consists of nurses and families working together to improve the success of the family and its members in adapting to normative and situational transitions as well as responses of health and illness. The purpose of this chapter is to present an overview of families and family nursing, theoretical frameworks, and strategies to assess and intervene with families in the community.

## Key Terms

cohabitation, p. 566

cue logic, p. 580

dual-career marriages, p. 566

dysfunctional families, p. 572

ecomap, p. 586

family, p. 568

Family Assessment Intervention Model, p. 583

family demographics, p. 565

family functions, p. 568

family health, p. 572

family nursing, p. 562

family nursing assessment, p. 583

family nursing theory, p. 573

family policy, p. 586

family resilience, p. 572

family structure, p. 568

Family Systems Stressor-Strength Inventory, p. 583

Friedman Family Assessment Model, p. 584

genogram, p. 586

Outcome Present-State Clinical Reasoning Model, p. 578

social policy, p. 588

*See Glossary for definitions*

## Chapter Outline

Challenges for Community-Oriented Nurses Working With Families

Family Demographics

*Marriage/Remarriage*

*Divorce*

*Cohabitation*

*Births*

*Single-Parent Families*

*Grandparent Households*

Definition of Family

*Family Functions*

*Family Structure*

Family Health

*Family Health, Nonhealth, and Resilience*

Four Approaches to Family Nursing

Theoretical Frameworks for Family Nursing

*Structure–Function Theory*

*Systems Theory*

*Developmental Theory*

*Interactionist Theory*

Working With Families for Healthy Outcomes

*Family Story*

*Cue Logic*

*Framing*

*Present State and Outcome Testing*

*Intervention and Decision Making*

*Clinical Judgment*

*Reflection*

Barriers to Practicing Family Nursing

Family Nursing Assessment

*Family Assessment Intervention Model Family Systems Stressor-Strength Inventory (FS³I)*

*Friedman Family Assessment Model*

*Summary of Family Assessment Models*

*Genograms and Ecomaps*

Social and Family Policy Challenges

## CHALLENGES FOR COMMUNITY-ORIENTED NURSES WORKING WITH FAMILIES

Each family is an unexplored mystery, unique in the ways it meets the needs of its members and society. Healthy and vital families are essential to the world's future because all family members are affected by what their families have invested in them or failed to provide for their growth and well-being. Families serve as the basic social unit of society.

An overview of issues facing families today shows that community-oriented nurses face several challenges in meeting the health needs of diverse and changing families. Given the immigration statistics and family demographic data, nurses need to be culturally competent, especially when one in ten Americans was born outside the United States and the birthrate is highest among foreign-born women living in the United States (U.S. Bureau of the Census, 2000). In addition, nurses are faced with health policy issues that address equal access to health care, tolerance, and fair immigration laws. See Box 24-1 for health issues associated with immigration from Russia.

Today, increases in the numbers of single-parent families and two-income-parent households stress child-rearing and child-caring capacities, as there are not enough affordable childcare resources. It appears that working women simply added a second "shift" to their lifestyles. The home and childcare are still considered the duty and responsibility of women. Although more men are involved in housework

## BOX 24-1  Health Issues Associated With Immigration From Russia

The impact of immigration on the American society is undeniable, especially on the health care system. According to the U.S. Bureau of the Census (2000), there have been 4.5 million recent immigrants, of which 243,000 were from Russia. The intricacy of immigration creates challenges both for the families who have emigrated and for the nurses who work with them, and the result can be unsatisfactory health care and decreased family health. It is important for nurses to know the factors that influence the health of these families. The limited review of literature presented here outlines the potential conflicts and health issues involved.

Challenges facing families who immigrate include adjustment to new societal rules, maintaining family cohesion, and accessing health care. In Russia, the management of health care follows socialistic rules, and the practice of nursing and medicine is a curative approach (Duncan and Simmons, 1996). In contrast, the health care system in the United States, as in most capitalist countries, favors a more preventative approach. Immigrants have to adapt to these changes and interact with health care resources that function by different rules and a different philosophy.

The prohibitive cost of health care, and specifically of health insurance, has forced immigrants to find ways to use health care resources that place stress on the U.S. health care system—for example, avoidance of routine health care, placing less value on preventative care, and accessing health care in emergency rooms. Individuals tend to approach health by using previously acquired health behaviors, which, in the case of immigrants, often results in a higher utilization of health clinics (Aroian et al, 1996, 2001; Duncan and Simmons, 1996). Socioeconomic characteristics, family support, health insurance, and differences in morbidity factors make the recent immigrant less likely than either native residents or less recent immigrants to receive timely health care (Leclere et al, 1994).

Nurses should not forget that traditions and family rituals are the bases of family cohesion and promote resilience. These rituals and former ways of life should be viewed by health professionals as a means to conserve the family's integrity, even though they may include behaviors that by Western standards would appear unhealthy—for example, heavy cigarette use, high alcohol intake, and dietary intake of high caloric foods (Duncan and Simmons, 1996). Western standards are not always applicable to families who do not value birth control and who consider being overweight an indicator of health (Duncan and Simmons, 1996).

Potential health problems can be linked to uncertain immunization status of children, preexisting diseases including undiagnosed mental health conditions, and long-term effects of environmental factors prior to the immigration (Smith, 1996). Duncan and Simmons (1996) reported that over 79% of immigrant Russians have had dental problems and are overweight, and that women between 18 and 40 years of age do not use birth control.

Nurses should not assume that Russian families would experience fewer stressors than other immigrants solely on the basis of their ethnicity. Even though a great majority of these immigrants are white, religion and circumstances related to immigration influence the families' ability to cope with the resettlement and acculturation processes (Aroian et al, 1996; Aroian et al, 2001; Wei and Spigner, 1994). The success of the immigration process depends on many factors, such as the belief systems, the cohesion, and the resiliency of the individuals and of the family (Aroian and Norris, 2000; Aroian et al, 1996, 2001; Leclere et al, 1994; Smith, 1996; Tran et al, 2000). Maladaptive behaviors and depression indicators are cross-generational events found in nonsupported families (Aroian et al, 1996; Leclere et al, 1994; Smith, 1996) and in older adult Russian-speaking immigrants who live alone (Tran et al, 2000). Depression of family members is the most frequent response to the changes associated with departure from homelands (Aroian and Norris, 1999; Tran et al, 2000).

The complexity and range of problems and behaviors associated with the immigration of Russian families are vast. The ability of Russian families to positively experience the immigration process is influenced by the original causes of emigration, their conditions of resettlement, and their mental and physical health on entry into the United States. When support is lacking, families are less likely to efficiently access available resources (Aroian et al, 1996; Duncan and Simmons, 1996; Leclere et al, 1994). Nurses should be sensitive to the fact that use of health care is influenced by behaviors acquired before immigration. It is crucial for nurses to refrain from trying to change the behavior patterns of Russian families, as this could destabilize their unity and potentially cause distress throughout the generations.

Aroian KJ, Norris AE: Somatization and depression among former Soviet immigrants, *J Cult Divers* 6(3):93-101, 1999; Aroian KJ, Norris AE: Resilience, stress, and depression among Russian immigrants to Israel, *West J Nurs Res* 22(1):54-67, 2000; Aroian KJ, Spitzer A, Bell M: Family stress and support among former Soviet immigrants, *West J Nurs Res* 18(6):655-674, 1996; Aroian J et al: Health and social service utilization among elderly immigrants from the former Soviet Union, *J Nurs Scholarsh* 33(3):265-271, 2001; Duncan L, Simmons M: Health practices among Russian and Ukrainian immigrants, *J Community Health Nurs* 13(2):129-137, 1996; Leclere RB, Jensen L, Biddlecom AE: Health care utilization, family context, and adaptation among immigrants to the United States, *J Health Social Behav* 35:370-384, 1994; Smith L: New Russian immigrants: health, problems, practices and values, *J Cult Divers* 3(3):68-73, 1996; Tran TV et al: Living arrangement, depression, and health status among elderly Russian-speaking immigrants, *J Gerontol Social Work* 33(2):63-77, 2000; U.S. Bureau of the Census: *Characteristics of the foreign born by place of birth.* Retrieved January 28, 2002 from http://www.census.gov/popluation/www/socdemo/foreign/p20-534.html#bi, updated 2000; Wei C, Spigner C: Health status and clinic utilization among refugees from Southeast Asia and the former Soviet Union, *J Health Educ* 25(5):266-273, 1994.

and childcare, more men also have abandoned their families and failed to provide court-ordered child support after divorce. There is reason to predict that role options in families will continue to become more flexible. There is also reason to believe that families will always have a gender-based division of labor. Even though divorce has leveled off, and some say it is decreasing, the rate remains high. Therefore many children live at a below-poverty level, especially in single-mother households.

The status of children in families has changed, and the changes have not all been to the advantage of the children. Although some argue that the key change is the absence of fathers, the major structural change is the poverty that affects children in single-parent homes. Families are not declining because of divorce, working mothers, and lower fertility. They are declining because American society continues to ignore the needs of an important proportion of its children. Many children do not get immunizations, are not fed or clothed, do not get health care, and live in dangerous environments (Gelles, 1995, p. 508).

The new morbidities that plague American families are substance abuse, early and risky sexual behaviors, intimate-partner violence, and homelessness. The chronic diseases outlined in the Healthy People 2010 objectives require lifestyle changes that are difficult to achieve with lasting results. The Healthy People 2010 box lists objectives that address families.

## FAMILY DEMOGRAPHICS

**Family demographics** is the study of family and household structures and the events that alter that structure (Teachman, Polonko, and Scanzoni, 1987). The importance of family demographics for nurses is the use of these data to forecast and predict developmental changes and stresses experienced by families so that possible solutions can be identified for family problems. In this chapter some demographic trends are described that affect community-oriented nurses.

There is an ongoing argument in the literature about whether there is a decline of the American family—that is, the nuclear family of dad, mom, and biological or adopted children (Bengtson, 2001). In part, this is accounted for by the decline in family households compared to nonfamily households. Family households consist of a householder and one or more people living together related by birth, marriage, or adoption (Simmons and O'Neill, 2001). In the 2000 census, family households made up 68% of the total households, with 76% of those family households composed of married couples (Simmons and O'Neill, 2001). The changes in family households have been in married couples with their own children, down from 40% in 1970 to 24% in 2000, and in other family households, growing from 11% in 1970 to 16% in 2000 (Fields and Casper, 2001). The category of married couples without children has remained relatively stable (Fields and Casper, 2001). These changes have led others to suggest that the definition of the nuclear family has been too narrow and limited to the modern industrial society (Stacey, 1996). The average size of all households has declined since 1970 from 3.14 to 2.62 persons per household (Fields and Casper, 2001).

It is important for nurses to keep themselves informed and up to date about demographic trends pertaining to children and families. Many family types other than those presented in this chapter can be identified, such as single households with no children, child-free couples, gay and lesbian couples, and intergenerational households. Such knowledge is essential so that nurses can identify high-risk populations, such as children living in poverty, children of working mothers who care for themselves (latchkey children), and

---

## Healthy People 2010 | Objectives Targeting Families

**1-6** Reduce the proportion of families that experience difficulties or delays in obtaining health care or do not receive needed care for one or more family members

**7-7** Increase the proportion of health care organizations that provides patient and family education

**8-18** Increase the proportion of persons who live in homes tested for radon concentrations

**8-19** Increase the number of new homes constructed to be radon resistant

**8-22** Increase the proportion of persons living in pre-1950s housing that have tested for the presence of lead-based paint

**8-23** Reduce the proportion of occupied housing units that are substandard

**9-12** Reduce the proportions of married couples whose ability to conceive or maintain a pregnancy is impaired

**11-1** Increase the proportion of households with access to the internet at home

**15-4** Reduce the proportion of persons living in homes with firearms that are loaded and unlocked

**15-25** Reduce residential fire deaths

**19-18** Increase food security among U.S. households and in so doing reduce hunger

**29-9** Increase the use of appropriate personal protective eyewear in recreational activities and hazardous situations around the home

From U.S. Department of Health and Human Services: *Healthy people 2010: national health promotion and disease prevention objectives,* ed 2, Washington, DC, 2000, U.S. Government Printing Office.

older adult women living alone. Changing demographics have implications for planning health, developing community resources, and becoming politically active, so that scarce funds and resources can be made available for health services needed by the growing and diverse population.

## Marriage/Remarriage

Marriage remains a popular American ideal. At the present time, more than 90% of Americans marry during their lifetime (Kreider and Fields, 2002). In 1996, 54% of men and 60% of women were in first-time marriages, whereas 13% of men and women had been married twice and 3% had been married three or more times (Kreider and Fields, 2002).

Until the 1970s, bereavement, the leading cause of remarriage, was replaced with divorce (Coleman, Ganong, and Fine, 2000). Over 50% of divorced people remarry (Kreider and Fields, 2002). Whereas gender was previously a leading factor in remarriage rates, recently the person who initiated the divorce has been found to be more a significant factor (Sweeney, 2002). That is, women who initiate divorce are more likely to remarry than women who were the noninitiators. However, with increasing age, women's (but not men's) opportunities to remarry declines (Sweeney, 2002). The length of time between divorce and remarriage is less than 4 years (Coleman et al, 2000). Although some persons remarry more than once, remarriages contracted by adults over 40 years of age may be more stable than first marriages (Coleman et al, 2000).

Two additional trends in marriage are worth noting: increased age for first marriage and interracial marriages. Since the beginning of the twentieth century, the median age for both sexes at the time of first marriage has increased steadily. At the beginning of the twenty-first century, the median age of first marriage for women was 25.1 years and 26.8 years for men (Fields and Casper, 2001). On the basis of adult and teen attitudes toward family issues, this trend has been projected to continue (Thornton and Young-DeMarco, 2001). Between 1970 and 2000, interracial marriages increased from 310,000 to 1,464,000 according to the U.S. Bureau of the Census (*World Almanac & Book of Facts,* 2002). That is, interracial marriages went from less than 1% to 2.6% of the total U.S. marriages in 30 years.

**Dual-career marriages,** or marriages where both partners work, have increased as more women enter the labor force. In a decade review of the work and family literature, Perry-Jenkins, Repetti, and Crouter (2000) discussed issues related to dual-career marriages: quality of childcare, work environment, impact of occupational stress on families, and multiple roles. Dual employment positively affects children, if it includes involvement in parenting, appropriate supervision, and quality childcare. The work environment affects families differently, depending on mediating variables. For example, a positive relationship has been shown between mothers' workplace complexity and the creation of a positive home environment for children. Autonomy, self-supervision, working with people, and

problem solving have predicted decreases in child behavior problems. Short-term and long-term job stress have different effects on the family, depending on mediating variables such as the parents behavior and their perception of stress. Multiple roles have been characterized as energizing people, but further research is needed before conclusions can be drawn (Perry-Jenkins et al, 2000).

## Divorce

Divorce can be said to be increasing, declining, or remaining stable, depending on the time referent. Divorce rates in the 1970s and into the mid 1980s climbed to 5.0/1000, but around 1985 through the 1990s they began to decline to 4.3/1000 (U.S. Bureau of the Census, 2001). In 1996, the median length of a marriage for divorcing couples was 7.8 years for men and 7.9 years for women (Kreider and Fields, 2002). Davidson and Moore (1996) identified factors that lead to divorce as spousal behavior, inability to manage conflict, sexual incompatibility, and poor quality of marriage. They summarized the following effects on the divorced family:

- Adjustment depends on a supportive positive response from parents and married friends.
- Men experience more severe initial responses after divorce, but women have a longer recovery period.
- Divorce is more devastating and lasts longer for the children than for the parents.
- Female children appear to be less vulnerable to divorce, but they actually internalize their stress as evidenced by lowered self-esteem and depression later.
- Many courts base custody on the best interests of the child.
- Both parents are responsible for child support.

The characteristics of people who divorce vary by race, religion, and educational level. The divorce rate for African Americans is higher than for whites, Hispanic Americans, or Asian and Pacific Islander Americans (Kreider and Fields, 2002; Teachman, Tedrow, and Crowder, 2000). Protestants have a higher divorce rate than Catholics. Women and men with at least a bachelor's degree are less likely to divorce than those who have a high school degree or less (Kreider and Fields, 2002).

## Cohabitation

One of the most dramatic changes in family structure has been **cohabitation,** or living together before marriage. Seltzer (2000) suggests that people cohabit for three reasons: some cohabitants would marry but do not for economic reasons; others seek a more equalitarian relationship; and others use cohabitation as a trial period to negotiate and assess whether to marry. The increase in cohabitation crosses all education groups for whites, African Americans, and Hispanic Americans, but the increase was greater for non-Hispanic whites and for those with a high school degree or less (Seltzer, 2000).

In the 2000 U.S. Census, 3.8 million households (7.6 million people) reported cohabitation. Fifty-eight percent of the women were less than 34 years old, whereas 53% of the men were less than 34 years old (Fields and Casper, 2001). Seltzer (2000) suggested that, with the aging of the population, cohabitation may be of increasing importance among older persons. In cohabiting relationships, 21% of the women were two or more years older than the men, whereas in marriages only 12% of wives are older than their husbands. Forty-nine percent of the women and 44% of the men had some college education (Fields and Casper, 2001). Forty-one percent of cohabitation families report having children, and these represent 5% of all children in the United States and 17% of all children living with unmarried parents (Fields and Casper, 2001).

Attempts have been made to examine the effects of cohabitation on children. Poverty and maternal parenting have been examined. Carlson and Danziger (1998) examined cohabitation and children in poverty and found that although the second income raised some families out of poverty, it affected the overall poverty rates minimally because of the low percentage of children in this category. As cohabitation increases, the effect of a second income is expected to increase. Thomson et al (2001) found that although mothers yell and spank or hit their children less when cohabitating or remarrying, they provide less supervision. Both Thomson et al (2001) and Seltzer (2000) agreed that cohabitation ends more quickly than marriage and therefore could have a negative effect on children, depending on their developmental stage.

> ### ( WHAT DO YOU THINK?
> Cohabitation before marriage does not increase or decrease the probability of divorce.

## Births

Birthrates in the United States declined during the 1990s, from 4158/1000 women who have children to 3959/1000 (U.S. Bureau of the Census, 2001). In the United States, there has been a trend to delay the birth of the first child and to have fewer children. The average age of the mother changed during the past 20 years, with fewer young mothers and more older mothers (U.S. Bureau of the Census, 2001). The increase in the number of children born to unmarried women continues to climb. In 1999, it is estimated that 33% of all births were to unmarried mothers, compared with 28% in 1990 (U.S. Bureau of the Census, 2001). The largest increase has been in unmarried women between 20 and 24 years of age, with data now being reported on women 35 and older (U.S. Bureau of the Census, 2001). At the same time, births to teenaged mothers declined from 12.8% in 1990 to 12.3% in 1999. Factors contributing to nonmarital childbearing in the United States include marriage patterns, sexual activity, contraceptive use, abortion (Ventura and Bachrach, 2000), and attitudes toward families (Thornton and Young-DeMarco, 2001)

## Single-Parent Families

In 2000, there were approximately 9.7 million single-mother households and just over 2 million single-father households (Fields and Casper, 2001). In 1996, 16.7 million children (28% of all children) lived with unmarried parents (Fields and Casper, 2001). The number of single-parent households varies by ethnicity. In 1996, 57% of African-American children lived with unmarried parents (Fields and Casper, 2001). The most important increase in the number of single-parent families involves single-mother households, which jumped from 11% in 1970 to 22% in 1990; father-only families jumped from 1% to 3% during that same time (Fields and Casper, 2001).

Single-parent mothers made some progress with poverty in the 2000 U.S. Census, going from 27.8% in 1999 to 24.7% in 2000. Looking at these data by race demonstrates that white single-parent mothers had a poverty rate of 16.9% (setting a record low), Hispanic single-parent mothers had a poverty rate of 34.2%, and African-American single-parent mothers had a poverty rate of 34.6% (Dalaker, 2001). Although some of these figures are encouraging, they still leave single-parent mothers in more poverty than single fathers or married couples.

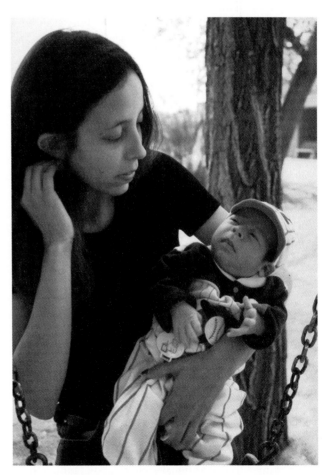

A young single mother with her infant son.

## Grandparent Households

The number of children who live with a grandparent increased from 3 million in 1970 to 5.1 million in 1996 (Fields and Casper, 2001). Of the 5.1 million, 3.1 million live with a grandparent without either of their parents present in the household (Fields and Casper, 2001). This was the fastest-growing group from 1992 to 1997 (Bryson and Casper, 1999). This change has altered the traditional supportive role of grandparenting to that of primary childrearing.

## DEFINITION OF FAMILY

The definition of *family* is critical to the practice of nursing. Family has traditionally been defined using the legal notions of relationships such as biological/genetic blood ties, adoption, guardianship, or marriage. Since the 1980s, a broader definition of family has been promulgated that moved beyond the traditional blood, marriage, and legal constrictions.

**Family** refers to two or more individuals who depend on one another for emotional, physical, and/or financial support. The members of the family are self-defined (Hanson, 2001a). Nurses working with families should ask people who they consider to be their family and then include those members in health care planning. The family may range from traditional notions of the nuclear and extended family to such "post-modern" family structures as single-parent, step-, and same-gender families, and friends.

**DID YOU KNOW?**

Most nursing students tend to have a narrow view of family based on their own experiences with their family of origin. Therefore it is important to study family nursing to broaden your understanding of other family variations.

## Family Functions

Throughout history, a number of functions traditionally have been performed by families (Hanson, 2001a). Six of these **family functions** are summarized:

1. Families exist to achieve financial survival. Families are economic units to which all members contribute and from which all family members benefit.
2. Families exist to reproduce the species.
3. Families provide protection from hostile forces.
4. Passing along the culture, including religious faith, is an important function for families.
5. Families educate (socialize) their young.
6. Families confer status in society.

Historically, families that performed all of these six functions were considered healthy and good. In contemporary times, the traditional functions of families have changed. The financial function of families has changed so

that family members do not need each other to stay financially healthy as much as they did in the past. Many married couples are electing to be child free rather than to reproduce. Families depend on other agencies, such as law enforcement, to provide safety, and other agencies are involved in the passing of the religious faith (e.g., churches or synagogues). Education (the socialization function) is relegated to the schools. Family names are no longer needed to confer status. The relationship function has become important in contemporary families, thus putting a great deal of pressure on how people get along and their level of satisfaction. The health function has become more evident because it is the basis of a lifetime of physical and mental health or the lack thereof. Thus functions that served families have evolved and changed: some have become more important and others less so (Patterson, 2002b).

**WHAT DO YOU THINK?**

All families have secrets. Some information gleaned from families may be exaggerated, minimized, or withheld.

## Family Structure

**Family structure** refers to the characteristics and demographics (sex, age, number) of individual members who make up family units. More specifically, the structure of a family defines the roles and the positions of family members (Box 24-2).

Family structures have changed over time. The great speed at which changes in family structure, values, and relationships are happening makes working with families at the beginning of the twenty-first century exciting and challenging. As social norms have become more tolerant of a range of choices in relation to managing one's life, there is no longer a general consensus that the traditional nuclear family model, consisting of father, mother, and children, is the only right model. There is no "typical" family model. As a consequence, there is a growing number of family and household types. For example, the single-mother household may be represented by the unmarried, teenage mother with an infant (unplanned pregnancy), the divorced mother with one or more children, or the career-oriented woman in her late thirties who elects to have a baby and remain single.

An individual may participate in a number of family life experiences over a lifetime (Figure 24-1). For example, a child may spend the early, formative years in the family of origin (mother, father, siblings); experience some years in a single-parent family because of divorce; and participate in a stepfamily relationship when the single parent who has custody remarries.

This same child as an adult may experience several additional family types: cohabitation while completing a de-

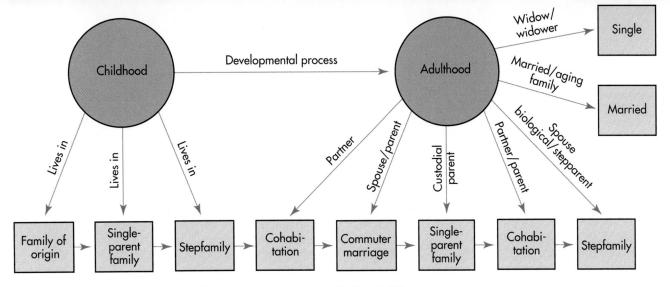

**Figure 24-1** An individual's family life experiences.

| BOX 24-2 | **Family and Household Structures** |
| --- | --- |

**MARRIED FAMILY**
- Traditional nuclear family
- Dual-career family
- Spouses reside in same household
- Commuter marriage
- Husband/father away from family
- Stepfamily
- Stepmother family
- Stepfather family
- Adoptive family
- Foster family
- Voluntary childlessness

**SINGLE-PARENT FAMILY**
- Never married
- Voluntary singlehood (with children, biological or adopted)
- Involuntary singlehood (with children)
- Formerly married
- Widow (with children)
- Divorced (with children)
- Custodial parent
- Joint custody of children
- Binuclear family

**MULTIADULT HOUSEHOLD (WITH OR WITHOUT CHILDREN)**
- Cohabitating couple
- Communes
- Affiliated family
- Extended family
- New extended family
- Home-sharing individuals
- Same-sex partners

sired education, and then a commuter marriage while developing a career. As an adult, the individual may divorce and become a custodial parent. The adult may eventually cohabit with another partner and finally marry another partner who also has children. As couples age, they have to address issues of the aging family, and subsequently the woman may become an older single widow. Nurses work with various families representing different structures and living arrangements.

Prospects for families in this twenty-first century are numerous. New family structures that are currently experi-

mental will emerge as everyday "natural" families (e.g., families in which the members are not related by blood or marriage, but who provide the services, caring, love, intimacy, and interaction needed by all persons to experience a quality life).

## FAMILY HEALTH

The meaning of family health is not precise and lacks consensus, despite the increased focus on family health within the nursing profession. The term *family health* is often used interchangeably with the concepts of family functioning,

## Families in Canada

Karon Janine Foster, R.N., B.Sc.N., M.N., Lecturer, Faculty of Nursing, University of Toronto

### TYPES OF FAMILIES

Most Canadians live in some type of family setting. The number of families has continued to increase (Statistics Canada, 2002a) Married-couple families are still the most common form, with 6.4 million in 2001 (Statistics Canada, 2002b). The number of traditional nuclear families, composed of two parents and children, continues to decline, whereas the number of families with no children living at home continues to rise (Statistics Canada, 2002c).

Common law families have increased 20% since 1995, with 1.2 million reported in 2001 (Statistics Canada, 2002b). In fact, 39% of all 20- to 29-year-olds living as couples are common law families (Milan, 2000). A majority of young Canadians choose common law as their first union (Statistics Canada, 2002b). Common law families continue to be less stable than married couple families, and about half of common law unions dissolve after 5 years (Milan, 2000).

For the first time, census data were collected on same-sex common law families. A total of 34,200 same-sex common law couples were identified, with a higher number of male same-sex couples than female (Statistics Canada, 2002c). Ontario was the province with the greatest number of same-sex couples. These data have begun to paint a picture of these types of families, but they may underrepresent the actual number of same-sex families in Canada. Recent challenges in provincial appeal courts in Ontario, British Columbia, and Quebec have challenged the legal definition of marriage, as it currently discriminates against same-sex couples and prohibits them from marriage. The court challenges argue that this is a violation of their rights on the basis of the Canadian Charter of Rights and Freedoms. The federal Ministry of Justice is to begin public consultation on the definition of marriage. If this consultation results in changes to the definition, same-sex couples may be able to legally marry and the structure of Canadian families will continue to change.

The number of single-parent families rose to 1.3 million in 2001 and women head more than 83% of these families (Statistics Canada, 2002c). Divorced persons account for 58% of single-parent families, and births outside of a relationship account for 22% (Milan, 2000). Quebec has the highest number of single parents.

With divorce or dissolution of common law unions and the formation of new relationships, the number of stepfamilies continues to grow, with 503,000 reported in 2001 (Statistics Canada, 2002b). Stepfamilies account for 12% of all families with children (Statistics Canada, 2002b). Four out of 10 families are blended families.

Blended families include a child from one of the spouses plus a new child born to the couple, or children from previous unions of both spouses.

One quarter of all households are one-person families (Statistics Canada, 2002c). Seniors, particularly women, are the individuals most likely to live on their own. Statistics from 2001 showed that 38% of women over 85 years old live on their own (Statistics Canada, 2002c).

An emerging trend is the number of three-generation households. In one decade (1986 to 1996), the number of these families increased from 150,000 to 208,000 (Milan, 2000). With an aging population, longer life expectancy, and immigration, this type of family will continue to increase.

Another trend is the increase in young adults living in the parental home. Statistics from 2001 show 41% of young adults (ages 20 to 29 years) now live in the parental home (Statistics Canada, 2002c). Higher tuition costs in postsecondary education, delayed age of marriage, cultural practices, and the economic recessions of 1991 and 1996 account for changes in this family structure (Boyd and Norris, 1999; Statistics Canada, 2002c).

### BIRTHRATES

Canadian families are smaller than they were 20 years ago. Since 1997, the average number of persons per family has been 3.0 in couple families (including married and common law couples), and 2.5 in single-parent families (Statistics Canada, 2000d). A declining birthrate has contributed to the smaller size of families. Canada's birthrate has decreased considerably over the past 40 years, from a rate of over 25 births per 1000 people to 10.8 births per 1000 people in 2000 (Statistics Canada, 2000). Many women now marry at a later age and delay having children until they are older and established in their careers. In 1997, 32% of first-time births were to women 30 years or older (Ministry of Industry, 2002). Women have an average of 1.5 children; this is the lowest fertility rate in Canadian history and below the replacement rate (Ministry of Industry, 2002).

### MARRIAGE AND DIVORCE RATES

Changes in marriage and divorce rates have influenced the structure of the Canadian family. The number of marriages has fallen since 1998, from 152,820 to 113,841 in 2002 (Statistics Canada, 2002e). Most first-time couples are delaying marriage until their late thirties. In 1999, the average age of brides was 31.3 years, and for grooms, 33.8 years (Statistics Canada, 2003). Between 1971 and 1997, the rate of remarriage increased from 15% to 34% (Milan, 2000). In 1997, 34% of marriages involved a divorcee and in half of these unions both partners were divorcees (Milan, 2000). The divorce rate has dropped since 1985, when the divorce laws changed. The crude divorce rate in 2000 was 2.3 divorces per 1000 people, compared to 3.6 in 1987 (Statistics Canada, 2002f). Divorce rates are highest among young adults in their late twenties.

### LOW-INCOME FAMILIES

A major concern for health professionals is the number of families who exist on low incomes. Single mothers have the lowest incomes, and childhood poverty remains a serious issue. Refer to the Canadian content box in Chapter 32 for further discussion.

### WORKING MOTHERS

Canadian mothers continue to be employed outside the home. In 1999, approximately 70% of women with children were working full-time. In the past 23 years, there has been a sharp increase, from 37% to 66%, in the number of women with children under the age of 3 years employed full-time (Zukewich, 2000). Mothers with school-age children are the most likely to be employed full-time. Working mothers must juggle the responsibilities of family and a job, which impacts on family life. Approximately one mother in three reported being stressed for time because of the complexity of her roles (Zukewich, 2000). Affordable and accessible childcare remains an issue for working families.

### GOVERNMENT BENEFITS FOR FAMILIES

In Canada, there are several benefits to assist families. Under the Employment Insurance Act, maternity and parental benefits are available to eligible parents. Since December 31, 2000, parents with a natural or adopted infant are eligible for parental benefits for 1 year. Revenue Canada offers other tax benefits to assist families with children. These include the Child Tax benefit for low-income families, the Goods and Services Tax credit, childcare expenses, equivalent-to-spouse deduction, tuition and education transfers, and medical expenses. For families with special needs children, there is also the disability tax credit, and caregiver and dependent person benefits.

### References

Boyd M, Norris D: The crowded nest: young adults at home, *Canadian Social Trends* 52:2-5, 1999.

Finnie R: The dynamics of poverty in Canada: what we know, what we can do, *C.D. Howe Institute Commentary* 145(Sept), 2000.

Government of Canada: *Services for children: guide to government of Canada services for children and their families,* pp 6-7, Ottawa, 2001, Minister of Public Works and Government Services.

Lindsay C: Seniors: a diverse group aging well, *Canadian Social Trends* 52:24-56, 1999.

Milan A: One hundred years of families, *Canadian Social Trends* 56:2-13, 2000.

Ministry of Industry: Births, *Health Rep* 13(2), 2002.

Statistics Canada: *Population, density, births and deaths for selected countries,* Ottawa, 2000, Statistics Canada, available at www.statcan.ca/english/Pgdb/demo01.htm (or go to www.statcan.ca and search for document name).

Statistics Canada: *Census families: number, and average size 1971-2000,* retrieved July 4, 2002a, from www.statcan.ca/english/Pgdb/famil40a.htm (or go to www.statcan.ca and search for document name).

Statistics Canada: Changing conjugal life in Canada, *The Daily* July 11, 2002b, retrieved from www.statcan.ca/Daily/English/020711/d020711a.htm, (or go to www.statcan.ca, The Daily, and search for document name).

Statistics Canada: *Profile of Canadian families and households: diversification continues,* 2002c, retrieved from www.statcan.ca/English/IPS/data/96F0030XIE2001003.htm (or go to www.statcan.ca and search for document name).

Statistics Canada: *Census families: numbers, average size, husband-wife and lone parent families,* 2002d, retrieved from www.statcan.ca/english/Pgdb/famil40b.htm (or go to www.statcan.ca and search for document name).

Statistics Canada: *Marriages: 1998-2002,* 2002e, retrieved from www.statcan.ca/english/Pgdb/famil04.htm (or go to www.statcan.ca and search for document name).

Statistics Canada: Divorces, *The Daily,* Dec 2, 2002f, retrieved from www.statcan.ca/Daily/English/021202/d021202f.htm (or go to www.statcan.ca, The Daily, and search for document name).

Statistics Canada: Marriages, *The Daily,* Feb 6, 2003, retrieved from www.statcan.ca/Daily/English?030206/d030206c.htm (or go to www.statcan.ca, The Daily, and search for document name).

Zukewich N: Paid and unpaid work. In *Women in Canada: a gender based statistical report: 2000,* Ottawa, 2000, Minister of Industry.

*Canadian spelling is used.*

healthy families, and familial health. Hanson (2001a, p. 6) defines **family health** as "a dynamic changing relative state of well-being which includes the biological, psychological, spiritual, sociological, and cultural factors of the family system."

This biopsychosociocultural–spiritual approach refers to individual members as well as the family unit as a whole entity and the family within the community context. An individual's health (the wellness and illness continuum) affects the functioning of the entire family, and in turn the family's functioning affects the health of individuals. Thus assessment of family health involves simultaneous assessment of individual family members, the family system as a whole, and the community in which the family is imbedded.

## Family Health, Nonhealth, and Resilience

Health professionals have tended to classify clients and their families into two groups: "good families" and "bad families" in need of psychosocial evaluation and intervention (Satariano and Briggs, 1999, p. 317). The term *family health* implies mental health rather than physical health. In recent years, a popular term for nonhealthy families is **dysfunctional families,** also called noncompliance, resistant, or unmotivated–phrases that label families who are not functioning well with each other or in the world. The labeling of a family as dysfunctional does not, however, allow for families to change, and it obstructs any kind of intervention; this and similar terms need to be dropped from the nursing language. Families are neither all good nor all bad; rather, all families have both strengths and difficulties. All families have seeds of resilience. Nurses should view family behavior on a continuum of need for intervention. Box 24-3 shows the levels of prevention for a family experiencing child abuse.

*Families with strengths, functional families,* and *resilient families* are terms often used to refer to healthy families that are doing well. There has been some research about healthy families, but it is clear that this research focuses on relational needs. This means that in healthy families, the basic survival needs are already met and they can move to a higher hierarchy of need, such as relational and self-fulfillment needs. According to Carter and McGoldrick (1998), the traits ascribed to healthy families are based solely on attachment and are affectionate in nature. Studies have identified traits of healthy families as well as family stressors that are useful for nurses to include in their assessment (Curran, 1983, 1985). Box 24-4 shows characteristics of families who are healthy and functioning well in society.

The most recent concept described in the family literature pertains to family resilience. **Family resilience** has been defined as the ability to withstand and rebound from adversity (Hawley, 1996, 2000; Patterson, 2002a,b; Walsh, 1996, 2002). According to Walsh (2002), health care professionals should work with families to find new possibilities in a problem-saturated situation and to help them overcome impasses to change and growth. This is a positive focus on bringing out the best to enhance family functioning and well-being. "The basic premise guiding this approach is that stressful crisis and persistent challenges influence the whole family, and in turn, key family processes mediate the recovery and resilience of vulnerable members as well as the family unit" (Walsh, 2002, p. 130). Family resilience is an important outcome when nurses look at family stressors and assess family strengths. Nurses have a responsibility to help families withstand and rebound from adversity.

---

**BOX 24-3 Examples of Levels of Prevention for Child Abuse**

**PRIMARY PREVENTION**

Child development programs for families at risk for child abuse, such as single-parent households.

**SECONDARY PREVENTION**

Child development and behavior management for families who have not yet abused their children, but whose children are brought to the attention of social authorities for aggressive behavior problems.

**TERTIARY PREVENTION**

Family therapy for abusive families; removal of children from the home.

---

**BOX 24-4 Characteristics of Healthy Families**

1. The family tends to communicate well and listen to all members.
2. The family affirms and supports all of its members.
3. Teaching respect for others is valued by the family.
4. The family members have a sense of trust.
5. The family plays together, and humor is present.
6. All members interact with each other, and a balance in the interactions is noted among the members.
7. The family shares leisure time together.
8. The family has a shared sense of responsibility.
9. The family has traditions and rituals.
10. The family shares a religious core.
11. Privacy of members is honored by the family.
12. The family opens its boundaries to admit and seek help with problems.

---

Modified from Hanson SMH: *Family health care nursing: theory, practice and research,* ed 2, Philadelphia, 2001a, Davis.

# FOUR APPROACHES TO FAMILY NURSING

Central to the practice of family nursing is conceptualizing and approaching the family from four perspectives, as discussed in the following paragraphs. All have legitimate implications for family nursing assessment and intervention (Figures 24-2 and 24-3). The approaches that nurses use are determined by many factors, including the issues for which the individuals or families as a whole are seeking help, the environment in which they coexist with other family members and the community, the interaction among all of these factors, and of course the nurse resources available to deal with all of these factors.

**Family as the context.** The family has a traditional focus that places the individual first and the family second. The family as context serves as either a strength or a stressor to individual health and illness issues. A nurse using this focus might ask an individual client, "How has your diagnosis of insulin-dependent diabetes affected your family?" or "Will your need for medication at night be a problem for your family?"

**Family as the client.** The family is primary and individuals are secondary. The family is seen as the sum of individual family members. The focus is concentrated on each individual as they affect the family as a whole. From this perspective, a nurse might say to a family member who has just become ill, "Tell me about what has been going on with your own health and how you perceive each family member's response to your mother's recent diagnosis of liver cancer."

**Family as a system.** The focus is on the family as client, and the family is viewed as an interactional system in which the whole is more than the sum of its parts. This approach focuses on individual members and the family as a whole at the same time. The interactions among family members become the target for nursing interventions (e.g., the interactions among both parents and children, and between the parental hierarchy). The systems approach to families always implies that when something happens to one family member, the other members of the family system are affected, and vice versa. Questions nurses ask when approaching the family as a system are "What has changed between you and your spouse since your child's head injury?" or "How do you feel about the fact that your son's long-term rehabilitation will affect the ways in which the members of your family are functioning and interact with one another?"

**Family as a component of society.** The family is seen as one of many institutions in society, along with health, education, and religious and financial institutions. The family is a basic or primary unit of society, as are all the other units, and they are all a part of the larger system of society. The family as a whole interacts with other institutions to receive, exchange, or give services. Community-oriented nurses who are family nurses have derived many of their tenets of practice from this component of society,

because they focus on the interface between families and community agencies.

# THEORETICAL FRAMEWORKS FOR FAMILY NURSING

**Family nursing theory** is an evolving synthesis of the scholarship from three different traditions: family social science, family therapy, and nursing (Figure 24-4). Currently, there is no single theory or conceptual framework from any one of these fields that fully describes the relationships and dynamics and can be used to understand and intervene with families. Thus an integrated approach drawn from all three bodies of knowledge is necessary for the theory, practice, research, and education of family nursing. One theoretical perspective does not provide nurses with enough knowledge to assess and intervene with families. Therefore nurses must draw on multiple theories to work effectively with families.

Of the three categories of theory, the family social science theories are the most well developed and informative with respect to how families function, the environment–family interchange, interactions within the family, how the family changes over time, and the family's reaction to health and illness. Therefore, in this chapter, only family social science theories are reviewed, and examples are given of how nurses use them in family nursing practice.

Within the family social science tradition, four conceptual approaches have dominated the field of marriage and family: structure–function theory, systems theory, developmental theory, and interactionist theory (White and Klein, 2002). These theories are constantly evolving and being tested, which helps to make this knowledge base stronger and more user friendly for working with families.

## Structure–Function Theory

The structure–function framework from a social science perspective defines families as social systems. Families are examined in terms of their relationship with other major social structures (or institutions), such as health care, religion, education, government, and the economy. This theory looks at the arrangement of members within the family, relationships between the members, and the roles and relationships of the individual members to the whole family (Artinian, 1994; Hanson and Kaakinen, 2001). The primary focuses are to determine how family patterns are related to other institutions in society and to consider the family in the overall structure of society. Emphasis is placed on the how the structure supports basic functions of families, or vice versa. Families as aggregates in society are studied by looking at their status and role. Family theorists use this approach to understand the social or family system and its relationship to the overall social system in the community. This approach describes the family as open to outside influences, yet at the same time the family maintains its boundaries. The family is seen as passive

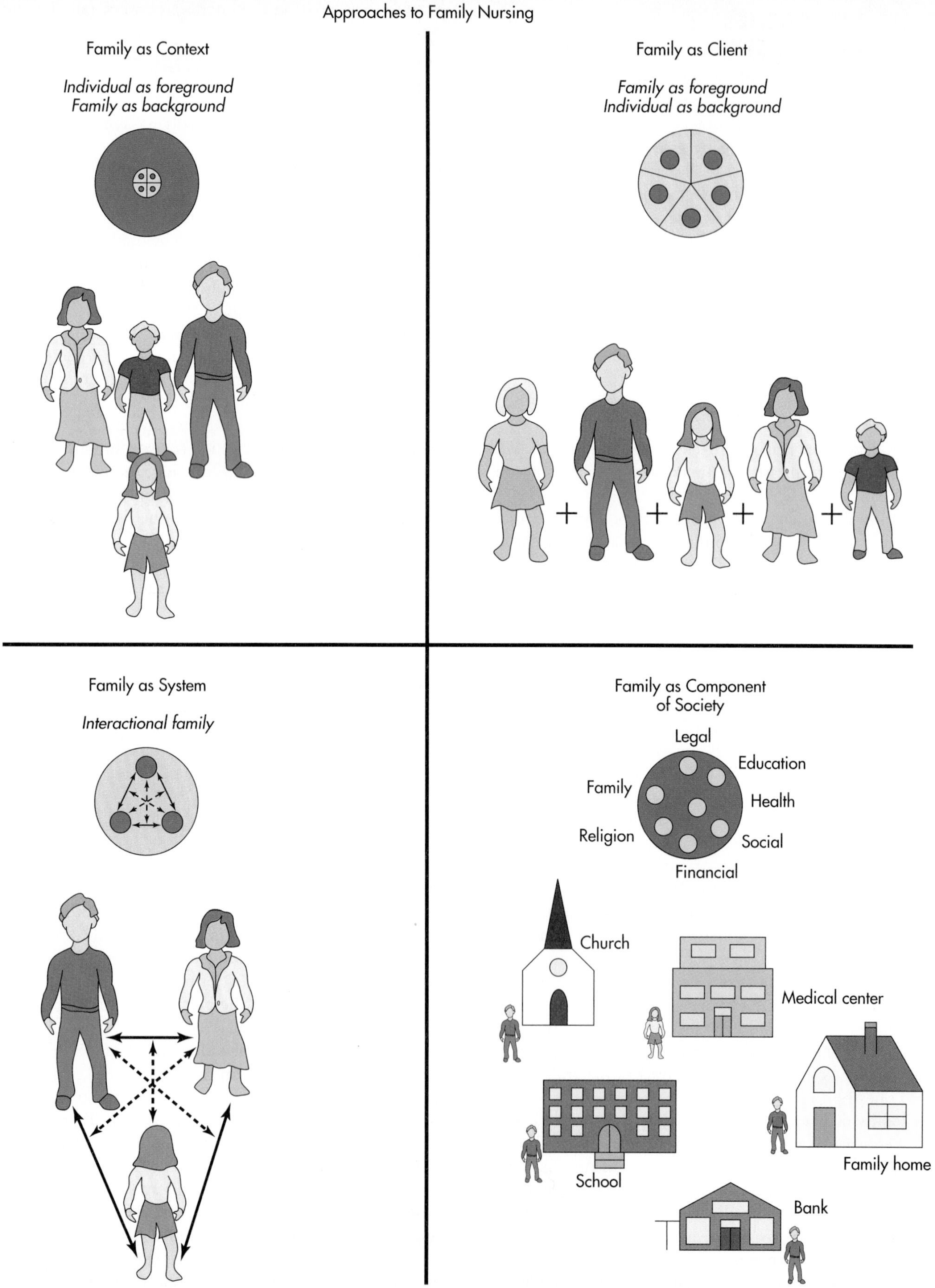

Approaches to Family Nursing

Family as Context

*Individual as foreground*
*Family as background*

Family as Client

*Family as foreground*
*Individual as background*

Family as System

*Interactional family*

Family as Component
of Society

Legal
Education
Family
Health
Religion
Social
Financial

Church
Medical center
School
Family home
Bank

**Figure 24-2** Approaches to family nursing. *(From Hanson SMH:* Family health care nursing: theory, practice, and research, *Philadelphia, 2001, Davis.)*

and adapting to the system rather than being an agent of change. Assumptions include the following:

- A family is a social system with functional requirements.
- A family is a small group that has basic features common to all small groups.
- Social systems, such as families, accomplish functions that serve the individuals in addition to those that serve society.
- Individuals act within a set of internal norms and values that are learned primarily in the family socializing process.

Nurses refer to this model when they talk about the structure, forms, or type of family, such as single-parent

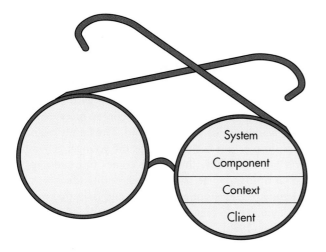

**Figure 24-3** Four views of the family.

families, stepfamilies, nuclear families, or extended families. Other structural dimensions of families include role structure, value system, communication patterns, power structure, and support networks (Friedman, Bowden, and Jones, 2003). This is a useful framework for assessing families and health. Illness of a family member results in alteration of the family structure and function. If a single mother is ill, she cannot carry out her various roles, so grandparents or siblings may have to assume childcare responsibilities. Family power structures and communication patterns are affected by the illness of a parent. Family assessment includes determining if changes resulting from health issues influence the family's ability to carry out its functions. Sample assessment questions are "How did the death alter the family structure?" and "What family roles were changed with the onset of the chronic illness?" Interventions become necessary when a change in the family structure alters the family's ability to function. Examples of interventions using this model include helping families use existing support structures and helping families modify the way they are organized so that role responsibilities can be distributed.

The major strength of the structure–function theory to family nursing is its comprehensive approach that views families in the broader community in which they live. The major weakness of this approach is the static picture of family, which does not allow for dynamic change over time.

## Systems Theory

The systems approach to understanding families was influenced by theory derived from physics and biology. A system is composed of a set of interacting elements; each

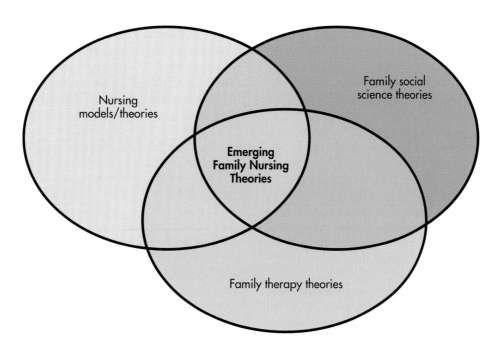

**Figure 24-4** Theory-based family nursing. *(Modified from Hanson SMH, Kaakinen JR, Friedman MM: In Friedman MM: Family nursing: research, theory, and practice, Stamford, Conn, 1998, Appleton & Lange.)*

system can be identified and is different from the environment in which it exists. An open system exchanges energy and matter with the environment (negentropy), whereas a closed system is isolated from its environment (entropy). Systems depend on both positive and negative feedback to maintain a steady state (homeostasis). Seeking therapy when the marital relationship is strained is an example of using negative feedback to maintain a steady state. Assumptions of the systems theory include the following:

- Family systems are greater than and different from the sum of their parts.
- There are many hierarchies within family systems and logical relationships between subsystems (e.g., mother–child, family–community).
- Boundaries in the family system can be open, closed, or random.
- Family systems increase in complexity over time, evolving to allow greater adaptability, tolerance to change, and growth by differentiation.
- Family systems change constantly in response to stresses and strains from within and from outside environments. There are structural similarities in different family systems (isomorphism).
- Change in one part of a family system affects the total system.
- Causality is modified by feedback; therefore causality is ever moving and does not exist in the real world.
- Family systems patterns are circular rather than linear; change must be directed toward the cycle.
- Family systems are an organized whole; therefore individuals within the family are interdependent.
- Family systems have homeostasis features to maintain stable patterns that can be adaptive or maladaptive.

The family systems theory encourages nurses to view clients as participating members of a family. Nurses using this theory determine the effects of illness or injury on the entire family system. Emphasis is on the whole rather than on individuals. Nursing assessment of family systems includes assessment of individual members, subsystems, boundaries, openness, inputs and outputs, family interactions, family processing, and adapting or change abilities. Assessment questions include "Who is in the family system?" and "How has one member's critical illness affected the entire family system?" Interventions need to assist individual, subsystem, and whole-family functioning. Some nursing strategies using this approach include establishing a mechanism for providing families with information about their family members on a regular basis and discussing ways to provide for a normal family life for family members after someone becomes ill.

The major strength of the systems framework is that it views families from both a subsystem and suprasystem approach. That is, it views the interactions within and between family subsystems as well as the interaction between families and the larger supersystems, such as community and world. The major weakness of the systems framework

is that the focus is on the interaction of the family with other systems rather than on the individual, which is sometimes more important.

## Developmental Theory

Individual developmental theory has been central to nursing of people across the life span. This approach looks at the family system over time through different phases that can be predicted, and through family transitions based on norms.

Duvall and Miller (1985) presented a synthesis of family developmental concepts. They take the principles of individual development and apply them to the family as a unit. The stages of family development are based on the age of the eldest child. Overall family tasks are identified that need to be accomplished for each stage of family development. Developmental concepts include moving to a different level of functioning, implying progress in a single direction. Family disequilibrium and conflicts are described as occurring during transition periods from one stage to another. The family has a predictable natural history designated by stages, beginning with the simple husband–wife pair. The family becomes more complex with the addition of each new child. The family again becomes simpler and less complex as the younger generation leaves home. Finally, the family comes full circle to the original husband–wife pair. At each family lifecycle stage, the family has developmental needs and tasks that must be performed. These concepts are further refined by Duvall and Miller (1985).

Developmental theory is an attempt to integrate the smaller scale (interactive framework) and larger scale (structural/functional framework) analyses of these two approaches while viewing the family as an open system in relation to structures in society. Developmental theory explains and predicts the changes that occur to people or to groups over time. Achievement of family developmental tasks helps individual members to accomplish their tasks. This framework assists nurses in anticipating clinical problems in families and in identifying family strengths. The framework also serves as a guide to nurses while they assess the family's developmental stage, the extent to which the family is fulfilling the tasks associated with its respective stage, the family's developmental history, and the availability of resources essential for performing developmental tasks.

In conducting an assessment of families using the developmental model, several questions can be asked: "Where does this family fit on the continuum of the family lifecycle?" "What are the developmental tasks that are not being accomplished?" Nursing intervention strategies that derive from the developmental perspective try to help individuals and families understand the growth and development stages and to help families deal with the normal transition periods between developmental periods (e.g., tasks of the school-age family member versus tasks of the adolescent family member).

Family nurses must recognize that in every family there are both individual and family developmental tasks that need to be accomplished for every stage of the individual or family lifecycle that are unique to that particular group.

Other basic assumptions of systems theory include the following:

- Families change and develop in different ways because of internal and environmental stimulation.
- Developmental tasks are goals worked toward rather than specific jobs completed all at once.
- Each family is unique in its composition and the complexity of age or role expectations and positions.
- Individuals and families are a function of their history as well as of the current social structure.
- Families have enough in common despite the way they develop over the family life span.
- Families may arrive at similar developmental levels through different processes.

The major strength of this approach is that it provides a basis for forecasting what a family will be experiencing at any period in the family lifecycle (e.g., role transitions, family structure changes). The major weakness of the model is that it was developed at a time when the traditional nuclear family was emphasized. However, Friedman et al (2003) explore family lifecycle or career stages in divorced families, stepparent families, and domestic-partner relationships. The perfect progress of families from marriage through death is not a current reality. What happens to the stages of the individual or family lifecycle when there is a divorce, death, adoption, and the other multiple forms that we now call family?

## Interactionist Theory

Interactionist theory views families as units of interacting personalities and examines the symbolic communications by which family members relate to one another. Within the family, each member occupies positions to which a number of roles are assigned. Members define their role expectations in each situation through their perceptions of the role demands. Members judge their own behavior by assessing and interpreting the actions of others toward them. The responses of others in the family serve to challenge or reinforce family members' perceptions of the norms of role expectations (Bomar, 1996). Central to the interactionist approach is the process of role taking. Every role exists in relation to some other role, and interaction represents a dynamic process of testing perceptions about each others' roles. The ability to predict other family members' expectations for one's role enables each member to have some knowledge of how to react in the role and indicates how other members will react to performing the role.

George Herbert Mead (1934) is credited with synthesizing previous work to bring together mind, self, and society as major concepts in the school known as symbolic interactionism. He describes the human mind's capacity to organize and control responses by selecting one option over another (reflection) and to derive meaning from symbols and gestures while interacting with others. The self emerges from these interactions with others and is a symbolic object in the mind's eye, apart from the body or from other objects or persons. A person derives the symbolic self from their social group and setting. Changes made in the social order mandate earlier changes in self. For example, family violence cannot be abolished until the "selves" making up society see these practices as criminal acts that violate individuals and families.

Some of the major assumptions are as follows:

- Complex sets of symbols having common meanings are acquired through living in a symbolic environment.
- Individuals distinguish, evaluate, and assign meaning to symbols.
- Behavior is influenced by meanings of symbols or ideas rather than by instincts, needs, or drives; therefore the meaning an individual assigns to symbols is important to understanding behavior.
- The self continues to change and evolve through introspection caused by experience and activity.
- The evolving self has several dimensions: the physical body and characteristics and a complex social self. The "me" is a conventional, habitual self that consists of learned, repetitious responses. The "I" is spontaneous to the individual.
- Individuals are actors as well as reactors; they select and interpret the environment to which they respond.
- Individuals are born into a dynamic society.
- The nature of the infant is determined by the environment and responses to the infant rather than by a predisposition to act in a certain way (genetic versus environmental influences are continually being questioned).
- Individuals learn from the culture and become the society.
- Individuals' behavior is a product of their history, which is continually being modified by new information.

Assessment of families using the interactionist theory emphasizes interaction between and among family members and family communication patterns about health and illness behaviors appropriate for different roles. Nurses intervene with strategies focused on the following (Bomar, 1996):

1. Effectiveness of communications among members
2. Ability to establish communication between nurses and families
3. Clear and concise messages between members
4. Similarities between verbal and nonverbal communication patterns
5. Directions of the interaction

Nurses can center their attention on how family members interact with one another, so this approach is useful in explaining family communication, roles, decision making, and problem solving (Friedman et al, 2003).

The major strength of this approach is the focus on internal processes within families, such as roles, conflict, status, communication, responses to stress, decision making, and socialization. Processes rather than end products of social interactions are the major focus; thus this framework has been used by many nurse scholars. The major weakness is that it is broad and there is lack of agreement about concepts and assumptions of the theory, which has made it difficult to refine. Interactionists consider families to be comparatively closed units with little relationship to the outside society.

The most critical aspect of understanding multiple theories is that they provide a framework for understanding families. Theories or models offer the nurse options or different ways to intervene and support families to achieve health.

---

**HOW TO   Assess a Family Process**

Assessment of families requires an organized plan before you see the family. This plan includes the following:

1. Why are you seeing the family?
2. Who will be present during the interview?
3. Where will you see the family and how will the space be arranged?
4. What are you going to be assessing?
5. How are you going to collect the data?
6. What are you going to do with the information you find?

---

## WORKING WITH FAMILIES FOR HEALTHY OUTCOMES

The goal of collaborating with families is to focus care, interventions and services to achieve the best possible outcome. The **Outcome Present-State Testing Model** (OPT) is a dynamic, systematic clinical reasoning process that emphasizes outcome of care (Pesut and Herman, 1999). Building on the traditional nursing process model, OPT emphasizes organizing care around the keystone issue that is challenging family health. By directing care to resolve the keystone family issue, a ripple effect will occur that results in resolving many peripheral problems. The OPT approach is an outcome-driven model of care. Nurses focus on collaboration with the family to achieve the most desirable outcome.

OPT consists of the following steps, which have been adapted specifically to work with family as client:

1. *Family story.* The family story provides essential information about individual family members and the family as a whole. Getting the family (client) story represents the data collection process. Nurses collect data about the family via a variety of methods (e.g., interviewing the family client, chart review, process logs, phone logs, phone conversations with other professionals, previous visits with the family, school records).

2. *Cue logic.* The nurse places the data into meaningful clusters of evidence. The clusters of evidence identify problems that are influencing the family's adaptation in the given circumstances. Nurses make connections or see relationships between the sets or clusters of data in order to identify the "keystone" or foundation problem affecting the family. By focusing on the keystone issue of concern, the nursing care will have a positive ripple affect, thereby resolving the direct and indirect issues confronting the family health. The keystone issue provides the direction for collaboration with the family in designing the outcome and interventions. The keystone issue is specifically stated as a family nursing diagnosis.

3. *Framing.* The role of the nurse is to help the family understand the present state and determine the best possible outcome. It is in this step that nurses think about the family story through the frame of multiple theory-based approaches, some of which were described earlier. By framing the problem from a theory, potential outcomes can be considered given the whole picture of the family client.

4. *Present state and desired outcome.* The keystone issue is stated as the present problem that needs to be resolved. The outcome is stated in a positive language. By placing side by side the present state with the desired outcome, evaluation criteria become more clear; in OPT, this step is called *testing.* It is these criteria that the nurse will consider to determine if the outcome is being achieved, partially achieved, or not achieved.

5. *Interventions and decision making.* The nurse and family work in a partnership to design and implement a plan of action based on the identified outcome.

6. *Clinical judgment.* Nurses make clinical judgments. If the plan of action is resulting in the achievement of the identified outcome, the nurse may decide to continue with the plan of care or that it is time to put plans in place to terminate the nurse–family partnership. If the outcome is not being achieved or is being partially achieved, it is critical that nurses step outside the situation or event to evaluate and reflect on the whole picture. In essence, the nurse needs to reenter the client story and the OPT process again.

7. *Reflection.* Nurses engage in purposeful, deliberate reflection to learn from the experience and build schemas or mental patterns of client stories—clusters of evidence, keystone issues, outcomes and interventions. This is the critical thinking aspect that

paves the way for nurses to move from novice to expert practitioners.

A more detailed discussion of the OPT model using case scenarios is presented later.

## Family Story

Nurses gather information about and from the family to determine the keystone health concern of the family. Data collection begins when an actual or potential problem is identified by a source, which may be the family, the physician, a school nurse, or a caseworker. Several examples follow:

1. A family is referred to the home health agency because of the birth of the newest family member. In that district, all births are automatically followed up with a home visit.
2. A family calls the Visiting Nurse Association to request assistance in providing care to a family member with a terminal illness.
3. A school nurse is asked to conduct a family assessment by a teacher who noticed that the student has frequent absences and demonstrated significant behavior changes in the classroom.
4. A physician requests a family assessment for a child who has failure to thrive.

The assessment process and data collection begins as soon as the referral occurs. Sources of pre-encounter data the nurse gathers include the following:

- *Referral source.* The information collected from the referral source includes data that leads to identification of a problem for this family. Demographic information and subjective and objective information may be obtained from the referral source.
- *Family.* A family may identify a health care concern and seek help. During the initial intake or screening procedure, valuable information can be collected from the family. Information is collected during phone interaction with the family member, even when calling to set up the initial appointment. This information might include family members' views of the problem, surprise that the referral was made, reluctance to set up the meeting, avoidance in setting up the interview, or recognizing that a referral was made or that a probable health care concern exists.
- *Previous records.* Previous records may be available for review before the first meeting between the nurse and the family. Often, a record release for information is necessary to obtain family or individual records.

Before contacting the family to arrange for the initial appointment, the nurse decides the best place to meet with the family, which might be in the home, clinic, or office. Often this decision is dictated by the type of agency with which the nurse works (e.g., home health is conducted in the home), or the mental health agency may choose to have the family meet in the neighborhood clinic office.

Advantages to meeting in the family home include viewing the everyday family environment. Also, family members are likely to feel more relaxed and thereby demonstrate typical family interactions. Meeting with a family in their home emphasizes that the problem is the responsibility of the whole family and not one family member. Conducting the interview in the home may increase the probability of having more family members present. There are two important disadvantages of meeting in the family's home. Their home may be the only sanctuary or safe place for the family or its members to be away from the scrutiny of others. Meeting with a family on their ground requires the nurse to be highly skilled in communication by setting limits and guiding the interaction.

Conducting the family appointment in the office or clinic allows easier access to other health care providers for consultation. An advantage of using the clinic may be that the family situation is so intense that a more formal, less personal setting may be necessary for the family to begin discussion of emotionally charged issues. A disadvantage of not seeing the everyday family environment is that it may reinforce a possible culture gap between the family and the nurse.

After the decision is made regarding where to meet the family, the nurse contacts the family. It is important to remember that the family gathers information about the nurse from this initial phone call to arrange a meeting, so the nurse should be confident and organized. After the introduction, the nurse concisely states the reason for requesting the family visit and encourages all family members to attend the meeting. Several possible times, including late afternoon or evening, for the appointment can be offered, which allows the family to select the most convenient time for all members to be present.

### HOW TO Set an Appointment With the Family

Data collection starts immediately upon referral to the nurse. The following are suggestions that will make the process of arranging a meeting with the family easier:

1. Remember that the assessment is reciprocal and the family will be making judgments about you when you call to make the appointment.
2. Introduce yourself and the purpose for the contact.
3. Do not apologize for contacting the family. Be clear, direct, and specific about the need for an appointment.
4. Arrange a time that is convenient for all parties and gets the most family members present.
5. Confirm place, time, date, and directions.

## Cue Logic

As nurses gather information about the family, they begin to place the information into meaningful datasets that help them see the whole family (as the client) in context, called **cue logic.** Nurses organize information into logical groups (or clusters) to determine the most important keystone issue challenging the family health. One of the most important pieces of information provided by the referral source is the focus, or the cluster of cues or symptoms, that leads them to believe that a problem might exist. However, it is important to view the family with an open approach as the central issue identified by the referral source may not be the actual keystone issue but may be a peripheral problem that contributes to the keystone issue. See, for example, the following case study:

The Raggs family is referred to the home health clinic by a physician for medication management. Sam, a 73-year-old husband, has been a diabetic for 13 years and has developed insulin-dependent diabetes mellitus. He is being discharged from the hospital. The potential area of concern that prompted the referral was the administration of insulin. After the initial meeting with the family, the nurse finds that administration of the medication is not the central issue for Sam and his wife, Rose. The keystone issue is managing his nutrition. The inference of the referral source was that the family knew how to manage the dietary aspects of diabetes because Sam had had a form of diabetes for 13 years.

If the keystone family issue is not accurately identified, the family and the nurse will collect data, design interventions, and implement plans of care that do not meet the most pressing family's needs. The importance of identifying the keystone family issue and making an accurate family nursing diagnosis is demonstrated by comparing the following two scenarios:

**Scenario 1:** The hypothesized keystone issue for the Raggs family was identified by the referral source: Is insulin being administered correctly by the Raggs family? On the basis of this keystone issue, the nurse collected only information that pertained to that single problem. The family nursing diagnosis was *Lack of family knowledge* related to the administration of insulin secondary to a new diagnosis of insulin-dependent diabetes as evidenced by (1) verbal statements of concern about giving injections, (2) difficulty drawing up the accurate amount of insulin, and (3) questions about the storage of insulin. This nursing diagnosis focuses further data collection and plan for interventions on (1) the psychomotor skills of family members necessary to give the insulin injection, (2) the correct amount of insulin to give according to blood glucose level, and (3) the correct storage and handling of the medication and the equipment. By not looking at the whole family, the nurse based the keystone family nursing diagnosis on a single problem confronting the family—administration of medication. (Figure 24-5 shows an example of linear clinical reasoning.)

**Scenario 2:** The nurse conducts the family assessment by focusing on the whole family client story and asks the following keystone question: What is the best way to ensure that the Raggs family understands how to manage the new diagnosis of insulin-dependent diabetes? After collecting and clustering the evidence

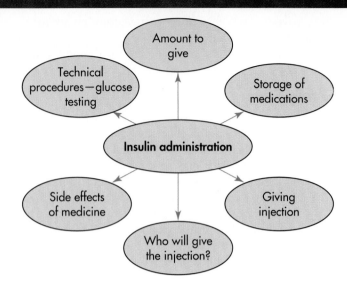

**Figure 24-5** Scenario 1: Keystone issue is *Lack of knowledge* related to medications administration. An example of linear problem-solving reasoning.

into logical groupings, the family nursing diagnosis identified was *Lack of family knowledge* related to nutrition management of a family member who has been newly diagnosed with insulin-dependent diabetes. Administration of the medication is only one aspect of the health problem confronting the Raggs family.

Asking a broader question allows the nurse to view the whole picture of the family dealing with this specific health concern and results in a more comprehensive holistic data-collection process. More evidence was collected in this case scenario because more options for possible interventions were considered concurrently in the clustering of the data. Areas of data collection for this nursing diagnosis were (1) administration of medication, (2) nutritional management, (3) blood glucose monitoring, (4) activity/exercise, (5) coping with a changed diagnosis, and (6) knowledge of pathophysiology of diabetes. The keystone issue for the family centered on nutritional management, which ultimately affects the administration of medication. (Figure 24-6 shows an example of complex clinical reasoning.)

## Framing

The major difference between these two scenarios was the way the nurse framed the question while listening to the family client story. In the first scenario, the nurse asked a question that allowed only one aspect of the family health to be considered. This type of step-by-step linear problem-solving process is tedious and time consuming, and it is likely to cause error in identifying the most pressing (or keystone) family nursing diagnosis. In the second scenario, the nurse asked a question that allowed critical thinking about several options concurrently. The nurse gathered information from the referral source, conducted an assessment of the impact of the new diagnosis

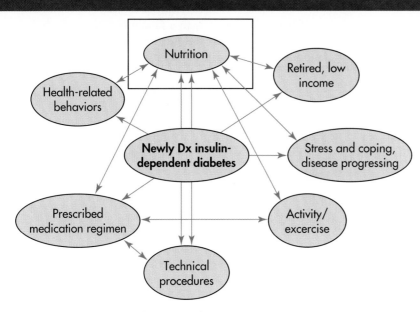

**Figure 24-6** Scenario 2. Keystone issue is *Lack of knowledge* related to nutrition management. An example of complex relationships between issues affecting the whole family because of the new diagnosis.

on the whole family, and made a clinical judgment that had a more far-reaching effect on the health outcome of the family.

The keystone family issue needs to be stated in a way that matches the nursing classification system used in the agency. Nursing classification systems related to families include the North American Nursing Diagnosis Association system (NANDA, 2001), the Omaha system (Martin and Scheet, 1992), the *Diagnostic and Statistical Manual of Mental Disorders* (American Psychiatric Association, 2000), and the *International Classification of Disease* (American Medical Association, 1997). After the keystone family diagnosis has been identified and verified with the family, the next steps are determining the present state, the outcome, and the testing evaluation criteria that will be used to determine if the outcome has been achieved.

## Present State and Outcome Testing

On the basis of the keystone issue, the present state of the health issue challenging the family is clearly identified. The nurse works with the family to determine a realistic outcome, which depends on the ability of the family to successfully adapt to the health issue, which in turn depends on the family's strengths, the pattern of family response in similar past situations, and the trajectory of the family health care problem. The nurse can predict the course of events or the pattern of change expected given information about the family. The types of outcomes possible depend on the focus of the problem for the individual and the family as a whole. The outcome may be directed at preventing a potential problem, minimizing the problem, stabilizing it, or recognizing it as a deteriorating problem. The outcome is the opposite of the presenting problem and should be stated in positive language. A case example showing the importance of focusing on the outcome follows:

**Scenario 3:** The home hospice nurse has been working with the Brush family for 3 weeks. The family consists of the following members: Dylan (the father), Myra (the mother), William (10 years old), Jessica (7 years), and Beatrice (Myra's 73-year-old mother).

*Family story:* Beatrice, Myra's mother, was diagnosed with terminal liver cancer 4 weeks ago. The Brush family agreed that Beatrice should live with them and be cared for in their home until her death. Beatrice has other children who live in the same city. The hospice nurse, in collaboration with the Brush family, identified the following keystone family diagnosis: *Family role conflict* related to the maternal grandmother moving into her daughter's home after being diagnosed with terminal liver cancer. Myra showed her role conflict by stating, "Sometimes I do not know who I am—daughter, nurse, mother, or wife." The outcome is family role sharing, which will be evaluated by statements that describe minimized role strain and spreading the caregiver role among the extended family members.

The nurse, who understands systems theory, knows that what affects one member of the family affects all members of the family. One of the strengths of the family is agreement that caring for the dying grandmother in the home is the right ethical choice for them. Disrupting the family and their expected roles will be short term because the grandmother will probably not live for more than 4 months. The family has a strong internal and external support system. The extended family is willing to be involved in Beatrice's care. The area of change to be experienced by the family members is family roles and the expected behaviors of each family member. The course of events is short term, but Myra's role conflict may increase as her caregiver role becomes more intense as her mother gets worse. The type of outcome is to mobilize resources to minimize Myra's role conflict.

The Brush family story was viewed through the frame of systems theory and the following interventions were implemented: (1) assisting the family in the role negotiation of tasks and who performs them, (2) educating family members so they can safely care for Beatrice, (3) providing respite care for all family members involved in the care process, and (4) referring the case to home hospice.

## Intervention and Decision Making

During the intervention and decision-making step, it is important for nurses to recognize that the family has the right to make its own health decisions. The role of the nurse is to offer guidance to the family, provide information, and assist in the planning process. The nurse and family work in a partnership to design and implement a plan of action on the basis of the identified outcome.

The nurse may assist the family by (1) providing direct care, which the family cannot; (2) removing barriers to needed services, which helps the family to function; and (3) improving the capacity of the family to act on its own behalf and to assume responsibility (Friedman et al, 2003). Decision making can be based on compiling nursing interventions by category (as in the Nursing Intervention Classification [NIC] system), on the Omaha System, or on levels of prevention.

## Clinical Judgment

In making clinical judgments or evaluating the outcome, nurses engage in critical thinking. When an outcome is not achieved, the nurse and the family work together to determine the barriers. Family apathy and indecision are known to be barriers in family nursing (Friedman et al, 2003). Friedman et al (2003) also identified the following nurse-related barriers to achieving the outcome: (1) nurse-imposed ideas, (2) negative labeling, (3) overlooking family strengths, and (4) neglecting cultural or gender implications. Family apathy may occur because of value differences between the nurse and the family, because it is overcome with a sense of hopelessness, because it views the problems as too overwhelming, or because its members have a fear of failure. Additional factors to be considered are that the family may be indecisive because they cannot determine which course of action is better, because they have an unexpressed fear or concern; or because they have a pattern of making decisions only when faced with a crisis.

An important part of the judgment step in working with families is the decision to terminate the relationship between the nurse and the family. Termination is phasing out the nurse from family involvement. When termination is built into the interventions, the family benefits from a smooth transition process. The family is given credit for the outcomes of the interventions that they helped design. Strategies often used in the termination component are decreasing contact with the nurse, extending invitations to the family for follow-up, and making referrals when appropriate. The termination should include a summative evaluation meeting, in which the nurse and family put a formal closure to their relationship.

When termination with a family occurs suddenly, it is important for the nurse to determine the forces bringing about the closure. The family may be initiating the termination prematurely, which requires a renegotiating process. The insurance or agency requirements may be placing a financial constraint on the amount of time the nurse can work with a family. Regardless of how termination comes about, it is an important aspect in working with families.

## Reflection

The last step in the OPT clinical reasoning model is for nurses to engage in critical, creative, and concurrent reflection about the case. This step has three distinct parts. One is to reflect on the client outcome that is, or is not, being achieved. The second purpose of reflection is to add the details of this case to the nurse's mental file (or library of knowledge), and the third purpose is to engage in self-judgment. By stepping outside the action and viewing the whole picture, including the self, nurses get a different perspective on the problem facing the family (Pesut and Herman, 1999, pp. 36-38). Seeing the whole picture from outside the action increases the options for action.

## THE CUTTING EDGE

A genetic revolution is underway that is having major impact on nurses and families. The human genome project (HGP) began in the mid 1980s and is an international research program. The HGP is more than just mapping genes; it addresses issues confronting difficult ethical and psychosocial questions. As HGP rapidly unfolds, mapping our 100,000 genes, families are being confronted with deterministic predictions about their fate.

Feetham S: Families and the genetic revolution: implications for primary health care, education and research, *Families, Systems and Health: Journal of Collaborative Family Health Care,* 17(1):27-42, 1999; Rolland JS: Families and genetic fate: a millennial challenge, *Families, Systems and Health: The Journal of Collaborative Family Health Care* 17(1): 123-132, 1999.

## BARRIERS TO PRACTICING FAMILY NURSING

Many barriers exist that affect the practice of family nursing in a community setting. Two significant barriers to family nursing are the narrow definition of family used by health care providers and social policymakers and the lack of consensus of what is a healthy family. Other barriers to practicing family nursing are summarized by Hanson (2001a):

- Until the last decade, most practicing nurses had little exposure to family concepts during their undergraduate education and have continued to practice using the individual focus. Family nursing was viewed as "common sense" and not a theory-based nursing approach.

- There has been a lack of good comprehensive family assessment models, instruments, and strategies in nursing.
- Nursing has strong historical ties with the medical model, which views families as structure and not central to individual health care.
- The traditional charting system in health care has been oriented to the individual.
- The medical and nursing diagnosis systems used in health care are disease centered, and diseases are focused on individuals.
- Insurance carriers have traditionally based reimbursement and coverage on the individual, not on a family unit.
- The hours during which health care systems provide services to families are at times of day when family members cannot accompany one another.

These and other obstacles to family nursing practice are slowly shifting. Nurses must continue to lobby for changes that are more conducive to caring for the family as a whole.

## FAMILY NURSING ASSESSMENT

**Family nursing assessment** is the cornerstone of family nursing interventions. By using a systematic process, family problem areas are identified and family strengths are emphasized as the building blocks for interventions and to facilitate family resiliency. Building the interventions with family-identified problems and strengths allows for equal family and provider commitment to the solutions and ensures more successful interventions. Two family assessment models and approaches are presented: the **Family Assessment Intervention Model** and the **Family Systems Stressor-Strength Inventory** (FS³I) (Hanson, 2001b; Hanson and Kaakinen, 2001; Hanson and Mischke, 1996), and the Friedman family assessment model and short form (Friedman et al, 2003). Genograms and ecomaps are presented as family assessment strategies that provide a clear, concise picture of intergenerational patterns and social supports or direction of family stress. Nurses are encouraged to select the model and strategy that provides the best fit to their particular philosophy and practice, or they can use a combination of both (see the case study in Appendix H.3).

### NURSING TIP

Assessment is interactive. As you are evaluating families, they are evaluating you.

## Family Assessment Intervention Model and Family Systems Stressor-Strength Inventory (FS³I)

The Family Assessment Intervention Model is based on an extension of Betty Neuman's Neuman Health Care Systems Model and uses a family-as-client approach (Hanson, 2001b; Hanson and Mischke, 1996; Neuman, 1995; Reed, 1993). This model reflects a systems approach. In this model, families are subject to the tensions produced when stressors (see arrows in Figure 24-7), in the form of problems, penetrate their defense system. The family's reaction depends on how deeply the stressor penetrates the family unit and how capable the family is of adapting to maintain its stability. The lines of resistance protect the family's basic structure, which includes the family's functions and energy resources. The core contains the patterns of family interactions and unit strengths. The basic family structure must be protected at all costs or the family will cease to exist. Reconstituting or adapting is the work the family undertakes to preserve or restore impaired family stability after stressors penetrate the family lines of defense, altering usual family functions. The model addresses three areas:

1. Health promotion, wellness activities, problem identification, and family factors at lines of defense and resistance
2. Family reaction and stability at lines of defense and resistance
3. Restoration of family stability and family functioning at levels of prevention

The basic assumptions for this family-focused model are listed in Box 24-5.

An assessment instrument based on this model was developed and named the Family Systems Stressor-Strength Inventory (FS³I) (Hanson, 2001b). The FS³I is a family health assessment/measurement instrument that provides for quantitative and qualitative input by all family members and the nurse. It focuses on identifying stressful situations occurring in families and the strengths families use to maintain health functioning despite their problems. The FS³I is divided into three sections: (1) family systems stressors: general, (2) family stressors: specific, and (3) family system strengths. See Appendix H for the forms.

The data collected by this instrument determine the level of prevention/intervention needed: primary, secondary, and tertiary (Pender, 1996). The primary prevention mode focuses on movement of the individual and family toward a positively balanced state of increased health or health promotion activities. Primary interventions include providing families with information about their strengths, supporting their coping and functioning abilities, and encouraging attempts toward wellness through family education. Secondary prevention modes address actions necessary to attain system stability after the family system has been invaded by stressors or problems. Secondary interventions include helping the family members handle their problems, helping them find and use

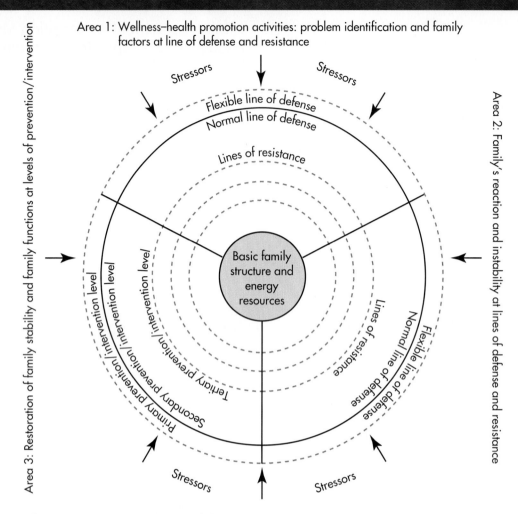

**Figure 24-7** Family Assessment Intervention Model (see text for elaboration). *(From Hanson SMH, Mischke KM: Family health assessment and intervention. In Bomar PJ, editor: Nurses and family health promotion: concepts, assessments, and interventions, Philadelphia, 1996, Saunders; modified from the Neuman Health Care Systems Model.)*

appropriate treatment, and intervening in crises. The tertiary prevention mode includes those actions instituted to maintain systems stability. Tertiary intervention strategies are initiated after treatment has been completed and may include coordination of care after discharge from the hospital or rehabilitation services.

In summary, the FS³I focuses on two concepts of family health: family stressors and family strengths. It provides nurses with entry into the family system to gather data useful for nursing intervention.

## Friedman Family Assessment Model

The **Friedman Family Assessment Model** (Friedman et al, 2003) draws heavily on the structure–function framework and on developmental and systems theory. The model takes a broad approach to family assessment, which views families as a subsystem of society. The family is viewed as an open social system. The family's structure (organization) and functions (activities and purposes) and the family's relationship to other social systems are the focus of this approach.

This assessment approach is important for family nurses because it enables them to assess the family system as a whole, as part of the whole of society, and as an interaction system. The general assumptions for this model are shown in Box 24-6.

The guidelines for the Friedman assessment model consist of six broad categories of interview questions:

1. Identifying data
2. Developmental family stage and history
3. Environmental data
4. Family structure, including communication, power structures, role structures, and family values
5. Family functions, including affective, socialization, and health care
6. Family coping

Each category has several subcategories. There are both long and short forms of this assessment tool (see Friedman et al, 2003).

In summary, this approach was developed to provide guidelines for family nurses who are interviewing a family

---

**BOX 24-5   Basic Assumptions for Family Assessment Intervention Model**

1. Although every family system is unique, each is a composite of commonly understood factors, or innate characteristics, with a normal range of responses contained within a basic structure.

2. Many known, unknown, and universal environmental stressors exist. Each differs in its potential for disturbing a family's usual stability level, or normal line of defense. The particular interrelationships of family variables—physiologic, psychological, sociocultural, developmental, and spiritual—can at any time affect the degree to which a family is protected by the flexible line of defense against possible reaction to one or more stressors.

3. Over time, each family or family system has evolved a normal range of responses to the environment, referred to as a normal line of defense, or a usual wellness/stability state.

4. When the cushioning, accordion-like effect of the flexible line of defense is no longer capable of protecting the family system against an environmental stressor, the stressor breaks through the normal line of defense.

5. The family, whether in a state of wellness or illness, is a dynamic composite of the interrelationships of

variables. Wellness is on a continuum of available energy to support the system in its optimal state.

6. Implicit within each family system is a set of internal resistance factors, known as lines of resistance, which function to stabilize and return the family to the usual wellness state (normal line of defense), or possibly to a higher level of stability, after the family has reacted to and recovered from an environmental stressor reaction.

7. Primary prevention relates to general knowledge that is applied in family assessment and intervention in identifying and mitigating risk factors associated with environmental stressors to prevent possible reaction.

8. Secondary prevention relates to symptoms after reaction to stressors, appropriate ranking of intervention priorities, and treatment to reduce their noxious effects.

9. Tertiary prevention relates to the adjustive processes taking place as reconstitution begins and maintenance factors move the client back in a circular manner toward primary prevention.

10. The family is in dynamic, constant energy exchange with the environment.

---

Based on data from Berkey KM, Hanson SMH: *Pocket guide to family assessment and intervention,* St Louis, 1991, Mosby; Neuman B, editor: The Neuman Systems Model, ed 3, Norwalk, Conn, 1995, Appleton & Lange.

---

to gain an overall view of what is going on in the family. The questions are extensive, and it may not be possible to collect all the data in one visit. All the categories may not be pertinent to every family.

## Summary of Family Assessment Models

Each family nursing assessment model and approach creates a different database on which to plan interventions. The family assessment intervention model and the FS³I measure very specific dimensions and give a microscopic view of family health. The Friedman Family Assessment Model is more broad and general. It is particularly useful for viewing families in their communities (see Appendix H.2). Examples of completed family assessment tools are in the case study presented in Appendix H.3. Many other resources are available for assessing and measuring families. Refer to this book's website at http://evolve.elsevier.com/Stanhope for a list of resources for family assessment and measurement. In addition, Yingling et al (1998) presented a unique way to assess global family functioning.

---

**BOX 24-6   Assumptions Underlying Friedman's Family Assessment Model**

1. The family is a social system with functional requirements.

2. A family is a small group possessing certain generic features common to all small groups.

3. The family as a social system accomplishes functions that serve the individual and society.

4. Individuals act in accordance with a set of internalized norms and values that are learned primarily in the family through socialization.

---

From Friedman MM, Bowden VR, Jones EG: *Family nursing: theory and practice,* ed 5, Upper Saddle River, NJ, 2003, Prentice Hall.

## Genograms and Ecomaps

The **genogram** and **ecomap** are essential components of any family assessment, and they should be used concurrently with any of the assessment approaches just described.

### Genogram

The genogram displays pertinent family information in a family tree format that shows family members and their relationships over at least three generations (McGoldrick, Gerson, and Shellenberger, 1999; De Maria, Hof, and Weeks, 1999). The genogram shows family history and patterns of health-related information, which is a rich source of information for planning interventions. The identified client and his or her family are highlighted on the genogram. Genograms enhance nurses' abilities to make clinical judgments and connect them to family structure and history.

A form that can be used for developing genograms is depicted in Figure 24-8, and the symbols most often used in a genogram are shown in Figure 24-9. An outline for a brief genogram interview is presented in Box 24-7, with genogram interpretive categories in Box 24-8. A sample of a three-generation genogram is depicted and discussed in the case study in Appendix H.3. The health history for all family members (morbidity, mortality, onset of illness) is important information for family nurses and can be the focus of analysis of the family genogram. Most families are cooperative and interested in completing the genogram, which does not have to be completed in one sitting. The genogram becomes a part of the ongoing health care record.

### Ecomap

The ecomap is a visual diagram of the family unit in relation to other units or subsystems in the community. The ecomap serves as a tool to organize and present factual information and thus allows the nurse to have a more holistic and integrated perception of the family situation. The ecomap shows the nature of the relationships among family members, and between family members and the community; it is an overview of the family, picturing both the important nurturing and the important stress-producing connections between the family and the world. The nurse starts with a blank ecomap, which consists of a large circle with smaller circles around it (Figure 24-10). The identified client and his or her family are placed in the center of the large circle. The outer smaller circles around the family unit represent significant people, agencies, or institutions in the family's environment that interact with the family members (Hanson, 2001b). The nature and quality of the relationships, and the direction of energy flow between the family members and the subsystems are shown by different connecting lines.

The ecomap serves as a tool to organize and present information, allowing the nurse to have a more holistic and integrated perception of the family situation. Not only does it portray the present situation but it can also be used to set goals for the future by encouraging connection and exchange with individuals and agencies in the community (see Figure 24-10). A more detailed discussion of ecomapping can be found in Hanson (2001b) and McGoldrick et al (1999). An example of a completed ecomap is shown in the case study in Appendix H.3.

> **( NURSING TIP**
>
> Too much disclosure during the early contacts between the family and nurse may scare the family away. Slow the process down and take time to build trust.

## SOCIAL AND FAMILY POLICY CHANGES

As professionals, nurses are accountable for participating in the development of legislation and **family policy.** Government actions that have a direct or indirect effect on families are called family policy. All government actions, whether at the local, county, state, or national level, affect

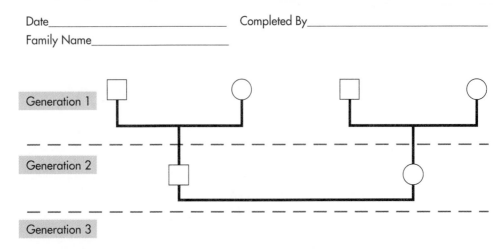

Date_____     Completed By_____

Family Name_____

Generation 1

Generation 2

Generation 3

**Figure 24-8** Genogram form. *(Modified from McGoldrick M, Gerson R:* Genograms in family assessment, *New York, 1985, Norton.)*

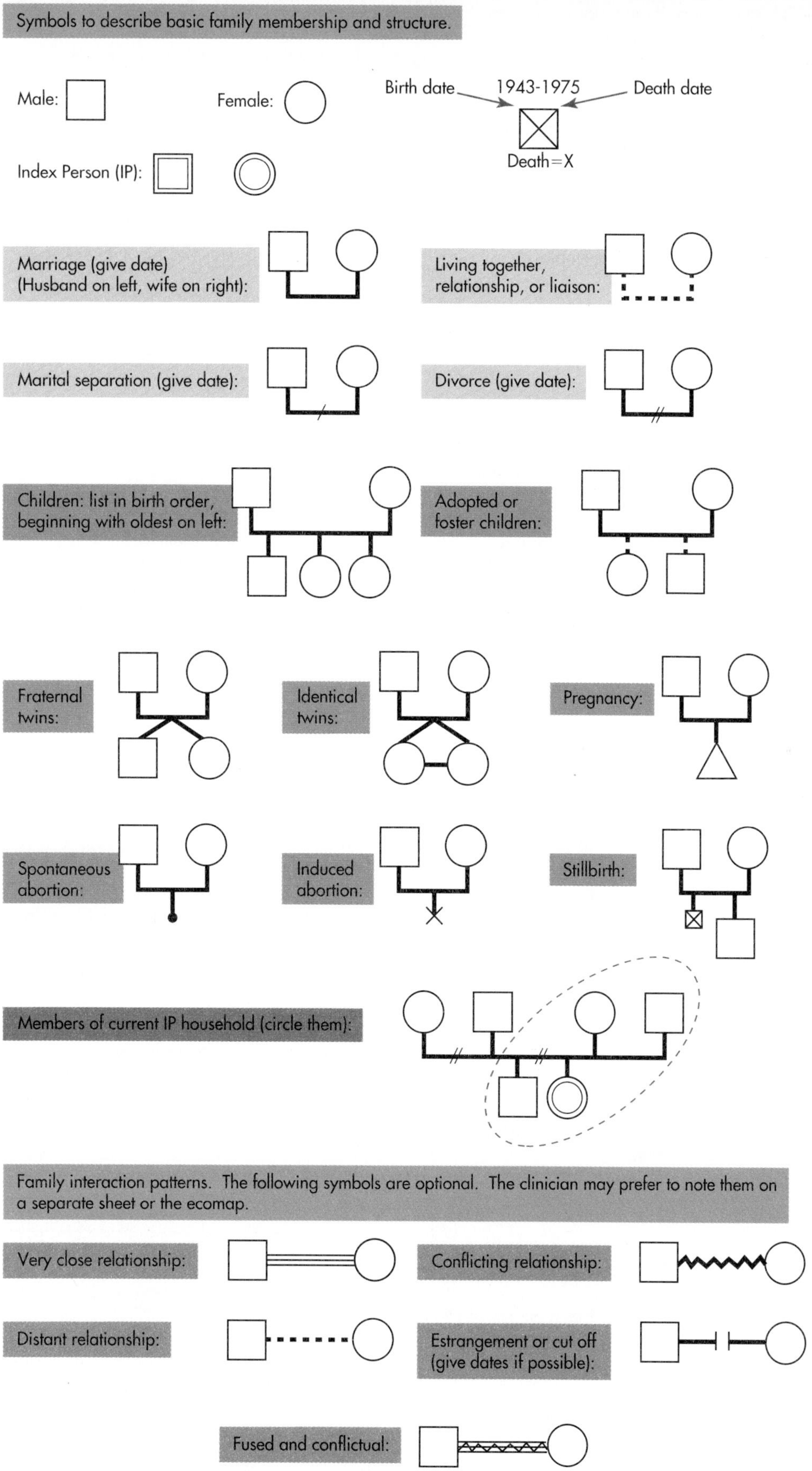

Symbols to describe basic family membership and structure.

Male: ☐    Female: ○    Birth date → 1943-1975 ← Death date

Index Person (IP): ☐    ◎    Death=X

Marriage (give date) (Husband on left, wife on right):

Living together, relationship, or liaison:

Marital separation (give date):

Divorce (give date):

Children: list in birth order, beginning with oldest on left:

Adopted or foster children:

Fraternal twins:

Identical twins:

Pregnancy:

Spontaneous abortion:

Induced abortion:

Stillbirth:

Members of current IP household (circle them):

Family interaction patterns. The following symbols are optional. The clinician may prefer to note them on a separate sheet or the ecomap.

Very close relationship:

Conflicting relationship:

Distant relationship:

Estrangement or cut off (give dates if possible):

Fused and conflictual:

**Figure 24-9** Genogram symbols. *(Modified from McGoldrick M, Gerson R:* Genograms in family assessment, *New York, 1985, Norton.)*

*Continued*

Medical history. Since the genogram is meant to be an orienting map of the family, there is room to indicate only the most important factors, such as major or chronic illnesses and problems. Include dates in parentheses where possible. Use diagnostic labels where available (e.g., cancer, stroke, schizophrenia).

Other family information of special importance may also be noted:

1. Ethnic background and migration date
2. Religion or religious change
3. Education
4. Occupation or unemployment
5. Military service
6. Retirement
7. Trouble with law
8. Physical abuse or incest
9. Obesity
10. Chemical use (smoking, alcohol, marijuana, etc.)
11. Dates when family members left home (e.g., LH '74)
12. Current location of family members

It is useful to have a space at the bottom of the genogram for notes on *other key information*. This would include date of original genogram, critical events, changes in the family structure since the genogram was made, hypotheses, and other notations of major family issues or changes. Notations should always be dated and kept to a minimum since every extra piece of information on a genogram complicates it and therefore diminishes its readability.

**Figure 24-9, cont'd** Genogram symbols. *(Modified from McGoldrick M, Gerson R:* Genograms in family assessment, *New York, 1985, Norton.)*

---

**BOX 24-7  Outline for a Genogram Interview**

For each person on the genogram, the nurse should determine which of the following information to include on the genogram. The information should be relevant to the issues the family is facing.

- First name
- Age
- Date of birth
- Occupation
- Health problems
- Cause of death
- Dates of marriages, divorces, separations, commitments, cohabitation, and remarriages
- Education level
- Ethnic or religious background

Modified from McGoldrick M, Gerson R: *Genograms in family assessment,* New York, 1985, Norton.

---

**BOX 24-8  Genogram Interpretive Categories**

The following areas are important to note in the family genogram:

1. Family structure: nuclear, blended, single-parent household, gay/lesbian relationship, cohabitation, divorces, and separations
2. Sibling subsystem group: birth order, sex, distance between ages of children
3. Patterns of repetition: patterns across the generations related to family structure, behaviors, health problems, relationships, violence, abuse, poverty
4. Life events: repeated similar events across generations, such as transitions, traumas

Modified from McGoldrick M, Gerson R: *Genograms in family assessment,* New York, 1985, Norton.

---

the family either directly or indirectly. The range of **social policy** decisions that affect families is vast, such as health care access and coverage, low-income housing, social security, welfare, food stamps, pension plans, affirmative action, and education. "Although all government polices affect families, in both negative and positive ways, the United States has no overall, official explicit family policy" (Zimmerman, 1992, p. 4). Most government policy indirectly affects families. The Family Leave legislation passed in the 1990s by the U.S. Congress is an example of a type of family policy that has been positive for families. A family member may take a defined amount of leave for family events (e.g., births, deaths) without fear of losing his or her job.

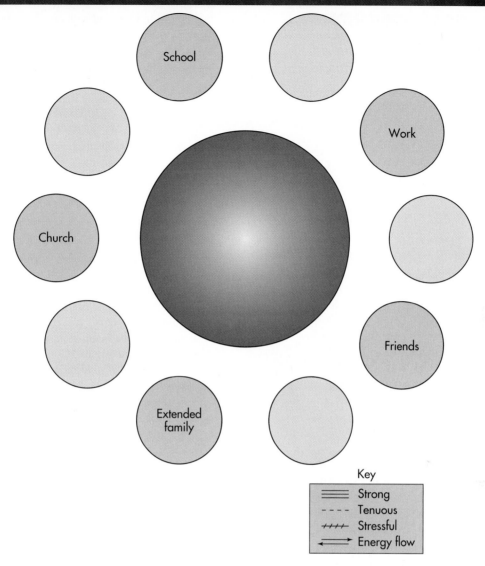

**Figure 24-10** Ecomap form. *(Modified from Friedman MM, Bowden VR, Jones EG:* Family nursing: research and practice, ed 5, *Upper Saddle River, NJ, 2003, Prentice Hall.)*

Public or social policy involves "the use by a regime of its resources to intervene into the accustomed behavior of some of its citizens to produce more or less of that behavior" (Ilchman and Uphoff, 1983). The challenges of social policy for families are numerous. Given the current debate as to what constitutes a family, social policies may specify a definition that is not consistent with the family's own definition. Examples include reproductive issues (e.g., a surrogate mother decides she wants to keep the baby) or issues involving care of older adults (e.g., a niece wants to institutionalize an older demented aunt because the aunt's children are not available).

Reproductive health policy challenges include the current debate on the use of fetal stem cells for research and ultimately as treatment for a variety of diseases. Who owns the placenta and who gets to decide whether it will be used in research? In vitro fertilization has recently caused significant dissent in the judicial system: a couple decides to divorce, but who owns the frozen embryos and who de-

cides their fate? If the mother gets the embryos, is the father legally and financially responsible for the child once it is born? If a woman receives donated sperm and gives birth to a child with significant health problems, who is financially responsible?

As the older generation increases in size, several social policies may be impacted. Will Medicare pay for prescription drugs or will seniors continue to purchase additional insurance? Health care policy is continually in the news. Foster care policies give preference to family members but reimburse differently for family and nonfamily foster care. Flu immunization is creating social challenges: recently, the method of distributing flu vaccine did not anticipate a limited supply of the vaccine. Healthy middle-class people were able to walk into the grocery store and obtain a vaccination, whereas the most vulnerable seniors in nursing homes had yet to receive a supply of vaccine.

The demise of the World Trade Center on September 11, 2001, and the subsequent fear of bioterrorism further raises

## Evidence-Based Practice

Bean, Crane, and Lewis (2002) conducted a content analysis of 440 studies to look at their attention to U.S. ethnic groups. Articles were analyzed according to ethnic population of interest, topic of study, implications for professionals, funding source, and demographic characteristics. Their findings showed an increase in sensitivity and a dedication to ethnic diversity in family science literature. They reported progress in researching African-American and Latino families. However, other ethnic groups are not well researched. Fewer than 16% of the studies focused on other ethnic groups. Only one fourth of the studies were found to make specific recommendations.

**Nurse Use:** These findings raise questions about the ability to generalize nursing interventions to families. This is a serious issue for social/family policymakers, because a policy made for families of one culture may not apply to families of another culture.

Bean RA, Crane DR, Lewis TL: Basic research and implications for practice in family science: a content analysis and status report for US ethnic groups, *Family Relations: Interdisc J Appl Family Stud* 51(1):15-21, 2002.

issues regarding immunization. Will the United States require smallpox vaccines as it did in the past? Who will accept financial responsibility if there is an adverse event because of the vaccination? Will a vaccination be developed for anthrax, and if so who will receive it? If there is a bioterrorist attack, who will receive first access to prevention and treatment? Access, distribution, and manufacturing of vaccines will all be issues in the event of bioterrorism.

Insurance for health care is currently a social policy challenge and will continue to be one in the near future. As health care costs continue to climb, who will receive services and how will those decisions be made? Will we prepare for the future by protecting our children, or will we provide health care services only to those who can afford to pay? Already, baby boomers are choosing to continue working part-time after 65 just for the insurance benefits.

Clearly, community-oriented nurses need to be actively involved in policy that affects families. Families depend on community health nurses to serve as a buffer between social policy and how these policies affect the everyday lives of their clients.

## Practice Application

The idealized family portrayed in the media during the twentieth century consists of a working father, a mother who stays home, and their children. Many families today compare their turbulent, hectic lives with those of the fictionalized past and find their situations wanting.

**A.** Did the idealized version of the traditional family ever really exist?

**B.** Some people believe that American families are in decline, and others believe that families are healthy. What do you think?

**C.** What do you think is happening with American families and what do you think the future will bring?

**D.** What are the implications for the practice of family community nursing?

Answers are in the back of the book.

## Key Points

- Families are the context within which health care decisions are made. Nurses are responsible for assisting families in meeting health care needs.
- Family nursing is practiced in all settings.
- Family nursing is a specialty area that has a strong theoretical base and is more than just common sense.
- Family demographics is the study of structures of families and households as well as events that alter the family, such as marriage, divorce, births, cohabitation, and dual careers.
- Demographic trends affecting the family include the older age of individuals when they marry, increase in interracial marriages, frequent remarriage of divorced people, increase in dual-career marriages, increase in number of children from maritally disrupted families, high divorce rate that has leveled off, dramatic increase in cohabitation, increased number of children who spend time in a single-parent family, delay of childbirth, increase in number of children born to women who are single or who have never married, and increase in number of children who live with grandparents.
- Traditionally, families have been defined as nuclear: mother, father, and young children. There is a variety of family definitions, such as a group of two or more, a unique social group, and two or more persons joined together by emotional bonds.
- The six functions performed by families are economic survival, reproduction, protection, cultural heritage, socialization of young, and conferring status.
- Family structure refers to the characteristics, sex, age, and number of the individual members who make up the family unit.
- Family health is difficult to define, but it includes the biological, psychological, sociologic, cultural, and spiritual factors of the family system.
- There are four approaches to viewing families: family as context, family as client, family as a system, and family as a component of society.
- Structure–function frameworks view the family as a social system with members who have specific roles and functions.

- Systems theory describes families as a unit of the whole composed of members whose interactional patterns are the focus of attention.
- Family development is one theoretical framework used to study families. This approach emphasizes how families change over time and focuses on interactions and relationships among family members.
- Interactional framework focuses on the family as a unit of interacting personalities and examines the communication processes by which family members relate to one another.
- Nurses should ask clients whom they consider to be family and then include those members in the health care plan.
- The OPT nursing process is a dynamic, systematic, organized method of critically thinking about the family.
- The purpose of the initial family meeting is to identify the health concerns of the family.
- The family nursing diagnosis is based on the keystone issue.
- The role of the nurse is to help the family understand the present state and determine the best possible outcome.
- It is important for the nurse to recognize that the family has the right to make its own health decisions.
- Two family assessment models and approaches are the family assessment intervention model and the Family Systems Stressor-Strength Inventory (FS³I) and the Friedman Family Assessment Model.
- The Friedman Family Assessment Model takes a macroscopic approach to family assessment, which views the family as a subsystem of society.
- The FS³I measures very specific dimensions and gives a microscopic view of health.
- The whole family picture is enhanced by merging data from both assessment tools.
- Genograms and ecomaps are essential components of any family assessment.
- All government actions, whether at the local, county, state, or national level, affect the family.

## Clinical Decision-Making Activities

1. Select six or more health professionals and ask them to define family. Analyze the responses for common points and differences. Write your own definition of family.
2. Define family nursing.
3. Discuss how family as client fits into nursing practice.
4. Form small groups and discuss the implications of family demography and demographic trends for nursing.
5. Characterize the different family structures and household arrangements represented in your community. This information may be available from

various sources, such as the health department, schools, other social and welfare agencies, and census data. Be specific.

6. Identify five barriers to practicing family nursing in a community setting. How can you check that these are real barriers?
7. Describe how a family assessment is different from an individual client assessment. What makes these differences complex?
8. Discuss the importance of determining the keystone issue for a family. How can you verify the issue?
9. What kind of difficulties might you experience when arranging for a meeting with a family? Are you considering the family's input?
10. Discuss factors to be considered when determining the place to conduct a family assessment interview. Include pros and cons of each meeting place.
11. How would you select which family assessment tool to use? How can you test the differences?
12. Describe and compare the Family Systems Stressor-Strength Inventory (FS³I) assessment tool and the Friedman Family Assessment Model. What evidence are you using to determine the differences?
13. Draw your own family genogram and ecomap. Discuss how they are used in family nursing.
14. Discuss the role of nursing related to family policy. Be specific about issues related to family culture.
15. Summarize and contrast the four family social science theories. Be specific.
16. Break into small groups and have students discuss the family in terms of the four family social science theories. Examine different situations when one theory is more appropriate to use than another.

## Additional Resources

These related resources are found either in the appendix at the back of this book or on the book's website at **http://evolve.elsevier.com/Stanhope.**

### Appendixes

Appendix H.2 Friedman Family Assessment Model (short form)

### *evolve* Evolve Website

Appendix A.1 Schedule of Clinical Preventive Services

Appendix H.1 Family Systems Stressor-Strength Inventory

Appendix H.3 Case Example of Family Assessment

WebLinks: Healthy People 2010

List of Family Assessment Tools

# References

American Medical Association: *International classification of diseases: clinical modifications* (ICD-9-CM), Vols 1 and 2, 9th revision, Dover, Del, 1997, AMA.

American Psychiatric Association: *Diagnostic & statistical manual of mental disorders (DSM-IV-TR),* ed 4, Washington, DC, 2000, APA.

Aroian KJ, Norris AE: Somatization and depression among former Soviet immigrants, *J Cult Divers* 6(3):93-101, 1999.

Aroian KJ, Norris AE: Resilience, stress, and depression among Russian immigrants to Israel, *West J Nurs Res* 22(1):54-67, 2000.

Aroian KJ, Spitzer A, Bell M: Family stress and support among former Soviet immigrants, *West J Nurs Res* 18(6):655-674, 1996.

Aroian J et al: Health and social service utilization among elderly immigrants from the former Soviet Union, *J Nurs Scholarsh* 33(3):265-271, 2001.

Artinian NT: Selecting model to guide family assessment, *Dimens Crit Care Nurs* 14(1):4, 1994.

Bean RA, Crane DR, Lewis TL: Basic research and implications for practice in family science: a content analysis and status report for US ethnic groups, *Family Relations: Interdisc J Appl Family Stud* 51(1):15-21, 2002.

Bengtson VL: Beyond the nuclear family: the increasing importance of multigenerational bonds, *J Marriage Family* 63:1-16, 2001.

Berkey KM, Hanson SMH: *Pocket guide to family assessment and intervention,* St Louis, Mo, 1991, Mosby.

Bomar P: *Nurses and family health promotion: concepts, assessment, and interventions,* ed 2, Philadelphia, 1996, Saunders.

Boyd M, Norris D: The crowded nest: young adults at home, *Canadian Social Trends* 52:2-5, 1999.

Bryson K, Casper LM: *Coresident grandparents and grandchildren, current populations reports: special studies,* P23-198, U.S. Department of Commerce, U.S. Census Bureau, Washington, DC, 1999, U.S. Government Printing Office.

Carlson M, Danziger S: *Cohabitation and the measurement of child poverty,* Poverty Measurement Working Papers, U.S. Census Bureau, pp 1-8, 1998, U.S. Government Printing Office.

Carter B, McGoldrick M: The family life cycle and family therapy: an overview. In Carter B, McGoldrick M, editors: *The changing family life cycle: a framework for family therapy,* New York, 1998, Gardner Press.

Coleman M, Ganong L, Fine M: Reinvestigating remarriage: another decade of progress, *J Marriage Family* 62:1288-1307, 2000.

Curran D: *Traits of a healthy family,* Minneapolis, 1983, Winston Press.

Curran D: *Stress and the healthy family,* Minneapolis, 1985, Winston Press.

Dalaker J: *Poverty in the United States: 2000,* U.S. Census Bureau, Department of Commerce, 2001, U.S. Government Printing Office.

Davidson JK, Moore NB: *Marriage and family: change and continuity,* Boston, 1996, Allyn & Bacon.

De Maria R, Weeks G, Hof L: *Focused genograms,* New York, 1999, Taylor and Francis.

Duncan L, Simmons M: Health practices among Russian and Ukrainian immigrants, *J Community Health Nurs* 13(2):129-137, 1996.

Duvall EM, Miller BC: *Marriage and family development,* ed 6, New York, 1985, Harper & Row.

Feetham S: Families and the genetic revolution: implications for primary health care, education and research, *Families, Systems and Health: Journal of Collaborative Family Health Care,* 17(1):27-42, 1999.

Fields J, Casper LM: *American's families and living arrangements,* P20-537, U.S. Census Bureau, Department of Commerce, pp 1-16, 2001, U.S. Government Printing Office.

Finnie R: The dynamics of poverty in Canada: what we know, what we can do, *C.D. Howe Institute Commentary* 145(Sept), 2000.

Friedman MM: *Family nursing: research, theory and practice,* ed 4, Norwalk, Conn, 1998, Appleton & Lange.

Friedman MM, Bowden VR, Jones EG: *Family nursing: research, theory and practice,* ed 5, Upper Saddle River, NJ, 2003, Prentice Hall.

Gelles RJ: *Sociology: an introduction,* ed 5, New York, 1995, McGraw-Hill.

Government of Canada: *Services for children: guide to government of Canada services for children and their families,* pp 6-7, Ottawa, 2001, Minister of Public Works and Government Services.

Hanson SMH: Family health care nursing: an overview. In Hanson SMH: *Family health care nursing: theory, practice and research,* ed 2, Philadelphia, 2001a, Davis.

Hanson SMH: Family nursing assessment and intervention. In Hanson SMH: *Family health care nursing: theory, practice, and research,* Philadelphia, 2001b, Davis.

Hanson SMH, Kaakinen J: Theoretical foundations for family nursing. In Hanson SMH: *Family health care nursing: theory, practice, and research,* Philadelphia, 2001, Davis.

Hanson SMH, Mischke KM: Family health assessment and intervention. In Bomar PJ, editor: *Nurses and family health promotion: concepts, assessments and interventions,* ed 2, Philadelphia, 1996, Saunders.

Hawley DR: Toward a definition of family resilience: integrating life-span and family perspectives, *Family Process* 35:283-298, 1996.

Hawley DR: Clinical implications of family resilience, *Am J Fam Ther* 28:101-116, 2000.

Ilchman WF, Uphoff NT: Public policy and organizational theory. In Hall RH, Quinn RE, editors: *Organizational theory and public policy,* Beverly Hills, Calif, 1983, Sage.

Kreider RM, Fields JM: *Number, timing and duration of marriages and divorces: 1996,* P1-20, U.S. Census Bureau, Department of Commerce, 2002, U.S. Government Printing Office.

Leclere RB, Jensen L, Biddlecom AE: Health care utilization, family context, and adaptation among immigrants to the United States, *J Health Social Behav* 35:370-384, 1994.

Lindsay C: Seniors: a diverse group aging well, *Canadian Social Trends* 52:24-56, 1999.

Martin K, Scheet M: *The Omaha system: application for community health nursing,* Philadelphia, 1992, Saunders.

McGoldrick M, Gerson R: *Genograms in family assessment,* New York, 1985, Norton.

McGoldrick M, Gerson R, Shellenberger S: *Genograms: assessment and intervention,* ed 2, New York, 1999, Norton.

Mead G: *Mind, self and society,* Chicago, 1934, University of Chicago Press.

Milan A: One hundred years of families, *Canadian Social Trends* 56:2-13, 2000.

Ministry of Industry: Births, *Health Rep* 13(2), 2002.

Neuman B, editor: *The Neuman systems model,* ed 3, Norwalk, Conn, 1995, Appleton & Lange.

North American Nursing Diagnosis Association: *Nursing diagnoses: definitions and classifications, 2000-2001,* Philadelphia, 2001, NANDA.

Patterson JM: Integrating family resilience and family stress theory, *J Marriage Fam* 64(5):349-360, 2002a.

Patterson JM: Understanding family resilience, *J Clin Psychol* 58(3):233-246, 2002b.

Pender N: *Health promotion in nursing practice,* Stamford, Conn, 1996, Appleton & Lange.

Perry-Jenkins M, Repetti RL, Crouter AC: Working and family in the 1990s, *J Marriage Fam* 62:981-998, 2000.

Pesut D, Herman J: *Clinical reasoning: the art and science of critical and creative thinking,* Boston, 1999, Delmar.

Reed KS: *Betty Neuman: the Neuman systems model,* Newbury Park, Calif, 1993, Sage.

Rolland JS: Families and genetic fate: a millennial challenge, *Families, Systems and Health: The Journal of Collaborative Family Health Care* 17(1):123-132, 1999.

Satariano HJ, Briggs NJ: The good family syndrome. In Wegner GD, Alexander RJ: *Readings in family nursing,* ed 2, Philadelphia, 1999, Lippincott.

Seltzer JA: Families formed outside of marriage, *J Marriage Fam* 62:1247-1268, 2000.

Simmons R, O'Neill G: *Households and families: 2000,* P1-8, U.S. Census Bureau, Department of Commerce, 2001, U.S. Government Printing Office.

Smith L: New Russian immigrants: health, problems, practices and values, *J Cult Divers* 3(3):68-73, 1996.

Stacey J: *In the name of the family: rethinking family values in the postmodern age,* Boston, 1996, Beacon Press.

Statistics Canada: *Population, density, births, and deaths for selected countries,* Ottawa, 2000, Statistics Canada, available at www.statcan.ca/english/Pgdb/demo01.htm (or go to www.statcan.ca and search for document name).

Statistics Canada: *Census families: number, and average size 1971-2000,* retrieved July 4, 2002a, from www.statcan.ca/english/Pgdb/famil40a.htm (or go to www.statcan.ca and search for document name).

Statistics Canada: Changing conjugal life in Canada, *The Daily* July 11, 2002b, retrieved from www.statcan.ca/Daily/English/020711/d020711a.htm, (or go to www.statcan.ca, The Daily, and search for document name).

Statistics Canada: *Profile of Canadian families and households: diversification continues,* 2002c, retrieved from www.statcan.ca/English/IPS/data/96F0030XIE2001003.htm (or go to www.statcan.ca and search for document name).

Statistics Canada: *Census families: numbers, average size, husband-wife and lone parent families,* 2002d, retrieved from www.statcan.ca/english/Pgdb/famil40b.htm (or go to www.statcan.ca and search for document name).

Statistics Canada: *Marriages: 1998-2002,* 2002e, retrieved from www.statcan.ca/english/Pgdb/famil04.htm (or go to www.statcan.ca and search for document name).

Statistics Canada: Divorces, *The Daily,* Dec 2, 2002f, retrieved from www.statcan.ca/Daily/English/021202/d021202f.htm (or go to www.statcan.ca, The Daily, and search for document name).

Statistics Canada: Marriages, *The Daily,* Feb 6, 2003, retrieved from www.statcan.ca/Daily/English?030206/d030206c.htm (or go to www.statcan.ca, The Daily, and search for document name).

Sweeney MM: Remarriage and the nature of divorce, *J Fam Issues* 33(3):410-440, 2002.

Teachman JD, Polonko KA, Scanzioni J: Demography of the family. In Sussman MB, Steinmetz SK, editors, *Handbook of marriage and the family,* New York, 1987, Plenum Press.

Teachman JD, Tedrow LM, Crowder KD: The changing demography of America's families, *J Marriage Fam* 62:1234-1246, 2000.

Thomson E et al: Remarriage, cohabitation, and changes in mothering behavior, *J Marriage Fam* 63:370-380, 2001.

Thornton A, Young-DeMarco L: Four decades of trends in attitudes toward family issues in the United States: the 1960s through the 1990s, *J Marriage Fam* 63:1009-1037, 2001.

Tran TV et al: Living arrangement, depression, and health status among elderly Russian-speaking immigrants, *J Gerontol Social Work* 33(2):63-77, 2000.

U.S. Bureau of the Census: *Characteristics of the foreign born by place of birth.* Retrieved January 28, 2002 from http://www.census.gov/popluation/www/socdemo/foreign/p20-534.html#bi, updated 2000.

U.S. Bureau of the Census: *Statistical abstract of the United States,* section 2, *Vital statistics,* P57-88, 2001.

U.S. Department of Health and Human Services: *Healthy people 2010: understanding and improving health,* ed 2, Washington DC, 2000, U.S. Government Printing Office.

Ventura SJ, Bachrach CA: Nonmarital childbearing in the United States, 1940-99, *Natl Vital Stat Rep* 48(6):1-39, 2000.

Walsh F: The concept of family resilience: crisis and challenge, *Fam Process* 35(3):261-281, 1996.

Walsh F: A family resilience framework: innovative practice applications, *Fam Relat* 51:130-137, 2002.

Wei C, Spigner C: Health status and clinic utilization among refugees from Southeast Asia and the former Soviet Union, *J Health Educ* 25(5):266-273, 1994.

White JM, Klein DN: *Family theories: an introduction,* ed 2, Thousand Oaks, Calif, 2002, Sage.

*World Almanac & Book of Facts:* Interracial married couples in the U.S., 1960-2000, p 882, New York, 2002, World Almanac Books.

Yingling L et al: *GARF: assessment source book: using the DSM-IV global assessment of relational functioning,* Washington DC, 1998, Brunner/Mazel.

Zimmerman S: *Family policies and family well-being: the role of political culture,* Newbury Park, Calif, 1992, Sage International.

Zukewich N: Paid and unpaid work. In *Women in Canada: a gender based statistical report: 2000,* Ottawa, 2000, Minister of Industry.

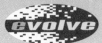
# Chapter 25

# Family Health Risks

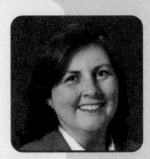

### Debra Gay Anderson, Ph.D., R.N.C.

Debra Gay Anderson is currently an associate professor of nursing at the College of Nursing of the University of Kentucky in Lexington. She is a certified public health nurse who has provided health care for homeless and other vulnerable populations. Dr. Anderson has taught public health, epidemiology, and research courses at the graduate and undergraduate levels. Her program of research, publications, and presentations are primarily about vulnerable populations, with a focus on vulnerable women. Dr. Anderson completed a family nursing postdoctoral fellowship at Oregon Health Sciences University.

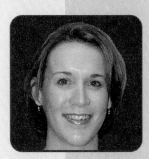

### Heather Ward, R.N., M.S.N.

Heather Ward graduated from Asbury College in 1999 with a bachelor's degree in biology, and from the University of Kentucky in 2000 with a bachelor of science in nursing degree. After working in intensive care, she returned to the University of Kentucky to obtain a master's degree in nursing through the family nurse practitioner program in 2003. While in the master's degree program, Heather worked as a research assistant to Dr. Anderson, participating in grant and manuscript preparation and poster presentations at the national conference of the American Public Health Association.

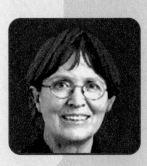

### Diane C. Hatton, R.N., C.S., D.N.Sc.

Diane Hatton is a certified clinical nurse specialist in community health nursing. She is a professor at the Hahn School of Nursing and Health Science, where she teaches courses related to community health nursing and qualitative research methods. Dr. Hatton's research program focuses on health and health care access for vulnerable populations, including homeless women and children.

## Objectives

After reading this chapter, the student should be able to do the following:

1. Analyze the various approaches to defining and conceptualizing family health
2. Analyze the major risks to family health
3. Analyze the interrelationships among individual health, family health, and community health
4. Explain the relevance of knowledge about family structures, roles, and functions for family-focused, community-oriented nursing
5. Discuss the implications of policy and policy decisions, at all governmental levels, on families
6. Explain the application of the nursing process (assessment, planning, implementation, evaluation) to reducing family health risks and promoting family health

A focus on the family is vital in promoting the health of individuals as well as the health of the community (Bomar, 1996; Nightingale et al, 1978). The family as a client unit is basic to the practice of community-oriented nursing, and nurses are responsible for promoting healthy families in society. Families in the twenty-first century continue to be more diverse. The purpose of this chapter is to make the reader aware of influences, both individual and societal, that place families at risk for poor health outcomes, and to discuss how positive outcomes for families can be accomplished.

First, it is important to place the family in the context of the twenty-first century. Americans tend to idealize *family* and wish for a return to family values and a golden time for families. However, that time of idealized families never occurred (Coontz, 1997). Instead of looking into the past and wishing for a time when families were cohesive, a look at the future is needed to recognize the weaknesses that families have, and to build on their strengths. Rather than arguing for a return to the traditional family (male breadwinner and woman at home), serious discussions are needed about how to make today's diverse families succeed (Coontz, 1997). These discussions can lead to policy

*The authors acknowledge the work of Carol Loveland-Cherry in previous editions.*

## Key Terms

behavioral risk, p. 606
biological risk, p. 600
contracting, p. 611
economic risk, p. 604
empowerment, p. 612
family crisis, p. 598
family health, p. 597
health risk appraisal, p. 598

health risk reduction, p. 598
health risks, p. 598
home visits, p. 607
in-home phase, p. 610
initiation phase, p. 608
life-event risk, p. 601
policy, p. 595
postvisit phase, p. 610

previsit phase, p. 608
risk, p. 596
social risks, p. 602
termination phase, p. 610
transitions, p. 601
*See Glossary for definitions*

## Chapter Outline

Early Approaches to Family Health Risks
*Health of Families*
*Health of the Nation*
Concepts in Family Health Risk
*Family Health*
*Health Risk*
*Health Risk Appraisal*

Health Risk Reduction
*Life Events*
*Family Crisis*
Major Family Health Risks and Nursing
   Interventions
*Family Health Risk Appraisal*
Community-Oriented Nursing Approaches
   to Family Health Risk Reduction

Home Visits
Contracting With Families
Empowering Families
Community Resources
*Family Policy*

decisions that have a positive effect on single-parent families, remarried and stepfamilies, gay and lesbian families, grandparent-headed families, and ethnically diverse families. Building support for families within society will lead to healthier families. Therefore, nurses should be involved in community assessment, planning, development, and evaluation activities that emphasize family issues and how to sustain families.

**Policy** is one method nurses can use to influence family health. Family policy means anything that is done by the government that directly or indirectly affects families. Family policy demonstrates a government's understanding of families and its role in promoting their health. The United States is beginning to develop specific "family policies" that either directly or indirectly affect families. Each state, as well as regions within states, has programs and laws related to family services. Although responsibility of the federal government in family programs and other sectors is shared with lower levels of government, health disparities have grown, and many families are without health insurance or adequate coverage (U.S. Department of Health and Human Services [USDHHS], 2000). The United States would benefit from a cohesive family policy to enhance the well-being of families. Policy is discussed in more detail in Chapter 8.

In establishing health objectives for the nation, an emphasis has been placed on both health promotion and risk reduction. Reducing the risks to segments of the population is a direct way of improving the health of the general population. Specific risks have been identified and related to specific objectives. The family is both an important environment affecting the health of individuals and a social unit whose health is basic to that of the community and the larger population. It is within the family that health values, health habits, and health risk perceptions are developed, organized, and performed. Individuals' health behaviors are affected by and acted out within the family environment, the larger community, and society. In the same manner, it is in the context of community norms and values that family health habits are developed, and they are developed on the basis of availability and accessibility. For example, in a television commercial for an over-the-counter stimulant, a man is featured who is able to coach his child's basketball team, work at a rehabilitation center, and work as a borough inspector for the city, and he is pursuing a college degree at night. The commercial credits the drug for providing the man with the energy needed to be successful in all of these areas. The message is clear: you can, and must, do it all, and taking drugs to succeed is a viable option. The health risks to individual and family health are affected by the societal norms—in this example, the norm is increasing productivity through drugs.

To intervene effectively and appropriately with families to reduce their health risk and thereby promote their health, it is necessary to understand family structure and functioning, family theory, nursing theory, and models of health risk (see Chapters 9, 14, and 24). However, it is necessary to go beyond the individual and the family and understand the complex environment in which the family exists. Increasing evidence of the effects of social, biological, economic, and life events on health requires a broader approach to addressing health risks for families. Pender (2002) identified six categories of risk factors: genetics, age, biological characteristics, personal health habits, lifestyle, and environment. In this chapter, health risks in these six categories for families are identified and analyzed, and approaches to reducing these risks are discussed. Options for structuring nursing interventions with families to decrease health risks and to promote health and well-being are explored.

## EARLY APPROACHES TO FAMILY HEALTH RISKS

### Health of Families

Historically, study of the family in health and illness focused on three major areas: (1) the effect of illness on families, (2) the role of the family in the cause of disease, and (3) the role of the family in its use of services. In his classic review of the family as an important unit, Litman (1974) pointed out the important role that the family (as a primary unit of health care) plays in health and illness and emphasized that the relationship between health, health behavior, and family "is a highly dynamic one in which each may have a dramatic effect on the other" (Litman, 1974, p. 495). Mauksch (1974) proposed the idea of distinguishing between family health and individual health. Pratt's (1976) examination of the role of the family in health and illness included the role of family health in promoting behavior. Pratt proposed the *energized family* as being an ideal family type that was most effective in meeting health needs. The energized family is characterized by promoting freedom and change, active contact with a variety of other groups and organizations, flexible role relationships, equal power structure, and a high degree of autonomy in family members. Doherty and McCubbin (1985) proposed a family health and illness cycle with six phases, beginning with family health promotion and risk reduction and continuing through the family's vulnerability to illness, their illness response, their interaction with the health care system, and finally their ways of adapting to illness.

### Health of the Nation

Increased attention has been given to improving the health of everyone in the United States. As a result of major public health and scientific advances, the leading causes of morbidity and mortality shifted from infectious diseases to chronic diseases, accidents, and violence, all of which have strong lifestyle and environmental components. A population-focused study in Alameda County, California, (Belloc and Breslow, 1972) demonstrated relationships between seven lifestyle habits and decreased morbidity and mortality. These habits were (1) sleeping 7 to 8 hours daily, (2) eating breakfast almost every day, (3) never or rarely eating between meals, (4) being at or near recommended height-adjusted weight, (5) never smoking cigarettes, (6) moderate or no use of alcohol, and (7) regular physical activity. These lifestyle health habits are still important for improved health in the twenty-first century.

A growing body of literature supports the notion that lifestyle and the environment interact with heredity to cause disease. In response to these findings and the to limited effect of medical interventions on the growing incidence and prevalence of injuries and chronic disease, the government launched a major effort to address the health status of the population. Part of this effort was a report by the Division of Health Promotion and Disease Prevention of the Institute of Medicine that examined the critical components of the physical, socioeconomic, and family environments related to decreasing risk and promoting health (Nightingale et al, 1978). The Surgeon General's Report on Health Promotion and Disease Prevention (Califano, 1979) described the risks to good health. Health objectives for the nation were established and then evaluated and restated for the year 2000 and again for 2010 (USDHHS, 2000).

The notion of **risk,** a factor predisposing or increasing the likelihood of ill health, takes on increased importance. Specific attention is paid to those environmental and behavioral factors that lead to ill health with or without the influence of heredity. Reducing health risks is a major step toward improving the health of the nation. Although the family is considered an important environment related to achieving important health objectives, limited attention has been given to (or research done on) family health risk and the role of society in promoting healthy families. The Healthy People 2010 box shows objectives that relate to families.

## CONCEPTS IN FAMILY HEALTH RISK

Two things motivate individuals to participate in health behaviors. One is a desire to promote one's own health, using "behaviors directed toward increasing the level of well-being and actualizing the health potential of individuals, families, communities and society" (Pender, 2002, p. 7). The second is a desire to protect health, using those behaviors "directed toward decreasing the probability of specific illness or dysfunction in individuals, families, and communities, including active protection against unnecessary stressors" (Pender, 2002, p. 7). An individual can reduce health risk by engaging in health protecting and health promoting behaviors.

Understanding family health risk requires an examination of several related concepts: family health, family health risk, risk appraisal, risk reduction, life events, lifestyle, and family crisis. These concepts will be defined and discussed. It important to remember that *health* can be defined in a number of ways, and it is defined by individuals within their own culture and value system.

## Family Health

Family theorists refer to healthy families but generally do not define family health. Based on the variety of perspectives of family (see Chapters 9, 14, and 24), definitions of healthy families can be derived within the guidelines of any one of the frameworks. For example, within the perspective of the developmental framework, **family health** can be defined as possessing the abilities and resources to accomplish family developmental tasks. Thus the accomplishment of stage-specific tasks is one indicator of family health.

From the perspective of Neuman Systems Model (1995), family health is defined in terms of system stability as characterized by five interacting sets of factors: physiologic, psychological, sociocultural, developmental, and spiritual. Neuman Systems Model is a wellness-oriented model in which the nurse uses strengths and resources to keep the system stable while adjusting to stress reactions that lead to health change and wellness. In other words, this model focuses on family wellness in the face of change. In this model, the client family is seen as a whole system with the five interacting factors. Because change is inevitable in every family, Neuman Systems Model proposes that families have a flexible external line of defense, a normal line of defense, and an internal line of resistance. When a life event is big enough to contract the flexible line of defense (a protective mechanism) and breaks through the normal line of defense, the family feels stress. The degree of wellness is determined by the amount of energy it takes for the system to become and remain stable. When more energy is available than is being used, the system remains stable. Examples of energy building characteristics in this system are social support, resources, and prevention (or avoidance) of stressors. Nurses can use preventive health care both to reduce the possibility that a family encounters a stressor

and to help strengthen the family's flexible line of defense (see Chapter 9). The following clinical example applies the Neuman Systems Model to one family's situation:

The Harris family consists of Ms. Harris (Gloria), 12-year-old Kevin, 8-year-old Leisha, and Ms. Harris's mother, 75-year-old Betty. Kevin was recently diagnosed with insulin-dependent diabetes mellitus, and the family was referred by the endocrinology clinic to the public health nursing service at the local health department to work with the family in adjusting to the diagnosis.

The focus of Neuman Systems Model would be to assess the family's ability to adapt to this stressful change and then focus on their strengths in the stabilizing process. The *five interacting variables* would be an important component of the assessment:

- *Physiologic:* Is the Harris family physically able to deal with Kevin's illness? Is everyone else in the family currently healthy? Are there current health stressors?
- *Psychological:* How well will the family be able to deal with the illness psychologically? Are their relationships stable and healthy? Are there any memories of other family members with diabetes?
- *Sociocultural:* How will the sociocultural variable come into play in Kevin's illness? Does the family have social support? Are the treatment and diagnosis culturally sensitive? Can family members support each other?
- *Developmental:* How will Kevin's development as a preadolescent be affected by diabetes? How will the family's development change? How will Kevin's diagnosis affect Leisha?
- *Spiritual:* How will the family's spiritual beliefs be affected by the diagnosis? What effect will they have on his treatment and willingness to adhere to therapy?

## Health Risk

Several factors contribute to the development of healthy or unhealthy outcomes. Clearly, not everyone exposed to the same event will have the same outcome. The factors that determine or influence whether disease or other unhealthy results occur are called **health risks.** Controlling health risks is done through disease prevention and health promotion efforts. Health risks can be classified into general categories. Healthy People 2010 (USDHHS, 2000) identifies major categories: inherited biological risk, including age-related risks, social and physical environmental risk, and behavioral risk. Each of these categories of risk is discussed later in terms of family health risk, under Major Family Health Risks and Nursing Interventions.

Although single risk factors can influence outcomes, the combined effect of accumulated risks is more than the sum of the individual effects. For example, a family history of cardiovascular disease is a single biological risk factor that is affected by smoking (a behavioral risk that is more likely to occur if other family members also smoke) and by diet and exercise. Diet and exercise are influenced by family and society's norms. People in the Northwest and West are more likely to eat heart-healthy diets and to exercise than people who live in the Midwest and South; thus communities in the Northwest and West are often more supportive of exercise and bicycle paths and diets lower in fat than communities in other parts of the United States. The combined effect of a family history, family behavioral risks, and society's influences is greater than the sum of the three individual risk factors (smoking, diet, and exercise).

## Health Risk Appraisal

**Health risk appraisal** refers to the process of assessing for the presence of specific factors in each of the categories that have been identified as being associated with an increased likelihood of an illness, such as cancer, or *an unhealthy event,* such as an automobile accident. Several techniques have been developed to accomplish health risk appraisal, including computer software programs and paper-and-pencil instruments. One technique is the Youth Behavioral Health Risk Appraisal instrument of the Centers for Disease Control and Prevention (CDC, 2001). The general approach is to determine whether a risk factor is present and to what degree. On the basis of scientific evidence, each factor is weighted, and a total score is derived. This appraisal method provides an individual score that can be examined as a whole within the family, thus appraising the health risks that are likely to be experienced by other members of the family. Additional research is needed to determine if the individual appraisals can be used to determine family risk.

## Health Risk Reduction

**Health risk reduction** is based on the assumption that decreasing the number of risks or the magnitude of risk will result in a lower probability of an undesired event. For example, to decrease the likelihood of adolescent substance abuse, family behaviors such as parents not drinking, alcohol not available in the home, and family contracts related to alcohol and drug use may be useful. Health risks can be reduced through a variety of approaches, such as those just described. It is important to note the specific risk and the family's tolerance of it. Pender (2002) provides examples of different kinds of risks:

- Voluntarily assumed risks are tolerated better than those imposed by others.
- Risks over which scientists debate and are uncertain are more feared than risks on which scientists agree.
- Risks of natural origin are often considered less threatening than those created by humans.

Thus risk reduction is a complex process that requires knowledge of the specific risk and the family's perceptions of the nature of the risk.

## Life Events

*Life events* can increase the risk for illness and disability. These events can be categorized as either normative or nonnormative. *Normative events* are those that are generally expected to occur at a particular stage of development or of the life span. Normative events can be identified from the stages of the family lifecycle (Carter and McGoldrick, 1999; Wright LM, 2000) (Table 25-1).

> ### WHAT DO YOU THINK?
> Governmental priority for funding health risk reduction and health promotion programs, including assistance programs, would have greater benefit to the population's health than funding for illness activities.

Examples of normative events are a child leaving home to go to college, retirement from work, and starting a first job. *Nonnormative events,* in contrast, are those that are unpredictable (e.g., family move related to job market, divorce, death of a child). Furthermore, life events, especially when more than one event occurs, can result in a family crisis under certain conditions.

## Family Crisis

A **family crisis** occurs when the family is not able to cope with an event and becomes disorganized or dysfunctional. When the demands of the situation exceed the resources of the family, a family crisis exists. When families experience a crisis or a crisis-producing event, they attempt to gather their resources to deal with the demands created by the situation. Burr and Klein (1994) differentiate between family resources and family coping strategies. The former are the resources, such as money and extended family, that a family has available to them. The latter are the "active processes and behaviors families actually try to do to help them manage, adapt, or deal with the stressful situation" (Burr and Klein, 1994, p. 129). Thus if a family were to experience an unexpected illness in the main wage earner, family resources might include financial assistance from relatives or emotional support. Family coping strategies, in contrast, would include whether the family was able to ask a relative to loan them emergency funds or was able to talk with relatives about the worries they were experiencing.

## Table 25-1    Family Life Cycle Stages

| FAMILY LIFE CYCLE STAGES | KEY PRINCIPLES FOR EMOTIONAL TRANSITION PROCESS | SECOND-ORDER CHANGES IN FAMILY STATUS REQUIRED TO PROCEED DEVELOPMENTALLY |
|---|---|---|
| Leaving home; single young adults | Accepting emotional and financial responsibility of self | • Differentiation of self in relation to family of origin<br>• Development of intimate peer relationships<br>• Establishment of self as related to work and financial independence |
| The joining of families through marriage; the new couple | Commitment to new system | • Formation of marital system<br>• Realignment of relationships with extended families and friends to include spouse |
| Families with young children | Accepting new members into system | • Adjusting marital system to make space for child(ren)<br>• Joining in child rearing, financial, and household tasks<br>• Realignment of relationships with extended family to include parenting and grandparenting roles |
| Families with adolescents | Increasing flexibility of family boundaries to include children's independence and grandparents' frailties | • Shifting of parent-child relationships to permit adolescent to move in and out of system<br>• Refocus on midlife marital and career issues<br>• Beginning shift toward caring for older generation |
| Launching children and moving on | Accepting a multitude of exits from and entries into the family system | • Renegotiation of marital system as a dyad<br>• Development of adult-to-adult relationship between grown children and their parents<br>• Realignment of relationships to include in-laws and grandchildren<br>• Dealing with disabilities and death of parents (grandparents) |
| Families in later life | Accepting the shifting of generational roles | • Maintaining own and couple functioning and interests in face of physiological decline; exploration of new familial and social role options<br>• Support for a more central role of middle generation<br>• Making room in the system for the wisdom and experience of the older generation, and supporting them without overfunctioning for them<br>• Dealing with loss of spouse, siblings, and other peers and preparing for own death<br>• Life review and integration |

Carter B, McGoldrick M: *The expanded family life cycle,* ed 3, Boston, 1999, Allyn and Bacon.

On the basis of the existing literature, Burr and Klein (1994) developed a three-level classification system of coping strategies, with seven major categories and 20 subcategories (Table 25-2).

It is important to note that the amount of support available to families in times of crisis from government and nongovernment agencies varies in different locales. In addition, the rules and conditions of support often differ and may inhibit families from seeking support, particularly if the conditions are demeaning.

## MAJOR FAMILY HEALTH RISKS AND NURSING INTERVENTIONS

As mentioned earlier, risks to a family's health arise in three major areas: biological, environmental, and behavioral. In most instances, a risk in one of these areas may

**Table 25-2    Burr and Klein's Conceptual Framework of Coping Strategies**

| HIGHLY ABSTRACT STRATEGIES | MODERATELY ABSTRACT STRATEGIES |
|---|---|
| 1. Cognitive | 1. Be accepting of the situation and others |
| | 2. Gain useful knowledge |
| | 3. Change how the situation is viewed or defined (reframe the situation) |
| 2. Emotional | 4. Express feelings and affection |
| | 5. Avoid or resolve negative feelings and disabling expressions of emotion |
| | 6. Be sensitive to others' emotional needs |
| 3. Relationships | 7. Increase cohesion (togetherness) |
| | 8. Increase adaptability |
| | 9. Develop increased trust |
| | 10. Increase cooperation |
| | 11. Increase tolerance of one another |
| 4. Communication | 12. Be open and honest |
| | 13. Listen to one another |
| | 14. Be sensitive to nonverbal communication |
| 5. Community | 15. Seek help and support from others |
| | 16. Fulfill expectations in organizations |
| 6. Spiritual | 17. Be more involved in religious activities |
| | 18. Increase faith or seek help from God |
| 7. Individual development | 19. Develop autonomy, independence, and self-sufficiency |
| | 20. Keep active in hobbies |

From Burr WR, Klein SR: *Reexamining family stress: new theory and research,* Thousand Oaks, Calif, 1994, Sage.

not be enough to threaten family health, but a combination of risks from two or more categories could be. For example, there may be a family history of cardiovascular disease, but often the health risk is increased by an unhealthy lifestyle. An understanding of each of these categories provides the basis for a comprehensive perspective on family health risk assessment and intervention.

Beginning with the Surgeon General's report (Califano, 1979), an emphasis on health promotion and disease prevention has focused on lifestyle patterns. Healthy People 2010 targets areas in health promotion, health protection, preventive services, and surveillance and data systems to describe age-related objectives (USDHHS, 2000). Included in the area of health promotion are physical activity and fitness, nutrition, tobacco use, use of alcohol and other drugs, family planning, mental health and mental disorders, and violent and abusive behavior. Health protection activities include issues related to unintentional injuries, occupational safety and health, environmental health, food and drug safety, and oral health. Preventive services, designed to reduce risks of illness, include maternal and infant health, heart disease and stroke, cancer, diabetes and other chronic disabling conditions, human immunodeficiency virus (HIV) infection, sexually transmitted diseases, immunization for infectious diseases, and clinical preventive services. The interrelationships among the various groups of risk are clear when the objectives for the nation are considered. Most of the national health objectives are based on

individual risk factors; some relate to families, work, school, and communities.

## Family Health Risk Appraisal

Assessment of family health risk requires many approaches. As in any assessment, the first and most important task is to get to know the family, their strengths, and their needs (see Chapter 24). This section focuses on appraisal of family health risks in the areas of biological and age-related risk, social and physical environmental risk, and behavioral risk. Healthy People 2010 (USDHHS, 2000) defines health and the risk categories (see p. 597).

### Biological and Age-Related Risk

The family plays an important role in both the development and the management of a disease or condition. Several illnesses have a family component that can be accounted for by either genetics or lifestyle patterns. These factors contribute to the **biological risk** for certain conditions. Patterns of cardiovascular disease, for example, can often be traced through several generations of a family. Such families are said to be at risk for cardiovascular disease. How or whether cardiovascular disease is found in a family is often influenced by the lifestyle of the family. Consistent research evidence supports the positive effects of diet, exercise, and stress management on preventing or delaying cardiovascular disease. The development of hypertension can be managed by following a low-sodium diet, maintaining a normal weight, exercising regularly, and employing effective stress management techniques, such as meditation. Diabetes mellitus is another disease with a strong genetic pattern, and the family plays a major role in the management of the condition. Family patterns of obesity increase the risk in individuals for a number of conditions, including heart disease, hypertension, diabetes, some types of cancer, and gallbladder disease (USDHHS, 2000). It is often difficult to separate biological risks from individual lifestyle factors.

**Transitions** (movement from one stage or condition to another) are times of potential risk for families. Age-related or **life-event risks** often occur during transitions from one developmental stage to another. Transitions present new situations and demands for families. These experiences often require that families change behaviors, schedules, and patterns of communication; make new decisions; reallocate family roles; learn new skills; and identify and learn to use new resources. The demands that transitions place on families have implications for the health of the family unit and individual family members and can be considered as life-event risks. How well prepared families are to deal with a transition depends on the nature of the event. If the event is normative, or anticipated, then it is possible for families to identify needed resources, make plans, learn new skills, or otherwise prepare for the event and its consequences. This kind of anticipatory preparation can increase the family's coping ability and lessen stress and negative outcomes. If, on the other hand, the event is nonnormative, or unexpected, families have little or no time to prepare and the outcome can be increased stress, crisis, or even dysfunction. Table 25-1 lists family stages and the developmental tasks associated with each stage.

Several normative events have been identified for families. The developmental model organizes these events into stages and identifies important transition points. It provides a useful framework for identifying normative events and preparing families to cope successfully with related demands. The developmental tasks associated with each stage identify the types of skills families need. The kinds of normative events families experience are usually related to the addition or loss of a family member, such as the birth or adoption of a child, the death of a grandparent, a child moving out of the home to go to school or take a job, or the marriage of a child. There are health-related responsibilities associated with each of these tasks. For example, the birth or adoption of a child requires that families learn about human growth and development, parenting, immunizations, management of childhood illnesses, normal childhood nutrition, and safety issues.

Nonnormative events present different kinds of issues for families. Unexpected events can be either positive or negative. A job promotion or inheriting a substantial sum of money may be unexpected but are usually positive events. More often, nonnormative events are unpleasant, such as a major illness, divorce, the death of a child, or loss of the main family income.

Regardless of whether a life event is normative or nonnormative, it is often a source of stress for families. Several theoretical frameworks have been developed to examine the processes of family stress and coping. Perhaps the most widely used is the ABC-X model. The model was originally developed by Hill (1949) and was based on work with families separated by war. In the model, crisis (X) was proposed to be a product of the nature of the event (A), the family's definition of the event (B), and the resources available to the family (C). Doherty and McCubbin (1985) extended the model to the Double ABC-X model to encompass the period after the initial crisis and introduced the idea of a pile-up of stressors. Adaptation or maladaptation by the family is proposed to be determined by the pile-up of stressors (Aa), the family's perception of the crisis (Bb), and new resources and coping strategies (Cc).

Burr and Klein (1994) challenged this step-by-step view of families and stress and coping. They advocated a more systems-oriented concept of family stress. They pointed out that families develop a series of processes to manage or transform inputs to the system (e.g., energy, time) to outputs (e.g., cohesion, growth, love) known as *rules of transformation*. Over time, families develop these patterns in enough quantity and variety to handle most changes and challenges; this is referred to as *requisite variety of rules of transformation*. However, when families do not have an adequate variety of rules to allow them to respond to an event, the event becomes stressful. Rather than being able to deal with the situation, they fall into a pattern of trying to figure out what it is they need to do, and the usual tasks of the family are not adequately addressed. Rules that were implicit in the family are now reconsidered and redefined.

Furthermore, Burr and Klein's family stress theory proposes three levels of stress: level I is change "in the fairly specific patterns of behavior and transforming processes" (e.g., change in who does which household chores); level II is change "in processes that are at a higher level of abstraction" (e.g., change in what are defined as family chores); and level III is changes in highly abstract processes (e.g., family values) (Burr and Klein, 1994, pp. 44-45). Coping strategies can be identified to address each level of stress that families go through in sequence, if necessary (see the Evidence-Based Practice box about a study of 50 families).

## Biological Health Risk Assessment

One of the most effective techniques for assessing the patterns of health and illness in families is the genogram (Bahr, 1990) (see Chapter 24 for further discussion and an example). Briefly, a genogram is a drawing that shows the family unit of immediate interest and includes several generations using a series of circles, squares, and connecting lines. Basic information about the family, relationships in the family, and patterns of health and illness can be obtained by completing the genogram with the family. As shown in Figure 25-1, a square indicates a male, a circle indicates a female, and an X through either a square or a circle indicates a death. Marriage is indicated by a solid horizontal line and offspring/children by a solid vertical line. A broken horizontal line indicates a divorce or separation. Dates of birth, marriage, death, and other important events can be indicated where appropriate. Major illness or conditions can be listed for each individual family member. Patterns can be quickly assessed and provide a guide for the health interviewer about health areas that need further exploring

The genogram in Figure 25-1 was completed for the fictional Graham family. Some of the interesting health patterns that can be seen from the genogram are the repetition of hypertension, adult onset diabetes, cancer, and hypercholesterolemia. Completing a genogram requires interviews with as many family members as possible. Bahr suggests that a family chronology, a timeline of family events over three generations, be completed to extend the genogram.

A more intensive and quantitative assessment of a family's biological risk can be achieved through the use of a standard family risk assessment. Because such assessments involve other areas in addition to biological risk, one will be described later, after the description of assessment of other types of risk.

Both normative and nonnormative life events pose potential risks to the health of families. Even events that are generally viewed as being positive require changes and can place stress on a family. The normative event of the birth of a child, for example, requires considerable changes in family structures and roles. Furthermore, family functions are expanded from previous levels, requiring families to add new skills and establish additional resources. These changes can in turn result in strain and, if adequate resources are not available, stress. Therefore, to adequately assess life risks, both normative and nonnormative events occurring in the family need to be considered. Community-level support groups have been successful in assisting families in dealing with a variety of stressful situations and crises (e.g., Families Anonymous, Bereaved Parents, Parents and Friends of Lesbian and Gay Persons, Single Parents) that arise from both life events and age-related events. Nurses have been instrumental in developing and moderating such groups.

## Environmental Risk

The importance of **social risks** to family health is gaining increased recognition (see Chapters 7 and 15). Living in high-crime neighborhoods, in communities without adequate recreation or health resources, in communities that have major noise pollution or chemical pollution, or in

### Evidence-Based Practice

Using the results of a study of 50 families who had experienced a variety of stressors, Burr and Klein (1994) examined the changes experienced under stress in nine areas of family life: marital satisfaction, family rituals and celebrations, quality of communication, family cohesion, functional quality of the executive subsystem, quality of the emotional atmosphere, management of daily routines and chores, contention, and normal family development versus changed or arrested development. The results of the study support that families did use the proposed strategies, both the helpful ones and the harmful ones, with significant differences between men and women on 10 of the 80 strategies. Women tended to use a wider range of strategies, and men tended to use more of the harmful strategies. The results supported the sequencing and developmental nature of families' use of strategies in acute stressor situations but

not in chronic stressor situations. Thus the pattern was evident in stresses, such as bankruptcy, but not in families with a child with a chronic condition.

**Nurse Use:** Results of this work provide direction for community health nursing intervention with families over the life span. The three levels share similarities with Neuman's (1995) flexible lines of defense (level I change), normal line of defense (level II change), and lines of resistance (level III change). On the basis of the Neuman Systems Model, primary prevention strategies (e.g., parenting classes) would be appropriate for dealing with level I change; secondary prevention strategies (e.g., crisis intervention) for dealing with level II change; and tertiary prevention strategies (e.g., family therapy) for dealing with level III change.

Burr WR, Klein SR: *Reexaming family stress: new theory and research,* Thousand Oaks, Calif, 1994, Sage; Neuman B: *The Neuman Systems Model,* ed 4, Norwalk, Conn, 1995, Appleton & Lange.

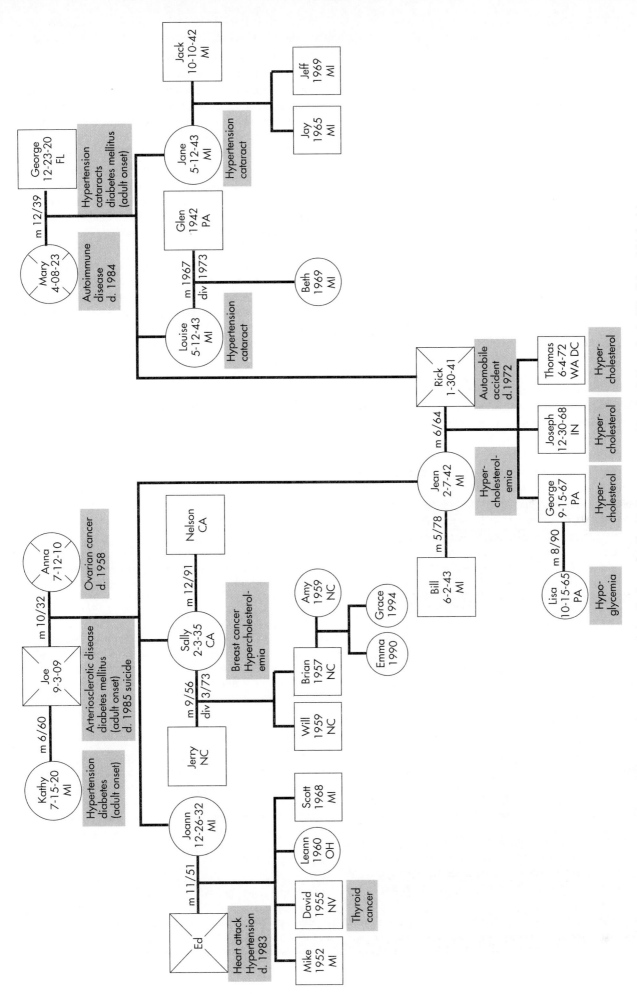

**Figure 25-1** Family genogram of the Graham family. *(Developed by Carol Loveland-Cherry for the fifth edition of this book.)*

other high-stress environments increases a family's health risk. One social stress is discrimination, whether racial, cultural, or other. The psychological burden resulting from discrimination is itself a stressor, and it adds to the effects of other stressors. The implication of these examples of risky social situations is that they contribute to the stressors experienced by the families. If adequate resources and coping processes are not available, breakdowns in health can occur.

The poor are at greater risk for health problems (see Chapter 32). **Economic risk,** which is related to social risk, is determined by the relationship between family financial resources and the demands on those resources. Having adequate financial resources means that a family is able to purchase the necessary commodities related to health. These include adequate housing, clothing, food, education, and health or illness care. The amount of money that a family has available is relative to situational, cultural, and social factors. A family may have an income well above the poverty level, but because of a devastating illness in a family member, they may not be able to meet financial demands. Likewise, families from ethnic populations or families with same-sex parents frequently experience discrimination in finding housing. Even if they find housing, they may not be welcome and may be harassed, resulting in increased stress.

Unfortunately, not all families have access to health care insurance. For families at the poverty level, programs such as Medicaid are available to pay for health and illness care. Families in the upper income brackets usually have health insurance through an employer, or they can afford to either purchase health insurance or pay for health care out of pocket. An increasing number of middle income families have major wage earners in jobs that do not have health benefits. These people often do not have enough income to purchase health care but earn too much money to qualify for public assistance programs. Consequently, many families have financial resources that allow them to maintain a subsistence level but that limit the quality of their purchasing power. Illness care may be available but not preventive care; food high in fat and calories may be affordable, whereas fresh fruit and vegetables are not. Nutritious diets are important in preventing illness and promoting health. For example, a U.S. Department of Agriculture (USDA) study examined the effects of its WIC nutrition program for women, infants, and children. They found that for "every $1.00 spent on a pregnant woman in its Women, Infants and Children (WIC) program, $1.77 to $3.13 was saved in Medicaid costs during her child's first 60 days of life" (Greer, 1995, p. 6).

## Environmental Risk Assessment

Assessment of environmental health risk is less well defined and developed. Information on relationships that the family has with others such as relatives and neigh-

## Evidence-Based Practice

Whitley et al (2001) examined the physical and mental health status and health-related behaviors of 100 African-American grandmothers who were the primary caregivers for their grandchildren ($n$ = 2.5 grandchildren). The study assessed the grandmothers' physical health conditions using two standardized instruments: the Short Form-36 General Health Survey (SF-36) (Ward and Sherbourne, 1992) and the Healthier People, Health Risk Appraisal (HRA) (Hutchins, 1991). To obtain additional physical health data, registered nurses (RNs) gathered the following information from each grandmother: blood pressure, weight, cholesterol count, and glucose levels.

The results of the study indicated that the grandmothers experienced only moderate interference with their many activities of daily living as a result of health or emotional factors. However, serious health risks were identified. The health data from the RNs revealed that 23% of the grandmothers were diabetic, 54% had hypertension, 22% had high cholesterol, and 80% were at least 20% overweight. Fifty-two percent of the grandmothers said that they had experienced one or more serious personal losses during the year, and 45% perceived their health as being fair or poor. In contrast, a lack of emotional support was found to be a problem with only 18% of the sample and the grandmothers reported that their emotional health was equal to or better than that of the general population.

The findings of this study suggest that African-American grandmothers may have difficulty meeting the demands of parenting on a long-term basis without the support of others, specifically in relation to their physical health. With the health risks identified, longevity and quality of life will be in jeopardy if health habits are not changed.

It is important that culturally sensitive educational interventions are developed for population groups. Even though these grandmothers have a strong desire to fulfill the parental role in the children's lives, there is a potential for these grandmothers to develop serious health problems in later years.

**Nurse Use:** Health problems could disrupt the secure home environment that the grandmothers have worked to establish for the children. The onset of many of these problems may be avoided or at least delayed with interventions from the community that would provide needed health and social services to support these families.

Whitley DM, Kelley SJ, Sipe TA: Grandmothers raising grandchildren: are they at increased risk of health problems? *Health Soc Work* 26:105-114, 2001.

bors; their connections with other social units—church, school, work, clubs, and organizations; and the flow of energy, positive or negative, can be assessed through the use of an ecomap (see Chapter 24 for further discussion and an example).

An ecomap represents the family's interactions with other groups and organizations, accomplished using a series of circles and lines. The family of interest (the Graham family in Figure 25-2) is represented by a circle in the middle of the page; other groups and organizations are then

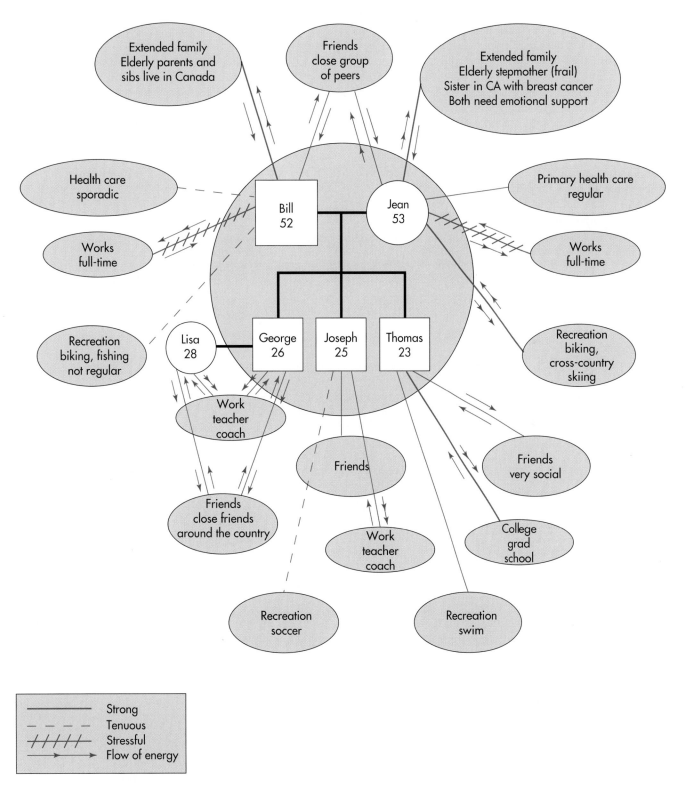

**Figure 25-2** Ecomap of the Graham family. *(Developed by Carol Loveland-Cherry for the fifth edition of this book.)*

indicated by other circles. Lines, representing the flow of energy, are drawn between the family circle and the circles representing other groups and organizations. An arrowhead at the end of each line indicates the direction of the flow of energy (into or out of the family), and the darkness of the line indicates the intensity of the energy. The Graham family ecomap indicates that much of the family energy goes into work (also a source of stress for the parents). Major *sources* of energy for the Grahams are their immediate and extended families and friends.

In addition to the support network shown by the ecomap, other aspects of social risk include characteristics of the neighborhood and community where the family lives. A nurse who has worked in the general geographic area may already have done a community assessment (see Chapter 15) and have a working knowledge of the neighborhood and community. It is important, however, for the nurse to obtain information from the family to understand their perceptions of the community.

Information about the origins of the family is useful to understand other social resources and stressors. Information about how long the family has lived in their current location and the immigration patterns of the family and their ancestors provides insight into the pressures they experience.

Economic risk is one of the foremost predictors of health. Families often consider financial information private, and both the nurse and the family may be uncomfortable when discussing finances. It is not necessary to know actual family income except in certain instances when it is necessary to determine whether families are eligible for programs or benefits. It is useful to know whether the family's resources are adequate to meet their needs. It is important to understand that the family may be quite comfortable with their finances and standard of living, which may be different from those of the health care provider. The provider should not try to push financial values onto the family. In terms of health risk, it is important to understand the resources that families have to obtain health/illness care; adequate shelter, clothing, and food; and access to recreation. Families with limited resources may qualify for programs such as Medicaid, Aid to Dependent Families, WIC, or Maternal Support Systems/Infant Support Systems. Families with wage earners with medical benefits and those with enough income are usually able to afford adequate health care. Unfortunately, in a growing number of families, the main wage earner is employed but receives no medical benefits and the salary is not sufficient for health promotion or illness-related care. This is a policy issue for which nurses are very capable of drafting legislation and providing testimony related to the stories of families in their caseloads. (See Chapter 8 for a discussion of policy involvement by nurses.)

## Behavioral (Lifestyle) Risk

Personal health habits continue to contribute to the major causes of morbidity and mortality in the United States (see Chapter 14). The pattern of personal health habits and **behavioral risk** defines individual and family lifestyle risk. The family is the basic unit within which health behavior—including health values, health habits, and health risk perceptions—is developed, organized, and performed. Families maintain major responsibility for determining what food is purchased and prepared, setting sleep patterns, planning family activities, setting and monitoring norms about health and health risk behaviors, determining when a family member is ill, determining when health care should be obtained, and carrying out treatment regimens. In 1999, more than half of all deaths in the United States were attributed to heart disease or cancer, both of which identify diet as a major causative factor (USDHHS, 2000). General guidelines from the USDHHS and the USDA include eating a variety of foods; maintaining healthy weight; choosing a diet low in fat and cholesterol, including plenty of vegetables, fruits, and grain products; limiting use of sugars, salt, and sodium; and consuming alcohol only in moderation.

Multiple health benefits of regular physical activity have been identified; regular physical exercise is effective in promoting and maintaining health and preventing disease. Among the benefits of regular physical activity are increased muscle strength, endurance, and flexibility; management of weight; prevention of colon cancer, stroke, and back injury; and prevention and management of coronary heart disease, hypertension, diabetes, osteoporosis, and depression (USDHHS, 2000). Families can structure time and activities for family members. It is helpful when the community in which they live promotes exercise by having accessible parks and walking or biking paths that help families select activities that provide moderate, regular physical exercise, rather than sedentary activities in the home setting.

Substance use and abuse is a major contributor to morbidity and mortality in the United States. Tobacco use has been identified as the single most preventable cause of death. It has been associated with several types of cancer, coronary heart disease, low birthweight, premature births, sudden infant death syndrome, and chronic obstructive pulmonary disease. Furthermore, passive smoke has been linked to disease in nonsmokers and children. Drug use, including alcohol, is a major social and health problem. In 2001, 41% of traffic deaths were alcohol related (National Cancer Institute, 2001; National Highway Traffic Safety Administration, 2002). Drug use is associated with transmission of HIV, fetal alcohol syndrome, liver disease, unwanted pregnancy, delinquency, school failure, violence, and crime. The literature consistently identifies the effects of family factors, such as family closeness, families doing activities together, and behavior modeled in the family as decreasing the risk of substance use in children.

Although violence and abusive behavior are not limited to families, the amount of intrafamilial violence is thought to be underestimated. It is difficult to collect data and obtain accurate statistics on family violence because the issue is so sensitive for families. Evidence supports the intergenerational nature of violence and abuse—that is, abusers were often abused as children.

## Behavioral (Lifestyle) Health Risk Assessment

Families are the major source of factors that can promote or inhibit positive lifestyles. They regulate time and energy and the boundaries of the system. A number of tools exist for assessing individuals' lifestyle risks, but few are available for assessing family lifestyle patterns. Although assessment of individual lifestyle contributes to determining the lifestyle risk of a family, it is important to look at risks for the family as a unit. One approach is to identify family patterns for each of the lifestyle components included in Healthy People 2010. In the areas of health promotion, health protection, and preventive services, lifestyle can be assessed in several dimensions. From the literature on health behavior research, the critical dimensions include the following:

- Value placed on the behavior
- Knowledge of the behavior and its consequences
- Effect of the behavior on the family
- Effect of the behavior on the individual
- Barriers to performing the behavior
- Benefits of the behavior

It is important to assess the frequency, intensity, and regularity of specific behaviors. It also is important to evaluate the resources available to the family for implementing the behaviors. Thus items for assessment of physical activity include the value that a family places on physical activity, the hours that a family spends in exercise, the kinds of exercise the family does, and resources available for exercise.

## COMMUNITY-ORIENTED NURSING APPROACHES TO FAMILY HEALTH RISK REDUCTION

### Home Visits

Nurses work with families in a variety of settings, including clinics, schools, support groups, and offices. However, an important aspect of the community-oriented nurse's role in reducing health risks and promoting the health of populations has been the tradition of providing services to families in their homes.

### Purpose

**Home visits** give a more accurate assessment of the family structure, the natural or home environment, and behavior in that environment, than do clinical visits. Home visits

also provide opportunities to identify both barriers and supports for reaching family health promotion goals. The nurse can work with the client directly to adapt interventions to match resources. Visiting the family in their home may also contribute to the family's sense of control and active participation in meeting their health needs. The majority of the studies evaluating home visits have focused on the maternal–child population (Bradley and Martin, 1994; Kang et al, 1995; Olds et al, 1998).

Home visiting programs are receiving increased attention and provide a broad range of services to achieve a variety of health-related goals. In a long-term follow-up project of current adolescents whose unmarried mothers received pre- and postnatal nursing visits at home (Olds et al, 1998), researchers found that these teens had fewer instances of running away, fewer arrests, fewer convictions and violations of probation, fewer sexual partners over a lifetime, fewer cigarettes smoked per day, and fewer days having consumed alcohol in the previous 6 months, when compared with a group of teens whose mothers had not received the nurse visits. Additionally, the parents of the nurse-visited children reported fewer behavioral problems related to the use of alcohol and drugs. Long-term effects of home visits are positive and are shown to be cost effective for society. As a result, several states have reinstituted home visits for high-risk families. If the home visit is to be a valuable and effective intervention, careful and systematic planning must occur.

### Advantages and Disadvantages

The effectiveness of health promotion services in the home has been critically reexamined by agencies such as health departments and visiting nurses associations (Barnes-Boyd, Norr, and Nacion, 1998; Olds et al, 1998). Advantages include client convenience, client control of the setting, providing of an option for those clients unwilling or unable to travel, the ability to individualize services, and a natural, relaxed environment for the discussion of concerns and needs. Costs are a major disadvantage. The cost of previsit preparation, travel to and from the home, time spent with one client, and postvisit preparation is high. Many agencies have actively explored alternative modes of providing service to families, particularly group interventions (see Chapter 23). The important issue is determining which families would benefit the most and how home visits can most effectively be structured and scheduled. With increasing demands for home health care, the home visit is again becoming a prominent mode for delivery of nursing services (see the Evidence-Based Practice box about the 15-year follow-up study).

### Process

The components of a home visit are summarized in Table 25-3. The phases include the initiation phase, the previsit

**Table 25-3  Phases and Activities of a Home Visit**

| PHASE | ACTIVITY |
| --- | --- |
| I. Initiation phase | • Clarify source of referral for visit<br>• Clarify purpose for home visit<br>• Share information on reason and purpose of home visit with family |
| II. Previsit phase | • Initiate contact with family<br>• Establish shared perception of purpose with family<br>• Determine family's willingness for home visit<br>• Schedule home visit<br>• Review referral and/or family record |
| III. In-home phase | • Introduce self and professional identity<br>• Interact socially to establish rapport<br>• Establish nurse–client relationship<br>• Implement nursing process |
| IV. Termination phase | • Review visit with family<br>• Plan for future visits |
| V. Postvisit phase | • Record visit<br>• Plan for next visit |

a result of case-finding activities. The **initiation phase** is the first contact between the nurse and the family. It provides the foundation for an effective therapeutic relationship. Subsequent home visits should be based on need and mutual agreement between the nurse and the family. Frequently, nurses are not sure of the reason for the visit. This carries with it the potential for the visit to be compromised and to come aimlessly or abruptly to a premature halt. Regardless of the reason for making a home visit, it is necessary that the nurse be clear about the purpose for the visit and that this purpose or understanding be shared with the family.

### Previsit Phase

The **previsit phase** has several components. For the most part, these are best accomplished in order, as presented in the How To box.

The possibility exists that the family may refuse a home visit. Less experienced nurses or students may mistakenly interpret this as a personal rejection. Families make decisions about when and which outsiders are allowed entry into their homes. The nurse needs to explore the reasons for the refusal; there may be a misunderstanding about the reason for a visit, or there may be a lack of information

phase, the in-home phase, the termination phase, and the postvisit phase. Building a trusting relationship with the family client is the cornerstone of successful home visits. Five skills are fundamental to effective home visits: observing, listening, questioning, probing, and prompting. The need for these skills is evident in all phases of the home visit process.

### Initiation Phase

Usually, a home visit is initiated as the result of a referral from a health or social agency. However, a family may request services, or the nurse may initiate the home visit as

- First, if at all possible, the nurse should contact the family by telephone before the home visit to introduce self, to identify the reason for the contact, and to schedule the home visit. A first telephone contact should be a maximum of 15 minutes. The nurse should give name and professional identity—for example, "This is Karen Smith. I'm a community health nurse from the Fayette County Health Department."

- The family should be informed of how they came to the attention of the nurse—for example, as the result of a referral or a contact from observations or records in the school setting. If a referral has been received, it is important and useful to ascertain whether the family is aware of the referral.

- A brief summary of the nurse's knowledge about the family's situation will allow the family to clarify their needs. For example, the nurse might say, "I understand that your baby was discharged from the hospital yesterday and that you requested some assistance with learning more about how to care for your baby at home."

- A visit should be scheduled as soon as possible. Letting the family know agency hours available for visits, the approximate length of the visit, and the purpose of the visit are helpful to the family in determining when to set the visit. Although the length of the visit may vary, depending on circumstances, approximately 30 minutes to 1 hour is usual.

- If possible, the visit should be arranged when as many family members as possible will be available for the entire visit. It is also important for the nurse to tell the client about any fee for the visit and subsequent visits and possible methods for payment.

- The telephone call can terminate with a review by the nurse of the time, place, and purpose for the visit and a means for the family to contact the nurse in case they need to verify or change the time for the visit or to ask questions. If the family does not have a telephone, another method for setting up the visit can be used. A note can be dropped off at the family home or sent by mail informing the family of when and why the home visit will occur and providing a way for the family to contact the nurse if necessary.

about services. The contact may be terminated as requested if the nurse determines that either the situation has been resolved or services have been obtained from another source, and if the family understands that services are available and how to contact the agency if desired. However, the nurse should leave open the possibility of future contact. There are instances when the nurse will be mandated to persist in requesting a home visit because of legal obligations, such as follow-up of certain communicable diseases.

Before visiting a family, the nurse should review the referral or, if this is not the first visit, the family record. If there is a time lapse between the contact and the visit, a brief telephone call to confirm the time often prevents the nurse from finding no one at home.

An issue that may arise either in approaching the family home or once the family has opened the door to the nurse is that of personal safety. Nurses need to examine personal fears and objective threats to determine if safety is indeed an issue. Certain precautions can be taken in known high-risk situations. Agencies may provide escorts for nurses or have them visit in pairs; readily identifiable uniforms may be required; or a sign-out process indicating timing and location of home visits may be used routinely. Home visits are generally very safe; however, as with all worksites, the possibility of violence exists. Therefore the nurse needs to use caution. If a reasonable question exists about the safety of making a visit, the visit should not be made.

The nurse should be aware that families may feel that they are being checked up on, that they are seen as being inadequate or dysfunctional, or that their privacy is being impinged on. Nursing services, especially those from health departments, have been identified by the public as being "public services" for needy families or those with inadequate funds to pay for care. These potential areas of concern underlie the need for sensitivity on the part of the nurse, the need for clarity in information regarding the reason for visits, and the need to establish collaborative, trusting relationships with the family.

Another factor that may affect the nature of the home visit is whether the visit is viewed as voluntary or required (Byrd, 1995). A *voluntary* home visit (visit requested by the client) is characterized by easier entry for the nurse, client-controlled interaction, an informal tone, and mutual discussion of frequency of future visits. In contrast, the client may feel little need for *required* home visits (often legally mandated). Entry may be difficult for the nurse; the interaction may be nurse controlled; there may be a more formal, investigatory tone to the visit with distorted nurse–client communication; and there may be no mutual discussion of frequency of future visits.

The changing nature of the American family can make it difficult to schedule visits during what have been traditional agency hours. The number of working single-parent or dual-income, two-parent families is increasing, which means that families have more demands on their time. Even if one parent is at home during the usual workday, the ideal is to work with the entire family unit. This often is not possible because of conflict between agency hours and school or work schedules. It may be possible to schedule a visit at the beginning or end of a day to meet with working or school-age members. In some parts of the country, agencies are reconsidering traditional hours and Monday through Friday visits. These issues are important to assess and address during the previsit phase so the nurse and the family will be better prepared for the visit.

Culture influences a person's interpretation of and response to health care (Purnell and Paulanka, 2003). It is important for health care providers to recognize each person's unique perspectives as legitimate. However, given the diversity of the United States and the diversity within cultural groups, it is impossible to cover every group extensively. Instead, practitioners need to take the responsibility to learn about their client's culture as they prepare for visits with families or communities.

### In-Home Phase

The actual visit to the home constitutes the **in-home phase** and affords the nurse the opportunity to assess the family's neighborhood and community resources, as well as the home and family interactions. The actual home visit includes several components. Once at the family home, the nurse provides personal and professional identification and tells the client the location of the agency. Then, a brief social period allows the client to assess the nurse and establish rapport. The next step is a description by the nurse of his or her role, responsibilities, and limitations. Another important component of the home visit is to determine the client's expectations.

The major portion of the home visit is concerned with establishing the relationship and implementing the nursing process. Assessment, intervention, and evaluation are ongoing. What then occurs in the home visit is determined by the reason for the visit. Some reasons for visits are listed in Box 25-2.

It is important that the nurse be realistic about what can be accomplished in a home visit. In some situations, one visit may be all that is possible or appropriate. In this instance, needs and the resources available to meet them are explored with the family, and it is determined whether further services are desired or indicated. If further services are indicated and the nurse's agency is not appropriate, the nurse can assist the family in identifying other services available in the community and can help in initiating referrals. Although it is not unusual to have only one home visit with a family, often multiple visits are made. The frequency and intensity of home visits vary not only with the needs of the family but also with the eligibility of the family for services as defined by agency policies and priorities. It is realistic to expect an initial assessment and at least the beginning of building a relationship to occur on a first visit.

Families may or may not be able to control interruptions during the visit. Telephones ring, pets join in the visit, people come and go, and televisions are left on. The nurse can ask that for a limited time televisions be turned off or that other disruptive activities be limited. Families may be so used to the background noises and routine activities that they do not recognize them as being potentially disruptive.

### Termination Phase

When the purpose of the visit has been accomplished, the nurse reviews with the family what has occurred and what

---

**BOX 25-2 Reasons for the Home Visit**

Nursing interventions may include some or all of the 17 resources identified by the Minnesota Department of Health Section of Public Health Nursing:
- Advocacy
- Case management
- Coalition building
- Collaboration
- Community organizing
- Consultation
- Counseling
- Delegated medical treatment and observations
- Disease investigation
- Health teaching
- Outreach/case findings
- Policy development
- Provider education
- Referral and follow-up
- Screening
- Social marketing
- Surveillance

From Keller LO et al: Population-based public health nursing interventions: a model from practice, *Public Health Nurs* 15(3):207, 1998.

---

has been accomplished. This is the major focus of the **termination phase,** and it provides a basis for planning further home visits. Ideally, termination of the visit and, ultimately, termination of service begins at the first contact with the establishment of a goal or purpose. If communication has been clear to this point, the family and nurse can now plan for future visits, specifically the next visit. Planning for future visits is part of another issue: setting goals and planning service. Contracting is a constructive approach to working with clients and is receiving increasing attention by health professionals. The purpose and components of contracting with clients are discussed later.

### Postvisit Phase

Even though the nurse has now concluded the home visit and left the client's home, responsibility for the visit is not complete until the interaction has been recorded. A major task of the **postvisit phase** is documenting the visit and services provided. Agencies may organize their records by families. That is, the basic record may be a "family" folder with all members included. However, often this does not occur, although it is useful for the family history and background. More often, each family member has a separate record, and other family members' records are cross-referenced. This is because the focus often shifts from the family to the individual. Consequently, nursing diagnoses, goals, and interventions are directed toward individual family members rather than the family unit.

Record systems and formats vary from agency to agency. The nurse needs to become familiar with the particular system used in the agency. All systems should include a database; a nursing diagnosis and problem list; a plan, including specific goals; actual actions and interventions; and evaluation. These are the basic elements needed for legal and clinical purposes. The format may consist of narratives; flow sheets; problem-oriented medical records (POMR); subjective, objective, assessment plans (SOAP); or a combination of formats. It is important that recording be current, dated, and signed.

Be sure to use theoretical frameworks that are appropriate to the family-centered nursing process. For example, a nursing diagnosis of *Ineffective mothering skill* related to lack of knowledge of normal growth and development is an individual-focused nursing diagnosis. *Inability for family to accomplish stage-appropriate task of providing safe environment for preschooler* related to lack of knowledge and resources is a family-focused nursing diagnosis based on knowledge of the developmental approach to families. At times, it may be necessary to present information for a specific family member. However, the emphasis should be on the individual as a member of, and within the structure of, the family.

## Contracting With Families

Increasingly, health professionals look at working with clients in an interactive, collaborative style. This approach is consistent with a more knowledgeable public and the recent self-care movement in the United States. However, it may not be consistent with other cultures that look to health care providers for more direct guidance; therefore, it is important to determine the family's value system before assuming that contracting will work.

**Contracting,** which is making an agreement between two or more parties, involves a shift in responsibility and control toward a shared effort by client and professional as opposed to an effort by the professional alone. The premise of contracting is family control. It is assumed that when the family has legitimate control, their ability to make healthful choices is increased. This active involvement of the client is reflected in several nursing models—for example, that of Orem (1995). Contracting is a strategy aimed at formally involving the family in the nursing process and jointly defining the roles of both the family members and the health professional.

### Purposes

The nursing contract is a working agreement that is continuously renegotiable and may or may not be written. It may be either a contingency or a noncontingency contract. A *contingency contract* states a specific reward for the client after completion of the client's portion of the contract; a *noncontingency contract* does not specify rewards. The implied rewards are the positive consequences of reaching the goals specified in the contract.

### Table 25-4 Phases and Activities in Contracting

| PHASE | ACTIVITY |
|---|---|
| I. Beginning phase | • Mutual data collection and exploration of needs and problems<br>• Mutual establishing of goals<br>• Mutual development of a plan |
| II. Working phase | • Mutual division of responsibilities<br>• Mutual setting of time limits<br>• Mutual implementation of plan<br>• Mutual evaluation and renegotiation |
| III. Termination phase | • Mutual termination of contract |

For family health risk reduction, it is essential that the contract be made with all responsible and appropriate members of the family. Involving only one individual is not sufficient if the goal is family health risk reduction, which requires a total family system effort and change. Scheduling a visit with all family members present may require extra effort; if meeting with the entire family is not possible, each family member can review a contract, give input, and sign it. This allows active participation by all family members without the necessity of finding a time when everyone involved can be present.

### Process of Contracting

Contracting is a learned skill on the part of both the nurse and the family. All persons involved need to know the purpose and process of contracting. There are three general phases: beginning, working, and termination. The three phases can be further divided into eight sets of activities, as summarized in Table 25-4.

The first activity is collection and analysis of data, and it involves both the family and the nurse. An important aspect of this step is obtaining the family's view of the situation and its needs and problems. The nurse can present his or her observations, validate them with the family, and obtain the family's view.

It is important that goals be mutually set and realistic. A pitfall for nurses and clients who are new to contracting is to set overly ambitious goals. The nurse should recognize that there may be discrepancies between professional priorities and those of the client and determine whether negotiating is required. Because contracting is a process characterized by renegotiating, the goals are not static.

Throughout the process, the nurse and family continually learn and recognize what each can contribute to meeting health needs. The exploring of resources allows both parties to become aware of their own and one another's strengths and requires a review of the nurse's skills and knowledge, the family support systems, and community resources.

Developing a plan to meet the goals involves specifying activities, prioritizing goals, and selecting a starting point. Next, the nurse and the family need to decide who will be responsible for which activities. Setting time limits involves deciding on a deadline for accomplishing (or evaluating progress toward accomplishing) a goal and the frequency of contacts. At the agreed-on time, the nurse and family together evaluate the progress in both process and outcome. The contract can be modified, renegotiated, or terminated on the basis of the evaluation.

## Advantages and Disadvantages of Contracting

Contracting takes time and effort and may require the family and nurse to reorient their roles. Increased control on the part of the family also means increased responsibility. Some nurses may have difficulty relinquishing the role of the controlling expert professional. Contracts are not always successful, and contracting is neither appropriate nor possible in some cases. Some clients do not want to have this kind of involvement; they prefer to defer to the "authority" of the professional. Included in this group are individuals with minimal cognitive skills, those who are involved in an emergency situation, those who are unwilling to be more active in their care, and those who do not see control or authority for health concerns as being within their domain. Some of these clients may learn to contract; others never will.

The nursing process does not necessarily provide an active role for the family as a client; the assumption that a need exists is based on professional judgment only, and it is also assumed that changes can and should be made within the family unit. Contracting is one alternative approach that depends on the value of input from both nurse and family, on the competency of the family, on the family's ability to be responsible, and on the dynamic nature of the process. This not only allows for but also requires continual renegotiating. Although it may not be appropriate in all situations or with all families, contracting can give direction and structure to health risk reduction and health promotion in families.

## Empowering Families

Approaches for helping individuals and families assume an active role in their health care should focus on **empowerment** rather than enabling or help giving (Rodwell, 1996). Help-giving interventions do not always have positive outcomes for clients. If families do not perceive a situation as a problem or need, offers of help may cause resentment. Help giving also may have negative consequences if there is not a match between what is expected and what is offered. A nurse's failure to recognize a family's competencies and to define an active role for them can lead to the family's dependency and lack of growth. This can be frus-

trating for both the nurse and the family. For families to become active participants, they need to feel a sense of personal competence and a desire for and willingness to take action. Definitions of empowerment reflect three characteristics of the empowered family seeking help:

- Access and control over needed resources
- Decision-making and problem-solving abilities
- The ability to communicate and to obtain needed resources

The last characteristic refers to the fact that families may need to learn how to identify sources of help, how to contact agencies, how to ask critical questions, and how to negotiate with agencies to have family needs met. These characteristics generally reflect a process by which people (individuals, families, organizations, or communities) take control of their own lives. The outcomes of empowerment are positive self-esteem, the ability to set and reach goals, a sense of control over life and change processes, and a sense of hope for the future (Rodwell, 1996). Box 25-3 shows prevention strategies applied to families.

Empowerment requires a viewpoint that often conflicts with the views of many helping professions, including nursing. Empowerment's underlying assumption is one of a partnership between the professional and the client as opposed to one in which the professional is dominant. Families are assumed to be either competent or capable of becoming competent. This implies that the professional is not an unchallenged authority who is in control. Empowerment promotes an environment that creates opportunities for competencies to be used. Finally, families need to identify that their actions result in behavior change. A nursing intervention that incorporates the principles of empowerment is directed toward the building of nurse–family partnerships that emphasize health risk reduction and health promotion. The nurse's approach to the family should be positive and focused on competencies rather than on problems or deficits. The interventions need to be consistent with family cultural norms and the family's perception of the problem. Rather than making decisions for the family, the nurse supports the family in

---

**BOX 25-3  Prevention Strategies Applied to Families**

**PRIMARY PREVENTION**

Completing a family genogram and assessing health risks with the family to contract for family health activities to prevent diseases from developing.

**SECONDARY PREVENTION**

Using a behavioral health risk survey and identifying the factors leading to obesity in the family.

**TERTIARY PREVENTION**

Developing a contract with the family to change nutritional patterns to reduce further complications from obesity.

primary decision making and bolsters their self-esteem by recognizing and using family strengths and support networks. Interventions that promote desired family behaviors increase family competency and decrease the need for outside help, resulting in families' seeing themselves as being actively responsible for bringing about desired changes. The goal of an empowering approach is to create a partnership between the nurse and the family characterized by cooperation and shared responsibility.

## COMMUNITY RESOURCES

Families have varied and complex needs and problems. The nurse is often involved in mobilizing several resources to effectively and appropriately meet family health promotion needs. Although the specific resources vary from community to community, general types can be identified. Government resources such as Medicare, Medicaid, Aid to Families with Dependent Children, Supplementary Security Income, Food Stamps, and WIC are available in most communities. These programs primarily provide support for basic needs (e.g., illness/health care, nutritional needs, funds for housing and clothing), and funds are based on meeting eligibility criteria.

In addition to government agencies providing health-related services to families, most communities have voluntary (nongovernmental) programs. Local chapters of such organizations as the American Cancer Society, the American Heart Association, the American Lung Association, and the Muscular Dystrophy Association provide education, support services, and some direct services to individuals and families. These agencies provide primary prevention and health promotion services, as well as screening programs and assistance after the disease or condition is diagnosed. Local social service agencies, such as Catholic Social Services, provide direct services such as counseling to families. Other voluntary organizations provide direct service (e.g., shelters for homeless or battered individuals, substance abuse counseling and treatment, Meals on Wheels, transportation, clothing, food, furniture).

Health resources in the community may be proprietary, voluntary, or public. In addition to private health care providers, nurses should be aware of voluntary and public clinics, screening programs, and health promotion programs.

Identifying resources in a community requires time and effort. One valuable source is the telephone book. Often community service organizations, such as the local chamber of commerce and health department, publish community resource listings. Regardless of how the resource is identified, the nurse must be familiar with the types of services offered and any requirements or costs involved. If this information is not available, the nurse can contact the resource.

Locating and using these systems often requires skills and patience that many families lack. Nurses work with families to identify community resources, and as client advocates they help families learn to use resources. This may involve sharing information with families, rehearsing with families what questions to ask, preparing required materials, making the initial contact, and arranging transportation. The appropriateness and effectiveness of resources should be evaluated with families afterward. It is important to remember that navigating the maze of resources is often difficult for the nurse. If a family is in crisis or does not have a phone or a home base from which to call or receive return calls, this process is even more difficult, and their sense of helplessness may be increased. Therefore the nurse's assistance, while promoting the family's sense of empowerment, is both necessary and complex.

## Family Policy

This chapter ends where it began, with a discussion of the nurse's role in policy development and implementation. Florence Nightingale, Lillian Wald, and Mary Breckenridge were all strongly involved nurses who advocated for families and influenced policy to improve the health of families and consequently the health of communities. Building on the gains made by these influential women is essential. Families are affected by the rules and values of society in general. If families—all families—are valued, the community will be strong and connected. If any family is neglected and not supported, the community will be weak and disconnected.

## THE CUTTING EDGE

In 2002 the Supreme Court ruled that an employer has the right to designate family medical leave, when appropriate, whether or not the employee requests this designation for a leave of absence from work.

## ◾ Practice Application

The initial contact between a community-oriented nursing service and a family provides limited information, and the situation that develops may be much more complex than anticipated. The following example, based on an actual case, illustrates the issues and approaches outlined in this chapter.

The Fayette County Health Department was notified that Amy Cress, age 16, had been referred by the school counselor at the local high school for prenatal supervision. Amy was 4 months pregnant, in apparently good health, in the tenth grade, and living at home with her mother, stepfather, and younger sister. The family lived in a rural area outside of a small farming community. The father of the baby also lived in the community and continued to see Amy on a regular basis. The referral information provided the nurse with a beginning, but limited, assessment of the family situation.

**A.** What would you do first as the nurse assigned to this family?

**B.** How would you help this family empower themselves to take responsibility for this situation?

**C.** After the initial contact, how would you extend the assessment to the entire family system?

**D.** Would you contract with this family? How? On what terms?

**Answers are in the back of the book.**

## Key Points

- The importance of the family as a major client system for community-oriented nurses in reducing health risks and promoting the health of individuals and populations is well documented.
- The family system is a basic unit within which health behavior, including health values, health habits, and health risk perceptions, is developed, organized, and performed.
- Knowledge of family structure and functioning, family theory, nursing theory, and models of health behavior are fundamental to implementing the nursing process with families in the community.
- Nurses need to go beyond the individual and family, and to understand the complex environment in which the family functions, to be effective in reducing family health risks. Categories of risk factors that are important to family health are biological risk, environmental risk (including economic factors), and behavioral risk.
- Several factors contribute to the experience of healthy/unhealthy outcomes. Not everyone exposed to the same event will have the same outcome. The factors that influence whether disease or other unhealthy results occur are called health risks. The accumulated risks are synergistic; their combined effect is more than the sum of the individual effects.
- An important aspect of nursing's role in reducing health risk and promoting the health of populations has been the tradition of providing services to individual families in their homes.
- Home visits afford the opportunity to gain a more accurate assessment of the family structure and behavior in the natural environment. Home visits also provide opportunities to make observations of the home environment and to identify both barriers and supports to reducing health risks and reaching family health goals.
- Increasingly, health professionals have come to look toward working with clients in a more interactive, collaborative style.
- Contracting, which is making an agreement between two or more parties, involves a shift in responsibility and control, from the professional alone to a shared effort by client and professional.
- Families have varied and complex needs and problems. The nurse often mobilizes several resources to effectively and appropriately meet family health needs.

- Policy development and implementation is an important skill that the nurse uses to improve the health of families and thus improve the health and livability of communities.

## Clinical Decision-Making Activities

1. Select one of the Healthy People 2010 objectives and identify how biological risk (including age-related risk), environmental risk (including economic risk), and behavioral risk contribute to family health risks for that objective. Give examples.
2. Select three to four families (hypothetically or from actual situations) that represent different ethnic and socioeconomic backgrounds. Complete a family genogram and ecomap for each family, and identify and compare major health risks. Summarize your findings.
3. Select one or more agencies in which community-oriented nurses work, and examine the agency and nursing philosophies and objectives with emphasis on individual care, family care, illness care, risk reduction, and health promotion. If you were to accept a position with this agency, what approach to family risk reduction would you be required to use? Is there a better way?
4. Identify three public health problems in your community, and discuss the implications of these problems for the health of families. How did you arrive at your conclusions?
5. Identify three health problems common to families in your community, and discuss the implications of the problems for the health and/or health care resources of the community. What strategies might you use to address the health problems?

## Additional Resources

These related resources are found either in the appendix at the back of this book or on the book's website at **http://evolve.elsevier.com/Stanhope.**

### Appendixes

Appendix H.2 Friedman Family Assessment Model (Short Form)

### *evolve* Evolve Website

Appendix A.1 Schedule of Clinical Preventive Services
Appendix H.1 Family Systems Stressor-Strength Inventory
Appendix H.3 Case Example of Family Assessment
List of Family Assessment Tools
WebLinks: Healthy People 2010

# References

Bahr KS: Student responses to genogram and family chronology, *Family Relat* 39(3):243, 1990.

Barnes-Boyd C, Norr KF, Nacion KW: Evaluation of an interagency home visiting program to reduce postneonatal mortality in disadvantaged communities, *Public Health Nurs* 13(3):201, 1998.

Belloc NB, Breslow L: Relationship of physical health in a general population survey, *Am J Epidemiol* 93:329, 1972.

Bomar PJ, editor: *Nurses and family health promotion: concepts, assessment, and interventions,* Baltimore, 1996, Williams & Wilkins.

Bradley PJ, Martin J: The impact of home visits on enrollment patterns in pregnancy-related services among low-income women, *Public Health Nurs* 11(6):392, 1994.

Burr WR, Klein SR: *Reexamining family stress: new theory and research,* Thousand Oaks, Calif, 1994, Sage.

Byrd ME: The home visiting process in the contexts of the voluntary vs. required visit: examples from fieldwork, *Public Health Nurs* 12(3):196, 1995.

Califano JA Jr: Healthy people: the surgeon general's report on health promotion and disease prevention, Washington, DC, 1979, U.S. Government Printing Office.

Carter B, McGoldrick M: *The expanded family life cycle,* ed 3, Boston, 1999, Allyn and Bacon.

Coontz S: *The way we really are: coming to terms with America's changing families,* New York, 1997, Basic Books.

Doherty WJ, McCubbin HI: Family and health care: an emerging arena of theory, research and clinical intervention, *Family Relat* 34(1):5, 1985.

Greer C: Something is robbing our children of their future, *Parade Magazine,* March 5, pp 4-6, 1995.

Hill R: *Families under stress,* New York, 1949, Harper.

Hutchins EB: *Health risk appraisal,* Decatur, Ga, 1991, The Healthier People Network.

Kang R et al: Preterm infant follow-up project: a multi-site field experiment of hospital and home intervention programs for mothers and preterm infants, *Public Health Nurs* 12(3):171, 1995.

Keller LO et al: Population-based public health nursing interventions: a model from practice, *Public Health Nurs* 15(3):207, 1998.

Litman TJ: The family as a basic unit in health and medical care: a social behavioral overview, *Soc Sci Med* 8:495, 1974.

Mauksch HO: A social science basis for conceptualizing family health, *Soc Sci Med* 8:521, 1974.

National Cancer Institute: *Cancer facts: environmental tobacco smoke,* available at http://cis.nci.nih.gov/fact/3_9.htm, 2001.

National Highway Traffic Safety Administration, U.S. Department of Transportation: *Traffic safety facts 2001: alcohol,* Washington, DC, 2002, NHTSA, available at http://www-nrd.nhtsa.gov.

Neuman B: *The Neuman Systems Model,* ed 4, Norwalk, Conn, 1995, Appleton & Lange.

Nightingale EO et al: *Perspectives on health promotion and disease prevention in the United States,* Washington, DC, 1978, Institute of Medicine, National Academy of Sciences.

Olds D et al: Long-term effects of nurse home visitation on children's criminal and antisocial behavior: 15-year follow-up of a randomized trial, *JAMA* 280:1238-1244, 1998.

Orem DE: *Nursing: concepts of practice,* ed 5, St Louis, Mo, 1995, Mosby.

Pender NJ: *Health promotion in nursing practice,* ed 4, Stamford, Conn, 2002, Appleton & Lange.

Pratt L: *Family structure and effective health behavior,* Boston, 1976, Houghton-Mifflin.

Purnell LD, Paulanka BJ: *Transcultural health care: a culturally competent approach,* ed 2, Philadelphia, 2003, Davis.

Rodwell CM: An analysis of the concept of empowerment, *J Adv Nurs* 23:305, 1996.

U.S. Department of Health and Human Services: *Healthy people 2010: understanding and improving health,* ed 2, Washington, DC, 2000, USDHHS, Public Health Service.

Whitley DM, Kelley SJ, Sipe TA: Grandmothers raising grandchildren: are they at increased risk of health problems? *Health Soc Work* 26:105-114, 2001.

Wright LM: *Nursing and families: a guide to family assessment and intervention,* ed 3, Philadelphia, 2000, Davis.

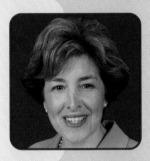
# Child and Adolescent Health

**Marcia K. Cowan, R.N., M.S.N., C.P.N.P.**

Marcia K. Cowan has been working as a pediatric nurse practitioner for 12 years in private practice. She consults with community day-care centers and coordinates a community weight management program for children and adolescents. Other community-oriented positions include working as a public health nurse, home health, school nurse practitioner, and discharge planner for newborns in intensive care. She has been an instructor in pediatrics at the University of Alabama in Birmingham.

## Objectives

After reading this chapter, the student should be able to do the following:

1. Describe significant physical and psychosocial developmental factors characteristic of the child and adolescent population
2. Examine the role of the nurse and discuss appropriate nursing interventions that promote and maintain the health of children and adolescents, both as individuals and as members of the community
3. Discuss major health problems of children and adolescents
4. Discuss two current issues, environmental hazards and complementary therapies, and their effects on child health
5. Describe the role of the community-oriented nurse with specific at-risk populations in the community

Walt Disney identified the greatest natural resource of any nation as the minds of its children. The future of the world depends on how well it cares for its youth. If this population is to thrive, it must be nurtured in an appropriate environment. Focusing on the health needs of children increases the chances that future adults will value and practice healthy lifestyles. Community-oriented nurses have two major roles in the area of child and adolescent health:

1. The nurse provides direct services to children and their families: assessing, managing care, education, and counseling.
2. Nurses are involved in the assessment of the community and the establishment of programs to ensure a healthy environment for this population.

The community-oriented nurse has the opportunity to teach healthy lifestyles to children and caregivers and to provide family-centered care in the ambulatory setting. This chapter provides information on the assessment of children and adolescents and activities to promote health. The content includes principles of growth and development from birth through adolescence and major health problems seen in this population. Two current issues, complementary therapies and environmental toxins, and their effects on children's health are reviewed. Two delivery programs are presented to show how nurses work with specific populations in communities. Healthy People 2010 objectives are used as a framework for focusing on needs of children in the community.

## STATUS OF CHILDREN

There were 84 million children through age 21 in the United States in 2000, representing almost one third of the population (U.S. Bureau of the Census, 2000). More than one third of them live in low-income families. The child poverty rate in the United States is two to three times higher than in most major Western industrialized nations. Trends include an increase in the working poor in all regions of the country. One in three families with children has inadequate housing or cannot afford housing. One in three children lives in single-parent households. This number increases to one out of two for minority children. Children who are living with unmarried mothers are more likely to be poor than children living with married partners (Children's Defense Fund, 2001).

One in seven children has no health insurance. This includes 1.3 million teenagers (National Center for Health Statistics [NCHS], 2002). To combat this problem, the U.S.

## Key Terms

**accommodation**, p. 626
**adolescent period**, p. 623
**assimilation**, p. 626
**attention deficit disorder**, p. 638
**attention deficit disorder with hyperactivity**, p. 638
**body mass index**, p. 632
**cognitive development**, p. 626
**complementary and alternative medicine**, p. 641

**development**, p. 617
**growth**, p. 617
**homeless child syndrome**, p. 645
**immunization**, p. 630
**infancy**, p. 618
**neonatal period**, p. 618
**preschool period**, p. 619
**psychosocial development**, p. 624
**puberty**, p. 623

**scheme**, p. 626
**school-age period**, p. 622
**secondhand smoke**, p. 639
**sudden infant death syndrome**, p. 637
**toddler period**, p. 619

*See Glossary for definitions*

## Chapter Outline

Status of Children
Child Development
*Physical Growth and Development: Neonate to Adolescent*
*Psychosocial Development*
*Cognitive Development*
Nutrition
*Factors Influencing Nutrition*
*Nutritional Assessment*
*Nutrition During Infancy*
*Nutrition During Childhood*
*Adolescent Nutritional Needs*
Immunizations

*Barriers*
*Immunization Theory*
*Recommendations*
*Contraindications*
*Legislation*
Major Health Problems
*Obesity*
*Injuries and Accidents*
*Acute Illness*
*Sudden Infant Death Syndrome*
*Chronic Health Problems*
*Alterations in Behavior*
*Tobacco Use*

Current Issues
*Environmental Health Hazards*
*Complementary and Alternative Medicine*
Models for Delivery of Health Care to Vulnerable Populations
*Home-Based Service Programs*
*Programs for Homeless Families*
Progress Toward Child Health: National Health Objectives
Role of the Community-Oriented Nurse in Child and Adolescent Health

Congress passed the Child Health Insurance Program (CHIPS) legislation in 1999 to cover children for basic preventive services and episodic illness services for underserved children. The number of uninsured children is stable and is not rising as was originally projected.

In 1994, 3.1 million children were abused or neglected, with 2000 deaths. This is a number that is often underreported because it is difficult to prove. Abuse occurs in all income, racial, and ethnic groups. The number of cases is increasing significantly (Children's Defense Fund, 2001). At either end of the age spectrum, children are at great risk. One out of six infants is born to a mother who did not receive prenatal care. Although infant mortality rates are decreasing, one out of 139 babies dies in the first year of life. The mortality rate for minority infants is twice that of white infants (NCHS, 2002).

Currently, one out of three children and teens is 1 year or more behind in school. In 1999, 1 million teenagers became pregnant, most unintentionally (see Chapter 34). Sexually transmitted diseases and genital carcinomas are increasing among teens. Each year, 500,000 to 1.5 million teenagers run away or are forced out of their homes. More than half are 15 to 16 years of age. About one out of eight teenagers leaves high school before graduation. One out of eleven 16- to 19-year-olds is detached, not in school or working. Juveniles 12 to 17 years of age commit one fourth of violent crimes. Of all violent crimes, teenagers are most often the victims (NCHS, 2002).

> **DID YOU KNOW?**
>
> One third of the uninsured children in the United States are eligible for Medicaid programs.

## CHILD DEVELOPMENT
### Physical Growth and Development: Neonate to Adolescent

**Growth** is the measurable aspect of the individual's size; **development** involves the observable changes in the individual. A unique feature of the pediatric population is the ongoing process of growth and development, resulting in physical, cognitive, and emotional changes. Health visits or well-child checkups are scheduled at key ages to monitor these processes. Nursing assessments include

**Table 26-1 Guidelines for Well-Child Care**

| | AGE (MO) | | | | | | | AGE (YR) | | | | | |
|---|---|---|---|---|---|---|---|---|---|---|---|---|---|
| | 2 | 4 | 6 | 9 | 12 | 15 | 18 | 2 | 3 | 4-6 | 7-9 | 10-13 | 14-21 |
| **General Physical Examination** | | | | | | | | | | | | | |
| Complete physical | * | * | * | * | * | * | * | * | * | * | * | * | * |
| Height, weight | * | * | * | * | * | * | * | * | * | * | * | * | * |
| Head circumference | * | * | * | * | * | * | * | * | * | | | | |
| Blood pressure | | | | | | | | | * | * | * | * | * |
| Vision | s | s | s | s | s | s | s | s | * | * | * | * | * |
| Hearing | s | s | s | s | s | s | s | s | s | * | * | * | * |
| Developmental | * | * | * | * | * | * | * | * | * | * | * | * | * |
| **Laboratory Tests** | | | | | | | | | | | | | |
| Hct/Hb | | | | * | | | | | | * | | * | |
| Urinalysis | | | | | | | | | | * | | * | |
| Cholesterol screen | | | | | | | | | c | c | | c | c |
| Lead level | | | | | * | | | | | * | | | |
| Pap smear | | | | | | | | | | | | | |
| STDs screen | * | | | | | | * | * | | | | ^ | ^ |
| **Anticipatory Guidance** | | | | | | | | | | | | | |
| Feeding/nutrition | * | * | * | * | * | * | * | * | * | * | * | * | * |
| Growth/development | * | * | * | * | * | * | * | * | * | * | * | * | * |
| Behavior | * | * | * | * | * | * | * | * | * | * | * | * | * |
| Safety/poisons/injury | * | * | * | * | * | * | * | * | * | * | * | * | * |
| Sexual behaviors | | | | | | | | | | | a | a | a |
| Substance abuse | | | | | | | | | | | a | a | a |
| Physical activity | | | | | | | | | | a | a | a | a |

Modified from American Academy of Pediatrics: *Guidelines for health supervision III: American Academy of Pediatrics guide to clinical preventive services,* Elk Grove Village, Ill, 1997, AAP.
*a,* As appropriate for age; *c,* based on assessment of family risk factors; *Hct/Hb,* hematocrit, hemoglobin; *s,* subjectively determined by behavioral observations, formal assessment as determined by history; *STDs,* sexually transmitted diseases; *,* recommendations vary according to state guidelines and individual risk; *^,* annually if sexually active.

growth and health status, developmental level, and the quality of the parent–child relationship. Table 26-1 identifies recommendations for schedules and components of well-child assessments as recommended by the American Academy of Pediatrics (AAP) and the Schedule of Clinical Preventive Services (see Appendix A.1). The nurse needs to be aware of issues of concern at each age.

Assessment strategies and tools, common concerns and problems, and specific interventions for each age-group are further discussed in Appendix E, and they can be found on the text's website at http://evolve.elsevier.com/Stanhope.

### Focus of Assessment

#### Neonates

The **neonatal period** extends from birth to 1 month of age. It is a time of transition. Physiologic stabilizing and rapid growth highlight this time. The nurse assesses the stability of the neonate by physical examination that includes recording of vital signs and weight (see the evolve website).

The parents are learning how to meet the needs of the baby, and the nurse assesses their ability to respond to the neonate's needs. Feeding, elimination, and sleep patterns are frequently issues of concern. The goal of care is to support the family as they increase their caregiving skills (Table 26-2).

The nurse may provide care for newborns discharged from the hospital at 24 hours of age. The nurse should be aware of factors that place the infant at risk, and of danger signs indicating the need for referral (see the evolve website).

#### Infants

**Infancy** extends from 1 month to 1 year. During this time, rapid growth continues. Nurses identify and intervene in situations when the infant is at risk because of health or socioeconomic problems. Nursing interventions include

## Table 26-2 Assessing the Neonate

| ASSESSMENT | FOCAL POINTS | NURSING IMPLICATIONS |
|---|---|---|
| Physical | • Assess stabilization of transition<br>• Assess vital signs<br>  • Temperature: 98.6° to 99.5° F (37° to 37.5° C) rectally<br>  • Heart rate: 120 to 140 beats/min<br>  • Respiratory rate: 40 to 60 breaths/min<br>• Assess for growth<br>  • Weight gain ½ to 1 ounce/day (15 to 30 g)<br>  • Length ½ to 1 in/mo (1.2 to 2.5 cm)<br>  • Head circumference: 0.6 in/mo (1.5 cm)<br>• Assess for normal variations and minor abnormalities (see evolve website)<br>• Screening (generally performed before nursery discharge): phenylketonuria (PKU), hypothyroid, sickle cell anemia, galactosemia, hearing | • Identify deviations and refer as needed<br>• Teach cord care, circumcision care, bathing, diaper area and skin care, temperature-taking techniques, normal variations of color, activity patterns, and variations in respiratory patterns<br>• Teach signs of illness and how to contact health care provider |
| Nutrition | • Assess feeding behaviors and parent comfort with feeding technique<br>• Assess adequacy of caloric intake based on weight gain and output | • Teach feeding techniques including breastfeeding, formula preparation, burping, and positioning<br>• Identify concerns related to getting enough to eat, spitting up, gas, and colic |
| Elimination | • Urine output: at least 6 to 8 wet diapers/day<br>• Stool patterns vary from several times per day to every 3 to 4 days<br>• Loose to firm consistency is normal<br>• Straining with bowel movements is common | • Educate and reassure parents about normal elimination patterns |
| Sleep | • Assess sleep patterns (high variability between active and quiet babies); average 16 hr per day | • Encourage supine sleep position<br>• Offer strategies to encourage night sleep |
| Development | • Observe responses to tactile, auditory, taste, and visual stimuli<br>• Note ability to self-quiet, reflex responses, habituate, and state transition | • Identify behaviors showing individuality, competence, consolability, and responsiveness<br>• Adapt caregiving strategies to match temperament |
| Safety | • Dependency on caregiver for safety | • Offer anticipatory guidance for well-child care and immunizations<br>• Discuss falls, car seat, water temperature, and fire safety in the home |

monitoring of growth and development, with particular attention to feeding, sleeping, elimination, development, and safety (Table 26-3).

The second half of infancy brings major accomplishments in gross motor activities. Rolling, sitting, pulling up, and walking bring safety concerns. Parents should be

given anticipatory guidance in these areas (see the evolve website).

### Toddlers and Preschoolers

The **toddler period** consists of the second and third years of life. The **preschool period** encompasses ages 3 to 5 years. Slowing and stabilizing growth are hallmarks of this period as reflected by changes in appetite and eating patterns. Increased physical ability and independence force parents to deal with discipline issues. The number of acute illnesses increases.

Children test limits, seeking rules and trying to make sense of the world. Negativism and aggressive behaviors upset parents and caregivers but are often a result of the

### DID YOU KNOW?

Many parents think that their child should be potty trained by 2 years of age. Only 4% of children are actually potty trained by age 2. By age 2½, 22% are trained; 60% by age 3; and 80% by age 3½.

**Table 26-3   Assessing the Infant**

| ASSESSMENT | FOCAL POINTS | NURSING IMPLICATIONS |
|---|---|---|
| Physical | • Continued assessment of stabilization of organ systems<br>• Vital signs<br>  • Heart rate: 115 to 130 beats/min<br>  • Respiratory rate: 20 to 40 breaths/min<br>• Growth<br>  • Weight gain:<br>    • First 6 months: 6 to 8 oz/wk (180 to 240 g)<br>    • Second 6 months: 3 to 4 oz/wk (90 to 120 g)<br>  • Length increase:<br>    • First 6 months: 1 in/mo (2.5 cm)<br>    • Second 6 months: $\frac{1}{2}$ in/mo (1.25 cm)<br>• Tooth eruption begins at average of 6 mo<br>• Primary series of immunizations<br>• Hearing: turns to sounds, babbles<br>• Vision: increased tracking of objects | • Anticipatory guidance about acute illness; risk factors include day care, smoke exposure, and poor hand hygiene<br>• Discuss risks/benefits of immunizations<br>• Refer abnormal physical findings |
| Nutrition | • Assess feeding patterns and techniques<br>• Identify parent concerns<br>• Addition of solids at 6 mo<br>• Breastfeeding or formula throughout the first year of life with weaning to a cup around 12 mo<br>• Fluoride source identified | • Introduction of new foods with progression from spoon feeding to soft finger foods<br>• Introduction of cup |
| Elimination | • Urine output continues to be at least 6 to 8 wet diapers/day<br>• Stools are soft to firm; easily passed; varying from daily to every few days | • Educate and reassure parents about normal elimination patterns |
| Sleep | • 3 months: 70% sleep 8 hr at night with two naps during the day<br>• 6 months: 80% sleep 8 hr at night with variable naps during the day<br>• 12 months: 90% sleep 8 to 12 hr at night with average of one 2-hr nap during the day | • Teaching strategies to promote falling asleep independently, self-comfort techniques, and bedtime routines |
| Development | • Development proceeds in cephalocaudal progression<br>• Behaviors progress from reflexive and involuntary to purposeful and voluntary<br>• Reaching, holding, mouthing, activities of the hands predominate during early infancy<br>• Rolling and sitting occur during middle infancy, with more shaking and banging of objects<br>• Pulling up, crawling, and walking occur during late infancy | • Anticipatory guidance includes education about attachment, stranger awareness, separation anxiety, and night wakening<br>• Encourage ways to play with the infant to encourage development |
| Safety | • Increasing gross and fine motor skills increase safety<br>• Environmental risks include lead exposure | • Educate about risks for falls, choking, aspiration, poison prevention, use of car seat, burn prevention<br>• Screen for lead toxicity if appropriate<br>• Offer anticipatory guidance for well-child care and immunizations |

child's frustrations. Discipline is important method of teaching self-control.

Toddlers and preschoolers are often around other children (e.g., at day-care centers), increasing exposure to viruses and bacteria. The child may have more episodes of acute illnesses, including upper respiratory infections, otitis media, and stomach viruses. Allergies may influence health. Children of this age often suffer from "runny, drippy" noses. Nurses monitor growth and development and offer anticipatory guidance about behavior and acute illness (Table 26-4) (see also the evolve website).

## Table 26-4 Assessing Toddlers and Preschool Children

| ASSESSMENT | FOCAL POINTS | NURSING IMPLICATIONS |
|---|---|---|
| Physical | • Assessment of organ systems: increased frequency of upper respiratory illness, otitis media, allergy symptoms, GI illness<br>• Vital signs<br>  • Heart rate: 100 to 110 beats/min<br>  • Respiratory rate: 20 to 40 breaths/min<br>  • Blood pressure: average 98/60 mm Hg<br>• Growth rate markedly decreased<br>• Weight gain averages 5 lb/yr (2.27 kg)<br>• Height increases 3 to 4 in/yr (7.6 to 10 cm)<br>• Dental: 20 primary teeth by age 2 yr<br>• Anterior fontanel closes by 18 mo<br>• Normal progression from bowlegs (12 to 18 mo) to knock-knees (18 to 24 mo) | • Anticipatory guidance about acute illness; risk factors include day care, smoke exposure, and poor hand hygiene<br>• Management of upper respiratory illness, GI viruses, otitis media, allergies<br>• Education about when to contact health care provider<br>• Refer abnormal physical findings<br>• Discuss risks/benefits of immunizations<br>• Cleaning and flossing of teeth; dental referral<br>• Vision screening age 3 yr and preschool<br>• Audiometry age 3 to 4 yr; sooner if concerns |
| Nutrition | • Slowing of growth results in decreased caloric needs and diminished appetite<br>• Obtain dietary history; food preferences and food jags are common<br>• Self-feeding skills increase | • Reassure with information related to growth needs and intake<br>• Encourage offering small, nutritious snacks frequently |
| Elimination | • Most children demonstrate readiness for toilet training between the ages of 2 and 3 yr<br>• Inappropriate emphasis on defecation may result in constipation | • Anticipatory guidance on cues for readiness, strategies to toilet train, and ways to discourage constipation or retention problems |
| Sleep | • By age 3 yr, most children sleep 8 to 12 hr at night, with an afternoon nap until age 3 to 5 yr<br>• Nightmares and night terrors may interrupt patterns of night sleep | • Provide guidance about routine and common problems<br>• Encourage bedtime routine |
| Development | • Toddler period<br>  • Increasing motor skills<br>  • Increasing autonomy and independence, with resulting periods of ambivalence<br>  • May show negativism and aggression when frustrated<br>  • Parallel play with peers<br>• Preschool period<br>  • Increasing verbal skills<br>  • Increasing initiative, but with difficulty with impulse control<br>  • Interacts more with peers, but this can lead to conflicts | • Developmental screening using standardized assessment tools, history, and observation<br>• Discipline strategies: effective use of time-out, ignoring negative behavior, rewarding positive behavior, avoiding conflict by distraction or timing of activities |
| Safety | • Increasing gross and fine motor skills, imitation, and independence increase risks for injury | • Provide anticipatory guidance related to climbing, falls, outdoor supervision, poison prevention, drowning, burns, guns, sunburn, and car seat |

GI, Gastrointestinal.

Examination of infants through preschoolers is easiest if the parent holds the child. It helps to offer the child a piece of examining equipment to handle. Showing the child how the equipment is used before using it on the child helps to alleviate fears. Describing what is happening may increase the child's confidence.

## School-Age Children

The **school-age period** begins at school entry and continues until the beginning of puberty, usually around 10 years of age. Physical growth is typically slow and steady. The focus shifts from family to peers as school fills more of the day (see the evolve website). The nurse should actively involve the child in the assessment and education process. Encouraging participation helps to model taking responsibility for making healthy lifestyle choices. Acute illnesses decrease during this time. School adjustment, peer relationships, and learning problems are issues to explore. Nurses assess growth and sexual development, dental health, sleep and eating patterns, immunization status, hearing, and vision (Table 26-5) (see Appendixes E.1 and E.2 and the evolve website).

Sports physicals are a common reason for seeking health care. Guidelines for sports safety should be dis-

### WHAT DO YOU THINK?

On Saturday morning television, there are an average of 20 to 25 violent acts per hour during cartoons. During the first hour of primetime network television, 75% of the shows include sexual talk or behavior. Should the government become involved in what is shown or in the development of ratings systems?

### Table 26-5   Assessing School-Age Children

| ASSESSMENT | FOCAL POINTS | NURSING IMPLICATIONS |
|---|---|---|
| Physical | • Decreasing number of acute illnesses<br>• Vital signs<br>  • Heart rate: 60 to 100 beats/min<br>  • Respiratory rate: 18 to 30 breaths/min<br>  • Blood pressure range: 90/60 to 108/66 mm Hg<br>• Growth rate stable<br>• Weight gain: 5 to 7 lb/yr (2.27 to 3 kg)<br>• Height increase: 2.5 in/yr (6 cm)<br>• Loss of primary teeth<br>• Vision: 20/20<br>• Skeletal growth: lengthening of legs and trunk, widening of thighs and shoulders | • Provide anticipatory guidance about normal growth patterns<br>• Identify deviant growth patterns<br>• Inspect number and condition of teeth, noting loss of deciduous teeth and eruption of permanent teeth<br>• Provide education on preventive dental care<br>• Identify dental problems |
| Nutrition | • Caloric needs increase with periods of increased growth<br>• Average requirements: 2400 to 2800 kcal/day<br>• Capable of selecting and preparing own meals<br>• Vulnerable to advertising<br>• Tends to have strong food preferences<br>• Tends to snack frequently | • Obtain diet history<br>• Provide education about balanced diet, healthful snacks, need for breakfast, and exercise needs<br>• Identify eating disorders |
| Sleep | • Obtain history of sleep requirements<br>• Ideal sleep: 9 hr/night with regularity of schedule | • Identify deviant sleep patterns<br>• Provide counseling on meeting sleep requirements |
| Development | • Increasing coordination of fine and gross motor skills, including eye–hand coordination<br>• Increasing intellectual competency with transition from concrete to abstract conceptualization<br>• Moving from egocentrism<br>• Time of intense competition between peers in school and activities<br>• Needs successful experiences | • Involve child in discussions<br>• Provide anticipatory guidance about safety, independence, peer pressure, and conformity<br>• Assess school performance<br>• Identify need to provide opportunities for successful experiences |
| Safety | • Involve child in education | • Sports safety, including protective equipment<br>• Bicycle safety: helmets, road rules<br>• Seat belts |

cussed (Box 26-1). Another important issue involves television viewing. Television time is inactivity. Program content may be inappropriate. Parents need to limit the time spent watching, to select programs carefully, to view programs with children, and to discuss content (see the evolve website).

*Adolescents*

The **adolescent period** refers to ages 11 through 21. **Puberty** refers to the biological changes that occur during this time, including the growth spurt and the development of secondary sexual characteristics. Both growth hormone and sex steroids mediate the growth spurt. The duration of the growth spurt averages 24 to 36 months, ending with epiphyseal closure. The onset varies with the individual and includes increases in both height and weight. Breast bud is the first sign of sexual development for a majority of girls. Testicular enlargement is the first for a majority of boys (see the evolve website).

Emotional and cognitive changes also occur during this progression toward maturity and independence. These processes may start before physical changes and may last beyond the end of growth. Emotional growth is as variable as biological growth and occurs with periods of development and regression. The process of change may involve a great deal of stress for families, although most adolescents cope well with the conflicts (Neinstein, 1996) (Figure 26-1). Some topics for parents to consider in the overall health of their adolescent are listed in Box 26-2.

Physical illness declines during adolescence. Injury and violence are the leading causes of morbidity and mortality. Studies of early and middle adolescents report increasing sexual activity, multiple sex partners, pregnancy, and sexually transmitted diseases (Centers for Disease Control and Prevention, 1996). Experimentation with alcohol, smoking, and drugs occurs at younger ages than it used to. Screening and education may prevent health problems during this period. The *Guidelines for Adolescent Preventative Services* (GAPS), released by the American Medical Association (GAPS Executive Committee, 1995), recommends yearly visits between ages 11 and 21 to identify adolescents who have considered or begun risky behaviors (Box 26-3). The goals of nursing care include early detection of physical, emotional, and behavioral problems. Nurses

---

**BOX 26-1    Guide to Sports Safety**

- Children should be grouped according to weight, size, maturation, and skill level.
- Qualified and competent persons should be available for supervision during games and practices.
- Adequate and appropriate-size equipment should be available.
- Goals should be developmentally and physically appropriate for the child.

---

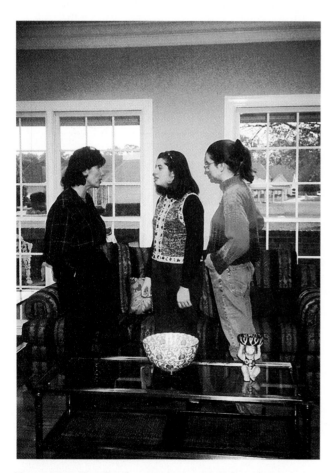

**Figure 26-1** Conflict between parents and teenagers is normal as teenagers experience physical and emotional growth processes.

---

**BOX 26-2    Topics for Health Guidance for Parents of Adolescents**

- Adolescent development—physical, sexual, and emotional
- Signs and symptoms of health problems and emotional distress
- Parenting behaviors that promote healthy adolescent adjustment
- Parents as role models
- Importance of discussing health-related behaviors
- Importance of family activities
- Methods for helping the adolescent avoid potentially risky behaviors
- Motor vehicle accidents
- Weapons
- Removing weapons and medicines as suicide precautions
- Monitoring social and recreational activities for use of tobacco, alcohol, drugs, and sexual behavior

promote healthy lifestyle choices and update immunizations (Table 26-6). Strategies to increase communication with adolescents are identified in the How To box. GAPS also recommends parental guidance visits during early and middle adolescence.

## Psychosocial Development

The child's growth process includes **psychosocial development.** The work of Erik Erikson focuses on the interaction of emotional, cultural, and social forces on personality development. Personality development culminates in the achievement of ego identity, which involves accepting oneself and having the skills for healthy functioning in society. Erikson believed that development is a continual process that occurs in distinct stages. At each stage, a developmental crisis requires resolving. Although a child never completely finishes all the developmental tasks in a given stage, some degree of mastery and comfort must be achieved before proceeding successfully to the next stage. As internal conflicts are resolved, there is new orientation to self and society. This sets the stage for the next conflict. Each crisis emerges from the mastery of the previous stage. All new development is rooted in prior experiences. Difficulty resolving the crisis will cause problems progressing through the subsequent stages. Table 26-7 lists the stages.

---

**BOX 26-3   Guidelines for Adolescent Preventative Services (GAPS) Annual Assessment**

- **Screen:** Hypertension, hyperlipidemia, eating disorders/body image
- **Interview:** Abuse of tobacco, alcohol, drugs; sexual behaviors; depression/suicide risks; emotional, physical, or sexual abuse; learning or school problems

---

**HOW TO   Communicate With Adolescents**

- Identify what issues remain confidential.
- Move from less personal to more personal topics.
- Use open-ended questions.
- Use matter-of-fact style.
- Acknowledge that discussion of sensitive subjects may cause uncomfortable feelings.
- Talk in terms that adolescents understand.
- Use nonjudgmental responses.
- Listen.
- Obtain information from the adolescent directly; plan on time with the adolescent without the parent for interview.
- Depersonalize questions (e.g., "Many teenagers go to parties where drugs are used. Do you?").

---

**Table 26-6   Assessing Adolescents**

| ASSESSMENT | FOCAL POINTS | NURSING IMPLICATIONS |
|---|---|---|
| Physical | • Decreasing number of acute illnesses<br>• Vital signs<br>  • Heart rate: 55 to 110 beats/min<br>  • Respiratory rate: 16 to 20 breaths/min<br>  • Blood pressure range: 110/66 to 120/76 mm Hg<br>• Growth spurt may last 24 to 36 mo and occurs for girls between 9½ and 14 yr and for boys between 10½ and 16 yr<br>• Weight gain varies<br>  • Boys: 12.5 to 29 lb (5.7 to 13.2 kg)<br>  • Girls: 10 to 23 lb (4.6 to 10.6 kg)<br>• Height increases<br>  • Boys: 10 to 11 in (26 to 28 cm)<br>  • Girls: 9 to 11 in (23 to 28 cm)<br>• Loss of primary teeth completed; addition of wisdom teeth<br>• Vision 20/20<br>• Growth of reproductive organs | • Provide anticipatory guidance about normal growth patterns<br>• Identify deviant growth patterns<br>• Inspect number and condition of teeth, noting loss of deciduous teeth and eruption of permanent teeth<br>• Educate about preventive dental care<br>• Identify dental problems<br>• Address issues of sexuality (including abstinence, physical and emotional changes, peer pressure verses option to decline, responsibility for sexual behaviors)<br>• Provide information on preventing pregnancy and sexually transmitted diseases |

Based on data from Millonig VL: *The pediatric nurse practitioner certification review guide,* Potomac Md, 1990, Health Leadership Associates; Neinstein L: *Adolescent health care: a practical guide,* ed 3, Philadelphia, 1996, Williams & Wilkins.

**Table 26-6    Assessing Adolescents—cont'd**

| ASSESSMENT | FOCAL POINTS | NURSING IMPLICATIONS |
|---|---|---|
| Physical—cont'd | • Skeletal growth: mass doubles<br>• Fat deposits and muscle mass increase<br>• Skin: increase of acne<br>• Hair growth: axillary and pubic; boys: facial, chest, and extremities<br>• Development of secondary sexual characteristics (Tanner staging)<br>  • Girls: menarche averages $12\frac{1}{4}$ yr; Tanner stage 3 to 4<br>  • Boys: ejaculation Tanner stage 3; fertility Tanner stage 4 | • Teach breast and testicular self-examination<br>• Immunizations<br>• Screening for hypertension<br>• Screen adolescents at risk for hyperlipidemia |
| Nutrition | • Caloric needs increase with periods of increased growth; average requirements:<br>  • Boys: 3000 kcal/day<br>  • Girls: 2100 kcal/day<br>• Capable of selecting and preparing own meals<br>• Increased occurrence of eating disorders: anorexia, bulimia, pica, obesity | • Obtain diet history<br>• Educate about balanced diet, healthful snacks, need for breakfast, and exercise needs<br>• Identify eating disorders, obesity, and problems with body image<br>• Refer as appropriate |
| Sleep patterns | • Obtain history of sleep requirements<br>• Ideal sleep: 9 hr/night with regularity of schedule | • Identify deviant sleep patterns<br>• Provide counseling on meeting sleep requirements |
| Development | • Early adolescence (10-13 yr): focus on body changes and comparison to peers; beginning separation from parents and challenging authority<br>• Middle adolescence (14-17 yr): increasing involvement with peers and independence from family; sexual exploration<br>• Late adolescence (18-21 yr): concern with future plans; likely to be involved in committed intimate relationship | • Discuss school performance<br>• Identify plans for future including school, work, relationships with family and peers, life skills<br>• Strategies to improve communication skills<br>• Strategies for anger management and conflict resolution without violence<br>• Strategies for handling independence |
| Safety | • Injury and accidents are the leading cause of morbidity and mortality in this age-group<br>• Risk-taking behaviors result from feelings of invincibility, challenging authority, and seeking peer approval | • Educate about tobacco and substance abuse, including alcohol, steroids, and over-the-counter substances<br>• Educate about safety: driving, sports (including protective equipment), seat belts, firearms |

**Table 26-7    Erikson's Stages of Ego Development**

| AGE | PSYCHOSOCIAL CONFLICT | RESOLUTION |
|---|---|---|
| 0-1 yr | Trust/mistrust | Sense of hope |
| 2-3 yr | Autonomy/shame or doubt | Self-confidence and self-control |
| 4-5 yr | Initiative/guilt | Independence |
| 6-11 yr | Industry/inferiority | Competence |
| 12-18 yr | Identity/identity diffusion | Sense of self/loyalty |

Sahler OJZ, Wood BL: Theories and concepts of development as they relate to pediatric practice. In Hoekelman R et al, editors: *Primary pediatric care*, ed 3, St Louis, Mo, 1997, Mosby.

## Cognitive Development

The work of Jean Piaget is widely used to understand the process of **cognitive development.** According to Piaget, learning results from actively manipulating objects and information, followed by a mental processing of the event. As the child interacts with the environment, new objects and problems are discovered. The child creates mental schemes or thought patterns to understand the encounter. The **scheme** is the action pattern and the mental basis for the action. It permits the child to receive information from the world, make sense of it, and predict future events. Development occurs as the schemes increase in scope and complexity.

**Assimilation** is the process of integrating new experiences into existing schemes. When new information cannot fit into the existing schemes, the child must modify schemes or develop new schemes. This process is **accommodation.** The general thought process or mental activity is an operation.

Piaget identified four stages of cognitive development that represent increasing problem-solving ability (Table 26-8). A transition period with combinations of behaviors exists between the stages. The nurse must understand characteristics of cognitive ability at each stage to work effectively with the child and family (Piaget, 1969).

## NUTRITION

Promoting good nutrition and dietary habits is a key to maintaining child health. The first 6 years are the most important for developing sound lifetime eating habits. The quality of nutrition has been widely accepted as an important influence on growth and development. It is now becoming recognized for an important role in disease prevention.

Atherosclerosis begins during childhood. Other diseases, such as obesity, diabetes, osteoporosis, and cancer, may have early beginnings also (Forbes, 1997). Healthy People 2010 objectives include reducing obesity, improving the quality of the diet, and increasing cardiovascular fitness (U.S. Department of Health and Human Services [USDHHS], 2000a). Educating children and their families is an appropriate way to accomplish these objectives. Low-income and minority families are at increased risk for poor nutrition, but all groups show poor dietary patterns.

## Factors Influencing Nutrition

The child and family both provide a range of variables that influence nutritional habits. Ethnic, racial, cultural, and socioeconomic factors influence what the parents eat and how they feed their children. The child brings individual issues to the nutritional arena, such as slow eating, picky patterns, food preferences, food allergies, acute or chronic health problems, and changes with acceleration and deceleration of growth. Parents often have unrealistic expectations of what children should eat. Table 26-9 offers guidelines to daily requirements for all ages.

## Nutritional Assessment

Physical growth serves as an excellent measure of adequacy of the diet. For children younger than 3 years old, height, weight, and head circumference, plotted on appropriate growth curves at regular intervals, allow assessment of growth patterns. Good nutritional intake supports physical growth at a steady rate (Figure 26-2).

A 24-hour diet recall by the parent is a helpful screening tool to assess the amount and variety of food intake. If the recall is fairly typical for the child, the nurse can compare the intake with basic recommendations for the child's age. It is important to ask about parent's concerns regarding diet. It is also helpful to look at the family's meal patterns. An important part of nutrition assessment includes exercise. Behavior problems that occur during meals may also be an issue.

## Nutrition During Infancy

The first year of life is critical for growth of all major organ systems of the body. Most of the brain growth that occurs during the life span occurs during infancy. The digestive and renal systems are immature at birth and during early infancy. Certain nutrients are not handled well. Energy needs are high. Nutrition during this time influences how an infant will grow and thrive.

### Types of Infant Feeding

Breast milk is the preferred method of infant feeding. Breast milk provides appropriate nutrients and antibodies for the infant. Breastfed infants have fewer illnesses and allergies. If breastfeeding is not chosen, commercially prepared formulas are an acceptable alternative. Although evaporated milk with added sugar has been used in the past as a low-cost alternative to breast milk, it is now discouraged. Errors in mixing and the lack of vitamins and minerals have been common problems.

The method of feeding is a choice that parents should make with guidance and education. The advantages and disadvantages of breast, formula, and combination feeding should be discussed with the parents.

Nurses should be prepared to instruct and support parents in the feeding method of their choice. For breastfeeding, teaching topics include comfortable position, appropriate techniques, feeding frequency, the let-down reflex, care of breasts, and length of feedings. The mother's feelings about nursing her infant and the presence or absence of family support are important to success. For bottle-feeding, parents need instruction about preparation and care of equipment and formula, position, frequency, and amount of feeding. Parents may need to discuss their feelings about the method of feeding.

### Supplements

Current recommendations from the American Academy of Pediatrics indicate that the iron in breast milk is highly available to the infant. Breastfed infants do not require iron supplementation. Infants who are not breastfed should be

## Table 26-8  Piaget's Stages of Cognitive Development

| STAGE | AGE | CHARACTERISTICS | EXAMPLE |
|---|---|---|---|
| Sensorimotor | 0-8 mo | • Reflex behaviors become purposeful | • Moves fist while grasping rattle; repeats action to shake rattle for the sound it makes |
| | 8-18 mo | • Object permanence: objects and people exist when not present | • Looks for hidden toy or cries for mother when she leaves |
| | 18-24 mo | • Symbolism: objects can represent other objects; words can represent objects; beginning of mental representation: think before doing action | • Gets an object from another room; knows mentally what object is even if not seen and can think about getting it before acting |
| Preoperation | 2-7 yr | • Self-awareness: aware of self as separate from events in environment; development of a sense of vulnerability<br>• Egocentric: inability to take other's view<br>• Symbolism: language is literal; blending of real world and fantasy; increasing complexity of symbolic play<br>• Irreversibility: cannot reverse an action or situation<br>• Finalism: every event has direct cause and every question has direct answer<br>• Centration: focuses on only one aspect of situation<br>• Magical thinking: not a clear sense of what is real; confuses coincidence with causation | • Asks questions to learn about environment<br>• Develops fears as unable to separate reality from things seen on television or heard<br>• Learns from imitation<br>• Nightmares seem real<br>• Cannot retrace steps of situation to look for lost thing<br>• Changing shape changes toy: rolling out a ball of clay makes it bigger<br>• Fascination with monsters and superheroes to cope with sense of vulnerability |
| Concrete operation | 7-11 yr | • Learns by manipulation of objects<br><br>• Classification: orders objects by characteristics<br>• Conservation: understands that properties of objects remain the same despite change of appearance<br>• Egocentricity: considers other view point<br>• Internal regulation: able to send messages to self | • Has better understanding of time, place, number<br>• Enjoys collections because of the ability to group and classify<br>• Ability to understand beyond the literal meanings of words<br><br>• Increasing use of humor, riddles, jokes<br>• Participates in group games; peer relationships important<br>• Increasing ability to apply relationships, build on previous experiences, and make inferences as long as the ideas involve concrete or physical objects |
| Formal operation | 11-19 yr | • Hypothesizes: uses propositional thinking, which does not require experience with the problem<br>• Considers alternative explanation for same phenomenon<br>• Considers alternative frames of reference<br>• Tests hypothesis with deductive reasoning<br>• Synthesizes and integrates concepts to other schemes<br>• Works with abstract ideas<br>• Reflective, futuristic thinking | • Ability to perform scientific process<br>• Follows train of thought to a logical conclusion<br>• Idealism may interfere with reality<br>• Begins to form personal rules and values |

Sahler OJZ, Wood BL: Theories and concepts of development as they relate to pediatric practice. In Hoekelman R et al, editors: *Primary pediatric care,* ed 3, St Louis, Mo, 1997, Mosby; Modified from Piaget J: *The psychology of the child,* New York, 1969, Basic

**Table 26-9** Daily Dietary Guidelines: Childhood and Adolescence

| FOOD GROUP | 1 TO 3 YEARS | | 4 TO 6 YEARS | | 7 TO 12 YEARS | | ADOLESCENT | |
|---|---|---|---|---|---|---|---|---|
| | SERVINGS/ DAY | SERVING SIZE | SERVINGS/ DAY | SERVING SIZE | SERVINGS/ DAY | SERVING SIZE | SERVINGS/ DAY | SERVING SIZE |
| **Dairy** | 2-3 | 1/2 c | 2 | 3/4 c | 2-3 | 1 c | 2-3 | 1 c |
| 1 serving = milk 1/2 c cheese 1/2 oz yogurt 1/3 c pudding 1/2 c | | | | | | | | |
| **Protein** | 2 | 1 oz | 2 | 2 oz | 2 | 2 oz | 2-3 | 2 oz |
| 1 oz lean meat= 1 egg or 1 oz cheese or 2 T peanut butter or 1/4 c cottage cheese or 1/2 c dried peas or beans | | | | | | | | |
| **Vegetables/fruits** | 4-5 | 3-4 T (1/4 c) | 4-5 | 4-6 T (1/2 c) | at least 5 | 1/3-1/2 c | at least 5 | 1/2 c |
| 1 small fruit = 1/2 c juice or 1/2 c cut fruit | | | | | | | | |
| **Breads/cereals** | 3-4 | 1/2 slice | 4 | 1/2 slice | 6-11 | 1 slice | 6-11 | 1 slice |
| 1 slice= 1/2 c cereal or 1 oz cold cereal or 1/2 c pasta or 2-3 crackers | | | | | | | | |

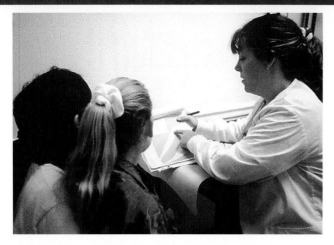

**Figure 26-2** A nurse explains the growth patterns on a growth chart to a child and her mother.

given a commercial formula that is fortified with iron. Addition of iron to formula has reduced the incidence of anemia and does not cause stomach symptoms. After 4 to 6 months of age, iron needs are further met by the introduction of iron-fortified cereals.

Fluoride at 0.25 mg/day is recommended for infants who drink ready-to-feed formula or formula mixed with water from a supply containing less than 0.3 parts per million (ppm) of fluoride. Fluoride is currently started at 6 months of age and maintained until 16 years of age. Fluoride is not recommended for breastfed infants whose mothers have a fluoridated water supply (AAP Committee on Nutrition, 1998).

Several recent reports have indicated an increase in the occurrence of rickets (Gummer-Strawn, 2001). Vitamin D supplementation is recommended for breastfed infants at risk for rickets. Box 26-4 shows strategies to prevent rickets at the three levels of prevention.

### Introduction of Solid Foods and Juice

Current trends include the introduction of solids between 4 and 6 months of age and juice at 6 months. There is no nutritional, developmental, or psychological advantage to starting earlier. Studies have not shown that cereal helps a baby sleep longer. Parents need to know the risks of feeding solids too early:

• The incidence of constipation is greater when solid food intake is too high.

• Early introduction of solids may lead to overfeeding and obesity.

• There is a greater possibility of food allergy because immunoglobulin A (IgA) production is insufficient for solid foods until closer to 6 months.

• If the infant lowers milk intake because of filling up on solids or juices, there may be an imbalance of nutrients.

Once parents have decided to start solids, nurses can help them plan a schedule for starting appropriate foods.

Dry cereal fortified with iron is a useful starter food because of the ease of digestion (see the evolve website).

At 1 year of age, the infant may be changed from formula to whole milk. Skim, low fat, and 2% milk are not recommended for babies less than 2 years of age because of inadequate fat and caloric content (AAP Committee on Nutrition, 1998).

## Nutrition During Childhood

The skill and desire to self-feed begins at approximately 1 year of age. The parents' role begins to shift at this time toward providing a balanced, healthy range of foods as the child assumes more independence. Growth rate and caloric needs decrease during this time. Nurses can best assist parents by offering information on daily needs and healthy food choices. Suggestions for children might include the following:

• Frequent, small meals may be better accepted.

• Offer a balanced diet incorporating variety and foods that the child likes.

• Limit milk intake to the recommendations for the child's age.

• Consider the child's development and safety; avoid nuts, popcorn, grapes, and similar foods to decrease risk of aspiration in young children.

• Encourage children to help with food selection and preparation as appropriate to developmental skills.

• Generally, vitamin and iron supplements are not necessary.

• Avoid using food as a punishment or reward.

Fat content in the diet should be restricted to less than 30% beginning at 2 years of age, with no more than 10% of the total calories coming from saturated fats. Studies show that children as young as 2 to 6 years of age have diets higher in total fats and in saturated fats than recommended.

In general, the family diet does not contain enough fiber-rich foods or fruits and vegetables. Diets of school-age children have been shown to be low in calcium. Children also need regular physical activity. Observations of children indicate that they are too sedentary. The entire family may benefit from suggestions to modify the diet:

- Choose low-fat protein sources: plant proteins, such as beans, peas, and wholegrain products or lean cuts of meat, chicken, or fish, with visible fat trimmed.
- Broil, bake, stir-fry, or poach foods rather than frying.
- Use polyunsaturated and monounsaturated fats found in nuts, seeds, nut butters, wheat germ, and vegetable oils.
- Decrease salt, sugar, and fats.
- Increase complex carbohydrates: breads, grains, cereals.
- Increase fruits and vegetables to at least five servings per day, especially green and orange vegetables and citrus fruits.
- Use low-fat dairy products.
- Increase calcium intake through low-fat dairy products, calcium-fortified products, and supplements if necessary.
- Maintain regular activity (e.g., exercise, sports, household chores) and limit television viewing.

Remind parents that they are teaching children lifelong strategies to prevent illness and promote good health (AAP Committee on Nutrition, 1998).

## Adolescent Nutritional Needs

The preadolescent and adolescent years are a time of increased growth that is accompanied by increases in appetite and nutritional requirements. Caloric and protein requirements increase for boys 11 to 18 years of age. Girls have an increased protein need but a decreased caloric need during the same age span. The iron needed by the adolescent is nearly double that needed by adults.

Adolescent nutritional needs are influenced by physical alterations and psychosocial adjustments. Teenagers are often free to eat when and where they choose. Eating habits acquired from the family are dropped. Food away from home is a major source of nutrition. Fad foods and diets are prominent. Accelerated growth and poor eating habits make the adolescent at risk for poor nutritional health. Adolescents have the most unsatisfactory nutritional status of all age-groups. Deficiencies in iron, vitamins, calcium, riboflavin, and thiamine are most common (Neinstein and Schack, 1996).

Nurses can initiate activities that promote improved nutritional status. Such activities include the following:

- Providing information on good nutrition in individual or group sessions
- Diet assessment
- Educational activities that focus on effects of fad foods and diets
- Supplying a list of "at-risk" nutrients

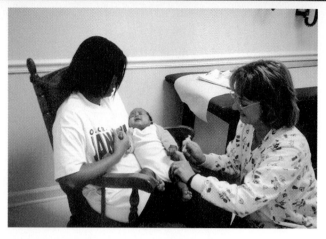

**Figure 26-3** An infant receives a regularly scheduled immunization.

- Providing a daily food guide (see Table 26-9)
- Suggesting snacks and "on the run" foods that supply essential nutrients
- Teaching the relationship of good nutrition to healthy appearance

## IMMUNIZATIONS

Increasing **immunization** coverage for children has been one of the most successful areas of the Healthy People objectives. Currently, 82% of children have been fully vaccinated with diphtheria, tetanus, and acellular pertussis (DTaP) and 90% with the other basic vaccines (USDHHS, 2000b). Routine immunization of children has been very successful in the prevention of selected diseases. The ultimate challenge is making sure that children receive immunizations (Figure 26-3).

## Barriers

Cost and convenience are two critical issues that affect whether children are immunized. Successful programs combine low-cost or free immunizations provided at accessible times and locations. It is important to urge parents to obtain immunizations for their children, and to focus on the issue at every opportunity.

## THE CUTTING EDGE

It is projected that by 2020, the cost of the recommended series of childhood immunizations will be $1200 per child. This is a projected increase of 200% over the 2001 cost of $400 per child. The projected costs are based on the probability of the introduction of seven new vaccines. This will be a major challenge to the universal vaccine goals.

Vaccine fears prevent children from getting immunized. Media stories giving attention to the dangers of vaccines, thimerosal issues, and the recall of the rotavirus vaccine raised parents' concerns about the safety of vaccines. No studies demonstrate an association between immunizations and autism, sudden infant death syndrome, multiple sclerosis, arthritis, diabetes, neurologic disabilities, deafness, cancer, or acquired immunodeficiency syndrome (AIDS). Parents question the need to vaccinate because the incidence of vaccine-preventable diseases is low. However, Japan, Great Britain, and Sweden stopped the use of the pertussis vaccine, and within 5 years there were epidemic levels of the disease and rising death rates (Offit and Bell, 1999).

Thimerosol is a mercury-containing preservative used in many vaccines. In 1999, a study suggested that the thimerosol levels were unsafe. The CDC and AAP recommended removing the preservative. Both organizations reported that there was no evidence of any harm to children since the first use of thimerosol in the 1930s. The manufacturer recalled rotavirus vaccine after a short period of use. There was some indication that it increased the risk for intussusception in those who received the vaccine. Although these events caused concerns about vaccine safety for some parents, there is no convincing evidence to stop using the current vaccines (Offit and Bell, 1999).

## Immunization Theory

The goal of immunization is to protect by using immunizing agents to stimulate antibody formation (see Chapter 38 for types of immunity). Immunizing agents for active immunity are in the form of toxoids and vaccines. A toxoid is a bacterial toxin (e.g., from the bacteria that cause tetanus and diphtheria) that has been heated or chemically treated to decrease virulence but not antibody-producing ability. Vaccines are suspensions of attenuated (live) or inactivated (killed) microorganisms. Examples include pertussis (inactivated bacteria); measles, mumps, and rubella (live attenuated virus); and hepatitis B (inactivated virus).

The neonate receives placental transfer of maternal antibodies. This natural passive immunity lasts for about 2 months. Protection is temporary and is only to diseases to which the mother has adequate antibodies. The immune system of both term and preterm infants is capable of adequate antibody response to immunizations by 2 months of age. Generally, this is the recommended age to start immunizations. (Exception: the hepatitis B series begins at birth.)

The interval between immunizations is important to the immune response. After the first injection, antibodies are produced slowly and in small concentrations (the primary response). When subsequent injections of the same antigen are given, the body recognizes the antigen and antibodies are produced much faster and in higher concen-

tration (the secondary response). Because of this secondary response, once an initial immunization series has been started, it does not need to be restarted if interrupted, regardless of the length of time elapsed. Once the initial series is completed, boosters are required at appropriate intervals to maintain an adequate concentration of antibodies. Further information about immunizing agents is available on the evolve website.

## Recommendations

Immunization recommendations rapidly change as new information and products are available. Two major organizations are responsible for guidelines: the American Academy of Pediatrics (AAP) and the U.S. Public Health Service's Advisory Committee on Immunization Practices (ACIP). Current recommendations for children and adolescents can be found on the evolve website. The main goal of the guidelines is to provide flexibility to ensure that the largest number of children will be immunized. All health care providers are urged to assess immunization status at every encounter with children and to update immunizations whenever possible.

## Contraindications

There are relatively few contraindications to giving immunizations. Minor acute illness is not a contraindication. Immunizations should be deferred with moderate or acute febrile illnesses because the reactions may mask the symptoms of the illness. The side effects of the immunization may be accentuated by the illness.

People with the following conditions are not routinely immunized and require medical consultation: pregnancy, generalized malignancy, immunosuppressive therapy or immunodeficiency disease, sensitivity to components of the agent, or recent administration of immune serum globulin, plasma, or blood.

## Legislation

The National Childhood Vaccine Injury Act became effective in 1988. It requires providers to advise parents and clients about the risks and benefits of the immunizing agent as well as possible side effects. Informed consent is recommended. Vaccine information statements (VIS) are used for this purpose.

Provisions for reporting adverse reactions to specific vaccines are also covered in this act (AAP, 2000). This program allows compensation for vaccine-related events. Since enactment lawsuits have been reduced, drug manufacturers have less of a liability burden (AAP, 2000).

Vaccines for Children (VFC) is an entitlement program enacted in 1995. It was designed to provide free vaccines to eligible children. This program includes children on Medicaid, children without health insurance, Native Americans, and those whose health insurance does not cover immunizations. This program is limited in scope, but it reflects an expanding focus on prevention.

## MAJOR HEALTH PROBLEMS

### Obesity

Obesity among the youth of the nation has reached epidemic proportions. Healthy People objectives have addressed youth fitness and obesity since 1990, yet the numbers continue to rise (Table 26-10).

Overweight is defined by using **body mass index** (BMI), which is a ratio of weight to height. The National Health and Nutrition Examination Survey (NHANES) III data of 1994 showed that 63% of men and 55% of women were overweight (USDHHS, 2000b). The risks for childhood obesity increase were related to obesity in the parents. If both parents are obese, the child has an 80% chance of being obese. The numbers of obese children and teenagers remained at 4% to 7% for years. The number more than doubled between 1980 and 1999. Now at least one out of three of the nation's youth have a BMI greater than 85% for their age. At least 70% will become overweight adults. The obesity rates are even higher in Native American, Hispanic, and African-American groups. Lower socioeconomic groups and urban settings have been associated with higher rates (Greger and Edwin, 2001).

The medical consequences of obesity vary. Obese children and teens have an increased prevalence of hypertension, respiratory problems, hyperlipidemia, bone and joint difficulties, hyperinsulinemia, and menstrual problems. The psychosocial disadvantages of overweight in the young may include teasing, scholastic discrimination, low self-esteem, and negative body image. There is a downward spiral of overweight, poor self-image, increasing isolation, and decreasing activity, which together lead to increasing overweight. Long-term risks include cardiovascular disease, diabetes, and cancer. Obesity is estimated to consume 6% of the national health care dollars (Greger and Edwin, 2001).

High-fat diets and inactivity are the major contributors to obesity. The American diet in general tends to be high in fat, calories, and sugar, with generous serving sizes. School lunches and *fast-food* meals tend to be oversized and nutritionally poor. Vending machines with *junk food* choices are becoming common in schools. Colas and sugary fruit punch add empty calories.

Snacking on high-sugar and high-fat foods is a problem pattern. Advertising directed at children glorifies poor food choices.

Television and computer time contributes to a sedentary lifestyle. NHANES III showed that 20% of American children participate in fewer than three sessions of vigorous activity per week. More than 60% of teenagers do not exercise regularly. Only one third of schools offer daily physical education. Typically, very little time in physical education classes is devoted to exercise (USDHHS, 2000b).

Interventions need to be based on goals of lifestyle changes for the entire family. The goal is to modify the way the family eats, exercises, and plans daily activities. Strategies for working with families are discussed in Box 26-5. The goal of managing weight in children and adolescents is to normalize weight. This may involve just slowing the rate of weight gain, allowing them to "grow" into their

---

**Table 26-10   Prevalence of Overweight Among U.S. Youth**

| AGE | 1963-1980 | 1988-1994 | 1999 |
|---|---|---|---|
| 6 to 19 yr | 4% to 7% | 11% | 13% to 14% |

From U.S. Department of Health and Human Services: *Healthy people 2010: national health promotion and disease prevention objectives,* ed 2, Washington, DC, 2000, U.S. Government Printing Office.

---

### BOX 26-5   Guidelines for Managing Childhood Obesity

- Set goals related to healthier lifestyle, not dieting.
- Keep objectives realistic and obtainable.
- Modify family eating habits to include low-fat food choices. Serve calorically dense foods that incorporate the food guide pyramid: whole grains, fruits, vegetables, lean protein foods, and low-fat dairy products.
- Encourage family members to stop eating when they are satisfied. Encourage recognizing hunger and satiation cues.
- Schedule regular times for meals and snacks. Include breakfast and do not skip meals.
- Have low-calorie, nutritious snacks ready and available. Avoid having empty-calorie junk foods in the home.
- Encourage keeping food intake and activity diaries.
- Promote physical activity. Make daily exercise a priority. Encourage family participation. Find ways to make the activity fun. Include peers.
- Limit television viewing. Do not allow snacking while watching TV.
- Scale back computer time. Replace sedentary time with hobbies, activities, and chores.
- Recognize healthier food choices when eating out. Order broiled, roasted, grilled, or baked items. Split orders or take home "doggie bags."
- Praise and reward children for the progress they make in reaching nutrition and activity goals. Emphasize the unique positive qualities of each child.
- Understand the genetic features of the child's/adolescent's body type. Acceptance of the "rounder" child may be a part of reaching health goals.

weight. Improved dietary habits, increased physical activity, improved self-esteem, and improved parent relationships are appropriate goals.

Healthy People 2010 objectives include improving the nutritional status and physical activity patterns of the nation's youth. Community-oriented nurses can use the following interventions to accomplish these goals in the community.

1. Provide physical education in schools. Work with community school systems to increase the number of students participating in physical education classes. Ensure that time is spent engaged in physical activity. Encourage introduction and participation in activities that are lifetime sports. Add information about physical activity in health education classes.
2. Provide safe places for activity. Work with community groups and schools to increase access to facilities, improve playgrounds, provide access to school and community facilities after school hours, and offer exercise programs classes and sports activities at reasonable costs and convenient times for working families.
3. Identify those who are overweight and at risk for overweight. Provide screening for at-risk populations. Ensure that health care providers are screening for growth parameters. Offer health fairs in the community. Provide screening at day-care and school facilities.
4. Educate the community about nutrition. Ensure that schools are offering nutrition education as part of curriculum. Enlist restaurants and grocery stores to participate in programs to help people make healthier food choices. Host healthy food fairs.
5. Initiate weight management programs that incorporate diet and lifestyle education need to be available and affordable.
6. Identify populations at risk within the community on the basis of cultural or ethnic practices. Begin educational programs designed to target these groups.

## Injuries and Accidents

Injuries and accidents are the most important cause of disease, disability, and death among children. Injuries are the number one cause of death for children up to age 21 years in the United States. Each year, 20% to 25% of all children have a serious problem related to accidents or injuries. Most are preventable.

The highest incidence is among poor children, urban African-American children, and Native Americans (NCHS, 2002). Reducing injuries from unintentional causes, as well as violence and abuse, is a goal of Healthy People 2010. To implement prevention strategies, nurses need to understand the developmental factors that place this population at risk. Two areas of focus are reduction of gun violence and safe recreation areas.

Motor vehicle accidents are the leading cause of death among children and teenagers. One fourth of those deaths involved drunk drivers. Two thirds of the children who are killed in motor vehicle accidents are unrestrained. Surveys show that 20% of infants and 40% of children and teens are unrestrained in cars (Figure 26-4). At least 80% of children who do use seat belts or are in car seats are restrained incorrectly (National Center for Injury Prevention and Control [NCIPC], 2000). Motor vehicle accidents include not only automobile collision but also pedestrian injury. Drowning and burns account for most of the other deaths; poisons and falls also contribute heavily. Development is an important issue in identifying risks to children. Table 26-11 lists the three leading injury causes of death by age.

### Developmental Considerations

#### Infants

Infants have the second highest injury rate of all groups of children. Their small size contributes to some types of injury. The small airway may be easily occluded. The small body fits through places where the head may be entrapped. Infants are handled on high surfaces for the convenience of the caregiver, placing them at great risk for falls. In motor vehicle accidents, small size is a great disadvantage and

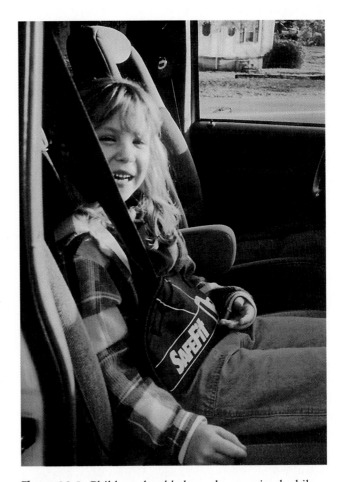

**Figure 26-4** Children should always be restrained while riding in a vehicle.

**Table 26-11   Types of Injury Causing Death, by Age-Group***

| LESS THAN 1 YEAR | 1 TO 4 YEARS | 5 TO 14 YEARS | 15 TO 20 YEARS |
|---|---|---|---|
| Aspiration | Fires/burns | Pedestrian | Motor vehicle accident |
| Homicide | Drowning | Motor vehicle accident | Suicide |
| Motor vehicle accident | Motor vehicle accident | Drowning | Homicide |

National Center for Health Statistics: *FASTATS* [on-line], 2002, available at www.cdc.gov/nchs.
*Listed in order of frequency.

increases the risk for crushing or being propelled into surfaces. Immature motor skills do not allow for escape from injury, placing them at risk for drowning, suffocating, and burns.

### Toddlers and Preschoolers

This population experiences a large number of falls and poisonings. They are active, and their increasing motor skills make supervision difficult. They are inquisitive and have relatively immature logic abilities.

---

**WHAT DO YOU THINK?**

Most states have enacted laws allowing health care providers to treat adolescents in certain situations without parental consent. These include emergency care, substance abuse, pregnancy, and birth control. All 50 states recognize the mature minors doctrine. This allows youths 15 years of age and older to give informed medical consent if it is apparent that they are capable of understanding the risks and benefits and if the procedure is medically indicated.

If a minor can give consent, is there also an obligation to maintain confidentiality when providing health care? Three premises guide health care providers. (1) It is thought that adolescents may not seek health care if they believe that their parents will be notified. (2) Many providers note that the client is the adolescent, not the parent. (3) Federal and state statutes and professional ethical standards support confidentiality for adolescents. In most situations, it is important to provide confidentiality. At certain times, release of information should occur despite the adolescent's desire for confidentiality. These include legal situations (e.g., physical abuse) or if the minor poses a danger to self or others (English, 1996).

Sandy, a 15-year-old, has revealed to the nurse that she has become sexually active with her boyfriend. She has no interest in any form of birth control. The nurse wants to involve her parents, but Sandy does not want them to know. What are the issues? What are Sandy's rights? What strategies could the nurse use in this situation?

### School-Age Children

The school-age group has the lowest injury death rate. At this age, it is difficult to judge speed and distance, placing them at risk for pedestrian and bicycle accidents. There are 180,000 emergency department visits per year for bicycle injury, most involving head trauma. Universal use of bicycle helmets would prevent deaths. Peer pressure often inhibits the use of protective devices such as helmets and limb pads. Sports and athletic injuries are increased in this age group (NCIPC, 2000).

### Adolescents

Injury accounts for 75% of all deaths during adolescence. Risk taking becomes more conscious at this time, especially among boys. The death and serious injury rates for boys are three times higher than for girls. Adolescents are at the highest risk of any age-group for motor vehicle deaths, drowning, and intentional injuries. Use of weapons and drug and alcohol abuse play an important role in injuries in this age group (Neinstein, 1996). There are 17 youth homicides per day. Youth gangs are more violent and seem to be increasing in prevalence. Suicide is the third leading cause of death among youths between the ages of 15 and 24 years (NCIPC, 2000). Poor social adjustment, psychiatric problems, and family disorganization increase the risk for suicide.

## Prevention Strategies

Health care provider offices, school, and day-care facilities provide opportunities to teach children, adolescents, and their families prevention of injuries. Safety can be incorporated into required health education courses. The Healthy People 2010 objectives target head injuries, motor vehicles, fires/smoke alarms, falls, drowning, and poisonings. Community-sponsored car seat and seat belt safety checks and safety fairs are another way to educate families. Injury prevention should be addressed at all health visits.

### Reducing Gun Violence

Each day in the United States, 13 children are killed and 30 are wounded in gun-related accidents, suicides, and homicides. Witnessing gun violence or knowing the victims affects other children indirectly. More than 135,000 children carry guns to school, many obtained in their own homes. At least 50% of the families in this country report owning guns, many of which are stored loaded. In a national survey, one third of teens and preteens reported that they could obtain a gun (USDHHS, 2000b).

Consequences of gun violence are serious. Permanent, debilitating physical injuries are sustained. Little is known about the emotional effects of being a victim of or witnessing acts of violence, but it has been proposed that the effects are long lasting. The financial burden of treatment and rehabilitation is high and often not completely compensated by insurance payments.

Characteristics associated with gun violence include history of aggressive behaviors, poverty, school problems, substance abuse, poverty, and cultural acceptance of violent behavior. Interventions must begin early and address each of these factors.

The Healthy People 2010 objectives seek to reduce the number of high school students who carry weapons. Nurses can actively participate in efforts to reduce gun violence among young people in the following ways (Havens and Zink, 1994):

- Urge legislators to support gun control legislation. Numerous legislative actions have been proposed limiting the sale of handguns to minors and restricting possession of guns in schools. The Brady Bill authorized a waiting period for handgun purchases, raised licensing fees for gun dealers, and required police notification of multiple gun purchases.
- Collaborate with schools to develop programs to discourage violence among children.
- Initiate community programs focusing on gun storage and safety at school.
- Support families' efforts to obtain supervision of their children after school.
- Identify populations at risk for violence and target aggression or anger management.
- Support community efforts to enhance family stability and promote self-esteem. This is vital to decreasing violence.

*Promoting Safe Playgrounds and Recreation Areas*
Schools, day-care centers, and community groups often need guidance toward developing safe places for children to play. One child is injured on a playground every 2½ minutes. Each year, over 66,000 children sustain severe injuries. The most frequent injuries are falls, and three fourths of them involve head injuries (NCIPC, 2000) (Figure 26-5).

The U.S. Consumer Product Safety Commission has published guidelines for playground safety. Guidelines cover structure, materials, surfaces, and maintenance of equipment (Box 26-6). The developmental skills of specific ages are incorporated, as well as recommendations for physically challenged children. Nurses can use these guidelines to help the community establish standards for play areas.

Nurses share responsibility in the prevention of accidents and injuries in the pediatric population. Assessment

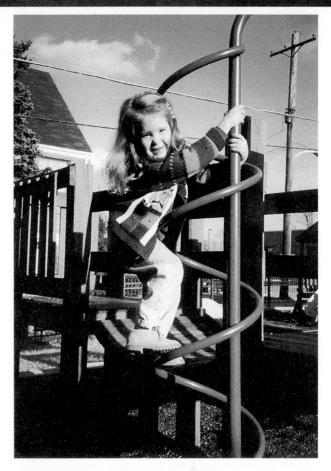

**Figure 26-5** Playground injuries are frequent among young children.

**BOX 26-6 Guidelines for Playground Safety**

- Playgrounds should be surrounded by a barrier to protect children from traffic.
- Activity centers should be distributed to avoid crowding in one area.
- Surfaces should be finished with substances that meet Consumer Product Safety Commission (CPSC) regulations for lead.
- Durable materials should be used.
- Sand, gravel, wood chips, and wood mulch are acceptable surfaces for limiting the shock of falls.
- Equipment should be inspected regularly for protrusions that could puncture skin or entangle clothes.
- Not recommended are multiple-occupancy swings, animal swings, rope swings, and trampolines.

Data from Swartz MK: Playground safety, *J Pediatr Health Care* 6(3):161, 1992.

---

BOX 26-7  **Injury Prevention Topics**

- Car restraints, seat belts, air-bag safety
- Preventing fires, burns
- Poison prevention
- Preventing falls
- Preventing drowning; water safety
- Bicycle safety
- Safe driving practices
- Sports safety
- Pedestrian safety
- Gun control
- Decreasing gang activities
- Substance abuse prevention

---

BOX 26-8  **Nursing Guide: Home Management of Gastrointestinal Virus (GIV) in Children**

- Education regarding expected course of the illness: GIV is usually self-limited, with vomiting lasting 1 to 2 days and diarrhea lasting up to 7 to 10 days.
- Progressive diet management: NPO for 3 to 4 hours; sips of oral electrolyte solution every 5 to 10 minutes for 2 hours; clear liquids (primarily oral electrolyte solution) for the rest of the day; bland, easily digested foods (BRAT diet: banana, rice, applesauce, toast) for the next 24 to 48 hours.
- Fever management with antipyretic agent if needed (avoid aspirin).
- Monitor for signs of dehydration: urination less than usual; parched, dry mouth and mucous membranes; poor skin turgor; sunken eyes with no tears; irritability; lethargy. Give instructions on seeking further care.
- Prevention of spread: instructions on hand-hygiene technique.

---

of the characteristics of the child, family, and environment identifies risk factors. Interventions include anticipatory guidance, modifying the environment, and safety education. Education should focus on age-appropriate interventions based on knowledge of leading causes of death and risk factor. Topics to consider are listed in Box 26-7 (see also the evolve website).

## Acute Illness

Infection is the most significant cause of illness in infants and children. Infectious diseases, whether bacterial or viral in origin, are usually associated with a variety of symptoms: fever, upper respiratory symptoms, generalized discomfort and malaise, loss of appetite, rash, vomiting, and diarrhea. Most are self-limited and can be handled by the family at home with interventions to prevent complications. The nurse may need to identify whether the child can be managed at home on the basis of the severity of symptoms and the family's ability to provide care. The nurse may be involved in developing a home care plan. Also, the nurse teaches the family about the illness and prevention of its spread. Nursing interventions for home care of a child with a gastrointestinal virus are shown in Box 26-8.

Infectious diseases may be more serious in younger children and infants. Neonates, because of their immunologic immaturity, are more susceptible to bacterial illness with spread to multiple organ systems, called sepsis. Children of all ages are at risk for invasion of the spinal fluid, or meningitis. The morbidity and mortality rates of these forms of infection vary with the age of the child, causative organism, severity of the illness, and timeliness of treatment. The nursing role includes early identification and referral, support of the family during the treatment phase, and follow-up care as indicated. Preventive measures include family education in hygiene and identification of environmental sources of infection (see the evolve website).

Day-care centers and schools provide an environmental framework for the child and adolescent population. One out of three young children less than 6 years of age is enrolled in day care. Studies have shown that these children are 18 times more likely to acquire infectious diseases than children who are not in day care (Children's Defense Fund, 2001). Most of the diseases for the older child and adolescent originate in school. The nurse can establish programs and serve as a resource to day-care centers and schools for infection control practices:

- Nurses can provide information regarding illness and injury prevention for childcare providers and teachers to improve health and safety.
- Centers and schools may need assistance in developing standards for hygiene, sanitation, and disinfection to prevent the spread of disease. This may include hand hygiene, food preparation, and cleaning of toys and equipment.
- Requirements for immunizations of both children and staff may need to be established.
- Guidelines for care of sick children should be developed.
- Staff members may benefit from educational programs on infectious diseases (see the Evidence-Based Practice box)
- Health education should be incorporated into the school curriculum for older children and adolescents. The students should be encouraged to participate in identifying the content and presentation of the material.

Nurses are in a key position to consult with these populations and serve as a resource for program development.

## Evidence-Based Practice

Data were gathered to determine if an instructional program for childcare could significantly reduce the spread of infectious diseases in the test center. In a test group of 3- to 5-year-olds and their teachers, classes were held on germs and hand hygiene. A similar control group maintained their usual hand-hygiene practices. During 21 weeks, including cold and flu season, the test group had significantly fewer colds than the control group.

**Nurse Use:** Past research suggests that children in center care are 18 more times as likely to become ill than children who stay at home. This study demonstrates a way to improve those statistics. Nurses who are in a position to consult with schools and day-care centers can develop educational strategies that are age appropriate and may make a difference in illness in their community.

Niffenegger JP: Proper handwashing promotes wellness in child care, *J Pediatr Health Care* 11:1.1997.

The Evidence-Based Practice box discusses a study involving hand-hygiene practices in a child care center.

## Sudden Infant Death Syndrome

Sudden death may occur in infants with a specific disorder such as meningitis or a chronic illness. When no specific cause of death can be determined, the death is labeled **sudden infant death syndrome** (SIDS). Each year, over 5000 infants die of SIDS in the United States, making it the most common cause of death during the first year of life. Few factors can be used to predict the occurrence. Most deaths occur between 1 and 5 months of age, although SIDS may occur up to 1 year of age. Only a small number of infants who died of SIDS experienced a previous episode of cyanosis or apnea. Cardiorespiratory monitoring has not been shown to decrease the incidence. SIDS occurs more often in preterm and low-birth-weight infants and possibly in infants with upper respiratory tract infections. SIDS also occurs more often in male infants and in low socioeconomic groups. Maternal cigarette smoking increases the risk three to four times. The risk to siblings is unclear at present. Studies show that the prone sleeping position and tight swaddling may increase the risk. The incidence has decreased 38% since the supine sleep position has been promoted. There is no test to identify infants who may die, making this a frustrating clinical problem (Brooks, 1997).

When an infant dies, the family requires tremendous support. The nurse provides empathetic support and assists the family as they progress through the grief process and deal with siblings and other family members. Referral to support groups may be helpful.

Nursing interventions for SIDS include teaching of the following prevention strategies:
- Supine position for healthy infants
- No parental smoking
- Improved access to prenatal and postnatal health care
- Teaching and providing close follow-up care for high-risk groups
- Improved use of baby monitors for selected infants

## Chronic Health Problems

Improved medical technology has increased the number of children surviving with chronic health problems. Examples include Down syndrome, spina bifida, cerebral palsy, asthma, diabetes, congenital heart disease, cancer, hemophilia, bronchopulmonary dysplasia, and AIDS. Despite the differences in the specific diagnoses, the families have complex needs and similar problems. Several variables exist to assess for each child and family:
- Is the condition stable or life threatening?
- What is the actual health status?
- What is the degree of impairment to the child's ability to develop?
- What types of treatments and therapy are required, and with what frequency?
- How often are health care visits and hospitalizations required?
- To what degree are the family routines disrupted?

The common issues of chronic health problems include the following:
- All children and adolescents with chronic health problems need routine health care. The same issues of pediatric health promotion and health care need to be addressed with this group.
- Ongoing medical care specific to the health problem needs to be provided. Examples include monitoring for complications of the health problem, specific medications, dietary adjustments, and therapies such as speech, physical, or occupational therapy. Ongoing evaluation of the effectiveness of treatment protocols is critical.
- Care is often provided by multiple specialists. There is a need for coordinating the scheduling of visits, tests, or procedures and the treatment regimen.
- Skilled care procedures are often required and may include suctioning, positioning, medications, feeding techniques, breathing treatments, physical therapy, and use of appliances.
- Equipment needs are often complex and may include monitors, oxygen, ventilators, positioning or ambulation devices, infusion pumps, and suction machines.
- Educational needs are often complex. Communication between the family and team of health care providers and teachers is essential to meet the child's health and educational needs.
- Safe transportation to health care services and school must be available. Several barriers exist,

including family resources, location, ability to be fitted appropriately in car restraint systems, and the amount and size of supportive equipment.

- Financial resources may not be adequate to meet the needs.
- Behavioral issues include the effect of the condition on the child's behavior as well as on other family members. Chronic health problems may put stress on relationships.

Nursing interventions in the primary care setting with a child diagnosed with asthma serve as a model for pediatric chronic health problems. There are 8.1 million children up to age 18 with asthma, representing an increase of 75% from 1980 to 1994 (NCHS, 2002). Preschool children are increasingly among the newly diagnosed cases. Low-income and minority groups, especially Hispanic and African-American youth, are more likely to be hospitalized or to die from asthma. Box 26-9 lists nursing guidelines for asthmatic children. Healthy People 2010 objectives include reduction of asthma-related deaths and morbidity by improved management and education of the condition. Community-oriented strategies for asthma management include the following:

- Education programs for families of children and adolescents who have asthma
- Development of home and environmental assessment guides to identify triggers
- Education and outreach efforts in high-risk populations to aid in case finding (e.g., in areas with low in-

come, high unemployment, and substandard housing, where there is exposure to secondhand smoke)
- Development of clean air policies within the community (e.g., no burning of leaves, presence of smoke-free zones)
- Improving access to care for asthmatic patients (e.g., developing clinic services with consistent health care providers to decrease emergency department use)
- Assessment of schools and day-care centers for asthma "friendliness" (Box 26-10)

## Alterations in Behavior

Behavioral problems in the child and adolescent are highly variable and may include eating disorders, attention problems, substance abuse, elimination problems, conduct disorders and delinquency, sleep disorders, and school maladaptation. A healthy self-concept is supported by positive interactions with others. Problem behaviors may provide negative feedback, which may generate low self-esteem. A child's coping mechanisms are influenced by the individual developmental level, temperament, previous stress experiences, role models, and support of parents and peers. Maladaptive coping mechanisms present as problem behaviors. Inappropriate behaviors may lead to further physical or developmental problems.

Managing behavior problems commonly requires the following:

- Understanding the relationship between self-concept and self-esteem issues
- A family-centered approach
- Involving a multidisciplinary teams in care

**Attention deficit disorder** (ADD) and **attention deficit disorder with hyperactivity** (ADHD) interventions are presented as a model for nursing management of a behavior problem (Box 26-11). There are over 3 million children and adolescents diagnosed with ADD or ADHD (NCHS, 2002). ADD is a combination of inattention and impulsiveness, and it may include hyperactivity inappropriate for the age of the child. ADD frequently includes low self-

---

### BOX 26-9  Nursing Guide: Asthma in Children

Family teaching includes the following:
- Disease process and complications
- Warning signs
- Medications: purpose and administration techniques
- Equipment: cleaning and use
- Trigger avoidance
- Exercise planning: type (intensity, duration), monitoring, coordination with family patterns and school activity
- Smoking prevention: additive effects to disease
- Review action plan
- Review emergency plan
- Coordination of services: primary care provider, school staff, pharmacy, provider of durable medical equipment
- Referral to support groups, camps for psychosocial needs, community education groups, educational websites
- Referral for qualification for state or federal programs (e.g., Children's Specialty Services)

---

### BOX 26-10  School Survey for Asthma "Friendliness"

- Is the school free from tobacco smoke?
- How is the air quality? Reduce or eliminate allergens or irritants (mold, dust mites, roaches, strong chemical odors)
- Is there a school nurse?
- How are medications administered to students?
- Are there emergency plans for taking care of students with asthma?
- Have the staff and students been taught about asthma and how to help a student with asthma?
- Are there good options for safe participation in physical education class?

esteem, labile mood, low frustration tolerance, temper out-bursts, and poor academic skills. The evaluation is based on symptoms. Diagnosis is made by excluding other disorders. Symptoms vary with the severity of the problem, and interventions range from simple to complex. A familial tendency exists; several members of a family may be affected. Treatment involves a family focus and includes health professionals and educators (Miller and Castellanos, 1998). ADD may coexist with learning disabilities and emotional disorders. This population is often overrepresented in statistics related to accidents, substance abuse, unemployment, criminal justice system, and divorce. Community-oriented interventions with this population include programs to improve stress management skills, problem-solving skills, impulse control, and interpersonal relationships. Strategies include the following:

- Self-help programs and guides
- Intensive summer camps
- Parent workshops
- Behavior counseling through mental health centers
- School-based intervention programs

Healthy People 2010 objectives related to ensuring mental health services can help guide interventions for this population.

## Tobacco Use

Smoking has been identified as the most important preventable cause of morbidity and mortality in the United States, yet 50 million Americans smoke. Smoking is associated with cardiovascular disease, cancer, and lung disease. **Secondhand smoke,** smoke exhaled or given off by a burning cigarette, is toxic. Approximately 3000 nonsmokers die each year of lung cancer as a result of secondhand smoke (USDHHS, 2000b). Parents often do not understand or believe the effects of smoking on children. Children exposed to secondhand smoke experience increased episodes of ear and upper respiratory tract infections. Children of smokers are more likely to smoke. Teenagers who become smokers are rarely able to quit (Brown, 2002). About half of all teenagers who smoke regularly will die from smoking-related disease (NCHS, 2002).

The number of teenagers who smoke has increased since 1990, and they are starting younger. As many as 6 million teenagers and 100,000 preteens smoke on a daily basis (NCHS, 2002). Tobacco industry advertising has increased through use of advertisements in the media, on billboards, and in sponsorship of sporting events. Cigarette advertisements appear in "teen" magazines, and companies offer logo products that appeal to children. More than 80% of a group of 6-year-old children were able to associate a picture of Joe Camel with cigarettes. Although 46 states have laws prohibiting the sale of cigarettes to minors, restrictions are not enforced. Minors have been able to purchase tobacco products 46% to 88% of the time (MacKenzie, Bartecchi, and Schrier, 1994). See the Evidence-Based Practice box about cigarette smoking.

Interventions to discourage smoking focus on the parent, the child or adolescent, and public policy. Parents should be

---

**BOX 26-11  Nursing Guide: Attention Deficit Disorder**

- **Assessment:** History, physical, parent/family assessment, learning and psychoeducational evaluations.
- **Behavioral modifications:** Home and school: teaching families techniques to support clear expectations, consistent routines, positive reinforcement for appropriate behavior, and time out for negative behaviors.
- **Classroom modifications:** Consulting with family and teachers to meet individual needs for remediation or alternative instruction methods if necessary; structuring activities to respond to the child's needs.
- **Support:** Referral to family therapy, support groups, or mental health services to assist development of positive coping behaviors.
- **Medications:** Consulting with physician to monitor for therapeutic and adverse effects
- **Follow-up:** Assessing at 3- to 6-month intervals when stable; dynamic process affected by relationships with others; behaviors will change with age; problem may persist through adulthood.

Modified from Miller KJ, Castellanos FX: Attention deficit/hyperactivity disorders, *Pediatr Rev* 19:11, 1998.

---

### Evidence-Based Practice

A randomized community trial indicates that a campaign to reduce youth access to tobacco can have a significant effect on teen smoking rates. Fourteen communities were randomly assigned to intervention or control groups. The communities in the intervention group participated in a 32-month program to change ordinances, merchant policies and practices, and law enforcement practices to reduce access. The communities used various ways to raise public awareness about the issue, including letter and petition drives and media campaigns. The prevalence of smoking climbed sharply in the control communities during the campaign. The increase in teen smoking in the intervention communities was less pronounced. Teens in the intervention communities reported that it had become more difficult to purchase cigarettes in the community.

**Nurse Use:** These results support community interventions as a way to decrease smoking in the teenage population.

Forster JL et al: *Am J Public Health* 88:1193, 1998.

offered educational programs dealing with the negative effects of smoking on children, interventions to stop smoking, and ways to create a smoke-free environment. Behavior modification techniques should be incorporated.

Antismoking programs directed toward children and teenagers are more successful if the focus is on short-term effects rather than on long-term effects. Developmentally, children and teenagers cannot visualize the future to imagine the consequences of smoking. The immediate health risks and the cosmetic effects should be emphasized. Teaching should include how advertising puts pressure on people to smoke. Music, sports, and other activities, including stress-reducing techniques, should be encouraged. Teaching social skills to resist peer pressure is critical.

Nurses should become politically active in the area of smoking. Banning tobacco advertising, enforcing restrictions of sale to minors, increasing funds for antismoking education, and restriction of public smoking may reduce the incidence of smoking. Insurers should be encouraged to reimburse smoking cessation therapies.

Community-based interventions can be based on Healthy People 2010 objectives and include the following:
- Working with schools to provide tobacco-free environments, including all school facilities, property, vehicles, and school events
- Working with schools to provide prevention curricula in elementary, middle, and secondary schools
- Working with health care providers to ensure that they are inquiring about and advising reduction of secondhand smoke exposure
- Working with health care providers to ensure that they are advising smoking cessation and providing strategies to assist in cessation

**WHAT DO YOU THINK?**

Taxes should be increased on tobacco products to provide funding for health care programs and to discourage young people from smoking.

**Table 26-12  Common Environmental Agents Hazardous to Children**

| TOXINS | SOURCES |
|---|---|
| **Heavy Metals** | |
| Lead | Paint, dust, soil, cookware, occupational exposure, hobbies, plumbing solder |
| Mercury | Thermometer/sphygmomanometer breakage, environmental contamination, folk remedies, fish |
| Arsenic | Food, water |
| Polychlorinated biphenyls | Food |
| **Air Pollutants** | |
| Combustion by-products: carbon monoxide, nitrous dioxide, sulfur dioxide | Space heaters, woodstoves, fireplaces, natural gas, engine exhaust (industrial and automotive) |
| Ozone | Power plants, engine and automotive exhaust |
| Radon | Ubiquitous radon gas, found in basement and first floor of buildings |
| Molds | Food, outdoor and indoor environments with excessive moisture |
| Particulate matter | Dust mites, cockroach particles, animal dander |
| Asbestos | Buildings |
| Nicotine, benzene tars, carbon monoxide, other carcinogens | Environmental tobacco smoke |
| Volatile organic compounds: hydrocarbons: methyl alcohol, formaldehyde | New and renovated buildings, mobile homes, paint products, cleaning agents, furniture, carpets, building materials |
| **Pesticides** | |
| Insecticides: organic chlorines | Food, soil, plants, water, air (spraying) |
| **Herbicides** | |
| Nitrites, nitrates | Water |

Modified from American Academy of Pediatrics Committee on Environmental Health: *Pediatric environmental health,* Elk Grove Village, Ill, 1999, AAP.

- Working with community merchants to enforce minors' access laws (see Evidence-Based Practice box)

## CURRENT ISSUES

### Environmental Health Hazards

The environment directly affects the health of children. Growth, size, and behaviors place the pediatric population at greater risk for damage from toxins. Lead poisoning is the most common environmental health hazard. Pesticides and poor air quality also pose serious risks. Indoor air pollutants increased as houses were built "tightly" to conserve energy, and as more chemicals were used in production (AAP, 1999). Common toxins and sources of pediatric exposure are listed in Table 26-12.

Growing tissues absorb toxins readily. Developing organ systems are more susceptible to damage. Smaller size means increased concentration of toxins per pound of body weight. The fact that children are short exposes them to lower air spaces, where heavy chemicals tend to concentrate. Outdoor play, especially during summer months, increases the opportunity for exposure to air pollutants. The type of play involves running and breathing hard, which increases the volumes inhaled. Chewing and mouthing behaviors offer contact to toxins such as lead. Playing on the floor increases exposure to chemicals in rugs and flooring. Rolling in grass results in pesticide exposure. Playground materials may be treated with chemicals. Exposure risks for adolescents are similar to those for adults and are primarily through work, school, and hobbies.

Populations at greatest risk include children with respiratory diseases and low income. Children with asthma and other respiratory problems are at risk from poor air quality and chemical irritants. The problems increase in urban and industrialized areas where pollutant levels are high. Low-income populations are more likely to have substandard housing. Poor nutritional status increases the risk of complications. Screening and treatment may be delayed if there is limited access to health care. Low-income neighborhoods have been shown to have higher levels of contaminants in the water source than the general population. They are also noted to be located closer to waste areas (AAP, 1999).

It is critical to assess environmental health hazards during health care visits (Box 26-12). Referral for treatment may be necessary. Counseling families on risk reduction is important.

Community-oriented nurses identify environmental problems within the community. They target at-risk populations and participate in community interventions (Table 26-13 has examples). Bringing screening programs into neighborhoods at risk may facilitate early case finding and interventions.

Lobbying efforts and education can bring public policy changes to make the environment healthier. The case presentation in Box 26-13 gives an example of how a school environment can lead to health problems.

### Complementary and Alternative Medicine

An increasing number of people use **complementary and alternative medicine** (CAM) for health promotion and disease prevention, although exact numbers are unclear. CAM therapies share elements of wellness, self-healing, and healthy lifestyle. Lines between traditional and nontraditional therapies are beginning to blur as some CAM therapies become more mainstream. Traditional providers are incorporating CAM therapies into practice as more research showing positive effects becomes available. CAM therapies are listed in Box 26-14.

Over 65% to 80% of the world's population use non-Western medicine for their health care needs. Herbal preparations are the most frequently used therapies in the world. Approximately one third of the adults in the United States and one fifth in Canada report using some form of CAM. It is estimated that this represents only a small proportion of actual use. A recent study reveals that 11% of children who were being seen by a traditional health care provider had received services from a nontraditional provider. Up to one third of pediatric patients have used CAM, and more than two thirds of families are treating children with chronic illness with nonconventional therapy. Parents choose CAM therapy because of concerns about the effects of conventional medicine and a belief in the safety of herbal products. Cultural, ethnic, and spiritual traditions influence decisions (Spigelblatt, 1997).

Over one third of children's visits to complementary providers are to chiropractors. Spinal manipulation is believed to improve immune responses. Chiropractors

---

**BOX 26-12  Environmental Hazard Assessment**

- Home and other buildings visited regularly, including schools and day care
- Age
- Basement
- Mobile home
- Remodeling or renovation
- Heat source
- Pesticide use
- Hobbies involving toxic substances
- Parental or adolescent occupational exposure
- Reside near industry, waste areas, highways, or polluted areas
- Smoke exposure
- Dietary sources of toxins
- Breastfeeding
- Water source
- Dietary supplements or ethnic remedies

**Table 26-13    Prevention Strategies Applied to Environmental Hazards**

| PREVENTION STRATEGIES | EXAMPLES |
|---|---|
| **Primary** | |
| Identification of at-risk populations | • Substandard housing communities<br>• Children with asthma |
| Health education about environmental risks | • Poison prevention<br>• Responses to poor air quality alerts |
| Formation of public health policies | • Air/water quality standards<br>• Safety inspections: playgrounds, schools, recreation centers<br>• Monitoring lead/radon levels in buildings |
| Research to assess impact of environmental hazards on the pediatric population | • Developing reference ranges/biological markers to assess toxic levels in children |
| **Secondary** | |
| Early detection, treatment, and referral for management of environmental toxins | • Removal of at-risk persons when lead/radon hazards are detected<br>• Assessment of lead levels of populations of at-risk children with treatment of individuals as indicated |
| **Tertiary** | |
| Restoration of environment/occupants to healthful state | • Asbestos/lead abatement of buildings<br>• Radon remediation of homes<br>• Decontamination of waste sites<br>• Replacement of heating, ventilation, air conditioning systems with mold<br>• Chelating agents for individuals with lead/mercury toxic levels |

Modified from Burns C, Dunn A, Sattler B: Resources for environmental health problems, *J Pediatr Health Care* 16:3, 2002.

---

**BOX 26-13    Case Presentation: "Sick School"**

Students in a middle school in Oregon were noted to have a high rate of absenteeism and illness. There was an unusually high incidence of headaches, asthma, upper respiratory tract illness, and many other health complaints. Test scores were lower than in previous years. Radon levels had been recorded as very high for 10 years by inspection teams, but the results were never reported to the school. A teacher ran a radon test and reported the levels to the school system. The school district found high levels of carbon dioxide in the air and high lead levels in the school drinking fountain. In addition to the high radon levels, there was an unacceptable level of mold in the building as a result of water leaks. Many agencies were involved in the cleanup of the school and the assessment and care of the children and staff. The lowered test scores were probably caused by poor attendance and poor health of the students. Long-term consequences include a higher risk for cancer. It is important for health care providers and school officials to consider the possibility of the school as a source of community illness.

Modified from Sahler OJZ, Wood BL: Theories and concepts of development as they relate to pediatric practice. In Hoekelman R et al, editors: *Primary pediatric care,* ed 3, St Louis, 1997, Mosby.

---

provide well-child care. They treat children for acute and chronic problems, such as respiratory problems, ear infections, enuresis, and colic. Homeopathic care accounts for 25% of visits to CAM providers. Homeopathy provides preparations for specific symptoms, such as teething, colic, sleep problems, and earaches. No scientific studies offer data to support the effectiveness of chiropractic or homeopathic care for pediatric diseases.

About 10% of CAM visits are to acupuncturists. Acupuncture has shown to be promising in the area of pain management, including childhood cancers. Naturopathy accounts for another 10% of visits. Naturopathy uses dietary management and supplements, healthy lifestyle, and herbal preparations. Large numbers of families treat themselves with herbs and nutritional supplements and are not represented in the reported visits (Spigelblatt,

## BOX 26-14 Complementary Therapies in Pediatrics

**BIOCHEMICAL**
- Herbs
- Vitamins
- Dietary supplements

**LIFESTYLE**
- Diet/nutrition
- Exercise
- Environmental changes
- Mind–body therapies
  - Biofeedback
  - Relaxation
  - Hypnosis
  - Meditation/spiritual

**BIOCHEMICAL**
- Massage
- Spinal adjustment
- Music therapy

**BIOENERGETIC**
- Acupuncture/acupressure
- Therapeutic touch
- Prayer/spiritual
- Homeopathy
- Meditation
- Aromatherapy

## BOX 26-15 Herbal Preparations Contraindicated for Children

- Borage
- Chaparral
- Coltsfoot
- Comfrey
- Ephedra (ma huang)
- Germander
- Gordolobo
- Heliotropes
- Jin bu huan
- Monkshood/wolfsbane/aconite
- Rattlebox
- Sassafras
- Bee pollen (anaphylaxis in asthmatics)

Modified from Blosser C: Complementary medicine. In Burns CG et al, editors: *Pediatric primary care*, ed 2, Philadelphia, 2000, Saunders.

1997). Some products are extremely safe for children. Others are potentially fatal.

Parents may assume that herbs and supplements are safe because they are natural products. Many of the herbs and supplements follow the same biochemical pathways as traditional medicines. The dosages are not defined. The amount of reactive agent varies depending on the part of the plant used, when it was harvested, and the method of preparation. The biochemical reaction is not defined in some cases, or poorly understood in others. Therapies used in the pediatric and adolescent population are listed at the end of the chapter. The list points out the paucity of research in this area. Clearly more studies need to be done to help families make informed choices.

The Dietary Supplement Health and Education Act of 1994 requires cautionary labels on all dietary supplements containing herbs. The U.S. Food and Drug Administration (FDA) does not approve marketing claims. Dietary supplements, including herbs, are not tested for safety or effectiveness. U.S. Pharmacopeia (USP) standards for purity and potency are voluntary. Many states have licensing boards for nontraditional providers, but there are no national credentialing requirements or standards (Blosser, 2000).

There are many concerns about the use of CAM for children. There are few scientific studies that support complementary therapies. Providers may not have the appropriate training to recognize pediatric problems. CAM may delay starting treatments of serious medical conditions. Some CAM providers discourage the immunization of children. Herbs and homeopathic preparations are not regulated for dose concentration or purity. There have been reports of contamination with pesticides, heavy metals, and alcohol. Effects on growing children with immature organ systems are poorly understood. Several available products are considered dangerous and are not recommended for children (Box 26-15).

Despite the concerns, several therapies are being carefully researched and show efficacy in pediatric care. Relaxation and biofeedback therapies are successful for children with migraine headaches, with abdominal pain, or undergoing painful procedures. Music therapy improves physical functioning and learning abilities for children with learning disabilities, Down syndrome, and ADHD. Some herbal remedies and dietary supplements are showing efficacy in controlled studies. Melatonin has been helpful for treating sleep problems in children with ADHD. Evening primrose oil proved effective for management of eczema. Massage therapy shows exciting results for infants, children, and adolescents in controlled studies (Table 26-14). The National Institutes of Health created the Office of Alternative Medicine in 1992 to promote research into complementary therapies (Blosser, 2000).

Nurses need to become familiar with complementary therapies used by families in the community. Nurses should

## Table 26-14 Efficacy of Massage Therapy for Pediatric Disorders

| PEDIATRIC DISORDERS | USES |
|---|---|
| Preterm infants | • Better weight gain<br>• Shorter hospital stay<br>• Increased responsiveness |
| Autism/attention deficit disorder with hyperactivity | • Improved attentiveness and learning |
| Juvenile rheumatoid arthritis | • Decreased pain |
| Posttraumatic stress syndrome/depression | • Decreased stress and anxiety |
| Eating disorders | • Improved eating patterns<br>• Improved self-image<br>• Decreased anxiety |
| Diabetes/asthma | • Improved clinical parameters |

Modified from Field T: Massage therapy: more than a laying on of hands, *Contemp Pediatr* 16:5, 1999.

---

### BOX 26-16 Resources for Complementary Therapies

| | |
|---|---|
| Office of Alternative Medicine/National Institutes of Health | http://www.altmed.od.nih.gov |
| Food and Drug Administration | http://www.fda.gov |
| American Holistic Nurses' Association | (919) 787-0116 |
| World Health Organization Collaborating Center for International Drug Monitoring | http://www.who.int/dap/drug-info.html |
| PDR for Herbal Medicines | http://www.pdr.com |
| University of Pittsburgh: The Alternative Medicine Homepage | http://www.pitt.edu |
| Rosenthal Center for Complementary and Alternative Medicine | http://www.cpmcnet.columbia.edu/dept/rosenthal/ |
| Longwood Herbal Task Force/Children's Hospital, Boston | http://www.mcp.edu/herbal/ |

---

ask about their use when assessing children. They should foster open discussion with a nonjudgmental approach. Families are likely to turn to nurses for information regarding safety and efficacy of therapies. The following questions should be explored:

- Is the therapy effective? What is the desired outcome?
- Is the therapy safe? What are the risks and benefits?
- Are there interactions with other medications or treatments prescribed?
- Why did the family choose this method of treatment?
- Are there other CAM therapies that may be useful?

Nurses also need to determine what resources are available in communities. They need to be aware of the types of providers and their experience with children and adolescents. They also need to know the cultural and ethnic backgrounds of families in the community to become attuned to some of the traditional remedies in use. One of the remedies used in the Hispanic culture for abdominal pain is pennyroyal oil, which may produce hepatitis. Educational programs in the community could address this issue through the schools and health clinics. Resources for more information about CAM therapies are listed in Box 26-16.

## MODELS FOR DELIVERY OF HEALTH CARE TO VULNERABLE POPULATIONS

Nurses are in a position to work with specific populations through programs targeting the health care needs of those at risk. In the following paragraphs, two strategies for common pediatric concerns in the community are described. One is a nursing intervention that can be used in the home, and the second targets the needs of homeless persons.

### Home-Based Service Programs

Home-based service programs vary in goals and target populations. In general, home visiting programs increase use of available community resources by bringing the services into the home or neighborhood or by promoting awareness of resources (Box 26-17).

Programs may consist of professional and trained lay people forming a team to provide services. Home-based programs have been shown to decrease preterm and low-birth-weight deliveries, improve parenting capabilities, enhance lives of disabled children, promote early hospital discharge, and decrease health care costs (Balinsky, 1999). Home care by nurses to facilitate the transition to home from the newborn intensive care unit has been shown to decrease the length of hospital stay and decrease the read-

## BOX 26-17  Community Resources for Children's Health Care

- Children's service clinics
- Well-child clinics
- Immunization clinics
- Infectious disease clinics
- Children's Specialty Services
- Family violence/child abuse centers
- School health programs
- Headstart
- Parents Anonymous
- Crisis hotlines
- Community education classes
- Early intervention/developmental services
- Childbirth education classes
- Breastfeeding support groups
- Parent support groups
- Family planning clinics
- Women, infant's, and children programs (WIC)
- Medicaid
- Youth employment/training programs

mission rate (Swanson and Naber, 1997). The Santa Cruz County Public Health Department implemented a home visit follow up program for premature infants. They provide a 7- to 12-month program to help family members feel comfortable and competent in their roles as parents and caregivers. Nurses provide care and education to optimize cognitive, emotional, and physical development (Santa Cruz, 2002).

## Programs for Homeless Families

Actual numbers of homeless children and adolescents are difficult to determine. Estimates vary from 200,000 to 800,000 children and adolescents. Families comprise the fastest growing segment of the homeless population; 25% to 40% of homeless are families, often a single mother with two or three children (NCHS, 2002). The destructive effects of homelessness on health increase with longer duration of homelessness and greater disruption of support systems. Children in homeless situations are often not immunized and suffer from poor nutrition. There is limited or no access to health care. Often there is increased exposure to environmental hazards, violence, and substance abuse. The combination of health problems, environmental dangers, and stress is referred to as the **homeless child syndrome** (Baunoli, 1996).

Children experience chronic illness, such as tuberculosis, asthma, anemia, and chronic otitis media. Hospitalizations are more frequent in this population. Behavioral

problems may exist, such as sleep disorders, withdrawal, aggression, and depression. School performance problems may arise from lack of regular attendance. Many of the children demonstrate developmental delays as a result of the lack of an appropriate environment to foster development.

The nurse may be involved in outreach programs combining health care workers and community members to take health care services to the homeless. Identifying a consistent team to provide continuity of care on a regular basis is important. The family is often removed from its network of neighbors, friends, relatives, and the usual health care providers. Emphasis should be placed on preventive and follow-up care and immediate problems. Services include physical examinations, behavioral and developmental assessments, nutritional support, screening tests, and immunizations (Baunoli, 1996).

## PROGRESS TOWARD CHILD HEALTH: NATIONAL HEALTH OBJECTIVES

States, cities, and communities throughout the country are using Healthy People 2010 objectives to develop health promotion programs and services. The focus is the families, neighborhoods, schools, and workplaces, which are the environments where change can occur. Race, ethnic group, sex, and economic status influence the level of health. Results, in terms of progress toward objectives, in specific child and adolescent areas developed for the year 2000 are reviewed in Table 26-15 (USDHHS, 2000a). Youth objectives discussed in this chapter are listed in the Healthy People 2010 box.

### WHAT DO YOU THINK?

The number of children with health insurance is decreasing. Should insurance companies be required to sell "children only" policies for families who cannot afford the cost of premiums for the entire family?

## ROLE OF THE COMMUNITY-ORIENTED NURSE IN CHILD AND ADOLESCENT HEALTH

A major goal of the Healthy People 2010 objectives is improving access to health care for children, specifically for preventive services and immunizations. Community-oriented nurses have the exciting opportunity to focus on this goal. They practice in a variety of settings, including community health centers, school-based clinics, and home health programs. They provide care through well-child clinics, immunization programs, federally mandated programs (such as the nutrition program for women, infants, and children, or WIC), or specific state-funded programs, such as Headstart. Access to care remains a significant issue. As the nation struggles to deal with this issue, solutions will probably include expanding the role of nurses

## Table 26-15  Final Report of Healthy People 2000 Objectives: Pediatric Applications

| OBJECTIVE | MOVING TOWARD GOAL | MOVING AWAY FROM GOAL |
|---|---|---|
| Fewer people overweight | | X |
| More people exercising regularly | X | |
| Fewer youths beginning to smoke | X | |
| Decreased alcohol use at 12-17 yr of age | X | |
| Decreased drug use at 12-17 yr of age | | X |
| Fewer teen pregnancies | | X |
| Fewer homicides and assault injuries | | X |
| Decreased suicide rate in adolescents | | X |
| Decreased weapon carrying and physical fighting in adolescents | X | |
| Fewer unintentional injuries and deaths | X | |
| Increased use of car safety restraints | X | |
| No children with elevated blood lead levels | X | |
| Fewer children with dental caries | X | |
| Fewer newborns of low birth weight | | X |
| Decreased infant mortality | X | |
| Fewer sexually transmitted diseases | X (except genital herpes) | |
| Higher immunization levels | X | |
| No barriers to preventive services | | X |

Modified from U.S. Department of Health and Human Services: *Healthy people 2000: final review,* Washington, DC, 2000a, USDHHS.

---

## Healthy People 2010 | Objectives Focused on Youth

### 7. EDUCATION AND COMMUNITY-BASED PROGRAMS

7-2  Increase the proportion of middle, junior high, and senior high schools that provide comprehensive school health education to prevent health problems in the following areas: unintentional injury; violence; suicide; tobacco use and addiction; alcohol or other drug use; unintended pregnancy; HIV/AIDS and STD infection; unhealthy dietary patterns; inadequate physical activity; and environmental health.

7-11  Increase the proportion of local health departments that have established culturally appropriate and linguistically competent community health promotion and disease prevention programs for racial and ethnic minority populations

### 8. ENVIRONMENTAL HEALTH

8-11  Eliminate elevated blood lead levels in children

8-18  Increase the proportion of persons who live in homes tested for radon concentrations

8-20  Increase the proportion of the nation's primary and secondary schools that have official school policies ensuring the safety of students and staff from environmental hazards, such as chemicals in special classrooms, poor indoor air quality, asbestos, and exposure to pesticides

8-22  Increase the proportion of persons living in pre-1950s housing that have tested for the presence of lead-based paint

8-25  Reduce exposure of the population to pesticides, heavy metals, and other toxic chemicals, as measured by blood and urine concentrations of the substances of their metabolites

### 14. IMMUNIZATIONS AND INFECTIOUS DISEASE

14-22  Achieve and maintain effective vaccination coverage levels for universally recommended vaccines among young children

14-24  Increase the proportion of young children who receive all vaccines that have been recommended for universal administration for at least 5 years

### 15. INJURY/VIOLENCE PREVENTION

15-3  Reduce firearm-related deaths

From U.S. Department of Health and Human Services: *Healthy people 2010: national health promotion and disease prevention objectives,* ed 2, Washington, DC, 2000, U.S. Government Printing Office.

## Healthy People 2010 | Objectives Focused on Youth—cont'd

### 15. INJURY/VIOLENCE PREVENTION—cont'd

15-14  Reduce nonfatal unintentional injuries

15-20  Increase use of child restraints in cars

15-32  Reduce homicides

15-38  Reduce physical fighting among adolescents

15-39  Reduce weapon carrying by adolescents on school property

### 16. MATERNAL, INFANT, AND CHILD CARE

16-3  Reduce deaths of adolescents and young adults

### 19. NUTRITION AND OVERWEIGHT

19-3  Reduce the proportion of children and adolescents who are overweight or obese

19-5  Increase the proportion of persons aged 2 years and older who consume at least two daily servings of fruit

19-6  Increase the proportion of persons aged 2 years and older who consume at least three daily servings of vegetables, with at least one third being dark green or deep yellow vegetables

19-7  Increase the proportion of persons aged 2 years and older who consume at least six daily servings of grain products, with at least three being whole grains

19-8  Increase the proportion of persons aged 2 years and older who consume less than 10% of calories from saturated fat

19-9  Increase the proportion of persons aged 2 years and older who consume no more than 30% of calories from fat

19-15  Increase the proportion of children and adolescents aged 6 to 19 years whose intake of meals and snacks at schools contributes proportionally to good overall dietary quality

### 22. PHYSICAL ACTIVITY AND FITNESS

22-6  Increase the proportion of adolescents who engage in moderate physical activity for at least 30 minutes on 5 or more of the previous 7 days

22-7  Increase the proportion of adolescents who engage in vigorous physical activity that promotes cardiorespiratory fitness 3 or more days per week for 20 or more minutes per occasion

22-8  Increase the proportion of the nation's public and private schools that require daily physical education for all students

22-10  Increase the proportion of adolescents who spend at least 50% of school physical education class time being physically active

### 24. RESPIRATORY DISEASES

24-1  Reduce asthma deaths

24-2  Reduce hospitalizations for asthma

24-3  Reduce hospital emergency department visits for asthma

24-6  Increase the proportion of persons with asthma who receive formal patient education, including information about community and self-help resources, as an essential part of the management of their condition

24-7  Increase the proportion of persons with asthma who receive appropriate asthma care according to the National Asthma Education and Prevention Program guidelines

### 27. TOBACCO USE

27-2  Reduce tobacco use by adolescents

27-3  Reduce initiation of tobacco use among children and adolescents

27-7  Increase tobacco use cessation attempts by adolescent smokers

27-9  Reduce the proportion of children who are regularly exposed to tobacco smoke at home

27-11  Increase smoke-free and tobacco-free environments in schools, including all school facilities, property, vehicles, and school events

27-14  Reduce the illegal buy rate among minors through enforcement of laws prohibiting the sale of tobacco products to minors

27-16  Eliminate tobacco advertising and promotions that influence adolescents and young adults

---

and the settings for practice. The nursing process and a knowledge base of the factors unique to this population provide a framework of care. Nursing, through developing and coordinating community services and through formation of public policies, promotes the well-being of children within the community. Assessments are made to identify the needs and target populations at risk (Figure 26-6). Programs based on the needs of specific at-risk populations are developed for the delivery of health care.

The nursing plan of care includes three major components. The first is the managing of actual or potential health problems. The second involves both education and anticipatory guidance. This enables families to understand what to expect in the areas of growth and development as well as social, emotional, and cognitive changes. The nurse offers information to promote healthy lifestyles and to prevent health problems and accidents. A third role is case management or coordination of care. For example, the nurse coordinates referrals to community agencies, other health care services or providers, or assistance programs. Box 26-17 lists community resources.

Evaluation of care has always been a critical part of the nursing process. It is a necessity in the current health care environment, with health care payers requiring the justifying of the cost of health care services. Nurses identify and document positive outcomes from the interventions. This may include objectives such as increased knowledge or observable changes in behaviors.

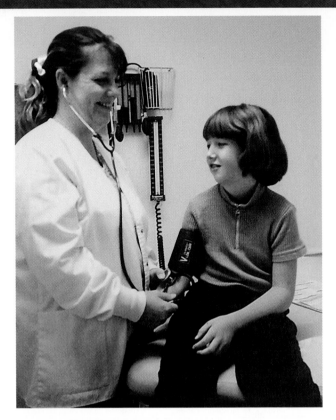

**Figure 26-6** A child gets her blood pressure taken during a well-child care assessment.

## Practice Application

John D. is a 9-year-old brought to the clinic by his mother for follow-up of an emergency department visit five nights ago for an episode of asthma. John has a history of recurrent episodes of wheezing and respiratory distress occurring on a regular basis since he was 4 years old. Until 4 or 5 months ago, John was under good control using a combination of bronchodilators and cromolyn sodium inhalers on a prescribed protocol, based on peak flow meter readings. His mother reports that over the past few months, John has been uncooperative about his asthma. He refuses to use his flow meter and would not use his maintenance medication at school. During this episode, he even refuses to use his bronchodilator at school, although he is still "sick." Mrs. D. is very frustrated and states that she just "can't understand him at all." She reports no changes at home or at school. John is an excellent student, who gets along well with peers, participates in many activities and sports, and normally is very cooperative with both parents. He frequently "picks on" his sister, but his mother perceives this as appropriate. Mrs. D. does admit that, because the weather has been so rainy, she has smoked inside the house a few times.

The clinic nurse reviews this information with the nurse practitioner who is John's health care provider.

They review findings from his assessment. Physical examination is unremarkable except for evidence of an upper respiratory tract infection and peak flow readings in the clinic of 60% to 80% of his expected baseline. His medication orders from the emergency department are appropriate for his condition and include albuterol and cromolyn sodium inhalations tid to qid using a spacer device. John is fairly knowledgeable about his asthma and the treatment regimen, but he has "forgotten" some of the information he learned when he first started his treatment. He admits that he does not go to the office to use his inhalers at school but does not reveal why.

A. Which of the following actions would be the most appropriate for the nurse?
1. Discuss the need to change medications with the nurse practitioner, as John seems unable to stay well on the current regimen.
2. Advise John and his mother that he must use his albuterol and cromolyn sodium inhalers. Review the pathophysiology of asthma, how the medications work, and orders for administration. Schedule a follow-up visit to see how well he is doing.
3. Ask John what could be done to make it easier for him to use his medications. Set up a contract with John, allowing him a reward system for compliance with his asthma protocol. Review asthma information using hands-on activities and games.
4. Refer John to an asthma specialist because he is having problems with control.

B. In talking with John's mother, the nurse should stress the importance of her smoking outside. In addition to the risks of secondhand smoke, Mrs. D. needs to know which of the following?
1. John will sense that she does not love him if she smokes inside.
2. John learns by observing role models. She models noncompliance with the treatment plan when she "breaks the rules."
3. If she is to smoke inside, she should do it when John is asleep so he will not be aware of the problem.
4. When the weather is bad, smoking is acceptable in the house as long as there is adequate ventilation.

C. The nurse refers the family to the regional asthma support program through the American Lung Association. He receives information about an asthma summer camp and names of children his age with asthma. Identify principles of development of school-age children that support this intervention.

D. John's immunization record was reviewed. He has had OPV #4, DTaP #5, MMR #1, and a PPD (age 4). What immunizations, if any, does he need at this time?

*Answers are in the back of the book.*

## Key Points

- Physical growth and development is an ongoing process resulting in physical, cognitive, and emotional changes that affect health status.
- Good nutrition is essential for healthy growth and development, and it influences disease prevention in later life. The adolescent population is at greatest risk for poor nutritional health.
- Immunizations are successful in prevention of selected diseases. Barriers to immunizing children are parental concerns, cost, and inconvenience.
- Pyschosocial development is subject to the interaction of emotional, cultural, and social forces. Resolving crises at each stage of development is important for mastery of skills needed to accept oneself and to function in society.
- Cognitive development follows an orderly process of increasing complexity of thought and action patterns. Understanding the child's cognitive level is the basis of effective interventions.
- The family is critical to the growth and development of the child. Social support has a powerful influence on successful parenting.
- Accidents and injuries are the major cause of health problems in the child and adolescent population. Most are preventable. Nurses have a major role in anticipatory guidance and prevention.
- Minimizing complications of the major health risks to the pediatric and adolescent population follows the goals of Healthy People 2010 initiatives.
- Families are turning to complementary therapies, but the efficacy of many has not been established.
- The pediatric population is vulnerable to environmental hazards. Decreasing exposure and remediation of problems is an important area for community-oriented nurses.
- Nurses are involved in strategies to meet the needs of the pediatric population in the community.
- Home-based service programs have been successful in providing care for at-risk populations.
- Children of homeless families are at risk for health problems, environmental dangers, and stress.
- Community programs to provide health care for the homeless may decrease those risks.

## Clinical Decision-Making Activities

1. Develop a plan of immunization for a 5½ year old who has had one DTaP, Hib, and OPV. Be specific about due dates for immunizations.
2. Develop a screening program for children and adolescents who live in a low-income older neighborhood with a large percentage of Hispanic residents. What risk factors would you consider in the process?
3. Plan a survey of a school district to determine its "friendliness" to children with chronic health problems. What would you do to implement changes?
4. Develop a plan of nursing care for a family who has a 12-year-old child with spina bifida and a family with a 12-year-old child with leukemia. Note the commonalities.
5. Develop a nutritional program for (1) mothers who are breastfeeding their infants, (2) a group of 5-year-olds in a kindergarten class, and (3) a group of high school sophomores. What factors do these programs have in common? How do they differ?
6. Administer a safety survey (e.g., the Injury Prevention Program [TIPP] from the American Academy of Pediatrics, or develop your own) to assess the home environment of a 6-month-old and a 5-year-old. Develop a plan of education and anticipatory guidance for the family. How would you apply this information to a larger population?

## Additional Resources

These related resources are found either in the appendix at the back of this book or on the book's website at **http://evolve.elsevier.com/Stanhope.**

### evolve Evolve Website

ACIP 2002 General Recommendations on Immunization

Accident Prevention in Children

Appendix A.1 Schedule of Clinical Preventive Services

Appendix D.2 Herbs and Supplements Used for Children and Adolescents

Appendix E.1 Vision and Hearing Screening Procedures

Appendix E.2 Screening for Common Orthopedic Problems

Common Concerns and Problems of First Year (Neonate and Infant)

Common Concerns and Problems of Toddler and Preschool Years

Common Behaviors of School-Age Child and Adolescent

Development Behaviors: School-Age Children

Development Characteristics: Summary for Children

Feeding and Nutrition Guidelines for Infants

*Continued*

## Additional Resources—cont'd

### Evolve Website—cont'd

Health Problems of School-Age Child and Adolescent

Healthy People 2010

Identification of At-Risk Newborns

Immunization Schedule for Children and Adolescents

Infant Reflexes

Infant Stimulation

Normal Variations and Minor Abnormalities in Newborn Physical Characteristics

Recommended Immunization Schedules for Children Not Immunized in First Year of Life

Recommended Immunizations for Specific At-Risk Populations

Summary of Rules for Childhood Immunizations

Tanner Stages of Puberty

WebLinks

## References

American Academy of Pediatrics: *Guidelines for health supervision III: American Academy of Pediatrics guide to clinical preventive services,* Elk Grove Village, Ill, 1997, AAP.

American Academy of Pediatrics: *2000 Red book: report of the committee on infectious diseases,* ed 24, Elk Grove Village, Ill, 2000, AAP.

American Academy of Pediatrics Committee on Environmental Health: *Pediatric environmental health,* Elk Grove Village, Ill, 1999, AAP. American Academy of Pediatrics Committee on Nutrition: *Pediatric nutrition handbook,* ed 4, Elk Grove Village, Ill, 1998, AAP.

Balinsky W: Pediatric home care: reimbursement and cost benefit analysis, *J Pediatr Health Care* 13:6, 1999.

Banouli J: *Homelessness in America,* Phoenix, 1996, Onyx.

Blosser C: Complementary medicine. In Burns CG et al, editors: *Pediatric primary care,* ed 2, Philadelphia, 2000, Saunders.

Brooks JG: Sudden infant death syndrome. In Hoekelman R et al, editors: *Primary pediatric care,* ed 3, St Louis, Mo, 1997, Mosby.

Brown ML: The effects of environmental tobacco smoke on children: information and implications for PNP's, *J Pediatr Health Care* 15:6, 2002.

Burns C, Dunn A, Sattler B: Resources for environmental health problems, *J Pediatr Health Care* 16:3, 2002.

Centers for Disease Control and Prevention: Youth risk surveillance, 1995, *MMWR Morb Mortal Wkly Rep* 43, 1996.

Children's Defense Fund: *The state of America's children: yearbook* [on-line], 2001, available at www.childrensdefense.org.

English A: Understanding legal aspects of care. In Neinstein L: *Adolescent health care: a practical guide,* ed 3, Philadelphia, 1996, Williams & Wilkins.

Field T: Massage therapy: more than a laying on of hands, *Contemp Pediatr* 16:5, 1999.

Forbes GB: Nutrition. In Hoekelman R et al, editors: *Primary pediatric care,* ed 3, St Louis, Mo, 1997, Mosby.

Forster JL et al: *Am J Public Health* 88:1193, 1998.

GAPS Executive Committee, Department of Adolescent Health: *American Medical Association guidelines for adolescent preventative services,* recommendations monograph, Chicago, 1995, AMA.

Greger N, Edwin CM: Obesity: a pediatric epidemic, *Pediatr Ann* 30:11, 2001.

Gummer-Strawn L: *The incidence of rickets in the U.S: final report—vitamin D expert panel meeting,* Centers for Disease Control and Prevention, Atlanta, 2001, CDC.

Havens DMH, Zink RL: A pediatric nurse practitioner call to arms: new solutions needed for nation's growing public health problem, *J Pediatr Health Care* 8:3, 1994.

MacKenzie TD, Bartecchi CE, Schrier MD: The human costs of tobacco use, *N Engl J Med* 330:14, 1994.

Miller KJ, Castellanos FX: Attention deficit/hyperactivity disorders, *Pediatr Rev* 19:11, 1998.

National Center for Health Statistics: *FASTATS* [on-line], 2002, available at www.cdc.gov/nchs.

National Center for Injury Prevention and Control: *Fact sheet* [on-line], 2000, available at www.cdc.gov/ncipc.

Neinstein L: *Adolescent health care: a practical guide,* ed 3, Philadelphia, 1996, Williams & Wilkins.

Neinstein LS, Schack LE: Nutrition. In Neinstein L: *Adolescent health care: a practical guide,* ed 3, Philadelphia, 1996, Williams & Wilkins.

Niffenegger JP: Proper handwashing promotes wellness in child care, *J Pediatr Health Care* 11:1, 1997.

Offit PA, Bell LM: *Vaccines: what every parent should know,* New York, 1999, IDG Books Worldwide.

Piaget J: *The psychology of the child,* New York, 1969, Basic Books.

Redlener I: Health care for homeless children: special circumstances. In Green M, Haggerty RJ, editors: *Ambulatory pediatrics,* ed 4, Philadelphia, 1991, Saunders.

Sahler OJZ, Wood BL: Theories and concepts of development as they relate to pediatric practice. In Hoekelman R et al, editors: *Primary pediatric care,* ed 3, St Louis, Mo, 1997, Mosby.

Santa Cruz County Public Health Department: 2002, available at www.santacruzhealth.org.

Spigelblatt L: Alternative medicine: a pediatric conundrum, *Contemp Pediatr* 14:8, 1997

Swanson S, Naber M: Neonatal integrated home care: nursing without walls, *Neonatal Netw* 16:7, 1997.

Swartz MK: Playground safety, *J Pediatr Health Care* 6(3):161, 1992.

U.S. Bureau of the Census: Index of census 2000, available at http://ftp2.census.gov/census_2000/.

U.S. Department of Health and Human Services: *Healthy people 2000: final review,* Washington, DC, 2000a, USDHHS.

U.S. Department of Health and Human Services: *Healthy people 2010: understanding and improving health,* ed 2, Washington, DC, 2000b, U.S. Government Printing Office.

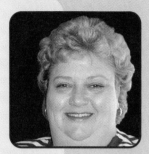

## Chapter 27

# Women's Health

### Lisa M. Kaiser, R.N., M.S.N., Ph.D.(c)

Lisa Kaiser began practicing community-oriented nursing in the mid 1980s when she began working in home health care. Much of her home health care practice involved women's health, specifically in mom–baby programs. Ms. Kaiser is currently a part-time associate faculty member at National University of La Jolla, California. She teaches community nursing at the baccalaureate level as well as community-focused courses in the graduate program. Ms. Kaiser is a doctoral candidate at the Hahn School of Nursing and Health Sciences at the University of San Diego, where she has been a research fellow on a federally funded grant examining health behaviors among homeless women.

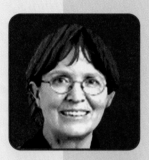

### Diane C. Hatton, R.N., C.S., D.N.Sc.

Diane Hatton is a certified clinical nurse specialist in community health nursing. She is a professor at the Hahn School of Nursing and Health Science where she teaches courses related to community health nursing and qualitative research methods. Dr. Hatton's research program focuses on health and health care access of vulnerable populations including homeless women and children.

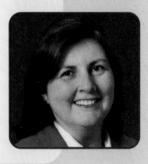

### Debra Gay Anderson, Ph.D., R.N.C.

Debra Gay Anderson is currently an associate professor of nursing at the College of Nursing of the University of Kentucky in Lexington. As a certified public health nurse, she has provided health care for homeless and other vulnerable populations. Dr. Anderson has taught public health, epidemiology, and research courses at the graduate and undergraduate levels. Her program of research, publications, and presentations are primarily on vulnerable populations with a focus on vulnerable women.

## Objectives

After reading this chapter, the student should be able to do the following:

1. Analyze how women's health is embedded in their communities
2. Discuss how the women's movement in the United States has affected women's health
3. Define the term *women's health*
4. Describe the health status of women in the United States
5. Discuss the leading causes of death among women in different ethnic/racial groups
6. Discuss selected health concerns of U.S. women
7. Identify health disparities among special groups of women
8. Analyze how health policy and legislation have influenced women's health

This chapter examines the health of women in the United States. Definitions of women's health, historical perspectives (including the women's health movement), relevant legislation, health policy, and Healthy People 2010 objectives that target women are considered. The chapter addresses women's health status, including mortality and morbidity, and explores the health disparities that exist among special groups of women in the United States. Although health issues relevant to women, such as violence, are covered elsewhere in this text, this chapter briefly describes these topics as they specifically relate to women's health. Trends in programs and services for women as well as access to health care are analyzed. The chapter avoids laundry lists of various diseases and instead emphasizes the context in which women experience health. Women's health is "embedded in their communities," not just in their individual bodies (Ruzek, Olesen, and Clarke, 1997, p. 13). Thus the chapter analyzes the factors in society that interact with each other to influence the distribution of health and disease among women.

## DEFINITIONS

Historically, at the beginning of the twentieth century, discussions surrounding **women's health** centered on repro-

## Key Terms

**anorexia**, p. 668
**bulimia**, p. 668
**caregiver**, p. 654
**caregiver burden**, p. 654
**Family and Medical Leave Act**, p. 654
**female genital mutilation**, p. 663
**gestational diabetes mellitus**, p. 665

**health**, p. 653
**menopause**, p. 663
**obesity**, p. 668
**Office of Women's Health**, p. 655
**Personal Responsibility and Work Opportunity Reconciliation Act**, p. 655
**preconceptual counseling**, p. 662

**Temporary Assistance for Needy Families**, p. 655
**unintended pregnancy**, p. 654
**women's health**, p. 652
**Women's Health Equity Act**, p. 655
**women's health movement**, p. 653
*See Glossary for definitions*

## Chapter Outline

Definitions
Historical Perspectives on Women's Health
Health Policy and Legislation
Health
*Mortality*
*Morbidity*
Women's Health Concerns
*Reproductive Health*
*Menopause*
*Osteoporosis*

*Female Genital Mutilation*
*Cardiovascular Disease*
*Diabetes Mellitus*
*Mental Health*
*Cancer*
*HIV/AIDS*
*Women and Weight Control*
Health Disparities Among Special Groups of Women
*Women of Color*

*Incarcerated Women*
*Lesbians*
*Women With Disabilities*
*Impoverished Women*
*Older Women*
Alternative/Complementary Therapies
U.S. Preventive Services Recommendations

duction and women's roles as mothers. In the 1920s with the birth control movement in its initial stages, women's health expanded to address family planning and reproductive health. The dominant point of view during these times reflected the biomedical model that emphasized disease. Today, women's health advocates have widened this framework by including many social, psychological, cultural, political, economic, and biological factors that influence women's health. The American Academy of Nursing's Expert Panel on Women's Health (1996) argued that women's health encompasses the entire life span, and that women's health care includes health promotion, disease prevention, maintenance, and restoration. This panel of nursing experts also identified fundamental features of excellent women's health care (Box 27-1).

In this chapter, the discussion also uses the basic definition of **health** from the World Health Organization (WHO): "a state of complete physical, mental, and social well-being, and not merely the absence of disease or infirmity" (WHO, 2001). From this broad perspective, the complexities of women's lives—their educational levels, income, culture, ethnicity/race, and a host of other identities and experiences—shape their health. In sum, women's health is created in complex, interactive ways (Ruzek et al, 1997).

# HISTORICAL PERSPECTIVES ON WOMEN'S HEALTH

The **women's health movement** had its seeds in the women's movement. The first Women's Right's Convention, organized by Elizabeth Cady Stanton, was held in Seneca Falls, New York in 1848, and the participants called it one of the most courageous acts on record. The attendees presented and adopted a Declaration of Sentiments that pointed out areas of life where women were treated unjustly (National Women's History Project, 2002). The declaration demanded changes in law, social custom, and attitudes. The speeches and documents born in this convention became the first organized feminist movement in the United States (Hoffert, 1995).

After women won the right to vote in 1920, the organized women's movement took several directions. A visiting nurse, Margaret Sanger, initiated one of the most influential movements in women's health. Sanger led the birth control movement endorsing a woman's right to be educated about family planning. In 1921, Sanger organized the American Birth Control League, which later evolved into the Federation of Planned Parenthood in 1942. Despite Sanger's work with women and birth control, it was not until the landmark Supreme Court decision, *Griswold v. Connecticut*

BOX 27-1  Features of Excellent Health Care for Women

- Grounded in an awareness of everyday women's lives
- Reflective of the diversity of women
- Oriented to comprehensive care across the life span
- Incorporated in a range of services
- Delivered by a range of health care providers
- Accessible to all women

Modified from American Academy of Nursing: Women's health and women's health care: recommendations of the 1996 AAN expert writing panel on women's health, *Nurs Outlook* 45(1):7-15, 1996.

BOX 27-2  Goals of the Institute of Medicine Unintended Pregnancy Campaign

1. Improve knowledge about contraception, unintended pregnancy, and reproductive health
2. Increase access to contraception
3. Explicitly address the major roles that feelings, attitudes, and motivation play in using contraception and avoiding unintended pregnancy
4. Develop and scrupulously evaluate a variety of local programs to reduce unintended pregnancy
5. Stimulate research to (1) develop new contraceptive methods for both men and women, (2) answer important questions about how best to organize contraceptive services, and (3) understand more fully the determinants and antecedents of unintended pregnancy

Modified from Institute of Medicine, Committee on Unintended Pregnancy: *The best intentions,* Washington, DC, 1995, National Academy Press.

in 1965 that the U.S. Supreme Court made birth control legal for married couples. Fortunately, Sanger lived to see this historic turn of events. She died a few months later in 1966 (Katz, 2001).

The woman's movement enjoyed a resurgence in the 1960s—a second wave of activism. Several events highlighted this era: President John Kennedy's establishment of the President's Commission on the Status of Women in 1961, the publishing by Betty Friedan in 1963 of *The Feminist Mystique,* the passage of title VII of the 1964 Civil Rights Act that banned sexual discrimination in the workplace, and the development of the National Organization for Women (NOW) in 1966. In 1972, Congress passed the Equal Rights Amendment; however, it failed to become part of the U.S. Constitution because the required number of states did not ratify it (National Women's History Project, 2002).

In 1973, a powerful Supreme Court made a decision that came to be commonly known as *Roe v. Wade.* This landmark case addressed a woman's right to have an abortion. In 1976, Congress passed the Hyde Amendment which excluded payment for abortions for low-income women through Medicaid; however, in cases of rape or incest, federal funding is allowed for the termination of pregnancy (American Civil Liberties Union [ACLU], 2002). Unintended pregnancies remain a major problem for U.S. women. In 1995, the Institute of Medicine (IOM) reported that nearly 60% of all pregnancies were unintended in the United States (IOM, 1995). Consequently, a campaign to reduce **unintended pregnancies** was mounted; it stressed the five core goals depicted in Box 27-2. More recently, Healthy People 2010 has addressed this issue as well in its objective 9-1: Increase the proportion of intended pregnancies from 51% to 70% (U.S. Department of Health and Human Services [USDHHS], 2000).

In 1974, the National Women's Health Network began to monitor national health policy. This organization serves as a clearinghouse and advocates for women's health, and it has played an important role in the development of pol-icy and legislation. Thus the women's movement that began in Seneca Falls many years ago has evolved today into a national movement that encompasses women's health.

## HEALTH POLICY AND LEGISLATION

Four pieces of important federal legislation have influenced women's health and their lives in their communities: the **Family and Medical Leave Act** (FMLA) of 1993, the Personal Responsibility and Work Opportunity Reconciliation Act of 1996, legislation establishing the Office of Women's Health, and the Women's Health Equity Act of 1990. The FMLA has affected one of the primary roles of women in society—that of caregiver. Women have a long history of providing care for others, but this role has expanded as the aging population increases in society. Women frequently provide unpaid care for their family members, such as children, grandchildren, partners, and aging parents. Estimates are that 72% of the unpaid family **caregivers** are women and that the majority of these women are midlife daughters or daughters-in-law (Robinson, 1997). Often, these women find themselves caring for aging parents at the same time they are caring for their young families. Women caregivers' multiple roles and responsibilities are frequently coupled with financial strain. This situation can lead them to experience **caregiver burden.** A number of factors, including socioeconomic conditions, resources of the caregiver, and specific stressors, can influence the intensity of this burden (Hoffman and Mitchell, 1998).

The FMLA provides job protection and continuous health benefits, where applicable, for eligible employees who need extended leave for their own illness or to care for a family member. FMLA allows 12 weeks of leave per year for personal or family health conditions, including adoptions or births (U.S. Department of Labor, 2002). The FMLA has provided assistance to many women caring for family members, but much still needs to be done. The financial consequences for aging women who must place their husbands in long-term care facilities, wages lost by women who must leave work to take family members to health-related appointments, and the profound isolation experienced by many women caregivers are among the issues that continue to warrant attention.

In 1996, Congress passed the **Personal Responsibility and Work Opportunity Reconciliation Act,** commonly known as *welfare reform*. This law targeted women who received public assistance and changed the previous Aid to Families with Dependent Children (AFDC) to **Temporary Assistance for Needy Families** (TANF)—a work program that mandates that women heads-of-household find employment to retain their benefits. The law sought to reduce federal spending. As states now find their budgets shrinking, their resources for TANF benefits also diminish. Women's advocates have argued that the TANF program presents serious health risks for U.S. families headed by women. They have noted that the jobs that low-income women find in the United States have meager salaries that do not pull them out of poverty. In addition, many women applied for AFDC in the past when they escaped from domestic violence situations. With the new law, women may be reluctant to apply for TANF with its restrictions, including the initiation of child support enforcement, especially if they believe their abusive partners will discover their place of residence. Therefore, as a consequence of this policy change, safety for these women has become a major concern (Stevens, 2000; U.S. Department of Health and Human Services [USDHHS], 1997).

In 2001, the 107th Congress established the **Office of Women's Health** (OWH) within the Department of Health and Human Services (USDHHS). Its charge is to serve as the federal government's champion for women's health issues, and to address inequities in research, health services, and education that have traditionally placed women at risk (USDHHS, Office on Women's Health [OWH], 2003). The intent is to coordinate these services and help eliminate disparities in health status as well as to support culturally sensitive programs that provide health education to various groups of women.

In years past, women were not extensively involved in clinical research, and this exclusion has limited what is known about their health. At the same time, some argue that researchers who did recruit and use impoverished inner-city women in their clinical research trials may have exploited them. However, generally women's health has not been on the forefront of health-related research. Rather, most clinical health research has pertained to health problems found in men (Narrigan et al, 1997).

To address this situation, in 1985 the National Institutes of Health (NIH) established a policy for including women in biomedical and behavioral research, and in 1990 Congress passed the **Women's Health Equity Act** (WHEA) intended to reduce the inequities in research between men and women. In this same year, Congress asked the Government Accounting Office (GAO) to study the guidelines related to inclusion of women in research and consequently established the Office of Research on Women's Health as the focal point for women's research at NIH (Pinn, 1998). With these guidelines in place, many researchers are hopeful that future research projects will address the many health concerns that are unique to women.

The community-oriented nurse serves in a unique position for advocacy and support of health legislation and policy that support women and their physical, mental, and social well-being. Advocacy can be accomplished in a variety of ways, such as by lobbying, public speaking, grassroots activities, and staying abreast of proposed legislation that potentially influences the health of women, their families, and communities.

## HEALTH

Health throughout women's life spans is closely related to their communities. Many factors, such as the food they eat, the work they perform, their exposures to toxic agents, their substance use, and the injuries they encounter are linked to their social and physical environments. Violence in their communities, available health services, employment opportunities, wages, and transportation are also among the factors that influence women's health (American Academy of Nursing, 1996).

Although most of the objectives of Healthy People 2010 can be applied to women, 28 focus areas are more

## THE CUTTING EDGE

The Office on Women's Health (OWH) within the Department of Health and Human Services (USDHHS) celebrated its tenth anniversary on December 3, 2001, with a ceremony to unveil a Women's Health Time Capsule to honor the progress made in women's health in the twentieth century.

The Time Capsule contains items that document how preventive health efforts and health communications have evolved over the last century. Other items that have improved women's quality of life, such as information on state-of-the-art diagnosis and treatment of the diseases that most affect women today, were included. Additionally, personal articles that demonstrate women's continued interest in beauty and body image have been placed in the Time Capsule.

It was buried on the grounds of the National Institutes of Health during Women's Health Week in 2002 and is to be opened in the year 2100.

**Healthy People 2010** | Selected Objectives Related to Women's Health

1-1  Increase the proportion of persons with health insurance to 100%

2-9  Reduce the overall number of cases of osteoporosis among adults aged 50 years and older from 10% to 8%

3-3  Reduce the breast cancer death rate from 27.7 deaths per 100,000 to 22.2 per 100,000

3-4  Reduce uterine cervical cancer death rate from 3.0 deaths per 100,000 to 2.0 per 100,000

3-11  Increase the number of women who receive a Pap test

3-13  Increase the proportion of women age 40 years and older who have received a mammogram within the preceding 2 years from 67% to 70%

9-1  Increase the proportion of intended pregnancies from 51% to 70%

9-5  Increase the proportion of health care providers who provide emergency contraception

13-17  Reduce new cases of perinatally acquired HIV infection

15-35  Reduce the annual rate of rape or attempted rape from 0.7 per 1000 to 0.8 per 1000

16-4  Reduce maternal deaths from 7.1 deaths per 100,000 live births to 3.3 per 100,000 live births

16-5  Reduce maternal illness and complications due to pregnancy

16-6  Increase the proportion of pregnant women who receive early and adequate prenatal care

16-17  Increase abstinence from alcohol, cigarettes, and illicit drugs among pregnant women

16-18  Increase the proportion of mothers who breast-feed their babies

19-13  Reduce anemia among low-income pregnant females in their third trimester from 29% to 20%

19-14  Reduce iron deficiency among pregnant females

25-6  Reduce the proportion of females who have ever required treatment for pelvic inflammatory disease (PID) from 8% to 5%

25-16  Increase the proportion of sexually active females age 25 years and under who are screened annually for genital chlamydial infections

25-17  Increase the proportion of pregnant females screened for sexually transmitted diseases (including HIV infection and bacterial vaginosis) during prenatal health care visits, according to recognized standards

27-6  Increase smoking cessation during pregnancy from 14% to 30%

From U.S. Department of Health and Human Services: *Healthy people 2010: national health promotion and disease prevention objectives,* ed 2, Washington, DC, 2000, U.S. Government Printing Office.

specifically targeted to this population (see the Healthy People 2010 box). This section of the chapter addresses selected health status indicators that reflect the well-being of U.S. women, taking into account the objectives from 2010. Discussion includes morbidity and mortality statistics as well as consideration of selected health problems that have particular relevance for women in the United States. These health problems are, as previously noted, embedded in women's communities.

## Mortality

The life expectancy of U.S. women is lower than that of women in 18 other developed countries (Table 27-1). In 1999, the life expectancy for U.S. women of all races at birth was 79.4 years, whereas for men it was 73.9 years. Although women live longer than men, they are more likely to use health services and report greater rates of disability (Centers for Disease Control and Prevention [CDC], National Center for Health Statistics [NCHS], 2001).

Life expectancy for women varies among ethnic/racial groups in the United States. For white women, the average life expectancy in 1999 was 79.9 years, and for African-American women, 74.7 years. Among all racial/ethnic groups combined, if a woman lives to age 65, she can then expect to live 19.1 years longer, whereas a man of 65 can expect to live 16.1 years longer. White women at age 65 can expect to live 19.2 years longer, whereas African-American women can expect to live 17.3 years longer (CDC, NCHS, 2001).

Not only are there disparities in the life expectancies of various groups of U.S. women but the leading causes of death also differ by racial/ethnic group (Table 27-2) (CDC, NCHS, 2001). These differences reflect the health challenges faced by women in certain racial/ethnic groups, who have varying mortality rates for diseases such as heart disease, cancer, accidents, chronic obstructive pulmonary disease, and human immunodeficiency virus (HIV) infection, or acquired immunodeficiency syndrome (AIDS). Early researchers thought genetics caused these differences in health status. Today, however, many scientists argue that these differences are caused by more than biological divisions in these populations. Although biological factors, such as genetics, may play a part in these health differences, it is more likely that a complex interplay between biology and socially determined exposure leads to population differences in health (Williams, 2002).

Researchers have observed these disparities in almost every area of health. For instance, white women have a higher incidence rate of breast cancer (114/100,000) than do African-American women (100/100,000). However,

## Table 27-1 Life Expectancy at Birth for Women, Ranked by Countries, 1996

| COUNTRY | LIFE EXPECTANCY (YR) |
|---------|----------------------|
| Japan | 83.6 |
| France | 82.9 |
| Switzerland | 82.3 |
| Spain | 82.0 |
| Italy | 81.9 |
| Sweden | 81.8 |
| Canada | 81.4 |
| Norway | 81.3 |
| Australia | 81.1 |
| Finland | 80.8 |
| Greece | 80.7 |
| Netherlands | 80.6 |
| Austria | 80.4 |
| Belgium | 80.2 |
| Germany | 80.2 |
| United Kingdom | 79.7 |
| New Zealand | 79.6 |
| United States | 79.1 |

From U.S. Department of Health and Human Services, Centers for Disease Control and Prevention, National Center for Health Statistics: *Health, United States, 2001 with urban and rural health chartbook,* 2001, available at http://www.cdc.gov/nchs/data/hus/hus01.pdf.

African-American women have higher mortality rates from breast cancer than do white women. Scientists speculate that these differences reflect lower rates of early detection and limited treatment for African-American women (Satcher, 2001). Similarly, for all sites of cancer combined and for each age-group, white women have the higher incidence rates whereas African-American women have the higher cancer death rates (Edwards et al, 2002). Again, these findings probably reflect lower rates of detection and more limited treatment for African-American women.

## Morbidity

When considering all ages, surveys show that women report about the same amount of limitation of activity caused by chronic conditions as men do (12.4% of women compared to 12.6% of men). However, when looking at reports from adults over the age of 65, 16.4% of women report some limitation of activity whereas only 9.2% of men do. Thus these limitations begin to widen as women and men age—also, women live longer (CDC, NCHS, 2001).

Although only a slightly higher percentage of women of all ages rate their health as either fair or poor (9.2%) when compared to men (8.6%), women are more likely than men to make visits to physicians' offices and emer-

gency departments, and to have home visits. In 1999, 88% of women reported such visits in the past 12 months compared to only 77% of men (CDC, NCHS, 2001). Many scholars in the area of women's health have analyzed the use of health services by women as compared to men over the years and have argued that a number of complex factors come into play, such as type of service, increased use for childbirth and other health encounters related to reproductive health, levels of education, and women's longer life spans (Woods, 1995).

### WHAT DO YOU THINK?

Research demonstrates that social support has a positive influence on how people manage illness and on the effects of illness in their everyday lives. Women in rural areas have a distinct disadvantage in accessing support groups because of their widely dispersed geographic locations, coupled with the challenges that travel imposes on those with chronic illness. Do you think urban women have more opportunities for social support?

## WOMEN'S HEALTH CONCERNS

### Reproductive Health

Women often use health care services for reproductive issues or problems, and nurses are frequently the health professionals they encounter. A number of Healthy People 2010 objectives address areas related to women's reproductive health, including increasing the number of pregnancies that are intended rather than unintended (objective 9-1); increasing the proportion of health care providers who provide emergency contraception (objective 9-5); reducing new cases of perinatally acquired HIV infection (objective 13-7); reducing maternal death, illness, and complications due to pregnancy (objectives 16-4, 16-5, and 16-6); increasing the number of pregnant women who receive prenatal care (objective 16-6); increasing abstinence from alcohol, cigarettes, and illicit drugs among pregnant women (objective 16-17); increasing the number of mothers breastfeeding their babies (objective 16-18); reducing anemia among low-income pregnant women (objective 19-13); reducing iron deficiency among pregnant females (19-14); increasing the number of pregnant females screened for sexually transmitted diseases (objective 25-17); and increasing smoking cessation during pregnancy (objective 27-6) (see the Healthy People 2010 box).

Community-oriented nurses are in a unique position to advocate for policies that increase women's access to services for reproductive health. In addition, many nurses discuss contraception with women of childbearing age. Contraceptive counseling requires accurate knowledge of current contraceptive choices and a nonjudgmental approach. The goal of contraceptive counseling is to ensure

*Text continued on p. 662*

## HOW TO    Provide High-Quality Women's Health Services

- Include women of various ages, ethnic groups, and socioeconomic status when planning women's health programs.
- Identify the specific health needs of targeted communities before planning programs.
- Provide comprehensive women's services. At a minimum, include gynecologic and reproductive services, health education programs, general medical services, shelter resources for women and children, transportation, translation, multicultural counseling, and a referral network.
- Learn about women's unique responses to health issues.
- Provide culturally relevant outreach to inform women about the magnitude of threats to health from smoking, poor diet, and lack of exercise.
- Work to reduce inducements to substance abuse and aggression toward women conveyed in films, television, and music.
- Support community programs aimed at reducing violence.
- Improve cultural and linguistic competence of health professionals.

- Develop new and effective ways to induce girls and women to engage in physical activity throughout life.
- Participate in partnerships and community coalitions to develop women's health services in nontraditional settings (e.g., churches, schools, workplaces, and beautician shops).
- Affiliate with other community-based organizations to provide services such as childcare and education completion programs.
- Integrate women's service programs with childcare programs to develop family health services.
- Seek ways to control and diminish the rising prevalence of depression in women (e.g., stress management, support groups, and assertiveness training).
- Strive to expand women's access to HIV/AIDS prevention counseling and treatment programs.
- Participate in the development of data collection strategies for population groups that have not been adequately monitored, such as lesbians and impoverished and less-educated women.
- Ensure that all health-related programs take into account women's needs, particularly single mothers, minorities, lesbians, and women in prison.

Modified from U.S. Department of Health and Human Services, Public Health Service: *Healthy people: progress review: women's health,* 1998, available at http://odphp.osophs.dhhs.gov/pubs/hp2000/PROGRVW/women/women. htm.

### Table 27-2    Leading Causes of Death Among U.S. Females, 1999

| CAUSES | NUMBER OF DEATHS | PERCENTAGES (%) |
|---|---|---|
| **Whites** | | |
| All causes | 1,056,013 | |
| 1. Diseases of the heart | 327,533 | 31 |
| 2. Malignant neoplasms | 229,842 | 22 |
| 3. Cerebrovascular diseases | 89,960 | 8 |
| 4. Chronic lower respiratory diseases | 57,735 | 5 |
| 5. Influenza and pneumonia | 32,413 | 0.3 |
| 6. Unintentional injuries | 29,347 | 0.2 |
| 7. Alzheimer's disease | 29,292 | 0.2 |
| 8. Diabetes mellitus | 29,094 | 0.2 |
| 9. Nephritis, nephritic syndrome, and nephrosis | 14,409 | 0.1 |
| 10. Septicemia | 13,798 | 0.1 |
| **African Americans** | | |
| All causes | 139,361 | |
| 1. Diseases of the heart | 40,998 | 29 |
| 2. Malignant neoplasms | 29,101 | 20 |
| 3. Cerebrovascular diseases | 10,990 | 7 |

From U.S. Department of Health and Human Services, Centers for Disease Control and Prevention: National Center for Heath Statistics, U.S., 2001.

## Table 27-2 Leading Causes of Death Among U.S. Females, 1999—cont'd

| CAUSES | NUMBER OF DEATHS | PERCENTAGES (%) |
| --- | --- | --- |
| **African Americans—cont'd** | | |
| 4. Diabetes mellitus | 7168 | 5 |
| 5. Unintentional injuries | 3955 | 2 |
| 6. Nephritis, nephritic syndrome, and nephrosis | 3703 | 2 |
| 7. Chronic lower respiratory diseases | 3415 | 2 |
| 8. Septicemia | 3203 | 2 |
| 9. Influenza and pneumonia | 3051 | 2 |
| 10. Human immunodeficiency virus (HIV) disease | 2400 | 1 |
| **Native Americans and Native Alaskans** | | |
| All causes | 5220 | |
| 1. Diseases of the heart | 1102 | 21 |
| 2. Malignant neoplasms | 887 | 17 |
| 3. Unintentional injuries | 437 | 8 |
| 4. Diabetes mellitus | 402 | 8 |
| 5. Cerebrovascular diseases | 310 | 6 |
| 6. Chronic liver disease and cirrhosis | 214 | 4 |
| 7. Chronic lower respiratory diseases | 209 | 4 |
| 8. Influenza and pneumonia | 168 | 3 |
| 9. Nephritis, nephritic syndrome, and nephrosis | 115 | 2 |
| 10. Septicemia | 88 | 1 |
| **Asians and Pacific Islanders** | | |
| All causes | 15,345 | |
| 1. Malignant neoplasms | 4176 | 27 |
| 2. Diseases of the heart | 3942 | 26 |
| 3. Cerebrovascular diseases | 1621 | 10 |
| 4. Diabetes mellitus | 625 | 4 |
| 5. Unintentional injuries | 586 | 4 |
| 6. Chronic lower respiratory diseases | 407 | 3 |
| 7. Influenza and pneumonia | 380 | 2 |
| 8. Nephritis, nephritic syndrome, and nephrosis | 282 | 2 |
| 9. Essential (primary) hypertension/hypertensive renal disease | 197 | 1 |
| 10. Septicemia | 196 | 1 |
| **Hispanic Americans** | | |
| All causes | 45,749 | |
| 1. Diseases of the heart | 12,312 | 27 |
| 2. Malignant neoplasms | 9565 | 21 |
| 3. Cerebrovascular diseases | 3098 | 6 |
| 4. Diabetes mellitus | 2847 | 6 |
| 5. Unintentional injuries | 2072 | 4 |
| 6. Chronic lower respiratory diseases | 1312 | 3 |
| 7. Influenza and pneumonia | 1154 | 3 |
| 8. Certain conditions originating in the perinatal period | 961 | 2 |
| 9. Chronic liver disease and cirrhosis | 829 | 2 |
| 10. Nephritis, nephritic syndrome, and nephrosis | 770 | 2 |

## Women's Health in Canada

Karon Janine Foster, R.N., B.Sc.N., M.Ed., Lecturer, Faculty of Nursing, University of Toronto

In 1999, females represented more than 50% of the Canadian population (Lindsay, 2000). Women 35 to 54 years old composed the greatest number of women, and senior women are the fastest growing segment. These changing demographics will have an impact on the health care system, as women live longer with more years of chronic illnesses and use health care services at a greater rate than men.

### LIFE EXPECTANCY AND CAUSES OF DEATH

Canadian women have seen their life expectancy improve. They can now expect to live to age 81, although the life expectancy for Aboriginal women is 76 (Normand, 2000; Tait, 2000). Since 1990, the death rate for women has fallen 4% and in 1997 was 522 deaths per 100,000 women (Statistics Canada, 1997). Heart disease and cancer account for more than 50% of deaths among women (Normand, 2000). For women under 30, motor vehicle accidents, heart disease, and respiratory conditions are the leading causes of death. For women between 30 and 60, cancer and heart disease are the leading causes. For women 65 years and older, it is heart disease, lung cancer, and cerebrovascular disease. Breast cancer is the leading cause of cancer deaths in women less than 60 years old, and lung cancer is the leading cause in women over 60.

### CHRONIC CONDITIONS AND HEALTH CONCERNS

In 1998-1999, the chronic diseases with the highest incidence for women were nonarthritic back problems, arthritis/rheumatism, migraines, allergies, hypertension, and urinary incontinence (Normand, 2000; Statistics Canada, 2002a). Other health problems include asthma, cataracts, heart disease, ulcers, cancer, diabetes, sexually transmitted diseases, and human immunodeficiency virus (HIV) infections. Women 75 years and older have higher rates of arthritis/rheumatism, hypertension, and cancer. Younger women report migraines and allergies as common problems. Nine percent of women in 1998-1999 reported chronic pain that affected their activities of daily living, with senior women the most affected (Statistics Canada, 2002c). Women experience more depression than men. About 6% of women have experienced a depressive episode (Federal, Provincial, Territorial Advisory Committee on Population Health, 1999). In 1997, there were 10 suicides per 100,000 women aged 45 to 54 (Federal, Provincial, Territorial Advisory Committee on Population Health, 1999). Women 40 to 49 years are at greatest risk for committing suicide. Aboriginal women have a suicide rate of 35 suicides per 100,000 women (Tait, 2000). A growing concern among health professionals is the increasing number of obese Canadians. The Canadian Community Health Survey for 2000-2001 reported that 15% of Canadians are obese, with a body mass index (BMI) over 30 (Statistics Canada, 2002c). Rates of obesity are greatest for women between 45 and 64 years old (Statistics Canada, 2001a).

### HEALTH CARE PRACTICES

In 1996-1997, approximately 95% of women reported visiting a health care professional at least once a year (Normand, 2000). Women over 65 years visited health professionals more frequently than younger women. General practitioners, specialists, and dentists were the health professionals most commonly seen. Women were also more likely to be hospitalized than men; women over 75 years were most frequently hospitalized and for longer periods of time.

Alternative health care is a growing trend in Canada. Nineteen percent of women consulted alternative health care providers such as chiropractors, massage therapists, acupuncturists, and naturopaths in 1998-1999 (Millar, 2001). Women 25 to 64 years old were most likely to use alternative care providers. Factors such as cultural practices, educational and income levels, chronic conditions or chronic pain, and attitudes to self-care were predictors of alternative health care use (McClennon-Leong and Ross-Kerr, 1999; Millar, 2001). The Canadian Cancer Society recommends that women between 50 and 69 be screened with a mammogram every 2 years, receive a clinical breast examination by a trained professional at least every 2 years, and do regular breast self-examinations. In 1996-1997, 60% of women over 35 years reported having a mammogram at least once; 46% of this sample had undergone one in the past year, and 75% had had a clinical breast examination (Normand, 2000). Breast screening clinics are available in all provinces and territories. The Canadian Cancer Society recommends that all sexually active women be regularly screened with a Pap smear every 3 years. As of 1998-1999, 76% of women 18 to 69 years old were screened with a Pap within 3 years, but 10% had never received one (Statistics Canada, 2002d).

### LIFESTYLE PRACTICES

Lifestyle factors such as smoking, alcohol use, diet, and physical activity also influence the health of women. Cigarette smoking is a risk factor for heart disease, cerebrovascular disease, and cancer. The percentage of Canadian women who smoke has declined in the past 15 years. In 2000-2001, 19.4% of women reported smoking daily, and women between 35 and 44 were the group that most frequently reported daily smoking (Statistics Canada, 2000b).

Alcohol consumption is associated with injuries and many diseases. In 1998-1999, 45% of females over 12 reported consuming an alcoholic beverage at least once a month (Normand, 2000). The most frequent regular drinkers were 20- to 24-year-old women.

Physical activity has both physical and mental benefits as well as contributing to prevention of disease.

Since 1994, women have increased their level of physical activity, so that now 41% of women reported being physically active (Statistics Canada, 2002b). Older women and women with chronic health problems are more sedentary. However, women are less physically active than men.

## FEDERAL GOVERNMENT INITIATIVES

In 1999, the Federal Minister of Health released Health Canada's *Women's Health Strategy.* The goal of this strategy is to improve the health of women in Canada by enhancing the responsiveness of the health system to women and women's health. The following objectives are listed in the strategy (Health Canada, 1999):

- Ensure that Health Canada policies and programs are responsive to sex and gender differences and to women's health needs
- Increase knowledge and understanding of women's health and women's health needs
- Support the provision of effective health services to women
- Promote good health through preventive measures and the reduction of risk factors that most imperil the health of women

To support these objectives, five federally funded Centers of Excellence for Women's Health across Canada have been established. These centers are responsible for generating new knowledge about women's health. As well, they support the Canadian Women's Health Network (CWHN), which represents 70 organizations across the provinces and territories. CWHN provides a website to offer women valuable on-line resources. Another activity includes health promotion and disease prevention activities such as more extensive screening to reduce cervical cancer mortality and morbidity.

In summary, women's life expectancy has improved in Canada; however, cancer and heart disease pose major threats to the health of women. Preventive health practices, lifestyle changes, and a variety of health promotion strategies need to be used to address these threats. The federal government has recognized the importance of women's health and has developed a strategy to improve the health of Canadian women.

## References

Federal, Provincial, Territorial Advisory Committee on Population Health: *Toward a healthy future: second report on health of Canadians,* Ottawa, 1999, Publications Canada

Health Canada: *Women's health strategy,* Ottawa, 1999, retrieved July 14, 2002, from www.hc-sc.gc.ca/english/women/womenstrat.htm.

Lindsay C: The female population. In *Women in Canada, 2000: a gender-based statistical report,* Ottawa, 2000, Minister of Industry.

McClennon-Leong J, Ross-Kerr J: Alternative health care options in Canada, *Can Nurse* 95(10):26-30, 1999.

Millar W: Patterns of use: alternative health care practitioners, *Health Rep* 13(1):9-21, 2001.

Normand J: The health of women. In *Women in Canada 2000: a gender-based statistical report,* pp 47-83, ed 4, Ottawa, 2000, Minister of Industry.

Statistics Canada: *Selected leading causes of death by sex,* 1997, retrieved July 4, 2002 from www.statcan.ca/english/Pgdb/health36.htm (also available at www.statcan.ca, choose Canadian statistics, and search for document name).

Statistics Canada: *National population health survey overview 1996/97,* Ottawa, 1998, Health Statistics Division.

Statistics Canada: *Alcohol consumption by sex, age-group, and level of education, 1998/99,* Ottawa, 1999, retrieved July 23, 2002 from www.statcan.ca/English/Pgdb/health05a.htm (also available at www.statcan.ca, choose Canadian statistics, and search for document name).

Statistics Canada: Taking risks and taking care, *Health Reports* 12(3):11-20, 2001a.

Statistics Canada: *Percentage of smokers in population 2000-2001,* Ottawa, 2001b, retrieved July 23, 2002 from www.statcan.ca/english/Pgdb/health07b.htm (also available at www.statcan.ca, choose Canadian statistics, and search for document name).

Statistics Canada: *How healthy are Canadians? a summary 2001 annual report,* pp 1-5, Ottawa, 2002a, Canadian Institute for Health Information.

Statistics Canada: Canadian community health survey: a first look, *The Daily* Ottawa, May 8, 2002b, retrieved from www.statcan.ca/Daily/English/020508/d020508a.htm (also available at www.statcan.ca, choose *The Daily,* and search for document name).

Statistics Canada: Pain or discomfort that affects activities, *Health Indicators* #1, 2002c, retrieved September 13, 2002, from www.statcan.ca/english/freepub/82-221-XIE/00502/tables/html/1274.htm (also available at www.statcan.ca, choose Canadian statistics, and search for document name).

Statistics Canada: Pap smears, *Health Indicators* #1, 2002d, retrieved from www.statcan.ca:80/english/freepub/82-221-XIE/00601/high/tables/htmltablesP3231.htm (also available at www.statcan.ca, choose Canadian statistics, and search for document name).

Tait H: Aboriginal women's health. In *Women in Canada 2000: a gender-based statistical report,* pp 247-259, Ottawa, 2000, Ministry of Industry.

*Canadian spelling is used.*

that women have appropriate instruction to make informed choices about reproduction. The choice of method depends on many factors including the woman's health, frequency of sexual activity, number of partners, and plans to have future children. No method provides a 100% guarantee against pregnancy or disease. The only 100% guarantee is not having intercourse, or abstinence (USDHHS, OWH, 2000).

The problem of unintended pregnancy exists among adolescents as well as adult women. Nurses must use caution and not assume that any woman is fully informed about contraception and that the method is used correctly and consistently. Because of the efforts of women's advocates such as Margaret Sanger, U.S. women have a wide array of contraceptives from which to choose today (Table 27-3).

Many women's health advocates have argued for expanding prenatal care to include **preconceptual counseling** (Earls, 1998; Kogan et al, 1998). Preconceptual counseling addresses risks before conception and includes education, assessment, diagnosis, and interventions. The purpose is to reduce or eliminate health risks for women and infants. For example, estimates are that 4000 pregnancies in the United States each year result in an infant born with spina bifida or anencephaly. Research has shown that intake of folic acid can significantly reduce the occurrence of these very serious and often fatal neural tube defects by 50% to 70%. Current estimates indicate that only 21% of women between the ages of 15 and 44 years consume at least 400 µg of folic acid per day from supplements or food sources—the amount recommended to prevent neural

---

### Table 27-3   Contraceptive Methods

**Barrier Methods**

| | |
|---|---|
| Male condom | Prevents direct contact with semen, infectious genital secretions, and genital lesions; except for abstinence, most effective method to reduce infection from HIV/AIDS; nonprescription; 86% estimated effectiveness |
| Female condom | Approved by FDA in 1993; nonprescription; 79% estimated effectiveness |
| Diaphragm | Dome-shaped rubber disk that covers the cervix; needs to be sized by a health professional; prescription; 80% estimated effectiveness |
| Cervical cap | Sized by a health professional; fits around the cervix; prescription; 60% to 80% estimated effectiveness |

**Vaginal Spermicides**

| | |
|---|---|
| Foam, cream, jelly, film, suppository, tablets | Contain sperm-killing chemicals; nonprescription; 74% estimated effectiveness |

**Hormonal Methods**

| | |
|---|---|
| Oral contraceptives | Most popular form of reversible birth control in the United States; prescription; 95% estimated effectiveness |
| Emergency contraceptives | Used when standard contraceptives have failed or no contraceptives used; prescription; 75% effective |
| Injectable progestins | Injection every 3 months; prescription; 99% estimated effectiveness |
| Implantable progestins | Surgically implanted under the skin of the upper arm; prescription; 99% estimated effectiveness |

**Intrauterine Device (IUD)**

| | |
|---|---|
| IUD | Mechanical device inserted into uterus by health professional; prescription; 98% to 99% estimated effectiveness |

**Traditional Methods**

| | |
|---|---|
| Fertility awareness | "Natural family planning" or periodic abstinence (i.e., not having sexual intercourse on days of the menstrual cycle when pregnancy is likely); instructions/knowledge and monitoring of body functions required; effectiveness estimates vary |

**Surgical Sterilization**

| | |
|---|---|
| Female sterilization | Blocks fallopian tubes; requires surgery; 99% estimated effectiveness |
| Male sterilization | Tying or cutting the male vas deferens; 99% estimated effectiveness |

From U.S. Department of Health and Human Services, Office on Women's Health, National Women's Health Information Center: *Birth control methods,* 2000, available at http://www.4woman.gov/faq/birthcont.htm; U.S. Food and Drug Administration: *Protecting against unintended pregnancy: a guide to contraceptive choices,* 2000, available at http://www.fda.gov/fdac/features/1997/babytabl.html.

tube defects. Healthy People 2010 objective 16-6 addresses increasing to 80% the proportion of pregnancies begun with an optimal folic acid level. However, research shows a continuing lack of awareness about the importance of taking folic acid supplements among women in low socioeconomic groups. The Centers for Disease Control and Prevention (CDC) has launched a national campaign to educate women of reproductive age about the importance of folic acid prior to conception. Nurses can promote increased awareness of folic acid intake among targeted women in their communities, and they can educate health care professionals who serve these women as well (Ahluwalia and Daniel, 2001; CDC, National Center on Birth Defects, 2002; USDHHS, OWH, 2000).

Another concern critical to preconception awareness is exposure to substances including alcohol. A major preventable cause of birth defects, mental retardation, and neurodevelopmental disorders is fetal exposure to alcohol during pregnancy. The American Academy of Pediatrics (AAP, 2000) noted that exposure to alcohol in utero is linked to a number of neurodevelopmental problems called alcohol-related neurodevelopmental disorder and alcohol-related birth defects. Children with these health problems can have lifelong disabilities. The recommendation of the AAP is abstinence from alcohol for women who plan to become pregnant or who are pregnant. Research shows that since 1995, the rates of alcohol use during pregnancy have decreased; however, binge drinking and frequent drinking have not declined and exceed the Healthy People 2010 targets (CDC, 2002). Nurses can participate in campaigns that print and broadcast advertisements informing women of childbearing age that drinking during pregnancy can cause birth defects.

In addition, it is critical for nurses to work toward eliminating factors associated with an increased incidence of substance use during pregnancy. For example, nursing research has shown that women who experience abuse during pregnancy have an increased incidence of substance use as well as psychosocial stress (Curry, 1998). To adequately address substance use during pregnancy, therefore, nursing interventions also need to address intimate partner violence.

Also related to women's reproductive health is access to prenatal care. Many argue that prenatal care is associated with improved birth outcomes. In the United States, estimates for the year 2000 indicated that, in general, 83.2% of women receive prenatal care in their first trimester. Four percent received late or no care. Only 69% of mothers of ages 15 to 19 received first trimester care and 7.2% of these teen mothers received late or no care (CDC, NCHS, 2002). For many women, barriers to prenatal care include lack of transportation, cumbersome bureaucratic systems, and health professionals who refuse to treat Medicaid patients (Roberts et al, 1998). Other barriers include crowded clinics and lack of childcare. Again, nurses can serve as advocates not only to encourage their clients to utilize prenatal care services but also to work toward the establishment of services that are accessible, affordable, and available to all pregnant women.

## Menopause

**Menopause,** also referred to as the *change* or *change of life*, is the time when the levels of the hormones estrogen and progesterone change in a woman's body. This change leads to the cessation of menstruation. The decline in these hormone levels has effects on a variety of functions. These effects can be seen in changes in the vaginal and urinary tract, the cardiovascular system, bone density, libido, sleep patterns, memory, and emotions (USDHHS, National Institute on Aging [NIA], 2001). A common complaint from women is the phenomenon known as hot flashes.

Women's attitudes toward menopause vary greatly and are influenced by culture, age, support, and the recounted experiences of other women. Menopause has been viewed on a continuum from a normal progression of aging to a disease state or time of imbalance or ill health.

Treatment for the unpleasant side effects of menopause has traditionally been with hormone replacement therapy (HRT). Recently, the NIH announced that they have stopped a major clinical trial examining the benefits of hormone replacement therapy for healthy menopausal women because of the increased risk for invasive breast cancer (NIH, 2002). The researchers also found increases in the rates of coronary heart disease, stroke, and pulmonary embolism in women taking HRT compared to those taking a placebo. The use of HRT remains controversial.

## Osteoporosis

It is estimated that one out of every two American women over the age of 50 will experience an osteoporosis-related fracture in her lifetime (USDHHS, NIA, 2001). Approximately 13.8 billion dollars per year is spent on the treatment of these conditions (USDHHS, NIA, 2001).

It is thought that the falling level of estrogen contributes to the loss of bone. Now, with the changes in beliefs about the risks involved in HRT, other measures designed to thwart the progression of osteoporosis will receive more attention. Primary prevention activities aimed at women need to include the importance of diets that are rich in calcium and vitamin D. Exposure to sunlight for 20 minutes a day is recommended as an alternative source of vitamin D. Exercise, especially weight-bearing activities such as walking, running, stair climbing, and weight lifting, improve bone density.

## Female Genital Mutilation

Common in many African countries and certain Asian and Middle Eastern countries, **female genital mutilation** (FGM) is a practice that is centuries old. Banned in the early 1990s in Somalia, FGM is now at an all-time high in that country because of that country's preoccupation with civil war. According to the WHO, there is approximately a 98% rate of genital cutting in Somalia today. Justification for FGM is related to tradition,

---

**BOX 27-3    Objectives of the Inter-African Committee (IAC)**

- Initiate establishment of National Committees and assist local organizations in developing appropriate policies and programs related to harmful traditional practices
- Work with governments, international organizations, and donors to develop and evaluate policies, laws, and programs that protect and promote the bodily integrity of women and young girls
- Develop local and international communication and advocacy activities for addressing harmful traditional practices
- Build national and international networks
- Develop national nongovernmental organization support, training, and capacity building

---

power inequities, and the compliance of women to community norms or law (Bosch, 2001). This practice is considered an important part of a woman's access to marriage and childbearing.

FGM can take several forms ranging from the excision of the clitoris with partial or total removal of the labia minora, to the severe form in which the labia majora are fused following the removal of the clitoris and labia minora (Bosch, 2001). These procedures are associated with morbidity related to substantial complications such as hemorrhage, infection, tetanus, and septicemia. Long-term effects of FGM include impaired urinary and menstrual functioning, chronic genital pain, cysts, neuromas, ulcers, urinary incontinence, and infertility (Ford, 2001). Increasingly, women who have been mutilated are immigrating to the United States. Thus nurses need to be familiar with the practices of immigrants in their communities and with state statutes related to FGM.

In 1998, the WHO estimated that almost 137 million women of all ages had undergone some form of FGM. Estimates are that every year 2 million girls are at risk for this devastating procedure (Bosch, 2001). Since the early 1980s, the WHO has proposed laws that would prohibit FGM in all countries. In May 2000, in Guinea Conakry, after the government had approved a law banning FGM, the excisors abandoned their work tools during a symbolic, public ceremony. In July 2001, the European Parliament Women's Rights Committee condemned FGM as a serious violation of human rights and as an act of violence against women (Bosch, 2001). Headquartered in Ethiopia, the Inter-African Committee (IAC) is the first nongovernmental organization to address the problems of harmful traditional practices such as FGM (Women's International Network, 2002). The objectives of this organization are described in Box 27-3.

## Cardiovascular Disease

Cardiovascular disease (CVD) ranks first among all disease categories for women who are discharged from the acute care setting. According to the American Heart Association (2002), CVD is responsible for 43.3% of deaths among women in America as well as in most developed countries. It is estimated that over 240,000 women die of heart attacks each year. African-American women have a higher incidence of CVD than white women. Taylor, Hughes, and Garrison (2002) suggest that the most notable feature of the CVD epidemic in the United States is the difference in morbidity and mortality rates that exists between white women and women of color. Rural African-American women have higher mortality rates with wide ranges per county from 124 to 1275 per 100,000 in areas with a low population density, for example, the Mississippi Delta region (Taylor et al, 2002).

Many factors predispose women to CVD. Physical factors that are thought to contribute to the development of CVD include smoking, high blood cholesterol levels, diabetes mellitus, obesity, hypertension, diets high in fat and low in fiber, and physical inactivity (Gerhard-Herman, 2002; Oliver-McNeil and Artinian, 2002). The relationship between hormone replacement therapy and CVD is under much debate. It had been thought that HRT had a positive effect on the incidence of CVD. However, in a recent clinical trial, enough CVD events occurred that researchers stopped the study on the basis of the deteriorating risk-to-benefit ratio (Writing Group for the Women's Health Initiative Investigators, 2002).

Sociocultural factors have a significant influence on women and CVD. It is known that a lower socioeconomic class correlates with low levels of knowledge and understanding about health, limited health maintenance and preventive care, and decreased access to care.

The key to addressing this alarming epidemic is education aimed at risk factor modification. Nurses need to be aware of the fact that heart disease is not a health problem just for men. Needed information about the various factors that influence the development of CVD can be accomplished through prevention and outreach activities (Box 27-4).

Intervention efforts should reflect the diversity of age, environment, and ethnicity. Identifying those at risk through a careful family history assessment can alert the nurse to situations that might place an individual at a higher level of risk. The U.S. Preventive Services Task Force Guide to Clinical Preventive Services (2001) suggests that screening women older than age 45 years for lipid disorders would identify nearly all those women who are at high risk for CVD.

## Diabetes Mellitus

In the Third National Health and Nutrition Examination Survey (NHANES III), it was noted that as a group, today's women are more obese and less physically active, which increases their risk for diabetes. These risk factors are more prevalent in women than in men. In 1995, there were more women than men in the world with diabetes (73 versus 62 million). Developed countries have more

BOX 27-4 Levels of Prevention as Related to Cardiovascular Disease in Women

**PRIMARY PREVENTION**

Collaborating with a variety of organizations such as the American Heart Association to design and implement interventions aimed at reducing women's risk for cardiovascular disease.

**SECONDARY PREVENTION**

Screening activities such as blood cholesterol and blood pressure monitoring are examples of secondary prevention.

**TERTIARY PREVENTION**

Developing a community-based exercise program for a group of women who have cardiovascular disease.

women with diabetes than developing countries (King, Aubert, and Herman, 1998).

In the United States, diabetes is a potentially debilitating disease. Women account for approximately 52% of all people over the age of 20 with diabetes (Beckles and Thompson-Reid, 2002). Black (2002) suggests that diabetes is an epidemic in the United States. She states that diabetes in women is more difficult to control and often results in more devastating outcomes. It is thought that certain sociocultural roles that women hold, such as "keeper of the culture," for example, the planning and preparing of traditional family meals may directly affect a woman's vulnerability to diabetes.

The socioeconomic status of women with diabetes is lower than that of women without diabetes. Given the opportunity, women with higher education may make decisions differently, have greater access to health care and have a higher standard of living, all which greatly impact health and health outcomes (Beckles and Thompson-Reid, 2001).

When compared to their non-Hispanic, white counterparts, minority women have consistently higher rates of diabetes (Beckles and Thompson-Reid, 2001). Studies demonstrate that minorities have a higher incidence of microvascular complications associated with diabetes, including renal failure and lower extremity amputations. Unequal access to health care might explain these differences in the complication rates. However, a recent study examined the disparities in diabetic complications among ethnic groups that had similar insurance coverage, and the ethnic disparities persisted (Karter et al, 2002). The authors felt that their results suggested a genetic origin or the contribution of unmeasured environmental factors.

Many complications are associated with diabetes: heart disease, stroke, hypertension, retinopathy, kidney disease, neuropathies, amputations, dental disease, and gestational diabetes. Given that gestational diabetes is a complication specific to women, it will be discussed in more detail.

**Gestational diabetes mellitus** (GDM) is a condition characterized by carbohydrate intolerance that is first identified or develops during pregnancy. Approximately 2% to 5% of all pregnancies in the United States are complicated with gestational diabetes (Beckles and Thompson-Reid, 2001). This complication is of concern as it affects the health of both the pregnant women and her unborn child. These women have a 25% to 45% greater risk for recurrence of diabetes in subsequent pregnancies as well as the development of diabetes later in life.

"Women are more likely to develop gestational diabetes if they are older, have a higher pre-pregnancy weight, high body mass index, or weight gain in young adulthood, have a high parity or history of a previous adverse pregnancy, or have preexisting hypertension, or a family history of diabetes" (Rowley et al, 2001, p. 73).

During their pregnancy, these women are also at greater risk for complications such as preeclampsia, caesarean section, and infection. Typically, the prevalence of GDM is determined on the basis of data from the universal screening of pregnant women.

Nurses are in a position to have a positive effect on the lives of women with diabetes. Reducing the morbidity and mortality of diabetes and enhancing the quality of life for these individuals is a key area of focus for public health. Two approaches that can be taken are (1) health care system interventions for optimizing care for persons with diabetes, and (2) diabetes self-management education interventions that are community based (CDC, 2001).

Assessing for a history of GDM in women, especially women of color, is important. Focusing on family history as well as on the personal health history provides an opportunity for the community nurse to identify those at high risk.

Primary prevention activities include interventions aimed at educating women about diabetes, nutrition and the risks of obesity, smoking, and physical inactivity. Community interventions that address healthy eating, exercise, and weight reduction benefit women who are at risk for diabetes. Screening for diabetes is an example of secondary prevention. Screening activities include a fingerstick blood glucose test or a full glucose tolerance test. Screening is also accomplished through a thorough history and physical examination. Nurses need to be well versed in understanding the health disparities among women in order to target those at greater risk. Tertiary prevention includes activities that are aimed to reduce the complications of the disease process. Examples of tertiary prevention for women with diabetes include intense monitoring of blood glucose levels, modification of diet and or medications as indicated, and efforts to prevent long-term complications such as those mentioned previously.

## Mental Health

Although both men and women suffer from mental illness, women experience certain conditions more often than men. In the United States, for example, depression and anxiety disorders are twice as likely to affect women as men, and women experience eating disorders nine times as often as men (National Institute of Mental Health, 2002). Depression is a particularly serious problem for women. The WHO concluded that depression is the leading cause of disease burden for women in both developing and developed regions of the world (Murray and Lopez, 1996).

A number of factors contribute to depression in women. Researchers are exploring how biological factors, including genetics and gonadal (sex) hormones, affect women's increased risk for depression. Other scientists are focusing on how psychosocial factors such as life stress, trauma, and interpersonal relationships contribute to women's depression (Mazure, Keita, and Blehar, 2002).

Nursing scholars have also documented the conditions under which women experience depression. For example, long-term consequences of intimate partner violence often involve depression and posttraumatic stress disorder (Campbell, 2002). Campbell argues that the global incidence of depression could be due to the experiences of women as a result of domestic violence, but this premise remains to be tested. Other researchers have found traumatic life events and sexual orientation may be poorly understood risk factors for depression (Matthews et al, 2002). Some scholars suggest that health professionals must use caution not to "medicalize" all the unhappiness in the lives of women; instead, they should explore the restrictive roles that women play in society that may lead to depression (Wright and Owen, 2001).

Noting women's increased risk for depression, the U.S. Preventive Services Task Force (2002) recommends screening for depression in adults when there are adequate systems in place to make an accurate diagnosis as well as to provide effective treatment and follow-up. Two screening questions are recommended: (1) "Over the past two weeks have you felt down, depressed, or hopeless?" (2) "Over the past two weeks have you felt little interest or pleasure in doing things?" Risk factors for depression include being female, family history of depression, unemployment, and chronic disease. Nurses can encourage health professionals in their communities to screen and treat depression among women and to work for other services that decrease stress and generally improve the mental well-being of women (Box 27-5).

## Cancer

Cancers are noted to be the second leading cause of death among all women. Cancer of the lung is the leading cause of cancer deaths, followed by cancer of the breast and colorectal cancers (CDC, NCHS, 2001). Researchers speculate that cancer rates among women have increased because of the larger number of women between 50 and 74 years old. Across all ages, however, death rates from cancers in women have decreased (Edwards et al, 2002). Overall, white women have a higher incidence of all cancers, whereas African-American women have a higher mortality rate for all cancers (Edwards et al, 2002). Although it is known that women suffer from other cancers, especially

---

**BOX 27-5  Example of Community-Based Intervention**

The Women to Women Project, established in Montana through a partnership between the College of Nursing at Montana State University and the Burns Telecommunications Center was designed to offer support to rural women using a community-based approach. The project offered a mechanism for providing support with telecommunications and computer technology. The overall goals of the project are to offer this support in a social context to rural women with chronic illness, and to compare their results with those of women who do not use technology as a support tool.

A variety of psychosocial outcome measures were applied to both groups of women to examine differences between the groups. Although data collection and analysis is still underway, powerful implications for nursing practice have been identified.

This project could serve as a basis for developing an expanded model of social support to other aggregates and underserved populations. This project was designed to meet the needs of those who are geographically isolated, but it could easily address the needs of those who are socially isolated for various causes. It also has implications for community-oriented nurses as they move to a new era of providing preventive health care services to populations in disembodied environments of care.

Modified from Weinert D: Social support in cyberspace for women with chronic illness, *Rehab Nurs* 25:4, 2000.

---

ones that are unique to women such as cervical and ovarian cancer, the discussion that follows addresses the top three cancers that lead to illness and death in women.

A diagnosis of cancer is a life-changing event and is considered a life transition. A woman is confronted with many decisions that often leave her feeling overwhelmed and out of control. A cancer diagnosis changes how a woman feels about her body and how she relates to and interacts with others (Spira and Kenemore, 2001).

Ethnicity plays a role in both the occurrence and death rates attributed to cancers among women. As noted, white women have the highest occurrence rates for all cancers but African-American women have the highest death rates for all cancers (Edwards et al, 2002). This is attributed to the barriers that women of color have in accessing health care and preventive services, which reinforces the health-related disparities found among women in the United States.

Lung cancer is linked to cigarette smoking. From a global perspective, by the year 2020 it is thought that tobacco will kill more people than any other disease including HIV (Murray and Lopez, 1996). According to the CDC, NCHS (2001), more young white women aged 18 to 34 smoke than their African-American counterparts. However, after the age

**Table 27-4  Incidence of HIV/AIDS in U.S. Adult Women and Female Adolescents**

| RACE/ETHNICITY | CASES PER 100,000 | RATE (%) |
| --- | --- | --- |
| White, not Hispanic | 1895 | 2 |
| African-American, not Hispanic | 6545 | 46 |
| Hispanic | 1855 | 14 |
| Asian/Pacific Islander | 77 | 2 |
| Native American/Native Alaskan | 68 | 8 |
| **Total** | 10,459 | 9 |

From Centers for Disease Control and Prevention, National Center for HIV, STD, and TB Prevention: *HIV/AIDS surveillance in women,* L264 slide series through 2000, 2002b, available at http://www.cdc.gov/hiv/graphics/images/l264/l264-1.htm.

of 35, more African-American women smoke. Smoking is considered a preventable health risk. Primary prevention aimed at young girls and highlighting the effects of smoking would be one avenue for nurses to employ in the battle against smoking.

The incidence of breast cancer is higher in white women than in African-American women, but the death rate for African-American women with breast cancer is higher than that for white women. Breast cancer is the second leading cause of cancer deaths among all women. Screening activities (the secondary level of prevention), such as mammography, clinical breast examination, and self-breast examination, make a difference in the mortality rates among these women. Early detection often means cure, whereas late detection typically ensures a limited prognosis. The differences in the outcomes between women of color and white women point to issues associated with early detection, access to health care and follow-up by a regular care provider (Schulz et al, 2002).

The third leading cause of cancer death in women is colorectal cancer. This cancer is typically found in women over the age of 75, and the 5-year relative survival rate is about 60%. Among all people who have had colorectal cancer in the past decade, African-American women have had the highest occurrence and death rates (Edwards et al, 2002). Primary prevention and early detection are the key to the survivability of women with colorectal cancer. Nurses can provide interventions that inform women of their risks, the signs and symptoms to be aware of, and screening opportunities in their communities.

## HIV/AIDS

As the HIV/AIDS epidemic has continued to plague the United States, the populations affected by the epidemic have shifted. Women accounted for only 14% of the HIV/AIDS cases reported in 1992, but by the first half of 2000, that percentage had grown to 26%. Looking back to 1985, the proportion of all cases among adult and adolescent women has more than tripled (7% in 1985; 25% in 1999) (CDC, National Center for HIV, STD, and TB Prevention, 2002a, b).

Once again, research shows disparities in the ethnic/racial distribution of HIV/AIDS in U.S. women. In 1999, among women between the ages of 25 and 44, HIV/AIDS was the fifth leading cause of death, and it was the third leading cause of death for African-American women in the same age-group. In 2000, the number of reported cases in Hispanic women was about equal to the number in white women, but the number of cases was seven times higher in Hispanic women (Table 27-4) (CDC, National Center for HIV, STD, and TB Prevention, 2002a, b).

The most common way that HIV/AIDS is transmitted to U.S. women is through heterosexual contact, which accounted for 64% of cases in 2000. One third of the cases were attributed to injection drug use. However, regional differences do exist. For example, in 2000, in the northeastern United States, women reported injection drug use as the source of their exposure more often than heterosexual contact. The cases in the Midwest and West were nearly equally distributed between these two sources of exposure, whereas in the South, women typically reported heterosexual contact (CDC, National Center for HIV, STD, and TB Prevention, 2002b).

Those women who acquired HIV/AIDS from heterosexual transmission had often had sex with an injection drug user. Women who have used injection drugs themselves are certainly at risk for infection. Women who use noninjection drugs, such as methamphetamines and crack cocaine, and those who trade sex for money and/or drugs, are also at high risk (CDC, National Center for HIV, STD, and TB Prevention, 2002a).

In 2000, over 45,000 women of childbearing age (15 to 44 years) in the United States had AIDS. Additionally, estimates from the 34 areas with name-based confidential surveillance indicated that 29,682 women in this same age-group had HIV infection. These latter numbers probably underestimate the actual number of HIV-infected women because the data include only those whose positive HIV test was reported to a health department. Many infected women may not have been tested, and many women reside in states that do not have HIV case surveillance in place (CDC, National Center for HIV, STD, and TB

Prevention, 2002b). These women represent a particularly important population, and nurses are in a strategic position to develop programs to prevent perinatal HIV transmission to their children. The latter route of transmission accounts for virtually all new HIV infections in children.

Women with HIV/AIDS require specific health and social services to reduce the burden of their disease. They require services that integrate both prevention and treatment of HIV/AIDS as well as any comorbidities such as other sexually transmitted diseases and substance use (CDC, National Center for HIV, STD, and TB Prevention, 2002a). In addition, nurses can serve as advocates by focusing not only on the high risk behaviors of individual women but also on the factors in their communities that lead to injection drug use and sexual exposure to the HIV virus. Interventions to improve education, employment opportunities, and adequate housing as well as to decrease drug use, isolation, and poverty can have a critical impact on this epidemic.

## Women and Weight Control

American women spend a great deal of time, energy, and money in the never-ending pursuit of the body beautiful. In 1998, the NIH began utilizing the calculated body mass index (BMI) to define overweight and **obesity** in individuals. BMI is the relationship of body weight and height. It is calculated using the following formula: BMI equals body weight (in pounds) divided by height (in inches squared), multiplied by 703 (or, in metric units, $kg/m^2$) (USDHHS, 2001).

BMI is now the medical standard for the determination of obesity and overweight. A BMI of 30 or greater represents obesity (USDHHS, National Institute of Diabetes and Digestive and Kidney Diseases, 2001). Overweight and obesity have been grouped as leading health indicators in Healthy People 2010.

The number of overweight women in the United States is on the rise. Those with a lower socioeconomic status are 50% more likely to be obese than those with a higher socioeconomic status (USDHHS, 2001). In general the prevalence of overweight and obesity is greater among women of color. As an example, the proportion of Hispanic women who are overweight or obese is 70%, compared to non-Hispanic African-American women who average 69%, and white non-Hispanic women who average 47% (USDHHS, 2001).

Obesity is a major health concern among women as it is linked to the development of diabetes, hypertension, cardiovascular disease, and other medical problems. The nurse can provide education about the risks to health of weight and obesity. The educational offerings can be fashioned after a community health model utilizing the levels of prevention to establish effective interventions for women at risk for weight control issues.

Because obesity in women is such a stigma in Western culture, women are at high risk for suffering adverse social and psychological consequences of obesity. Even as children, women begin to fear obesity. These consequences can include social as well as financial discrimination. More women enter weight loss programs for their perceived loss of attractiveness than for health concerns. Recently, Southwest Airlines has adopted a policy requiring overweight individuals who take up too much room on the airplane, to purchase an additional seat.

In today's American culture, being thin is often identified with competence, success, control, power, and sexual attractiveness. The culture's focus and preoccupation with the thinness and shape of women can be seen in the media and entertainment, where beautiful is equated with very thin women. These idealistic and often unrealistic images perpetuate women's dissatisfaction and preoccupation with their bodies. According to Devlin (2001), as many as 66% of women are dissatisfied with their body weight. Research has consistently documented that more women than men are dissatisfied with their bodies. Often women of normal weight and those who are considered to be underweight view their bodies as too large. People frequently associate obesity with laziness and a lack of will power. Obesity in women is a stigma in the U.S. culture.

In the past two decades, reports of eating disorders have increased. Many women are unhappy with their current shape and weight but in actuality only a few of them go on to develop a serious eating disorder. The most common eating disorders seen in women are anorexia nervosa and bulimia. **Anorexia** is defined as a fear of gaining weight coupled with disturbances in perceptions of the body. Excessive weight loss is the most noticeable clue. Individuals with anorexia rarely complain of weight loss because they view themselves as normal or overweight. Many of these women struggle with psychological problems, including depression, obsessive symptoms, and social phobias.

**Bulimia** is characterized by a persistent concern with the shape of the body along with body weight, recurrent episodes of binge eating, a loss of control during these binges, and use of extreme methods to prevent weight gain, such as purging, strict dieting, fasting, use of laxatives or diuretics, or vigorous exercise (NIMH, 2001).

### DID YOU KNOW?

In a recent study examining women and weight, magazine covers told an interesting story. Of magazines most often read by women, 78% contained some message about female body appearance on the cover, whereas none of the 53 magazines read often by men displayed messages on the cover about male body images.

Bulimia is observed across all weight categories, but most women who have bulimia are within a normal weight range. Although bulimia is considered less dangerous medically than anorexia, electrolyte imbalance and dehydration can create serious physical complications such as cardiac dysrhythmias.

Nurses are in a key position to include assessment for eating disorders and referral for treatment into their routine clinical practices. The goal of the nurse is to identify not only women with eating disorders, but also those women at risk for developing eating problems. Through a comprehensive physical and psychosocial assessment, as well as a history of dietary practices, the nurse may be able to identify women with eating disorders and provide appropriate referrals. Nurses should promote healthy eating habits and regular physical activity as a weight control strategy. At a population level, nurses can discourage advertising that promotes exceptionally thin bodies for women. They can also promote exercise and healthy eating programs in their communities.

## HEALTH DISPARITIES AMONG SPECIAL GROUPS OF WOMEN

### Women of Color

Women of color represent approximately 29% of all women in the United States (U.S. Bureau of the Census, Population Estimates Program, 2001). These women come from the five major ethnic/racial groups depicted in Figure 27-1. Considerable debate exists over whether *race* or *ethnicity* is the more appropriate term when talking about these groups. Some argue that ethnicity is more appropriate, while others argue that when race is not used, the health effect of racism is minimized.

Moreover, using the major groups of women as shown in Figure 27-2 does not capture many of the subgroups of women in U.S. society. For example, subgroups include recent immigrants, who may not view themselves among these racial/ethnic groups and can even be undercounted in the census (Stover, 2002). Rural women are another unique subgroup not captured by the five major groups; estimates are that 20% of U.S. women live in rural areas and 16% of rural dwellers are in nonwhite groups. Rural women of color have special health-related situations including geographic and informational isolation, few services, limited transportation, and poverty (Hargraves, 2002).

Women of color experience many of the same health problems as their white counterparts. However, as a group they have poorer health, access fewer health care services,

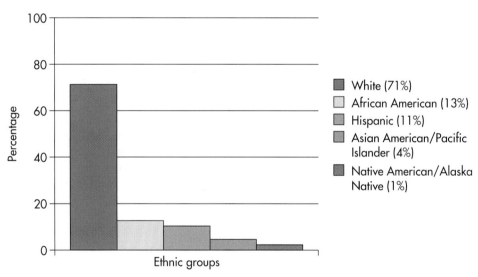

**Figure 27-1** Distribution of U.S. women in racial/ethnics groups.

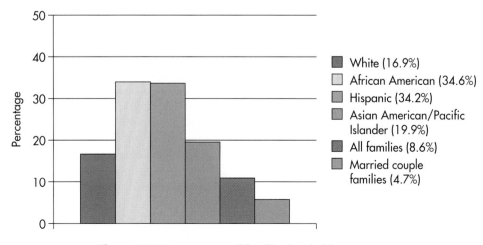

**Figure 27-2** Poverty rate of families headed by women.

suffer disproportionately from earlier deaths, receive fewer preventive health services, and are underinsured (Cornelius, Smith, and Simpson, 2002; Satcher, 2001). The process of addressing these disparities is daunting. The intent is to close the gap in health disparities while preserving the richness and unique influences of various cultures. Evidence suggests that ensuring access to a regular health care provider is the key to meeting the preventive health care needs of women of color (Cornelius et al, 2002). Many providers do not incorporate preventive screenings into their practice; therefore, nurses can target interventions designed to address preventive health issues. In particular, culturally sensitive and gender-sensitive programs are needed for communities with women of color.

### NURSING TIP

Because of the known health disparities experienced by women of color, preventive services targeted at women should address diversity and cultural awareness throughout the entire program planning process.

## Incarcerated Women

Incarcerated women represent an increasing issue for nurses in the United States. Although the rate of incarceration for men exceeds that of women, the rate doubled for women between the years 1986 and 1997 (U.S. Department of Justice, 1999).

The Bureau of Justice reports that for every 100,000 women in the United States, there were 110 female inmates. Although female incarceration rates are lower than male rates at all ages, both rates reveal considerable racial and ethnic disparities. African-American/non-Hispanic women had a prison and jail rate of 380/100,000, which is three times higher than that of Hispanic women (117/100,000) and six times than that of white women (63/100,000). Moreover, all age-groups of African-American non-Hispanic, and Hispanic women reflected these disparities (U.S. Department of Justice, 1999) (Box 27-6).

## Lesbians

Lesbians have been considered a hidden but special population in many ways, partly because of the social stigma associated with lesbianism coupled with the fear of discrimination. The social environments that lesbians share may influence their behaviors and produce patterns of both negative and positive health habits that influence their health status (Aaron et al, 2001, p. 974).

Several social factors have been identified as potential contributors to the risk factors that lesbian and bisexual women are faced with, such as "depending on bars as a social gathering place, non-traditional female roles, a wider acceptance of diverse body shapes and sizes, and discrimination" (Aaron et al, 2001, p. 974).

Current studies on lesbians have typically included women who consider themselves either gay or bisexual.

---

### BOX 27-6 Population-Level Intervention

Welcome Home Ministries is an innovative program developed in southern California by a nurse/minister to ease the transition for women from jail (population) to life on the "outside." In the program, a registered nurse and formerly incarcerated women help others recently released make this adjustment. The program is based on research in which women reported histories of poverty, physical and emotional abuse, addiction (usually to crystal methamphetamine), and repeated incarceration. Many also report grief over their lives and especially over their children. The program includes a protocol for jail visitations to women prisoners by formerly incarcerated women and transportation of newly released women to new homes on release. All women are encouraged to participate in gatherings where they support and encourage one another. Struggles of transition and successes are shared and goals are set to help women remain healthy and drug free.

Modified from Parsons ML, Warner-Robbins C: Holistic nursing on the front lines, *Am J Nurs* 102(6):73-77, 2002.

---

Findings indicate that lesbians and bisexual women in the United States are found to have a higher prevalence of several risk factors than their heterosexual counterparts with regard to smoking, alcohol use, and lack of preventative cancer screening (Rosenberg, 2001). Compounding these problems is research evidence suggesting that many health care providers still feel that lesbians are sick, abnormal, immoral, perverse, and dangerous, and lesbian clients report feelings of rejection and alienation in the health care system (Stevens, 1994). In the negative stories that these women tell, *facelessness, feelings of intrusion,* and *abandonment* are just a few of the words describing their experiences with health care (Stevens, 1994).

To improve the health of lesbian women, services that address their unique needs are warranted. Safe places where these women are able to voice their concerns and receive effective health promotion, disease prevention, and treatment are critical. Nurses can work as advocates to reduce stereotypes and discrimination toward lesbian women.

## Women With Disabilities

According to the Office on Women's Health (OWH), there are 26 million American women who live with some type of disability (USDHHS, 2002). The varying conditions that comprise disability make women's roles more challenging. Many disabling conditions and diseases disproportionately affect women, as reflected in the U.S. Census Bureau's findings that 20.7% of women of all ages are disabled as compared to 18.6% of men of all ages (1997).

Many issues surround women with disabilities. Concerns associated with health, aging, civil rights, abuse, and independent living are examples of the types of problems facing them. The Center for Research on Women With Disabilities (CROWD), based at Baylor College of Medicine, actively addresses these concerns. In a study examining the issues that disabled women face, CROWD (1999) identified themes that were categorized into six domains: sense of self, relationship issues, information about sexuality, sexual functioning, abuse, and general and reproductive health.

Sense of self, or how women see themselves, includes self-concept, self-esteem, locus of control, sexual identity, and body image (Nosek and Hughes, 2001). After a disabling accident that resulted in paraplegia, one woman shared that she felt like a child again, and was, in fact treated like one, losing all identity of herself as a women (Schriempf, 2001). This persistent stereotyping and treatment of disabled women as asexual and dependent is a major barrier to addressing their needs.

A women's sexual identity is usually something that is taken for granted. Societal attitudes equate women as sexual beings by their overall appearance and desirability to men. Women with disabilities identify those attitudes as barriers in achieving their sexual potential (USDHHS, OWH, 2003). Physical problems impose many barriers to sexual activity in women with disabilities, and this is compounded by the reluctance of health care providers to address the topic. Older women with disabilities may have had inadequate information about sexual issues, and they may be too embarrassed to ask questions related to their specific concerns.

Although all women are subjected to violence and abuse, women with disabilities are thought to endure abuse for longer periods of time than their nondisabled counterparts and are also more likely to suffer abuse at the hands of caregivers and personal assistants (Curry, Hassouneh-Phillips, and Johnston-Silverberg, 2001). It is thought that between 51% and 79% of disabled women experience sexual abuse (CDC, 1999). Determining the actual prevalence of abuse among disabled women is difficult, as public records such as police reports do not indicate if the victim is disabled.

Nurses can develop an awareness of the many health-related issues facing disabled women in society. Care should be taken to recognize the physical barriers that prevent women from accessing health care, such as structures that are not accessible despite the Americans With Disabilities Act (ADA) recommendations. Some women are physically unable to position themselves on examination tables, posing a challenge in providing routine gynecologic exams.

Nurses are positioned to act in a variety of roles such as an advocate, educator, and case manager. Having knowledge about appropriate community resources is the key in identifying services geared toward meeting these women's needs. Developing health promotion programs targeted at this vulnerable, high-risk group will assist in promoting health and well-being among this growing population.

## Impoverished Women

Unfortunately, many U.S. women do not have the resources to achieve a basic level of health. Although poverty rates dropped in 2000, many in the United States, particularly women, remain poor, with women's earnings at only 76% of men's (U.S. Department of Labor, 2001). Poverty is a special problem for *head-of-household* women. Female-householder families have grown from 10% in 1959 to 17% in 2000. Of U.S. female-householder families with no husband present, 24.7% were poor in contrast to 4.7% of married couples. Poverty among head-of-household women also reflects the disparities that exist in the United States between various ethnic/racial groups, as female-headed African-American and Hispanic families suffer disproportionately higher rates of poverty than other families (see Figure 27-2). African-American female-householder families have a poverty rate of 34.6%. Hispanic female-householder families have a rate of 34.2% (U.S. Census Bureau, Current Population Reports, 2001; U.S. Census Bureau, 2002).

Some U.S. politicians have proposed that unless women marry, they will remain poor (Dionne, 2002). However, Williams (2002) counters this argument by noting that in other developed countries with substantial public services, such as Sweden, female head-of-household families do not experience the same rates of poverty as they do in the United States. Many factors make it difficult for these women to rise out of poverty. In an account of her effort to work at minimum wage jobs and try to get by, Ehrenreich (2002) concludes that because of low wages and high rents, a single woman in good health, who has a car, can barely support herself in a minimum-wage job in the United States.

Ehrenreich argues that in addition to increasing the incomes of U.S. workers, public services that include adequate health insurance, childcare, housing, and efficient public transportation are needed. To support the interests of low-income women, nurses can effect change in these services by participating in debates with health policy-makers at local, state, and national levels (Salsberry et al, 1999).

Women who subsist below the poverty line are at great risk for becoming homeless. According to the U.S. Conference of Mayors (2001), single women made up 14% of the homeless population in 2001. In addition, women frequently head the families that comprise 40% of the homeless population (U.S. Conference of Mayors, 2001). Homeless women experience health problems at rates greater than women in the general population. For example, Bassuk et al (1996) found in a study of homeless mothers that they had a higher lifetime prevalence of major depressive disorder, posttraumatic stress disorder, and substance use disorders. They had lower physical functioning and a higher prevalence of chronic health conditions. These women generally have few economic resources, social supports, and higher rates of violent abuse throughout their life spans.

Other researchers have shown that low-income women, and in particular, low-income mothers, rate their health below the norms for the general population and report a

## Evidence-Based Practice

The purpose of this quantitative study was "to examine the impact that various levels of support from substance users and non-users have on homeless women's psychosocial profiles, health and health behaviors, and use of health services" (Nyamathi, 2000, p. 318). This study examined 1302 homeless women's support systems and their resulting outcomes of support. A homeless woman was defined as one who had stayed the previous night in a shelter, hotel, motel, or home of a relative or friend. Also, women who did not know where they would be living in the next 60 days were included.

Researchers made appointments with the study participants and conducted a structured, face-to-face interview composed of a collection of questionnaires or instruments. Demographic data including age, ethnicity, education, marital status, number of children, adult history of victimization, duration of homelessness, and number of times homeless were gathered. Additionally, the researchers measured the women's social support, substance use, sexual risk behavior, self-esteem, coping profile, life satisfaction, psychological symptoms, health status, and use of health services. More than half reported that they had no support person, which reflected their social isolation and the health risks that are common in this population.

**Nurse Use:** Women with primary support from non-drug-using persons had greater strengths (higher levels of self-esteem, life satisfaction, and active, problem-focused coping), less anxiety and depression, and a greater likelihood of having participated in a drug treatment program at some time. In contrast, women who reported primary support from individuals still using substances appeared to be as vulnerable as those women who reported having no support. Clearly, more support did not translate into better outcomes for the women if the support came from substance users.

Nyamathi A et al: Type of social support among homeless women: its impact on psychosocial resources, health and health behaviors, and use of health services, *Nurs Res* 49(6):318-326, 2000.

significant level of depression. Moreover, the health scores reported by low-income mothers reflect an inability to work as required by the welfare reform initiatives (Salsberry et al, 1999). Research also demonstrates that impoverished women are at increased risk for domestic violence, and that many women who receive welfare report having experienced domestic violence. Consequently, these women are more likely than other women to suffer from both physical and mental health problems. Thus economic independence is an essential factor for all women's safety and future (Lyon, 2002).

## Older Women

Women make up the largest proportion of the older population in the United States. In 2000, 58% of those aged 65 and older were women, and 70% of those 85 and older. In 2030, the overall size of the older population is expected to double, and one out of five people will be 65 or older. In 2000, those 85 and older made up approximately 2% of the total population—this fastest-growing subgroup of the population will comprise 5% of the population in 2050 (Table 27-5) (Federal Interagency Forum on Aging Related Statistics, 2000; U.S. Bureau of the Census, 2000).

Research shows that older women, especially women of color and from lower socioeconomic groups, experience higher rates of chronic illness and disability than their white and more affluent counterparts. Women with lower-level educations, with lower incomes, and who are enrolled in Medicare programs are more likely to report fair or poor health than women from higher socioeconomic groups. Low-income and less-educated women report not only more chronic illness but more symptoms, including severe pain from arthritis, than their white and more affluent counterparts (Bierman and Clancy, 2001).

To improve the health of older women, community health nursing programs need to address these racial/ethnic and socioeconomic disparities. The improvement of preventive services and the management of chronic conditions are imperative. However, it will also be necessary to consider older women's socioeconomic status, educational levels, and racial/ethnic backgrounds to adequately address their health needs.

## COMPLEMENTARY AND ALTERNATIVE THERAPIES

In July, 2002 the National Heart, Lung, and Blood Pressure Institute (NHLBI) called a halt to a clinical study of combined hormone replacement therapy (HRT) for the management of menopausal symptoms because of the increased risk of breast cancer, blood clots, CVD, and stroke associated with HRT. The fear of these side effects has led many women to seek alternative approaches for the management of their menopausal symptoms.

Women experiencing menopause frequently report symptoms including hot flashes, vaginal dryness, and irregular menses. Alternative therapies are those actions that are taken by women instead of HRT. Complementary therapies are those that are taken to augment (or as a complement to) HRT. The listing of alternative/complementary therapies for menopausal symptoms can be an endless task, but Box 27-7 provides common examples. However, the American College of Obstetricians and Gynecologists (ACOG) (2001) notes that there is little research evidence to support the efficacy of these therapies. Based only on

## Table 27-5 Age Projections for U.S. Women

| YEAR | MEAN AGE | 65 AND OVER (× 1000) | 85 AND OVER (× 1000) |
|---|---|---|---|
| 2000 | 37.7 | 20,362 | 3018 |
| 2010 | 39.1 | 22,749 | 3882 |
| 2020 | 40.3 | 30,185 | 4437 |
| 2030 | 41.4 | 39,166 | 5716 |
| 2040 | 41.9 | 43,167 | 8945 |
| 2050 | 42.0 | 45,710 | 11,921 |

From U.S. Bureau of the Census, Population Projections Program, Population Division: *Projections of the total resident population by 5-year age groups, and sex with special age categories,* 2000, available at http://www.census.gov/population/projections/nation/summary/np-t3-a.txt.

## BOX 27-7 Examples of Alternative/Complementary Therapies for Menopausal Symptoms

- Herbal remedies (ingested as tinctures or teas)
- Acupuncture
- Acupressure
- Massage therapy
- Healing touch
- Aromatherapy
- Guided imagery
- Chiropractic healing

## BOX 27-8 Prevention Checklist for Women 25 and Older

- Dental health
- Regular dental examinations
- Floss, brush with fluoride toothpaste daily
- Health screening
- Blood pressure
- Height and weight
- Lipid disorders (women 45 and older)
- Papanicolaou (Pap) test (all women sexually active with a cervix)
- Colorectal cancer (women age 50 and older)
- Mammogram (women age 40 and older)
- Problem drinking
- Rubella serology or vaccination (women of child-bearing age)
- Chlamydia (sexually active women age 25 and younger; women over 25 with new or multiple sex partners)
- Chemoprophylaxis
- Multivitamin/folic acid (women planning or capable of pregnancy)
- Immunizations
  - Tetanus-diphtheria (Td) boosters
  - Rubella (women of childbearing age)
  - Pneumococcal vaccine (65 and older)
  - Influenza (annually for women 65 and older or at risk)

U.S. Preventive Services Task Force, Agency for Healthcare Research and Quality: *Guide to preventive services,* ed 3, 2000, available at http://www.ahcpr.gov/clinic/cps3dix.htm.

consensus and expert opinion, the ACOG concludes that in the short term (<2 years), soy and isoflavones, St. John's wort, and black cohosh may be helpful in managing menopausal symptoms.

## U.S. PREVENTIVE SERVICES RECOMMENDATIONS

The U.S. Preventive Services Task Force (2000) recommends preventive services that individuals should receive in primary care settings. This task force reviews the scientific evidence available and makes decisions about what particular services are appropriate in clinical settings. Its recommendations that apply to women, particularly those 25 and older, are summarized in Box 27-8.

Women's health is a growing area of interest for community-oriented nurses. By considering the environment within which women's health is experienced, one can see that women's health is *embedded in their communities* not just in their individual bodies. Health disparities exist among women. The way women of color experience health is different from the way their white counterparts experience it; this is attributable to a variety of issues, among them poverty, barriers in accessing health care, and knowledge deficits. Many populations of women, such as lesbians, older women, incarcerated women, impoverished women, and disabled women, are at a higher risk for health concerns than the general population. Legislation has helped shed light on the needs of women through the establishment of the Office of Women's Health and the passage of the Women's Health Equity Act.

## Practice Application

During her clinical time in community nursing, Laura accompanied Marie, her preceptor, on an initial home visit to a young woman named Josie. Josie, a 20-year-old single woman, had gone to the Public Health Center the previous week for a gynecologic exam because she thought she might have some sort of infection. At the health center, Josie mentioned to the clinic nurse that she did not have any food in the house. After the examination, the clinic nurse made a referral to the Women's Resource Service Center for a home visit and perhaps inclusion into their case management program.

When Marie and Laura arrived at Josie's apartment, they immediately noted that the living areas were devoid of furniture except for a soiled mattress on the floor of the living room. Dirty clothing was on the floor; empty take-out food sacks and trash littered the area. The kitchen area was also dirty, with evidence of cockroach infestation.

Marie and Laura noticed that Josie appeared to be uncomfortable and had difficulty interacting with either of them. Marie explained that they were there because the nurse at the clinic had asked them to come by and if there was any way that they might help her with her health care needs and living situation. Immediately, Josie began to cry. She had been with her abusive boyfriend until about 3 weeks ago when she kicked him out. Marie and Laura were able to learn that since that time, Josie had been prostituting as a way to survive. She was frightened and thought that her boyfriend was going to return and harm her. She also feared that she was pregnant.

On the basis of this situation, what potential actions might Laura and her preceptor Marie take?

**A.** Make an appointment for Josie to return to the woman's clinic for pregnancy testing.
**B.** Suggest that she focus on cleaning up her apartment, reminding her of the hazards of spoiled food.
**C.** Refer her to a safe-house shelter as a victim of domestic violence.
**D.** Make a referral for food delivery from a local church.

**Answers are in the back of the book.**

## Key Points

- Women's health is embedded not only in their individual bodies but also in their communities.
- Societal factors influence the distribution and of health and disease among women.
- Women's health advocates have widened the framework of women's health by including many social, psychological, cultural, political, economic, and biological factors.
- The complexities of women's lives—their educational levels, income, culture, ethnicity/race, and a host of other identities and experiences—shape their health.
- Estimates are that 72% of the unpaid family caregivers are women and that the majority of these women are midlife daughters or daughters-in-law.
- In 2001, the 107th Congress established the Office of Women's Health (OWH), which works to address inequities in research, health services, and education that have traditionally placed women at risk.
- The life expectancy of U.S. women is lower than that of women in 18 other developed countries.
- The problem of unintended pregnancy exists among adolescents as well as adult women.
- Prenatal care is associated with improved birth outcomes.
- Women's attitudes toward menopause vary greatly and are influenced by culture, age, support, and the experiences of other women passed on to them in recounted stories.
- In July of 2001, the European Parliament Women's Rights Committee condemned female genital mutilation as a serious violation of human rights and as an act of violence against women.
- Cardiovascular disease ranks first among all disease categories for women who are discharged from the acute care setting.
- When compared to their non-Hispanic, white counterparts, minority women have consistently higher rates of diabetes.
- Approximately 2% to 5% of all pregnancies in the United States are complicated with gestational diabetes.
- The World Health Organization has concluded that depression is the leading cause of disease burden for women in both developing and developed regions of the world.
- Overall, white women have a higher incidence rate for all cancers, whereas African-American women have a higher mortality rate for all cancers.
- In 2000, over 45,000 U.S. women of childbearing age (15 to 44) had AIDS.
- Women with a lower socioeconomic status are 50% more likely to be obese than those with a higher socioeconomic status.
- Women of color represent approximately 29% of all women in the United States.
- The Bureau of Justice reports that for every 100,000 women in the United States, there are 110 female inmates.

- Findings indicate that lesbians and bisexual women in the United States have a higher prevalence of several risk factors (smoking, alcohol use, lack of preventive cancer screening) than their heterosexual counterparts.
- According to the Office on Women's Health, there are 26 million American women who live with some type of disability.
- Poverty among female heads of households reflects the disparities that exist in the United States between various ethnic/racial groups; female-headed African-American and Hispanic families suffer higher rates of poverty than do other families.
- Research shows that older women, especially women of color and from lower socioeconomic groups, experience higher rates of chronic illness and disability than their white and more affluent counterparts.
- It is estimated that one out of every two American women over the age of 50 will experience an osteoporosis-related fracture in her lifetime.

## Clinical Decision-Making Activities

1. Interview three women, each from a different culture, about their experiences accessing health care. Are there differences in their stories about how they meet their health care needs? Do variances in ethnicity and culture present barriers to accessing health care?
2. Review current legislation that deals with women's health. Note patterns or trends in the issues that are being considered by the Senate or the House of Representatives. Are there obvious gaps in legislation that adversely affect women's health?
3. Considering breast cancer, apply the levels of prevention to women in underserved areas. Describe approaches to meeting their health care, social, and psychological needs. What barriers might prevent an effective program addressing breast cancer?
4. Contact your local public health office to determine what services are available for women. Identify community resources and agencies targeted for women. How do these organizations communicate their services to women in the community?
5. Propose a community-based intervention for women with HIV. Describe various program components such as goals and objectives, evaluation methods, and program outcomes.

## Additional Resources

These related resources are found either in the appendix in the back of this book or on the book's website at **http://evolve.elsevier.com/Stanhope.**

### evolve Evolve Website

Appendix A.1 Schedule of Clinical Preventive Services
Immunization Information
WebLinks: Healthy People 2010

## References

Aaron DJ et al: Behavioral risk factors for disease and preventive health practices among lesbians, A*m J Public Health* 91(6):972-975, 2001.

Ahluwalia IB, Daniel KL: Are women with recent live births aware of the benefits of folic acid? *MMWR Morb Mortal Wkly Rep* 50(RR-6):3, 2001.

American Academy of Nursing: Women's health and women's health care: recommendations of the 1996 AAN expert writing panel on women's health, *Nurs Outlook* 45(1):7-15, 1996.

American Academy of Pediatrics: Fetal alcohol syndrome and alcohol-related neurodevelopmental disorders, *Pediatrics* 106(2):358, 2000.

American Civil Liberties Union: *Public funding for abortion,* 2002, available at http://www.aclu.org/library/funding.html.

American College of Obstetricians and Gynecologists: *Use of botanicals for management of menopausal symptoms,* 2001, available at http://www.acog.org/from_home/publications/misc/pb028.htm.

American Heart Association: *Facts about women and cardiovascular disease,* 2002, available at http://216.185.112.5/presenter.jhtml?identifier=2876.

Bassuk EL et al: The characteristics and needs of sheltered homeless and low-income housed mothers, *JAMA* 276(8):640-646, 1996.

Beckles GLA, Thompson-Reid PE: Socioeconomic status of women with diabetes—United States, 2000, *JAMA* 287(19):2496, 2002.

Beckles GLA, Thompson-Reid PE, editors: *Diabetes and women's health across the life span: a public health perspective,* Atlanta, 2001, U.S. Department of Health and Human Services, National Center for Chronic Disease Prevention and Health Promotion.

Bierman AS, Clancy CM: Health disparities among older women: identifying opportunities to improve quality of care and functional health outcomes, *J Am Med Women's Assoc* 56(4):155-160, 2001, available at http://jamwa.amwa-doc.org/vol56/56_4_1a.htm.

Black SA: Diabetes, diversity, and disparity: what do we do with the evidence? *Am J Public Health* 92(4):543, 2002.

Bosch X: Female genital mutilation in developed countries, *Lancet* 358:1177-1178, 2001.

Campbell JC: Health consequences of intimate partner violence, *Lancet* 359:1331, 2002.

Center for Research on Women With Disabilities: *National study of women with physical disabilities,* 1999. available at http://www.bcm.tmc.edu/crowd/national_study/SPECIALS.htm.

Centers for Disease Control and Prevention: Strategies for reducing morbidity and mortality from diabetes through health-care interventions and diabetes self-management education in community settings: a report on recommendations of the Task Force on Community Preventative Services, *MMWR Morb Mortal Wkly Rep* 50(RR-15):1-15, 2001.

Centers for Disease Control and Prevention: Alcohol use among women of childbearing age—United States, 1991-1999, *MMWR Morb Mortal Wkly Rep* 51(13):273, 2002.

Centers for Disease Control and Prevention, National Center for Health Statistics: *Health, United States,* 2001, available at http://www.cdc.gov/nchs/products/pubs/pubd/hus/tables/2001/01hus028.pdf.

Centers for Disease Control and Prevention, National Center for Health Statistics: *Prenatal care,* 2002, available at http://www.cdc.gov/nchs/fastats/prenatal.htm

Centers for Disease Control and Prevention, National Center for HIV, STD, and TB Prevention: *HIV/AIDS among U.S. women: minority and young women at continuing risk,* 2002a, available at http://www.cdc.gov/hiv/pubs/facts/women.htm.

Centers for Disease Control and Prevention, National Center for HIV, STD, and TB Prevention: *HIV/AIDS surveillance in women,* L264 slide series through 2000, 2002b, available at http://www.cdc.gov/hiv/graphics/images/l264/l264-1.htm.

Centers for Disease Control and Prevention, National Center for Injury Prevention and Control: *Sexual violence against people with disabilities,* 1999, available at http://www.cdc.gov/ncipc/factsheets/disabvi.htm.

Centers for Disease Control and Prevention, National Center on Birth Defects and Developmental Disabilities: *The folic acid national campaign,* 2002, available at http://www.cdc.gov/ncbddd/folicacid/folcamp.htm.

Cornelius LJ, Smith PL, Simpson GM: What factors hinder women of color from obtaining preventive health care? *Am J Public Health* 92(4):535-539: 2002.

Curry MA: The interrelationships between abuse, substance use, and psychosocial stress during pregnancy, *J Obstet Gynecol Neonat Nurs* 27(6):692, 1998.

Curry MA, Hassouneh-Phillips D, Johnston-Silverberg A: Abuse of women with disabilities: an ecological model and review, *Violence Against Women* 7(1):50-79, 2001.

Devlin MJ: Body image in the balance, *JAMA* 286:2159, 2001.

Dionne EJ: The welfare-marriage wars, *The Washington Post,* Feb 26, 2002.

Earls F: Positive effects of prenatal and early childhood interventions, *JAMA* 14:1271, 1998.

Edwards BK et al: Annual report to the nation on the status of cancer, 1973-1999, featuring implications of age and aging on U.S. cancer burden, *Cancer* 94(10):2766-2792, 2002.

Ehrenreich B: *Nickel and dimed,* New York, 2002, Holt.

Federal Interagency Forum on Aging Related Statistics: Older Americans 2000: key indicators of well-being, 2000, available at http://www.agingstats.gov/chartbook2000/Population1-9.pdf.

Federal, Provincial, Territorial Advisory Committee on Population Health: *Toward a healthy future: second report on health of Canadians,* Ottawa, 1999, Publications Canada

Ford N: Tackling female genital cutting in Somalia, *Lancet* 358:1179, 2001.

Gerhard-Herman M: Cardiovascular disease in women, *Female Patient* 27:25-29, 2002.

Hargraves M: Elevating the voices of rural minority women, *Am J Public Health* 92:514-515, 2002.

Health Canada: *Women's health strategy,* Ottawa, 1999, retrieved July 14, 2002, from www.hc-sc.gc.ca/english/women/womenstrat.htm.

Hoffert SD: *When hens crow,* Bloomington, 1995, Indiana University Press.

Hoffman RL, Mitchell AM: Caregiver burden: historical development, *Nurs Forum* 33(4):5-11, 1998.

Institute of Medicine, Committee on Unintended Pregnancy: *The best intentions,* Washington, DC, 1995, National Academy Press.

Karter AJ et al: Ethnic disparities in diabetic complications in an insured population, *JAMA* 287(19):2519, 2002.

Katz E: *Margaret Sanger: biographical sketch,* 2001, available at http://www.nyu.edu/projects/sanger/ms-bio.htm.

King H, Aubert RE, Herman WH: Global burden of diabetes, 1995-2025, *Diabetes Care* 21(9):1414, 1998.

Kogan MD et al: The changing pattern of prenatal care utilization in the United States, 1981-1995, using different prenatal care indices, *JAMA* 279(20):1623-1628, 1998.

Lindsay C: The female population. In *Women in Canada, 2000: a gender-based statistical report,* Ottawa, 2000, Minister of Industry.

Lyon E: Poverty, welfare, and battered women: what does the research tell us? *Violence Against Women Online Resources,* 2002, available at http://www.vaw.umn.edu/Vawnet/welfare.htm.

Matthews AK et al: Prediction of depressive distress in a community sample of women: the role of sexual orientation, *Am J Public Health* 92:1131, 2002.

Mazure CM, Keita GP, Blehar MC: *Summit on women and depression: proceedings and recommendations,* Washington, DC, 2002, American Psychological Association, available at www.apa.org/pi/wpo/women&depression.pdf.

McClennon-Leong J, Ross-Kerr J: Alternative health care options in Canada, *Can Nurse* 95(10):26-30, 1999.

Millar W: Patterns of use: alternative health care practitioners, *Health Rep* 13(1):9-21, 2001.

Murray CJ, Lopez AD: *Global burden of disease,* Cambridge, Mass, 1996, Harvard University Press.

Narrigan D et al: Research to improve women's health: an agenda for equity. In Ruzek SB, Olesen VL, Clarke AE, editors: *Women's health: complexities and differences,* Columbus, 1997, Ohio State University Press.

National Center for Complementary and Alternative Medicine: *Alternative therapies for managing menopausal symptoms,* 2002, available at nccam.nih.gov.

National Institute of Diabetes and Digestive and Kidney Diseases: *Understanding adult obesity,* 2001, available at http://www.niddk.nih.gov.

National Institutes of Health, National Heart, Lung, and Blood Pressure Institute: NHLBI *stops trial of estrogen plus progestin due to increased breast cancer risk, lack of overall benefit,* available at http://www.nhlbi.nih.gov/new/press/02-07-09.htm.

National Institute of Mental Health: *Eating disorders: facts about eating disorders and the search for solutions,* 2001, available at www.nimh.nih.gov/publicat/eatingdisorder.cfm#ed2.

National Institute of Mental Health: *Women's mental health consortium,* 2002, available at http://www.nimh.nih.gov/wmhc/index.cfm.

National Women's History Project: *Living the legacy: the women's rights movement 1848-1998,* 2002, available at http://www.legacy98.org/move-hist.html.

Normand J: The health of women. In *Women in Canada 2000: a gender-based statistical report,* pp 47-83, ed 4, Ottawa, 2000, Minister of Industry.

Nosek MA, Hughes RB: Psychospiritual aspects of sense of self in women with physical disabilities, *J Rehabil* 67(1):20-25, 2001.

Nyamathi A et al: Type of social support among homeless women: its impact on psychosocial resources, health and health behaviors, and use of health services, *Nurs Res* 49(6):318-326, 2000.

Oliver-McNeil S, Artinian NT: Women's perceptions of personal cardiovascular risk and their risk-reducing behaviors, *Am J Crit Care* 11(3):221-227, 2002.

Parsons ML, Warner-Robbins C: Holistic nursing on the front lines, *Am J Nurs* 102(6):73-77, 2002.

Pinn VW: The NIH Office of Research on Women's Health goals and recent activities, *JAMWA* 53:1, 1998.

Roberts RO et al: Barriers to prenatal care: factors associated with late initiation of care in a middle-class midwestern community, *J Family Pract* 47:1, 1998.

Robinson KM: Family care giving: who provides the care, and at what cost? *Nurs Econ* 15(2):243, 1997.

Rosenberg J: Lesbians are more likely than U.S. women overall to have risk factors for gynecologic and breast cancer, *Fam Plann Perspect* 33(4):183-184, 2001.

Rowley DL et al: In Beckles GLA, Thompson-Reid PE, editors: *Diabetes and women's health across the life span: a public health perspective,* Atlanta, 2001, U.S. Department of Health and Human Services, National Center for Chronic Disease Prevention and Health Promotion.

Ruzek SB, Olesen VL, Clarke AE: *Women's health: complexities and differences,* Columbus, 1997, Ohio State University Press.

Salsberry PJ et al: Self-reported health status of low-income mothers, *Image J Nurs Scholar* 31(4):375, 1999.

Satcher D: American women and health disparities, *J Am Med Women's Assoc* 56(4):131-133, 2001.

Schriempf A: (Re)fusing the amputated body: an interactionist bridge for feminism and disability, *Hypatia* 16(4):53-79, 2001.

Schulz MA et al: Outcomes of a community-based three-year breast and cervical cancer screening program for medically underserved, low income women, *J Am Acad Nurse Pract* 14(5):219, 2002.

Spira M, Kenemore E: Cancer as a life transition: a relational approach to cancer wellness in women, *Clin Soc Work J* 30(2):173, 2001.

Statistics Canada: *Selected leading causes of death by sex,* 1997, retrieved July 4, 2002 from www.statcan.ca/english/Pgdb/health36.htm (also available at www.statcan.ca, choose Canadian statistics, and search for document name).

Statistics Canada: *National population health survey overview 1996/97,* Ottawa, 1998, Health Statistics Division.

Statistics Canada: *Alcohol consumption by sex, age-group, and level of education, 1998/99,* Ottawa, 1999, retrieved July 23, 2002 from www.statcan.ca/English/Pgdb/health05a.htm (also available at www.statcan.ca, choose Canadian statistics, and search for document name).

Statistics Canada: Taking risks and taking care, *Health Reports* 12(3):11-20, 2001a.

Statistics Canada: *Percentage of smokers in population 2000-2001,* Ottawa, 2001b, retrieved July 23, 2002 from www.statcan.ca/english/Pgdb/health07b.htm (also available at www.statcan.ca, choose Canadian statistics, and search for document name).

Statistics Canada: *How healthy are Canadians? a summary 2001 annual report,* pp 1-5, Ottawa, 2002a, Canadian Institute for Health Information.

Statistics Canada: Canadian community health survey: a first look, *The Daily,* Ottawa, May 8, 2002b, retrieved from www.statcan.ca/Daily/English/020508/d020508a.htm (also available at www.statcan.ca, choose *The Daily,* and search for document name).

Statistics Canada: Pain or discomfort that affects activities, *Health Indicators* #1, 2002c, retrieved September 13, 2002, from www.statcan.ca/english/freepub/82-221-XIE/00502/tables/html/1274.htm (also available at www.statcan.ca, choose Canadian statistics, and search for document name).

Statistics Canada: Pap smears, *Health Indicators* #1, 2002d, retrieved from www.statcan.ca:80/english/freepub/82-221-XIE/00601/high/tables/htmltablesP3231.htm (also available at www.statcan.ca, choose Canadian statistics, and search for document name).

Stevens PE: Lesbians' health-related experiences of care and noncare, *West J Nurs Res* 16(6):639-659, 1994.

Stevens PE: A nursing critique of US welfare system reform, *Adv Nurs Sci* 23(2):1-11, 2000.

Stover GN: Colorful communities: toward a language of inclusion, *Am J Public Health* 92:512-514, 2002.

Tait H: Aboriginal women's health. In *Women in Canada 2000: a gender-based statistical report,* Ottawa, 2000, Ministry of Industry, pp 247-259.

Taylor HA, Hughes GD, Garrison RJ: Cardiovascular disease among women residing in rural America: epidemiology, explanations, and challenges, *Am J Public Health* 92(4):548-551, 2002.

U.S. Bureau of the Census: *Americans with disabilities,* 1997, accessed 2002, http://www.census.gov/hhes/www/disable/sipp/disab97/asc97.html.

U.S. Bureau of the Census, Current Population Reports: *Poverty in the United States: 2000* (series P60-214), Washington, DC, 2001, U.S. Government Printing Office.

U.S. Bureau of the Census, Current Population Survey: *Poverty 2000,* accessed 2002, available at http://www.census.gov/hhes/www/poverty00.html.

U.S. Bureau of the Census, Population Estimates Program, Population Division: *Resident population estimates of the United States by sex, race, and Hispanic origin*, 2001, available at http://eire. census.gov/popest/archives/national/ nation3/intfile3-1.txt.

U.S. Bureau of the Census, Population Projections Program, Population Division: *Projections of the total resident population by 5-year age groups, and sex with special age categories*, 2000, available at http://www.census.gov/population/ projections/nation/summary/np-t3-a.txt.

U.S. Conference of Mayors: *A status report on hunger and homelessness in America's cities 2001*, 2001, available at http://www.usmayors.org/uscm/ hungersurvey/2001/hungersurvey2001.pdf.

U.S. Department of Health and Human Services, Centers for Disease Control and Prevention, National Center for Health Statistics: *Health, United States, 2001 with urban and rural health checkbook*, 2001, available at http://www. cdc.gov/nchs/data/hus/hus01.pdf.

U.S. Department of Health and Human Services: *Welfare reform implementation informational package*, 1997, available at http://www.acf.dhhs.gov/news/welfare/ wrpack.htm.

U.S. Department of Health and Human Services: *Healthy people 2010: understanding and improving health*, ed 2, Washington, DC, 2000, U.S. Government Printing Office.

U.S. Department of Health and Human Services: *The surgeon general's call to action to prevent and decrease overweight and obesity in 2001*, 2001, available at www.surgeongeneral.gov/library.

U.S. Department of Health and Human Services, National Institute on Aging: *Menopause: one woman's story, every woman's story: a resource for making healthy choices*, n.d., available at http:// www.nia.nih.gov/health/pubs/menopause/ menopause.pdf.

U.S. Department of Health and Human Services, National Institute of Diabetes and Digestive and Kidney Diseases: *Understanding adult diabetes*, 2001, available at http://www.niddk.nih.gov/ health/nutrit/pubs/unders.htm.

U.S. Department of Health and Human Services, Office on Women's Health: *Women with disabilities*, accessed April 2003 at http://www.4women.gov/wwd/ wwd.cfm?page=80.

U.S. Department of Health and Human Services, Office on Women's Health, National Women's Health Information Center: *Birth control methods*, 2000, available at http://www.4woman.gov/faq/ birthcont.htm.

U.S. Department of Health and Human Services, Public Health Service: *Healthy people: progress review: women's health*, 1998, available at http://odphp.osophs. dhhs.gov/pubs/hp2000/PROGRVW/ women/women.htm.

U.S. Department of Justice, Bureau of Justice Statistics: *Correctional populations by gender*, 1999, available at http:// www.ojp.usdoj.gov/bjs/glance/cpgend. htm.

U.S. Department of Labor, Bureau of Labor Statistics: Women's earnings 76 percent of men's in 2000, *Monthly Labor Review*, 2001, available at http://www. bls.gov/opub/ted/2001/sept/wk1/art02. htm.

U.S. Department of Labor: *Elaws—FMLA advisor,* 2002, available at http://www.elaws.dol.gov/fmla/wren/s1.htm.

U.S. Food and Drug Administration: *Protecting against unintended pregnancy: a guide to contraceptive choices,* 2000, available at http://www.fda.gov/fdac/features/1997/babytabl.html.

U.S. Preventive Services Task Force, Agency for Healthcare Research and Quality: *Guide to Preventive Services,* ed 3, 2000, available at http://www.ahcpr.gov/clinic/cps3dix.htm.

U.S. Preventive Services Task Force, Agency for Healthcare Research and Quality: *Guide to preventive services: screening for lipid disorders,* 2001, available at http://www.ahcpr.gov/clinic/cps3dix.htm.

U.S. Preventive Services Task Force, Agency for Healthcare Research and Quality: *Screening for depression,* 2002, available at http://www.ahcpr.gov/clinic/3rduspstf/depression/depresswh.pdf.

Weinert C: Social support in cyberspace for women with chronic illness, *Rehab Nurs* 25:4, 2000.

Williams DR: Racial/ethnic variations in women's health: the social embeddedness of health, *Am J Public Health* 92(4):588-597, 2002.

Women's International Network: Genital and sexual mutilation of females, *Women's Int Network News* 28(2):61, 2002.

Woods NF: Women and their health. In CI Fogel, NF Woods, editors: *Women's health care,* pp 1-22, Thousand Oaks, Calif, 1995, Sage.

World Health Organization, *WHO definition of health,* 2001, available at http://www.who.int/m/topicgroups/who_organization/en/index.html.

Wright N, Owen S: Feminist conceptualizations of women's madness: a review of the literature, *J Adv Nurs* 36:143, 2001.

Writing Group for the Women's Health Initiative Investigators: Risks and benefits of estrogen plus progestin in healthy postmenopausal women, *JAMA* 288(3):321-323, 2002.

# Men's Health

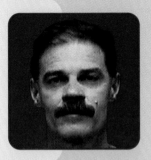

**Thomas Kippenbrock,
R.N., M.S.N., Ed.D.**

Thomas Kippenbrock became involved in men's health when his practice of nursing began in the 1970s. His interest in clinical practice started with acute care and expanded to population-focused men's health care. He has researched, lectured, and written on the topic of men's health for the last two decades.

## Objectives

After reading this chapter, the student should be able to do the following:

1. Identify legislation affecting men's health
2. Explain the unique aspects of developmental stages and tasks that affect young and middle-aged men
3. Discuss risk factors and their consequences on men's health
4. Understand how the lifestyles that men lead affect their health
5. Identify legislation affecting men's health
6. Describe the nurse's role in maintaining and promoting men's health
7. Describe the advanced practice nurse's role in men's health

Males are physiologically more vulnerable than females. More male infants die at birth. More men die of cardiovascular, liver, and chronic pulmonary diseases, as well as cancers, accidents, and suicide. Males have a shorter life span. Many explanations exist for such gender differences in health outcomes: genetics, risk-taking behaviors, stressors, ignoring warning signs. This chapter discusses men's health by reviewing developmental stages of men, identifying men's health problems and needs, and exploring the nurse's role in maintaining and promoting men's health in the community.

Men's health, as a separate and distinct practice of care, is at an early developmental level. Men's health goes beyond care of the prostate, genitalia, sexual dysfunction, and associated diseases. Today's focus is on the entire person, requiring a holistic approach.

This chapter also addresses the goals of Healthy People 2010 (U.S. Department of Health and Human Services [USDHHS], 2000). Two goals, increasing quality and years of healthy life and eliminating health disparities by focusing on the unique health needs of men, will be addressed in this chapter. Health promotion strategies are described to help men deal effectively with the leading causes of death affecting them. In addition, nursing interventions are discussed that are designed to assist men in taking advantage of preventive services that they tend to overlook to a greater extent than do women. The strategies described in this chapter illustrate the many ways in which the Healthy People 2010 goals and objectives can be applied to men.

## HOW MEN DEFINE HEALTH

Although men and women have similar ideas about health, there are some distinct differences. Most people view health as being closely associated with well-being. Both men and women define health comprehensively and refer to it as a state or condition of being, and they often relate this condition to capacity, performance, and function.

Health is grounded in a sense of self and the physical body, and both are tied to conceptions of past and future actions. When men are asked about health, they look at physical, mental, and emotional well-being. Also, they believe the state of self has the potential to affect the state of others. Many men believe health is individualized. This means one person's idea of health and well-being may differ from another's thoughts of being healthy. Men frequently refer to healthiness as *keeping* or *being in control* and *minding* one's body. Men seem to imagine themselves as having *power over* their relationship to their bodies. Men speak about their bodies as though they *belong* to them in the same way an object belongs to them (Saltonstall, 1993).

Today, the health care focus is changing: it used to be on diseases and their treatments, but now it is on disease prevention and identification of needs. This preventive focus is a wise one: men are an unmistakably high-risk

## Key Terms

**assaultive violence**, p. 691
**body maintenance**, p. 694
**development**, p. 682
**digital rectal examination**, p. 688
**generativity versus stagnation**, p. 682

**intimacy versus isolation**, p. 682
**men's health nurse practitioner**, p. 695
**moral development**, p. 683
**prostate cancer**, p. 688
**psychosocial development**, p. 682

**testicular cancer**, p. 689
**testicular self-examination**, p. 689
*See Glossary for definitions*

## Chapter Outline

How Men Define Health
The Health Status of Men in the United States
Male Development
*Psychosocial*
*Moral*
Men's Health and Mortality
Gender Differences
Cultural Differences
Leading Causes of Men's Deaths

*Heart and Cardiovascular Diseases*
*Cancer*
*Accidents*
*Pulmonary Diseases*
*Suicide*
*Assaults*
*Alcohol-Induced Disorders*
*Human Immunodeficiency Virus*
Men's Health Practices in Everyday Life

The Community-Oriented Nurse's Role
   in Men's Health
*Educator*
*Client Advocate*
*Case Manager*
*Men's Health Nurse Practitioner*

## THE CUTTING EDGE

A men's health hotline is offered by the former U.S. Secretary of Health, Dr. C. Edward Koop. Learn more about men's health issues at www.drkoop.com.

group. They frequently engage in compensatory, aggressive, and risk-taking behavior predisposing them to illness, injury, and even death.

Men tend to avoid medical help as long as possible, leading to serious health problems. With the exception of orthopedics and pediatrics, women use medical specialties more often than men (Davidson and Daly, 2000; Steele, 2000). Men need to openly express their health care concerns. Health care professionals can help men examine their concerns by encouraging them to discuss nonhealth problems as well as health care problems, and by promoting preventive health care. Although some men are apprehensive about intimate interaction with professionals, strategies can be employed to reduce men's anxiety. Nurses can remove physical barriers separating themselves from the client, use handouts and other written information to support oral instructions, and show a genuine interest in men's needs.

## THE HEALTH STATUS OF MEN IN THE UNITED STATES

The 1990s saw considerable attention on health reform, with economics playing a key role (see Chapter 5). Both men and women will be affected by changes in health care. Review of past health care legislation affecting men may provide clues to where future legislation is headed. Rules and regulations on elder care, work-related injuries, and veterans' services have affected men's health.

Most Americans turning 65 years old are eligible for Medicare, part A, which provides hospital insurance, skilled nursing, home health care, and hospice care. Disabled men are also eligible for these benefits. Currently, millions of men participate in this government-operated insurance plan. Medicare, part B, which requires subscribers to pay a monthly fee, provides 80% of coverage on other medical-related expenses such as physician costs.

In 1983, to hold down the spiraling cost of Medicare, a prospective payment system was established by amendments to the Social Security Act (see Chapter 5). The system provides diagnostic billing categories for almost all U.S. hospitals reimbursed by Medicare.

The Worker's Compensation Act (WCA) and Americans with Disabilities Act (ADA) (Office of Human Resource Management, 2003; Rumrill, 2001) were two significant laws affecting men's health because of the high occupational accident rate. The WCA required all industrial employers to carry worker's compensation for their employees in case of job-related injuries; however, some nonprofit organizations are exempt. Worker's compensation insurance pays for an employee's partial lost wages and medical costs encountered. If the employee is permanently disabled, the worker is entitled to additional compensation.

ADA was designed to protect people from being discriminated against in the workplace; this means employers are prohibited from discriminating against qualified disabled individuals in hiring, promotion, job assignment, discharge, compensation, and all other "terms, conditions, and privileges" of employment (Rumrill, 2001). An ADA-qualified individual is defined as a person with a disability who meets the skill, experience, education, and other job-related requirements of a position held or desired and who, with or without a reasonable accommodation, can perform the essential functions of a job. If a person is injured on the job, the employer has to look at all the circumstances and evaluate how the employee may be taken care of after the injury.

With more men assuming parenting and elder caregiver roles, the Family and Medical Leave Act (U.S. Department of Labor, 2003) offers opportunities to meet family responsibilities. An eligible employee is entitled to a maximum of 12 weeks for the birth of a child, to care for an ill child or spouse, to adopt or accept a foster or an adoptive child, and last, for his recovery from a serious health condition. When the person's leave is over, he is entitled to return to work in the same or an equivalent position with the same or equivalent pay scale and benefits. During the leave, the employer is not required to pay the employee, although vacation time, personal time off, or sick leave can be used. Other benefits such as life insurance and health insurance will continue; however, the employer is required to pay only for the employee.

The effects of war have influenced men's health care legislation. Until the Vietnam era, most American veterans were men. Since the mid 1970s, women have entered the armed forces and are eligible for veterans' benefits. Nevertheless, the majority of veterans are men. Health-related veterans' benefits include hospital and nursing home care, counseling for stress trauma, alcohol and drug treatments, prosthetic services, outpatient pharmacy services, and dental services. Other entitlements include a pension program.

## MALE DEVELOPMENT

### Psychosocial

**Development** is a process of human change in structure, thoughts, or behaviors as a consequence of biological or environmental factors. Usually, these changes are progressive and cumulative, and they are not as rapid in adults as they are in children. Because adult men and women follow similar developmental patterns, developmental theorists have not typically separated the sexes.

Erikson (1968) explained the **psychosocial development** of adults as stages in which a person's capacities or experiences dictate major life adjustments in his or her so-

cial environment or self. The following overview of psychosocial development focuses on men during their young and middle adulthood.

### Young Adulthood

Erikson labels the young adulthood stage (between 20 and 45 years) **intimacy versus isolation.** During this stage, each person must establish a secure personal identity. Once this task is accomplished, the person is able to form intimate and loving relationships (Box 28-1 summarizes the tasks in this stage). The young male adult begins to focus on developing close relationships with others and eventually choosing a mate. These relationships lead to his forming a family and pursuing a career. Two periods of reevaluation occur, first at about 30 years and again at 40 years, during which the person closely examines his goals and accomplishments. This may be a crisis period for men, and they may decide to make changes in their lives.

### Middle Adulthood

Erikson labels the middle adulthood stage (40 to 65 years) **generativity versus stagnation.** This stage focuses on contributions to the next generation. Men are involved in sharing, nurturing, and contributing to the growth of others (Box 28-2 summarizes the tasks in this stage). Middle adulthood has been typically defined as being a period of stability; yet many men undergo a transition period equal to or greater than the one they experienced in adolescence. In 1933, the psychiatrist Jung noted a gradual personality change in which men search their inner selves for a greater meaning in their lives. At this time, they may begin to acknowledge *tender feelings* and to be more expressive. Marriage and the spousal relationship are the best predictors of male midlife satisfaction and perceived stress reduction. Thus a redefinition of husband and father roles may occur. Men also must cope with the physical changes that occur during this time.

## Moral

Over time, society has changed from hunting and gathering to farming, manufacturing, and service. In prehistoric

---

### BOX 28-1 Tasks of the Young Adult Man

1. To develop an intimate relationship with another
2. To choose a mate
3. To establish a role as husband or father or both
4. To manage a household independent of his parents' home and care
5. To develop a career or vocation
6. To continue development of a social structure
7. To develop a community role focusing on citizenship
8. To develop a lifestyle suitable to his philosophy on life

times, human's need to hunt and kill game was essential for survival; however, with the discovery of machines, energy, and agriculture, the need to kill should cease. Yet humans continue to kill and commit crimes against humanity. Questions about human moral development can be explained by reviewing related theory. This chapter explores why some men resort to violence.

Kohlberg (1984) focused on the **moral development** of the individual. As a person reasons and thinks about moral issues and problems, the individual should become motivated to develop new and broader viewpoints. People do not lose the insight they gained earlier but instead build on it. Kohlberg divided moral development into stages or levels of reasoning (Box 28-3). The stages are hierarchical. Progression usually occurs, with advancement from one stage to the next; however, individuals may regress to a previous stage. Stage advancement does not depend on physical maturity. The typical movement through stages is an orderly process from a focus on self to the larger society and universal principles.

## MEN'S HEALTH AND MORTALITY

In the United States, men's life expectancy at all ages is one of the lowest in developed countries, and it is much lower than that of women (Table 28-1). The Japanese infant can expect to outlive the U.S. infant by almost

---

### BOX 28-2  Tasks of the Middle-Aged Adult Man

1. To promote a deep relationship with the spouse or partner
2. To nurture and share in the growth of children and the next generation
3. To adjust to physical changes
4. To reassess himself and his career goals
5. To achieve desired goals in life and career
6. To find acceptable leisure activities
7. To cope with the empty-nest syndrome

---

### BOX 28-3  Stages of Morality

**STAGE I: PRECONVENTIONAL MORALITY**

The individual is guided by rules dictating good or bad, right or wrong. The individual translates these rules into physical or hedonistic consequences of action such as rewards, favors, and physical power over others.

**STAGE II: CONVENTIONAL MORALITY**

Usually in the teens, the individual shifts from unquestioning obedience to a concern for "good" motives. Assumptions about family, groups, and society as valuable in themselves occur in this stage. Conforming to personal and social expectations, as well as to the concepts of loyalty, support, maintenance, and championing order, results in this stage.

**STAGE III: UNIVERSAL PRINCIPLES**

The individual is concerned with individuals' rights and social contracts apart from his or the group's needs. The individual is concerned with consistent, comprehensive ethical principles.

---

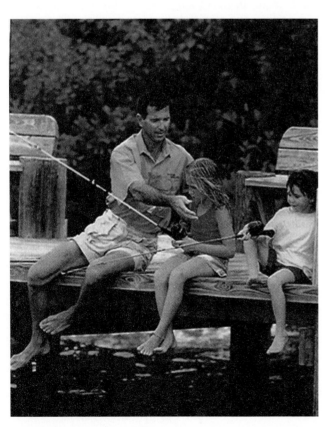

During the young adulthood stage, men generally focus on marriage and family issues.

---

| Table 28-1  Life Expectancies for Men and Women in Selected Countries | | |
|---|---|---|
| COUNTRY | MEN (YR) | WOMEN (YR) |
| United States | 73.9 | 79.4 |
| Canada | 76.1 | 81.8 |
| France | 74.2 | 82.0 |
| Netherlands | 75.0 | 80.7 |
| Norway | 75.2 | 81.1 |
| Sweden | 76.3 | 80.8 |
| Japan | 76.8 | 82.9 |

*Statistical Yearbook 2000,* New York, 2000, The United Nations.

## Men's Health in Canada

Karon Janine Foster, R.N., B.Sc.N., M.Ed., Lecturer, Faculty of Nursing, University of Toronto

### LIFE EXPECTANCY AND CAUSES OF DEATH

Canadian men have seen their life expectancy improve over the past 40 years. Today, a male child can expect to live to age 75. The disability-free life expectancy (the years a person can expect to live without significant disability) for men in 1997 was 65.5 years (Statistics Canada, 2002a). The death rate for men fell 8% from 1990 and is now 848 deaths/100,000 men (Statistics Canada, 1997a, 2002a). The major killers of men are heart disease, cancer, and cerebrovascular disease (Statistics Canada, 2002a). In men ages 20 to 44, the leading causes of death are suicide and injuries from motor vehicle accidents, followed by human immuno-deficiency virus (HIV) and cancer. For men ages 45 to 64, the leading causes of death are cancer, circulatory disease, and suicide. Lung cancer and ischemic heart disease are the major threats to men of this age. For men over 65, the order is reversed, with circulatory disease killing more men than cancer. Ischemic heart disease, lung cancer, and stroke are the main causes of death for this age-group. Suicide and falls are also significant causes of death for those over 65 years.

In 1997, mortality rates for men were 229.7 deaths per 100,000 of the total population by cancer, 230.8/100.000 by heart disease, and 52.8/100,000 by cerebrovascular disease (Statistics Canada, 1997b). In the same year, male suicides accounted for 19.5/100,000 (Statistics Canada, 1997b). The most common cancer deaths in men are due to lung cancers, followed by prostate and colorectal cancers (Statistics Canada, 2002a). Ischemic heart disease and cerebrovascular diseases are the leading causes of circulatory deaths.

### CHRONIC CONDITIONS AND HEALTH CONCERNS

Surveys done in 1998-1999 showed approximately 52% of men suffer from a chronic health condition (Normand, 2000). The chronic diseases with the highest incidence for men were nonarthritic arthritis/rheumatism, back problems, hypertension, heart disease, asthma, migraines, and allergies (Normand, 2000; Statistics Canada, 2002a). Other health problems include bronchitis, diabetes, cancer, skin cancer, and a rising incidence of prostate cancer. Men 65 years and older have higher incidence rates of arthritis/rheumatism, heart disease, and cancer. Hypertension is one of the major chronic illnesses reported in men, and it is also a risk factor for cardiovascular disease. Injuries requiring medical attention are more frequent in males. In 2000-2001, 10% of males reported injuries requiring medical attention (Statistics Canada, 2002b). Men most commonly reported injuries to the back and spine, with

the highest percentage of these injuries occurring at work or school, followed closely by sports and leisure activities. More than 70% of men over 75 years experienced an activity-limiting injury due to falls in 1996/1997 (Wilkins, 1999). Recent data shows falls were the fifth leading cause of hospitalization in men (Wilkins, 1999). Depression can also cause admission to hospital and suicide. In 1996/1997, 3% of men reported experiencing an episode of clinical depression, with those in age-groups 18 to 19 and 35 to 44 most likely to experience a depressive episode (Normand, 2000).

A growing concern among health professionals is the increasing number of obese Canadians. Obesity is a factor in heart disease, diabetes, and cancer. The Canadian Community Health Survey 2000/2001 reported that 15% of Canadians, or 2.8 million people, are obese, on the basis of a body mass index (BMI) over 30 (Statistics Canada, 2002c). Obesity rates have increased more in men than women, with 16% of men considered obese. Men in the age-group 55 to 64 accounted for the greatest increase in obesity (Statistics Canada, 2002c).

### HEALTH CARE PRACTICES

Approximately 66% of men report visiting a health care professional at least once per year (Statistics Canada, 2002a). Men over 65 years visited health professionals more frequently than younger men. General practitioners, dentists, and specialists were the health professionals most commonly seen, whereas chiropractors were the alternative health care service providers most frequently consulted. Since 1994, there has been a slight increase in men's use of alternative health care services. Men 25 to 64 were the most likely to consult an alternative care provider. The hospitalization rate for men in 1998/1999 was 9000 per 100,000. Men were most frequently hospitalized for circulatory disease, followed by digestive tract and respiratory diseases (Normand, 2000). The incidence of prostate cancer has fallen only slightly and it is the second leading cause of cancer deaths in men, with 4300 reported in 2001 (National Cancer Institute, 2001). Early screening is important to control this disease, and the Canadian Cancer Society's recommendations for periodic examinations include a yearly digital rectal examination for men over 40 years.

### LIFESTYLE PRACTICES

Lifestyle factors such as smoking, alcohol use, diet, and physical activity influence the health of men. Cigarette smoking is a risk factor for heart disease, stroke, and cancer. The percentage of Canadian men who smoke has declined sharply in the past 15 years. In 2000/2001,

23.5% of boys and men over 12 reported smoking daily (Statistics Canada, 2001b). Men 20 to 34 were the most likely to smoke daily. Teenagers are the most likely group to start smoking.

Alcohol consumption is associated with injuries and is a risk factor in many diseases. In 1998/1999, 48% of men consumed alcohol at least once a week (Statistics Canada, 2001a). Men aged 25 to 44 were the most frequent drinkers. Binge drinking, the consumption of more than five drinks at one sitting, is a phenomenon more common in men than in women. Twenty-four percent of men indicated binge drinking at least once a month (Statistics Canada, 2002a). Younger men, 18 to 24 years old, were the group with the highest binge drinking. Responsible use of alcohol is an issue that health professionals working with young adults continue to promote.

Physical activity is promoted as a behaviour to prevent disease and maintain health. Men are more physically active in their leisure time than women. Canadian men have gradually become more physically active: in 1997 to 1998, 25% of men were physically active (Statistics Canada, 2001a).

## GOVERNMENTAL LEGISLATION AND MEN'S HEALTH

Men experience risks to their health from exposure to hazardous materials in their work, and from work-related injuries. Occupational health is a provincial responsibility, and government monitoring of health and safety is carried out by different agencies in each province. Employers are required to provide information about substances in the workplace that are hazardous to a worker's health through the Workplace Hazards Management Information System (WHMIS) program. Compensation for injuries that occur during employment is provided through the Workplace Safety Insurance Board.

Men with biological and adopted children are eligible for parental leave, which allows an opportunity to adjust to parenthood. Health care and support services are available to Canadian veterans through the Federal Department of Veterans Affairs.

In summary, men's life expectancy has improved in Canada. However, cancer, heart disease, and respiratory disease pose major threats to the health of men. Health professionals need to continue to encourage men to make lifestyle changes and incorporate a variety of health promotion strategies into their practice in order to address these health threats.

## References

Millar W: Patterns of use: alternative health care practitioners, *Health Rep* 13(1):9-21, 2001.

National Cancer Institute of Canada: *Canadian cancer statistics* 2001, Toronto, 2001, NCIC.

Normand J: The health of women. In *Women in Canada 2000: a gender-based statistical report,* pp 47-83, Ottawa, 2000, Minister of Industry.

Statistics Canada: *Age standardized mortality rates, 1997,* 1997a, retrieved July 2002 from www.statcan.ca/english/Pgdb/health30b.htm (also available at www.statcan.ca, choose Canadian statistics, and search for document name).

Statistics Canada: *Selected leading causes of death by sex, 1997,* 1997b, retrieved July 2002 from www.statcan.ca/english/Pgdb/health36.htm (also available at www.statcan.ca, choose Canadian statistics, and search for document name).

Statistics Canada: Taking risks and taking care, *Health Rep* 12(3):11-20, 2001a.

Statistics Canada: *Percentage of smokers in population 2000-2001,* 2001b, retrieved July 2002 from www.statcan.ca/english/Pgdb/health07b.htm (also available at www.statcan.ca, choose Canadian statistics, and search for document name).

Statistics Canada: *High blood pressure 2000-2001,* 2001c, retrieved July 2002 from www.statcan.ca/english/Pgdb/health03.htm (also available at www.statcan.ca, choose Canadian statistics, and search for document name).

Statistics Canada: *How healthy are Canadians? a summary 2001 annual report,* pp 1-6, Ottawa, 2002a, Health Statistics Division.

Statistics Canada: Injuries causing limitations of normal activities, by age-group, sex, and household population aged 12 and over (catalogue #82-221-XIE), *Health Indicators* 2002(1), 2002b, available at www.statcan.ca/english/freepub/82-221-XIE/01002/tables/html/12181.htm (also available at www.statcan.ca, choose Canadian statistics, and search for "injuries causing limitations").

Statistics Canada: Canadian community health survey: a first look, *The Daily,* May 8, pp 1-6, 2002c, retrieved from www.statcan.ca/Daily/English/020508/d020508a.htm (also available at www.statcan.ca, choose *The Daily,* and search for the document name).

Wilkins K: Health care consequences of falls for seniors, *Health Rep* 10(4):47-55, 1999.

*Canadian spelling is used.*

3 years, but once again the Japanese women outlive the men (Statistical Yearbook, 2000).

For American adolescents (15 to 24 years old) and early adult men (25 to 34 years), death rates are more than twice those of men in Japan and the Netherlands. In addition, American men ages 45 to 54 years rank second highest in death rates among the 13 developed countries; but interestingly, mortality has significantly declined for American men of ages 45 to 54 years. The least progress toward mortality decline is in the men's age-group of 25 to 34 years. Accidents, homicides and other violence, cancers, circulatory system diseases, and infectious and parasitic diseases account for most deaths in developed countries. American men rank high in all areas except parasitic disease. The good news is that there has been a decline in men's ischemic heart disease in the United States; however, American men's and women's heart disease mortalities are still among the highest in the world (USDHHS, 2000b).

## GENDER DIFFERENCES

Among whites, the death rates of male neonates, post-neonates, and infants are higher than those of females and males combined. Among African-American babies, the death rates of males are also higher than those of females and males combined (Table 28-2) (Hoyert et al, 2001).

At the other end of the life span, men have a shorter life expectancy than women. Government data reveal that the U.S. life expectancy for men at birth was a record high in 1999 but considerably fewer years than for women. The gender differences are 6.9 years for African Americans and 5.3 years for whites. In 1999, the age-adjusted death rate for men (1061 per 100,000) of all races was 1.4 times that of women (743 per 100,000) (Hoyert et al, 2001).

Men do engage in more risk-taking behaviors than women. This is particularly true with behaviors involving physical challenges or illegal behavior. Men drink more alcohol than women, which may explain men's higher mortalities from accidents, liver cirrhosis, and some types of cancer. Men's jobs are more hazardous, resulting in more job-related accidents. Men are also exposed to more industrial carcinogens. Other areas contributing to gender differences in morbidity or mortality may include stress responses, genetics, physiologic differences, environmental factors, and presence or absence of preventive behavior.

---

**Table 28-2  Death Rates (per 100,000) for Selected Groups of Infants**

| AGE | WHITES | | AFRICAN AMERICANS | |
|---|---|---|---|---|
| | MALES | MALES AND FEMALES | MALE | MALES AND FEMALES |
| Neonates to 4 weeks | 419 | 355 | 1071 | 879 |
| 1 month | 215 | 159 | 521 | 436 |
| Infants to 1 year | 635 | 515 | 1591 | 1315 |

Hoyert DL et al: Deaths: final data for 1999, *Natl Vital Stat Rep* 49(8):1-113, 2001.

---

**Table 28-3  Leading Causes of Men's Death, and Comparisons to Women (per 100,000)**

| CAUSE OF DEATH | MEN | | WOMEN | | MALE-TO-FEMALE RATIO |
|---|---|---|---|---|---|
| | DEATH RATE | RANK | DEATH RATE | RANK | |
| Heart disease | 328.1 | 1 | 220.9 | 1 | 1.4 |
| Cancer | 251.6 | 2 | 169.0 | 2 | 1.5 |
| Cerebrovascular disease | 62.4 | 3 | 60.5 | 3 | 1.0 |
| Chronic lower respiratory | 58.1 | 4 | 38.2 | 4 | 1.5 |
| Accidents (unintentional injuries) | 50.6 | 5 | 22.7 | 5 | 2.2 |
| Diabetes mellitus | 25.0 | 7 | 19.5 | 7 | 1.5 |
| Influenza and pneumonia | 28.0 | 6 | 20.8 | 6 | 1.3 |
| Alzheimer's disease | 14.0 | 10 | 17.6 | 8 | 0.8 |
| Nephritis, nephritic syndrome, nephrosis | 16.2 | 9 | 11.2 | 9 | 1.4 |
| Septicemia | 11.1 | 12 | 9.5 | 10 | 1.2 |
| Intentional self-harm (suicide) | 18.2 | 8 | 4.1 | 12 | 4.4 |
| Chronic liver disease and cirrhosis | 13.7 | 11 | 6.1 | 11 | 2.2 |

Anderson RN: Deaths: leading causes for 1999, *Natl Vital Stat Rep* 49(Suppl):11, 2001.

HOW TO  Assess Chest Pain

| | Angina | Myocardial infarction |
|---|---|---|
| Onset | Sudden or gradual | Sudden |
| Duration | Usually longer than 15 min | 30 to 120 min |
| Location | Substernal, or anterior chest; however, not sharply localized | Same as angina |
| Radiation | Back, neck, arms, jaw, abdomen, or fingers | Jaws, neck, back, shoulder, and one or both arms |
| Quality and intensity | Mild to moderate tightness, pressure described as squeezing and crushing | Persistent and severe pressure; described like angina pain |

Often, differences are related to a combination of these factors.

Similarities and differences exist as to the leading causes of death among men and women (Table 28-3). Heart disease and cancer are by far the leading causes of mortality for both sexes. The most prominent differences are for intentional self-harm (suicides), assaults (homicides), liver diseases, and accidents. For example, suicides are more than four and one-half times higher; homicides are more than three times higher; and accidents and liver diseases are more than two times higher. Men and women have similar death rates from cerebrovascular disease, influenza/pneumonia, diabetes, Alzheimer's disease, septicemia, and renal diseases, so they will not be discussed here, even though they are leading causes of death for men.

## CULTURAL DIFFERENCES

Men's health status differs between the various cultures and races. In the general population, mortality is higher for African Americans than for whites. When analyzing the leading causes of death, death rates for African-American men exceed those for white men in 12 of the 15 leading causes: cardiovascular diseases, cancers, cerebrovascular disease, accidents, diabetes mellitus, influenza/pneumonia, nephritis, septicemia, chronic liver diseases, hypertension, and assaults.

For the Hispanic population, the age-adjusted death rate was also higher for men than for women. In an analysis of leading causes of death, the death rates for Hispanic men exceed those for non-Hispanic men in only three of the 15 leading causes: diabetes mellitus, chronic liver diseases, and assaults (Hoyert et al, 2001).

## LEADING CAUSES OF MEN'S DEATHS
### Heart and Cardiovascular Diseases

For men, heart disease is the leading cause of death. The age-adjusted death rate for men who died of heart disease in 1999 was 328 per 100,000 population, accounting for 30% of all men's deaths. This health statistic is unquestionably significant in young and middle-aged men. For men 35 to 44 years of age, the heart disease death rate is 2.4 times higher than for women; for men 45 to 54 years of age, the death rate is 2.8 times higher than for women; and for 55- to 64-year-old men, the death rate is 2.3 higher than for women of the same age categories (Table 28-4) (Anderson, 2001).

Coronary heart disease (CHD) is the leading cause of morbidity and mortality in the United States despite the decline during the last three decades. Over 12.6 million American people are diagnosed with CHD, and 7.5 million of these people have myocardial infarctions. About 450,000 men die annually from CHD, accounting for one third of all deaths (American Heart Association, 2002). (See the How To box about assessing chest pain.)

Gaziano (1998) identified two factors that will contribute to future heart disease statistics in the United States. One factor is the anticipated increase in the older population, which will result in more incidents of cardiovascular disease. Several physiologic changes occur as a person ages, including an increase in the size of the heart. The biggest changes take place on the left side of the heart, or the pumping side. Heart mass increases 1 to 1.5 grams/year between ages 30 and 90 years. However, the heart may atrophy if the person has extended illness. Aging results in valve and vascular changes, and systolic blood pressure rises because the blood vessels are less compliant.

| Table 28-4 | Heart Disease Rates (per 100,000) for Young and Middle-Aged Men and Women | | |
|---|---|---|---|
| AGE-GROUP | MEN | WOMEN | MALE-TO-FEMALE RATIO |
| 35-45 yr | 43.3 | 17.6 | 2.4 |
| 45-54 yr | 145.7 | 51.9 | 2.8 |
| 55-64 yr | 391.6 | 167.5 | 2.3 |

Anderson RN: Deaths: leading causes for 1999, *Natl Vital Stat Rep* 49(Suppl):11, 2001.

## Evidence-Based Practice

There have been testimonials that alternative therapies have reduced heart disease symptoms. It is estimated that more than 100,000 U.S. residents have received a chelating agent, ethylenediamine triacetic acid (EDTA), in combination with oral vitamins and minerals to treat ischemic heart disease. At a cost of $4000 per serial treatment, that results in a $400 million national health cost.

To study the efficacy of chelation therapy, a double-blind, randomized, placebo-controlled trial was conducted to determine the effect of EDTA on exercise-induced ischemic threshold and the quality of life. One group received 40 mg/kg of EDTA for 3 hours per treatment, twice a week for 15 weeks. The other group received an intravenous placebo. Both groups took multivitamins.

**Nurse Use:** The results indicated there were no beneficial effects of chelation therapy, when compared to the placebo, as measured by exercise time to ischemia, exercise capacity, and quality of life.

Knudtson ML, Wyse DG, Galbraith PD: Chelation therapy for ischemic heart disease: a randomized controlled trial, *JAMA* 287(4):481-486, 2002.

---

The other factor affecting the prevalence of heart disease is found in the very young. Evidence from the Bogalusa heart study identified children and young adults had traditional risk factors related to arteriosclerosis in the aorta and coronary arteries. This means that cardiovascular changes can occur at much younger ages than ever thought. In autopsies of 86 white males, 52 African-American males, and 66 females, researchers found that the extent of aortic and coronary artery vessels with fatty streaks and fibrous plaques increased with age among children and young adults. Among the cardiovascular risk factors found in the dead subjects, body mass index, systolic and diastolic blood pressures, and serum concentrations of total cholesterol, triglycerides, low-density-lipoprotein cholesterol, and high-density-lipoprotein cholesterol were strongly associated with the extent of lesions in the aorta and coronary arteries. In addition, cigarette smokers had more lesions than nonsmokers (Berenson and Sathanur, 1998).

Over time, decline in the age-adjusted rates of CHD and strokes has been attributed both to improved treatment and to primary and secondary prevention among middle-aged and older people. Anti smoking efforts, screening for hypertension and high blood cholesterol levels, and improved treatments for acute myocardial infarctions had direct results in recent CHD declines. Hunink et al (1997) reported that 25% of the decline in CHD mortality was the result of primary prevention, while more of the decline was explained by improved CHD client man-

agement through a combination of risk factor reduction and treatments. Interventions to decrease lipoproteins by diet or lipid-lowering medications explains about one third of the CHD mortality, showing that interventions are sometimes negative. Many men participate in alternative therapies for heart disease. Outcomes and examples are provided in Box 28-4.

## Cancer

Malignant neoplasms are the second leading cause of death for men of all ages. The age-adjusted death rate is 251 per 100,000 population, accounting for 24% of all men's deaths in the United States (Hoyert et al, 2001). The cancers that most significantly affect men are prostate, testicular, and skin.

### Prostate Cancer

The second most common cancer among U.S. men, after pulmonary neoplasms, with a reported age-adjusted death rate of 29 per 100,000 population, is **prostate cancer** (Hoyert et al, 2001). The risk for prostate cancer increases with each decade after 50 years of age and is highest among men 75 years and older. The death rates among African-American men were more than twice those among white men, and the lowest rates were among Asian Americans. The decline in death rates for whites and Asians was approximately twice the decrease for African Americans, Hispanics, and Native Americans (Garguiullo et al, 2002).

The exact cause of prostatic cancer is unknown. Genetics, hormones, diet, environment, and viruses have all been implicated as risk factors. Early diagnosis is essential because treatment is usually unsuccessful later. One diagnostic problem is the lack of symptoms; thus the cancer may be advanced before detection.

The two most commonly used early diagnostic methods are an annual **digital rectal examination** (DRE) and the serum prostate-specific antigen (PSA). DRE can detect palpable masses. The presence of asymmetry, induration or a firm nodule is a sign of cancer. Men consider the examination painful and avoid the procedure; however, the test is inexpensive and results are quick. PSA is a serum protease used to detect nonpalpable and recurrent prostrate lesions. Measurements that are shown to increase over time are more important than an elevated one-time result (Pobursky, 1995). Other forms of testing include transrectal ultrasounds, radiographic assessment, computerized tomography, magnetic resonance imaging, and biopsy.

More frequent examinations are recommended for men who are considered at risk. Men are considered to be at risk if they have (1) continuing urinary symptoms with a family history of prostatic cancer and (2) benign prostatic hypertrophy or a partial prostatectomy.

Treatment options include a wait-and-monitor period. Continued assessment of urine, DRE, and PSA is used in the early cancer stage. More intense treatment may include one or more of the following: radiation therapy, hormonal therapy, pharmacologic management, and surgical man-

## BOX 28-4   Alternative and Complementary Treatments for Heart Disease

Herbal products for treatment of heart disease are being studied and results are being reported at alternative and complementary medicine conferences. Herbal manufacturers make no claim their herbs cure or treat heart diseases. Consequently, the U.S. Food and Drug Administration (FDA) does not classify them as medicines and thus they are not regulated nor is their production supervised. Because external evaluations are not common industrial practices, the herbs could be laced with heavy metals and other toxins, or they could simply be a placebo. The following herbs are commonly taken for heart disease. People buy and ingest herbs with the hope of controlling cholesterol, weight, and blood pressure, which are risk factors for heart disease. The therapeutic outcomes for treatment of heart disease using alternative therapies are very limited, as shown in the table (Torpy, 2002).

**COMPLEMENTARY THERAPY FOR HEART DISEASE: HERBALISM**

| Herb | Intended purpose | Outcome |
|---|---|---|
| Garlic | To reduce low-density-lipoprotein (LDL) cholesterol | Inconsistent effects |
| | Antihypertensive | Not effective |
| Gugulipid | To reduce low-density-lipoprotein (LDL) cholesterol | Reduction of 15% to 20% |
| Vitamin C | Antihypertensive | Unclear effect |
| Ma huang | Obesity | Weight loss with palpitations and chest pain |

Modified from Torpy JM: Integrating complementary therapy into care, *JAMA* 287:306-307, 2002.

---

agement. Even though survival rates have improved, it is still necessary to continue to educate men concerning the risks and the need for regular examinations. Garguiullo et al. (2002) reported a 5-year survival rate of 95% for white men and 88% for African-American men.

Closely related and a precursor to prostate cancer is benign prostatic hyperplasia (BPH). Aging is the major risk factor for BPH. By 60 years of age, more than 50% of men will experience BPH. This rate increases to 90% by 85 years of age. In fact, one in four U.S. men will require treatment of symptomatic BPH by 80 years (Epperly and Moore, 2000). Symptoms may include frequency of urination, nocturia, urgency, straining to urinate, hesitancy in urination, weak or intermittent stream, and feeling of incomplete emptying. Prostate enlargement does not necessarily correlate with the severity of the symptoms or the amount of restriction to urine flow. Complications include urinary retention, renal insufficiency, urinary tract infections, hematuria, and bladder stones.

Symptom assessment may be done using a self-administered questionnaire called the American Urological Association Symposium Index (Madsen and Bruskewitz, 1995). This questionnaire consists of six symptom-related questions and one quality-of-life question. The symptoms (including most of those just listed) are scored from 0 (not at all) to 5 (almost always). The total score can range from 0 (asymptomatic) to 35 (highly symptomatic). The quality-of-life question has six possible responses ranging from delighted to terrible. Additional diagnostic tests are also used to reach a diagnosis. These include uroflometry, postvoid residual urine, pressure flow studies, and urethrocystoscopy.

## Testicular Cancer

**Testicular cancer** is a commonly found solid tumor malignancy in men 15 to 35 years of age. Jemal et al (2002)

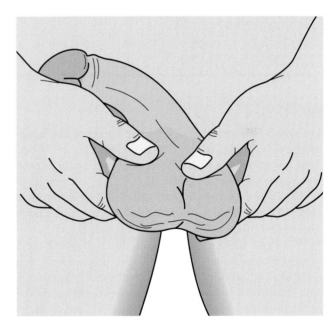

**Figure 28-1** Performing a testicular self-examination.

reported an estimated 7500 new cases and 400 deaths in 1 year. The etiology of this cancer, testicular germ cell, is unknown. Many possible explanations exist, such as age, family history, endocrine and genetic disorders, the human immunodeficiency virus (HIV), cryptorchidism (undescended testicles), and occupational factors.

The most common presenting symptom is a painless, firm scrotal mass or swelling accidentally discovered. Low back pain may result with retroperitoneal lymph node involvement. Unfortunately 64% of men do not do **testicular self-examination** (TSE) to detect this cancer (Wynd, 2002) (Figure 28-1).

Modeling and guided practice should be components of a comprehensive testicular educational program. A program should consist of audiovisual aids and pamphlets, followed by step-by-step procedures and return demonstrations (see the How To box on TSE). This approach results in men having an increased comfort level about performing the procedure and doing it more often. If tumors are found, the most common form of management is retroperitoneal lymph node dissection and chemotherapy for metastases larger than 3 cm.

> **HOW TO**    **Perform a Step-by-Step Monthly Testicular Self-Examination**
>
> 1. Perform the TSE while taking a warm bath or shower.
> 2. Roll each testicle between your thumb and fingers using warm hands. *Testicles should be egg-shaped, 4 cm in the longer dimension, and similar in size; they should have a rubbery texture; the left dangles lower than the right.*
> 3. Check the epididymis. *It should be soft and slightly tender.*
> 4. Check the spermatic cord. *It should have a firm, smooth, tubular structure.*

## Skin Cancer

The three main types of skin cancer are basal and squamous cell carcinomas and malignant melanomas. When these are combined, skin cancers rank fifth among newly reported cancers in men, with 30,100 cases, compared to 23,500 to women (Jemal et al, 2002). The death rate for men (3.4/100,000 population) is much higher than that for women (1.9/100,000 population) (Hoyert et al, 2001).

Prolonged sun exposure and high ultraviolet B rays cause skin cancer. Red-, blond-, or light-brown-haired men with light complexions or freckles are the most susceptible. Also, men with a history of long-term occupational or recreational sun exposure, such as farmers, construction workers, sailors, swimmers, surfers, and sunbathers, are at high risk.

Malignant melanoma is the deadliest form of skin cancer and the incidence is rising worldwide (Figure 28-2). This cancer can metastasize to the brain, lungs, bones, liver, and other areas of the skin with generally fatal results.

Prevention includes decreasing exposure to direct sunlight, especially between the peak hours of 10 A.M. and 3 P.M. Men should wear protective clothing and use a sunblock with an SPF rating of at least 15 when outside. Regular skin inspection and assessment are also important. Early diagnosis and treatment improve the chances of recovery.

## Accidents

The fourth leading cause of death in men of all ages is accidental death, with an age-adjusted death rate of 50.6 per 100,000 population. This death rate is significantly higher for men than for women of certain ages. For example, the male accident death rate peaks at 59 per 100,000 population in the 20- to 24-year-old age-group, compared to 17.6 for women in the same age-group. In fact, the accident death rates for men are twice those for women among 18- to 44-year-olds (Anderson, 2001).

### Fatal Accidents

Men are at greater risk for fatal occupational injuries than women. Injuries in construction and mining are two of the leading fatal occupational injuries. Other fatal injuries occur in manufacturing, wholesale trade, and agriculture.

Death rates from injury differ notably by sex. Among males, these rates increase with age. For boys between 1 and 4 years old, the death rate by drowning is twice that of girls. Among 5- to 14-year-old children, boys are at greater risk for other water accidents and more likely to die in a motor vehicle accident than girls. The injury death rates for 15- to 24-year-old males are three to four times those of females (USDHHS, 2000a).

### Nonfatal Accidents

An estimated 3.3 million persons age 16 years of age or older were treated for occupational injuries in emergency departments. This equates to an average annual rate of 2.8 injuries per 100 full-time employees (FTEs). An analysis of male to female injuries reveal rates of 3.3 per 100 FTEs for men (69% of total injuries) compared to 2.1 per 100 FTEs for women. An evaluation of the age-groups showed the most frequent injury rate for 18- to 19-year-old men (6.2 per 100 FTEs) and then for 20- to 24-year-old men (5.9 per 100 FTEs). In comparison, the most frequent rates in women were for 18- to 19-year-old women (2.7 per 100 FTEs) and 20- to 24-year-old women (2.6 per 100 FTEs). About 27% of the nonfatal injuries were sprains and strains, followed by

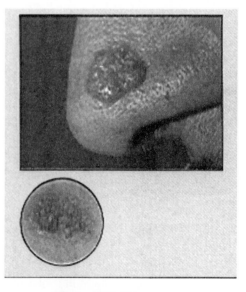

**Figure 28-2** Skin cancer.

lacerations (22%) and contusions/abrasions/hematomas (20%) (Surveillance for nonfatal occupational injuries, 1998).

## Pulmonary Diseases

Chronic lower respiratory diseases such as bronchitis, emphysema, and asthma are the fifth leading cause of age-adjusted death among men. Men have a greater chance of dying from chronic pulmonary problems than women. Also, the death rate from respiratory system cancer is higher in men (67.1 per 100,000) than in women (45.0 per 100,000) (Hoyert et al, 2001).

Smoking is a definite risk factor for pulmonary disease. Historically, men have used tobacco more heavily than women; however, this trend is changing. In 1955, approximately 65% of men 18 years old and older smoked cigarettes compared, to 25% of women. Most recently, overall smoking reduction has occurred more sharply for men (27.6%) than for women (22%) (Centers for Disease Control and Prevention, 1999).

There are also cultural differences in smoking rates. Winkleby et al (1999) found white boys and girls had an increase in smoking rates at 14 to 17 years of age, followed by a doubling for white women and a tripling for white men between the ages of 18 and 24. Hispanic boy's smoking rates were comparable to those of white boys through age 17, but they only doubled between the ages of 18 and 24, compared to younger age-groups. There was also a substantial increase in smoking for African-American men in the 18- to 24-year-old age-group.

### WHAT DO YOU THINK?

It is clear that tobacco use in any form has detrimental effects on personal health. Current legislation has limited or banned smoking in public places. These policies have been criticized by smokers who cite the "common courtesy approach" as being effective.

## Suicide

Some of the most significant health differences between men and women occur in the mental health domain. The age-adjusted suicide rate in men is 18.2 per 100,000 population, compared with 4.1 for women, representing nearly a fivefold gender difference. Suicide is the eighth leading cause of death overall for men; high-risk groups are men 15 to 34 years old (the third leading cause) and men 35 to 44 years old (the fourth leading cause) (Anderson, 2001; Hoyert et al, 2001).

Men are more likely to make a serious attempt to kill themselves than to use a suicide attempt as a cry for help. Firearms are the most common method of suicide, and 79% of all firearm suicides are committed by white men. Furthermore, white men over 85 have the highest suicide rate (59/100,000) of all age-groups (National Institute of Mental Health [NIMH], 1999).

Suicide, and the grief it causes family members and friends, can often be prevented. Community-oriented nurses can often identify men at risk for suicide. Table 28-5 shows the suicidal risk factors. Despite the widespread use of telephone crisis lines, school-based intervention programs, and antidepressive medications, high rates of suicide continue. All suicide attempts should be taken seriously. The nursing goal is to detect risk factors, promote safety, prevent self-harm, make appropriate referrals, and help people back to health.

## Assaults

Men are also prone to engage in dangerous and risky behavior, such as carrying weapons and fighting. The age-adjusted homicide death rate for men is 9.4 per 100,000 population, compared with 2.9 for women. Homicides are the 14th leading cause of death in men of all ages. More significantly, the death rate data are four to six times higher in men than in women at selected age-groups. For example, in the 15- to 19-year-old age-group, the male assault death rate is 17.2 per 100,000 compared to 3.6 for women; the rate peaks to 26.2 for men compared to 5.2 for women in the 20- to 24-year-old age-group, and remains lopsided in the 25- to 35-year-old age-group, where it is 17.8 versus 4.6 (Anderson, 2001).

**Assaultive violence** is the threat or attempt to strike another aimed at causing fatal or nonfatal injury, whether successful or not, provided the target is aware of the danger (National Center for Injury Prevention and Control,

| Table 28-5 | Suicide Risk Factors |
| --- | --- |
| **FACTOR** | **EFFECT OF FACTOR** |
| Gender | Men use more violent means and have a higher completed suicide rate than women. |
| Marital status | Unmarried men have a greater risk than married men. |
| Employment | Unemployed men are at greater risk. |
| Previous attempts | Men with more than one attempt have a much higher chance of attempting it again. One quarter to one half of deaths are by people who have made previous attempts. |
| Family history | A positive family history increases the risk of suicide. |
| Medical illness | Men suffering from terminal illness or other medical conditions are at high risk. |

2000). The assaulter must be reasonably capable of carrying through the attack. Assaultive violence is both a criminal wrong, for which one may be charged and tried, and a civil wrong, for which the target may sue for damages due to the assault, including for mental distress. Rates of assaultive violence are largely influenced by broad-scale social forces, such as poverty, lack of opportunity, that operate independently of human cognition.

Multiple reasons are cited for violent behavior. For example, brain dysfunction is associated with irregularities in the limbic system, the part of the brain that regulates emotions and motivation and is associated with violence. Other causes of dysfunction include organic brain disease, psychosis, depression, mental retardation, and brain tumors.

Violence is associated with social, economic, cultural, and environmental factors that contribute to assaults. Poverty and inner-city residency have also been shown to be strongly associated with violent victimization (see Chapter 37). An analysis of race reveals African-American, Hispanic, and Native American men assault death rates are much higher than those of white men for the 15- to 34-year-old age-groups. For example, the homicide death rate for African-American males 15 to 19 years old is 63, for Hispanic it is 29.4, for Native Americans 18.7, and for white men 8.7/100,000. Furthermore, for African-American men 20 to 24 years old, the homicide death rate is 110, for Hispanics 40, for Native Americans 23, and for white men 12/100,000 (Anderson, 2001). One example of health-related problems related to gun ownership is workplace homicides. Examples can be found in daily newspapers or by listening to the television news.

Little is known about the long-term effects men experience following sexual assaults. Nurses need to understand violent crimes and develop prevention and educational programs for assisting the male victim. Until such programs are available, nurses must continue to support and provide counseling for the male victim who demonstrates emotional distress.

Violence is a public health emergency. Solutions are complex but are believed to be reachable. First, nurses need to identify signs and symptoms of violent behavior. The practitioner should be concerned about a man who is excessively restless and agitated; he may pace up and down or start pounding on walls, doors, furniture, and other objects. He may appear angry and tense by clenching his teeth, jaw, and fists. His voice may become loud, and he may use profanity. He may become argumentative by refusing to follow directions and making threats. Another sign to watch for includes impulsive behaviors. Alcohol and drug abuse and psychiatric disorders are highly associated with violent behavior. Finally, the most predictive indicator of violence is a history of aggressive behavior and family violence.

## Alcohol-Induced Disorders

In the Special Report to the U.S. Congress on Alcohol and Health (2000), the USDHHS reported approximately 14 million Americans meet the diagnostic criteria for alcohol abuse or alcoholism. This is equal to 7.4% of the population. Furthermore, the USDHHS reported there is a relationship between alcohol and crimes. Of the 11.1 million annual victims of violent crimes, 27% reported that the offender had a drinking problem.

An evaluation of gender differences reveals the men's age-adjusted death rate from alcohol-induced causes was 3.6 times the rate for women (Hoyert et al, 2001).

Chronic liver disease and cirrhosis are health hazards associated with alcohol abuse. Age-adjusted death rates from alcohol abuse demonstrate striking differences between men and women: 13.7 per 100,000 for men compared with 6.1 for women. African-American men have an even higher death rate of 15.1, compared to 6.4 for African-American women, and the rate for Hispanic men is 23.0 compared to 8.5 for Hispanic women. Comparisons of races in the 55- to 60-year-old age-group revealed that death rates related to alcohol were 80/100,000 among Native American men, 45/100,000 among African-American men, and 34/100,000 among whites (Anderson, 2001; Hoyert et al, 2001).

Patterns of alcohol, tobacco, and drug use established during the teen years often persist into adulthood and contribute to mortality and morbidity. Alcohol is closely associated with several negative aspects of society: suicide, violent crime, birth defects, and domestic and sexual abuse. Rivara et al (1997) found alcohol and illicit drug use were associated with increased risk of violent deaths in the home. Males drinking and using drugs accounted for the majority of the homicide (63%) and suicide victims (72%).

Motor vehicle accidents among teenage drivers are a leading cause of death, and a significant percentage of the deaths are alcohol related. Elder and Shults (2002) found the highest rate of alcohol-related fatal crashes occurred with the 21- to 24-year-old age group (16 per 100,000 population), followed by 18- to 20-year-olds (14 per 100,000 population) and 16- to 17-year-olds (6 per 100,000).

Alcohol has harmful effects on the male reproductive system. Alcohol use is associated with low testosterone and altered levels of additional reproductive hormones. Also, researchers investigated several potential mechanisms for alcohol's damage. These mechanisms are related to alcohol metabolism, alcohol-related cell damage, and other hormonal reactions associated with alcohol consumption. Chronic alcohol use in male rats also has been shown to affect their reproductive ability and the health of their offspring (Emanuele and Emanuele, 2001).

In the United States, alcohol consumption is a major drug problem. Nurses must start educating the younger population about the effects of alcohol. One focal point is the message to *stop underage drinking*. Even though alcohol use under 21 years of age is illegal in most states, alcohol is easily accessible. Education is the best prevention at this time (Box 28-5).

## BOX 28-5  Population Intervention for Alcohol-Related Injuries

A population-based alcohol reduction intervention can reduce men's deaths. Holder et al. (2000) demonstrated that a coordinated, comprehensive, population-based intervention can reduce young men's high-risk alcohol consumption patterns (such as binge drinking, drinking and driving, and underage drinking), which are linked to vehicular accidents and homicides. Community-oriented nurses can plan interventions targeted to reduce high-risk drinking and alcohol-related injuries and assaults. The community interventions consisted of five prevention strategies: (1) to mobilize the community to support the project through community coalitions and media advocacy; (2) to advise alcohol distributors and retailers to develop policies to reduce intoxication and drunk driving; (3) to reduce underage access by advising retailers to stop selling alcohol to men under 21; (4) to increase the actual and perceived risk of arrest for drunk driving; and (5) to assist the community in developing local restriction of alcohol through zoning laws.

Other strategies that the nurse can work with the community to implement include (1) buying state-of-the-art breath-testing technology; (2) encouraging police to conduct roadside checks to detect drinking and driving; and (3) encouraging police to conduct sting operations to enforce responsible beverage distribution.

Modified from Holder HD et al: Effect of community-based interventions on high-risk drinking and alcohol-related injuries, *JAMA* 284(18):2341-2347, 2000.

## Human Immunodeficiency Virus

Although HIV has not made the top 15 for all causes of U.S. deaths for many years, the disease continues to be a major U.S. and worldwide health concern. However, HIV is a leading cause of death in the United States for young and middle-age men. The disease is the seventh leading cause of death for the 20- to 24-year-old age-group and the sixth leading cause for the age-group of 25 to 54. Furthermore, there is a wide difference in death rates between men and women. For all ages and all races, the age-adjusted men's death rate is 8.4 per 100,000 population, whereas for women it is 2.6 per 100,000. After the late 1990s, the U.S. epidemic shifted from white men to African-American and Hispanic men. Evaluating race and gender, the African-American male death rate is highest at 82.7, followed by Hispanic males at 28 and white males at 13.2/100,000 for the 35- to 44-year-old age-group. Even higher are the death rates in the 45- to 54-year-old age-group for African-American men (89.3) and Hispanic men (24.9) (Anderson, 2001; Hoyert et al, 2001). Furthermore, death rates for males from HIV and acquired immunodeficiency syndrome (AIDS) around the world far outnumber those for women on every continent except sub-Saharan Africa.

### DID YOU KNOW?

If a person with HIV or AIDS knowingly infects another person, it may be considered a criminal offense.

Men must evaluate their behavior and fight this infectious disease. Men's behaviors result in their having higher infection rates than women. Men drink more alcohol, inject more illegal drugs, and use other substances that lead to unsafe sex. For example, 80% of the world's people who inject drugs are men. This risky behavior accounted for 36% of the total U.S. AIDS cases and 22% of the new cases in 1999. Men by and large have more sex partners; therefore, they transmit the virus to more people than women. Unprotected sex initiated by men accounts for the highest risk factor category for the infection. For example, the data reveal that for all ages and all races, men who have sex with men account for 40% of the new HIV cases. Among young men, 75% of the HIV cases come from men having sex with men (American Association for World Health, 2000).

The American Association for World Health recommends that men become active in combating the proliferation of HIV. Men need to change their beliefs about themselves and share these thoughts with the younger generation. In the U.S. culture, men feel pressure to exert their manhood, which means being physically and emotionally detached, dominating others, and being invulnerable and virile. However, this self-image leads to unhealthy behaviors resulting in infectious diseases.

The following manhood stereotypes lead to higher incidence of HIV:
- Real men take risks.
- Real men use drugs.
- Real men have more sex.
- Real men have multiple sex partners.
- Safe sex is unmanly.
- Real men don't visit health professionals when they are sick.
- Real men don't seek help for problems.
- Real men don't take care of children.

There are two community-oriented approaches in the battle to prevent HIV: (1) uninfected men should focus on keeping themselves from becoming infected, and (2) HIV-positive men should focus on preventing opportunistic infections. Box 28-6 has recommendations for avoiding HIV infection.
- Abstinence from sexual intercourse is the surest way to avoid becoming infected.
- Do not have sex with someone if you are not sure of his or her health status.
- Commit to a monogamous relationship with a person free of HIV.
- Use only new latex condoms and only water-based lubricant.

**BOX 28-6**   **Three Levels of Prevention for HIV**

**PRIMARY PREVENTION**

The nurse advises men who have sex with other men to use a new latex condom during oral or anal sex. In group and individual counseling about HIV, the nurse indicates to clients that they should not share needles, syringes, razors, or toothbrushes.

**SECONDARY PREVENTION**

The nurse advises an infected man to swallow all of his highly active antiretroviral therapy (HAART) medication on schedule. The nurse advises a man who had unprotected sex to be tested with a standard enzyme-linked immunosorbent assay (ELISA), followed by a confirmatory Western blot test.

**TERTIARY PREVENTION**

The nurse teaches men newly diagnosed with HIV to exercise regularly, eat a balanced nutritious diet, sleep at least 8 hours a day, and stop or limit alcohol. The nurse advises clients not to donate blood, plasma, or organs.

- Unprotected anal sex is extremely risky, especially if you or your partner has previously engaged in high-risk sex behavior.
- Always use sterile injection supplies.
- Seek treatment for substance abuse.
- Do not share needles, syringes, or other injection supplies.
- Seek personal counseling about your low self-esteem.

## MEN'S HEALTH PRACTICES IN EVERYDAY LIFE

Men and women both have biological and physiologic needs for rest, exercise, and food consumption to maintain health. However, they differ on health priorities. Women listed food first, then exercise, and then rest. Men emphasized exercise first, then sleep, and food last. Men emphasized the nutrient quality of food; women focused on the food's calories rather than its nutrient quality. Men perceived body maintenance activities as essential to producing health and emphasized sports and outdoor activities for better body maintenance. Furthermore, men viewed the body as a medium of action; function and capacity were of paramount importance.

The concept of **body maintenance** has two components: the inner and the outer body. Inner refers to optimal functioning, performance, and capacity to do things. Outer refers to appearance, movement within social space, and having the potential to be heard and touched. Men discern the inner body in terms of function and capacity. They would rather look at how they went through the day, what they accomplished, and what kind of physical shape

they are in so they can perform. Less attention is given to having good color and skin tones.

Men need to look at themselves and develop a plan to stay healthy by becoming knowledgeable about health and their own bodies. Along with knowledge comes desire to be healthy. In addition, men need to set health-related goals and develop an action plan. With the support of the nursing profession, men can take responsibility for changing and maintaining healthier lifestyles. Healthy People 2010 suggests objectives that will enhance men's health (see the Healthy People 2010 box). Table 28-6 summarizes men's biological and psychosocial health care needs.

## THE COMMUNITY-ORIENTED NURSE'S ROLE IN MEN'S HEALTH

Community-oriented nurses have knowledge and skills that enable them to assess, diagnose, plan, implement, and evaluate the care of men. Nurses using a range of skills and in a variety of roles work with men in diverse communities ranging from isolated agricultural regions to densely populated cities. The roles of educator, client advocate, case manager, and men's health nurse practitioner are discussed.

### Educator

The goal of patient education is to provide knowledge and skills for learning new behaviors or changing unhealthy behaviors. The educator's goal is to improve or maintain the health status of men. When the community-oriented nurse encounters men in the clinics, health departments, or their homes, a teaching opportunity exists. The myth about men not being receptive to health information is not substantiated by research.

### Client Advocate

The goal of client advocacy is to ensure that men's long-term health care needs are met. The goal for the advocacy role is to inform and support men in their health care decisions. The nurse needs to become knowledgeable about the health care options and to support the patient in his decisions. For example, after a myocardial infarction, a man needs to be informed about his treatment options, (e.g., diet, exercise, drugs, therapy, stress reduction, and surgical interventions). The nurse should assist him in seeing his options so that he can make effective and cost-conscious decisions.

> **NURSING TIP**
>
> Use the therapeutic communication skills of empathy and respect when gathering information from men about their health.

### Case Manager

Being a case manager in men's health means more than just coordinating patient services. The role involves prob-

## Healthy People 2010 | Objectives Related to Men's Health

### 3. CANCER

3-5 Reduce the colorectal cancer death rate

3-7 Reduce the prostate cancer death rate

3-8 Reduce the rate of melanoma cancer deaths

3-9 Increase the proportion of persons who use at least one of the following protective measures that may reduce the risk of skin cancer: avoid the sun between 10 A.M. and 4 P.M., wear sun-protective clothing when exposed to sunlight, use sunscreen with a sun protective factor (SPF) of 15 or higher, and avoid artificial sources of ultraviolet light

3-12 Increase the proportion of adults who receive a colorectal cancer screening examination

### 9. FAMILY PLANNING

9-6 Increase male involvement in pregnancy prevention and family planning efforts

### 12. HEART DISEASE AND STROKE

12-1 Reduce coronary heart disease deaths

12-2 Increase the proportion of adults aged 20 years and older who are aware of the early warning symptoms and signs of a heart attack and the importance of accessing rapid emergency care by calling 911

12-7 Reduce stroke deaths

12-9 Reduce the proportion of adults who are aware of the early warning symptoms and signs of a stroke

12-11 Increase the proportion of adults with high blood pressure who are taking action (e.g., losing weight, increasing physical activity, and reducing sodium intake) to help control their blood pressure

### 13. HUMAN IMMUNODEFICIENCY VIRUS

13-2 Reduce the number of new AIDS cases among adolescent and adult men who have sex with men

13-3 Reduce the number of new AIDS cases among females and males who inject drugs

13-4 Reduce the number of new AIDS cases among adolescent and adult men who have sex with men and inject drugs

13-6 Increase the proportion of sexually active persons who use condoms

13-8 Increase the proportion of substance abuse treatment facilities that offer HIV/AIDS education, counseling, and support

### 15. INJURY AND VIOLENCE PREVENTION

15-3 Reduce firearm-related deaths

15-4 Reduce nonfatal unintentional injuries

15-15 Reduce deaths caused by motor vehicle crashes

15-32 Reduce homicides

15-37 Reduce physical assaults

### 18. MENTAL HEALTH AND MENTAL DISORDERS

18-1 Reduce the suicide rate

### 26. SUBSTANCE ABUSE

26-1 Reduce deaths and injuries caused by alcohol- and drug-related motor vehicle crashes

26-3 Reduce drug-induced deaths

26-7 Reduce intentional injuries resulting from alcohol- and illicit-drug–related violence

### 27. TOBACCO USE

27-1 Reduce tobacco use by adults

27-2 Reduce tobacco use by adolescents.

From U.S. Department of Health and Human Services: *Healthy people 2010: national health promotion and disease prevention objectives,* ed 2, Washington, DC, 2000, U.S. Government Printing Office.

lem solving and managing men's health care services in a supportive, effective, and efficient manner. The American Nurses Association (1988) described the nursing care manager's role as "a health care delivery process whose goals are to provide quality health care, decrease fragmentation, enhance the client's quality of life, and contain cost." The role of the case manager is structured to the client's needs.

## Men's Health Nurse Practitioner

Bozett and Forrester, in 1989, argued that men's health care needs are not being met by physicians. Typically, men choose not to communicate their health concerns to physicians. In the office and clinics, pleasantries and shallow comments are exchanged, and critical health care concerns are avoided. Physicians rarely give their male patients adequate time for reflective discussion and thoughtful communications about their health needs. Furthermore,

physicians focus on pathologic findings and "cure" treatments. Prevention and health promotion activities are not high priorities.

A **men's health nurse practitioner** (MHNP) can alleviate some of these concerns. This advanced practice role can deliver comprehensive men's health care, assessing and managing minor health problems as well as acute and chronic conditions. The functions and roles of the MHNP include conducting histories and physical examinations, ordering and interpreting diagnostic studies, prescribing medications and treatments, providing health maintenance care, promoting positive health behaviors and self-care, and collaborating with physicians and other health professionals. Effective interpersonal skills and empathetic listening are important communication skills the nurse practitioner can use to facilitate men discussing their health concerns.

## Table 28-6　Men's Health Care Needs

| | BIOLOGICAL | PSYCHOSOCIAL | COMBINATION |
|---|---|---|---|
| Expression | | Desire to communicate with others about health care concerns | |
| Support | | Support from others about certain sex roles and lifestyles that influence their physical and mental health | |
| Respect and dignity | | | Attention from professionals regarding factors that may cause illness or affect a man's expression of illness, including occupational factors, leisure patterns, and interpersonal relationships |
| Health-seeking knowledge and behaviors | Information about their body's functions, what is normal and abnormal, what action to take, and the contributions of proper nutrition and exercise<br>Self-care instruction including testicular and genital self-examinations<br>Physical examination and history taking, including sexual and reproductive health and illness across the life span | | |
| Holistic medical care and availability | | Adjustment of health care system to men's occupational constraints related to time and location of health care | Treatment for problems of couples, including interpersonal problems, infertility, family planning, sexual concerns, and sexually transmitted diseases |
| Parental guidance | | Help with fathering (e.g., being included as a parent in care of children)<br>Help with fathering as a single parent—in particular, with a child of the opposite sex, in addressing the child's sexual development and concerns | |
| Coping | | Recognition that feelings of confusion and uncertainty in a time of rapid social change are normal and may mark onset of healthy adaptation to change | |
| Fiduciary | | Financial ways to obtain the preceding needs | |

# Practice Application

Analyze the following case. Focus on the issues of how men define health, the developmental patterns and the health practices of men, and a nursing care plan.

John, a 29-year-old white man with a wife and three children, was employed as a sales representative in a small, rural community. His health was excellent except for injuries sustained in a car accident several years ago that required three blood transfusions. After the accident, John returned to work, thinking he was fully recovered. His business success continued, and he was well respected by employers, co-workers, and community leaders.

Years after the accident, John became ill with pneumonia and required hospitalization. While he was hospitalized, a blood test discovered HIV. John and his family decided to keep his condition confidential so he could live the rest of his life as normally as possible.

When John returned to work, his co-workers seemed distant and they avoided him. He began to receive threatening telephone calls telling him to leave town, and his car was spray-painted with derogatory words. Clearly, there had been a breach of confidentiality. John later discovered his hospital file was marked "AIDS" in large red letters. Furthermore, he learned that nurses had refused to care for him while he was hospitalized and that he was the focus of dinner conversation throughout the hospital.

John's circumstances worsened, and he felt isolated and rejected. He was eventually fired from work, losing health insurance for himself and his family. His wife divorced him. All his accumulated savings were depleted. He could not pay his hospital bills, and he filed for bankruptcy.

John is now homeless. His symptoms have progressed. He has a fever, tachypnea, lymphadenopathy, night sweats, and diarrhea. A friend has suggested he visit the local clinic, but John is reluctant to speak about his disease. He is extremely fatigued and whispers softly. He refuses any governmental services. However, you, the nurse in the public health clinic, are able to convince him to enter the homeless shelter across the street for the night. You ask him to return to the clinic in the morning.

  A. What information do you want to collect?
  B. What data might you collect, and what nursing diagnoses might be relevant?
  C. What short-term goals are appropriate for the first clinic visit?
  D. What long-term goals do you want to plan with John?
  E. What social and health agencies would you consult in planning for John's care?
  F. What outcome criteria should you use to evaluate the effectiveness of your plans and interventions?

**Answers are in the back of the book.**

# Key Points

- Men are physiologically the more vulnerable sex, demonstrated by shorter life spans and a higher infant mortality.
- Men's psychosocial and moral development continues through young and middle adulthood.
- Life expectancy of men in the United States is one of the lowest in developed countries.
- Men engage in more risk-taking behaviors such as physical challenges and illegal behaviors than do women.
- The most significant death rate differences between men and women are related to AIDS, suicide, homicide, and accidents.
- Men tend to avoid diagnosis and treatment of illnesses that may result in serious health problems.
- Legislation has been enacted that is helpful to men in the areas of elder care, worker's compensation, Americans with disabilities, family and medical leaves, and veterans.
- The men's health nurse practitioner is an advanced practice role focusing on the comprehensive health needs of men.

# Clinical Decision-Making Activities

1. Interview six men ranging in age from 21 to 70 years and ask them to list what they believe are health risk factors for them, what activities they regularly engage in that promote health, and what changes they believe they should make to improve their own health and reduce any existing risk factors. How do their answers compare to the recommendations from the Clinical Preventive Services Guidelines? (See Appendix A.1.)
2. Using the information gathered in the preceding activity, design a plan for health promotion for each man who is interviewed using the man's lifestyle, occupation, interest in social and recreational activities, income level, health risks, limitations in activities, and medical conditions. Review this plan with the man and determine how effectively it fits his perception of what he might do to ensure a healthier state. How would you contract with him to implement the plan?
3. Using the information gathered from the interviews and from the design of the health plan, determine at which developmental level the man is functioning. Is the level consistent with the age of the man? What do you know about developmental studies that relate to men?
4. Because morbidity and mortality data indicate that women live longer than men in the United States, interview 10 women ranging in age from 21 to 70 years and compare their health status, health risks, and participation in health-promoting behaviors

with those of the 10 men who were interviewed to see what differences exist that might explain the different life expectancies. Explain what you find.

5. Using the leading causes of men's death described in this chapter, design a diet for men from two different cultural groups in the United States that would promote health and reduce the risks from their leading causes of death. Be specific.

6. Because violence, suicide, and accidents are major causes of mortality for men in the United States, look at your community and describe the leading risk factors for violence, suicide, and accidents. Assess each category separately. Use statistical data to document incidence. What agencies exist in the community to help prevent death or disability from these three risk factors? What services do the agencies offer?

**Additional Resources**

These related resources are found either in the appendixes at the back of this book or on the book's website at **http://evolve.elsevier.com/Stanhope.**

**evolve Evolve Website**

Appendix A.1 Schedule of Clinical Preventive Services
Immunization Information
WebLinks: Healthy People 2010

# References

American Association for World Health: *World AIDS day 2000,* Washington, DC, 2000, ANA.

American Heart Association: *2002 heart and stroke statistical update,* Dallas, Tex, 2003, AHA

American Nurses Association: *Nursing care management,* Kansas City, Mo, 1988, ANA.

Anderson RN: Deaths: leading causes for 1999, *Natl Vital Stat Rep* 49(Suppl): 11, 2001.

Berenson GS, Sathanur R: Association between multiple cardiovascular risk factors and atherosclerosis in children and young adults, *N Engl J Med* 338(23):1650-1656, 1998.

Bozett FW, Forrester DA: A proposal for men's health nurse practitioner, *Image J Nurs Schol* 21:158-161, 1989.

Centers for Disease Control and Prevention: Achievements in public health, 1990-1999: tobacco use—United States, 1900-1999, *MMWR Morb Mortal Wkly Rep* 48(43):986-993, 1999.

Davidson K, Daly T: The extent to which partnership status of older men influences their health needs perceptions. *Gerontologist* 2:28, 2000.

Elder RW, Shults RA: Involvement by young drivers in fatal alcohol-related motor-vehicle crashes, *MMWR Morb Moral Wkly Rep* 51:1089-1091, 2002.

Emanuele MA, Emanuele N: Alcohol and the male reproductive system, *Alcohol Res Health* 25(4):282-287, 2001.

Epperly TD, Moore KE: Health issues in men: common genitourinary disorders, *Am Family Physician* 61:3657-3664, 2000.

Erikson E: *Identity: youth and crisis,* New York, 1968, Norton.

Garguiullo P et al: Recent trends in mortality rates for four major cancers, by sex and race/ethnicity—US, 1990-1998, *JAMA* 287(11):1391-1392, 2002.

Gaziano JM: When should heart disease prevention begin? *N Engl J Med* 338:(23):1690-1693, 1998.

Hill G, Hill K: *Real life dictionary of the law,* General Publishing Group, available at http://dictionary.law.com/.

Holder HD et al: Effect of community-based interventions on high-risk drinking and alcohol-related injuries, *JAMA* 284(18):2341-2347, 2000.

Hoyert DL et al: Deaths: final data for 1999, *Natl Vital Stat Rep* 49(8):1-113, 2001.

Hunink GM et al: The recent declines in mortality from coronary heart disease, 1980-1990: the effect of secular trends in risk factors and treatment, *JAMA* 277(7):535-542, 1997.

Jemal A et al: Cancer statistics, 2002, *CA Cancer J Clin* 52(1):23-27, 2002.

Jung CG: *Modern man in search of a soul,* New York, 1933, Harcourt Brace Jovanovich.

Knudtson ML, Wyse DG, Galbraith PD: Chelation therapy for ischemic heart disease: a randomized controlled trial, *JAMA* 287(4):481-486, 2002.

Kohlberg L: *Psychology of moral development: the nature and validity of moral stages,* San Francisco, 1984, Harper.

Madsen FA, Bruskewitz RC: Clinical manifestation of benign prostatic hyperplasia, *Urol Clin North Am* 22:291-298, 1995.

Millar W: Patterns of use: alternative health care practitioners, *Health Rep* 13(1):9-21, 2001.

National Cancer Institute of Canada: *Canadian cancer statistics 2001,* Toronto, 2001, NCIC.

National Center for Injury Prevention and Control, Centers for Disease Control and Prevention: *Youth violence,* Atlanta, 2003, available at www.cdc.gov.

National Institute of Mental Health: *Suicide facts, completed suicides: U.S. 1999,* 1999, available at www.nimh. nih.gov/research/suifact.htm.

Normand J: The health of women. In *Women in Canada 2000: a gender-based statistical report,* pp 47-83, Ottawa, 2000, Minister of Industry.

Office of Human Resource Management, Worker's Compensation Fund, 2003, available at: http://www.intranet. au.edu/hrm/workman.html.

Pobursky J: Prostrate cancer: detection and treatment options, *Today's OR Nurse* 17:5-9, 1995.

Rivara F et al: Alcohol and illicit drug abuse and the risk of violent death in the home, *JAMA* 278:569-575, 1997.

Rumrill P: Reasonable accommodations and the Americans With Disabilities Act: it's all about communication, *J Voc Rehab* 16:235-236, 2001.

Saltonstall R: Healthy bodies, social bodies: men's and women's concepts and practices of health in everyday life, *Soc Sci Med* 36:7, 1993.

*Statistical Yearbook, 1997,* New York, 2000, The United Nations.

*Statistical Yearbook, 2000,* New York, 2000, The United Nations.

Statistics Canada: *Age standardized mortality rates, 1997,* 1997a, retrieved July 2002 from www.statcan.ca/english/Pgdb/health30b.htm (also available at www.statcan.ca, choose Canadian statistics, and search for document name).

Statistics Canada: *Selected leading causes of death by sex, 1997,* 1997b, retrieved July 2002 from www.statcan.ca/english/Pgdb/health36.htm (also available at www.statcan.ca, choose Canadian statistics, and search for document name).

Statistics Canada: Taking risks and taking care, *Health Rep* 12(3):11-20, 2001a.

Statistics Canada: *Percentage of smokers in population 2000-2001,* 2001b, retrieved July 2002 from www.statcan.ca/english/Pgdb/health07b.htm (also available at www.statcan.ca, choose Canadian statistics, and search for document name).

Statistics Canada: *High blood pressure 2000-2001,* 2001c, retrieved July 2002 from www.statcan.ca/english/Pgdb/health03.htm (also available at www.statcan.ca, choose Canadian statistics, and search for document name).

Statistics Canada: *How healthy are Canadians? a summary 2001 annual report,* pp 1-6, Ottawa, 2002a, Health Statistics Division.

Statistics Canada: Injuries causing limitations of normal activities, by age-group, sex, and household population aged 12 and over (catalogue #82-221-XIE), *Health Indicators* 2002(1), 2002b, available at www.statcan.ca/english/freepub/82-221-XIE/01002/tables/html/12181.htm (also available at www.statcan.ca, choose Canadian statistics, and search for "injuries causing limitations").

Statistics Canada: Canadian community health survey: a first look, *The Daily,* May 8, pp 1-6, 2002c, retrieved from www.statcan.ca/Daily/English/020508/d020508a.htm (also available at www.statcan.ca, choose *The Daily,* and search for the document name).

Steele C: Short and long-term stability and change in older men's health following spousal bereavement, *Gerontologist* 2:28, 2000.

Surveillance for nonfatal occupational injuries treated in hospital emergency department: US, 1996, *MMWR Morb Mortal Wkly Rep* 47:302-306, 1998.

Torpy JM: Integrating complementary therapy into care, *JAMA* 287:306-307, 2002.

U.S. Department of Health and Human Services: *Health, United States 1999,* Hyattsville, Md, 2000b, Centers for Disease Control and Prevention, NCHS.

U.S. Department of Health and Human Services: *Healthy people 2010: understanding and improving health,* ed 2, Washington, DC, 2000a, U.S. Government Printing Office.

U.S. Department of Health and Human Services: *Special report to the U.S. Congress on alcohol and health,* ed 10, Washington, DC, 2000c, U.S. Government Printing Office.

U.S. Department of Labor: *Work injuries and illnesses by selected characteristics,* Washington, DC, 2003, Bureau of Labor Statistics.

Wilkins K: Health care consequences of falls for seniors, *Health Rep* 10(4):47-55, 1999.

Winkleby MA et al: Ethnic variation in cardiovascular disease risk factors among children and young adults, *JAMA* 282(11):1006-1013, 1999.

Wynd CA: Testicular self-examination in young adult men, *J Nurs Scholarsh* 34(3):251-255, 2002.

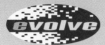
# Health of Older Adults

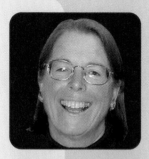

**Cynthia J. Westley, R.N.C., M.S.N., A.N.P.(c)**
Cynthia J. Westley is a community care manager in the University of Virginia Health System. She develops, implements, and evaluates programs related to the continuum of care supporting the health of older adults and individuals with chronic illness.

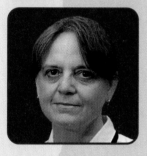

**Kathleen Ryan Fletcher, R.N., M.S.N., A.P.R.N.-B.C., G.N.P.**
Kathleen Ryan Fletcher is the administrator of senior services in the University of Virginia Health Systems in Charlottesville. She is involved in the development, implementation, and evaluation of interdisciplinary geriatric services throughout a continuum of care. Kathy has been with the University of Virginia since 1986.

## Objectives

After reading this chapter, the student should be able to do the following:

1. Describe the changing demography of older adults in the United States
2. Define terms commonly used to refer to older adults
3. Discuss various biological, psychosocial, and developmental theories of aging
4. Identify the multidimensional influences on aging and how these affect the health status of older adults
5. Detail the components of a comprehensive health assessment of an older adult
6. List chronic health problems often experienced by older adults
7. Describe several community-based models for gerontological nursing practice
8. Examine role opportunities in gerontological nursing for community-oriented nurses

The growth of the population ages 65 and older in the United States has steadily increased since the beginning of the twentieth century. In 1900, approximately 4% of the population was over age 65; today, older adults account for nearly 13% of the U.S. population. In the year 2030, the percentage of individuals over age 65 is projected to be about 25%. In the year 2000, there were 50,454 centenarians (individuals 100 years and older), and the number is expected to increase to about 500,000 in 2030. Reflecting the general U.S. population, the older U.S. population is more racially diverse than in the past. The effect this demographic shift has had on nursing practice in all settings is considerable. Estimates are that two thirds of a nurse's career today is spent working with older adults (Simon, Fletcher, and Francis, 1998). Because most health care for these clients is delivered outside the acute care setting, community-oriented nurses in particular have been providing nursing care to an increased proportion of older adults, which calls for specialized knowledge, skills, and abilities in gerontology.

This chapter begins by describing the demographic profile of older adults living in the United States and giving some introductory terminology. The multidimensional influences of aging and disease are then presented, followed by a detailed description of the gerontological assessment skills needed by the nurse. The chapter concludes with a discussion of role opportunities for practicing gerontology in the community.

## DEMOGRAPHICS

An individual born in 1900 could expect to live to be about 47 years old. A newborn in 1996 could expect to live to be about 76 years old. The older population numbered 35 million in 2000. Figure 29-1 shows the growth in older age groups between 1990 and 2000 (U.S. Bureau of the Census, 2001). The oldest old (those over age 85) are the fastest growing subgroup. The longer an individual lives, the more likely that person will live even longer. Persons reaching age 65 have an average life expectancy of an additional 18 years. Future growth projections reveal that by the year 2030, when the baby boom generation reaches age 65, there will be about 70 million older adults. That number represents more than twice the number in society today.

## Key Terms

advance medical directives, p. 709
ageism, p. 703
aging, p. 703
basic activities of daily living, p. 701
caregiver, p. 705
chronic illness, p. 707
durable medical power of attorney, p. 709
ego-integrity versus despair, p. 704
five Is, p. 709

geriatrics, p. 703
gerontological nursing, p. 703
gerontology, p. 703
instrumental activities of daily living, p. 701
life review, p. 704
living will, p. 709
long-term care facilities, p. 713
neglect, p. 709

older persons abuse, p. 709
Patient Self-Determination Act, p. 709
respite care, p. 711
three Ds, p. 709
wellness, p. 715
*See Glossary for definitions*

## Chapter Outline

Demographics
Definitions
Theories of Aging
*Biological Theories*
*Psychosocial Theories*
*Developmental Theories*
Multidimensional Influences on Aging

Components of a Comprehensive Health Assessment
Chronic Health Concerns of Older Adults in the Community
*Ethical and Legal Issues*
*Family Caregiving*
Community-Based Models for Gerontological Nursing

*Nursing Roles*
*Community Care Settings*
Role Opportunities for Nurses: Health Promotion, Disease Prevention, and Wellness

A closer look at the demographics of this generation today reveals a sex ratio of 145 women for every 100 men. Women outlive men by about 7 years, an advantage that is suspected to be biological. Minority populations today represent about 15% of all older adults, with projections that the minority composition will double by the year 2030. The western and southern regions of the United States are experiencing the most growth in total and older adult population.

Most older adults live in a noninstitutional community setting, and a majority (67%) of them live with someone else (Figure 29-2). About 4.5% live in a nursing home, a likelihood that increases significantly as one ages. For example, for persons in the 65- to 74-year-old age group, the percentage of individuals in a nursing home is 1%; it increases to 5% for persons ages 75 to 84, and to 18% for those over age 85. Older adults as a whole are not an affluent group. Of those reporting income to the Internal Revenue Service in 1996, 40% reported an annual income of less than $10,000.

Chronological age is an arbitrary way to project health care needs, and in this population there is a wide difference in state of health. The age of 65 has been used as a benchmark since 1935, when Franklin D. Roosevelt used it in eligibility criteria for Social Security. This seemed reasonable at the time, as most individuals did not live long enough to collect Social Security. As life expectancy has increased, however, consideration has been given to increasing the age of eligibility. Although using chronological age is limiting, some projections in the realm of physical function and prevalence of chronic illness can be made. More than half of people over age 65 report having difficulty in carrying out **basic activities of daily living** (ADLs, such as bathing, dressing, eating) and **instrumental activities of daily living** (IADLs, such as preparing meals, taking medications, managing money), with a disproportionate share of individuals with disability in the older age groups. In 1997, more than half (54.5%) of the older population reported having at least one disability of some type. As shown in Figure 29-3, the percentages with disabilities and a need for assistance with ADLs and IADLs increase sharply with age.

In 1999, 26.1% of older persons self-assessed their health as fair or poor compared to 9.2% for all persons. African Americans (41.6%) and Hispanics (35.1%) were

**Population 65 Years and Over by Age and Sex: 1990 and 2000**

(Numbers in thousands. For information on confidentiality protection, nonsampling error, and definitions, see *www.census.gov/prod/cen2000/doc/sfl.pdf.*)

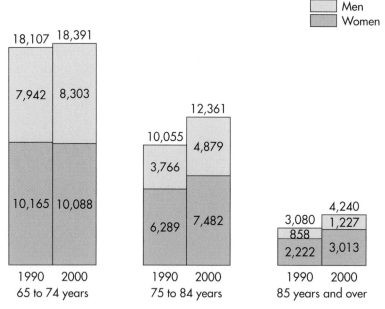

**Figure 29-1**  Population 65 years and over, by age and sex: 1990 and 2000. (Numbers in thousands. For information on confidentiality protection, nonsampling error, and definitions, see www.census.gov/prod/cen2000/doc/sfl.pdf.) *(From U.S. Bureau of the Census:* Census 2000, summary file 1: 1990 census of population, general population characteristics, *United States.)*

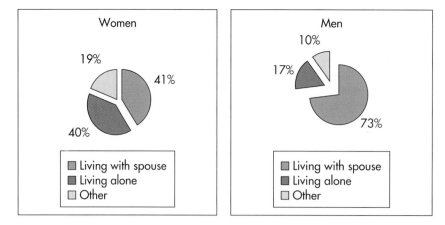

**Figure 29-2**  Living arrangements of persons 65 and over. *(Based on data from U.S. Bureau of the Census:* America's families and living arrangements: population characteristics, *June 2001, Current Population Reports, P20-537, Washington, DC, 2000, U.S. Government Printing Office;* The 65 years and over population: 2000, *Census 2000 brief, October, 2001, Washington, DC, 2000, U.S. Government Printing Office.)*

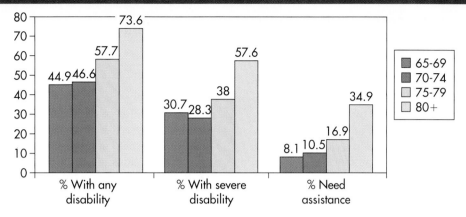

**Figure 29-3** Percent with disabilities by age, 1997. *(From: Administration on Aging: A profile of older Americans, 2001, available at www.aoa.dhhs.gov/aoa/stats/profile2001/.2.html.)*

more likely to rate their health as fair or poor than older whites (26%). The last few years of an older adult's life are often spent in declining physical functioning. A goal for nurses is to help older adults maximize functional status and minimize functional decline. Health promotion and disease prevention strategies must be emphasized in older adults.

---

**WHAT DO YOU THINK?**

Surveys documenting the functional status rating of an individual by the nurse, the caregiver, and the clients themselves often differ. What factors cause the different perspectives in measuring and noting functional status?

---

## DEFINITIONS

**Aging,** if defined purely from a physiologic perspective, is as a process of deterioration of body systems. This definition is clearly inadequate to describe the multidimensional aging process. Aging can be more appropriately defined as the total of all changes that occur in a person with the passing of time. Influences on how one ages come from several domains that include the physiologic, psychological, sociologic, and spiritual processes. The physiologic declines associated with aging have been easier to understand than aging as a process of growth and development.

Myths associated with aging have evolved over time. Some of the common myths involve the perception that all older adults are infirm or senile and cannot adapt to change or learn new behaviors or skills. These myths are easily debunked by those who run marathons, learn to use the internet, and are vibrant members of society. **Ageism** is the term used for prejudice about older people. Prejudice may be obvious or subtle. Ageism fosters a stereotype that does not allow older adults to be viewed realistically.

Changing demographics have facilitated the recognition of the special needs for older persons and the expansion of knowledge about the aging process. **Gerontology** is the specialized study of the processes of growing old. **Geriatrics** is the study of disease in old age. The American Nurses Association (ANA) encourages the use of the broader term *gerontological nursing* to refer to the specialized nursing of older adults that encompasses the perspectives of both health and illness. **Gerontological nursing** is the specialty of nursing concerned with assessment of the health and functional status of older adults, planning and implementing health care and services to meet the identified needs, and evaluating the effectiveness of such care (Lueckenotte, 2000).

## THEORIES OF AGING

There is no one definition of aging; however, circadian rhythms and metabolic clocks suggest that metabolic age is a more accurate measure of status than chronological age. Aging begins with conception and occurs continuously over time. Lack of a clear definition of aging leads to the development of many theories that attempt to explain a variety of influences on what we know is a complex process. Although it is inevitable that all persons will age, individuals age at different rates.

Hayflick (1994) noted, "Aging is not merely the passage of time. It is the obvious biological events that occur over a span of time. There is no perfect definition of aging, but, as with love and beauty, most of us know it when we experience it or see it." No one theory or definition can explain the process of aging. Thus biological, psychosocial, and developmental theories of aging have been developed.

## Biological Theories

These theories have a central theme of change. They are explained on molecular, cellular, and systemic levels. Genetics effects occur at all levels. Great strides are being made in understanding changes in aging; however, many questions remain unanswered. An individual theory may not totally answer the questions of aging but may attempt to explain the forces within the body that affect the aging process.

Other biological influences such as environment and nutrition need consideration as well. The daily ingestion of or contact with many substances can produce unhealthy changes. These include smoke and other air pollutants, mercury, lead, arsenic, and pesticides. What is eaten also can have a significant influence on aging. Too many, too few, or too poor in quality nutrients can negatively influence aging. Attention has been given to the influence of nutritional supplements on the aging process. It is important for nurses to keep an open mind to clients' desire for information. Information should be grounded in objective research, and clients should be educated to be careful consumers.

## Psychosocial Theories

Psychologists study personality, development, heredity, environmental influences, intelligence, memory, and psychogenic disorders. Sociologists study attitudes, family structures, economic influences, cultural differences, and political influences. In the study of aging, they come together to address the effect of behavior of older adults on aging.

Disengagement theory, developed over 40 years ago (Cumming and Henry, 1961), states that society and individuals disengage in mutual withdrawal, allowing the individual to become more self-focused and balanced. This is contrasted to the activity theory. Activity theory states that it is important to maintain regular roles and activities that are both social and solitary and to develop new roles to substitute for lost roles. Most normal older persons do make choices, influenced by past experiences, to maintain a high level of activity.

Continuity theory focuses on the relationship between continued, consistent activity; coping abilities; and life satisfaction. Past experiences, decisions, and behaviors determine the predisposition to make present and future choices. Patterns of personality and coping are developed in early adulthood and continue into later life as an individual adapts to life changes (Havighurst, Neugarten, and Tobin, 1968).

Humanistic theorists, such as Carl Rogers and Abraham Maslow, give a holistic view of development that tries to account for different human experiences. Humanistic theory views people as unique, self-determined, worthy of respect, and guided by a variety of basic human needs. Rogers believed that the process of becoming a fully functioning adult is aided throughout life by important relationships that provide unconditional positive regard (Berger, 1994). Maslow thought that an individual's behavior was motivated by universal needs that range from the most basic (food, sleep, safety) to the highest need for self-actualization (Maslow, 1968).

There is a complex interaction between culture, health status, socioeconomic status, and personality influences on aging. When performing an assessment, the nurse must consider the client's current situation and social network, as well as past history of coping behavior, and must try to not make assumptions based on the individual's chronological age.

## Developmental Theories

Aging is a process, and all individuals must perform certain developmental tasks at different stages of life. Clark and Anderson (1967) characterized developmental tasks as an internal change process. They refer to adaptive tasks as the externalization of that internal process. Their theory demonstrates that although aging has positive and negative consequences, individuals continue to adjust and adapt by the following:

- Recognition of aging and definition of limitations
- Redefinition of physical and social life space
- Substitution of alternative sources of need satisfaction
- Reassessment of criteria for evaluation of the self
- Reintegration of values and life goals

Erik Erikson's (1959) stages of development are widely cited as a way of viewing development across the life span. His eighth stage, **ego-integrity versus despair,** describes the process of examining one's own life in relationship to humanity and the world. A sense of failure can lead to despair, depression, and fear of death rather than acceptance and satisfaction.

The process of **life review** involves recalling past life experiences in an attempt to believe that one's life has had meaning and to prepare for death without fear. Reminiscence can help maintain self-esteem and reaffirms a sense of identity (Burnside and Haight, 1994). Egan (1996) developed a reminiscing game to help players share their life philosophy and early memories. Nurses can use tools like this and can employ active listening techniques to help clients validate their lives, resolve conflicts, and complete the tasks of aging.

Numerous predictable and unpredictable events occur in an individual's life. Even as the complexity and individuality of aging is acknowledged, it is necessary to organize the process through theories. Theories can provide a useful framework as long as the nurse maintains an appreciation for the individuality of each older adult client.

## MULTIDIMENSIONAL INFLUENCES ON AGING

The client experiences aging in many ways: physiologically, psychologically, sociologically, and spiritually. Physiologic changes occur in all body systems with the passing of time. There is considerable variation between individuals in how and when these processes occur, and there is variation in the degree of aging within the various body systems in the same individual. Table 29-1 highlights physiologic changes seen with the aging of body systems, and the nursing implications of these changes. The effect of these physiologic changes overall result in a diminished physiologic reserve, a decrease in homeostatic mechanisms, and a decline in immunologic response. No known intrinsic psychological changes occur with aging. The personality and developmental theories noted previously imply certain expectations and behaviors related to later life; however, these are

## Table 29-1  Physiologic Age-Related Changes in Body Systems

| SYSTEM | AGE-RELATED CHANGE | IMPLICATION FOR NURSING |
|---|---|---|
| Skin | Skin thins | Skin breakdown and injury |
| | Atrophy of sweat glands | Increased risk of heat stroke |
| | Decrease in vascularity | Frequent pruritus, dry skin |
| Respiratory | Decreased elasticity of lung tissue | Reduced efficiency of ventilation |
| | Decreased respiratory muscle strength | Atelectasis and infection |
| Cardiovascular | Decrease in baroreceptor sensitivity | Orthostatic hypotension and falls |
| | Decrease in number of pacemaker cells | Increased prevalence of dysrhythmias |
| Gastrointestinal | Dental enamel thins | Periodontal disease |
| | Gums recede | Swallowing dysfunction |
| | Delay in esophageal emptying | Constipation |
| | Decreased muscle tone | Altered peristalsis |
| Genitourinary | Decreased number of functioning nephrons | Modifications in drug dosing may be required |
| | Reduced bladder tone and capacity | Incontinence more common |
| | Prostate enlargement | May compromise urinary function |
| Neuromuscular | Decrease in muscle mass | Decrease in muscle strength |
| | Decrease in bone mass | Osteoporosis, increased risk of fracture |
| | Loss of neurons/nerve fibers | Altered sensitivity to pain |
| Sensory | Decreased visual acuity, depth perception, adaptation to light changes | May pose safety issues |
| | Loss of auditory neurons | Hearing loss may cause limitation in activities |
| | Altered taste sensation | May change food preferences and intake |
| Immune | Decrease in T cell function | Increased incidence of infection |
| | Appearance of autoantibodies | Increased prevalence of autoimmune disorders |

not specific or discrete. The influences of the environment and culture on personal development and maturation are substantial and further limit the ability of the nurse to predict how an individual ages psychologically.

Some known and some disputed changes in brain function over time may influence cognition and behavior. Reaction speed and psychomotor response is somewhat slower, which can be related to the neurologic changes that occur with aging. This is demonstrated particularly during timed tests of performance, where speed is an influencing variable. It has also been demonstrated in simulated tests of driving skills, where speed of response, perception, and attention slow with age. Typically, older individuals can learn and perform as well as younger individuals, though they may be slower and it may take them longer to accomplish a specific task.

Intellectual capacity does not decline with age as was previously thought. An age-associated memory impairment, benign senescent forgetfulness, involves very minor memory loss. This is not progressive and does not cause dysfunction in daily living. Reassurance is important for the older adult and families, as anxiety often exacerbates the problem of mild memory impairment. Memory aides (e.g., mnemonics, signs, notes) may help the client compensate for this type of impairment.

There are many external influences on mental health and aging, particularly those associated with loss and change. Adapting and coping responses of even the most resilient individuals will be challenged when successive losses and changes occur within a relatively short period. The later years for many older adults mark a period of changing social dynamics. Most older people continue to respond to life situations as they did earlier in their lives. Old age does not bring about radical changes in beliefs and values but may bring about abrupt changes over which they have little control. How individuals stay involved in activities and with people who bring their lives meaning and support is a major factor that can contribute to ongoing health and vitality. Depression is a factor in the ability of a person to cope with these changes. Box 29-1 is a geriatric depression scale.

Higher socioeconomic status, income, and education tend to be reflected in large and different types of social networks (Ebersole and Hess, 2001). For example, families typically remain involved with aging parents, with estimates that over 5 million are involved in some type of parent care as a caregiver. A **caregiver** is defined as one who provides unpaid, informal care to an older adult who requires help with ADLs and personal needs.

Although most of the multidimensional influences of aging are marked by decline and loss, it is almost never too

---

**BOX 29-1    Geriatric Depression Scale**

Use the following questionnaire to determine a client's degree of depression. Instruct the client, "Choose the best answer for how you felt the past week."

| | | |
|---|---|---|
| 1. Are you basically satisfied with your life? | Yes | No* |
| 2. Have you dropped many of your activities and interests? | Yes* | No |
| 3. Do you feel that your life is empty? | Yes* | No |
| 4. Do you often get bored? | Yes* | No |
| 5. Are you hopeful about the future? | Yes | No* |
| 6. Are you bothered by thoughts you can't get out of your head? | Yes* | No |
| 7. Are you in good spirits most of the time? | Yes | No* |
| 8. Are you afraid that something bad is going to happen to you? | Yes* | No |
| 9. Do you feel happy most of the time? | Yes | No* |
| 10. Do you often feel helpless? | Yes* | No |
| 11. Do you often get restless and fidgety? | Yes* | No |
| 12. Do you prefer to stay at home, rather than going out and doing new things? | Yes* | No |
| 13. Do you frequently worry about the future? | Yes* | No |
| 14. Do you feel you have more problems with memory than most? | Yes* | No |
| 15. Do you think it is wonderful to be alive now? | Yes | No* |
| 16. Do you often feel downhearted and blue? | Yes* | No |
| 17. Do you feel pretty worthless the way you are now? | Yes* | No |
| 18. Do you worry a lot about the past? | Yes* | No |
| 19. Do you find life very exciting? | Yes | No* |
| 20. Is it hard for you to get started on new projects? | Yes* | No |
| 21. Do you feel full of energy? | Yes | No* |
| 22. Do you feel that your situation is hopeless? | Yes* | No |
| 23. Do you think that most people are better off than you are? | Yes* | No |
| 24. Do you frequently get upset over little things? | Yes* | No |
| 25. Do you frequently feel like crying? | Yes* | No |
| 26. Do you have trouble concentrating? | Yes* | No |
| 27. Do you enjoy getting up in the morning? | Yes | No* |
| 28. Do you prefer to avoid social gatherings? | Yes* | No |
| 29. Is it easy for you to make decisions? | Yes | No* |
| 30. Is your mind as clear as it used to be? | Yes | No* |

*Each answer indicated by an asterisk counts 1 point. Scores between 15 and 22 suggest mild depression; scores above 22 suggest severe depression. A 15-item short-form includes questions 1-4, 7-10, 12, 14, 17, and 21-23. On the short form, scores between 5 and 9 suggest depression; scores above 9 generally indicate depression.

---

From Yesavage JA et al: Development and validation of a geriatric depression screening scale: a preliminary report. *J Psychiatr Res* 17(1):37-49, 1983.

---

late to begin benefiting from healthy habits such as smoking cessation, sensible diet, and exercise. Some age-related changes are reversible: with encouragement, clients can recover lost function and decrease health risks. It has been suggested that there is an increased spiritual awareness and consciousness as one ages and that religion is a powerful cultural force in the lives of older clients. Spirituality refers to the need to transcend physical, psychological, and social identities to experience love, hope, and meaning in life. Religious affiliations and religious rituals are one aspect of spirituality that can include other activities and relationships. Caring for pets and plants or experiencing nature through a walk in the woods can also foster spiritual growth. Physical and functional impairments and fear of death may challenge one's spiritual integrity. Having a strong sense of spirituality enables individuals who are physically and functionally dependant on others to avoid despair by appreciating that they are still capable of giving, and deserving of receiving, love, respect, and dignity.

## COMPONENTS OF A COMPREHENSIVE HEALTH ASSESSMENT

Assessing the health status of older clients poses challenges because of the wide variability in their health. It is important to look at the many dimensions of health on a continuum. If one looks at the physiologic, psychological, sociologic, and spiritual domains, the older adult may be at various points on the health continuum. For example, an individual may demonstrate successful psychological aging through adapting and coping while experiencing a physio-

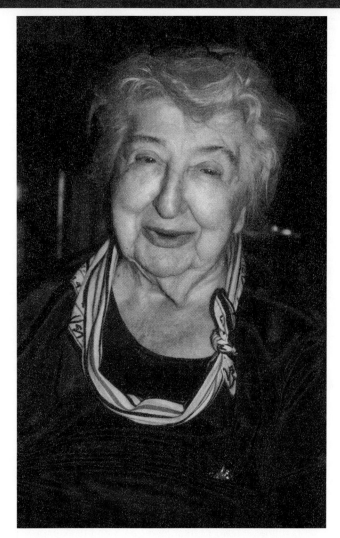

Although now in a wheelchair, this 88-year-old former operating room nurse still enjoys each day to its fullest.

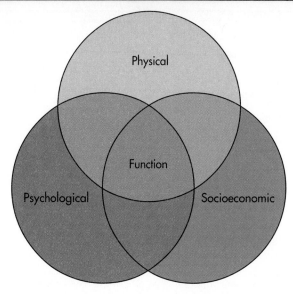

**Figure 29-4** Kane's conceptualization of central function. *(From Kane RL, Ouslander JG, Abrass IB:* Essentials of clinical geriatrics, *ed 4, New York, 1999, McGraw-Hill.)*

logically terminal disease or significant functional impairment. The nurse intervenes appropriately in each of these domains to help the client age successfully in each of these domains.

Effective care of clients by the nurse requires an accurate assessment of their health status. The goal of this care is to optimize health status and function and to minimize health decline and functional deterioration. Central to the comprehensive assessment is a functional assessment (Figure 29-4). A comprehensive geriatric assessment differs from a standard medical evaluation by including nonmedical issues, emphasizing functional ability and quality of life, and emphasizing interdisciplinary teams.

Finding a good assessment instrument that reflects all of these domains and yet is reasonable in terms of length is important. The multidimensional functional assessment of the Older American Resources and Services (OARS) organization is a lengthy and comprehensive tool designed to evaluate most of the domains just mentioned. The tool is designed to evaluate ability, disability, and the functional capacity level. Five dimensions are considered for assessment: social resources, economic resources, physical health, mental health, and ADLs. Each component uses a quantitative rating scale. At the conclusion of the assessment, a cumulative impairment score (CIS) is established. Once problems are assessed through a multidimensional process, the nurse uses the nursing process to diagnose and intervene in the problems (see Chapter 15).

## CHRONIC HEALTH CONCERNS OF OLDER ADULTS IN THE COMMUNITY

Chronic illnesses occur over a long period with occasional acute exacerbations and remissions. They can affect multiple systems and can be expensive and discouraging. The prevalence of chronic disease rises with the lengthening of the life span and the increasing availability of highly technical medical care. Until the late 1930s, illnesses were generally caused by bacteria or parasites. With antibiotics, immunizations, and public health measures, these diseases have decreased in Western nations and other health problems have become more common. Table 29-2 shows the prevalence of chronic conditions for men and women. Not only do chronic conditions cause disability and activity restriction but they often require frequent hospitalizations for exacerbations.

Health care in general is oriented toward acute illness. In **chronic illness,** cure is not expected, so nursing activities need to be more holistic, addressing function, wellness, and psychosocial issues. With chronic illness, the focus is on *healing* (a unique process resulting in a shift in the body–mind–spirit system) rather than *curing* (elimination

**Table 29-2    Percentages of Persons Age 70 or Older Who Report Having Selected Chronic Conditions—1995**

|  | ARTHRITIS | DIABETES | CANCER | STROKE | HYPERTENSION | HEART DISEASE |
|---|---|---|---|---|---|---|
| Total | 58.1 | 12.0 | 19.4 | 8.9 | 45.0 | 21.4 |
| Men | 49.5 | 12.9 | 23.4 | 10.4 | 40.5 | 24.7 |
| Women | 63.8 | 11.5 | 16.7 | 7.9 | 48.0 | 19.2 |
| 70 to 74 | 54.4 | 13.4 | 18.5 | 7.1 | 43.7 | 18.9 |
| 75 to 79 | 58.3 | 12.6 | 20.2 | 8.7 | 44.9 | 22.0 |
| 80 to 84 | 61.4 | 11.0 | 20.2 | 10.4 | 47.8 | 23.0 |
| 85 or older | 64.1 | 8.0 | 19.0 | 13.2 | 45.2 | 25.4 |
| Non-Hispanic—white | 57.9 | 10.9 | 21.0 | 8.6 | 44.0 | 22.0 |
| Non-Hispanic—black | 67.2 | 20.4 | 9.1 | 12.2 | 58.7 | 18.5 |
| Hispanic | 50.2 | 17.4 | 10.5 | 9.6 | 42.0 | 17.0 |

NOTE: Hispanics may be of any race. These data refer to the civilian noninstitutionalized population.
From National Center for Health Statistics: *Supplement on aging and second supplement on aging,* appendix 14, Washington, DC, 1997, U.S. Government Printing Office.

of the signs and symptoms of disease). Eliopoulos (2001) lists the following goals for chronic care:

- Maintain or improve self-care capacity
- Manage the disease effectively
- Boost the body's healing abilities
- Prevent complications
- Delay deterioration and decline
- Achieve highest possible quality of life
- Die with comfort, peace, and dignity

Chronic illness requires a shift in perspective compared with the rapid onset and focus on curing of an acute problem. The focus is on the development of self-management skills. The nurse is in partnership with the client, paying attention to the client's self-concept and self-esteem as well as to the resources that are needed to manage the disease outside the medical system. Goals for care are structured to help clients adjust their day-to-day choices to maintain the highest level of functional ability possible within the limits of their conditions. The motivation to make lifestyle choices necessary to cope with chronic illness stems from the fear of death; disability; pain; and negative effects on work, family, or activity. Redeker (1988) developed the health belief model to explain how individuals decide whether a choice is worth making. According to this model, knowledge of a medical condition does not affect compliance as much as personal thoughts and feelings and a therapeutic alliance with health care providers.

One way clients are taking more control of their own health is through the use of self-care or complementary and alternative health strategies. Older Americans are seeking out health information about complementary and alternative therapies and how to integrate them with their medical care. The nurse needs to have some knowledge about different therapies—some of which are legitimate and some fads—because the older person with chronic ill-

**BOX 29-2    Types of Alternative Medicine Commonly Used in the Elderly**

- Chelation therapy is used to treat atherosclerosis and other chronic degenerative diseases through intravenous infusions of ethylenediaminetetraacetic acid (EDTA) accompanied by vitamins, minerals, and other supplements.
- Chiropractic medicine focuses on the spine as integrally involved in maintaining health and balance. It is primarily used to treat lower back and neck pain.
- Naturopathy is a philosophy and way of life that emphasizes the body's ability to heal itself by the use of nutritional counseling, homeopathy, herbs, massage, yoga, hydrotherapy, fresh air, etc., and a general avoidance of drugs and surgery.
- Acupuncture is the practice of inserting needles into specific points along the body's meridian system to treat disease, relieve pain, and balance the flow of energy in the body.

From Jonas WB, Levin JS: *Essentials of complementary and alternative medicine,* Philadelphia, 1999, Lippincott Williams & Wilkins.

ness is especially vulnerable to fads (Box 29-2). Especially with cancer treatment, alternatives are seen as an integral part of the treatment of symptoms such as pain. The nurse should not make specific recommendations but have an open mind, encouraging the client to discuss self-care strategies used and determine how these strategies are supporting or hindering the client's health. A branch of the National Institutes of Health, the National Center for Complementary and Alternative Medicine, seeks to support rigorous research and provide information to the public and professionals on which modalities work and which do not, and why. The evidence that can be found on their website (http://nccam.nih.gove/) can help the nurse provide assistance to patients who are considering their various treatment options.

Tierney, McPhee, and Papadakis (2002) outline chronic conditions that can adversely affect the aging experience. These are intellectual impairment, immobility, instability, incontinence, and iatrogenic drug reactions, called the **five Is.** Their **three Ds** of intellectual impairment are dementia (progressive intellectual impairment), depression (mood disorder), and delirium (acute confusion).

Immobility is most often caused by degenerative joint disease and results in pain, stiffness, loss of balance, and psychological problems. Fear of falling is a major cause of immobility. This is related to instability, which results in 30% of falls each year.

Urinary incontinence often contributes to institutional care. Because it may also result in social isolation, it is difficult to estimate the number of individuals affected by, and the cost of, incontinence. It is important to address continence routinely in the assessment process, identify the type of incontinence, and intervene appropriately.

Iatrogenic drug reactions result from changes in the older individual's absorption, metabolism, and excretion processes that lead to altered responses to drugs. Many take numerous medicines, increasing the chance of drug reactions.

> ### WHAT DO YOU THINK?
>
> The average older adult in the community has 11 different prescriptions filled each year. What are some of the hazards of this situation?

## Ethical and Legal Issues

Ethical issues regarding the care and treatment of older adults arise regularly. As the population continues to age and technologic advances continue to be developed, complex ethical and legal questions will continue to increase. The most common of these issues involve decision making—assessment of the ability of the client to make decisions, the appropriate surrogate decision maker, disclosure of information to make informed decisions, level of care needed on the basis of function, and termination of treatment at the end of life.

One often-overlooked concern of older persons is that of abuse. **Older person abuse** encompasses physical, psychological, financial, and social abuse or violation of an individual's rights (McKenna, 1997). Abuse consists of the following:

- The willful infliction of physical pain or injury
- Infliction of debilitating mental anguish and fear
- Theft or mismanagement of money or resources
- Unreasonable confinement or the depriving of services

**Neglect** refers to the failure of a caregiver to provide services that are necessary for the physical and mental health

of an individual. Older persons can make independent choices with which others may disagree. Their right to self-determination can be taken from them if they are declared incompetent. Exploitation is the illegal or improper use of a person or their resources for another's profit or advantage. During the assessment process, nurses need to be aware of contradictions between injuries and the explanation of their cause, dependency issues between client and caregiver, and substance abuse by the caregiver. Nearly all 50 states have enacted mandatory reporting laws and have instituted protective service programs. The local social services agency or area agency on aging can help with information on reporting requirements.

The **Patient Self-Determination Act** of 1991 requires those providers receiving Medicare and Medicaid funds to give clients written information regarding their legal options for treatment choices if they become incapacitated. A routine discussion of **advance medical directives** can help ease the difficult discussions faced by health care professionals, family, and clients. The nurse can help an individual complete a values history instrument. These instruments ask questions about specific wishes regarding different medical situations. This clarifying process leads to completion of advance directives to document these preferences in writing. There are two parts to the advance directives. The **living will** allows the client to express wishes regarding the use of medical treatments in the event of a terminal illness. A **durable medical power of attorney** is the legal way for the client to designate someone else to make health care decisions when he or she is unable to do so. A do-not-resuscitate order (DNR) is a specific order from a physician not to use cardiopulmonary resuscitation.

> ### DID YOU KNOW?
>
> The Omnibus Budget Reconciliation Act of 1987 (OBRA 87) spells out the following rights of older adults:
> - To individualized care
> - To be free from discrimination
> - To privacy
> - To freedom from neglect and abuse
> - To control one's own funds
> - To sue
> - To freedom from physical and chemical restraint
> - To be involved in decision making
> - To vote
> - To have access to community services
> - To raise grievances
> - To obtain a will
> - To enter into contracts
> - To practice the religion of one's choice
> - To dispose of one's own personal property

State laws vary widely regarding the implementation of these tools, so it is important to consult a knowledgeable source for information. It is also important to involve the family, and especially the designated decision maker or agent, in these discussions, so that everyone is clear about the client's choices.

## Family Caregiving

Eighty-five percent of all older adults live in homes, either alone, with spouses, or with other family or friends. Female spouses represent the largest group of family caregivers. Stress, strain, burden, and burnout are words that are used to reflect the negative effects of family caregiving.

Issues involve the work itself, past and present relationships, the effect on others, and the caregivers' lifestyle and well-being. It is estimated that at least 5 million adults are providing direct care to an older adult relative at any given time, with another 44 to 45 million assuming some type of responsibility for an older relative. For many families, the caregiving experience is positive, rewarding, and fulfilling. Nursing intervention can facilitate good health for older persons and their caregivers, and can contribute to meaningful family relationships during this period. Eliopoulos (2001) uses the acronym "TLC" to represent these interventions for caregivers:

- **T** = Training in care techniques, safe medication use, recognition of abnormalities, available resources
- **L** = Leaving the care situation periodically to obtain respite and relaxation and maintain the caregiver's normal living needs
- **C** = Care for the caregivers themselves through adequate sleep, rest, exercise, nutrition, socialization, solitude, support, financial aid, and health management

## COMMUNITY-BASED MODELS FOR GERONTOLOGICAL NURSING

### Nursing Roles

Communities are where people live, work, and socialize. Often, older people can remain in the setting of their choice by modifying their environment and obtaining support services. Community health settings include public health departments, nurse-managed health centers, ambulatory care clinics, and home health agencies. The cultural values of the community shape lifestyle and influence health status. Legislation that affects the health care system is a product of that culture. In 2000, the organization that administers Medicare and Medicaid changed its name from Health Care Financing Administration (HCFA) to Center for Medicare and Medicaid Services (CMS). Dramatic changes have occurred since the Social Security Act was enacted in 1935 (Table 29-3).

Demographic changes in this country include an ever-growing population of older adults. Most of these individuals wish to stay in their own homes and communities and will be frequent consumers of health services. Nurses are involved in direct care, providing self-care information, supervision of paraprofessionals, or collaborating with other disciplines to provide the most appropriate, high-quality, cost-effective care at the most appropriate level and location. Services are provided on a continuum of care, as detailed in Box 29-3.

A knowledge of community resources is a fundamental part of caring for the older adult in any community. The nurse assesses the need for and helps develop the resources. Every community has an area agency on aging that coordinates planning and delivery of needed services, and it can be a good resource for the nurse. Figure 29-5 shows an example of a home safety evaluation tool developed by an area agency on aging that is used by community nurses. Most communities have an information and referral system, as well as a public directory of services available.

---

**NURSING TIP**

Older adults are at increased risk for infection. Prevention in the community includes encouraging routine hand hygiene and adapting universal precautions specifically to the practice setting.

---

## Community Care Settings

### Senior Centers

Senior centers were developed in the early 1940s to provide social and recreational activities. Now many centers are multipurpose, offering recreation, education, counseling, therapies, hot meals, and case management, as well as health screening and education. Some even offer primary care services. Nurses have a unique opportunity to provide services to a group of older persons who wish to remain independent in the community.

An example of a senior nutrition site that has begun to expand services to include primary care is the Geriatric Assessment and Intervention Team (GAIT). The GAIT initiative is an example of a community-sponsored program that seeks and visits vulnerable older persons (Jefferson Area Board for Aging, 1998). The GAIT initiative is an example of a community-sponsored program that seeks out and goes to vulnerable older adults. The team consists of a nurse practitioner, a case manager, and a geriatric social worker who use the rural nutrition site as a home base. Their goal is to improve access to appropriate health care with an emphasis on health promotion and disease prevention.

### Adult Day Health

Adult day health is for individuals whose mental or physical function requires them to get more health care and supervision. It serves as more of a medical model than the se-

## Table 29-3 Health Care–Related Political Events Relevant to Older Adults' Health

| DATE | EVENT | IMPACT |
|------|-------|--------|
| 1935 | Social Security Act signed | Increases financial security |
| 1948 | Hospital Construction and Facilities Act (Hill-Burton) | Provides funds for construction of long-term care facilities |
| 1950 | First National Conference on Aging in Washington, D.C. | Beginning of federal policy and national attention to problems of older adults |
| 1963 | Kennedy formed President's Council on Aging; designated May as Older Americans' Month | |
| 1965 | Older Americans Act Social Security Act Amendments | Mandates comprehensive services by states |
| | Medicare (Title XVIII) | National medical insurance for all older adults |
| | Medicaid (Title XIX) | Federal/state program to increase medical services for poor and disabled; more nursing homes and federal regulations |
| | Title XX | In-home services for indigent through Social Services |
| 1972 | Medicare reform | Professional Standards Review Organizations to review hospital services for overuse Intermediate care facilities reimbursed New regulations |
| 1973 | Older Americans Act | Establishes area agencies on aging to coordinate amendment's services Increases public transportation to rural areas, concentrating on older adults and disabled Establishes National Clearing House for Aging |
| 1976 | Title V of Older Americans Act | Appropriates funds for multipurpose Senior Centers |
| 1981 | Omnibus Reconciliation Act (OBRA) | Provides funds for community, preventive programs leading to growth in home health services |
| 1982 | Tax Equity and Fiscal Responsibility Act (TEFRA) | Introduces idea of prospective payment for Medicare instead of fee-for-service |
| 1983 | Diagnostic related groups (DRGs) | Hospital prospective payment plan to control Medicare costs |
| 1987 | New OBRA laws | Increase standards of care in nursing homes Establish ombudsman programs |
| 1990 | Americans With Disabilities Act | Prohibits discrimination against disabled individuals |
| 1991 | Patient Self-Determination Act | Increases importance of advance directives |
| 1996 | Health Insurance Portability and Accountability Act | Safeguards health coverage for people who change jobs Establishes medical savings accounts for medical and long-term expenses |
| 1997 | Balanced Budget Act | Establishes Medicare + Choice program to expand choices through managed care companies Changes reimbursement for long-term care and home health to prospective payment Increases preventive services offered |
| 1998 | Prospective Payment System (PPS) | Impacts reimbursement by consolidating care into one payment |
| 2001 | National Family Caregiver Support Program | Provides federal support to help ease the burden of caregivers |

nior center, and often individuals return home to their caregivers at night. Some settings offer **respite care** for short-term overnight relief for caregivers. This provides caregivers the opportunity to work or have personal time during the day. Often, support groups for caregivers are offered by nurses.

## Home Health

Home health can be provided by multidisciplinary teams. Nurses provide individual and environmental assessments, direct skilled care and treatment, and short-term guidance and instruction. Nurses often function independently in the home and must rely on their own resources and knowledge

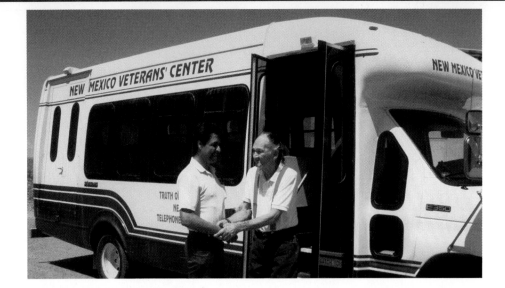

This older adult man lives in a residential center for veterans.

---

**BOX 29-3** **Available Options for Care of Older Adults**

**IN THE HOME**
- Home safety assessment and equipment
- Meals on Wheels
- Homemaker and chore services
- Telephone reassurance/friendly visitor
- Personal emergency response system
- Pharmacies/grocers that deliver
- Area Agency on Aging services
- State health, legal, social service departments
- Adult protective services—city social services
- Home health aide
- Home health nurses and therapists
- Hospice

**IN THE COMMUNITY**
- Specialized transportation for disabled
- Multipurpose senior centers
- Health screenings, health fairs
- Congregate meal sites
- Community mental health clubhouses
- Adult day health care
- Respite care
- Community nursing clinics

- Comprehensive geriatric medical service
- Medicare and Medicaid health maintenance organizations
- Caregiver or disease-focused support groups
- Case/disease management
- Health promotion/self-care classes

**IN SPECIAL HOUSING**
- Elder Cottage Housing Opportunity (ECHO)
- Home sharing
- Accessory apartments
- Foster home
- Group home
- Assisted living facility
- Life care community
- Retirement village
- Intermediate care facility
- Skilled nursing facility
- Rehabilitation hospital
- Subacute unit/hospital
- Acute care hospital
- State mental hospital

---

to improvise and adapt care to meet the client's unique physical and social circumstances. They work closely with the family and other caregivers to provide necessary communication and continuity of care. CMS requires that home health agencies electronically report data from an assessment tool, the Outcome and Assessment Information Set (OASIS).

### Hospice

Hospice represents a philosophy of caring for and supporting life to its fullest until death occurs. The hospice team encourages the client and family to jointly make decisions to meet physical, emotional, spiritual, and comfort needs (see palliative care in the Content Resources section of the evolve website).

## JABA Home Safety Evaluation

### 1. EXTERIOR ENTRANCES AND EXITS
- [ ] Note condition of walk and drive surface; existence of curb cuts
- [ ] Note handrail condition, right and left sides
- [ ] Note light level for driveway, walk, porch
- [ ] Check door threshold height
- [ ] Note ability to use knob, lock, key, mailbox, peephole, and package shelf
- [ ] Do door and window locks work?

### 2. INTERIOR DOORS, STAIRS, HALLS
- [ ] Note height of door threshold, knob and hinge types; clear width door opening; direction that door swings
- [ ] Note presence of floor level changes
- [ ] Note hall width, adequate for walker/wheelchair
- [ ] Determine stair flight run: straight or curved
- [ ] Note stair rails: condition, right and left side
- [ ] Examine light level, clutter hazards
- [ ] Note floor surface texture and contrast

### 3. BATHROOM
- [ ] Are basin and tub faucets, shower control, and drain plugs manageable?
- [ ] Are hot water pipes covered?
- [ ] Is mirror height appropriate, sitting and standing?
- [ ] Note ability to reach shelf above, below basin
- [ ] Note ability to step in and out of the bath and shower
- [ ] Can resident use bath bench in tub or shower?
- [ ] Note toilet height; ability to reach paper, flush; come from sit to stand posture
- [ ] Is space available for caregiver to assist?

### 4. KITCHEN
- [ ] Note overall light level, task lighting
- [ ] Note sink and counter heights
- [ ] Note wall and floor storage shelf heights
- [ ] Are undersink hot water pipes covered?
- [ ] Is there under counter knee space?
- [ ] Is there a nearby surface to rest hot foods on when removed from oven?
- [ ] Note stove control location (rear or front)

### 5. LIVING, DINING, BEDROOM
- [ ] Chair, sofa, bed heights allow sitting or standing?
- [ ] Do rugs have nonslip pad or rug tape?
- [ ] Chair available with arm rests?
- [ ] Able to turn on light, radio, TV, place a phone call from bed, chair, and sofa?

### 6. LAUNDRY
- [ ] Able to hand wash and hang clothes to dry?
- [ ] Able to access automatic washer/dryer?

### 7. TELEPHONE AND DOOR
- [ ] Phone jack location near bed, sofa, chair?
- [ ] Able to get to phone, dial, hear caller?
- [ ] Able to identify visitors, hear doorbell?
- [ ] Able to reach and empty mailbox?
- [ ] Wears neck/wrist device to obtain emergency help?

### 8. STORAGE SPACE
- [ ] Able to reach closet rods and hooks, open bureau drawers?
- [ ] Is there a light inside the closet?

### 9. WINDOWS
- [ ] Opening mechanism at 42 inches from the floor?
- [ ] Lock accessible, easy-to-operate?
- [ ] Sill height above floor level?

### 10. ELECTRIC OUTLETS AND CONTROLS
- [ ] Sufficient outlets?
- [ ] Outlet height, wall locations
- [ ] Low vision/sound warnings available?
- [ ] Extension cord hazard?

### 11. HEAT, LIGHT, VENTILATION, SECURITY, CARBON MONOXIDE, WATER TEMP CONTROLS
- [ ] Are there smoke/$CO_2$ detectors and a fire extinguisher?
- [ ] Thermometer displays easily readable?
- [ ] Accessible environmental controls?
- [ ] Pressure balance valve available?
- [ ] Note rooms where poor light level exists
- [ ] Able to open windows, slide patio doors?
- [ ] Able to open drapes or curtains?

### COMMENTS:
_____
_____
_____
_____
_____

Used with permission by Jefferson Area Board for Aging, Charlottesville, Virginia.

**Figure 29-5** Jefferson Area Board for Aging: Home safety assessment.

## Assisted Living

Assisted living covers a wide variety of choices, from a single shared room to opulent independent living accommodations in a full-service, life-care community. The differences are related to the type and extent of the amenities provided and the contract signed for them. The role of the nurse varies depending on the philosophy and leadership of the management of the facility. The nurse generally provides assessment and interventions, medication review, education, and advocacy.

## Long-term Care

Nursing homes, or **long-term care facilities** as they are often called, house only about 5% of the older population at a given time; however, 25% of those over 65 years old will spend some time in a nursing home. Nursing homes provide a safe environment, special diets and activities, routine personal care, and the treatment and management of health care needs for those needing rehabilitation, as well as for those needing a permanent supportive residence. Like hospitals, nursing homes are paid using the prospective payment model based on the nursing assessment. The nurse uses a tool called the Minimum Data Set (MDS) to document the assessment and outcome of treatment.

---

### Evidence-Based Practice

The Mobile Health Unit was implemented to increase access to nursing services, to improve and/or maintain functional status and health status, and to increase health promotion behaviors of rural older adults experiencing difficulty obtaining health care because of illness, transportation problems, or financial factors. For 222 project participants, 1773 encounters were completed, with a mean number of visits per individual of 7.9. Participants in the project demonstrated increased breast and cervical cancer screenings; increased immunization rates for influenza, pneumonia, and tetanus; and decreased use of the emergency room.

**Nurse Use:** This project represents an alternative model of health care delivery in a rural area with limited resources and health care providers.

Alexy BB, Elnitsky CL: Rural mobile health unit: outcomes, *Public Health Nurs* 15(1):3, 1998.

---

### Rehabilitation

Rehabilitation is a combination of physical, occupational, psychological, and speech therapy to help debilitated persons maintain or recover their physical capacities. Rehabilitation is typically needed for older adults after a hip fracture, stroke, or prolonged illness that results in serious deconditioning.

Creative models for nurses have been established in the various settings described. The Visiting Nurse Association (VNA) of Springfield, Massachusetts, uses the Geriatric Resource Nurse model (Francis, Fletcher, and Simon, 1998). Originally developed in the acute care setting, the VNA tailored this model to home care. The VNA prepared nurses interested in geriatrics with the knowledge, skills, and abilities necessary to become resource nurses to the home care staff. The Program of All-Inclusive Care for the Elderly (PACE) is a capitated demonstration program authorized by Medicare to keep individuals in the community as long as medically, socially, and financially possible. An interdisciplinary team assesses patient needs, develops a care plan, and integrates primary care and other services.

Nursing homes are increasingly contracting with physician/nurse practitioner teams who have gerontological expertise to provide primary care to nursing home residents. Examples of effective models include Evercare (Ryan, 1999) and the Fallon Health Systems (Burl et al, 1998). The advanced practice gerontological nurse practitioner, in addition to providing primary care, also frequently educates the nursing staff on gerontological issues.

---

### THE CUTTING EDGE

The geriatric resource nurses at the University of Virginia developed self-learning modules in geriatric care for older clients. The SPPICEES mnemonic addresses eight distinct modules, each targeting a common area of health concern for older adults across health care settings. The mnemonic stands for sleep, problems with eating and nutrition, pain, immobility, confusion, elimination, older adult mistreatment, and skin. For more information, contact krf9d@virginia.edu.

---

## ROLE OPPORTUNITIES FOR NURSES: HEALTH PROMOTION, DISEASE PREVENTION, AND WELLNESS

Community-oriented nurses focus on the prevention of disease and the promotion and maintenance of health. To achieve these goals, nurses are involved in client and community education, counseling, advocacy, and care management. The overall goal is improving the health of the individual and the community through collaborative practice with other members of the health care team. Achieving this goal involves the nurse in all three levels of prevention. Examples of preventive activities for the older person in the community are shown in Box 29-4.

The nurse should be familiar with the guidelines for preventive services and screening activities for individuals 65 years of age and older (see Appendixes I.1 and I.2). Many evidence-based resources are available for nurses who are working with the older population (Box 29-5).

Healthy People 2010 (U.S. Department of Health and Human Services, 2000) offers direction through measures for reducing and preventing unnecessary disease, disability, and death across the life span. The goals are increasing the quality and years of healthy life for Americans, and eliminating health disparities among Americans. The Healthy People 2010 box lists the objectives related to adults age 65 and older. Health promotion activities involve behaviors that positively affect a person's health status. The government's Put Prevention Into Practice program is designed to help health care professionals structure their preventive activities. Although many older adults enjoy good health, many live with chronic conditions and need support to maximize their strengths.

The term **wellness** was coined by Travis (1977) to help bring to mind the idea of health as holistic rather than merely the absence of disease or illness. It includes the physical, emotional, mental, and spiritual components of a person. With this approach to chronic illness, it is possible for individuals to maintain their own optimal level of wellness along a continuum, as shown in Figure 29-6 (Ebersole and Hess, 2001). The traditional way of looking at health as either present or absent is less helpful for the older person. More appropriate is the positive approach of addressing risk factors that affect the experience of chronic illness. Travis (1977) outlines five dimensions of wellness:

1. Self-responsibility: The core of wellness, encouraging self-help strategies, taking control of health and life choices, and partnering with health care providers rather than abdicating control
2. Nutritional awareness: Learning about the selection and preparation of food and developing eating habits that lead to a more balanced, nutritionally appropriate diet
3. Physical fitness: Involving aerobic capacity, body structure, body composition, balance, muscle flexibility, and muscle strength
4. Stress management: Developing new attitudes and ways to cope with events in life that seem beyond control and that cause negative physical and mental problems
5. Environmental sensitivity: Influencing one's personal room/home space; physical earth issues of conservation and pollution; and social components of government, economics, and culture

Although persons do slow down and become more susceptible to disease as aging occurs, it is the advances in prevention and wellness measures that delay the onset of debilitating disease and functional decline and increase the years of quality life. Nurses can provide health education and screening and other wellness programs for individuals and groups in all settings. Another important role for nurses is participating in research related to the outcomes of care and cost effectiveness of different health promotion programs.

The aging population is creating a major shift in the health care needs of the present and future. There are many myths about the older population. People age at different rates and have different cultural and religious values that influence their health care choices. Controlling national health care expenditures is a major issue. New directions in health care for older adults means significant changes in social, political, and economic policies and structures (Corbin and Cherry, 1997). Nurses are in a position to influence these changes. As no one holds a crystal ball to tell where these changes will lead, having knowledge and being involved, flexible, and creative will help. It is to nurses that older adults turn for advice and counseling about the confusing array of services and choices available. Nurses must be role models for positive attitudes toward and advocates for the unique needs of older adults in different community settings.

## Healthy People 2010 | Selected Objectives for Adults Aged 65 and Older

**1-9** Reduce hospitalization rates for three ambulatory-care-sensitive conditions—pediatric asthma, uncontrolled diabetes, and immunization-preventable pneumonia and influenza in older adults

**1-15** Increase the proportion of persons with long-term care needs who have access to the continuum of long-term care services

**1-16** Reduce the proportion of nursing home residents with a current diagnosis of pressure ulcers

**2-1** Increase the mean number of days without severe pain among adults who have chronic joint symptoms

**2-2** Reduce the proportion of adults with chronic joint symptoms who experience a limitation in activity due to arthritis

**2-3** Reduce the proportion of all adults with chronic joint symptoms who have difficulty in performing two or more personal care activities, thereby preserving independence

**2-8** Increase the proportion of persons with arthritis who have had effective, evidence-based arthritis education as an integral part of the management of their condition

**2-9** Reduce the overall number of cases of osteoporosis

**2-10** Reduce the proportion of adults who are hospitalized for vertebral fractures associated with osteoporosis

**3-5** Reduce the colorectal cancer death rate

**3-13** Increase the proportion of women aged 40 years and older who have received a mammogram within the preceding 2 years

**6-3** Reduce the proportion of adults with disabilities who report feelings such as sadness, unhappiness, or depression that prevent them from being active

**6-4** Increase the proportion of adults with disabilities who participate in social activities

**6-5** Increase the proportion of adults with disabilities reporting sufficient emotional support

**6-11** Reduce the proportion of people with disabilities who report not having the assistive devices and technology needed

**7-12** Increase the proportion of older adults who have participated during the preceding year in at least one organized health promotion activity

**12-6** Reduce hospitalizations of older adults with heart failure as the principal diagnosis

**12-8** Increase the proportion of adults who are aware of the early warning symptoms and signs of a stroke

**12-10** Increase the proportion of adults with high blood pressure whose blood pressure is under control

**12-14** Reduce the proportion of adults with high total blood cholesterol levels

**17-3** Increase the proportion of primary care providers, pharmacists, and other health care professionals who routinely review with their patients with chronic illnesses or disabilities all new prescribed and over-the-counter medicines

**17-5** Increase the proportion of patients who receive verbal counseling from prescribers and pharmacists on appropriate use and potential risks of medications

**19-17** Increase the proportion of physician office visits made by patients with a diagnosis of cardiovascular disease, diabetes, or hyperlipidemia that include counseling or education related to diet and nutrition

**21-4** Reduce the proportion of older adults who have had all their natural teeth extracted

**21-7** Increase the proportion of adults who, in the past 12 months, report having had an examination to detect oral and pharyngeal cancer

**21-11** Increase the proportion of long-term care residents who use the oral health care system each year

**22-4** Increase the proportion of adults who perform physical activities that enhance and maintain muscular strength and endurance

**22-5** Increase the proportion of adults who perform physical activities that enhance and maintain flexibility

**27-1** Reduce tobacco use by adults

**28-5** Reduce visual impairment due to diabetic retinopathy

**28-6** Reduce visual impairment due to glaucoma

**28-7** Reduce visual impairment due to cataract

**28-10** Increase the use of vision rehabilitation services and adaptive devices by people with visual impairments

From U.S. Department of Health and Human Services: *Healthy people 2010: national health promotion and disease prevention objectives,* ed 2, Washington, DC, 2000, U.S. Government Printing Office.

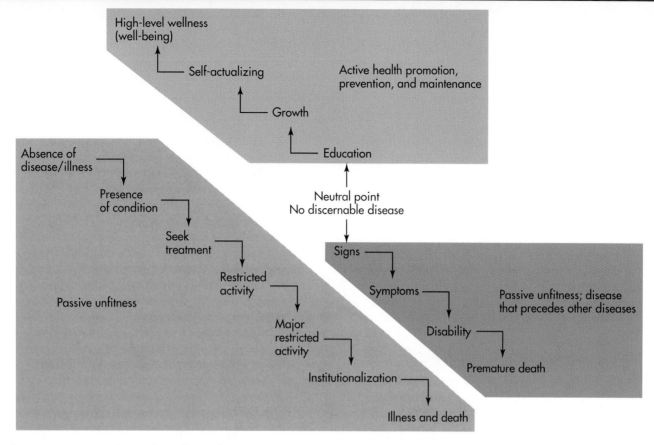

**Figure 29-6** Comparison of a wellness–health continuum with the traditional medical continuum. *(From Ebersole P, Hess P: Toward healthy aging: human needs and nursing response, ed 6, St Louis, Mo, 2003, Mosby.)*

## Practice Application

Mrs. Eldridge, a 79-year-old widow, was reported by neighbors and the administrator of the senior high-rise residence where she lives to the nurse who visited residents there. Mrs. Eldridge lives alone, and no one had been observed coming or going from her apartment recently. When Mrs. Eldridge was seen by her neighbors, she appeared self-neglected and did not appear to recognize her neighbors.

When the nurse made a visit to the apartment, Mrs. Eldridge answered the door. She was pleasant but there was an odor of stale urine. The nurse validated the unkempt appearance of both Mrs. Eldridge and the apartment. Even though Mrs. Eldridge was hesitant and unsure in her answers, the history revealed medical problems. A son and daughter-in-law lived in the next county and phoned at least once a week; their number was taped to the table by the phone. Several pill bottles were observed on the kitchen counter with the names of a local physician and pharmacist.

The nurse noted that both Mrs. Eldridge and her clothes were dirty, and that she moved without aids and appeared steady on her feet. The kitchen was littered with

unwashed dishes and empty frozen-food boxes, which Mrs. Eldridge could not recall being bought or having been delivered. A billfold with several bills was lying open on the kitchen counter, as well as an uncashed Social Security check.

A. What should the nurse do about the situation she found?
1. Call adult protective services and get an emergency order to put Mrs. Eldridge in a nursing home.
2. Call Mrs. Eldridge's son and see if his mother can move in with him since she cannot take care of herself.
3. Complete a physical and mental examination to first determine the cause of Mrs. Eldridge's situation.
4. Call Mrs. Eldridge's pharmacist to see what medications she is taking.
5. Call Mrs. Eldridge's son to discuss the situation with him and to make plans with him and his mother for her future.

B. What factors make this a difficult situation?

**Answers are in the back of the book.**

## Key Points

- The population aged 65 years and older in the United States is steadily growing, accompanied by an increase in chronic conditions, greater demand for services, and strained health care budgets.
- Most older adults live in the community. The last few years of life often represent functional decline. Nurses strive to help the person maximize functional status and minimize costs through direct care and appropriate referral to community resources.
- Nurses address the chronic health concerns of older adults by focusing on maintaining or improving self-care and preventing complications to maintain the highest possible quality of life.
- Assessing the older adult incorporates physical, psychological, social, and spiritual domains. Individual and community-focused interventions involve all three levels of prevention through collaborative practice.

## Clinical Decision-Making Activities

1. Describe your impression of a typical older adult and compare it with the demographic information given in this chapter. Illustrate what you mean by your impression.
2. From the Practice Application for this chapter, identify an example of a theory of aging and an example of ageism, and write at least two nursing diagnoses. Be exact.
3. Think about television or movie portrayals of aging you have seen and identify both positive and negative ways older adults are shown. Be specific.
4. Interview an older member of your family, and ask him or her to list any health problems, and to rate his or her health on a scale of 1 to 10 (with 10 being the highest). Ask him or her to describe a typical day's activities. Keep a 24-hour dietary recall. What does this tell you about this person's risks or strengths related to aging? Compare the answers to what you have learned in this chapter.
5. From the information you obtained in activity 4, do the following:
   a. Devise screening recommendations for your relative. Explain why you chose these recommendations.
   b. Derive at least one nursing diagnosis. Why did you choose this one?
   c. What theory of aging best fits your relative? Explain.
6. Interview a peer about his or her attitude toward aging, and determine whether this attitude involves any myths about aging. Describe what you can do to aid in overcoming the myths and examples of ageism that are pervasive in society.
7. Visit a senior center in your community. Observe the physical characteristics of the participants, activities they are doing or planning, the food served, and the safety and comfort features available. Ask the participants what they like and do not like about the services, and what other community services they are using. Ask them what kinds of problem they have encountered in attempting to access community services in general and the senior center specifically. How did they overcome the barriers? How can you help?
8. Discuss how the perceptions of nurses who work in long-term care institutions may be different from the perceptions of those who work in the hospital. How could we check that the different perceptions are real?

# References

Alexy BB, Elnitsky CL: Rural mobile health unit: outcomes, *Public Health Nurs* 15(1):3, 1998.

Berger KS: *The developing person through the life span,* ed 3, New York, 1994, Worth.

Burl JB et al: Geriatric nurse practitioners in long-term care: demonstration of effectiveness in managed care, *J Am Geriatr Soc* 46:506, 1998.

Burnside I, Haight B: Reminiscence and life review: therapeutic interventions for older people, *Nurse Pract* 19(4):55-61, 1994.

Clark M, Anderson PB: *Culture and aging: an anthropological study of older Americans,* Springfield, Ill, 1967, Thomas.

Corbin J, Cherry J: Caring for the aged in the community. In Swanson E, Tripp-Reimer T, editors: *Chronic illness and the older adult,* New York, 1997, Springer.

Cumming E, Henry H: *Growing old: the process of disengagement,* New York, 1961, Basic Books.

Ebersole P, Hess P: *Geriatric nursing and healthy aging,* St Louis, Mo, 2001, Mosby.

Egan DE: The reminiscing game, *Pennsylvania Nurse* 50(2):22, 1996.

Eliopoulos C: *Gerontological nursing,* ed 5, Philadelphia, 2001, Lippincott.

Erikson EH: *Identity and the lifecycle,* New York, 1959, International Press.

Francis D, Fletcher K, Simon L: The geriatric resource nurse model of care: a vision for the future, *Nurs Clin North Am* 33(3)481, 1998.

Havighurst RL, Neugarten BL, Tobin SS: Disengagement and patterns of aging. In Neugarten BL, editor: *Middle age and aging,* Chicago, 1968, University of Chicago.

Hayflick L: *How and why we age,* New York, 1994, Ballantine Books.

Jefferson Area Board for Aging: *Your pathway to health: senior wellness network and a geriatric assessment intervention team* [brochure], Charlottesville, Va, 1998, JABA.

Jonas WB, Levin JS: *Essentials of complementary and alternative medicine,* Philadelphia, 1999, Lippincott Williams & Wilkins.

Kane RL, Ouslander JG, Abrass IB: *Essentials of clinical geriatrics,* ed 4, New York, 1999, McGraw-Hill.

Leipzig RM: That was the year it was: an evidence-based clinical geriatric update, *J Am Geriatr Soc* 46:1040-1049, 1998.

Lueckenotte A: *Gerontologic nursing,* ed 2, St Louis, 2000, Mosby.

Maslow A: *Toward a psychology of being,* ed 2, Princeton, NJ, 1968, Van Nostrand.

McKenna LS: Older adults abuse: preparing to identify and intervene in health care, *Home Care Provid* 2(1):30, 1997.

National Center for Health Statistics: *Supplement on aging and second supplement on aging,* Appendix 14, Washington DC, 1997, U.S. Government Printing Office.

Redeker N: Health beliefs and adherence in chronic illness, *Image J Nurs Scholarsh* 29(1):31, 1988.

Rudberg M et al: Guidelines, practice policies, and parameters: the case for geriatrics, *J Am Geriatr Soc* 42:665-669, 1994.

Ryan J: Collaboration between the nurse practitioner and physician in long-term care. In Fletcher K, editor: The nurse practitioner in long-term care, *Lippincott's Primary Care Practice* April/May, 1999.

Simon L, Fletcher K, Francis D: The geriatric resource model of care: a vision for the future. In Abraham I, Fulmer T, Milisen K, editors: Advances in geriatric nursing, *Nurs Clin North Am* 33:3:481, 1998.

Taler G: Clinical practice guidelines: their purposes and uses, *J Am Geriatr Soc* 44:1108-1111, 1996.

Tierney LM, McPhee SJ, Papadakis MA: *Current medical diagnosis and treatment,* ed 41, East Norwalk, Conn, 2002, Appleton & Lange.

Travis J: *Wellness workbook: a guide to high level wellness,* Mill Valley, Calif, 1977, Wellness Resource Center.

U.S. Bureau of the Census: *Age 2000,* brief C2KBR/01-12, Washington, DC, 2001, U.S. Government Printing Office.

U.S. Department of Health and Human Services: *Healthy people 2010: understanding and improving health,* ed 2, Washington, DC, 2000, U.S. Government Printing Office.

Yesavage JA et al: Development and validation of a geriatric depression screening scale: a preliminary report, *J Psychiatr Res* 17(1):37-49, 1983.

# Chapter 30

http://evolve.elsevier.com/Stanhope

# The Physically Compromised

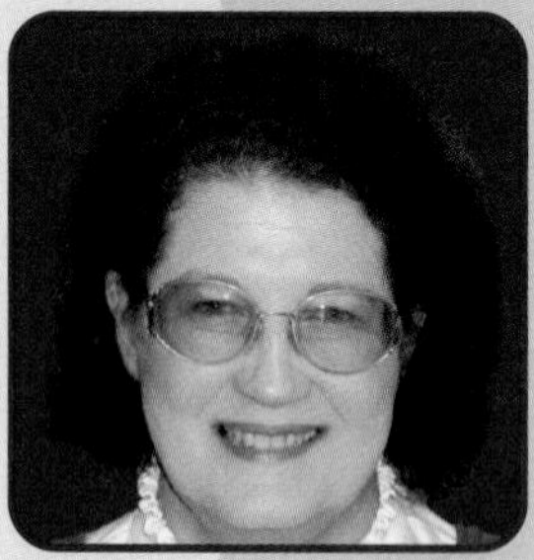

**Mary Ann McClellan, M.N., C.P.N.P., A.R.N.P.**

Mary Ann McClellan is an assistant professor teaching in the nurse practitioner program at the College of Nursing at the University of Oklahoma. Her bachelor's degree in nursing is from Texas Woman's University, her master's degree in nursing is from the University of Washington, and her certificate as a pediatric nurse practitioner is from the University of Texas at Arlington. She has experience as a public health staff nurse, a district supervisor, and a maternal child health consultant, and she practices part-time as a pediatric nurse practitioner.

## Objectives

After reading this chapter, the student should be able to do the following:

1. Define selected terms related to being physically compromised
2. Discuss implications of being developmentally disabled, handicapped, disabled, impaired, or chronically ill
3. List six conditions that may cause a person to become physically compromised
4. Compare the effects of being physically compromised on the individual, the family, and the community
5. Describe the implications of being physically compromised for selected (rural, low-income, worksite) populations
6. Discuss selected issues for those who are physically compromised (abuse, health promotion)
7. Discuss the objectives of Healthy People 2010 and Healthy Communities 2010 as they relate to physical compromise
8. Examine the nurse's role in caring for people who are physically compromised

Early public health nursing emphasized home care of the sick and the poor, prevention of communicable diseases, and conditions of hygiene in the home and the community. Federal funding in the 1960s allowed state and local health departments to expand services to include the following: secondary prevention through early detection of selected chronic diseases (e.g., cancer, glaucoma), family planning services to improve the health of mothers and children, and expanded community health nursing services to those who were mentally handicapped. Home health care through the Medicare program increased at about the same time. These changes, along with laws affecting handicapped and developmentally disabled people and many of the objectives of Healthy People 2010 and the Healthy Cities movement (see Chapter 17), have led to more opportunities for nurses to work with families and other community groups that have members who are physically compromised in some manner.

This chapter defines several terms related to being physically compromised, discusses the scope of the problem, and describes the effects of disabling conditions on individuals, families, and communities. It discusses the relationships between these problems, Healthy People 2010 and Healthy Communities 2010 specific objectives, and the concepts of Healthy Cities. Of special importance is the nurse's role and interventions with individuals, families, and communities in dealing with or preventing these health problems.

## DEFINITIONS AND CONCEPTS

This chapter's topic is so broad that definitions of several related terms are necessary. The term **developmental disability** relates to the functioning of a person and comes from the Rehabilitation, Comprehensive Services, and Developmental Disabilities Amendments of 1978 (Public Law 95-602): A **severe, chronic disability** of a person is a condition with the following characteristics:

- It relates to a mental or physical impairment or a combination of mental and physical impairments.
- It occurs before the person reaches age 22.

## Key Terms

**Americans With Disabilities Act**, p. 737
**chronic disease**, p. 723
**developmental disability**, p. 720
**developmental stifling**, p. 723
**disability**, p. 721

**disorder**, p. 721
**dual diagnosis**, p. 723
**functional limitations**, p. 721
**handicap**, p. 722
**impairment**, p. 721

**physically compromised**, p. 723
**severe chronic disability**, p. 720
**work disability**, p. 724
*See Glossary for definitions*

## Chapter Outline

Definitions and Concepts
Scope of the Problem
Effects of Being Physically Compromised
*Effects on the Individual*
*Effects on the Family*
*Effects on the Community*

Special Populations
*Low-Income Populations*
Selected Issues
*Abuse*
*Health Promotion*
*Complementary and Alternative Medicine*

Healthy People 2010 Objectives
Healthy Cities/Healthy Communities
Role of the Nurse
Legislation

- It is likely to continue indefinitely.
- It results in substantial functional limits in three or more areas of major life activity.
- It reflects the person's need for a combining and sequencing of special interdisciplinary or basic care, treatment, or other services that are of lifelong or extended duration and are individually planned and coordinated.

### NURSING TIP

Major life activities refer to self-care, receptive and expressive language, learning, mobility, self-direction, capacity for independent living, and financial sufficiency.

A **disability** "is any restriction or lack (resulting from an impairment) of ability to perform an activity in the manner or within the range considered normal for a human being" (Badley, 1993, p. 163) at a specific age (Heerkens et al, 1994). The medical model has dominated the definition of a disability. Other models and definitions include such areas as interactions and relationships between the individual, society, and the environment (Imrie, 1997; Orr and Schkade, 1997; Peters, 1996). In addition, culture has been considered (Banja, 1996). An **impairment** "is any loss or abnormality of psychological, physiological or anatomical structure or function. 'Impairment' is more inclusive than **'disorder'** in that it covers losses, e.g., the loss of a leg is an impairment, but not a disorder" (Badley, 1993, p. 162).

**Functional limitations** are essentially descriptions of functions such as hearing, seeing, grasping, moving, climbing, and reading. Emphasis is placed on the level of function rather than on the purpose of the activity, so that functional limitation can be associated with the disability. For example, an impairment in the strength or range of motion of the arm could lead to functional limitations in grasping or reaching. These in turn could give rise to disabilities—for example, an inability to reach up to high shelves, get dressed, perform hair care, or cook (Badley, 1993).

**Handicap** refers to social implications for a person who is impaired or disabled. A handicap is a disadvantage for a given individual with an impairment or a disability that limits or prevents the fulfillment of a role that is normal for that individual. Handicap reflects the value attached to an individual's situation or experience by others when it departs from the norm, and the individual's performance or status and the expectations of the individual himself or of the particular group of which he is a member (Badley, 1993).

In psychiatry, the phrase **dual diagnosis** generally means a substance abuse disorder concurrent with a mental illness disorder (Stuart and Laraia, 2001). For clients with developmental disabilities, dual diagnosis usually means that a mental illness disorder is present simultaneously with mental retardation (Reber and Borcherding, 1997). It is also possible for nurses to care for clients who have dual diagnoses involving physical limitations.

The term **developmental stifling** primarily refers to a symptom pattern of developmental deficiencies unrelated to medical problems. It can occur when a parent perceives a child as being especially vulnerable and seeks professional care by describing the child's behaviors and developmental level as a greater problem than they are. Consequently, the parent reinforces lower functioning in the child, stifling the child's intellectual and emotional development (Elder and Kaplan, 2000). A child with a physical disability can also be at risk for impairment from developmental stifling if the parent perceives the child to be more vulnerable than he really is.

**Chronic disease,** or illness, refers to any long-lasting condition or illness. Disease processes (e.g., diabetes mellitus, cancer, tuberculosis) or a congenital or an acquired condition (e.g., Down syndrome, severe burns, amputation of a limb), are examples of chronic diseases. Therefore concepts related to disabilities, handicaps, impairments, and functional limitations may apply to individuals with a chronic disease or other conditions. For nurses working with these clients, the onset, course, outcome, and degree of limitation are important factors to assess in deciding the meaning of the disease to individuals and the families.

A person who is **physically compromised** may have any of the conditions listed in Box 30-1.

## SCOPE OF THE PROBLEM

Nurses provide care for individuals who are physically compromised, for their families, for the populations and subpopulations that they make up, and for the communities in which they live. The nurse must remember that some clients prefer to be regarded as being physically challenged or physically compromised, whereas others may think such terms minimize the importance of the needs and problems of people who are disabled. See the website at http://evolve. elsevier.com/ Stanhope for selected assessment tools for use with people who are physically compromised.

People may be physically compromised from many different causes. Three major categories of such causes are injuries, developmental disabilities, and chronic diseases

---

**BOX 30-1  Rankings of Causes of Disabilities Among Civilian Noninstitutionalized Persons Aged ≥18 Years, United States, 1999**

1. Arthritis or rheumatism
2. Back or spine problem
3. Heart trouble/hardening of the arteries
4. Lung or respiratory problem
5. Deafness or hearing problem
6. Limb/extremity stiffness
7. Mental or emotional problem
8. Diabetes
9. Blindness or vision problems
10. Stroke
11. Broken bone/fracture
12. Mental retardation
13. Cancer
14. High blood pressure
15. Head or spinal cord injury
16. Learning disability
17. Alzheimer's disease/senility/dementia
18. Kidney problems
19. Paralysis
20. Missing limbs
21. Stomach/digestive problems
22. Epilepsy
23. Alcohol or drug problem
24. Hernia or rupture
25. AIDS or AIDS-related condition
26. Cerebral palsy
27. Tumor/cyst/growth
28. Speech disorder
29. Thyroid problems

Other (the total number in this category actually places the category as #3 in this list.)

From Centers for Disease Control and Prevention: Prevalence of disabilities and associated health conditions among adults— United States, 1999, *MMWR Morb Mortal Wkly Rep* 50(7):120-125, 2001.

---

(Figure 30-1). As Figure 30-1 indicates, some of these conditions may occur at different ages and stages of development of the individual. Therefore the effects on the person's life are influenced by the timing as well as by the severity of the condition. Several specific conditions and inherited problems can cause disability. These include genetic disorders, acute and chronic illnesses, violence, tobacco use, lack of access to health care, and failure to eat correctly, exercise reg-

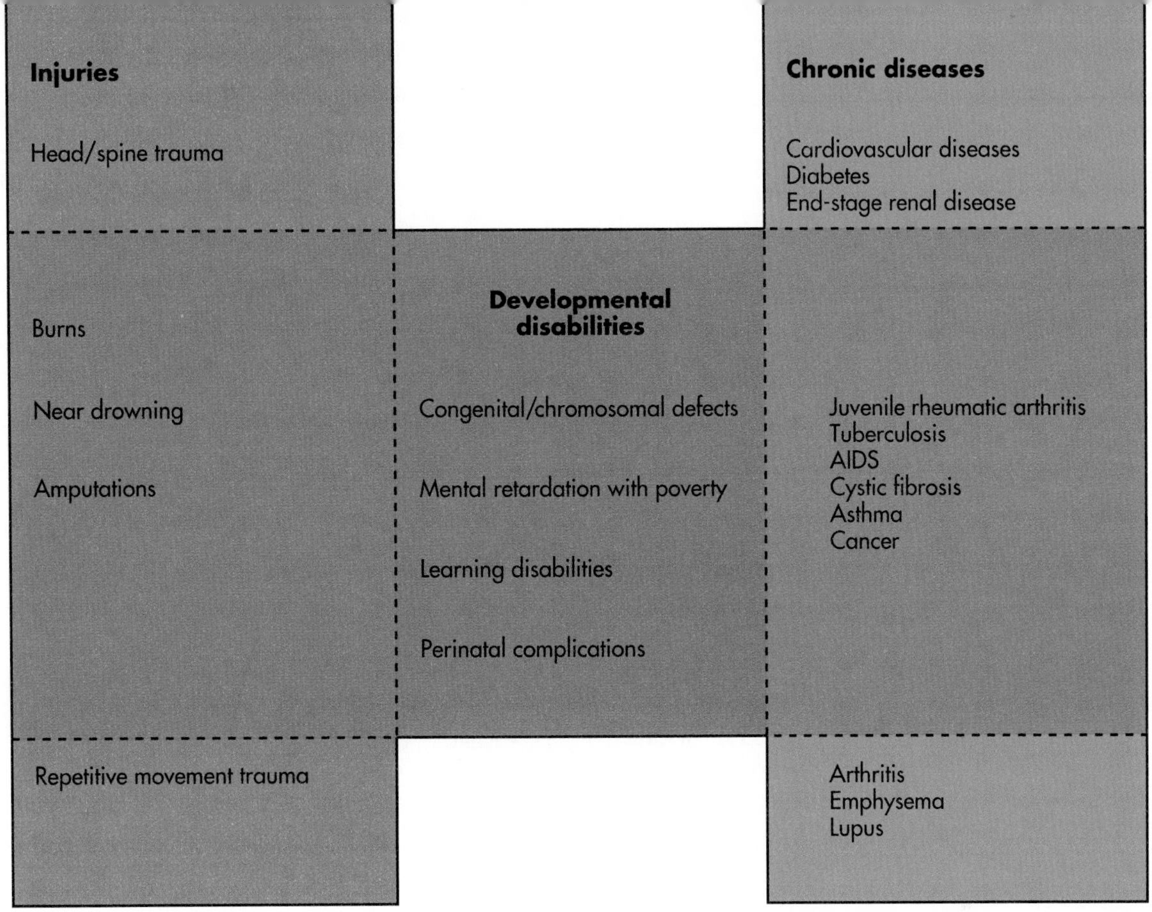

## Injuries

Head/spine trauma

Burns

Near drowning

Amputations

Repetitive movement trauma

## Developmental disabilities

Congenital/chromosomal defects

Mental retardation with poverty

Learning disabilities

Perinatal complications

## Chronic diseases

Cardiovascular diseases
Diabetes
End-stage renal disease

Juvenile rheumatic arthritis
Tuberculosis
AIDS
Cystic fibrosis
Asthma
Cancer

Arthritis
Emphysema
Lupus

**Figure 30-1** Examples of conditions related to being physically compromised.

ularly, or manage stress effectively. Other causes include perinatal complications, injuries, substance abuse, environmental problems, and unsanitary living conditions.

One example includes both tobacco use and environmental problems. In 1996, cigarette smoking prevalence was added to the nationally notifiable health problems to be reported to the Centers for Disease Control and Prevention (CDC) by states. Approximately 15 million children and adolescents were exposed to cigarette smoke in their homes in 1996 (CDC, 1997a). The WebLinks on http://evolve.elsevier.com/Stanhope list national organizations with information about disabilities.

Box 30-1 lists selected causes of disabilities ranked by prevalence in adults in the United States from the Survey of Income and Program Participation (SIPP) in 1999. The people reporting these causes identified difficulty with functional limitations (except for speech, hearing, or vision), activities of daily living (ADLs), instrumental ADLs (IADLs), the inability to do housework or to work at a job or business. This list came from people who had one primary cause of disability and as many as two other causes of disabilities from the list of 30 conditions (CDC, 2001).

According to the 2000 U.S. Census, there were 29.7 million people 5 years old and older, or 19% of the total population, with some type of disability. Of these, 8%, or 5.2 million, were ages 5 to 20 years. Between the ages of 21 and 64 years, 30.6 million were disabled, of whom 57% were employed. Of the 14.0 million people 65 years and older, 42% had disabilities.

### DID YOU KNOW?

The percentages of residents of Arkansas, Kentucky, Missouri, and West Virginia 5 years and older with disabilities were the highest in the country (U.S. Bureau of the Census, 2002).

By definition, developmental disabilities start before age 22 and continue throughout the person's lifetime. There are no specific statistics on total numbers of children's developmental disabilities in this country. According to the CDC and the National Center on Birth Defects and Developmental Disabilities (2002a), about 17% of children less than 18 years old have a developmental disability. Although the cause of a disability in a particular child may be unknown, about 2% of school-age children in the United States have serious developmental disabilities such as cerebral palsy or mental retardation. These children require supportive care or special education services. Education departments at the state and federal levels spend approximately $36 billion a year for special education programs for those ages 3 to 18 years old with developmental disabilities (CDC and National Center on Birth Defects and Developmental Disabilities, 2002a). The states reported providing services to 107,591 students with multiple disabilities during the 1998-1999 school year (National Information Center for Children and Youth with Disabilities, 2001).

Although data about disabilities among adults are also inadequate, there has been a continued decline between 1982 and 1994 in the prevalence of disability in those over 65 years, from 24.9% to 21.3% (Manton, Corder, and Stallard, 1997). The national long-term care surveys of the 1980s showed widening differences in disability between African-American and white older adult populations. Institutional care for the same groups was about the same (Clark, 1997). Liao et al (1999) found that those with higher income had less illness and disability and a better quality of life in their last years.

**Work disability,** the inability to perform work for 6 months or more because of a mental, physical, or other health condition (CDC, 1993), costs billions of dollars each year in lost wages and direct and indirect medical costs. In 2000, full-time workers ages 16 to 64 with work disabilities averaged $33,109 in earnings. In contrast, workers without such disability averaged $43,269. Also, 72% of those 16 to 64 years old with work disabilities had high school diplomas in 2001. The proportion of people 16 to 64 years old with work disabilities who have college degrees was even less, 11% (U.S. Bureau of the Census, 2002). Thus the effects of personal income on the functional status and early retirement of those with chronic diseases is significant (Kington and Smith, 1997).

## EFFECTS OF BEING PHYSICALLY COMPROMISED

The extent to which the physically compromised individual may need extra support, care, and services from the family unit and the community is shown in Box 30-2. Understanding these relationships is best grasped by starting with the stresses placed on the individual.

### Effects on the Individual

The Disability and Health Team of the CDC has determined that people who have disabilities are more likely than those without disabilities to have had two immunizations and a continuing source of health care. However, they are also more likely to be obese and to smoke cigarettes, and less likely to have health insurance and to take part in physical activity three times each week (CDC and National Center on Birth Defects and Developmental Disorders, 2002a).

Health care tends to be organized around medical diagnoses rather than an individual's degree and kind of functional strengths and limitations. However, the effects

---

**BOX 30-2    Potential Effects of Being Physically Compromised: Individuals, Families, and Communities**

**INDIVIDUAL**
- Related health problems (e.g., nutrition, oral health, hygiene, limited activity/stamina)
- Self-concept/self-esteem
- Life expectancy and risk for infection and secondary injury
- Developmental tasks; change in role expectations

**FAMILY**
- Stress on family unit
- Need for use of external resources to help family meet their role expectations
- Options limited in use of any discretionary income
- Social stigma

**COMMUNITY**
- Need/demand to reallocate resources
- Discomfort or fear due to lack of knowledge of disability
- Need to comply with legislation
- Services provided by health department, health care providers
- Need for other services beyond medical diagnosis (e.g., transportation)

---

of being physically compromised vary with the cause of the disability, the person's resilience, the severity of limitations, and other factors (Turner-Henson and Holaday, 1995). Because it is not possible to discuss here every cause of being physically compromised, some of the effects will be discussed, instead, from a life span perspective.

### Children: Infancy Through Adolescence

The wide variety of effects related to cause is best shown by looking at some specific examples. For example, infants and children, even those whose parents have accepted their need for gastrostomies, usually have poor growth and development. Better nutrition often improves the children's general health. They seem more alert and responsive. However, past negative experiences with oral feedings may result in continued facial defensiveness. For example, they may turn away from parents' kisses (Thorne, Radford, and McCormick, 1997). In addition, children with significant sensory deficits (e.g., hearing or vision impairments) are at risk for social isolation, cognitive and neuropsychological impairment, and developmental delays (Burns et al, 2000).

Chronic health conditions can also result in increased risk for additional health problems. Dosa, Boeing, and Kanter (2001) found that children with chronic health problems were three times more likely to have unscheduled admissions to an intensive care unit than children who were previously healthy. In another study, researchers identified children who were more likely to have functional limitations after cardiac surgery for congenital heart defects (Limperopoulos et al, 2001). These were children with microcephaly prior to or after surgery, and children who had had other abnormalities before open heart surgery or a delay in elective surgical corrections of the heart defects.

Social implications for children who are chronically ill are important. School-age children who are chronically ill may be discriminated against in their school systems, peer groups, and communities, and by government institutions. A study by Cole, Roberts, and McNeal (1996) looked at schoolchildren's perceptions of imaginary chronically ill peers with diabetes mellitus, asthma, acquired immunodeficiency syndrome (AIDS), or cystic fibrosis. The fourth-, fifth-, and sixth-grade students thought all of the diseases were contagious and had difficulty accepting children who had them as peers. Such results showed a need for early childhood education about those with chronic diseases.

Realistic needs of children's chronic health problems may cause embarrassment for them. For example, students who have ostomies or renal disease might need to leave classrooms or other school settings quickly to go to the bathroom. Having to explain this need could call unwanted attention to them and their diseases (Kliebenstin and Brome, 2000).

The effects on adolescents may vary with the time of onset of the physical problem. For example, in one study the researchers found that older adolescents tended to worry less, to have better quality-of-life scores, and to have lower diabetes impact scores than younger adolescents (Faro, 1999). For some conditions in adolescents, results of the effects of the health problem may vary in different studies. Snethen, Broome, and Bartels (2001) found that the majority of adolescents with end-stage renal disease had more positive outlooks about their lives than previous studies had shown. Adolescents who are physically compromised may be like their healthier peers in many ways. For example, adolescents who are developmentally delayed vary in employment rates. Adolescents' sociodemographic characteristics are often more important in successful employment than are their disabilities (Rimmerman et al, 1996). Adolescents who have chronic health problems are found to be as sexually active as their well peers. The visibility of the chronic conditions does not seem to affect the adolescents' sexual behavior (Suris et al, 1996).

### Transitions

Predictable transition points in a child's development can be difficult for those with disabilities and for their families. Children's first words, first steps, and first days at school are important events. These may highlight the differences between what is "normal" and what children's true abilities are (Mallory, 1996).

Of special concern is the change to adulthood by adolescents with disabilities. Parents often begin worrying about this issue when their children are between 5 and 10 years old. That is the age range in which the permanence of the disability is clearer. Many students with disabilities do not complete high school, have poor success in college, and are unemployed (Brown and Nourse, 1997). There is likely to be variation in success rates depending on such factors as the type of children's disabilities and the socioeconomic level of their families.

### Adults

Even with appropriate medical or surgical treatment, sequelae of the childhood health problem can persist into adulthood, affecting the quality of life of the affected individual. For example, Zebrack et al (2002) found that survivors of Hodgkin's and non-Hodgkin's lymphoma and of childhood leukemia were at greater risk for depression and somatic complaints as young adults if they were female, were of low socioeconomic status, and had received intensive chemotherapy.

Other conditions known to have major effects on the adult population include injuries that may lead to early death. The cost of low back pain, sometimes resulting from repeated microtrauma, is estimated to be about $85 billion a year in the United States. The effects of low back pain vary from minor inconvenience to major disability and psychosocial dysfunction in the person and his family (Simmonds, Kumar, and Lechelt, 1996). Older adults with fragility fractures are much more likely to die in the 6 months after a fracture. Hip fractures also increase the likelihood of repeated hospitalizations, the need for help with ADLs, and the need to enter a nursing home for the first time. The effects of fragility fractures are worsened by the presence of preexisting chronic diseases (Cooper, 1997; Wolinsky, Fitzgerald, and Stump, 1997). Furthermore, an individual's poor psychological status can increase the degree of disability more than would be expected on the basis of the physical problem itself. Hardiness and depression in an individual can affect the severity of a disability (Cataldo, 2001).

Other factors that affect the course of chronic illness in adults include their previous problem-solving skills and their ability to manage tasks related to their conditions and to development. Alcohol and drug use, living arrangements, insurance, prescription drug spending, the physical environment, the use of assistive equipment, and sexuality are all factors that affect adult responses to chronic illness (International Seminar on Women and Disability, 1997; Kochhar and Scott, 1997; Mueller, Schur, and O'Connell, 1997; Satariano, 1997; Verbrugge, Rennert, and Madans, 1997).

In older adults, chronic disease and factors such as loss, dependency, and loneliness can instigate malnutrition, reinforcing declining health (Chen, Schilling, and Lyder, 2001). In regard to ADLs among older adults, the progression of the loss of abilities was first walking, followed by bathing, transferring, dressing, toileting, and feeding. Women outlive men, just as in the well population, but are disabled for a significantly longer time (Dunlop, Hughes, and Manheim, 1997).

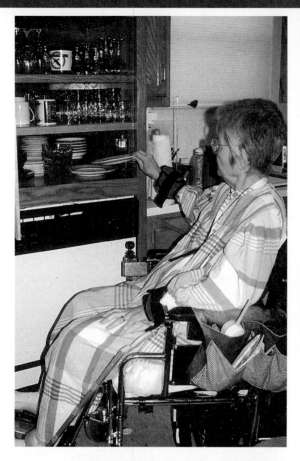
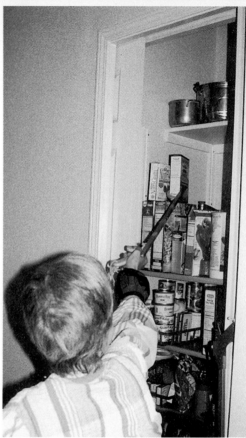
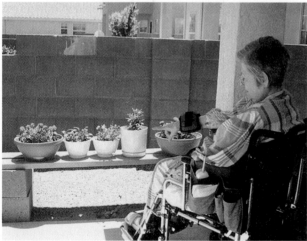
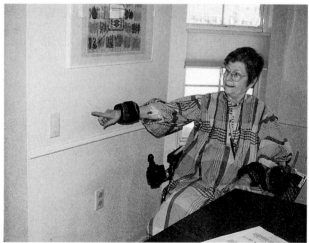

This disabled woman is able to live in and maintain her own home, including growing plants and flowers, with the help of easy-access devices and lower light fixtures and cabinets.

## Effects on the Family

Most people who are physically compromised are cared for at home by one or more family members. As many as one out of every seven adults in the United States may be caring for relatives or friends. More than one in five of these caregivers is a woman aged 35 to 64. About one third of this care may be given to people who are older adults (Marks, 1996). Figure 30-2 depicts some of the issues and concerns that occur when a family member is disabled and shows the effect of the disability on the family unit. As Figure 30-2 shows, the entire family system is affected when one of its members is disabled.

### Children: Infancy Through Adolescence

Many children with chronic illnesses or defects survive conditions that would have been fatal 20 years ago. However,

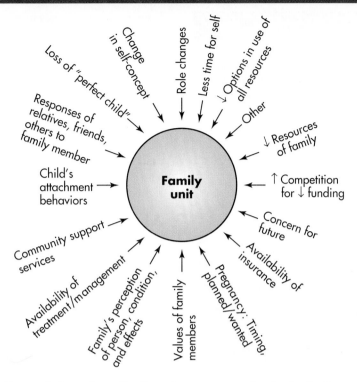

**Figure 30-2** Factors influencing a family unit when a member is physically compromised.

a child's disability may have long-term effects on the primary caregiver, usually the mother, and on the marital relationship. Mothers of severely brain-injured children describe these children and themselves as "different people" after the accident (Guerriere and McKeever, 1997).

In families with a child with a disability, the mother is most often the primary caregiver and, after the child, the focus of most research and support efforts. Fathers may feel left out and even denied support (Feudtner, 2002). Mothers' perceptions of the effect that their chronically ill children have on their families directly affect maternal mental health (Ireys and Silver, 1996). The family's response to a child's disability may also affect the child. If the family and mother have a positive psychological adjustment, so will the child. The school is often an area of conflict for parents of children with disabilities. One study reports differences in parent and teacher ratings of adaptive behavior in children with disabilities. The teachers' ratings were higher than those of the parents (Voelke, 1997). There is a need for a greater array of community and support services for children with disabilities who have behavior problems (Floyd and Gallagher, 1997).

Effects on siblings may vary with the particular disorder of the disabled children. If the disorder is emotional or communicative rather than physical, siblings may have difficulty adjusting (Fisman et al, 1996). In a recent review of more than 40 studies on the effects of chronically ill children on their siblings, Williams (1997) found that about 60% reported an increased risk of adjustment for siblings; 30% reported no risk. About 10% showed

### Evidence-Based Practice

This article describes the need for and development of the TIMDAC (the thematic instrument for measuring death anxiety in children). No tool before this existed to measure death anxiety of children with HIV/AIDS that was culturally sensitive to African-American and Hispanic (Latino) populations. The test uses projective technique with four colored pictures to interview children. The child tells a story about each picture. Death anxiety–related (DAR) and non–death anxiety–related (NDAR) responses are totaled. A death anxiety profile is created from this process. Interrater reliability in the final study was .80. However, the authors pointed out that studying the construct validity of an instrument is ongoing, especially with projective techniques.

**Nurse Use:** Children with life-threatening illnesses have less psychological damage when the family communicates openly about the disease. Therefore nurses need to support family openness in discussing the meaning of the illness with the child.

Emotional needs of HIV-infected and AIDS-diagnosed children should be investigated clinically. Nurses need to listen to these children's anxieties about and perceptions of death.

Ireland M, Malgady RG: Thematic instrument for measuring death anxiety in children (TIMDAC), *J Pediatr Nurs* 14(1):28, 1999.

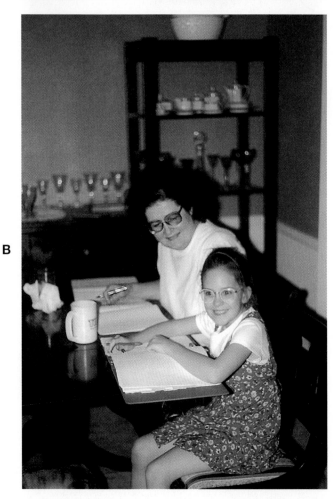

**A,** An at-risk infant girl who was 1 month premature and delivered by cesarean section because of abruption. This child's Apgar scores were 1 at one minute of age and 3 at five minutes of age. **B,** The same child at 10 years of age. She is profoundly hearing impaired. Her parents' commitment has helped her to be mainstreamed successfully, and she is able to do her own homework.

both positive and negative effects of having a disabled sibling.

Families with an infant who needs technologically assisted care at home may have home-health nurses present 12 to 18 hours each day. The presence of these non–family members may add stress to the family (Murphy, 1997). Going through such life-threatening, prolonged illnesses as leukemia in a child is stressful for the whole family. Some of these children may show such problems as posttraumatic stress, depression, anxiety, and learning problems. The parents of such children seem to be affected even more (Stuber, 1996).

### Adults

Physically compromised adults affect the family in various ways. For example, the financial effect of having a disabled family member may be worse if that person has been the main source of family income. Other concerns related to children living in a home with one or more disabled adults are risks for accidental injuries and the potential for behavioral problems (Gates and Lackey, 1998). Developmentally delayed adults pose special concerns for their parents who worry about the future of these adult children as the parents themselves age (Mengel, Marcus, and Dunkle, 1996).

Family members who are caregivers for physically compromised adults are most likely to be spouses or daughters of the affected individuals. Family caregivers are often poorly trained and at risk for injury (Brown and Mulley, 1997). Furthermore, primary informal caregivers commonly experience depression (Miller, 2002).

Pruchno, Patrick, and Burant (1997) confirmed that African-American mothers of adult children with disabilities experience greater caregiver burden and caregiver satisfaction than do white mothers. The meaning to a family of a member's disability is affected by that family's cultural background. Cultural implications and differences are found in the following areas (McCallion, Janicki, and Grant-Griffin, 1997):

- How disability is perceived
- Who are "family"
- Who provides care
- How the family makes decisions
- What family members think of each other
- What support families receive from friends and their community
- Why the family moved
- Cultural values important to family members
- Family willingness to accept services from outside the family
- The family's first language
- The family's concerns about service providers

## Effects on the Community

The presence of physically compromised people and their families in a community may have far-reaching effects on all aspects of community life. The community may be called on to respond in new ways to these citizens, especially as a result of federal laws affecting those who are disabled (U.S. Department of Justice, Civil Rights Division, Disability Rights Section, 2001).

## Children: Infancy Through Adolescence

The inclusion of children with complex medical problems in the New York City school system has created the need for skilled services of at least 150 nurses. A special curriculum to ensure these skills was developed by the school system (Lipper et al, 1997).

Children who are chronically ill or disabled and who enter school for mainstream education need more support from the community. Properly modified regular education can meet the learning needs of many students with disabilities (Terman et al, 1996). However, increased resources and support for regular classrooms, increased teacher training, and committed local school systems are requirements to successfully include children with disabilities.

Public schools must evaluate their effectiveness with students who are disabled, which adds to the cost of educating children. Education of local pediatricians and nurses helps to attain supportive and knowledgeable collaboration for the development of early intervention programs in the schools.

Transition points in children's lives require the investment of additional community resources. Parents feel highly involved in decisions about their disabled children in inclusive school environments. Teachers are generally positive about parent involvement. Both groups learn to value the need for shared commitment among all those involved (Bennett, DeLuca, and Bruns, 1997). Contact, books about disabled children, and discussions about attitudes can help preschool-age children develop positive attitudes and acceptance of people with disabilities (Favazza and Odom, 1997).

## Adults

One of the most visible ways in which those with disabilities affect their communities is through the changes that become necessary to accommodate access to buildings. The effects on facilities at hotels and motels to accommodate people with disabilities have been varied. Upscale lodgings are more likely to be accessible; however, some economy chains are recognized as having consistently accessible facilities (England, 1996). Increasing awareness of needs of library patrons with disabilities has changed some services. One area of limitation has been the use of adaptive technology that permits disabled users to search a library's online catalog and databases (Nelson, 1996).

The managed care system has seemingly failed to recognize basic characteristics of chronic disease and disability and the services needed to care for these clients. Persons with chronic conditions are the fastest-growing, costliest, and most complex group receiving health care (Bringewatt, 1996). Sources of costs for chronic health

problems include poor psychosocial adjustment and increased demands for screening of communicable diseases (Watt et al, 1997). Tuberculosis is an example of a communicable disease that is also a chronic health problem of varying severity.

People with disabilities affect the Medicaid and Medicare systems (Davis and O'Brien, 1996). Medicare data show that persons with disabilities have more functional limitations, poorer health status, and lower incomes, and they experience more barriers to health care than older adult Medicare beneficiaries. Information from Medicaid shows that a significant increase in the Medicaid disabled population has led to the young disabled outnumbering the Medicaid-eligible older adults. Medicaid serves an increasingly younger disabled population.

The way people with developmental disabilities affect their communities may be influenced by changes in Medicaid. It is expected that fewer people will be covered by Medicaid in the future and this will increase the burden of care on the communities in which these people live.

## SPECIAL POPULATIONS
### Low-Income Populations

Physically compromised individuals often experience poverty, as do other special population groups: single parents and their children, the aged, the unemployed, and members of racial and ethnic minorities. Persons with low income have less access to health care throughout their lives and are less likely to participate in all levels of prevention. Therefore they are at greater risk for the onset of disabling conditions and for more rapid progression of disease processes. Those in poverty are also at greater risk for disabling conditions resulting from lifestyle, such as injuries, tobacco abuse, and inadequate nutrition.

People who are disabled and in poverty are less likely to have the resources to provide for their special needs. Those who are physically compromised are often unemployed, even though they may be able to work and are seeking jobs. Employers may be reluctant to hire people whose conditions may increase health insurance costs. Therefore lack of insurance through the work setting further limits access to health care by those who are physically compromised.

The prevalence of chronic illness among U.S. youths is a significant public health concern. The lack of transition services for these youths fosters major delays in further education, vocational rehabilitation, and employment. For these and other reasons, many youths with chronic health problems must cope with the additional burden of poverty (Ireys et al, 1996). Other factors that affect low-income, physically compromised clients' access to needed services are inadequate transportation, lack of coordination of care, and limited locally available services for those who cannot pay for them. Figure 30-3 provides an illustration of the relationship between poverty and disabilities.

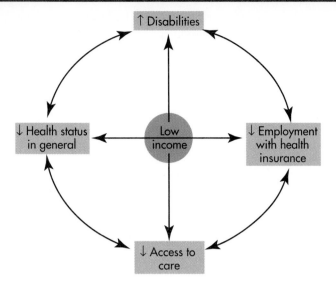

**Figure 30-3** Relationships of poverty and disability.

## SELECTED ISSUES

### Abuse

Most of the literature on abuse of those who are physically disabled is related to children and older adults. However, nurses need to understand state laws about reporting suspected abuse of the disabled of any age.

For adults, abuse associated with physical disability has been identified as occurring after the disability. One study about abuse by informal and formal personal caregivers of women who were physically and/or cognitively disabled found several major themes in interviewing the study participants. They concluded that women who are disabled can effectively prevent or manage abuse with experience, appropriate resources, and support (Saxton et al, 2001).

In children, physical disability may result from abuse or neglect, or abuse may occur after the onset of disability. A form of child abuse, Münchausen's by proxy syndrome, may present as a developmental disability or with neurologic symptoms, especially seizure activity. Several studies have shown that adults and children who are developmentally delayed are at higher risk for sexual abuse than the general public.

Much has been written about characteristics of abusers and the children and older adults who are abused. The interaction between the environment, the victim, and the abuser seems to be most important. Figure 30-4 includes several factors to consider. For example, those who are physically compromised and who are in group residences or must travel long distances in buses may be at risk for abuse from a variety of possible predators. Such potential victims seem to be especially at risk if they cannot communicate (Porter, Yuille, and Bent, 1995). Children with cerebral palsy or other conditions affecting their appearance, gait, and mobility are a vulnerable group. As they are more likely to be victimized by their peers, they need spe-

### Evidence-Based Practice

Mothers of 708 mainly at-risk infants were interviewed in their homes soon after their babies' discharge from the hospital. These children were at risk as a result of low birth weight, congenital defects, maternal age (14 to 17 years), or other medical and social problems. The interview included items thought to be related to the ecologic model of child maltreatment from behavior domains of the child, family, social, and parent. State (North Carolina) child abuse and neglect central registry data were tracked every 6 months until these children became 4 years old.

Some of the predisposing risk factors found soon after birth would still predict child maltreatment reports through 4 years of age. Generally, families with low levels of support had a higher risk of being reported for child maltreatment. Those families with higher levels of mothers' being depressed and/or with life-event stress and low social support had up to 4 times the risk of being reported for child maltreatment.

**Nurse Use:** Nurses need to include assessment of social support for the mother and family, especially when caring for high-risk children.

Ongoing, periodic monitoring and support by community health nurses can identify developing problems, reinforce effective parental behavior and problem solving, and help the client access formal or informal community support services.

Kotch JB: Predicting child maltreatment in the first 4 years of life from characteristics assessed in the neonatal period, *Child Abuse Negl* 23(4):305, 1999.

cial support and protection at school and in other settings with groups of children (Dawkins, 1996).

Breakdowns in parent–child interactions often result from the lack of maternal/caregiver knowledge of the young children's cues or of the limited capacity of some children with disabilities to stimulate their caregivers. Nurses can facilitate caregiver–child interactions by interpreting the child's cues (Hadadian, 1996).

Of special interest to nurses is the concern that the services developed to help children with disabilities may contribute to their increased risk for abuse. For example, depersonalizing potential victims is a critical factor in making violence toward them acceptable. One study found that nurses used the term "baby" with parents of full-term healthy newborns. The same nurses used the more distancing term "infant" with parents whose newborns had disabilities (Sobsey, 1997).

Children's disabilities are unlikely to be identified if the child must enter a state's child protection system—another way to depersonalize the child. This could mean that children do not receive all the care that they need, or, in many

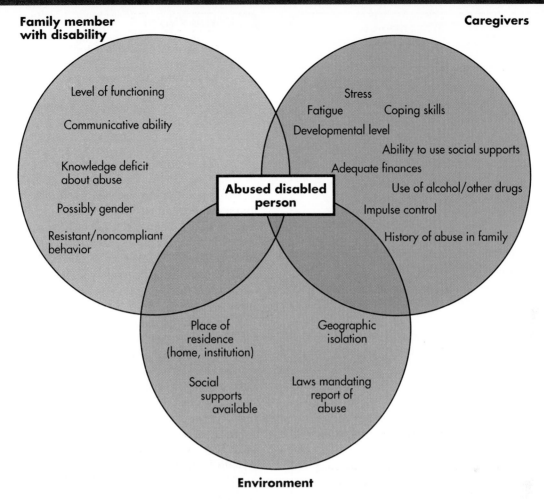

**Figure 30-4** Factors influencing the abuse of those who are physically compromised.

cases, that consideration is given only to the living situation's ability to protect and care for them, whereas the special education needs of the abused or neglected children are not taken into account. Often, routine lack of compliance with special education on the part of the involved school system is a major problem (Bonner, Crow, and Hensley, 1997; Weinberg, 1997).

There is limited research on abuse of people who are physically compromised and its many effects on the abused person. Nevertheless, nurses' comprehensive approach to health problems promotes their ability to consider multiple factors in these situations.

## Health Promotion

Health promotion usually focuses on the primary prevention of conditions that may lead to disability (e.g., smoking cessation to prevent lung cancer). Actually all three levels of prevention apply to physically compromised clients (Box 30-3). They do need information and counseling for health-promoting behaviors for secondary prevention of the progress of a condition or added pathology (Rimmer and Braddock, 2002). For example, a child with a serious congenital heart defect does not need the added insult of

increased respiratory infections from exposure to secondhand cigarette smoke.

Health promotion is a multidimensional concept that applies to all individuals regardless of disability. Strategies are needed to expand the knowledge base of health promotion for those who are physically compromised. Research, partnerships, and communication with those who have disabilities and among health care professionals are recommended (Fowler, 1997). Persons with chronic disability have frequently defined themselves in terms of their physical problems and sick role. Davidhizar and Shearer (1997) state that a client may be diagnosed with a physical illness, a chronic illness, or a disability and still work to attain high-level wellness by functioning in an integrated way with the environment. Health promotion programs for those with disabilities should have goals of reducing complications (fractures, malnutrition, pressure ulcers), maintaining optimal functional independence, providing opportunities for recreation, and improving quality of life by decreasing environmental barriers to healthful living (Rimmer, 1999).

Many health promotion and disease prevention needs are similar across the life span (e.g., exercise, diet, avoidance

## BOX 30-3  Levels of Prevention for Physically Compromised Clients

### PRIMARY PREVENTION

- Educate community residents about behaviors during pregnancy that will reduce the risk of having a baby with a disability.
- Push for a congressional mandate for addition of folic acid to cereals in the United States to reduce neural tube defect in infants.
- Promote exercise and physical fitness programs in schools to lessen obesity in that population and decrease incidence of dysmetabolic syndrome.

### SECONDARY PREVENTION

- Initiate early detection actions to identify any chronic or disabling condition.
- Initiate blood pressure screening programs to identify those at risk for strokes or heart damage as soon as possible.
- Push programs for earliest detection of cancer (e.g., mammography, malignant melanoma), as comorbidities are more common with cancers detected later.

### TERTIARY PREVENTION

- Take action to maintain or increase functional abilities for persons who have a physically compromising condition.
- Encourage exercise programs for sedentary clients with osteoporosis, to reduce the likelihood of fractures.
- Initiate a diabetes type I education program for children and parents, with a focus on disease management and prevention of disease complications.

### DID YOU KNOW?

Mexican Americans 65 years and older with type II diabetes mellitus have a greater prevalence and health burden from the disease than do non-Hispanic and African Americans of the same age group. This is especially true among older adult men (Black, Ray, and Markides, 1999).

---

of excess substance use, and injury prevention.) However, specific problems and interventions to deal with these needs vary according to age, specific disabling condition, and developmental status. For example, nutritional needs of premature infants are related to obtaining adequate energy, protein, fat, vitamins, and minerals. An older adult with type II diabetes mellitus may be concerned primarily with reducing the risk of experiencing a myocardial infarction.

Because one of the most important needs of those with disabilities is appropriate nutrition, nurses may consult with dietetics professionals or refer clients to them for assistance. For example, a client with Down syndrome may need a lower caloric intake than a nondisabled persons of the same age. A dietitian could provide information or counseling about managing this need (Cloud, 1997).

Tertiary prevention for clients with developmental disabilities who are in residential facilities is enhanced by involvement of a dietitian (Hogan and Evers, 1997). Families and professionals can work together to meet the nutritional needs of children with disabilities and chronic health care problems. Doing so before a child becomes severely malnourished or a family becomes dysfunctional is possible with such an approach (Secrist-Mertz et al, 1997).

A large body of research about exercise science has been published in the last 30 years. However, little information is available on the activity patterns and physiologic responses to exercise in people with disabilities. The availability of such information would be helpful to nurses in counseling those with disabilities.

A variety of smoking cessation treatments are effective as secondary prevention with the disabled as with well populations. These treatments can be used with groups of smokers who have chronic illnesses (Wewers and Ahijevych, 1996).

It is especially important to establish lifelong, health-promoting behaviors in children who are disabled. Unfortunately, parents may be so overwhelmed by caring for such children that this aspect of care is not considered. Furthermore, health promotion and disease protection for those who are physically compromised have often not been emphasized in primary care or in rehabilitation. Table 30-1 summarizes issues that limit access to health care and health promotion for those who are physically compromised (Gans, Mann, and Becker, 1993).

As an example, women who are disabled generally receive screening and preventive care comparable to that of women who are not disabled. Exceptions are women who have significant mobility deficits of the lower extremities. They are much less likely to receive Papanicolaou smears, mammograms, and inquiries from health care providers about smoking (Iezzoni et al, 2001).

Access to physicians' offices can be improved in the following areas (Jones and Tamari, 1997):

- Transportation and entrance to the facility

### WHAT DO YOU THINK?

Nurses should participate in analyzing various types of data (e.g., traffic accident patterns) to identify problems that could be improved with public health approaches or interventions.

**Table 30-1  Impediments to Primary Health Care of the Physically Compromised**

| ISSUES | EXAMPLES |
|---|---|
| Transportation | May not be able to drive; limited flexibility in public/private transportation; may need specially equipped van |
| Access to clinic or office | Entrances, halls, restrooms may all be inadequate. Examination tables, scales, life-support equipment unavailable or inappropriate. Increased time needed for disabled client's visit. |
| Inadequate care from primary care providers | Limited or no training in primary care needs or health promotion of those with disabilities; lack of understanding reasons that those with disabilities often delay treatment until at crisis levels; limited ability to distinguish between progress in a disability and different, new health problems |
| Information given to clients | Often unavailable or available to only few specialists; may not have been given basic health information in school; most have never received comprehensive rehabilitation |
| Finances | Health maintenance or promotion costly; cost of good food, and someone to obtain and prepare it; exercise; transportation; fees of facilities and assistance with exercise |
| Personal assistance | Needed by some with disabilities for most basic health activities, hygiene, laundry |

Based on data from Gans BM, Mann NR, Becker BE: Delivery of primary care to the physically challenged, *Arch Phys Med Rehabil* 74(12-S):S15, 1993; Nosek MA: Primary care issues for women with severe disabilities, *J Women's Health* 1(4):245, 1992.

- Entrance to the office
- Waiting rooms
- Restrooms
- Examination rooms
- General building features

## Complementary and Alternative Medicine

People with disabilities and their caregivers can feel helpless and frustrated when conditions are labeled as incurable by the usual treatments of Western medicine. The label may be especially accurate for conditions of chronic pain and those that are terminal. In addition, cultural backgrounds of various people may influence their belief in and use of alternative methods to maintain or improve health (Dokken and Sydnor-Greenberg, 2000).

The National Center for Complementary and Alternative Medicine (NCCAM) in the National Institutes of Health classifies alternative medical treatments as mind–body medicine, alternative medical systems, lifestyle and disease prevention, biologically based treatments, manipulative and body-based systems, biofield, and bioelectronics (see www.nccam.nih.gov). Several chronic health problems have been identified as being treated by various alternative medicine methods. Examples include shark cartilage for cancer (biologically based treatments) (Dokken and Sydnor-Greenberg, 2000); ephedra, or ma huang, used for asthma (biologically based treatments) (Pettit, 2002); and osteopathic manipulative therapy (OMT) or chiropractic for rheumatic diseases (manipulative and body-based systems) (Fiechtner and Brodeus, 2002).

Nurses working in health promotion programs for populations with disabilities need to explore these groups' beliefs and understanding of conventional and unconventional therapies for their health problems. Nurses also need to be aware of the comorbidities associated with their client groups' chronic health problems for which the clients may use alternative treatments (Kanning, 1999). Also, nurses need to understand potential problems and known benefits of alternative therapies. For example, glucosamine has been shown to benefit those with arthritis or other joint damage. Nurses can best help their clients by exploring and discussing their use of alternative treatment methods. For example, "Are you doing anything else for your health (or health problems)?" can introduce the topic without the potentially judgmental term *alternative treatment*. This topic should be considered an ongoing one in contacts with groups in health promotion programs.

## HEALTHY PEOPLE 2010 OBJECTIVES

Healthy People 2010 objectives can be found at http://evolve.elsevier.com/Stanhope. Clearly, many of the national health goals that apply to people without disabling conditions also apply to people who are physically compromised.

Of the 467 objectives in Healthy People 2010, 207 include recommendations applicable to people with disabilities. For the first time, a Healthy People plan has a chapter (Chapter 6) that specifically focuses on the health promotion and general well-being of children and adults with disabilities across their life spans (see the Healthy People 2010 box).

Examples of recent reports on surveillance results, with implications for disability prevention or management, include those on the incidence of birth defects in the United States and toy-related injuries among U.S. children and teenagers (1997c). Surveillance activities include identifying

**Healthy People 2010** | Objectives for People With Disabilities

6-1 Include in the core of all relevant Healthy People 2010 surveillance instruments a standardized set of questions that identify "people with disabilities"
6-2 Reduce the proportion of children and adolescents with disabilities who are reported to be sad, unhappy, or depressed
6-3 Reduce the proportion of adults with disabilities who report feelings such as sadness, unhappiness, or depression that prevents them from being active
6-4 Increase the proportion of adults with disabilities who participate in social activities

6-5 Increase the proportion of adults reporting sufficient emotional support
6-6 Increase the proportion of adults reporting satisfaction with life
6-8 Eliminate disparities in employment between working-age adults with and without disabilities
6-10 Increase the proportion of health and wellness and treatment program and facilities that provide full access for people with disabilities
6-11 Reduce the proportion of people who report not having the assistive devices and technology needed

From U.S. Department of Health and Human Services: *Healthy people 2010: understanding and improving health,* ed 2, Washington, DC, 2000, U.S. Government Printing Office.

children with fetal alcohol syndrome (FAS) and those who were seriously hearing impaired (CDC, 1997b). Nurses need to use preventive-care practices to reduce the complications and disability from chronic disease.

## HEALTHY CITIES/HEALTHY COMMUNITIES

The Healthy Cities movement of the World Health Organization was the forerunner of Healthy Communities (Duhl, 2000). In 1996, the Coalition for Healthier Cities and Communities (CHCC) was formed. The purposes of this group are to be a resource link, a voice for public policy, and a facilitator of nationwide Healthy Communities efforts (Norris and Pittman, 2000). Nurses working with people with disabilities can access information from this coalition at www.healthycommunities.org.

Families are grounded in the communities in which they live. Informal support networks, or systems, are key factors in assisting families. Also, community-based family support intervention has been shown to have the positive effect of promoting the adjustment of children with selected chronic health problems (Chernoff et al, 2002).

A city can be considered healthy if it meets the following requirements:

1. The ability to meet developmental needs (food, clothing, shelter), functional and aesthetic needs, communication and networks, ecologic considerations, and attention to competing priorities for creation of a stable infrastructure
2. The flexibility to cope with change or crisis
3. The competence that makes it possible for individuals or groups to use the city
4. The ability to perform its educational role, which is defined as learning that permits questions, is free from prejudiced opinions, and is open to the possibility that there are different ways of viewing a problem

To ensure these requirements for a healthy city, the following Healthy Communities principles are needed for all residents (Lee, 2000):
- Broad definition of health
- Broad definition of community
- Shared vision from community values
- Quality of life addressed for everyone
- Diverse citizen participation and widespread community ownership
- Focus on "systems change"
- Building capacity using local assets and resources
- Benchmarking and measurement of progress and outcomes

These requirements apply to all citizens, including those who are physically compromised. One of the major elements of the Healthy Cities project, as described in Chapter 17, is the understanding that the health of communities and the health of people who live in them depend on the environment.

## THE CUTTING EDGE

Healthy Cities can help members of their communities promote their own health through community-wide campaigns supporting physical activity (Task Force on Community Preventive Services, 2002). Approaches and messages informing about and supporting physical activity can be developed for specific groups with disabilities.

The greatest obstacles faced by people with disabilities are often attitudinal ones. Programs that place responsibility for rehabilitation and integration within the community can foster a better understanding of the issues. Until significant progress is made in this area, problems of access in communities that ignore those with disabilities will continue (Peat, 1997).

The Institute of Medicine (1996) has recommended that government public health agencies develop the capacity to identify and work in partnership with all the agencies that influence a community's health. This approach could emphasize the involvement of such established institutions and agencies as local hospitals and health departments (Burger et al, 1998). Nurses working with individuals or populations who are physically compromised can be a member of the partnership.

## ROLE OF THE NURSE

Many factors influence the role of the nurses who work with physically compromised people. These factors include the community's awareness of those who are disabled and its commitment to their health needs. The agencies in which nurses work have particular influence. The structure and priorities of an agency determine whether a nurse will carry a general caseload or focus on service to a special population. If funding sources are dedicated to particular programs (e.g., tuberculosis control, maternal–child health services), care for those who are physically compromised may be dispersed throughout several program areas and may be difficult to identify.

In dealing with those who are physically compromised, the nurses' roles may further change as the focus varies between the levels of individuals, families, groups, or entire communities. For example, the nurses may be caregivers and apply the nursing process and principles of epidemiology at any of these levels. This may include, among other things, assessing, implementing, and evaluating technical care for ventilator-dependent clients at home.

A second role long associated with community-oriented nursing is that of educator. Educators provide clients at any level with sufficient knowledge to enable them to decide on the most appropriate behavior for their own needs. Nurses may provide an entire community with information about reducing disability by decreasing a specific cause, such as spinal cord injury. The closely related counseling role is of value in that clients learn to improve their problem-solving skills as the nurses guide them.

Community-oriented nurses' roles as advocates for individuals and families or groups of those who are physically compromised are especially important. An advocate is someone who speaks on behalf of others who are unable to speak for themselves. One of the potential problems with this role is that nurses may unintentionally foster excessive dependence by individuals, families, or other groups. Nurses focus on using advocacy to support those who need this service. At the same time, observing nurses' data-collecting and negotiating skills can serve as models for clients who are capable of using such knowledge. For example, nurses might advocate a school environment that is adapted to the specific needs of children who are wheelchair mobile but who do not necessarily have to be limited to their chairs, without explicitly telling the children when they should use their wheelchairs. Nurses may help family caregivers of disabled individuals by validating that the caregivers' own basic needs are being sacrificed and by identifying ways that this problem can be moderated.

As referral agents, nurses maintain current information about agencies whose services are of potential use to those

---

**HOW TO**  **Promote Appropriate Use of Asthma Medications by Children**

A. Collaborate/coordinate efforts with health care provider managing child's asthma.
  1. Personnel in all areas in which child uses drugs need to be informed of regimen.
  2. Be aware of factors that could affect adherence to regimen:
     a. Prolonged therapy
     b. Medications used prophylactically
     c. Delayed consequences of nonadherence
     d. Drugs expensive, hard to use
     e. Family concerns about side effects
     f. Adherence less likely with mild or severe asthma; most likely with moderate asthma
     g. Child with cognitive or emotional problems
     h. Poorly functioning family
     i. Strong alternative health beliefs
     j. Multiple caregivers
B. Assess child's adherence to regimen.
  1. Count pills; float test for remaining amount in inhalers (gross estimate).
  2. Ask child, "In an average week, how many puffs of your inhaler do you actually get?"
  3. Refill history from pharmacist (information can be obtained from child's health care provider)
C. Interventions
  1. Educate child, parents, and other caregivers.
  2. Encourage adaptation of regimen to family's needs.
     a. Health care provider may need additional information about family situation.
     b. Signed, dated, written permission to exchange information with such a provider is needed.
  3. Encourage consideration of acceptability of medication to child, family.
  4. Be encouraging, caring, supportive, and willing to work with family.
  5. Follow-up and monitor progress closely, including school attendance, when appropriate.
  6. Consider home visits (e.g., to assess/manage environmental triggers).
  7. Identify an "asthma partner" (i.e., another adult besides parents when they do not reliably monitor child).
  8. Use a contract for adherence.
  9. In extreme cases, especially with young and/or ill children, consider reporting family to child protective services for medical neglect.

who are disabled. Referral, one of the most important functions of nurses, is the process of directing clients to the resources that can meet their needs. For self-directed clients and families, information about an agency's services, phone number, and address may be adequate. For families with little understanding of how systems work for a developmentally delayed child, more specific guidance and case conferences with the local schools may be necessary to coordinate the child's health-related and educational needs.

As primary care providers, those who make essential care universally accessible, nurses may be the most logical persons to ensure that primary prevention for other health problems (e.g., communicable diseases) and information about health promotion are made available to clients who are physically compromised. On a more individualized basis, the case manager role means meeting the needs of clients by developing a plan of care to reach that goal. Nurses may see to it that others carry out the plan and then be responsible for evaluating the plan's effectiveness. For example, clients who have been disabled through complications of diabetes mellitus may have several immediate problems, such as adjusting to the amputation of one or more limbs, learning strategies for better management, and compliance to slow progress of other complications. Nurses (as case managers) will develop plans with clients and families to meet those needs and establish time frames to evaluate specific outcomes.

In the coordinator role, nurses are not responsible for developing overall plans of client care. Instead, responsibilities include assisting clients and families by organizing and integrating the resources of other agencies or care providers to meet clients' needs most efficiently. For example, with the families' agreement, nurses may arrange for them to see social workers on the same day that they bring their children to be followed up in a pediatric cardiology clinic.

Nurses perform the functions of collaborators by taking part in joint decision making with clients, families, groups, and communities. Collaboration may, of course, be part of community-oriented nurses' role with other care providers, too. This role is of particular importance as nurses seek to involve those who are physically disabled in community-level decisions that affect their lives. An example is working with agencies or groups who make decisions about community housing for those who are physically compromised.

The role of nurses as case finders is historically a basic part of community-oriented nursing. Nurses identify individuals with disabilities who need services they are not currently receiving. Developmental, vision, and hearing screening of young children by nurses are examples of ways in which this role is carried out. It is important to bear in mind that, although the nurses' efforts are for particular clients, the focus of case finding is on monitoring the health status of entire groups or communities. Case

finding of tuberculosis may indicate the increase in a population of this chronic disease, which is also a communicable disease. Nurses may also identify those who are members of vulnerable populations and who are not yet physically compromised. Such people may have limited or no access to health promotion or disease prevention services, or they may be unaware of those for which they are eligible.

Nurses may function as change agents at all levels, including the health care delivery system. A change agent is one who originates and creates change. This process includes identifying a need for change, enlightening and motivating others as to this need, and starting and directing the proposed change. Nurses may function in the role by helping to obtain more appropriate health care services for those who are physically compromised.

## LEGISLATION

One nurse who works with physically compromised clients may have a general caseload of clients of all ages, whereas another, such as a school nurse, may see clients in a specific age group. A nurse's need to know about laws related to specific groups will vary with the population that is the nurse's focus of care. Box 30-4 summarizes categories of historically significant federal legislation designed to benefit those who are disabled.

The United States Department of Justice provides *A Guide to Disability Rights Law* (2001), an overview of federal civil rights laws designed to ensure equal opportunity for people with disabilities. This guide is available at www.

---

### BOX 30-4 Categories of Federal Legislation for Those With Disabilities

**EDUCATION**
- Early childhood special education
- Elementary and Secondary Education Act and amendments
- Vocational education for those who are disabled

**REHABILITATION**
- Vocational
- Medical, including Medicare and Medicaid
- Rehabilitational

**SERVICES**
- Economic assistance
- Facility construction and architectural design
- Deinstitutionalization and independent living
- Civil rights and advocacy

Based on data from National Information Center for Children and Youth with Disabilities: *NICHCY News Digest* 1(1):12, 1991.

usdoj.gov/crt/ada/publicat.htm. The document is also available in large print, Braille, audiotape, and computer disk from this website.

Rehabilitation services were originally developed through legislation for veterans of World War I. In time, others who were physically compromised were regarded less as sources of embarrassment to their families and more as citizens who should participate as fully as possible in all aspects of society. This change in attitudes is reflected in major laws being passed. For example, the **Americans With Disabilities Act** of 1990 (ADA), PL 101-336 and subsequent amendments, has had far-reaching effects on the civil rights of those in the community who are physically compromised. Significantly, this act includes all of the following:

- Persons who have a physical or mental impairment that substantially limits one or more of the major life activities of the individual
- Persons who have a record of such an impairment
- Persons who are perceived or regarded as having a disability

Examples include someone with a condition that is not presently disabling (e.g., hypertension or a mild congenital deformity).

Herr (1997) describes the Individuals with Disabilities Education Act of 1990 as a rare piece of landmark legislation. Everyone concerned needs to maintain the effectiveness of such legislation so that school systems will be fair and provide administrative equity to all. Actions can include the following:

1. Promoting the fundamental principle that "all means all," because all children with disabilities must be educated
2. Leveling the "playing field" by retaining the balance of due process safeguards to prevent abuses and infringements of rights
3. Respecting partnerships and the orderly process that the act promotes now
4. Understanding the interrelated role of advocacy and monitoring to ensure compliance with the law
5. Strengthening the act to help children with disabilities and their families to live productive lives

Nurses are in positions to provide advocacy for these children by supporting such actions.

For older adults, the ADA and the adoption of living wills and related protections by various states are important recent legislative changes. These support the legal rights of older adults and disabled people in attempting to live as normal lives as possible and to make their own decisions about serious or terminal illnesses (Slavitt and LaBant, 1996).

In addition, most states and many large cities and counties have their own laws prohibiting discrimination on the basis of disability. Such laws sometimes offer greater protection to employees by extending coverage to smaller employers, by using more expansive definitions of disability than those used under the ADA, and by expanding the duty to accommodate to require that employers assist employees with disabilities to move to new positions for which they are qualified. As such, it is important for nurses to be familiar with the state law in the area in which they practice and how it may affect employer obligations to employees with disabilities (Pennell and Johnson, 1997). Considering the potential significance of major legislation for nurses' practice, it may be necessary to provide or obtain continuing education on the topic.

The ADA has been an effective means of addressing allegations of employer discrimination brought forward by people with seizure disorders. However, it has not increased the number of people with disabilities who are employed. In combination with employer education and rehabilitation counseling, legislative protection can help those with epilepsy to be more successful in pursuing employment opportunities (Troxell, 1997).

The Federal Rehabilitation Act of 1973 and the ADA have given physically impaired athletes the legal means to challenge medical sports participation decisions. Health care providers who work with physically compromised individuals must recognize the potential conflict between medical safety recommendations and the expanded legal rights of these individuals. Prospective athletes, after being fully informed about risks of participation in sports, have greater responsibility in the decision-making process (Nichols, 1996).

There have been recent changes in the types of legal ways to correct violations that inhibit a student's right to free appropriate public education (FAPE). For example, there has been increased use of compensating education–educational services allowed despite a student's being beyond the age of eligibility because of past violations of the right to FAPE. In addition, courts have increasingly considered monetary damages for "mental distress" or "pain and suffering" as potential remedies for people with disabilities who are judged to have been denied FAPE (Katsiyannis and Maag, 1997). Nurses may be in positions to emphasize to school systems and to parents of children with disabilities that compliance with the Individuals with Disabilities Education Act (IDEA) and other related laws is more cost effective in the long run.

In 1986, part H was added to the IDEA, expanding coverage to include infants and toddlers from birth to age 2. Many of these children have multiple, serious health problems. Early intervention specialists, including nurses, are being faced with do-not-resuscitate (DNR) orders without specific legal guidance. All children with special health care needs should have clear emergency procedures and guidelines within their Individual Family Service Plan (IFSP) at school. All involved staff should be informed of the program's policies for emergency procedures, including DNR orders, and should be trained in appropriate interventions.

Assisted suicide of people with disabilities is an area with many ethical, legal, and practice considerations for health care providers. Part of the discussion focuses on whether physician-assisted suicide should be considered as part of a medical treatment continuum. Another consideration is the possibility that viewing assisted suicide as a public health issue may provide insight into preventive measures to lower risk factors. This can also improve the lives of members of the community who are disabled (Blanck, Kirschner, and Bienen, 1997).

Both federal and state legislation and rules and regulations have implications for nurses working with those who are disabled. Nurses must remember that other state and federal laws and rules and regulations are applicable for all citizens. For example, some states have wrongful death laws that specify who must be consulted and who can make decisions about the type of resuscitation to be used and under what circumstances.

## Practice Application

A referral was made to a public health department from a nearby regional level III neonatal intensive care unit (NICU) regarding discharge plans for a developmentally delayed infant. The infant, Joel, was born at 27 weeks of gestation and had remained in intensive care for 7 months. His hospital course was complicated by hyaline membrane disease, bronchopulmonary dysplasia, and intraventricular hemorrhage. At the time of discharge, Joel was receiving neither supplemental oxygen nor medications and was taking all of his feedings orally. There were strong indications of spastic diplegia, and he was diagnosed as having severe retinopathy of prematurity with the expectation of eventual blindness.

Family financial resources were extremely limited. Although Medicaid coverage was available for subsequent needs, the family owed over $100,000 to the hospital. Joel's grandmother would babysit while Mary, Joel's mother, finished high school. Joel's father, who was also 17 years old and unemployed, had not been active with Mary and her mother in the hospital discharge planning program. His involvement with Mary and Joel was expected to be minimal. The hospital was seeking a home evaluation before discharge.

What would you consider to be the first step in completing the home evaluation?

---

**Answer is in the back of the book.**

## Key Points

- The community-oriented health nurse has numerous opportunities to influence the development of disabling conditions through health promotion, especially health education for parents who might be at high risk for having a disabled child, for children at risk for accidents and injuries, and for adults with chronic illnesses who might prevent disability through careful health practices.

- Many of the Healthy People 2010 objectives apply to physically compromised individuals, their families, and communities.

- Physically compromised people need to participate in health promotion to prevent the onset of a new health disruption, to strengthen their well-functioning aspects, and to prevent further deterioration of their health problem.

- Nursing interventions for physically compromised clients requires attention to their health, as well as to the environment in which they live.

- Nurses influence policy decisions that affect the health and well-being of physically compromised individuals.

- Nurses must know both federal and state laws pertaining to disabilities to most effectively assist clients and their families.

## Clinical Decision-Making Activities

1. Divide the class or the clinical group into two teams and debate the following: Children with developmental disabilities should or should not be mainstreamed into classrooms with nondisabled children.

2. During a home visit first to an adult and then to a child who has a chronic illness that leaves them physically compromised, answer the following questions:
   a. Could this disability have been prevented? If so, what steps could a nurse have taken to provide health promotion activities that would have prevented the occurrence of the disability condition?
   b. What role, if any, does the environment play in the onset of this compromising health condition?
   c. What preventive activities are currently needed to assure the highest possible quality of life for this person?

3. For the next week, look at each building that you enter and consider the following:
   a. What accommodations have been made to allow physically compromised people to enter this building?
   b. What accommodations should still be made?
   c. Who should pay for these architectural accommodations?

4. Spend one day following your usual schedule using either crutches or a wheelchair, so you can understand better what it means to be physically compromised.

5. Using a telephone book or community resource directory for your town, identify all agencies whose scope of work is devoted to assisting physically compromised individuals and their families.

## Additional Resources

These related resources are found either in the appendix at the back of this book or on the book's website at **http://evolve.elsevier.com/Stanhope.**

### Appendixes

Appendix I.1 Instrumental Activities of Daily Living (IADLs) Scale

### evolve Evolve Website

Appendix A.1 Schedule of Clinical Preventive Services

Appendix C.2 The Living Will Directive

Assessment Tools for Communities With Physically Compromised Members

Assessment Tools for Families With Physically Compromised Members

Assessment Tools for Physically Compromised Individuals

Immunization Schedules

WebLinks: Healthy People 2010

# References

Badley EM: An introduction to the concepts and classifications of the international classification of impairments, disabilities, and handicaps, *Disabil Rehabil* 15(4):161-163, 1993.

Banja JD: Ethics, values, and world culture: the impact on rehabilitation, *Disabil Rehabil* 18(6):279, 1996.

Bennett T, DeLuca D, Bruns D: Putting inclusion into practice: perspectives of teachers and parents, *Exceptional Children* 64(1):115, 1997.

Black SA, Ray LA, Markides KS: The prevalence and health burden of self-reported diabetes in older Mexican Americans: findings from the Hispanic established populations for epidemiological studies of the elderly, *Am J Public Health* 89(4):546, 1999.

Blanck P, Kirschner K, Bienen L: Socially assisted dying and people with disabilities: some emerging legal, medical, and policy implications, *Ment Phys Disabil Law Rep* 21(4):538, 1977.

Bonner BL, Crow SM, Hensley LD: State efforts to identify maltreated children with disabilities: a follow-up study, *Child Maltreatment* 2(1):52, 1997.

Bringewatt RJ: Integrating care for people with chronic conditions, *Creative Nurs* 2(2):7, 1996.

Brown AR, Mulley GP: Injuries sustained by caregivers of disabled elderly people, *Age Aging* 26(1):21, 1997.

Brown P, Nourse SW: Moving from school to adult life, *Phys Med Rehabil Clin North Am* 8(2):359, 1997.

Burger A et al: Healthy valley 2000, *Am J Public Health* 88(5):821, 1998.

Burns CE et al: *Pediatric primary care,* ed 2, Philadelphia, 2000, Saunders.

Cataldo JK: The relationships of hardiness and depression to disability in institutionalized older adults, *Rehabil Nurs* 26(1):28-33, 2001.

Centers for Disease Control and Prevention: Prevalence of work disability, United States, 1990, *MMWR Morb Mortal Wkly Rep* 42(39):757, 1993.

Centers for Disease Control and Prevention: State-specific prevalence of cigarette smoking among adults, and children's and adolescents' exposure to environmental tobacco smoke, *MMWR Morb Mortal Wkly Rep* 46(44):1038, 1997a.

Centers for Disease Control and Prevention: Surveillance for fetal alcohol syndrome using multiple sources—Atlanta, Georgia, 1981-1989, *MMWR Morb Mortal Wkly Rep* 46(47):1118, 1997b.

Centers for Disease Control and Prevention: Toy-related injuries among children and teenagers—United States, 1996, *MMWR Morb Mortal Wkly Rep* 46(50):1185, 1997c.

Centers for Disease Control and Prevention: Prevalence of disabilities and associated health conditions among adults—United States, 1999, *MMWR Morb Mortal Wkly Rep* 50(7):120-125, 2001.

Centers for Disease Control and Prevention: *Healthy people 2010—changing national health priorities,* 2002, available at http//www.cdc.gov/ncbddd/dh/schp.htm.

Centers for Disease Control and Prevention, National Center on Birth Defects and Developmental Disabilities: *Developmental disabilities: about developmental disabilities,* 2002a, available at http://www.cdc.gov/ncbddd/dd/default.htm.

Centers for Disease Control and Prevention, National Center on Birth Defects and Developmental Disabilities: *Healthy people 2010: leading health indicator data for people with disabilities,* 2002b, available at http://www.cdc.gov/ncbddd/dh/hpleading.htm.

Chen CC, Schilling LS, Lyder CH: A concept analysis of malnutrition in the elderly, *J Adv Nurs* 36(1):131-142, 2001.

Chernoff RG et al: A randomized, controlled trial of a community-based support program for families of children with chronic illness: pediatric outcomes, *Arch Pediatr Adolesc Med* 156(6):533-539, 2002, available at http://archpedi.ama-assn.org/issues/v156n6/rfull/poal1379.html.

Clark DO: US trends in disability and institutionalization among older blacks and whites, *Am J Public Health* 87(3):328, 1997.

Cloud HH: Expanding roles for dietitians working with persons with developmental disabilities, *J Am Dietet Assoc* 97(2):129, 1997.

Cole KL, Roberts MC, McNeal RE: Children's perceptions of ill peers: effects of disease, grade, and impact variables, *Child Health Care* 25(2):107, 1996.

Cooper C: The crippling consequences of fractures and their impact on quality of life, *Am J Med* 103(2A):12S, 1997.

Davidhizar R, Shearer R: Helping the client with chronic disability achieve high-level wellness, *Rehabil Nurs* 22(3):131, 1997.

Davis MH, O'Brien E: Profile of persons with disabilities in Medicare and Medicaid, *Health Care Financ Rev* 17(4):179, 1996.

Dawkins JL: Bullying, physical disability and the pediatric patient, *Dev Med Child Neurol* 38(7):603, 1996.

Dokken D, Sydnor-Greenberg N: Exploring complementary and alternative medicine in pediatrics: parents and professionals working together for new understanding, *Pediatr Nurs* 26(4):383-390, 2000.

Dosa NP, Boeing NM, Kanter RK: Excess risk of severe acute illness in children with chronic health conditions, *Pediatrics* 107(3):499-504, 2001.

Duhl LJ: A short history and some acknowledgments, *Public Health Rep* 115(2,3):116-117, 2000.

Dunlop DD, Hughes SL, Manheim LM: Disabilities in activities of daily living: patterns of change and a hierarchy of disability, *Am J Public Health* 87(3):387, 1997.

Elder JH, Kaplan EB: Developmental stifling: an emerging symptom pattern, *Issues Compr Pediatr Nurs* 23:49-57, 2000.

England D: Accessibly inn-correct, *Accent on Living* 41(3):26, 1996.

Faro B: The effect of diabetes on adolescents' quality of life, *Pediatr Nurs* 25(3):247-253, 286, 1999.

Favazza PC, Odom SL: Promoting positive attitudes of kindergarten-age children toward people with disabilities, *Exceptional Children* 63(3):405, 1997.

Feudtner C: Grief-love: contradictions in the lives of fathers of children with disabilities, *Arch Pediatr Adolesc Med* 156(7):643, 2002.

Fiechtner JJ, Brodeus RR: Manual and manipulation techniques for rheumatic disease, *Med Clin North Am* 86(1):83-96, 2002.

Fisman S et al: Risk and protective factors affecting the adjustment of siblings of children with chronic disabilities, *J Am Acad Child Adolesc Psychiatry* 35(11):1532, 1996.

Floyd FJ, Gallagher EM: Parental stress, care demands, and use of support services for school-age children with disabilities and behavior problems, *Fam Relat* 46(4):359, 1997.

Fowler SB: Health promotion in chronically ill older adults, *J Neurosci Nurs* 29(1):39, 1997.

Gans BM, Mann NR, Becker BE: Delivery of primary care to the physically challenged, *Arch Phys Med Rehabil* 74(12-S):S15, 1993.

Gates MF, Lackey NR: Youngsters caring for adults with cancer, *Image J Nurs Scholar* 30(1):11-15, 1998.

Guerriere D, McKeever P: Mothering children who survive brain injuries: playing the hand you're dealt, *J Soc Pediatr Nurses* 2(3):105, 1997.

Hadadian A: Attachment relationships and its significance for young children with disabilities, *Infant-Toddler Interven* 6(1):1, 1996.

Heerkens YF et al: Impairments and disabilities—the difference: proposal for adjustment of the international classification of impairments, disabilities, and handicaps, *Phys Ther* 74(5):430, 1994.

Herr SS: Reauthorization of the Individuals with Disabilities Education Act, *Ment Retard* 35(2):131, 1997.

Hogan SE, Evers SE: A nutritional rehabilitation program for persons with severe physical and developmental disabilities, *J Am Dietet Assoc* 97(2):162, 1997.

Iezzoni LI et al: Use of screening and preventive services among women with disabilities, *Am J Med Qual* 16(4):135-144, 2001.

Imrie R: Rethinking the relationships between disability, rehabilitation, and society, *Disabil Rehabil* 19(7):263, 1997.

Institute of Medicine: *Healthy communities: new partnerships for the future of public health,* Washington, DC, 1996, National Academy Press.

International Seminar on Women and Disability: Abstracts, *Sexual Disabil* 15(1):11, 1997.

Ireland M, Malgady RG: Thematic instrument for measuring death anxiety in children (TIMDAC), *J Pediatr Nurs* 14(1):28, 1999.

Ireys HT, Silver EJ: Perception of the impact of child's chronic illness: does it predict maternal mental health? *Dev Behav Pediatr* 17(2):77, 1996.

Ireys HT et al: Schooling, employment, and idleness in young adults with serious physical health conditions: effects of age, disability status, and parental education, *J Adolesc Health* 19(1):25, 1996.

Jones KE, Tamari IE: Making our offices universally accessible: guidelines for physicians, *Canad Med Assoc J* 156(5):647, 1997.

Kanning M: Complementary and alternative therapies for rheumatic diseases I, *Rheum Clin North Am* 25(4):823-831, 1999.

Katsiyannis A, Maag JW: Ensuring appropriate education: emerging remedies, litigation, compensation, and other legal considerations, *Exceptional Children* 64(4):451, 1997.

Kington RS, Smith JP: Socioeconomic status and racial and ethnic differences in functional status associated with chronic diseases, *Am J Public Health* 87(5):805, 1997.

Kliebenstein MA, Brome ME: School re-entry for the child with chronic illness: parent and school personnel perceptions, *Pediatr Nurs* 26(6):579-582, 2000.

Kochhar S, Scott CG: Living arrangements of SSI recipients, *Soc Sec Bull* 60(1):18, 1997.

Kotch JB: Predicting child maltreatment in the first 4 years of life from characteristics assessed in the neonatal period, *Child Abuse Negl* 23(4):305, 1999.

Lee P: Health communities: a young movement that can revolutionize public health, *Public Health Rep* 115(2,3):114-115, 2000.

Liao Y et al: Socioeconomic status and morbidity in the last years of life, *Am J Public Health* 89(4):569, 1999.

Limperopoulos C et al: Functional limitations in young children with congenital heart defects after cardiac surgery, *Pediatrics* 108(6):1325-1331, 2001.

Lipper EG et al: Partnerships in school care: meeting the needs of New York City schoolchildren with complex medical conditions, *Am J Public Health* 87(2):291, 1997.

Mallory BL: The role of social policy in life cycle transitions, *Exceptional Children* 62(3):213, 1996.

Manton KG, Corder L, Stallard E: Chronic disability trends in elderly United States populations: 1982-1994, *Proc Nat Acad Sci USA* 94(6):2593, 1997.

Marks NF: Caregiving across the life span, *Fam Relat* 45(1):27, 1996.

McCallion P, Janicki M, Grant-Griffin L: Exploring the impact of culture and acculturation on older families caregiving for persons with developmental disabilities, *Fam Relat* 46(4):347, 1997.

Mengel MH, Marcus DB, Dunkle RE: "What will happen to my child when I'm gone?" a support and education group for aging parents as caregivers, *Gerontologist* 36(6):816-820, 1996.

Miller ET: Targeting interventions for primary informal caregivers of adults with cognitive and physical losses, *Rehabil Nurs* 27(2):46-51, 79, 2002.

Mueller C, Schur C, O'Connell J: Prescription drug spending: the impact of age and chronic disease status, *Am J Public Health* 87(10):1626, 1997.

Murphy KE: Parenting a technology assisted infant: coping with occupational stress, *Social Work Health Care* 24 (3-4):113, 1997.

National Information Center for Children and Youth With Disabilities: *NICHCY News Digest* 1(1):12, 1991.

National Information Center for Children and Youth With Disabilities: *Severe and/or multiple disabilities,* 2002, available at http://www.nichcy.org/pubs/factshe/fs10txt.htm.

National Institutes of Health, National Center for Complementary and Alternative Medicine: See information at http://www.nccam.nih.gov.

Nelson PP: Library services for people with disabilities: results of a survey, *Bull Med Librar Assoc* 84(3):397, 1996.

Nichols AW: Sports medicine and the Americans With Disabilities Act, *Clin J Sport Med* 6(3):190, 1996.

Norris T, Pittman M: The Healthy Communities movement and the coalition for healthier cities and communities, *Public Health Rep* 115(2,3):118-125, 2000.

Nosek MA: Primary care issues for women with severe disabilities, *J Women's Health* 1(4):245, 1992.

Orr C, Schkade J: The impact of the classroom environment on defining function in school-based practice, *Am J Occupat Ther* 51(1):64, 1997.

Peat M: Attitudes and access: advancing the rights of people with disabilities, *Can Med Assoc J* 156(5):657, 1997.

Pennell FE, Johnson J: Legal and civil rights aspects of vocational rehabilitation, *Phys Med Rehabil Clin North Am* 8(2):245, 1997.

Peters DJ: Disablement observed, addressed, and experienced: integrating subjective experience into disablement models, *Disabil Rehabil* 18(12):593, 1996.

Pettit JL: Alternative medicine: ephedra, *Clin Rev* 12(10):46-48, 2002.

Porter S, Yuille JC, Bent A: A comparison of the eyewitness accounts of deaf and hearing children, *Child Abuse Negl* 19(1):51-61, 1995.

Pruchno R, Patrick JH, Burant CJ: African-American and white mothers of adults with chronic disabilities: caregiving burden and satisfaction, *Fam Relat* 46(4):335, 1997.

Reber M, Borcherding BG: Dual diagnosis. In Batshaw ML, editor: *Children with disabilities,* ed 4, pp 405-424, Baltimore, 1997, Paul H. Brooks.

Rimmer JH: Health promotion for people with disabilities: the emerging paradigm shift from disability prevention to prevention of secondary conditions, *Phys Ther* 79(5):495-502, 1999.

Rimmer JH, Braddock D: Health promotion for people with physical, cognitive, and sensory disabilities: an emerging national priority, *Am J Health Promot* 16(4):220-224, 2002.

Rimmerman A et al: Job placement of urban youth with developmental disabilities: research and implications, *J Rehabil* 62(1):56, 1996.

Satariano WA: The disabilities of aging: looking to the physical environment, *Am J Public Health* 87(3):331, 1997.

Saxton M et al: "Bring my scooter so I can leave you": a study of disabled women handling abuse by personal assistance providers, *Violence Against Women* 7(4):393-417, 2001.

Secrist-Mertz C et al: Helping families meet the nutritional needs of children with disabilities: an integrated model, *Children's Health Care* 26(3):151, 1997.

Simmonds MJ, Kumar S, Lechelt E: Psychosocial factors in disabling low back pain: causes or consequences? *Disabil Rehabil* 18(4):161, 1996.

Slavitt EB, LaBant TM: Living and leaving life on one's own terms: certain legal rights of older adults and persons with disabilities, *Topics Stroke Rehabil* 2(4):44, 1996.

Snethen JA, Broome ME, Bartels J: Adolescents' perception of living with end-stage renal disease, *Pediatr Nurs* 27(2):159-167, 2001.

Sobsey D: Letter to editor, *Child Abuse Negl* 21(9):819, 1997.

Stuart GW, Laraia MT: *Principles and practice of psychiatric nursing,* ed 7, St Louis, Mo, 2001, Mosby.

Stuber ML: Psychiatric sequelae in seriously ill children and their families, *Psychiatr Clin North Am* 19(3):481, 1996.

Suris JC et al: Sexual behavior of adolescents with chronic disease and disability, *J Adolesc Health* 19(2):124, 1996.

Task Force on Community Preventive Services: Recommendations to increase physical activity in communities, *Am J Prev Med* 22(45):67-72, 2002.

Terman DL et al: Special education for students with disabilities: analysis and recommendations, *Future Children* 6(1):4, 1996.

Thorne SE, Radford MJ, McCormick J: The multiple meanings of long-term gastrostomy in children with severe disability, *J Pediatr Nurs* 12(2):89, 1997.

Troxell J: Epilepsy and employment: the Americans with Disabilities Act and its protections against employment discrimination, *Med Law* 16(2):375, 1997.

Turner-Henson A, Holaday B: Daily life experiences for the chronically ill: a life-span perspective, *Fam Community Health* 17(4):1, 1995.

U.S. Department of Health and Human Services: *Healthy people 2010: understanding and improving health*, ed 2, Washington, DC, 2000, U.S. Government Printing Office.

U.S. Department of Justice, Civil Rights Division, Disability Rights Section: *A guide to disability rights law*, 2001, available at www.usdoj/gov/crt/ada/publicat.htm.

U.S. Bureau of the Census: *Facts and features, 2002*, available at http://www.census.gov/Press-Release/www/2002/cb02ff11.html.

Verbrugge LM, Rennert C, Madans JH: The great efficacy of personal and equipment assistance in reducing disability, *Am J Public Health* 87(3):384, 1997.

Voelke S: Discrepancies in parent and teacher ratings of adaptive behavior of children with multiple disabilities, *Ment Retard* 35(1):10, 1997.

Watt S et al: Age, adjustment and costs: a study of chronic illnesses, *Soc Sci Med* 44(10):1483, 1997.

Weinberg LA: Problems in educating abused and neglected children with disabilities, *Child Abuse Negl* 21(9):889, 1997.

Wewers ME, Ahijevych KL: Smoking cessation interventions in chronic illness, *Annu Rev Nurs Res* 14:75, 1996.

Williams PD: Siblings and pediatric chronic illness: a review of the literature, *Int J Nurs Stud* 34(4):312, 1997.

Wolinsky FD, Fitzgerald JF, Stump TE: The effect of hip fracture on mortality, hospitalization, and functional status: a prospective study, *Am J Public Health* 87(3):398, 1997.

Zebrack BJ et al: Psychological outcomes in long-term survivors of childhood leukemia, Hodgkin's disease, and non-Hodgkin's lymphoma: a report from the Childhood Cancer Survivor Study, *Pediatrics* 110(1):42-52, 2002.

# Part 6

Vulnerability:
Community-Oriented
Nursing Issues
for the Twenty-first
Century

The twenty-first century has begun and the complexity of health and social problems is increasing. Community health problems remain more a societal problem than an individual problem. Solutions will require an integrated social and health care approach that begins with a commitment to primary health care. Primary health care involves a partnership between public health and primary care to address the problems of the society as well as of the individual.

Communities increasingly experience significant problems as a result of conditions that are often expensive and hard to treat: violence against people and property, unresolved mental health illnesses, abuse of substances among people of all groups, teen pregnancy, and an increasing number of people who are disenfranchised from society. Personal resources and access to health and social services are limited for these populations. The chapters in Part 6 present a discussion of the most common problems seen in communities.

The stage is set with a discussion of the concept of vulnerability and the implications for communities of the growing number of vulnerable people. Poverty and homelessness are two conditions that have profound effects on the health of individuals, families, and communities. The growing community health problems arising from increased rates of teen pregnancy, and the implications of the growing migrant population in cities and rural areas across the country are highlighted. Problems that are on the increase include mental health issues, substance abuse, interpersonal violence and abuse, and communicable diseases such as HIV, hepatitis, and sexually transmitted diseases.

# Vulnerability and Vulnerable Populations: An Overview

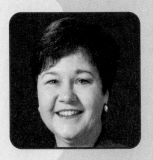

**Juliann G. Sebastian, A.R.N.P., Ph.D., F.A.A.N.**
Juliann G. Sebastian developed an interest in community-oriented nursing while obtaining her B.S.N. degree, when she provided care to vulnerable populations in rural Appalachia. Since then, she has cared for a range of vulnerable populations across the life span and in a variety of settings. Currently, she directs the University of Kentucky's College of Nursing Academic Clinical Program, in which faculty, staff, and students serve many vulnerable populations in community-based settings. As part of that role, she co-directs, with Dr. Marcia Stanhope, an integrated nurse-managed center that provides population-focused care to vulnerable populations such as homeless adults, uninsured children, families and adults, and high-risk adolescents.

## Objectives

After reading this chapter, the student should be able to do the following:

1. Define what is meant by vulnerable populations
2. Analyze trends that have influenced the development of vulnerability among certain population groups and social attitudes toward vulnerability
3. Analyze the effects of public policies on vulnerable populations and on reducing health disparities experienced by these populations
4. Examine the multiple individual and social factors that contribute to vulnerability
5. Evaluate strategies that can be used by public and community health nurses to improve the health status and eliminate health disparities of vulnerable populations

This chapter introduces the concept of vulnerability and the nursing roles for meeting the health needs of vulnerable population groups. Selected population groups who are more vulnerable than others to poor health outcomes are described. Public policies that have influenced vulnerable groups and the effects of these policies are explored. The nature of vulnerability is analyzed, and factors that predispose people to vulnerability, outcomes of vulnerability, and the cycle of vulnerability are described. Community-oriented nursing interventions are designed to help break the cycle of vulnerability. Numerous interventions are possible at the individual, family, group, community, and population levels. This chapter details the nurse's use of the nursing process with vulnerable population groups and presents case examples throughout and at the end to clarify these ideas.

## PERSPECTIVES ON VULNERABILITY

### Definition

"Vulnerable populations are defined as social groups who have an increased relative risk or susceptibility to adverse health outcomes" (Flaskerud and Winslow, 1998, p. 69). In health care, **risk** is an epidemiologic term meaning that some people have a higher probability of illness than others. In the familiar concept of the epidemiologic triangle, the agent, host, and environment interact to produce illness or poor health. The model for the natural history of disease explains how certain aspects of physiology and the environment, including personal habits, social environment, and physical environment, make it more likely that one will develop particular health problems (Valanis, 1999). For example, a smoker is at risk for developing lung cancer because cellular changes occur with smoking. However, not everyone who is at risk develops health problems. Some individuals are more likely than others to develop the health problems for which they are at risk. These people are more *vulnerable* than others. The web of causation model better explains what happens in these situations. A **vulnerable population group** is a subgroup of the population that is more likely to develop health problems as a result of exposure to risk or to have worse outcomes from these health problems than the rest of the population. Vulnerability is a global concern, with different populations being more vulnerable in different countries. Box 31-1 explains that vulnerable populations have poorer health than others.

According to the web of causation model of health and illness (Valanis, 1999), the interaction between numerous

## Key Terms

**advocacy**, p. 750
**barriers to access**, p. 752
**brokering health services**, p. 768
**case finding**, p. 749
**case management**, p. 768
**comprehensive services**, p. 750
**culturally appropriate health care**, p. 750
**cumulative risks**, p. 747
**cycle of vulnerability**, p. 760
**differential vulnerability hypothesis**,
p. 747
**disadvantaged**, p. 748
**disenfranchisement**, p. 759

**distribution effects**, p. 752
**empowerment**, p. 764
**enabling**, p. 755
**federal poverty level**, p. 754
**health disparities**, p. 748
**health field concept**, p. 759
**health literacy**, p. 757
**human capital**, p. 754
**iterative assessment process**, p. 761
**linguistically appropriate health care**,
p. 750
**market model**, p. 755
**outreach**, p. 749

**priority population groups**, p. 748
**resilience**, p. 754
**risk**, p. 746
**risk marker**, p. 748
**social Darwinism**, p. 756
**social isolation**, p. 758
**social justice**, p. 750
**socioeconomic status gradient**, p. 754
**threshold model of poverty**, p. 754
**vulnerable population group**, p. 746
**waiver**, p. 750
**wrap-around services**, p. 749
*See Glossary for definitions*

## Chapter Outline

Perspectives on Vulnerability
*Definition*
*Examples of Vulnerable Groups*
*Health Disparities*
*Trends Related to Caring for Vulnerable
Populations*
Public Policies Affecting Vulnerable
Populations
*Landmark Legislation*
*Implementation Issues*
*Effects of Insurance on Health Care for
Vulnerable Populations*
Factors Contributing to Vulnerability
*Socioeconomic Resources*
*Poverty*
*Health Status*

*Health Risk*
*Marginalization*
Outcomes of Vulnerability
*Poor Health Outcomes and Health Disparities*
*Chronic Stress*
*Hopelessness*
*Cycle of Vulnerability*
Community-Oriented Nursing Approaches
to Care
*Core Functions of Public Health*
*Essential Services*
Assessment Issues
*Nursing Conceptual Approaches*
*Socioeconomic Considerations*
*Physical Health Issues*
*Biological Issues*

*Psychological Issues*
*Lifestyle Issues*
*Environmental Issues*
Planning and Implementing Care
for Vulnerable Populations
*Roles of the Nurse*
*Client Empowerment and Health Education*
*Levels of Prevention*
*Strategies for Promoting Healthy Lifestyles*
*Healthy People 2010 Objectives and Healthy
People in Healthy Communities Guidelines*
*Comprehensive Services*
*Resources for Vulnerable Populations*
*Case Management*
Evaluation of Nursing Interventions With
Vulnerable Populations

---

### ❮ DID YOU KNOW?

Vulnerable populations are more susceptible to poor outcomes from health risks (Flaskerud and Winslow, 1998). They experience disparities in access to care and health status compared with the population as a whole.

---

causal variables creates a more potent combination of factors predisposing an individual to illness (see Chapter 11 for more information on epidemiology). One way of thinking about this is that not only are more independent variables (e.g., causal factors) present, but these variables interact, resulting in a higher probability of illness. This means that the relative risk for illness or poor health outcome is greater for vulnerable populations (Aday, 1997). Members of vulnerable groups often have **cumulative risks,** or combinations of

risk factors (Nichols, Wright, and Murphy, 1986) that make them more sensitive to the adverse effects of individual risk factors that others might be able to overcome. Vulnerability implies that certain people are more sensitive to risk factors than others (O'Connor, 1994). Those who are at risk but not as likely to develop the health problem are more resilient than their more vulnerable counterparts. Being at risk for a certain health problem is necessary for development of that problem, but it is not sufficient. It also seems to be necessary to possess other characteristics that increase one's vulnerability before the health problem actually develops. For example, vulnerable population groups are those who are not only particularly sensitive to risk factors but also possess multiple, cumulative risk factors. This is referred to as the **differential vulnerability hypothesis** (Aday, 2001).

Some populations have certain nonmodifiable characteristics that may be most appropriately described as *risk*

---

**BOX 31-1    Vulnerable Population Groups of Special Concern to Nurses**

- Poor and homeless persons
- Pregnant adolescents
- Migrant workers and immigrants
- Severely mentally ill individuals
- Substance abusers
- Abused individuals and victims of violence
- Persons with communicable disease and those at risk
- Persons who are HIV positive or have hepatitis B virus or sexually transmitted disease

---

*markers* (Appel, Harrell, and Deng, 2002). A **risk marker** is a screening variable that may be associated with a higher prevalence of a disease but does not directly affect or cause morbidity and mortality as a risk factor would do. An example of this is race. Although race has been thought of as a nonmodifiable risk factor, it may be that it is simply associated with other factors that actually do influence the development and natural history of a disease (Appel et al, 2002).

## Examples of Vulnerable Groups

Vulnerable individuals and families often have multiple risk factors. For example, nurses work with pregnant adolescents who are poor, have been abused, and are substance abusers. Nurses also work with substance abusers who test positive to human immunodeficiency virus (HIV) and to hepatitis B virus (HBV), as well as those who are severely mentally ill. Community-oriented nurses work with homeless and marginally housed individuals and families. They also provide care for migrant workers and immigrants. Any of these groups may be victimized by abuse and violence. Box 31-1 lists vulnerable population groups. Each of these groups is discussed in detail in Chapters 32 through 39.

Priority population groups differ in other countries. **Priority population groups** are groups targeted by national governments for special emphasis in health care goals because their health status is particularly poor. In Canada, Aboriginal Indians and people who live in remote rural areas of northern Canada need special attention to reduce health disparities. The infant mortality rate for Canada as a whole was 6.1 per 1000 live births in 1995. By comparison, the infant mortality rates for the Yukon and the Northwest Territories in Canada were 12.8 and 13.0 per 1000 live births (Statistics Canada, 1998). In New Zealand, the Maori people suffer poorer health status than the rest of the country (Woodward and Kawachi, 2000). This is thought to result at least in part from socioeconomic and environmental conditions.

This chapter highlights some of the problems that the vulnerable populations just described have with access to care, quality and appropriateness of care, and health outcomes. Chapters 32 to 39 describe these vulnerable populations in more detail.

## Health Disparities

Nurses, other public health professionals, and policymakers target health care interventions toward vulnerable population groups in part because these groups suffer from disparities in access to care, uneven quality of care, and the poorest health outcomes. **Health disparities** refer to the wide variations in health services and health status between certain population groups. Both Healthy People 2010 (U.S. Department of Health and Human Services, 2001a) and Healthy People in Healthy Communities (USDHHS [USDHHS], 2001b) highlight vulnerable population groups and illness prevention and health promotion objectives for them. Because of the continuing disparities in health status between certain demographic subgroups of people living in the United States and those who have adequate care, a major effort is underway to eliminate the less-than-adequate care experienced by some groups as defined by "age, gender, race or ethnicity, education or income, disability, geographic location or sexual orientation" (USDHHS, 2001a, p. 11).

In 1998, President Clinton initiated a program to decrease health disparities in six areas for members of racial and ethnic minority populations. The Presidential Initiative on Race recognized that although the health of Americans improved throughout the 1990s, certain racial and ethnic minority populations continued to experience a higher than average burden from poor health. The groups that were targeted in this initiative are African Americans, Hispanics, Native Americans, Native Alaskans, and Asian–Pacific Islanders. These groups are expected to "grow as a proportion of the total U.S. population; therefore, the future health of America as a whole will be influenced substantially by success in improving the health of these racial and ethnic minorities" (Hamburg, 1998, p. 372). Clinton's initiative was expanded in Healthy People 2010 with the elimination of health disparities cited as one of two overarching goals for the nation. Twenty-eight focal areas in Healthy People 2010 emphasize access, chronic health problems, injury and violence prevention, environmental health, food safety, health communication, health educational programming, and individual health-related behaviors.

Furthermore, the description of population subgroups affected by health disparities was broadened to include other demographic characteristics beyond race and ethnicity alone. Healthy People 2010 targets health disparities in groups characterized by "age, gender, race or ethnicity, education or income, disability, geographic location or sexual orientation" (USDHHS, 2001a, p. 11).

Healthy People 2010 is an implementation guide for all federal and most state health initiatives, with a special emphasis on promoting systematic approaches to eliminating health disparities experienced by underserved and disadvantaged populations. **Disadvantaged** populations are those that have fewer resources for promoting health and treating illness than the average person in the United States. For example, a family or individual below the federal poverty line would be considered disadvantaged in terms of access to economic resources. These groups are considered vulnerable because of the combination of risk factors, health status, and lack of the resources needed to access health care and mitigate risk factors (Flaskerud et al, 2002).

Examples of areas that show health disparities across population groups are infant mortality, childhood immunization rates, and disease-specific mortality rates. In 1995, African Americans had an infant mortality rate of 14.6 per 1000 live births, compared with 6.3 for whites, and 5.3 for Asian Americans or Pacific Islanders (Hamburg, 1998). Each of the target populations in President Clinton's initiative had lower childhood immunization rates than whites in 1996 (Hamburg, 1998). African Americans have significantly higher death rates from prostate and breast cancer and from heart disease than non-Hispanic whites living in the United States. Hispanics have higher mortality rates from diabetes than non-Hispanic whites living in the United States. Race and ethnicity are not thought to be the causes of these disparities, although research is underway to determine biological susceptibilities by race, ethnicity, and gender. Rather, poverty and low educational levels are more likely to contribute to social conditions in which disparities develop. People who are poor often live in unsafe areas, work in stressful environments, have less access to healthy foods and opportunities for exercise, and are more likely to be uninsured or underinsured (USDHHS, 2001a).

## Trends Related to Caring for Vulnerable Populations

Disparities in the health status of certain population groups compared with the majority population has focused public and professional attention on strengthening the health services available to vulnerable populations. However, in the United States, the national goal to eliminate health disparities (USDHHS, 2001a) is occurring at a time when health care costs are rising, costs of employer-provided health insurance are increasing, and federal, state, and local budgets are strained to provide human services. Although these particular concerns are unique at this time, over the years there have been different focuses for care of vulnerable populations. An analysis of these trends can help nurses learn from lessons of the past and develop new approaches best suited for the contemporary environment. Box 31-2 delineates trends related to caring for vulnerable populations.

During colonial times, persons with chronic physical or mental conditions were cared for in their own communities. Later, the social reforms of the nineteenth century led to institutional care for many of these individuals. In the twenty-first century, there is a renewed emphasis on caring for vulnerable population groups in the community through partnerships between groups such as public

---

**BOX 31-2  Trends Related to Vulnerable Populations**

- Growth in disparity between socioeconomically advantaged and disadvantaged populations around the world
- Community-based care and interorganizational partnerships
- Outreach and case finding
- Comprehensive health care and social services in workplaces, schools, faith-based organizations
- Social justice activism and advocacy
- Culturally and linguistically appropriate care
- Partnerships between public and private payers

---

health, managed care, and community groups (Sebastian, 1999). This has been referred to as "community-oriented managed care" (Aday, 1997, p. 16).

Many of the vulnerable population groups described in this chapter and in Chapters 32 to 39 have less access to health services than other groups. The trend is toward more outreach and case finding to make access easier (American Academy of Nursing, 1992). **Outreach** is an approach to making health care more easily available to certain populations by implementing health education, counseling, or support services in places where people normally congregate, such as places of worship, schools, workplaces, and community centers. **Case finding** occurs when community-oriented nurses design methods for finding populations and individuals especially in need of services. A related trend is to develop culturally and linguistically appropriate forms of outreach and care delivery to more effectively promote the health of these populations (Bushy, 1999). For example, in African-American communities in the United States, one of the most effective locations for outreach and community education is the neighborhood church or mosque. The American Cancer Society program, Sister to Sister, involves African-American women going door to door in African-American neighborhoods and providing individualized education about the importance of breast cancer screening.

There is also a trend toward providing more comprehensive, family-centered services when treating vulnerable population groups. It is important to provide comprehensive, family-centered, "one-stop" services. Providing multiple services during a single clinic visit is an example of one-stop services. If social and economic assistance are also provided and included in interdisciplinary treatment plans, services can be more responsive to the combined effects of social and economic stressors on the health of special population groups. This situation is sometimes referred to as providing **wrap-around services,** in which comprehensive health services are available and social and economic services are "wrapped around" these services.

It is helpful to provide comprehensive services in locations where people live and work, including schools, churches, neighborhoods, and workplaces. **Comprehensive services** are health services that focus on more than one health problem or concern. For example, some nurses use mobile outreach clinics to provide a wide array of health promotion, illness prevention, and illness management services in migrant camps, schools, and local communities. A single client encounter might focus on an acute health problem such as influenza, but it may also include health education related to diet and exercise, counseling related to smoking cessation, and a follow-up appointment for immunizations once the influenza has resolved. The shift away from hospital-based care includes a renewed commitment to the public health services that vulnerable populations need to prevent illness and promote health (Baker et al, 1994; Fielding and Halfon, 1994), such as reduction of environmental hazards and violence and assurance of safe food and water.

---

### DID YOU KNOW?

Vulnerable populations are often most effectively served by making a comprehensive set of services available in one place and at one time. If a mother brings a child to a community clinic for a simple acute problem, it may be a good time to check to see if the child has up-to-date immunizations. Siblings who might be present could also be evaluated for immunization status at the same time and each child provided with the necessary immunizations, assuming none are contraindicated.

---

Community-oriented nurses focus more explicitly on advocacy and social justice concerns. **Advocacy** refers to that set of actions one undertakes on behalf of another. Nurses may function as advocates for vulnerable populations by working for the passage and implementation of policies that will result in improved public health services for these populations. Examples would be a nurse who serves on a local coalition for uninsured people, and one who works toward development of a plan for sharing the provision of free or low-cost health care by local health care organizations and providers.

**Social justice** refers to providing humane care and social supports for the most disadvantaged members of society (Linhorst, 2002). Nurses who function in advocacy roles and facilitate change in public policy are intervening to promote social justice. Because many of the determinants of health are beyond an individual's control, the interventions needed are likewise beyond what a single person can do (Woodward and Kawachi, 2000). Nurses can function as advocates for policy changes to improve social, economic, and environmental factors that predispose vulnerable populations to poor health.

Community-oriented nurses also want to provide **culturally** and **linguistically appropriate health care** (Bushy, 1999). Healthy People 2010 (USDHHS, 2001a) discusses the need for culturally sensitive and linguistically competent care. Linguistically appropriate health care means communicating health-related assessment and information in the recipient's primary language when possible and always in a language the recipient can understand.

A major shift in providing care for certain vulnerable populations in the United States is the increasing reliance on private managed care by Medicaid and Medicare. Many states now have 1115 waivers from the federal government that permit them to test innovative approaches to organizing care for Medicaid beneficiaries (Epstein, 1997). With an 1115 **waiver,** a particular state is allowed to waive certain usual Medicaid requirements in order to test unique approaches to providing health care in specific local areas. These waivers have been used in most cases to develop various forms of managed care arrangements for all or part of the Medicaid beneficiaries in a state. An advantage of the waivers is that they allow states to develop strategies that work best in their local communities, rather than mandating that all states use the same model.

Some vulnerable populations are such high financial risks and have such unique needs that their care is contracted to specialty groups. For example, mental health and substance abuse services are often contracted out to behavioral managed care firms. These contracts are referred to as *carve outs* because the care for a specific population has been carved out of an overall managed care plan for all other clinical populations. Other groups whose care may be carved out are older adults, disabled populations, and children with special health care needs. Care also may be carved out as part of a block grant, in which funds are given in a block to a local region that focuses on a broad area, such as maternal and child health. Block grants are intended to enable local areas to have more control in deciding how to spend funds so that they can respond to local needs and conditions. In one city, funds from a block grant broadly focused on energy and home heating were used to help support a homeless shelter.

The situation in Canada differs because control of local health care decisions rests largely at the provincial government level rather than at the federal level. This permits responsiveness to local conditions and needs. A major challenge in today's health care environment is developing flexible new care delivery strategies for high-risk populations that are responsive to local cultural mores and social context, and that result in improved clinical outcomes at an affordable cost.

A disadvantage of mandated managed care for Medicaid enrollees is that studies have shown that the majority of beneficiaries remain on Medicaid less than a year (Carrasquillo et al, 1998), severely limiting the continuity of care that is available to them. One of the primary reasons for leaving Medicaid is a change in work status. Although this has important benefits, if the individual chooses a managed care plan at a new place of employment, the likelihood is that he or she will also be required to select a new primary care provider from that particular company's panel of providers.

A second and related set of disadvantages relates to cultural variations across groups who normally receive Medicaid. Native Americans may find that policies associated with Medicaid managed care plans require them to choose primary care providers who are not part of the Indian Health Service (IHS) (Wellever, Hill, and Casey, 1998). These providers may be far from the individual's home and may not allow for the culturally appropriate practices that are accepted within the IHS. Native Americans are also likely to believe that having their care managed by a group outside the IHS interferes with their tribal authority. These problems can be handled by customizing requirements for the needs of the special population group (Wellever et al, 1998).

## NURSING TIP

Nurses demonstrate respect to clients of different cultural backgrounds by learning about the cultural norms, values, and traditions of the groups within a particular community. Being fluent in a second language is especially important. Nurses who work in communities with a large Hispanic population find it useful to be fluent in Spanish. Similarly, nurses who work with people who are deaf should consider learning sign language.

---

> **BOX 31-3 Legislation That Has Affected Vulnerable Population Groups in the United States**
>
> **LEGISLATION THAT PROVIDED DIRECT AND INDIRECT FINANCIAL SUBSIDIES TO CERTAIN VULNERABLE POPULATION GROUPS**
> - Social Security Act of 1935
> - Medicare and Medicaid Social Security Act amendments of 1965
> - State Child Health Insurance Program amendment, 1998
>
> **LEGISLATION THAT PROVIDED FINANCIAL SUPPORT FOR BUILDING HEALTH CARE FACILITIES**
> - Hill-Burton Act of 1946
> - Community Mental Health Centers Act of 1963
> - Stewart B. McKinney Homeless Assistance Act of 1988
>
> **LEGISLATION THAT AFFECTED HOW HEALTH CARE RESOURCES WERE USED**
> - National Health Planning and Resources Development Act of 1974
> - Tax Equity and Fiscal Responsibility Act of 1982
> - Federal Balanced Budget Act of 1997

## PUBLIC POLICIES AFFECTING VULNERABLE POPULATIONS

### Landmark Legislation

Public policy is shaped by legislation that specifies the general directions for government bodies to take. Even though laws may relate to only a certain proportion of the population, they tend to have a ripple effect and result in other groups following the general intent of the law. As seen in Box 31-3, various pieces of landmark legislation have affected vulnerable population groups throughout the twentieth century.

Three of these pieces of legislation provided direct and indirect financial subsidies to certain vulnerable groups. The Social Security Act created the largest federal support program for older adult and poor Americans in history. This act sought direct payments to eligible individuals to ensure a minimal level of support for people at risk for problems resulting from inadequate financial resources. Later, the Medicare and Medicaid amendments to the Social Security Act of 1965 provided for the health care needs of older adult, poor, and disabled people who might be vulnerable to impoverishment resulting from high medical bills, or to poor health status from inadequate access to health care. These acts created third-party health care payers at the federal and state levels. Title XXI of the Social Security Act, enacted in 1998, provides for the State

Child Health Insurance Program (CHIP) to provide funds to insure currently uninsured children. In addition to CHIP, new outreach and case-finding efforts will enroll eligible children in Medicaid. "Taken together, these two approaches will seek to provide health insurance for at least half of the 10 million uninsured children in this country" (Hamburg, 1998, p. 375).

Three of the other laws created financial support for building health facilities, thereby improving access to health services for vulnerable groups. The Hill-Burton Act of 1946 provided financial support to build hospitals that would provide care to indigent people. The Community Mental Health Centers Act of 1963 funded construction of community mental health centers and training of mental health professionals who provided community-based care for the severely mentally ill individuals who were discharged from state mental hospitals. This overall policy of deinstitutionalization from mental hospitals was also included in the act and is similar to the current trend to treat more people in their communities and homes rather than in institutions. A policy that encourages more community-based care also requires that the community-based services that people need be developed and implemented. Finally, the Stewart B. McKinney Homeless Assistance Act of 1988 resulted in money for clinics and a wide variety of educational and social services for homeless individuals and families.

The other three pieces of legislation, the National Health Planning and Resource Development Act of 1974, the Tax Equity and Fiscal Responsibility Act of 1982, and the Balanced Budget Act of 1997, influenced the use of resources for providing health services. The National Health Planning and Resource Development Act was intended to provide local mechanisms for planning which types of health services and facilities were really needed so that duplication of expensive facilities and services would be avoided. The goal was to reduce the increasing cost of health services; this would indirectly influence access for vulnerable population groups by making health services more affordable. Also, part of the planning process included community health needs assessment, with the goal of providing balanced services so all would have access to the care they needed.

The Tax Equity and Fiscal Responsibility Act (TEFRA) of 1982 focused on the cost of health services but did so in a very different way. This act was designed to limit the rapid increase in health care costs, but it did not focus on community planning. Instead, TEFRA mandated that payment for hospital services for all Medicare patients would no longer be done on a retrospective cost basis; that is, the Health Care Financing Administration (HCFA) would no longer simply pay the bills that were submitted to them for Medicare enrollees. Now, the HCFA would pay for services on a prospective basis. The agency did this by developing a list of common medical diagnoses (diagnosis-related groups, or DRGs) and determining what they would pay for the care of people with these diagnoses. If hospitals provided services that cost more than the amount indicated on the list, those hospitals lost money. This led to an increased emphasis on shorter hospital stays, more emphasis on identifying cost-effective treatments, and more emphasis on community-based care and care in the home. This was difficult for certain vulnerable groups, such as the homeless, who did not have the same level of resources and support to continue with the care necessary after discharge.

A similar shift in payment occurred with the stipulations related to home health in the Balanced Budget Act of 1997. In an attempt to curb the rapid growth in spending on home health and financial fraud in that industry, the Health Care Financing Administration (now the Centers for Medicare and Medicaid Services [CMS]) instituted prospective payment for home health services. More stringent regulations, related to which services will be reimbursed and for how long, may limit access to care for certain vulnerable groups, such as frail older adults, chronically ill individuals whose care is largely home based, and people who are HIV positive. The goal is to ensure that care is appropriate, rather than to limit access. Nurses and other health care providers must work even more closely with families to determine the kinds of services needed to foster self-care, and the optimal timing of these services. The Balanced Budget Act of 1997 also reduced payments for services for Medicare beneficiaries, with the result that some providers have chosen to no longer treat Medicare beneficiaries. This means that those whose health needs may be high (some chronically ill and older adult persons) may have limited access to care.

## Implementation Issues

Once a law is passed, it must be put into place before it will have a substantial effect on the public. Often, unanticipated problems occur during the implementation phase. These problems sometimes mean that the "letter of the law" is followed but that the intentions of the law are not met. For example, the Community Mental Health Centers Act intended to move treatment of severely mentally ill people into the communities so they would have better outcomes. However, the community supports necessary to help this population were not always adequate, so many eventually lost contact with families and jobs and became homeless (Institute of Medicine, 1988). Another example of an unanticipated outcome is the effects that increasingly strict immigration and border control policies have had on the flow of illegal immigrants into the United States. Mexican immigrants, in particular, have chosen to cross southern U.S. borders at increasingly risky locations, arriving in the country sick and injured. Another effect of policies that reduced benefits to legal immigrants was the creation of a new, underserved population without equal access to public health and welfare services (Freedberg and McLeod, 1998).

Implementation problems also occur because the law has unintended effects on other groups that lawmakers did not anticipate. These are called distribution effects. **Distribution effects** are seen in the criticisms that mental hospitals do not discharge people quickly because the administrators and staff have much to lose. Staff lost jobs and administrators lost perquisites, such as homes and their own personal staff, as censuses dropped (Torrey et al, 1990).

Even though laws such as Medicaid and the McKinney Act were passed to support care for vulnerable groups, some vulnerable individuals and families still do not have adequate access to care. Friedman (1994) argues that nonfinancial **barriers to access** include subtle and often unintentional discrimination. Barriers to access are policies and financial, geographic, or cultural features of health care that make services difficult to obtain or so unappealing that people do not wish to seek care. Examples include offering services only on weekdays without providing evening or weekend hours for working adults, being uninsured or underinsured, not having reasonably convenient or economical transportation, or providing services only in English and not in the population's primary language.

Subconscious discrimination can result in an inadequate number of providers who are willing to treat certain racial groups and people with certain diagnoses, such as HIV. Discrimination against certain diagnoses can influence which conditions insurers are willing to pay for. Other nonfinancial barriers include having inadequate providers in rural areas and certain sections in urban areas, and cultural barriers such as the inability of many vulnerable groups to manage the health care system (Friedman, 1994). One study (Gifford and Bettenhausen, 1997) found that receptionists in physicians' offices responded differently over the telephone to young women on Medicaid, thereby subtly creating barriers to access. Culturally ineffective communication patterns between clinicians and patients of different races may contribute to lower levels of referrals (Einbinder and Schulman, 2000). Thus, even though laws have been passed to increase access to health services by vulnerable groups, inequities still exist for these populations because of attitudes.

## Effects of Insurance on Health Care for Vulnerable Populations

Lack of insurance is a major contributing factor to limited access to health care for vulnerable populations. These populations may be uninsured or underinsured. Some may be eligible for public insurance such as Medicaid, Medicare, or the State Children's Health Insurance Program (SCHIP). Because the eligibility limits for Medicaid are so stringent in many states, many people who cannot afford to purchase private insurance may be uninsured. In other cases, people whose insurance is paid by employers may not be able to afford the deductibles and co-payments included in their benefits policies. These people are underinsured.

### WHAT DO YOU THINK?

Who should assume responsibility for providing health services to vulnerable populations? Providers sometimes close their practices to people on Medicaid or Medicare because providers feel they cannot afford to provide care to people whose insurers reimburse at levels below what it costs to provide care.

Minority populations who are uninsured experience greater disparities in access to health care than uninsured white populations (Hargraves, 2002). This same study found that minority populations have lower incomes than whites. The study's author speculates that because whites have more financial resources they are less disadvantaged by lack of health insurance than minority populations.

In many areas, the growth of public managed care (i.e., Medicaid and Medicare managed care options) has reduced access to the personal health services for individuals (e.g., primary care clinics in health departments). In some cases, the competition for clients in heavy managed care markets has made it more attractive to private clinics and physicians' offices to provide the personal care services that some public health departments formerly provided because they can obtain payment for these services. On the other hand, in some situations clinicians have closed their practices to new Medicaid patients because the low reimbursement rates make it difficult to cover the costs of care. Some public

health departments have eliminated personal health services and focus on providing population-focused services only, such as communicable disease control, environmental services, and managing public food and water supplies (Aiken and Salmon, 1994). In this way, many public health departments are refocusing on the core functions of public health (i.e., assessment, policy, and assurance).

However, not all private health agencies choose to provide vulnerable populations with services, and many are concerned that disparities in health care access and outcomes could grow even greater. Aiken and Salmon (1994) explain that vulnerable populations are more expensive to treat, because they possess multiple, cumulative risks and require special service delivery considerations (e.g., to help overcome transportation problems or provide culturally competent care). Managed care organizations possess strong incentives to control costs by keeping their enrollees healthy. These groups may prefer to care for the healthiest people rather than those who are most vulnerable and, in fact, may find this necessary to remain financially solvent. As noted earlier, one approach that is used to manage care for high-risk populations is to contract their care to specialty organizations (referred to as *carve outs*). These specialty organizations often develop innovative approaches to caring for these high-risk populations.

For example, one school of nursing contracted with its regional Medicaid office to provide a new care delivery program for families with medically fragile children. This was a family program that aimed to strengthen families who had children with high-risk health problems. Nurse practitioners and a clinical nurse specialist provided primary care, urgent care, health education, health coaching, family counseling and support, and case management for families in the program. Most care was provided in the home. However, program staff also worked with clients in hospitals, clinics, and physicians' offices to facilitate seamless care delivery.

## FACTORS CONTRIBUTING TO VULNERABILITY

Vulnerability results from the combined effects of limited resources, poor health, and high levels of risk factors (Flaskerud and Winslow, 1998). Figure 31-1 highlights the kinds of resources that vulnerable populations may lack. It shows the interactions between limitations in physical and environmental resources, personal resources (or human capital), and biopsychosocial resources (e.g., presence of illness and genetic predispositions) (Aday, 2001). Poverty, limited social support, and working in a hazardous environment are examples of limitations in physical and environmental resources. People with preexisting illnesses, such as those with communicable or infectious diseases, or those with chronic illnesses such as cancer, heart disease, or chronic airway disease, have less physical ability to cope with stressors than those without such physical problems.

**Social status**

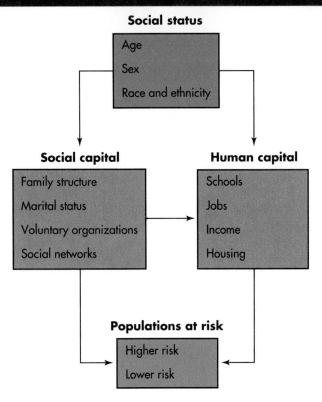

**Figure 31-1** Predictors of populations at risk. *(From Aday LA:* At risk in America: the health and health care needs of vulnerable populations in the United States, ed 2, *San Francisco, 2001, Jossey-Bass.)*

**Human capital** refers to all of the strengths, knowledge, and skills that give each individual the potential to live a productive, happy life. People with little education have fewer choices about employment, housing, and lifestyle than those with higher levels of education.

Vulnerability is multidimensional; that is, several factors contribute to vulnerability. Resource limitations, poor health status, health risks, and marginalization are the factors emphasized in this chapter. Figure 31-2 illustrates the dynamic interactions between these factors. It is important to emphasize, however, that vulnerability is not simply a state of deficiency. Rather, it is dynamic and can be counteracted by acquiring the resources necessary to function more easily in contemporary society and by fostering **resilience.** Resilience is the characteristic of being able to recover from problems and of possessing a sense of inner strength. Nursing interventions focus on helping vulnerable populations acquire the resources needed for better health and reduction of risk factors. In particular, public and community health nurses should focus on changing the social, economic, and environmental precursors to health problems, and function as community change advocates for vulnerable populations. Figure 31-3 shows one model for targeting interventions for vulnerable population groups. In this model, interventions such as case finding, health education, and policy making related to improving

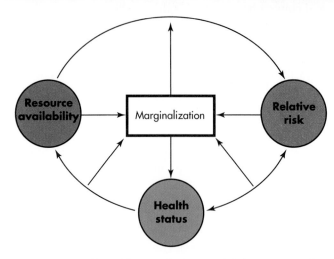

**Figure 31-2** Vulnerable population: social dynamics and outcomes. *(Modified from Flaskerud JH, Winslow BJ: Conceptualizing vulnerable populations health-related research,* Nurs Res *47(2):70, 1998.)*

health for vulnerable populations are all appropriate interventions for nurses.

## Socioeconomic Resources

Lack of adequate social, educational, and economic resources predisposes people to vulnerability. Poverty, a primary cause of vulnerability, is a growing problem in the United States (Northam, 1996; Pesznecker, 1984), as is income inequality between the richest and poorest segments of the population (Erickson, 1996). Poverty is a relative state. The federal definition of poverty is used to develop eligibility criteria for entitlement and other programs. According to Healthy People 2010, roughly 1 of every 11 people in the United States has an income below the federal poverty level (USDHHS, 2001a). In 1998, the **federal poverty level** for a family of four was $16,450 for all states except Hawaii, Alaska, and the District of Columbia (Superintendent of Documents, 1998). However, many people who earn just a little more than the federal poverty level are ineligible for assistance programs yet are unable to manage their living expenses. Poverty causes vulnerability by making it more difficult for people to function in society and by limiting people's access to the resources for living a healthy life.

However, living just above or just below the poverty level is only a rough measure of the relationship between socioeconomic status and health. This type of approach is called the **threshold model of poverty** (Adler and Ostrove, 1999). Research has found a correlation between individual indicators of socioeconomic status (e.g., income, education, occupational status) and a range of health indicators (e.g., morbidity and mortality resulting from various health problems). This correlation is called the **socioeconomic status gradient.** The shape of the gradient seems to

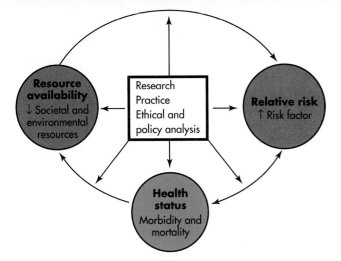

**Figure 31-3** Vulnerable populations conceptual model for research and practice. *(Modified from Flaskerud JH, Winslow BJ: Conceptualizing vulnerable populations health-related research,* Nurs Res *47(2):70, 1998.)*

vary across countries based on the extent to which the country has an egalitarian social structure and whether it is industrialized (Adler and Ostrove, 1999). Finally, not only do individual-level measures of socioeconomic status seem to matter, but also population-level measures make a difference. Income inequality across groups is related to morbidity and mortality and reduced life expectancy (Adler and Ostrove, 1999).

It is often difficult for a young family with an employed father in the home to obtain financial support from social services, even if the father is earning less money than the family needs. This family is considered near poor; sometimes, in these situations, families decide they would be better off financially if the fathers were absent because they become eligible for welfare. Vulnerability results from families' efforts to do what is necessary to manage even when it is disruptive to the family system. Box 31-4 lists various types of poverty.

The gap between the rich and the poor increased in the latter part of the twentieth century in the United States, corresponding to a decrease in federal assistance for the poor (Erickson, 1996). In 1979, 11.4% of the U.S. population lived in poverty, whereas in 1989, 31.5% were poor (Shugars, O'Neill, and Bader, 1991). Poverty is a global problem. The gap between rich and poor countries, as well as between social strata within the developing countries in particular, widened during this century (de la Barra, 1998). "The concentration of wealth has increased annually since 1991" (de la Barra, 1998, p. 47). This depletes human potential worldwide and creates economic, political, and cultural instability, all of which influence health. For example, children in the poorest sections of Accra, Ghana, have three times the risk for infectious disease mortality and twice the risk for respiratory mortality as children in

wealthier sections. Children under the age of 5 who live in poor sections of Sao Paulo, Brazil, have mortality rates from infectious and respiratory diseases that are four times higher than those living in wealthier sections (de la Barra, 1998).

Persons who do not have the financial resources to pay for medical care are considered medically indigent. They may be self-employed or they may work in small businesses and be unable to afford health benefits. Some people have inadequate health insurance coverage. This may be because their deductibles and co-payments are so high they have to pay for most expenses out of pocket, or because few conditions or services are covered. In these situations, poverty in its relative sense causes vulnerability because uninsured and underinsured people are less likely to seek preventive health services because of the expense and are more likely to suffer the consequences of preventable illnesses.

Currently, health care reimbursement policies are based more on a market model than on a human service model. This type of model perpetuates inequities in service availability and accessibility. The **market model** assumes that people who have the resources to purchase services are the ones entitled to those services. Furthermore, a market model assumes that consumers have the information and opportunity to make free choices about where to purchase services. Individuals unable to purchase services must somehow not be "fit" to receive services. Ambivalent attitudes toward the poor may result partly from professional opinions regarding enabling behavior. The concept of **enabling** comes from the literature on addictions and refers to the behavior of people in the dependent person's environment who make it possible for the addiction to continue, such as covering up and "making things right."

Some think that the presence of loose eligibility criteria for health and social services enables individuals to maintain patterns of dependency. Moccia and Mason (1986) observed that social Darwinism is a subtle social value in the United States. **Social Darwinism** refers to the idea of survival of the fittest in relationship to their ability to purchase goods and services. Social Darwinism conflicts with the belief that at least some basic level of health care is a right and should be provided regardless of ability to pay. The two perspectives reflect the controversy in health care reform over how involved the government should be in providing health and social services to vulnerable groups.

One of the problems that results from this idea, whether intended or not, is that policies that reflect this posture reinforce a cycle that may be almost impossible for people living in poverty to break (Curtin, 1986). For example, groups who are unable to afford adequate preventive services are likely to develop more chronic diseases, which further deplete the human potential in those groups. This is referred to as a drain on human capital, where human capital means that the potential of all people in the community is a valuable resource. Depletion of health status results in decreased human capital and limits the abilities of group members to obtain employment, seek advanced education, or behave in ways that improve their situations. Poor health leads to reduced human capital, and reduction in human capital leads to higher overall levels of health risks (Aday, 2001). Ultimately the whole community suffers if the potential of its members is limited.

## Poverty

Economic status is strongly related to health (Adler et al, 1997; USDHHS, Public Health Service, 1998). People who are poor are more likely to live in hazardous environments that are overcrowded and have inadequate sanitation, work at high-risk jobs, have less nutritious diets, and have multiple stressors, because they do not have the extra resources to manage unexpected crises and may not even have adequate resources to manage daily life (de la Barra, 1998; Erickson, 1996). Figure 31-4 shows the relationship between perceptions of poor health and household income: as income increases, people are more likely to think their health is good. Poverty often reduces an individual's access to health care. In the developed countries of the world, this is more likely to be a problem for those just above the poverty line who are not eligible for public support, whereas in developing countries, poverty is correlated with decreased access to health care. Children who are raised in poverty may be less able to develop resilience and more likely to be depressed later in life (Adler et al, 1997). In fact, income and education may have some influence on poor health status beyond individual health risk behaviors. Income and education by themselves predict poorer self-perceptions of health status (Lantz et al, 2001). It is important for nurses to understand that certain populations are vulnerable to poor health not only be-

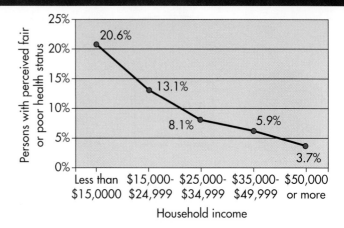

**Figure 31-4** Percentage of persons with perceived fair or poor health status by household income, United States, 1995 *(From U.S. Department of Health and Human Services: Healthy people 2010: understanding and improving health, ed 2, Washington, DC, 2000, U.S. Government Printing Office.)*

cause of controllable individual behaviors but also because of social and economic conditions.

Although race has been correlated with poor health outcomes, poverty seems to be a key causal factor for minority populations. Figure 31-5 shows the relationship between race and ethnicity and poverty by type of household. Female-headed households, and in particular those of African-American and Hispanic descent, are more likely to live in poverty than others. In a study of the widening gap in life expectancy between African Americans and whites in the United States, researchers concluded that the causes of the differences were related to low socioeconomic status rather than race (Kochanek, Maurer, and Rosenberg, 1994). It may also be that race and economic status interact in some situations, and that relationships between race and economic status vary by disease (Adler et al, 1997). In one study, income inequality between African-American and white populations and the degree of residential segregation were strongly associated with premature mortality (Cooper et al, 2001). The authors argue that "institutionalized racism" (p. 464) contributes to some poorer health outcomes for African Americans.

Poverty is more likely to affect women, children, and older adults, with over 80% of those in poverty being in these groups (Erickson, 1996). These populations are already vulnerable to poor health outcomes, and adding the stressors associated with poverty increases the effect of vulnerability. Adolescent pregnancy is a key contributing factor to familial cycles of poverty. Teenagers from poor families, or who are homeless or runaway, are more likely to get pregnant (Fullerton et al, 1997). Adolescents who choose to keep and raise their infants are more likely to remain poor themselves. With increased social acceptability of out-of-wedlock pregnancy (Pierre and Cox, 1997), a large proportion of teenage mothers do choose to keep and raise their children

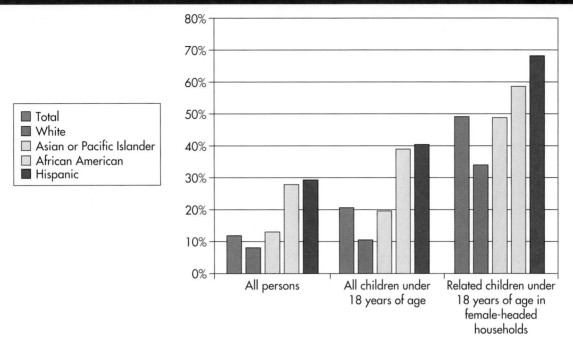

**Figure 31-5** Percentage of persons below the poverty level by race and ethnicity and type of household, United States, 1996. *(From U.S. Department of Health and Human Services:* Healthy people 2010: understanding and improving health, *ed 2, Washington, DC, 2000, U.S. Government Printing Office.)*

(Yoos, 1987). This often results in interrupted education for one or both of the parents, limited job opportunities, expenses associated with child rearing, and a long-term cycle of economic problems that affect both the parents and their children (Koniak-Griffin and Turner-Pluta, 2001). The teenage mother is often a single parent, with even more economic consequences. Economic problems are worsened by the many health problems associated with adolescent pregnancy.

Single-parent families headed by women are more likely to live in poverty than two-parent families (Federal Interagency Forum on Child and Family Statistics, 2000; Lutenbacher, 2002), and children in these families are more likely to be abused. This seems to result in part from the interactions between a mother's history of abuse, feelings of maternal depression, and anger over everyday stressors (Lutenbacher, 2002).

Education plays an important role in health status. Although education is related to income (Adler and Ostrove, 1999), educational level seems to influence health separately. Higher levels of education may provide people with more information for making healthy lifestyle choices. More highly educated people are better able to make informed choices about health insurance and providers. Education may also influence perceptions of stressors and problem situations and give people more alternatives. Finally, education and language skills affect health literacy; "**Health literacy** is a measure of patients' ability to read, comprehend and act on medical instructions. Poor health literacy is common among racial and

ethnic minorities, older adult persons, and patients with chronic conditions, particularly in public sector settings" (Schillinger et al, 2002, p. 475).

The interactions among multiple socioeconomic stressors make people more susceptible to risks than others with more financial resources who may cope more effectively. In the following example, Felicia's situation illustrates how living environment and practical problems such as transportation and cost interact to make people who are poor particularly vulnerable to health problems.

Felicia is a 22-year-old single mother of three children whose primary source of income is Aid to Families with Dependent Children. She is worried about the future because she will no longer be eligible for welfare by the end of the year. She has been unable to find a job that will pay enough for her to afford childcare. Her friend, Maria, said that Felicia and her children could stay in Maria's trailer for a short time, but Felicia is afraid that her only choice after that will be a shelter.

Felicia recently took all three children with her to the health department because 15-month-old Hector needed immunizations. Felicia was also concerned about 5-year-old Martina, who had had a fever of 100° to 101° F on and off for the past month. Felicia and her friends in the trailer park think that some type of hazardous waste from the chemical plant next door to the park is making their children sick. Now that Martina was not feeling well, Felicia was particularly concerned. However, the health department nurse told her that no appointments were available that day and that she would need to bring Martina back to the clinic on the next day. Felicia left discouraged because it was so difficult for her to get all three children ready and on the bus to go to the health department, not to mention the expense. She thought maybe Martina just had a cold and she would wait a little longer before bringing her back. However, she wanted to take care of Martina's problem before losing her medical card. Felicia is desperate to find a way to manage her money problems and take care of her children.

Extreme poverty, in the form of homelessness, affects women, children, and minorities more often than others (Erickson, 1996). Thirty percent of the homeless in the United States are families, and "85% of those families are headed by women of whom the majority are minorities" (Erickson, 1996, p. 165). Those who are homeless or marginally housed have even fewer resources than poor people who have adequate housing. Homeless and marginally housed people must struggle with heavy demands as they try to manage daily life. These individuals and families do not have the advantage of shelter and must cope with finding a place to sleep at night and to stay during the day, as well as finding food, before even thinking about health care. In fact, many of the health care needs of homeless individuals are related to their regular search for shelter and food. For example, homeless individuals often have foot problems from constant walking, hypothermia from exposure to the cold, and exacerbations of chronic health problems because they have no place to store their medications, cannot always find nutritious meals, and cannot maintain a healthy balance of rest and activity because of vagrancy laws that prohibit loitering in one place for a prolonged time (Sebastian, 1985).

Like economic status, **social isolation** is strongly related to vulnerability (Aday, 2001). A study of gay men with acquired immunodeficiency syndrome (AIDS) (Rabkin et al, 1993) found that the men were optimistic, did not deny the severity of their illnesses, and displayed high levels of psychological resilience. The researchers attributed this to the fact that almost all the men reported having confidants, or "someone who was 'there' for them" (p. 167). Similarly, Hogan and DeSantis (1994) reported that adolescents who had experienced the death of a sibling were helped when they felt that their friends were "there for them." Not only does access to a strong social support network help buffer the negative impact of certain stressors for individuals, but social capital facilitates healthy community functioning (Kawachi, 1999). Social capital is the level of cooperation and trust in a community and refers to the extent to which people have concern for others in the community and work together to solve common problems and promote quality of life in the community.

## Health Status

Changes in normal physiologic status predispose individuals to vulnerability. This may result from disease processes, such as in someone with one or more chronic diseases. Infection with HIV is a good example of a pathophysiologic situation that increases vulnerability to opportunistic infections such as *Mycobacterium avium* complex

because of immunodeficiency. Chapter 39 describes HIV, hepatitis, and sexually transmitted diseases (STDs) in detail. Physiologic alterations may also result from accidents, injuries, or congenital problems leading to mental or physiologic disability. Older adults often exhibit vulnerability because of both age-related physiologic changes and multiple chronic illnesses, and resulting in limitations in functional status and loss of independence. Chapter 29 discusses elder health. Physically compromised individuals are another example of a vulnerable group, as discussed in Chapter 30.

Vulnerable groups may share certain physiologic and developmental characteristics that predispose them to unique risks. Among these, age is probably the most central variable. It has long been known that clients at the extreme ends of the age continuum are less able physiologically to adapt to stressors. For example, infants of substance-abusing mothers risk being born addicted and having severe physiologic problems and developmental delays. Older adults are more likely to develop active infections from communicable diseases such as tuberculosis (TB), and they generally have more difficulty recovering from infectious processes than younger people because of their less effective immune systems. Chapter 36 discusses substance abuse, and Chapter 38 describes communicable disease risk.

Certain individuals are vulnerable at particular ages because of the interaction between crucial developmental characteristics and socioeconomic tensions. For example, adolescent girls (especially those under age 14 years) are more likely to deliver low-birth-weight infants than women in their twenties (Simpson et al, 1997), probably because of physiologic variables, although socioeconomic conditions may play an equally important role (Koniak-Griffin and Turner-Pluta, 2001). An inability to afford prenatal care, a lack of awareness of the existence of or importance of prenatal care, and a tendency to seek such care later in pregnancy than older mothers also contribute to poor pregnancy outcomes of adolescents. Chapter 33 describes adolescent pregnancy in more detail.

## Health Risk

Vulnerable populations not only experience multiple, cumulative risks, but they also seem to be particularly sensitive to the effects of those risks. Risks may originate in environmental hazards (e.g., lead exposure from peeling, lead-based paint) or social hazards (e.g., crime and violence), in personal behavior (e.g., diet and exercise habits), or from biological or genetic makeup (e.g., congenital addiction or compromised immune status). Members of vulnerable populations often have comorbidities, or multiple illnesses, with each affecting the other. Risk factors may interact with each other, creating a more hazardous situation. For example, perceptions of discrimination have been linked with stress and with one health-risk behavior in particular—smoking by African-American adolescent girls (Guthrie et al, 2002). Health risks may be related to basic needs. In one study, homeless youths in Canada were found to be highly uncertain about their access to food and to have little or no control over the type and quality of food they ate (Dachner and Tarasuk, 2002). These elements of multiple risk factors, cumulative effects of risk factors, and low thresholds for risk must be addressed when assessing the needs of vulnerable populations and designing services for them.

## Marginalization

Vulnerable populations may be marginalized with respect to the population as a whole. This means that their problems may not be visible to the larger populace and that they may have limited power for acquiring the resources they need. Moccia and Mason (1986) stated that poverty is a power issue because it involves a lack of control over critical resources needed to function effectively in society. In contemporary American society, money is one of the most critical resources; insufficient financial means put individuals in dependent positions and further removes control over choices between available options. In addition, having insufficient financial resources limits the degree of participation many have in making decisions that will affect them, thus limiting their potential to influence even the kinds of options available to them. In the past, community health planning was often unintentionally patriarchal. Health professionals thought they knew better than lay people which health needs were most important and the best ways to provide services to meet those needs. This belief is changing because community health professionals emphasize working as partners with vulnerable groups.

The **health field concept** explains how limited control over one's own health is part of vulnerability. This concept was developed by LaFramboise (1973, cited in Dever, Sciegaj, and Wade, 1988, p. 26) and expanded by Lalonde (1974, also cited in Dever et al, 1988, p. 26). Individual control of health is only one factor in a comprehensive model of health in which biology, environment, and the health care system make up the remaining three focuses. According to the health field concept, individuals share control and responsibility for their health status with society as a whole.

People typically choose their own health-promoting or potentially health-damaging behaviors. Although individuals do not control their biological heritage, they share some responsibility for the heritage they pass on to their offspring (e.g., through the effects that prenatal health and maternal lifestyle have on infant health). Society determines the types of health services and the types of reimbursement mechanisms available as well as environmental hazards. Thus the health field concept explains how health status is affected by both individual factors (individual and biology) and broader societal factors (environment and health care system). The health of people with AIDS, for example, is affected not only by their own health behaviors but also by the fact that they may lose access to medications and laboratory tests when their insurance policies are cancelled.

In many cases, aspects of the physical and social environment that adversely affect the health status of vulnerable populations are beyond their control and are the responsibility of society. For example, communities sometimes find it difficult to locate group homes for severely mentally ill clients in residential neighborhoods despite the emphasis on providing care for these individuals in more normal environments. Neighbors may fear mentally ill people, or they may worry that their property values will drop. If group homes are located in poor neighborhoods, residents are more likely to be victims of crime, to be exposed to environmental hazards such as air pollutants, and to feel ostracized. Some argue that the best way to reduce the health disparities experienced by vulnerable populations is to provide the economic, educational, and social supports needed by these populations, reduce the environmental hazards they face, and develop health-promoting public policies (Flaskerud et al, 2002).

One aspect of marginalization is **disenfranchisement.** This refers to a feeling of separation from mainstream society in which the person does not have an emotional connection with any group in particular or with the larger social fabric in general. In addition to perceived disenfranchisement, certain groups such as the poor, the homeless, and migrant workers may essentially be "invisible" to society as a whole and forgotten in health and social planning. Disenfranchisement suggests that vulnerable groups do not have the social supports necessary to effectively manage an emotionally and physically healthy lifestyle. Many vulnerable individuals have limited formal support networks because they do not have well-established linkages with formal organizations in their communities, such as churches and schools. They may also have few informal sources of support, such as family, friends, and neighbors. For example, homeless individuals are often isolated and have few people whom they can call on for assistance. Certainly not all vulnerable groups lack sources of social support. Nurses should remember that although disenfranchisement is part of being vulnerable for many, strong support from churches, family, and neighbors may be advantages that some vulnerable individuals can draw on, even though they may feel disenfranchised from society as a whole.

Thus, in many ways, vulnerable groups have limited control over potential and actual health needs. Because these groups are in the minority, they are more disadvantaged than others because typical health planning focuses on the majority. Ironically, the traditional public health emphasis on the utilitarian value of "the greatest good for the greatest number" places vulnerable populations at a disadvantage. Disadvantage also results from lack of resources that others may take for granted. Vulnerable groups have limited social and economic resources with which to manage their health care. The family resiliency model predicts that families who have access to adequate resources can more effectively withstand stressors (McCubbin and McCubbin, 1991). For example, women sometimes choose to tolerate domestic violence rather than risk losing a place for themselves and their children to live. Women who are among the working poor are more likely to become homeless when they leave an abusive partner. They may not have adequate financial resources to pay for a place to live when they lose their partners' income. In their epidemiologic study of the effects of undesirable life events, McLeod and Kessler (1990) found that lower socioeconomic status resulted in "pervasive disadvantages inherent in the lives of persons who occupy lower-status positions" (p. 169).

## OUTCOMES OF VULNERABILITY

Outcomes of vulnerability may be negative, such as lower health status than the rest of the population, or they may be positive with effective interventions. For example, culturally competent, family-focused, community-oriented health nursing interventions may improve vulnerable populations' health status and provide such groups with the tools and resources to promote their own health.

### Poor Health Outcomes and Health Disparities

Vulnerable populations often have worse health outcomes than more advantaged populations in terms of morbidity and mortality. This means that they experience health disparities. Health disparities occur in the areas of access to care, quality of care and cultural and linguistic appropriateness of care, and health status (USDHHS, 2001a). These groups have a high prevalence of chronic illnesses, such as hypertension, and high levels of communicable diseases, such as TB, HBV, STDs, and upper respiratory illnesses, including influenza. They have high mortality rates from crime and violence, including domestic violence. For example, clinicians at the Montefiore Health Care Outreach Team for the Homeless (Plescia et al, 1997), located in the Bronx in New York City, found that the most common diagnoses from 1992 to 1995 were well-child and well-adult care, need for immunizations, chemical dependence, and upper respiratory infections. They also found a heavy emphasis on social issues. Other types of health outcomes that deserve further study in vulnerable populations include functional status, overall perception of physical and emotional well-being, quality of life, and satisfaction with health services. There is some evidence that vulnerable groups wait longer to obtain appointments to see a clinician, and that they perceive the communications with their clinicians as less than desirable (Agency for Healthcare Research and Quality, 2002). Nursing interventions should target strategies aimed at increasing resources or reducing health risks in order to reduce health disparities between vulnerable populations and populations with more advantages (Flaskerud et al, 2002).

### Chronic Stress

Poor health creates stress as individuals and families try to manage health problems with inadequate resources. For example, if someone with AIDS develops one or more opportunistic infections and is either uninsured or underinsured, that person and the family and caregivers will have more difficulty managing than if the individual had adequate insurance. Vulnerable populations cope with multiple stressors, so managing multiple stressors creates a sort of "cascade effect," with chronic stress likely to result. This can lead to feelings of hopelessness.

### Hopelessness

Hopelessness results from an overwhelming sense of powerlessness and social isolation. For example, substance abusers who feel powerless over their addiction and who have isolated themselves from the people they care about may believe that no way exists to change their situation. Feelings of hopelessness contribute to a continuing **cycle of vulnerability** by creating feelings of limited control over one's health and socioeconomic condition.

### Cycle of Vulnerability

The factors that predispose people to vulnerability and the outcomes of vulnerability create a cycle in which the outcomes reinforce the predisposing factors, leading to more negative outcomes. Unless the cycle is broken, it is difficult for vulnerable populations to change their health status. Public and community-oriented health nurses identify areas where they can work with vulnerable populations to break the cycle. The nursing process guides nurses in assessing vulnerable individuals, families, groups, and communities; developing nursing diagnoses of their strengths and needs; planning and implementing appropriate therapeutic nursing interventions in partnership with the vulnerable clients; and evaluating the effectiveness of interventions.

## COMMUNITY-ORIENTED NURSING APPROACHES TO CARE

### Core Functions of Public Health

The core functions of public health are assessment, policy, and surveillance. These functions refer to actions initiated on behalf of a group or population, rather than with individuals. However, these functions parallel the stages of the nursing process. Assessment of groups is similar to assessment of individuals. Policy development and implementation can occur within organizations or at local, state or national levels. Policies are population-level interventions, much like interventions targeted toward individuals. A major difference is that policies create conditions that affect many people, such as healthy workplaces, health-promoting community resources (e.g., bike paths, safe places for walking), and laws related to seat belts, to name just a few examples. Policy interventions may be interpreted more broadly to include developing programs and initiatives for populations, such as home-visiting programs for adolescent mothers (Koniak-Griffin and Turner-Pluta, 2001), support groups for caregivers of people with Alzheimer's disease, health literacy programs for newly settled immigrants, and health education programs for schoolchildren. Another example is developing health-related public service announcements or other ways of providing health messages to large groups. Surveillance refers to evaluation and monitoring to ensure that policies and programs are implemented as intended, that unplanned changes are managed effectively, and that goals and objectives are met. Each of these three core functions is similar to those in the nursing process, with the key distinction being their emphasis on assessing, planning, implementing, and evaluating health services for groups and populations. Many activities in which community-oriented nurses engage with and on behalf of vulnerable populations are based on these core functions and represent forms of social advocacy and promotion of social justice for these groups.

## Essential Services

Ten services have been identified as essential public health services that ensure that the core functions of public health are being carried out (USDHHS, 2001b). These services include monitoring community health status, identifying community health hazards, providing people with the education and tools to promote health and prevent illness and injury, mobilizing community partnerships to solve community health problems, developing policies and plans to solve community health problems, and evaluating community health services and outcomes. Community-oriented nurses design their population-level assessment, policy, and surveillance strategies to eliminate health disparities of vulnerable population groups in the 10 essential services of public health.

## ASSESSMENT ISSUES

Box 31-5 lists guidelines for assessing members of vulnerable population groups, whether individuals, families, or larger groups. The following discussion expands on the points listed in that box.

## Nursing Conceptual Approaches

Nursing assessment of vulnerable populations may be organized around any nursing conceptual framework that takes into account the multiple stressors experienced by these groups and the particular difficulties they have managing their health. The approaches of Neuman (Fawcett, 2001), Roy (Fawcett, 2002), and Orem (Denyes et al, 2001) are particularly appropriate to use with vulnerable populations. Neuman's focus on identifying stressors and lines of resistance is a useful framework for organizing a nursing assessment, because vulnerable populations experience multiple, overlapping stressors. Roy's emphasis on health-promoting modes of adaptation helps the nurse emphasize client strengths that are resources for coping with stressors. Orem's self-care approach directs the nurse to assess the client's self-care needs and abilities so that therapeutic nursing interventions can target self-care deficits. These three nursing models are consistent with Pesznecker's (1984) adaptational model of poverty, which states that poor persons possess both individual and group factors, past experiences, and coping skills that, when combined with environmental factors such as stressors and stigma, lead to either healthy or unhealthy adaptive responses. Mediating factors such as public policy and social support can influence whether health-promoting or health-damaging adaptive responses are more likely. Pesznecker's model is particularly relevant to vulnerable populations, so nurses should consider using nursing conceptual frameworks that expand on this model as the basis for client assessment.

Because members of vulnerable populations often experience multiple stressors, nursing assessment must balance the need to be comprehensive with the ability to focus only on information that the nurse has a need for and that the client is willing to provide. The discussion that follows focuses on assessment of individual clients and families and on assessment of entire vulnerable population groups. With individuals and families, assessment can be intrusive and tiring, so it is important that the nurse have a reason to obtain the data before asking the client. This means that assessing becomes an **iterative assessment process,** involving progressively more depth as the nurse refines hypotheses about the nursing diagnosis.

## Socioeconomic Considerations

Vulnerable populations often have limited socioeconomic resources. Assessment should include questions about the clients' perceptions of socioeconomic resources, including identifying people who can provide support and financial resources. Support from other people may include information, caregiving, emotional support, and help with activities of daily living, such as transportation, shopping, and babysitting. Financial resources may include the extent to which the client can pay for health services and medications, as well as questions about eligibility for third-party payment. It is important to assess the extent to which individuals, families, groups, and populations can afford basic necessities such as food, safe housing, clean water, and reliable transportation. The nurse should ask the client about the perceived adequacy of both formal and informal support networks.

## Physical Health Issues

Often, nurses see individual clients in clinic settings. These clients may be concerned about specific problems, which should be the initial priority. However, because vulnerable populations often find it difficult to seek routine health promotion and illness prevention services, nurses should take the opportunity to explain to clients the value of preventive assessment. If clients agree, nursing assessment should include evaluation of clients' preventive health needs, including age-appropriate screening tests, such as immunization status, blood pressure, weight, serum cholesterol, Papanicolaou smears, breast examinations, mammograms, prostate examinations, glaucoma screening, and dental evaluations. It may be necessary to make referrals to have some of these tests done for clients. Assessment should also include preventive screening for physical health problems for which certain vulnerable groups are at a particularly high risk. For example, HIV-positive persons should be evaluated regularly for their T4

**BOX 31-5   Guidelines for Assessing Members of Vulnerable Population Groups**

**SETTING THE STAGE**

- Create a comfortable, nonthreatening environment.
- Learn as much as you can about the culture of the clients you work with so that you will understand cultural practices and values that may influence their health care practices.
- Provide culturally and linguistically competent assessment by understanding the meaning of language and nonverbal behavior in the client's culture.
- Be sensitive to the fact that the individual or family you are assessing may have other priorities that are more important to them. These might include financial or legal problems. You may need to give them some tangible help with their most pressing problem before you will be able to address issues that are more traditionally thought of as health concerns.
- Collaborate with others as appropriate; you should not provide financial or legal advice. However, you should make sure to connect your client with someone who can and will help them.

**NURSING HISTORY OF AN INDIVIDUAL OR FAMILY**

- You may have only one opportunity to work with a vulnerable person or family. Try to complete a history that will provide all the essential information you need to help the individual or family on that day. This means that you will have to organize in your mind exactly what you need to ask, and no more, and why the data are necessary.
- It will help to use a comprehensive assessment form that has been modified to focus on the special needs of the vulnerable population group with whom you work. However, be flexible. With some clients, it will be both impractical and unethical to cover all questions on a comprehensive form. If you know that you

are likely to see the client again, ask the less pressing questions at the next visit.

- Be sure to include questions about social support, economic status, resources for health care, developmental issues, current health problems, medications, and how the person or family manages their health status. Your goal is to obtain information that will enable you to provide family-centered care.
- Does the individual have any condition that compromises his or her immune status, such as AIDS, or is the individual undergoing therapy that would result in immunodeficiency, such as cancer chemotherapy?

**PHYSICAL EXAMINATION OR HOME ASSESSMENT**

- Again, complete as thorough a physical examination (on an individual) or home assessment as you can. Keep in mind that you should collect only the data for which you have a use.
- Be alert for indications of physical abuse, substance use (e.g., needle marks, nasal abnormalities), or neglect (e.g., being underweight or inadequately clothed).
- You can assess a family's living environment using good observational skills. Does the family live in an insect- or rat-infested environment? Do they have running water, functioning plumbing, electricity, and a telephone?
- Is perishable food (e.g., mayonnaise) left sitting out on tables and countertops? Are bed linens reasonably clean? Is paint peeling on the walls and ceilings? Is ventilation adequate? Is the temperature of the home adequate? Is the family exposed to raw sewage or animal waste? Is the home adjacent to a busy highway, possibly exposing the family to high noise levels and automobile exhaust?

cell counts and for common opportunistic infections, including TB and pneumonia. Intravenous drug users should be evaluated for HBV, including liver palpation and serum antigen tests as necessary. Alcoholic clients should also be asked about symptoms of liver disease and evaluated for jaundice and liver enlargement. Severely mentally ill clients should be assessed for the presence of tardive dyskinesia, indicating possible toxicity from their antipsychotic medications. Chapters 32 to 39 provide more specific details about physical health assessment for vulnerable groups.

## Biological Issues

Vulnerable populations should be assessed for congenital and genetic predisposition to illness and either receive education and counseling as appropriate or be referred to other health professionals as necessary. For example, pregnant adolescents who are substance abusers should be re-

ferred to programs to help them quit using addictive substances during their pregnancies and ideally after delivery of their infants as well. Pregnant women over age 35 should be informed about amniocentesis testing to determine if genetic abnormalities exist in the fetus. Specialized counseling about treatment and anticipatory guidance regarding the infant's needs can be provided by an advanced practice nurse or a physician. Screening may be done as part of health fairs provided at places where people live (e.g., neighborhoods, community centers, shelters), work, pray (faith communities), or play (recreational settings).

## Psychologic Issues

Vulnerable family groups should be assessed for the extent of stress the family may be experiencing and the presence of healthy or dysfunctional family dynamics. The nurse should also evaluate these families for effective communication patterns, caregiving capabilities, and the extent to which family developmental tasks are being met. Vulnerable individuals should be assessed for the presence of stressors, their usual coping styles, levels of self-efficacy (or the belief that one is capable of meeting life's challenges), their overall sense of well-being and level of self-esteem, and the presence of depression and anxiety (Berne et al, 1991; Pesznecker, 1984). It is important to be sensitive to cues that members of vulnerable groups are depressed, as this appears to be a prevalent problem and a critical predictor of risky behaviors such as abuse and violence (Lutenbacher, 2000; Sachs et al, 1999). Vulnerable individuals and families should be assessed for risks of or exposure to violence and abuse. Likewise, groups (such as a school population) should be evaluated for the presence of or potential for violence.

## Lifestyle Issues

Nurses should assess lifestyle factors of vulnerable individuals, families, and groups that may predispose them to further health problems. Lifestyle factors include usual dietary patterns, exercise, rest, and the use of drugs, alcohol, and caffeine. For example, many homeless individuals eat their meals either at shelters or at fast-food restaurants. Because of the unpredictability of meals and food availability, it is often difficult for them to eat a diet that is low in fat, cholesterol, and sodium, and it is particularly difficult to eat the recommended five servings of fruit and vegetables per day. Cultural preferences may also influence lifestyle and health risk behaviors.

## Environmental Issues

Vulnerable groups are more likely to be exposed to environmental hazards such as pollutants or carcinogens than other groups. Nurses should assess the living environment and neighborhood surroundings of vulnerable families and groups for environmental hazards such as lead-based paint, asbestos, water and air quality, industrial wastes, and the incidence of crime. Nurses must often establish partnerships with vulnerable groups to put changes into place, such as persuading a local industry to reduce the levels of effluents from their plants or working with local government and law enforcement to develop crime prevention programs.

## PLANNING AND IMPLEMENTING CARE FOR VULNERABLE POPULATIONS

In some situations, the nurse works with individual clients. In other cases, the nurse develops programs and policies for populations of vulnerable persons. In either case, planning and implementing care for members of vulnerable populations involves partnership between nurse and client. Nurses who direct and control the client's care cannot establish a trusting relationship and may inadvertently foster a cycle of dependency and lack of personal health control. In fact, the most important initial step is for nurses to establish that they are trustworthy and dependable. For example, nurses who work in a community clinic for substance abusers must overcome any suspicion that

---

### BOX 31-6 Nursing Roles When Working With Vulnerable Population Groups

- Case finder
- Health educator
- Counselor
- Direct care provider
- Population health advocate
- Community assessor and developer
- Monitor and evaluator of care
- Case manager
- Advocate
- Health program planner
- Participant in developing health policies

---

clients may have of them and eliminate any fears that they will manipulate them with "games."

## Roles of the Nurse

Nurses working with vulnerable populations may fill numerous roles, including those listed in Box 31-6. They identify vulnerable individuals and families through outreach and case finding. They encourage vulnerable groups to obtain health services, and they develop programs that respond to their needs. Nurses teach vulnerable individuals, families, and groups strategies to prevent illness and promote health. They counsel clients about ways to increase their sense of personal power and help them identify strengths and resources. They provide direct care to clients and families in a variety of settings, including storefront clinics (Aiken and Salmon, 1994), mobile clinics, shelters (Mayo, 1996), homes, neighborhoods (Jenkins and Torrisi, 1997), worksites, churches, and schools (Hacker, 1996). For example, a nurse in a mobile migrant clinic might administer a tetanus booster to a client who has been injured by a piece of farm machinery and may also check that client's blood pressure and cholesterol level during the same visit. A home-health nurse seeing a family referred by the courts for child abuse may weigh the child, conduct a nutritional assessment, and help the family learn how to manage anger and disciplinary problems. A nurse working in a school-based clinic may lead a support group for pregnant adolescents and conduct a birthing class. Nurses working with people being treated for TB monitor drug treatment compliance to ensure that they complete their full course of therapy (Frieden, 1994). Public and community-oriented health nurses serve as population health advocates and work with local, state, or national groups to develop and implement healthy public policy. They also collaborate with other community members and serve as community assessors and developers, and they monitor and evaluate care and health programs. Healthy People in Healthy Communities describes one approach for working collaboratively with communities to develop healthy communities and eliminate health disparities (USDHHS, 2001b). Nurses often function as case managers for vulnerable clients, making referrals and linking them with community services, and they serve as advocates. The nurse functions as an advocate when referring clients to other agencies, working with others to develop health programs, and influencing legislation and health policies that affect vulnerable populations.

## THE CUTTING EDGE

Nursing centers provide care for vulnerable populations. These centers often care for large numbers of uninsured and underinsured persons and focus on community health promotion. Nursing center directors are working with policymakers to develop new reimbursement strategies that will make it possible for these centers to remain financially solvent and to provide innovative forms of care to meet the special needs of vulnerable populations.

The nature of nurses' roles varies depending on whether the client is a single person, a family, or a group. For example, a nurse might teach an HIV-positive client about the need for prevention of opportunistic infections, or may help a family with an HIV-positive member understand myths about transmission of HIV, or may work with a community group concerned about HIV transmission among students in the schools. In each case, the nurse teaches how to prevent infectious and communicable diseases, and the size of the group and the teaching method is different. Box 31-7 lists principles for intervening with vulnerable populations. Box 31-8 lists examples of evidence-based interventions for vulnerable adolescents.

## Client Empowerment and Health Education

Nurses should help all vulnerable groups achieve a greater sense of personal **empowerment** through effective health education and facilitating acquisition of necessary resources, because one of the core dimensions of vulnerability is a perception of powerlessness, which can lead to hopelessness. Clients who feel empowered are more likely to be able to make their own decisions about health care and improve their health status. Nurses empower clients by helping them acquire the skills needed for healthy living and for being an effective health care consumer. For example, one of the first steps in helping abused individuals is to empower them so they can begin to help themselves. Nurses can do this through active listening, by letting clients know that what is happening to them is illegal and that all people have the right to be safe, and by reas-

suring them that their fears and concerns are normal (Chez, 1994). Chez also suggests helping clients make independent decisions and helping them recognize the strengths they can draw on to change the situation.

Health education is one key to working with vulnerable populations. Teach members of populations with low educational levels what they need to do to promote health and prevent illness rather than directing health education to groups that you *think* might be at high risk but have no evidence to support your perception. For example, in a study of cardiovascular disease risk for rural southern women, Appel et al (2002) found that only body mass index and educational level predicted risk for cardiovascular disease within this population. They recommended health education for all low-income rural Southern women and not just for particular racial groups. A new concern for public and community health nurses is whether the populations with whom they work have adequate health literacy to benefit from health education. It may be necessary to collaborate with an educator, an interpreter, or an expert in health communications to design messages that vulnerable individuals and groups can understand and use.

One way to foster empowerment is to ensure that health-promoting strategies are culturally and linguistically appropriate (Bushy, 1999). For example, culturally appropriate health education strategies ensure that information is provided in language that is meaningful to the group (semantic approach to cultural sensitivity) and that the cultural context is taken into account (instrumental approach to cultural sensitivity) as the educational program is designed (Bayer, 1994). Culturally appropriate health education strategies are based on respect for cultural diversity and demonstrate that the culture of the participants is respected. For example, when working with the homeless, it is important to build on the survival skills they have developed and to ensure that health programs reflect the fact that their first priority is usually survival. The culture of homelessness is oriented to the present, so a wide range of services should be available in a single location—"one-stop shopping" (Davis, 1996, p. 182). It is useful to collaborate with educators, health communications specialists, or health librarians to develop health education materials that are both culturally and linguistically appropriate and at the appropriate reading level for the population. Community-based health education programs, supplemented by the use of interpreters and specialists in the culture of the population, are effective interventions. Culturally and linguistically appropriate interventions may help reduce health disparities by making it easier for members of vulnerable population groups to receive and use health information and to incorporate health practices into personal cultural beliefs and lifestyles (Brach and Fraser, 2000).

Sometimes, the first step in empowering clients is when the nurse is an advocate for them, especially in the policy arena, where vulnerable populations may not always be represented. For example, in one community a nursing

## BOX 31-7 Principles for Intervening With Vulnerable Populations

### GOALS

- Set reasonable goals that are based on the baseline data you collected. Focus on eliminating disparities in health status among vulnerable populations and include realistic goals using Healthy People 2010 objectives as a guide.
- Work toward setting manageable goals with the client, whether the client is an individual, family, or community. Goals that seem unattainable may be discouraging.
- Set goals collaboratively with the client as a first step toward client empowerment.
- Set family-centered, culturally sensitive goals.
- Be sure to communicate with the client (individual, family, or group) in culturally and linguistically appropriate ways. Obtain the assistance of an interpreter if necessary.

### INTERVENTIONS

- Set up outreach and case-finding programs to help increase access to health services by vulnerable populations.
- Try to minimize the "hassle factor" connected with your interventions. Vulnerable groups do not have the extra energy, money, or time to cope with unnecessary waits, complicated treatment plans, or confusion. As your client's advocate, identify what hassles may occur and develop ways to avoid them. This may include providing comprehensive services during a single encounter, rather than asking the client to return for multiple visits. Multiple visits for more specialized aspects of the client's needs, whether individual or family, reinforce a perception that health care is fragmented and organized for the professional's convenience rather than the client's.
- Work with clients to ensure that interventions are culturally sensitive and competent and linguistically appropriate. Arrange to have an interpreter available if English is not the population's first language.

- Focus on teaching clients skills in health promotion and disease prevention. Also, teach them how to be effective health care consumers. For example, role-play, asking questions in a physician's office with a client. Work with professional educators or health communications experts to help resolve literacy issues and deliver health messages in ways that members of the population are comfortable with.
- Enlist the involvement of peers (for adolescents) and community members as appropriate to help communicate health messages.
- Help clients learn what to do if they cannot keep an appointment with a health care or social service professional.
- Work with the media to design public service announcements about health.
- Design and implement health fairs in schools, workplaces, neighborhood centers, and faith-based organizations.

### EVALUATING OUTCOMES

- It is often difficult for vulnerable clients to return for follow-up care. Help your client develop self-care strategies for evaluating outcomes. For example, teach homeless individuals how to read their own tuberculosis skin test and give them a self-addressed, stamped card they can return by mail with the results.
- Remember to evaluate outcomes in terms of the goals you have mutually agreed on with the client. For example, one outcome for a homeless person receiving isoniazid therapy for TB might be that the person returns to the clinic daily for direct observation of the compliance with the drug therapy
- Also, evaluate outcomes using the indicators in the Healthy People 2010 objectives. This makes it easier to compare outcomes in terms of national priorities and across areas.

## BOX 31-8 Examples of Evidence-Based Interventions for Vulnerable Adolescents

- Home visiting programs for pregnant adolescents and adolescent mothers (Koniak-Griffin et al, 2000)
- Parenting classes for pregnant adolescents (Koniak-Griffin et al, 2000)
- Brief street outreach interventions related to sexual health promotion for homeless adolescents (Rew, Chambers, and Kulkarni, 2002)

- Health education curricula implemented in school settings (Browne et al, 2001)
- Use of peer counselors to reduce minority adolescent health risk behaviors (Browne et al, 2001)
- Public service announcements by adolescent peer leaders related to health risk behaviors (Browne et al, 2001)

Browne DC et al: Minority health risk behaviors: an introduction to research on sexually transmitted diseases, violence, pregnancy prevention and substance abuse, Matern Child Health J 5(4):215-224, 2001; Koniak-Griffin D et al: A public health nursing early intervention program for adolescent mothers: outcomes from pregnancy through 6 weeks postpartum, Nurs Res 49(3):130-138, 2000; Rew L, Chambers KB, Kulkarni S: Planning a sexual health promotion intervention with homeless adolescents, Nurs Res 51(3):168-174, 2002.

student learned that a social service agency had restrictive policies toward serving homeless alcoholic men. This was the primary agency that could provide shelter for these men, but their restrictive policies made it difficult for the men to obtain shelter as often as necessary. After advocating for the needs of this vulnerable population and persuading the agency to relax their policies, this nurse participated on the board of the agency to ensure that their policies continued to meet the needs. Providing shelter made it more likely that the men could get adequate rest, and could bathe and dress in clean clothes so they could look for jobs and become more self-sufficient.

## Levels of Prevention

Healthy People 2010 (USDHHS, 2001a) objectives emphasize improving health by modifying the individual, social, and environmental determinants of health. One way to do this is for vulnerable individuals to have a primary care provider who both coordinates health services for them and provides their preventive services. This primary care provider may be an advanced practice nurse or a primary care physician (e.g., a family practice physician). Another approach is for a nurse to serve as a case manager for vulnerable clients and, again, coordinate services and provide illness prevention and health promotion services.

One example of primary prevention is to give influenza vaccinations to vulnerable populations who are immunocompromised (unless contraindicated). Secondary prevention is seen in conducting screening clinics for vulnerable populations. For example, nurses who work in homeless shelters, prisons, migrant camps, and substance abuse treatment facilities should know that these groups are at high risk for acquiring communicable diseases. Both clients and staff need routine screening for TB. Screening homeless adults and providing isoniazid to those who test positive for TB are examples of secondary prevention (Tulsky et al, 2000) (Box 31-9). Tertiary prevention is conducting a therapy group with the residents of a group home for severely mentally ill adults. Nurses who work with abused women to help them enhance their levels of self-esteem are also providing tertiary preventive activities.

## Strategies for Promoting Healthy Lifestyles

Helping vulnerable persons develop healthy lifestyle behaviors requires great sensitivity by nurses. They should focus on identifying clients' priorities and helping them meet these priorities. For example, discussing exercise with a homeless person requires empathy and creativity. Often, vulnerable individuals and families are coping with crises, so the nurse must begin by using crisis intervention strategies. After the crisis has been managed, a trusting relationship is likely to exist between the nurse and client. This relationship forms the basis for health promotion interventions. Nurses must be sensitive to the lifestyles of their vulnerable clients and must develop methods of health promotion that recognize these lifestyle factors. For instance, Brennan's ComputerLink program for people with AIDS provides personal computers in the homes of

> **HOW TO** Coordinate Health and Social Services for Members of Vulnerable Populations
>
> Nurses who work with vulnerable populations often need to coordinate services across multiple agencies for members of these groups. It is helpful to have a strong professional network of people who work in other agencies. Effective professional networks make it easier to coordinate care smoothly and in ways that do not add to clients' stress. Nurses can develop strong networks by participating in community coalitions and attending professional meetings. When making referrals to other agencies, a phone call can be a helpful way to obtain information that the client will need for the visit. When possible, having an interdisciplinary, interagency team plan care for clients at high risk for health problems can be quite effective. It is crucial to obtain the clients' written and informed consent before engaging in this kind of planning because of confidentiality issues. The following list of tips can be helpful:
>
> - Be sure to involve clients in making decisions about the kinds of services they will find beneficial and can use.
> - Work with community coalitions to develop plans for service coordination for targeted vulnerable populations.
> - Collaborate with legal counsel from the agencies involved in the coalitions to ensure that legal and ethical issues related to care coordination have been properly addressed. Examples of issues to address include privacy and security of clinical data and ensuring compliance with the Health Insurance Portability and Accountability Act (HIPAA), contractual provisions for coordinating care across agencies, and consent to treatment from multiple agencies.
> - Develop policies and protocols for making referrals, following up on referrals and ensuring that clients receiving care from multiple agencies experience the process as smooth and seamless.

people with AIDS and enables them to obtain information about ways to maintain a high quality of life in the privacy of their homes (Brennan and Ripich, 1994). Another program was designed to encourage inner-city Latino families to increase their intake of low-fat milk (Wechsler and Wernick, 1992). This successful program included providing money-off coupons for low-fat milk, making it less costly for the families.

## Healthy People 2010 Objectives and Healthy People in Healthy Communities Guidelines

The Healthy People 2010 objectives emphasize increasing the number and quality of years of healthy life and eliminating health disparities through prevention and health promotion (USDHHS, 2001a). Objectives have been de-

## BOX 31-9 Levels of Prevention With Vulnerable Populations

**PRIMARY PREVENTION**

- Provide health teaching about balanced diet and exercise.
- Give influenza shots to people who are immuno-compromised or who live in high-risk environments, such as in shelters or in the streets.

**SECONDARY PREVENTION**

- Conduct screening clinics to assess for such things as tuberculosis.
- Develop a way for homeless individuals to read their TB skin test, if necessary, and to transfer the results back to the facility where the skin test was administered.
- Develop a portable immunization chart, such as a wallet card, that mobile population groups such as the homeless and migrant workers can carry with them.

**TERTIARY PREVENTION**

- Provide fluids and a place to rest for people with influenza.
- If someone tests positive for tuberculosis, immediately try to get the person on isoniazid.
- Provide directly observed medication therapy for people with active TB.

veloped for access, chronic conditions, community-based programs, environmental health, health communication, and health behaviors. Data have been compiled related to racial and ethnic minorities, and to people vulnerable to poor health by virtue of age and socioeconomic status. These data are to be used as baselines against which to measure progress toward achievement of the objectives. This makes it possible to track reductions in health disparities until the goal of eliminating the disparities is met.

Healthy People 2010 (USDHHS, 2001a) objectives include targets for improvement over baseline incidence and prevalence statistics on illness and health problems. Communities should determine local incidence and prevalence statistics and establish realistic targets for improvement.

Healthy People in Healthy Communities (USDHHS, 2001b) provides suggestions for communitywide strategies to develop and maintain healthier communities. These strategies use the MAP-IT approach, in which the focus is on building coalitions and improving community health through a wide range of community partnerships. These partnerships might include health professionals, business people, educators, politicians, and local community leaders, to name a few. MAP-IT is an acronym for mobilizing community resources, assessing, planning, implementing, and tracking results (USDHHS, 2001b). Community partnerships can be helpful to public health nurses who wish to intervene at the population level to improve the socioeconomic environment in which vulnerable populations live.

## Comprehensive Services

In general, more agencies are needed that provide comprehensive services with nonrestrictive eligibility requirements. Communities often have many agencies that restrict eligibility for their services to people most likely to benefit from those services, or they limit eligibility to make it possible for more people to receive services. For example, shelters may prohibit people who have been drinking alcohol from staying overnight and sometimes limit the number of sequential nights a person can stay. Food banks usually limit the number of times a person can receive free food. Agencies are frequently very specialized as well. For vulnerable individuals and families, this means that they must go to many agencies to find services for which they qualify and that meet their needs. This is so tiring and discouraging that people are sometimes willing to forgo help because it is just too difficult to obtain it.

## Resources for Vulnerable Populations

Nurses should know about community agencies that offer a variety of health and social services for vulnerable populations. They should also follow up with the client after the referral to ensure that the desired outcomes were achieved. Sometimes, excellent community resources may be available but impractical for clients because of transportation or reimbursement problems. Nurses should identify those problems that will interfere with clients' following through with referrals, and they should work with other team members to make referrals as convenient and realistic as possible. Although clients with social problems such as financial needs should be referred to social workers, nurses should understand the close connections between health and social problems and know how to work effectively with other professionals. A list of community resources can often be found in the telephone book, and many communities have publications that list them. Examples of agency resources found in most communities are as follows:

- Health departments
- Community mental health centers
- American Red Cross and other voluntary organizations
- Food and clothing banks
- Missions and shelters
- Nurse-managed neighborhood clinics
- Social service agencies such as Travelers' Aid and Salvation Army
- Church-sponsored health and social service assistance

Two other important categories of resources for vulnerable populations are their own personal coping skills and social supports (Aday, 2001). These groups must often be quite resourceful and creative to manage in the face of multiple stressors. Nurses should work with clients to help them identify their own personal strengths and draw on those strengths when managing their health needs. Also, clients may be able to depend on informal support networks. Even though social isolation is a problem for many

## Healthy People 2010 | Goals for Vulnerable Populations

The following are examples of objectives that community-oriented nurses who work with vulnerable populations might want to note:

**1-5** Increase the proportion of persons with a usual primary care provider

**18-7** Increase the proportion of children with mental health problems who receive treatment

**18-9** Increase the proportion of adults with mental disorders who receive treatment

**18-13** Increase the number of states, territories, and the District of Columbia with an operational mental health plan that addresses cultural competence

**24-1d** Reduce asthma deaths

**25-11** Increase the proportion of adolescents who abstain from sexual intercourse or use condoms if currently sexually active

From U.S. Department of Health and Human Services: *Healthy people 2010: understanding and improving health,* ed 2, Washington, DC, 2000, U.S. Government Printing Office.

## Evidence-Based Practice

An ecologic view of health suggests that vulnerability results from the interaction between the social and economic environment and the resources available to populations living in that environment. This view suggests that the context in which vulnerable populations live is important, but it is not entirely clear what should be done (or how) to ameliorate the effects of a low socioeconomic status environment. This study was a secondary analysis of data from the California and New York State Departments of Health. Researchers hypothesized that there would be greater variability in those health problems that were more likely to be influenced by the socioeconomic environment and less likely to be influenced by genetics and health behaviors. For example, they expected to find that communicable diseases and accidents would show greater variation in counties with a low socioeconomic status. The researchers compared the mortality rates for a range of health outcomes (including homicide, suicide, acquired immunodeficiency syndrome [AIDS], pneumonia, chronic obstructive pulmonary disease, stroke, neoplastic disease, and accidents) to countywide socioeconomic status. They found the greatest variability in mortality rates from homicide,

AIDS, and cirrhosis. As expected, these health outcomes varied by county socioeconomic status, with the lower socioeconomic status counties having the highest mortality rates from these causes. Thus the hypotheses were supported, indicating that a relationship exists in variability of mortality from health problems that are especially sensitive to socioeconomic factors.

Although this correlational study of secondary data does not indicate what actions community-oriented nurses or other public health professionals should take to improve health, it does suggest that improving the socioeconomic status of a community may lead to improvements in health.

**Nurse Use:** Community-oriented nurses should consider interventions that enhance the population's ability to stay in school and to obtain jobs that provide a living wage. For example, providing reproductive education and strengthening adolescents' ability to delay pregnancy may boost high school graduation rates. Providing day care for high school and college students may be a tangible strategy for helping those adolescents who are already parents.

Karpati A et al: Variability and vulnerability at the ecologic level: implications for understanding the social determinants of health, *Am J Public Health* 92(11):1768-1772, 2002.

vulnerable clients, nurses should not assume that clients have no one who can help them.

## Case Management

**Case management** involves linking client with services and providing direct nursing services to clients, such as teaching, counseling, screening, and immunizing (Bower, 1992). Lillian Wald was the first nurse case manager. She linked vulnerable families with a variety of services to help them stay healthy (Buhler-Wilkerson, 1993). Aiken and Salmon

(1994) explain that "public health nurses represent the interface between personal health services and population-based health promotion" (p. 327). Linking, or **brokering health services,** is accomplished by making appropriate referrals and by following up with clients to ensure that the desired outcomes from the referral were achieved. Nurses are effective case managers in community nursing clinics, health departments, and case management programs where the focus includes both community and hospital care. Nurse case managers emphasize health promotion and ill-

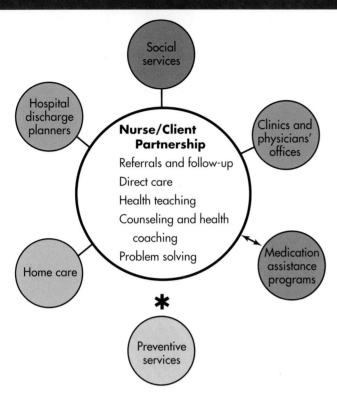

**Figure 31-6** The nurse as case manager for vulnerable populations.

ness prevention with vulnerable clients and focus on helping them avoid unnecessary hospitalization. Figure 31-6 illustrates the coordination and brokering aspect of the nurse's role as case manager for vulnerable populations.

## EVALUATION OF NURSING INTERVENTIONS WITH VULNERABLE POPULATIONS

Evaluation of therapeutic nursing interventions begins with client goals and objectives and focuses on the extent to which client health outcomes are achieved, whether clients are individuals, families, groups, or populations. Nurses may evaluate individual client goal achievement, the extent to which a vulnerable family achieved goals developed in partnership with the nurse, or the extent to which a nursing program achieved its objectives for a particular population. Evaluation takes place while providing care and gives the nurse a basis for revising therapeutic interventions to make them more effective. Evaluation also takes place when a case is closed or when a program is completed, and then it gives nurses data to use in providing care to similar clients or programs in the future. The types of client outcomes that may be evaluated include improved quality of life, improved indicators of physical health status (e.g., blood pressure, skin integrity, mobility), reduced depression or anxiety, improved functional status, increased levels of knowledge about health behaviors, and satisfaction with care. Nurses use a variety of scales to evaluate these outcome indicators; they sometimes interview clients or administer short questionnaires; and they use laboratory reports and results of health assessments to help evaluate goal achievement with individuals and clients. Incidence and prevalence data, survey data, and service utilization data are used to evaluate health programs for vulnerable populations.

## ◗ Practice Application

Assume that you are a nurse working in a free migrant health clinic. Ms. Nunio, a 46-year-old farmworker pregnant with her fifth child, comes in requesting treatment for swollen ankles. During your assessment, you learn that she was seen by the nurse practitioner at the local health department 2 months ago. The NP gave her some sample vitamins, but Ms. Nunio lost them because she has moved twice since that time. She has not received regular prenatal care and has no plans to do so because she does not have a green card and is worried that she will be deported. Her previous pregnancies were essentially normal, although she said she was "toxic" with her last child. Ms. Nunio is 5 feet 2 inches tall, weighs 190 pounds, and has a blood pressure of 160/90 with pitting edema of the ankles and a mild headache. She shares with you that she used to have "spells" when she lived in her home country and occasionally took medication because she was hearing voices.

You are aware that Ms. Nunio's situation, while acute, is not unusual in your community. The migrant farmworker population has grown in recent years and some of the families are beginning to accompany the primary wage earner in the household and settle in the community. Not all local residents are comfortable with this because they say that taxpayer money is being used to provide services for people who are not legal residents and who do not pay taxes. The situation is becoming tense and a few vocal community members have begun a drive to put forth a referendum addressing the issue. The nurses in your clinic have debated whether you should become involved in these local discussions and help raise community awareness of the health and social needs of the migrant farmworker population. Each of you understands that the immigration issues are complex and you respect local concerns, but you are also eager to be part of the solution.

Where should you and your colleagues begin to address the problems experienced by the migrant farmworker population (both legal immigrants and illegal aliens) and the local community's concerns?

A. Make a list of the issues and present it to the local city council.

B. Help develop the language for the referendum.

C. Mount vigorous opposition to the local group that is considering a referendum on the issues.

D. Gather data to describe the extent of the issues by meeting with local concerned citizens, migrant farmworkers, politicians and policymakers, and health care providers.

**Answers are in the back of the book.**

## Key Points

- Vulnerable populations are more likely to develop health problems as a result of exposure to risk or to have worse outcomes from those health problems than the rest of the population. Vulnerable populations are more sensitive to risk factors than those who are more resilient and are more often exposed to cumulative risk factors. These populations include poor or homeless persons, pregnant adolescents, migrant workers, severely mentally ill individuals, substance abusers, abused individuals, persons with communicable diseases, and persons with sexually transmitted diseases, including HIV and HBV.

- All countries have these special population groups that are more vulnerable to poor health than others. The identities of the groups vary across countries, depending on local political, economic, cultural, and demographic characteristics.

- Health care is increasingly moving into the community. This began with deinstitutionalization of the severely mentally ill population and is continuing today as hospitals reduce inpatient stays. Vulnerable populations need a wide variety of services, and because these are often provided by multiple community agencies, nurses coordinate and manage the service needs of vulnerable groups.

- Public policies sometimes provide financial assistance for vulnerable populations and sometimes provide money to build health facilities and train professionals to work with vulnerable groups. Unanticipated implementation problems often further disadvantage vulnerable populations. Health care reform policies are focused on controlling costs and may have the unintended effect of limiting services to vulnerable populations.

- The health field concept suggests that both individuals and society are responsible for health status. Individuals and groups may be vulnerable to social and health problems as a result of both their own actions and the policies and decisions made at the societal level. There are many dimensions to vulnerability, including limited control over one's own health, victimization, disenfranchisement, disadvantaged status, powerlessness, and cumulative health risks.

- Socioeconomic problems, including poverty and social isolation, physiologic and developmental aspects of age, poor health status, and highly stressful life experiences, predispose people to vulnerability. Vulnerability can become a cycle, where the predisposing factors lead to poor health outcomes, chronic stress, and hopelessness, and these outcomes in turn increase vulnerability.

- Nurses assess vulnerable individuals, families, and groups to determine which socioeconomic, physical, biological, psychologic, and environmental factors are problems for clients. They work as partners with vulnerable clients to identify client strengths and needs and develop intervention strategies designed to break the cycle of vulnerability.

- Community-oriented nursing roles seen when working with vulnerable populations include health teacher, counselor, direct care provider, case manager, advocate, health program planner, and participant in developing health policies. Nurses focus on empowering clients to prevent illness and promote health, and they work to achieve the Healthy People 2010 national health objectives with vulnerable populations. Nurses link clients with resources in the community and monitor client outcomes to ensure that community referrals are effective.

- Evaluation of therapeutic nursing interventions with vulnerable populations occurs both during and after service delivery. Results of evaluations are used to make revisions in nursing care, with the ultimate goal of improving client outcomes.

## Clinical Decision-Making Activities

1. Vulnerability implies that certain populations have both a higher relative risk for illness because of the presence of multiple risk factors and a greater sensitivity to the effects of individual risk factors. Identify populations in your community that you think are more vulnerable to poor health than others. List the risk factors members of these populations are more likely to have, and identify the prevalence of these risk factors in your community. Discuss with your classmates or a nurse in a clinical agency the effect you believe these risk factors are having on the health of vulnerable populations in your community. Analyze whether members of these special populations seem to be more sensitive to the effect of the risk factors than the population as a whole. What are some of the complexities that are related to these issues?

2. Examine health statistics and demographic data in your geographic area to determine which vulnerable groups predominate in your area. Look through your phone book for examples of agencies that you think provide services to these vulnerable groups. Make appointments with key individuals in several of these agencies to discuss the nature of their target population, the types of services provided, and the reimbursement mechanisms for these services. Various class members should visit different agencies and then share their results during class. On the basis of your findings, identify gaps or overlaps in services provided to vulnerable groups in your community. Try to be specific and delineate the political and economic reasons for the gaps and overlaps. What might be some ways to manage these gaps and overlaps to help clients receive the services they need?

3. Debate with your class the nature and extent of services that you believe should be made available to the homeless. Defend your position regarding "en-

abling" and "worthiness." What evidence have you used in constructing your arguments?

4. Health care spending accounts for about 14% of the gross domestic product (GDP). Most people do not want to spend any more of the GDP on health care. Assuming then that the amount of money available to spend on health care is fixed at any point in time, explain what proportion of that money you think the federal government should spend on prevention and treatment of AIDS, substance abuse, severe mental illness, and breast cancer. What criteria did you use to arrive at your conclusions? What research evidence supports your position?

5. To what extent do you think economic issues and social values play a role in the way that health services are offered to vulnerable population groups? Explain why you think the population as a whole should or should not pay for care for vulnerable groups. Read the article by Grey (1994) in the reference list on the development of health services for migrant workers for an example of this debate. Base your argument on the concept of social justice.

6. Discuss the types of assistance you might provide to the following clients:
   a. A chronically homeless, pregnant, 33-year-old, mildly mentally retarded woman and her unemployed boyfriend
   b. A 14-year-old runaway girl who is earning money through prostitution and has a drug habit
   c. A 22-year-old woman with four children who is receiving welfare and whose boyfriend smokes crack cocaine
   d. An HIV-positive woman with no family and few friends who is trying to make plans for someone to care for her three children after her death
   e. A 56-year-old alcoholic male migrant farmworker whose TB skin test just came back positive

   What kinds of nursing needs do these clients have in common? Analyze the dimensions of vulnerability described in this chapter in terms of how these

clients may possess these characteristics and how you, as a nurse, can help them break out of the cycle of vulnerability. In what ways would you choose to function as an advocate for the vulnerable populations represented by these individuals?

7. Examine the pros and cons of school-based reproductive care for adolescents. What does the research literature say about the optimal ways to provide such care? What are the ethical issues involved in providing reproductive information to adolescents, with or without parental consent? Check state and federal legal requirements related to privacy and confidentiality of personal health information in these situations. How would public health nurses be expected to balance confidentiality concerns of teens in school-based clinics, with parental interest in their children's health information?

8. Interview nurses at a health department to identify which personal care services they provide to vulnerable populations and which population-based services they provide. Discuss their opinions about whether personal care services should be provided only by private agencies. Analyze this issue from the perspectives of the core functions of public health, access to care for vulnerable populations, and cost effectiveness of care provided by public health departments as compared with private agencies. Include research support for your arguments.

## Additional Resources

These related resources are found either in the appendix at the back of this book or on the book's website at **http://evolve.elsevier.com/Stanhope.**

***evolve*** **Evolve Website**

WebLinks: Healthy People 2010

## References

Aday LA: Vulnerable populations: a community-oriented perspective, *Fam Community Health* 19(4):1-18, 1997.

Aday LA: *At risk in America: the health and health care needs of vulnerable populations in the United States,* ed 2, San Francisco: Jossey-Bass, 2001.

Adler NE, Ostrove JM: Socioeconomic status and health: what we know and what we don't, *Ann NY Acad Sci* 896:3-15, 1999.

Adler NE et al: Socioeconomic inequalities in health: no easy solution. In Lee PR, Estes CL, editors: *The nation's health,* ed 5, pp 18-31, Sudbury, Mass, 1997, Jones and Bartlett.

Agency for Healthcare Research and Quality: *Statistical brief #3: children's health care quality, fall 2000,* Rockville, Md, 2002, available at http://www.meps.ahrq.gov/papers/st3/stat03.htm.

Aiken LH, Salmon ME: Health care workforce priorities: what nursing should do now, *Inquiry* 31(3):318-329, 1994.

American Academy of Nursing Expert Panel Report: Culturally competent health care, *Nurs Outlook* 40(6):277-283, 1992.

Appel SJ, Harrell JS, Deng S: Racial and socioeconomic differences in risk factors for cardiovascular disease among southern rural women, *Nurs Res* 51(3):140-147, 2002.

Baker EL et al: Health reform and the health of the public: forging community health partnerships, *JAMA* 272(16):1276-1282, 1994.

Bayer R: AIDS prevention and cultural sensitivity: are they compatible? *Am J Public Health* 84(6):895-898, 1994.

Berne AS et al: A nursing model for addressing the health needs of homeless families, *Image J Nurs Scholar* 22(1):8-13, 1991.

Bower KA: *Case management by nurses,* Kansas City, Mo, 1992, American Nurses' Association.

Brach C, Fraser I: Can cultural competency reduce racial and ethnic disparities? A review and conceptual model, *Med Care Res Rev* 57(Suppl. 1):181-217, 2000.

Brennan PF, Ripich S: Use of a home-care computer network by persons with AIDS, *Int J Technol Assess Health Care* 10(2):258-272, 1994.

Browne DC et al: Minority health risk behaviors: an introduction to research on sexually transmitted diseases, violence, pregnancy prevention and substance abuse, *Matern Child Health J* 5(4):215-224, 2001.

Buhler-Wilkerson K: Bringing care to the people: Lillian Wald's legacy to public health nursing, *Am J Public Health* 83(12):1778-1786, 1993.

Bushy A: The need for cultural-linguistic competent care for families with special health problems. In Sebastian J, Bushy A, editors: *Special populations in the community: advances in reducing health disparities,* Gaithersburg, Md, 1999, Aspen.

Carrasquillo O et al: Can Medicaid managed care provide continuity of care to new Medicaid enrollees? an analysis of tenure on Medicaid, *Am J Public Health* 88(3):464, 1998.

Chez N: Helping the victim of domestic violence, *Am J Nurs* 94(7):32-37, 1994.

Cooper RS et al: Relationship between premature mortality and socioeconomic factors in black and white populations of US metropolitan areas, *Public Health Rep* 116(5):464-473, 2001.

Curtin L: Throwaway people? *Nurs Manag* 17(12):7-8, 1986.

Dachner N, Tarasuk V: Homeless "squeegee kids": food insecurity and daily survival, *Soc Sci Med* 54(7):1039-1049, 2002.

Davis RE: Tapping into the culture of homelessness, *J Prof Nurs* 12(3):176-183, 1996.

de la Barra X: Poverty: the main cause of ill health in urban children, *Health Educ Behav* 25(1):46-59, 1998.

Denyes MJ et al: Self-care: a foundational science, *Nurs Sci Q* 14(1):48-54, 2001.

Dever GEA, Sciegaj M, Wade TE: Creation of a social vulnerability index for justice in health planning, *Fam Community Health* 10(4):23-32, 1988.

Einbinder LC, Schulman KA: The effect of race on the referral process for invasive cardiac procedures, *Med Care Res Rev* 57(Suppl. 1):162-180, 2000.

Epstein AM: Medicaid managed care and high quality: can we have both? *JAMA* 278(19):1617-1621, 1997.

Erickson GP: To pauperize or empower: public health nursing at the turn of the 20th and 21st centuries, *Public Health Nurs* 13(3):163-169, 1996.

Fawcett J: The nurse theorists: 21st century updates—Betty Neuman, interview by Jacquelin Fawcett, *Nurs Sci Q* 14(3):211-214, 2001.

Fawcett J: The nurse theorists: 21st century updates—Sister Callista Roy, interview by Jacquelin Fawcett, *Nurs Sci Q* 15(4):308-310, 2002.

Federal Interagency Forum on Child and Family Statistics: *America's children: key national indicators of well-being,* Washington, DC, 2000, U.S. Government Printing Office.

Fielding J, Halfon N: Where is the health in health system reform? *JAMA* 272(16):1292-1296, 1994.

Flaskerud JH, Winslow BJ: Conceptualizing vulnerable populations health-related research, *Nurs Res* 47(2):69-78, 1998.

Flaskerud JH et al: Health disparities among vulnerable populations: evolution of knowledge over five decades in nursing research publications, *Nurs Res* 51(2):74-85, 2002.

Freedberg L, McLeod RG: The other side of the law: despite all efforts to curb it, immigration is rising, *San Francisco Chronicle* Oct 13, 1998.

Frieden TR: Tuberculosis control and social change, *Am J Public Health* 84(11):1721-1723, 1994.

Friedman E: Money isn't everything: nonfinancial barriers to access, *JAMA* 271(19):1535-1538, 1994.

Fullerton D et al: Preventing unintended teenage pregnancies and reducing their adverse effects, *Qual Health Care* 6(2):102-108, 1997.

Gifford BD, Bettenhausen KL: Physicians' receptiveness to teen Medicaid recipients seeking office-based prenatal care, *Fam Community Health* 20(2):70-79, 1997.

Grey MR: The medical care programs of the Farm Security Administration, 1932 through 1947: a rehearsal for national health insurance? *Am J Public Health* 84(10):1678-1687, 1994.

Guthrie BJ et al: African American girls' smoking habits and day-to-day experiences with racial discrimination, *Nurs Res* 51(3):183-190, 2002.

Hacker K: Integrating school-based health centers into managed care in Massachusetts, *J School Health* 66(9):317-321, 1996.

Hamburg M: Eliminating racial and ethnic disparities in health: response to the Presidential initiative on race, *Public Health Rep* 113(July/Aug):372-375, 1998.

Hargraves JL: The insurance gap and minority health care, 1997-2001, *Center for Studying Health System Change Tracking Report* 2:1-4, 2002.

Hogan NS, DeSantis L: Things that help and hinder adolescent sibling bereavement, *West J Nurs Res* 16(2):132-153, 1994.

Institute of Medicine: *Homelessness, health, and human needs,* Washington, DC, 1988, National Academy Press.

Jenkins M, Torrisi D: Community partnership primary care case study: Abbottsford Community Health Center, *Nurse Pract Forum* 8(1):21-27, 1997.

Karpati A et al: Variability and vulnerability at the ecologic level: implications for understanding the social determinants of health, *Am J Public Health* 92(11):1768-1772, 2002.

Kawachi I: Social capital and community effects on population and individual health, *Ann NY Acad Sci* 896:120-130, 1999.

Kochanek KD, Maurer JD, Rosenberg HM: Why did black life expectancy decline from 1984 through 1989 in the United States? *Am J Public Health* 84(6):938-944, 1994.

Koniak-Griffin D, Turner-Pluta C: Health risks and psychosocial outcomes of early childbearing: a review of the literature, *J Perinat Neonatal Nurs* 15(20):1-17, 2001.

Koniak-Griffin D et al: A public health nursing early intervention program for adolescent mothers: outcomes from pregnancy through 6 weeks postpartum, *Nurs Res* 49(3):130-138, 2000.

Lantz PM et al: Socioeconomic disparities in health change in a longitudinal study of U.S. adults: the role of health risk behaviors, *Soc Sci Med* 53:29-40, 2001.

Linhorst DM: Federalism and social justice: implications for social work, *Soc Work* 47(3):201-208, 2002.

Lutenbacher M: Perceptions of health status and relationship with abuse history and mental health in low-income single mothers, *J Fam Nurs* 6(4):320-340, 2000.

Lutenbacher M: Relationships between psychosocial factors and abusive parenting attitudes in low-income single mothers, *Nurs Res* 51(3):158-167, 2002.

Mayo K: Community collaboration: prevention and control of tuberculosis in a homeless shelter, *Public Health Nurs* 13(2):120-127, 1996.

McCubbin MA, McCubbin HI: Family stress theory and assessment: the resiliency model of family stress, adjustment, and adaptation. In McCubbin HI, Thompson AI, editors: *Family assessment inventories for research and practice,* Madison, Wisc, 1991, University of Wisconsin.

McLeod JD, Kessler RC: Socioeconomic status differences in vulnerability to undesirable life events, *J Health Soc Behav* 31:162-172, 1990.

Moccia P, Mason DJ: Poverty trends: implications for nursing, *Nurs Outlook* 34(1):20, 1986.

Nichols J, Wright LK, Murphy JF: A proposal for tracking health care for the homeless, *J Community Health* 11(3):204-209, 1986.

Northam S: Access to health promotion, protection, and disease prevention among impoverished individuals, *Public Health Nurs* 13(5):353-364, 1996.

O'Connor FW: A vulnerability-stress framework for evaluating clinical interventions in schizophrenia, *Image J Nurs Scholar* 26(3):231-237, 1994.

Pesznecker B: The poor: a population at risk, *Public Health Nurs* 4(1):237-249, 1984.

Pierre N, Cox J: Teenage pregnancy and prevention programs, *Curr Opin Pediatr* 9(4):310-316, 1997.

Plescia M et al: A multidisciplinary health care outreach team to the homeless: the 10-year experience of the Montefiore Care for the Homeless Team, *Fam Community Health* 20(2):58-69, 1997.

Rabkin JG et al: Resilience in adversity among long-term survivors of AIDS, *Hosp Community Psychiatry* 44(2):162-167, 1993.

Rew L, Chambers KB, Kulkarni S: Planning a sexual health promotion intervention with homeless adolescents, *Nurs Res* 51(3):168-174, 2002.

Sachs B et al: Potential for abusive parenting by rural mothers with low birth weight children, *Image J Nurs Scholar* 31:21-25, 1999.

Schillinger D et al: Association of health literacy with diabetes outcomes, *JAMA* 288(4):475-482, 2002.

Sebastian JG: Homelessness: a state of vulnerability, *Fam Community Health* 8(3):11-24, 1985.

Sebastian JG: Population-based and community-focused approaches to vulnerability and disadvantage. In Sebastian J, Bushy A, editors: *Special populations in the community: advances in reducing health disparities,* Gaithersburg, Md, 1999, Aspen.

Shugars DA, O'Neill EH, Bader JD, editors: *Healthy America: practitioners for 2005, an agenda for U.S. health professional schools,* Durham, NC, 1991, Pew Health Professions Commission.

Simpson CC et al: Preventing pregnancy in early adolescence: identifying risks, *Adv Nurse Pract* 5(4):22-26, 1997.

Statistics Canada: *Infant mortality rates, 1998,* retrieved Dec 8, 1998 from www.statcan.ca/english/Pgdb/health21.htm.

Superintendent of Documents: Annual update of the HHS poverty guidelines, *Federal Register* 63(36), 1998.

Torrey EF et al: *Care of the seriously mentally ill: a rating of state programs,* ed 3, Washington, DC, 1990, Public Health Citizen Health Research Group and the National Alliance for the Mentally Ill.

Tulsky JP et al: Adherence to isoniazid prophylaxis in the homeless: a randomized controlled trial, *Arch Intern Med* 160:697-702, 2000.

U.S. Department of Health and Human Services: *Healthy people 2010: understanding and improving health,* Pittsburgh, Penn, 2001a, U.S. Government Printing Office.

U.S. Department of Health and Human Services: *Healthy people in healthy communities: a community planning guide using healthy people 2010,* Pittsburgh, Penn, 2001b, U.S. Government Printing Office.

U.S. Department of Health and Human Services, Public Health Service: *Health, United States,* Washington, DC, 1998, U.S. Government Printing Office.

Valanis B: *Epidemiology in health care,* ed 3, Stamford, Conn, 1999, Appleton & Lange.

Wechsler H, Wernick SM: A social marketing campaign to promote low-fat milk consumption in an inner-city Latino community, *Public Health Rep* 107(2):202-207, 1992.

Wellever A, Hill G, Casey M: Medicaid reform issues affecting the Indian Health Care System, *Am J Public Health* 88(2):193-195, 1998.

Woodward A, Kawachi I: Why reduce health inequalities? *J Epidemiol Community Health* 54:923-929, 2000.

Yoos L: Perspectives on adolescent parenting: effect of adolescent egocentrism on the maternal-child interaction, *J Pediatr Nurs* 2(3):193, 1987.

# Chapter 32

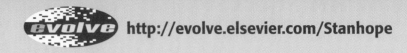

# Poverty and Homelessness

**Christine Di Martile Bolla, R.N., D.N.Sc.**
Christine Di Martile Bolla began her community health nursing career as a home health nurse in 1986. Her client population was high-risk mothers and infants. She began teaching community health nursing in 1990 and later changed the focus of her (and her students') practice to vulnerable populations. Dr. Bolla and her students have worked extensively with homeless women and children in the San Francisco Bay Area in California. Dr. Bolla currently is a clinical assistant professor in the Department of Nursing at San Francisco State University.

## Objectives

After reading this chapter, the student should be able to do the following:

1. Analyze the concept of poverty
2. Discuss nurses' perceptions about poverty and health
3. Describe the social, political, cultural, and environmental factors that influence poverty
4. Discuss the effects of poverty on the health and well-being of individuals, families, and communities
5. Analyze the concept of homelessness
6. Discuss nurses' perceptions about homelessness and health
7. Describe the social, political, cultural, and environmental factors that influence homelessness
8. Discuss the effects of homelessness on the health and well-being of individuals, families, and communities
9. Discuss nursing interventions for poor and homeless individuals

American society values self-reliance, individual responsibility, and personal accountability. Although our societal values are important and have contributed to our strength as a nation, these cultural expectations make it difficult to garner public support for programs targeted to persons who are unable to live independent, successful lives. Interventions aimed at improving the plight of poor and/or homeless persons have, historically, generated heated debates concerning individual versus societal responsibility. These debates over social versus individual responsibility for poverty and homelessness are constrained by issues of power, politics, economics, and ethics.

Community-oriented nurses encounter poor persons, families, and aggregates in a variety of settings, such as private homes, congregate living situations, schools, churches, clinics, and meal sites. To provide effective care for individuals, families, and aggregates living in **poverty,** nurses need to understand the issues related to poverty and homelessness, which include historical, social, political, economic, biological, psychological, and spiritual dimensions. To appreciate the concepts of poverty and homelessness, it is important to begin with an honest self-examination of personal beliefs, values, and **personal knowledge.** Next, develop an appreciation for the history of public responses to poor and homeless persons, and the relationship of this history to contemporary public and personal debates. The nurse must identify health care needs, barriers to care, and essential health care services for poor and homeless individuals, families, and aggregates. To provide effective nursing interventions, the nurse needs to understand the epidemiology, health problems, and risk factors associated with poverty as well as funding sources and existing programs for this vulnerable aggregate (Aday, 2001).

This chapter describes the many ways that poverty and homelessness affect the health status of individuals, families, and communities and suggests effective nursing intervention strategies for poor and homeless aggregates. The concepts of poverty and homelessness are examined in historical, economic, political, and spiritual contexts.

*The author wishes to acknowledge the contributions of Teresa Acquaviva and Jeanette Lancaster to the content of this chapter in previous editions.*

## Key Terms

consumer price index, p. 777
crisis poverty, p. 784
cultural attitudes, p. 776
deinstitutionalization, p. 785
Elizabethan poor laws, p. 775
Federal Income Poverty Guidelines, p. 777
gentrification, p. 785
historical factors, p. 775
homelessness, p. 783

Interagency Council on the Homeless,
p. 788
media discourses, p. 776
near poor, p. 777
neighborhood poverty, p. 777
persistent poverty, p. 777
personal beliefs, p. 775
personal knowledge, p. 774
poverty, p. 774

Poverty Threshold Guidelines, p. 777
Stewart B. McKinney Homeless
Assistance Act of 1994, p. 783
Temporary Assistance to Needy Families,
p. 777
Women, Infants, and Children, p. 777
*See Glossary for definitions*

## Chapter Outline

Concept of Poverty
*Personal Beliefs and Values*
*Historical Context of Public Attitudes Toward
Poor Persons*
*Cultural Attitudes and Media Discourses*
Defining and Understanding Poverty
*Social and Cultural Definitions of Poverty*
*Political Dimensions*
*Environmental Perspectives*

Poverty and Health: Effects Across the Life
Span
*Childbearing Women and Poverty*
*Children and Poverty*
*Deadbeat Parents*
*Older Adults and Poverty*
*The Community and Poverty*
Understanding the Concept of Homelessness
*Personal Beliefs, Values, and Knowledge*

*Clients' Perceptions of Homelessness*
*Homelessness in the United States*
*How Many People Are Homeless?*
*Causes of Homelessness*
Effects of Homelessness on Health
*Homelessness and At-Risk Populations*
*Prevention and Preventive Services*
*Federal Programs for the Homeless*
Role of the Nurse

## CONCEPT OF POVERTY

Individual perceptions of poverty and poor persons are rooted in social, political, cultural, and environmental factors. Personal beliefs, social values, personal knowledge of poverty, cultural attitudes, media portrayals, and **historical factors** influence our understanding of poverty in the United States. It is important for nurses to be aware of their values and beliefs concerning poor and homeless persons.

### Personal Beliefs and Values

To be effective, nurses must recognize and acknowledge the personal beliefs, values, and knowledge that form their worldviews and influence the way they practice. **Personal beliefs** are ideas about the world that an individual believes to be true. Personal beliefs are rooted in societal values. Personal beliefs about poor persons in the United States are influenced by societal/cultural values of personal responsibility, individual autonomy, and personal accountability. Societal values evolve over time.

### Historical Context of Public Attitudes Toward Poor Persons

Public perceptions of poor persons and individual attitudes regarding what should be done for the poor can be traced to **Elizabethan poor laws.** In seventeenth century England, being poor was no disgrace because nearly everyone lived in poverty. Therefore people often shared what they had with one another and frequently banded together to help those whose luck had taken a downturn. With the advent of the industrial revolution, however, populations became increasingly mobile. Increased migration from rural areas to urban industrial townships brought with it questions of whom among the downtrodden should be helped. In short, how could society distinguish poor persons deserving assistance from those who did not (Katz, 1989)?

Society changed to adapt to the industrial revolution. Elizabethan poor laws, established in the seventeenth century, considered those persons who were born within the boundaries of the community deserving of assistance. A traveler who needed assistance was shipped back to his or her original community. Differentiating the deserving from the undeserving poor became more complex during the industrial revolution. Persons who were down-and-out were classified as deserving of assistance if their poverty was considered to be beyond their control. Widowed women, orphaned children, laborers who were injured on the job, persons with chronic illness not caused by personal failure were considered deserving of public assistance. Alcoholics, prostitutes, mentally ill persons, and those considered to be lazy were the undeserving poor, and they were denied assistance (Katz, 1989).

Societal responses to poverty and homeless persons are rooted in these historical issues. It is important to also consider the effects of cultural attitudes and media discourses on societal responses to poverty and homelessness.

## Cultural Attitudes and Media Discourses

**Cultural attitudes** are the beliefs and perspectives that a society values. Perspectives regarding individual responsibility for health and well-being are influenced by prevailing cultural attitudes. **Media discourses,** or views, involve communication of thoughts and attitudes through literature, film, art, television, and newspapers. Media images of persons on welfare influence, and are influenced by, cultural attitudes and values. For example, criminals in films and television programs are often portrayed as poor, desperate persons. Poor persons are often cast as lazy, shiftless folk. These media images influence what we believe to be true about poor persons.

---

**HOW TO  Test Values and Beliefs About Poverty**

Nurses should ask themselves the following questions about poverty and persons living in poverty:
1. What do I believe to be true about being poor?
2. What do I personally know about poverty?
3. How have family and friends influenced my ideas about being poor?
4. Have I ever personally been poor?
5. How have media images of poor persons helped to shape our images of poverty and poor persons?
6. What do I feel when I see a hungry child? a hungry adult?
7. Do I believe that people are poor because they just don't want to work? Or do I believe that society has a significant influence on one's becoming poor?
8. What really causes poverty?
9. What do I really think can be done to prevent poverty and homelessness?

---

These issues may seem abstract, but individuals can make the discussion more concrete by considering questions that test their own values and beliefs. Nurses can evaluate their beliefs, values, and knowledge about poverty by considering the following clinical situations:
- You are doing health screening at a homeless shelter and one of the clients asks you for money for bus fare. Do you give it to her?
- You are in the home of an older adult client whose kitchen is covered with roaches. What are your obligations in terms of the client's home environment? Where do you sit if he offers you a chair?
- You are making a visit to an especially unclean home. What do you do if the client offers you some food?
- What interventions would you initiate for an aggregate of poor or homeless families in a local shelter?

- How could you effectively advocate for a group of medically indigent men?

There are no easy answers to these questions. However, nurses' behaviors in these situations influence their relationships with clients who are poor. Nurses' behaviors in these situations are influenced by all of the issues just presented.

In addition to personal beliefs, values, and knowledge, nurses should consider how nursing theories and theories from other disciplines influence the care they provide to persons living in poverty (Paille, Pilkington, 2002). Many nursing theories are based on the assumption that human beings have inherent dignity and worth. Some theories view the human being as a system in continuous interaction with the environment. Other theories suggest that the human being is continuous with, and inseparable from, the environment. In community-oriented nursing, the concepts of person, health, environment, and nursing are reconceptualized to encompass a population focus. The concept of environment may include economics, power, class, race, politics, sexual orientation, and access to health care (Diez Roux, 2001; Stevens, 1989).

Nursing is based on valuing individuals, promoting health, respecting and restoring human dignity, and improving the quality of life of individuals, families, and aggregates (Jacobs, 2001). Conflicts in values, beliefs, and perceptions often arise when nurses work with persons from different social, cultural, and economic backgrounds. A lack of agreement between the professional's and the client's perceptions of need can lead to conflict. As a result of this conflict, clients may fail to follow the prescribed treatment protocol; the nurse may then inaccurately interpret the client's behavior as resistance, lack of cooperation, or noncompliance.

Nurses should evaluate clients and aggregates in the context of environment to develop effective nursing interventions. Treating medical problems alone is inadequate. Instead, care must be multidimensional and include biological, psychological, social, environmental, economic, and spiritual factors.

## DEFINING AND UNDERSTANDING POVERTY

More than 40 million persons have incomes below the federal poverty level (National Coalition for the Homeless, 1998a), and 20.5% of America's young children live in poverty. Persons living in poverty, however, are not a homogeneous group. It is essential to listen closely to clients to individualize their care and to avoid making inappropriate assumptions concerning their needs. In addition, the fears and misconceptions of health care providers related to poverty can create barriers that prevent them from fully engaging in relationships with those who come from different socioeconomic and cultural backgrounds. By taking the time to know clients by name and to listen to the stories of their lives, nurses begin the process of breaking down the barriers of fear, isolation, uncertainty, and the unknown

## Social and Cultural Definitions of Poverty

Social definitions of poverty vary. Olsen (1999) states that current measures are no longer valid for measuring and defining poverty for various groups. As discussed in Chapter 31, poverty refers to having insufficient financial resources to meet basic living expenses. These expenses include costs of food, shelter, clothing, transportation, and medical care. People who are poor are more likely to live in dangerous environments, to work at high-risk jobs, to eat less nutritious foods, and to have multiple stressors. Multiple stressors for poor persons include employment issues, inadequate housing, lack of affordable day care, and societal indifference (Berne et al, 1997).

Meanings and perceptions of poverty can differ across cultures. Whereas most Western cultures view poverty negatively, other cultures respect the poor. Many of the differences in perceptions of poor and underserved groups are rooted in religious and political differences. Meanings of lower socioeconomic status can also vary among various groups within a culture. Hsieh (2002) found that perceptions of lower socioeconomic status differed by level of education and age, with the less educated and older individuals having a more positive perception of their quality of life when compared with younger, more educated persons.

For years, income level has been used as the criterion that determines whether someone is poor. Although income continues to be the measurement of choice, the federal *poverty* guidelines have been renamed **Federal Income Poverty Guidelines.** Income is also a qualifying factor for a variety of programs, such as federal housing subsidies, **Temporary Assistance to Needy Families** (TANF, formerly called AFDC); medical assistance, food stamps, **Women, Infants, and Children** (WIC), and Head Start.

Poverty is a power issue, according to some authors, because it involves a lack of control over critical resources needed to function effectively in society. The federal government uses two terms to discuss poverty: poverty thresholds and poverty guidelines. The **Poverty Threshold Guidelines** are issued by the U.S. Bureau of the Census and are used primarily for statistical purposes. The federal income guidelines are issued by the U.S. Department of Health and Human Services (USDHHS) and are used to determine whether a person or family is financially eligible for assistance or services under a particular federal program. The federal income guidelines are updated annually to be consistent with the **consumer price index** (CPI). The CPI is a measure of the average change over time in the prices paid by urban consumers for a fixed market basket of consumer goods and services (Gibson, 1998).

Many people who earn slightly more than the government-defined income levels (Table 32-1) are unable to meet living expenses and are not eligible for government assistance programs. In a family of four, for example, whose annual income is considered above the defined income level of

| Table 32-1 Poverty Thresholds for 2001, by Size of Family (Including Related Children Under 18 Years of Age) | |
| --- | --- |
| SIZE OF FAMILY UNIT | INCOME GUIDELINE ($) |
| 1 | 9214 |
| 2 | 11,859 |
| 3 | 13,853 |
| 4 | 18,267 |
| 5 | 22,029 |
| 6 | 25,337 |
| 7 | 29,154 |
| 8 | 32,606 |
| 9 or more | 39,223 |

From U.S. Bureau of the Census: *Current population survey,* Washington, DC, 2002, U.S. Government Printing Office.

$18,267, the adult family members would not qualify for Medicaid in some states (U.S. Bureau of the Census, 2002). As discussed in Chapter 31 persons and families whose income is above the federal income guidelines but insufficient to meet living expenses are often called the **near poor.**

Social scientists often use the terms *persistent poverty* and *neighborhood poverty* to describe types of poverty. **Persistent poverty** refers to individuals and families who remain poor for long periods and who pass poverty on to their descendants. **Neighborhood poverty** refers to geographically defined areas of high poverty, characterized by dilapidated housing and high levels of unemployment. Although the social definitions used to describe and identify various types of poverty are interesting, they are not sufficient. For nurses, the most significant factor is being able to accept and respect clients and attempt to understand how their life situations influence their health and well-being. Being poor is one variable that must be measured against the presence of other variables that may increase or decrease the negative effects of poverty.

## Political Dimensions

Poverty in the United States was not recognized as a social problem before the Civil War (Katz, 1989). The prevalent attitude during that time was that poverty was an individual's problem, and poor individuals had only themselves to blame. Generally, society did not assume responsibility for alleviating the plight of the poor. However, the post–Civil War industrialized society changed this attitude. Widespread unemployment, undesirable working conditions, insufficient wages, and substandard housing forced a rethinking of public responsibility for the poor (Wilson, 1990). Many laws concerning public health and housing were passed. This social reform movement led to an early interest in urban poverty research (Bremner, 1956; Miller, 1966). Despite influences of the depression of the 1930s and national discussion of New Deal legislation, such as the Social Security Act of 1935, the public's interest in the plight of the poor was not sustained (Wilson, 1990).

A resurgence of political activity on behalf of disadvantaged groups occurred during the late 1950s and early 1960s. In 1959 the Kerr-Mills Act increased funds for health care for aged persons (Fine, 1998). In 1961 President Kennedy approved a pilot food program in response to the hunger he observed on the campaign trail (Price, 1994). In 1963 President Kennedy instructed his administration to develop a major policy effort to combat poverty. After Kennedy's assassination, President Johnson sustained the interest in the antipoverty campaign. Johnson established the War on Poverty in 1964, which emphasized job-training programs and community organization and involvement (Pilisuk and Pilisuk, 1976; Wilson, 1990). In 1964 the Social Security Administration established the income level of the official poverty line. Individuals and families with incomes below the federal poverty line were considered to be living in poverty. In 1965 the Medicare amendments to the Social Security Act were passed. After 1965 considerable research focused on poverty as it related to education, health, housing, the law, and public welfare (Wilson, 1990).

Policy changes during the 1980s led to an emphasis on defense spending rather than on social programs. Jargowsky and Band (1998) noted that a series of events in the 1980s, such as the visibility of the homeless and the media attention on an underclass of individuals, seemed to blame the person for being poor. Jargowsky and Band argued, instead, that poverty is the result of the economic environment in an urban area, and it is influenced by the degree that an area has a wide division in income levels and races.

During the 1990s, record numbers of people received welfare benefits. Concern about the increasing numbers of

---

### WHAT DO YOU THINK?

Opinions and beliefs about welfare differ among recipients, taxpayers, politicians, economists, health care providers, and others. Some people believe that welfare benefits are inadequate, whereas others argue that welfare breeds dependency and illegitimacy. Families receiving welfare benefits also have differing views.

The political debate in the 1990s was whether to abolish or to reform welfare. Aid to Families with Dependent Children (AFDC) was replaced with the Temporary Assistance to Needy Families (TANF) program. What is the relationship between welfare reform and health? What implications does welfare reform have on community-oriented nurses working in the community? How would you have redesigned the welfare system? What issues will emerge in the first decade of the twenty-first century?

---

persons receiving public assistance stimulated enthusiasm for reform of health care and the welfare system (Zedlewski, 2002). In 1996, a bill creating the Temporary Assistance for Needy Families (TANF) program was enacted. This welfare reform legislation replaced the Aid to Families with Dependent Children (AFDC) program with a program of temporary welfare benefits. Under TANF, recipients of benefits are provided with benefits for a limited time and are required to find jobs and/or to enroll in job-training programs. Overall poverty has declined following welfare reform. Unfortunately, the economic status of many families who were forced from welfare to work has declined. Because persons working full-time for minimum wage do not receive other types of government compensation, they have incomes below the federal poverty level (Zedlewski, 2002).

## Environmental Perspectives

The causes of poverty are complex and interrelated. In recent decades the number of adult and older adult Americans living in poverty has decreased, whereas the number of women and children living in poverty has increased. The following factors affect the growing number of poor persons in the United States:

- Decreased earnings
- Increased unemployment rates
- Changes in the labor force
- Increase in female-headed households
- Inadequate education and job skills
- Inadequate antipoverty programs
- Inadequate welfare benefits
- Weak enforcement of child support statutes
- Dwindling Social Security payments to children
- Increased numbers of children born to single women

As the fiscal characteristics of most industrialized nations have changed from industrial economies to service economies, job opportunities have increasingly excluded workers who do not have, at a minimum, a high school education (Freudenberg, 2000). Many manufacturing jobs do not pay sufficient salary to support a family. Also, many jobs at the lower end of the pay scale do not include health care or retirement benefits.

## POVERTY AND HEALTH: EFFECTS ACROSS THE LIFE SPAN

The number of persons living in poverty in the United States increased by almost 26%, from 25.4 million to 31.9 million, between 1970 and 1988. By 1996, 36.5 million Americans lived in poverty (Dalaker and Naifeh, 1998). By the year 2000, 31 million Americans (11.3%) lived in poverty (U.S. Bureau of the Census, 2000).

Poverty directly affects health and well-being. Persons living in poverty and in near-poverty have higher rates of chronic illness, higher infant morbidity and mortality, shorter life expectancy, more complex health problems, and more significant complications and physical limitations resulting from chronic disease. Chronic health problems having a higher incidence among poor persons include asthma, diabetes, and hypertension. Hospitalization rates for poor persons are three times those for persons with higher incomes (Ensign and Santelli, 1998).

These poor health outcomes are often secondary to barriers that impede access to health care, such as inability to pay for health care, lack of insurance, geographic location, language, maldistribution of providers, transportation difficulties, inconvenient clinic hours, and negative attitudes of health care providers toward poor clients. Access to health care is especially difficult for the working poor. Many employers, especially those paying low or minimum wage, do not provide health care insurance for their employees. Persons working for these employers are ineligible for most public health insurance programs, and they are often unable to obtain affordable health care.

## Childbearing Women and Poverty

Poverty, while presenting a significant obstacle to health across the life span, has an especially negative effect on women of childbearing age. Women living in poverty have lower levels of physical functioning, as well as higher reported levels of bodily discomfort, than women in higher socioeconomic groups. Prevalence rates for ulcer disease, asthma, and anemia are significantly higher among women living in poverty. Poor women also report significantly more risk behaviors for infection with human immunodeficiency virus (HIV) than more affluent women (Weinreb et al, 1998a).

Poverty has significant effects on adolescent women. Poor teens are four times more likely than nonpoor teens to have below-average academic skills. Regardless of their race, poor teens are nearly three times as likely to drop out of school as their nonpoor counterparts. Teenage women who are poor and who have below-average skills are more likely to have children than nonpoor teenage women. Poor pregnant women are more likely than other women to receive late or no prenatal care and to deliver low-birth-weight babies, premature babies, or babies with birth defects (Stein, Lu, Gelberg, 2000).

Welfare reform will most likely affect the health and well-being of childbearing women and their families. For example, the Personal Responsibility and Work Opportunity Reconciliation Act of 1996 requires more families to work to receive assistance. This requirement forces legislators to target funding for childcare subsidies to families going from welfare to work but decreases the amount of funding available for other working poor women and their children. Changes in welfare policy are generally propelled by the goals of adults. Unfortunately, two thirds of those receiving cash benefits are children (National Center for Children and Poverty, 1998a).

## Children and Poverty

Many American children are members of the 5H club. They are hungry, homeless, hugless, hopeless, and without

health care (Elders, 1994). The 2000 poverty rate of 16.2% for children is higher than that for any other age-group. Moreover, poverty among young African-American and Hispanic children is more than three times that of white, non-Hispanic children (Table 32-2). Poverty among children (newborn to age 5 years) has increased in all racial and ethnic groups, as well as in all urban, suburban, and rural geographic areas.

## Deadbeat Parents

Under current federal law, noncustodial parents are required to provide financial support to their children. Current child support policies are designed to provide financial security to children, prevent single-parent families from entering the welfare system, help single-parent families get off welfare as quickly as possible, and decrease welfare expenditures (Waller and Plotnick, 1999). Individual states are responsible for locating nonsupporting custodial parents, establishing paternity, and enforcing financial responsibility. In most states, government involvement in locating noncustodial parents begins when the custodial parent applies for TANF.

An important criticism of the current system is that public expectations of financial responsibility for noncustodial parents are based on an assumption that the noncustodial parent is working full-time. Unfortunately, many low-income parents were never married, and many have intermittent work histories. Current policy requires the custodial parent to assign all financial support from the noncustodial parent to the state to equal the amount that the family receives from the welfare system. In response to these regulations, many low-income parents often make private, informal arrangements for child support payments. Under these verbal arrangements, the noncustodial parent pays the custodial parent directly.

Although the term *deadbeat dad* was created for fathers who do not contribute to the financial support of their children, the number of custodial single fathers is increasing. Noncustodial mothers are equally responsible under the law to provide for the economic well-being of their children; thus the term *deadbeat parent* is more gender-sensitive and appropriate.

Changes in welfare policy can affect family income, parenting behaviors, and children's access to services

---

**Table 32-2  Poverty Rates for Children in the United States by Ethnic Group**

| ETHNIC GROUP | PERCENTAGE IN POVERTY |
|---|---|
| African American | 30 |
| Latino | 28 |
| White | 9 |

National Center for Children in Poverty: *Child poverty fact sheet,* March, New York, 2002, Columbia University.

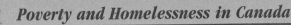

## POVERTY

Poverty is a major health and social issue and one of the most important determinants affecting the health and well-being of a nation. In Canada, many are just one paycheck, a divorce, or an illness away from being poor. There is no official poverty line in Canada. The poverty threshold levels used by Statistics Canada are low-income cut-offs (LICO), which are based on a sustenance concept of poverty and calculated on expenditure patterns. Individuals are considered poor if 55% of their income is spent on food, shelter, and clothing. Those living in poverty in Canada are mainly children, women, older adults, and the aboriginal population.

One child in five (18.5% of all children) experiences poverty; this figure has decreased from one in six in 1989 (Campaign 2000, 2002a). Although the United Nations Human Development Index rates Canada as one of the best countries to live in, UNICEF ranks Canada only 17 out of 23 countries in its treatment of the poor. In fact, the gap between the privileged and the disadvantaged children in Canada is among the most marked in the industrialized world. In 2000, both two-parent families and female-led-lone-parent families continued to fall deeper into poverty. Between 1984 and 1999, the average net worth of the top 20% of couples with children increased by 43%, whereas for families at the bottom of the income scale, net wealth fell by more than 51% (Canadian Council on Social Development, 2002). Poverty in children is strongly associated with lower health status (lower birth weight, chronic illness, and disabilities) and other health and social issues. Being poor has severe consequences for a child's emotional development, as living in substandard housing, not having enough to eat or adequate clothing, and not having access to play and recreation facilities all impact on the child's emotional well-being. Increased incidence of family dysfunction, child abuse and neglect, and child and parental depression are also effects of poverty (Canadian Public Health Association, 1997a).

In Canada, women are at a higher risk for poverty than men: in 1999, the poverty rate was 17.5% for women and 13.2% for men over the age of 18. Although the overall poverty rate for seniors in Canada continues to decrease, falling to 17.7% in 1999, the poverty rate for older adult women increased from 47.9% in 1998 to 48.5% in 1999 (National Council of Welfare, 1999). Social programs, including the federal Old Age Security, the Guaranteed Income Supplement, the Spouse's Allowance, and the Canada/Quebec Pension Plan, and income supplements provided by five provinces and territories are strongly associated with the decreased poverty rate in the older adult population. Health effects that are associated with poverty in the older adult population include activity limitations and exacerbations of chronic illness and disease.

The aboriginal population is the most economically disadvantaged group in Canada and poverty is widespread. This population includes status and nonstatus Indians living on and off reserves, as well as the Metis and Inuit people. The poverty rate for aboriginal people, whether living on or off the reserve, is almost 1 in 2 (50%), which is three times the overall poverty rate in Canada, and these people are four times more likely to experience hunger than nonaboriginal people (Campaign 2000, 2002b). More than 25% of aboriginal families with young children are headed by single parents, and 39% of aboriginal single mothers earn less than $12,000 per year (Canadian Council on Social Development, 2002). The aboriginal people have a lower health status, lower life expectancy, and increased morbidity and mortality rates (including infant mortality rate, and fire and accidental deaths) than the overall Canadian population (Health Canada, 2002).

## HOMELESSNESS

Homelessness, whether a cause or a consequence of ill health, has emerged as a fundamental health issue for Canadians. Homelessness has been linked to poverty, changes in the housing market, and changes in the delivery of mental health services. As in the United States, the shift of mental health services from institutions to

(National Center for Children and Poverty, 1998b). Decreases in family income can result in an increase in the number of children living in extreme poverty and will increase parental stress. Increased parental stress can have a negative effect on the well-being of children. Welfare changes that deny social and health services to the poor have negative effects on the health and well-being of poor children.

Young children (0 to 5 years of age) are at highest risk for the most harmful effects of poverty. Shore (1997) examined the effects of inadequate nutrition on brain development. According to Shore, sound nutrition during the first years of life is crucial for emotional and intellectual development. Unfortunately, many children live in poverty during their early childhood years. Nearly one in six children in the United States lived in poverty in 2000. According to recent research, the brain is directly affected by environmental stimulation during a critical time that extends from the prenatal period through early childhood (National Center for Children in Poverty, 1997a). Several risk factors appear to impede cognitive development in young children, including inadequate nutrition (Brown and Pollitt, 1996), maternal substance abuse (Mayes, 1996), maternal depression (Petterson and Albers, 2001), exposure to environmental

the community (deinstitutionalization) in the Canadian health care system is a significant cause of homelessness. Among the homeless of Canada are adolescents (street youths), persons living with mental illness, and aboriginal people. The most alarming demographic change noted among the homeless is the rapid growth of the number of homeless women and children (Canadian Public Health Association, 1997b). In 2000, it was estimated that between 35,000 and 40,000 people were homeless in Canada (Murphy, 2000). Although there has been no recent report on the national state of homelessness, regional reports, research studies, and community agency reports have provided compelling evidence that there has been a substantial increase in homelessness across Canada.

The most common health issues associated with homelessness include communicable diseases such as tuberculosis, HIV/AIDS and other sexually transmitted diseases, severe infections, musculoskeletal disease, dental problems, assault, mental health and suicide, increased drug and substance use, and decreased access to health services.

### POVERTY AND HOMELESSNESS INITIATIVES

The increase in poverty and homelessness has prompted all levels of government in Canada (federal, provincial, and municipal) to respond. Lobby efforts, from a variety of stakeholders and interest groups including nursing representation, were instrumental in the appointment of a Minister of Labour and Federal Coordinator on Homelessness and the creation of the National Homelessness Initiative (NHI). The NHI is a 3-year program totalling $753 million that includes a shelter-enhancement program, an urban aboriginal strategy, a youth homelessness component, a community partnerships initiative, and a residential rehabilitation program (NHI, 2002). At the local level, many community agencies continue to implement programs such as food banks, healthy children programs, and interventions for the homeless, including street patrols, cold-weather alert systems involving shelters, and mobile health units.

In May 2002, Canada joined other nations in New York to sign the United Nations Declaration "A World Fit for Children" that calls for each nation to develop a na-

tional action plan. In 1990, Canada signed the International Covenant on Economic, Social and Cultural Rights guaranteeing everyone's right to an adequate standard of living, including adequate food, clothing, and housing. Currently, minimal efforts are directed toward improving living standards or advancing economic policies. Therefore, all levels of government need to ensure that future social policy initiatives and resource allocation address the growing social disparities in Canadian society, including poverty, homelessness, and job insecurity.

### References

Campaign 2000: *Poverty amidst prosperity: building a Canada for all children,* Toronto, 2002a, Author, available at www.campaign2000.ca.

Campaign 2000: *The UN Special Session on Children: putting promises into action—a report on a decade of child and family poverty in Canada,* May 2002, Toronto, Author, 2002b, available at www.campaign2000.ca.

Canadian Council on Social Development: *The progress of Canada's children: 2002 highlights,* Ottawa, 2002, Author, available at www.ccsd.ca.

Canadian Public Health Association: *Health impacts of social and economic conditions: implications for public policy,* Ottawa, 1997a, Author, available at www.cpha.ca.

Canadian Public Health Association: *1997 Position paper in homelessness and health,* Ottawa, 1997b, Author, available at www.cpha.ca.

Health Canada: *Healthy Canadians: a federal report on comparable health indicators,* Ottawa, 2002, Author, available at www.healthcanada.ca.

Murphy B: *On the street: how we created homeless,* Ottawa, 2000, Author.

National Council of Welfare: *Poverty profile 1999,* Ottawa, 1999, Author, available at www.ncwcnbes.net.

UNICEF: *Child poverty in rich nations, Innocenti Report Card, June 2000,* 2000, available at www.unicef.org.

*Canadian spelling is used.*

toxins (Preslow et al, 2001), trauma and abuse (Streeck-Fischer and van der Kolk, 2000), and quality of daily care (Burchinal, Lee and Ramey, 1989). Unfortunately, poor children have greater exposure to these identified risk factors (National Center for Children in Poverty, 1997a).

The document *Healthy People 2010* (USDHHS, 1998) acknowledges the effects of low income and low educational and occupational levels on infant mortality, prematurity, low birth weight, birth defects, and infant deaths. Other effects are listed in Box 32-1. Poverty also increases the likelihood of chronic disease, injuries, traumatic death, developmental delays, poor nutrition, inadequate immu-

nization levels, iron deficiency anemia, and elevated blood lead levels. Furthermore, children of poverty are more likely than nonpoor children to be hungry and suffer from fatigue, dizziness, irritability, headaches, ear infections, frequent colds, weight loss, inability to concentrate, and increased school absenteeism (Brown and Pollitt, 1996; U.S. Department of Commerce, 1996).

## Older Adults and Poverty

In 2000, an estimated 10.2% of older adults (65 years and over) lived in poverty (Institute for Research on Poverty, 2002). This figure represents a decrease in the poverty rate

- Blacks (22.1%) and Hispanics (21.1%) have poverty rates far higher than the national average.
- The poverty rate for families headed by single women is the highest of all family groups (24.7%, compared with 4.7% for families in which men are present).
- Among black and Hispanic families headed by women, the poverty rate is nearly 35%.
- Among the states, New Mexico has the largest percentage of persons living in poverty (19.3% in 2000).
- Connecticut, Iowa, Maryland, Minnesota, and New Hampshire have the lowest poverty rates of all the states (below 8% in 2000).

From U.S. Bureau of the Census, *Poverty in the United States, 2000,* Washington, DC, 2000, U.S. Government Printing Office.

for this age-group. The decrease is a consequence of improvements in Social Security and the Supplemental Security Income Program. Certain groups of older adults, however, continue to be vulnerable to the effects of poverty. Older African Americans, for example, are at significantly greater risk for chronic and nutrition-related diseases than older white adults (Schoenberg and Gilbert, 1998).

Older adults living in poverty are disproportionately more likely to have poor health outcomes than their more affluent counterparts. Studies comparing selected characteristics of persons living in geographic areas of concentrated affluence with those of persons living in areas of concentrated poverty show that affluence has a significant protective effect on the health of older adults (Waitzman and Smith, 1998). Prevalence rates for chronic illness and

### BOX 32-1 The Effects of Poverty on the Health of Children

- Higher rates of prematurity, low birth weight, and birth defects
- Higher infant mortality rates
- Increased incidence of chronic disease
- Increased incidence of traumatic death and injuries
- Increased incidence of nutritional deficits
- Increased incidence of growth retardation and developmental delays
- Increased incidence of iron deficiency anemia
- Increased incidence of elevated blood lead levels
- Increased incidence of infections
- Increased risk for homelessness
- Decreased opportunities for education, income, and occupation

chronic illness complications, general morbidity, poor dental health, and overall mortality are significantly greater among poor older adults (Persson et al, 1998; Waitzman and Smith, 1998). Moreover, poor older adults are more likely to seek acute crisis care rather than preventive health care. Older adults are particularly at risk because they may be alone and unable to manage their personal affairs. Many older adults are eligible for benefits but do not know how to access them.

## NURSING TIP

A client's advice to nurses caring for the poor:
- Treat the poor like everyone else.
- Do not be condescending.
- Do not make it obvious that someone is poor.
- Do not prejudge; ask if someone wants to pay on their bill.
- Remember that people can't always pay for their medicine.
- Suggest programs that might help, such as food banks, churches, and clothing centers.
- Poor people need a lot of support.
- Many poor people need help to learn how to promote their own health given a paucity of resources.

## The Community and Poverty

Poverty can affect both urban and rural communities. A number of characteristics describe poor communities. For example, poorer neighborhoods have more minority residents and single-parent families, higher rates of unemployment, and lower wage rates. Residents of poor neighborhoods are also more likely to be victims of crime, substance abuse, racial discrimination, and police brutality. Differences in quality and level of education also exist. Health care is less available to residents of poor neighborhoods. Housing conditions in some areas are deplorable, with many families living in run-down shacks or condemned apartment buildings. Residents living in poverty are often exposed to environmental hazards, such as inadequate heating and cooling, exposure to rain and snow, inadequate water and plumbing, and the presence of pests and other vermin (Jargowsky and Band, 1998).

Being poor affects the health and well-being of individuals, families, and communities. Poverty is a part of the pic-

## THE CUTTING EDGE

Poverty and homelessness are affected by the employment rate. When companies close or relocate, workers often go long periods of time without a steady income.

ture, not the whole picture. Being poor is a health risk factor that should be assessed; however, nurses need to examine individual and community strengths, resources, and sources of support. Poverty and homelessness are affected by the employment rate. When companies close or relocate, workers often go long periods without income.

## UNDERSTANDING THE CONCEPT OF HOMELESSNESS

Understanding the concept of **homelessness** similarly requires considerable reflection and analysis. Several variables, such as personal beliefs, personal/societal values, cultural norms, political debate, and personal knowledge/experience influence the nurse's perception of homelessness. The life stories of homeless clients can help nurses understand this significant public health problem.

### Personal Beliefs, Values, and Knowledge

Poverty can lead to homelessness. Homelessness, like poverty, is a complex concept. Although people who have never been homeless cannot truly understand what it means to be homeless, nurses can increase their sensitivity regarding homeless clients and aggregates by exploring their own personal beliefs, values, and knowledge of homelessness. The questions in the How To box prompt this constructive self-evaluation.

### Clients' Perceptions of Homelessness

People who live on the street are the poorest of the poor. They are often perceived by those more fortunate as faceless, nameless, invisible, inaudible entities. As nurses begin to work with homeless groups and to know their clients by name, they can begin to appreciate the humanity of homeless clients and engage in therapeutic relationships. There are many paths to homelessness. Morrell-Bellai, Goering, and Boydell (2000) conducted in-depth, semistructured interviews with 29 homeless adults to learn about reasons for becoming and remaining homeless. These researchers identified macro-level and personal vulnerability factors.

---

> ### HOW TO  Evaluate the Concept of Homelessness
>
> - What is it like to live on the streets?
> - What issues might confront a young mother and her children inside a homeless shelter?
> - How is it that people are so poor that they have no place to go?
> - What really causes homelessness?
> - How do you respond to the person on the street asking for money to buy a sandwich or catch a bus?
> - How is your response different (or not) when a young mother with children asks you for money?
> - How do you react to the smell of urine in a stairwell or elevator?

---

The Evidence-Based Practice box lists the factors involved in both categories.

### Homelessness in the United States

According to the **Stewart B. McKinney Homeless Assistance Act** of 1994, a person is considered homeless who "lacks a fixed, regular, and adequate night-time residence and . . . has a primary nighttime residency that is: (A) a supervised publicly or privately operated shelter designed to provide temporary living accommodations; (B) an institution that provides a temporary residence for individuals intended to be institutionalized; or (C) a public or private place not designed for, or ordinarily used as, a regular sleeping accommodation for human beings" (National Coalition for the Homeless, 1998a, p. 1). This definition generally refers to persons who are homeless on the streets, in shelters, or who face eviction within 1 week.

### How Many People Are Homeless?

Point prevalence (counting the number of persons who are homeless at a particular point in time) has been the traditional method used to estimate the number of homeless persons in the United States. However, many public health professionals have questioned the accuracy of the

---

> ### Evidence-Based Practice
>
> **BECOMING AND REMAINING HOMELESS: A QUALITATIVE INVESTIGATION**
>
> **Purpose:** To identify reasons for becoming and remaining homeless
>
> **Study Group:** Twenty-nine homeless adults
>
> **Method:** In-depth, semistructured interviews
>
> **FINDINGS**
>
> Individuals become and remain homeless as a result of factors at the *macro-level* and factors related to *personal vulnerability.*
>
> **Macro-level factors**
> Poverty
> Unemployment
> Inadequate welfare payments
> Lack of affordable housing
>
> **Personal vulnerability factors**
> Childhood abuse/neglect
> Mental illness
> Inadequate support networks
> Substance abuse
>
> **Nurse Use:** Identify factors in the community that could contribute to homelessness. Identify ways to intervene. If possible, initiate interventions.
>
> ---
>
> Morrell-Bellai T, Goering PN, Boydell KM: Becoming and remaining homeless: a qualitative investigation, *Issues Ment Health Nurs* 21(6):581-604, 2000.

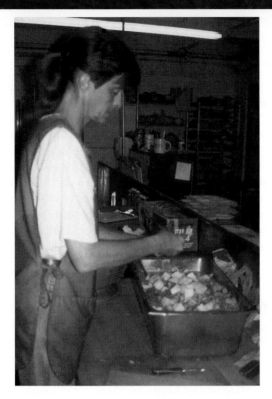

Increasingly, women, many with children, are becoming part of the homeless population. This woman is a resident in a homeless shelter where residents help with the cooking, laundry, and other chores.

point prevalence method (Link et al, 1994; Phelan and Link, 1999).

It is difficult to report accurately the number of homeless persons in any community. Counts of visible homeless persons are used to generate statistics related to homelessness in the United States. For example, people living in homeless shelters, eating in soup kitchens, or sleeping on sidewalks and in parks are part of the estimates of homeless people at any given time. Precise calculation of the number of homeless persons at a point in time is complicated by several factors:

- Homeless persons are often hard to locate because many sleep in boxcars, on roofs of buildings, in doorways, or under freeways. Others stay temporarily with relatives. Figures given by statisticians fail to include these "invisible" persons.
- Once located, many homeless persons refuse to be interviewed or deliberately hide the fact that they are homeless.
- Some persons experience short intervals of homelessness or have intermittent homeless episodes. They are harder to identify at any specific time.
- It is difficult to generalize from one location to another. For example, the patterns of homelessness differ in large versus small cities, and in urban versus rural areas.

It appears that homelessness may be much more widespread than statistics generally indicate (Phelan and Link,

1999). Link et al (1994) studied homelessness using random number dialing and telephone interviews. Respondents were asked if they had been homeless during the last 5 years, how long they were homeless, and where they slept during homeless episodes. Data indicated that the point prevalence method understated the number of homeless individuals and did not accurately describe the characteristics of homeless persons.

The concept of homelessness includes two broad categories. The first encompasses persons living in **crisis poverty.** These are people whose lives are generally marked by hardship and struggle. For them, homelessness is often transient or episodic. Persons living in crisis poverty often resort to brief stays in shelters or other temporary accommodations. Their homelessness may result from lack of employment opportunities, lack of education, obsolete job skills, or domestic violence. Such issues lead to persistent poverty and need to be addressed along with efforts to find stable housing.

Persons in the second category, persistent poverty, are chronically homeless men and women, many of whom have mental or physical disabilities. This is the group that is most frequently identified with homelessness in the United States. Physical and mental disabilities in this group often coexist with alcohol and other drug abuse, severe mental illness, other chronic health problems, and/or chronic family difficulties. These people lack money and family support, they often end up living on the streets, and their homelessness is often persistent. Members of this group need economic assistance, rehabilitation, and ongoing support.

Many homeless people previously had homes and managed to survive on limited incomes. Today's homeless include people of every age, sex, ethnic group, and family type. Surprisingly, the single homeless tend to be younger and better educated than stereotypes would suggest. Many are long-standing residents of their communities and have some history of job success (National Coalition for the Homeless, 1998b). Box 32-2 summarizes the characteristics of America's homeless.

Homeless people are found in both rural and urban areas. Many sleep at night in shelters that they must vacate during the day. This means that during the day, they sit or stand on the street, in parks, alleys, shopping centers, libraries, and in places such as trash bins, cardboard boxes, or under loading docks at industrial sites. They may also seek shelter in public buildings, such as train and bus stations. Those who do not sleep in shelters may sleep in single-room-occupancy hotels, all-night movie theaters, abandoned buildings, and vehicles.

Rural communities, despite their peaceful images, are not immune to homelessness. The extent of the problem is more often disguised than in the urban areas because rural people are often more likely to help one another. Therefore family and friends often provide temporary housing to their neighbors who have no place to live. Homeless individuals and families living in rural areas suffer from the same types of health problems as their urban counterparts (Craft-Rosenberg, Powel and Culp, 2000).

## BOX 32-2  Who Are America's Homeless?

- Families
- Children
- Single women
- Female heads of household
- Adults who are unemployed, earn low wages, or are migrant workers
- People who abuse alcohol or other substances
- Abandoned children
- Adolescent runaways
- Older adults with no place to go and no one to care for them
- Persons who are mentally ill
- Vietnam War–era veterans

From *Health: United States, 1998*, USDHHS Publication No. (PHS) 08-1232, Washington, DC, 1998, U.S. Government Printing Office.

## Causes of Homelessness

Most people move into homelessness gradually. Once they give up their own dwellings, they move in with family or friends. Only when all other options are exhausted do people go to shelters or seek refuge on the streets. Many factors contribute to the increasing numbers of homeless persons, including a growing number of people living in poverty, a decrease in the number of affordable housing units, emergency demands on income, gentrification of neighborhoods, alcohol and drug addiction, and a decrease in the number of transitional treatment facilities for deinstitutionalized mentally ill individuals (Arno et al, 1996; Culhane, Averyt, and Hadley, 1997; de la Barra, 1998).

As noted previously, the percentage of people living below the poverty level has increased. Changes in the housing market have also had a profound negative effect on many persons who were marginally meeting their financial obligations. The move to upgrade urban housing, or **gentrification,** began with a positive intent that unfortunately led to negative consequences for many of the former residents of urban areas. During the 1980s, the supply of low-income housing dropped by about 2.5 million units; simultaneously, a large increase occurred in the need for low-income housing units. Historically, urban neighborhoods provided homes for older adults and poor persons. As neighborhoods were modernized, former residents were often unable to afford either to use existing housing in the old neighborhoods or to relocate to new housing elsewhere. In many older neighborhoods, people who are now homeless previously lived in single-room-occupancy (SRO) buildings where they rented rooms on a long-term basis. Urban renewal eliminated many of the SROs and left a more attractive, better-maintained neighborhood that became unaffordable for its former residents. A poignant example of the effects of urban gentri-

fication on the poor recently occurred in Oakland, California, where the condemnation and closure of the Hotel Royal, combined with decreased availability of other similarly priced SRO hotels, forced the majority of its residents to become homeless (Fagan, 1998). One of the tenants said, "I hate those fleas, I hate the cold, I hate that they haven't fixed up this disgusting place I have to live in. But even more, I hate how they are just tossing us on the street without hardly any notice; this isn't what you'd call great, but at least it was home. Until now" (Fagan, 1998, p. A20).

**Deinstitutionalization** of chronically mentally ill individuals from public psychiatric hospitals increased the number of homeless persons. Deinstitutionalization intended to replace large state psychiatric hospitals with community-based treatment centers. The goal was for clients to have shorter stays in mental health facilities and move into appropriately designed and readily available community-based care. Unfortunately, those hospitals were often either downsized or closed, and federal and state governments failed to allocate the needed funds to provide community-based services. Furthermore, few of the intended community mental health centers were ever built. According to statistics from the National Coalition for the Homeless (1998a), 38% of single homeless adults suffer from a significant mental illness.

## EFFECTS OF HOMELESSNESS ON HEALTH

Homelessness is correlated with poor health outcomes. Homeless individuals suffer significantly greater incidences of acute and chronic illness, acquired immunodeficiency syndrome (AIDS), and trauma (Busen and Beech, 1997). Even though they are at higher risk of physiologic problems, homeless persons have greater difficulty accessing health care services (Gillis and Singer, 1997). Health care is usually crisis oriented and sought in emergency departments, and those who access health care have a hard time following prescribed regimens (Gelberg and Doblin, 1996).

An insulin-dependent diabetic man who lives on the street may sleep in a shelter. His ability to get adequate rest, exercise, take insulin on a schedule, eat regular meals, or follow a prescribed diet is virtually impossible. How does one purchase an antibiotic without money? How is a child treated for scabies and lice when there are no bathing facilities? How does an older adult with peripheral vascular disease elevate his legs when he must be out of the shelter at 7 A.M. and on the streets all day? These health problems are often directly related to poor access to preventive health care services. Healthy People 2010, a national prevention initiative, expands upon previous versions by increasing awareness and the demand for preventive health services. Healthy People 2010 goals related to access to care are listed in the Healthy People box.

In addition to facing challenges related to self-care, homeless people usually give lower priority to health promotion and health maintenance than to obtaining food and shelter. They spend most of their time trying to survive. Just getting money to buy food is a major chore.

## Healthy People 2010 | Access to Care

National goals for improving access to care that affect poor and homeless people are:

**1-1** Increase the proportion of persons with health insurance

**1-4** Increase the proportion of persons who have a specific source of ongoing care

**1-6** Reduce the proportion of families that experience difficulties or delays in obtaining health care, or who do not receive needed care for one or more family members

From U.S. Department of Health and Human Services: *Healthy people 2010: national health promotion and disease prevention objectives,* ed 2, Washington, DC, 2000, U.S. Government Printing Office.

---

### Table 32-3  Common Health Problems of Homeless Persons

**PSYCHOSOCIAL**

- Depressive symptoms
- Mental/psychiatric illness
- Alcohol/substance abuse

**INFECTIOUS**

- HIV/AIDS
- TB/MDR TB
- Other infectious diseases

**OTHER**

- Trauma
- COPD
- Musculoskeletal problems
- Foot problems
- Malnutrition

- Preterm birth
- Low birth weight
- Decreased access to care
- Increased ED utilization rates

---

*AIDS,* Acquired immunodeficiency syndrome; *COPD,* chronic obstructive pulmonary disease; *ED,* emergency department; *HIV,* human immunodeficiency virus; *MDR TB,* multidrug-resistant tuberculosis; *TB,* tuberculosis.

Culhane DP, Averyt JM, Hadley TR: The rate of public shelter admission among Medicaid-reimbursed users of behavioral health services, *Psychiatr Serv* 48(3):390, 1997; Darmon N et al: Dietary inadequacies observed in homeless men visiting an emergency shelter in Paris, *Public Health Nutr* 4(2):155-161, 2001; Hwang SW: Homelessness and health, *CMAJ* 164(2):229-233, 2001; Kamieniecki GW: Prevalence of psychological distress and psychiatric disorders among homeless youth in Australia, *Aust N Z J Psychiatry* 35(3):352-358, 2001; Stein JA, Lu MC, Gelberg L: Severity of homelessness and adverse birth outcomes, *Health Psychol* 19(6):524-534, 2000.

---

persons. Disorders caused by exposure include hypothermia and heat-related illnesses, such as heat stroke. The prevalence of diabetes, poor skin integrity, chronic disease, nutritional deficits, trauma, and use and abuse of alcohol and illicit drugs compounds the effects of exposure. Because they produce decreased sensitivity to hot and cold, the use of street drugs can lead to hyperthermia or hypothermia (Brickner et al, 1996).

Cardiovascular and respiratory diseases in the homeless population include peripheral vascular disease, hypertension, tuberculosis, pneumonia, and chronic obstructive pulmonary diseases. Homeless persons spend many hours on their feet and often sleep in positions that compromise their peripheral circulation. Hypertension is exacerbated by high rates of alcohol abuse and high sodium content of foods served in fast-food restaurants, shelters, and other meal sites. Crowded living conditions put homeless persons at risk for exposure to viruses and bacteria that cause pneumonia and tuberculosis. In addition, high rates of tobacco, alcohol, and illicit drug use diminish immune response and contribute to an increased prevalence of chronic obstructive pulmonary disease in homeless persons (White et al, 1997).

AIDS is also a growing concern among the homeless population. The seroprevalence of HIV infection in the homeless is estimated to be at least double that found in the general population. The use of intravenous drugs and sexual assault are other risk factors. Homeless persons with AIDS tend to develop more virulent forms of infectious diseases, to have longer hospitalizations, and to have less access to treatment (Fournier and Carmichael, 1998; Gelberg and Doblin, 1996).

Trauma is a significant cause of death and disability in the homeless population. Major trauma includes gunshot wounds, stab wounds, head trauma, suicide attempts, and fractures. Minor trauma includes bruises, abrasions, concussions, sprains, puncture wounds, eye injuries, and cellulitis (Heffron, Skipper, and Lambert, 1997).

As mentioned, deinstitutionalization has contributed to the growing number of homeless persons who suffer from mental illnesses, including schizophrenia and affective disorders. The prevalence of alcohol and substance abuse compounds the effects of mental illness. Many homeless persons were mentally ill before becoming

Although some homeless persons are eligible for entitlement programs, such as TANF, WIC, or Social Security, others must beg for money, sell plasma or blood products, steal, sell drugs, or engage in prostitution.

Some of the health problems accompanying homelessness include hypothermia, infestations, peripheral vascular disease, hypertension, respiratory infections, tuberculosis, AIDS, trauma, and mental illness (White et al, 1997). Table 32-3 lists significant health problems of homeless

homeless, whereas others develop acute mental distress as a result of being homeless. Although treatment modalities may exist, homeless persons are often unable to gain access to mental health treatment facilities. Barriers to treatment include lack of awareness of treatment options, lack of available space in treatment facilities, inability to pay for treatment, lack of transportation, nonsupportive attitudes of service providers, and lack of coordination of services (Dennis, Steadman, and Cocozza, 2000).

In addition to its effects on physical health, homelessness also affects psychological, social, and spiritual well-being. Becoming homeless means more than losing a home, or a regular place to sleep and eat; it also means losing friends, personal possessions, and familiar surroundings. Homeless persons live in chaos, confusion, and fear. Many describe experiencing loss of dignity, low self-esteem, lack of social support, and generalized despair.

## Homelessness and At-Risk Populations

Being homeless affects health across the life span. Imagine the effect of homelessness on pregnancy, childhood, adolescence, or older adulthood; each group has different needs. Nurses must be aware of the unique needs of homeless clients at every age.

Homeless pregnant women are at high risk for complex health problems. Pregnancy outcomes for homeless pregnant women are significantly poorer than for pregnant women in the general population. Pregnant homeless women present several challenges. They have higher rates of sexually transmitted diseases, higher incidences of addiction to drugs and alcohol, poorer nutritional status, and a higher incidence of poor birth outcomes (i.e., lower birth weight and lower Apgar scores). Although homeless women who are pregnant are at increased risk for pregnancy complications, they have less access to prenatal care. Severity of homelessness has been shown to significantly predict lower birth weight and preterm births, even for homeless women receiving regular prenatal care (Stein et al, 2000).

The health problems of homeless children, although similar to those of poor children, often have more serious consequences. Homeless children have poorer health than children in the general population, and they experience more symptoms of acute illness, such as fever, ear infection, diarrhea, and asthma than their housed counterparts (Weinreb et al, 1998b). Homeless children living on the streets in urban areas are at greatest risk of poor health (de la Barra, 1998). Menke and Wagner (1998) compared mental health, physical health, and health care practices of homeless, previously homeless, and nonhomeless school-age children; they found that homeless children demonstrated higher levels of anxiety, were significantly more depressed, and were at higher risk for physical and mental health problems than poor children who were not homeless. Homeless children are at greater risk for inadequate nutrition, which can lead to delayed growth and development, failure to thrive, or obesity. Homeless children also experience higher rates of school absenteeism, academic failure, and emotional and behavioral maladjustments. The stress of homelessness can be manifested in behaviors such as withdrawal, depression, anxiety, aggression, regression, and self-mutilation. Homeless children may have delayed communication, more mental health problems, and histories of abuse, and they are less likely to have attended school than their housed counterparts (Cumella, Grattan, and Panos, 1998).

Statistics related to the number of homeless adolescents are often subsumed under the title *homeless children*. Homeless adolescents living on the streets exhibit greater risk-taking behaviors, poorer health status, and decreased access to health care than teens in the general population (Ensign and Santelli, 1997). In addition, homeless adolescents are at high risk of contracting serious communicable diseases, such as AIDS and hepatitis B, and are more likely to use alcohol and illicit substances. Homeless teens often have histories of runaway behavior, physical abuse, and sexual abuse (Busen and Beech, 1997). Once on the streets, many homeless adolescents exchange sex for food, clothing, and shelter. In addition to the increased risk of sexually transmitted diseases and other serious communicable diseases, homeless adolescent girls who exchange sex for survival are at high risk for unintended pregnancy (Rew, 1996). A study comparing homeless adolescents with domiciled teens found that homeless youths initiated sexual activity at an earlier age, were less likely to use contraception at first sexual experience, were twice as likely to have been pregnant, had more sex partners, and were twice as likely to have visited an emergency room in the past 12 months (Ensign and Santelli, 1998). Homeless youths have higher rates of depression, lower self-esteem, more suicidal ideation, and poorer overall health than their domiciled counterparts (Unger et al, 1997).

Homeless older adults are the most vulnerable of the impoverished older adult population. They have lived in long-standing poverty, have fewer supportive relationships, and are likely to have become homeless as a result of catastrophic events. Life expectancy for homeless older adults is significantly lower than for older, housed adults (Hwang, 2001). Permanent physical deformities, often secondary to poor or absent medical care, are common among homeless older adults. Homeless older adults suffer from untreated chronic conditions, including tuberculosis, hypertension, arthritis, cardiovascular disease, injuries, malnutrition, poor oral health, and hypothermia (Schoenberg and Gilbert, 1998). As with younger homeless persons, older adults who are homeless must focus their energy on survival, leaving little time for health promotion activities.

Homelessness has a deleterious effect on the health of persons across the life span. Community-oriented nurses must be able to identify the precursors to homelessness and anticipate the effects of homelessness on physical, emotional, and spiritual well-being.

## Prevention and Preventive Services

Understanding levels of prevention related to homelessness is vital for community-oriented nurses working with persons living in poverty. Community-oriented nurses accept the political and social commitments necessary to promote primary, secondary, and tertiary prevention related to vulnerable populations. Often, this commitment involves investing time outside the traditional areas of nursing practice. Community-oriented nurses must continue to advocate for affordable housing, community outreach services, preventive health services, and other assistance programs for poor and homeless persons.

### Preventive Services

Preventive services related to homelessness include providing affordable, adequate housing. Aday (2001) identifies three major types of effective housing modalities for prevention of homelessness and its complications: low-income, supportive, and emergency housing. *Low-income housing* refers to affordable housing that is available to all persons. Unfortunately, recent federal policy in the United States indicates a reversal in commitment to affordable housing for all Americans. *Supportive housing* refers to subsidized housing for vulnerable population groups, such as persons with physical and mental disabilities, women and children who are victims of abuse, and alcohol and drug users. *Emergency housing* refers to shelters for persons who are already homeless. Emergency housing is especially important for prevention of health problems for persons who are recently homeless (Aday, 2001).

### Levels of Prevention and the Community-Oriented Nurse

It is difficult to separate services for homelessness into primary, secondary, and tertiary levels of prevention because interventions related to homelessness can be assigned to more than one level. Affordable housing, for example, may qualify as primary prevention, but it could also be an important secondary or tertiary preventive intervention (Box 32-3).

Primary preventive services include affordable housing, housing subsidies, effective job training programs, employer incentives, preventive health care services, multisystem case management, birth control services, safe sex education, needle exchange programs, and counseling programs. Nurses can form networks with other health professionals to educate policymakers and the public about the value of these preventive services. These programs could prevent homelessness from occurring at all, which would prevent many of its devastating sequelae.

Secondary preventive services target persons on the very verge of homelessness as well as those who are newly homeless. Examples include supportive and emergency housing, targeted case management, housing subsidies, soup kitchens and meal sites, and comprehensive physical and mental health services. Nurses can work with homeless and near-homeless aggregates to provide education about existing services and strategies for influencing public policy that will provide more comprehensive services for homeless and near-homeless persons.

Tertiary prevention for homelessness includes comprehensive case management, physical and mental health services, emergency shelter housing, needle exchange programs, and drug and alcohol treatment. An important prerequisite for population-focused practice is a sound understanding of the sociopolitical milieu in which problems occur. Nurses can influence politicians and other policymakers at the federal, state, and local levels about the plight of vulnerable homeless populations in their community.

## Federal Programs for the Homeless

A tremendous need exists for comprehensive, affordable, and accessible care for the nation's homeless population. The federal government officially became involved with meeting the needs of the homeless in 1987 with the passage of the Stewart B. McKinney Homeless Assistance Act (PL 100-77). Title 11 of the McKinney Act provided funding for outpatient health services; however, the monies for these services were not large, and many needs go unmet. The McKinney Act grants homeless children the same access to education as permanently housed children. This act also created the **Interagency Council on the Homeless** (ICH) to coordinate and direct federal homeless activities.

The ICH is made up of the heads of 16 federal agencies that have programs or activities for the homeless. The general goals of the ICH are to improve federal programs for the homeless through better coordination and linkages, decreasing the amount of documentation required to qualify for benefits. By targeting the most vulnerable segments of the homeless population, the ICH intends to influence the problem of homelessness. Children are a priority for the ICH.

Homeless families with children are eligible to receive shelter and nutrition assistance from the U.S. Department of Agriculture's WIC program. Persons receiving WIC benefits receive vouchers entitling them to free nutritious foods and infant formulas from local grocers. The TANF program can be a key source of income for homeless families.

Unfortunately, health care for homeless persons tends to be fragmented and limited in scope. Some of the most useful health care programs for the homeless begin with grants from private funding agencies, such as the Robert Wood

---

### BOX 32-3  Levels of Prevention Related to Poverty and Homelessness

**PRIMARY PREVENTION**
Provide health education in the local area for prevention of diseases related to multiuse of needles.

**SECONDARY PREVENTION**
Screen patients for early detection of drug use and the possibility of multiple users of needles; screen for diseases that may result from injection drug use: HIV, hepatitis, and other bloodborne diseases.

**TERTIARY PREVENTION**
Implement more systematic programs for needle exchange; begin treatment for any diseases that are detected.

Johnson Foundation and the Pew Charitable Trusts. Projects funded by these agencies have followed sound public health principles by encouraging community involvement, public/private partnerships, and commitment to outreach. Most of these projects rely heavily on nurse practitioners and physician assistants to deliver care in collaboration with physicians, nurses, and social workers. In recent years, many schools of nursing have received funding from the Division of Nursing in the USDHHS to establish nurse-managed centers for the homeless. Both faculty and students provide a range of services in these centers.

## ROLE OF THE NURSE

Nurses have a critical role in the delivery of health care to poor and homeless people. To be effective, nurses need strong physical and psychosocial assessment skills, current knowledge of available resources, and an ability to convey respect, dignity, and value to each person. Nurses need to be able to work with poor and homeless clients to promote, maintain, and restore health. Nurses must be prepared to look at the whole picture: the person, the family, and the community interacting with the environment. The following strategies are important to consider when working with homeless individuals, families, and aggregates:

- *Create a trusting environment.* Trust is essential to the development of a therapeutic relationship with poor or homeless persons. Many clients and families have been disappointed by their interactions with health care and social systems; they are now mistrustful and see little hope for change. By following through and doing what they say they will do, nurses can establish trusting relationships with clients. If the answer to a question is unknown, an appropriate response might be, "I don't know the answer, but I will try to find out. Let me make a few phone calls and I will let you know Friday." Reliability helps to build the foundation for a trusting relationship.
- *Show respect, compassion, and concern.* Poor and homeless clients are defeated so often by life's circumstances that they may feel that they do not deserve attention. Listen carefully and empathize with clients so that they believe that they are worthy of care. Too often, poor and homeless persons are not treated with respect and dignity by health and social services workers. Since clients respond well to nursing interactions that demonstrate respect, it is helpful to use reflective statements that convey acceptance and understanding of their situation.
- *Do not make assumptions.* A comprehensive and holistic assessment is crucial to identifying underlying needs. Just because a young mother with three preschool children misses a clinic appointment does not mean that she does not care about the health of her children. She may not have transportation, one child may be sick, or she may be sick. Find out the reason for the absence and help solve the problem.
- *Coordinate a network of services and providers.* The multiple and complex needs of poor and homeless people make working with them exceedingly challenging. Many ser-

vices exist, but often the people who could benefit are unaware of their existence. Developing a coordinated network of providers involves conducting a thorough assessment of the service area to identify federal, state, and local services available for poor and homeless clients. Where are the food banks? Where can you get clothing? What programs are available in the local churches and schools? How do people access these services? What are the eligibility requirements? How helpful are the people who work at the service agencies? What service is provided to eligible individuals and families? Nurses can identify these services and help link families with appropriate resources. In addition, a thorough assessment of available services for homeless persons in a nurse's service area can identify significant gaps in essential services. Once these gaps are identified, nurses serving as case managers can work with other health care providers and with community members to advocate for necessary services for homeless clients.

- *Advocate for accessible health care services.* Poverty and homelessness create a number of barriers that prevent access to health care services. Nurses can advocate for accessible and convenient locations of health care services. Neighborhood clinics, mobile vans, and home visits can bring health care to people unable to access care. Coordinating services at a central location often improves client compliance because it reduces the stress of getting to multiple places. Many homeless shelters and transitional housing units have clinics on site. These multiservice centers provide health care, social services, day care, drug and alcohol recovery programs, and comprehensive case management. Multiservice models are usually multidisciplinary. For example, midlevel practitioners (NPs and PAs), community-oriented nurses, social workers, psychologists, child psychologists, and administrative personnel might provide a network of support for clients in shelters and low-income housing facilities.
- *Focus on prevention.* Nurses can use every opportunity to provide preventive care and health teaching. Important health promotion (primary prevention) topics include child and adult immunization, and education regarding sound nutrition, foot care, safe sex, contraception, and prevention of chronic illness. Screening for health problems such as tuberculosis, diabetes, hypertension, foot problems, and anemia is an important form of secondary prevention. Know what other screening and health promotion services are available in the target area, such as nutrition programs, job-training programs, educational programs, housing programs, and legal services. All these services may be included in a comprehensive plan of care.
- *Know when to walk beside the client and when to encourage the client to walk ahead.* This area is often difficult for the nurse to implement. Nursing interventions range from extensive care activities to minimal support. At times, nursing actions include providing encouragement and support, or providing information. At other times,

## HOW TO Apply Case Management Strategies to Working With the Homeless

- Determine available services and resources.
- Determine missing resources and develop creative solutions for service deficiencies.
- Integrate and use clinical skills.
- Establish long-term therapeutic relationships with families.
- Enhance the family's personal coping skills, survival skills, and resourcefulness.
- Facilitate service delivery on behalf of the family.
- Guide the family toward the use of appropriate community resources.
- Communicate and collaborate with professionals from multiple service systems.
- Advocate for the development of creative solutions.
- Participate in policy analysis and political activism.
- Manipulate and modify the environment as needed.
- Connect with local, state, and federal legislators.

nurses may actually call a pediatrician to set up an appointment for a sick child and may call again to see that the appointment was kept. Nurses assess for the presence of strengths, problem-solving ability, and coping ability of an individual or family while providing information on where and how to gain access to services. For example, a local hospital may provide free mammograms for uninsured women. Women who qualify for this free service may not take advantage of it because they are afraid that they may have breast cancer. Nurses can find out about this important service, inform the women of the service, teach them about the importance of preventive care, and assess and deal with fear and anxiety. The challenge for the nurse becomes choosing whether to schedule the appointments for the women or to simply provide them with a referral sheet, knowing that many will not follow through. The choice is not clear, but the goal is to make available a needed screening intervention without taking away the woman's right to decide what to do for herself.

- *Develop a network of support for yourself.* Caring for poor and homeless persons is challenging, rewarding, and at times exhausting. It is important to find a source of personal strength, renewal, and hope. The people you encounter are often looking to you to maintain hope and provide encouragement. Discover for yourself what restores and encourages you. For some nurses it is poetry, music, painting, or weaving. For others it is a walk in a peaceful place, a weekend retreat, a good run, a workout at the gym, or meeting with other nurses who are engaged in the same work. Be attentive to your own needs, and create the time and space to restore your spirit.

## ■ Practice Application

Tonya, a single mother with AIDS, lives in an apartment with seven other family members and her children, who are HIV positive. Tonya does not often keep her children's numerous appointments at the immunology clinic. How do you respond?

  **A.** Make an unsolicited telephone call or visit to Tonya and her family to let them know they are important and that you are thinking about them.
  **B.** Call child protective services to report her failure to keep her children's appointments because she is noncompliant and neglectful of her children.
  **C.** Do a more thorough assessment to determine why appointments are missed.

**Answer is in the back of the book.**

## ■ Key Points

- Poverty and homelessness affect the health status of people.
- To understand the concepts of poverty and homelessness, consider your personal beliefs and attitudes, clients' perceptions of their condition, and the social, political, cultural, and environmental factors that influence poverty and homelessness.
- The definition of poverty varies depending on the source consulted. The federal government defines poverty on the basis of income, family size, age of the head of household, and number of children under 18 years of age. Those who are poor insist that poverty has less to do with income and more to do with a lack of family, friends, love, and support.
- Factors leading to the growing number of poor persons in the United States include decreased earnings, diminishing availability of low-cost housing, increases in the number of households headed by women (women's incomes are traditionally lower than men's), inadequate education, lack of marketable job skills, welfare reform, and reduced Social Security payments to children.
- Poverty has a direct effect on health and well-being across the life span. Poor persons have higher rates of chronic illness, higher infant morbidity and mortality, shorter life expectancy, and more complex health problems.
- Child poverty rates remain twice as high as those for adults. Children in single-parent homes are twice as likely to be poor as those who live in homes with two parents. Younger children (0 to 5 years) are at highest risk for developmental delays and damage caused by inadequate nutrition or lack of health care.
- Poverty affects both urban and rural communities. The poorer the neighborhood, the greater is the proportion of residents who are members of minority groups.

- At present, the following groups often constitute the homeless in both rural and urban areas: families, single mothers, single women, recently unemployed persons, substance abusers, adolescent runaways, mentally ill individuals, and single men.
- Factors contributing to homelessness include an increase in the number of persons living in poverty, diminishing availability of low-cost housing, increased unemployment, substance abuse, lack of treatment facilities for mentally ill persons, domestic violence, and family situations causing children to run away.
- The complex health problems of homeless persons include inability to get adequate rest, exercise, and nutrition; exposure; infectious diseases; acute and chronic illness; infestations; trauma; and mental health problems.
- Nurses have a critical role in the delivery of care to persons who are poor and homeless. Nurses bring to each client encounter the ability to assess the client in context, and to intervene in ways that restore, maintain, or promote health.
- In addition to interactions with individuals who are poor or homeless, nurses use the nursing process to assess and diagnose, and to plan, implement, and evaluate population-focused interventions.

## Clinical Decision-Making Activities

1. Examine health statistics and demographic data to identify the rate of poverty and homelessness in your geographic area. What resources and agencies are available in your area to support homeless persons? What services are available from federal, state, and local sources? Identify a specific geographic region and assess this target area in terms of services for poor and homeless persons. Do a literature search to identify recommended state-of-the-art interventions for poor and homeless persons. Compare the recommended programs and interventions with those available in your target area. How does your area measure up? Give some specific recommendations about how you would fill the gaps.
2. Examine the specific programs identified in the preceding assessment. How do those who need services access them? Working with other students, make appointments with key persons in the agencies identified to find out what each agency offers, which particular aggregate is served, how clients access the services, who is eligible, how the agency receives funding, and what methods are used to evaluate the agency's ability to meet the needs of its targeted aggregates. Give some examples.
3. Identify nurses in your community who work with the homeless or with other vulnerable groups. Invite these nurses to come to a class meeting to share their experiences. What constitutes a typical workday? What are the rewards and challenges of working with vulnerable populations? How do they deal with the frustrations and challenges of their work? What advice might they offer to students working with vulnerable aggregates? What programs do they recommend? How would you advocate for vulnerable aggregates in your practice?
4. Imagine yourself as a nurse working in a homeless shelter or making a home visit to a family in an impoverished neighborhood. How have your life experiences and education prepared you (or not) for these situations?
5. Discuss welfare reform with other students. How does our welfare system work? Who receives welfare? Who is eligible for benefits? How do people apply for welfare? What are the strengths and weaknesses of welfare reform in the United States? What are the financial and personal costs of welfare reform? Identify federal and state senators and representatives in your districts. Where do they stand on the issue of welfare reform? Give details of your ideas for changing our welfare system.

## Additional Resources

These related resources are found either in the appendix at the back of this book or on the book's website at **http://evolve.elsevier.com/Stanhope.**

**evolve   Evolve Website**

WebLinks: Healthy People 2010

## References

Aday LA: *At risk in America,* ed 2, San Francisco, 2001, Jossey-Bass.

Arno PS et al: The impact of housing status on health care utilization of persons with HIV disease, *J Health Care Poor Underserved* 7(1):36, 1996.

Berne AS et al: A nursing model for addressing the health needs of homeless families. In Spradley BW, Allender JA, editors: *Readings in community health nursing,* ed 5, Philadelphia, 1997, Lippincott-Raven.

Bremner RH: *From the depths: the discovery of poverty in the United States,* New York, 1956, University Press.

Brickner PW et al: *Health care of homeless people,* New York, 1996, Springer.

Brown L, Pollitt E: Malnutrition, poverty and intellectual development, *Sci Am* 274(2):38, 1996.

Burchinal M, Lee M, Ramey C: Type of day care and preschool intellectual development in disadvantaged children, *Child Dev* 60(1):128, 1989.

Busen NH, Beech B: A collaborative model for community-based health care screening of homeless adolescents, *J Prof Nurs* 13(5):316, 1997.

Campaign 2000: *Poverty amidst prosperity: building a Canada for all children,* Toronto, 2002a, Author, available at www.campaign2000.ca.

Campaign 2000: *The UN Special Session on Children: putting promises into action—a report on a decade of child and family poverty in Canada,* May 2002, Toronto, Author, 2002b, available at www.campaign2000.ca.

Canadian Council on Social Development: *The progress of Canada's children: 2002 highlights,* Ottawa, 2002, Author, available at www.ccsd.ca.

Canadian Public Health Association: *Health impacts of social and economic conditions: implications for public policy,* Ottawa, 1997a, Author, available at www.cpha.ca.

Canadian Public Health Association: *1997 position paper in homelessness and health,* Ottawa, 1997b, Author, available at www.cpha.ca.

Culhane DP, Averyt JM, Hadley TR: The rate of public shelter admission among Medicaid-reimbursed users of behavioral health services, *Psychiatr Serv* 48(3):390, 1997.

Cumella S, Grattan E, Panos V: The mental health of children in homeless families and their contact with health, education, and social services, *Health Soc Care Community* 6(5):331-342, 1998.

Craft-Rosenberg M, Powel SR, Culp K: Health status and resources of rural homeless women and children, *West J Nurs Res* 22(8):863-878, 2000.

Dalaker J, Naifeh M: U.S. Bureau of the Census, *Current Population Reports,* Series P60-201, Poverty in the United States, Washington, DC, 1998, U.S. Government Printing Office.

Darmon N et al: Dietary inadequacies observed in homeless men visiting an emergency shelter in Paris, *Public Health Nutr* 4(2):155-161, 2001.

de la Barra X: Poverty: the main cause of ill health in urban children, *Health Educ Behav* 25(1):46, 1998.

Dennis DL, Steadman HJ, Cocozza JJ: The impact of federal systems integration initiatives on services for mentally ill homeless persons, *Ment Health Serv Res* 2(3):165-174, 2000.

Diez Roux AV: Investigating neighborhood and area effects on health, *Am J Public Health* 91(11):1783-1789, 2001.

Elders J: "An urban health crisis," Keynote address presented at Mothers and Children 1994, Washington, DC, 1994.

Ensign J, Santelli J: Shelter-based homeless youth: health and access to care, *Arch Pediatr Adolesc Med* 151(8):817, 1997.

Ensign J, Santelli J: Health status and service use: comparison of adolescents at a school-based health clinic with homeless adolescents, *Arch Pediatr Adolesc Med* 152(1):20, 1998.

Fagan K: Resident hotel's 60 tenants evicted: Oakland calls Hotel Royal a health hazard, *San Francisco Chronicle,* p. A20, May 14, 1998.

Fine S: The Kerr-Mills Act: medical care for the indigent in Michigan, 1960-1965, *J Hist Med Allied Sci* 53(3):285-316, 1998.

Flynn L: The health practices of homeless women: a causal model, *Nurs Res* 46(2):72, 1997.

Fournier AM, Carmichael C: Socioeconomic influences on the transmission of human immunodeficiency virus infection: the hidden risk, *Arch Fam Med* 7(3):214, 1998.

Freudenberg N: Health promotion in the city: a review of current practice and future prospects in the United States, *Annu Rev Public Health* 21:573-503, 2000.

Gelberg L, Doblin BH: Ambulatory health services provided to low-income and homeless adult patients in a major community health center, *J Gen Intern Med* 11(3):156, 1996.

Gibson S: *Understanding the consumer price index: answers to some questions,* Washington, DC, 1998, U.S. Bureau of Labor Statistics.

Gillis LM, Singer J: Breaking through the barriers: healthcare for the homeless, *J Nurs Admin* 27(6):30, 1997.

Health Canada: *Healthy Canadians: a federal report on comparable health indicators,* Ottawa, 2002, Author, available at www.healthcanada.ca.

*Health: United States, 1998,* USDHHS Publication No. (PHS) 08-1232, Washington, DC, 1998, U.S. Government Printing Office.

Heffron WA, Skipper BJ, Lambert L: Health and lifestyle issues as risk factors for homelessness, *J Am Board Fam Pract* 10(1):6, 1997.

Hsieh CM: Trends in financial satisfaction: does poverty make a difference? *Int J Aging Hum Dev* 54(1):15-30, 2002.

Hunter JK et al: Factors limiting evaluation of health care programs for the homeless, *Nurs Outlook* 45(5):224, 1997.

Hwang SW: Homelessness and health, *CMAJ* 164(2):229-233, 2001.

Institute for Research on Poverty: *Who is poor?* 2002, available at http://www.ssc.wisc.edu/irp.

Jacobs BB: Respect for human dignity: a central phenomenon to philosophically unite nursing theory and practice through consilience of knowledge, *ANS Adv Nurs Sci* 24(1):17-35, 2001.

Jargowsky MP, Band MJ: Ghetto poverty: basic questions. In Lynn KE, Mc Geary M, editors: *Inner city poverty in the United States,* Washington, DC, 1998, National Academy Press.

Kamieniecki GW: Prevalence of psychological distress and psychiatric disorders among homeless youth in Australia, *Aust N Z J Psychiatry* 35(3):352-358, 2001.

Katz MB: *The undeserving poor: from the war on poverty to the war on welfare,* New York, 1989, Pantheon Books.

Link BG et al: Lifetime and five year prevalence of homeless in the United States, *Am J Public Health* 84(12):1907, 1994.

Mayes L: *Early experience and the developing brain: the model of prenatal cocaine exposure.* Paper presented at the invitational conference, brain development in young children: new frontiers for research, policy and practice, Chicago, June 12, 1996, University of Chicago.

Menke EM, Wagner JD: A comparative study of homeless, previously homeless, and never homeless school-aged children's health, *Issues Compr Pediatr Nurs* 20(3):153, 1998.

Miller HP: *Poverty American style,* Belmont, Calif, 1966, Dadsworth.

Morrell-Bellai T, Goering PN, Boydell KM: Becoming and remaining homeless: a qualitative investigation, *Issues Ment Health Nurs* 21(6):581-604, 2000.

Murphy B: *On the street: how we created homeless,* Ottawa, 2000, Author.

National Center for Children and Poverty: *Anticipating the effects of federal and state welfare changes on systems that serve children,* New York, 1998a, Columbia University.

National Center for Children and Poverty: *How welfare reform can help or hurt children,* New York, 1998b, Columbia University.

National Center for Children in Poverty: *Poverty and brain development in early childhood,* New York, 1997a, Columbia University.

National Center for Children in Poverty: *Young children in poverty fact sheet,* New York, 1997b, Columbia University.

National Center for Children in Poverty: *Child poverty fact sheet,* March, New York, 2002, Columbia University.

National Coalition for the Homeless: *How many people experience homelessness?* Fact sheet #3, Washington DC, 1998a, NCH.

National Coalition for the Homeless: *Why are people homeless?* Fact Sheet #1, Washington DC, 1998b, NCH.

National Council of Welfare: *Poverty profile 1999,* Ottawa, 1999, Author, available at www.ncwcnbes.net.

Olsen KA: Application of experimental poverty measures to the aged, *Soc Security Bull* 62(3):3-19, 1999.

Paille M, Pilkington FB: The global context of nursing: a human becoming perspective, *Nurs Sci Q* 15(2):165-170, 2002.

Persson RE et al: Oral health and medical status in dentate low-income older adults, *Spec Care Dentist* 18(2):70, 1998.

Petterson SM, Albers AB: Effects of poverty and maternal depression on early childhood development, *Child Dev* 72(6):1794-1813, 2001.

Phelan JC, Link BG: Who are "the homeless"? Reconsidering the stability and composition of the homeless population, *Am J Public Health* 89(9):1334-1338, 1999.

Pilisuk M, Pilisuk P: *How we lost the war on poverty,* New Jersey, 1976, Transaction Books.

Preslow BL et al: Environmental health and antisocial behavior: implications for public health, *J Environ Health* 63(9):9-19, 2001.

Price J: More mouths, more money, *Washington Times,* p. A6, April 19, 1994.

Rew S: Health risks of homeless adolescents: implications for holistic nursing, *J Holist Nurs* 14(4):348, 1996.

Schoenberg NE, Gilbert GH: Dietary implications of oral health decrements among African-American and white older adults, *Ethnic Health* 3(1-2):59, 1998.

Shore R: *Rethinking the brain: new insights into early development,* New York, 1997, Families and Work Institute.

Stein JA, Lu MC, Gelberg L: Severity of homelessness and adverse birth outcomes, *Health Psychol* 19(6):524-534, 2000.

Stevens PE: A critical social reconceptualization of environment in nursing: implications for methodology, *ANS Adv Nurs Sci* 11(4):56-68, 1989.

Streeck-Fischer A, van der Kolk BA: Down will come baby, cradle and all: diagnostic and therapeutic implications of chronic trauma on child development, *Aust N Z J Psychiatry* 34(6):903-918, 2000.

Unger JB et al: Homeless youths and young adults in Los Angeles: prevalence of mental health problems and the relationship between mental health and substance abuse disorders, *Am J Psychol* 25(3):371, 1997.

UNICEF: *Child poverty in rich nations, Innocenti Report Card, June 2000,* 2000, available at www.unicef.org.

U.S. Bureau of the Census, *Poverty in the United States, 2000,* Washington, DC, 2000, U.S. Government Printing Office.

U.S. Bureau of the Census: *Current population survey,* Washington, DC, 2002, U.S. Government Printing Office.

U.S. Department of Commerce: *Dynamics of economic well-being: who stays poor? who doesn't? Current population reports: household economic studies,* Washington, DC, 1996, U.S. Department of Commerce.

U.S. Department of Health and Human Services: *Leading indicators for Healthy People 2010: a report from the HHS group on sentinel objectives,* Washington, DC, 1998, USDHHS, Public Health Service.

U.S. Department of Health and Human Services: *Healthy people 2010: national health promotion and disease prevention objectives,* ed 2, Washington, DC, 2000, U.S. Government Printing Office.

Waitzman NJ, Smith KR: *Separate but unequal: the effects of economic segregation on mortality in metropolitan America,* Washington, DC, 1998, U.S. Bureau of the Census, U.S. Government Printing Office.

Waller W, Plotnick R: *Child support and low-income families: perceptions, practices, and policy,* San Francisco, 1999, Policy Institute of California.

Weinreb L et al: Health characteristics and medical service use: patterns of sheltered homeless and low-income housed mothers, *J Gen Intern Med* 13(6):389, 1998a.

Weinreb L et al: Determinants of health and service use patterns in homeless and low-income housed children, *Pediatrics* 102(3 Pt 1):554, 1998b.

White MC et al: Association between time homeless and perceived health status among the homeless in San Francisco, *J Community Health* 22(4):271, 1997.

Wilson WJ: *The truly disadvantaged: the inner city, the underclass, and public policy,* Chicago, 1990, University of Chicago Press.

Zedlewski SR: Family economic resources in the post-reform era, *Future Child* 12(1):120-145, 2002.

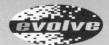
# Migrant Health Issues

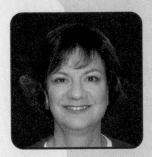

**Marie Napolitano, R.N., Ph.D., F.N.P.**

Marie Napolitano is an associate professor and the coordinator of the Family Nurse Practitioner program at Oregon Health and Science University. She has had 17 years of clinical practice and funded research with migrant farm-workers and their families. Her areas of expertise include consultation and teaching regarding cultural content with immigrant and Hispanic populations. She is a member of the Migrant Clinicians' Network and the American Public Health Association's Caucus on Refugee and Immigrant Health.

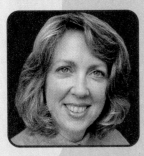

**Kim Dupree Jones, Ph.D., R.N., F.N.P.**

Kim Dupree Jones is a researcher in chronic pain and a family nurse practitioner. She is a member of the faculty in the School of Nursing and the School of Medicine at Oregon Health and Science University. Dr. Jones's specific areas of interest are exercise physiology and neuroendocrine physiology, particularly in at-risk populations, such as low-income persons, women, and those with limited access to health care. She is currently the principal investigator on a clinical trial entitled Maximizing Exercise Efficacy in Fibromyalgia, funded by the National Institutes of Health (NIH). She is also the co-investigator on an NIH-funded study to examine regional versus widespread pain in women after breast cancer surgery.

## Objectives

After reading this chapter, the student should be able to do the following:

1. Define the term *migrant farmworker* and discuss the difficulties in investigating this population
2. Describe common health problems of the migrant farmworker and farmworker families
3. Examine the barriers to migrant farmworkers and their families in securing health care
4. Evaluate successful programs that encourage health promotion among migrant farmworkers and their families
5. Analyze the role of the nurse in planning and providing care to migrant farmworkers and their families
6. Recommend legislation that would improve the lives and working conditions of migrant farmworkers and their access to health care services
7. Describe the cultural needs of migrant farmworkers and their families, and list methods of providing culturally based nursing care through assessment, planning, intervention, and evaluation

Imagine yourself attempting to deliver treatment to a toddler in a migrant camp whose throat culture was positive for pertussis. The camp is located in an isolated rural community. The toddler lives in a trailer with her parents and siblings and extended family members (13 individuals). The family must also be treated as contacts. No one speaks English, so you have an interpreter with you. The family is just returning from picking strawberries all day in the fields, and they are tired and hungry. The family is willing to give medicine to the toddler because she is sick; however, they do not understand why the rest of them must take the medicine also, because they are not sick. The family tells you that they will not be able to take the noon dose because they have no water with them at work.

Walking to the drinking barrel will take too long, and they will lose income. As a nurse, what would you do?

Nurses need to inform themselves about the culture, lifestyle, and health picture of the populations they serve. Migrant and seasonal farmworkers are an economically disadvantaged working group of individuals and families. Although the availability and affordability of food in the United States depends on these individuals, their economic and social status has not changed significantly over the past several decades. Estimates of the numbers of migrant and seasonal farmworkers in the United States vary from 1 to 5 million; the estimate of the Office of Migrant Health was 4.2 million persons (U.S. Department of Health and Human Services [USDHHS], 1993). The wide range results from dif-

## Key Terms

common migrant health problems, p. 796    migrant lifestyle, p. 795        *See Glossary for definitions*
migrant farmworker, p. 795              pesticide exposure, p. 799
Migrant Health Act, p. 796             political advocate, p. 803


## Chapter Outline

Migrant Lifestyle                    *Pesticide Exposure*                 *Health Beliefs and Practices*
*Housing*                            *Other Specific Health Problems*     Health Promotion and Illness Prevention
Health and Health Care               Children and Youths                 Role of the Nurse
*Access to Health Care*              Cultural Considerations in Migrant Health Care
Occupational and Environmental Health  *Nurse–Client Relationship*
  Problems                           *Health Values*

ferences in the definition of a migrant, divergent methods of estimating numbers, and difficulties in counting mobile populations. Sixty-eight percent of migrant farmworkers are employed in eight states (in descending order: California, Texas, Florida, Washington, Michigan, Oregon, North Carolina, and Georgia) (Larson and Plascencia, 1993).

The composition of the migrant population varies from region to region. The majority of all migrant farmworkers are Latinos (70%); foreign-born workers comprise 60% of the population, and 96% of them are from Latin American countries (Mines, Gabbard, and Samadrick, 1993). Other workers include African Americans, Jamaicans, Haitians, Laotians, and Thais. Most migrant farmworkers are either American citizens or authorized to work in the United States. The number of undocumented workers has been estimated at around 20% of the migrant farmworker population (Mines, Gabbard, and Boccalandro, 1991). Certain parts of the agricultural industry rely heavily on these undocumented workers.

The Office of Migrant Health of the U.S. Public Health Service defines a **migrant farmworker** as an individual "whose principal employment is in agriculture on a seasonal basis, who has been so employed within the last 24 months and who establishes for the purpose of such employment a temporary abode" (Office of the Federal Registrar, 1994, p. 238). Seasonal farmworkers work cyclically in agriculture but do not migrate. Although migrant and seasonal farmworkers comprise two distinct populations, they do share many demographic, cultural, and occupational characteristics. Much of the available information on agricultural farmworkers does not distinguish between migrant and seasonal farmworkers. True migrant farmworkers probably account for about 40% of agricultural workers (Mines et al, 1993). Migrant farmworkers coming into the United States for work tend to settle in permanent locations eventually and seek other types of employment.

## MIGRANT LIFESTYLE

The way of life of a migrant farmworker, or the **migrant lifestyle,** is stressful. Leaving home every year, traveling, experiencing uncertainty about work and housing, isolation in new communities, and a lack of resources are considerable challenges. Most farmworkers earn an annual income below the federal poverty line (National Advisory Council on Migrant Health [NACMH], 1993), and approximately 50% earn annual incomes of less than $7500 per individual (Oliveira, Effland, and Hamm, 1993). Rarely do they receive other benefits such as workers' compensation, disability compensation, or health or retirement benefits.

Migrant farmworkers traditionally have followed one of three migratory streams: eastern, originating in Florida; midwestern, originating in Texas; and western, originating in California. However, as workers increasingly travel throughout the country seeking employment, these streams are becoming less distinct. The majority of migrant farmworkers are employed in field crops, orchards, nurseries, and canneries. The cyclic nature of agricultural work, along with its dependence on weather and economic conditions, results in considerable uncertainty for migrant farmworkers. These individuals and families leave their base home with the expectation of work at certain sites. Word of mouth, newspaper announcements, or previous employment lead them to work these sites. However, upon arrival, migrant farmworkers may find that other workers arrived first or that the crops are late, leaving them without employment.

### Housing

On arrival at a worksite, migrant farmworkers may not find any available housing, or the housing they find is too expensive or in poor condition. Housing conditions vary between states and localities. Housing for migrant farmworkers can be located in camps with cabins, trailers, or houses. However, migrant farmworkers will live in cars or tents, if

795

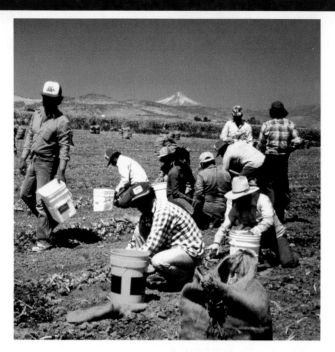

Migrant farmworkers working in fields.

necessary. National data on the type and quality of housing occupied by farmworkers are sparse. The Housing Assistance Council (HAC), a nonprofit organization whose mission is to improve affordable housing in rural areas around the country, found that, by federal standards, farmworker housing is crowded (National Center for Farmworker Health, 2001). Fifty men may live in one house, or three families may share a trailer. Often this occurs because housing is so expensive. Almost one third of migrant workers paid more than 30% of their total income for housing; those in the western stream paid up to 43% of their total income (Holden, 2001). Many also support a home-base household.

In addition to crowded conditions, housing may lack individual sanitation, bathing or laundry facilities, screens on windows, and fans or heaters. Housing may be located next to fields that have been sprayed by pesticides or where farming machinery poses a danger to children. Housing problems can run from peeling paint to broken windows to serious structural deficiencies (found in 22% of HAC housing units surveyed) (Holden, 2001). Poor-quality and crowded housing can contribute to a number of significant health problems such as tuberculosis, gastroenteritis, and hepatitis. Renting housing in rural areas is made almost impossible by barriers such as high rent, substantial rental deposits, long-term leases, lack of credit, discrimination, and a lack of rental units (Lopez, 1995). Federal programs provide some funds for farmworker housing, but they are insufficient to meet the demand. Increased funding and better coordination between agencies are needed.

## HEALTH AND HEALTH CARE

The National Migrant Resource Program for the Office of Migrant Health (1990) reports that in the United States the infant mortality rate for migrant farmworkers is 25% greater than the national average; furthermore, migrant farmworkers' life expectancy is 49 years as opposed to 75 years for white men. The poor health status of the migrant farmworker population and **common migrant health problems** have been cited in the literature (Dever, 1991; NACMH, 1995) and witnessed by the health professionals who care for these individuals. However, because it is difficult to study this population, a clear picture of their health problems is not available. Data obtained by Dever (1991) from four migrant health centers in Michigan, Indiana, and Texas showed that migrant farmworkers have more complex health problems than the general population. Multiple and complex health problems exist among 40% of all farmworkers who visit migrant health centers. Slesinger and Ofstead (1993) found that 33.6% of migrant farmworkers surveyed believed their health was fair or poor, compared to 9.4% of the U.S. population. Only 13.3% thought that their health was excellent, compared to 40.2% of the U.S. population (Box 33-1).

## Access to Health Care

The **Migrant Health Act** signed by President John Kennedy in 1962 is funded under Section 329 of the Public Health Service Act. The act provides primary and supplemental health services to migrant workers and their families. Today, migrant health centers serve over 600,000 individuals at more than 360 sites across the country (National Center for Farmworker Health [NCFH], 2001). However, it is estimated that these clinics serve less than 20% of the migrant farmworker population (NCFH, 2001).

"Farmworkers' unmet need for basic health care is not only a national disgrace, but also a national challenge" (USDHHS, 1993, p. 20). Migrant farmworkers experience limited access to health care. Financial, cultural, transportation, mobility, language, and occupational factors are frequently cited as the major barriers that limit their access to health care. Furthermore, access to dental, mental health, and pharmacy services is even more problematic (Adam, 1994; Mobed, Gold, and Schenker, 1992). Surveys indicate that only 12% to 15% of eligible migrants use clinic services (Decker and Knight, 1990; Galarneau, 1993; Helsinki Commission, 1993; USDHHS, 1993). Mull et al (2001) found that of 5597 farmworkers surveyed, 63.7% used hospital emergency departments or clinics as their usual source of care, 42% used private physicians, and 29.7% used migrant health clinics.

A lack of access to health care is of concern to migrant farmworkers themselves. They identified a lack of sufficient health care services (including specialty services and information regarding services), transportation needs, fear of immigration authorities, cost of services and medications, and information regarding such health problems as sexually transmitted diseases and human immunodeficiency virus (HIV) infection as particularly significant concerns (Perilla et al, 1998).

Factors that limit adequate provision of health care services include the following:

## BOX 33-1   What Migrants Say About . . .

### HEALTH AND HEALTH CARE

"What we have to do is reeducate our people and let them know that we have many rights to live and work and to educate and to have health care. And without health care, we cannot have the other three." Unidentified male farmworker, California

### WORK CONDITIONS

"We're used to working. We don't want to be given things. We just want to be respected and to be paid the salaries." Teresa, California

"Right now, because I'm here today [testifying at a hearing on work conditions], I may not have my job. Possibly I may not have my job tomorrow." José, California

### PESTICIDE EXPOSURE

"You go to the fields and you think that it's a foggy day because it's so pretty and it's white, but it's actually the chemicals that have been sprayed." Adelaide, California

"Pesticides presently occupy us tremendously during our work. We wear rubber gloves and that in itself creates a problem because it takes flesh, pieces of flesh from our hands." Guadalupe, California

### HOUSING

"My slogan is, there must be a way to build houses. I believe we have the right to live in a decent way. We are the labor force. It's like we are foreigners—I am a U.S. citizen.

Farmworkers come here with hope, but go home worse off than before." Unidentified male farmworker, Colorado

"We have no coolers in the summer and no heaters in the winter. Temperatures range up to 100 degrees in the summer and 30 degrees in the winter. We work out in the open for 12 or more hours and after working there for more than 12 hours, we have no place to rest. This creates a tremendous amount of frustration, not being able to provide the children with the minimum for comfort." Margarita, California

"The foremen even charged [the farmworkers] for sleeping under the trees." Teresa, California

### WOMEN

"Another thing I would like to mention is the way we are treated as women. As women we are discriminated with our co-workers because they see us as insignificant beings. The men think that they are superior." Maria, California

### CHILDREN AND YOUTH

"[The children] go out to the fields. They lay under the trees and there is a residue falling on the children. They are picking grapes, what happens? The sprayers are there with the residue falling on the children." Irma, Oregon

"We have worked in the fields! Well, I'm not very young but I've left some of my youth in the work." Juliana, Washington

From Galarneau C, editor: *Under the weather: farm worker health,* Austin, Tex, 1993, National Advisory Council on Migrant Health, Bureau of Primary Health Care, USDHHS.

---

- *Lack of knowledge about services.* Because of their isolation, migrant farmworkers lack the usual sources of information about available services, especially if they are not receiving public benefits.
- *Inability to afford care.* Medicaid, which is intended to serve the poor, is too often not available to migrant farmworkers, who may not remain in a geographic area long enough to be considered for benefits or may lose benefits when they relocate to a state with different eligibility standards. Their salaries may fluctuate by the month, resulting in ineligible periods.

### WHAT DO YOU THINK?

Substandard wages paid to migrant farmworkers allow Americans to pay less for their fruits and vegetables.

- *Availability of services.* The welfare reform legislation of 1996 changed the availability of federal services accessible to certain immigrants to this country (Mines, Gabbard, and Steinman, 1997). Immigrants are treated differently depending on whether they were in the United States before August 22, 1996, and depending on the category of immigrant status

to which they are assigned. As a result of this legislation, each state determined whether to fill any or part of the services gap to immigrants. Many legal immigrants and undocumented immigrants are ineligible for services such as Supplemental Security Income and food stamps. Overall, less than 20% of the total farmworker population is reached by public health funds (Helsinki Commission, 1993; Mines et al, 1997; National Association of Community Health Centers, 1991; National Farmworker Health Conference, 1998).

- *Transportation.* Health care services may be located a great distance from work or home, and transportation to and from sites may be unavailable. Transportation can be unreliable and expensive and most migrant farmworkers do not own their own vehicles (Mines et al, 1991). Privacy is compromised when migrant workers depend on employers to provide transportation to clinics (Casseta, 1994; Caudle, 1993; USDHHS, 1993).
- *Hours of services.* Many health services are available only during work hours; therefore seeking health care results in loss of earnings.
- *Mobility and tracking.* As migrant families move from job to job, their health care records do not typically

go with them, which leads to fragmented services in such areas as tuberculosis (TB) treatment, chronic illness management, and immunizations. For example, health departments are known to dispense TB medications on a monthly basis. Adequate treatment for TB requires 6 to 12 months of medication. When the migrant farmworker relocates, he or she must independently seek out new health services to continue medications. Furthermore, fear of immigration authorities may deter clients with TB from seeking continued health care (Asch, Leake, and Gerberg, 1994).

- *Discrimination.* Although migrant farmworkers and their families bring revenue into the community, they are often perceived as poor, uneducated, transient, and ethnically different. These perceptions foster acts of discrimination against them.
- *Documentation.* Many farmworkers and their families are legal residents of the United States. However, some workers are undocumented and not in compliance with Immigration and Naturalization Service regulations. Some illegal workers fear that securing services in a federally funded or state-funded clinic may lead to discovery and deportation.
- *Language.* The recruitment and retention of bicultural/bilingual health care provider staff is a priority of the National Farmworker Health Conference (1998).
- *Cultural aspects of health care.* (See Cultural Considerations in Migrant Health Care, later.)

## OCCUPATIONAL AND ENVIRONMENTAL HEALTH PROBLEMS

Agricultural work is the third most dangerous occupation in the United States (National Safety Council, 1996). Working conditions, chemical exposure, and use of machinery produce health risks for the migrant farmworkers who may be inadequately protected. A panel of experts convened by the National Institute of Occupational Safety and Health in 1995 identified occupational health risks for agricultural workers. These included musculoskeletal injuries, traumatic injuries, respiratory problems, dermatitis, infectious diseases, cancer, and eye problems (NACMH, 1995).

Injuries such as falls, cuts, and amputations are common in agricultural work (Bureau of Labor Statistics, 2000;

---

**DID YOU KNOW?**

In many states, workers' compensation benefits are not available to migrant farmworkers for on-the-job injuries.

Mines R, Gabbard S, Steinman A: *A profile of U.S. farm workers, demographics, household composition, income and use of services,* Washington DC, April, 1997, U.S. Department of Labor, Office of the Assistant Secretary for Policy, Commission on Immigration Reform.

---

Myers, 1997). Lack of a comprehensive surveillance system makes it difficult to know the extent of all injuries within the migrant population. Reported injuries have included fractures or sprains from falls from ladders or equipment; strains and sprains from prolonged stooping, heavy lifting, and carrying; amputations, deaths, and crush injuries from tractors, trucks, or other machinery; pesticide poisoning; electrical injuries; and drowning in ditches.

The physical demands of harvesting crops 12 to 14 hours a day take a toll on the musculoskeletal system. Stooping over to pick strawberries all day, reaching overhead while on a ladder to pick pears, lifting heavy crates with straight legs—all will cause pain by day's end. Back and neck pains were the most common types of chronic pain reported, and many workers leave or change jobs as a result (Strong and Maralani, 1998; Villarejo et al, 2000).

Naturally occurring plant substances or applied chemicals can cause irritation to the skin (contact dermatitis) or to the eyes (allergic or chemical conjunctivitis). Green tobacco sickness (dermal exposure to wet tobacco) was experienced by 50% of tobacco workers interviewed in North Carolina (Quandt et al, 2000). Infectious diseases caused by poor sanitary conditions at work and home, poor-quality drinking water, and contaminated foods take the form of acute gastroenteritis and zoonoses (Ciesielski et al, 1992; Wilk, 1993). Eye problems, secondary to exposure to chemicals, dust, and pollen, have been documented (Mines, Mullinax, and Saca, 2001; Myers, 1997; Villarejo et al, 2000). When unavailability of resources results in the lack of eye care, these individuals may develop chronic eye problems and even loss of vision. Cancer is another cited but not well documented health problem for migrant farmworkers, mainly because of their exposure to chemicals. A high prevalence of breast cancer, brain tumors, non-Hodgkin's lymphoma, and leukemia have been found in agricultural communities (Larson, 2001; Ray and Richards, 2001).

---

**WHAT DO YOU THINK?**

Benefits to migrants should be provided equitably in every state. Do you agree or disagree?

---

## Pesticide Exposure

The vast majority of the North American food supply is treated with pesticides. Organophosphate pesticides, which are the largest group of pesticides in current use, are known to be potential hazards (Villarejo and Baron, 1999; Von Essen and McCurdy, 1998). Farmworkers are exposed not only to the immediate effects of working in fields that are foggy or wet with pesticides but also to the unknown long-term effects of chronic exposure to pesticides. The migrant farmworker's dwelling also can be a major source of contamination for the worker and his family. The Environmental Protection Agency (EPA) and the Occupational Safety and Health Administration (OSHA) require that farmworkers be given information regarding pesticide safety. Studies have shown that migrant farmworkers may not receive this information or are receiving ineffectual training (Larson, 2000; Mines et al, 1997; Napolitano et al, 2002)

Acute health effects of **pesticide exposure** include mild psychological and behavioral deficits, such as memory loss, difficulty with concentration, mood changes, abdominal pain, nausea, vomiting, diarrhea, headache, malaise, skin rashes, and eye irritation. Acute severe pesticide poisoning can result in death (Moses, 1989). More chronic exposure may lead to cancer, blindness, Parkinson's disease, infertility or sterility, liver damage, and polyneuropathy and neurobehavioral problems (Moses, 1989; Zahm and Blair, 1993). Health professionals who are not educated in the recognition and treatment of pesticide illness may attribute the farmworker's symptoms and physical findings to other causes.

Although legislation is in effect to minimize pesticide risk, migrant farmworker families remain at high risk for exposure. Lack of resources for monitoring, culturally inappropriate educational methods, migrants' fear of reporting violations and being fired, and language differences are just a few of the barriers that hinder a safer pesticide environment for migrant farmworkers.

## Other Specific Health Problems

Dental disease ranks as one of the top five health problems for farmworkers aged 5 to 19 (Dever, 1991). Farmworkers of all ages consistently have more dental disease than the general population. In a 1999 California agricultural worker health survey, high rates of untreated caries, missing or broken teeth, and gingivitis were found (Villarejo et al, 2000). Inadequate knowledge of oral health and lack of access to care (and the resources to pay) were prevalent among those surveyed. Farmworkers do not seek dental care unless they have an oral emergency (Entwistle and Swanson, 1989); therefore they have no opportunities for

the dental education that occurs during regular dental visits. Funding to increase access to dental care has been insufficient to meet the needs of this population. Without insurance or personal resources, private dentistry is usually not an option for the farmworker. Those migrant health centers with dental care experience a high rate of utilization (Lombardi, 2001).

The incidence of TB is estimated to be higher among migrant farmworkers than in the general population (Centers for Disease Control and Prevention [CDC], 1992). TB is more common among immigrants from countries with higher rates of the disease (McCurdy, Arretz, and Bates, 1997), including migrants from Mexico, Haiti, and Southeast Asia. Frequently, the disease is resistant to commonly used antituberculosis drugs (CDC, 1992). The mobility of the migrant farmworkers and their lack of resources make it difficult to screen, treat, and monitor individuals and families for TB. Migrant farmworkers also experience increased respiratory problems such as chronic wheezing, coughing, and phlegm production (Garcia, Dresser, and Zerr, 1996).

Studies have found higher rates of HIV-seropositive individuals among migrant farmworkers than among persons born in the United States (CDC, 1992; Jones, 1992; Lyons, 1992), including women farmworkers who have been infected from heterosexual contact (Skjerkal, Misha, and Benavides-Vaello, 1996). Migrant farmworkers are at high risk for HIV because of their lack of education, low use of condoms, and social isolation, which can lead to drug abuse and multiple sexual contacts.

The mental health status of migrant farmworkers has only recently begun to be assessed, although this population is exposed to considerable stressors—especially the lack of support from family, friends, and community. High depression levels have been identified among migrant farmworkers and have been associated with such factors as high acculturative stress, low self-esteem, and discrimination (Hovey and Magana, 2000). Migrant farmworkers may be also at risk for developing anxiety-related disorders (Hovey and Magana, 2002). One study of migrant children in North Carolina (Kupersmidt and Martin, 1997) found alarmingly elevated levels of mental health problems. These included phobias, different types of anxiety, avoidance, and depression. Although minimal documentation is available, we have heard the complaint of "nervousness" many times from younger males while delivering primary care in migrant camps.

The duties and responsibilities of migrant women place them at risk for experiencing significant anxiety. In addition to working all day under the same conditions as the men, the women then return home to cook, clean, and take care of the children. Unfortunately, an unknown number of these women experience domestic violence. Two studies (Rodriguez, 1998; Van Hightower, Gorton, and DeMoss, 2000) have shown that approximately 20% of farmworker women surveyed reported physical abuse in the past year. Domestic violence is a major health problem with significant physical, emotional, and psychological

---

> **HOW TO** **Recognize the Symptoms of Pesticide Exposure**
>
> Symptoms of pesticide exposure vary according to the amount and length of time of exposure. Most body systems can be affected by pesticide exposure.
> - Symptoms of acute poisoning include neuromuscular symptoms (headache, dizziness, confusion, irritability, twitching muscles, muscle weakness), respiratory symptoms (shortness of breath, difficulty breathing, nasal and pharyngeal irritation), and gastrointestinal symptoms (nausea, vomiting, diarrhea, stomach cramps).
> - Symptoms of chronic exposure are related to illnesses such as cancers, Parkinson's disease, infertility or sterility, liver damage, polyneuropathy, and neurobehavioral problems.
>
> If symptoms of pesticide exposure are suspected, the nurse should develop a pesticide exposure history. A good example of an exposure form can be found at http://pesticide.umd.edu.

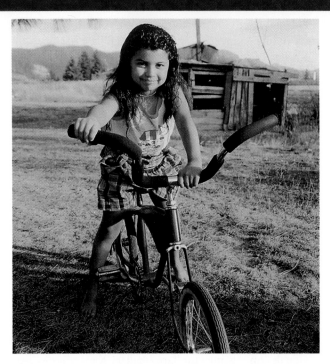

Children of migrant farmworkers experience many hardships. They may have to help with the agricultural work while trying to maintain their schoolwork and to fit into two different cultures. These efforts can be difficult, especially if the children frequently have to move or are often sick.

consequences. Because of the lack of access to care and information, migrant women may not receive prenatal care early or at all. The infant mortality rate is 25% higher for the migrant population than for the general population (National Center for Farmworker Health, 2001).

## CHILDREN AND YOUTHS

Migrant farmworker parents want a better future for their children. In fact, this strong desire was the catalyst for many farmworkers to leave their country of origin. These children often appear to the outsider as happy, outgoing, and inquisitive. On the surface, they may look like children in any other aggregate. However, these children often suffer from health care deficits, including malnutrition (vitamin A, iron), infectious diseases (upper respiratory infection, gastroenteritis), dental caries (due to prolonged use of the bottle, bottle propping, limited access to fluoride and dental care), inadequate immunization status, pesticide exposure, injuries, overcrowding and poor housing conditions, and disruption of their social and school life.

Children of migrant farmworkers may need to work for the family's economic survival. The number of migrant farmworker children under age 14 is unknown. According to the Fair Labor Standards Act, the minimum age that a child can work in agriculture is 14 years, although the age is 16 in other industries (Davis, 2001). Children 12 to 13 years of age can work on a farm with the parents' consent or if the parent works on the same farm, and children younger than 12 can work on a farm with fewer than seven full time workers (Davis, 2001). Some additional protections are provided to children by the majority of states, such as limiting the number of hours per day and per week.

Some adolescent farmworkers accompany their parents to work; however, others are either alone or have accompanied an uncle, a cousin, or a friend. These children are the most vulnerable to low wages; no education; social isolation; risks associated with alcohol, drug, and HIV; and occupational hazards. Although data are limited, fatal injuries to children who work in agriculture were found in one study to be 8.0 per 100,000 between 1991 and 1993, and nonfatal injuries were 1717 per 100,000 between 1990 and 1993 (Rivara, 1997). Machinery, drowning, and firearms/explosives were the three leading causes of deaths for farmworker children (Rivara, 1997).

### DID YOU KNOW?

Farmworker children are excluded from the protection of the 1938 Child Labor Act. Children as young as 10 years can work in the fields. Annually, 300 children die in work-related injuries, and 25,000 are injured (Helsinki Commission, 1993).

Federal law does not protect children from overwork and does not set limits related to the time of day when they work. Therefore children may work until late in the evenings or start very early in the mornings every day of the week if not protected by state law or if inadequately monitored. In Oregon in 2001, adolescent farmworkers shared that they were frequently too tired after working to do homework and to attend classes. Children of migrant farmworkers in general are likely to attend an average of 24 different schools by fifth grade (National Farmworker Health Conference, 1998). Frequent change of schools and constant fatigue set these children up for failure. It has been reported that only 55% of migrant children graduate from high school nationwide (National Center for Farmworker Health, 2001).

Some children of migrant farmworkers stay home to care for younger children. We have visited camps in Oregon where 8- to 10-year-old girls were caring for their siblings and for other children alone. The Migrant Head Start Program is a safe, healthy, and educative option for children 6 months to 5 years old. However, inadequate funding results in lack of services for all migrant children. The Migrant Education Program is a state and nationally sponsored summer school program for farmworkers' children over 5 years of age. However, this program also is not available to all eligible migrant youths.

Nurses can play an important role in the lives of migrant children as portrayed in the words of migrant children in southern Georgia. During focus groups, these children talked about the importance of nurses in their health and health care (Wilson, Pittman, and Wold, 2000). For example, one child stated, "the nurses teach you how to stay healthy, like good things to eat, how to stay safe, and how to learn in school," and another child said "the nurse also told us how to stay safe in our neighborhood, like staying away from people who drink and take drugs" (Wilson et al, 2000, p. 143).

## CULTURAL CONSIDERATIONS IN MIGRANT HEALTH CARE

To provide culturally competent care to migrant farmworkers, nurses need to appreciate and become more knowledgeable about the cultural backgrounds of these individuals. As the majority of migrant farmworkers are of Mexican descent, this section will focus on that culture.

Although certain health beliefs and practices have been identified with the Mexican culture, the nurse must remember that beliefs and practices differ between regions and localities of a country, and between individuals. Mexico is a multicultural country, and the cultural backgrounds of Mexican immigrants vary with their place of origin. Many indigenous groups in Mexico speak their own group dialect. Mexican immigrants may or may not understand or speak Spanish. Mexican immigrants who are less educated, with fewer economic resources, and from the rural areas tend to possess more traditional beliefs and practices.

### Nurse–Client Relationship

The nurse is considered an authority figure who should respect (respeto) the individual, be able to relate to the individual (personalismo), and maintain the individual's dignity (dignidad). Mexican individuals prefer polite, nonconfrontational relationships with others (simpatia). At times, because of simpatia, individuals and families may appear to understand what is being said to them (by nodding their heads), when in actuality they do not understand. The nurse should take measures to validate the understanding of these individuals. The Mexican individual expects to converse about personal matters (chit-chat) for the first few minutes of an encounter. They expect the nurse not to appear rushed and to be a good listener. Humor is appreciated, and touching as a caring gesture is seen as a positive behavior.

Health professionals may not be the first source of health care sought by Mexican clients, who may have consulted with knowledgeable individuals in their family or community (the popular arena of care) or with folk healers (the traditional arena of care). Examples of members of the popular arena are the señora or wise, older woman living in the community, one's grandmother (la abuela), and the local parish priest.

> **NURSING TIP**
>
> If you regularly work with Latino migrant workers, you will be able to be more helpful if you learn some key Spanish words and phrases.

### Health Values

Family, in general, is a significant component of a Mexican individual's health care and social support system. The woman in the household is considered to be the caretaker, and the man is considered to be the major decision maker. However, Mexican women in certain families have significant influence over most matters including health decisions. Grandmothers and sisters are highly significant to the wife in the immediate family. They provide advice, care, and support.

Not all Mexican immigrants have extended families in the United States. If family members are not present, communication may be maintained with family in Mexico. However, a support system for these individuals may be lacking.

Love of their children, rather than concern for their own health, may encourage migrant parents to adopt healthier lifestyles. One example is when the parents of a child with asthma choose to stop smoking (Perilla et al, 1998). In Oregon, when asked if they protected themselves from pesticide exposure, Mexican migrant parents responded negatively in general. However, they were willing to change their behaviors if, as a result, their children would be protected from pesticides (Napolitano et al, 2002).

The Mexican client may be more willing to follow the advice of another Mexican individual with a similar health problem than the advice of the health professional. For example, 12 Mexican women with diabetes in Oregon stated that their physicians followed the same routine during every visit for their diabetes (Napolitano, 1992). The physician would test their blood, change their medication, and lecture to them about diet and exercise. The women admitted to ignoring these instructions and being disillusioned with the physician. However, these women would ask other Mexican individuals with diabetes about their personal practices for diabetes, and in several cases, would adopt these practices. One woman, who was unable to differentiate between the symptoms of hyper- and hypoglycemia, would drink a bottle of grape juice when she felt her "sugar high."

Although the majority of Mexican immigrants may identify themselves as Catholics, many Mexican individuals belong to other churches. The individual's religion may influence health practices such as birth control; however, the nurse cannot assume that a Catholic, for example, would not use some method of birth control.

### Health Beliefs and Practices

In the Mexican culture, health may be considered a gift from God. Another common perception of health is that a healthy person is one who can continue to work and to perform daily activities independent of symptoms or diagnosed diseases. The nurse should understand that a Mexican individual who does not follow up with a clinic appointment may simply be capable of working that day. Mexican immigrants may believe that illness is a punishment from God and may cite this belief as a rationale for why therapies have not cured them. This more commonly occurs with chronic illnesses. Four other common folk illnesses that a nurse may encounter with the Mexican client are mal de ojo (evil eye), susto (fright), empacho (indigestion), and caida de mollera (fallen fontanel). Symptoms and

## Evidence-Based Practice

Data were evaluated from the Virginia Garcia Migrant Clinic's mobile van program in 2001. The purpose of the project was to describe the population seen, the types of health needs found, and the diagnoses, interventions, and referrals made by the project personnel. Of the 644 clients seen, 75% were male and 25% were female, with half the sample ranging in age from 19 to 30 years. Forty-five percent of the clients were evaluated by a primary care provider, and the remaining 55% received preventive services such as blood pressure screening and tetanus vaccine. The three most common diagnoses were skin infection, muscle strain/sprain, and upper respiratory infection. Medications and education were the major primary care interventions. Analgesics, antifungals, antibiotics, and antacids were the most common medications dispensed. Referrals were made for 83 clients; 68 of those were to the main clinic, and the others were to dental and eye clinics.

The mobile van program provides critical services and identifies both chronic and acute health problems. Unfortunately, client follow-up remains difficult. Further research is needed to test methods of follow-up.

**Nurse Use:** Because of the transient nature of the work of migrants, it is hard to provide continuity of care even when using resources such as a mobile van. Their lack of continuity of care and their exposure to injuries and illnesses puts them in a high risk category of patients.

Rodriguez R et al: *Mobile van program in Washington and Yamhill counties: migrant farmworkers health needs,* abstract from 129th annual meeting of the American Public Health Association, Atlanta, Ga, October 21-25, 2001.

---

### BOX 33-2 Levels of Prevention Related to Migrant Health Issues

**PRIMARY PREVENTION**

Teach migrant workers how to reduce exposure to pesticides.

**SECONDARY PREVENTION**

Conduct screening, such as urine testing for pesticide exposure.

**TERTIARY PREVENTION**

Initiate treatment for the symptoms of pesticide exposure such as nausea, vomiting, and skin irritation.

---

## THE CUTTING EDGE

The Migrant Clinicians' Network sponsors annual national migrant health fellowships for graduates of health professional programs. As an outcome of the ongoing commitment of the School of Nursing at the Oregon Health and Sciences University to providing academic and clinical experiences with migrant farmworker populations in Oregon, five nurse practitioner and midwifery graduates have been awarded this prestigious fellowship in the past 5 years. Information about these fellowships can be obtained at www.mcn.org.

---

treatments may vary depending on the individual's or family's origin in Mexico. Other cultural beliefs, relating to balance between hot and cold, pregnancy, and postpartum behaviors *(cuarentena)*, have been documented. When experiencing a folk illness, the traditional Mexican individual would prefer to seek care with a folk healer. The more common healers are the *curanderos, herbalistas,* and *espiritualistas*. The most commonly used herbs are chamomile *(manzanilla)*, peppermint *(yerba buena)*, aloe vera, cactus *(nopales)*, and *epazote*.

## HEALTH PROMOTION AND ILLNESS PREVENTION

The same principles for health promotion and prevention that apply to the general U.S. population apply also to migrant farmworkers. However, health promotion and disease prevention may be difficult concepts for migrant workers to embrace because of their beliefs regarding disease causality, their irregular and episodic contact with the

health care system, and their lower educational level (on average, sixth grade).

Health promotion begins by informing the farmworker family about health topics and the resources available to improve their health. Several migrant health programs have recruited migrant workers to serve as outreach workers and lay camp aides to assist in outreach and health education of the workers. Outreach, as defined by the Migrant Health Program, should "improve utilization of health services, improve effectiveness of health services, provide comprehensive health services, be accessible, be acceptable, and be appropriate to the population served" (USDHHS, 1993, p. 54). Outreach programs succeed because they recognize the diversity of this group and the need for flexibility in the provision of services. Because these outreach workers are members of the migrant community, they are trusted and know the culture and the language (Watkins and Larson, 1991). Nurses can be part of the planning and teaching for these programs.

## ROLE OF THE NURSE

Community-oriented nurses are in an ideal position to maximize health by attending to prevention at the primary, secondary, and tertiary levels (as defined in Chapter 14). As applied to the health of migrant and seasonal farmworkers,

## ENVIRONMENTAL HEALTH

8-13 Reduce pesticide exposures that result in visits to a health care facility

8-24 Reduce exposure to pesticides as measured by urine concentrations of metabolites

## IMMUNIZATIONS AND INFECTIOUS DISEASES

14-1 Reduce or eliminate indigenous cases of vaccine-preventable diseases

14-11 Reduce tuberculosis

14-12 Increase the proportion of all tuberculosis patients who complete curative therapy within 12 months

## MATERNAL, INFANT, AND CHILD HEALTH

16-6 Increase the proportion of pregnant women who receive early and adequate prenatal care

## OCCUPATIONAL SAFETY AND HEALTH

20-1 Reduce deaths from work-related injuries

20-2 Reduce work-related injuries resulting in medical treatment, lost time from work, or restricted work activity

20-8 Reduce occupational skin diseases or disorders among full-time workers

## ORAL HEALTH

21-10 Increase the proportion of children and adults who use the oral health care system each year

21-12 Increase the proportion of low-income children and adolescents who received any preventative dental service during the past year

## SEXUALLY TRANSMITTED DISEASES

25-8 Reduce HIV infections in adolescent and young adult females aged 13 to 24 years that are associated with heterosexual contact

From U.S. Department of Health and Human Services: *Healthy people 2010: national health promotion and disease prevention objectives,* ed 2, Washington, DC, 2000, U.S. Government Printing Office.

---

### BOX 33-3    Assessing Migrant Workers

Faculty members and community health nursing and family nurse practitioner students relocated to a rural southeastern U.S. county to provide health care to migrant farmworkers. During the 2-week immersion learning experience, we noted that migrant workers were most receptive to obtaining health services after 4 P.M. We also realized that a mobile health van located in the camps where the workers lived was used more often than a better-equipped migrant health care facility located farther away.

---

primary prevention activities include education for the prevention of infectious diseases such as HIV, measures to reduce pesticide exposure (Box 33-2), and immunizations in childhood and adulthood, especially for TB. Secondary prevention activities include urine screening for pesticide exposure, TB skin-testing, diabetes screening, and prenatal monitoring and diagnostic testing. Tertiary prevention includes rehabilitation for musculoskeletal injury, especially low back pain, and treatments for lead poisoning and anemia.

The health status of all people is a function of their ecology, or all that "touches" them. The nurse keeps a finger on the pulse of the community by remaining active in the political, social, religious, and employment areas that involve the client. The nurse can be a catalyst for change to continually assess farmworker needs, to direct efforts to obtain needed health care services, and to evaluate the success of those efforts. Acting as a community educator, knowledgeable about how to obtain the latest information and resources, the nurse can work to assess the infrastructure and needs of the community.

The Healthy People 2010 box lists the objectives that most closely relate to health promotion and disease prevention in migrant farmworkers. They were selected on the basis of occupational, lifestyle, and socioeconomic factors that place migrant farmworkers and their families at unique risk for suboptimal health.

Follow-up assessments by the nurse are critical. For example, the needs assessment might indicate inadequate child and adult immunizations, which may best be provided in the fields, camps, and schools. The nurse may create an immunization tracking system to share information with other counties and states as the farmworkers migrate (Box 33-3).

Nurses can take responsibility for the screening and monitoring of migrant farmworkers' health. Diseases such as TB, diabetes, and hypertension are frequently missed in a mobile population without access to care. Nurses can create programs for screening in migrant camps and other farmworker housing. After problems are identified and treated, nurses can monitor the success of medication regimes, preventive measures, and follow-up within the health care system. The nurse can provide culturally specific health promotion and disease prevention materials, as well as information about any further referral sources. Selected resources for the nurse working with migrant farmworkers can be found on this book's evolve website at http://evolve.elsevier.com/Stanhope.

Nurses can be social and **political advocates** for the migrant population. Educating communities about these individuals, collecting necessary data on their lives and health, and communicating with legislators and other policymakers at local, state, and national levels are needed actions that nurses are prepared to undertake, but there are barriers that must be overcome. It is clearly a challenge for nurses to make a difference in the health of migrant farmworkers and their families in rural communities where most full-time residents are well known to one other, where farmers hold the community purse strings, and where migrant workers are often exploited, discriminated against, and ostracized.

## Practice Application

Louisa is 17 years old and has spent most of her life as a migrant farmworker. Her family (her father and two siblings) work most of the year, traveling up the east coast of the United States and picking crops in season. She is presently picking tobacco in the southeastern United States. One evening after finishing her work, she asks to speak with Joan, a nurse who is with the medical van parked outside the trailer camp where Louisa and her family live. She is most concerned about a rash on her hands, arms, and chest. Joan notes that Louisa's eyes are red and she occasionally coughs. Louisa asks Joan for something for her rash. She wants treatment quickly, so the rash will go away and she will be able to work without scratching. Louisa seems to be in a great hurry and says she does not want her father to know she stopped by the van because he would be angry. While waiting for the nurse practitioner, Joan, who speaks fluent Spanish, asks if Louisa has any other problems. Initially hesitant, Louisa says she wishes she should go to school on a regular basis. She is most concerned about her brother and sister, ages 8 and 10, who work in the fields as well. She says they constantly cough and have been having breathing trouble, especially when her father smokes, when the wind blows dust around their trailer, and when picking crops soon after pesticides have been sprayed.

  A. Determine the additional information needed to complete an assessment of Louisa and her family. Recognizing the specific cultural concerns, how would you obtain this information?
  B. List community resources that might be available for Louisa and her family.
  C. Discuss potential barriers that may prevent access to health care and other services.

---

**Answers are in the back of the book.**

## Key Points

- A migrant farmworker is a laborer whose principal employment involves moving from farm to farm, planting or harvesting agricultural products and obtaining temporary housing.
- An estimated 3 to 5 million migrant farmworkers are in the United States. The number is controversial because of the inconsistency in defining farmworkers and limitations in obtaining data.

- The life expectancy of the migrant farmworker is 49 years, compared with 75 years for other U.S. residents.
- Health problems of migrant farmworkers are linked to their work environment, limited access to health services and education, and lack of economic opportunities.
- Migrant farmworkers are faced with uncertainty regarding work and housing, inadequate wages, unsafe working conditions, and lack of enforcement of legislation for field sanitation and safety regulations.
- Farmworkers are subject not only to the immediate effects of pesticides in the fields, but also to the unknown long-term effects of chronic exposure.
- When harvesting is completed, the farmworker is simultaneously homeless and unemployed. Forced migration to find employment leaves little time or energy to seek out and improve living standards.
- Children of migrant farmworkers may need to work for the family's economic survival.

## Clinical Decision-Making Activities

1. Outreach workers are generally hired by an agency, such as a health department; they provide education to migrant persons. Lay health promoters are often from a community of migrant people who also provide community-based education. Find out if both of these roles exist in your community. Interview or work with these workers for a few hours. Compare and contrast their roles. How are they complementary? How are they duplicative? How can they work together to maximize health? How are their approaches to education different? (For example, does one use a protocol or template while the other is led by community concerns?)
2. Interview community leaders to determine the presence of migrant farmworkers in your area. Gather information about migrant farmworkers by interviewing teachers, clergy, and politicians, and compare and contrast it with the information you obtain from migrant outreach workers, personnel from the Wage and Hour Bureau, Department of Labor personnel, and Migrant Head Start program employees.
3. In some areas of the United States, placement agencies specialize in helping businesses hire migrant workers. Determine whether an agency of this type exists in your area. If it does, interview a key person and ask how they recruit workers, how long workers typically stay in one location, what health screening they do, and who provides health services to the workers they place.
4. Determine eligibility for Medicaid and Temporary Assistance to Needy Families services. You may consult the county health department and the state office. Do migrant workers in your state qualify?

5. Design a clinic to provide health care to migrant workers in your area. What services would you provide? What hours would you operate? How would you staff the clinic?

6. The following are a few settings and RN-delivered services for migrant clients. Can you propose others?

   • Health departments (generally state and county funded) monitor communicable diseases, treat communicable outbreaks such as tuberculosis and pertussis.

   • Migrant camps (generally funded through migrant clinics or health departments) assess and triage, take vital signs, dispense medications (under protocol), educate, interview families (know families well), coordinate care in conjunction with health department RN.

   • Migrant clinics (generally federally funded) work with client's primary care provider, hold prenatal programs (both classes and home visits), handle diabetes intervention, and do follow-up.

**Additional Resources**

These related resources are found either in the appendix at the back of this book or on the book's website at **http://evolve.elsevier.com/Stanhope.**

*evolve* **Evolve Website**

Resources for the Nurse Working With Migrant Farmworkers

WebLinks: Healthy People 2010

# References

Adam V: Health status of vulnerable populations, *Ann Public Health* 15:487, 1994.

Asch S, Leake B, Gerberg L: Does fear of immigration authorities deter tuberculosis patients from seeking care? *West J Med* 161(4):373, 1994.

Bureau of Labor Statistics: *Workplace injuries and illnesses in 1999,* Washington DC, 2000, Bureau of Labor Statistics.

Cassetta R: Needs of migrant health workers challenge RNs, *Am Nurse* 6(6):34, 1994.

Caudle P: Providing culturally sensitive health care to Hispanic clients, *Nurse Pract* 18(12):40, 1993.

Centers for Disease Control and Prevention: *1990 tuberculosis statistics in the United States,* Atlanta, 1992, U.S. Department of Health and Human Services.

Ciesielski S et al: Intestinal parasites among North Carolina migrant farmworkers, *Am J Public Health* 82:1258-1262, 1992.

Davis S: Child labor, *Migrant health issues, monograph series,* October 2001, National Center for Farmworker Health.

Decker S, Knight L: Functional health assessment: a seasonal migrant farm worker community, *J Community Health Nurse* 7(3):141, 1990.

Dever A: *Profile of a population with complex health problems,* Austin, Tex, 1991, Migrant Clinicians' Network.

Entwistle B, Swanson T: Dental needs and perceptions of adult Hispanic migrant farmworkers in Colorado, *J Dent Health* July-Aug:286-292, 1989.

Galarneau C, editor: *Under the weather: farm worker health,* Austin, Tex, 1993, National Advisory Council on Migrant Health, Bureau of Primary Health Care, USDHHS.

Garcia F, Dresser K, Zerr A: Respiratory health of Hispanic migrant farm workers in Indiana, *Am J Ind Med* 29:23-32, 1996.

Helsinki Commission: *Migrant farm workers in the United States,* briefings of the Commission on Security and Cooperation in Europe, Washington, DC, 1993, U.S. Government Printing Office.

Holden C: *Survey of demand for the RHS farm labor housing,* Washington, DC, 2001, Housing Assistance Council.

Hovey J, Magana C: Acculturative stress, anxiety, and depression among Mexican immigrant farmworkers in the Midwest United States, *J Immigrant Health* 2:119-131, 2000.

Hovey J, Magana C: Cognitive, affective, and physiological expressions of anxiety symptomatology among Mexican migrant farmworkers: predictors and generational differences, *Community Ment Health J* 38(3):223-237, 2002.

Jones J: HIV-related characteristics of migrant workers in rural South Carolina, *Migrant Health Newsline* Mar/Apr, 1992.

Kupersmidt J, Martin S: Mental health problems of children of migrant and seasonal farm workers: a pilot study, *J Am Acad Child Adolesc Psychiatry* 36:224-232, 1997.

Larson A, Plascencia L: *Migrant enumeration project 1993,* Rockville, Md, 1993, Bureau of Primary Health Care.

Larson A: *An assessment of worker training under the Worker Protection Standard,* Washington, DC, 2000, EPA, Office of Pesticide Programs.

Larson A: Environmental/occupational safety and health, *Migrant health issues, monograph series,* October 2001, National Center for Farmworkers Health.

Lombardi G: Dental/oral health services, *Migrant health issues, monograph series,* October 2001, National Center for Farmworker Health.

Lopez N: Meeting the challenge: providing migrant farmworker housing, *Rural Voices* Fall:3-7, 1995.

Lyons M: Study yields HIV prevalence for New Jersey farmworkers, *Migrant Health Newsline* March/April, 1992.

McCurdy S, Arretz D, Bates R: Tuberculin reactivity among California Hispanic migrant farm workers, *Am J Ind Med* 33:600-605, 1997.

Mines R, Gabbard S, Boccalandro B: *Findings from the National Agricultural Worker's Survey 1990, a demographic and employment profile of perishable crop farm workers,* Washington, DC, 1991, U.S. Department of Labor, Office of Program Economics Research Report No. 1.

Mines R, Gabbard S, Samadrick R: *U.S. farmworkers in the post-IRCA period,* Washington DC, 1993, U.S. Department of Labor.

Mines R, Gabbard S, Steinman A: *A profile of U.S. farm workers, demographics, household composition, income and use of services,* Washington DC, April, 1997, U.S. Department of Labor, Office of the Assistant Secretary for Policy, Commission on Immigration Reform.

Mines R, Mullinax N, Saca L: *The Binational Farmworker Health Survey: an in-depth study of agricultural worker health in Mexico and the United States,* Davis, Calif, 2001, California Institute for Rural Studies.

Mobed IK, Gold E, Schenker M: Occupational health problems among migrant and seasonal farmworkers, *West J Med* 157(3):367, 1992.

Moses M: Pesticide-related health problems and farmworkers, *Am Assoc Occup Health Nurses J* 37:115-130, 1989.

Mull L et al: National farmworker database: establishing a farmworker cohort for epidemiologic research, *Am J Ind Med* 40:612-618, 2001.

Myers J: *Injuries among farmworkers in the United States, 1993,* DHHS (NIOSH) publication No. 97-115, Cincinnati, OH, 1997, Department of Health and Human Services.

Napolitano M: "Lived experiences of Oregon Mexican American women with diabetes and selected family members," unpublished dissertation, 1992, Oregon Health & Sciences University.

Napolitano M et al: Un lugar seguro para sus ninos: development and evaluation of a pesticide education video, *J Immig Health* 4(1):35-45, 2002.

National Advisory Council on Migrant Health: *Recommendations of the National Advisory Council on Migrant Health,* Rockville, Md, 1993, Department of Health and Human Services, Bureau of Primary Health Care.

National Advisory Council on Migrant Health: *Losing ground: the condition of farmworkers in America,* Rockville, Md, 1995, Department of Health and Human Services, Bureau of Primary Health Care.

National Association of Community Health Centers: *Medicaid and migrant farm worker families: analysis of barriers and recommendations for change,* Washington, DC, 1991, National Association of Community Health Centers.

National Center for Farmworker Health: Introduction, *Migrant health issues, monograph series,* 2001, National Center for Farmworker Health.

National Farmworker Health Conference: Houston, Tex, May 13-17, 1998, National Advisory Council on Migrant Health.

National Migrant Resource Program for the Office of Migrant Health: Bureau of Health Care Delivery and Assistance, Public Health Service, Health Resources and Services Administration, U.S. Department of Health and Human Services, 1990.

National Safety Council: *Accident facts,* Itasca, Ill, 1996, National Safety Council.

Office of the Federal Registrar: *Code of federal regulations,* Public Health Title 42, Chapter 1, Section 56.102, 1994.

Oliveira V, Effland J, Hamm S: *Hired farm labor use on fruit, vegetable, and horticultural specialty farms,* Washington DC, 1993, U.S. Department of Agriculture.

Perilla J et al: Listening to migrant voices: focus groups on health issues in South Georgia, *J Community Health Nurs* 15(4):251-263, 1998.

Quandt S et al: Migrant farmworkers and green tobacco sickness: new issues for an understudied disease, *Am J Ind Med* 37:307-315, 2000.

Ray D, Richards P: The potential for toxic effects of chronic, low dose exposure to organophosphates, *Toxicol Lett* 120:343-351, 2001.

Rivara F: Fatal and non-fatal farm injuries to children and adolescents in the United States, 1990-3, *Inj Prev* 3(3):190-194, 1997.

Rodriguez R: Clinical interventions with battered migrant farmworker women. In Campbell J, editor: *Empowering survivors of abuse,* Newbury Park, Calif, 1998, Sage.

Rodriguez R et al: *Mobile van program in Washington and Yamhill counties: migrant farmworkers health needs,* abstract from 129th annual meeting of the American Public Health Association, Atlanta, Ga, October 21-25, 2001.

Skjerkal K, Misha S, Benavides-Vaello S: A growing HIV/AIDS crisis among migrant and seasonal farmworker families, *Migrant Clinicians' Network Streamline* 2:1-3, 1996.

Slesinger D, Ofstead C: Economic and health care needs of Wisconsin migrant farmworkers, *J Rural Health* 9:138-148, 1993.

Strong M, Maralani V: *Farmworkers and disability: results of a national survey,* Berkeley, Calif, 1998, Berkeley Planning Associates.

U.S. Department of Health and Human Services: *Healthy people 2000: national health promotion and disease prevention objectives,* Washington, DC, 1991, USDHHS, Public Health Service.

U.S. Department of Health and Human Services: *1993 recommendations of the National Advisory Council on Migrant Health,* Austin, Tex, 1993, National Advisory Council on Migrant Health, National Migrant Resource Program.

U.S. Department of Health and Human Services: *1994 update to the recommendations of the National Advisory Council on Migrant Health,* Austin, Tex, 1994, National Advisory Council on Migrant Health, National Migrant Resource Program.

U.S. Department of Health and Human Services: *1998 update to the recommendations of the National Advisory Council on Migrant Health,* Austin, Tex, 1998, National Migrant Resource Program.

U.S. Department of Labor: *National agricultural worker's survey,* 1997, Office of the Assistant Secretary for Policy.

U.S. Department of Health and Human Services: *Healthy people 2010: national health promotion and disease prevention objectives,* ed 2, Washington, DC, 2000, U.S. Government Printing Office.

Van Hightower N, Gorton J, DeMoss C: Predictive models of domestic violence and fear of intimate partners among migrant and seasonal farm worker women, *J Fam Violence* 15(2):137-154, 2000.

Villarejo D, Baron S: The occupational health status of hired farm workers: state of the art reviews, *Occup Med* 14(3):613-635, 1999.

Villarejo D et al: *Suffering in silence: a report on the health of California's agricultural workers,* Davis, Calif, 2000, California Institute for Rural Studies.

Von Essen SG, McCurdy SA: Health and safety risks in production agriculture, *West J Med* 169:214-220, 1998.

Watkins E, Larson K: *Migrant lay health advisors: a strategy for health promotion, a final report,* Chapel Hill, NC, 1991, University of North Carolina.

Wilk V: Health hazards to children in agriculture, *Am J Ind Med* 24:283-290, 1993.

Wilson A, Pittman K, Wold J: Listening to the quiet voices of Hispanic migrant children about health, *J Pediatr Nurs* 15(3):137-147, 2000.

Zahm SH, Blair A: Cancer among seasonal farmworkers: an epidemiologic review and research agenda, *Am J Ind Med* 24:753-766, 1993.

# Chapter 34

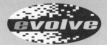 

# Teen Pregnancy

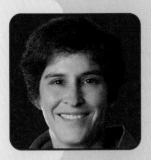

**Dyan A. Aretakis, R.N., F.N.P., M.S.N.**
Dyan A. Aretakis began her nursing practice in pediatrics at the University of Connecticut and at a regional residential facility for the mentally retarded. She went on to co-develop a model Teen Health Center at the University of Virginia Health System in 1990 and currently practices in and directs its daily and long-term programs. This program is unique because it provides a range of adolescent primary health care services as well as community and professional outreach programs.

## Objectives

After reading this chapter, the student should be able to do the following:

1. Discuss approaches that could be used in working with the adolescent client
2. Identify trends in adolescent pregnancy, births, abortions, and adoption in the United States
3. Discuss reasons that may affect whether a teenager becomes pregnant
4. Explain some of the deterrents to the establishment of paternity among young fathers
5. Develop nursing interventions for the prevention of pregnancy problems that adolescents are at risk for experiencing
6. Identify nursing activities that may contribute to the prevention of adolescent pregnancy

---

Teen pregnancy is an area of great public concern because of its significant effect on communities. Resources to support the special needs of pregnant teenagers are decreasing, and the costs of sustaining young families are prohibitive. Many teenagers who become pregnant are caught in a cycle of poverty, school failure, and limited life options. Even under the ideal circumstances of adequate finances, loving and supportive families, and good birth outcomes, a teen parent must circumvent her own necessary developmental tasks to raise her child.

There is neither a uniform reason that teens become pregnant nor a universally acceptable solution. The causes of teen pregnancy are diverse and affected by changing moral attitudes, sexual codes, and economic circumstances. Teen pregnancy places an enormous strain on the health care and social service systems. Social concern also is raised about the lost potential for young parents when pregnancy occurs, and the academic and economic disadvantages that their children will experience. Nurses are in

a key position to understand how teen pregnancy affects both the individual and the community. This chapter presents a variety of issues associated with teen pregnancy and proposes nursing interventions to promote healthy outcomes for individuals and communities.

## ADOLESCENT HEALTH CARE IN THE UNITED STATES

Adolescents are generally healthy, and when they seek health care it is for reasons different from those of adults or young children. The main causes of teen mortality are high-risk behaviors: motor vehicle accidents (usually including alcohol), homicide, suicide, and accidental injuries (such as falls, fires, or drowning). Teens often engage in behaviors that put them at risk for life-threatening diseases. For example, each year, one quarter of both new human immunodeficiency virus (HIV) infections and newly identified sexually transmitted diseases occur among adolescents. It is during the teen years that other behaviors are initiated (e.g., smoking, decreased activity, and poor nutrition) that can ultimately lead to poor health during the adult years. Working with teens requires that nurses provide health education and also influence behavior change that can significantly alter a young person's life.

Several national surveys highlighted the health issues facing adolescents. There have been some improvements in risk behaviors as well as a worsening of others. Among ninth to twelfth graders participating in the 1999 Youth

### DID YOU KNOW?

States spend more on the costs of supporting teen parents and their children than on preventing teen pregnancy. For example, in the Southern states, only a penny is invested in the primary prevention of pregnancy for every dollar spent on public programs to support families begun by teenagers.

## Key Terms

abortion, p. 810
adoption, p. 813
birth control, p. 809
coercive sex, p. 814
gynecologic age, p. 819
intimate partner violence, p. 817

low birth weight, p. 819
paternity, p. 814
peer pressure, p. 809
prematurity, p. 819
prenatal care, p. 817
repeat pregnancy, p. 821

sexual debut, p. 812
sexual victimization, p. 813
statutory rape, p. 814
weight gain, p. 819

*See Glossary for definitions*

## Chapter Outline

Adolescent Health Care in the United States
The Adolescent Client
Trends in Adolescent Sexual Behavior
    and Pregnancy
Background Factors
*Sexual Activity and Use of Birth Control*
*Peer Pressure and Partner Pressure*

*Other Factors*
Young Men and Paternity
Early Identification of the Pregnant Teen
Special Issues in Caring for the Pregnant Teen
*Violence*
*Initiation of Prenatal Care*
*Low-Birth-Weight Infants and Preterm Delivery*

*Nutrition*
*Infant Care*
*Repeat Pregnancy*
*Schooling and Educational Needs*
Teen Pregnancy and the Nurse
*Home-Based Interventions*
*Community-Based Interventions*

Risk Behavior Surveillance System, fewer teens reported carrying a weapon on school property, getting into physical fights, failing to wear a seat belt, and using smokeless tobacco. But other significant risk behaviors continued at high rates. Of ninth to twelfth graders, 50% reported current alcohol use (31% reported episodic heavy drinking); 34% of teens were current cigarette smokers; and 47% had tried marijuana (25% were current users and 11% tried before the age of 13). Seventeen percent of respondents had carried a weapon in the previous month (Centers for Disease Control and Prevention [CDC], 2000b). Mental health issues are also strongly associated with girls during the adolescent years: 18% of high school girls reported eating disorders of binging and purging, 20% had been victims of childhood physical and sexual abuse, and 25% experienced depression. Boys experienced similar mental health concerns but at slightly lower rates (Commonwealth Fund, 1997). Suicide was considered by 10% of girls and 7.5% of boys and attempted by 5% and 2%, respectively (Resnick et al, 1997).

Adolescents may not seek care for these problems for the following reasons: (1) access to health care may be hindered because of a limited number of professionals who have expertise in dealing with teenagers, (2) costs of care or availability of insurance may limit services, (3) adolescents need to believe that their visits are confidential before they will honestly reveal information, and (4) health care professionals must be able to discuss sensitive topics in a nonjudgmental and supportive manner and demonstrate a desire to work with youths. Nurses who want to promote the health of adolescents by providing anticipatory guidance about **peer pressure,** assertiveness, and future planning need to have knowledge of adolescent behaviors, health risks, and the social context in which they live. Involvement and education of the parents about youth culture and development serves to promote positive and supportive parenting of teens.

## THE ADOLESCENT CLIENT

Adolescents have limited experience of independently seeking health care. When they do seek care, it is often to discuss concerns about a possible pregnancy or to find a **birth control** method. These teens may also need assistance negotiating complex health care systems. Special approaches in both the client interview and subsequent client education are often warranted. The behavior of adolescents toward the nurse can range from mature and competent during one visit to hostile, rude, or distant at other times because behavior often reflects intense anxiety over what the teen is experiencing.

Because client interviews usually begin with evaluation of a chief complaint, teens need to know that their concerns are heard. Health care providers may have their own opinions about what teenagers need and may fail to take the chief complaint seriously. For example, when a teen expresses a desire to become pregnant, this should be discussed in depth even though the nurse may feel uncomfortable providing information to a teen about how to conceive. During the interview, the nurse can provide preconception counseling and emphasize the need to achieve good health and to establish a health-promoting lifestyle before pregnancy. Health risks to the mother, as well as to fetal development, can be discussed. Not only does information presented this way demonstrate that the nurse has heard what the teen is saying but also it allows the nurse to provide useful health information that may encourage the teen to examine her plans carefully, seriously, and maturely.

It is also important to pay attention to what the teen *fails* to verbalize. Knowledge of adolescent health care issues is valuable so that the nurse can anticipate other health concerns and provide an environment in which the adolescent feels safe about raising other concerns. By creating a caring and understanding atmosphere, the nurse can encourage the young person to discuss concerns about family violence, drugs, alcohol, or dating.

Discussing reproductive health care is a sensitive matter for both teens and many adults. Teens may have difficulty expressing themselves because of a limited sexual vocabulary or embarrassment resulting from their lack of knowledge. The nurse must recognize this potential deficit and embarrassment and assist teens by anticipating concerns. It is also important to allow teens to express themselves in their own language, which may include crude or offensive words. Nurses must learn about common slang expressions and common misconceptions so they do not miss important concerns that a teenager might have. The nurse can offer more appropriate terms once trust is established.

Teens may have difficulty discussing topics that provoke a judgmental reaction, such as discussing sexually transmitted diseases (STDs) (Box 34-1). It is important for the nurse to choose neutral words to elicit symptoms (e.g., "Has there been a change in your typical vaginal discharge?"). This approach also gives the nurse a chance to educate the young client about normal anatomy and physiology.

Considerable debate exists over whether adolescents should make reproductive health care decisions without their parents' knowledge. As seen in Box 34-2, the adolescent's right to privacy, and thus her right to contraceptive treatment, is federally protected. Obstacles to services do exist, however, and this may result in a teen not receiving contraceptive information and treatment. Obstacles can include lack of transportation to a health care facility, money to pay for services, or permission to leave school early to attend an appointment.

**Abortion** services for adolescents are not clearly defined. No federal protection is extended to adolescents requesting abortion services, and the adolescent's right to privacy and ability to give consent varies by state (Box 34-3). Confidential care to teenagers may mean the difference between preventing an unwanted pregnancy, an abortion, and a birth. This care can influence whether prenatal visits begin in the first trimester or in the second or third trimester. Teens have various reasons for pursuing confidential care, including seeking independence as well as serious and well-founded concerns about a parent's potential reaction (i.e.,

---

### BOX 34-1 Sexually Transmitted Diseases and Teen Pregnancy

Sexually transmitted diseases (STDs) affect 25% of sexually experienced teenagers each year. STDs are more easily transmitted to women than men and can be more difficult to detect. STD infections among women can contribute to infertility, cancer, and ectopic pregnancy. When a young woman is pregnant, these infections can cause premature rupture of membranes, premature labor, and postpartum infection. Also, the baby can be affected by all STDs in several ways: prematurity and low birth weight, febrile infection after delivery, long-term infection, and even death (e.g., exposure to viral infections such as human papilloma virus and herpes simplex virus).

The pregnant adolescent is at high risk for acquiring an STD because she may not be using contraceptives such as condoms. During the pregnancy, she will require periodic STD screening. STD education and counseling should accompany this screening. Information given should include ways to reduce risk, such as maintaining a mutually monogamous relationship and using latex condoms.

---

abuse of the teen). Once nurses recognize the reason for confidential care, they can work with teens to discuss reproductive health care needs with the family. To do so, first clarify family values about sexuality and family communication styles with the teen. In a dysfunctional family, referral to community agencies (e.g., child protective services, Al-Anon) may be necessary. However, the nurse may need to honor the adolescent's need for confidentiality for an unknown period and proceed with the usual interventions, such as pregnancy testing, options counseling, and referral for clinical care.

## TRENDS IN ADOLESCENT SEXUAL BEHAVIOR AND PREGNANCY

Each year 800,000 to 900,000 teens become pregnant, and more than half go on to have babies. Births to teenagers make up 12% of all births in the United States (American College of Obstetricians and Gynecologists [ACOG], 2000). The numbers of teens who become pregnant are generally identified in the following way: by age-group (younger than 15, ages 15 to 17, ages 18 to 19); by pregnancy outcomes (birth, induced abortion, or spontaneous abortion); by rates (number of pregnancies, births, and abortions per 1000 young women); and by race/ethnicity (African American, white, Hispanic/Latino). Teen birthrates increase by age, with the highest rates occurring among 19-year-olds. Pregnancy and birthrates increased steadily among teens of all ages from 1986 to 1991 and declined among teens of all ages and ethnicity from 1991 to 1997 (CDC, 2000a). Decreases from 25% to 22% were also noted in the teen repeat birth rate from 1991 to 1998 (ACOG, 2000). All these decreases are attributed to stabilization of the numbers of teens becoming sexually active, increased condom use, and

---

## THE CUTTING EDGE

The nurse who is knowledgeable about the increase in nongenital sexual behavior among younger teens can incorporate appropriate safer-sex messages into educational programs.

increased use of more effective and long-acting hormonal methods of birth control (CDC, 2000a). Over the last 36 years, rates and numbers of births to teens have fluctuated widely. The highest rates occurred in the 1960s and 1970s, followed by a drop to the lowest point in 1986 and since then rising and falling again (Moore et al, 1997).

Over 78% of teens are unmarried at the time of their child's birth, a number that has quadrupled since 1960 (ACOG, 2000). Healthy People 2010: Understanding and Improving Health (U.S. Department of Health and Human Services [USDHHS], 2000) has identified goals to reduce teen pregnancy and birthrates.

In 1996, 35% of pregnancies to teenagers were ended by elective abortion (ACOG, 2000). Elective abortion rates for teenagers increased from the time of legalization in 1973 until 1986. From 1986 to 1994, there was a 21% decrease in abortions to teens (Moore et al, 1997). This decrease was caused in part by decreases in the pregnancy rate but may also have resulted from laws that required parental notification or consent for minors requesting abortion services in some states. African-American and white teens choose abortion at similar rates. Adolescents who terminate their pregnancies by abortion differ from those who give birth in the following ways: they are more likely to complete high school, are more successful in school, have higher educational aspirations, and are more likely to come from a family of a higher socioeconomic status (Alexander and Guyer, 1993).

The United States leads the developed world in rates of teenage pregnancy, teen births, and teen abortions. Teens in Sweden have the highest rate of sexual activity (the United States is second), but they experience fewer pregnancies, births, and abortions. If these same comparisons are made with only white teens, the United States still leads in the number of pregnancies, births, and abortions. Comparisons with statistics in other countries suggest that much of this difference is caused by the limited use of contraceptives among teens, as well as a general ambivalence about providing comprehensive sexuality education at home and at school for children and adolescents in the United States (Hatcher et al, 1998).

## BACKGROUND FACTORS

Many adults have difficulty understanding why young people would jeopardize their careers and personal potential by becoming pregnant during the teen years. Adolescents, however, do not view the world in the same way adults do. Teens often feel invincible and therefore do not recognize any risk related to their behaviors or anticipate the consequences. That is, they may not believe that sexual activity will lead to pregnancy. When teens become pregnant, they do not think that the negative outcomes they are advised of could come true. Many teens believe that they are unique and different and that everything will work out fine. The developmental circumstances of adolescence, coupled with potential background disadvantages, can magnify the problems facing the pregnant and parenting teen. Pregnant teens often express the unrealistic attitude that they can do it all: school, work, parenting, and socializing.

**OBJECTIVES RELATED TO FAMILY PLANNING**

**9-7** Reduce pregnancies among adolescents

**9-8** Increase the proportion of adolescents who have never engaged in sexual intercourse before age 15 years

**9-9** Increase the proportion of adolescents who have never engaged in sexual intercourse

**9-10** Increase the proportion of sexually active, unmarried adolescents aged 15 to 17 years who use contraception that both effectively prevents pregnancy and provides barrier protection against disease

**9-11** Increase the proportion of young adults who have received formal instruction (before turning age 18 years) on reproductive health issues, including all of the following topics: birth control methods, safer sex to prevent HIV, prevention of STDs, and abstinence

**OBJECTIVES RELATED TO SEXUALLY TRANSMITTED DISEASES**

**25-1** Reduce the proportion of adolescent and young adults with *Chlamydia trachomatis* infections

**25-8** Reduce HIV infections in adolescents and young adult females aged 13 to 24 years that are associated with heterosexual contact

**25-11** Increase the proportion of adolescents who abstain from sexual intercourse or use condoms if currently sexually active

**25-26** Increase the proportion of sexually active females age 25 years and under who are screened annually for genital chlamydial infection

From U.S. Department of Health and Human Services: *Healthy people 2010: understanding and improving health,* ed 2, Washington, DC, 2000, U.S. Government Printing Office.

---

The characteristics of the teens who are giving birth are changing. A disproportionate number of teens who give birth are poor (more than three quarters), have limited educational achievements, and see few advantages in delaying pregnancy as they do not expect that their circumstances will improve at a later time (Whitman et al, 2001). Most teens report that their pregnancy was unplanned. They typically say they think a pregnancy should be delayed until people are older, have completed their education, and are employed and married (Hatcher et al, 1998). Their behaviors, however, do not support the opinions they express. In fact, some teens actually seem ambitious about becoming pregnant. Several factors that often contribute to pregnancy are discussed next.

## Sexual Activity and Use of Birth Control

The **sexual debut,** or first experience with intercourse, for a teen will have a significant impact on pregnancy risk. Although the percentage of sexually active teens today is much greater than it was in the 1970s, decreases over the last 5 years have been noted. In the ninth grade, 37% of students are sexually active, 48% by tenth grade, 58% by the eleventh grade, and 66% by the twelfth grade. Male students (12%) and African-American students (24%) were more likely than white, Hispanic/Latino, or female students to initiate sexual activity before age 13. African-American students (73%) are more likely to report a history of sexual activity, followed by Hispanic/Latino (57%) and white students (48%) (CDC, 2000b).

The Healthy People 2010 goal is to increase the proportion of adolescents who have never engaged in sexual intercourse to 88% by age 15 and to 75% by age 17 (baselines of 81% girls and 79% boys by age 15; 62% girls and 57% boys by age 17 (USDHHS, 2000b).

**DID YOU KNOW?**

In 1996, Congress passed the Personal Responsibility and Work Opportunity Reconciliation Act. This welfare reform package strives to discourage teen pregnancy and other nonmarital births in a variety of ways. Emphasis is on the primary prevention of pregnancy through abstinence education and discouraging sex before marriage. Furthermore, benefits may be withdrawn if adolescent parents do not live in an adult-supervised home and attend school.

Although more teens have begun using birth control in the past 10 years, there still is progress to be made; 78% of adolescent girls (Moore, Driscoll, and Lindberg, 1998) report use of birth control at first voluntary coitus. Male teens use condoms with increasing frequency (99% reported using condoms at some time during the past year) but not consistently. Overall, 44% of male teens use condoms consistently, with the greatest use reported by African-American male teens and the lowest use reported by Hispanic/Latino male teens (Moore et al, 1998). Half of all first-time pregnancies occur within 6 months of initiating intercourse (Hatcher et al, 1998). Teens harbor many myths that contribute to poor use of birth control, such as believing you cannot get pregnant the first time, and some teens have erroneous knowledge about a woman's fertile time. Failure to use birth control can also reflect teens' embarrassment in discussing this practice with partners,

**Table 34-1  Hormonal Birth Control Methods Used by Teenagers**

| METHOD | FAILURE WITH TYPICAL USE | PATTERN OF USE | COMMONLY REPORTED SIDE EFFECTS |
|---|---|---|---|
| Birth control pills | 5% | Take a pill daily | Nausea, menstrual irregularities, breast tenderness, weight gain |
| Depo-Provera | 0.3% | Intramuscular injection every 3 months | Menstrual irregularities, weight gain |
| Lunelle monthly combined contraceptive injection | Less than 0.2% | Intramuscular injection every month | Menstrual irregularities, weight change, breast tenderness, emotional lability, acne, nausea |
| Nuva-Ring combined contraceptive vaginal ring | 0.7% | Insert new ring vaginally for first 21 days of cycle and remove for 7 days | Headache, vaginal discomfort, nausea |
| Evra transdermal combined contraceptive patch | 1.2% | Attach new patch to skin weekly for 3 weeks, then remove for 7 days | Menstrual irregularities, headache, nausea, application site reactions, breast discomfort |

Data from Hatcher RA et al: *Contraceptive technology,* New York, 1998, Ardent Media; and *The Contraceptive Report,* 12(3):8-12, and 12(4):8, Houston, Tex, 2001, Emron, available at www.contraceptiononline.org.

friends, parents, and health care providers and the obstacles they encounter finding facilities that provide confidential and affordable birth control (Hatcher et al, 1998).

The earlier the sexual debut, the less likely a birth control method will be used, as younger teens have less knowledge and skill related to sexuality and birth control. School-based sex education can come too late or not at all. Birth control is usually discussed in the secondary-school curriculum, but this could be eighth grade in one school district and tenth in another; school curricula are not standardized. Younger teens may falsely believe that they are too young to purchase birth control methods such as condoms. Confidential reproductive health care services may be available for teens, but problems are still associated with transportation, school absences, and costs of care that ultimately restrict access to these services.

Inconsistent use of birth control can reflect teens' willingness to take risks, their dissatisfactions with available birth control methods, and their ambivalence about becoming pregnant. Real and perceived side effects of birth control methods can discourage use. Hormonal methods such as Depo-Provera (an intramuscular injection every 3 months) and the Nuva-Ring (a monthly vaginal ring) appeal to some women because the method is less directly tied to coitus. These newer methods may have nuisance-type effects (e.g., irregular bleeding or insertion into the vagina) that may be unappealing to young women. Table 34-1 describes hormonal birth control methods that would be appropriate for the adolescent to consider.

As noted earlier, the use of alcohol and other substances is common among adolescents and can contribute to unplanned pregnancy. Mood-altering effects may reduce inhibitions about engaging in intercourse and interfere with the proper use of a chosen birth control method.

## Peer Pressure and Partner Pressure

Peer pressure among teens is not a new phenomenon, but many of the influences have become more serious. Influence has expanded from fashion and language to cigarettes, substance abuse, sexuality, and pregnancy. Teens are more likely to be sexually active if their friends are sexually active (Bearman and Bruckner, 1999). Peers reinforce teen parenting by exaggerating birth control risks, discouraging abortion and **adoption,** and glamorizing the impending birth of the child.

Both young men and young women may think that allowing a pregnancy to happen verifies one's love and commitment for the other. In addition, young men from socioeconomically disadvantaged backgrounds may be more likely to say that fathering a child would make them feel more manly, and they are less likely to use an effective contraceptive (Marsiglio, 1993).

## Other Factors

Other factors influencing teen pregnancy are a history of **sexual victimization,** family structure, and parental influences. Pregnant teenagers have a greater likelihood of having been sexually abused during their lifetime, with rates recorded as high as 62% (Stock et al, 1997). Adolescent girls with a history of sexual abuse are at risk for earlier initiation of voluntary sexual intercourse, are less likely to use birth control, are more likely to use drugs and alcohol at first intercourse, and are more likely to have older sexual partners (Boyer and Fine, 1992). The youngest women are more likely to experience **coercive sex** (74% of women who had intercourse before age 14 reported that it was involuntary) (Moore et al, 1998). Young women may also become pregnant as a result of forced sexual intercourse. A history of sexual victimization will influence a young woman's ability to exert control over future sexual experiences, which will affect the use of birth control and rejection of unwanted sexual experiences. All these factors contribute to an increased risk for becoming pregnancy (Osborne and Rhodes, 2001). In addition, young women who have experienced a lifetime of economic, social, and psychological deprivation may think that a baby will bring joy into an otherwise bleak existence. Some mistakenly think that a baby can provide the love and attention that her family has not provided.

Family structure can influence adolescent sexual behavior and pregnancy. Adolescents raised in single-parent families are more likely to have intercourse and to give birth than those raised in two-parent families. This difference is striking: sexual activity will occur among 22% of girls from two-parent families and 44% of girls from other family situations. A similar difference is also seen in the likelihood of giving birth by age 20 (Moore et al, 1998).

Parenting styles can influence a young woman's risk for early sexual experiences and pregnancy. Parents who are extremely demanding and controlling or neglectful and who have low expectations are least successful in instilling parental values in their children. Parents who have high demands for their children to act maturely and who offer warmth and understanding with parental rules have children more likely to exhibit appropriate social behavior and to delay early sexual experiences and pregnancy. Children of parents who are neglectful are the most sexually experienced, followed by children of parents who are very strict. Furthermore, parents who discuss birth control, sexuality, and pregnancy with their children can positively influence delay of sexual initiation and effective birth control use. Parents who do not communicate about sexuality with their teens may find them more at risk for sexual permissiveness and pregnancy (Kirby, 2001b).

### WHAT DO YOU THINK?

In response to federal welfare reform recommendations, there has been a recent trend toward the enforcement of **statutory rape** laws by individual states. These laws make it a crime to have sexual contact with a person before the age of consent is reached (which varies among states). Supporters of this action think that it will discourage adult men from relationships with minors and consequently reduce teen pregnancy. Opponents believe that this strategy does not take into account the complex issues involved in teen pregnancy (such as poverty and limited opportunities for young women) and think it may do more to distance a father from involvement in his child's life.

## YOUNG MEN AND PATERNITY

One in 15 males becomes a father during the teen years. Although one third of the fathers of babies born to teens are also teens, more than half the fathers are between ages 20 and 24. Most fathers of babies born to adolescent mothers are 2 to 3 years older than the mother (Moore and Driscoll, 1997). Teen fathers face special challenges because of concomitant social problems and limited future plans or ability to provide support. There also may be an overlap between young fatherhood and delinquency. Young fathers who demonstrate law-breaking behaviors, alcohol or substance use, school problems, and aggressive behaviors may have difficulty developing a positive fathering role (Stouthamer-Loeber and Wei, 1998).

**Paternity,** or fatherhood, is legally established at the time of the birth for a teen who is married. However, it is more difficult to establish paternity among nonmarried couples. Some of the difficulty lies in the complexity of the specific state system for young men to acknowledge paternity. In some states, a young man may have to work with the judicial system outside of the hospital after the birth, and if he is under age 18, he may need to involve his parents.

Some young couples do not attempt to establish paternity and prefer a verbal promise of assistance for the teen mother and child. Although a verbal commitment may be acceptable when the child is born, the mother may become more inclined to pursue the establishment of paternity later when the relationship ends or for reasons related to financial, social, or emotional needs of the child. Young women who receive state or federal assistance (e.g., Aid for Dependent Children, Medicaid) may be asked to name the child's father so the judicial process can be used to establish paternity.

Young men react differently when they learn that their partner is pregnant. The reaction often depends on the nature of the relationship before the pregnancy. Many young men will accompany the young woman to a health care center for pregnancy diagnosis and counseling. A large percentage of young men will continue to accompany the young woman to some prenatal visits and may even attend the delivery. These young men may also want to and need to be involved with their children regardless of changes in their relationships with the teen mother. It is not unusual for a young man to be excluded or even rejected by the young woman's family (usually her mother). He may then begin to act as though he is disinterested when he may really feel that he cannot provide resources for his child or know how to take care of him or her (Rhein et al, 1997) (Figure 34-1).

Nurses can acknowledge and support the young man as he develops in the role of father. His involvement can positively affect his child's development and provide greater personal satisfaction for himself and greater role satisfaction for the young mother (Rhein et al, 1997). Young mothers who report less social support from their baby's father are more apt to be unhappy and distressed in the parenting role and consequently more at risk for abuse of their child (Zalenko et al, 2001). The immediate concerns revolve around his fi-

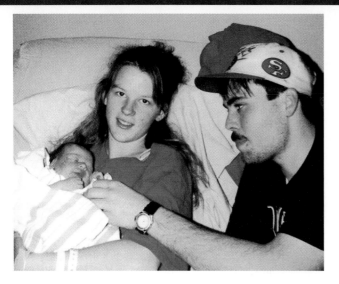

**Figure 34-1** It is important to include both the teen mother and the father in teaching about child development.

nancial responsibility, living arrangements, relationship issues, school, and work. Establishing an opportunity to meet with the young man and both families is helpful to clarify these issues and identify roles and responsibilities.

Young men who grow up in poor families are more likely to believe that fathering a child can make them feel manly, and they are more likely to be pleased with a pregnancy than their affluent counterparts. These young men are also less likely to use or to discuss birth control with a partner. Young men who had previously impregnated a young woman are more likely to feel and act this way (Marsiglio, 1993).

## EARLY IDENTIFICATION OF THE PREGNANT TEEN

Some teens delay seeking pregnancy services because they fail to recognize signs such as breast tenderness and a late period, as they are experiencing a variety of other pubertal changes. Most young women, however, suspect pregnancy as soon as a period is late. These young women may still delay seeking care since they falsely hope that the pregnancy will just go away. A teen also may delay seeking care to keep the pregnancy a secret from family members, who may pressure her to terminate the pregnancy, or because of fears about gynecologic examinations (Cartwright et al, 1993).

Nurses must be sensitive to subtle cues that a teenager may offer about sexuality and pregnancy concerns. Such cues include questions about one's fertile period or requests for confirmation that one need not miss a period to be pregnant. Once the nurse identifies the specific concern, information can be provided about how and when to obtain pregnancy testing. The nurse should determine how a teenager would react to the possible pregnancy before completing the test. If the test is negative, the nurse should take the opportunity to assess whether the young woman would consider counseling to prevent pregnancy. A follow-up visit

---

### BOX 34-4 Levels of Prevention Related to Teen Pregnancy

**PRIMARY PREVENTION**

Teach young people about sexual practices that will prevent untimely pregnancy.

**SECONDARY PREVENTION**

Provide services for early detection of teen pregnancy.

**TERTIARY PREVENTION**

Counsel the young person or young couple about available options, including keeping the baby (and making appropriate plans to care for the child), abortion, and adoption.

---

is important after a negative test to determine if retesting is necessary or if another problem exists.

In looking at teen pregnancy from the perspective of levels of prevention, several steps could be taken. These are shown in Box 34-4.

A young woman with a positive pregnancy test requires a physical examination and pregnancy counseling. It is advantageous to offer these at the same time so that the counseling is consistent with the findings of the examination. The purpose of the examination is to assess the duration and well-being of the pregnancy, as well as to test for sexually transmitted infection. The pregnancy counseling should include the following: information on adoption, abortion, and child-rearing; an opportunity for assessment of support systems for the young woman; and identification of the immediate concerns she might have.

The availability of affordable abortion services up to 13 weeks' gestation varies from community to community. Similarly, second-trimester services may be available locally or involve extensive travel and cost. The nurse should be knowledgeable about abortion services and provide information or refer the pregnant teenager to a pregnancy counseling service that can assist.

The pregnant teenager needs information about adoption, such as current policies among agencies that allow continued contact with the adopting family. Also, church organizations, private attorneys, and social service agencies provide a variety of adoption services with which the nurse should be familiar. Box 34-5 lists guidelines for adoption counseling. At this time, 8% of adolescent women age 17 and under relinquish custody of their infants (ACOG, 2000).

---

### NURSING TIP

An important counseling opportunity presents itself when a teen has a pregnancy test that is negative. Use this time to clarify a desire or disinterest in pregnancy and help empower her to influence her reproductive future.

## Teen Pregnancy in Canada

Karen Wade, R.N., B.N., M.Sc.N., Toronto Public Health
Jann Houston, B.Sc.N., M.Sc.N., Toronto Public Health

### ADOLESCENT SEXUAL BEHAVIOUR IN CANADA

Canadian data at the national level regarding adolescent and young adult sexual behaviour is quite limited (Maticka-Tyndale, Barrett, and McKay, 2000). The Canada, Youth, and AIDS study (King et al, 1988) surveyed 38,000 Canadian adolescents in grades 7, 9, 11, and first-year college or university to explore their sexual behaviours. Results revealed that 49% of grade 11 boys and 46% of grade 11 girls had been sexually active. The most recent Canadian survey data regarding sexual practices show that 68.5% of women and 70.5% of men age 20 to 24 reported having intercourse before the age of 20 (Maticka-Tyndale, 2001; National Population Health Survey 1996-1997, as cited in Maticka-Tyndale, McKay, and Barrett, 2001). A Canada-wide study currently in progress is updating the Canada, Youth, and AIDS study. Approximately 30,000 students in grades 7, 9, and 11 in each province and territory are being surveyed to explore the broader sociocultural determinants of sexual health as well as the interpersonal contexts of sexual risk taking in youth (Connop and Boyce, 2000).

Most Canadian adolescents have access to reproductive health care services (i.e., contraceptive information and services, sexually transmitted diseases [STDs] and human immunodeficiency virus [HIV] testing and treatment, prenatal and maternity services, and abortions) through Canada's universal health insurance system; however, the degree of access varies across the country. In some communities, clinical services are available both in school clinics and in other community-based clinics, whereas in other communities there are few or nonexistent services (Maticka-Tyndale et al, 2001).

Despite the availability of reproductive health care services, unprotected sexual activity is commonplace among Canadian youths, and it poses serious health threats, including STDs, HIV infection, and unplanned pregnancy.

Many sexually active teens do not use condoms or use them inconsistently (Hampton et al, 2001; Health Canada, 1997; Richardson et al, 1997; Thomas, DiCenso, and Griffith, 1998). Findings from the 1996 National Population Health Survey indicated that 80.8% of single, sexually experienced 15- to 19-year-old males and 69.8% of females reported using a condom the last time they had sexual intercourse (Maticka-Tyndale et al, 2001).

### TRENDS IN ADOLESCENT PREGNANCY IN CANADA

A comparison of teenage pregnancy rates for women of ages 15 to 19 in Canada, the United States, Sweden, France, and Great Britain in the mid 1990s revealed that the rate of teenage pregnancy in Canada is lower than that of the United States (which, at 84 per 1000 women, was the highest rate) but higher than that of several European countries. The lowest pregnancy rates were in France and Sweden, at 20 and 25 per 1000, respectively. Canada and Great Britain were in the middle at 46 and 47 per 1000, respectively. These rates include births and induced abortions but do not include spontaneous abortions or miscarriages (Darroch et al, 2001).

Dryburgh (2000) reviewed data related to teenage pregnancy in Canada from 1974 to 1997. The teenage pregnancy rate (the sum of live births, induced abortions, and fetal loss [miscarriages and stillbirths] for which administrative records were available, per 1000 female population aged 15 to 19) in Canada dropped overall from 53.7 per 1000 in 1974 to 42.7 per 1000 in 1997. The Canadian pregnancy rate in 1997 for 18- to 19-year-olds (68.9 per 1000) was more than double that of 15- to 17-year-olds (25.5 per 1000) (Health Statistics Division, Canadian Vital Statistics Database, Canadian Institute for Health Information, as cited in Dryburgh, 2000). The decrease in the Canadian teenage

*The views expressed in this box represent those of the writer and do not represent the views of the City of Toronto, Toronto Public Health.*

Pregnancy counseling requires that the nurse and young woman explore strengths and weaknesses for personal care and responsibility during a pregnancy and parenting. Young women vary in their interest in including the partner or their parents in this discussion. Issues to raise include education and career plans, family finances and qualifications for outside assistance, and personal values about pregnancy and parenting at this time in their life. Often it is difficult to focus on counseling in any depth at the time of the initial pregnancy testing results. A follow-up visit is usually more productive and should be arranged as soon as possible.

As decisions are made about the course of the pregnancy, the nurse is instrumental in referral to appropriate programs such as WIC (a supplemental food program for women, infants, and children), Medicaid, and prenatal services. The

young woman and her family also need to know about expected costs of care and, if there is a family insurance policy, whether it will cover the pregnancy-related expenses of a dependent child. For those without insurance, the family can apply for Medicaid or determine whether local facilities offer indigent care programs (e.g., Hill-Burton programs for assistance with hospital expenses). The nurse can also begin prenatal education and counseling on nutrition, substance abuse and use, exercise, and special medical concerns.

## SPECIAL ISSUES IN CARING FOR THE PREGNANT TEEN

Pregnant teenagers are considered high-risk obstetric clients. Many of the complications of their pregnancy result from poverty, late entry into prenatal care, and lim-

pregnancy rate began several years later than the one that occurred in the United States (Combes-Orme, 1993, and Alan Guttmacher Institute, 1999, both as cited in Dryburgh, 2000).

In 1974, the majority (66%) of teenage pregnancies in Canada ended in a live birth, whereas 26% of teens had therapeutic abortions and 8% had stillbirths or miscarriages (Wadhera and Millar, 1997). By 1997, with the decline in live births to teens, abortion became the most common outcome of teenage pregnancy (Health Statistics Division, Canadian Vital Statistics Database, Canadian Institute for Health Information, as cited in Dryburgh, 2000).

Teen pregnancy rates in Canada tend to be higher in the Prairie Provinces and the North than in other regions of the country. In 1997, the teenage pregnancy rate for 15- to 19-year-olds varied substantially, from less than 35 per 1000 in Newfoundland and New Brunswick to a high of 123.3 per 1000 in the Northwest Territories (Health Statistics Division, Canadian Vital Statistics Database, Canadian Institute for Health Information, as cited in Dryburgh, 2000).

It is important to note that teenage pregnancy rates may be underestimated for several reasons. Rates reflect the year in which the pregnancies ended, thus they do not include pregnancies that began at age 19 and ended at age 20. Teenagers who miscarry may not require medical attention. Those that do are frequently treated in outpatient settings and thus are not included in the hospital morbidity database. Abortions that occur in physicians' offices and in some American states are not included. Age is not reported for all abortions in all provinces, and the provincial distribution reflects only those cases for which age was known (Dryburgh, 2000).

### References

Connop HL, Boyce W: Announcements: national research project to build on Canada, Youth, and AIDS study, *Can J Human Sexual* 9(1):75, 2000.

Darroch JE et al: Differences in teenage pregnancy rates among five developed countries: the roles of sexual activity and contraceptive use, *Fam Plann Perspect* 33(6):244-250, 281, 2001.

Dryburgh H: Teenage pregnancy (Statistics Canada, Catalogue 82-003), *Health Rep* 12(1):9-19, 2000.

Hampton MR et al: Sexual experience, contraception, and STI prevention among high school students: results from a Canadian urban centre, *Can J Human Sexual* 10(3-4):111-126, 2001.

Health Canada: *Sexual risk behaviors of Canadians: bureau of HIV/AIDS and STD Epi Update Series,* Laboratory Center for Disease Control, Ottawa, Ont, 1997, Health Canada.

King A et al: *Canada, youth, and AIDS study,* Ottawa, Ont, 1988, Health Canada, Federal Centre for AIDS.

Maticka-Tyndale E: Sexual health and Canadian youth: how do we measure up? *Can J Human Sexual* 10 (1-2):1-17, 2001.

Maticka-Tyndale E, Barrett M, McKay A: Adolescent sexual and reproductive health in Canada: a review of national data sources and their limitations, *Can J Human Sexual* 9(1):41-65, 2000.

Maticka-Tyndale E, McKay A, Barrett M: *Teenage sexual and reproductive behaviour in developed countries: country report for Canada—occasional report No. 4,* New York, 2001, Alan Guttmacher Institute.

Richardson HRL et al: Factors influencing condom use among students attending high school in Nova Scotia, *Can J Human Sexual* 6(3):185-196, 1997.

Thomas BH, DiCenso A, Griffith L: Adolescent sexual behaviour: results from an Ontario sample—part II: adolescent use of protection, *Can J Public Health* 89(2):94-97, 1998.

Wadhera S, Millar WJ: Teenage pregnancies, 1974 to 1994 (Statistics Canada, Catalogue 82-003-XPB), *Health Rep* 9(3):9-17, 1997.

*Canadian spelling is used.*

ited knowledge about self-care during pregnancy. Nursing interventions through education and early identification of problems may dramatically alter the course of the pregnancy and the birth outcome.

## Violence

Teens are more likely to experience violence during their pregnancies than adult women. Age may be a factor in their greater vulnerability to potential perpetrators that include partners, family members, and other acquaintances. Violence in pregnancy has been associated with an increased risk for substance abuse, poor compliance with **prenatal care,** and poor birth outcome. In the case of partner violence, young women may be protective of their partners because of fear or helplessness. Eliciting this history from an adolescent is not easy. The nurse must inquire about violence at every visit. Frequent routine assessments are more revealing than a single inquiry at the first prenatal visit (Covington et al, 1997). Recent research has demonstrated that 21% of pregnant adolescents reported violence during the pregnancy, a rate greater than that reported by adult women (Covington et al, 1997). Violence that began during the pregnancy may continue for several years after, with increasing severity. Variations by ethnicity have also been observed during this postpartum period as **intimate partner violence** may peak at 3 months postpartum among African-American and Hispanic/Latino new mothers and at 18 months for white mothers

## BOX 34-5 Guidelines for Adoption Counseling

1. Assess your own thoughts and feelings on adoption. Do not impose your opinion on the decision-making process of teen mothers.
2. Be knowledgeable about state laws, local resources, and various types of adoption services.
3. Choose language sensitively. Examples follow:
    a. Avoid saying "giving away a child" or "putting up for adoption." It is more appropriate and positive to say "releasing a child for adoption," "placing for adoption," or "making an adoption plan."
    b. Avoid saying "unwanted child" or "unwanted pregnancy." A more appropriate term may be *unplanned pregnancy.*
    c. Avoid saying "natural parents" or "natural child," because the adopted parents would then seem to be "unnatural." The terms *biological parents* and *adopted parents* are more appropriate.
4. Assess when a discussion of adoption is appropriate. It can be helpful to begin with information on adoption, then explore feelings and concerns over time. Individuals will vary in how much they may have already considered adoption, and this will influence the counseling session.
5. Assess the relationship between the pregnant teen and her partner and what role she expects him to play. Discuss the reality of this.
6. It may be helpful for a pregnant teen to talk with other teens who have been pregnant, are raising a child, have released a child for adoption, or have been adopted themselves.
7. A young woman can be encouraged to begin writing letters to her baby. These can be saved or given to the child when released to the adoptive family.

Modified from Brandsen CK: *A case for adoption,* Grand Rapids, Mich, 1991, Bethany.

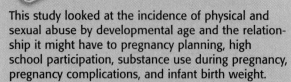

### Evidence-Based Practice

This study looked at the incidence of physical and sexual abuse by developmental age and the relationship it might have to pregnancy planning, high school participation, substance use during pregnancy, pregnancy complications, and infant birth weight.

The 559 ethnically diverse study participants were between the ages of 13 and 19 and receiving prenatal care at clinics in the Northwest. The teens were interviewed one time during their pregnancy. Abuse was measured by the abuse assessment screen, which has reported validity and reliability. Substance abuse was identified by confidential self-reporting, and information about pregnancy complications was determined from the medical records.

In this study, 37% of adolescents reported abuse in the past year and 14% during the pregnancy. The highest rates of abuse occurred during middle adolescence (ages 16 to 17) and dropped significantly by age 18. Although this study did not identify the perpetrator, it was assumed that in some cases it was a family member. The authors speculate that some abuse may decline at age 18 when some young women moved away from the family home. Deleterious pregnancy outcomes, such as low birth weight, were not increased among those reporting the greatest abuse. Overall, rates of abuse among pregnant teens were not as high as those reported by other studies. The authors conclude that more abuse will be reported by teens if screening is done multiple times throughout the pregnancy.

**Nurse Use:** To get accurate information from pregnant teens about this emotionally charged topic, it is important to screen for (that is, inquire about) abuse multiple times throughout the pregnancy.

Curry MA, Doyle BA, Gilhooley J: Abuse among pregnant adolescents: differences by developmental age, *MCN Am J Matern Child Nurs* 23(3):144, 1998.

(Harrykissoon, Rickert, and Wiemann, 2002). The nurse must observe for physical signs of abuse, as well as for controlling or intrusive partner behavior (see the Evidence-Based Practice box).

## Initiation of Prenatal Care

Pregnant adolescents differ remarkably from pregnant adults in initiation and compliance with prenatal care. Inadequate prenatal care has been negatively associated with health risks to both the mother and the fetus. In 1998, 7% of the pregnant 15- to 19-year-olds received late or no prenatal care, and 25% began care in the second trimester. This delay in receiving prenatal care is noted more frequently among African-American teens (ACOG, 2000). Teens report that the greatest barrier to care is real or perceived cost (Cartwright et al, 1993). Other barriers

include denial of the pregnancy, fear of telling parents, transportation, dislike of providers' care, and offensive attitudes among clinic staff toward pregnant teens (Cartoof, Klerman, and Zazveta, 1991; VanWinter and Simmons, 1990).

Once a teen is enrolled in prenatal care, the nurse becomes an important liaison between personnel at the clinical site and the young woman. Confusion and misunderstandings occur easily when teens do not understand what a health care provider says to them. Often these misunderstandings are based on lack of knowledge about basic anatomy and physiology. For example, a teen may be told as she gets close to term that the head of the baby is down and it can be felt. This is an alarming piece of information for a young woman who imagines the entire baby could just pop out any time!

Cooperation between the nurse and the clinical staff can also maximize the client's compliance with special health or nutritional needs. For example, a teen who has premature contractions may be placed on bed rest and instructed to increase fluids. The nurse who makes home visits can provide additional assessment of the teen's condition and can solve problems about self-care, hygiene, meals, and school.

## Low-Birth-Weight Infants and Preterm Delivery

Teens are more likely than adult women to deliver infants weighing less than 5½ pounds or to deliver before 37 weeks' gestation. In 1998, **low-birth-weight** babies represented 9.5% of all babies born to adolescents (ACOG, 2000). In 1998, 22% of all births to the youngest mothers, those under the age of 15, were preterm. These low-birth-weight and premature infants are at greater risk for death in the first year of life and are more at risk for long-term physical, emotional, and cognitive problems (USDHHS, 2000). For example, low-birth-weight and premature infants can be more difficult to feed and soothe. This challenges the limited skills of the young mother and can further strain relations with other members of the household, who may not know how to offer support or assistance.

The risk for low-birth-weight infants and premature births can be averted by the teen's early initiation into prenatal care. Although such births still occur, it is important to work closely with the teen mother as soon as she is identified as pregnant to try to promote compliance with prenatal care visits and self-care during the pregnancy. After the pregnancy, these infants and their mothers will benefit from frequent nursing supervision to ensure that their care is appropriate and that everyone in the home is coping adequately with the strain of a small infant.

## Nutrition

The nutritional needs of a pregnant teenager are especially important. First, the teen lifestyle does not lend itself to overall good nutrition. Fast foods, frequent snacking, and hectic social schedules limit nutritious food choices. Snacks, which account for approximately a third of a teen's daily caloric intake, tend to be high in fat, sugar, and sodium and limited in essential vitamins and minerals. Second, the nutritive needs of both pregnancy and the concurrent adolescent growth spurt require the adolescent to change her diet substantially. The growing teen must increase caloric nutrients to meet individual growth needs as well as allow for adequate fetal growth. Third, poor eating patterns of the teen and her current growth requirement may leave her with limited reserves of essential vitamins and minerals when the pregnancy begins. The nurse can assess the pregnant teenager's current eating pattern and provide creative guidance. For example, protein can be increased at fast-food establishments by ordering milkshakes instead of soft drinks and cheeseburgers or broiled chicken sandwiches instead of hamburgers. Snack foods can be purchased for eating on the way to school in the morning and for midmorning snacks (Story and Stang, 2000).

The recommended nutritional needs of the adolescent may depend on the **gynecologic age** of the teen—that is, the number of years between her chronological age and her age at menarche, as well as her chronological age. Young women with a gynecologic age of 2 or less years or under the age of 16 may have increased nutrient requirements because of their own growth. Furthermore, the younger and still-growing teen may compete nutritionally with the fetus. Fetuses may show evidence of slower growth in young women ages 10 to 16 years (Scholl, Hediger, and Schall, 1997; Story and Stang, 2000). The nurse, in collaboration with the WIC nutritionist, can determine the nutritional needs of the pregnant teenager to tailor education appropriately. Table 34-2 describes adolescent nutritional needs in pregnancy.

**Weight gain** during pregnancy is one of the strongest predictors of infant birth weight. Although precise weight gain goals in adolescence are controversial, pregnant adolescents who gain 25 to 35 pounds have the lowest incidence of low-birth-weight babies (Story and Stang, 2000). Younger teen mothers (ages 13 to 16), because of their own growth demands, may need to gain more weight then older teen mothers (ages 17 and over) to have the same-birth-weight baby. Differentiating the still-growing teen from the grown teen may not be possible in the clinic setting, so encouraging all teens to gain at the upper end of their weight goals may be the best approach (Lederman, 1997). Teenagers who begin the pregnancy at a normal weight should be counseled to begin weight gain in the first trimester and to average gains of 1 pound per week for the second and third trimesters (Story and Stang, 2000). Table 34-3 shows the recommendations established by the Institute for Medicine for adolescent gestational weight gain by pre-pregnant weight categories.

It is important for the nurse to assess the attitudes of the pregnant teen about weight gain and to follow her progress. Studies indicate that most teenagers view prenatal weight gain positively. However, teens who are overweight before pregnancy may have negative attitudes about weight gain (Story, 1997). Family support of the pregnant teen can be a strong influence in adequate weight gain and good nutrition during the pregnancy. Nutrition education should emphasize what accounts for weight gain and how fetal growth will benefit.

Iron deficiency is the most common nutritional problem among both pregnant and nonpregnant adolescent females (Story, 1997). The adolescent may begin a pregnancy with low or absent iron stores because of heavy menstrual periods, a previous pregnancy, growth demands, poor iron intake, or substance abuse. The increased maternal plasma volume and increased fetal demands for iron (especially in the third trimester) can further compromise the adolescent. Iron deficiency in pregnancy may contribute to increased **prematurity,** low birth weight, postpartum hemorrhage, maternal headaches, dizziness, shortness of breath, and so on (Story and Stang, 2000). The nurse can reinforce the need for the teen to take prenatal vitamins during pregnancy and after the baby's birth. Vitamins should contain

**Table 34-2  Adolescent Nutritional Needs During Pregnancy**

| NUTRIENT | DAILY REQUIREMENT DURING PREGNANCY* | FOOD SOURCE |
|---|---|---|
| Calcium | 1300 mg (decrease to 1000 mg for 19-year-olds) | Macaroni and cheese; Taco Bell chili cheese burrito; pizza; McDonald's Big Mac; puddings, milk, yogurt; also fortified juices, water, breakfast bars |
| Iron | 30 mg (recommendation is for 30 mg elemental iron as a daily supplement) | Meats, dried beans and peas, dark green leafy vegetables, whole grains, fortified cereal; absorption of iron from plant foods improved by vitamin C sources taken simultaneously |
| Zinc | 15 mg | Seafood, meats, eggs, legumes, whole grains |
| Folate (folic acid) | 0.6 mg (prenatal vitamins contain 0.4 to 1.0 mg of folic acid) | Green leafy vegetables, liver, breakfast cereals |
| Vitamin A | 800 μg | Dark yellow and green vegetables, fruits |
| Vitamin B$_6$ | 2.2 mg | Chicken, fish, liver, pork, eggs |
| Vitamin D | 5 μg | Fortified milk products and cereals |

*Higher ranges are especially important for the younger pregnant teen.

**Table 34-3  Gestational Weight Gain Recommendations for Adolescents***

| PRE-PREGNANT WEIGHT CATEGORIES† | RECOMMENDED TOTAL GAIN | | TRIMESTER 1 (lb) | TRIMESTERS 2 AND 3 (lb/wk) |
|---|---|---|---|---|
| | kg | lb | | |
| Underweight (BMI 19.8) | 12.5-18 | 28-40 | 5 | 1.0+ |
| Normal weight (BMI 19.9-26) | 11.5-16 | 25-35 | 3 | 1.0+ |
| Overweight (BMI 26-29) | 7.0-11.5 | 15-25 | 2 | 0.66+ |
| Very overweight (BMI 29) | 7.0-9.1 | 15-20 | 1.5 | 0.5+ |

*Very young adolescents (14 years of age or younger, or less than 2 years postmenarche) should strive for gains at the upper end of the range.
†BMI (body mass index) is calculated as weight (kg) per height (m) squared.
From Story M, Stang J, editors: *Nutrition and the pregnant adolescent: a practical reference guide,* Minneapolis, Minn, 2000, University of Minnesota, Center for Leadership, Education, and Training in Maternal and Child Nutrition.

30 to 60 mg elemental iron daily. The nurse should educate about iron-rich foods and foods that promote iron absorption, such as those containing vitamin C.

## Infant Care

Many adolescents have cared for babies and small children and feel confident and competent. Few teens are ever prepared, however, for the reality of 24-hour care of an infant. The nurse can help prepare the teen for the transition to motherhood while she is still pregnant. The trend toward early discharge from the hospital has made prenatal preparation even more important. The nurse can enlist the support of the teen's parents in education about infant care and stimulation. Young fathers-to-be would benefit from this education as well. Family values, practices, and beliefs about childcare may be deeply embedded and require the nurse to work gently and persuasively to challenge any that

may be detrimental to an infant (Wayland and Rawlins, 1997). For example, a family may believe that corporal punishment is a necessary component of child-rearing.

Adolescents often lack the self-confidence and knowledge required to positively interact with their infants (Diehl, 1997). They may also have unrealistic expectations about their children's development (Andreozzi et al, 2002); for example, they may expect their children to feed themselves at an early age or think that their children's behavior is more difficult than an adult mother might think. Teen parents often lack knowledge about infant growth and development, as seen in their limited verbal communication with their children, limited eye contact, and the tendency to display frustration and ambivalence as mothers (Leadbeater and Way, 2001; Whitman et al, 2001). Over time, adolescents can improve their ability to foster their children's emotional and social growth. Children of adolescent mothers have also been found to be at risk for academic and behavior problems in late childhood and adolescence (Diehl, 1997). These risks can be reduced when the teen mother receives professional intervention and supervision in the area of infant social and cognitive development (Whitman et al, 2001).

Abusive parenting is more likely to occur when the parents have limited knowledge about normal child development. It may also be more likely to occur among parents who cannot adequately empathize with a child's needs. Younger teens are particularly at risk for being unable to understand what their infant or child needs. This frustration may be exhibited as abusive behavior toward the child (Diehl, 1997). Teens who exhibit greater psychological distress or lack social supports should also be continuously assessed for child abuse risk by the nurse (Zelenko et al, 2001).

After the birth of the baby, the nurse should observe how the mother responds to infant cues for basic needs and distress. Specific techniques that the new mother can be instructed to use in early childcare are listed in the How To box. It is important to begin parenting education as early as possible. Adolescents who feel competent as parents have enhanced self-esteem, which in turn positively influences their relationship with their child (Diehl, 1997). Recognizing

---

### HOW TO Promote Interactions Between the Teen Mother and Her Baby

The nurse can make the following suggestions to the teen mother:

1. Make eye contact with your baby. Position your face 8 to 10 inches from your baby's face and smile.
2. Talk to your baby often. Use simple sentences, but try to avoid baby talk. Allow time for your baby to "answer." This will help your baby acquire language and communication skills.
3. Babies often enjoy when you sing to them, and this may help soothe them during a difficult time or help them fall asleep. Experiment with different songs and melodies to see which your baby seems to like.
4. Babies at this age cannot be spoiled. Instead, when babies are held and cuddled, they feel secure and loved.
5. Babies cry for many reasons and for no reason at all. If your baby has a clean diaper, has recently been fed and is safe and secure, he or she may just need to cry for a few minutes. What works to calm your baby may be different from other babies you have known. You can try rocking, gentle reassuring words, soft music, or quiet.
6. Make feeding times pleasant for both of you. Do not prop the bottle in your baby's mouth. Instead, you should sit comfortably, hold your baby in your arms, and offer the bottle or breast.
7. When babies are awake, they love to play. They enjoy taking walks and looking at brightly colored objects or pictures and toys that make noises, such as rattles and musical toys.

---

these good parenting skills and providing positive feedback help a young mother gain confidence in her role.

## Repeat Pregnancy

Teen mothers who experience a closely spaced second pregnancy, or **repeat pregnancy,** have poorer birth, educational, and economic outcomes. In 2000, 21% of teen births were a repeat birth (Papillo et al, 2002). Earlier studies showed that in some communities, repeat teen pregnancies occur as often as 35%. Additionally, young women having their first child before age 20 will average three children, whereas older mothers average two children (Whitman et al, 2001). The Healthy People 2010 goal is to reduce the percentage of closely spaced subsequent births (over 24 months) to 6% for women of all ages (USDHHS, 2000). Nurses should recognize which teens have risk factors for a second teen pregnancy: those from disadvantaged backgrounds, those from large families, those who are married, and those who discontinued their education after the delivery of the first child. Also, teens who reported a planned first pregnancy are more likely to have a second pregnancy within 24 months to complete their family. Parenting adolescents who return to school after the birth of their first child, regardless of prior school performance, are least likely to repeat a pregnancy and more likely to use birth control (Leadbeater and Way, 2001).

Discussions about family planning should be initiated during the third trimester of the current pregnancy. Contraceptive options should be reviewed, and the young woman should begin identifying the methods she is most likely to use. It is helpful to determine at this time the methods she has used in the past, her satisfaction or dissatisfaction, and reasons for use or nonuse. Many teens express unrealistic goals, such as "I am never going to have sex again" or "I need a break from guys," and they may erroneously believe that they are unable to conceive for some time after the delivery. After delivery, the nurse should follow up on the young woman's plan. Obstacles to obtaining contraceptives may exist, and the nurse can identify these and help problem solve with the new mother.

## Schooling and Educational Needs

Adolescents who become parents may have had limited school success before the pregnancy. However, coping with the demands of child-rearing coupled with the immaturity of the young mother may make school even less of a priority (Hofferth, Reid, and Mott, 2001). As noted previously, the potential for a closely spaced second birth may be lessened by a return to school. Federal legislation passed in 1975 prohibits schools from excluding students because they are pregnant. Greater emphasis is placed on keeping the pregnant adolescent in school during the pregnancy and having her return as soon as possible after the birth. Several factors may positively influence a young woman's return to school. These include her parents' level of education and their marital stability, small family size, whether there have been reading materials at home, whether her mother is employed, and whether the young woman is African American.

A practical challenge for young parents is locating and affording quality childcare; difficulties with this may prevent the highly motivated teenager from returning to high school. In the past 30 years, the percentage of parenting teens who return to high school and graduate has improved significantly. Attendance in college, now becoming the career requisite, is still less attainable to women who had children as teenagers than those who delayed childbearing (Hofferth et al, 2001; Leadbeater and Way, 2001).

Young women who have pregnancy complications may seek home instruction. This decision is made according to regulations issued by the state boards of education. Some young women have difficulty attending school because of the normal discomforts of pregnancy or because of social and emotional conflicts associated with the pregnancy. Teens who leave school without parental or medical excuses may face legal problems because of truancy. This increases the potential for them to become school dropouts. The nurse can determine if this has happened and try to coordinate with the school personnel (and school nurse, if one exists) to tailor efforts for a particular pregnant teen to keep her in school. Specific needs to be addressed include (1) using the bathroom frequently, (2) carrying and drinking more fluids or snacks to relieve nausea, (3) climbing stairs and carrying heavy bookbags, and (4) fitting comfortably behind stationary desks. Schools that are committed to keeping students enrolled are generally helpful and will assist in accommodating special needs.

## TEEN PREGNANCY AND THE NURSE

Nurses can influence teen pregnancy through appropriate interventions at home and in the community.

### Home-Based Interventions

Nurses can identify young women at risk for pregnancy in families currently receiving services. Younger sisters of pregnant teens are at a twofold-increased risk for becoming pregnant themselves (East and Felice, 1992). Anticipatory guidance that addresses sexuality issues can be offered to the parents of all preteens and teens during home visits to increase their knowledge and awareness.

Visiting the pregnant teen in her home allows the nurse to obtain an assessment of the facilities available at home for management of her pregnancy needs and suitability of the environment for her child. Some specific areas to assess are adequacy of heating and cooling, a source of water, cleanliness of the home, cooking facilities, and food storage. The nurse may find it more convenient for parents and other family members to participate in education and counseling sessions in their own home. Also, the need for financial assistance and other social service support may be more easily identified. Home visiting by nurses during a young woman's pregnancy can be critical in achieving compliance with antepartum goals around weight gain, good nutrition, and prenatal medical concerns (Figure 34-2).

When a teen pregnancy occurs, the family dynamics can shift. Families may go through stages of reactions. First, a crisis stage may occur, characterized by many emo-

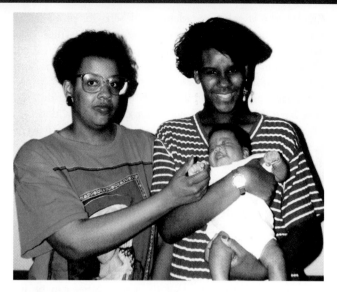

**Figure 34-2** Both the teen mother and the teen's own mother can be included in health teaching.

tions and conflict. By the third trimester, a honeymoon stage may occur, with greater acceptance and understanding of the teen and the impending birth. Finally, after the infant's birth, reorganization may occur, during which conflict may emerge again over issues of childcare and the young woman's role. The nurse can facilitate family coping and resolution of these stages by treating the family as client and assessing each person's role and strengths. Ultimately, family support for a teen parent can positively influence both mother and infant (Ruchala and James, 1997). A balance of moderate family guidance or supplementary care supports young mothers in their parenting role rather than replacing it (Whitman et al, 2001).

### Community-Based Interventions

Broad-based coalitions and planning councils are forming in many areas to facilitate a comprehensive approach to teen pregnancy. These groups usually include health care professionals, social workers, clergy, school personnel, businessmen, legislators, and members of other youth-serving agencies. The nurse can have a significant role on this team by participating in or organizing community assessments, public awareness campaigns, group education (for professionals, parents, and youths), and interdisciplinary programs for high-risk youths. Community acceptance is more likely when there is a broad base of support for activities directed at the reduction of teen pregnancy or reduction of consequences.

Research has evaluated years of pregnancy prevention programs. As less funding is available, programs must stand out to receive financial support. Research summaries that can be used by communities for strategic planning are available from the National Campaign to Prevent Teen Pregnancy (http://www.teenpregnancy.org), based in Washington, D.C. Four types of programs had the strongest evidence of effectiveness: HIV and sexuality education programs with a life skills component; clinic-based programs with a focus on sexual behavior; service learning programs that include both volunteer work and classroom discussions about the service; and programs that were multifaceted, with youth development components, health care services, and close relationships with staff (Kirby, 2001a).

The nurse can also be a valuable asset to schools. Family life education programs are strongly recommended or mandated in 46 states, and all 50 states recommend or mandate acquired immunodeficiency syndrome (AIDS) education (Kirby et al, 1994). Health teachers may call on nurses for educational materials or assistance with classroom instruction, especially in the areas of family planning, STDs, and pregnancy. Schools that do not have nurses may arrange to have a public health nurse available for health consultations with students during school hours. Schools may also request that nurses participate on their health advisory boards.

School-based clinics are operating in more than 400 middle and high schools in the United States. The services offered may include counseling, referrals, general health evaluations, and family planning. Some of these programs have been found to delay the onset of intercourse and increase the use of contraception (Kirby et al, 1994). The nurse can assist school systems to design these programs and can also refer young women in need of reproductive health care services.

### DID YOU KNOW?

Emergency contraception can reduce the risk for pregnancy by 75% when used within 72 hours after unprotected intercourse. Although this is an effective and safe method, a regularly used birth control method provides greater protection.

Nurses bring their knowledge about youth and reproductive behavior to any organization or group that has teens, their parents, or other professionals working with teens. Churches are becoming increasingly interested in addressing the needs of their youth, especially since teen sexual activity, pregnancy, and parenting are affecting more of their members.

## Practice Application

A local youth-serving agency requested the assistance of a community health nurse, Kristen, in the implementation of a new high school–based program for pregnant and parenting teen girls. The primary goal of the program is to keep these teens in school through graduation. The secondary goal is to provide knowledge and skills about healthy pregnancy, labor and delivery, and parenting. After delivery, students enrolled in this program were paid for school attendance and this money could be used to defray the costs of childcare.

A community health nurse was the ideal choice to conduct the educational sessions. The group met weekly during the lunch hour. The curriculum that was developed had topics from early pregnancy through the toddler years. Occasionally, Kristen brought in outside speakers such as a labor and delivery nurse or an early intervention specialist.

She also met individually with each enrolled student to provide case management services. Ideally, she would ensure that each student had a health care provider for prenatal care, that each was visited at home by a community health nurse, that each had enrolled in WIC and Medicaid if eligible, and that both the pregnant teen and her partner knew about other parenting and support groups.

One educational session that was particularly interesting was the discussion about the postpartum course—the 6 weeks after delivery. There were many lively discussions about labor experiences as well as some emotional discussions about the reality of coming home with a baby and changes in the relationship with their male partner. Many girls benefited from understanding the normalcy of postpartum blues, but one young woman recognized that she had a more serious and persistent depression and privately approached the community health nurse for assistance.

At the end of the first school year, the dropout rate for pregnant and parenting teens had been reduced by half, and preterm labor rates had also declined. The local school board and a local youth-serving agency joined together to provide financial support to continue this program for an additional 2 years. Kristen was asked to expand the educational programs and interventions she had developed.

What are some directions in which Kristen might expand the program? List four.

*Answers are in the back of the book.*

## Key Points

- The provision of reproductive health care services to adolescents requires sensitivity to the special needs of this age-group. This includes being knowledgeable about state laws regarding confidentiality and services for birth control, pregnancy, abortion, and adoption.
- Pregnant teenagers have a substantial percentage of the first births in the United States. They are more likely to deliver prematurely and have a baby of low birth weight. This risk can be reduced by early initiation of prenatal care and good nutrition.
- Factors that can influence whether a young woman becomes pregnant include a history of sexual victimization, family dysfunction, substance use, and failure to use birth control. Several factors may overlap.
- Nutritional needs during pregnancy can be challenged if the teenager has unhealthy eating habits and begins the pregnancy with limited reserves of vitamins and minerals. With education, the adolescent can make good food choices while still snacking or eating fast foods. Weight gain during pregnancy is a significant marker for a normal-weight baby.
- Young men need special attention and preparation as they become fathers. The interventions include

information about pregnancy and delivery, declaration of paternity, care of infants and children, and psychosocial support in this role.

- The pregnant teen will need support during her pregnancy and in child-rearing. Families may provide most of this support. However, many communities have a variety of services available for adolescents. These services include financial assistance for medical care, nutritional programs, and school-based support groups.
- Adolescent parents have unrealistic expectations about their children and consequently do not know how to stimulate emotional, social, and cognitive development. The children born to adolescents are at risk for academic and behavioral problems as they become older. Teens who receive education on normal development and childcare will be more likely to avert these problems with their children.
- During a pregnancy, teenagers are expected to attend school. Homebound instruction is reserved for those with medical complications. Teen mothers who return to school and complete their education after the birth of their child are less likely to have a repeat pregnancy. Problems finding childcare and the need to have an income can create an obstacle to school return.
- Community coalitions, which include nurses, can have a significant impact on teen pregnancy. These coalitions generally have diverse representation from the community, and therefore their activities meet with more community support.

## Clinical Decision-Making Activities

1. Become familiar with statistics on teen pregnancy, births, miscarriages, and abortions in your area.

Collect information also on utilization of prenatal care, low-birth-weight and premature deliveries, high school completion, and repeat pregnancies. Compare the trends in statistics to the impact and costs to the individual, her family, and the community.

2. Call or visit local schools and interview the school nurse or guidance counselors about teen pregnancy. Determine what resources are available through the schools for pregnancy prevention. Assess the family life education curriculum, and identify a teaching project for nursing students. Can pregnancy prevention and parenting education be incorporated into the learning objectives in the existing school curriculum?

3. Design and offer a childbirth preparation class for pregnant teens and their support persons. Include a plan for identifying potential participants, select a site that is accessible, and develop an evaluation method. Develop teaching tools that acknowledge adolescent development.

4. Assess reproductive health care services for young men in your community. Design an awareness campaign targeting young men on paternity issues and the prevention of pregnancy. Be specific about ways to bring in male role models and mentors.

### Additional Resources

These related resources are found either in the appendix at the back of this book or on the book's website at **http://evolve.elsevier.com/Stanhope.**

**evolve** **Evolve Website**

WebLinks: Healthy People 2010

## References

Alexander CS, Guyer B: Adolescent pregnancy: occurrence and consequences, *Pediatr Ann* 22(2):85, 1993.

American College of Obstetricians and Gynecologists: *Adolescent pregnancy facts,* Washington, DC, 2000, ACOG.

Andreozzi L et al: Attachment classifications among 18-month-old children of adolescent mothers, *Arch Pediatr Adolesc Med* 156:20, 2002.

Bearman P, Bruckner H: *Power in numbers: peer effects on adolescent girls' sexual debut and pregnancy,* Washington, DC, 1999, National Campaign to Prevent Preteen Pregnancy.

Boyer D, Fine D: Sexual abuse as a factor in adolescent pregnancy and child maltreatment, *Fam Plann Perspect* 24(1):4, 1992.

Brandsen CK: *A case for adoption,* Grand Rapids, Mich, 1991, Bethany.

Cartoof VG, Klerman LV, Zazveta VD: The effect of source of prenatal care on care-seeking behavior and pregnancy outcomes among adolescents, *J Adolesc Health* 12:124, 1991.

Cartwright PS et al: Teenagers' perceptions of barriers to prenatal care, *South Med J* 86(7):737, 1993.

Centers for Disease Control and Prevention: Pregnancy rates among adolescents—United States, 1995-1997, *MMWR Morb Mortal Wkly Rep* 49(27):605, 2000a.

Centers for Disease Control and Prevention: Youth risk behavior surveillance—United States, 1999, *MMWR Morb Mortal Wkly Rep* 49(SSO5):1, 2000b.

Commonwealth Fund: *The commonwealth fund survey of the health of adolescent girls,* New York, 1997, Commonwealth Fund.

Connop HL, Boyce W: Announcements: national research project to build on Canada, Youth, and AIDS study, *Can J Human Sexual* 9(1):75, 2000.

The contraceptive report, 12(3):8-12 and 12:4):8, Houston, Texas, 2001, Emron, available at www.contraceptiononline. org.

Covington DL et al: Improving detection of violence among pregnant adolescents, *J Adolesc Health* 21(1):18, 1997.

Curry MA, Doyle BA, Gilhooley J: Abuse among pregnant adolescents: differences by developmental age, *MCN Am J Matern Child Nurs* 23(3):144, 1998.

Darroch JE et al: Differences in teenage pregnancy rates among five developed countries: the roles of sexual activity and contraceptive use, *Fam Plann Perspect* 33(6):244-250, 281, 2001.

Diehl K: Adolescent mothers: what produces positive mother-infant interaction, *MCN Am J Matern Child Nurs* 22(2):89, 1997.

Dryburgh H: Teenage pregnancy (Statistics Canada, Catalogue 82-003), *Health Rep* 12(1):9-19, 2000.

East PL, Felice ME: Pregnancy risk among the younger sisters of pregnant and childbearing adolescents. *J Dev Behav Pediatr* 13(2):128-136, 1992.

Hampton MR et al: Sexual experience, contraception, and STI prevention among high school students: results from a Canadian urban centre, *Can J Human Sexual* 10(3-4):111-126, 2001.

Harrykissoon SD, Rickert VI, Wiemann CW: Prevalence and patterns of intimate partner violence among adolescent mothers during the postpartum period, *Arch Pediatr Adolesc Med* 156:325, 2002.

Hatcher RA et al: *Contraceptive technology,* New York, 1998, Ardent Media.

Health Canada: *Sexual risk behaviors of Canadians: bureau of HIV/AIDS and STD Epi Update Series,* Laboratory Center for Disease Control, Ottawa, Ont, 1997, Health Canada.

Hofferth S, Reid L, Mott F: The effects of early childbearing on schooling over time, *Fam Plann Perspect* 33(6):259, 2001.

King A et al: *Canada, youth, and AIDS study,* Ottawa, Ont, 1988, Health Canada, Federal Centre for AIDS.

Kirby D: *Emerging answers: research findings on programs to reduce teen pregnancy,* Washington, DC, 2001a, National Campaign to Prevent Teen Pregnancy.

Kirby D: Understanding what works and what doesn't in reducing adolescent sexual risk-taking, *Fam Plann Perspect* 33(6):276, 2001b.

Kirby D et al: School-based programs to reduce sexual risk behaviors: a review of effectiveness, *Public Health Rep* 109(3):339, 1994.

Leadbeater BJ, Way N: *Growing up fast, transitions to early adulthood of inner-city adolescent mothers,* Mahwah, NJ, 2001, Lawrence Erlbaum.

Lederman SA: Nutritional support for the pregnant adolescent. In Adolescent nutritional disorders prevention and treatment, *Ann NY Acad Sci* 817:304, 1997.

Marsiglio W: Adolescent males' orientation toward paternity and contraception, *Fam Plann Perspect* 25(1):22, 1993.

Maticka-Tyndale E: Sexual health and Canadian youth: how do we measure up? *Can J Human Sexual* 10(1-2):1-17, 2001.

Maticka-Tyndale E, Barrett M, McKay A: Adolescent sexual and reproductive health in Canada: a review of national data sources and their limitations, *Can J Human Sexual* 9(1):41-65, 2000.

Maticka-Tyndale E, McKay A, Barrett M: *Teenage sexual and reproductive behaviour in developed countries: country report for Canada—occasional report No. 4,* New York, 2001, Alan Guttmacher Institute.

Moore KA, Driscoll A: *Partners, predators, peers, protectors: males and teen pregnancy: new data analysed by the 1995 national survey of family growth,* Washington, DC, 1997, National Campaign to Prevent Teen Pregnancy.

Moore KA, Driscoll AK, Lindberg LD: *A statistical portrait of adolescent sex, contraception and childbearing,* Washington, DC, 1998, National Campaign to Prevent Teen Pregnancy.

Moore KA et al: *Facts at a glance,* Sponsored by the Charles Stewart Mott Foundation, Washington, DC, 1997, Child Trends.

National Abortion and Reproductive Rights Action League: *Supreme Court decisions concerning reproductive rights, a chronology: 1965-2001,* Washington DC, 2001, NARAL.

National Abortion and Reproductive Rights Action League Foundation: *Who decides? a state-by-state review of abortion and reproductive rights,* Washington, DC, 2002, NARAL.

Osborne LN, Rhodes JE: The role of life stress and social support in the adjustment of sexually victimized pregnant and parenting adolescents, *Am J Community Psychol* 29(6):833, 2001.

Papillo AR et al: *Facts at a glance,* Sponsored by the Charles Stewart Mott Foundation, Flint, Mich, Washington DC, 2002, Child Trends.

Resnick MD et al: Protecting adolescents from harm, *JAMA* 278(10):823, 1997.

Rhein LM et al: Teen father participation in child rearing: family perspectives, *J Adolesc Health* 21(4):244, 1997.

Richardson HRL et al: Factors influencing condom use among students attending high school in Nova Scotia, *Can J Human Sexual* 6(3):185-196, 1997.

Ruchala PL, James DC: Social support, knowledge of infant development and maternal confidence among adolescent and adult mothers, *J Obstet Gynecol Neonatal Nurs* 26(6):685, 1997.

Scholl TO, Hediger ML, Schall JI: Maternal growth and fetal growth: pregnancy course and outcome in the Camden study. In Adolescent Nutritional Disorders Prevention and Treatment, *Ann NY Acad Sci* 817:292, 1997.

Stock JL et al: Adolescent pregnancy and sexual risk taking among sexually abused girls, *Fam Plann Perspect* 29(5):200, 1997.

Story M: Promoting healthy eating and ensuring adequate weight gain in pregnant adolescents: issues and strategies. In Adolescent Nutritional Disorders Prevention and Treatment, *Ann NY Acad Sci* 817:321, 1997.

Story M, Stang J, editors: *Nutrition and the pregnant adolescent: a practical reference guide,* Minneapolis, Minn, 2000, University of Minnesota, Center for Leadership, Education, and Training in Maternal and Child Nutrition.

Stouthamer-Loeber M, Wei EH: The precursors of young fatherhood and its effect on delinquency of teenage males, *J Adolesc Health* 22(1):56, 1998.

Thomas BH, DiCenso A, Griffith L: Adolescent sexual behaviour: results from an Ontario sample—part II: adolescent use of protection, *Can J Public Health* 89(2):94-97, 1998.

U.S. Department of Health and Human Services: *Healthy people 2010: understanding and improving health,* ed 2, Washington, DC, 2000, U.S. Government Printing Office.

VanWinter JT, Simmons PS: A proposal for obstetric and pediatric management of adolescent pregnancy, *Mayo Clin Proc* 65:1061, 1990.

Wadhera S, Millar WJ: Teenage pregnancies, 1974 to 1994 (Statistics Canada, Catalogue 82-003-XPB), *Health Rep* 9(3):9-17, 1997.

Wayland J, Rawlins R: African American teen mothers' perceptions of parenting, *J Pediatr Nurs* 12(1):13, 1997.

Whitman RL et al: *Interwomen lives,* Mahwah, NJ, 2001, Lawrence Erlbaum.

Zelenko M et al: The child abuse potential inventory and pregnancy outcome in expectant adolescent mothers, *Child Abuse Negl* 25:1481, 2001.

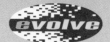
# Chapter 35

# Mental Health Issues

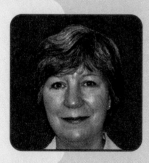

**Anita Thompson-Heisterman, M.S.N., R.N., C.S., F.N.P.**
Anita Thompson-Heisterman began practicing community mental health nursing in 1983 as a psychiatric nurse in a community mental health center. Her community practice has included clinical and management activities in a psychiatric home care service, a nurse-managed primary care center in public housing, and an outreach program for rural older adults. Currently she is a clinical instructor in the Division of Family, Community and Mental Health Systems at the University of Virginia School of Nursing.

## Objectives

After reading this chapter, the student should be able to do the following:

1. Describe the history of community mental health and make predictions about the future
2. Discuss essential mental health services and corresponding national objectives for healthier people
3. Analyze the status of the population that has mental illness in the United States
4. Evaluate standards, models, concepts, and research findings for use in community mental health nursing practice
5. Describe the role of the community mental health nurse with individuals and with groups at risk for psychiatric mental health problems
6. Apply the nursing process in community work with clients diagnosed with psychiatric disorders, families at risk for mental health problems, and populations at risk
7. Examine ways to improve the mental health of people who are at risk in a complex society

---

Providing community services and nursing care to people suffering from mental illness or emotional distress is a complex endeavor influenced by many individual and community factors and requiring a variety of approaches. Some of these factors are (1) the scope of emotional and mental disorders, (2) the uncertainty about specific cause, cure, and treatment for most severe mental disorders, (3) the severe chronic disabling nature of some mental disorders, and (4) the complexity of the community mental health services sector. The scarcity of resources compounds the problems and presents challenges in community mental health work.

Cultural beliefs and economics influence the amount and types of services and treatment available in countries. However, two universal truths exist: services for people with mental disorders are inadequate in all countries, and the impact of mental illness on families, communities, and

nations is profound. Therefore specialized knowledge and skills about severe mental illness and mental health problems are necessary for effective community and public health nursing practice. It is helpful to understand both the organization of mental health services from a historical perspective and the trends in current health care demands and delivery. Knowledge about populations at risk for psychiatric mental health problems and understanding illness outcomes in terms of biopsychosocial consequences are even more important. Finally, it is necessary to refine and broaden nursing process skills in treatment planning to include the impact of mental illness on families and communities.

This chapter focuses on the scope of mental disorders, development of community mental health services, current health objectives for mental health and mental disorders, and the role of the nurse in community settings. Conceptual frameworks useful in community mental health nursing practice are also presented. Because other chapters in this book are devoted to high-risk groups such as the homeless population and those with substance

*The author gratefully acknowledges the significant contributions to this chapter by Patricia Howard, this chapter's author in previous editions of this textbook.*

## Key Terms

**Americans With Disabilities Act**, p. 832
**assertive community treatment**, p. 834
**community mental health centers**, p. 828
**Community Support Program**, p. 828
**consumer**, p. 828
**consumer advocacy**, p. 828

**deinstitutionalization**, p. 832
**institutionalization**, p. 830
**mental health problems**, p. 828
**National Alliance for the Mentally Ill**,
   p. 828
**National Institute of Mental Health**, p. 828

**relapse management**, p. 833
**severe mental disorders**, p. 827
**systems theory**, p. 833
*See Glossary for definitions*

## Chapter Outline

Scope of Mental Illness in the United States
*Consumer Advocacy*
*Neurobiology of Mental Illness*
Systems of Community Mental Health Care
*Managed Care*
Evolution of Community Mental Health Care
*Historical Perspectives*
*Hospital Expansion, Institutionalization, and the
   Mental Hygiene Movement*
*Federal Legislation for Mental Health Services*

Deinstitutionalization
*Civil Rights Legislation for Persons With Mental
   Disorders*
*Advocacy Efforts*
Conceptual Frameworks for Community
   Mental Health
*Levels of Prevention*
Role of the Nurse in Community Mental
   Health
*Clinician*

*Educator*
*Coordinator*
Current and Future Perspectives in Mental
   Health Care
National Objectives for Mental Health Services
*Children and Adolescents*
*Adults*
*Adults With Serious Mental Illness*
*Older Adults*
*Cultural Diversity*

abuse problems, this chapter's focus is on the continuum of mental health problems encountered in communities, with an emphasis on populations who have long-term, severe mental disorders and groups who are most vulnerable to mental health problems.

## SCOPE OF MENTAL ILLNESS IN THE UNITED STATES

Mental health and illness can be viewed as a continuum. Mental health is defined in Healthy People 2010 (U.S. Department of Health and Human Services [USDHHS], 2000) as encompassing the ability to engage in productive activities and fulfilling relationships with other people, to adapt to change, and to cope with adversity. Mental health is an integral part of personal well-being, both family and interpersonal relationships, and contribution to community or society. Mental disorders are conditions that are characterized by alterations in thinking, mood, or behavior, which are associated with distress and/or impaired functioning (USDHHS, 2000). Mental illness refers collectively to all diagnosable mental disorders.

**Severe mental disorders** are determined by diagnoses and criteria that include degree of functional disability (American Psychiatric Association, 2000).

Mental disorders are indiscriminate. They occur across the life span and affect persons of all races, cultures, sexes, and educational and socioeconomic groups. In the United States, approximately 40 million adults (ages 18 to 64 years), or 22% of the population, have a mental disorder. At least one in five children and adolescents between ages 9 and 17 years has a diagnosable mental disorder in a given year, and about 5% of children and adolescents are extremely impaired by mental, behavioral, and emotional disorders. An estimated 25% of older people experience specific mental disorders, such as depression, anxiety, substance abuse, and dementia that are not part of normal aging. Alzheimer's disease, the primary cause of dementia, strikes between 8% and 15% of people over age 65. The number of cases in the population doubles every 5 years of age after age 60 and will increase as the population ages (USDHHS, 2000). Affective disorders include major depression and manic-depressive or bipolar illness. Although bipolar illness may only affect 1% of the population, a study done for the World Health Organization found major depression to be pervasive and the leading cause of disability among adults in developed nations such as the United States (Murray and Lopez, 1996). Nearly 7% of women and over 3% of men have major depression in any year. Anxiety disorders, including panic disorder, obsessive-compulsive disorder, posttraumatic stress disorder (PTSD), and phobias are more common than other mental disorders and affect as many as 19 million people in the United States annually (USDHHS, 2000). Schizophrenia affects more than 2 million people a year in the United States. Mental disorders can also be a secondary problem among people with other disabilities. Depression and anxiety, for example, occur more frequently among people with disabilities (USDHHS, 2000).

The impact of mental illness on overall health and productivity in the United States and throughout the world is often profoundly underrecognized. In the United States, mental illness is on a par with heart disease and cancer as a cause of disability (USDHHS, 2000). Despite the prevalence of mental illness, only 25% of persons with a mental disorder obtain help for their illness in any part of the health care system, and the majority of persons with mental disorders do not receive specialty mental health services at all. In comparison, between 60% and 80% of persons with heart disease seek and receive care. Of those aged 18 years and older getting help, about 15% receive help from mental health specialists. Of young people aged 9 to 17 years who have a mental disorder, 27% receive treatment in the health sector and an additional 20% of children and adolescents use mental health services only in their schools (USDHHS, 2000). Given this information, it is critical that community-oriented nurses recognize and provide health services for those with mental disorders in nontraditional community settings, such as schools.

In addition to diagnosable mental conditions, there is increasing awareness and concern regarding the public health burden of stress, especially following the terrorist attacks on the World Trade Center and the Pentagon on September 11, 2001. Strengthening the public health sector to respond to terrorism involves developing mental health responses as well as other defenses. Community mental health nurses (CMHNs) play an important role in identifying stressful events, assessing stress responses, educating communities, and intervening to prevent or alleviate disability and disease resulting from stress.

Although all of us are vulnerable to stressful life events and may develop **mental health problems,** persons with chronic and persistent mental illness have numerous problems. Many lack access to adequate health services, along with other resources such as housing. A myriad of accessible and coordinated services are needed to maintain people with chronic mental illness in the community, yet these often are not available. Despite the inadequacy of resources, advances have been made in the treatment of mental illness. These advances have been influenced by two major

movements: **consumer advocacy,** and better understanding of the neurobiology of mental illness (Foulkes, 2000; Keltner et al, 1998; Manderscheid and Henderson, 2001). A third movement, managed care, has influenced changes in the treatment of mental illness, and it appears this influence has had both positive and negative outcomes on access to mental health services (Hannon and Roth, 2001; Mowbry, Grazier, and Holter, 2002).

## Consumer Advocacy

Advocacy movements for people with mental illness, like those for other illnesses, came about to fulfill unmet needs. Specifically, the **National Alliance for the Mentally Ill** (NAMI) was the first **consumer** group to advocate for better services. This consumer advocacy group worked to establish education and self-help services for individuals and families with mental illness (Foulkes, 2000; Manderscheid and Henderson, 2001). Efforts of the NAMI gained momentum in the early 1980s. Subsequently, political groups and legislative bodies responded with direct support. One example of direct support was funding for the **Community Support Program** (CSP) by the **National Institute of Mental Health** (NIMH). The CSP provides grant monies to states to develop comprehensive services for persons discharged from psychiatric institutions Foulkes, 2000; (Manderscheid and Henderson, 2001). These and similar efforts have helped bring consumers, families, and professionals together to work toward improvement in the treatment and care of persons with mental illness.

## Neurobiology of Mental Illness

Mental illnesses are complex biopsychosocial disorders. Most of the emphasis in the past decade has been focused on the biological basis of mental illness. The 1990s were declared the "decade of the brain" (USDHHS, 1999) and great strides occurred through research in neurology, microbiology, and genetics in understanding the structural and chemical complexity of the brain. Consequently, more is now known about the functions of the brain than at any time in history. We have learned that the brain is not a static organ. The concept of brain plasticity demonstrates that new learning actually changes brain structure. For example, traumatic experiences change brain biochemistry, as do significant positive experiences (Mohr and Mohr, 2001; USDHHS, 1999). This information supports the notion that both experience and psychosocial factors have effects on etiology and on treatment of mental illnesses. Both somatic and psychosocial interventions need to be employed in the treatment of mental illness. In addition to research, neuroradiologic techniques aid diagnosis and treatment of people with psychiatric disorders. Angiography is used to screen for abnormalities of the vascular system, such as atherosclerosis and brain tumors, that can result in behavior changes. Diagnosis is also improved by using noninvasive scanning of the brain. Computed axial tomography (CAT) scans provide a cross-sectional view of the brain, whereas nuclear magnetic resonance (NMR) offers the advantage of imaging the brain from different planes. Still other techniques, such as positron emission tomography (PET) and single photon emission computed tomography (SPECT), provide information about cerebral blood flow and brain metabolism. The information gained from these advanced technologies can lead to better understanding about mental illness.

## THE CUTTING EDGE

Using noninvasive imaging techniques, scientists will be able to study the effects of different forms of psychotherapeutic interventions on the brain.

Discoveries in psychopharmacology have also revolutionized treatment of mental illness (Boyd, 2002; Manderscheid and Henderson, 2001). The new atypical antipsychotic drugs used in the treatment of schizophrenia have led to an improved quality of life for many, primarily because of fewer side effects. However, new side effects, including weight gain, insulin resistance, and dangerously high blood glucose levels, have created new concerns for consumers and providers (Lindenmayer, Nathan, and Smith, 2001; Seaburg, McLendon, and Doraiswamy, 2001). New antidepressant medications known as selective serotonin reuptake inhibitors (SSRIs) are now considered the first choice in the treatment of depression because they lead to good responses with fewer side effects. They are now widely prescribed by primary care physicians as well as psychiatrists. Paxil (paroxetine) in 2002 was one of the six most prescribed medications in the United States (Barry, 2002).

## WHAT DO YOU THINK?

Although psychopharmacology has dramatically improved the lives of people with severe mental illness, controversies exist about medication side effects and the costs of monitoring treatment. For example, side effects of antipsychotic drugs include central and peripheral nervous system manifestations. New or atypical antipsychotics have reduced some of these side effects but have caused weight gain, insulin resistance, and life-threatening hyperglycemia. Do the benefits offered by these medications justify their side effects?

## SYSTEMS OF COMMUNITY MENTAL HEALTH CARE

### Managed Care

Managed care is a system of managing health care to ensure access to appropriate and cost-effective services. Managed mental health care grew rapidly during the last decade. By 1999, 79% of Americans were enrolled in a managed health care plan (Mowbry et al, 2002). Initially a method to control costs and access to mental health care in the private insurance sector, managed care became a significant factor in public mental health, and by 1998, 54% of all Medicaid enrollees were in a managed mental health care plan (Mowbry et al, 2002). Consumer outcomes such as health status, quality of life, functioning, and satisfaction are just beginning to emerge at the advent of the new millennium (Manderscheid and Henderson, 2001). As one purpose of managed care is to control costs, often by substituting less costly services for more costly ones (Manderscheid and Henderson, 2001), the findings about consumer outcomes are critical. For example, community care is generally less costly than hospital care, although the provision of quality comprehensive services in the community is not inexpensive. Services must fit the needs of the consumer, and outcomes research can help guide care decisions.

## DID YOU KNOW?

Managed care programs tend to reduce coverage for inpatient hospital stays for mental illness. However, community survival for people with serious mental illness requires a broad range of well-coordinated services, including mental and physical health, housing assistance, substance abuse treatment for some, and social and vocational rehabilitation.

Changes continue to take place in the managed care arena. Although federal legislation was passed in 2002 ensuring parity for mental illness coverage in insurance plans, the implementation and the effects on managed care plans remains to be seen. The seemingly constant changes in mental health funding present challenges for nurses, who need to make judgments about the positive and negative outcomes of these changes on the people they care for before research findings that can be generalized to the population are readily available.

Mental health problems and mental disorders are treated by a variety of caregivers who work in diverse and loosely connected facilities. In the United States today, there are four major ways through which people receive mental health services. These are (1) the specialty mental health system, both public and private, (2) the general medical or primary care sector, (3) the human service sector, and (4) the voluntary support network, including advocacy groups (USDHHS, 1999). It is important for community-oriented nurses to understand that delivery of mental health services may occur in any of these systems. In fact, most older adults receive mental health services through the primary care sector, whereas most children and adolescents are served through human services that include schools (USDHHS, 1999). Those with resources, less severe mental health problems, and access to primary care are more likely to have their mental health needs addressed within the context of a visit to their primary care provider. Again because of the influence of managed care, access to a specialist, if indicated for psychiatric treatment, occurs via this route as well.

The community mental health model is the primary method of care for people with serious and persistent mental illness. Components of this model include team care, case management, outreach, and a variety of rehabilitative models to help prevent exacerbations of illness. In most states, the model is implemented through comprehensive **community mental health centers** (CMHCs), yet neither the model and its components nor the CMHCs are refined processes and systems of care. Rather, the model continues to evolve in this era of health care reform, as the CMHCs react to societal, political, and fiscal pressures. There is great variance in how each state and locality implements the model. As resources diminish, the focus narrows and many CMHCs are unable to provide services to populations other than those with serious and persistent mental illness. The community mental health model of care is not limited to the United States. Indeed it was developed in England as part of the social psychiatry movement of the 1940s and 1950s, and it is also used in western Europe, where integration with and funding of social services is more embraced than in the United States. The trend towards CMHCs is also evolving in many eastern countries. For example, in Hong Kong, mental health services were largely based in hospitals until the early 1990s; now community mental health nurses provide care in day and residential centers (Yip, 1998). Historically, both in the United States and abroad, reform movements influenced the development of mental health services and models of care whether they were located in hospital or community settings.

## EVOLUTION OF COMMUNITY MENTAL HEALTH CARE

### Historical Perspectives

The manner in which the community has perceived the etiology of mental and emotional illness across the ages has influenced the care and treatment of persons suffering from these disorders. These patterns were often cyclical. In ancient times, mental illness was viewed as resulting from supernatural forces and those afflicted were shunned. During the Greco-Roman era, mental and physical illnesses were seen as interrelated and resulting from physical conditions. Treatment was aimed at curing the disease by restoring balance. A return to a belief in supernatural etiologies occurred during the Middle Ages in Europe and continued in the colonies well into the eighteenth century. These beliefs resulted in poor treatment of the mentally ill, including incarceration, starvation, and torture (Boyd, 2002). Near the end of the eighteenth century, the revolution in mental health care known as Humanitarian Reform took place. This reform movement, influenced by Philippe Pinel (1759-1820) in France and Benjamin Rush (1745-1813) in America, led to hospital expansion, medical treat-

ment, and the community mental health movements (Boyd, 2002).

Before the Humanitarian Reform, persons with mental illness were often housed in jails because health and social services had not been developed. Even later, after the development of hospitals as a site of treatment, persons with mental disorders were neglected and mistreated. Although the first psychiatric hospital in the United States was built in Williamsburg, Virginia, in 1773, approximately 50 years passed before widespread construction of facilities in other states took place. One person in particular, Dorothea Dix, led reform efforts to correct inhumane practices (Boyd, 2002; Worley, 1997).

Dorothea Lynde Dix (1802-1887) focused attention on three populations: criminals, those with mental disorders, and victims of the Civil War (Worley, 1997). She said that people with mental disorders needed health and social services, and her efforts resulted in improved organization of mental health services. Her work led to the development of hospitals as the primary site of care, and she influenced standards for hospital administration and nursing care. Because of her lifetime efforts, often through political action, treatment for mentally infirm persons was altered on both the North American and European continents.

## Hospital Expansion, Institutionalization, and the Mental Hygiene Movement

Psychiatric hospitals constructed during the expansion era were located in rural areas and were intended for small numbers of clients. However, they soon became overcrowded with people who had severe mental disorders, with older adults, and with immigrants who were poor and unable to speak English (Boyd, 2002; Worley, 1997). Clients were essentially separated from the community and isolated from their families. Many were institutionalized for the rest of their lives, in response to both a continued fear of persons with mental disorders and a lack of community resources. **Institutionalization** of large numbers of people, combined with minimal information about cause, cure, and care, resulted in overcrowded conditions and exploitation of clients.

At the beginning of the twentieth century, institutional conditions were reported publicly in the United States by Clifford Beers, who had been hospitalized both in private and public mental hospitals (Boyd, 2002). Beers urged reform and influenced the founding of the National Committee for Mental Hygiene. During the mental hygiene movement, attention shifted to ideas about prevention, early intervention, and the influence of social and environmental factors on mental illness. These ideas about treatment also influenced the development of multidisciplinary approaches to treatment. The mental hygiene and community mental health movements increased understanding about mental illness.

Further understanding about the scope of mental illness was gained during the conscription process for the armed services in World War II. Many of the persons screened for military service during World War II were found to have neurologic and psychiatric mental health disorders. Even more military personnel required treatment for mental health problems associated with social and environmental stress during and after the war, not only in the United States but also in Europe, Russia, and Pacific Rim countries (Boyd, 2002). At the same time, the community mental health model continued to expand slowly while populations consisting of individuals with severe mental disorders and older adult persons with dementia grew larger in the state hospitals. Demands for mental health services in communities, combined with concerns about conditions of state psychiatric hospitals, prompted federal legislation that influenced development of the community mental health concept.

## Federal Legislation for Mental Health Services

The first major piece of legislation to influence mental health services in the United States was the Social Security Act in 1935. This act, created in response to economic and social problems of the era, shifted the responsibility of care for ill people from the state to the federal government. The federal government's role expanded when the demand for mental health services increased during and after World War II. Key points of legislation that influenced the development of community mental health services are summarized in Table 35-1.

In 1946, the National Mental Health Act was passed and the NIMH administered its programs (Boyd, 2002; Worley, 1997). Objectives included development of education and research programs for community mental

health treatment approaches. The act also included financial incentives for training grants to increase the number of professional workers, including nurses, in mental health services. Education and research programs materialized readily, along with advances in science and technology and the development of psychotropic medications (Boyd, 2002; Worley, 1997).

In 1955 the Mental Health Study Act was passed and the Joint Commission on Mental Illness and Health was established by the NIMH (Boyd, 2002). Members of the commission studied national mental health needs and submitted to Congress a report entitled Action for Mental Health. Recommendations of the report included continued development of research and education programs, early and intensive treatment for acute mental illness, and shifting the care of severely mentally ill persons away from the large hospitals to psychiatric wards in general hospitals and to community mental health clinics. Along with prevention and intervention, community services were to include aftercare services following hospitalization for individuals with major mental illness (Boyd, 2002). The shift in the locus of care from state hospitals to community systems was begun.

The Community Mental Health Centers Act (CMHC) was passed in 1963, and the CMHC concept was formalized. Federal funds were designated to match state funds to construct CMHCs and start programs. CMHCs were mandated to have five basic services: inpatient, outpatient, partial hospitalization, 24-hour emergency services, and consultation/education services for community agencies and professionals (Boyd, 2002). In addition, regulations encouraged states to offer diagnostic and rehabilitative

| Table 35-1 | Legislation That Influenced Community Mental Health Services | |
|---|---|---|
| **YEAR** | **LEGISLATION** | **FOCUS** |
| 1946 | National Mental Health Act | Education and research for mental health treatment approaches began (NIMH) |
| 1955 | Mental Health Study Act | Resulted in Joint Commission on Mental Illness and Health, which recommended transformation of state hospital systems and establishment of community mental health clinics |
| 1963 | Community Mental Health Centers Act | Marked beginning of community mental health centers concept and led to deinstitutionalization of large psychiatric hospitals |
| 1975 | Developmental Disabilities Act | Addressed the rights and treatment of people with developmental disabilities and provided foundation for similar action for individuals with mental disorders |
| 1977 | President's Commission on Mental Health | Reinforced importance of community-based services, protection of human rights, and national health insurance for mentally ill persons |
| 1978 | Omnibus Reconciliation Act | Rescinded much of the 1977 commission's provisions and shifted funds for all health programs from federal to state resources |
| 1986 | Protection and Advocacy for Mentally Ill Individuals Act | Legislated advocacy programs for mentally ill persons |
| 1990 | Americans With Disabilities Act | Prohibited discrimination and promoted opportunities for persons with mental disorders |

precare and aftercare services (Boyd, 2002). However, many CMHCs, especially those in poor and rural areas, were unable to generate adequate money for continuing their start-up programs. Funding did not follow the client to the community. The deinstitutionalization of persons with severe mental disorders was well underway before some of these shortcomings were recognized.

## DEINSTITUTIONALIZATION

**Deinstitutionalization** involved transitioning large numbers of people from state psychiatric hospitals to communities. The cost of institutional care was perhaps the main reason for the movement; other influences included the discovery of psychotropic medications and civil rights activism (Boyd, 2002; Lamb, 2001; Worley, 1997). The goal of deinstitutionalization was to improve the quality of life for people with mental disorders by providing services in the communities where they lived rather than in large institutions. To change the locus of care, large hospital wards were closed and persons with severe mental disorders were returned to the community to live. Many were discharged to the care of family members; others went to nursing homes. Still others were placed in apartments or other types of adult housing; some of these were supervised settings, and others were not.

Not surprisingly, as with any abrupt, dramatic change, problems related to unexpected service gaps between the hospitals and the CMHCs led to continuity-of-care problems. According to Mowbry, et al (2002), although deinstitutionalization was noble in conception, it was bankrupt in implementation. For example, families were not prepared for the treatment responsibilities they had to assume and yet few mental health systems offered them education and support programs. Although many older adult clients were admitted to nursing homes and personal care settings, education programs were seldom available for staff, who often lacked the skills necessary to treat persons with mental disorders. And finally, some clients found themselves in independent settings such as rooming houses and single-room occupancy hotels with little or no supervision. Clients, families, communities, and the nation suffered as poor living and social conditions were associated with mental disorders. Homelessness and placement of the mentally ill in jails and prisons also occurred (Lamb, 2001). These types of issues prompted additional legislation and advocacy efforts.

## Civil Rights Legislation for Persons With Mental Disorders

The development of CMHCs was based partially on the principle that persons with mental disorders had a right to treatment in the least restrictive environment (Boyd, 2002). Although CMHCs did prove less restrictive than institutions, they lacked necessary services. For example, people with severe mental disorders require daily monitoring or hospitalization during acute episodes of illness.

Even though hospital services were available, many individuals expressed their rights to refuse treatment and resisted admission. Also, transitional care following discharge for those persons who were admitted to hospitals was not available in most communities (Lamb, 2001). In addition to the right to refuse treatment, advocates for mentally ill individuals focused on such civil rights issues as segregated services, inhumane practices in psychiatric hospitals, and failure to include clients in treatment planning. Activism for minorities and handicapped persons also influenced civil rights legislation for persons with mental disorders. In particular, during the 1970s institutional conditions of persons with developmental handicaps prompted the Developmental Disabilities Assistance Act and the Bill of Rights Act (Wasserbauer, 1996). Other legislation shifted funding from the federal to the state level. The Mental Health Systems Act was repealed in 1980. This action limited the federal leadership role, shifted more costs back to the states from the federal government, and further impeded the implementation and provision of community mental health services (Sharfstein, 2000).

State systems of mental health services developed in diverse ways and were often inadequate. In general, individuals with severe mental disorders were vulnerable and neglected and either lacked or were unable to access health and social services. In an effort to offset these problems, in 1986 the federal Protection and Advocacy for Mentally Ill Individuals Act and the Mental Health Planning Act were legislated. Advocacy programs for mentally ill persons became part of the same state advocacy systems developed earlier under the Developmental Disability Act, and consumer involvement in CMHCs was mandated (Boyd, 2002). In spite of advocacy efforts and legislation, the CMHCs were unable to meet the increased and diverse demands for mental health services in their communities. The lack of services combined with concerns about discrimination against all people with disabilities led to additional legislation.

In 1990 the **Americans With Disabilities Act (ADA)** was passed. The ADA mandated that individuals with mental and physical disabilities not be discriminated against and be brought into the mainstream of American life through access to employment and public services (Boyd, 2002; Wasserbauer, 1996). History reveals that past legislation promoted the rights of persons with mental disorders, but litigation was also responsible for the lack of growth, if not the decline, in community mental health services. The community mental health nurse can advocate for clients to ensure equality in access to health services, housing, and employment.

## Advocacy Efforts

Consumers, defined as persons who are current or former recipients of mental health services, and their families have had a significant impact on mental health services. As in all areas of health care, the rights and wishes of consumers are important in planning and delivering services.

However, consumers of mental health services have traditionally had difficulty advocating for themselves. In the past, treatment programs often fostered passivity in clients and excluded them from the treatment planning process. In addition, family members were responsible for care in the home, but they lacked resources and even information about treatment (Foulkes, 2000). Like consumers, family members suffered from the stigma of mental illness and public attitudes that contributed to self-advocacy problems (Wahl, 1999). In contrast, self-advocacy and involvement in treatment planning fosters self-confidence, promotes participation in services, and may influence policy decisions. Consumer and family groups fostered these objectives (Foulkes, 2000; Wahl, 1999).

---

### BOX 35-1   Advocacy and Self-Help Organizations

- Community Support Program (CSP): A program of the U.S. Department of Health and Human Services (USDHHS), Substance Abuse and Mental Health Administration (SAMHA), Center for Mental Health Services (CMHS), that developed plans for a model continuum of care, offers grants for demonstration programs including community rehabilitation projects, and provided money to states for development of consumer and family services and advocacy efforts

- Consumer/Survivor Mental Health Research and Policy Work Group: An endeavor sponsored by the Mental Health Statistics Improvement Program of the CMHS to initiate consumer representation in activities of the National Association of State Mental Health Program Directors (NASMHPD)

- National Alliance for the Mentally Ill (NAMI): A family organization that promotes family support groups, education programs, public campaigns to reduce stigma, and advocacy for mental health policy and services at local and national levels

- NAMI Consumers' Council: A consumer advocacy group that advocates for improved and effective psychiatric services and consumer empowerment

- National Association of Psychiatric Survivors (NAPS): A consumer organization that advocates for such things as involuntary treatment and some forms of treatment like electroconvulsive therapy

- National Mental Health Association (NMHA): An organization aimed at improving mental health in the population at large, emphasizing prevention

- National Mental Health Consumers' Association (NMHCA): A consumer organization that advocates for improvements in the mental health system

See this book's website at http://evolve.elsevier.com/Stanhope for more information about these organizations.

---

Family members led self-advocacy efforts in the 1970s, when small groups organized to challenge and change mental health services. These early efforts resulted in the formation of the National Alliance for the Mentally Ill (NAMI), which today has both state and local affiliates. Soon, consumer groups formed to advocate for better services, changes in mental health policy, self-help programs in treatment, and empowerment. Several advocacy groups that support these consumer efforts are summarized in Box 35-1. In their assessment of resources, nurses can identify community advocacy and support groups.

## CONCEPTUAL FRAMEWORKS FOR COMMUNITY MENTAL HEALTH

The community mental health principles that are the underpinnings of practice include the right to mental health services delivered in the least restrictive environment, consumer involvement in treatment, advocacy, and rehabilitative services. Other useful theories to enhance understanding of the multidimensional aspects of community mental health nursing are those that encompass the full range of biopsychosocial frameworks. Theories and models that explain biological systems, personality, life span development, family dynamics, and stress and coping are all important components of community mental health. Principles consistent with nursing practice and community mental health are a focus on wellness or recovery, relapse prevention or **relapse management,** and helping the client reach a maximal level of function.

Another useful framework for community mental health practice is **systems theory,** which emphasizes the relationship between the elements of a unit and the whole. An understanding of the whole occurs through the examination of interactions and relationships that exist between the parts. A holistic view of system and subsystems can be applied in a variety of ways in community mental health practice. One example of a subsystem in a community is its cultural groups. Subsystems of the cultural groups are families; subsystems of the families are individuals. Using systems theory to explore the background, conditions, and context of situations will reveal information about the positive and negative forces that either promote or undermine the well-being of any unit in the system.

A concept useful to CMHN practice is the diathesis-stress model. This theory integrates the effects of biology and environment, or nature and nurture, on the development of mental illness (Boyd, 2002). Certain genes or genetic combinations produce a predisposition to a disorder. When an individual with a predisposition to a disorder is challenged by an environmental stressor, the expression of the mental disorder may result (Boyd, 2002). The integration of psychosocial and neurobiological paradigms is critical to the practice of psychiatric nursing (McCabe, 2002). Community-oriented nurses must recognize the effects of environment and biology on people and actively work to mitigate psychosocial as well as biological stressors.

## Levels of Prevention

Health promotion and illness prevention are fundamental to community mental health practice as well as to national objectives for mental health (USDHHS, 2000). Therefore the concepts of primary, secondary, and tertiary levels of prevention are useful in community mental health practice. Levels of prevention are described in Box 35-2.

Primary prevention refers to the reduction of health risks. It involves both health promotion and disease prevention (Worley, 1997). Health promotion strategies aim to enhance the well-being of healthy populations, whereas disease prevention strategies focus on the identification of populations at risk and conditions that have the potential to cause stress and illness. An example of mental health promotion is providing education about stress reduction techniques to senior citizens attending a health fair. An example of disease prevention is to provide mental health information in schools to adolescents on topics such as depression and eating disorders.

**NURSING TIP**

Nurses need to teach individuals and groups strategies to promote mental health and reduce stress.

Secondary prevention activities are aimed at reducing the prevalence or pathologic nature of a condition. They involve early diagnosis, prompt treatment, and limitation of disability (Worley, 1997). Many functions of the practitioner role are aimed at secondary prevention for individuals. These include providing individual and group psychotherapy, case management, and referral. Screening members of a community for depression during National Depression Screening Day is an example of population-based secondary prevention. Counseling, referral, and treatment interventions after traumatic incidents, such as terrorist attacks or natural disasters, are other community interventions.

Tertiary prevention efforts attempt to restore and enhance functioning. On a community level, tertiary prevention activities might include support of affordable housing, promotion of psychosocial rehabilitation programs, and involvement in advocacy and consumer groups for the mentally ill. Many nursing role activities in community mental health are aimed at tertiary prevention with individuals. They include monitoring illness symptoms and treatment responses, coordinating transition from the hospital to the community, and identifying respite care options for caregivers.

Relapse management is central to many of the programs and activities that enhance coping skills and competence. Effective modalities in community mental health in which the nurse participates are **assertive community treatment** (ACT) programs, psychosocial rehabilitation (clubhouses), and intensive case management. ACT programs differ from intensive case management approaches in that they are based more on a medical model and team approach and provide crisis and case management services 24 hours a day, 7 days a week. They are sometimes referred to as hospitals without walls (Schaedle et al, 2002). Intensive case management models vary across programs but generally include contact with clients several times a week by an individual case manager. Nurses have critical roles in both treatment programs, as they have the knowledge and skills to provide comprehensive biopsychosocial care.

For example, the nurse visits the client at home, checks medication, assesses physical and emotional functioning, and may take the client shopping for nutritional food. The nurse may accompany the consumer to the doctor's office and serve as an advocate for the client in this setting.

As case managers, nurses foster coping and competency aimed at managing illness symptoms with consumers, family members, and other caregivers. The aim of managing illness symptoms is to offset relapse and promote recovery. Since relapse management is a major goal of interventions in community mental health nursing, the Moller-Murphy Symptom Management Assessment Tool (MM-SMAT) may be especially useful during nursing process activities. The tool was developed to provide consumers, family members, and professionals with a recovery model and common framework for managing neurobiological disorders such as schizophrenia, bipolar disorder, and major depression (Moller and Murphy, 1997). Assessment of the frequency, intensity, and duration of symptoms for the purpose of identifying biological, environmental, and behavioral triggers that may lead to illness relapse helps the consumer manage the illness and promotes recovery. Examples of triggers are poor nutrition, poor social skills, hopelessness, and poor symptom management. Once triggers are identified, interventions aimed at fostering effective coping skills can be introduced to offset relapse of symptoms. For example, an intervention that may promote effective coping to offset social isolation is guiding the client to organized consumer group activities available in the community. Another is to promote consumer and family efforts at job training through community vocational agencies. Still another is to promote competency in family members by coordinating services that enhance their understanding of the illness, provide social support, and include respite when needed. Finally, medication management is an important intervention for offsetting relapse.

As previously discussed, scientific advances that led to the use of medications to treat mental illness revolutionized mental health care and services (Boyd, 2002). Atypical antipsychotics and new antidepressants with fewer side effects have further influenced mental health care in the community. Although these new drugs have dramatically improved the lives of many people with mental disorders, they are not without problems and are not a cure. The nurse has a critical role in monitoring side effects, detecting related health problems such as diabetes, and providing education and intervention. The most effective approaches combine medications with other relapse management approaches (Noordsy and O'Keefe, 1999). These include culturally sensitive social, behavioral, and psychotherapeutic interventions.

## ROLE OF THE NURSE IN COMMUNITY MENTAL HEALTH

The role of the nurse in community mental health was shaped both by the evolution of services and by the work of nursing pioneers. Development of a knowledge base for the nursing discipline and the further expansion of mental health care services to nontraditional community sites called for more advanced community based practitioners (American Nurses Association [ANA], 2000). Nursing practice standards reflect the values of the profession, describe the responsibilities of nurses, and provide direction for the delivery and evaluation of nursing care. These standards also describe the roles of nurses in both advanced and basic practice.

Advanced practice psychiatric nurses have had graduate-level education. The psychiatric nurse practitioner title and role have been expanded to encompass primary care and specialty knowledge and skills (Dyer et al, 1997; Flaskerud and Wuerker, 1999). They provide primary, secondary, and tertiary care to individuals, groups, families, adults, children, and adolescents. Depending on state laws, some prescribe medications and have hospital admission privileges. For example, the advanced practice nurse may see clients individually to provide psychotherapy, may prescribe medications, and may conduct physical examinations or

**BOX 35-3  Roles and Functions in Psychiatric/Mental Health Nursing Community Practice**

**ROLES**
- Clinician
- Educator
- Coordinator

**FUNCTIONS**
- Advocacy
- Case finding and referral
- Case management
- Community action and involvement
- Complementary interventions
- Counseling
- Crisis intervention
- Health promotion
- Health maintenance
- Health teaching
- Home visits
- Intake screening and evaluation
- Milieu therapy
- Promotion of self-care activities
- Psychiatric rehabilitation
- Psychobiological interventions

Modified from American Nurses Association, American Psychiatric Nurses Association, and International Society of Psychiatric Mental Health Nurses: *Scope and standards of psychiatric–mental health nursing,* Washington, DC, 2000, American Nurses Publishing.

coordinate this care with other providers in primary care settings. The blended nurse practitioner role has been a response to a shift in the health care system away from specialization and toward comprehensive services that address both physical and mental health problems (McCabe, 2002).

Nurses prepared at the undergraduate level provide basic primary, secondary, and tertiary services that are equally valuable. Specific roles and functions of nurses at the basic level (Box 35-3) are based on clinical nursing practice and standards (ANA, 2000). The functions suggest the overlapping roles of clinician, educator, and coordinator.

## Clinician

Objectives of the practitioner role are to help the client maintain or regain coping abilities that promote functioning. This involves using the nursing process to guide the diagnosis and treatment of human responses to actual or potential mental health problems (ANA, 2000). Role functions at the basic practitioner level include case management, counseling, milieu therapy, and psychobiological interventions with individuals and with groups. Clinician skills are used in a variety of settings including the home, and often with large groups of people in specific neighborhoods, schools, and public health districts. For example, many clients who have schizophrenia live in personal care homes. These clients require biopsychosocial interventions related to medication management, milieu management for improved social interaction, and assistance with self-care activities for community living such as use of public transportation (Moller and Murphy, 1997; Torrey and Wyzik, 2000). Also, the practitioner increasingly coordinates these activities with staff members in community settings. Therefore coordination of care is often the means for promoting treatment plan outcomes and enhancing quality of life for clients. These activities can support positive outcomes for others in the community at large.

For example, family members are a primary support system for individuals with schizophrenia. Whether the client lives in a personal care home, a family residence, or another setting, counseling family members and the client about the illness may offset the stressors of caregiving (Dixon et al, 2000). Moreover, educating the public may reduce the stigma and offset social isolation for both clients and families. For the community, implications of these basic-level functions may include public support for needed services and decreased costs of health care resulting from reduced hospitalization. As suggested in these examples, clinician and educator roles overlap.

## Educator

The educator role uses teaching–learning principles to increase understanding about mental illness and mental health. The educator role is foundational to health maintenance, health promotion, and community action. Teaching clients about illness symptoms and the benefits of medications promotes health maintenance and may reduce the risk for illness relapse (Moller and Murphy, 1997). Research supports similar education programs for family members to increase their ability to monitor illness symptoms and to identify events that lead to relapse (Czuchta and McCay, 2001; Dixon et al, 2000; Kane, Blank, and Hundley, 1999; Moller and Murphy, 1997). The nurse may facilitate a combined support and education group for parents of children with schizophrenia or for consumers with major mental illness in weekly sessions at the community mental health center. The CMHN, both at the basic and the advanced level, may be involved in developing educational groups and programs for consumers, families, and other providers either alone or in collaboration with other organizations such as the Mental Health Association or the National Alliance for the Mentally Ill.

At the community level, both formal and informal teaching is important. One important objective for mental health promotion is to teach positive coping skills. An example of an ineffective coping skill among individuals is overmedicating. Even when medications are properly used

in treatment, the nurse requires specialized knowledge about drug interactions, pharmacokinetics, and pharmacodynamics. Factors that influence pharmacokinetics include anatomic and physiologic changes that occur with aging or with coexisting mental and physical conditions. Use of nonprescription medication such as herbal remedies and over-the-counter drugs can influence pharmacokinetics. As one out of three persons uses nontraditional remedies (Beaubrun and Gray, 2000), and many of these are specific for psychiatric conditions, it is imperative that the nurses assess the use of these substances, be aware of interactions, and teach clients (Skiba-King, 2002).

> **◖ DID YOU KNOW?**
>
> Many people use herbal remedies such as ginkgo for memory improvement, valerian for sleep, and St. Johns wort for depression to self-treat mental health symptoms.

## Coordinator

Coordination of care is a basic principle of the multidisciplinary team approach in community mental health services. Yet there is often a lack of coordination as well as limited services in many communities. Therefore, at a minimum, the role of coordinator must include case finding, referral, and follow-up to evaluate system breakdown and deficits. Because of current system deficits, nurses in community mental health function as coordinators who carry out intake screening, crisis intervention, and home visits. The nurse coordinator also tries to improve the client's health and well-being by promoting independence and self-care in the least restrictive environment. For example, the nurse may teach the client how to fill a medication box or how to use relaxation techniques to reduce stress. Health teaching related to nutrition, smoking cessation, and sleep promotion are essential for consumers with mental illness. These functions are consistent with descriptions of clinical case management that emphasize continuity of care for individuals who need complex services (Farrell et al, 1999; Saraceno, 1997; Schaedle et al, 2002; Ziguras and Stewart, 2000).

To achieve these objectives and improve services, the nurse must work with a variety of professionals, including advanced practice nurses, social workers, physicians, psychologists, occupational and vocational therapists, and rehabilitation counselors. The nurse is often the advocate for the consumer who needs assistance making his or her needs clear and accessing both health and social services. Because nonlicensed paraprofessionals are frequently involved in direct care activities, their services must be directed, coordinated, and evaluated within the context of treatment planning. Finally, coordination also involves work with individuals who may not have formal preparation but who are essential for positive treatment outcomes. These individuals include family members, shelter volunteers, consumer support groups, and community leaders who can influence development of services. For example, the nurse can teach others about mental illness and effective interventions for times when symptoms become apparent and behaviors become difficult to manage. In the coordinator role, nurses can identify and influence health system effectiveness and ineffectiveness.

> **NURSING TIP**
>
> To assist your client in accessing community resources and services, it is as important to develop positive relationships with other community providers as it is with your clients.

## CURRENT AND FUTURE PERSPECTIVES IN MENTAL HEALTH CARE

Agreement is widespread that health care services are lacking both nationally and internationally. In the United States, large segments of the population do not have basic health care services or insurance to cover both expected and unexpected illnesses. Health insurance coverage for most Americans is linked to employment. In an economic recession when jobs are lost, insurance is often lost as well, and people are no longer able to afford health care (Manderscheid and Henderson, 2001). Also, consumers, family members, and health care providers are concerned about issues of basic treatment, continuity of care, housing, and costs for acute and long-term mental health services (Manderscheid and Henderson, 2001; Worley, 1997). Aging demographics as large numbers of baby boomers reach retirement and Medicare eligibility has focused concern on whether this resource will exist for older Americans. Therefore health care reform continues to be a major political, social, and economic issue. Significant alterations in the current health care delivery system, if they occur, will occur slowly. In the meantime, nurses working in communities must understand the models of care, the scope of mental illness, and the national health objectives designed to promote the health and welfare of persons with mental health problems.

Managed care, as described previously, will continue to have an effect on the delivery of mental health services (Manderscheid and Henderson, 2001). This will occur through a continued focus on providing services in primary care settings, through attempts to reduce inpatient stays, and through a more systematic evaluation of the outcomes of the care provided. The massive growth in managed care plans has dramatically reduced hospital stays but it is yet unclear whether it can be effective in providing care to those with long-term care needs (Mowbry et al, 2002; Sharfstein, 2000). As the public mental health system is the only remaining state and federally supported treatment system for a specific set of disorders, the use of managed care in this arena is of concern. Public monies could be spent on spurious programs not offering adequate services. This could lead to gaps in services and large holes in the safety net for vulnerable consumers suffering from mental illness.

Community mental health nurses are well positioned to be important providers in managed care because of their emphasis on wellness and health promotion, skills at teaching and case management, and lower cost for service. In communities, nurses practice primary, secondary, and tertiary prevention activities by conducting comprehensive client histories to determine health problems and interventions that improve quality of care and cost effectiveness. In home health settings, nurses screen for ineffective coping techniques such as use of alcohol or other substances to offset the stress of traumatic life events, thereby preventing further problems and costly care. They also screen for signs of psychiatric disorders in primary care and community health care settings. Community mental health services must include access to work and school settings for families and children. These types of nursing assessments and subsequent interventions may offset costly treatment in hospital settings.

Providing the range of community services necessary to handle persistent mental illness is difficult without sufficient funds for health and social services (Manderscheid and Henderson, 2001). Clearly, managed care has changed the mental health field, and more changes are anticipated. It is important for nurses and others working in CMHCs to recognize the impact of changes in funding, target populations, restructuring, and disagreements between professions, agencies, and levels of government. Such information enables nurses to advocate for adequate services to meet the needs of individuals with severe and persistent mental illness. Coddington (2001) recommends measures consistent with community-oriented nursing, such as agency networking, interagency collaboration, and building relationships to improve the quality of care for clients.

## NATIONAL OBJECTIVES FOR MENTAL HEALTH SERVICES

The goals of the community mental health movement are consistent with the health promotion and disease prevention objectives outlined in Healthy People 2010 (USDHHS, 2000). The Healthy People 2010 box illustrates the primary objectives of the national health agenda for mental health promotion and illness prevention. The objectives of Healthy People 2010 address both settings where people receive care (primary care, juvenile justice systems) and populations at risk (children, adults with mental illness, and older adults). Increasing cultural competency and consumer satisfaction with mental health services are further objectives of the national agenda for mental health.

The new millennium brought recognition of the importance of addressing mental health and mental illness as part of disease prevention. Murray and Lopez (1996) highlighted the recognition of the worldwide burden of mental illness, especially in developed countries, in a report for the World Health Organization. The status of mental

**Healthy People 2010** | Targeted National Health Objectives for Mental Health

**Goal:** Improve mental health and ensure access to appropriate, quality mental health services

**MENTAL HEALTH STATUS IMPROVEMENT**

18-1 Reduce suicide to less than 5 per 100,000
18-2 Reduce adolescent suicide attempts to 12-month average of 1%
18-3 Reduce proportion of homeless adults who have serious mental illness (SMI) to 19% from 25%
18-4 Increase employment of persons with SMI from 43% to 51%
18-5 Reduce eating disorder relapse rates

**TREATMENT EXPANSION**

18-6 Increase the number of people screened for mental disorders in primary care
18-7 Increase numbers of children treated for mental health problems
18-8 Increase number of juvenile justice facilities that screen new admissions for mental health problems

18-9 Increase treatment for adults with mental disorders, specifically SMI, schizophrenia, depression, and generalized anxiety disorders
18-10 Increase the proportion of adults receiving treatment who have co-occurring mental and substance abuse disorders
18-11 Increase proportion of communities with jail diversion programs for those with mental illness

**STATE ACTIVITIES**

18-12 Increase from 36 to 50 the number of states tracking consumer satisfaction with mental health services
18-13 Increase number of states with plans addressing cultural competence
18-14 Increase number of states from 24 to 50 that have screening, crisis intervention, and treatment services for older adults

From U.S. Department of Health and Human Services: *Healthy people 2010: national health promotion and disease prevention objectives,* Washington, DC, 2000, U.S. Government Printing Office.

health in the United States was further clarified by a landmark report from the surgeon general's office, "Mental Health, A Report of the Surgeon General" (USDHHS, 1999), followed by a report from the Surgeon General's Conference on Children's Mental Health in 2000. A national agenda for action described in Healthy People 2010 (USDHHS, 2000) made mental health one of the 10 leading health indicators, which are chosen on the basis of relevance as a broad public health issue.

Overall, the national goals are to improve mental health and ensure access to quality and appropriate mental health services. Approaches emphasize prevention, maintenance, and restoration of mental health and independent functioning. The standards address mental health conditions of concern across the life span and with specific populations. Community-oriented nurses can (1) promote the standards in the agencies where they are employed, (2) use the standards in community assessment activities, and (3) introduce information about the standards to other groups and agencies, including local consumer and family organizations, to help prioritize mental health concerns.

As indicated in the definitions at the beginning of this chapter, mental health is a dynamic process, influenced by both internal and external factors, that enables and promotes the individual's physical, cognitive, affective, and social functioning. In contrast, threats to mental health create stress that undermines relationships and diminishes the individual's ability to pursue and achieve life's goals. Values and beliefs influence the allocation of resources for

neighborhoods and schools and can contribute to or undermine the mental health of people in communities.

Mental health problems are manifested in many ways. Untoward incidents or even anticipated life events can diminish physical, cognitive, affective, and social functioning. For example, in most situations, either anticipated or unexpected death of a family member results in grief that may temporarily interrupt the functioning of surviving family members and produce mental distress. Given adequate support and adaptation, most persons resume their lifestyles following the death of a loved one in spite of the sadness that they are likely to experience. When people do not have adequate resources, or when bereavement is complicated because of the conditions of the situation, there is an increased risk for threats to the mental health of surviving family members. Important interventions with individuals experiencing sorrow and grief are to encourage roles and activities that promote comfort and reduce isolation. Death of a family member can affect survivors of different ages in various ways. Infants and youths may be deprived of significant nurturing and care that will result in long-term emotional deficits, whereas adults are at increased risk for stress related to role changes, and older adults are vulnerable to social isolation as relatives and friends die. In any of these situations, individual or group therapy may be indicated not only for the immediate situation but also for prevention of longer-term problems.

However, bereavement is not the only cause of diminished mental health. Other causes include but are not limited to physical health problems, disabilities resulting from trauma, exposure to violence in the neighborhood, job loss and unstable employment, and unanticipated environmental disasters that result in loss. Because multiple threats to mental health exist across the life span, it is useful to organize the study of problems according to life stages along life's continuum.

## Children and Adolescents

Healthy People 2010 objectives aim to increase the number of children screened and treated for mental health problems. Children are at risk for disruption of normal development by biological, environmental, and psychosocial factors that impair their mental health, interfere with education and social interactions, and keep them from realizing their full potential as adults (USDHHS, 2000). For example, children may develop depression after a loss, or behavior problems from abuse or neglect. Examples of environmental factors include crowded living conditions, violence, separation from parents, and lack of consistent caregivers. Veenema (2001) found exposure to community violence to be related to significant stress and depression in children. Types of mental health problems typically diagnosed during childhood are depression, anxiety, and attention deficit disorders. Examples of chronic disorders commonly seen are mental retardation, Down syndrome, and autism. These problems affect growth and development and influence mental health during adolescence.

Suicide is the third leading killer of young persons between ages 15 and 24, and in 90% of cases, there was a mental or substance abuse disorder (USDHHS, 2000). The second objective of Healthy People 2010 is to reduce the rate of suicide attempts by adolescents. Some of the risk factors for both adolescents and adults include prior suicide attempts, stressful life events, and access to lethal methods. In addition to depression and substance abuse, adolescent problems include conduct disorders and eating disorders.

Another objective of Healthy People 2010 is to reduce the relapse rates for persons with eating disorders. Many CMHNs do not directly work with persons with a primary eating disorder, but eating disturbances are frequently a symptom accompanying other conditions. As most children are not seen in the mental health system, an important role of the CMHN is to educate other community providers, teachers, parents, and children. School nurses are in an ideal position to provide primary, secondary, and tertiary interventions for children with eating disorders. Nutrition education, early recognition, intervention, referral, and follow-up can help prevent eating disorders from becoming severe and can prevent relapses. Community-oriented nurses can advocate in and beyond their communities for the provision of a nurse in all schools. This would increase the chances of early recognition of and treatment for persons with eating disorders.

There is recognition that effective service expansion for children, particularly for those with serious emotional dis-

turbances, depends on promoting collaboration across critical areas of support including schools, families, social services, health, mental health, and juvenile justice. Better services and collaboration for children with serious emotional disturbance and their families will result in greater school retention, decreased contact with the juvenile justice system, increased stability of living arrangements, and improved educational, emotional, and behavioral development. One of the objectives of Healthy People 2010 is to ensure that children in the juvenile justice system receive access to mental health assessment and treatment (USDHHS, 2000). Children and adolescents require a variety of mental health services, including crisis intervention and both short- and long-term counseling. Nurses working in community settings, well-child clinics, and home health can help to offset this problem through prevention, education, and including parents in program planning. Because many children and adolescents lack services or access to them, community mental health assessment activities are essential. Assessment activities include identifying types of programs available or lacking in places where children and adolescents spend time. Assessments should be performed in schools and in the homes of clients served, and also in day-care centers, churches, and organizations that plan and guide age-specific play and entertainment programs. Assessment data are essential for planning and developing programs that address mental health problems prevalent from the prenatal period through adolescence. Preventing problems during these developmental periods can reduce mental health problems in adulthood. Further interventions can be found in the How To box.

---

### HOW TO    Prevent a Culture of Youth Violence

Yearwood (2001) asked Dr. Bell, a nationally known community mental health psychiatrist, how youth violence could be prevented. He suggested community mental health providers work to do the following:

- Reestablish the village through the creation of coalitions and partnerships.
- Provide access to health care and mental health care to treat conditions associated with violent behavior.
- Improve bonding, attachment, and connectedness by supporting mothers and families.
- Improve self-esteem among youths by recognizing and building on strengths.
- Increase social skills by helping children learn to stop, think, and act.
- Reestablish the adult protective shield by educating and supporting parents.
- Minimize the effects of trauma through early intervention.

From Yearwood E: Is there a culture of youth violence? *J Child Adolesc Psychiatr Nurs* 15(1):35, 2001.

## Adults

Adults suffer from varied sources of stress that contribute to their mental health status. Sources of stress include multiple role responsibilities, job insecurity, and unstable relationships. These and other conditions can undermine mental health and contribute to serious mental illness, depression, anxiety disorders, and substance abuse. Objectives of Healthy People 2010 are aimed at helping adults access treatment in order to decrease associated human and economic costs and to reduce suicide rates (USDHHS, 2000).

At some time or another, virtually all adults will experience a tragic or unexpected loss, a serious setback, or a time of profound sadness, grief, or distress. Major depressive disorder, however, differs both in intensity and duration from normal sadness or grief. Depression disrupts relationships and the ability to function and can be fatal. Suicide was the ninth leading cause of death in the United States in 1996, and at least 90% of those who kill themselves have a mental or substance abuse disorder. Other risk factors include prior suicide attempts, stressful life events, and access to lethal methods (USDHHS, 2000). Women are twice as likely to experience depression, and women who are poor or unemployed are even more at risk for this condition (USDHHS, 2000). Research suggests that domestic violence can lead to posttraumatic stress disorder (PTSD) and major depression among women (Breslaw et al, 1997). Available medications and psychological treatment can help 80% of those with depression, yet only a minority seek help. Those with depression are more likely to visit a physician for some other reason, and the mental health condition may not be noted. Therefore it is imperative that community-oriented nurses in all settings recognize and screen for depression.

Anxiety disorders are common both in the United States, and elsewhere. An alarming 24% of the population will experience an anxiety disorder, many with overlapping substance abuse disorders. Anxiety disorders may have an early onset and are characterized by recurrent episodes of illness and periods of disability. Panic disorder and agoraphobia along with depression are associated with increased risks of attempted and completed suicide (USDHHS, 2000).

The lifetime rates of co-occurrence of mental disorders and addictive disorders are strikingly high. About one in five persons in the United States experiences a mental disorder in the course of a year, and nearly one in three adults who have a mental disorder in their lifetime also experiences a co-occurring substance (alcohol or other drugs) abuse disorder (USDHHS, 2000). Individuals with co-occurring disorders are more likely to experience a chronic course and to use services than are those with either type of disorder alone, yet the services are often fragmented and treatment occurs in different segments of the system.

How can nurses intervene? The general medical sector, including primary care clinics, hospitals, and nursing homes, has long been identified as the initial point of contact for many adults with mental disorders; for some, these providers may be the only source of mental health services. Early detection and intervention for mental health problems can be increased if persons presenting in primary care are assessed for mental health problems. Nurses who work in the general medical sector and in other community settings are in an ideal position to assess and detect mental health problems. Nurses conduct comprehensive biopsychosocial assessments and are often the professional most trusted with sensitive information by patients in these settings. The use of screening tools for depression, anxiety, substance abuse, and cognitive impairment can assist the nurse in early detection and intervention for mental health problems. Suicide can be prevented in many cases by early recognition and treatment of mental disorders, and by preventive interventions that focus on risk factors. Thus reduction in access to lethal methods and recognition and treatment of mental and substance abuse disorders are among the most promising approaches to suicide prevention (USDHHS, 2000). Nurses, long respected as community-oriented providers, can work with legislators for measures to limit access to weapons such as handguns.

## Adults With Serious Mental Illness

Objectives of Healthy People 2010 that address tertiary prevention and are targeted to persons with serious mental illness are to reduce the proportion of homeless adults who have serious mental illness and to increase their employment, and to decrease the number of adults with mental disorders who are incarcerated. Brief hospital stays and inadequate community resources have resulted in an increased number of persons with serious mental illness living on the streets or in jail. It is estimated that 7% of those in jail suffer from a mental illness (USDHHS, 2000). Some people arrested for nonviolent crimes could be better served if diverted from the jail system to a community-based mental health treatment program with linkage to mental health services. Approximately one quarter of homeless persons in the United States have a serious mental illness, and only 41% of persons with serious mental illness have any form of employment (USDHHS, 2000). At present, many people with severe mental disorders live in poverty because they lack the ability to earn or maintain a suitable standard of living. Even people who live with family caregivers or in supervised housing are at risk for inadequate services, because the long-term care they require frequently depletes human and fiscal resources. Modalities such as rehabilitation services, intensive case management, and persistent patient outreach and engagement strategies have been shown by research to be effective in helping persons with serious mental illness (Schaedle et al, 2002; Ziguras and Stewart, 2000) and in lowering rates of hospitalization (Salkever et al, 1999).

CMHNs are engaged in all forms of case management activities with persons with serious and persistent mental illness. They provide important case management services, coordinate resources for consumers, and function as important members of assertive community treatment (ACT) programs, which provide continuous assistance to persons with mental illness. Nurses by philosophy and training promote independent living and provide support and encouragement for persons to achieve a maximal level of wellness and function. Nurses recognize the importance of the mental health benefits of meaningful work that improves self-esteem and independence. Nursing interventions can be provided in shelters, soup kitchens, and other places where homeless persons receive food and protection.

## Older Adults

In the United States, the population over 65 years of age has steadily increased since the year 2000. As the life expectancy of individuals continues to grow, the number experiencing mental disorders of late life will increase. This trend will present society with unprecedented challenges in organizing financing and delivering effective preventative and treatment services for mental health in this population (USDHHS, 2000). Although many older people maintain highly functional lives, others have mental health deficits associated with normal sensory losses related to aging, failing physical health, difficulty performing activities of daily living, and social deprivation or isolation. Life changes related to work roles and retirement often result in reduced social contacts and support. Other previously described losses are associated with the death of a spouse, other family members, or friends. Reduced social networks and contacts brought about by these life events can influence mood and contribute to serious states of depression. However, depression is not a normal part of aging.

The depression rate among older adults is half that of younger people, but the presence of a physical or chronic illness increases rates of depression. Depression rates for older adults in nursing homes range from 15% to 25%. In the United States men between the ages of 65 and 74 continue to be in the highest risk category for suicide; men account for 80% of all suicides of those over age 65 (USDHHS, 2000). Alzheimer's disease and vascular conditions can cause a severe loss of mental abilities with behavioral manifestations. Twenty-five percent of those over age 85 have some form of dementia. All these conditions affect the mental health status of individuals and their family caregivers.

Older adults, because they may be dependent on others for care, are at risk for abuse and neglect. Healthy aging activities such as physical activity and establishing social networks improve the mental health of older adults. Older adults underutilize the mental health system and are more likely to be seen in primary care or to be recipients of care in institutions (USDHHS, 2000). The nurse can reach them by organizing health promotion programs through senior centers or other community-based settings. Home health care nurses can assess and intervene to protect those at risk for abuse and neglect, and mental health nurses can provide stress management education for nursing home staff. Stress management for caregivers and respite day-care

programs for an older adult family member can increase coping and prevent abuse. Nurses can advocate with health authorities and localities to increase awareness of the importance of meeting the mental health needs of this growing population.

Most family caregivers are women who care for a spouse, an aging parent, or a child with a long-term disabling illness. These caregivers are also at risk for health disruption. The impact of caregiving has been studied with persons who care for those with chronic illness, and with fathers of persons with schizophrenia (Howard, 1998) (see the Evidence Based-Practice box about caregiving fathers). Caregivers of persons with severely disabling mental disorders often have their mental health threatened by lack of social support (Doornbas, 2002), the stigma of the disease, and chronic strain (Czuchta and McCay, 2001). During stressful life events such as these, it is important for caregivers to know how to manage the many competing demands in their lives.

### Evidence-Based Practice

Fathers were the subjects of this study about caregiving for adult children with schizophrenia. Subjects were middle-aged and older adults. Cross-sectional data in the form of in-depth interviews were based on naturalistic inquiry. Findings of a previous study with maternal caregivers led to a description of the stages and concepts of life-long learning about how to live with a child who had schizophrenia. Findings of this study indicated that fathers too were engaged in a prolonged caregiving event. Three themes explained the extent to which these fathers engaged in caregiving: involvement in care, unresolved issues, and severity of the event.

**Nurse Use:** Home care services and transition programs (from the hospital to community services) are important for families with relatives who have severe mental disorders. Interventions with families should include education, respite services, and stress management.

Howard PB: The experience of fathers of adult children with schizophrenia, *Issues Ment Health Nurs* 19(2):399, 1998.

Activities to improve the mental health status of adults include public education programs, prevention approaches, and providing mental health services in primary care. Specific approaches to reduce stress include use of community support groups, education about lifestyle management, and worksite programs. Nevertheless, most programs currently available for adults, families, and caregivers with health problems primarily monitor or restore health rather than prevent problems. Therefore the nurse can refer family caregivers and others to organizations such the local Alliance for the Mentally Ill for group support services. In addition, many national organizations

**BOX 35-4  Examples of Sources of Information and Help for People With Mental Illness and Mental Health Problems**

- Alcoholics Anonymous
- Al-Anon
- American Anorexia/Bulimia Association
- American Association of Suicidology
- Anxiety Disorders Association of America
- Attention Deficit Information Network
- Children and Adults With Attention Deficit Disorder
- Depressive/Manic Depressive Association
- Gamblers Anonymous
- National Center for Post-Traumatic Stress Disorder
- National Center for Learning Disabilities
- Obsessive-Compulsive Foundation
- Overeaters Anonymous
- Schizophrenics Anonymous

See this book's website at http://evolve.elsevier com/ Stanhope for more information about these organizations.

designed for groups with specific problems (Box 35-4) have local chapters or information that can be accessed on the internet. Some state activities expand mental health services to older adults, and Healthy People 2010 aims to increase cultural competence within the mental health system.

## Cultural Diversity

To work effectively, health care providers need to understand the differences in how various populations in the United States perceive mental health and mental illness and treatment services. These factors affect whether people seek mental health care, how they describe their symptoms, the duration of care, and the outcomes of the care received. Research has shown that various populations use mental health services differently. They may not seek mental health services in the formal system, they may drop out of care, or they may seek care at much later stages of illness, driving the service costs higher (USDHHS, 2000). This pattern of use appears to be the result of a community-based mental health service system that is not culturally relevant, responsive, or accessible to select populations.

Although all socioeconomic and cultural groups have mental health problems, low-income groups are at greater risk because they often lack minimal resources for meeting basic physical and mental health needs (USDHHS, 2001). Caution is needed, however, when discussing differences among racial and ethnic groups in the rates of mental illness. Studies of the number of cases of mental health problems among racial and ethnic populations, while increasing in number, remain limited and often inconclusive. Discussion of the rates of existing cases must consider differences in how persons of different cultures and racial and ethnic groups perceive mental illness. Behavioral problems, which Western medicine views as signs of mental illness, may be assessed differently by individuals in various racial and ethnic groups. With this caution in mind, along with the recognition that sample sizes for racial and ethnic groups may be limited, examination of existing large-scale studies for mental health trends among racial and ethnic groups remains important.

### WHAT DO YOU THINK?

Does the manner in which people of different cultures describe emotional distress affect the detection and treatment of mental illness?

According to the surgeon general's report on culture, race, and ethnicity, the predominant minority populations in the United States are African Americans, Hispanics, Asian and Pacific Islander Americans, and Native Americans including Native Alaskans (USDHHS, 2001). Within each of these groups there is also much diversity, as they consist of subgroups with unique cultural differences. Therefore it is important to avoid simplification and overgeneralization in discussions about the characteristics and problems of minorities. Rather, it is critical to conduct community assessments to determine unique characteristics and factors that contribute to mental health needs within specific aggregates of the population. The information presented here is intended to stimulate thinking and awareness for developing nursing process activities in individual communities. Community assessments that include data about specific populations from organized agencies such as the Indian Health Service are important because assessment data guide role activities during all steps of the nursing process.

Community-oriented nurses provide a variety of primary, secondary, and tertiary prevention interventions with populations at risk that help meet the objectives for improving mental health. Consumers have historically influenced mental health services, and the health care industry increasingly is using consumer opinion to gain information on service needs and changes. The final objective of Healthy People 2010 is to increase state tracking of consumer satisfaction with mental health services. Nurses working within broad-based coalitions of consumers, families, other providers, and community leaders can help to achieve the goals of accessible, culturally sensitive, quality mental health services for all of our people.

### African Americans

African Americans make up 12% of the population in the United States and are represented in all socioeconomic groups, yet 22% live in poverty (USDHHS, 2001). Ethnic

## Evidence-Based Practice

Parents at a public health clinic were surveyed using a structured interview to determine their expectations about seeking mental health care for their children. These parents, most of whom were African American, reported a number of negative expectations. Barriers to seeking services included the stigma of mental disorders, a lack of trust in mental health providers, and a belief that services would be unavailable or unsatisfactory.

**Nurse Use:** The following points should be kept in mind by community-oriented nurses in the field of mental health:

- Nurses need to understand existing barriers that prevent people from seeking mental health services, and to design culturally sensitive approaches for vulnerable populations.
- Nurses can work to decrease the stigma of mental illness by educating minorities about the biological basis of many mental disorders.
- Designing services that integrate mental health services into primary care systems will help increase access and decrease barriers.
- Recruitment of a culturally diverse nursing workforce may increase trust in mental health providers.

Richardson LA: Seeking and obtaining mental health services: what do parents expect? *Arch Psychiatr Nurs* 15(5):223, 2001.

and racial minorities in the United States live in an environment of social and economic discrimination and inequality, which takes a toll on mental health and places them at risk for associated mental problems. African Americans are more likely to be exposed to, or to become victims of, violence, placing them at risk for the development of PTSD. They are overrepresented both in the homeless and in the correctional system populations, further increasing the risk of developing mental health problems (USDHHS, 2001). Although in the past they were less likely to commit suicide, the suicide rate of young African-American men is now equal to that of whites (USDHHS, 2001). Despite these issues, African Americans are less likely to use mental health services. Richardson (2001) found that a group of parents had significant negative expectations about mental health services (see the Evidence-Based Practice box about parents' expectations of mental health care). Nurses can promote the mental health of African Americans by integrating mental health care into primary care settings, providing services in community centers, collaborating with African-American faith communities, providing education to decrease the stigma, working toward the provision of safer communities, and

recruiting African Americans to work as community mental health providers.

## Hispanic Americans

Hispanic Americans are the second largest minority group in America, and by 2050 they are projected to make up 25% of the population (USDHHS, 2001). Although they live primarily in the southwestern regions of the country, many have migrated to states in the Southeast and Midwest. Migrant farmworkers are also an important subpopulation among Hispanics. As discussed in Chapter 33, migratory living patterns that are marked by low income, poor education, and lack of health services contribute to stressful living conditions. Nurses and nurse practitioners are the primary health care providers for migrant laborers; their roles include case management and interagency collaboration (Sandhaus, 1998). Collaboration includes networking and referral to community mental health agencies and advanced practice psychiatric nurses when either drug or alcohol abuse or mental illness is the primary health problem.

Hispanic Americans living in low-income urban areas are subject to many of the conditions described for low-income and disadvantaged African-American families. The surgeon general's report (USDHHS, 2001) indicates that recent Hispanic immigrants had lower rates of depression than those born in the United States. Rew et al (2001) found high rates of suicide thoughts and attempts among young Hispanic women. Significant relationships were found between suicide and having a family history of suicide, physical or sexual abuse, and environmental stress. These findings suggest serious stressful living conditions for both individuals and families. Nurses working with Hispanic families need knowledge and skill in both the language and cross-cultural therapies, and they also need to include consumers in planning and evaluating mental health service delivery (Lantican, 1998). This can be done by holding focus groups with the consumers.

## Asian and Pacific Islander Americans

Asian and Pacific Islander Americans can be characterized by a diverse and rapidly increasing population (USDHHS, 2001). This group includes both settled citizens and new refugees. The largest segment of this population lives in California. Whereas Asian and Pacific Islander Americans, like other minority groups, are represented in all socioeconomic strata, the lower-income groups include refugees and recent immigrants who are dealing with the displacement issues of loss, adjustment, and adaptation. Losses often involve forfeiture of family, traditions, and lifestyles for cultures that may seem alien. Adjustments and adaptations include those basic to daily living: learning new languages, laws, and monetary systems and locating support systems. Finding support systems includes becoming acquainted with the health care delivery system. Our knowledge of the mental health needs of this population is limited, as they have the lowest rates of utilization of mental health services of any cultural group (USDHHS, 2001). This avoidance of mental health care is associated with the stigma and shame related to having a mental disorder. Assessment, planning, and interventions with members of this diverse group must include information about their health beliefs, a key component in any program. This is the first step in providing culturally sensitive interventions.

### Native Americans

Native Americans represent 1.5% of the U.S. population. Although this is a small group, it is also diverse, with over 551 tribes and over 200 languages (USDHHS, 2001). Native Americans also appear to have significant rates of substance abuse, depression, and suicide (1.5 times the national rate), along with unintentional injury and homicide. They are exposed to violence at more than twice the national rate, which results in significant rates of PTSD (USDHHS, 2001). Use of mental health services has been difficult to determine, as only a small percentage of Native Americans use those provided by the Indian Health Service.

A promising intervention to address the needs of this diverse group is to build on the traditions of the specific tribe culture to foster identity and belongingness and enhance protective factors. A return to traditional values of community and group support has been shown to be effective in reducing rates of substance abuse (USDHHS, 2001). Nurses working with Native Americans need to learn the culture of the specific group and to plan culturally sensitive interventions at levels of primary, secondary, and tertiary prevention.

### Practice Application

Mr. B. is an 81-year-old white widowed man living in a rural area 20 miles from a small city. He was referred for an evaluation to the community-oriented outreach nurse by the nurse practitioner who saw him for an acute care visit for sinusitis at the primary care practice. She noted that he had lost weight and had begun to cry when talking about his wife who had died several years before. During the initial visit, the community-oriented nurse noted that Mr. B. weighed only 110 pounds, was not sleeping, had stopped going to church, and was quite anxious and sad about his finances, his limitations due to arthritis, his relationship with his 27-year-old stepson, Bart, and the possibility of nursing home placement.

The nurse conducted a suicide assessment, knowing that Mr. B. was at high risk due to his age, his mood, and the presence of guns in the home. He stated that he had considered shooting himself, but he was reluctant to have the rifles removed at the nurse's suggestion because Bart used the guns for hunting. Mr. B. agreed to a family meeting with his son, and Bart agreed to remove the guns from the house. Both Mr. B. and Bart needed significant education about the biological basis of depression and the efficacy of using a new antidepressant, along with support to treat his condition. Mr. B., like many

older adults, did not wish to see a psychiatrist or use the community mental health system. He did agree to a trial of antidepressant, however.

The community mental health nurse, through the primary care nurse practitioner, arranged for a prescription of an antidepressant (a selective serotonin reuptake inhibitor) that is safe for use with older adults, and Mr. B. started the medication within 2 weeks of the initial visit. In addition to medication and counseling, Mr. B. needed help with nutrition. As Bart was away 10 hours a day, at work in the city, Mr. B. was alone all day. Mr. B. was not able to prepare meals due to his arthritis. The nurse arranged with the local board for aging to provide home-delivered meals. This not only helped with nutrition but also gave Mr. B. a visit from the volunteer twice a week.

Mr. B. and Bart needed help with financial planning, as they did not want to lose the farm should Mr. B. need more assistance or nursing home placement in the future. The nurse arranged for them to talk with a social worker regarding long-term care planning.

In addition to addressing the immediate concerns, the nurse continued to provide weekly visits to Mr. B. for support and counseling, medication monitoring, and case management activities. Family meetings with Bart and Mr. B. to discuss mutual concerns were arranged every 2 months and as needed. The significant improvement of depressive symptoms (sleep, appetite, weight, mood) in Mr. B. were monitored not only clinically but also through use of a depression rating scale.

Psychological, physical, and social problems of older adults are closely intertwined and are best evaluated and treated by a multidisciplinary team. Psychiatric illness often presents first with physical symptoms, and physical limitations create further psychological distress. Older adults often prefer not to use formal mental health services, so careful assessment in primary care settings is critical to detect their mental health problems.

A. In addition to his son and the nurse, who else might notice if Mr. B.'s condition began to deteriorate?
B. What nursing measures are important in monitoring Mr. B.'s response to the antidepressant?
C. What secondary prevention measures were employed by the nurse?
D. What resources might be available for Bart should he need more information about depression?

**Answers are in the back of the book.**

### Key Points

- Reform movements and subsequent federal legislation influenced the development of the current community mental health model that includes team care, case management, prevention, and rehabilitation components of service.

- During the past decade, federal legislation in the United States focused on mainstreaming persons with mental disabilities into American life by legislating access to employment, services, and housing.
- Prevalence rates for mental health problems are very high, and people are at risk for threats to mental health at all ages across the life span. Low-income and minority groups are often at increased risk because they lack access to services and because programs may lack cultural sensitivity.
- National health objectives to promote health and services for persons who have mental health problems and severe mental disorders illustrate the scope of mental illness and provide direction for community mental health practice.
- Guidelines for attaining national health objectives were designed to help individuals at regional and local levels establish health priorities that include those for mental illness.
- Recent redefinitions of American Nurses Association standards provide a framework for the roles and functions of community mental health nurses.
- Frameworks that are useful in community mental health nursing include primary, secondary, and tertiary levels of prevention; biological theories including the effects of psychosocial factors on the brain, growth, and development; and rehabilitation and recovery models.

## Clinical Decision-Making Activities

1. For 1 week, keep a list of incidents related to mental health problems that you learn about in the local media. Categorize the incidents according to age, sex, and socioeconomic, ethnic, or minority status.
2. Visit a local shelter or organization that offers temporary protection for persons with mental disorders. Determine services that are available or lacking for children, women, and men.
3. Visit with representatives of your local self-help organizations for consumers to determine their needs and the adequacy of resources for people with severe mental disorders and their caregivers; determine gaps in services. Develop a list of the agencies in your community that provide direct or indirect services for those with mental illness and their families.

4. Interview a school nurse, an occupational health nurse, an emergency department nurse, or a hospice nurse in your community to discuss types of mental health problems they deal with in their practice settings. Determine resources that are available or lacking for primary, secondary, and tertiary prevention.
5. Interview a nurse working in a local community mental health agency to discuss roles, functions, programs, and resources available or lacking for primary, secondary, and tertiary prevention. Compare findings about prevention programs with information obtained from the preceding interview.
6. Visit a consumer-operated program or a psychosocial rehabilitation program. Interview members to learn how they view the services, and what resources are available or lacking in this setting.
7. Accompany a community mental health nurse on home visits to clients enrolled in an assertive community outreach program, and a psychiatric nurse in a home care agency. Compare and contrast how the services, funding, populations served, and philosophies of treatment differ.
8. As a class activity, arrange for a panel of speakers representing the minority populations described in this chapter. Discuss their views about the way culture shapes thinking about mental illness, and determine types of culturally sensitive services that are available or lacking in your community.
9. Review articles in at least four research journals to determine current research findings about mental disorders and mental health problems, and to compare nursing care in the United States with that of other countries.

### Additional Resources

These related resources are found either in the appendix at the back of this book or on the book's website at **http://evolve.elsevier.com/Stanhope.**

**evolve** **Evolve Website**

WebLinks: Healthy People 2010

## References

American Nurses Association, American Psychiatric Nurses' Association, and International Society of Psychiatric Mental Health Nurses: *Scope and standards of psychiatric–mental health nursing,* Washington, DC, 2000, American Nurses Publishing.

American Psychiatric Association: *Diagnostic and statistical manual of mental disorders,* ed 4-TR, Washington, DC, 2000, APA.

Barrio C: The cultural relevance of community support programs, *Psychiatr Serv* 51(17):879, 2000.

Barry P: Ads, promotions, drive up costs, *AARP Bulletin* 43(3):3, 2002.

Beaubrun G, Gray GE: A review of herbal medicines for psychiatric disorders, *Psychiatr Serv* 51(9):1130, 2000.

Boyd MA: *Psychiatric nursing: contemporary practice,* ed 2, Philadelphia, 2002, Lippincott Williams & Wilkins.

Breslaw N et al: Psychiatric sequelae of post-traumatic stress disorder in women, *Arch Gen Psych* 54:81, 1997.

Coddington DG: Impact of political, societal, and local influences on mental health center service providers, *Adm Policy Ment Health* 29(1):81, 2001.

Czuchta DM, McCay E: Help seeking for parents of individuals experiencing a first episode of schizophrenia, *Arch Psychiatr Nurs* 15(4):159, 2001.

Dixon L et al: Therapists' contacts with family members of persons with severe mental illness in a community treatment program, *Psychiatr Serv* 51(4):1449, 2000.

Doornbas MM: Family caregivers and the mental health system: reality and dreams, *Arch Psychiatr Nurs* 16(1):39, 2002.

Dyer JG et al: The psychiatric-primary care nurse practitioners: a futuristic model for advanced practice, *Arch Psychiatr Nurs* 11(1):2, 1997.

Farrell SP et al: Predicting whether patients receive continuity of care after discharge from state hospitals, *Arch Psychiatr Nurs* 13(6):279, 1999.

Flaskerud JH, Wuerker AS: Mental health nursing in the 21st century: a neuropsychiatric paradigm, *Issues Ment Health Nurs* 20(1):5, 1999.

Foulkes DF: Advocating for persons who are mentally ill: a history of mutual empowerment of patient and profession, *Adm Policy Ment Health* 27(5):353, 2000.

Hannon MJ, Roth D: Past and present insurance coverage in a public sector community mental health population, *Adm Policy Ment Health* 26(6):499, 2001.

Howard PB: The experience of fathers of adult children with schizophrenia, *Issues Ment Health Nurs* 19(2):399, 1998.

Kane C, Blank M, Hundley P: Care provision and community adjustment of rural consumers with serious mental illness, *Arch Psychiatr Nurs* 13(1):19, 1999.

Keltner NL et al: *Psychobiological foundations of psychiatric care,* St Louis, Mo, 1998, Mosby.

Lamb HR: Deinstitutionalization at the beginning of the new millennium. In Lamb HR, Wienberger LE, editors: *Deinstitutionalization: promise and problems—new directions for mental health services,* San Francisco, 2001, Jossey-Bass.

Lantican L: Mexican American clients' perceptions of services in an outpatient mental health facility in a border city, *Issues Ment Health Nurs* 19:125, 1998.

Lindenmayer JP, Nathan AM, Smith RC: Hyperglycemia associated with the use of atypical antipsychotics, *J Clin Psychiatry* 62(suppl 23):30-38, 2001.

Manderscheid RW, Henderson MJ, editors, Center for Mental Health Services: *Mental health, United States, 2000,* USDHHS publication No. (SMA) 01-3537, Washington, DC, 2001, U.S. Government Printing Office.

McCabe S: The nature of psychiatric nursing: the intersection of paradigm, evolution, and history, *Arch Psychiatr Nurs* 16(2):51, 2002.

Mohr WK, Mohr BD: Brain, behavior, connections and implications: psychodynamics no more, *Arch Psychiatr Nurs* 15(4):171, 2001.

Moller M, Murphy M: The three R's rehabilitation program: a prevention approach for the management of relapse symptoms associated with psychiatric diagnosis, *Psychiatr Rehabil J* 20(3):42, 1997.

Mowbry CT, Grazier WL, Holter M: Managed behavioral health care in the public sector: will it become the third shame of the states? *Psychiatr Serv* 53(2):157, 2002.

Murray CJL, Lopez AD, editors: *The global burden of disease: a comprehensive assessment of mortality and disability from diseases, injuries, and risk factors in 1990 and projected to 2020,* Cambridge, 1996, Harvard School of Public Health for WHO & World Bank.

Noordsy DL, O'Keefe C: Effectiveness of combining atypical antipsychotics and psychosocial rehabilitation in a community mental health center setting, *J Clin Psychiatry* 60(suppl 19):47, 1999.

Rew L et al: Correlates of recent suicide attempts in a tri-ethnic group of adolescents, *J Nurs Scholarsh* 33(4):361, 2001.

Richardson LA: Seeking and obtaining mental health services: what do parents expect? *Arch Psychiatr Nurs* 15(5):223, 2001.

Salkever D et al: Assertive community treatment for people with severe mental illness: the effects on hospital use and costs, *Health Serv Res* 34(2):577, 1999.

Sandhaus S: Migrant health: a harvest of poverty, *Am J Nurs* 98(9):52, 1998.

Saraceno B: Psychosocial rehabilitation as a public health strategy, *Psychiatr Rehabil* J 20(4):10, 1997.

Schaedle DSW et al: A comparison of expert's perspectives on assertive community treatment and intensive case management, *Psychiatr Serv* 53(2):207, 2002.

Seaburg HL, McLendon BM, Doraiswamy PM: Olanzapine associated severe hyperglycemia, ketonuria, and acidosis: case report and review of literature, *Pharmacotherapy* 21(11):1448, 2001.

Sharfstein SS: Whatever happened to community mental health? *Psychiatr Serv* 51(5):616, 2000.

Skiba-King EW: Vitamins, herbs and supplements: tools of empowerment, *J Psychosoc Nurs Ment Health Serv* 39(4):134, 2002.

Torrey WC, Wyzik P: The recovery vision as a service improvement guide for community mental health center providers, *Community Ment Health J* 36(2):209, 2000.

U.S. Department of Health and Human Services: *Mental health: a report of the surgeon general,* Rockville, Md, 1999, USDHHS.

U.S. Department of Health and Human Services: *Healthy people 2010: national health promotion and disease prevention,* ed 2, Washington, DC, 2000, U.S. Government Printing Office.

U.S. Department of Health and Human Services: *Mental health: culture, race, and ethnicity—supplement to mental health: a report of the surgeon general,* Rockville, Md, 2001, USDHHS.

Veenema TG: Children's exposure to community violence, *J Nurs Scholarsh* 33(2):162, 2001.

Wahl OF: Mental health consumers' experience of stigma, *Schizophr Bull* 25(3):467, 1999.

Wasserbauer LI: Psychiatric nurses' knowledge of the Americans With Disabilities Act, *Arch Psychiatr Nurs* 10(6):324, 1996.

Worley NK: *Mental health nursing in the community,* St Louis, Mo, 1997, Mosby.

Yearwood E: Is there a culture of youth violence? *J Child Adolesc Psychiatr Nurs* 15(1):35, 2001.

Yip KS: A historical review of mental health services in Hong Kong (1841 to 1995), *Int J Soc Psychiatry* 44(1):46, 1998.

Ziguras SJ, Stewart GW: A meta-analysis of the effectiveness of mental health case management over 20 years, *Psychiatr Serv* 51(11):1410, 2000.

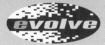

# Chapter 36

http://evolve.elsevier.com/Stanhope

# Alcohol, Tobacco, and Other Drug Problems in the Community

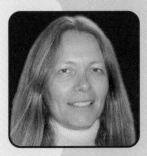

**Mary Lynn Mathre, R.N., M.S.N., C.A.R.N.**

Mary Lynn Mathre has 27 years of experience as an acute care nurse and has worked in the field of alcohol, tobacco, and other drugs for the past 17 years. Since 1991, she has worked as the addictions consult nurse for the University of Virginia Health System. This role has required much interaction with community resources to provide appropriate referrals and aftercare for the patient population. She is an active member of the International Nurses Society on Addictions and serves on the editorial board for the *Journal of Addictions Nursing,* the *Drug and Alcohol Professional* (a quarterly journal published in the United Kingdom), and the *Journal of Cannabis Therapeutics.*

## Objectives

After reading this chapter, the student should be able to do the following:

1. Analyze personal attitudes toward alcohol, tobacco, and other drug problems
2. Differentiate between the terms substance use, abuse, dependence, and addiction
3. Examine the differences between the major psychoactive drug categories
4. Explain the role of the nurse in primary, secondary, and tertiary prevention of alcohol, tobacco, and other drug problems as it relates to individual clients and their families
5. Evaluate the role of the nurse in primary, secondary, and tertiary prevention of alcohol, tobacco, and other drug problems as it relates to the community and national policies

Substance abuse is the number one national health problem, causing more deaths, illnesses, and disabilities than any other health condition. Almost 20% of all Medicaid hospital costs, and nearly one in four dollars of Medicare's inpatient hospital costs, are associated with substance abuse (Schneider Institute for Health Policy, 2001). Of the 2 million U.S. deaths each year, one quarter are attributed to alcohol, tobacco, and illicit drug use. There are approximately 13.6 million Americans who use illicit drugs and 51 million tobacco smokers. Of the 113 million Americans who used alcohol in the past month, 33 million (29%) were binge drinkers and 11 million (10%) were heavy drinkers (Schneider Institute for Health Policy, 2001). The substance abuser is not only at risk for personal health problems but may be a threat to the health and safety of family members, co-workers, and other members of the community.

Substance abuse and addiction affect all ages, races, sexes, and segments of society. As seen in the webLinks at http://evolve.elsevier.com/Stanhope, Healthy People 2010 (U.S. Department of Health and Human Services [USDHHS], 2000) lists tobacco as the third priority area, and alcohol and other drugs as the fourth priority area, with a total of 46 objectives, as well as related objectives in

other priority areas. The newer phrase of alcohol, tobacco, and other drug (ATOD) problems rather than substance abuse reminds us that alcohol and tobacco represent the major drugs of abuse when discussing substance abuse, drug addiction, or chemical dependency.

This chapter begins by providing a broad perspective of ATOD problems to clarify the relevant issues. A historical overview of ATOD problems and attitudes toward ATOD users and addicts is examined. Relevant terms are defined to decrease the confusion caused by frequent misuse of terms. The major drug categories are described, including information on commonly used substances and current ATOD use trends. The remainder of the chapter examines the role of the nurse in primary, secondary, and tertiary prevention and how the nurse can improve the outcomes for individuals, families, and communities with ATOD problems when using a harm reduction model. The reader is encouraged to consider possible nursing strategies to apply the Healthy People 2010 objectives for ATOD problems.

## ATOD PROBLEMS IN PERSPECTIVE

ATOD abuse and addiction can cause multiple health problems for individuals. Heavy ATOD use has been associated

## Key Terms

**addiction treatment**, p. 867
**Alcoholics Anonymous**, p. 868
**alcoholism**, p. 854
**blood alcohol concentration**, p. 854
**brief interventions**, p. 868
**codependency**, p. 866
**cross-tolerance**, p. 867
**denial**, p. 864
**depressants**, p. 854
**detoxification**, p. 866

**drug addiction**, p. 853
**drug dependence**, p. 852
**enabling**, p. 866
**fetal alcohol syndrome**, p. 865
**hallucinogens**, p. 859
**harm reduction**, p. 851
**inhalants**, p. 859
**injection drug users**, p. 865
**mainstream smoke**, p. 856
**polysubstance use or abuse**, p. 861

**prohibition**, p. 849
**psychoactive drugs**, p. 854
**set**, p. 859
**setting**, p. 859
**sidestream smoke**, p. 856
**stimulants**, p. 855
**substance abuse**, p. 852
**tolerance**, p. 854
**withdrawal**, p. 853

*See Glossary for definitions*

## Chapter Outline

ATOD Problems in Perspective
*Historical Overview*
*Attitudes and Myths*
*Paradigm Shift*
*Definitions*
**Psychoactive Drugs**
*Depressants*
*Stimulants*
*Marijuana*
*Hallucinogens*
**Predisposing/Contributing Factors**

*Set*
*Setting*
*Biopsychosocial Model of Addiction*
**Primary Prevention and the Role of the Nurse**
*Promotion of Healthy Lifestyles and Resiliency Factors*
*Drug Education*
**Secondary Prevention and the Role of the Nurse**
*Assessing for ATOD Problems*
*Drug Testing*

*High-Risk Groups*
*Codependency and Family Involvement*
**Tertiary Prevention and the Role of the Nurse**
*Detoxification*
*Addiction Treatment*
*Smoking Cessation Programs*
*Support Groups*
*Nurse's Role*
**Outcomes**

with many problems, including neonates with low birth weight and congenital abnormalities; accidents, homicides, and suicides; chronic diseases, such as cardiovascular diseases, cancer, and lung disease; violence; and family disruption. Factors that contribute to the substance abuse problem include lack of knowledge about the use of drugs; the labeling of certain drugs (alcohol, nicotine, and caffeine) as nondrugs; lack of quality control of illegal drugs; and drug laws that label certain drug users as criminals.

## Historical Overview

Psychoactive drug use has been part of most cultures since the beginning of humanity. Often a culture encourages use of some drugs while discouraging the use of others. Caffeine, alcohol, and tobacco are socially acceptable drugs in the United States and Canada, whereas other cultures prohibit their use. Conversely, marijuana, cocaine, and heroin use are not accepted in mainstream U.S. society, although these substances are considered sacred or beneficial and their use is accepted in various other cultures.

The United States' primary solution to various "drug problems" has been **prohibition.** During alcohol prohibition from 1920 to 1933, the United States experienced a sharp increase in violent crime and corruption among law officials secondary to the illicit marketing of alcohol. Distilled beverages were pushed because of the higher profit margin per bottle of liquor than for beer or wine. The high alcohol content in illicit moonshine caused severe health problems. The alcohol prohibition was eventually recognized as a failure and repealed (Rose, 1996).

Similar problems are occurring with the current war on drugs and the newer prohibition on marijuana, cocaine, and other drugs. An increase in both violent crime and reports of corruption among law officials as a result of the illicit market has become a major national problem. Stronger drugs are pushed because of their greater profits. In the past two decades, the U.S. war on drugs has escalated. New laws have created mandatory sentences for drug offenders, are destroying civil liberties, and are putting more resources into law enforcement than into drug education and treatment (Baum, 1997; Davis, 1998). As the drug war budget grows each year (more than $18 billion for 2001), approximately 70% of that budget goes to law enforcement and punishment, leaving only 30% for prevention and treatment (Office of National Drug Control Policy, 2001).

In recent years, many drug treatment centers have closed because insurance companies reduced their coverage for addiction treatment (Moyers, Casiato, and Hughes, 1998). Despite the effectiveness of many drug programs, many just as programs in public health and mental health, have reduced the range of services offered. Services most often are those dealing with education, mental health, social services, and drug rehabilitation.

The Physician Leadership on National Drug Policy (PLNDP) found that drug addiction can be treated with as much success as illnesses such as diabetes, hypertension, and asthma, and that treatment is much more cost effective than putting addicts in prison (Marwick, 1998) (Figure 36-1). A 3-year study by the National Center on Addiction and Substance Abuse closely examined the states' 1998 budgets to measure the impact of substance abuse and addiction on their health, social service, criminal justice, education, mental health, developmentally disabled, and other programs. Of the $620 billion total the states spent in 1998, $81.3 billion (13.1%) was used to deal with substance abuse and addiction. Of every such dollar the states spent, 96 cents went to shoveling up the wreckage caused by substance abuse and addiction and only 4 cents was used to prevent or treat it.

More specifically, for every $113 states spend on the consequences of substance abuse just for children, they only spent $1 on prevention and treatment for children (National Center on Addiction and Substance Abuse, 2001).

## Attitudes and Myths

Attitudes are developed through cultural learning and personal experiences. Attitudes toward ATOD problems are influenced by the way society categorizes drugs as either "good" or "bad." In the United States, good drugs are over-the-counter (OTC) or those prescribed by a health care provider, yet this makes them no less problematic or addictive. Bad drugs are the illegal drugs, and persons who use these drugs are considered criminals regardless of whether the drug has caused any problems.

Americans rely heavily on prescription and OTC drugs to relieve (or mask) anxiety, tension, fatigue, and physical or emotional pain. Rather than learning nonmedicinal methods of coping, many people choose the "quick fix" and take pills to deal with their problems or negative feelings.

Addicts are often viewed as immoral, weak-willed, or irresponsible persons who should try harder to help them-

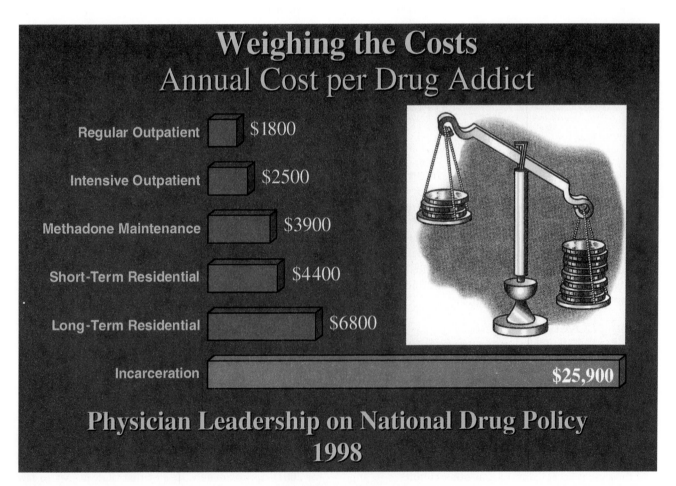

**Figure 36-1** Weighing the costs—annual cost per drug addict. *(Prepared by Physician Leadership on National Drug Policy [PLNDP] National Project Office, Brown University Center for Alcohol and Addiction Studies, Providence, RI, 1998.)*

selves. Although alcoholism was recognized as a disease by the American Medical Association in 1954, and drug addiction was recognized as a disease some years later, much of the public and many health care professionals have failed to change their attitudes and accept alcoholics and addicts as ill persons in need of health care.

---

**WHAT DO YOU THINK?**

Antiprohibitionists believe that the prohibition of drugs causes greater societal problems than the use of those drugs and that the government has no right to forbid adults from what they choose to ingest. Although antiprohibitionists are often called "legalizers," this label is misleading because it implies that by "legalizing" a drug, the government is condoning its use. Do you understand the difference between the terms? If some drugs should be prohibited, who should decide which drugs to prohibit? Should persons be incarcerated because they have consumed a prohibited drug?

---

Nurses must examine their attitudes toward ATOD use, abuse, and addiction before working with this health problem. To be therapeutic, the nurse must develop a trusting, nonjudgmental relationship with the client. Systematic assessment for ATOD problems is based on awareness that there may be problems with legal drugs as well as with illegal drugs. If the nurse's attitude toward a client with a drug abuse problem is negative or punitive, the issue may never be directly addressed or the client may be avoided. If the client senses the negative attitude of the health care provider, either by words or tone of voice, communication may cease and information may be withheld. To develop a therapeutic attitude, the nurse must realize that any drug can be abused, that anyone may develop drug dependence, and that drug addiction can be successfully treated.

Myths develop over years, and if myths are not questioned, many attitudes may be formed solely on the basis of fiction rather than fact. Some common myths are as follows: "An alcoholic is a skid row bum"—but less than 5% of persons with addictions fit this description. "If you teach people about drugs, they will abuse them"—although it is true that people may choose to use drugs if they have knowledge about them, it is more likely that people without knowledge about them will abuse them. "Addiction is a sin or moral failing"—addiction is recognized as a health problem involving biopsychosocial factors, and persons who use drugs do not do so with the intent to become addicted.

## Paradigm Shift

We can hope to see a major shift in how the United States conceptualizes ATOD problems in the new millennium. The old criminal justice model is based on stereotypes, misinformation, and punishment, and it uses war tactics to fight the drug users, addicts, and suppliers (fellow citizens).

Campaigns have been launched using the slogans "zero tolerance" for drug users, "just say no" to drugs, and striving for a "drug-free America"—all of which vilify the drug user or drug addict. The newest campaign, which has evolved since the bombing of the World Trade Centers in 2001, attempts to link drug users to terrorism. This punitive approach to illicit drug use hinders open communication between the health care professional and the drug user. Those who are abusing drugs, experiencing secondary health problems, or possibly becoming addicted may not seek help for fear of being arrested or confined.

The **harm reduction** model is a health care approach to ATOD problems initially used in Great Britain, the Netherlands, Germany, Switzerland, and Australia, and interest in it is spreading throughout Europe and in Canada. This new public health model is based on understanding that addiction is a health problem, that any psychoactive drug can be abused, that accurate information can help persons make responsible decisions about drug use, and that persons who have ATOD problems can be helped. This approach accepts the reality that psychoactive drug use is endemic, and it focuses on pragmatic interventions, especially education, to reduce the adverse consequences of drug use and get treatment for addicts. The United States has already taken a harm reduction approach with tobacco and alcohol. Educational campaigns are used to inform the public about the health risks of tobacco use. Warnings have appeared on tobacco product labels since 1967 as a result of the surgeon general's 1966 report on the dangers of smoking. In 1971, a ban on television and radio cigarette advertising was imposed. Cigarette smoking has decreased from 42% of the population in 1965 to 25% in 1997 (Schneider Institute for Health Policy, 2001). A federal report shows that smoking is on the decline among eighth and tenth graders. According to the report, 5.5% of eighth graders smoked in 2001, down from 7.4% the previous year. Among tenth graders, 12% smoked in 2001, down from 14% in 2000 (www.childstats.gov).

Education is beginning to address the dangers of alcohol abuse and to establish guidelines for safe alcohol use. Alcohol consumers are choosing lower-alcohol-content products such as beer and wine coolers rather than distilled products. Nurses have a responsibility to seek the underlying roots of various health problems and plan action that is realistic, nonjudgmental, holistic, and positive, and a harm reduction model for ATOD problems facilitates such an approach.

## Definitions

The terms *drug use* and *drug abuse* have virtually lost their usefulness because the public and government have narrowed the term *drug* to include only illegal drugs rather than including prescription, OTC, and legal recreational drugs. The current phrase *alcohol, tobacco, and other drugs* (ATOD) is a reminder that the leading drug problems involve alcohol and tobacco. The term *substance* broadens

## Use of Alcohol, Tobacco, and Other Drugs in Canada

Pat Sanagan, R.N., B.Sc.N., M.Ed.

The Canadian approach to substance abuse prevention endeavors to provide a balance among prevention, intervention, treatment, and legislation. Canada recognizes the multiple realities that can impact on drug use, such as poverty, racism, homelessness, and other systemic issues. Canada's drug strategy is to develop appropriate prevention and treatment programs along with programs to reduce supply and drug trafficking.

Health Canada's Drug Strategy and Controlled Substances Programme (1998) regulates controlled substances and promotes initiatives that reduce or prevent the harm associated with these substances and alcohol (see the Health Canada website www.hc-sc.gc.ca/hecs-sesc/hecs/dscs.htm). The programme also provides expert advice and drug analysis services to law enforcement agencies across the country. The programme includes the Office of Canada's Drug Strategy, the Office of Controlled Substances, the Office of Cannabis Medical Access, and the Drug Analysis Service. This programme's mandate is governed by the following legislation:

- The Controlled Drug and Substances Act
- The Canadian Centre on Substance Abuse Act
- The Food and Drug Act

### CANADIAN STATISTICS

The most recent report on drug use statistics in Canada—The Canadian Profile of 1999—indicates that Canadian patterns of use of alcohol and other drugs continue to be a potential source of problems (Canadian Centre on Substance Abuse [CCSA], 1999). Of particular note is binge-drinking—42.1% of past-year drinkers reported consuming five or more drinks on a single occasion (CCSA, 1999). In 2001, the rate of driving while impaired went up for the first time in 20 years, increasing by 7% (CCSA, 2001). Cannabis use either stayed the same or increased, depending on the jurisdiction. For example, in Ontario, cannabis use among students in grades 7 to 13 increased from 12.7% in 1993 to 29.3% in 1999 but stabilized over the next 2 years (29.8% in 2001) (Adlaf and Paglia, 2001). Canadian older adults continue to experience adverse

effects from prescribed and over-the-counter medications. Noncompliance with prescription instructions is the cause of 25% of hospital admissions for older adults and 23% of all nursing home admissions (Coambs et al, 1995; Lazarou, Pomerantz, and Corey, 1998).

The Canadian Tobacco Use Monitoring Survey (CTUMS) confirms that smoking rates continue to drop in Canada. The survey reveals that 5.4 million Canadians, or 22% of the population age 15 years and older, were smokers in the year 2001. This is the lowest overall level since regular monitoring of smoking began in 1965, when prevalence rates were at 50% of the population (CTUMS, 2001).

### CANADIAN RESPONSE

Canadian community health nurses are involved in health promotion and disease prevention related to substance use at the individual, family, aggregate, and community level. Strategies are targeted at primary, secondary, and tertiary prevention. Primary prevention includes development of programs and policies to support comprehensive health promotion, including education and skill-building, supportive environments, and community capacity-building. Strategies for secondary prevention include working with at-risk groups, developing appropriate and effective harm reduction programs, and assessment and referral interventions. A "best practice" compendium developed by Health Canada in 2001 identifies 14 prevention principles for effective programming to prevent and reduce substance use problems among youth (Health Canada, 2002). Tertiary prevention initiatives include collaboration with treatment centres to ensure comprehensive client aftercare, and advocacy to provide treatment options that recognize a range of needs.

### EMERGING SUBSTANCE USE ISSUES FOR CANADIAN COMMUNITY HEALTH NURSES

- *Cannabis.* After the release of the final report from the Senate Special Committee on Illegal Drugs ("Cannabis: Our Position for a Canadian Public

the scope to include alcohol, tobacco, legal drugs, and even foods. **Substance abuse** is the use of any substance that threatens a person's health or impairs social or economic functioning. This definition is more objective and universal than the government's definition of drug abuse, which is the use of a drug without a prescription or any use of an illegal drug. Although any drug or food can be abused, this chapter focuses on psychoactive drugs: drugs that affect mood, perception, and thought.

Drug dependence and drug addiction are often used interchangeably, but they are not synonymous. **Drug dependence** is a state of neuroadaptation (a physiologic change in the central nervous system [CNS]) caused by the chronic, regular administration of a drug; in drug dependence, continued use of the drug becomes necessary to prevent withdrawal symptoms (O'Brien, 1996). This happens when persons are given an opiate such as morphine on a regular basis for pain management. To prevent

Policy"), and the House of Commons Special Committee Report on the Non-Medical Use of Drugs ("Policy for a New Millennium: Working Together to Redefine Canada's Drug Strategy"), there may be changes to drug laws, particularly those addressing cannabis (Canadian Senate Report, 2002; House of Commons Committee Reports, 2002).

- *Fetal alcohol syndrome/fetal alcohol effects (FAS/FAE).* It is estimated that in Canada, at least one child is born with FAS each day, and initial studies suggest that the rates of FAS/FAE in some aboriginal communities may be significantly higher (see the Health Canada website at www.hc-sc. gc.ca).
- *Blood alcohol concentration and impaired driving.* A current debate concerning blood alcohol concentration (BAC) and driving suggests that the criminal code BAC limit should be reduced from 0.08% to 0.05% or lower (Solomon, 2002).
- *Human immunodeficiency virus (HIV), acquired immunodeficiency syndrome (AIDS), hepatitis C virus (HCV), and injection drug use (IDU).* The prevalence of HIV/AIDS and HCV in federal and provincial prisons has continued to increase since 1996. In particular, in Canada's federal prison system, the number of reported cases of HIV/AIDS rose from 14 in January 1989 to 159 in March 1996, and then to 217 in December 2000—an increase of 36% between 1996 and 2000. Even higher are hepatitis C rates. IDU and other drug use are believed to be a major cause of these increases (see Canadian HIV/AIDS Legal Network website at www.aidslaw.ca).

### References

Adlaf EM, Paglia A: Drug use among Ontario students, 1977-2001: Findings from the OSDUS, CAMH research document No. 10, Toronto, 2001, Centre for Addiction and Mental Health.

Canadian Centre for Justice Statistics: *Juristats,* Ottawa, 2001, CCJS.

Canadian Centre on Substance Abuse: *Proportions of crimes associated with alcohol and other drugs in Canada,* Ottawa, April 2002, CCSA.

Canadian Centre on Substance Abuse, Centre for Addiction and Mental Health: *Canadian profile, 1999,* Ottawa, 1999, CCSA.

Canadian Senate Report: *Cannabis: our position for a Canadian public policy,* Ottawa, 2002, Senate Special Committee on Illegal Drugs, available at http://www. parl.gc.ca/37/1/parlbus/commbus/senate/com-e/ ille-e/rep-e/summary-e.htm.

Canadian Tobacco Use Monitoring Survey: *Results from 2001,* Ottawa, 2001, Health Canada.

Coambs RB et al: *Health promotion research: review of the scientific literature on the prevalence, consequences, and health costs of noncompliance & inappropriate use of prescription medication in Canada,* Toronto, University of Toronto Press, 1995.

Health Canada: *Preventing substance use problems among young people: a compendium of best practices,* Ottawa, 1998, Health Canada. Updated information available at http://www.hc=sc.gc.ca/hecs.sesc.hecs/ dscs.htm.

House of Commons Committee: *Special Report on the Non-Medical Use of Drugs,* 2002, available at http://www.parl.gc.ca/InfoCom/CommitteeMain.asp? Language=E&CommitteeID=301&Joint=0 or by contacting Carol Chafe, Clerk, House of Commons, Room / piéce 605, éd., Wellington Bldg., Ottawa, Ontario, K1A OA6: snud@parl.gc.ca.

Lazarou J, Pomerantz BH, Corey PN: Incidence of adverse drug reactions in hospitalized patients, *JAMA* 279:1200-1205, 1998.

Solomon R: *Taking back our roads: a strategy to eliminate impaired driving in Canada,* Ottawa, 2002, MADD Canada.

WebLinks at http://evolve.elsevier.com/Stanhope to see Canadian websites related to drug, tobacco, and alcohol issues.

*Canadian spelling is used.*

**withdrawal** symptoms, the morphine should be gradually tapered rather than abruptly stopped.

**Drug addiction** is a pattern of abuse characterized by an overwhelming preoccupation with the use (compulsive use) of a drug, securing its supply, and a high tendency to relapse if the drug is removed. Frequently, addicts are physically dependent on a drug, but there also appears to be an added psychological component that causes the intense cravings and subsequent relapse. In general, anyone can develop a drug dependence as a result of regular administration of drugs that alter the CNS; however, only 7% to 15% of the drug-using population will develop a drug addiction. The process of becoming addicted is complex and related to several factors, including the addictive properties of the substance, family and peer influences, personality, age of first use, cultural and social factors, existing psychiatric disorders, and genetics (Schneider Institute for Health Policy, 2001).

**Alcoholism** is addiction to the drug called alcohol. Alcoholism and drug addiction are recognized as illnesses under a biopsychosocial model. Simply stated, the disease concept of addiction and alcoholism identifies them as chronic and progressive diseases in which a person's use of a drug or drugs continues despite problems it causes in any area of life–physical, emotional, social, economic, or spiritual.

## PSYCHOACTIVE DRUGS

Although any drug can be abused, ATOD abuse and addiction problems generally involve the **psychoactive drugs.** Because they can alter emotions, these drugs are used for enjoyment in social and recreational settings and for personal use to self-medicate physical or emotional discomfort. Psychoactive drugs are divided into categories according to their effect on the CNS and the general feelings or experiences the drugs may induce. The internet or a pharmacology text can provide detailed information on these drug categories (e.g., depressants, stimulants, and hallucinogens). Often, if persons cannot obtain their drug of choice, another drug from the same category will be substituted. For example, a person who cannot drink alcohol may begin using a benzodiazepine as an alternative because both are CNS depressants.

## Depressants

**Depressants** lower the body's overall energy level, reduce sensitivity to outside stimulation, and, in high doses, induce sleep. Low doses of depressants may produce a feeling of stimulation caused by initial sedation of the inhibitory centers in the brain. In general, depressants decrease heart rate, respiration rate, muscular coordination, and energy and dull the senses. Higher doses lead to coma and, if the vital functions shut down, death. Major categories include alcohol, barbiturates, benzodiazepines, and the opioids. Although the community-oriented nurse should be alert for abuse and addiction problems with many of the prescribed depressants, only alcohol and heroin will be reviewed.

### Alcohol

Alcohol (ethyl alcohol, or ethanol) is the oldest and most widely used psychoactive drug in the world. Approximately 65% of Americans of age 18 and older consume alcohol, and approximately 5.2% are alcohol dependent, 8% are problem drinkers, and 9.4% are at-risk drinkers (exceed the recommended guidelines) (Manwell et al, 1997). Alcohol abuse contributes to illness in each of the top three causes of death in the United States: heart disease, cancer, and stroke. The life expectancy of a person with alcoholism is reduced by 26 years (Schneider Institute for Health Policy, 2001).

Alcohol abuse costs billions of dollars in lost productivity, property damage, medical expenses from alcohol-related illnesses and accidents, family disruptions, alcohol-related violence, and neglect and abuse of children. In a study examining alcohol and interpersonal violence, results showed that approximately half of all violent episodes are drug related, with alcohol as the drug most often associated with violence (Cychosz, 1996). Chronic alcohol abuse exerts profound metabolic and physiologic effects on all organ systems. Gastrointestinal (GI) disturbances include inflammation of the GI tract, malabsorption, ulcers, liver problems, and cancers. Cardiovascular disturbances include cardiac dysrhythmias, cardiomyopathy, hypertension, atherosclerosis, and blood dyscrasias. CNS problems include depression, sleep disturbances, memory loss, organic brain syndrome, Wernicke-Korsakoff syndrome, and alcohol withdrawal syndrome. Neuromuscular problems include myopathy and peripheral neuropathy. Males may experience testicular atrophy, sterility, impotence, or gynecomastia, and females who consume alcohol during pregnancy may reproduce neonates with fetal alcohol syndrome (FAS) or fetal alcohol effects (FAE). Some of the metabolic disturbances include hypokalemia, hypomagnesemia, and ketoacidosis. Also, endocrine disturbances may result in pancreatitis or diabetes (National Institute on Alcohol Abuse and Alcoholism, 1997).

> ### ( NURSING TIP
>
> The National Institute on Alcohol Abuse and Alcoholism (1995) recommends the following limitations for persons who drink: For men, no more than two drinks per day. For women, no more than one drink per day. For persons over age 65, no more than one drink per day.

The concentration of alcohol in the blood is determined by the concentration of alcohol in the drink, the rate of drinking, the rate of absorption (slower in the presence of food), the rate of metabolism, and a person's weight and sex. The amount of alcohol the liver can metabolize per hour is equal to about $3/4$ ounce of whiskey, 4 ounces of wine, or 12 ounces of beer. Figure 36-2 shows the effects on the CNS as the **blood alcohol concentration** (BAC) increases. However, with chronic consumption, **tolerance** will develop, and a person can reach a high BAC with minimal CNS effects.

Sex affects the BAC because females have less alcohol dehydrogenase activity than men (except for males with chronic alcoholism). Because this enzyme detoxifies alcohol, a deficiency results in a higher bioavailability of alcohol. Consequently, females suffer the long-term effects of alcohol intake at much lower doses in a shorter time span (Gordon, 2002).

Alcohol use in moderation may provide health benefits by providing mild relaxation and lowering the serum cholesterol (Abramson et al, 2001). Controlled drinking organizations such as Moderation Management (www.moderation.

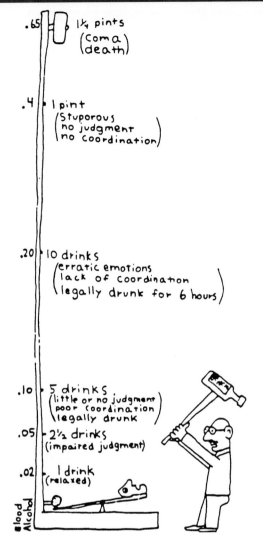

**Figure 36-2** Blood alcohol level and related CNS effects of a normal drinker (160-lb man) according to the number of drinks consumed in 1 hour. *(From Kinney J, Leaton G: Loosening the grip, ed 5, St Louis, Mo, 1995, Mosby.)*

org) provide guidelines for persons who want to have alcohol in their lives.

## Heroin

Heroin is one of the opioids. Opiates include the natural drugs found in the opium poppy, namely, opium, morphine, and codeine. Opioids are synthetic drugs, such as heroin (semisynthetic), meperidine, methadone, oxycodone, and propoxyphene, that mimic the effects of the natural opiates. Opiates are by far the most effective drugs for pain relief. When used for pain control, only approximately 0.1% of those patients will develop addiction, and therefore fear of addiction should not be used as a reason to undertreat pain.

The United States has approximately 600,000 to 800,000 heroin addicts, and more than 2 million people who have tried it (Gordon, 2001). Whereas typical heroin

addicts from the 1950s to the 1980s were primarily inner-city African-American men who were using it intravenously, trends have changed in the 1990s. Heroin today is purer and less expensive and use is spreading among the younger middle class and Hispanic Americans, who are often snorting or smoking this purer product (Castro et al, 1999; Stine and Kosten, 1999). A Caron Foundation study found that 90% of their admissions for heroin addiction were white, more than 50% were employed full-time, and almost 89% had a high school diploma or higher level of education. Also, over 70% of their adolescent admissions lived in suburban or rural locales (Gordon, 2001).

Tolerance develops quite readily with opioids and can reach striking levels. Tolerance to one opioid extends to other opioids, and thus cross-tolerance can occur. Physical dependence also develops quite quickly; less than 2 weeks of continuous use can cause withdrawal symptoms if the drug is not tapered. Chronic abuse of the opioids causes few physiologic problems except for constipation. The negative consequences result primarily from their illegal status.

## Stimulants

People use **stimulants** to feel more alert or energetic, as these drugs act by activating or exciting the nervous system. An increase in alertness and energy results as the stimulant causes the nerve fibers to release noradrenaline and other stimulating neurotransmitters. However, these drugs do not *give* the person more energy; they only make the body expend its own energy sooner and in greater quantities than it normally would.

If used carefully, stimulants are useful and have few negative health effects. The body must be allowed time to replenish itself after use of a stimulant. The cost for the "high" is the "down" state after the use of a stimulant: a feeling of sleepiness, laziness, mental fatigue, and possibly depression. Many persons abusing stimulants soon begin a vicious cycle of avoiding the down feeling by taking another dose, and they can become physically dependent on the stimulant to function. Common stimulants include nicotine, cocaine, caffeine, and amphetamines.

### Nicotine

One in five deaths in the United States is attributed to cigarettes. The Centers for Disease Control and Prevention (CDC) estimates an average of 430,700 deaths per year are caused by complications of cigarette smoking (Schneider Institute for Health Policy, 2001) (Figure 36-3). In 1993, more than 14% of Medicaid expenditures in all states were attributable to cigarette smoking.

Nicotine, the active ingredient in the tobacco plant, is a particularly toxic drug. To protect itself, the body quickly develops tolerance to the nicotine. If a person smokes regularly, tolerance to nicotine develops within hours, compared with days for heroin or months for alcohol. Pipes and cigars are less hazardous than cigarettes because the harsher smoke discourages deep inhalation. However,

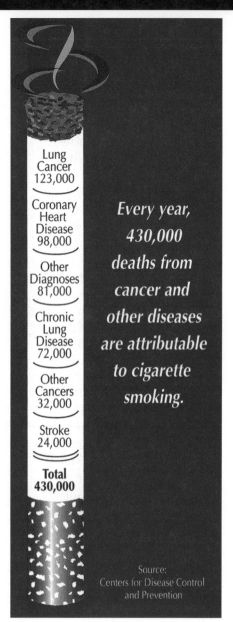

Every year, 430,000 deaths from cancer and other diseases are attributable to cigarette smoking.

Lung Cancer 123,000
Coronary Heart Disease 98,000
Other Diagnoses 81,000
Chronic Lung Disease 72,000
Other Cancers 32,000
Stroke 24,000
Total 430,000

Source: Centers for Disease Control and Prevention

**Figure 36-3** Cigarette smoking mortality. *(From Centers for Disease Control and Prevention, Atlanta, Ga.)*

## Evidence-Based Practice

African Americans disproportionately experience greater smoking-attributable morbidity and mortality. The smoking rate for inner-city African-American smokers is higher than in the general population (45% versus 25%) and they attempt to quit smoking more frequently, but their success rate at quitting is 34% lower. Using community outreach efforts, investigators recruited 600 urban, low-income African-American volunteers, of whom 70% were women. Average age of the sample was 44 years and average number of cigarettes smoked was 17 per day. Subjects were randomized to receive placebo or 150 mg of bupropion SR (one pill once daily for the first 3 days, then twice daily) for 7 weeks. All subjects received in-person and telephone contacts with African-American counselors.

After the 7 weeks of treatment, 36% of subjects taking bupropion SR and 19% of subjects taking placebo had not smoked. At 26 weeks, smoking cessation rates were 21% in the bupropion SR group and 13.7% in the placebo group. Self-reported cessation was verified through biochemical tests. In addition, by week 6, those taking bupropion SR had a greater mean reduction in depressive symptoms than those in the placebo group. After controlling for continuous abstinence, they also gained less weight than did subjects taking placebo.

When combined with professional counseling, bupropion SR helped lower-income African Americans quit smoking with fewer depressive symptoms and less weight gain, based on this randomized, controlled trial.

**Nurse Use:** Although the study had limitations (in that it included a high proportion of female subjects; it used volunteers, who are typically more motivated to quit; and all the subjects had access to professional counselors), it did indicate that clinical trials that focus on minority groups are critical for the development of appropriate interventions. Such strategies can be used in many communities.

Ahluwalia JS et al: Sustained-release bupropion for smoking cessation in African Americans: a randomized controlled trial, *JAMA* 288(4):468-474, 2002.

---

pipes and cigars increase the risk of cancer of the lips, mouth, and throat.

Smoke can be inhaled directly by the smoker **(main-stream smoke),** or it can enter the atmosphere from the lighted end of the cigarette and be inhaled by others in the vicinity **(sidestream smoke).** Sidestream smoke contains greater concentrations of toxic and carcinogenic compounds than mainstream smoke. An estimated 3000 annual lung cancer deaths are attributed to sidestream smoke, and more than 6000 annual deaths among children are linked in part to parental smoking (Schneider Institute for Health Policy, 2001). Smoking bans are being adopted with the intent to reduce the discomfort and health hazards among nonsmokers.

Nicotine is also used as chewing tobacco or snuff. Marketed as "smokeless tobacco," a wad is put in the mouth and the nicotine is absorbed sublingually. Higher doses of nicotine are delivered in the smokeless forms because the nicotine is not destroyed by heat. Nevertheless, this form is less addictive because nicotine enters the bloodstream less directly.

## Cocaine

Cocaine comes from the coca shrub found on the eastern slopes of the Andes mountains and has been cultivated by

South American Indians for thousands of years. The Indians chew a mixture of the coca leaf and lime to get a mild stimulant effect similar to coffee. By 1860 cocaine was isolated from the plant as a hydrochloride salt. It could be dissolved in water and used intravenously or orally when mixed in soft drinks. By the early 1900s, the common route of administration of the white powder was intranasal "snorting" (Weil and Rosen, 1998).

In the 1970s, "freebasing" was introduced. This involved making the hydrochloride salt a more volatile substance by using highly flammable substances such as ether to convert the powder to a crystal that could then be smoked in a pipe. By the early 1980s, another form of smokeable cocaine was introduced. Cocaine was dissolved in water, mixed with baking soda, and then heated to form rocks, or "crack." Intranasal cocaine has been a popular recreational drug among the rich and famous, but the cheaper crack form, sold in small quantities at $2 to $20, has become popular, particularly among inner-city black populations. In 1998, about 1.7 million Americans were current (at least once per month) cocaine users; this is about 0.8% of the population age 12 and older, with the highest rate of use among 18- to 25-year-olds (2%). Of the current cocaine users, about 437,000 used crack (National Institute on Drug Abuse, 2002).

> **WHAT DO YOU THINK?**
>
> More than 400,000 whites use cocaine, compared to 200,000 Hispanics and 48,000 African Americans (Marwick, 1998). However, 99% of the drug-trafficking defendants in the United States between 1985 and 1987 were African American (Baum, 1997).

Cocaine produces a feeling of intense euphoria, increased confidence, and a willingness to work for long periods. Smoking cocaine gives intense effects because the drug quickly reaches the brain through the blood vessels in the lungs. Cocaine's interaction with dopamine seems to be the basis for the addictive patterns. The extreme euphoria is believed to be caused by cocaine's effect of dopaminergic stimulation. Chronic administration can lead to neurotransmitter depletion (especially of dopamine), which results in an extreme dysphoria characterized by apathy, sadness, and anhedonia (lack of joy). Thus a cocaine user

> **DID YOU KNOW?**
>
> Cocaine, a vasoconstrictor, decreases cerebral blood flow by an average of 20% for men. A new study found no changes in cerebral blood flow for women during the follicular phase of their menstrual cycle (days 1-14 prior to ovulation) and a 10% decrease in flow during their luteal phase (days 15 to 28 after ovulation) (Kaufman et al, 2001).

can get caught up in a dangerous cycle of gaining an extreme high followed by an extreme low and avoiding that low by consuming more cocaine. Crack addiction develops rapidly and is expensive, with addicts needing between $100 and $1000 per day. Addicts soon learn that their ill health and drug use are related, but, overwhelmed by cravings, they may resort to criminal activities (theft or prostitution) to get the drug.

Street cocaine ranges in purity from 5% to 60% and may be cut with other drugs, such as procaine or amphetamine, or any white powder, such as sugar or baby powder. High doses can cause extreme agitation, paranoid delusions, hyperthermia, hallucinations, cardiac dysrhythmias, pulmonary complications, convulsions, and possibly death (Beers and Berkow, 1999).

## Caffeine

Caffeine is one of the most widely used psychoactive drugs in the world, with a U.S. daily per capita consumption of 211 mg. Caffeine in soft drinks and cold coffee drinks is becoming the drug of choice for American youth. New names such as Surge, Zapped, Jolt, and Outburst and slogans such as "slammin' a Dew" (for Mountain Dew) reflect the marketing strategy for "power" drinks aimed at teens (Cordes, 1998).

Caffeine is found in coffee, tea, chocolate, soft drinks, and various medications (Table 36-1). Moderate doses of caffeine from 100 to 300 mg per day increase mental alertness and probably have little negative effect on health. Higher doses can lead to insomnia, irritability, tremulousness, anxiety, cardiac dysrhythmias, GI disturbances, and headaches. Regular use of high doses can lead to physical dependence, and the withdrawal symptoms may include headaches, slowness, and occasional depression (Weinberg and Bealer, 2001)). Treating afternoon headaches with analgesics containing caffeine may in reality be preventing a withdrawal symptom from heavy morning coffee consumption.

## Amphetamines

Amphetamines are a class of stimulants similar to cocaine, but the effects last longer and the drugs are cheaper. Amphetamines have a chemical structure similar to adrenaline and noradrenaline and are generally used to decrease fatigue, increase mental alertness, suppress appetite, and create a sense of well-being. Historically, amphetamines have been issued to American soldiers and pilots to decrease fatigue and increase mental alertness. They are currently popular among truck drivers and college students.

These drugs are taken orally, intranasally, or by injection, or they are smoked. When taken intravenously, they quickly induce an intense euphoric feeling (a "rush"). The user may speed for several days (go on a "speed run") and then fall into a deep sleep for 18 or more hours ("crash"). "Ice," a smokeable form of crystallized methamphetamine, was introduced in the late 1980s as an alternative to crack because it can be easily manufactured and the effects last up to 24 hours. Methamphetamine use first appeared in

**Table 36-1    Caffeine Content in Commonly Consumed Substances**

| SUBSTANCE | CAFFEINE CONTENT (MG) |
|---|---|
| **Coffee (5 oz)** | |
| Brewed | 60-180 |
| Instant | 30-120 |
| Decaffeinated | 1-5 |
| **Chocolate** | |
| Cocoa (5 oz) | 2-20 |
| Semisweet (1 oz) | 5-35 |
| **Tea (5 oz)** | |
| Brewed | 20-90 |
| Iced | 67-76 |
| **Soft drinks (12 oz)** | |
| Colas | 40-45 |
| Mountain Dew | 53 |
| Orange soda, ginger ale, Sprite, 7 Up, and several fruit-flavored drinks | 0 |
| **Prescription Drugs** | |
| propoxyphene (Darvene) | 32.4 |
| Fiorinal | 40 |
| ergotamine (Cafergot) | 100 |
| **Over-the-Counter Drugs** | |
| Anacin | 32 |
| Excedrin | 65 |
| NoDōz | 100 |
| Vivarin | 200 |

Honolulu and western areas of the continental United States. Use increased in the 1990s in both rural and urban areas of the South and Midwest (National Institute on Drug Abuse, 1998a). In 1999, women made up 47% of the patients in addiction treatment programs who identified methamphetamine as their drug of choice (Curley, 2002).

Other drugs containing caffeine, ephedrine, or phenylpropanolamine (singly or in combination) are referred to as "look-alikes." These drugs gained market attention after access to amphetamines was controlled by prescription. These chemicals are often found in OTC cold remedies as a nasal decongestant and in diet pills (e.g., Dexatrim).

## Marijuana

Marijuana (*Cannabis sativa* or *C. indica*) is the most widely used illicit drug in the United States. It is estimated that 20 to 30 million Americans regularly use marijuana. Up to 60% of people between 18 and 25 years old have tried marijuana at some time. Use peaked among high school seniors in the late 1970s, when about 60% reported having used marijuana and nearly 11% reported daily use. By 1997, just fewer than 50% reported having used marijuana, and 5.8% were daily users (Cargo, 1998).

Compared with the other psychoactive drugs, marijuana has little toxicity and is one of the safest therapeutic agents known (Petro, 1997). However, because of its illegal status, there is no quality control, and a user may consume contaminated marijuana. Users enjoy a mild euphoria, a relaxed feeling, and an intensity of sensory perceptions. Side effects include dry and reddened eyes, increased appetite, dry mouth, drowsiness, and mild tachycardia. Adverse reactions include anxiety, disorientation, and paranoia.

### ( DID YOU KNOW?

Before the marijuana prohibition, cannabis was a popular plant grown for its fiber (hemp), seed (popular birdseed), oil, and medicinal as well as psychoactive properties. During World War II, the hemp fiber was so valuable that farmers were required to grow marijuana to ensure a supply. Hemp fiber and seeds do not contain enough active THC to produce any psychoactive effects, and these products are becoming available in the United States.

The greatest physical concern for chronic users is possible damage to the respiratory tract from smoking the drug. Tolerance can develop as well as physical dependence; however, the withdrawal symptoms are benign. Addiction can occur for some chronic users and is difficult to treat because the progression tends to be subtle.

### ( DID YOU KNOW?

Marijuana contains a group of compounds called cannabinoids. A synthetic oral preparation (dronabinol) of the primary psychoactive cannabinoid, delta-9-tetrahydrocannabinol (THC), is available by prescription as a schedule III drug. However, new research shows that other nonpsychoactive cannabinoids are believed to have more therapeutic value (Joy, Watson, and Benson, 1999).

Before the Marihuana Tax Act of 1937, tincture of *Cannabis* was listed in the U.S. Pharmacopoeia through 1941 for such ailments as migraines, spasticity, and dysmenorrhea and in the treatment of heroin or cocaine addiction. In 1970, marijuana was placed in the schedule I category of drugs by the passage of the Controlled Substances Act and since then has not been available for medicinal use. The only legal access to this medicine has been through the U.S. Food and Drug Administration's (FDA's) Compassionate Investigational New Drug Program. In 1992, this program was closed, and there are only seven remaining legal clients. In response to this complete prohibition, some health care organizations support access to this medication through formal resolutions, including 10 state nurses' associations (Arkansas, California, Colorado, Hawaii, Mississippi, North Carolina, New Jersey, New Mexico, New York, and Virginia as of 1998), and the American Public Health Association (American Public Health Association; 1996). Also, since 1996, nine states (Alaska, Arizona, California, Colorado, Hawaii, Maine, Nevada, Oregon, and Washington) and Washington, D.C., have passed laws allowing patients to use marijuana as medicine under the recommendation of their physician, but the federal government continues its total prohibition efforts (www.medicalcannabis.com).

## Hallucinogens

Also called psychedelics ("mind vision"), **hallucinogens** can produce hallucinations. Many of these drugs have been used for centuries in religious ceremonies and healing rituals and are used by many cultures to produce euphoria and as aphrodisiacs. For these drugs, the user's mood, basic emotional makeup, and expectations **(set)** along with the immediate surroundings **(setting)** influence the mental effects experienced by the user. The physical effects are more constant and consist of CNS stimulation.

The two broad chemical families of hallucinogens are the indole hallucinogens and those that resemble adrenalin and amphetamines. The indoles are related to hormones (serotonin) made in the brain by the pineal gland and include such drugs as lysergic acid diethylamide (LSD), psilocybin, mushrooms, and morning glory seeds. The second group lacks the chemical structure called the indole ring and includes peyote, mescaline, and MDMA (ecstasy). Phencyclidine (PCP) is in a class by itself. It is a potent anesthetic and analgesic with CNS stimulant, depressant, and hallucinogenic properties; its use was especially high in the 1980s. LSD is the most well known drug in the hallucinogen category, but MDMA will be discussed because it is currently a popular drug.

### MDMA (Ecstasy)

MDMA (Ecstasy) is a semisynthetic drug first patented by Merck Pharmaceuticals in 1914. It was not widely used until the late 1970s and early 1980s, when psychiatrists and psychotherapists began using it to facilitate psychotherapy. It is classified as a mood elevator that produces feelings of empathy, openness, and well-being. Taken orally, its effects are experienced in 20 to 40 minutes, with the peak effect at 60 to 90 minutes, ending after about 3 to 5 hours. Ecstasy has gained current popularity as a "club" drug used at all night "rave" dances. Deaths have occurred at these rave parties secondary to overheating. Some of these deaths have been listed as overdoses of Ecstasy, because it raises the body's temperature, pulse rate, and blood pressure. Harm reduction strategies such as having free water available and rooms for people to relax could help prevent such overdoses. An additional risk to illicit Ecstasy is adul-

teration of the drug by other more toxic drugs (Byard et al, 1998; Greer and Tolbert, 1998; www.DanceSafe.org).

## Inhalants

Inhalants are often among the first drugs that young children use. Young people, especially those between the ages of 7 and 17, are most likely to abuse inhalants. Recent surveys show that about 6% of American children have tried inhalants by the fourth grade, with use peaking around the eighth grade (National Institute on Drug Abuse, 2000).

The inhalants, which include gases and solvents, do not fit neatly into other categories. There are four categories of **inhalants:** volatile organic solvents, aerosols, volatile nitrites, and gases. These substances are inhaled ("huffed") from bottles, aerosol cans, or soaked cloth or put into bags or balloons to increase the concentration of the inhaled fumes and decrease the inhalation of other substances in the vapor (e.g., paint particles). See www.inhalants.org for examples of products in these categories and specific drug information. At least 100 children die each year from inhaling common household chemicals. "Sudden sniffing death" syndrome may occur, which appears to be related to acute cardiac dysrhythmia (National Institute on Drug Abuse, 2000). Dangers with administration of gases increase when inhaling directly from pressurized tanks because the gas is very cold and can cause frostbite to the nose, lips, and vocal cords. Also, if a gas such as nitrous oxide is not mixed with oxygen, the user may die from asphyxiation (www.inhalants.org).

## PREDISPOSING/CONTRIBUTING FACTORS

In addition to the specific drug being used, two other major variables influence the particular drug experience: set and setting (Weil and Rosen, 1998). To understand various patterns of drug use and abuse by individuals, all three factors (drug, set, and setting) should be considered.

### Set

Set refers to the individual using the drug, as well as that individual's expectations, including unconscious expectations, about the drug being used. A person's current health may alter a drug's effects from one day to the next. Some people are genetically predisposed to alcoholism or other drug addiction, and their chemical makeup is such that simply consuming the drug triggers the disease process. Persons with underlying mood disorders or other mental illness may try to self-medicate with psychoactive drugs. Sometimes their choice of drug exacerbates their symptoms; for example, a depressed person might consume alcohol and become more depressed.

With psychoactive drugs, the user may not notice any mind-altering effects with medicinal use. This may be the case for a child with cancer, for example, who uses marijuana to stop the nausea and vomiting secondary to the chemotherapy. However, an older person using marijuana for the same reason, who believes the stories that marijuana causes insanity, may experience an exacerbation of the sensory effects as a result of the expectations.

## Setting

Setting is the influence of the physical, social, and cultural environment within which the use occurs. Social conditions influence the use of drugs. The fast pace of life, competition at school or in the workplace, and the pressure to accumulate material possessions are daily stressors. Pharmaceutical, alcohol, and tobacco companies are continuously bombarding the public with enticing advertisements pushing their products as a means of feeling better, sleeping better, having more energy, or just as a "treat." People grow up believing that most of life's problems can be solved quickly and easily through the use of a drug.

For persons of a lower socioeconomic background and with minimal education or employment possibilities, many of life's opportunities may seem out of reach. For these people, psychoactive drug use may offer a way to numb the pain or escape from their hopeless reality. These people rarely seek relief through a physician's prescription or other therapeutic measures. Instead, they rely on alcohol or illicit drugs, which are more readily available. For some, illicit drug dealing may appear to be the only way out of the poverty and unemployment path.

## Biopsychosocial Model of Addiction

Many theories exist on the etiologic factors of addiction, and no consensus exists on specific causes. The underlying etiologic factors include the belief that addiction is a disease, a moral failing, a psychological disturbance, a personality disorder, a social problem, a dysbehaviorism, or a maladaptive coping mechanism. Different people develop addiction in different ways. For example, some alcoholics say, "I knew I was an alcoholic from my first drink; I drank differently than others." Others have no family history of addiction, but when stressed (chronic pain, significant losses, or abusive relationships resulting in low self-esteem) they find that drugs may temporarily relieve their stress. Over time, heavy use of one or more drugs to cope with the stress may lead to addiction. Current research focuses on the neurochemistry of addiction, which shows actual brain chemistry changes among addicts. The biopsychosocial model provides a framework for understanding addiction as being the result of the interaction of multiple factors.

## PRIMARY PREVENTION AND THE ROLE OF THE NURSE

The harm reduction approach to substance abuse focuses on health promotion and disease prevention. Primary prevention for ATOD problems includes (1) the promotion of healthy lifestyles and resiliency factors and (2) education about drugs and guidelines for use. Nurses are ideally prepared to use health promotion strategies such as promoting and facilitating healthy alternatives to indiscriminate, careless, and often dangerous drug use practices and providing education about drugs to decrease harm from irresponsible or unsafe drug use practices.

## Promotion of Healthy Lifestyles and Resiliency Factors

Assisting clients to achieve optimal health includes identifying interventions other than or in addition to the use of drugs whenever possible. Teaching assertiveness and decision-making skills helps clients increase self-responsibility for health and helps them increase their awareness of the various options.

Nagging health problems such as difficulty sleeping, muscle tension, lack of energy, chronic stress, and mood swings are common reasons people turn to medications, especially the psychoactive drugs. Nurses can help clients understand that medications mask problems rather than solving them. Stress reduction and relaxation techniques along with a balanced lifestyle can address these problems more directly than medications. Lack of sleep, improper diet, and lack of exercise contribute to many health complaints. Assisting clients to balance their rest, nutrition, and exercise on a daily basis can reduce these complaints. Nurses can provide useful information to groups, assisting the development of community recreational resources, or facilitating stress reduction, relaxation, or exercise groups. Nurses can help persons increase their awareness of drug-free community activities. The How To box lists community-based activities in which the nurse may become involved.

---

**HOW TO**    **Set Up Community-Based Activities Aimed at Substance Abuse Prevention**

- Increase involvement and pride in school activities
- Organize student assistant programs (students helping students)
- Organize a Students Against Drunk Driving (SADD) chapter
- Mobilize parental awareness and action groups (e.g., Mothers Against Drunk Driving [MADD])
- Increase availability of recreational facilities
- Encourage parental commitment to nondrinking parties
- Encourage religious institutions to convey nonuse messages, and provide activities associated with nonuse
- Curtail media messages that glamorize drug and alcohol use
- Support and reinforce antidrug-use peer-pressure skills
- Provide general health screenings, including ATOD use
- Collaborate with community leaders to solve problems related to crime, housing, jobs, and access to health care

Lack of educational opportunities, job training, or both can contribute to socioeconomic stress and poor self-esteem, which can lead to drug use to escape the situation. Nurses can help clients identify community resources and solve problems to meet basic needs rather than avoid them.

In addition to decreasing risk factors associated with ATOD problems, it is important to increase protective or resiliency factors. Prevention guidelines to teach parents and teachers how to increase resiliency in youths include the following strategies:

- Help them develop an increased sense of responsibility for their own success.
- Help them identify their talents.
- Motivate them to dedicate their lives to helping society rather than believing that their only purpose in life is to be consumers.
- Provide realistic appraisals and feedback; stress multicultural competence; encourage and value education and skills training.
- Increase cooperative solutions to problems rather than competitive or aggressive solutions.

The objectives in Healthy People 2010 (see the Healthy People 2010 box) provide guidance for ways to decrease the reliance on alcohol, drugs, and tobacco (USDHHS, 2000).

## Drug Education

ATOD problems include more than abuse of psychoactive drugs. Today more than 450,000 different drugs and drug combinations are available, and prescription drugs are involved in almost 60% of all drug-related emergency room visits and 70% of all drug-related deaths.

Nurses are experts in medication administration and understand the potential dangers of indiscriminant drug use and the inherent inability of drugs to cure all problems. Nurses can influence the health of clients by destroying the myth of good drugs versus bad drugs. This means teaching clients that no drug is completely safe and that any drug can be abused, and helping persons learn how to make informed decisions about their drug use to minimize potential harm.

Drug technology is growing, yet the public receives little information about how to safely use this technology. Harm reduction as a goal recognizes that people consume drugs and that they need to know about the use of drugs and risks involved in order to make responsible decisions about their drug use. Drug education should begin on an individual basis by reviewing the client's prescription medications. Because a physician or nurse practitioner has prescribed the medication, clients often presume there is little risk involved.

Is the client aware of any untoward interactions this drug may have with other drugs being used or with food? A common occurrence with drug users is the use of drugs from different categories used together or at different times to regulate how they feel, known as **polysubstance use** or **abuse.** For example, a person may drink alcohol when snorting cocaine to "take the edge off"; or some intravenous drug users

---

### Healthy People 2010 | Objectives Related to ATOD Use

26-9 Increase the age and proportion of adolescents who remain alcohol and drug free

26-10 Reduce past-month use of illicit substances

26-11 Reduce the proportion of persons engaging in binge drinking of alcoholic beverages

26-12 Reduce average annual alcohol consumption

26-13 Reduce the proportion of adults who exceed guidelines for low-risk drinking

26-14 Reduce steroid use among adolescents

26-15 Reduce the proportion of adolescents who use inhalants

26-16 Increase the proportion of adolescents who disapprove of substance use

26-17 Increase the proportion of adolescents who perceive great risk associated with substance abuse

27-1 Reduce tobacco use by adults

27-2 Reduce tobacco use by adolescents

27-3 Reduce initiation of tobacco use among children and adolescents

27-4 Increase the average age of first use of tobacco products by adolescents and young adults

27-5 Increase smoking cessation attempts by adult smokers

27-6 Increase smoking cessation during pregnancy

27-7 Increase smoking cessation attempts by adolescent smokers

27-8 Increase insurance coverage of evidence-based treatment for nicotine dependency

27-9 Reduce the proportion of children who are regularly exposed to tobacco smoke at home

27-10 Reduce the proportion of nonsmokers exposed to environmental tobacco smoke

27-11 Increase smoke-free and tobacco-free environments in schools, including all school facilities, property, vehicles, and events

27-12 Increase the proportion of worksites with formal smoking policies that prohibit smoking or limit it to separately ventilated areas

27-13 Establish laws on smoke-free indoor air that prohibit smoking or limit it to separately ventilated areas in public places and worksites

From U.S. Department of Health and Human Services: *Healthy people 2010: national health promotion and disease prevention objectives,* Washington, DC, 2000, U.S. Government Printing Office.

combine cocaine with heroin (speedball) for similar reasons. Polysubstance use can cause drug interactions that can have additive, synergistic, or antagonistic effects. Indiscriminant polysubstance abuse may lead to serious physiologic consequences and can be complicated for the health care professional to assess and treat.

People need to know what questions to ask regarding their personal drug use and should be encouraged to seek the answers to these questions before using any drug. Encouraging clients to ask questions regarding their drug use can increase their responsibility for personal health while increasing their awareness that drugs will alter their body chemistry. The How To box about determining the relative safety of a drug lists seven key pieces of information that clients should obtain before taking a drug/medication to decrease the possible harm from unsafe medication consumption.

---

( **HOW TO** **Determine the Relative Safety of a Drug for Personal or Client Use**

Before using a drug/medication always determine the following:
- The chemical being taken
- How and where the drug works in the body
- The correct dosage
- Whether there will be drug interactions, including interactions with herbal remedies
- If there are potential allergic reactions
- If there will be drug tolerance
- If the drug will produce physical dependence*

---

*Caution: Approximately 10% of the population may suffer from the disease of addiction. For them, responsible use of psychoactive drugs is limited because of their disease. They need to notify their physician of the addiction if use of psychoactive medicines is being considered as treatment.
From Miller M: *Drug consumer safety rules,* Mosier, Ore, 2002, Mothers Against Misuse and Abuse, available at www.mamas.org.

---

Nurses can identify various references and community resources available to provide the necessary information, and they can clarify the information. User-friendly reference texts are available that offer information about drug interactions among medications, other drugs (including alcohol, tobacco, marijuana, and cocaine), and other substances (food and beverages), and that serve as excellent guides for the nurse as well as for the client's personal and family use (Griffith and Moore, 2002; Rybacki and Long, 2002).

As people learn to ask questions about their prescription medications, the nurse can encourage them to ask the same questions about self-administered OTC and recreational drugs. This does not mean that nurses should encourage other drug use but rather that the potential harm

from self-medication can be reduced if clients have the necessary information to make more informed decisions.

As parents learn to seek information regarding their use of medications, they begin to act as role models for their children. It can be confusing for children and adolescents to be told to "just say no" to drugs while they see their parents or drug advertisements try to "quick fix" every health complaint with a medication.

The simple "just say no" approach does not help young people for several reasons. First, children are naturally curious, and drug experimentation is often a part of normal development (Shedler and Block, 1990). Second, children from dysfunctional homes often use drugs to get attention or to escape an intolerable environment. And finally, the "just say no" approach does not address the powerful influence of peer pressure (Lloyd-Richardson et al, 2002).

Drug education has moved into the school curriculum with Project DARE (Drug Abuse Resistance Education), the most widely used school-based drug-use prevention

---

### Evidence-Based Practice

This study examined how current practice in middle school substance use prevention programs compare with the recommended guidelines adapted from the Centers for Disease Control and Prevention guidelines for school-based tobacco use prevention guidelines.

In 1999, a questionnaire was mailed to a nationally representative sample of 1496 public and private schools with middle grades that reported having a substance abuse prevention program. An estimated 64% of the schools met four or more of the recommendations for school-based use prevention practice, and 4% met all seven recommendations. Schools were most likely to report having and enforcing substance use prevention policies (84.5%) and least likely to report training teachers in substance abuse prevention (17.9%). Most recommendations were implemented in schools that were public and had large enrollments, had greater perceived availability of resources, had greater school board and parental support for substance abuse prevention, and had hired a school substance abuse prevention coordinator.

**Nurse Use:** The low prevalence of a comprehensive substance use prevention program in U.S. middle schools may limit the potential effect of school programs on the prevalence of youth substance abuse. Teacher training is a critical aspect of the implementation of substance use prevention curricula, yet schools were least likely to meet this recommendation. This is a role that could easily and effectively be filled by a community-oriented school nurse.

Wenter DL et al: Comprehensiveness of substance use prevention programs in U.S. middle schools, *J Adolesc Health* 30(6):455-462, 2002.

program in the United States. This program uses law enforcement officers to teach the material, but recent studies find that it is less effective than other interactive prevention programs and may even result in increased drug use (Hallfors and Godette, 2002). Basic ATOD prevention programs for young people should combine efforts to increase resiliency factors with drug education. Nurses can serve as educators or as advisors to the school systems or community groups to ensure that all of these areas are addressed. Role playing is useful in teaching many of these skills.

## SECONDARY PREVENTION AND THE ROLE OF THE NURSE

To identify substance abuse and plan appropriate interventions, nurses must assess each client individually. When drug abuse, dependence, or addiction is identified, nurses must assist clients to understand the connection between their drug use patterns and the negative consequences on their health, their families, and the community.

## Assessing for ATOD Problems

Assessing for substance abuse problems should be included in health assessments. An assessment of self-medication practices as well as recreational drug use should be done at the time of the medication history. This puts all relevant drug use history together and aids in the assessment of drug use patterns. When working with a client over time, periodic assessment of drug use patterns will alert the nurse to any changes requiring intervention.

After obtaining a medication history, follow-up questions can determine if problems exist. For prescription drug use, is the client following the directions correctly? Nurses should inquire about any prescribed psychoactive drug use: How long has the client been taking the drug? Has the client increased the dosage or frequency above the prescription?

When assessing self-medication and recreational or social drug use patterns, nurses should determine the reason for use. Some underlying health problems (e.g., pain, stress, weight, or insomnia) may be alleviated by nonpharmaceutical interventions. Nurses should ask about the amount, frequency, and duration of use, and the route of administration of each drug. Box 36-1 shows the levels of prevention related to substance abuse.

### NURSING TIP

Think of "the 4 Hs" to remember what to ask when assessing drug use patterns: How taken (route), How much, How often, and How long.

To establish the presence of a substance abuse problem, determine if the drug use is causing any negative health consequences or problems with relationships, employment, finances, or the legal system. The How To box shows examples of questions to ask to determine the presence of socioeconomic problems that are often secondary to substance abuse.

If there is a pattern of chronic, regular, and frequent use of a drug, nurses should assess for a history of withdrawal symptoms to determine if there is physical dependence on the drug. A progression in drug use patterns and related problems warns about the possibility of addiction.

### BOX 36-1    Levels of Prevention Related to Substance Abuse

**PRIMARY PREVENTION**

Provide community education to teach healthy lifestyles; focus on how to resist getting involved in substance abuse.

**SECONDARY PREVENTION**

Institute early detection programs in schools, the workplace, and other areas in which people gather to determine the presence of substance abuse.

**TERTIARY PREVENTION**

Develop programs to help people reduce or end substance abuse.

### HOW TO    Assess Socioeconomic Problems Resulting From Substance Abuse

If the client admits to use of alcohol, tobacco, or other drugs, ask the following questions:

1. Do your parents, spouse, or friends worry or complain about your drinking or using drugs?
2. Has a family member gone for help about your drinking or using drugs?
3. Have you neglected family obligations as a result of drinking or using drugs?
4. Have you missed work because of your drinking or using drugs?
5. Does your boss complain about your drinking or using drugs?
6. Do you drink or use drugs before or during work?
7. Have you ever been fired or quit because of drinking or using drugs?
8. Have you ever been charged with driving under the influence (DUI) or being drunk in public (DIP)?
9. Have you ever had any other legal problems related to drinking and using drugs, such as assault and battery, breaking and entering, or theft?
10. Have you had any accidents while intoxicated, such as falls, burns, or motor vehicle accidents?
11. Have you spent your money on alcohol or other drugs instead of paying your bills (e.g., telephone, electricity, rent)?

**Denial** is a primary symptom of addiction. Methods of denial include lying about use, minimizing use patterns, blaming or rationalizing, intellectualizing, changing the subject, using anger or humor, and "going with the flow" (agreeing there is a problem, stating behavior will change, but not demonstrating any behavior changes). Suspect a problem if the client becomes defensive or exhibits other behavior indicating denial when asked about alcohol or other drug use.

## Drug Testing

During the 1980s, preemployment or random drug testing in the workplace gained popularity. Drug testing can be done by examining a person's urine, blood, saliva, breath (alcohol), or hair. The most common method of drug screening is urine testing. Urine testing indicates only past use of certain drugs, not intoxication. Thus persons can be identified as having used a certain drug in the recent past, but the degree of intoxication and extent of performance impairment cannot be determined with urine testing. Also, most drug-related problems in the workplace are related to alcohol, and alcohol is not always included in a urine drug screen. Other problems with urine testing include using it as a tool of intimidation, false positives, invasion of privacy, and not being cost effective (American Civil Liberties Union, 1999).

When is drug testing appropriate? Drug testing that follows documented impairment may help to substantiate the cause of the impairment, and thus it serves as a backup rather than the primary screening method. It is also useful for recovering addicts. Part of their treatment is to abstain from psychoactive drug use; therefore a urine test yielding positive results for a drug indicates a relapse.

Blood, breath, and saliva drug tests can indicate current use and amount. Any of these tests can help to determine alcohol intoxication, and they are often used to substantiate suspected impairment. A serum drug screen can be useful when overdose is suspected to determine the specific drug ingested. The testing of hair is gaining attention because the results can provide a long history of drug use patterns.

Employee assistance programs (EAPs) are being established in work settings, and at least 30% of U.S. workers have access to an EAP. Addiction or substance abuse is the most common personnel problem in most workplaces, accounting for 20% of voluntary EAP referrals and 50% of supervisory referrals to EAP (Curley, 2002). These programs can identify health problems among employees and offer counseling or referral to other health care providers as necessary. EAPs provide early identification of and intervention for substance abuse problems; they also offer services to employees to reduce stress and provide health care or counseling so that they may prevent substance abuse problems from developing. Nurses frequently develop and run these programs.

## High-Risk Groups

Identifying high-risk groups helps nurses design programs to meet specific needs and to mobilize community resources.

### Adolescents

The younger a person is when beginning intensive experimentation with drugs, the more likely dependence will develop. More than 40% of those who started drinking at age 14 or younger developed alcohol dependence, compared with 10% of those who began drinking at age 20 or older (Schneider Institute for Health Policy, 2001). Heavy drug use during adolescence can interfere with normal development. Note that Healthy People 2010 objectives 27-4 and 26-9 refer to delay of the initiation of use of tobacco, alcohol, and marijuana.

Reports from annual high school drug surveys monitor the national trends among youths, including data on lifetime use, recent use, and daily use. Regarding lifetime use from the 1997 survey, by the eighth grade 53.8% have tried alcohol, 47.3% smoked cigarettes, 22.6% tried marijuana, and 4.4% tried cocaine. By twelfth grade, about 81.7% have used alcohol, 65.4% smoked cigarettes, 49.6% used marijuana, and 8.7% tried cocaine (National Institute on Drug Abuse, 1998b). These figures are probably low in that they do not include high school dropouts.

Family-related factors (genetics, family stress, parenting styles, child victimization) appear to be the greatest variable that influences substance abuse among adolescents. The co-occurrence with psychiatric disorders (especially mood disorders) and behavioral problems is also associated with substance abuse among adolescents, leaving peer pressure as a less influential factor. Research suggests that successful social influence–based prevention programs may be driven by their ability to foster social norms that reduce an adolescent's social motivation to begin using ATOD. The most effective treatment approach for adolescents appears to be the use of family-oriented therapy (Weinberg et al, 1998).

### Older Adults

Older adults (65 years of age and older) represent 13% of the U.S. population and are the fastest growing segment of U.S. society, expected to represent 21% by the year 2030. They consume more prescribed and OTC medications than any other age-group. Approximately 27% of all tranquilizer prescriptions and 38% of hypnotic prescriptions in 1991 were written for older adults. Alcohol and prescription drug misuse affects as many as 17% of adults age 60 and older. Problems with alcohol consumption, including interactions with prescribed and OTC drugs, far outnumber any other substance abuse problem among older adults (Center for Substance Abuse Treatment, 1998).

The increased use of prescription drugs and alcohol by older adults may be related to coping problems. Problems of relocation, possible loss of independence, retirement, illness, death of friends, and lower levels of achievement contribute to feelings of sadness, boredom, anxiety, and loneliness. Factors such as slowed metabolic turnover of drugs, age-related organ changes, enhanced drug sensitivities, a tendency to use drugs over long periods, and a more frequent use of multiple drugs all contribute to greater negative consequences from drug use among older adults.

Often, alcohol abuse is not identified because its effects on cognitive abilities may mimic changes associated with normal aging or degenerative brain disease. Also, depression may simply be attributed to the more frequent losses rather than the depressant effects of alcohol, and the older adult may subsequently receive medical treatment for depression rather than alcoholism.

### Injection Drug Users (IDUs)

In addition to the problem of addiction, **injection drug users** (those who self-administer intravenously or subcutaneously) are at risk for other health complications. Intravenous (IV) administration of drugs always carries a greater risk of overdose because the drug goes directly into the bloodstream. With illicit drugs, the danger is increased because the exact dosage is unknown. In addition, the drug may be contaminated with other chemicals, such as sugar, starch, or quinine, that can cause negative consequences. Often IDUs make their own solution for IV administration, and any particles present can result in complications from emboli.

The sharing of needles has been a common practice among addicts. The spread of human immunodeficiency virus (HIV) through needle sharing is a public health risk. Hepatitis C and other bloodborne diseases can also be transmitted through contaminated needles. Infections and abscesses may develop secondary to dirty needles or poor administration techniques.

IDUs represent the most rapidly growing source of new cases of acquired immunodeficiency syndrome (AIDS), and they are at the greatest risk for spread of the virus in the heterosexual community. Half of all new HIV infection cases occur among IDUs, with a disproportionate impact on those in minority groups (Schneider Institute for Health Policy, 2001). Primarily because of this trend, emphasis is being placed on reducing the transmission of this disease through contaminated needles. Abstinence is ideal but unrealistic for many addicts. Using the harm reduction model, the nurse should provide education on cleaning needles with bleach between uses and about needle exchange programs to decrease the spread of the virus. Studies indicate that needle exchange programs have not increased injection drug abuse but have, in fact, increased the number of people entering treatment programs (Drug Scope, 2002).

### Drug Use During Pregnancy

Most drugs can negatively affect a fetus. Thus the use of any drug during pregnancy should be discouraged unless medically necessary. Healthy People 2010 objectives address this issue. **Fetal alcohol syndrome** has been identified as the third leading cause of birth defects and the most preventable form of mental retardation in the United States (Gordon, 2002). One study found that women who are depressed during their pregnancy are more likely to

binge drink. Thus depression screening and treatment as needed could be a useful adjunct to FAS/FAE intervention efforts (Larkby, Hanusa, and Kraemer, 2002). A Danish study of 24,768 women found an increasing risk of stillbirth with increasing moderate alcohol intake during pregnancy (Kesmodel et al, 2002).

> **◖ WHAT DO YOU THINK?**
>
> In some states, pregnant women who are using illicit drugs are reported to child protective services because of the potential harm to the fetus. Will this practice do more harm than good? What about women who drink alcohol or smoke cigarettes?

Another survey estimates that 12.4% of pregnant women drink alcohol, with 3.9% reporting binge drinking. Estimates of illicit drug use during pregnancy range from 1.3% of women aged 26 to 44 years to 12.9% of adolescent girls aged 15 to 17 years. Tobacco remains the most used addictive substance during pregnancy, with about 18.6% of pregnant women smoking (Gordon, 2002).

Despite the increased focus on drug abuse interventions, many pregnant women with drug problems do not receive the help they need. This may be a result of ignorance, poverty, lack of concern for the fetus, lack of available services, and fear of the consequences of revealing drug use. The fear of criminal prosecution may push addicted women farther away from the health care system, cause them to conceal their drug use from medical providers, and cause them to deliver their babies in out-of-hospital settings, thus further jeopardizing the pregnancy outcome (Gordon, 2002).

### Use of Illicit Drugs

The strategy of "just say no" to drugs is both simplistic and misleading. Indiscriminant use of "good" drugs has caused more health problems from adverse reactions, drug interactions, dependence, addiction, and overdoses than use of "bad" drugs. However, the war on drugs focuses on illicit drugs and punishes illicit drug users. The black market associated with illicit drug use puts otherwise law-abiding citizens in close contact with criminals, prevents any quality control of the drugs, increases the risk of AIDS and hepatitis secondary to needle sharing, and hinders health care professionals' accessibility to the abuser or addict.

Lack of quality control (unknown strength and purity) can cause unexpected overdoses or secondary effects of the impurities. A synthetic analog of fentanyl (3-methylfentanyl) marketed as "heroin" is 6000 times as potent as morphine. Unsafe administration (contaminated needles) leads to local and systemic infections. The high cost on the black market leads to crime to support the addiction.

## Codependency and Family Involvement

Drug addiction is often a family disease. One in four Americans experiences family problems related to alcohol abuse. One study found that 52.9% of Americans of age 18 years and older have a family history of alcoholism among first- or second-degree relatives (Dawson and Grant, 1998). People in a close relationship with the addict often develop unhealthy coping mechanisms to continue the relationship. This behavior is known as **codependency,** a stress-induced preoccupation with the addicted person's life, leading to extreme dependence and excessive concern with the addict (Talashek, Gerace, and Starr, 1994).

Strict rules typically develop in a codependent family to maintain the relationships: don't talk, don't feel, don't trust, don't lose control, and don't seek help from outside the family. Codependents try to meet the addict's needs at the expense of their own. Codependency may underlie many of the medical complaints and emotional stress seen by health care providers such as ulcers, skin disorders, migraine headaches, chronic colds, and backaches.

When the addicted person refuses to admit the problem, the family continues to adapt to emotionally survive the stress of the addict's irrational, inconsistent, and unpredictable behavior. Members of the family consequently develop various roles that tend to be gross exaggerations of normal family roles. Members cling irrationally to these roles, even when they are no longer functional.

One of the most significant roles a family member may assume is that of an enabler. **Enabling** is the act of shielding or preventing the addict from experiencing the consequences of the addiction. As a result, the addict does not always understand the cost of the addiction and thus is "enabled" to continue to use.

Although codependency and enabling are closely related, a person does not have to be codependent to enable. Anyone can be an enabler: a police officer, a boss or co-worker, and even a drug treatment counselor. Health care professionals who do not address the negative health consequences of the drug use with the addicted person are enablers.

The nurse can help families recognize the problem of addiction and help them confront the addicted member in a caring manner. Whether or not the addicted family member is agreeable to treatment, the family members should be given some guidance about the literature and services that are available to help them cope more effectively. The nurse can help identify treatment options, counseling assistance, financial assistance, support services, and (if necessary) legal services for the family members. Children of ATOD abusers or addicts are themselves at a greater risk for developing addiction and must be targeted for primary prevention.

## TERTIARY PREVENTION AND THE ROLE OF THE NURSE

The nurse is in a key position to help the addict and the addict's family. The nurse's knowledge of community resources and how to mobilize them can significantly influence the quality of care clients receive.

## Detoxification

**Detoxification** is the clearing of one or more drugs from the person's body and managing the withdrawal symptoms. Depending on the particular drug and the degree of dependence, the time required may range from a few days to several weeks. Because withdrawal symptoms vary (depending on the drug used) and range from uncomfortable to life threatening, the setting for and management of withdrawal depend on the drug used.

Drugs such as stimulants or opiates may produce withdrawal symptoms that are uncomfortable but not life threatening. Detoxification from these drugs does not require direct medical supervision, but medical management of the withdrawal symptoms increases the comfort level. On the other hand, drugs such as alcohol, benzodiazepines, and barbiturates can produce life-threatening withdrawal symptoms. These clients should be under close medical supervision during detoxification and should receive medical management of the withdrawal symptoms to ensure a safe withdrawal. Of those who develop delirium tremens from alcohol withdrawal, 15% may not survive despite medical management; therefore close medical management is initiated as the blood alcohol level begins to fall.

**DID YOU KNOW?**

Because of cost-containment efforts, more primary care providers and drug treatment programs use outpatient or home detoxification for persons requiring medical detoxification for alcohol withdrawal. Nurses can provide the necessary monitoring and evaluation of the client's health status in the home environment to reduce the risk of medical complications related to alcohol withdrawal, as well as to provide encouragement and support for the client to complete the detoxification.

A general rule in detoxification management is to wean the person off the drug by gradually reducing the dosage and frequency of administration. Thus a person with chronic alcoholism could be safely detoxified by a gradual reduction in alcohol consumption. In practice, however, the switch to another drug, usually a benzodiazepine, of-

**DID YOU KNOW?**

Auricular acupuncture (needles inserted in the ear) can be effective in treating withdrawal symptoms from various drugs and as an aid during substance abuse treatment and relapse prevention. It is a specific acupuncture technique that is quick, inexpensive, and safe. In some states, nurses who are trained in this technique can be certified to use it to help with substance abuse detoxification and treatment (Moner, 1996).

ten offers a safer withdrawal from alcohol as well as an abrupt end to the intoxication from the drug of choice. For example, chlordiazepoxide (Librium) is commonly used for alcohol detoxification.

## Addiction Treatment

Addiction treatment differs from the management of negative health consequences of chronic drug abuse, overdose, and detoxification. **Addiction treatment** focuses on the addiction process. The goal is to help clients view addiction as a chronic disease and assist them to make lifestyle changes to halt the progression of the disease. According to the disease theory, addicts are not responsible for the symptoms of their disease; they are, however, responsible for treating their disease. It is estimated that 18 million people who consume alcohol and almost 5 million who use illicit drugs need substance abuse treatment. However, less than one fourth of those who need treatment get it, for various reasons. On any given day, approximately 1 million persons receive treatment for alcohol or other drug addiction. In 2000, most clients (89%) were enrolled in some kind of outpatient program (Substance Abuse and Mental Health Services Administration, 2002).

Most treatment facilities are multidisciplinary because the intervention strategies require a wide range of approaches. Their programs involve interactions between the addict, family, culture, and community. Strategies include

medical management, education, counseling, vocational rehabilitation, stress management, and support services. The key to effective treatment is to match individual clients with the interventions most appropriate for them (National Institute on Drug Abuse, 1998c).

For those addicted individuals unwilling or unable to completely abstain from psychoactive drugs, other medications can assist them in abstaining from their drug of choice. Such is the case with methadone maintenance programs for treating heroin addiction. Methadone, when administered in moderate or high daily doses, produces a **cross-tolerance** to other narcotics, thereby blocking their effects and decreasing the craving for heroin. The advantages of methadone are that it is long acting, effective orally, and inexpensive and has few known side effects. The oral use of methadone offers a solution to the danger of the spread of AIDS and other bloodborne infections that commonly occur among needle-sharing addicts. Although not recognized as a cure for heroin (or other opiate) addiction, methadone maintenance is a harm reduction intervention because it reduces deviant behavior and introduces addicted persons to the health care system. This may ultimately lead to total abstinence.

Total abstinence is the most recommended treatment for ATOD addiction. People who are addicted to a particular drug (e.g., cocaine) are advised to abstain from the use of all psychoactive substances. The use of another drug may simply reinforce the craving for the original drug and cause relapse. More commonly, the addiction merely transfers to the replacement substance.

Treatment may be on an inpatient or outpatient basis. In general, the more advanced the disease is, the greater the need for inpatient treatment. Inpatient treatment programs usually last 28 days, although they may range from less than 1 week to 90 days. Once a person has completed detoxification (considered the first phase of the treatment process), the programs use counseling and group interaction to help the client stay clean long enough for the body chemistry to rebalance. This is often a difficult time for persons recovering from addictions because they may experience mood swings and difficulty sleeping and dealing with emotions.

The goal of the educational part of the programs is to provide information about the disease concept and how drugs affect a person physically and psychologically. Clients are informed of the various lifestyle changes that are recommended, and they learn about tools to assist them in making these changes. Discharge planning continues throughout treatment as clients build the support systems that they will need when they leave the controlled environment of a treatment center and face pressures and temptations (triggers) that may lead to relapse.

Long-term residential programs, also called halfway houses, have been developed to ease the person recovering from an addiction back into society. These facilities provide continued support and counseling in a structured

---

## THE CUTTING EDGE

GW Pharmaceuticals, a British pharmaceutical company operating under license from the UK Home Office, has developed an Advanced Dispensing System (ADS), a novel, secure drug dispensing technology. ADS has the potential to enhance a drug's safety, prevent diversion, provide greatly increased flexibility in prescribing patterns, monitor a patient's progress remotely, and provide information on natural patterns of consumption of prescribed drugs in the community.

ADS is a handheld device that dispenses a range of drugs and dosage forms contained within a proprietary medicinal cartridge format. The device communicates to the user in real time through a software system using existing telecommunication technologies.

GW has commenced a Home Office–endorsed collaboration with the National Addiction Centre in London to test its proprietary ADS for the administration of methadone and diamorphine in the treatment of drug addiction. The aim is to provide a better and more cost-effective means of treatment for Britain's estimated quarter of a million heroin addicts. If successful, the programme will extend to other countries in Europe and North America.

environment for persons needing long-term assistance in adjusting to a drug-free lifestyle. The residents are expected to secure employment and take responsibility in managing their financial obligations.

Outpatient programs are similar in the education and counseling offered, but they allow the clients to live at home and continue to work while undergoing treatment. This method is very effective for persons in the earlier stages of addiction who feel confident that they can abstain from drug use and have established a strong support network.

Most programs include family counseling and education. In addition, specific programs address the needs of various populations such as adolescents, women during pregnancy, specific ethnic groups, gays and lesbians, as well as health care professionals.

Recovery from addiction involves a lifetime commitment and may include periods of relapse. The addicted person must realize that modern medicine has not found a cure for addiction; therefore returning to drug use may ultimately reactivate the disease process.

## Smoking Cessation Programs

Included in the Healthy People 2010 objectives related to tobacco use are decreasing the incidence of smoking to 12% of the population from a 1998 baseline of 24%, and increasing the smoking cessation attempts to 75% from a 1998 baseline of 41%. Nurses can be active in smoking prevention programs for individuals as well as in community efforts to assist persons to quit smoking.

Nearly 35 million Americans try to quit smoking each year. Less than 10% of those who try to quit on their own are able to stop for a year. Studies show that significantly greater cessation rates occur for smokers receiving interventions than for those smokers who do not receive interventions. Interventions that involve medications and behavioral treatments appear most promising (Anderson et al, 2002).

Nicotine replacement therapy can be used to help smokers withdraw from nicotine while focusing their efforts on breaking the psychological craving or habit. Four types of nicotine replacement products are available: nicotine gum and skin patches are available over the counter, and nicotine nasal spray and inhalers are available by prescription. These products are about equally effective and can almost double the chances of successfully quitting. Other treatments include smoking cessation clinics, hypnosis, and acupuncture. The most effective way to get people to stop smoking and prevent relapse involves multiple interventions and continuous reinforcement, and most smokers require several attempts at cessation before they are successful. Many resources are available on smoking cessation programs and support groups, including those listed in Box 36-2.

## Support Groups

The founding of **Alcoholics Anonymous** (AA) in 1935 began a strong movement that recognized the important role of peer support in the treatment of a chronic illness. AA groups have developed throughout the world, and their success has led to the development of other support groups such as Narcotics Anonymous (NA) for persons with narcotic addictions and Pills Anonymous for persons with polydrug addictions. Similar programs have been developed for process addictions, such as Overeaters Anonymous and Gamblers Anonymous.

AA and NA help addicted people develop a daily program of recovery and reinforce the recovery process. The fellowship, support, and encouragement among AA members provide a vital social network for the person recovering from an addiction.

Al-Anon and Alateen are similar self-help programs for spouses, parents, children, or others involved in a painful relationship with an alcoholic (Nar-Anon for those in relationships with persons with narcotic addictions). Al-Anon family groups are available to anyone who has been affected by their involvement with an alcoholic person. The purposes of Alateen include providing a forum for adolescents to discuss family stressors, learn coping skills from one another, and gain support and encouragement from knowledgeable peers. Adult Children of Alcoholics (ACOA) groups are also available in most areas to address the recovery of adults who grew up in alcoholic homes and are still carrying the scars and retaining dysfunctional behaviors.

For some persons, the AA program places too much emphasis on a higher power or focuses too much on the negative consequences of past drinking. Women for Sobriety focuses on rebuilding self-esteem, a core issue for many women with alcoholic problems (www.womenforsobriety. org). Rational Recovery has a cognitive orientation and is based on the assumption that ATOD addiction is caused by irrational beliefs that can be understood and overcome (www.rational.org).

## Nurse's Role

Many people with alcoholism and drug addiction become lost in the health care system. If satisfactory care is not provided in one agency or the waiting list is months long, the person may give up rather than seek alternative sources of care. The nurse who knows the client's history, environment, support systems, and the local treatment programs can offer guidance to the most effective treatment modality (Littman and Ritterbusch, 1997). **Brief interventions** by health care professionals who are not treatment experts can be effective in helping ATOD abusers

---

**WHAT DO YOU THINK?**

Research has shown that antidepressants can help persons stop smoking. GlaxoWellcome has developed a specific drug, bupropion hydrochloride, for persons to use to help them stop smoking. Insurance companies do not pay for the use of this medicine.

---

**BOX 36-2  Smoking Cessation Resources**

American Cancer Society
1559 Clifton Rd. NE
Atlanta, GA 30329
1-800-ACS-2345
www.cancer.org
"Fresh Start" smoking cessation program

American Heart Association
7272 Greenville Ave.
Dallas, TX 75231-4596
(214) 373-6300
www.americanheart.org
"In Control: Freedom from Smoking" program

American Lung Association
1740 Broadway
New York, NY 10019
www.lungsusa.org
"Freedom From Smoking for You and Your Family"

Americans for Nonsmokers Rights
2530 San Pablo Ave., Suite J
Berkeley, CA 94702
(510) 841-3032
www.no-smoke.org

ASH (Action on Smoking and Health)
2013 H St. NW
Washington, DC 20006
(202) 659-4310
www.ash.org

Five Day Plan to Stop Smoking (general headquarters)
6553 California Ave. SW
Seattle, WA 98116-4448
(206) 935-5696
www.newstarthealthcare.com

The Foundation for a Smoke-Free America
P.O. Box 492028
Los Angeles, CA 90049-8028
www.tobaccofree.org

National Cancer Institute
NCI Public Inquiries Office, Suite 3036A
6116 Executive Blvd., MSC 8322
Bethesda, MD 20892-8322
(800) 4-CANCER

Office on Smoking and Health
U.S. Department of Health and Human Services
200 Independence Ave.
Washington, DC, 20201
(800) 232-1311
www.hhs.gov

SmokEnders
901 NW 133rd St., #A
Vancouver, WA 98685
(800) 828-4357
www.smokenders.com

For more information, see the WebLinks on this book's website at http://evolve.elsevier.com/Stanhope.

---

and addicts change their risky behavior. Brief interventions may convince the ATOD abuser or addict to reduce substance consumption or follow through with a treatment referral (Gentilello et al, 1999; Whitlock et al, 2002). Box 36-3 describes six elements commonly included in brief interventions, using the acronym FRAMES.

Strategies used with clients can vary depending on their readiness for change. Understanding the stages of change listed in Box 36-4 and recognizing which stage a client is in are important factors for determining which interventions and programs may be most helpful to the client (Center for Substance Abuse Treatment, 1997).

After the client has received treatment, the nurse can coordinate aftercare referrals and follow up on the client's progress. The nurse can provide additional support in the home as the client and family adjust to changing roles and the stress involved with such changes. The nurse can support addicted persons who have relapsed by reminding them that relapses may well occur, but that they and their families can continue to work toward recovery and an improved quality of life.

**BOX 36-3  Brief Interventions Using the FRAMES Acronym**

- **Feedback.** Provide the client direct feedback about the potential or actual personal risk or impairment related to drug use.
- **Responsibility.** Emphasize personal responsibility for change.
- **Advice.** Provide clear advice to change risky behavior.
- **Menu.** Provide a menu of options or choices for changing behavior.
- **Empathy.** Provide a warm, reflective, empathetic, and understanding approach.
- **Self-efficacy.** Provide encouragement and belief in the client's ability to change.

Modified from Bien TH, Miller WR, Tonigan JS: Brief interventions for alcohol problems: a review, *Addictions* 88:315, 1993.

---

**BOX 36-4** **Stages of Change**

**PRECONTEMPLATION**

At this stage, the person does not intend to change in the foreseeable future. The person is often unaware of any problem. Resistance to recognizing or modifying a problem is the hallmark of precontemplation.

**CONTEMPLATION**

At this stage, the individual is aware that a problem exists and is seriously thinking about overcoming it but has not yet made a commitment to take action. The nurse can encourage the individual to weigh the pros and cons of the problem and the solution to the problem.

**PREPARATION**

Preparation was originally referred to as *decision making*. At this stage, the individual is prepared for action and may reduce the problem behavior but has not yet taken effective action (e.g., cuts down amount of smoking but does not abstain).

**ACTION**

At this stage, the individual modifies the behavior, experiences, or environment to overcome the problem. The action requires considerable time and energy. Modification of the target behavior to an acceptable criterion and significant overt efforts to change are the hallmarks of action.

**MAINTENANCE**

In this stage, the individual works to prevent relapse and consolidate the gains attained during action. Stabilizing behavior change and avoiding relapse are the hallmarks of maintenance.

---

Modified from Prochaska JO, DiClemente CC, Norcross JC: In search of how people change: applications to addictive behaviors, *Am Psychol* 47(9):1102, 1992.

---

## OUTCOMES

Health promotion and risk reduction are basic concepts in community-oriented nursing. Promoting a healthy environment in the home and local community provide individuals and families a nurturing environment in which to achieve optimal health. Individuals with high self-esteem, access to health care, and information about the health risks related to drug use can be responsible for their personal health and make informed decisions about drug use. Nurses can assess the health of the community and its citizens, prioritize the needs, and identify local resources to collaborate with others to develop strategies that will improve the underlying health of the community.

Early identification and intervention for persons with ATOD problems can prevent many of the harmful physical, emotional, and social consequences that may occur if abuse continues and may also prevent abuse patterns from developing into addiction. The nurse needs to assess individual and community ATOD problems and target at-risk groups to develop strategies to increase assessment and pro-

vide appropriate interventions. Review the national health objectives (refer back to the Healthy People 2010 box) for the tobacco and substance abuse areas and note how many can be achieved with secondary prevention strategies.

A study of California drug treatment centers found that for every dollar spent on treatment, the public saves 7 dollars in health care and crime costs (National Opinion Research Center, 1994). Besides saving money, treatment helps addicted individuals and their families recover from the devastating effects of addiction. Addicts and their families often become hopeless and helpless while actively addicted. The nurse can offer hope in affirming the addict's self-worth and can be the bridge to community resources to assist in treatment and recovery.

Many of these expected outcomes for ATOD problems have been lessened because a lack of funding has resulted from federal strategies that focus on law enforcement and punishment rather than on education and treatment. The greatest challenge for nurses is to influence policy-makers to put the emphasis on health care for this major health problem.

## ■ Practice Application

Jane Doe, RN, is a home health case manager in a large, low-income housing area in her local community. She designs care plans and coordinates health care services for clients who need health care at home. She makes the initial visits to determine the level and frequency of care needed and then acts as supervisor of the volunteers and nurses' aids who perform most of the day-to-day care. Single-parent families are the norm, and drug dealing is commonplace in this housing area.

Jane made a home visit to Anne, a 26-year-old mother of three. Anne is taking care of her 62-year-old maternal grandfather, Mr. Jones, who is recovering from cardiac bypass surgery. He has a smoking history of two packs per day for almost 40 years. Since his surgery, he has decreased to one pack per day, but he refuses to quit. He had a history of alcohol dependence, reportedly consuming up to a fifth of liquor a day, and a history of withdrawal seizures. Four years ago, he went through alcohol detoxification, but he refused to stay at the facility for continued treatment, stating he could stay sober on his own. Since that time he has had several binge episodes, but Anne reports that he has not been drinking since the surgery. A widower for 5 years, Mr. Jones now lives with Anne.

Anne is a widow and has two sons, ages 3 and 9, and a daughter, age 5. The oldest son's father is an alcoholic who is currently incarcerated for manslaughter while driving under the influence of alcohol, and the father of her two youngest children was killed by a stray bullet in a cocaine bust 3 years ago. Years earlier, Anne and her husband had smoked crack cocaine for several months but both stopped when she became pregnant with their youngest child and remained cocaine free. Anne has been angry at the system and frightened of police officers ever since the drug raid in which her husband was killed. Other residents were also hurt, and less than $500 worth of cocaine was found three apartments away from hers.

Anne doesn't consume alcohol, but she smokes one to two packs per day. She quit smoking during her pregnancies but restarted soon after each birth.

A. What type of interventions can Jane provide for Mr. Jones regarding his smoking?

B. How can Jane help Anne cope with the potential risk of Mr. Jones's continuing to drink when he progresses to more independence?

C. How can Jane help Anne with her cigarette smoking?

D. Knowing that there is a genetic link to alcoholism and being aware of the high rate of drug problems in the housing area, how can Jane help prevent Anne and her children from developing substance abuse problems?

E. What problems seem greater because of the drug laws, and what can Jane do to help make the environment safer and more nurturing?

**Answers are in the back of the book.**

## Key Points

- Substance abuse is the number one national health problem, linked to numerous forms of morbidity and mortality.
- Harm reduction is a new approach to ATOD problems; it deals with substance abuse primarily as a health problem rather than as a criminal problem.
- All persons have attitudes about the use of drugs that influence their actions.
- Social conditions such as a fast-paced life, excessive stress, and the availability of drugs influence the incidence of substance abuse.
- Important terms to understand when working with individuals, groups, or communities for whom substance abuse is prevalent are *drug dependence, drug addiction, alcoholism, psychoactive drugs, depressants, stimulants, marijuana, hallucinogens,* and *inhalants.*
- Primary prevention for substance abuse includes education about drugs and guidelines for use, as well as the promotion of healthy alternatives to drug use either for recreation or to relieve stress.
- Nurses can play a key role in developing community prevention programs.
- Secondary prevention depends heavily on careful assessment of the client's use of drugs. Such assessment should be part of all basic health assessments.
- High-risk groups include pregnant women, young people, older adults, intravenous drug users, and illicit drug users.
- Drug addiction is often a family, not merely an individual, problem.
- Codependency describes a companion illness to the addiction of one person in which the codependent member is addicted to the addicted person.

- Brief interventions by a nurse can be as effective as treatment.
- Nurses are in ideal roles to assist with tertiary prevention for both the addicted person and the family.

## Clinical Decision-Making Activities

1. Read your local newspaper for 4 days and select stories that illustrate the effects of substance abuse on individuals, families, and the community.

2. For each of the stories in the newspaper related to substance abuse, describe preventive strategies that a nurse might have tried before the problem reached such a dire state.

3. Looking at your local community resources directory (or the telephone book), identify agencies that might serve as referral sources for individuals or families for whom substance abuse is a problem.

4. In groups of three to five students, discuss your personal attitudes toward drinking, smoking, and drug abuse. Discuss each category of substance abuse separately. Consider the following areas: sex, age, amount, time, occasion, place where substance abuse occurs, companions, motivation, and incentives.

5. Review popular magazine and television advertisements for alcohol, tobacco, and other medicines (e.g., sleep aids, analgesics, laxatives, stimulants). In small groups, discuss the messages conveyed in the advertisements, and discuss the implications of client education to reduce possible harm from misuse and abuse of these substances.

6. Attend an open AA or NA meeting and an Al-Anon meeting. Go alone if possible or with an alcoholic or a drug-addicted friend. As the members introduce themselves, give your first name and state, "I am a visitor." Plan to listen and do not attempt to take notes. Respect the anonymity of the persons present. Discuss your experiences later in a group.

7. In groups of four or five, review the national health objectives in Healthy People 2010 (see Appendix J) under Tobacco Use and under Substance Abuse. Pick an objective from each section, and brainstorm about possible community efforts a nurse could initiate to reach that objective.

## Additional Resources

These related resources are found either in the appendix at the back of this book or on the book's website at **http://evolve.elsevier.com/Stanhope.**

**evolve** Evolve Website

WebLinks: Healthy People 2010

# References

Abramson JL et al: Moderate alcohol consumption and risk of heart failure among older persons, *JAMA* 285(15):1971-1977, 2001.

Adlaf EM, Paglia A: *Drug use among Ontario students, 1977-2001: Findings from the OSDUS,* CAMH research document No. 10, Toronto, 2001, Centre for Addiction and Mental Health.

Ahluwalia JS et al: Sustained-release bupropion for smoking cessation in African Americans: a randomized controlled trial, *JAMA* 288(4):468-474, 2002.

American Civil Liberties Union: *Drug testing: a bad investment,* New York, 1999, ACLU.

American Public Health Association: Access to therapeutic marijuana/cannabis #9513, *Am J Public Health* 36(3):441, 1996.

Anderson JE et al: Treating tobacco use and dependence: an evidence-based clinical practice guideline for tobacco cessation, *Chest* 121(3):932-941, 2002.

Baum D: *Smoke and mirrors: the war on drugs and the politics of failure,* Boston, 1997, Little, Brown.

Beers MH, Berkow R, editors: *The Merck manual of diagnosis and therapy,* section 15: psychiatric disorders, chapter 195: drug use and dependence, Whitehouse Station, NJ, 1999, Merck.

Bien TH, Miller WR, Tonigan JS: Brief interventions for alcohol problems: a review, *Addictions* 88:315, 1993.

Byard RW et al: Amphetamine derivative fatalities in South Australia—is "Ecstasy" the culprit? *Am J Forensic Med Pathol* 19(3):261-265, 1998.

Canadian Centre for Justice Statistics: *Juristats,* Ottawa, 2001, CCJS.

Canadian Centre on Substance Abuse: *Proportions of crimes associated with alcohol and other drugs in Canada,* Ottawa, April 2002, CCSA.

Canadian Centre on Substance Abuse, Centre for Addiction and Mental Health: *Canadian profile, 1999,* Ottawa, 1999, CCSA.

Canadian Senate Report: *Cannabis: our position for a Canadian public policy,* Ottawa, 2002, Senate Special Committee on Illegal Drugs, available at http://www.parl.gc.ca/37/1/parlbus/commbus/senate/com-e/ille-e/rep-e/summary-e.htm.

Canadian Tobacco Use Monitoring Survey: *Results from 2001,* Ottawa, 2001, Health Canada.

Cargo S: Increases in teen drug use appear to level off, *NIDA Notes* 13(2):10, 1998.

Castro FG et al: *Ethnic and cultural minority groups, addictions: a comprehensive guidebook,* pp 499-526, New York, 1999, Oxford University Press.

Center for Substance Abuse Treatment: *A guide to substance abuse services for primary care clinicians,* treatment improvement protocol (TIP) series, No. 24, DHHS Publication No. (SMA) 97-3139, Washington, DC, 1997, U.S. Government Printing Office.

Center for Substance Abuse Treatment: *Substance abuse among older adults,* treatment improvement protocol (TIP) series, No. 26. USDHHS Publication No. (SMA) 98-3179. Washington, DC, 1998, U.S. Government Printing Office.

Coambs RB et al: *Health promotion research: review of the scientific literature on the prevalence, consequences, and health costs of noncompliance & inappropriate use of prescription medication in Canada,* Toronto, 1995, University of Toronto Press.

Cordes H: Generation wired: caffeine is the new drug of choice for kids, *The Nation* 266(15):11, 1998.

Curley B: *Discrimination against people in recovery rampant, advocates say,* Join Together Online, 8/14/2002, available at www.jointogether.org/sa.

Cychosz C: Alcohol and interpersonal violence: implications for educators, *J Health Educ* 27(2):73-77, 1996.

Davis AY: Masked racism: reflections on the prison industrial complex, *ColorLines* 1(1):1, 1998.

Dawson DA, Grant BF: Family history and gender: their combined effects on DSM-IV alcohol dependence and major depression, *J Stud Alcohol* 59(1):97-106, 1998.

Drug Scope: *Drug reforms range from the "impressively forward looking to the dangerously short-sighted,"* Press release, July 15, 2002, www.drugscope.org.uk.

Gentilello LM et al: Alcohol interventions in a trauma center as a means of reducing the risk of injury recurrence, *Ann Surg* 230(4):473-483, 1999.

Gordon SM: *Heroin: challenge for the 21st century,* Wernersville, Penn, 2001, Caron Foundation.

Gordon SM: *Women and addiction: gender issues in abuse and treatment,* Wernersville, Penn, 2002, Caron Foundation.

Greer G, Tolbert R: A method of conducting therapeutic sessions with MDMA, *J Psychoactive Drugs* 30(4):371-379, 1998.

Griffith WH, Moore SW: *Complete guide to prescription and nonprescription drugs,* New York, 2002, Body Press/Perigee.

Hallfors D, Godette D: Will the "principles of effectiveness" improve prevention practice? Early findings from a diffusion study, *Health Educ Res* 17(4):461-470, 2002.

Health Canada: *Preventing substance use problems among young people: a compendium of best practices,* Ottawa, 2002, Health Canada.

House of Commons Committee: *Special Report on the Non-Medical Use of Drugs,* 2002, available at http://www.parl.gc.ca/InfoCom/CommitteeMain.asp?Language=E&CommitteeID=301&Joint=0.

Joy JE, Watson SJ, Benson JA, editors: *Marijuana and medicine: assessing the science base,* Washington, DC, 1999, Institute of Medicine, National Academy Press.

Kaufman M et al: Cocaine-induced cerebral vasoconstriction differs as a function on sex and menstrual cycle phase, *Biol Psychiatry* 49(9):774-781, 2001.

Kesmodel U et al: Moderate alcohol intake during pregnancy and the risk of stillbirth and death in the first year of life, *Am J Epidemiol* 155(4):305-312, 2002.

Kinney J, Leaton G: *Loosening the grip,* ed 5, St Louis, Mo, 1995, Mosby.

Larkby C, Hanusa B, Kraemer K: The relation of depression and alcohol use among pregnant women, *Alcohol Clin Exp Res* 26(5 supplement): 28A, 2002.

Lazarou J, Pomerantz BH, Corey PN: Incidence of adverse drug reactions in hospitalized patients, *JAMA* 279:1200-1205, 1998.

Littman PS, Ritterbusch J: Tried, true, and new: public health nursing in a county substance abuse treatment system, *Public Health Nurs* 14(5):286-292, 1997.

Lloyd-Richardson EE et al: Differentiating stages of smoking intensity among adolescents: stage specific psychological and social influences, *J Consult Clin Psychol* 70(4):998-1009, 2002.

Manwell L et al: Tobacco, alcohol, and drug use in a primary care sample: 90 day prevalence and associated factors, *J Addict Dis* 17(1):67, 1997.

Marwick C: Physician leadership on national drug policy finds addiction treatment works, *JAMA* 279(15):1149, 1998.

Miller M: *Drug consumer safety rules,* Mosier, Ore, 2002, Mothers Against Misuse and Abuse, available at www.mamas.org.

Moner SE: Acupuncture and addiction treatment, *J Addict Dis* 15(3):79, 1996.

Moyers BD, Casiato T, Hughes K: "Moyers on addiction: close to home" (5-part video series), Princeton, NJ, 1998, Films for the Humanities and Sciences.

Mueller MD, Wyman JR: Study sheds new light on the state of drug abuse treatment nationwide, *NIDA Notes* 12(5):1, 1997.

National Center on Addiction and Substance Abuse: *Shoveling up: the impact of substance abuse on state budgets,* New York, 2001, Center on Addiction and Substance Abuse at Columbia University.

National Institute on Alcohol Abuse and Alcoholism: *The physician's guide to helping patients with alcohol problems,* Rockville, Md, 1995, NIAAA.

National Institute on Alcohol Abuse and Alcoholism: Alcohol's effect on organ function, *Alcohol Res World* 21(1):3, 1997.

National Institute on Drug Abuse: Comparing methamphetamine and cocaine, *NIDA Notes* 13(1):15, 1998a.

National Institute on Drug Abuse: Trends in drug use among 8th, 10th, and 12th graders, *NIDA Notes* 13(2):15, 1998b

National Institute on Drug Abuse: Drug addiction treatment conference emphasizes combining therapies, *NIDA Notes* 13(3):1, 1998c.

National Institute on Drug Abuse: *Research report series: inhalant abuse,* NIH Publication No. 00-3818, Rockville, Md, 2000, National Clearinghouse on Alcohol and Drug Information.

National Institute on Drug Abuse: *Infofax: crack and cocaine,* No. 13674, Rockville, Md, 2002, U.S. Department of Health and Human Services (www.nida.nih.gov/cocaine).

National Opinion Research Center: *Evaluating recovery services: the California drug and alcohol treatment assessment,* Chicago, 1994, Author.

O'Brien CP: Drug abuse and drug addiction. In Hardman JG, Limbird LE, editors: *Goodman & Gilman's pharmacological basis of therapeutics,* ed 9, New York, 1996, McGraw-Hill.

Office of National Drug Control Policy: *1999 National drug control strategy— 1999 budget summary,* available at www.whitehousedrugpolicy.gov/policy/99ndcsbudget.

Office of National Drug Control Policy: *National drug control budget, executive summary, fiscal year 2002,* Washington, DC, 2001, ONDCP.

Petro DJ: Pharmacology and toxicity of cannabis. In Mathre ML, editor: *Cannabis in medical practice: a legal, historical and pharmacological overview of the therapeutic use of marijuana,* Jefferson, NC, 1997, McFarland.

Prochaska JO, DiClemente CC, Norcross JC: In search of how people change: applications to addictive behaviors, *Am Psychol* 47(9):1102, 1992.

Rose KD: *American women and the repeal of prohibition,* New York, 1996, New York University Press.

Rybacki JJ, Long JW: *The essential guide to prescription drugs,* New York, 2002, Harper Perennial.

Schneider Institute for Health Policy: *Substance abuse: the nation's number one health problem: key indicators for health policy,* Princeton, NJ, 2001, Robert Wood Johnson Foundation.

Shedler J, Block J: Adolescent drug use and psychological health: a longitudinal inquiry, *Am Psychol* 45(5):612, 1990.

Solomon R: *Taking back our roads: a strategy to eliminate impaired driving in Canada,* Ottawa, 2002, MADD Canada.

Stine SM, Kosten TR: *Opioids, addictions: a comprehensive guidebook,* pp 141-161, New York, 1999, Oxford University Press.

Substance Abuse and Mental Health Services Administration: *National survey of substance abuse treatment services,* Rockville, Md, 2002, SAMHSA.

Talashek ML, Gerace LM, Starr KL: The substance abuse pandemic: determinants to guide interventions, *Public Health Nurs* 11(2):131, 1994.

From U.S. Department of Health and Human Services: *Healthy people 2010: national health promotion and disease prevention objectives,* Washington, DC, 2000, U.S. Government Printing Office.

U.S. Department of Health and Human Services: *Healthy people 2010: understanding and improving health,* ed 2, Washington, DC, 2000, U.S. Government Printing Office.

Weil A, Rosen W: *Chocolate to morphine: understanding mind-active drugs,* Boston, 1998, Houghton Mifflin.

Weinberg BA, Bealer BK: *The world of caffeine: the science and culture of the world's most popular drug,* New York, 2001, Routledge.

Weinberg NZ et al: Adolescent substance abuse: a review of the past 10 years, *J Am Acad Child Adolesc Psychiatry* 37(3):252, 1998.

Wenter DL et al: Comprehensiveness of substance use prevention programs in U.S. middle schools, *J Adolesc Health* 30(6):455-462, 2002.

Whitlock EP et al: Evaluating primary care behavioral counseling interventions: an evidence-based approach, *Am J Prev Med* 22(4):267-284, 2002.

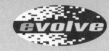
# Violence and Human Abuse

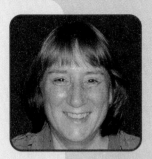

## Kären M. Landenburger, R.N., Ph.D.

Kären M. Landenburger is an associate professor of nursing at the University of Washington, Tacoma. She received her Ph.D. in nursing and her postdoctoral training in women's health from the University of Washington. Her area of expertise in community/public health nursing is the health and functioning of communities and populations, with an emphasis on community partnerships and community assessment. She is working on identifying field methods to use in collecting data on communities and populations. Her current research and practice focus on violence against women. She is involved on community and state levels in the education of health professionals about domestic violence as a social issue and about the needs of women who seek care. Currently, she is collaborating with Asian-American Pacific Islander communities, particularly the women, regarding domestic violence. She is a member of the Nursing Network on Violence Against Women and the Nursing Research Consortium on Violence and Abuse.

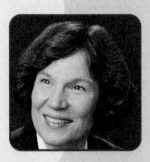

## Jacquelyn C. Campbell, Ph.D., RN, F.A.A.N.

Jacquelyn C. Campbell is the Anna D. Wolf Endowed Professor and associate dean for faculty affairs in the Johns Hopkins University School of Nursing with a joint appointment in the Bloomberg School of Public Health. Her B.S.N., M.S.N., and Ph.D. are from Duke University, Wright State University, and the University of Rochester schools of nursing. She has been conducting advocacy policy work and research in the area of domestic violence since 1980. Dr. Campbell has been the principle investigator on nine major National Institutes of Health, National Institute of Justice, and Centers for Disease Control and Prevention research grants and has published more than 120 articles and five books on this subject. She is an elected member of the Institute of Medicine and the American Academy of Nursing, a member of the congressionally appointed U.S. Department of Defense Task Force on Domestic Violence, and a member of the board of directors of the Family Violence Defense Fund and the House of Ruth Battered Women's Shelter.

## Objectives

After reading this chapter, the student should be able to do the following:

1. Discuss the scope of the problem of violence in American communities
2. Examine at least three factors existing in most communities that influence violence and human abuse
3. Identify at least three types of community facilities that can help prevent violence
4. Identify indicators of potential child abuse
5. Define the four general types of child abuse: neglect, physical, emotional, and sexual
6. Discuss abuse of older adults as a growing community health problem
7. Evaluate the roles that nurses can assume with rape victims
8. Analyze primary preventive nursing interventions for community violence
9. Evaluate the different responses that a nurse would expect to see in a battered woman from the beginning of the abuse until after the relationship has ended
10. Discuss the principles of nursing intervention with violent families
11. Describe specific nursing interventions with battered women

The word *violence* comes from the Latin *violare*, meaning to violate, injure, or rape. Indeed, violence is a violation, with both emotional and physical effects. Unfortunately, the United States has the fifth highest homicide rate in the world. Newspaper headlines and television reports are filled with news of violence. Although considerable progress has been made in decreasing rates of death from all other causes since 1940, the risk of assault and homicide in the United States has increased (U.S. Department of Health and Human Services [USDHHS], 1999). The violence in our streets and in our homes threatens the health and well-being of our entire population.

It is not clear from research if violence stems from an innate aggressive drive or it is primarily learned behavior. Clearly, all human beings have the capability for violence,

## Key Terms

**assault**, p. 879
**child abuse**, p. 884
**child neglect**, p. 884
**emotional abuse**, p. 884
**emotional neglect**, p. 884
**forensic**, p. 880
**homicide**, p. 878
**incest**, p. 885

**intimate partner violence**, p. 885
**neglect**, p. 882
**older adult abuse**, p. 887
**physical abuse**, p. 882
**physical neglect**, p. 884
**posttraumatic stress disorder**, p. 880
**rape**, p. 879
**sexual abuse**, p. 882

**spouse abuse**, p. 885
**suicide**, p. 881
**survivors**, p. 880
**violence**, p. 875
**wife abuse**, p. 885
*See Glossary for definitions*

## Chapter Outline

Social and Community Factors Influencing
 Violence
*Work*
*Education*
*Media*
*Organized Religion*
*Population*
*Community Facilities*

Violence Against Individuals or Oneself
*Homicide*
*Assault*
*Rape*
*Suicide*
Family Violence and Abuse
*Development of Abusive Patterns*
*Types of Family Violence*

Nursing Interventions
*Primary Prevention*
*Secondary Prevention*
*Tertiary Prevention: Therapeutic Intervention
 With Abusive Families*
Violence and the Prison Population
Clinical Forensic Nursing

yet some entire societies are basically nonviolent (Counts, Brown, and Campbell, 1999). Therefore it is important to understand under what conditions aggression and violence are increased and, conversely, what keeps them in check and promotes nonviolent conflict resolution.

Violence is a community health nursing concern. Significant mortality and morbidity result from violence. Communities across the United States are concerned about crime and violence rates. Medical, nursing, psychology, and social service professionals have been slow to develop a response to violence that is part of their daily professional lives. As a result, the estimated 4 million victims of violence annually may not receive the best care possible. In addition, the extent of their pain that could have been avoided by community health prevention efforts is

unknown. Nurses can take a more active role in the development of community responses to violence, public policy, and needed resources.

**Violence** is generally defined as those nonaccidental acts, interpersonal or intrapersonal, that result in physical or psychological injury to one or more persons. Violent behavior is predictable and thus preventable, especially with community action. Strategies have been developed in schools to prevent various forms of violence (Horton, 2001; Peterson, Larson, and Skiba, 2001). The identification of poverty, urban crowding, and racial inequality as factors that lead to violence can serve as a starting point for social change and subsequently a change in the level of societal violence (Sampson, 2001). An increase in home-based services (Leventhal, 2001), the evaluation of current practices such as protection orders (Carlson, Harris, and Holden, 1999), and media campaigns (Gandy, 2001) are all examples of methods to prevent violence. Violence is a major cause of premature mortality and life-long disability, and violence-related morbidity is a significant factor in health care costs. Violence is the twelfth leading cause of death in the United States and the sixth leading cause of premature mortality (USDHHS, 1999). A section of the Healthy People 2010 objectives is devoted to violence.

This chapter examines violence as a public health problem and discusses how nurses can help individuals, families, groups, and communities cope with and reduce violence and abuse. Nurses work with clients in a wide variety of settings, including the home. Since they are in key positions to detect and intervene in community and family violence, nurses need to understand how community-level influences can affect all types of violence.

## SOCIAL AND COMMUNITY FACTORS INFLUENCING VIOLENCE

Many factors in a community can support or minimize violence. Changing social conditions, multiple demands on people, economic conditions, and social institutions influence the level of violence and human abuse. The following discussion of selected current social conditions helps to explain factors that influence violent behavior.

### Work

Productive and paid work is an expectation in mainstream American society. Work can be fulfilling and contribute to a sense of well-being; it can also be frustrating and unfulfilling, contributing to stress that may lead to aggression and violence. Unemployment is also associated with violence both within and outside the home.

When jobs are repetitive, boring, and lacking in stimulation, frustration mounts. Some work environments discourage creativity and reward conformity and "following the rules." In many work settings, people try to get ahead regardless of the cost to others. Workers often go home feeling physically and psychologically drained. They may have worked at a backbreaking pace all day only to be yelled at by the boss for what seemed like a trivial oversight. It is hard to separate feelings generated at work from those at home.

For example, a father arrives home feeling tired, angry, and generally inadequate because of a series of reprimands from his boss. Soon after he sits down, his 4-year-old son runs through the house pretending to fly a wooden airplane. After about three loud trips past his father, who keeps shouting for the child to be quiet and go outside, the airplane hits the father in the head. The father may hit the boy out of frustration and anger.

During economic downturns, people hesitate to give up jobs that are frustrating, boring, or stressful. Family needs may necessitate that they keep the hated job. They feel trapped and may resent those who depend on them. This frustration and resentment may lead to violence.

Unemployment may precipitate aggressive outbursts. The inability to secure or keep a job may lead to feelings of inadequacy, guilt, boredom, dissatisfaction, and frustration. Unemployment does not fit the image of the ideal man in American society, and these men are more likely to be violent both within and outside the family (Catalano, Novaco, and McConnell, 1997; McCloskey, 2001). In a recent study of intimate partner homicide of women, the male partner's unemployment was the only demographic risk factor that increased the risk of murder (by 350%) over and above prior domestic violence (Campbell et al, in press).

Young, minority men have the highest rates of unemployment in the United States, ranging upward to 50% even in times of prosperity. This group also has the highest rate of violence. They live in a world of oppression, with lack of opportunity and enormous anger. They believe they are pushed out of mainstream society and are on the receiving end of the fallout of policies that ignore their dilemmas and give them no stake in mainstream America. Most analyses conclude that the differential rates of violence between African-Americans and whites in the United States have more to do with economic realities, such as poverty, unemployment, and overcrowding, than with race (Kauffman and Joseph-Fox, 1996; Sampson, 2001; True and Guillermo, 1996).

## Education

In recent years, schools have assumed many responsibilities traditionally assigned to the family. Schools teach sexual development, discipline children, and often serve as a place to "dump" children who have no other place to go. Large classes often mean that teachers spend more time and energy monitoring and disciplining children than challenging and stimulating them to learn. In large classes, children who do not conform to norms of expected behavior are often isolated. The nonconforming child is simply removed from the classroom because time is not available to help the child learn alternative ways of behavior.

It is ironic that parents often punish children for hitting or biting other children by spanking them. Corporal punishment is also still used in many U.S. schools. Such punishment only reinforces the child's tendency to strike out at others. Schools are often places where the stressors and frustrations that can contribute to violence are rampant, and violence is learned rather than discouraged; yet school can be a powerful contributor to nonviolence. Classes can help adolescents learn peaceful conflict resolution and the issues of date rape and help young children deal with the threat of sexual abuse (Hilton et al, 1998; Reis, 1997). Parents can be advised of the availability of such programs, and school boards should be urged to adopt them into the curriculum.

## Media

The media can be instrumental in campaigns against violence. Recent television programs, both documentaries and dramatizations, and print articles have heightened public awareness about family violence (Klein et al, 1997). Abused women and rape victims have especially benefited from media attention, which tends to lessen the stigma of such victimization. The media are also useful in publicizing services. However, the media have often served as a source of frustration to poor persons in U.S. society, as a cause of public apathy, and as a model of violence to be emulated.

Television, movies, newspapers, and magazines show happy, fun-loving people. Television parades all the wonders money can provide; yet for many Americans, the hope of buying many of these nonessentials seems unrealistic. Such polarization between what is available and what is possible provides fertile ground for the development of abusive patterns. Frustration, unfilled dreams, and unmet wishes are often handled through hurting someone who cannot fight back.

The media cater to children by advertising products to buy and things to do. Parents may get angry when their children request the foods, toys, and clothes they see on television, in magazines, or in newspapers or hear advertised on the radio. In addition, many toys and video games encourage violence through play.

Too often, the media portray the world as a violent place. When the public is convinced that violence is rampant, there are two possible results. People may become blasé about violence and no longer feel outraged and galvanized to action when terrible things happen in their community. On the other hand, some become frightened of their neighbors, isolate themselves, and refuse to become involved when someone needs help. Neither response is useful in any community action program.

Hitting, kicking, stabbing, and shooting are seen daily as ways to handle anger and frustration. By the age of 18 years, the average child has seen 1800 murders and countless acts of nonfatal violence on television. Often in these acts of violence, the good guys conquer the bad ones. Thus violence is often seen as justified when the perpetrator views the cause to be worthy. Frequent violent television viewing by children has been associated with aggressive behavior in longitudinal research (Simmons, Stalsworth, and Wentzel, 1999). On the other hand, the media can be a powerful force for increasing public awareness of various forms of violence and what can be done to address them (Klein et al, 1997).

## Organized Religion

Historically, a seemingly contradictory relationship exists between abuse and religion. For example, many religious groups uphold the philosophy of "spare the rod, spoil the child." Also, some faiths uphold the victimization of people with their disapproval of divorce. Family members may stay together, although they are at emotional or physical war with one another, because of religious commitments (Fortune, 2001).

Although churches have been slow to recognize domestic violence, some changes are taking place. Issues of male domination over women have become a major issue of discussion in some church groups, whereas in other groups women continue to be blamed for abuse that they sustain. Clergy need to be taught about the nature and dynamics of violence in the family, about religious messages and the potential for support, and about the need for collaboration between the church and advocates for the prevention of domestic violence. In religious groups where there is collaboration with advocates against abuse to children, women, and elders, there is a greater recognition of the harm of abuse and the clarity of the role of the clergy in dealing with abuse (Cooper-White, 1996; Wolff et al, 2001).

## Population

A community's population can influence the potential for violence. Density, poverty, and diversity, particularly racial tension and overt racism, contribute to violence (Evans and Taylor, 1995; Hampton and Yung, 1996).

High-population-density communities can positively or negatively influence violence. Those with a sense of cohesiveness may have a lower crime rate than areas of similar size that lack social and cultural groups to support unity among members. Bonds formed among church groups, clubs, and professional organizations may promote harmony among members. Such groups provide members an opportunity to talk about stressors rather than to respond through violence. For example, residents of public housing often form neighborhood associations to deal with situations common to many or all residents. Tension can often be released in a productive way through projects carried out by the association.

Some high-population areas experience a community feeling of powerlessness and helplessness rather than one of cohesiveness. Lack of jobs and low-paying jobs result in feelings of inadequacy, despair, and social alienation. Social alienation and exclusion from opportunities can lead to decreased social cohesion and increased violence (Moore and Harrisson, 1995; Wilkinson, 1997). Fear and apathy may cause community residents to withdraw from social contact. Withdrawal can foster crime because many residents assume someone else will report suspicious behavior, or they fear reprisals for such reports.

Youths often attempt to deal with feelings of powerlessness by forming gangs. Poverty and lack of education appear to be the overriding risk factors. A number of these young adults have attempted to deal with their feelings by turning to crime against people and property to release frustration. In many cities, these gangs have been highly destructive. Unfortunately, many programs have focused on family functioning, using secondary prevention through intervention with families, rather than focusing on primary prevention and the primary issues leading to gang membership (Winfree, Esbensen, and Osgood, 1996).

Other high-population areas may be characterized by a sense of confusion, resulting in disintegration and disorganization. These areas often have transient populations who have limited physical or emotional investment in the community. Lack of community concern allows crime and violence to go unchecked and may become a norm for the area. Also, as crime increases, residents who are able to move leave the area. This increases community disintegration because the residents who leave are often the most capable members of the population.

The potential for violence also tends to increase among highly diverse populations. Differences in age, socioeconomic status, ethnicity, religion, or other cultural characteristics may disrupt community stability. Highly divergent groups may not communicate effectively and neither accept nor understand one another. Many such groups become hostile and antagonistic toward one another. Each group may see the other as different and not belonging. The alienated group may become the focal point for the others' frustrations, anger, and fears. Racism, classism, and heterosexism are examples of major causes of community disintegration resulting in a vicious cycle of dishonesty, distrust, and hate.

## Community Facilities

Communities differ in the resources and facilities they provide to residents. Some are more desirable places to live, work, and raise families and have facilities that can reduce the potential for crime and violence. Recreational facilities such as playgrounds, parks, swimming pools, movie theaters, and tennis courts provide socially acceptable outlets for a variety of feelings, including aggression.

Spectator sports, such as football or hockey, also allow members of the community to express feelings of anger and frustration. However, viewing sports can encourage a sense of violence as participants hit or shove one another.

Although the absence of such facilities can increase the likelihood of violence, their presence alone does not prevent violence or crime. These facilities are adjuncts and resources that residents can use for pleasure, personal enrichment, and group development.

Familiarity with factors contributing to a community's violence or potential for violence enables nurses to recognize them and intervene accordingly. It is the nurse's responsibility to work with the citizens and agencies of the community to correct or improve deficits.

## VIOLENCE AGAINST INDIVIDUALS OR ONESELF

The potential for violence against individuals (e.g., murder, robbery, rape, and assault) or oneself (e.g., suicide) is directly related to the level of violence in the community. Persons living in areas with high rates of crime and violence are more likely to become victims than those in more peaceful areas. The major categories of violence addressed in this chapter are described in terms of the scope of the problem in the United States and underlying dynamics.

### Homicide

**Homicide** is the eleventh leading cause of death for all Americans, and the number one cause of death for young (age 15 to 34 years) African-American men and women (USDHHS, 1999). However, the African-American homicide rate has decreased significantly since 1970, whereas the white homicide rate has increased slightly (Bureau of Justice Statistics, 1997; USDHHS, 1999). Although the data are not adequate, it also appears that Hispanic-American men have a much higher rate of homicide than non–Hispanic-American whites. Homicide is increasing the most among adolescents, but even among very young children in the United States homicide occurs at an alarming rate. The National Child Abuse and Neglect Data System (NCANDS) reported that in 1997 that there were an estimated 1196 child fatalities, or 1.7 children per 100,000 in the general population. Seventy-seven percent were children 3 and under (USDHHS, 2002b). Only 13% to 15% of all homicides in the United States are caused by strangers (Riedel, 1998). When strangers are involved, many of these homicides are related to the illegal substance–abuse network.

The majority of homicides, however, are perpetrated by a friend, acquaintance, or family member during an argument. Therefore prevention of homicide is at least as much an issue for the public health system as for the criminal justice system (Rosenberg and Fenley, 1991).

## Homicide Within Families

At least 13% of the homicides in the United States occur within families (Bachman, 1994), and half of these occur between spouses. These numbers, however, do not include unmarried couples who are living together or those who are either divorced or estranged, a group at higher risk. Husbands or ex-husbands made up about 75% of the perpetrators in spousal homicides, and self-defense is involved approximately seven times as often when wives kill their husbands than vice versa (Bachman, 1994; Campbell, 1995).

An alarming aspect of family homicide is that small children often witness the murder or find the body of a family member. No automatic follow-up or counseling of these children occurs through the criminal justice or mental health system in most communities. These children are at great risk for emotional turmoil and for becoming involved in violence themselves.

The underlying dynamics of homicide within families vary greatly from those of other murders. Homicide within families is most often preceded by abuse of a family member (Campbell, Sharps, and Glass, 2000). Thus prevention of family homicide involves working with abusive families. In fact, in a recent study of intimate partner homicide of women, 47% of the women who were killed had been seen in a health care setting during the year before they were killed by their husband or boyfriend or ex-partner (Sharps et al, 2001). Nurses have a duty to warn family members of the possibility of homicide when severe abuse is present, just as they warn of the hazards of smoking (Campbell, 1995). Other nursing care issues are further discussed under Family Violence and Abuse in this chapter.

## Assault

The death toll from violence is indeed staggering, yet the physical injuries and emotional costs of **assault** are equally important issues in terms of the acute health care system and both public health nursing and home health care. At least 100 nonfatal assaults occur for each homicide that occurs in the United States (USDHHS, 1999). Thirty-nine percent of females and 24% of males reported injury related to physical assault (Tjaden and Thoennes, 2000). The greatest risk factor for an individual's victimization through violence is age, and youths are at significantly higher risk. Whereas more males than females are victims of homicide and assault, women are more likely to be victimized by a relative, especially a male partner (Bachman, 1994). Sometimes the difference between a homicide and an assault is only the response time and the quality of emergency transport and treatment facilities. The same community measures used to address homicide are also useful to combat assault. Also, nurses often see assaulted persons in home health care with long-term health problems such as head injuries, spinal cord injuries, and stomas from abdominal gunshot wounds. In addition to physical care, nurses must also address the emotional trauma re-sulting from a violent attack by helping victims talk through their traumatic experience to try to make some sense of the violence, and by referring them for further counseling if anxiety, sleeping problems, or depression persists after the assault.

## Rape

Currently, **rape** is one of the most underreported forms of human abuse in the United States. Although the number of rapes reported to law enforcement agencies has decreased since 1993, only a third of victims or survivors report rape or sexual assault to a law enforcement agency. One of six women and 1 of 33 men are victims of rape. The rates of completed and attempted rape are almost equivalent. The incidence of rape exceeds the prevalence of rape victims because some victims experience more than one rape in a twelve-month period (Tjaden and Thoennes, 2000). In 1992, there were 84 rapes per 100,000 women, the lowest since 1976 (U.S. Department of Justice, 1997). Victim reporting of rape has improved. Hospital, emergency personnel, and police have better protocols for victims of rape. Although the collection of information leading to prosecution is emphasized, the protocols try to ensure respectful and supportive treatment for victims.

Another important factor is the recognition of date and marital rape. The majority of violence against women is intimate partner violence. In the National Violence Against Women Survey (Tjaden and Thoennes, 2000), 64% of rapes, physical assaults, and stalkings were committed against women by either current or former intimate partners. Official recognition of rape regardless of a victim's relationship to the perpetrator has led to an increased number of women reporting rape. Rape also happens to men, especially boys and young men, but the statistics on the incidence of male rape vary. A major problem in obtaining statistics is that the definition of rape adopted by the Federal Bureau of Investigation for compiling the Uniformed Crime Reports is limited to penile-vaginal penetration only (Koss and Harvey, 1991). It appears that the emotional trauma for a male rape victim is at least as serious as that for a woman.

For reported rapes, cities constitute higher risk areas than do rural areas, and the hours between 8 P.M. and 2 A.M., weekends, and the summer are the most critical times. In about half of rapes, the victim and the offender meet on the street, whereas in other cases the rapist either enters the victim's home or somehow entices or forces the victim to accompany him.

Prevention of rape, like that of other forms of human abuse, requires a broad-based community focus for educating both the community as a whole and key groups such as police, health providers, educators, and social workers. Rape rates and community-level variables such as community approval and legitimization of violence (e.g., violent network television viewing and permitting corporal punishment in schools) appear related and underscore the need for community-level intervention (Donat and D'Emilio, 1997).

## Attitudes

The first priority is to change attitudes about rape and about victims or survivors. Rape is a crime of violence, not a crime of passion. The underlying issues are hostility, power, and control rather than sexual desire. The defining issue is lack of consent of the victim. When a woman or man refuses any sexual activity, that refusal means "no." People have the right to change their mind, even when they seemed initially agreeable. Pressure from physical contact, threats, or deliberate inducement of drug or alcohol intoxication is a violation of the law. The myths that women say "no" to sex when they really mean "yes" and that the victims of rape are culpable because of the way they dress or act must end. On college campuses, negative attitudes toward acquaintance or date rape are slow to change. Women on college campuses underreport allegations of rape because of issues of confidentiality and fear of being discredited (Koss and Cook, 1998).

## Pornography

Although there is evidence of a relationship between the viewing of pornographic material showing violence against women and aggressive sexual behavior (Cottle et al, 1997; Kimmel, 1996; Russell, 1995a), it is not clear if the relationship is causal. In other words, our current research does not yet prove that viewing pornography occurs before sexual aggressiveness or that young men who are sexually violent tend to watch pornography. Some experts also maintain that it is watching violent rather than erotic pornography that may be a risk factor for sexual assault. However, there is enough current evidence on the subject to recommend keeping violent pornography illegal, especially for minors. Prevention also involves providing information to women about self-protection, including self-defense procedures, avoiding high-risk locations, and safeguarding one's home against unwanted entry.

## Victim or Survivor?

During the act of rape, **survivors** are often hit, kicked, stabbed, and severely beaten. It is this violence that most traumatizes the person because of the fear for her life and her helplessness, lack of control, and vulnerability.

People react to rape differently, depending on their personality, past experiences, background, and support received after the trauma. Some cry, shout, or discuss the experience. Others withdraw and fear discussing the attack. During the immediate as well as the follow-up stages, victims tend to blame themselves for what has happened. It is important while working with rape victims to help them identify the issues behind self-blame. Although fault should not be placed on survivors, they should be taught to take control, learn assertiveness, and therefore believe that they can take certain actions to prevent future rapes. Survivors need to talk about what happened and to express their feelings and fears in a nonjudgmental atmosphere. Nonjudgmental listening is important.

In any psychological trauma, the right to privacy and confidentiality is of the utmost importance. Victims should be given privacy, respect, and assurance of confidentiality. They also should be told about health care procedures conducted immediately after the rape and should be linked with proper resources for ease of reporting. Nurses often provide continuous care once the victim enters the health care system. Because many victims deny the event once the initial crisis is past, a single-session debriefing should be completed during the initial examination. The physical assessment, examination, and debriefing should be carried out by specially trained providers (Aiken and Speck, 1995).

In most states, nurses trained in sexual assault examination (SANE nurses, a subspecialty of **forensic** nursing) perform the physical examination in the emergency department to gather evidence (e.g., hair samples, skin fragments beneath the victim's fingernails, evidence from pelvic exams using colposcopy) for criminal prosecution of sexual assault (Ledray and Simmelink, 1997). This is an important nursing intervention because physicians may be impatient with the time required for this procedure; nurses can take advantage of this opportunity to provide therapeutic communication. Nurses can be trained to conduct the examination, and their evidence is credible and effective in resultant court proceedings (Ledray and Simmelink, 1997). Nurses can lobby for changes in hospital policies and state laws to make this strategy a reality in all states.

Rape is a situational crisis for which advance preparation is rarely possible. Therefore nursing efforts are directed toward helping victims cope with the stress and disruption of their lives caused by the attack. Counseling focuses on the crisis and the concomitant fears, feelings, and issues involved. Nurses can help survivors learn how to regroup personal forces. If **posttraumatic stress disorder** (PTSD) has developed, professional psychological or psychiatric treatment is indicated.

Many rape victims need follow-up mental health services to help them cope with the short- and long-term effects of the crisis. The time after a rape is one of disequilibrium, psychological breakdown, and reorganization of attitudes about the safety of the world. Common, everyday tasks often tax a person's resources. Many individuals

> ### DID YOU KNOW?
>
> Forty to forty-five percent of physically abused women are also being forced into sex. This has implications for the prevention of unintended and adolescent pregnancies, human immunodeficiency virus (HIV), acquired immunodeficiency syndrome (AIDS), and sexually transmitted diseases (STDs), as well as for women's healthy sexuality and self-esteem.

forget or fail to keep appointments. Therefore nurses can make appropriate referrals and obtain permission from the victim to remain in contact through telephone conversations. In this manner, the ongoing needs of the victim can be assessed and support, encouragement, and resources can be offered as needed (Koss and Harvey, 1991).

## Suicide

In 1998, **suicides** were committed by 30,575 people in the United States. Approximately 671,000 visits to hospital emergency departments resulted from self-inflected injuries. The number of actual suicides in addition to attempted suicides reflects the gravity of the problem. The risk for death by suicide is greater than for death by homicide (National Center for Injury Prevention and Control, 2001). Although more women attempt suicide, rates are higher for men, older adults, non-Hispanic whites, and Native Americans/Alaskan Natives (Centers for Disease Control and Prevention, 1997). Suicide is four times more frequent among whites than among African Americans. Affluent and educated people have higher rates of suicide than do the economically and educationally disadvantaged. The presence of a gun in the home is an important risk factor for suicide as well as homicide (Kellerman, Rivara, and Rushforth, 1993).

Boys and young men between the ages of 15 to 19 were five times more likely to commit suicide than females. They are seven times more likely to commit suicide between the ages of 20 to 24 than their female counterparts (National Center for Injury Prevention and Control, 2001). Leading risk factors for adolescent suicide are mental illness including depression, severe stress, incest, and extrafamilial sexual and physical abuse, and increased access to firearms (Eggert et al, 1994; Hernandez, Lodico, and DiClemente, 1993; O'Carroll et al, 2001). An important risk factor for actual and attempted suicide in adult women is spousal abuse (Stark and Flitcraft, 1991).

Nurses need to be involved in the reduction of suicide and the care for victims, including the community, the family, and individuals. On a community level, nurses can be involved in a coordinated response to the prevention of suicide and the care of attempted suicides. Through their roles in public health and school nursing, they can be involved in the development of policies and protocols for suicide across the life span. Nursing care may focus on family members and friends of suicide victims. Survivors often feel angry toward the dead person yet frequently turn the anger inward. Likewise, survivors often question their own liability for the death. The impact of suicide can affect family, friends, co-workers, and the community. Survivors may have difficulty dealing with their feelings toward the dead person. They may have difficulty concentrating and may limit their social activities because it is often difficult for both survivors and their friends to talk about the suicide. Nurses can help survivors cope with the trauma of the loss and make referrals to a counselor or support groups.

## FAMILY VIOLENCE AND ABUSE

Family violence, including sexual abuse, emotional abuse, and physical abuse, causes significant injury and death. These three forms tend to occur together as part of a system of coercive control. Generally, violence within families is perpetrated by the most powerful against the least powerful. Intimate partner violence is directed primarily toward wives (although they may physically fight back). In the National Violence Against Women Survey, 25% of women compared to 8% of men experienced violence in a partnered relationship (Tjaden and Thoennes, 1998).

Recognizing the battered child or spouse in the emergency department is relatively simple after the fact. It is unfortunate that, by the time medical care is sought, serious physical and emotional damage may have been done. Nurses are in a key position to predict and deal with abusive tendencies. By understanding factors contributing to the development of abusive behaviors, nurses can identify abuse-prone families.

## Development of Abusive Patterns

Factors that characterize people who become involved in family violence include upbringing, living conditions, and increased stress. Understanding how these factors influence the development of abusive behavior can help the nurse deal with abusive families.

### Upbringing

Of all the factors that characterize the background of abusers, the most predictably present is previous exposure to some form of violence (Markowitz, 2001). As children, abusers were often beaten themselves or witnessed the beating of siblings or a parent. Children raised in this way learn that violence is a suitable mechanism for managing conflict.

For both men and women, witnessing abuse as children was associated with abuse of one's children in the future (Markowitz, 2001; Mihalic and Elliott, 1997). Childhood physical punishment teaches children to use violent conflict resolution as an adult. A child may learn to associate love with violence because a parent is usually the first person to hit a child. Children may think that those who love them also are those who hit them. The moral rightness of hitting other family members thus may be established when physical punishment is used to train children, especially when it is used more than occasionally. These experiences predispose children ultimately to use violence with their own children.

As well as having a history of child abuse themselves, people who become abusers tend to have hostile personality styles and be verbally aggressive. They have often learned these characteristics from their own childhood experiences. Their parents may have set unrealistic goals, and when the children failed to perform accordingly, they were criticized, demeaned, punished, and denied affection. These children may have been told how to act, what to do, and how to feel, thereby discouraging the development of normal attachment, autonomy, problem-solving skills, and creativity (Briere et al, 1996). Children raised in this way grow up feeling unloved and worthless. They may want a child of their own so that they will feel assured of someone's love.

To protect themselves from feelings of worthlessness and fear of rejection, abused children form a protective shell and grow increasingly hostile and distrustful of others. The behavior of potential abusers reflects a low tolerance for frustration, emotional instability, and the onset of aggressive feelings with minimal provocation. Because of their emotional insecurity, they often depend on a child or spouse to meet their needs of feeling valued and secure. When their needs are not met by others, they become overly critical. Critical, resentful behavior and unrealistic expectations of others lead to a vicious cycle. The more critical these people become, the more they are rejected and alienated from others. Abusive individuals tend to perceive that the target of their hostility is "out to get" them. These distorted perceptions can be detected when parents talk about an infant crying or keeping them up at night "on purpose" (Briere et al, 1996).

### Increased Stress

A perceived or actual crisis may precede an abusive incident. Because crisis reinforces feelings of inadequacy and low self-esteem, a number of events often occur in a short time to precipitate abusive patterns. Unemployment, strains in the marriage, or an unplanned pregnancy may set off violence.

The daily hassles of raising young children, especially in an economically strained household, intensify an already stressed atmosphere for which an unexpected and difficult event provokes violence. Stressful life events, poverty, and the number of small children are often associated with family violence (Lambert and Firestone, 2000; Mohr, 1999). Crowded living conditions may also precipitate abuse. The presence of several people in a small space heightens tensions and reduces privacy. Tempers flare because of the constant stimulation from others.

Social isolation is associated with abuse in families (Briere et al, 1996). Such isolation reduces social support, decreasing a family's ability to deal with stressors. The problem may be intensified if a violent family member tries to keep the family isolated to escape detection. Therefore, when a family misses clinic or home visit appointments, nurses need to keep in mind that abuse may be present. Nurses can encourage involvement in community activities and can help neighbors reach out to neighbors to help prevent abuse.

Frequent moves disrupt social support systems, are associated with an overall increased stress level, and tend to isolate people, at least briefly. Mobility can have a serious negative effect on the abuse-prone family. These families do not readily initiate new relationships. They rely on the family for support. Resources may be unfamiliar or inac-

cessible to them. Because frequent moving may be both a risk factor for abuse and a sign of an abusive family trying to avoid detection, nurses should assess such families carefully for abuse.

## Types of Family Violence

Because various forms of family violence and violence outside the home often occur together, nurses who detect child abuse should also suspect other forms of family violence. When older adult parents report that their (now adult) child was abused or has a history of violence toward others, the nurse should recognize the potential for elder abuse. **Physical abuse** of women is frequently accompanied by **sexual abuse** both inside and outside the marital relationship. Severe wife abusers may have a history of other acts of violence. Families who are verbally aggressive in conflict resolution (e.g., using name calling, belittling, screaming, and yelling) are more likely to be physically abusive. Although the various forms of family violence are discussed separately, they should not be thought of as totally separate phenomena.

No member of the family is guaranteed immunity from abuse and neglect. Spouse abuse, child abuse, abuse of older adults, serious violence among siblings, and mutual abuse by members all occur. Although these examples are not inclusive, they demonstrate the scope of family violence.

### Child Abuse

The most recent published national survey projected that 879,000 children and adolescents were subjected to **neglect,** medical neglect, physical and sexual abuse, and emotional maltreatment in the year 2000 (USDHHS, 2002a). Of these children, 19% were victims of physical abuse, 10% were sexually abused, and 8% were psychologically maltreated. This is probably a conservative figure, as only the most severe cases are reported. The number of children who are reported as victims of maltreatment has decreased steadily from 1993 to 1999 from a level of 15.3 per 1000 children in the population to 11.8 per 1000, and then there was a slight increase in 2000 to 12.2 per 1000 children in the population. The victims were equally distributed between boys and girls except in the realm of sexual abuse, where female children were four times more likely to be sexually abused than male children (USDHHS, 2002a).

Many children each year witness domestic violence (Peled, 1996). Children witnessing domestic violence may experience PTSD (Kilpatrick, Litt, and Williams, 1997). In addition, children who live in a home where violence takes place between their parents are more likely to be abused themselves (Salzinger et al, 2002). Risk factors for children who are abused include a number of parental factors such as strain on the economic resources of the family, lack of social support, and problems with substance abuse. Some of the risk factors are identified in Box 37-1. Children who witness abuse may react differently according to their age, level of development, and sex. Regardless of these factors,

## BOX 37-1  Risk Factors for Child Abuse

Ask the following questions to determine if risk factors are present.

1. What are the ages of the parents?
2. Does the child come from a single-parent household or a family with a large number of children?
3. Do the parents have the financial resources to care for a child?
4. Are the parents communicative with each other and the nurse?
5. Is there a support network that is willing to offer assistance?
6. Does the mother of the child seem frightened of her partner?
7. Does either of the parents have a history of child abuse?
8. Do the parents have knowledge about child development?
9. Does either parent or both have problems with substance abuse?
10. Does the child suffer from recurrent injuries or unexplained illnesses?

Barnett OW, Miller-Perrin CL, Perrin RD: *Family violence across the lifespan: an introduction,* Thousand Oaks, Calif, 1997, Sage; Sedlak AJ, Broadhurst DD: *Executive summary of the Third National Incidence Study of Child Abuse and Neglect,* U.S. Department of Health and Human Services, Administration for Children and Families, Administration on Children, Youth and Families, National Center on Child Abuse and Neglect, Washington, DC, 1996, National Clearinghouse on Child Abuse and Neglect; Widom CS, Hiller-Sturmhöfel S: Alcohol abuse as a risk factor for and consequence of child abuse, *Alcohol Res Health* 25(1):52-57, 2001.

## HOW TO  Identify Potentially Abusive Parents

The following characteristics in couples expecting a child constitute warning signs of actual or potential abuse.

- Denial of the reality of the pregnancy, as seen in a refusal to talk about the impending birth or to think of a name for the child
- An obvious concern or fear that the baby will not meet some predetermined standard: sex, hair color, temperament, or resemblance to family members
- Failure to follow through on the desire for an abortion
- An initial decision to place the child for adoption and a change of mind
- Rejection of the mother by the father of the baby
- Family experiencing stress and numerous crises so that the birth of a child may be the last straw
- Initial and unresolved negative feelings about having a child
- Lack of support for the new parents
- Isolation from friends, neighbors, or family
- Parental evidence of poor impulse control or fear of losing control
- Contradictory history
- Appearance of detachment
- Appearance of misusing drugs or alcohol
- Shopping for hospitals or health care providers
- Unrealistic expectations of the child
- Verbal, physical, or sexual abuse of mother by father, especially during pregnancy
- Child is not biological offspring of male stepfather or mother's current boyfriend
- Excessive talk of needing to "discipline" children and plans to use harsh physical punishment to enforce discipline

the child's reactions are influenced by the severity and frequency of the abuse witnessed (Ryan and King, 1997).

The presence of child abuse signifies ineffective family functioning. Abusive parents who recognize their problem are often reluctant to seek assistance because of the stigma attached to being considered a child abuser.

Children are frequent victims of abuse because they are small and relatively powerless. In many families, only one child is abused. Parents may identify with this particular child and be especially critical of the child's behavior. In some cases, the child may have certain qualities, such as looking like a relative, being handicapped, or being particularly bright and capable, that provoke the parent.

Parents with low social support, a tendency toward depression, multiple stress factors, and a history of abuse are at risk for abusing their children (Kotch et al, 1999). Abusive parents often have unrealistic expectations of a child's developmental abilities. They tend to have little involvement with and show minimal warmth toward their child (Brown et al, 1998). Parents who abuse their children

use physical discipline more frequently. The discipline can be in the form of physical punishment and verbal abuse (Jackson et al, 1999). The nurse must not only teach normal parental behavior but also address the underlying emotional needs of the parents. These parents often experience pain and poor emotional stability and need intervention as much as their children. Following are some of the behavioral indicators of potentially abusive parents.

### Foster Care

When child abuse is discovered, the child is often placed in a foster home. It is unfortunate that there is not enough good foster care for all abused children, and many foster care situations are also abusive. Abused children generally want to return to their parents, and the goal of most agencies is to keep natural families together as long as it is safe for the child. However, a family preservation approach is not always effective in keeping children safe (Chalk and King, 1998). Many times the nurse's role involves helping to monitor a family in which a formerly abused child is returned after a time in foster care. Keen judgment and close collaboration with social services are necessary in these situations. The nurse must ensure the safety of the child while working with the parents in an empathetic way. The nurse's goal is to enhance their parenting skills, not to be viewed as yet another watchdog.

Another point to keep in mind about abusive parents is that their desire to replace a child who has been removed by the courts because of abuse is a normal response to the grief of losing a child. Rather than regarding another pregnancy as a sign of continued poor judgment or pathologic behavior, the pregnancy can be perceived by the nurse as an opportunity for intensive intervention to prevent the abuse of the expected child. Generally, the parents are eager to avoid further problems if enlisted as partners in the project.

### Indicators of Child Abuse

It is essential that nurses recognize the physical and behavioral indicators of abuse and neglect. **Child abuse** ranges from violent physical attacks to passive neglect. Violence such as beating, burning, kicking, or shaking may

---

**HOW TO** Recognize Actual or Potential Child Abuse

Be alert to the following:
- An unexplained injury
- Skin: burns, old or recent scars, ecchymosis, soft tissue swelling, human bites
- Fractures: recent, or older ones that have healed
- Subdural hematomas
- Trauma to genitalia
- Whiplash (caused by shaking small children)
- Dehydration or malnourishment without obvious cause
- Provision of inappropriate food or drugs (alcohol, tobacco, medication prescribed for someone else, foods not appropriate for the child's age)
- Evidence of general poor care: poor hygiene, dirty clothes, unkempt hair, dirty nails
- Unusual fear of nurse and others
- Considered to be a "bad" child
- Inappropriate dress for the season or weather conditions
- Reports or shows evidence of sexual abuse
- Injuries not mentioned in history
- Seems to need to take care of the parent and speak for the parent
- Maternal depression
- Maladjustment of older siblings

---

lead to severe physical injury. Passive neglect may result in insidious malnutrition or other problems. Abuse is not limited to physical maltreatment but includes **emotional abuse** such as yelling at or continually demeaning and criticizing the child. Children who come from a family where there is intimate partner violence are at greater risk for physical and psychological abuse and child neglect (McGuigan and Pratt, 2001; Rumm et al, 1999).

Emotional abuse involves extreme debasement of feelings and may result in the child feeling inadequate, inept, uncared for, and worthless. Victims of emotional abuse learn to hide their feelings to avoid incurring additional scorn. They may act out by performing poorly in school, becoming truant, and being hostile and aggressive. Children who are abused or who witness domestic violence can suffer developmentally (Wolak and Finkelhor, 1998). Often adolescents run away from home as a direct result of domestic violence (Nadon, Koverola, and Schludermann, 1998).

Physical symptoms of physical, sexual, or emotional stress may include hyperactivity, withdrawal, overeating, dermatologic problems, vague physical complaints, stuttering, enuresis (bladder incontinence), and encopresis (bowel incontinence). It is ironic that bedwetting is often a trigger for further abuse, which creates a particularly vicious cycle. When a child displays physical symptoms without clear physiological origin, ruling out the possibility of abuse should be part of the nurse's assessment process.

### Child Neglect

The two categories of **child neglect** are physical and emotional. **Physical neglect** is defined as failure to provide adequate food, proper clothing, shelter, hygiene, or necessary medical care. Physical neglect is most often associated with extreme poverty (Gillham et al, 1998).

In contrast, **emotional neglect** is the omission of basic nurturing, acceptance, and caring essential for healthy personal development. These children are largely ignored or in many cases treated as nonpersons. Such neglect usually affects the development of self-esteem. It is difficult for a neglected child to feel a great deal of self-worth because the parents have not demonstrated that they value the child.

Neglect is more difficult to assess and evaluate than abuse because it is subtle and may go unnoticed. Astute observations of children, their homes, and the way in which they relate to their caregivers can provide clues of neglect.

### Sexual Abuse

Child abuse also includes sexual abuse. Approximately one of four female children and one of ten males in the United States will be subject to some form of sexual abuse by the time they reach 18 years of age. The exact prevalence is difficult to obtain because not all children have the cognitive ability to describe these experiences (Kendall-Tackett and Marshall, 1998). This abuse ranges from unwanted sexual touching to intercourse. The majority of childhood sexual abuse is perpetrated by someone the child knows and trusts. Between one third and one half of all sexual abuse involves a family member (Russell, 1995b). Although sexual abuse is perpetrated by all categories of caregivers, a child's risk for abuse is higher with stepparents or nonrelated caregivers (Gelles, 1998). Adults that children and parents are inclined to trust, such as coaches, scout leaders, and even priests, have been reported sexual abusers. The long-term effects of sexual abuse are depression, sexual disturbances, and substance abuse (Carlson et al, 1997).

Research has shown that many of the characteristics of physically abusive and sexually abusive parents, such as unhappiness, loneliness, and rigidity, are shared by both groups (Brown et al, 1998). However, sexually abusive parents report fewer family problems and a more positive view of the child than do physically abusive parents.

Father–daughter incest is the type of **incest** most often reported. Although mother–son incest takes place, the incidence remains quite small (Ehrmin, 1996). Many cases of parental incest go unreported because victims fear punishment, abandonment, rejection, or family disruption if they acknowledge the problem. Incest occurs in all races, religious groups, and socioeconomic classes. Incest is receiving greater attention because of mandatory reporting laws, yet all too often its incidence remains a family secret.

Because nurses are often involved in helping women deal with the aftermath of incest, it is crucial to understand the typical patterns and the long-term implications. A typical pattern is as follows. The daughter involved in paternal incest is usually about 9 years of age at the onset and is often the oldest or only daughter. The father seldom uses physical force. He most likely relies on threats, bribes, intimidation, or misrepresentation of moral standards, or he exploits the daughter's need for human affection (Phelan, 1995).

Nurses must be aware of the incidence, signs and symptoms, and psychological and physical trauma of incest. Green (1996) identified clusters of affective symptoms, including low self-esteem, depression, and intrusive imagery. Somatic symptoms include headaches, eating and sleeping disorders, menstrual problems, and gastrointestinal distress. Other symptoms include difficulties in social situations, especially in forming and maintaining close relationships with men, and behavioral symptoms such as substance abuse and sexual dysfunction. Children often try to avoid or escape the abusive behavior. Avoidance can take the form of either behavioral or mental reactions, such as dressing to cover one's body or pretending that the abuse is not taking place. The child can escape either physically by running away or emotionally by withdrawing into other activities and thereby placing the sexual abuse in the background (Darlington, 1996).

Adolescents may display inappropriate sexual activity or truancy or may run away from home. Running away is usually considered a sign of delinquency; however, an adolescent who runs away may be using a healthy response to a violent family situation. Therefore the assessment should ask about sexual and physical abuse at home and plan appropriate intervention.

The effects of childhood sexual abuse can be mitigated by continual professional support. At different developmental stages, children may need assistance to overcome negative feelings about their own sexuality (Beitchman et al, 1993). Adult survivors of sexual abuse often have significant health problems that need to be addressed in terms of the ongoing effects of their childhood and adult experiences (Draucker, 1997; Green, 1995).

## Abuse of Female Partners

Although women do abuse men, by far the greater proportion of what is often discussed as **spouse abuse** or domestic violence is actually **wife abuse.** At least 1.5 million women are battered and/or raped by their male partner each year in the United States (Tjaden and Thoennes, 1998). Neither the term *wife abuse* nor the term *spouse abuse* takes into account violence in dating or cohabiting relationships or violence in same-sex relationships. **Intimate partner violence** is a more inclusive term to refer to all kinds of violence between partners, and all adults should be assessed for violence in their primary intimate relationship. The incidence of violence in same-sex relationships is considered to be the same as in heterosexual relationships (Renzetti, 1997). The abuse of female partners has the most serious community health ramifications because of the greater prevalence, the greater potential for homicide (Campbell, 1995), the effects on the children in the household, and the more serious long-term emotional and physical consequences.

Victims of child abuse and individuals who saw their mothers being battered are at risk of using violence toward an intimate partner, whether one is male or female (Mihalic and Elliott, 1997). However, using evidence of a violent childhood to identify women at risk of abuse is less useful, because abuse cannot be predicted on the basis of characteristics of the individual woman. It is the violent background of an abusive male, combined with his tendencies to be possessive, controlling, and extremely jealous, that is most predictive of abuse. Substance abuse is also associated with battering, although it cannot be said to cause the violence.

### Signs of Abuse

Battered women often have bruises and lacerations of the face, head, and trunk of the body. Attacks are often carefully inflicted on parts of the body that can easily be disguised by clothing. This pattern of proximal location of injuries (breasts, abdomen, upper thighs, and back) rather than distal and patterned injuries (in various stages of healing, in particular configurations matching the body part or object used as a weapon) is characteristic of abuse (Campbell and Sheridan, in press). When a woman has a black eye or bruises about the mouth, the nurse should ask, "Who hit you?" rather than, "What happened to you?" The latter implies that the nurse is neither knowledgeable nor comfortable with violence, and this may prompt the woman to fabricate a more acceptable cause of her injury.

Once abused, women tend to exhibit low self-esteem and depression (Campbell et al, 1997). They have more physical health problems than other women, specifically symptoms such as chronic pain (back, head, abdominal), neurologic problems, problems sleeping, gynecologic symptoms, urinary tract infections, and chronic gastrointestinal problems (Campbell, 2002; Eby et al, 1995). Although the focus tends to be on the victim of the abuse, it is important to note that there are health consequences to the perpetrator as well. These physical and mental health consequences incur health care costs that are preventable (Gerlock, 1999).

### Abuse as a Process
Nursing research by both Landenburger (1998) and Campbell et al (1998) suggests that there is a process of response to battering over time wherein the woman's emotional and behavioral reactions change. At first there is a great need to minimize the seriousness of the situation. The violence usually starts with a slight shove in the middle of a heated argument. All couples fight, and if there is any physical aggression, both the man and the woman tend to blame the incident on something external such as a particularly stressful day at work or drinking too much. The male partner usually apologizes for the incident, and as with any problem in a relationship, the couple tries to improve the situation. Although marital counseling may be useful at this early stage, it is generally contraindicated at all other stages because of the risk to the woman's safety. Unfortunately, abuse tends to escalate in frequency and severity over time, and the man's remorse tends to lessen. The risk is such that women who try to leave an abusive relationship are at significant risk for homicide (Campbell, 1995).

Because women have often been taught to take responsibility for the success of a relationship, they usually go through a period in which they tend to change their behavior to end the violence. They may even blame themselves for infuriating their spouse. Women who blame themselves for provoking the abuse are more likely to have low self-esteem and be depressed than those who do not blame themselves. Some women experience a moral conflict between their need to leave an abusive relationship and their sense that it is their responsibility to maintain relationships (Belknap, 1999). Women find that no matter what they do, the violence continues. During this period, the woman tries to hide the violence because of the stigma attached. She tries to placate her spouse and feels she is losing her sense of self (Landenburger, 1998). She is also typically concerned about her children whether she leaves or stays.

Some abuse escalates to the point that the woman is kept in terror, similar to a prisoner of war (Okun, 1986). She is constantly subjected to emotional degradation, absolute financial dependency, sadistic physical and sexual violence, and control of all her activities. She may fear for her life and that of her children. She is in terror that her partner will try to kill her, her children, or both if she attempts to leave. This fear is, in fact, often justified. Clinically, she may experience learned helplessness, traumatic stress syndrome, or both, and she will need intensive therapy. She may kill herself or her abuser to escape because she sees no other way out (Campbell, 1995). Because of the severity of the abuse, a woman may flee to a shelter to obtain physical safety for herself and her children (Humphreys and Neylan, 1999). As a woman tries to leave, the risk of homicide increases, creating a catch-22: the women feels she will die regardless of whether she stays or leaves the relationship. A nurse encountering severe abuse needs to consider the safety of the woman and her children as the priority. The woman will need an order of protection, a legal document specifically designed to keep the woman's abuser away from her. She will also need help in getting to a safe place, such as a wife abuse shelter in an anonymous location. At the very least, the woman must design a carefully thought-out plan for escape and arrange for a neighbor or an adolescent child to call the police when there is another violent episode.

The more frequently encountered battered woman is one who has tried several times to leave. Each attempt to leave is a gathering of resources, a trial of her children's ability to survive without a father, and a testing of her partner's promises to reform. When and if it becomes clear that he is not going to change and she has the emotional support and the financial resources to do so, she will end the relationship. Often this will involve using a shelter for abused women or individual advocacy and support groups and/or the criminal justice system. A woman often experiences violence while in an abusive relationship and after she has left such a relationship. Successful attempts at leaving abusive relationships may still end in a woman's not being able to collect resources acquired while in the relationship (Kurz, 1996). Regardless of the risk, women have hope for ending the abuse and have the requisite strength to leave abusive relationships (Merritt-Gray and Wuest, 1995).

An alternative to ending the relationship is the male partner's attendance at programs for batterers. These programs have been shown to be most effective if they are court mandated and if the man's underlying values about women are addressed, as well as his violence (Dutton, 1995). Abused women need affirmation, support, reassurances of the normalcy of their responses, accurate information about shelters and legal resources, and brainstorming about possible solutions. These needs can be met by other women in similar situations and by professionals such as nurses (Campbell, 1998). Women should not be pushed into actions they are not ready to take.

After the abuse has ended, a period of recovery ensues. This includes a normal grief response for the relationship that has ended and a search for meaning in the experience (Landenburger, 1998). Thus a formerly battered woman who is feeling depressed and lonely after the relationship has ended is exhibiting a normal response for which support is needed.

### Intimate Partner Sexual Abuse

Campbell and Soeken (1999) report that 45% of battered women are also forced into sexual encounters. The nurse must carefully assess for this form of violence in women in ongoing relationships. Also, between 10% and 14% of all American women have been raped within a marriage. This sexual abuse is usually but not always accompanied by physical abuse.

The notion that men have a right to force their wives to have sex comes from traditional English law that stated that a woman gave irrevocable and perpetual consent to her husband on marriage to have sex whenever and however he wanted. Marital rape was not considered a crime in all of the United States until 1993 (Yllo, 1999). Serious physical and emotional damage has been documented from marital rape. Often women who have come to emergency departments because of abuse have not been screened for forced sex because the issue is considered too intrusive (Campbell and Soeken, 1999). Therefore, like intimate partner violence in the past, marital rape remains a private issue.

There is also an alarming incidence of date rape, the dynamics of which may parallel marital rape. Adolescent boys are more like to perpetrate sexual dating violence than girls (Malik, Sorenson, and Aneshensel, 1997). Young women who have been victims of dating violence experience low self-esteem, depression, anger, and irritability (Shapiro and Schwarz, 1997).

To assess for sexual assault, the question "Have you ever been forced into sex you did not wish to participate in?" should be used in all nursing assessments to see if marital rape, date rape, or rape of a male has occurred.

### Abuse During Pregnancy

Battering during pregnancy has serious implications for the health of both women and their children. Approximately one of six pregnant women is physically battered during pregnancy, with a larger proportion (20%) of adolescents abused during pregnancy than adult women. Although abuse during pregnancy occurs across ethnic groups, white women experience a significantly higher severity of abuse than African-American or Hispanic women (McFarlane and Parker, 1994). These women are at risk for spontaneous abortion, premature delivery, low-birth-weight infants, substance abuse during pregnancy, and depression (McFarlane, Parker, and Soeken, 1994). Abuse before pregnancy often precedes abuse during pregnancy (see the Evidence-Based Practice box). A man's control of contraception, a form of abusive controlling, may lead to unintended pregnancy and subsequent abuse. In addition, a man's refusal to use of a condom places a woman at an increased risk of sexually transmitted diseases, including infection with human immunodeficiency virus (HIV) (Campbell and Campbell, 1995; Eby et al, 1995).

### Evidence-Based Practice

Nursing researchers evaluated the safety behaviors of equal numbers of Hispanic, African-American, and white women abused during pregnancy (*n* = 132) who received a 10-minute nursing intervention for domestic violence three times during pregnancy. There was a significant increase in each of the 15 safety behaviors (such as hiding money and car keys, asking neighbors to call the police, removing weapons) over time, with the largest increase after the first intervention (outcomes were measured twice during pregnancy and three times in the postpartum year).

**Nurse Use:** Because one out of six women is abused during pregnancy, nurses need to provide this tested intervention to increase safety for the women and their infants.

McFarlane J et al: Safety behaviors of abused women after an intervention during pregnancy, *J Obstet Gynecol Neonat Nurs* 27(1):64, 1998.

Generally, the same dynamics of coercive control operate when a woman is battered during pregnancy. In one in-depth study of 76 battered women, about one third (36%) said that they were subject to the same abuse whether or not they were pregnant. About 20% escaped abuse during pregnancy, although they were abused again after the baby was born. Another 35% indicated that their perception of the reason for abuse during pregnancy was that their partner was jealous of or angry at the baby (Campbell et al, 1998). It could be anticipated that this group of infants would be at particularly high risk of child abuse after they are born. The main difference found between women who were battered during pregnancy and those who were not was that those women battered during pregnancy had been battered more frequently and severely previous to their pregnancy (Campbell et al, 1998). The clear implication is that all pregnant women should be assessed for abuse at each prenatal care visit, and postpartum home visits should include assessment for child abuse and partner abuse. In as many as 77% of families where there is severe wife abuse, there is also child abuse (Straus and Gelles, 1990).

### Abuse of Older Adults

**Older adult abuse** is a form of family violence that is becoming more apparent. About 3% to 6% of senior citizens suffer from some form of abuse, neglect, or exploitation (Comijs et al, 1998). Like spouse abuse and child abuse, most cases of older adult abuse go unreported. As with other forms of human abuse, older adult maltreatment includes emotional, sexual, and physical neglect, as well as physical and sexual violence; financial abuse and violation of rights are particular issues for elders. A major difference is that experts and the public agree that a single incidence of maltreatment connotes elder abuse (Hudson and Carlson, 1998).

### Types of Older Adult Abuse

Older adults are neglected when others fail to provide adequate food, clothing, shelter, and physical care and to meet physiological, emotional, and safety needs. Older adult neglect either through lack of care or improper care can be considered criminal neglect. In addition, violation of an older adult's rights, medical abuse, and abandonment are considered elder abuse (Kleinschmidt, 1997). Older adults are also at risk for financial abuse through fraud, coercion to relinquish property rights, and money mismanagement (Wilber and Reynolds, 1996).

Roughness in handling older adults can lead to bruises and bleeding into body tissues because of the fragility of their skin and vascular systems. It is often difficult to determine if the injuries of older adults result from abuse, falls, or other natural causes. Careful assessment both through observation and discussion can help in determining the cause of injuries. Other physical abuse occurs when caregivers impose unrealistic toileting demands, and when the special needs and previous living patterns of the person are ignored.

Older adults can also be abused with regard to nutrition. They may be given food that they cannot chew or swallow or that is contraindicated because of dietary restrictions. Caregivers may overlook food preferences or social or cultural beliefs and patterns about food. Older adults may become undernourished if they can neither prepare their own food nor eat the food that is prepared for them.

Caregivers occasionally give older adults medication to induce confusion or drowsiness so that they will be less troublesome, will need less care, or will allow others to gain control of their financial and personal resources. Once medicated, older adults have few ways to act on their own behalf.

The most common form of psychological abuse is rejection or simply ignoring older adults. This kind of treatment conveys that they are worthless and useless to others. Older adults may subsequently regress and become increasingly dependent on others, who tend to resent the imposition and demands on their time and lifestyles. The pattern becomes cyclical: the more regressed the person becomes, the greater the dependence. Further, older adult's past accomplishments and present abilities are not consistently acknowledged, causing them to feel even less capable. Indicators of actual or potential older adult abuse follow.

### Precipitating Factors for Older Adult Abuse

Caregivers abuse older adults for a variety of reasons. Older family members may impose a physical, emotional, or financial burden on the caregiver, leading to frustration and resentment. In another scenario, earlier family patterns may now be reversed—that is, the older adult may have formerly been the abuser (Baron and Welty, 1996).

---

> **HOW TO** **Identify Potential or Actual Older Adult Abuse**
>
> - Financial mismanagement
> - Withdrawal and passivity
> - Depression
> - Unexplained or repeated physical injuries
> - Untreated health problems such as decubitus ulcers
> - Poor nutrition
> - Unexplained genital infections
> - Physical neglect and unmet basic needs
> - Social isolation
> - Rejection of assistance by caregiver
> - Lack of compliance to health regimens
>
> ---
>
> Baron S, Welty A: Elder abuse, *J Gerontol Soc Work* 25(1/2):33, 1996; Butler RN: Warning signs of elder abuse, *Geriatrics* 54(3):3-4, 1999; Wilber KH, Reynolds SL: Introducing a framework for defining financial abuse of the elderly, *J Elder Abuse Negl* 8(2):61-80, 1996.

Many people tend to think of abused older adults as dependent on others for their care. A factor that increases the risk of older adult abuse is the dependency of a significant other on the older adult (Baron and Welty, 1996). Spouses who batter continue to abuse as they age. Therefore, many female abused older adults are battered women who have become old. Additionally, children who have lived in abusive households learn that behavior. Thus, although it is important to assess for elder abuse when older adults are in need of care from family members, all older adults should be assessed for abuse.

Confused and frail older adults are a high-risk group for abuse. Large numbers of frail older adults, many with serious physical or mental impairments, live in the community and are cared for by their families. Also, those with cognitive impairments such as Alzheimer's disease and other dementias have a greater risk for physical abuse than older adults with other illnesses. These illnesses place a high burden on the caregiver, with subsequent caregiver depression (Lachs et al, 1997). Living with and providing care to a confused older adult is difficult. The round-the-clock tasks often exhaust family members. In addition, patients with Alzheimer's may become verbally and even physically aggressive as part of their illness, which may trigger retaliatory violence. Family stress increases as members must work harder to fulfill their other responsibilities in addition to the needs of the older adults.

In addition, when families are planning to take care of an older family member at home, nurses must help them fully evaluate that decision and prepare for the stressors that will be involved. A plan for regular respite care is essential. Strategies for the primary and secondary prevention of abuse of older adults include victim support groups, senior advocacy volunteer programs, and training for providers working with older adults (Wolf, Pillemer, and Wilson, 1994).

Elderly people need to retain as much autonomy and decision-making ability as possible. Nurses have many ways to detect elder abuse, and they have the skills and responsibility for discovering it, giving treatment, and making referrals. Many families who care for older adult members exhaust their resources and coping ability. Nurses can help them find new sources of support and aid.

# NURSING INTERVENTIONS
## Primary Prevention

To prevent violence and human abuse, a community approach is essential. First, the community can take a stand against violence and make sure their elected officials and the local media consider nonviolence a priority. Public education programs can educate communities about different forms of violence and ways to get help and intervene (www.FVPF.org; Klein et al, 1997). Nurses as community advocates can help with this process. In the legislative arena, laws are needed to outlaw physical punishment in schools and marital rape. State laws can enforce mandatory arrest for abusers, which has been shown to decrease repeat offenses, at least for men who are employed and well connected in their communities (Edleson and Tolman, 1992). Court-mandated batterer intervention that is carefully monitored by the community has also been found to increase the effectiveness of such intervention.

Strong community sanctions against violence in the home can reduce abuse levels (Counts et al, 1999). Neighbors can watch what is happening and work together to address problems in other families; this is not an invasion of privacy but a sign of community cohesiveness. Nurses can work with advocate groups to make sure police deal with assault within marriage as swiftly, surely, and severely as assault between strangers. Nurses can encourage others to interfere when they see children beaten in a grocery store, notice that an older adult is not being properly cared for, see a neighborhood bully beat up his classmates, or hear a neighbor hitting his wife.

Second, people can take measures to reduce their vulnerability to violence by improving the physical security of their homes and learning personal defense measures. Nurses can encourage people to keep windows and doors locked, trim shrubs around their homes, and keep lights on during high-crime periods. Many neighborhoods organize crime watch programs and post signs to that effect. Other signs indicate that certain homes will assist children who need help; these homes are identified by the sign of a hand, usually posted in a window. Other neighbors informally agree to monitor one another's property and safety. Also, many law enforcement agencies evaluate homes for security and teach individual or neighborhood safety programs. Individuals install home security systems, participate in personal defense pro-grams such as judo or karate, and purchase firearms for their protection.

Unfortunately, handguns are far more likely to kill family members than intruders (Kellerman et al, 1993). Firearm accidents are a leading cause of death for young children, and handguns kept in the home are unfortunately easy to use in moments of extreme anger with other family members or in extreme depression. The majority of homicides between family members and most suicides involve a handgun. Nursing assessments should include a question about guns kept in the home. The family should be made aware of the risk that a handgun holds for family members. If the family thinks that keeping a gun is necessary, safety measures should be taught, such as keeping the gun unloaded and in a locked compartment, keeping the ammunition separate from the gun and also locked away, and instructing children about the dangers of firearms. Lobbying for handgun-control laws is a primary prevention effort that can significantly decrease the rate of death and serious injury caused by handguns in the United States.

### Assessment for Risk Factors

Identification of risk factors is an important part of primary prevention. Although abuse cannot be predicted with certainty, several factors influence the onset and support the continuation of abusive patterns. Nurses can identify potential victims of abuse because they see clients in a variety of settings. Factors to include in an assessment for individual or family violence, or for potential family violence, are categorized by Logan and Dawkins as illustrated in Figure 37-1 (Logan and Dawkins, 1986). Both individual and familial factors must be assessed within the context of the larger community (Gelles, 1997; Gullotta and McElhaney, 1999; Tajima, 2002). Factors that must be included are found in Box 37-2.

> **WHAT DO YOU THINK?**
>
> Most experts on violence agree that all women entering the health care system should be asked about domestic violence and sexual assault experience; yet men are also victimized by violence, even though little is known about their responses to such experiences. Some experts think that health care professionals should ask men if they are perpetrators of violence as a secondary prevention activity, reasoning that if identified early, such behavior may be more amenable to interventions. Others are concerned that since it is not certain what health care system interventions are most effective for male perpetrators or victims of violence, it is premature to do routine screening. There is also some concern that perpetrators of domestic violence or child abuse may become angry if asked about their violent behavior and retaliate against the family member.

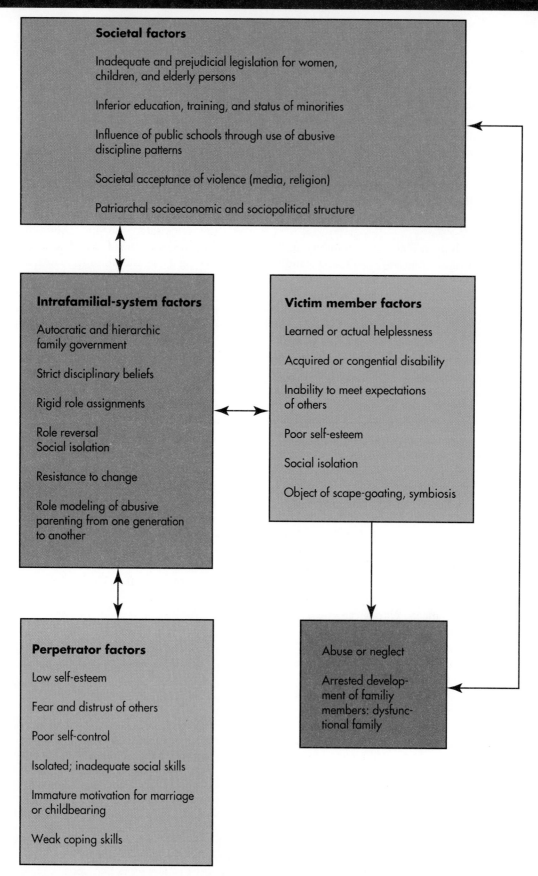

**Figure 37-1** Factors to include when assessing an individual's or a family's potential for violence.

## BOX 37-2  Assessing for Violence in a Community Context

### INDIVIDUAL FACTORS

- Signs of physical abuse (abrasions, contusions, burns)
- Physical symptoms related to emotional distress
- Developmental and behavioral difficulties
- Presence of physical disability
- Social isolation
- Decreased role performance within the family, and in job or school-related activities
- Mental health problems such as depression, low self-esteem, and anxiety
- Fear of intimate others
- Substance abuse

### FAMILIAL FACTORS

- Economic stressors
- Presence of some form of family violence
- Poor communication
- Problems with child rearing
- Lack of family cohesion
- Recurrent familial conflict
- Lack of social support networks
- Poor social integration into the community
- Multiple changes of residence
- Access to guns
- Homelessness

### COMMUNITY CHARACTERISTICS

- High crime rate
- High levels of unemployment
- Lack of neighborhood resources and support systems
- Lack of community cohesiveness

## BOX 37-3  Levels of Prevention Related to Violence

### PRIMARY PREVENTION

Strengthen individual and family by teaching parenting skills.

### SECONDARY PREVENTION

Reduce or end abuse by early screening; teach families how to deal with stress and how to have fun and enjoy recreation.

### TERTIARY PREVENTION

When signs of abuse are evident, refer client to appropriate community organizations.

## BOX 37-4  Prevention Strategies for Violence

### PREVENTION STRATEGIES AT THE INDIVIDUAL/FAMILY LEVEL AND AT THE COMMUNITY LEVEL

**Individual and Family Levels**

- Assessment during routine examination (secondary)
- Assessment for marital discord (secondary)
- Education on developmental stages and needs of children (primary)
- Counseling for at-risk parents (secondary)
- Teaching parenting techniques (primary)
- Assistance with controlling anger (secondary)
- Treatment for substance abuse (tertiary)
- Teach stress-reduction techniques (primary)

**Community Level**

- Develop policy
- Conduct community resource mapping
- Collaborate with community to develop systemic response to violence
- Develop media campaign
- Develop resources such as transition housing and shelters

## Individual and Family Strategies for Primary Prevention

Primary prevention of violence can take place through community, family, and individual interventions (Boxes 37-3 and 37-4). Nurses, in their work in schools, community groups, employee groups, day-care centers, and other community institutions, can foster healthy developmental patterns and identify signs of potential abuse. For example, nurses may take part in media campaigns that identify risk factors for abuse. Nurses can be at the forefront of developing after-school programs and late-night programs that support young people in using their energies toward positive goals and in developing a constructive support network. Through capacity mapping of community resources, nurses can assist in identifying community needs (see the Nursing Tip box). The identification of strengths and weaknesses can assist in

### NURSING TIP

It is not difficult to assess for intimate partner violence. You might use the following questions:

- Is somebody hurting you?
- You seem frightened by your partner. Has he hurt you?
- Did someone you know do this to you?

determining future goals and needed interventions for the good of the community.

Primary prevention of abuse includes strengthening individuals and families so they can cope more effectively with multiple life stressors and demands, and reducing the destructive elements in the community that support and encourage violence. Providing support and psychological enrichment to at-risk individuals and families often prevents the onset of health disruption. For example, nurses can strengthen and teach parenting abilities. Basic skills such as diapering, feeding, quieting, and even holding and rocking a baby can be the focus of a class or home or clinic visit. Parents also need to learn acceptable and effective ways to discipline children so that limits are maintained without causing the child emotional or physical harm.

Mutual support groups are valuable for new parents, families with special children, or abused people themselves. Such groups have variable formats and can provide information, support, and encouragement. Nurses can help begin such groups or can actually serve as group leaders. Chapter 23 describes the role of the nurse in working with community groups.

## Secondary Prevention

When abuse occurs, nurses can initiate measures to reduce or terminate further abuse. Both developmental and situational crises present opportunities for abusive situations to develop. On a community level, nurses must form collaborative relationships to provide health services for battered women (Campbell et al, 1999). Researchers must work effectively with community agencies to use current research to screen for domestic violence and to use model treatments that have a positive effect on decreasing domestic violence (Edleson and Bible, 1998; Hausman, Spivak, and Prothrow-Stith, 1995).

Nurses can be primary leaders in the development of screening practices in the health care arena. The development of training programs for health care providers can be an effective step in identifying and treating victims of violence. Nurses can work closely with shelters in identifying the needs of individuals who seek sanctuary from abusive situations.

On a family level, nursing intervention can help family members discuss problems and seek ways to deal with the tension that led to the abusive situations. Injured persons must be temporarily or permanently placed in a safe location. Secondary preventive measures are most useful when potential abusers recognize their tendency to be abusive and seek help. For children, there is often a need for 24-hour child protection services or caregivers who can take care of the child until the acute family or individual crisis is resolved. Respite care is extremely important in families with frail older adult family members. Telephone crisis lines can be used to provide immediate emergency assistance to families.

Effective communication with abusive families is important. Typically, these families do not want to discuss their problems and many are embarrassed to be involved in an abusive situation. Often a lot of guilt is involved. Effective communication must be preceded by an attitude of acceptance. It is often difficult for nurses to value the worth of an individual who willfully abuses another. The behavior, not the person, must be condemned.

Additionally, families do not always know how to have fun. Nurses can assess how much recreation is integrated into the family's lifestyle. Through community assessment, nurses know what resources and facilities are available and how much they cost. Families may need counseling about the value of recreation and play in reducing tension and appropriately channeling aggressive impulses.

## Tertiary Prevention: Therapeutic Intervention With Abusive Families

Although it may be hard to form a trusting relationship with abusive families, nurses can act as a case manager, coordinating the other agencies and activities involved. Principles of giving care to families who are experiencing violence include the following:
- Intolerance for violence
- Respect and caring for all family members
- Safety as the first priority
- Absolute honesty
- Empowerment

Nurses must clearly indicate that any further violence, degradation, and exploitation of family members will not be tolerated, but that all family members are respected, valued human beings. However, everyone must understand that the safety of every family member is the first priority.

Abusers often fear they will be condemned for their actions, so it is often difficult to make and maintain contact with abusive families. Although nurses convey an attitude of caring and concern for them, families may doubt the sincerity of this concern. They may avoid being home at the scheduled visit time out of fear of the consequences of the visit or an inability to believe that anyone really wants to help them. If the victim is a child, parents may fear that the nurse will try to remove the child.

Nurses are mandatory reporters of child abuse, even when only suspected, in all states. They are also mandatory reporters of elder abuse and abuse of other physically and cognitively dependent adults as well as of felony assaults of anyone in most states. The mandatory reporting laws also protect reporters from legal action on cases that are never substantiated. Even so, physicians and nurses are sometimes reluctant to report abuse. They may be more willing to report abuse in a poor family than in a middle-class one, or they may think that an older adult or child is better off at home than in a nursing home or foster home. Referral to protective service agencies should be viewed as enlisting another source of help, rather than an automatic step toward removal of the victim or criminal justice action. This same attitude can be communicated to families, so that reporting is done with families rather than without their knowledge and prior input. Absolute honesty about what will be reported to officials, what the family can expect, what the nurse is entering into records, and what the nurse is feeling is essential.

To further empower the family, the nurse needs to recognize and capitalize on the violent family's strengths, as well as to assess and deal with its problems. The nurse must use a nurse–family partnership rather than a paternalistic or authoritarian approach. Families can often generate many of their own solutions, which tend to be more culturally appropriate and individualized than those the nurse generates. Victims of direct attack need information about their options and resources and reassurance that abuse is unfortunately rather common and that they are not alone in their dilemma. They also need reassurance that their responses are normal and that they do not deserve to be abused. Continued support for their decisions must be coupled with nursing actions to ensure their safety.

## Nursing Actions

The nurse can meet the family's therapeutic needs in a variety of ways. Besides referral to appropriate community agencies, nurses can act as role models for the family. During clinic and home visits, nurses can demonstrate constructive adult–child interactions. Nurses often teach mothers childcare skills such as proper feeding, calming a fretful child, effective discipline, and constructive communication.

Nurses can demonstrate good communication skills and discipline by teaching both parents and children in a calm, respectful, and informative manner. Caregivers, especially those caring for children, handicapped people, or older adults, may need to learn age-appropriate expectations. It is unreasonable to expect a 14-month-old infant to differentiate between right and wrong. Children at this age do not deliberately annoy caregivers by breaking delicate pieces of china. Likewise, a person with poor sphincter control does not willingly soil clothes or bedding.

Role modeling can be used with abuse victims of all ages. When providing nursing care to abused spouses or to older adults, nurses can demonstrate communication skills, conflict resolution, and skill training. For example, adult children often become abusive toward their older parents when they become frustrated in trying to care for them. During home visits, nurses can show how to physically and psychologically care for the relative. The nurse can work with caregivers to help them develop approaches that are acceptable to the individual older adult. Assessment, creativity, and critical thinking help the nurse, family, and client learn how to meet client and family needs without causing undue stress and frustration.

The emotional investment and sheer drain of energy required to effectively work with abusers and victims of abuse cannot be disregarded. Abusers present difficult clinical challenges because of their reluctance to seek help or to remain actively involved in the helping process.

Referral is an important component of tertiary prevention. Nurses should know about available community resources for abuse victims and perpetrators. Some of these

**BOX 37-5  Common Community Services**

- Child protective services
- Child abuse prevention programs
- Adult protective services
- Parents Anonymous
- Wife abuse shelter
- Program for children of battered women
- Community support group
- 24-hour hotline
- Legal advocacy or information
- State coalition against domestic violence
- Batterer treatment
- Victim assistance programs
- Sexual assault programs

resources are listed in Box 37-5. If attitudes and resources are inadequate, it is often helpful to work with local radio and television stations and newspapers to provide information about the nature and extent of human abuse as a community health problem. This also helps to acquaint people with available services and resources. Frequently, people do not seek services early in an abusive situation because they simply do not know what is available to them. Ideally, a program or plan for abused people begins with a needs assessment to identify potential clients and to determine how to effectively serve this group. Nurses can help to get programs started and provide public education.

## Nursing Interventions Specific to Female Partner Abuse

Women in abusive relationships most often seek care for injuries in an emergency setting, a physician's office, or a prenatal clinic. These women may be seeking assistance for injuries sustained during physically abusive episodes (Dearwater et al, 1998), but even more often they are in the health care system for other health problems. Despite the overall incidence of battering and its resultant physical and emotional health problems for women, health professionals, even those in emergency departments, often fail to identify abused women and are often seen as paternalistic, judgmental, insensitive, and less effective and helpful than they could be.

**NURSING TIP**

Capacity mapping can be both an approach and a tool for community assessment. It is an approach to planning based on building on community strengths rather than responding to deficits. As a tool, it is a method for identifying talents, skills, and resources within a community.

Because of the stigma involved, women and health care providers may hesitate to initiate discussion about abuse. However, the majority of battered women say they would have liked to talk about the issue with a health care professional if they were asked (King and Ryan, 1996). Because abuse develops slowly, starting with minor psychological abuse and building to more severe physical incidents, it often goes unrecognized by victims and health care providers alike until a severe episode occurs.

The quality of health care that a battered woman receives often determines whether she follows through with referrals to legal, social service, and health care agencies. In emergency departments, at least 15% of adult female clients have been physically or sexually abused by a partner or ex-partner (Dearwater et al, 1998). Care in the emergency department is often fragmented and necessarily oriented toward life-and-death situations. Therefore women may not be adequately assessed and often receive little or no specific emotional support or intervention. A cycle persists in which women seek care and receive either no interventions or ineffective interventions. This cycle perpetuates feelings of anger and inadequacy in health care providers, resulting in blame placed on women for their lack of compliance to remedies offered.

Managed care and clinic settings may be the best places to routinely screen for domestic violence. Between 10% and 25% of adult women in these primary care settings have been physically abused within the last year (Campbell, 1998). If battered women can be identified in those settings, perhaps effective interventions can be provided that will prevent the kind of serious injury that later results in emergency department visits or even a homicide (see the Evidence-Based Practice box on p. 887).

However, some battered women hesitate to identify themselves as victims of domestic violence for several reasons. They may fear that revelation will further jeopardize their safety by increasing the violence, and they may also feel that it will increase their sense of shame and humiliation. This hesitation to speak out often makes it difficult for health care professionals to identify the battered woman. In addition, the nature of the systems in which victims of violence introduce themselves can be barriers. Emergency departments, clinics, managed care settings, and health departments are busy places. Staff members work hard to maintain the functioning of these facilities. Sometimes it is difficult in such chaotic settings for staff members to realize their importance as the first or only health provider to recognize violence in their clients' lives, and that women need them to take the time to deal with this issue (Senter, 1993).

Studies have found that only a small percentage of battered women in emergency departments and other health care settings were identified as such and treated for the abuse, despite the significant prevalence (Dearwater et al, 1998). Battered women present for treatment in a number of ways, including physical complaints (such as not being able to sleep or chronic pain) related to the chronic stress of living in an abusive situation or to old injuries. They may be unaware of the relationship of their symptoms to the violence in their lives. Therefore professional nursing organizations (American Nurses Association; Emergency Nurses Association; Association of Women's Health, Obstetric and Neonatal Nurses; American College of Nurse-Midwives) recommend that all women be routinely screened for domestic violence each time they come to a health care setting. For the battered woman and the staff to begin to make the connection between her life situation and the presenting complaints, the nurse needs to ask direct questions in a supportive, open, and concerned manner (Hattendorf and Tollerud, 1997).

### Assessment

Assessment for all forms of violence against women should therefore take place for all women entering the health care system. The assessment should be ongoing and confidential. A thorough assessment gathers information on physical, emotional, and sexual trauma from violence, risk for future abuse, cultural background and beliefs, perceptions of the woman's relationships with others, and stated needs. The assessment should be conducted in private. Other adults who are present should be directed to the waiting area and told that it is policy that initially women are seen alone. Women should be asked directly if they were in an abusive relationship as a child or are currently in an abusive relationship as an adult. They should also be asked if they have ever been forced into sex that they did not wish to participate in. Shame and fear often make disclosure difficult. Verbal acknowledgment of the situation and emotional and physical support assist women in talking about past or current circumstances.

Women can be categorized into three groups: no, low, or moderate to high risk. Women with no signs of current or past abuse are considered at no risk. However, future visits should include questioning a woman about whether there have been any changes in her life or whether she has additional information or questions about topics discussed at previous visits. If there is a new intimate partner in her life, she should again be screened for abuse. The abuse assessment screen (AAS) is a four-question screen that has been successfully used in almost every kind of health care setting and can be downloaded from the Nursing Network on Violence Against Women International (NNVAWI) website (www.nnvawi.org).

Women at low risk show no evidence of recent or current abuse. Education that helps a woman gain perspective on her situation and her needs should be discussed. Resource materials including group and individual formats can be suggested. The risk level should be recorded, and preventive measures and teaching should be documented.

Assessment of moderate to high risk includes evaluation of a woman's fear for both psychological and physical abuse. Lethality potential should be assessed (Campbell, 1995) and can be done with the danger assessment, also available at the NNVAWI website. Risk factors for lethality include behaviors such as stalking or frequent harassment, threats or an escalation of threats, use of weapons or threats with weapons, excessive control and jealousy, and forced sex. Statements from an abuser such as "If I can't have you, no one can" should be taken seriously. In all cases, a history of abuse and alcohol and drug use should be collected and carefully documented. The determined risk level should also be documented along with any past or present physical evidence of abuse from prior or current assault; this evidence should be photographed, shown on a body map, or described narratively. It is important that the assailant be identified in the record; this can take the form of either quotes from the woman or subjective information. These records can be very important for women in future assault or child custody cases, even if the woman is not ready to make a police report at the present time.

Immediate care for a woman in a potentially harmful or present abusive situation involves the development of a safety plan. A woman can be assisted to look at the options available to her. Shelter information, access to counseling, and legal resources should be discussed. If a woman wants to return to her partner, she can be helped in the development of plans that can be carried out if the abuse continues or becomes more serious.

Whenever there is evidence of sexual assault within the prior 24 to 48 hours, a rape kit examination should be performed. Lists of resources such as rape crisis clinics and support groups for survivors of physical and emotional abuse should be made available.

### Prevention

Prevention, public policy, and social attitudes are intertwined. Our society has taken a major step toward the secondary prevention of abuse through the establishment of programs that encourage women and children to speak about their experiences. Nurses need to support these programs further by believing the experiences they are told. In the development of laws that punish child and woman abuse, society has given some support to the victims of abuse. Often, however, the victims are again victimized by disbelief of their experiences, a devaluing of the effects of these assaults, and a focus on assisting the perpetrators of the crimes. Primary prevention includes a social attitudinal change. Both girls and boys need to be taught human values of interdependence, respect for human life, and a commitment to empathy and strength in the development of the human species regardless of sex, race, or socioeconomic status. We must urge continued progress toward eliminating the feminization of poverty and ensuring gender parity in economic resources. In addition, local communities must make it clear that violence against women is not tolerated by eliminating pornography, mandating arrests of abusers, and creating a general climate of nonviolence.

Abused women need assistance in making decisions and taking control of their lives. Community-oriented nurses, prenatal nurses, planned parenthood, primary care, and emergency department nurses are involved with women when they can be screened for the presence or absence of abuse. Mechanisms for screening women who are either abused or at risk for abuse are available (Soeken et al, 1998). To intervene effectively, nurses must understand abuse as a cumulative process that must be examined as a continuum within the context of a relationship. During this process, the abuse, the relationship, and a woman's view of changes within herself require time-specific interventions. Women are often blamed and held responsible for the abuse inflicted on them by their male partners (Landenburger, 1998). When this happens, either they are assisted in a way that discounts their feelings and further devalues them, or the abuse is ignored.

### Strategies Addressing Education for Health Professionals

A variety of strategies have been reported that address the knowledge deficit of health practitioners on abuse issues. The National March of Dimes Birth Defects Foundation has sponsored a variety of training sessions for health professionals and produced an excellent training manual that addresses violence against women and battering during pregnancy (McFarlane and Parker, 1994). The recommended nursing intervention was tested experimentally, and the safety behaviors of battered women who received the intervention increased significantly throughout the pregnancy and 1 year after the birth (McFarlane et al, 1998).

Campbell et al (2001) demonstrated that a system change model of training and environmental change for emergency departments (EDs) was an effective means of increasing staff's knowledge and attitudes about domestic violence and women's satisfaction with care in the ED. After inception of a hospital-based family violence program housed in an urban ED, Sheridan (1998) demonstrated that the number of identified positive and probable battered women rose from 242 in 1986 to 337 in 1987—approximately a 40% increase in identification. The program included ongoing inservice training of all emergency department personnel including nonmedical support staff (i.e., unit secretaries, housekeepers, and security guards), as well as daily chart audits and telephone follow-up calls.

## VIOLENCE AND THE PRISON POPULATION

Sexual assault is commonplace in U.S. prisons. Few studies have been conducted on the prevalence of sexual assault in the female population. The prevalence is higher in the male population than in the female prison population. For women, the context in which sexual assault takes place is not clearly understood. Browne, Miller, and Maguin (1999) report that women in prison have a history of violence that is much greater than that of the general population of women. The majority of women who have experienced abuse in prison have a history of experiencing multiple types of abuse as a child and as an adult (Bradley and Davino, 2002; Leonard, 2001). Currently, a significant number of women are imprisoned for killing their male partners. Prior to committing homicide, many of these women tried to utilize the social resources available to them. For many of these women, the homicide of their partners was an act of desperation that resulted from a system that failed to support them in remaining safe in their own homes. Nurses working in prisons must be aware of the complex histories of the prison population. It is essential to develop resources that can respond to the multiple social needs of prisoners. Discharge planning for women leaving prison is essential, as is assisting them to identify transition behaviors and resources that will decrease the likelihood of violence.

## CLINICAL FORENSIC NURSING

Clinical forensic nursing is a relatively new specialty that has an interesting history and pattern of development. This field is defined as the "application of clinical and scientific knowledge to questions of law and the civil or criminal investigation of survivors of traumatic injury and/or patient treatment involving court-related issues" (Lynch, 1993, p. 8). John Butts, chief medical examiner for Alberta, Canada, established in 1975 a program using registered nurses as medical examiner investigators. He did this because he saw that nurses had a good education in medical terminology and pharmacology, and they had the ability to be sensitive and communicate effectively with grieving families. As has been shown in this chapter, trauma as a result of violence is a growing public health problem. Many people who survive trauma are considered to be living forensic patients in contrast to earlier descriptions of forensics that dealt primarily with death.

Forensic means pertaining to the law. Currently, forensic specialists evaluate and assess victims of rape, drug and alcohol addiction, domestic violence, assaults, automobile or pedestrian accidents, incest, medical malpractice, and the injuries associated with food and drug tampering (Lynch, 1995; Sheridan, 2001). Although much of the work in forensic nursing occurs in the ED, there is clearly a community-oriented nursing role in primary prevention as well as in follow-up of clients seen.

A client who is admitted to a hospital with traumatic injuries should be evaluated as to the potentially forensic nature of the injuries. The response to victims of assault includes a number of steps (Box 37-6). The nurse most often comes in contact with police, victims, and perpetrators of violence or crime in the emergency department. The nurse provides a vital link between the investigative process, health care, and the court (Lynch, 1995). There are specific actions that nurses should take when they come in contact with victims. It is important that evidence be collected in such a way that the collection itself protects rather than destroys or alters the evidence. For example, when cutting a shirt off a victim who has been shot in the chest, be sure to not cut through the bullet hole in the shirt. Rather, cut to the side of the hole to protect the point of origin of the bullet for later criminal investigation.

---

**BOX 37-6** **Emergency Response to Assault Victims**

1. Use standardized medical treatment and forensic protocols
2. Assess for sexual assault (using "forced sex" terminology rather than "rape" or "sexual assault"), and call sexual assault nurse examiner if appropriate
3. Support privacy of assault victim
4. Explain procedures clearly to the assault victim
5. Document location, date, and time of assault
6. Collect evidence in a systematic format; take pictures if necessary
7. Take care not to destroy evidence while giving care
8. Maintain chain of evidence
9. Maintain evidence integrity
10. Document the following:
    a. Injuries
    b. Emotional state
    c. Medical history
    d. Victim's account of assault
11. Identify and refer to resources to be used after the assault

Ledray LE: *Sexual assault nurse examiner: development and operation guide,* Washington, DC, 1999, U.S. Department of Justice, available at http://www.ojp. usdoj.gov/ovc/publications/infores/sane/saneguide.pdf; Parnis D, DuMont J: Examining the standardized application of rape kits: an exploratory study of post-sexual assault professional practices, *Health Care Women Int* 23:846-853, 2002.

---

The most common types of evidence are clothing, bullets, bloodstains, hairs, fibers, and small pieces of material such as fragments of metal, glass, paint, and wood. Lynch (1995) provides detailed guidelines about how to process clothing: what to look for, how to document what is found, how to remove the clothes and preserve them, and how to determine who should have custody of the clothes. She also describes what is called the chain of custody, which means who gets control of items that may provide evidence about what happened. She gives an in-depth description of wound characteristics and how they should be handled.

According to Lynch (1995, pp. 496-497), implementation of the clinical forensic nursing role includes the ability to do the following:

- Develop the appropriate forensic protocols in compliance with accreditation standards
- Triage clients at risk for forensic injuries
- Report to proper legal agencies
- Document, collect, and preserve evidence
- Secure evidence and maintain the chain of custody

- Serve as liaison between the health care institution, law enforcement agencies, and medical examiner/coroner, and make referrals when medical treatment and/or crisis intervention is required

Maintaining an index of suspicion is important. Community-oriented nurses, like their colleagues in the emergency department, have many opportunities to observe for signs of violence and to determine if the injuries occurred from natural or unnatural causes. Prevention is a key antiviolence strategy. Nurses should observe for injuries, listen for conversation that would suggest that violence is present in the family or that the potential for violence is great, and be aware of risk factors and compare them to the characteristics of the people with whom they work. It is believed that violence is underreported, and this may be particularly true for rape. For this reason, assessment, observation, and evaluation must always be present.

## Practice Application

Mrs. Smith, a 75-year-old bedridden woman, consistently became rude and combative when her daughter, Mary, attempted to bathe her and change her clothes each morning. During a home visit, Mary told the nurse, Mrs. Jones, that she had gotten so frustrated with her mother on the previous morning that she had hit her. Mary felt terrible about her behavior. She stressed that her mother's incontinence made it essential that she be kept clean; her clothes had to be changed every day for her own safety and physical well-being.

    A. How should Mrs. Jones respond to this disclosure?
    B. What specific nursing actions should be taken?
    C. What ongoing services does the nurse need to provide?

---

**Answers are in the back of the book.**

## Key Points

- Violence and human abuse are not new phenomena, but they have increasingly become community health concerns.
- Communities throughout the United States are angry and frustrated about increasing levels of violence.
- Nurses can evaluate and intervene in incidents of community and family violence; to intervene effectively, the nurse must understand the dynamics of violence and human abuse.
- Factors influencing social and community violence include changing social conditions, economic conditions, population density, community facilities, and institutions within a community, such as organized religion, education, the mass communication media, and work.
- The potential for violence against individuals or against oneself is directly related to the level of violence in the community. Identification and correc-

tion of factors affecting the level of violence in the community constitute one way of reducing violence against family members and other individuals.

- Violence and abuse of family members can happen to any family member: spouse, older adult, child, or developmentally disabled person.
- People who abuse family members were often themselves abused and react poorly to real or perceived crises. Other factors that characterize the abuser are the way the person was raised and the unique character of that person.
- Child abuse can be physical, emotional, or sexual. Incest is a common and particularly destructive form of child abuse.
- Spouse abuse is usually wife abuse. It involves physical, emotional, and, frequently, sexual abuse within a context of coercive control. It usually increases in severity and frequency and can escalate to homicide of either partner.
- Nurses are in an excellent position to identify potential victims of family abuse because they see clients in a variety of settings, such as schools, businesses, homes, and clinics. Treatment of family abuse includes primary, secondary, and tertiary prevention and therapeutic intervention.

## Clinical Decision-Making Activities

1. For 1 week, keep a log or diary related to violence.
   a. Make a note of each time you feel as though you are losing your temper. Consider what it might take to cause you to react in a violent way.
   b. Think back. When was the last time you had a violent outburst? What precipitated it? What were your thoughts? What were your feelings? How might you have handled the situation or those feelings without reacting in a violent way?
   c. During this same week, make note of the episodes of violent behaviors you observe. For example, do parents hit children in the supermarket? What seems to precipitate such outbursts? What alternatives might exist for reacting in a less violent way?
2. If you learned, after a careful assessment of your community, that family violence is a significant community health problem, what plan of action might you take to intervene? Remember that the goal is to promote health. Outline a plan of action with objectives, timetables, implementation strategies, and evaluation plans for intervening in family violence in your community.
3. Complete a partial community assessment to determine the actual incidence and types of violence in your community.
4. What resources are available in your community for victims of violence? Interview a person who works in an agency that seeks to aid victims of violence.

What is the role of the agency? Do its services seem adequate? Who is eligible? Is there a waiting list? What is the fee scale?

5. Cut out all stories about violence in your local newspaper every day for 2 weeks. Note the patterns. Is the majority of the violence perpetrated by strangers or family members? How are the victims portrayed? What kinds of families are involved? What kinds of stories and families get front-page treatment rather than a few lines in the back of the paper?

**Additional Resources**

These related resources are found either in the appendix at the back of this book or on the book's website at **http://evolve.elsevier.com/Stanhope.**

**evolve Evolve Website**

WebLinks: Healthy People 2010

## References

Aiken MM, Speck PM: Sexual assault and multiple trauma: a sexual assault nurse examiner (SANE) challenge, *J Emerg Nurs* 21(5):466, 1995.

Bachman R: *Violence against women: a national crime victimization survey report,* Washington, DC, 1994, U.S. Department of Justice, Office of Justice Programs, Bureau of Justice Statistics.

Barnett OW, Miller-Perrin CL, Perrin RD: *Family violence across the lifespan: an introduction,* Thousand Oaks, Calif, 1997, Sage.

Baron S, Welty A: Elder abuse, *J Gerontol Soc Work* 25(1/2):33, 1996.

Beitchman JH et al: a review of the long-term effects of child sexual abuse, *Child Abuse Negl* 16:101-118, 1993.

Belknap RA: Why did she do that? issues of moral conflict in battered women's decision making, *Issues Ment Health Nurs* 20:387-404, 1999.

Bradley RG, Davino KM: Women's perceptions of the prison environment: when prison is "The safest place I've ever been," *Psychol Women Q* 26:351-359, 2002.

Briere J et al: *The APSAC handbook on child maltreatment,* Thousand Oaks, Calif, 1996, Sage.

Brown J et al: A longitudinal analysis of risk factors for child maltreatment: findings of a 17-year prospective study of officially recorded and self-reported child abuse and neglect, *Child Abuse Negl* 22:1065-1078, 1998.

Browne A, Miller B, Maguin E: Prevalence and severity of lifetime physical and sexual victimization among incarcerated women, *Int J Law Psychiatry* 22:301-322, 1999.

Bureau of Justice Statistics: *Criminal victimization 1996,* Washington, DC, 1997, U.S. Department of Justice.

Butler RN: Warning signs of elder abuse, *Geriatrics* 54(3):3-4, 1999.

Campbell JC: *Assessing dangerousness: potential for further violence of sexual offenders,* Newbury Park, Calif, 1995, Sage.

Campbell JC: *Empowering survivors of abuse: health care, battered women and their children,* Newbury Hills, Calif, 1998, Sage.

Campbell JC: Health consequences of intimate partner violence, *Lancet* 359(9314):1331-1336, 2002.

Campbell JC, Campbell D: The influence of abuse on pregnancy intention, *Women's Health Issues* 5(4):214-223, 1995.

Campbell JC, Sharps PW, Glass NE: Risk assessment for intimate partner homicide. In Pinard GF, Pagani L, editors: *Clinical assessment of dangerousness: empirical contributions,* pp. 136-157, New York, 2000, Cambridge University Press.

Campbell JC, Sheridan DJ: Domestic violence assessment. In Jarvis C, editor: *Physical examination and health assessment,* ed 4, St. Louis, 2004, Mosby.

Campbell JC, Soeken KL: Forced sex and intimate partner violence, *Violence Against Women* 5:1017-1035, 1999.

Campbell JC et al: Predictors of depression in battered women, *Violence Against Women* 3(3):271-293, 1997.

Campbell JC et al: Voices of strength and resistance: a contextual and longitudinal analysis of women's responses to battering, *J Interpers Violence* 13:743-762, 1998.

Campbell JC et al: Collaboration as a partnership, *Violence Against Women* 5:1140-1157, 1999.

Campbell JC et al: An evaluation of a system-change training model to improve emergency department response to battered women, *Acad Emerg Med* 8(2):131-138, 2001.

Campbell JC et al: Risk factors for femicide in abusive relationships: results from a multi-site case control study, *Am J Public Health* (in press).

Carlson MJ, Harris SD, Holden GW: Protective orders and domestic violence: Risk factors for abuse, *J Family Violence* 14(2):205-226, 1999.

Carlson RB et al: A conceptual framework for the long term psychological effects of traumatic childhood abuse, *Child Maltreatment* 2(3):272, 1997.

Catalano R, Novaco R, McConnell W: A model of the net effect of job loss on violence, *Violence Victims* 16(1):1440-1447, 1997.

Centers for Disease Control and Prevention: Regional variations in suicide rates—United States, 1990-1994, *MMWR Morb Mortal Wkly Rep* 46(34):789, 1997.

Chalk R, King PA: *Violence in families: assessing prevention and treatment programs,* Washington, DC, 1998, National Academy Press.

Comijs HC et al: Risk indicators of elder mistreatment in the community, *J Elder Abuse Negl* 9(4):67-76, 1998.

Cooper-White P: An emperor without clothes: the churches' views about treatment of domestic violence, *Pastoral Psychol* 45(1):3-20, 1996.

Cottle CE et al: Conflicting ideologies and the politics of pornography. In O'Toole LL, Schiffman JR, editors: *Gender violence: interdisciplinary perspectives,* New York, 1997, New York University Press.

Counts D, Brown J, Campbell J: *To have and to hit: cultural perspectives on wife beating,* Chicago, Ill, 1999, University of Illinois Press.

Darlington Y: Escape as a response to childhood sexual abuse, *J Child Sexual Abuse* 5(3):77-93, 1996.

Dearwater S et al: Prevalence of domestic violence treated in a community hospital emergency department, *JAMA* 280(5):433, 1998.

Donat PL, D'Emilio N: A feminist redefinition of rape and sexual assault: historical foundations and change. In O'Toole LL, Schiffman JR, editors: *Gender violence: interdisciplinary perspectives,* New York, 1997, New York University Press.

Draucker CB: Impact of violence in the lives of women: restriction and resolve, *J Ment Health Nurs* 18:559-586, 1997.

Dutton DG: *The domestic assault of women,* Newton, Mass, 1995, Allyn and Bacon.

Eby KK et al: Health effects of experiences of sexual violence for women with abusive partners, *Health Care Women Int* 16:563-576, 1995.

Edleson JL, Bible AL: *Forced bonding or community collaboration.* Paper presented at the National Institute of Justice Annual Conference on Criminal Justice Research and Evaluation: Viewing Crime and Justice from a Collaborative Perspective, Washington, DC, July 28, 1998, revised September, 1998.

Edleson JL, Tolman RM: *Intervention for men who batter,* Newbury Park, Calif, 1992, Sage.

Eggert LL et al: Prevention research program: reconnecting at-risk youth, *Issues Ment Health Nurs* 15(2):107, 1994.

Ehrmin JT: No more mother blaming: a feminist nursing perspective on the mother's role in father–daughter incest, *Arch Psychiatr Nurs* 10(4):252-260, 1996.

Evans JP, Taylor J: Understanding violence in contemporary and earlier gangs: an exploratory application of the theory of reasoned action, *J Black Psychol* 21(1):71, 1995.

Fortune MM: Religious issues and violence against women. In Renzetti CM, Jeffery L, Bergen RK, editors: *Sourcebook on violence against women,* Thousand Oaks, Calif, 2001, Sage.

Gandy OH: Racial identity, media use, and the social construction of risk among African Americans, *J Black Studies* 31(5):600-618, 2001.

Gelles RJ: *Intimate violence in families,* ed 3, Thousand Oaks, Calif, 1997, Sage.

Gelles RJ: The youngest victims: violence toward children. In Bergen RK, editor: *Issues in intimate violence,* Thousand Oaks, Calif, 1998, Sage.

Gerlock A: Health impact of domestic violence, *Issues Ment Health Nurs* 20:373-385, 1999.

Green AH: Comparing child victims and adult survivors: clues to the pathogenesis of child sexual abuse, *J Am Acad Psychoanal* 23:655-670, 1995.

Green AH: Overview of child sexual abuse. In Kaplan SJ, editor: *Family violence: a clinical and legal guide,* Washington, DC, 1996, American Psychiatric Press.

Gillham B et al: Unemployment rates, single-parent density, and indices of child poverty: their relationship to different categories of child abuse and neglect, *Child Abuse Negl* 22:79-90, 1998.

Gullota TP, McElhaney SJ, editors: *Violence in homes and communities,* Thousand Oaks, Calif, 1999, Sage.

Hampton RL, Yung BR: Violence in communities of color: where we were, where we are, and where we need to be. In Hampton RL, Jenkins P, Gullotta TP, editors: *Preventing violence in America,* Thousand Oaks, Calif, 1996, Sage.

Hattendorf J, Tollerud TR: Domestic violence: counseling strategies that minimize the impact of secondary victimization, *Perspect Psychiatr Care* 33(1):14-23, 1997.

Hausman AJ, Spivak H, Prothrow-Stith D: Evaluation of a community-based youth violence prevention project, *J Adolesc Health* 17:353-359, 1995.

Hernandez JT, Lodico M, DiClemente RJ: The effects of child abuse and race on risk taking in male adolescents, *J Natl Med Assoc* 85(8):593, 1993.

Hilton NZ et al: Antiviolence education in high schools, *J Interpers Violence* 13(6):726-742, 1998.

Horton A: The prevention of school violence: new evidence to consider, *J Human Behav Soc Environ* 4(1):49-59, 2001.

Hudson MF, Carlson JR: Elder abuse: expert and public perspectives on its meaning, *J Elder Abuse Negl* 9(4):77-97, 1998.

Humphreys J, Neylan T: Trauma history of sheltered battered women, *Issues Ment Health Nurs* 20:319-332, 1999.

Jackson S et al: Predicting abuse-prone parental attitudes, and discipline practices in a nationally representative sample, *Child Abuse Negl* 23:15-29, 1999.

Kauffman J, Joseph-Fox YK: American Indian and Alaska Native Women. In Bayne-Smith M, editor: *Race, gender, and health,* Thousand Oaks, Calif, 1996, Sage.

Kellerman AL, Rivara RP, Rushforth NB: Gun ownership as a risk factor for homicide in the home, *N Engl J Med* 329:1084-1091, 1993.

Kendall-Tackett K, Marshall R: Sexual victimization of children: incest and child sexual abuse. In Bergen RK, editor: *Issues in intimate violence,* Thousand Oaks, Calif, 1998, Sage.

Kilpatrick KL, Litt M, Williams LM: Post-traumatic stress disorder in child witnesses to domestic violence, *Am J Orthopsychiatry* 67:639-644, 1997.

Kimmel MS: Does censorship make a difference? an aggregate empirical analysis of pornography and rape, *J Psychol Human Sexual* 8(3):1, 1996.

King MC, Ryan J: Woman abuse: the role of nurse mid-wives in assessment, *J Nurse Midwifery* 41(6):436-441, 423-427, 1996.

Klein E et al: *Ending domestic violence: changing public perceptions/halting the epidemic,* Newbury Park, Calif, 1997, Sage.

Kleinschmidt KC: Elder abuse: a review, *Ann Emerg Med* 30:463-472, 1997.

Koss MP, Cook SL: Facing the facts: date and acquaintance rape are significant problems for women. In Bergen RK, editor: *Issues in intimate violence,* Thousand Oaks, Calif, 1998, Sage.

Koss MP, Harvey MR: *The rape victim: clinical and community intervention,* ed 2, Newbury Park, Calif, 1991, Sage.

Kotch JB et al: Predicting child maltreatment in the first 4 years of life from characteristics assessed in the neonatal period, *Child Abuse Negl* 23:305-319, 1999.

Kurz D: Separation, divorce and woman abuse, *Violence Against Women* 2:63-81, 1996.

Lachs MS et al: Risk factors for reported elder abuse and neglect: a nine year observational cohort survey, *Gerontologist* 37:469-474, 1997.

Lambert LC, Firestone JM: Economic context and multiple abuse techniques, *Violence Against Women* 6(1):49-67, 2000.

Landenburger K: Exploration of women's identity: clinical approaches with abused women—empowering survivors of abuse: health care, battered women and their children, Newbury Hills, Calif, 1998, Sage.

Ledray LE: *Sexual assault nurse examiner: development and operation guide,* Washington, DC, 1999, U.S. Department of Justice, available at http://www.ojp.usdoj.gov/ovc/publications/infores/sane/saneguide.pdf.

Ledray LE, Simmelink K: Sexual assault: clinical issues—efficacy of SANE evidence collection: a Minnesota study, *J Emerg Nurs* 23(1):75, 1997.

Leonard ED: Convicted survivors: comparing and describing California's battered women inmates, *Prison J* 81(1):73-86, 2001.

Leventhal JM: The prevention of child abuse and neglect: successfully out of the blocks, *Child Abuse Negl* 25(4):431-439, 2001.

Logan BB, Dawkins CE: *Family-centered nursing in the community,* Menlo Park, Calif, 1986, Addison-Wesley.

Lynch VA: Forensic nursing: diversity in education and practice, *J Psychosoc Nurs* 31(11):7-8, 1993.

Lynch VA: Clinical forensic nursing: a new perspective in the management of crime victims from trauma to trial, *Crit Care Nurs Clin North Am* 7(3):497, 1995.

Malik S, Sorenson SB, Aneshensel CS: Community and dating violence among adolescents: perpetration and victimization, *J Adolesc Health* 21:291-301, 1997.

Markowitz FE: Attitudes and family violence: linking intergenerational and cultural theories, *J Fam Violence* 16:205-218, 2001.

McCloskey LA: The "Medea complex" among men: the instrumental abuse of children to injure wives, *Violence Victims* 16(1):19-37, 2001.

McFarlane J, Parker B: *Abuse during pregnancy: a protocol for prevention and intervention,* White Plains, NY, 1994, March of Dimes Birth Defects Foundation.

McFarlane J, Parker B, Soeken K: Abuse during pregnancy: effects on maternal complications and birthright in adult and teenage women, *Obstet Gynecol* 84(3):323, 1994.

McFarlane J et al: Safety behaviors of abused women after an intervention during pregnancy, *J Obstet Gynecol Neonat Nurs* 27(1):64, 1998.

McGuigan WM, Pratt CC: The predictive impact of domestic violence on three types of child maltreatment, *Child Abuse Negl* 25:869-883., 2001.

Merritt-Gray M, Wuest J: Counteracting abuse and breaking free: the process of leaving revealed through women's voices, *Health Care Women Int* 16:399-412, 1995.

Mihalic SW, Elliott D: A social learning theory model of marital violence, *J Family Violence* 12:21-47, 1997.

Mohr WK: Family violence: toward more precise and comprehensive knowing, *Issues Ment Health Nurs* 20:305-317, 1999.

Moore R, Harrisson S: In poor health: socioeconomic status and health chances—a review of the literature, *Soc Sci Health* 1(4):221, 1995.

Nadon SM, Koverola C, Schludermann EH: Antecedents to prostitution: childhood victimization, *J Interpers Violence* 13(2):206, 1998.

National Center for Injury Prevention and Control: *Injury fact book,* November 2001, Centers for Disease Control and Prevention.

O'Carroll PW et al: Interviewing suicide "descendents": a fourth strategy for risk factor assessment, *Suicide Life-Threatening Behav* 32(supplement):3-6, 2001

Okun LE: *Woman abuse: facts replacing myths,* Albany, NY, 1986, State University of New York Press.

Parnis D, DuMont J: Examining the standardized application of rape kits: an exploratory study of post-sexual assault professional practices, *Health Care Women Int* 23:846-853, 2002.

Peled E: Secondary victims no more: refocusing intervention with children. In Edleson JL, Eisikovits ZC, editors: *Future interventions with battered women and their families: visions for policy, practice, and research,* Thousand Oaks, Calif, 1996, Sage.

Peterson RL, Larson J, Skiba R: School violence prevention: current status and policy recommendations, *Law Pol* 23(3):345-371, 2001.

Phelan P: Incest and its meaning: the perspectives of fathers and daughters, *Child Abuse Negl* 19:7-24, 1995.

Reis B: *Safe schools report of the anti-violence documentation project from the safe schools coalition of Washington—will you be there for every child?* Seattle, Wash, 1997, Safe Schools Coalition of Washington.

Renzetti CM: Violence in lesbian and gay relationships. In O'Toole LL, Schiffman JR, editors: *Gender violence: interdisciplinary perspectives,* New York, 1997, New York University Press.

Riedel M: Counting stranger homicides, *Homicide Studies* 2:206, 1998.

Rosenberg ML, Fenley MA, editors: Violence in America: a public health approach, New York, 1991, Oxford.

Rumm PD et al: Identified spouse abuse as a risk factor for child abuse, *Child Abuse Negl* 24:1375-1381, 1999.

Russell DEH: Pornography and rape: a causal model, *Prevent Human Serv* 12(2):45, 1995a.

Russell DEH: The prevalence, trauma, and sociocultural cause of incestuous abuse of females: a human rights issue. In Rolf K et al, editors: *Beyond trauma: cultural and societal dynamics,* New York, 1995b, Plenum.

Ryan J, King MC: Child witness of domestic violence: principles of advocacy, *Clin Excellence Nurse Pract* 1:47-57, 1997.

Salzinger A et al: Effects of partner violence and physical child abuse on child behavior: a study of abused and comparison children, *J Fam Violence* 17:23-52, 2002.

Sampson RJ: Crime and public safety: insights from community-level perspectives on social capital. In Saegert S, Thompson JP, Warren MR, editors: *Social capital and poor communities,* New York, 2001, Russell Sage Foundation.

Sedlak AJ, Broadhurst DD: *Executive summary of the Third National Incidence Study of Child Abuse and Neglect,* U.S. Department of Health and Human Services, Administration for Children and Families, Administration on Children, Youth and Families, National Center on Child Abuse and Neglect, Washington, DC, 1996, National Clearinghouse on Child Abuse and Neglect.

Senter S: *Program planning manual for implementing a response to domestic violence in hospital emergency departments,* Seattle, Wash, 1993, Seattle-King County Department of Public Health.

Shapiro BL, Schwarz JC: Date rape: its relationship to trauma symptoms and sexual self-esteem, *J Interpers Violence* 12:407-419, 1997.

Sharps PW et al: Health care provider's missed opportunities for preventing femicide, *Prevent Med* 33:373-380, 2001.

Sheridan D: Health care based programs for domestic violence survivors. In Campbell J: *Empowering survivors of abuse: health care, battered women and their children,* Newbury Park, Calif, 1998, Sage.

Sheridan D: Treating survivors of intimate partner abuse: forensic identification and documentation. In Olshaker JS, Jackson MC, Smock WS, editors: *Forensic emergency medicine,* Philadelphia, 2001, Lippincott Williams & Wilkins.

Simmons B, Stalsworth K, Wentzel H: Television violence and its effect on young children, *Early Childhood Educ J* 26(3):149-153, 1999.

Soeken K et al: The abuse assessment screen: a clinical instrument to measure frequency, severity, and perpetrator of abuse against women. In Campbell JC, editor: *Beyond diagnosis: changing the health care response to battered women and their children,* Newbury Park, Calif, 1998, Sage.

Stark E, Flitcraft A: Spouse abuse. In Rosenberg ML, Finley MA: *Violence in America,* New York, 1991, Oxford.

Straus MA, Gelles RJ: Physical violence in American families: risk factors and adaptations to violence in 8,145 families, New Brunswick, NJ, 1990, Transaction.

Tajima EA: Risk factors for violence against children, *J Interpers Violence* 17(2):122-149, 2002.

Tjaden P, Thoennes N: *Prevalence, incidence and consequences of violence against women: findings from the National Violence Against Women Survey,* National Institute of Justice Centers for Disease Control and Prevention Research Brief, November 1-16. Washington, DC, 1998, U.S. Department of Justice.

Tjaden P, Thoennes N: *Full report of the prevalence, incidence, and consequences of violence against women: findings from the National Violence Against Women Survey,* National Institutes of Justice Centers for Disease Control and Prevention, November, Washington, DC, 2000, U.S. Department of Justice.

True R, Guillermo T: Asian/Pacific Islander American women. In Bayne-Smith M, editor: *Race, gender, and health,* Thousand Oaks, Calif, 1996, Sage.

U.S. Department of Health and Human Services: *Healthy people 2010: national health promotion and disease prevention objectives,* ed 2, Washington, DC, 2000, USDHHS, Public Health Service.

U.S. Department of Health and Human Services, Administration on Children, Youth and Families: *Child maltreatment 2000,* Washington, DC, 2002a, U.S. Government Printing Office.

U.S. Department of Health and Human Services: *National child abuse and neglect data system (NCANDS) summary of key findings from calendar year 2000,* retrieved May 26, 2002, from http://nccanch.acf.hhs.gov/pubs/factsheets/canstats.cfm

U.S. Department of Justice: *Sex offenses and offenders: an analysis of data on rape and sexual assault* (NCJ-163392), Washington, DC, 1997, Bureau of Justice Statistics.

Widom CS, Hiller-Sturmhöfel S: Alcohol abuse as a risk factor for and consequence of child abuse, *Alcohol Res Health* 25(1):52-57, 2001.

Wilber KH, Reynolds SL: Introducing a framework for defining financial abuse of the elderly, *J Elder Abuse Negl* 8(2):61-80, 1996.

Wilkinson RG: Comment: income, inequality, and social cohesion, *Am J Public Health* 87(9):1540, 1997.

Winfree LT, Esbensen F, Osgood DW: Evaluating a school-based gang-prevention program, *Eval Rev* 20(2):181, 1996.

Wolak J, Finkelhor D: Children exposed to partner violence. In Jasinski JL, Williams LM, editors: *Partner violence: a comprehensive review of 20 years of research,* Thousand Oaks, Calif, 1998, Sage.

Wolf RS, Pillemer K, Wilson NL: What's new in elder abuse programming, *Gerontologist* 34(1):126, 1994.

Wolff DA et al: Training clergy: the role of the faith community in domestic violence, *J Religion Abuse* 2(4):47-62, 2001.

Yllo K: Wife rape, *Violence Against Women* 5:1059-1063, 1999.

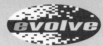 

# Chapter 38

# Infectious Disease Prevention and Control

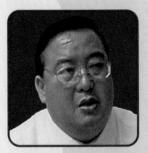

**Francisco S. Sy, M.D., Dr.P.H.**
Francisco S. Sy taught infectious disease epidemiology at the University of South Carolina School of Public Health for 15 years. Today he is a senior health scientist in the Division of HIV/AIDS Prevention of the National Center for HIV, STD and TB Prevention at the Centers for Disease Control and Prevention. Dr. Sy is a clinical associate professor of family and preventive medicine at the University of South Carolina School of Medicine.

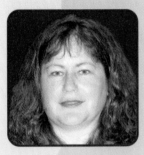

**Susan C. Long-Marin, D.V.M., M.P.H.**
Susan C. Long-Marin developed an interest in infectious disease and public health while she was in the Philippines as a Peace Corps Volunteer in the 1970s. Training in veterinary medicine further increased her respect for the ingeniousness of microbes and the importance of primary prevention. Today she manages the epidemiology program of an urban county health department in Charlotte, North Carolina, that is adjusting to serve a growing and rapidly changing population from a variety of racial, ethnic, and national backgrounds.

## Objectives

After reading this chapter, the student should be able to do the following:

1. Discuss the current impact and threats of infectious diseases on society
2. Explain how the elements of the epidemiologic triangle interact to cause infectious diseases
3. Provide examples of infectious disease control interventions at the three levels of public health prevention
4. Explain the multisystem approach to control of communicable diseases
5. Define surveillance and discuss the functions and elements of a surveillance system
6. Discuss the factors contributing to newly emerging or reemerging infectious diseases
7. Discuss the illnesses most likely to be associated with the intentional release of a biological agent
8. Discuss issues related to obtaining and maintaining appropriate levels of immunization against vaccine-preventable diseases
9. Describe issues and agents associated with foodborne illness and appropriate prevention measures
10. Define the bloodborne pathogen reduction strategy, universal precautions

---

The topic of infectious diseases includes the discussion of a wide and complex variety of organisms; the pathology they may cause; and their diagnosis, treatment, prevention, and control. This chapter presents an overview of the communicable diseases with which community and public health nurses deal most often. Diseases are grouped according to descriptive category (by mode of transmission or means of prevention) rather than by individual organism (e.g., *Escherichia coli*) or taxonomic group (e.g., viral, parasitic). Detailed discussion of sexually transmitted diseases, human immunodeficiency virus (HIV), acquired immunodeficiency syndrome (AIDS), viral hepatitis, and tuberculosis is provided in Chapter 39. Although not all infectious diseases are directly communicable from person to person, the terms *infectious diseases* and *communicable diseases* are used interchangeably throughout this chapter.

## DID YOU KNOW?

Antibiotics are not effective against viral diseases, a fact found unacceptable to many clients looking for relief from the misery of a cold or flu. The inappropriate prescribing of antibiotics contributes to the growing problem of infectious agents that have developed resistance to once powerful antibiotics.

## Key Terms

**acquired immunity**, p. 906
**active immunization**, p. 906
**agent**, p. 905
**common vehicle**, p. 906
**communicable disease**, p. 905
**communicable period**, p. 906
**disease**, p. 906
**elimination**, p. 911
**emerging infectious diseases**, p. 908
**endemic**, p. 907
**environment**, p. 906

**epidemic**, p. 907
**epidemiologic triangle**, p. 905
**eradication**, p. 911
**herd immunity**, p. 906
**horizontal transmission**, p. 906
**host**, p. 905
**incubation period**, p. 906
**infection**, p. 906
**infectiousness**, p. 906
**natural immunity**, p. 906
**nosocomial infection**, p. 928

**pandemic**, p. 907
**passive immunization**, p. 906
**resistance**, p. 906
**severe acute respiratory syndrome**, p. 907
**surveillance**, p. 907
**universal precautions**, p. 928
**vector**, p. 906
**vertical transmission**, p. 906
*See Glossary for definitions*

## Chapter Outline

Historical and Current Perspectives
Transmission of Communicable Diseases
*Agent, Host, and Environment*
*Modes of Transmission*
*Disease Development*
*Disease Spectrum*
Surveillance of Communicable Diseases
*Elements of Surveillance*
*Surveillance for Agents of Bioterrorism*
*List of Reportable Diseases*
Emerging Infectious Diseases
*Emergence Factors*
*Examples of Emerging Infectious Diseases*
Prevention and Control of Communicable
   Diseases
*Primary, Secondary, and Tertiary Prevention*

*Role of Nurses in Prevention*
*Multisystem Approach to Control*
Agents of Bioterrorism
*Anthrax*
*Smallpox*
Vaccine-Preventable Diseases
*Routine Childhood Immunization Schedule*
*Measles*
*Rubella*
*Pertussis*
*Influenza*
Food-Borne and Waterborne Diseases
*Ten Golden Rules for Safe Food Preparation*
*Salmonellosis*
Escherichia coli *O157:H7*
*Waterborne Disease Outbreaks and Pathogens*

Vector-Borne Diseases
*Lyme Disease*
*Rocky Mountain Spotted Fever*
*Prevention and Control of Tick-Borne Diseases*
Diseases of Travelers
*Malaria*
*Food-Borne and Waterborne Diseases*
*Diarrheal Diseases*
Zoonoses
*Rabies (Hydrophobia)*
Parasitic Diseases
*Intestinal Parasitic Infections*
*Parasitic Opportunistic Infections*
*Control and Prevention of Parasitic Infections*
Nosocomial Infections
Universal Precautions

## HISTORICAL AND CURRENT PERSPECTIVES

In 1900, communicable diseases were the leading causes of death in the United States. By 2000, improved nutrition and sanitation, vaccines, and antibiotics had put an end to the epidemics that once ravaged entire populations. In 1900, tuberculosis caused 11.3% of all deaths in the United States and was the second leading cause of death. In 1999, although tuberculosis was no longer on the list of leading causes of death, this formerly often fatal disease caused 0.03% of all deaths (Centers for Disease Control and Prevention [CDC], 2001a). As individuals live longer, chronic diseases—heart disease, cancer, and stroke—have replaced infectious diseases as the leading causes of death.

Infectious diseases, however, have not vanished. They are still the number one cause of death worldwide. In the United States, infectious diseases account for 25% of all physician visits each year (CDC, 1994). Organisms once susceptible to antibiotics are becoming increasingly drug resistant and may result in vulnerability to diseases thought no longer a threat. And in the twenty-first century, infectious diseases have become a means of terrorism.

New killers are emerging, and old familiar diseases are taking on different, more virulent characteristics. Consider the following recent developments. The advent of the AIDS epidemic in the 1980s reminds us of plagues from the past and challenges our ability to contain and control infection like no other disease in this century. AIDS and injury are the leading killers of persons 25 to 44 years of age. Legionnaire's disease and toxic shock syndrome, unknown in the mid-twentieth century, have become part of common vocabulary. The identification of infectious agents causing Lyme disease and ehrlichiosis has provided two new tick-borne diseases to worry about. In the summer of 1993 in the southwestern United States, healthy young adults were stricken with a mysterious and unknown but often fatal respiratory disease that is now known as hantavirus pulmonary syndrome. A severe, invasive strain of *Streptococcus pyogenes* group A drew public attention in 1994, referred to by the press as the "flesh-eating" bacteria. Consumption of improperly cooked hamburgers and unpasteurized apple juice contaminated with a highly toxic strain of *E. coli* (*Escherichia coli* 0157:H7) caused illness and death in children across the country. In 1996, 10 states had outbreaks of diarrheal disease traced to imported fresh berries. The implicated organism in these outbreaks, *Cyclospora cayetanensis* (a coccidian parasite), was first diagnosed in humans in 1977 (CDC, 1996a). Also in 1996, the fear that "mad cow disease" (bovine spongiform encephalopathy, or BSE) could be transferred to humans through beef consumption led to the slaughter of thousands of British cattle and a ban on the international sale of British beef. Although never seen in the United States, BSE has now been reported in Europe and Japan as well as Great Britain. Variant Creutzfeldt-Jakob disease (vCJD), which attacks the brain with fatal results, is the disease hypothesized but not yet proven to result from eating beef infected with the transmissible agent that causes BSE (CDC, 2002a). Vancomycin-resistant *Staphylococcus aureus* (VRSA) was reported in 1997; previously, vancomycin had been considered the only effective antibiotic against methicillin-resistant *S. aureus* (MRSA). Ebola hemorrhagic fever, a sporadic but highly fatal virus unknown to most people 25 years ago, is now the subject of movies and best-selling books. A 2002 outbreak in Gabon and the Republic of the Congo killed 79% of the affected individuals. And in 1999, the first western hemisphere activity of West Nile virus, a mosquito-transmitted illness that can affect livestock, birds, and humans, occurred in New York City. By 2002, West Nile virus, believed to be carried by infected birds and possibly mosquitoes in cargo containers, had spread across the United States as far west as California and was reported in Canada and Central America as well. And in early 2003, severe acute respiratory syndrome (SARS), a previously unknown disease of undetermined etiology and no definitive treatment, frightened us into canceling trips to China and Hong Kong and avoiding people who had recently returned from Asia, while we watched on television residents in outbreak-affected countries go about their daily business wearing surgical-style masks.

Worldwide, infectious diseases are the leading killer of children and young adults, accounting for more than 13 million deaths a year, and for half of all deaths in devel-

---

## Healthy People 2010 | Objectives Related to Communicable Diseases

**14-1** Reduce or eliminate indigenous cases of vaccine-preventable disease

**14-4** Reduce bacterial meningitis in young children

**14-5** Reduce invasive pneumococcal infections

**14-7** Reduce meningococcal disease

**14-8** Reduce Lyme disease

**14-11** Reduce tuberculosis

**14-12** Increase the proportion of all tuberculosis patients who complete curative therapy within 12 months

**14-13** Increase the proportion of contacts and other high-risk persons with latent tuberculosis infection who complete a course of treatment

**14-14** Reduce the average time for a laboratory to confirm and report tuberculosis cases

**14-15** Increase the proportion of international travelers who receive recommended preventive services when traveling in areas of risk for select diseases: hepatitis A, malaria, and typhoid

**14-16** Reduce invasive early onset group B streptococcal disease

**14-17** Reduce hospitalizations caused by peptic ulcer disease in the United States

**14-18** Reduce the number of courses of antibiotics for ear infections for young children

**14-19** Reduce the number of courses of antibiotics prescribed for the sole diagnosis of the common cold

**14-22** Achieve and maintain effective vaccination coverage levels for universally recommended vaccines among young children

**14-23** Maintain vaccination coverage levels for children in licensed day-care facilities and children in kindergarten through the first grade

**14-24** Increase the proportion of young children who receive all vaccines that have been recommended for universal administration for at least 5 years

**14-26** Increase the proportion of children who participate in fully operational population-based immunization registries

**14-27** Increase routine vaccination coverage levels of adolescents

**14-29** Increase the proportion of adults who are vaccinated annually against influenza and ever vaccinated against pneumococcal disease

**14-30** Reduce vaccine-associated adverse events

From U.S. Department of Health and Human Services: *Healthy people 2010: national health promotion and disease prevention objectives,* ed 2, Washington, DC, 2000, U.S. Government Printing Office.

oping countries. Of these infectious disease deaths, 90% result from six causes: pneumonia, diarrheal diseases, tuberculosis, malaria, measles, and HIV/AIDS (Institute of Medicine [IOM], 2001). It is estimated that in the United States, 90,000 people per year die from microbial causes, not including AIDS-associated illnesses (McGinnis and Foege, 1993). The economic burden of infectious diseases is staggering. In the United States, the annual cost of infections caused by the growing problem of antibiotic resistant bacteria is estimated to be between $4 and $5 billion (IOM, 1998). Hospitalization for food-borne illnesses is estimated at over $3 billion per year, with an additional cost of $8 billion in lost productivity (CDC, 2002b). Yearly, direct health care provider charges for AIDS are estimated at $5.8 billion, and more than $4.5 billion may be added to health costs each year by infections acquired during hospitalization (CDC, 1998a).

Because of the morbidity, mortality, and associated cost of infectious diseases, the national health promotion and disease prevention goals outlined in Healthy People 2010 list a number of objectives for reducing the incidence of these illnesses (see the Healthy People 2010 box). An objective for reducing salmonellosis and other food-borne infections is found in the section on food and drug safety. Although infectious diseases may not be the leading cause of death in the United States at the beginning of the twenty-first century, they continue to present varied, multiple, and complex challenges to all health care providers. Nurses must know about these diseases to effectively participate in diagnosis, treatment, prevention, and control.

## TRANSMISSION OF COMMUNICABLE DISEASES

### Agent, Host, and Environment

The transmission of **communicable diseases** depends on the successful interaction of the infectious agent, the host, and the environment. These three factors make up the **epidemiologic triangle** (Figure 38-1) as discussed in Chapter 11. Changes in the characteristics of any of the factors may result in disease transmission. Consider the following examples. Not only may antibiotic therapy eliminate a specific pathologic agent but it may also alter the balance of normally occurring organisms in the body. As a result, one of these agents overruns another, and disease, such as a yeast infection, occurs. HIV performs its deadly work not by directly poisoning the host but by destroying the host's immune reaction to other disease-producing agents. Individuals living in the temperate climate of the United States do not contract malaria at home, but they may become infected if they change their environment by traveling to a climate where malaria-carrying mosquitoes thrive. As these examples illustrate, the balance among agent, host, and environment is often precarious and may be unintentionally disrupted. In the twenty-first century, the potential results of such disruption requires attention as advances in science and technology, destruction of natural

habitats, explosive population growth, political instability, and a worldwide transportation network combine to alter the balance among the environment, people, and the agents that produce disease.

### Agent Factor

Four main categories of infectious agents can cause infection or disease: bacteria, fungi, parasites, and viruses. The individual **agent** may be described by its ability to cause disease and by the nature and the severity of the disease. *Infectivity, pathogenicity, virulence, toxicity, invasiveness,* and *antigenicity,* terms commonly used to characterize infectious agents, are defined in Box 38-1.

### Host Factor

A human or animal **host** can harbor an infectious agent. The characteristics of the host that may influence the

---

**BOX 38-1  Six Characteristics of an Infectious Agent**

- **Infectivity:** The ability to enter and multiply in the host.
- **Pathogenicity:** The ability to produce a specific clinical reaction after infection occurs.
- **Virulence:** The ability to produce a severe pathologic reaction.
- **Toxicity:** The ability to produce a poisonous reaction.
- **Invasiveness:** The ability to penetrate and spread throughout a tissue.
- **Antigenicity:** The ability to stimulate an immunologic response.

---

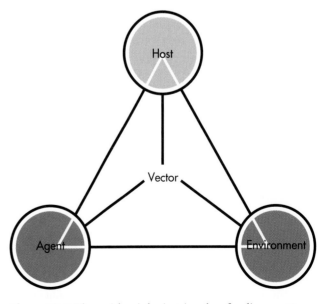

**Figure 38-1** The epidemiologic triangle of a disease. *(From Gordis L:* Epidemiology, *Philadelphia, 1996, Saunders.)*

spread of disease are host resistance, immunity, herd immunity, and infectiousness of the host. **Resistance** is the ability of the host to withstand infection, and it may involve natural or acquired immunity.

**Natural immunity** refers to species-determined, innate resistance to an infectious agent. For example, opossums rarely contract rabies. **Acquired immunity** is the resistance acquired by a host as a result of previous natural exposure to an infectious agent. Having measles once protects against future infection. Acquired immunity may be induced by active or passive immunization. **Active immunization** refers to the immunization of an individual by administration of an antigen (infectious agent or vaccine) and is usually characterized by the presence of an antibody produced by the individual host. Vaccinating children against childhood diseases is an example of inducing active immunity. **Passive immunization** refers to immunization through the transfer of specific antibody from an immunized individual to a nonimmunized individual, such as the transfer of antibody from mother to infant or by administration of an antibody-containing preparation (immune globulin or antiserum). Passive immunity from immune globulin is almost immediate but short-lived. It is often induced as a stopgap measure until active immunity has time to develop after vaccination. Examples of commonly used immunoglobulins include those for hepatitis A, rabies, and tetanus.

**Herd immunity** refers to the immunity of a group or community. It is the resistance of a group of people to invasion and spread of an infectious agent. Herd immunity is based on the resistance of a high proportion of individual members of a group to infection. It is the basis for increasing immunization coverage for vaccine-preventable diseases. Higher immunization coverage will lead to greater herd immunity, which in turn will block the further spread of the disease.

**Infectiousness** is a measure of the potential ability of an infected host to transmit the infection to other hosts. It reflects the relative ease with which the infectious agent is transmitted to others. Individuals with measles are extremely infectious; the virus spreads readily on airborne droplets. A person with Lyme disease cannot spread the disease to other people (although the infected tick can).

### Environment Factor

The **environment** refers to all that is external to the human host, including physical, biological, social, and cultural factors. These environmental factors facilitate the transmission of an infectious agent from an infected host to other susceptible hosts. Reduction in communicable disease risk can be achieved by altering these environmental factors. Using mosquito nets and repellants to avoid bug bites, installing sewage systems to prevent fecal contamination of water supplies, and washing utensils after contact with raw meat to reduce bacterial contamination are all examples of altering the environment to prevent disease.

## Modes of Transmission

Infectious diseases can be transmitted horizontally or vertically. **Vertical transmission** is the passing of the infection from parent to offspring via sperm, placenta, milk, or contact in the vaginal canal at birth. Examples of vertical transmission are transplacental transmission of HIV and syphilis. **Horizontal transmission** is the person-to-person spread of infection through one or more of the following four routes: direct/indirect contact, common vehicle, airborne, or vector borne. Most sexually transmitted diseases are spread by direct sexual contact. Enterobiasis, or pinworm infection, can be acquired through direct contact or indirect contact with contaminated objects such as toys, clothing, and bedding. **Common vehicle** refers to transportation of the infectious agent from an infected host to a susceptible host via food, water, milk, blood, serum, saliva, or plasma. Hepatitis A can be transmitted through contaminated food and water, hepatitis B through contaminated blood. Legionellosis and tuberculosis are both spread via contaminated droplets in the air. **Vectors** can be arthropods such as ticks and mosquitoes or other invertebrates such as snails that can transmit the infectious agent by biting or depositing the infective material near the host.

## Disease Development

Exposure to an infectious agent does not always lead to an infection. Similarly, infection does not always lead to disease. Infection depends on the infective dose, the infectivity of the infectious agent, and the immunocompetence of the host. It is important to differentiate infection and disease, as clearly illustrated by the HIV/AIDS epidemic. **Infection** refers to the entry, development, and multiplication of the infectious agent in the susceptible host. **Disease** is one of the possible outcomes of infection, and it may indicate a physiologic dysfunction or pathologic reaction. An individual who tests positive for HIV is infected, but if that person shows no clinical signs, he is not diseased. Similarly, if an individual tests positive for HIV and also exhibits clinical signs of AIDS, he is both infected and diseased.

---

**DID YOU KNOW?**

Discovered only in 1983, an infectious agent, *Helicobacter pylori,* is now recognized as the major factor in peptic ulcer disease.

---

Incubation period and communicable period are not synonymous. **Incubation period** is the time interval between invasion by an infectious agent and the first appearance of signs and symptoms of the disease. The incubation periods of infectious diseases vary from between 2 and 4 hours for staphylococcal food poisoning to between 10 and 15 years for AIDS. **Communicable period** is the interval during which an infectious agent may be transferred directly or indirectly from an infected person to another person. The period of communicability for influenza is 3 to 5 days after the clinical onset of symptoms. Hepatitis B–infected persons are infectious many weeks before the onset of the first symptoms and remain infective during the acute phase and chronic carrier state, which may persist for life.

## Disease Spectrum

Persons with infectious diseases may exhibit a broad spectrum of disease that ranges from subclinical infection to severe and fatal disease. Those with subclinical or inapparent infections are important from the public health point of view because they are a source of infection but may not be receiving the care that those with clinical disease are receiving. They should be targeted for early diagnosis and treatment. Those with clinical disease may exhibit localized or systemic symptoms and mild to severe illness. The final outcome of a disease may be recovery, death, or something in between, including a carrier state, complications requiring extended hospital stay, or disability requiring rehabilitation.

At the community level, the disease may occur in endemic, epidemic, or pandemic proportion. **Endemic** refers to the constant presence of a disease within a geographic area or a population. Pertussis is endemic in the United States. **Epidemic** refers to the occurrence of disease in a community or region in excess of normal expectancy. Although people tend to associate large numbers with epidemics, even one case can be termed epidemic if the disease is considered previously eliminated from that area. For example, one case of polio, a disease considered eliminated from the United States, would be considered epidemic. **Pandemic** refers to an epidemic occurring worldwide and affecting large populations. HIV/AIDS is both epidemic and pandemic, as the number of cases is growing rapidly across various regions of the world as well as in the United States. SARS is an emerging infectious disease and a recent example of a pandemic.

### Severe Acute Respiratory Syndrome (SARS)

In February 2003, the world learned of a mysterious respiratory disease primarily infecting travelers and health care workers in Southeast Asia. Thought at first to be a form of influenza, the illness was soon recognized as an atypical and sometimes deadly pneumonia, transmitted easily through close contact, and seemingly unresponsive to treatment with antibiotics and antivirals. Initially confined to mainland China, this disease of unknown etiology and no respect for national borders spread to Hong Kong and then quickly to Hanoi, Singapore, and Toronto, prompting the World Health Organization (WHO) to release a rare emergency travel advisory that heightened surveillance of patients with atypical pneumonia around the globe. Intense international investigation revealed that **severe acute respiratory syndrome,** or SARS, as this illness came to be called, was associated with a new strain of coronavirus.

Three months after the first official news of SARS, over 8000 cases with more than 700 deaths had been reported to WHO from 28 countries. Efforts around the world are concentrated on developing a reliable diagnostic test and a vaccine. A very large number of individuals infected by SARS can be traced back to unrecognized cases in hospitals, suggesting that prompt identification and isolation of symptomatic people is the key to interrupting transmission. (The information and updates on SARS can be obtained at the WHO's SARS website: http://www.who.int/csr/sars/archive/2003_04_11/en/#events.)

## SURVEILLANCE OF COMMUNICABLE DISEASES

During the first half of the twentieth century, the weekly publication of national morbidity statistics by the U.S. Surgeon General's Office was accompanied by the statement, "No health department, state or local, can effectively prevent or control disease without knowledge of when, where, and under what conditions cases are occurring" (CDC, 1996b). **Surveillance** gathers the who, when, where and what; these elements are then used to answer why. A good surveillance system systematically collects, organizes, and analyzes current, accurate, and complete data for a defined disease condition. The resulting information is promptly released to those who need it for effective planning, implementation, and evaluation of disease prevention and control programs.

### Elements of Surveillance

Infectious disease surveillance incorporates and analyzes data from a variety of sources. Box 38-2 lists 10 commonly used data elements.

### Surveillance for Agents of Bioterrorism

In the wake of September 11, 2001, heightened emphasis has been placed on surveillance for any disease that might be associated with the intentional release of a biological agent. The concern is that, because of the interval between exposure and disease, a covert release may go unrecognized

---

**BOX 38-2    Ten Basic Elements of Surveillance**

1. Mortality registration
2. Morbidity reporting
3. Epidemic reporting
4. Epidemic field investigation
5. Laboratory reporting
6. Individual case investigation
7. Surveys
8. Utilization of biological agents and drugs
9. Distribution of animal reservoirs and vectors
10. Demographic and environmental data

and without response for some time if the resulting outbreak closely resembles a naturally occurring one. Health care providers are asked to be alert to (1) temporal or geographic clustering of illnesses (people who attended the same public gathering or visited the same location), especially those with clinical signs that resemble an infectious disease outbreak—previously healthy people with unexplained fever accompanied by sepsis, pneumonia, respiratory failure, rash, or flaccid paralysis; (2) an unusual age distribution for a common disease (e.g., chicken pox–like disease in adults without a child source case); and (3) a large number of cases of acute flaccid paralysis such as that seen in *Clostridium botulinum* intoxication. Although more active infectious disease surveillance is being encouraged because of the potential for bioterrorism, the positive benefit is increased surveillance for other communicable diseases as well. Such heightened surveillance can just as easily warn of a community outbreak of salmonellosis or influenza (CDC, 2001b).

Nurses are frequently involved at different levels of the surveillance system. They play important roles in collecting data, making diagnoses, investigating and reporting cases, and providing information to the general public. Examples of possible activities include investigating sources and contacts in outbreaks of pertussis in school settings or shigellosis in day care; tuberculosis (TB) testing and contact tracing; collecting and reporting information pertaining to notifiable communicable diseases; and providing morbidity and mortality statistics to those who request them, including the media, the public, service planners, and grant writers.

## List of Reportable Diseases

Requirements for disease reporting in the United States are mandated by state rather than federal law. The list of reportable diseases varies by state. State health departments, on a voluntary basis, report cases of selected diseases to the CDC in Atlanta, Georgia. The 58 diseases presently included in the National Notifiable Diseases Surveillance System (NNDSS) at the CDC are listed in Box 38-3 (CDC, 2002c). The NNDSS data are collated and published weekly in the *Morbidity and Mortality Weekly Report* (MMWR). Final reports are published annually in the *Summary of Notifiable Diseases* (CDC, 1996a).

## EMERGING INFECTIOUS DISEASES

### Emergence Factors

**Emerging infectious diseases** are those in which the incidence has actually increased in the past two decades or has the potential to increase in the near future. These emerging diseases may include new or known infectious diseases. Consider the following examples. Identified only in 1976 when sporadic outbreaks occurred in Sudan and Zaire, Ebola virus is a mysterious new killer with a frightening mortality rate that sometimes reaches 90%, has no known treatment, and has no recognized reservoir in nature. It appears to be transmitted through direct contact with bodily secretions and as such can potentially be contained once cases are identified. Why outbreaks occur is not understood. Ebola is an example of new viruses that may appear as civilization intrudes farther and farther into previously uninhabited natural environments, changing the landscape and disturbing ecologic balances that may have existed unaltered for hundreds of years.

Closer to home, hantavirus pulmonary syndrome was first detected in 1993 in the Four Corner area of Arizona and New Mexico, when a mysterious and deadly respiratory disease appeared to target young, healthy Native Americans. The disease was soon discovered to be a variant of, but to exhibit different pathology from, a rodent-borne virus previously known only in Europe and Asia. Transmission is thought to occur through aerosolization of rodent excrement. One explanation for the outbreak in the Southwest is that an unseasonably mild winter led to an unusual increase in the rodent population; more people than usual were exposed to a virus that had until that point gone unrecognized in this country. Infection in Native Americans first brought attention to hantavirus pulmonary syndrome because of a cluster of cases in a small geographic area, but no evidence suggests that any ethnic group is particularly susceptible to this disease. Hantavirus pulmonary syndrome has now been diagnosed in sites across the United States. The best protection against this virus seems to be avoiding rodent-infested environments.

Not only is HIV/AIDS a relatively new disease but the resultant immunocompromise is largely responsible for the rising numbers of previously rare opportunistic infections such as cryptosporidiosis, toxoplasmosis, and *Pneumocystis* pneumonia. HIV may have existed in isolated parts of sub-Saharan Africa for years and emerged only recently into the rest of the world as the result of a combination of factors including new roads, increased commerce, and prostitution. Tuberculosis is a familiar face turned newly aggressive. After years of decline, it has resurged as a result of infection secondary to HIV/AIDS and development of multidrug resistance.

West Nile virus (WNV) was first identified in Uganda in 1937. There are two lineages, one in Africa that seems to be enzootic (i.e., related to animals in a particular vicinity) and that does not result in severe human illness, and a second associated with clinical human encephalitis that has been seen in Africa, Asia, India, Europe, and now North America. How WNV first arrived in the United States may never be known, but the answer most likely involves infected birds or mosquitoes. Because the virus is new in this country, and the outbreak of 2002 caused numerous deaths, WNV has garnered a great deal of media attention. However, for the majority of people, infection with WNV results in no clinical signs or only mild flulike symptoms. In a small percentage of individuals—usually the young, the old, and the immunocompromised—a more severe, potentially fatal encephalitis may develop.

## BOX 38-3  Nationally Notifiable Infectious Diseases

1. Acquired immunodeficiency syndrome (AIDS)
2. Anthrax
3. Botulism
   - Food-borne
   - Infant
   - Other (wound and unspecified)
4. Brucellosis
5. Chancroid
6. *Chlamydia trachomatis*, genital infections
7. Cholera
8. Coccidioidomycosis
9. Cryptosporidiosis
10. Cyclosporiasis
11. Diphtheria
12. Ehrlichiosis
    - Human granulocytic
    - Human monocytic
    - Human, other or unspecified
13. Encephalitis, arboviral
    - California serogroup, viral
    - Eastern equine
    - Powassan
    - St. Louis
    - Western equine
    - West Nile
14. Enterohemorrhagic *Escherichia coli*
    - 0157:H7
    - Shiga toxin positive, serogroup non-0157
15. Giardiasis
16. Gonorrhea
17. *Haemophilus influenzae*, invasive disease
18. Hansen disease (leprosy)
19. Hantavirus pulmonary syndrome
20. Hemolytic uremic syndrome, postdiarrheal
21. Hepatitis, viral, acute
22. Hepatitis A, acute
23. Hepatitis B, acute
24. Hepatitis B virus, perinatal infection
25. Hepatitis C, non-A, non-B, acute
26. HIV infection
    - Adult (13 years)
    - pediatric (<13 years)
27. Legionellosis
28. Listeriosis
29. Lyme disease
30. Malaria
31. Measles
32. Meningococcal disease
33. Mumps
34. Pertussis
35. Plague
36. Poliomyelitis, paralytic
37. Psittacosis
38. Q fever
39. Rabies
    - Animal
    - Human
40. Rocky Mountain spotted fever
41. Rubella
42. Rubella, congenital syndrome
43. Salmonellosis
44. Shigellosis
45. Streptococcal disease, invasive, group A
46. Streptococcal toxic shock syndrome
47. *Streptococcus pneumoniae*, drug-resistant, invasive
48. *Streptococcus pneumoniae*, invasive in children <5 years
49. Syphilis
    - Primary
    - Secondary
    - Latent
    - Early latent
    - Late latent
    - Latent, unknown duration
    - Neurosyphilis
    - Late, nonneurologic
50. Syphilis, congenital
    - Syphilitic stillbirth
51. Tetanus
52. Toxic shock syndrome
53. Trichinosis
54. Tuberculosis
55. Tularemia
56. Typhoid fever
57. Varicella (deaths only)
58. Yellow fever

From Centers for Disease Control and Prevention: Notice to readers: changes in national notifiable diseases list and data presentation, *MMWR Morb Mortal Wkly Rep* 51(01):9-10, 2002c.

NOTE: Although chicken pox is not a nationally notifiable disease, the Council of State and Territorial Epidemiologists (CSTE) recommends reporting of cases of chicken pox via the National Notifiable Diseases Surveillance System (NNDSS).

After first appearing in New York City in 1999, the virus spent several years quietly spreading up and down the East Coast without remarkable morbidity or mortality. This situation changed abruptly in the summer of 2002, when WNV was reported across the country and was accompanied by significant avian, equine, and human mortality. By the fall of 2002, over 3000 human cases with more than 180 deaths had been recorded. Especially hard hit were Illinois, Louisiana, Ohio, and Michigan (CDC, 2002d). The explanation for these periodic outbreaks is speculated to result from a complex interaction of multiple factors, including weather—hot, dry summers followed by rain, which influenced mosquito breeding sites and population growth. Since the mid 1990s, outbreaks of WNV involving humans and horses appear to have increased in frequency in Europe, the Middle East, and the United States, with an apparent increase in severity of human disease and an accompanying high mortality rate in birds (Peterson and Roehrig, 2001). Because the ecology of WNV is not fully understood, the future pattern and nature of the virus in this country is uncertain; preventing human infection will continue to be a challenge for the foreseeable future. Currently, an equine vaccine exists and work is underway in developing vaccines for both birds and humans.

Several factors, operating singly or in combination, can influence the emergence of these diseases (Table 38-1) (CDC, 1994). Except for microbial adaptation and changes made by the infectious agent, such as those likely in the emergence of *E. coli* 0157:H7, most of the emergence factors are consequences of activities and behavior of the human hosts, and of environmental changes such as deforestation, urbanization, and industrialization. The rise in households with two working parents has increased the

number of children in day care, and with this shift has come an increase in diarrheal diseases such as shigellosis. Changing sexual behavior and illegal drug use influence the spread of HIV/AIDS as well as other sexually transmitted diseases. Before the use of large air-conditioning systems with cooling towers, legionellosis was virtually unknown. Modern transportation systems closely and quickly connect regions of the world that for centuries had little contact. Insects and animals as well as humans may carry disease between continents via ships and planes. Immigrants, legal and illegal, as well as travelers bring with them a variety of known and potentially unknown diseases. To prevent and control these emerging diseases, effective ways to educate people and change their behavior and to develop effective drugs and vaccines must be developed. Also, current surveillance systems must be strengthened and expanded to improve the detection and tracking of these diseases.

## Examples of Emerging Infectious Diseases

Examples of emerging and resurgent infectious diseases around the world are shown in Figure 38-2 (CDC, 1994). Selected emerging infectious diseases, including a brief description of the diseases and symptoms they cause, their modes of transmission, and causes of emergence are listed in Table 38-2.

## PREVENTION AND CONTROL OF COMMUNICABLE DISEASES

Communicable disease can be prevented and controlled. The goal of prevention and control programs is to reduce the prevalence of a disease to a level at which it no longer poses a major public health problem. In some cases, diseases may even be eliminated or eradicated. The goal of

**Table 38-1  Factors That Can Influence the Emergence of New Infectious Diseases**

| CATEGORIES | SPECIFIC EXAMPLES |
|---|---|
| Societal events | Economic impoverishment, war or civil conflict, population growth and migration, urban decay |
| Health care | New medical devices, organ or tissue transplantation, drugs causing immunosuppression, widespread use of antibiotics |
| Food production | Globalization of food supplies, changes in food processing and packaging |
| Human behavior | Sexual behavior, drug use, travel, diet, outdoor recreation, use of child care facilities |
| Environmental | Deforestation/reforestation, changes in water ecosystems, flood/drought, famine, global changes (e.g., warming) |
| Public health | Curtailment or reduction in prevention programs, inadequate communicable disease infrastructure surveillance, lack of trained personnel (epidemiologists, laboratory scientists, vector and rodent control specialists) |
| Microbial adaptation | Changes in virulence and toxin production, development of drug resistance, microbes as co-factors in chronic diseases |

From Centers for Disease Control and Prevention: *Addressing emerging infectious disease threats: a prevention strategy for the U.S.*, Atlanta, 1994, CDC.

**elimination** is to remove a disease from a large geographic area such as a country or region of the world. **Eradication** is the irreversible termination of all transmission of infection by extermination of the infectious agents worldwide (Last, 2001). The WHO officially declared the global eradication of smallpox on May 8, 1980 (Evans, 1985). After the successful eradication of smallpox, the eradication of other communicable diseases became a realistic challenge. The WHO adopted resolutions for eradication of paralytic poliomyelitis and dracunculiasis (guinea worm infection) from the world by the year 2000. This goal was not reached, but substantial progress has been made. In 2001, 480 cases of polio caused by wild-type virus were reported from 10 polio-endemic countries, compared to 350,000 reported cases from 125 countries in 1988. The Americas were certified polio free in 1994 (an outbreak in Haiti and the Dominican Republic in 2000 was vaccine derived), the western Pacific in 2000, and Europe in 2002 (WHO, 2002). Although most of the world has been certified dracunculiasis free, this disease remains a significant public health problem in Africa, especially in Sudan (CDC, 2000a).

## Primary, Secondary, and Tertiary Prevention

There are three levels of prevention in public health: primary, secondary, and tertiary. In prevention and control of infectious disease, primary prevention seeks to reduce the incidence of disease by preventing it before it happens, and in this it is often assisted by government. Many interventions at the primary level, such as federally supplied vaccines and "no shots, no school" immunization laws are population based because of public health mandate. Nurses deliver many of these childhood immunizations in public and community health settings, check immunization records in day-care facilities, and monitor immunization records in schools.

The goal of secondary prevention is to prevent the spread of disease once it occurs. Activities center on rapid identification of potential contacts to a reported case. Contacts may be (1) identified as new cases and treated, or (2) determined to be possibly exposed but not diseased and appropriately treated with prophylaxis. Public health disease control laws also assist in secondary prevention because they require investigation and prevention measures for individuals affected by a communicable disease report or outbreak. These laws can extend to the entire community if the exposure potential is deemed great enough, as could happen with an outbreak of smallpox or epidemic influenza. Much of the communicable disease surveillance and control work in this country is performed by community-oriented nurses. Whereas many infections are acute, with either recovery or death occurring in the short term, some exhibit chronic courses (AIDS) or disabling sequelae (leprosy).

Tertiary prevention works to reduce complications and disabilities through treatment and rehabilitation. Box 38-4

---

> **WHAT DO YOU THINK?**
>
> Refusal of preventive health care to undocumented residents may prove a threat to the public's health.

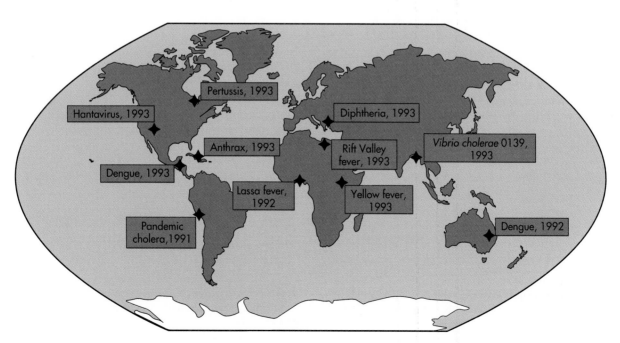

**Figure 38-2** Examples of emerging and resurgent infectious diseases in the 1990s. *(From Centers for Disease Control and Prevention: Addressing emerging infectious disease threats: a prevention strategy for the US, Atlanta, 1994, CDC.)*

**Table 38-2   Examples of Emerging Infectious Diseases**

| INFECTIOUS AGENT | DISEASES/ SYMPTOMS | MODE OF TRANSMISSION | CAUSES OF EMERGENCE |
|---|---|---|---|
| *Borrelia burgdorferi* | Lyme disease: rash, fever, arthritis, neurologic and cardiac abnormalities | Bite of infective *Ixodes* tick | Increase in deer and human populations in wooded areas. |
| *Escherichia coli* 0157:H7 | Hemorrhagic colitis, thrombocytopenia, hemolytic uremic syndrome | Ingestion of contaminated food, especially undercooked beef and raw milk | Likely to be caused by a new pathogen. |
| Ebola-Marburg viruses | Fulminant, high mortality, hemorrhagic fever | Direct contact with infected blood, organs, secretions, and semen | Unknown. |
| *Legionella pneumophila* | Legionnaires' disease: malaise, myalgia, fever, headache, respiratory illness | Air-cooling systems, water supplies | Agent had caused illness in the past, but was only recognized/identified because a large group of people were infected, resulting in several deaths, and CDC, on investigation, isolated the organism. Probably was the cause of many isolated incidences of respiratory infection in which an agent was never identified. Similar to hantavirus in this country, which was first recognized because of a group outbreak in the four-corners area of New Mexico. |
| Hantavirus | Hemorrhagic fever with renal syndrome, pulmonary syndrome | Inhalation of aerosolized rodent urine and feces | Human invasion of virus's ecologic niche. |
| Human immunodeficiency virus (HIV-1) | HIV infection, AIDS/HIV disease, severe immune dysfunction, opportunistic infections | Sexual contact with or exposure to blood or tissues of infected persons; perinatal | Urbanization, lifestyle changes, drug use, international travel, transfusions, transplant. |
| Human papillomavirus | Skin and mucous membrane lesions (warts); strongly linked to cancer of the cervix and penis | Direct sexual contact, contact with contaminated surfaces | Newly recognized; changes in sexual lifestyle. |
| Cryptosporidium | Cryptosporidiosis: infection of epithelial cells in gastrointestinal and respiratory tracts | Fecal–oral, person-to-person, waterborne | Development near watershed areas; immunosuppression. |
| *Pneumocystis carinii* | Acute pneumonia | Unknown; possibly airborne or reactivation of latent infection | Immunosuppression. |
| West Nile virus | No clinical signs to mild flulike symptoms to fatal encephalitis | Bite of infected mosquitoes; infected birds serve as reservoirs | International travel and commerce. |

Based on data from Centers for Disease Control and Prevention: Addressing emerging infectious disease threats: a prevention strategy for the United States executive summary, *MMWR Morb Mortal Wkly Rep* 43(RR-7):1, 1994; Ledeberg J, Shope RE, Oaks SC: *Emerging infections: microbial threats to health in the US*, Washington, DC, 1992, National Academy Press; Peterson LR, Roehrig JT: West Nile virus: a re-emerging global pathogen, *Emerg Infect Dis* 7(4):612-614, 2001.

has examples of communicable disease prevention and control interventions at the three levels of prevention.

## Role of Nurses in Prevention

Prevention is at the center of public and community health, and nurses perform much of this work. Examples of such involvement include delivery of immunization for vaccine-preventable disease, especially childhood immunization and the monitoring of immunization status in clinic, day-care, school, and home settings. Nurses work in communicable disease surveillance and control, teach and monitor bloodborne pathogen control, and advise on prevention of vector-borne disease. They teach methods for responsible sexual behavior, screen for STDs, and provide HIV counseling and testing. They screen for TB, identify TB contacts and deliver directly observed TB treatment in the community.

## Multisystem Approach to Control

Communicable diseases represent an imbalance in the harmonious relationship between the human host and the environment. This state of imbalance provides the infectious agent an opportunity to cause illness and death in the human population. Given the many factors that can disrupt the agent–host–environment relationship, a multisystem approach to control of communicable diseases (Table 38-3) must be developed (Wenzel, 1998).

> **NURSING TIP**
>
> When dealing with a communicable disease that has outbreak potential, include family members and close contacts as well as the sick person when developing a treatment and prevention plan.

## AGENTS OF BIOTERRORISM

September 11, 2001, made real the specter of terrorism on American soil. The anthrax attacks that followed further highlighted the possibilities for the intentional release of a biological agent, or bioterrorism. The CDC suggests that biological agents most likely to be employed in a bioterrorist attack are those that both have the potential for high mortality and can be easily disseminated, with the results of major public panic and social disruption. Six infectious agents are considered of highest concern: anthrax *(Bacillus anthracis)*, plague *(Yersinia pestis)*, smallpox (variola major), botulism *(Clostridium botulinum)*, tularemia *(Francisella tularensis)*, and selected hemorrhagic viruses (filoviruses and arenaviruses).

## Anthrax

Until the fall of 2001, anthrax was more commonly a concern of veterinarians and military strategists than the general public. In the days following September 11, the news of deaths caused by letters deliberately contaminated with anthrax and transmitted through the postal service profoundly changed our view of this infectious disease. Anthrax is an acute disease caused by the spore-forming bacterium *Bacillus anthracis*. Historical speculation suggests that anthrax may have caused the biblical fifth and sixth plagues of Exodus as well as the Black Bane of Europe in the 1600s. Of special note is that anthrax in 1881 became the first bacterial disease for which immunization was available. More commonly seen in cattle, sheep, and goats, anthrax in modern times has rarely and sporadically affected humans (Cieslak and Eitzen, 1999).

## CANADIAN NOTIFIABLE DISEASE LIST

In Canada, each province legislates its own list of reportable diseases. The list of national notifiable diseases is agreed on by consensus among provincial and federal health authorities through the Advisory Committee on Epidemiology (ACE). The following list indicates the diseases that are reported by each province to Health Canada (Population and Public Health Branch, 2002).

- Acquired immuno-deficiency syndrome (AIDS)
- Amoebiasis
- Botulism
- Brucellosis
- Campylobacteriosis
- Chancroid
- Chicken pox
- Cholera
- Diphtheria
- Genital chlamydia
- Giardiasis
- Gonococcal infections
- Gonococcal ophthalmia neonatorum
- *Haemophilus influenzae* type B
- Hepatitis A
- Hepatitis B
- Hepatitis C
- Hepatitis non-A, non-B
- HIV
- Legionellosis
- Leprosy
- Listeriosis (all types)
- Malaria
- Measles
- Meningitis, pneumococcal
- Meningitis, other bacterial
- Meningitis, viral
- Meningococcal infections
- Mumps
- Paratyphoid
- Pertussis
- Plague
- Poliomyelitis
- Rabies
- Rubella
- Rubella, congenital
- Salmonellosis
- Shigellosis
- Syphilis, congenital
- Syphilis, early latent
- Syphilis, early symptomatic
- Syphilis, other
- Tetanus
- Trichinosis
- Tuberculosis
- Typhoid
- Verotoxigenic *E. coli*
- Yellow fever

## INFECTIOUS DISEASES

### Meningococcal Disease

In 1999 in Canada, there were 203 reported cases of meningococcal infections. Since 1990, group B has been the most common cause of meningococcal disease in the Americas. Community outbreaks of group C disease, affecting school and college-age youths, have occurred with increasing frequency in Canada and the United States since 1990 (Population and Public Health Branch, 2002).

### Tuberculosis (TB)

Although Canada has one of the lowest reported incidences of TB in the world, the disease is important in certain high-risk populations, including aboriginal peoples, foreign-born residents from countries with a high prevalence of TB, disadvantaged inner-city populations, and those with HIV infection. In 1999, there were 1807 reported cases of TB in Canada. Two priorities in Canada are close surveillance of the TB–HIV co-epidemic and TB drug resistance (Population and Public Health Branch, 2002). An important strategy being implemented in certain Canadian jurisdictions is direct observed therapy. This approach ensures that individuals take the prescribed course of therapy, and public health staff can also help to assist clients to obtain the health care and social support they need.

## VACCINE-PREVENTABLE DISEASES

### Measles, Mumps, and Rubella

The National Advisory Committee on Immunization (NACI) recommends that all children receive a first dose of a combined vaccine against measles, mumps, and rubella (MMR) at 12 months of age, and a second dose at either 18 months or at 4 to 6 years (NACI, 2002). Since the introduction of this two-dose schedule in 1996, reported measles cases in Canada have dropped from 2361 in 1995 to 29 in 1999. There are approximately 500 cases of mumps reported in Canada each year. The overall incidence of rubella in Canada has remained low; however, outbreaks continue to occur in certain geographic centres (Population and Public Health Branch, 2002).

### *Haemophilus influenzae* Type B (HiB)

In the early 1990s, HiB was the most common cause of bacterial meningitis in Canada. Since the introduction of a new vaccine in 1992, the number of cases in Canada has decreased by more than 70%. In 1999 there were 30 reported cases of HiB in Canada (Population and Public Health Branch, 2002).

### Pertussis

Since the introduction of the vaccine in 1943, rates of pertussis have decreased over 90% in Canada. In 1999, Canada had 6096 reported cases of pertussis (Population and Public Health Branch, 2002). Only acellular vaccines are now available in Canada (NACI, 2002).

---

The views expressed in this box represent those of the writer and do not represent the views of the City of Toronto, Toronto Public Health.

## Influenza

Influenza occurs in Canada every year, generally during the late fall and winter. Canada, like other countries, has been affected by major influenza pandemics. The NACI recommends that priority be given to ensuring annual vaccination of people at high risk of influenza-related complications, those capable of transmitting influenza to individuals at high risk, and those providing essential community services. Because of the significant morbidity and societal costs associated with influenza, healthy adults and children who wish to protect themselves from influenza should be encouraged to receive the vaccine (NACI, 2002).

## IMMUNIZATION

In Canada, immunization cannot be made mandatory because of the Canadian Constitution. Only three provinces (out of 10 provinces and three territories) require proof of immunization for school entrance. The delivery of immunization services also varies in Canada, although immunization is provided free to all citizens. In some provinces and territories, the public health care system administers all childhood immunizations and in others private physicians provide the immunization with vaccine ordered from local public health units (Laboratory Centre for Disease Control, 1996). The NACI recommends the following Canadian vaccination schedule for infants and children (NACI, 2002):

| Age at vaccination | DTaP[1] | IPV | HiB[2] | MMR | Td[3] or dTap[10] | Hep B[4] (3 doses) | V | PC | MC |
|---|---|---|---|---|---|---|---|---|---|
| Birth | | | | | | | | | |
| | | | | | | Infancy or preadolescence (9-13 years) | | | |
| 2 months | X | X | X | | | | | X[8] | X[9] |
| 4 months | X | X | X | | | | | X | X |
| 6 months | X | (X)[5] | X | | | | | X | X |
| 12 months | | | | X | | | X[7] | X | |
| 18 months | X | X | X | (X)[6] | | | | | |
| 4-6 years | X | X | | (X)[6] | | | | | |
| 14-16 years | | | | | X[10] | | | | X[9] |

1. DTaP: Diphtheria, tetanus, pertussis (acellular) vaccine
2. Hib: *Haemophilus influenzae* type B conjugate vaccine
3. Td: Tetanus and diphtheria toxoid, adult type with reduced diphtheria toxoid
4. Hep B: Hepatitis B vaccine can be routinely given to infants or preadolescents, depending on the provincial/territorial policy. A two-dose schedule for adolescents is also possible.
5. IPV: Inactivated poliovirus vaccine. This dose is not used routinely but can be included for convenience.
6. MMR: Measles, mumps and rubella vaccine. A second dose of MMR is recommended, at least 1 month after the first dose is given. For convenience, options include giving it with the next scheduled vaccination at 18 months of age or with school entry vaccinations (4 to 6 years, depending on the provincial/territorial policy), or at any intervening age that is practical.
7. V: Varicella. Children aged 12 months to 12 years should receive one dose of varicella vaccine. Individuals 13 years of age or older should receive two doses at least 28 days apart.
8. PC: Pneumococcal conjugate vaccine. Recommended schedule, number of doses, and subsequent use of the vaccine depend on the age of the child when vaccination is begun.
9. MC: Meningococcal C conjugate vaccine. Recommended schedule and number of doses of vaccine depends on the age of the child.
10. dTap: Tetanus and diphtheria toxoid, acellular pertussis, adolescent/adult type with reduced diphtheria and pertussis components

### References

Laboratory Centre for Disease Control, Health Protection Branch: *Canadian national report on immunization,* Ottawa, 1996, Health Canada.

National Advisory Committee on Immunization: *Canadian immunization guide,* ed 6, Ottawa, 2002, Canadian Medical Association.

Population and Public Health Branch: *Notifiable diseases on-line,* Ottawa, 2002, Health Canada, available at http://dsol-smed.hc-sc.gc.ca/dsol-smed/ndis.

*Canadian spelling is used.*

**Table 38-3    A Multisystem Approach to Communicable Disease Control**

| GOAL | EXAMPLE |
|---|---|
| Improve host resistance to infectious agents and other environmental hazards | Improved hygiene, nutrition, and physical fitness; increased immunization coverage; provision of chemoprophylaxis and chemotherapy; stress control and improved mental health |
| Improve safety of the environment | Improved sanitation, provision of safe water and clean air; proper cooking and storage of food; control of vectors and animal reservoir hosts |
| Improve public health systems | Increased access to health care; adequate health education; improved surveillance systems |
| Facilitate social and political changes to ensure better health for all people | Individual, organizational, and community action; legislation |

Modified from Wenzel RP: Control of communicable diseases: overview. In Wallace RB, editor: *Public health and preventive medicine*, ed 14, Stamford, Conn, 1998, Appleton & Lange.

Anthrax is a clever organism that perpetuates itself by forming spores. When animals dying from anthrax suffer terminal hemorrhage and infected blood comes into contact with the air, the bacillus organism sporulates. These spores are highly resistant to disinfection and environmental destruction and may remain in contaminated soil for many years. In the United States, anthrax zones are said to follow the cattle drive trails of the 1800s. Sometimes referred to as woolhandler's disease, anthrax has commonly posed the greatest risk to people who work directly with dying animals, such as veterinarians, or those who handle infected animal products such as hair, wool, and bone or bone meal, or products made from these materials such as rugs and drums. Products made from infected materials may transmit this disease around the world. Person-to-person transmission is rare (Chin, 2000).

Anthrax disease may manifest in one of three syndromes: cutaneous, gastrointestinal, and respiratory or inhalational. Cutaneous anthrax, the form most commonly seen, occurs when spores come in contact with abraded skin surfaces. Itching is followed in 2 to 6 days by the development of a characteristic black eschar, usually surrounded by some degree of edema and possibly secondary infection. The lesion itself usually is not painful. If untreated, infection may spread to the regional lymph nodes and bloodstream, resulting in septicemia and death. The fatality rate for untreated cutaneous anthrax is between 5% and 20% but if appropriately treated, death seldom occurs. Before 2001, the last cutaneous case in the United States was reported in 1992. Gastrointestinal anthrax is considered very rare and occurs from eating undercooked contaminated meat.

Inhalational anthrax is also considered rare, usually having been seen in occupational exposure such as hide tanning or bone processing. Before 2001, the last case reported in the United States was in 1976. Initially, symptoms are mild and nonspecific and may include fever, malaise, mild cough, or chest pain. These symptoms are followed 3 to 5 days later, often after an apparent improvement, by fever and shock, rapid deterioration, and death. Untreated cases of inhalational anthrax are fatal; treated cases may show as high as a 95% fatality rate if treatment is initiated after 48 hours from the onset of symptoms.

Because of factors such as the ability for aerosolization, the resistance to environmental degradation, and a high fatality rate, inhalational anthrax has long been considered to have an extremely high potential for being the single greatest biological warfare threat (Cieslak and Eitzen, 1999). An accidental release from a biological research institute in Sverdlovsk, Russia, in 1979 resulted in the documented death of 66 individuals and demonstrated the capacity of this organism as a weapon. Manufacture and delivery of the spores have been considered a challenge because of a tendency for the spores to clump. During 1998 in the United States, more than two dozen anthrax threats (letters purporting to be carrying anthrax) were made. None of them were real. The events of the fall of 2001, when 11 people were sickened and five died from deliberate exposure by an unknown hand, have shown that the threat of anthrax as a weapon of bioterror is all too real.

Any threat of anthrax should be reported to the Federal Bureau of Investigation and to local and state health departments. Anthrax is sensitive to a variety of antibiotics including the penicillins, chloramphenicol, doxycycline, and the fluoroquinolones. In cases of possible bioterrorism activity, individuals with a credible threat of or confirmed exposure, or at high risk of exposure, are immediately started on antibiotic prophylaxis, preferably fluoroquinolones. Immunization is recommended as well. People who have been exposed are not contagious, so quarantine is not appropriate (Chin, 2000).

## Smallpox

Formerly a disease found worldwide, smallpox has been considered eradicated since 1979. The last known natural

> **HOW TO** **Distinguish Chicken Pox From Smallpox**
>
> Despite the availability of a vaccine, chicken pox is still a common disease of childhood and may be seen in suscepti-
> ble adults as well. Although many health care providers are familiar with chicken pox, most have never seen a case of
> smallpox. Because of the potential for smallpox to be used as a bioweapon, the CDC suggests that nurses and other
> practitioners familiarize themselves with the differences in presentation between the two diseases. The rash pattern for
> each disease is distinctive, but it has been observed that in the first 2 to 3 days of development, the two may be indis-
> tinguishable. Infectious disease texts and posters provide a pictorial description. If a smallpox infection is suspected,
> the local health department should be notified immediately.
>
> **Chickenpox (varicella)**
> Sudden onset with slight fever and mild constitutional
> symptoms (both may be more severe in adults)
> Rash is present at onset
>
> Rash progression is maculopapular for a few hours, vesicular
> for 3-4 days, followed by granular scabs
>
> Rash is "centripetal" with lesions most abundant on the
> trunk or areas of the body usually covered by clothing
> Lesions appear in "crops" and can be at various stages in
> the same area of the body
> Vesicles are superficial and collapse on puncture; mild
> scarring may occur
>
> **Smallpox (historical variola major)**
> Sudden onset of fever, prostration, severe body aches, and
> occasional abdominal pain and vomiting, as in influenza
> Clear-cut prodromal illness, rash follows 2-4 days after fever
> begins decreasing
> Progression is macular, papular, vesicular, and pustular, fol-
> lowed by crusted scabs that fall off after 3-4 weeks if pa-
> tient survives
> Rash is "centrifugal" with lesions most abundant on the face
> and extremities
> Lesions are all at same stage in all areas
>
> Vesicles are deep-seated and do not collapse on puncture;
> pitting and scarring are common
>
> From Chin J, editor: *Control of communicable diseases manual,* ed 17, Washington, DC, 2000, American Public Health Association;
> Henderson DA: Smallpox: clinical and epidemiologic features, *Emerg Infect Dis* 5(4):537-539, 1999.

death from smallpox occurred in Somalia in 1977. The
United States stopped routinely immunizing for smallpox
in 1982. The only documented existing virus sources are
located in freezers at the CDC in Atlanta and a research
institute in Novosibirsk, Russia. Controversy exists over
the destruction of these viral stocks, and despite an earlier
call by WHO for destruction in 2002, this date has been
postponed to allow for additional research needed should
clandestine supplies fall into terrorist hands.

Smallpox has been identified as one of the leading candidate agents for bioterrorism. Susceptibility is 100% in
the unvaccinated (those vaccinated before 1982 are not
considered protected) and the fatality rate is estimated at
20% to 40% or higher. Vaccinia vaccine, the immunizing
agent for smallpox, is available through the CDC and is
effective even after exposure (CDC, 2001a). Because of the
potential for bioterrorism and the fact that many health
care providers have never seen this disease, it is important
to become familiar with the clinical and epidemiologic
features of smallpox and how it is differentiated from
chickenpox (see the How To box).

## VACCINE-PREVENTABLE DISEASES

Vaccines are one of the most effective methods of preventing and controlling communicable diseases. The
smallpox vaccine, which left distinctive scars on so many
shoulders, is no longer in general use because the smallpox
virus has been declared totally eradicated from the world's
population. Despite threats of bioterrorism, there are no

plans to reintroduce universal smallpox immunization
with existing vaccine because of potential side effects.
Diseases such as polio, diphtheria, pertussis, and measles,
which previously occurred in epidemic proportions, are
now controlled by routine childhood immunization. They
have not, however, been eradicated, so children need to be
immunized against these diseases. In the United States,
"no shots, no school" legislation has resulted in the immunization of most children by the time they enter
school. However, many infants and toddlers, the group
most vulnerable to these potentially severe diseases, do not
receive scheduled immunizations on time despite the
availability of free vaccines. Surveys show inner-city children from minority and ethnic groups to be particularly at
risk for incomplete immunization. Healthy People 2010
contains several objectives about obtaining and maintaining appropriate levels of immunization in all age groups.

Because many children receive their immunizations at
public health departments, nurses play a major role in the
effort to increase immunization coverage of infants and
toddlers. Public health nurses track children known to be
at risk for underimmunization and call or send reminders
to their parents. They help avoid missed immunization
opportunities by checking the immunization status of
every young child encountered, whether the clinic or
home visit is related to immunization or not (see the
Evidence-Based Practice box). In addition, they organize
immunization outreach activities in the community that
deliver immunization services; provide answers to parents'

## Evidence-Based Practice

Researchers asked if increased parent awareness through case management would result in parental demand for immunizations, and thus providers would miss fewer opportunities to immunize during child health visits. To answer this question, a group of Los Angeles African-American newborns and their families were assigned randomly to either a case management or a control group and observed through the child's first birthday. Families in the case management group were regularly visited and telephoned, educated on the importance and safety of immunizations, and encouraged to request immunizations from their providers. Control group families received no extra education or attention.

After children turned 1 year, parents were interviewed and provider records were examined. Of children whose records were reviewed, missed opportunities occurred at more than 50% of all health visits. Home visits and parent education were only minimally associated with reducing missed opportunities. Missed opportunities occurred more often with private than public providers, and more often at visits for acute illness than at well-child visits.

**Nurse Use:** Missed opportunities to immunize are determined primarily by factors controlled by the provider. The immunization history of every child presenting for a child health visit should be assessed, and immunization should be considered if contraindications are not present.

Community-oriented nurses, who contact families for a variety of reasons during and outside child health visits, are in an excellent position to assess immunization status and encourage immunization when needed.

Wood D: Reducing missed opportunities to vaccinate during child health visits: how effective are parent education and case management? *Arch Pediatr Adolesc Med* 152(3):238, 1998.

questions and concerns about immunization; and educate parents about why immunizations are needed, about inappropriate contraindications to immunization, and about the importance of completing the immunization schedule on time.

## Routine Childhood Immunization Schedule

Routine immunization against the following 11 diseases is recommended for children in the United States: hepatitis B, diphtheria, pertussis, measles, mumps, rubella, polio, *Haemophilus influenzae* type B meningitis, varicella (chicken pox), and *Streptococcus pneumoniae*-related illnesses (CDC, 2002e). The recommended vaccine schedule is a rather complex and frequently changing document that makes continuing adjustments for the latest research and recommendations. The newest addition is the pneumococcal conjugate vaccine (PCV), licensed in 2000 to prevent diseases caused by *Streptococcus pneumoniae,* including pneumonia, sinusitis, meningitis, and acute otitis media (CDC, 2000b). To the undoubted relief of parents who feared days of work lost to caring for children miserable with chicken pox, the varicella vaccine was licensed for general use in 1995. In 1996, acellular pertussis transformed the former diphtheria, pertussis, and tetanus combination from DTP to DTaP, and in 1999, orally delivered live polio vaccine (OPV) was totally replaced in the schedule by inactivated polio vaccine (IPV). Measles, mumps, and rubella (MMR) remain in combination but are now given at as early as 12 months. Because most of these vaccines require three to four doses, they ideally should begin when an infant reaches 2 months of age in order to achieve recommended immunization levels by 2 years of age. Additional doses may be required before a child enters school and at adolescence or on entering college. Booster doses of tetanus should be given every 10 years. The Advisory Committee on Immunization Practices, the American Academy of Pediatrics, and the American Academy of Family Physicians regularly update recommended immunization schedules. Examples of other vaccines available for use in special circumstances include those against hepatitis A, influenza, meningococcal meningitis, plague, rabies, and yellow fever.

## Measles

Measles is an acute, highly contagious disease that, although considered a childhood illness, is often seen in the United States in adolescents and young adults. Symptoms include fever, sneezing and coughing, conjunctivitis, small white spots on the inside of the cheek (Koplik's spots), and a red, blotchy rash beginning several days after the respiratory signs. Measles is caused by the rubeola virus and is transmitted by inhalation of infected aerosol droplets, or by direct contact with infected nasal or throat secretions or with articles freshly contaminated with the same nasal or throat secretions. Its very contagious nature, combined with the fact that people are most contagious before they are aware they are infected, makes measles a disease that can spread rapidly through the population. Infection with measles confers lifelong immunity (Chin, 2000).

Measles and malnutrition form a deadly combination for many children in the developing world. Despite the introduction in 1963 of a live attenuated measles vaccine that is safe, effective, and widely available, measles is still endemic in many countries and results in as many as 800,000 deaths per year. Much of this mortality is preventable by immunizing all infants (CDC, 2002f).

Immunization has dramatically decreased measles cases in the United States to the point that, in March 2000, a panel of experts declared measles no longer endemic in the United States (CDC, 2000c). Before introduction of the vaccine in 1963, 200,000 to 500,000 cases of measles were reported yearly, but by 1983 reported cases had fallen to an all-time low of less than 1500. In the late 1980s, the incidence of measles began to climb again, with more than 55,000 cases reported between 1989 and 1991. This increase resulted from low immunization rates among preschool children and was countered with efforts to increase immunization rates and the routine use of two doses of measles vaccine for all children. Except for outbreaks in 1994 that occurred predominantly among high school and college-age persons, many of whom had not received two doses of measles vaccine, reported measles cases have dropped continuously since 1991 (CDC, 1997). In 2000, only 86 confirmed cases were reported to the CDC, the lowest number reported since measles became a nationally reportable disease in 1912 (CDC, 2002e).

With first-dose vaccine coverage of preschool children at greater than 90% and schools in 49 states requiring two doses of vaccine, the pattern of infection has shifted from underimmunization of infants and school-age children to disease acquired from other countries. Of the 86 measles cases reported in 2000, 62% were documented as being imported or linked to imported cases. Because these imported cases did not result in large outbreaks, it appears that vaccination efforts in this country have been successful in increasing herd immunity against measles. Groups who remain at greatest risk for infection are those who do not routinely accept immunization, such as people with religious or philosophical objections, students in schools that do not require two doses of vaccine, and infants in areas where immunization coverage is low. The exposure of these groups to an imported case could result in a major outbreak (CDC, 2002e).

Healthy People 2010 calls for the sustained elimination of indigenous cases of vaccine-preventable disease. Efforts to meet this goal will require (1) rapid detection of cases and implementation of appropriate outbreak control measures, (2) achievement and maintenance of high levels of vaccination coverage among preschool-age children in all geographic regions, (3) continued implementation and enforcement of the two-dose schedule among young adults, (4) the determination of the source of all outbreaks and sporadic infections, and (5) cooperation among countries in measles control efforts. Nurses receive reports of cases, investigate them and initiate control measures for outbreaks, and use every opportunity to immunize adolescents and young adults who lack documentation of two doses of measles vaccine. Nurses who work in regions where undocumented residents are common, where groups obtain exemption from immunization on religious grounds, where preschool coverage is low, and/or where international visitors are frequent need to be especially alert for measles cases and the need for prompt outbreak control among particularly susceptible populations.

## Rubella

The rubella (German measles) virus causes a mild febrile disease with enlarged lymph nodes and a fine, pink rash that is often difficult to distinguish from measles or scarlet fever. In contrast to measles, rubella is only a moderately contagious illness. Transmission is through inhalation of or direct contact with infected droplets from the respiratory secretions of infected persons. Children may show few or no constitutional symptoms, whereas adults usually experience several days of low-grade fever, headache, malaise, runny nose, and conjunctivitis before the rash appears. Many infections occur without a rash (Chin, 2000).

Since the introduction of a vaccine in 1969, cases of rubella in the United States have fallen precipitously, from 57,686 to less than 300 in 1999, a decrease of more than 99% (CDC, 2001c). And with this decrease at the end of the twentieth century has come a shift in the epidemiology of the disease. Although still considered a childhood illness, rubella increasingly occurs in adolescents and young adults. From 1997 to 1999, approximately 80% of cases were reported in individuals between 15 and 44 years old. Among people of Hispanic ethnicity, the percentage of reported cases increased from 19% in 1991 to 77.6% in 1999. When children are well immunized, infections in older populations become more important. Until recently, outbreaks in adolescents and adults were often seen in institutions, universities, and the military, but now they are appearing in the workplace and the community. Immigration may play a large role in this shift in age-group, ethnicity, and outbreak location, as rubella is increasingly seen in young male Hispanics, ages 15 to 44, who come from countries without or with newly introduced rubella control programs. Unimmunized immigrants do not necessarily import disease, but their unimmunized status leaves them vulnerable to infection once they arrive (CDC, 2000b).

For many years, because it caused only a mild illness, rubella was considered to be of minor importance. Then, in 1941, the link between maternal rubella and certain congenital defects was recognized, and the disease suddenly assumed major public health significance. Congenital rubella syndrome (CRS) occurs in up to 90% of infants born to women who are infected with rubella during the first trimester of pregnancy (Chin, 2000). Rubella infection, in addition to causing intrauterine death and spontaneous abortion, may result in anomalies that can affect single or multiple organ systems. Defects include cataracts, congenital glaucoma, deafness, microcephaly, mental retardation, cardiac abnormalities, and diabetes mellitus. Of the 24 cases of reported CRS during 1997 to 1999, 83.3% were born to Hispanic mothers (CDC, 2000b).

Eliminating rubella and CRS will require many of the same efforts discussed for measles, including achievement and maintenance of high rates of immunization among preschoolers, emphasizing early detection and outbreak control, taking advantage of opportunities such as high school and college entrance to immunize susceptible adolescents, and extending immunization opportunities to religious groups that traditionally do not seek health care. Because of the large percentage of cases reported in Hispanic communities, outreach to adolescents and young adults, especially women of childbearing age, from countries that may have only recently begun to vaccinate routinely against rubella is of critical importance.

## Pertussis

Pertussis (whooping cough) begins as a mild upper respiratory infection that progresses to an irritating cough that within 1 to 2 weeks may become paroxysmal (a series of repeated violent coughs). The repeated coughs occur without intervening breaths and can be followed by a characteristic inspiratory "whoop." Pertussis is caused by the bacterium *Bordetella pertussis* and is transmitted via an airborne route through contact with infected droplets. It is highly contagious and considered endemic in the United States. Vaccination against pertussis, delivered in combination with diphtheria and tetanus, is a part of the routine childhood immunization schedule. Treatment of infected individuals with antibiotics such as erythromycin may shorten the period of communicability but does not relieve symptoms unless given early in the course of the infection. A 2-week treatment with antibiotics is recommended for family members and close contacts of infected individuals, regardless of immunization status (Chin, 2000).

Before the development of a whole-cell vaccine in the 1940s, pertussis resulted in hundreds of thousands of cases and thousands of deaths per year, the majority of cases occurring in children under 5 years. After vaccine licensure, reported cases in the United States steadily declined, hitting a record low of just over 1000 in 1976. However, beginning in the early 1980s, pertussis cases have shown cyclic increases every 3 to 4 years. From 1997 to 2000, over 29,000 cases were reported (CDC, 2002g).

Immunization coverage of U.S. children, 19 to 35 months of age, was estimated to be between 77% and 90% during the 1990s. The licensure and recommendation of a less reactogenic acellular vaccine (DTaP) in 1996 may have decreased some parental reluctance to vaccinating their children against pertussis. This hesitation resulted from the frequency of minor adverse reactions to the whole-cell pertussis vaccine, as well as publicity surrounding infrequent but serious adverse reactions and the inaccurate suggestion that pertussis vaccine could result in permanent neurologic damage (Marwick, 1996).

Pertussis in very young children, especially those less than 6 months, is attributed to being under- or unimmunized because of age. Cases in older children result largely from underimmunization, and in adolescents and adults with histories of complete immunization, cases are thought to be the result of waning immunity. Cases in adolescents and adults have been increasing, with 49% of reported cases during 1997 to 2000 occurring in this age-group, a greater than 60% increase over the 1994 to 1996 reporting period. Some of this adult and adolescent increase is the result of improved reporting and increased awareness. However, the fact that the percent of cases in fully immunized 1- to 4-year-olds decreased and in 5- to 9-year-olds remained stable while incompletely or nonimmunized infant cases increased by 11% suggests an actual rise in pertussis

circulation. The increase in adolescent and adult pertussis is alarming not because of increased morbidity—their cases are often mild or inapparent—but because they serve as a reservoir of infection for infants, especially those less than 6 months, who are the most vulnerable to pertussis (55.5 cases/100,000 in 1997 to 2000) and the most likely to suffer complications resulting in hospitalization and death.

Although natural infection with pertussis results in permanent immunity, immunization through vaccination does not. Pertussis vaccines are not labeled for use in individuals older than 6 years; catching up children who are missing doses and boostering for waning immunity are not presently options for preventing outbreaks. The routine boostering of adults for pertussis is under discussion. Prevention efforts should be directed at maintaining high rates of immunization coverage, increasing awareness of pertussis in adolescents and adults, and promptly implementing treatment and control in the face of outbreaks (CDC, 2002f).

Nurses may expect periodic outbreaks of pertussis because of its cyclical nature. Working with the community to maintain the highest possible levels of immunization coverage can minimize these occurrences. Because of the contagious nature of pertussis, nurses play a major role in limiting transmission during outbreaks by ensuring appropriate treatment of family members, classmates, and other close contacts.

## Influenza

Influenza is a viral respiratory infection often indistinguishable from the common cold or other respiratory diseases. Transmission is airborne and through direct contact with infected droplets. Unlike many viruses that do not survive long in the environment, the flu virus is thought to survive for many hours in dried mucus. Outbreaks are common in the winter and early spring in areas where people gather indoors such as in schools and nursing homes. Gastrointestinal and respiratory symptoms are common. Because symptoms do not always follow a characteristic pattern, many viral diseases that are not influenza are often called flu. The most important factors to note about influenza are its epidemic nature and the mortality that may result from pulmonary complications, especially in older adults.

There are three types of influenza viruses: A, B, and C. Type A is usually responsible for large epidemics, whereas outbreaks from type B are more regionalized; type C epidemics are less common and usually result in only mild illness. Influenza viruses often change in the nature of their surface appearance or their antigenic makeup. Types B and C are fairly stable viruses, but type A changes constantly. Minor antigenic changes are referred to as antigenic drift, and they result in yearly epidemics and regional outbreaks. Major changes such as the emergence of new subtypes are called antigenic shift; these occur only with type A viruses. Antigenic shift and drift lead to epidemic outbreaks every few years and pandemic outbreaks every 10 to 40 years.

Mortality rates associated with epidemics may be higher than those in nonepidemic situations (Chin, 2000).

In 1997 in Hong Kong, the first known cases of human illness associated with an avian influenza virus, A (H5N10), were reported. Referred to in the press as Hong Kong bird flu, this virus appears to have been transmitted to people through contact with infected poultry. As a result of this association, Hong Kong officials ordered the slaughter of all chickens in and around Hong Kong, which appears to have stopped the spread of this disease. No cases were reported outside Hong Kong, and despite recurring outbreaks of avian flu, no further outbreaks of A (H5N10) have been reported. Although investigation of this disease did not rule out the possibility of human to human transmission, the fact that it did not spread more readily among a population essentially without antibodies to this virus suggests that it is not being efficiently transmitted between people (CDC, 1998b).

The preparation of influenza vaccine each year is based on the best possible prediction of what type and variant of virus will be most prevalent that year. Because of the changing nature of the virus, yearly immunization is necessary and in the United States is given in early fall before the flu season begins. Immunization is highly recommended for older adults, individuals with chronic respiratory disease, and those with other chronic disease conditions that impair the immune system, as well as health care workers and anyone involved in essential community services. Although immunization is recommended for the previously mentioned groups, any individual may benefit from this protection. Flu shots do not always prevent infection, but they do result in milder disease symptoms. Because of small quantities of egg protein found in the vaccine, individuals with egg sensitivity should consult their physician to determine if immunization should be administered.

Unlike the immunizations for childhood diseases, flu shots are largely targeted at an adult population. Although influenza is often self-limiting in the healthy population, serious complications, particularly viral and bacterial pneumonias, can be deadly to older adults and those debilitated by chronic disease. Since 80% to 90% of all influenza-associated deaths in the United States occur in people age 65 and older, it is important to couple influenza immunization of this population with immunization against pneumococcal pneumonia (Chin, 2000).

Amantadine and rimantadine offer effective chemoprophylaxis against type A but not type B influenza. The use of these drugs should be considered in the nonimmunized or groups at high risk of complications such as older adults in institutions or nursing homes when an appropriate vaccine is not available or as a supplement when immediate maximum protection against type A influenza is required (Chin, 2000).

Healthy People 2010 targets increasing the proportion of the population vaccinated annually against influenza and ever vaccinated against pneumococcal disease. Public health nurses often spearhead influenza immunization campaigns that target older adults. Examples include conducting flu clinics at polling places during elections or at community centers and churches during "senior vaccination Sundays." Inhabitants of residences and nursing homes for older adults are at risk, as influenza can spread rapidly with severe consequences through such living arrangements. As with children, nurses should check immunization history and encourage immunization for every adult encountered in a clinic or home visit.

# FOOD-BORNE AND WATERBORNE DISEASES

Food-borne illness, or "food poisoning," is often categorized as food infection or food intoxication. Food infection results from bacterial, viral, or parasitic infection of food and includes salmonellosis, hepatitis A, and trichinosis. Food intoxication results from toxins produced by bacterial growth, chemical contaminants (heavy metals), and a variety of disease producing substances found naturally in certain foods such as mushrooms and some seafood. Examples of food intoxications are botulism, mercury poisoning, and paralytic shellfish poisoning. Table 38-4 presents some of the most common agents of food intoxication, their incubation period, source, symptoms, and pathology. Although it is not a hard-and-fast rule, food infections are associated with incubation periods of 12 hours to several days after ingestion of the infected food, whereas intoxications become obvious within minutes to hours after ingestion. Botulism is a clear exception to this rule, with an incubation period of a week or more in adults. The expression *ptomaine poisoning*, often used when discussing food-borne illness, does not refer to a specific causal organism.

It is estimated that in the United States 76 million illnesses, 325,000 hospitalizations, and 5000 deaths occur from food-borne illnesses each year (Mead, 1999). Of identified agents, *Salmonella* and *Campylobacter* are most frequently involved with illness; *Salmonella*, *Listeria*, and *Toxoplasma*, with deaths. FoodNet is a CDC sentinel surveillance system targeting seven states and collecting information on seven bacterial and two parasitic agents. Confirmed food-borne outbreaks are reported by states to the CDC through the Food-borne Disease Outbreak Surveillance System; on average, 1300 outbreaks have been reported every year since 1998. In June 2001, the CDC launched an Electronic Food-borne Outbreak Reporting System (EFORS).

In recent years, publicity has surrounded the deaths of children who ate undercooked fast-food hamburgers containing a virulent strain of *E. coli;* nationwide outbreaks of diarrheal disease from *Cyclospora*-contaminated Guatemalan raspberries; outbreaks of hepatitis A in schoolchildren who consumed tainted frozen strawberries; and salmonella infections associated with uncooked poultry and eggs. Although the very young, the very old, and the very debilitated are most susceptible, anyone can acquire food-borne illness regardless of socioeconomic status, race, sex, age, occupation, education, or area of residence. However, a new, particularly susceptible population is emerging as a result of the increasing older adult population, the growing numbers of

**Table 38-4 Commonly Encountered Food Intoxications**

| CAUSAL AGENT | INCUBATION PERIOD | DURATION | CLINICAL PRESENTATION | ASSOCIATED FOOD |
|---|---|---|---|---|
| *Staphylococcus aureus* | 30 min to 7 hr | 1-2 days | Sudden onset of nausea, cramps, vomiting, and prostration, often accompanied by diarrhea; rarely fatal | All foods, especially those likely to come into contact with food-handlers' hands that may be contaminated from infections of the eyes and skin |
| *Clostridium perfringens* (strain A) | 6-24 hr | 1 day or less | Sudden onset of colic and diarrhea, maybe nausea; vomiting and fever unusual; rarely fatal | Inadequately heated meats or stews; food contaminated by soil or feces becomes infective when improper storage or reheating allows multiplication of organism |
| *Vibrio parahemolyticus* | 4-96 hr | 1-7 days | Watery diarrhea and abdominal cramps; sometimes nausea, vomiting, fever, and headache; rarely fatal | Raw or inadequately cooked seafood; period of time at room temperature usually required for multiplication of organism |
| *Clostridium botulinum* | 12-36 hr, sometimes days | Slow recovery, maybe months | Central nervous system signs; blurred vision, difficulty in swallowing and dry mouth, followed by descending symmetrical flaccid paralysis of an alert person; "floppy baby" in infant; fatality <15% with antitoxin and respiratory support | Home-canned fruits and vegetables that have not been preserved with adequate heating; infants have become infected from ingesting honey |

Based on data from Chin J, editor: *Control of communicable diseases manual,* ed 17, Washington, DC, 2000, American Public Health Association.

immunocompromised individuals (resulting from chemotherapy, immunosuppressive drugs, and AIDS), and the larger numbers of children surviving debilitating illness. At the same time the centralized food production and processing system with its widespread distribution network increases the potential for any contamination to result in a large-scale food-borne disease outbreak. Public health officials think that the number of reported cases of food-borne illness vastly underestimates the true number of cases, and that the number of food-borne outbreaks is likely to increase.

## Ten Golden Rules for Safe Food Preparation

Protecting the nation's food supply from contamination by all virulent microbes is a complex issue that will be incredibly costly and time consuming to address. However, much food-borne illness, regardless of causal organism, can be prevented easily through simple changes in food preparation, handling, and storage to destroy or denature contaminants and prevent their further spread. Because these measures are so important in preventing food-borne disease, Healthy People 2010 has included an objective directed toward them, and the WHO has developed the

**THE CUTTING EDGE**

Irradiation of meat and poultry is one option being used to prevent outbreaks of food-borne disease.

"Ten Golden Rules for Safe Food Preparation" presented in Box 38-5 (Chin, 2000).

## Salmonellosis

Salmonellosis is a bacterial disease characterized by sudden onset of headache, abdominal pain, diarrhea, nausea, sometimes vomiting, and almost always fever. Onset is typically within 48 hours of ingestion, but the clinical signs are impossible to distinguish from other causes of gastrointestinal distress. Diarrhea and lack of appetite may persist for several days, and dehydration may be severe. Although morbidity can be significant, death is uncommon except among infants, older adults, and the debilitated. The rate of infection is highest among infants and small children. It is estimated that only a small proportion of cases are recognized clinically and that only 1% of clinical cases are reported. The number of salmonella infections yearly may actually number in the millions (Chin, 2000).

Outbreaks occur commonly in restaurants, hospitals, nursing homes, and institutions for children. The transmission route is eating food derived from an infected animal or contaminated by feces of an infected animal or person. Meat, poultry, and eggs are the foods most often associated with salmonellosis outbreaks. Animals are the common reservoir for the various *Salmonella* serotypes, although infected humans may also fill this role. Animals are more likely to be chronic carriers. Reptiles such as iguanas have been implicated as *Salmonella* carriers, along with pet turtles, poultry, cattle, swine, rodents, dogs, and cats. Person-to-person transmission is an important consideration in day-care and institutional settings.

## *Escherichia coli* 0157:H7

*Escherichia coli* 0157:H7 belongs to the enterohemorrhagic category of *E. coli* serotypes that produce a strong cytotoxin that can cause a potentially fatal hemorrhagic colitis. This pathogen was first described in humans in 1992 following the investigation of two outbreaks of illness that were associated with consumption of hamburger from a fast-food restaurant chain. Undercooked hamburger has been implicated in several outbreaks, as have roast beef, alfalfa sprouts, unpasteurized milk and apple cider, municipal water, and person-to-person transmission in day-care centers. Infection with *E. coli* 0157:H7 causes bloody diarrhea, abdominal cramps, and, infrequently, fever. Children and older adults are at highest risk for clinical disease and complications. Hemolytic uremic syndrome is seen in 5% to 10% of cases and may result in acute renal failure. The case fatality rate is 3% to 5% (Chin, 2000).

Hamburger often appears to be involved in outbreaks because the grinding process exposes pathogens on the surface of the whole meat to the interior of the ground meat, effectively mixing the once-exterior bacteria thoroughly throughout the hamburger so that searing the surface no longer suffices to kill all bacteria. Tracking the contamination is complicated by the fact that hamburger is often made of meat ground from several sources. The best protection against this pathogen, as with most food-borne agents, is to thoroughly cook food before eating it.

## Waterborne Disease Outbreaks and Pathogens

Waterborne pathogens usually enter water supplies through animal or human fecal contamination and frequently cause enteric disease. They include viruses, bacteria, and protozoans. Hepatitis A virus is probably the most publicized waterborne viral agent, although other viruses may also be transmitted by this route (enteroviruses, rotaviruses, and paramyxoviruses). The most important waterborne bacterial diseases are cholera, typhoid fever, and bacillary dysentery. However, other *Salmonella* types, *Shigella*, *Vibrio*, and various coliform bacteria including *E. coli* 0157:H7 may be transmitted in the same manner. In the past, the most important waterborne protozoans have been *Entamoeba histolytica* (amebic dysentery) and *Giardia lamblia*, but recent outbreaks of cryptosporidiosis in municipal water, such as that which resulted in diarrheal outbreaks that crippled the city of Milwaukee in 1993, have pushed *Cryptosporidium* into the debate over how to best safeguard municipal water supplies. Protozoans do not respond to traditional chlorine treatment as do enteric and coliform bacteria, and their small size requires special filtration.

The CDC defines an outbreak of waterborne disease as an incident in which two or more persons experience similar illness after consuming water that epidemiologic evidence implicates as the source of that illness. Only a single incident is required in cases of chemical contamination. The CDC and the Environmental Protection Agency

(EPA) maintain a collaborative surveillance program for collection and periodic reporting of data on the occurrence and causes of waterborne disease outbreaks.

## VECTOR-BORNE DISEASES

Vector-borne diseases refer to illnesses for which the infectious agent is transmitted by a carrier, or vector, usually an arthropod (mosquito, tick, fly), either biologically or mechanically. With *biological transmission,* the vector is necessary for the developmental stage of the infectious agent. An example is the mosquitoes that carry malaria. *Mechanical transmission* occurs when an insect simply contacts the infectious agent with its legs or mouth parts and carries it to the host. For example, flies and cockroaches may contaminate food or cooking utensils.

Vector-borne diseases commonly encountered in the United States are those associated with ticks, such as Lyme disease *(Borrelia burgdorferi),* ehrlichiosis *(Ehrlichia chafeensis),* and Rocky Mountain spotted fever *(Rickettsia rickettsii).* Nurses who work with large immigrant populations or with international travelers may encounter malaria and dengue fever, both carried by mosquitoes. Most recently in the news, West Nile virus is an example of endemic mosquito-borne viruses which include St. Louis, LaCrosse, and western and eastern equine encephalitis. Plague *(Yersinia pestis)* is carried by fleas of wild rodents. More rarely seen are babesiosis *(Babesia microti),* tularemia *(Francisella tularensis),* and Q fever *(Coxiella burnetii),* all associated with ticks.

### Lyme Disease

Parents in Lyme, Connecticut, concerned about the unusual incidence of juvenile rheumatoid arthritis in their children, were the first to bring attention to this tick-borne infection that now bears their town's name. First described in 1975, Lyme disease became a nationally notifiable disease in 1991 and is now the most common vector-borne disease in the United States, with over 15,000 cases reported per year (CDC, 2002h). The causative agent, the spirochete *Borrelia burgdorferi,* was identified in 1982. Lyme disease is transmitted by ixodid ticks that are associated with white-tailed deer *(Odocoileus virginianus)* and the white-footed mouse *(Peromyscus leucopus).* Lyme disease usually occurs in summer during tick season, and it has been reported throughout the United States, with 95% of cases concentrated in rural and suburban areas of the northeast, mid-Atlantic, and north-central states, particularly Wisconsin and Minnesota.

The clinical spectrum of Lyme disease can be divided into three stages. Stage I is characterized by erythema chronicum migrans, a distinctive skin lesion often called a bull's-eye lesion because it begins as a red area at the site of the tick attachment that spreads outward in a ringlike fashion as the center clears. About 50% to 70% of infected persons develop this lesion 3 to 30 days after a tick bite. The skin lesion may be accompanied or preceded by fever, fatigue, malaise, headache, muscle pains, and a stiff neck, as well as tender and enlarged lymph nodes and migratory joint pain.

Most clients diagnosed in this early stage respond well to 10 to 14 days of oral tetracycline or penicillin.

If not treated during this first stage, Lyme disease can progress to stage II, which may include additional skin lesions, headache, and neurologic and cardiac abnormalities. Clients who progress to stage III have recurrent attacks of arthritis and arthralgia, especially in the knees, that may begin months to years after the initial lesion. The clinical diagnosis of classic Lyme disease with the distinctive skin lesion is straightforward. Illness without the lesion is more difficult to diagnose, because serologic tests are more accurate in stages II and III than in stage I (Chin, 2000).

### Rocky Mountain Spotted Fever

Contrary to its name, Rocky Mountain spotted fever (RMSF) is seldom seen in the Rocky Mountains and most commonly occurs in the southeast, Oklahoma, Kansas, and Missouri. The infectious agent is *Rickettsia rickettsii.* The tick vector varies according to geographic region. The dog tick, *Dermacentor variabilis,* is the vector in the eastern and southern United States. RMSF is not transmitted from person to person. It is thought that one attack confers lifelong immunity.

Clinical signs include sudden onset of moderate to high fever, severe headache, chills, deep muscle pain, and malaise. About 50% of cases experience a rash on the extremities that spreads to most of the body. Many cases of what has been referred to as "spotless" RMSF may actually be caused by recently identified forms of human ehrlichiosis, another tick-borne infection. RMSF responds readily to treatment with tetracycline. Definitive diagnosis can be made with paired serum titers. Because early treatment is important in decreasing morbidity and mortality, treatment should be started in response to clinical and epidemiologic considerations rather than waiting for laboratory confirmation (Chin, 2000).

### Prevention and Control of Tick-Borne Diseases

Healthy People 2010 targets reducing the incidence of Lyme disease in all states to less than 7.7 cases per 100,000 population. A vaccine for Lyme disease, recommended for use by persons living in high-risk areas, was licensed in 1998; however, in 2002, the manufacturer withdrew it from the commercial market. Measures for preventing exposure to ticks include reducing tick populations, avoiding tick-infested areas, wearing protective clothing when outdoors (long sleeves and long pants tucked into socks), using repellants, and immediately inspecting for and removing ticks when returning indoors. Researchers are looking at the effectiveness of using tick-killing acaricides in rodent bait boxes and at deer feeding stations in areas where Lyme disease is highly concentrated. Ticks require a prolonged period of attachment (6 to 48 hours) before they start blood-feeding on the host; prompt tick discovery and removal can help prevent transmission of disease. Ticks should be removed with steady, gentle traction on tweezers applied to the head parts of the tick. The tick's body should not be squeezed during the removal process to avoid infection that could be transmitted from resultant tick feces and tissue juices (Walker and Raoult, 2000). When outdoors, permetherin sprayed on clothing and tick repellents containing diethyltoluamide (DEET) can offer effective protection; use of DEET should be avoided on children under 2 years because of reports of significant toxicity, including skin irritation, anaphylaxis, and seizures.

## DISEASES OF TRAVELERS

Individuals traveling outside the United States need to be aware of and take precautions against potential diseases to which they may be exposed. Which diseases and what precautions depends on the individual's health status, the travel destination, the reason for travel, and the length of travel. Persons who plan to travel in remote regions for an extended period may need to consider rare diseases and take special precautions that would not apply to the average traveler. Consultation with public health officials can provide specific health information and recommendations for a given situation.

On return from visiting exotic places, travelers may bring back with them an unplanned souvenir in the form of disease. Therefore, in a presenting client, a history of travel should always be closely considered. Even the apparently healthy returned traveler, especially one who was in a tropical country for some time, should undergo routine screening to rule out acquired infections. Likewise, refugees and immigrants may arrive with infectious disease problems ranging from helminthic infections to diseases of major public health significance, such as tuberculosis, malaria, cholera, and hepatitis. Community-oriented nurses may find themselves dealing with these diseases, as refugees and immigrants, especially the undocumented, are often treated through the public health system.

## Malaria

Caused by the bloodborne parasite *Plasmodium*, malaria is a potentially fatal disease characterized by regular cycles of fever and chills. Transmission is through the bite of an infected *Anopheles* mosquito. The word *malaria* is based on an association between the illness and the "bad air" of the marshes where the mosquitoes breed. Malaria is an old disease that first appears in recorded history in 1700 B.C. China. Worldwide, malaria is the most prevalent vector-borne disease occurring in over 100 countries. More than 40% of the world's population is considered at risk; 90% of cases occur in Africa. There is no vaccine available to protect against this disease, which affects from 300 to 500 million people a year and results in over 2 million deaths, half in children under the age of 5 (WHO, 1997).

Malaria prevention depends on protection against mosquitoes and appropriate chemoprophylaxis. Drug resistance is an increasing problem in combating malaria. Of the four causes of human malaria, *Plasmodium ovale* and *Plasmodium vivax* result in disease that can progress to re-

lapsing malaria, and *P. vivax* is increasingly drug resistant. *Plasmodium falciparum* causes the most serious malarial infection and is highly drug resistant. Thus decisions about antimalarial drugs must be tailored individually on the basis of the type of malaria in the specific area of the country to be visited, the purpose of the trip, and the length of the visit. The CDC and the WHO publish guides on the status of malaria and recommendations for prophylaxis on a country-by-country basis. At this time, there is no one drug or drug combination known to be safe and efficacious in preventing all types of malaria. Antimalarials are generally started a week to several weeks before leaving the country and are continued for 4 to 6 weeks after returning. Despite appropriate prophylaxis, malaria may still be contracted. Travelers should be advised of this fact and urged to seek immediate medical care if they exhibit symptoms of cyclical fever and chills up to 1 year after returning home. Immigrants and visitors from areas where malaria is endemic may become clinically ill after entering this country. Approximately 1500 cases of malaria in travelers and immigrants are reported in the United States every year. In addition, during the past 15 years, over 80 people have contracted locally transmitted malaria (CDC, 2002i).

## Food-Borne and Waterborne Diseases

As in this country, much food-borne disease abroad can be avoided if the traveler eats thoroughly cooked foods prepared with reasonable hygiene; eating foods from street vendors may not be a good idea. Trichinosis, tapeworms, and fluke infections, as well as bacterial infections, result from eating raw or undercooked meats. Raw vegetables may act as a source of bacterial, viral, helminthic, or protozoal infection if they have been grown with or washed in contaminated water. Fruits that can be peeled immediately before eating such as bananas are less likely to be a source of infection. Dairy products should be pasteurized and appropriately refrigerated.

Water in many areas of the world is not potable (safe to drink), and drinking this water can lead to infection with a variety of protozoal, viral, and bacterial agents including amoebae, *Giardia*, *Cryptosporidium*, hepatitis, cholera, and various coliform bacteria. Unless traveling in an area where the piped water is known to be safe, only boiled water (boiled for 1 minute), bottled water, or water purified with iodine or chlorine compounds should be consumed. Ice should be avoided, as freezing does not inactivate these agents. If the water is questionable, choose coffee or tea made with boiled water, carbonated beverages without ice, beer, wine, or canned fruit juices.

## Diarrheal Diseases

Travelers often suffer from diarrhea, so much so that colorful names, such as Montezuma's revenge, *turista*, and Colorado quickstep, exist in our vocabulary to describe these bouts of intestinal upset. Some of these diarrheas do not have infectious causes and result from stress, fatigue, schedule changes, and eating unfamiliar foods.

Acute infectious diarrheas are usually of viral or bacterial origin. *E. coli* probably causes more cases of traveler's diarrhea than all other infective agents combined. Protozoan-induced diarrheas such as those resulting from *Entamoeba* and *Giardia* are less likely to be acute, and they more commonly present once the traveler returns home. Travelers need to pay special attention to what they eat and drink.

## ZOONOSES

A zoonosis is an infection transmitted from a vertebrate animal to a human under natural conditions. The agents that cause zoonoses do not need humans to maintain their life cycles; infected humans have simply somehow managed to get in their way. Means of transmission include animal bites, inhalation, ingestion, direct contact, and arthropod intermediates. This last transmission route means that some vector-borne diseases may also be zoonoses. Other than vector-borne diseases, some of the more common zoonoses in the United States include toxoplasmosis *(Toxoplasma gondii)*, cat-scratch disease *(Bartonella henselae)*, brucellosis *(Brucella* species), listeriosis *(Listeria monocytogenes)*, salmonellosis *(Salmonella* serotypes), and rabies (family Rhabdoviridae, genus *Lyssavirus).*

## Rabies (Hydrophobia)

One of the most feared of human diseases, rabies has the highest case fatality rate of any known human infection, essentially 100%. In the 1970s, three cases of presumed rabies recovery were reported. All had received preexposure or postexposure prophylaxis. Since that time, despite the intensive medical care available in the United States, no survivors have been reported. A significant public health problem worldwide with as many as 50,000 deaths a year, mostly in developing countries, rabies in humans in the United States is a rare event because of the widespread vaccination of dogs begun in the 1950s. Today, the major carriers of rabies in the United States are not dogs but wild animals—raccoons, skunks, foxes, coyotes, and bats. Small rodents, rabbits and hares, and opossums rarely carry rabies. Epidemiologic information should be consulted for information on the potential carriers for a given geographic region. When the virus spreads from wild to domestic animals, cats are often involved. Of the 32 human cases of rabies reported in the United States since 1990, 24 were acquired in this country and have been associated with insectivorous bats; the six acquired outside the county were associated with bites from dogs (CDC, 2000d).

Rabies is transmitted to humans by introducing virus-carrying saliva into the body, usually via an animal bite or scratch. Transmission may also occur if infected saliva comes into contact with a fresh cut or intact mucous membranes. Rabies is found in neural tissue and is not transmitted via blood, urine, or feces. Airborne transmission has been documented in caves with infected bat colonies. Transmission from human to human is theoretically possible but has not been documented except for six cases of rabies acquired by receiving corneal transplants harvested from individuals who died of undiagnosed rabies. Guidelines for organ donation now exist to prevent this possibility (Beck and Rupprecht, 2000).

The best protection against rabies remains vaccinating domestic animals—dogs, cats, cattle, and horses. If an individual is bitten, the bite wound should be thoroughly cleaned with soap and water and a physician consulted immediately. Suspicion of rabies should exist if the bite is from a wild animal or an unprovoked attack from a domestic animal. Even when there is no suspicion of rabies, a physician should be contacted, as tetanus or antibiotic prophylaxis may be indicated.

No successful treatment exists for rabies once symptoms appear, but if given promptly and as directed, postexposure prophylaxis with human rabies immune globulin and rabies vaccine can prevent the development of the disease. Three products are licensed for use as rabies vaccine in the United States: human diploid cell vaccine (HDCV), rabies vaccine adsorbed (RVA), and purified chick embryo cell (PCEC) culture (RabAvert) (CDC, 1999). The vaccine is administered in a series of five 1-ml doses injected into the deltoid muscle. Reactions to the vaccine are fewer and less serious than with previously used vaccines. Individuals who deal frequently with animals, such as zookeepers, lab workers, and veterinarians, may choose to receive the vaccine as preexposure prophylaxis. The decision to administer the vaccine to a bite victim depends on the circumstances of the bite and is made on an individual basis.

Recommendations for providing postexposure prophylaxis treatment are provided by the Advisory Committee for Recommendations on Immunization Practices and are available through local public health officials or the CDC. In general, cats and dogs that have bitten someone and have verified rabies vaccinations are confined for 10 days for observation. Treatment is initiated only if signs of rabies are observed during this period. If the animal is known or suspected to be rabid, treatment begins immediately. If the animal is unknown to the victim and escapes, public health officials should be consulted for help in deciding whether treatment is indicated. With wild animal bites, treatment is begun immediately. With bites from livestock, rodents, and rabbits, treatment is considered on an individual basis. Decisions to treat become more complicated for possible nonbite exposure to saliva from known infected animals, and again public health officials are helpful in making these treatment decisions (CDC, 1999).

## PARASITIC DISEASES

Parasitic diseases are more prevalent in developing countries than in the United States because of tropical climate and inadequate prevention and control measures. A lack of cheap and effective drugs, poor sanitation, and a scarcity of funding lead to high reinfection rates even when control programs are attempted. Parasites are classified into four groups: nematodes (roundworms), cestodes

## Table 38-5 Selected Parasite Categories

| CATEGORY | PARASITE AND DISEASE |
|---|---|
| Intestinal nematodes | *Ascaris lumbricoides* (roundworm)<br>*Trichuris trichiura* (whipworm)<br>*Ancylostoma, Necator* (hookworm),<br>*Enterobius vermicularis* (pinworm) |
| Blood and tissue nematodes | *Wuchereria bancrofti* (filariasis)<br>*Onchocerca volvulus* (river blindness) |
| Cestodes | *Taenia solium* (pork tapeworm)<br>*Taenia saginata* (beef tapeworm) |
| Trematodes | *Schistosoma* species (schistosomiasis) |
| Protozoans | *Giardia lamblia* (giardiasis)<br>*Entamoeba histolytica* (amebiasis)<br>*Plasmodium* species (malaria)<br>*Leishmania* species (leishmaniasis)<br>*Trypanosoma* species (African sleeping sickness, Chagas' disease)<br>*Toxoplasma gondii* (toxoplasmosis) |

Based on data from Brown H, Neva FA: *Basic clinical parasitology,* ed 6, Norwalk, Conn, 1994, Appleton & Lange.

(tapeworms), trematodes (flukes), and protozoa (single celled animals). Nematodes, cestodes, and trematodes are all referred to as helminths. Table 38-5 presents examples of diseases caused by parasites from these groups.

Nurses and other health professionals should be aware of the growing numbers of reported parasitic infections in the United States. The following list includes factors that may be contributing to this rise in detection (Kappus et al, 1994).

- International travel
- Immigration of persons from developing countries
- Incidence of AIDS with secondary parasitic opportunistic infections such as *Pneumocystis carinii* pneumonia, cryptosporidiosis, and toxoplasmosis
- Recognition of *Giardia* and *Cryptosporidium* as common infectious agents in day-care centers and waterborne disease outbreaks
- Incidence and recognition of sexually transmitted parasitic enteric infections acquired through oral–anal sex
- Recognition of *Cryptosporidium* species as pathogens in immunocompetent individuals resulting from improvement in stool examination techniques

## Intestinal Parasitic Infections

Enterobiasis (pinworm) is the most common helminthic infection in the United States, with an estimated 42 million cases a year. Pinworm infection is seen most often among children and is most prevalent in crowded and institutional settings. Pinworms resemble small pieces of white thread and can be seen with the naked eye. Diagnosis is usually accomplished by pressing cellophane tape to the perianal region early in the morning. Treatment with oral vermicides results in a cure rate of 90% to 100%.

A study by state diagnostic laboratories found intestinal parasites in 20% of 216,275 stool specimens examined. The most commonly identified parasites were *Giardia lamblia, Entamoeba histolytica, Trichuris trichiura* (whipworm), and *Ascaris lumbricoides* (roundworm) (Kappus et al, 1994). The opportunities for widespread indigenous transmission of these intestinal parasites are limited because of improved sanitary conditions in this country. Effective drug treatment is available for these intestinal parasitic infections.

## Parasitic Opportunistic Infections

Some of the common parasitic opportunistic infections in clients with AIDS and others who are immunocompromised include *Pneumocystis carinii* pneumonia (PCP), cryptosporidiosis, microsporidiosis, and isosporiasis. *P. carinii* is found in the lungs and can cause severe pneumonia in immunocompromised individuals; immunocompetent persons are unaffected. PCP is seen is in as many as 80% of clients with AIDS. Effective drugs for treatment and prophylaxis of PCP are available, including trimethoprim-sulfamethoxazole and pentamidine isethionate (Martinez, Suffredini, and Masur, 1998).

*Cryptosporidium, Microsporidium,* and *Isospora belli* are intestinal protozoans that cause diarrheal disease and are transmitted by fecal–oral contact. The AIDS epidemic has brought about an increased incidence of illness due to these organisms. From 15% to 20% of refractory unexplained diarrhea in AIDS clients may be due to microsporidiosis. An estimated 10% to 15% of AIDS clients in this country, and as many a 30% to 50% around the world, have developed chronic cryptosporidiosis. In the United States, infection with *I. belli* among AIDS clients is rare (about 1%), but 15% to 20% of Haitian and African clients may be infected. There is currently no consistently effective drug treatment approved by the U.S. Food and Drug Administration (FDA) for cryptosporidiosis or microsporidiosis. Trimethoprim-sulfamethoxazole is effective for isosporiasis (DeVita, Hellman, and Rosenberg, 1997).

## Control and Prevention of Parasitic Infections

Correct diagnosis by nurses and other health care workers allows the provision of appropriate treatment and client education for preventing and controlling parasitic infections. Diagnosis of parasitic diseases is based on history of travel, characteristic clinical signs and symptoms, and the use of appropriate laboratory tests to confirm the clinical diagnosis. Knowing what specimens to collect, how and when to collect, and what laboratory techniques to use are all important in establishing a correct diagnosis. Effective drug treatment is available for most parasitic diseases. The high cost of the drugs, drug resistance, and toxicity are some of the common therapeutic problems. Measures for prevention and control of parasitic diseases include early diagnosis and treatment, improved personal hygiene, safer sex practices, community health education, vector control, and improvements in sanitary control of food, water, and waste disposal.

## NOSOCOMIAL INFECTIONS

**Nosocomial infections** are those acquired during hospitalization or developed within a hospital setting. They may involve patients, health care workers, visitors, or anyone who has contact with a hospital. Invasive diagnostic and surgical procedures, broad-spectrum antibiotics, and immunosuppressive drugs, along with the original underlying illness, leave hospitalized patients particularly vulnerable to exposure to virulent infectious agents from other patients and indigenous hospital flora from health care staff. In this setting, the simple act of performing hand hygiene before approaching every patient becomes critical. Each year, hospital-acquired infections may affect as many as 2 million people, result in 88,000 deaths, and add 5 billion dollars to health costs (CDC, 2000e). In addition, nosocomial infections have a high likelihood of involving and contributing to antibiotic resistance. The CDC maintains the National Nosocomial Infection Surveillance (NNIS) system, the only source of national data on the epidemiology of nosocomial infections in the United Sates.

Infection control practitioners play a key role in hospital infection surveillance and control programs. Without a qualified and well-trained person in this position, the infection control program is ineffective. Over 95% of infection control practitioners are nurses. Their common job titles are infection control nurse, infection control coordinator, and nurse epidemiologist.

## UNIVERSAL PRECAUTIONS

In 1985, in response to concerns regarding the transmission of HIV infection during health care procedures, the CDC recommended a **universal precautions** policy for all health care settings. This strategy requires that blood and body fluids from *all clients* be handled as if infected with HIV or other bloodborne pathogens. When in a situation where potential contact with blood or other body fluids exists, health care workers must always perform hand hygiene and wear gloves, masks, protective clothing, and other indicated personal protective barriers. Needles and sharp instruments must be used and disposed of properly (CDC, 1989). The CDC also made recommendations for preventing transmission of HIV and hepatitis B during medical, surgical, and dental procedures (CDC, 1991).

## ■ Practice Application

The rising numbers of foreign-born residents in communities that did not previously have large immigrant populations provides a challenge to those involved with communicable disease control, especially in outbreak situations. Language barriers, specific cultural practices, and undocumented status all contribute to opportunities for infection as well as presenting obstacles to prevention and control. It is common for diseases such as tuberculosis, brucellosis, measles, hepatitis B, and parasitic infections to originate in other countries and be diagnosed only after arrival in the United States. People coming from countries without, with newly established, or with poorly enforced vaccination programs may be unimmunized. These people are particularly susceptible to infection in outbreak situations. For example, many people coming from Latin America have not been immunized against rubella. Differences in cultural practices can lead to outbreaks of food-borne illness. Listeriosis outbreaks have been traced to the use of unpasteurized milk in cottage industry cheese production.

In the face of a single infectious disease report or an outbreak situation, when working with communities whose members speak little English, it is vital (1) to have a means of communication, (2) to be able to provide a culturally appropriate message, and (3) to have an established level of trust. Ideally, these requirements are addressed before an outbreak occurs, allowing a prompt and efficient response when immediate action is needed.

A. What would be a useful first step in building trust with a largely non–English-speaking immigrant community?
- Hold a health fair in the community.
- Provide incentives to use health department services.
- Identify trusted community leaders such as religious leaders and ask their help in developing a plan.
- Distribute a brochure in the target community language.

B. What might best encourage undocumented residents to respond to a request to be immunized during an outbreak situation?
- Using an already established public health program to provide interpreter services, making it clear that proof of immigration status is not required for services
- A request in the newspaper in the language of the targeted individuals
- Involving trusted community leaders in making the request
- Emphasizing to the individuals the severity of the consequences if immunization does not occur

C. What means of communication would work best when targeting largely non–English-speaking communities of recent immigrants?
- Newspaper articles in target language

- Radio announcements in target language
- Fliers in target language posted in the community
- Announcements from trusted community leaders

D. How would public health officials best go about developing information to effectively reach a largely non–English-speaking community of recent immigrants?

- Use the services of the local university communications department.
- Ask community leaders to work with translators and prevention specialists to develop messages using their own words.
- Hire a professional to translate an existing well-developed English-language brochure.
- Use brochures provided by the state health department.

---

**Answers are in the back of the book.**

## Key Points

- The burden of infectious diseases is high in both human and economic terms. Preventing these diseases must be given high priority in our present health care system.
- The successful interaction of the infectious agent, host, and environment is necessary for disease transmission. Knowledge of the characteristics of each of these three factors is important in understanding the transmission, prevention, and control of these diseases.
- Effective intervention measures at the individual and community levels must be aimed at breaking the chain linking the agent, host, and environment. An integrated approach focused on all three factors simultaneously is an ideal goal to strive for but may not be feasible for all diseases.
- Health care professionals must constantly be aware of vulnerability to threats posed by emerging infectious diseases. Most of the factors causing the emergence of these diseases are influenced by human activities and behavior.
- Communicable diseases are preventable. Preventing infection through primary prevention activities is the most cost-effective public health strategy.
- Health care professionals must always apply infection control principles and procedures in the work environment. They should strictly practice the universal blood and body fluid precautions strategy to prevent transmission of HIV and other bloodborne pathogens.
- Effective control of communicable diseases requires the use of a multisystem approach focusing on improving host resistance, improving safety of the environment, improving public health systems, and facilitating social and political changes to ensure health for all people.
- Communicable disease prevention and control programs must move beyond providing drug treatment and vaccines. Health promotion and education aimed at changing individual and community behavior must be emphasized.
- Nurses play a key role in all aspects of prevention and control of communicable diseases. Close cooperation with other members of the interdisciplinary health care team must be maintained. Mobilizing community participation is essential to successful implementation of programs.
- The successful global eradication of smallpox proved the feasibility of eradication of communicable diseases. As professionals and concerned citizens of the global village, health care workers must support the current global eradication campaigns against poliomyelitis and dracunculiasis.

## Clinical Decision-Making Activities

1. Ride with a nurse who makes home visits. Discuss living situations and other risk factors that may contribute to the development of infectious diseases, as well as possible points where the nurse may intervene to help prevent these diseases, such as checking the immunization status of all individuals in the household. What are realistic interventions and how much responsibility should a nurse take in attempting to affect the living situation?
2. To become familiar with the reportable diseases that are a problem in your community, look at how many cases have been reported during the past month, 6 months, and year. Contrast these numbers with national and state statistics. How is your county or city different from or similar to these larger jurisdictions? If different, what environmental, political, or demographic features may contribute to this difference?
3. Spend time with the persons who are responsible for reporting and investigating communicable disease in your community. Discuss types of surveillance conducted and outbreak procedures that may accompany the reporting of some of these diseases. If possible, go on an outbreak investigation. Would the existing surveillance systems and outbreak control policies be sufficient in the case of a bioterrorism event?
4. Review the demographic profile of your community including trends from the past 10 years and projections for the next decade. Pay special attention to growth patterns of particular populations such as racial and ethnic groups or specific age-groups (e.g., children under 18, adults 65 and older). How do changes in these populations affect the delivery of interventions for infectious disease control such as immunization?

5. Visit a clinic that serves a refugee, immigrant, or migrant labor population to observe the infectious diseases commonly seen in these groups. Compare and contrast this visit with a visit to a clinic that serves an inner-city population and a visit to a clinic that serves a rural population. How are the infectious disease control issues different and/or similar for these varied populations?

6. Sit in a clinic waiting room for immunization services and talk with parents about their concerns and the barriers they may perceive in obtaining immunizations for their children. How can this information be used to better facilitate immunization services?

7. Spend time with a school nurse to see what infectious diseases are routinely encountered in the educational setting. Discuss risk factors for disease in school-age youths and the strategies employed to prevent infectious diseases in this age-group. Do school policies support the strategies needed for the prevention of infectious diseases in students?

8. Visit a day-care center. Observe potential situations for the communication of infectious diseases and discuss with the director the steps taken to prevent and control infection, including immunization requirements and procedures for hand hygiene and food preparation. Does the center have specific infection control policies and procedures, and do the staff appear to be following them?

## Additional Resources

These related resources are found either in the appendix at the back of this book or on the book's website at **http://evolve.elsevier.com/Stanhope.**

*evolve* **Evolve Website**

WebLinks: Healthy People 2010

## References

Beck TP, Rupprecht CE: Rabies virus. In Mandell GL, Bennett JE, Dolin R, editors: *Principles and practice of infectious diseases,* ed 5, New York, 2000, Churchill Livingstone.

Brown H, Neva FA: *Basic clinical parasitology,* ed 6, Norwalk, Conn, 1994, Appleton & Lange.

Centers for Disease Control and Prevention: Guidelines for prevention of transmission of HIV and hepatitis B virus to health care and public safety workers, *MMWR Morb Mortal Wkly Rep* 38(S-6):1, 1989.

Centers for Disease Control and Prevention: Recommendations for preventing transmission of HIV and hepatitis B virus to patients during exposure-prone invasive procedures, *MMWR Morb Mortal Wkly Rep* 40(RR-8):1, 1991.

Centers for Disease Control and Prevention: *Addressing emerging infectious disease threats: a prevention strategy for the U.S.,* Atlanta, 1994, CDC.

Centers for Disease Control and Prevention: *MMWR Morb Mortal Wkly Rep,* 43(RR-7):1, 1994.

Centers for Disease Control and Prevention: Outbreaks of *Cyclospora cayetanensis* infection—United States, 1996, *MMWR Morb Mortal Wkly Rep* 54(25):549, 1996a.

Centers for Disease Control and Prevention: Notifiable disease surveillance and notifiable disease statistics—United States, June 1946 and June 1996, *MMWR Morb Mortal Wkly Rep* 45(25):530, 1996b.

Centers for Disease Control and Prevention: Measles—United States, 1996 and the interruption of indigenous transmission, *MMWR Morb Mortal Wkly Rep* 46(11):242, 1997.

Centers for Disease Control and Prevention: Preventing emerging infectious diseases: a strategy for the 21st century—overview of the updated CDC plan, *MMWR Morb Mortal Wkly Rep* 47(RR15):12, 1998a.

Centers for Disease Control and Prevention: Update: isolation of avian influenza A (H5N1) viruses from humans—Hong Kong, 1997-1998, *MMWR Morb Mortal Wkly Rep* 46(52, 53):1245, 1998b.

Centers for Disease Control and Prevention: Human rabies prevention—United States, 1999: recommendations of the Advisory Committee on Immunization Practices, *MMWR Morb Mortal Wkly Rep* 48(RR-1):1-21, 1999.

Centers for Disease Control and Prevention: Progress toward global dracunculiasis eradication, *MMWR Morb Mortal Wkly Rep* 49(32):731-735, 2000a.

Centers for Disease Control and Prevention: Preventing pneumococcal disease among infants and young children: recommendations of the Advisory Committee on Immunization Practices (ACIP), *MMWR Morb Mortal Wkly Rep* 49(RR09):1-38, 2000b.

Centers for Disease Control and Prevention: Measles, rubella, and congenital rubella syndrome—United States and Mexico, 1997-1999, *MMWR Morb Mortal Wkly Rep* 49(46):1048-1050, 2000c.

Centers for Disease Control and Prevention: Human rabies—California, Georgia, Minnesota, New York, and Wisconsin—2000, *MMWR Morb Mortal Wkly Rep* 49(49):1111-1115, 2000d.

Centers for Disease Control and Prevention: *Hospital infections cost U.S. billions of dollars annually,* Atlanta, 2000e, CDC, Media Relations, available at http://www.cdc.gov/od/oc/media/pressrel/r2k0306b.htm.

Centers for Disease Control and Prevention: *Reported tuberculosis in the United States 2000,* Atlanta, 2001a, CDC.

Centers for Disease Control and Prevention: Recognition of illness associated with the intentional release of a biologic agent, *MMWR Morb Mortal Wkly Rep* 50(41):893-897, 2001b.

Centers for Disease Control and Prevention: Control and prevention of rubella: evaluation and management of suspected outbreaks, rubella in pregnant women, and surveillance for congenital rubella syndrome, *MMWR Morb Mortal Wkly Rep* 50(RR-12):1-23, 2001c.

Centers for Disease Control and Prevention: *New variant CJD fact sheet,* Atlanta, 2002a, CDC, available at http://www.cdc.gov/ncidod/diseases/cjd/cjd_fact_sheet.htm.

Centers for Disease Control and Prevention: *Programs in brief: food safety,* Atlanta, 2002b, CDC, available at http://www.cdc.gov/programs/infect2.htm.

Centers for Disease Control and Prevention: Notice to readers: changes in national notifiable diseases list and data presentation, *MMWR Morb Mortal Wkly Rep* 51(01):9-10, 2002c.

Centers for Disease Control and Prevention: *West Nile count 10/24/2002,* Atlanta, 2002d, CDC, Office of Communications, Media Relations, available at http://www.cdc.gov/od/oc/media/wncount.htm.

Centers for Disease Control and Prevention: Notice to readers: recommended childhood immunization schedule, *MMWR Morb Mortal Wkly Rep* 49(RR05):1-2, 2002e.

Centers for Disease Control and Prevention: Measles—United States, 2000, *MMWR Morb Mortal Wkly Rep* 51(06):120-123, 2002f.

Centers for Disease Control and Prevention: Pertussis—United States 1997-2000, *MMWR Morb Mortal Wkly Rep* 51(04):73-76, 2002g.

Centers for Disease Control and Prevention: Lyme disease—United States, 2000, *MMWR Morb Mortal Wkly Rep* 51(02):29-31, 2002h.

Centers for Disease Control and Prevention: *Protecting the nation's health in an era of globalization: CDC's global infectious disease strategy,* Atlanta, 2002i, CDC.

Chin J, editor: *Control of communicable diseases manual,* ed 17, Washington, DC, 2000, American Public Health Association.

Cieslak TJ, Eitzen EM Jr: Clinical and epidemiologic principles of anthrax, *Emerg Infect Dis* 5(4):552-555, 1999.

DeVita VT, Hellman S, Rosenberg SA, editors: *AIDS: etiology, diagnosis, treatment and prevention,* ed 4, Philadelphia, 1997, Lippincott-Raven.

Evans AS: The eradication of communicable diseases: myth or reality? *Am J Epidemiol* 122(2):199, 1985.

Henderson DA: Smallpox: clinical and epidemiologic features, *Emerg Infect Dis* 5(4):537-539, 1999.

Institute of Medicine: *Antimicrobial drug resistance: issues and options—workshop report,* Washington, DC, 1998, National Academy Press.

Institute of Medicine: *Emerging infectious diseases from the global to the local perspective—workshop report,* Washington, DC, 2001, National Academy Press.

Kappus KD et al: Intestinal parasitism in the U.S.: update on a continuing problem, *Am J Trop Med Hyg* 50(6):705, 1994.

Laboratory Centre for Disease Control, Health Protection Branch: *Canadian national report on immunization,* Ottawa, 1996, Health Canada.

Last JM, editor: *A dictionary of epidemiology,* ed 4, New York, 2001, Oxford University Press.

Ledeberg J, Shope RE, Oaks SC: *Emerging infections: microbial threats to health in the US,* Washington, DC, 1992, National Academy Press.

Martinez A, Suffredini AF, Masur H: Pneumocystis carinii disease in HIV-infected persons. In Wormser GP, editor: *AIDS and other manifestations of HIV infection,* ed 3, Philadelphia, 1998, Lippincott-Raven.

Marwick C: Acellular pertussis vaccine is licensed for infants, *JAMA* 276(7):516, 1996.

McGinnis JM, Foege WH: Actual causes of death in the U.S., *JAMA* 270(18):2207, 1993.

Mead PS, et al: Food-related illness and death in the United States, *Emerg Infect Dis* 5(5):607-625, 1999.

National Advisory Committee on Immunization: *Canadian immunization guide,* ed 6, Ottawa, 2002, Canadian Medical Association.

Neva FA, Brown H: *Basic clinical parasitology,* ed 6, Norwalk, Conn, 1994, Appleton & Lange.

Peterson LR, Roehrig JT: West Nile virus: a re-emerging global pathogen, *Emerg Infect Dis* 7(4):612-614, 2001.

Population and Public Health Branch: *Notifiable diseases on-line,* Ottawa, 2002, Health Canada, available at http://dsol-smed.hc-sc.gc.ca/dsol-smed/ndis.

U.S. Department of Health and Human Services: *Healthy people 2010: national health promotion and disease prevention objectives,* Washington, DC, 2000, U.S. Government Printing Office.

Walker DH, Raoult D: Rickettsia rickettsii and other spotted fever group rickettsiae. In Mandell GL, Bennett JE, Dolin R, editors: *Principles and practice of infectious diseases,* ed 5, New York, 2000, Churchill Livingstone.

Wenzel RP: Control of communicable diseases: overview. In Wallace RB, editor: *Public health and preventive medicine,* ed 14, Stamford, Conn, 1998, Appleton & Lange.

Wood D: Reducing missed opportunities to vaccinate during child health visits: how effective are parent education and case management? *Arch Pediatr Adolesc Med* 152(3):238, 1998.

World Health Organization: World malaria situation in 1994, *Wkly Epidemiol Rec* 72(36):269-273, 1997.

World Health Organization: Press Release—Europe achieves historic milestone as region is declared polio-free, Geneva, Switzerland, WHO, Information Office, June 21, 2002.

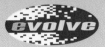
# Chapter 39

# Communicable and Infectious Disease Risks

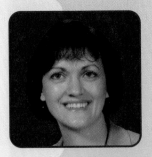

**Patty J. Hale, R.N., Ph.D., F.N.P.**

Patty J. Hale has worked as a public health nurse in Wisconsin and Virginia. She has consulted on HIV/AIDS and communicable diseases to numerous organizations, including schools, employers, and the World Health Organization. In addition to teaching nursing and environmental health courses, she directs health programs for a grant funded by the U.S. Department of Housing and Urban Development that is based on the Asset-Based Community Development Model (ABCD) in Lynchburg, Virginia.

## Objectives

After reading this chapter, the student should be able to do the following:

1. Describe the natural history of human immunodeficiency virus (HIV) infection and appropriate client education at each stage
2. Explain the clinical signs of selected communicable diseases
3. Evaluate the trends in incidence of HIV, STDs, hepatitis, and tuberculosis, and identify groups that are at greatest risk
4. Analyze behaviors that place people at risk of contracting selected communicable diseases
5. Evaluate nursing activities to prevent and control selected communicable diseases
6. Explain the various roles of nurses in providing care for those with selected communicable diseases

---

Knowledge about the risk of communicable diseases has changed dramatically in recent years. For example, in the decades following the development of antibiotics in the 1940s, **sexually transmitted diseases (STDs)** were considered to be a problem of the past. The recent emergence of new viral STDs and antibiotic-resistant strains of bacterial STDs have posed new challenges. Left unchecked, STDs can cause poor pregnancy outcomes, infertility, and cervical cancers. There is also the problem of co-infection, with one STD increasing the susceptibility to other STDs, such as human immunodeficiency virus (HIV).

This concern about infectious diseases has prompted the development of standards for STDs, HIV and acquired immunodeficiency syndrome (AIDS), hepatitis, and tuberculosis in the Healthy People 2010 report. The Healthy People 2010 box shows some objectives used to evaluate progress toward decreasing communicable diseases by the year 2010.

Several communicable diseases and all STDs are acquired through behaviors that can be avoided or changed, and thus intervention efforts by nurses have focused on disease prevention. Prevention can take the form of vaccine administration (as with hepatitis A and hepatitis B), early detection (of tuberculosis, for example), or teaching clients about abstinence or safer sex. Individuals who live with these chronic infections can transmit them to others.

This chapter describes selected communicable diseases and their nursing management. It concludes with implications for community-oriented nursing care in primary, secondary, and tertiary prevention.

## HUMAN IMMUNODEFICIENCY VIRUS INFECTION

**Human immunodeficiency virus** (HIV) infection and acquired immunodeficiency syndrome (AIDS) have had an enormous political and social impact on society. Many controversies have arisen over many aspects of HIV. The public's fears about HIV and the attitude of blaming patients for their infections have resulted in discrimination. These beliefs are magnified by the fact that this disease has commonly afflicted two groups who have been largely scorned by society: homosexuals and injection drug users (Herek, Capitanio, and Widaman, 2002). Debates have arisen over how to control disease transmission and how to pay for related health services. An ongoing debate involves whether clean needles should be distributed to injection drug users to prevent the spread of HIV.

## Key Terms

acquired immunodeficiency syndrome, p. 934

chlamydia, p. 942

directly observed therapy, p. 955

genital herpes, p. 943

genital warts, p. 943

gonorrhea, p. 938

hepatitis A virus, p. 944

hepatitis B virus, p. 944

hepatits C virus, p. 946

HIV antibody test, p. 935

HIV infection, p. 934

human immunodeficiency virus, p. 932

human papillomavirus, p. 943

incidence, p. 936

incubation period, p. 934

injection drug use, p. 936

nongonococcal urethritis, p. 943

partner notification, p. 950

pelvic inflammatory disease, p. 942

perinatal HIV transmission, p. 936

prevalence, p. 936

sexually transmitted diseases, p. 932

syphilis, p. 942

tuberculosis, p. 947

*See Glossary for definitions*

## Chapter Outline

Human Immunodeficiency Virus Infection

*Natural History of HIV*

*Transmission*

*Epidemiology of HIV/AIDS*

*HIV Surveillance*

*HIV Testing*

*Perinatal/Pediatric HIV Infection*

*AIDS in the Community*

*Resources*

Sexually Transmitted Diseases

*Gonorrhea*

*Syphilis*

*Chlamydia*

*Herpes Simplex Virus 2 (Genital Herpes)*

*Human Papillomavirus Infection*

**Hepatitis**

*Hepatitis A Virus*

*Hepatitis B Virus*

*Hepatitis C Virus*

**Tuberculosis**

*Epidemiology*

*Diagnosis and Treatment*

**Nurse's Role in Providing Preventive Care for Communicable Diseases**

*Primary Prevention*

*Secondary Prevention*

*Tertiary Prevention*

Economic costs of HIV/AIDS result from premature disability and treatment. The fact that 88% of afflicted persons are between the ages of 20 and 49 years results in disrupted families and lost creative and economic productivity at a period of life when vitality is the norm. The health care delivery costs of this group are supported primarily by Medicaid and Medicare. Many people with HIV qualify for Medicaid or Medicare because they are indigent or fall into poverty when paying for health care over the course of the illness. Estimates of individuals' health care costs per year are $20,000 to $24,700, which means $6.7 to 7.8 billion annually for the United States (Hellinger and Fleishman, 2000).

The Ryan White Comprehensive AIDS Resource Emergency (CARE) Act was passed in 1990 to provide services for persons with HIV infection (Centers for Disease Control and Prevention [CDC], 1997b). This program continues to provide funds for health care in the geographic areas with the largest number of AIDS cases. Health services that are covered include emergency services, services for early intervention and care (sometimes including coverage of health insurance), and drug reimbursement programs for HIV-infected individuals. The AIDS Drug Assistance Programs (ADAPs) are awards that pay for medications on the basis of the estimated number of persons living with AIDS in the individual state (U.S. Department of Health and Human Services, 2002).

## Natural History of HIV

The natural history of HIV includes three stages: the primary infection (within about 1 month of contracting the virus), followed by a period when the body shows no symptoms (called clinical latency), and a final stage of symptomatic disease (Pantaleo et al, 1997).

Upon HIV entering the body, a person may experience a flulike syndrome referred to as a primary infection or acute retroviral syndrome. This may go unrecognized. The body's CD4+ white blood cell count drops for a brief time when the virus is most plentiful in the body. The immune system increases antibody production in response to this initial infection, which is a self-limiting illness. The symptoms are lymphadenopathy, myalgias, sore throat, lethargy, rash, and fever (Pantaleo et al, 1997). Even if the client seeks medical care at this time, the antibody test at this stage is usually negative, so it is often not recognized as HIV.

After a variable period of time, commonly from 6 weeks to 3 months, HIV antibodies appear in the blood.

## Healthy People 2010 | Objectives Related to Communicable Diseases

**13-1** Reduce AIDS among adolescents and adults

**13-2** Reduce the number of new AIDS cases among adolescent and adult men who have sex with men

**13-3** Reduce the number of new AIDS cases among females and males who inject drugs

**13-4** Reduce the number of new AIDS cases among adolescent and adult men who have sex with men and inject drugs

**13-5** Reduce the number of cases of HIV infection among adolescents and adults

**13-6** Increase the proportion of sexually active persons who use condoms

**13-11** Increase the proportion of adults with tuberculosis (TB) who have been tested for HIV

**13-12** Increase the proportion of adults in publicly funded HIV counseling and testing sites who are screened for common bacterial sexually transmitted diseases (STDs) (chlamydia, gonorrhea, and syphilis) and are immunized against hepatitis B virus

**13-13** Increase the proportion of HIV-infected adolescents and adults who receive testing, treatment, and prophylaxis, consistent with current Public Health Service treatment guidelines

**13-14** Reduce deaths from HIV infection

**13-15** Extend the interval of time between an initial diagnosis of HIV infection and AIDS diagnosis in order to increase years of life of an individual infected with HIV

**13-16** Increase years of life of an HIV-infected person by extending the interval of time between an AIDS diagnosis and death

**13-17** Reduce new cases of perinatally acquired HIV infection

**14-2** Reduce chronic hepatitis B virus infections in infants and young children (perinatal infections)

**14-3** Reduce hepatitis B

**14-6** Reduce hepatitis A

**14-9** Reduce hepatitis C

**14-10** Increase the proportion of persons with chronic hepatitis C infection identified by state and local health departments

**14-11** Reduce tuberculosis

**14-12** Increase the proportion of all tuberculosis patients who complete curative therapy within 12 months

**14-28** Increase hepatitis B vaccine coverage among high-risk groups

**25-1** Reduce the proportion of adolescents and young adults with *Chlamydia trachomatis* infections

**25-2** Reduce gonorrhea

**25-3** Eliminate sustained domestic transmission of primary and secondary syphilis

**25-4** Reduce the proportion of adults with genital herpes infection

**25-5** Reduce the proportion of persons with human papillomavirus (HPV) infection

**25-6** Reduce the proportion of females who have ever required treatment for pelvic inflammatory disease (PID)

**25-7** Reduce the proportion of childless females with fertility problems who have had an STD or who have required treatment for PID

**25-8.1** Reduce HIV infections in adolescent and young adult females aged 13 to 24 years that are associated with heterosexual contact

**25-19** Increase the proportion of all sexually active transmitted disease clinic patients who are being treated for bacterial STDs (chlamydia, gonorrhea, and syphilis) and who are offered provider referral services for their sex partners

**26** Reduce neonatal consequences from maternal STDs, including chlamydial pneumonia, gonococcal and chlamydial ophthalmia neonatorum, laryngeal papillomatosis (from human papillomavirus infection), neonatal herpes, and preterm birth and low birth weight associated with bacterial vaginosis

**26-1** Increase the proportion of adolescents who abstain from sexual intercourse or use condoms if currently sexually active

**26-2** Increase the proportion of sexually active females aged 25 years and under who are screened annually for genital chlamydia infections

**26-3** Increase the proportion of pregnant females screened for STDs (including HIV infection and bacterial vaginosis) during prenatal health care visits, according to recognized standards

From U.S. Department of Health and Human Services: *Healthy people 2010: understanding and improving health,* ed 2, Washington, DC, 2000, U.S. Government Printing Office.

Although most antibodies serve a protective role, HIV antibodies do not. However, their presence helps in the detection of **HIV infection** because tests show their presence in the bloodstream.

If left untreated, 80% to 90% of HIV-infected persons will survive about 10 years (Chin, 2000). During this prolonged **incubation period,** clients have a gradual deterioration of the immune system and can transmit the virus to others. The use of highly active antiretroviral therapy (HAART) has greatly increased the survival time of persons with HIV/AIDS.

**Acquired immunodeficiency syndrome** (AIDS) is the last stage on the long continuum of HIV infection and may result from damage caused by HIV, secondary cancers, or opportunistic organisms. AIDS is defined as a disabling or life-threatening illness caused by HIV; it is diagnosed in a person with a CD4+ T-lymphocyte count of less than 200/mL with documented HIV infection. Infectiousness, the ability to infect others, appears to increase as immune function decreases and patients become more ill. Infectiousness is also believed to be high immediately after infection (Chin, 2000).

Many of the AIDS-related opportunistic infections are caused by microorganisms that are commonly present in healthy individuals but do not cause disease in persons with an intact immune system. These microorganisms proliferate in persons with HIV/AIDS because of a weakened immune system. Opportunistic infections may be caused by bacteria, fungi, viruses, or protozoa. The most common opportunistic diseases are *Pneumocystis carinii* pneumonia and oral candidiasis. On January 1, 1993, an expanded case definition for AIDS was implemented to include pulmonary tuberculosis, invasive cervical cancer, or recurrent pneumonia (CDC, 1992).

In 2000, the case definition was further revised to include HIV nucleic acid tests (DNA or RNA) that were not available in 1993. This laboratory evidence is sufficient to identify HIV/AIDS and is useful in diagnosing infants. The previous definition of AIDS-defining conditions and evidence of immunosuppression are still used as evidence of AIDS (CDC, 1999a).

Tuberculosis, an infection that is becoming more prevalent because of HIV infection, can spread rapidly among immunosuppressed individuals. Thus HIV-infected individuals who reside in close proximity to one another, such as in long-term care facilities, prisons, drug treatment facilities, or other settings, must be carefully screened and deemed noninfectious before admission to such settings. Tuberculosis is covered in more depth later in this chapter.

## Transmission

HIV is transmitted through exposure to blood, semen, vaginal secretions, and breast milk (Levy, 1998). HIV is not transmitted through casual contact such as touching or hugging someone who has HIV infection. HIV is also not transmitted by insects, coughing, sneezing, office equipment, or sitting next to or eating with someone who has HIV infection. Except for those persons who had blood or other body fluid exposure or sexual or needle-sharing contact with an infected person, no one has developed infection (CDC, 1994a). The modes of transmission are listed in Box 39-1. The exposure categories of AIDS are shown in Figure 39-1.

Potential donors of blood and tissues are screened through interviews to assess for a history of high-risk activities, and with the **HIV antibody test.** Blood or tissue is not used from individuals who have a history of high-risk behavior or who are HIV infected. In addition to being screened, coagulation factors used to treat hemophilia and other blood disorders are made safe through heat treatments to inactivate the virus. Screening has significantly reduced the risk of transmission of HIV by blood products and organ donations. It is estimated that the odds of contracting HIV infection through receiving a blood transfusion are 1 in 450,000 units of blood transfused (Levy, 1998).

When a client has an STD infection such as chlamydia or gonorrhea, the risk of HIV infection increases, and HIV may also increase risk for other STDs. This may result

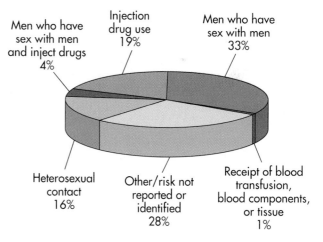

**Figure 39-1** Adult AIDS cases by exposure category from June 2000 through June 2001, United States. *Note:* The category "other/risk not reported" includes three children who were exposed to HIV-infected blood; one child was infected after intentional inoculation with HIV-infected blood, and two children were exposed to HIV-infected blood in a household setting. The category "receipt of blood transfusion, components, or tissue" includes 41 adults and adolescents and two children who developed AIDS after receiving blood screened negative for HIV antibody. Thirteen additional adults developed AIDS after receiving tissue organs or artificial insemination from HIV-infected donors. Four of the 13 received tissue, organs, or artificial insemination from a donor who was negative for HIV antibody at the time of donation. *(Data from Centers for Disease Control and Prevention:* HIV/AIDS Surveillance Report *13[1]:12, 2001b.)*

### BOX 39-1 Modes of Transmission of Human Immunodeficiency Virus (HIV)

HIV can be transmitted in the following ways:
- Sexual contact, involving the exchange of body fluids, with an infected person
- Sharing or reusing needles, syringes, or other equipment used to prepare injectable drugs
- Perinatal transmission from an infected mother to her fetus during pregnancy or delivery, or to an infant when breastfeeding
- Transfusions or other exposure to HIV-contaminated blood or blood products, organs, or semen

from any of the following: open lesions providing a portal of entry for pathogens; STDs decreasing the host's immune status, resulting in a rapid progression of HIV infection; and HIV changing the natural history of STDs or the effectiveness of medications used in treating STDs (Institute of Medicine [IOM], 1997).

The nurse serves as an educator about the modes of transmission, as well as a role model for how to behave toward and provide supportive care for those with HIV infection. An understanding of how transmission does and does not occur will help family and community members feel more comfortable in relating to and caring for persons with HIV (see Box 39-1).

## Epidemiology of HIV/AIDS

Nurses must identify the trends of HIV infection in the populations they serve, so that they can screen clients who may be at risk and can adequately plan prevention programs and illness care resources. For example, knowing that AIDS disproportionately affects minorities assists the nurse in setting priorities and planning services for these groups. Factors such as geographic location, age, and ethnic distribution are tracked to more effectively target programs.

Since the first cases of AIDS were identified in 1981, the total reported number of persons living with AIDS/HIV in the United States has grown to 466,023 in 2001 (CDC, 2001b). Note that this number reflects only those who are living; it does not include those who have died. Although epidemiologic evidence shows a decline in the number of persons newly infected with HIV, the **prevalence** of AIDS increased 7.9% from 1999 to 2000, reflecting increased life expectancy from the use of antiretroviral therapy.

Initially, the groups with the highest **incidence** of HIV infection were homosexual and bisexual men, injection drug users and their sexual partners, and hemophiliacs (CDC, 1989). Figure 39-1 shows the exposure categories for persons diagnosed with AIDS for 2000 to 2001. Although men who have sex with men (MSM) still make up the largest group with AIDS in the United States, the

number of persons contracting HIV through heterosexual transmission is increasing at a faster rate. Heterosexual transmission has surpassed **injection drug use** as the primary mode of HIV transmission in women, with 39% reporting heterosexual exposure and 23% reporting injection drug use in 2000 to 2001 (CDC, 2001b).

The distribution of pediatric AIDS reflects the infection rate in women. The number of perinatally acquired AIDS cases has decreased dramatically because of prenatal care that includes HIV testing, zidovudine drug therapy for the mother, and cesarean delivery. The **perinatal HIV transmission** rate early in the epidemic before treatment became available was between 16% and 25%. During 2000-2001, perinatal transmission rates of under 2% were achieved (CDC, 2001d).

Between 1996 and 2000, adult cases of AIDS incidence decreased in all ethnic categories. As depicted in Table 39-1, AIDS has disproportionately affected minority groups. African Americans made up approximately 12% of the total U.S. population according to the 2000 census, but they represented 48.8% of those reported to have AIDS and 52% of those with HIV infection (CDC, 2001b). This overrepresentation is associated with economically poor, marginalized populations composed of persons who are likely to be urban residents, may use injection drugs, and may use prostitution to obtain illicit drugs (Aral, 1996).

The geographic distribution of AIDS is clustered in urban areas. Regionally, the eastern United States and the U.S. territory of Puerto Rico report the highest rates (CDC, 2001b). States with an AIDS prevalence greater than 25 per 100,000 population in 2000 and 2001 were Florida, New York, Maryland, Delaware, and the District of Columbia (CDC, 2001b).

## HIV Surveillance

Study of diagnosed cases of AIDS does not reveal current HIV infection patterns because of the long interval between infection with HIV and the onset of clinical disease. Moreover, the effectiveness of antiretroviral drugs given

---

**Table 39-1 HIV Infection Cases by Sex and Race/Ethnicity Reported Through June 2001, From 36 Areas With Confidential HIV Infection Reporting**

| RACE/ETHNICITY | MALES | FEMALES | TOTAL |
|---|---|---|---|
| White, non-Hispanic | 44,514 | 9681 | 54,196 |
| Black, non-Hispanic | 47,575 | 8147 | 75,689 |
| Hispanic | 9448 | 2629 | 12,553 |
| Asian/Pacific Islander | 445 | 81 | 597 |
| Native American/Alaskan Native | 660 | 41 | 905 |
| Total* | 104,050 | 41,694 | 145,753 |

*Totals include 1813 persons whose race/ethnicity is unknown.
From Centers for Disease Control and Prevention: *HIV/AIDS Surveillance Report* 13(1), 2001b.

early in the HIV infection before symptoms start provides impetus for early identification of infection. Thus several experts, including the CDC, have called for mandatory reporting of HIV-positive status by name in all 50 states (CDC, 1999a). AIDS is a reportable condition by name of client within the United States. However, the reporting of HIV infection varies among states. All states report HIV infection either by name or by code, except Washington, California, Pennsylvania, and the District of Columbia. As of June 2001, 34 states had begun name-based HIV reporting of adults and children in addition to the existing name-based AIDS surveillance systems (CDC, 2001b). Opponents express concerns about the government's ability to maintain confidential registries and about potential invasions into personal lives, particularly as related to housing, employment, and insurance discrimination.

## HIV Testing

The HIV antibody test is the most commonly used screening test for determining infection. This test does just as its name implies: it does not reveal whether an individual has AIDS, nor does it isolate the virus. It does indicate the presence of the antibody to HIV. The most commonly used form of this test is the enzyme-linked immunosorbent assay (EIA). The EIA effectively screens blood and other donor products. In cases of false-positive results, a confirmatory test, the Western blot, is used to verify the results. False-negative results may also occur after infection and before antibodies are produced. Sometimes referred to as the window period, this can last from 6 weeks to 3 months.

Testing for HIV infection is offered at health department STD clinics and family planning clinics, primary care offices, and freestanding HIV-counseling and HIV-testing sites. Voluntary screening programs for HIV may be either confidential or anonymous: the process for each is unique. Confidential testing involves reporting the person's name and address; this information is considered privileged. With anonymous testing, the client is given an identification code number that is attached to all records of the test results. Demographic data such as the person's sex, age, and race may be collected, but there is no record of the client's name and address. An advantage of anonymous testing may be that it increases the number of people who are willing to be tested, because many of those at risk are engaged in illegal activities. The anonymity eliminates their concern about the possibility of arrest or discrimination.

## Perinatal/Pediatric HIV Infection

Perinatally acquired AIDS accounts for nearly all HIV infection in children and can occur during pregnancy, labor and delivery, or breastfeeding. However, the effectiveness of zidovudine therapy in pregnant women in preventing transmission from mother to fetus or infant has made pediatric HIV rates decline sharply. On the basis of the effectiveness of zidovudine treatment, it is recommended that HIV testing be a routine part of prenatal care and that

all pregnant women be tested for HIV (CDC, 2001d). HIV prevention in women must remain the primary focus of efforts to reduce pediatric HIV infection.

**( DID YOU KNOW?**

Measures that prevent STDs also prevent a woman from having a baby. Current research is focused on developing products that prevent infection without killing or blocking sperm.

If left untreated, the clinical picture of pediatric HIV infection involves a shorter incubation period than in adults, and symptoms may occur within the first year of life. The physical signs and symptoms in children are also different from those in adults. These include failure to thrive, diarrhea, developmental delays, and bacterial infections such as otitis media and pneumonia.

Detection of HIV infection in infants of infected mothers is through different tests from those used in children over 18 months of age. The EIA test is not valid because it tests for antibodies, which in the infant reflect passively acquired maternal antibodies. Thus a diagnosis of HIV infection in early infancy requires the use of other tests, such as HIV culture or polymerase chain reaction (PCR) results (CDC, 2001d).

Despite having an infected mother, many children do not acquire AIDS. However, one or both parents may die due to HIV infection. The families of many children with AIDS are impoverished, with limited financial, emotional, social, and health care resources. The added strain of this illness makes many individuals and families unable to provide for the emotional, physical, and developmental needs of affected children.

## AIDS in the Community

AIDS is a chronic disease, so individuals continue to live and work in the community. Persons with AIDS have bouts of illness interspersed with periods of wellness when they are able to return to school or work. When ill, much of their care is provided in the home. The nurse teaches families and significant others about personal care and hygiene, medication administration, standard precautions to ensure infection control, and healthy lifestyle behaviors such as adequate rest, balanced nutrition, and exercise.

The Americans With Disabilities Act of 1990 and other laws protect persons with HIV/AIDS against discrimination in housing, at work, and in other public situations. In 1998, the Supreme Court ruled that antidiscrimination protection also covered HIV-infected persons who were asymptomatic (CDC, 2001b). Policies regarding school and worksite attendance have been developed by most states and localities on the basis of these laws. These policies provide direction for the community's response when an individual develops HIV infection. Among the roles of the nurse are identifying resources such as social and financial support services and interpreting school and work policies.

Nurses can assist employers by educating managers about how to deal with ill or infected workers to reduce the risk of breaching confidentiality or wrongful actions such as termination. Revealing a worker's infection to other workers, terminating employment, and isolating an infected worker are examples of situations that have resulted in litigation between employees and employers. The CDC supports workplace issues through programs offered by its Business and Labor Resource Service. See resources on the evovle website at http://evolve.elsevier.com/Stanhope.

Children who are HIV infected should attend school because the benefit of attendance far outweighs the risk of transmitting or acquiring infections. None of the cases of HIV infection in the United States have been transmitted in a school setting. Decisions regarding educational and care needs should be based on an interdisciplinary team that includes the child's physician, public health personnel, and the child's parent or guardian (CDC, 1996b).

---

**DID YOU KNOW?**

Because of impaired immunity, children with HIV infection are more likely to get childhood diseases and suffer serious sequelae. Therefore DPT (diphtheria, pertussis, tetanus), IPV (inactivated polio virus), and MMR (measles, mumps, rubella) vaccines should be given at regularly scheduled times for children infected with HIV. HiB (*Haemophilus influenzae* type B), hepatitis B, pneumococcus, and influenza vaccines may be recommended after medical evaluation.

---

Individual decisions about risk to the infected child or others should be based on the behavior, neurological development, and physical condition of the child. Attendance may be inadvisable in the presence of cases of childhood infections, such as chicken pox or measles, within the school, because the immunosuppressed child is at greater risk of suffering complications. Alternative arrangements, such as homebound instruction, might be instituted if a child is unable to control body secretions or displays biting behavior.

## Resources

As the number of individuals with HIV/AIDS has increased, services to meet these needs has grown. Voluntary and faith-based service organizations, such as community-based organizations or AIDS support organizations, have developed in some localities to address these needs. These services may include counseling, support groups, legal aid, personal care services, housing programs, and community education programs. Nurses collaborate with workers from community-based organizations in the client's home and may serve to advise these groups in their supportive work.

The federal government and many organizations have established toll-free numbers and websites to provide in-

formation. Box 39-2 presents contact numbers for several of these organizations.

## SEXUALLY TRANSMITTED DISEASES

The number of new cases (the incidence) of some STDs, such as syphilis, has been declining recently, whereas the numbers of others, such as herpes simplex and chlamydia, continue to increase. It is estimated that actual rates of STDs are twice the reported rate. Because of the impact of STDs on long-term health and the emergence of eight new STDs since 1980, continued attention to their prevention and treatment is vital (IOM, 1997).

The common STDs listed in Table 39-2 are grouped by whether their cause is bacterial or viral. The bacterial infections include gonorrhea, syphilis, and chlamydia. Most of these are curable with antibiotics, with the exception of the newly emerging antibiotic-resistant strains of gonorrhea.

STDs caused by viruses cannot be cured. These are chronic diseases resulting in a lifetime of symptom management and infection control. The viral infections include herpes simplex virus and human papillomavirus (HPV), also referred to as genital warts. The hepatitis A and hepatitis B viruses, which may also be transmitted via sexual activity, are discussed later in this chapter.

### Gonorrhea

*Neisseria gonorrhoeae* is a gram-negative intracellular diplococcal bacterium that infects the mucous membranes of the genitourinary tract, rectum, and pharynx. It is transmitted through genital–genital contact, oral–genital contact, and anal–genital contact.

**Gonorrhea** is identified as either uncomplicated or complicated. Uncomplicated gonorrhea refers to limited cervical or urethral infection. Complicated gonorrhea includes salpingitis, epididymitis, systemic gonococcal infection, and gonococcal meningitis. The signs and symptoms of infection in males are purulent and copious urethral discharge and dysuria, although it is estimated that 10% to 20% of males are asymptomatic.

Gonococcal infection may be asymptomatic, and then treatment is not sought and it continues to be spread to others through sexual activity. Some individuals, even when symptomatic, continue to be sexually active and infect others (Hook and Handsfield, 1999).

Up to 40% of those infected with gonorrhea are co-infected with *Chlamydia trachomatis* (CDC, 1998b). Therefore selection of a treatment that is effective against both organisms, such as doxycycline or azithromycin, is recommended (CDC, 1998b).

Gonorrhea rates declined until 1998, when the rate increased and since has remained unchanged (Division of STD Prevention, 2001). Prior to 1998, the decline was the result of the testing of asymptomatic women and follow-up with their partners to prevent reinfection. Although the reported number of cases in the United States in 1996 was just under 300,000, the CDC estimates the actual number of annual cases to be 600,000 (CDC, 1998b). The differ-

*Text continued on p. 942*

**Table 39-2  Summary of Sexually Transmitted Diseases**

| DISEASE/PATHOGEN | INCUBATION | SIGNS AND SYMPTOMS | DIAGNOSIS | TREATMENT | NURSING IMPLICATIONS |
|---|---|---|---|---|---|
| **Bacterial** | | | | | |
| Chlamydia: *Chlamydia* | 3-21 days | *Male:* Nongonococcal urethritis (NGU); painful urination and urethral discharge; epididymitis *Female:* None or muco-purulent cervicitis (MPC), vaginal discharge; if untreated, progresses to symptoms of PID: diffuse abdominal pain, fever, chills | Tissue culture; Gram stain of endocervical or urethral discharge: presence of PMNs without gram-negative intracellular diplococci suggests NGU | One of the following treatments:<br>• Doxycycline 100 mg PO bid × 7 days<br>• Azithromycin 1 g PO × 1<br>• Erythromycin 500 mg qid × 7 days<br>• Ofloxacin 300 mg PO bid × 7 days<br>• Doxycycline—effective and cheap<br>• Azithromycin—good because single dose is sufficient | Refer partners of past 60 days; counsel client to use condoms and to avoid sex until therapy is complete and symptoms are gone in both client and partners; medication teaching<br>Annual screening recommended for all sexually active women under 25, and women over 25 if new or multiple sexual partners |
| Gonorrhea: *Neisseria gonorrhoeae* | 3-21 days | *Male:* Urethritis, purulent discharge, painful urination, urinary frequency; epididymitis *Female:* None, or symptoms of PID | Culture of discharge; Gram stain of urethral discharge, endocervical or rectal smear | One of the following treatments:<br>• Ceftriaxone 125 mg IM × 1<br>• Ciprofloxacin 500 mg PO × 1 (not used in Hawaii or California because of resistant strains)<br>• Ofloxacin 400 mg PO × 1<br>• Cefixime 400 mg PO × 1<br>• Levofloxacin 250 mg. PO × 1<br>If chlamydial infection is not ruled out, give azithromycin 1 g PO × 1 | Refer partners of past 60 days; return for evaluation if symptoms persist; counsel client to use therapy until complete and symptoms are gone in both client and partners; medication teaching |

From Centers for Disease Control and Prevention: Sexually transmitted diseases treatment guidelines 2002, *MMWR Morb Mortal Wkly Rep* 51:(RR-6), 2002.

*AIDS,* Acquired immunodeficiency syndrome; *CSF,* cerebrospinal fluid; *DNA,* deoxyribonucleic acid; *EIA.* enzyme-linked immunosorbent assay; *FTA-ABS,* fluorescent treponemal antibody absorption test; *MHA-TP,* microhemagglutination—*Treponema pallidum; Pap,* Papanicolaou; *PID,* pelvic inflammatory disease; *PMN,* polymorphonuclear neutrophil; *VDRL,* Venereal Disease Research Laboratory test for syphilis.

*Continued*

**Table 39-2  Summary of Sexually Transmitted Diseases—cont'd**

| DISEASE/PATHOGEN | INCUBATION | SIGNS AND SYMPTOMS | DIAGNOSIS | TREATMENT | NURSING IMPLICATIONS |
|---|---|---|---|---|---|
| **Bacterial—cont'd** | | | | | |
| Syphilis: *Treponema pallidum* | 10-90 days | Primary: Usually single, painless chancre; if untreated, heals in a few weeks | Visualization of pathogen on darkfield microscopic examination; single painless ulcer (chancre); FTA-ABS or MHA-TP, VDRL (reactive 14 days after appearance of chancre) | Penicillin G 2.4 million U, IM once. If penicillin allergy:<br>• Doxycycline 100 mg PO bid × 2 weeks<br>• Tetracycline 500 mg qid × 14 days<br>Tetracycline hydrochloride should not be administered to pregnant women or those with neurosyphilis or congenital syphilis | Counsel to be tested for HIV; screen all partners of past 3 months; reexamine client at 3 and 6 months |
| | 6 weeks to 6 months | Secondary: Low-grade fever, malaise, sore throat, headache, adenopathy, and rash | Clinical signs of secondary syphilis | | |
| | Within 1 year of infection | Early latency: Asymptomatic, infectious lesions may recur | VDRL: FTA-ABS or MHA-TP | Early latent: Benzathine penicillin G 2.4 million U, IM once | |
| | After 1 year from date of infection<br>Late active:<br>• 2 to 40 years<br>• 20-30 years<br>• 10-30 years | Late latency: Asymptomatic; noninfectious except to fetus of pregnant women<br>Gummas of skin, bone, mucous membranes, heart, liver<br>CNS involvement: Paresis, optic atrophy<br>Cardiovascular involvement: Aortic aneurysm, aortic value insufficiency | Lumbar puncture, CSF cell count, protein level determination and VDRL | Late latent: Benzathine penicillin G 7.2 million U total in three doses of 2.4 million U each<br>In general, penicillins are prescribed in varying doses depending on diagnosis | |
| **Viral** | | | | | |
| Human immunodeficiency virus (HIV) | 4 to 6 weeks | Possible: Acute mononucleosis-like illness (lymphadenopathy, fever, rash, joint and muscle pain, sore throat) | HIV antibody test: EIA or the Western blot test; OraSure (new test, SmithKline Beecham)—an oral HIV-1 antibody testing system—test results in about 3 days | Prophylactic administration of zidovudine (ZDV) immediately after exposure may prevent seroconversion | HIV education and counseling |
| | Seroconversion: 6 weeks to 3 months<br>AIDS: month to years (average, 11 years) | Appearance of HIV antibody<br>Opportunistic diseases: most commonly *Pneumocystis carinii* pneumonia, oral candidiasis, Kaposi's sarcoma | CD4+ T-lymphocyte count of less than 200/μL with documented HIV infection, or diagnosis with clinical manifestation of AIDS as defined by the CDC | Asymptomatic infection with HIV-1 and CD4+ counts ≤500/mm³:<br>Treat with ZDV 500-600 mg/day; treatment can be held in those with asymptomatic infection and CD4+ counts between 500 and 200/mm³ until symp- | HIV education and counseling; partner referral for evaluation; medication education; assessment and referral<br>Men who have sex with men should be tested annually for HIV, chlamydia, syphilis, and gonorrhea |

| Disease | Incubation | Signs | Treatment | Patient Education |
|---|---|---|---|---|
| *(continued)* | | | toms appear or CD4+ counts rise Symptomatic infection: Start ZDV 20 mg q8h; alternatives to ZDV: didanosine (ddI), stavudine (d4t), zalcitabine (ddC), and combination of ZDV and ddI; additional treatments necessary for opportunistic infections | |
| Genital warts: human papillomavirus (HPV) | 4-6 weeks most common; up to 9 months | Often subclinical infection; painless lesions near vaginal openings, anus, shaft of penis, vagina, cervix; lesions are textured, cauliflower appearance; may remain unchanged over time | Visual inspection for lesions; Pap smear; hybrid capture 2 HPV DNA test; colposcopy | No cure; one third of lesions will disappear without topical treatment *Patient-applied:* Topical podofilox 0.5% or imiquimod 5% cream *Provider administered:* Podophyllum resin 10%-25%, or trichloroacetic acid 80%-90%—repeat weekly if needed; cryotherapy with liquid nitrogen, laser, or surgical removal | Warts and surrounding tissues contain HPV, so removal of warts does not completely eradicate virus; examination of partners not necessary, as treatment is only symptomatic; condom use may reduce transmission; medication application |
| Genital herpes: herpes simplex virus 2 (HSV-2) | 2-20 days; average, 6 days | Vesicles, painful ulceration of penis, vagina, labia, perineum, or anus; lesions last 5-6 weeks and recurrence is common; may be asymptomatic | Presence of vesicles; viral culture (obtained only when lesions present and before they have scabbed over) | No cure; treatment may be episodic or suppressive for frequent recurrence Episodic treatment: acyclovir 800 mg PO bid × 5 days, or acyclovir 200 mg five times a day × 5 days, or valacyclovir 1 g PO qd × 5 days | Refer partners for evaluation; teach client about likelihood of recurrent episodes and ability to transmit to others even if asymptomatic; condom use; annual Pap smear |

From Centers for Disease Control and Prevention: Sexually transmitted diseases treatment guidelines 2002, *MMWR Morb Mortal Wkly Rep* 51:(RR-6), 2002.
*AIDS,* Acquired immunodeficiency syndrome; *CSF,* cerebrospinal fluid; *DNA,* deoxyribonucleic acid; *EIA,* enzyme-linked immunosorbent assay; *FTA-ABS,* fluorescent treponemal antibody absorption test; *MHA-TP,* microhemagglutination—*Treponema pallidum; Pap,* Papanicolaou; *PID,* pelvic inflammatory disease; *PMN,* polymorphonuclear neutrophil; *VDRL,* Venereal Disease Research Laboratory test for syphilis.

ence between the actual cases and reported cases occurs because gonorrhea may be unreported by health care providers, and because clients who are asymptomatic do not seek treatment and are therefore not identified. Groups with the highest incidence of gonorrhea are African Americans, persons living in the southern United States, and persons 15 to 24 years of age (Division of STD Prevention, 2001).

The number of antibiotic-resistant cases of gonorrhea in the United States has risen at an alarming rate. Penicillin-resistant gonorrhea was first identified in 1976 when 15 cases were reported (Phillips, 1976). By 1990, 64,972 resistant cases were reported (J. Blount, personal communication, January 18, 1991). After resistance to penicillin was identified, a strain of tetracycline-resistant *N. gonorrhoeae* developed. Antibiotics that have been effective against both penicillin- and tetracycline-resistant gonorrhea are now showing less effectiveness. Resistance to fluoroquinolones, specifically ciprofloxacin, has been identified in Hawaii, as well as resistance to the antibiotic azithromycin in Kansas City (CDC, 2000a). Treatment failures for gonorrhea are to be reported to the CDC in order to stay abreast of emerging resistance. Additionally, studies to document antibiotic resistance continue in specific localities.

The increase in antibiotic-resistant infections is partially attributed to the indiscriminate or illicit use of antibiotics as a prophylactic measure by persons with multiple sexual partners (Zenilman et al, 1988). To ensure proper treatment and cure, those diagnosed with gonorrheal infection should return for health care if symptoms persist, have their partner evaluated for infection, and remain sexually abstinent until antibiotic therapy is completed (CDC, 1998b).

The development of **pelvic inflammatory disease** (PID) is a risk for women who remain asymptomatic and do not seek treatment. PID is a serious infection involving the fallopian tubes (salpingitis) and is the most common complication of gonorrhea but may also result from chlamydia infection. Its symptoms include fever, abnormal menses, and lower abdominal pain, but PID may not be recognized because the symptoms vary among women. PID can result in ectopic pregnancy and infertility related to fallopian-tube scarring and occlusion. It may also cause stillbirths and premature labor. It has been estimated that the cost of the complications resulting from PID is more than $3.5 billion annually (IOM, 1997).

## Syphilis

**Syphilis** is caused by a member of the treponemal group of spirochetes called *Treponema pallidum*. It infects moist mucosal or cutaneous membranes and is spread through direct contact, usually by sexual contact or from mother to fetus. In sexual transmission, microscopic breaks in the skin and mucous membranes during sexual contact create a point of entry for the bacteria (Chin, 2000).

After peaking to a 40-year high in 1988, the rates of primary and secondary syphilis in 2000 were at their lowest since 1941 when reporting began (Division of STD Prevention, 2001). The low rate coupled with the concen-

tration of infections in specific geographic areas has led to the development of a plan to eliminate syphilis from the United States.

The clinical signs of syphilis are divided into early and late stages. Latency, a period when an individual is free of symptoms, may occur during the early and late stages. As defined by the United States Public Health Service, the early stage is the first full year after infection and includes the primary, secondary, and early latent stages. The late stage is the time after this first year and includes late latency and tertiary syphilis. During latency, there are no clinical signs of infection, but the person has historical or serologic evidence of infection. The possibility of relapse remains.

### Primary Syphilis

When syphilis is acquired sexually, the bacteria produce infection in the form of a chancre at the site of entry. The lesion begins as a macula, progresses to a papule, and later ulcerates. If left untreated, this chancre persists for 3 to 6 weeks and then heals spontaneously (Musher, 1999).

### Secondary Syphilis

Secondary syphilis occurs when the organism enters the lymph system and spreads throughout the body. Signs include rash, lymphadenopathy, and mucosal ulceration. Symptoms of secondary syphilis include sore throat, malaise, headaches, weight loss, variable fever, and muscle and joint pain.

### Tertiary Syphilis

Tertiary syphilis may involve the complications of blindness, congenital damage, cardiovascular damage, or syphilitic psychoses. Another potential outcome of tertiary syphilis is the development of lesions of the bones, skin, and mucous membranes, known as gummas. Tertiary syphilis usually occurs several years after initial infection and is rare in the United States because the disease is usually cured in its early stages with antibiotics. Tertiary syphilis does, however, remain a major problem in developing countries.

### Congenital Syphilis

Congenital syphilis rates have declined dramatically, but the effects are devastating. Syphilis is transmitted transplacentally and if untreated can cause premature stillbirth, blindness, deafness, facial abnormalities, crippling, or death. Signs include jaundice, skin rash, hepatosplenomegaly, or pseudoparalysis of an extremity. Treatment consists of penicillin given intravenously or intramuscularly (CDC, 1998b).

## Chlamydia

**Chlamydia** infection results from the bacterium *Chlamydia trachomatis*. It infects the genitourinary tract and rectum of adults and causes conjunctivitis and pneumonia in neonates. Transmission occurs when mucopurulent discharge from infected sites, such as the cervix or urethra, comes into contact with the mucous membranes of a noninfected person. Like gonorrhea, the infection is often asymptomatic in women and, if left untreated, can result in PID. When symptoms of chlamydial infection are present in women, they include dysuria, urinary frequency, and purulent vaginal discharge. In men the urethra is the most common site of infection, resulting in **nongonococcal urethritis** (NGU). The symptoms of NGU are dysuria and urethral discharge. Epididymitis is a possible complication.

Chlamydia is the most common reportable infectious disease in the United States (Division of STD Prevention, 2001). Because it causes PID, ectopic pregnancy, infertility, and neonatal complications, it is a major focus of preventive efforts (CDC, 1997a). Rates of chlamydia have increased in recent years, partly because of improved diagnosis and reporting. Risk factors that positively correlate with chlamydial infection are age less than 25 years, inconsistent use of barrier contraceptives, multiple sexual partners, and a history of infection with other STDs (United States Preventive Services Task Force, 2002). The high frequency of chlamydial infections in individuals infected with gonorrhea requires that effective treatment for both organisms be given when a gonorrheal infection is identified (CDC, 1998a).

## Herpes Simplex Virus 2 (Genital Herpes)

Herpes viruses infect genital and nongenital sites. Herpes simplex virus 1 (HSV-1) primarily causes nongenital lesions such as cold sores that may appear on the lip or mouth. Herpes simplex virus 2 (HSV-2) is the primary cause of **genital herpes.**

As is true for other viral STDs, there is no cure for HSV-2 infection, and it is considered a chronic disease. The virus is transmitted through direct exposure and infects the genitalia and surrounding skin. After the initial infection, the virus remains latent in the sacral nerve of the central nervous system and may reactivate periodically with or without visible vesicles.

Signs and symptoms of HSV-2 infection include the presence of painful lesions that begin as vesicles and ulcerate and crust within 1 to 4 days. The first episode is typically longer and is usually characterized by more lesions than seen in subsequent infections. Lesions may occur on the vulva, vagina, upper thighs, buttocks, and penis and have an average duration of 11 days (Figure 39-2). The vesicles can cause itching and pain and may be accompanied by dysuria or rectal pain. Although the ability to pass the infection to others is higher with active lesions, some individuals can spread the virus even when they are asymptomatic. Approximately 50% of people experience a prodromal phase. This may include a mild, tingling sensation up to 48 hours before eruption, or shooting pains in the buttocks, legs, or hips up to 5 days before eruption (Corey and Wald, 1999).

A national survey has identified that one in five Americans is infected with genital herpes, and that it has increased 20% in the last 30 years (Fleming et al, 1997). The number of people who become infected annually is estimated to be 724,000, and because it is incurable, the preva-

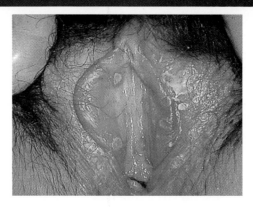

**Figure 39-2** Herpes genitalis. *(From Habif TP: Clinical dermatology: a color guide to diagnosis and therapy, ed 3, St Louis, Mo, 1996, Mosby.)*

lence has increased (Fleming et al, 1997). Because a large number of people have no symptoms and thus HSV-2 is difficult to identify, the prevalence is likely to be underrated.

The consequences of HSV-2 are of particular concern for women and their children. HSV-2 infection is linked with the development of cervical cancer. There is also an increased risk of spontaneous abortion and risk of transmission to the newborn during vaginal delivery (Brown et al, 1997). The clinical infection in infants may present as liver disease, encephalitis, or infection limited to the skin, eyes, or mouth (Chin, 2000). A pregnant woman who has active lesions at the time of giving birth should have a cesarean delivery before the rupture of amniotic membranes to avoid fetal contact with the herpetic lesions, whereas those who have no clinical evidence of herpes lesions should be delivered vaginally. A small number of infants are infected in utero (Corey and Wald, 1999).

## Human Papillomavirus Infection

**Human papillomavirus** (HPV), also called **genital warts,** can infect the genitals, anus, and mouth. Transmission of HPV occurs through direct contact with warts that result from HPV. However, HPV has been detected in semen, and exposure to the virus through body fluids is also possible. Genital warts are most commonly found on the penis and scrotum in men and the vulva, labia, vagina, and cervix in women. They appear as textured surface lesions, with what is sometimes described as a cauliflower appearance. The warts are usually multiple and vary between 1 and 5 mm in diameter. They may be difficult to visualize, so careful examination is required.

The number of new cases annually of genital HPV infection is estimated to be 500,000 to 1 million (IOM, 1997). Estimates are that about 16% of women are infected with genital HPV (Koutsky and Kiwiat, 1999). As with genital herpes, the actual prevalence is difficult to ascertain because it is not a reported disease, and many infections are subclinical.

Complications of HPV infection are especially serious for women. The link between HPV infection and cervical cancer has been established and is associated with specific types of the virus. In 80% to 90% of cases of cervical cancer, evidence of HPV has been found in the tumor (Chin, 2000). HPV infection is exacerbated in both pregnancy and immune-related disorders, which are believed to result from a decrease in cell-mediated immune functioning. HPV may infect the fetus during pregnancy and can result in a laryngeal papilloma that can obstruct the infant's airway. Genital warts may enlarge and become friable during pregnancy, and therefore surgical removal may be recommended.

Because there is no cure for HPV, the goal of therapy is to eliminate the lesions. Genital warts spontaneously disappear over time, as do skin warts. However, because the condition is worrisome for the client and HPV may lead to the development of cervical neoplasia, treatment of the lesions through surgical removal, cytotoxic agents, or immunotherapies is often used.

**DID YOU KNOW?**

The challenge of HPV prevention is that condoms do not necessarily prevent infection. Warts may grow where barriers, such as condoms, do not cover and skin-to-skin contact may occur.

## HEPATITIS

Viral hepatitis refers to a group of infections that primarily affect the liver. These infections have similar clinical presentations but different causes and characteristics. Brief profiles of the types of hepatitis are presented in Table 39-3.

## Hepatitis A Virus

**Hepatitis A virus** (HAV) is most commonly transmitted through the fecal–oral route. Sources may be water, food, or sexual contact. The virus level in the feces appears to peak 1 to 2 weeks before symptoms appear, making individuals highly contagious before they realize they are ill.

Hepatitis A infection is one of the most frequently reported vaccine-preventable diseases, despite the availability of the vaccine since 1995. Persons most at risk for HAV infection are travelers to countries with high rates, children living in areas with high rates of HAV infection, injection drug users, men who have sex with men, and persons with clotting disorders or chronic liver disease.

Hepatitis A is found worldwide. In developing countries where sanitation is inadequate, epidemics are not common because most adults are immune from childhood infection. In countries with improved sanitation, outbreaks are common in day-care centers whose staff must change diapers, among household and sexual contacts of infected individuals, and among travelers to countries where hepatitis A is endemic. In the United States, cases are most common among schoolchildren. In many outbreaks, one individual is the source of an infection that may become community-

wide. In other cases, hepatitis A is spread through food contaminated by an infected food-handler, contaminated produce, or contaminated water. The source of infection may never be identified in as many as 25% of outbreaks.

Children are often infected but show no symptoms, so they play an extremely important role in HAV transmission and are a source of infection for others. The reported incidence of HAV in the United States is highest among children 5 to 14 years old, with about one third of reported cases being in children under 15 years old. Rates are also highest in the western United States and among Alaskan Natives and American Indians (CDC, 1999b).

The clinical course of hepatitis A ranges from mild to severe and often requires prolonged convalescence. Onset is usually acute, with fever, nausea, lack of appetite, malaise, and abdominal discomfort followed after several days by jaundice. Each year in the United States, about 100 people die from acute liver failure resulting from HAV (CDC, 1999b).

Appropriate sanitation and personal hygiene remain the best means of preventing infection. The HAV vaccine is recommended for those who travel frequently or for long periods to countries where the disease is endemic. In cases of exposure through close contact with an infected individual or contaminated food or water, an injection of prophylactic immune globulin (IG) is indicated. IG should be given as soon as possible, but within 2 weeks of exposure. Candidates for IG administration are listed in Box 39-3 (Chin, 2000).

## Hepatitis B Virus

The number of new cases of **hepatitis B virus** (HBV) in the United States increased by 37% between 1979 and 1989 (CDC, 1991). Since the use of the HBV vaccine, the numbers have fallen dramatically—from 10.65 cases per 100,000 persons in 1987 to 4.01 cases per 100,000 in 1996 (CDC, 1997c). The groups with the highest prevalence are users of injection drugs, persons with STDs or multiple sex partners, immigrants and refugees and their descendants who came from areas where there is a high endemic rate of HBV, health care workers, hemodialysis clients, and inmates of long-term correctional institutions.

The HBV is spread through blood and body fluids and, like HIV, is referred to as a bloodborne pathogen. It has the same transmission properties as HIV, and thus individuals should take the same precautions to prevent spread of both HIV and HBV. A major difference is that HBV remains alive outside the body for a longer time than does HIV and thus has greater infectivity. The virus can survive for at least 1 week dried at room temperature on environmental surfaces, and thus infection control measures are paramount in preventing transmission from client to client (CDC, 1990a; CDC, 1997c).

Infection with HBV results in either acute or chronic HBV infection. The acute infection is self-limited, and individuals develop an antibody to the virus and successfully eliminate the virus from the body. They subsequently have

**Table 39-3  Viral Hepatitis Profiles**

| | HEPATITIS A | HEPATITIS B | HEPATITIS C | HEPATITIS D | HEPATITIS E | HEPATITIS G |
|---|---|---|---|---|---|---|
| Incubation period | Average, 30 days; range, 15-50 days | Average, 75 days; range, 40-120 days | Average, 45 days; range, 17-175 days | Average, 28 days; range, 14-43 days | Average, 40 days; range, 15-60 days | Unknown |
| Mode of transmission | Fecal-oral, waterborne, sexual | Bloodborne, sexual, perinatal | Primarily bloodborne; also sexual and perinatal | Superinfection or co-infection of hepatitis B case | Fecal-oral | Bloodborne; may facilitate other strains of viral hepatitis to progress more rapidly |
| Incidence | 125,000-200,000 cases/yr in the U.S. | 140,000-320,000 cases/yr in the U.S. | 28,000-180,000 cases/yr in the U.S. | 7500 cases/yr in the U.S. | Low in the U.S., epidemic outbreaks worldwide | 0.3% of all acute viral hepatitis |
| Chronic carrier state? | No | Yes, 0.1%-15% of cases | Yes, 85% or more of cases | Yes, 70%-80% of cases | No | Yes, 90%-100% of cases |
| Diagnosis | Serologic test (anti-HAV), viral isolation | Serologic tests (HBsAg), viral isolation | Serologic texts (anti-HCV) | Serologic tests (anti-HDV), liver biopsy | Serologic tests (anti-HEV) | None currently |
| Sequelae | No chronic infection | Chronic liver disease; liver cancer | Chronic liver disease; liver cancer | Chronic liver disease; liver cancer | No chronic infection | Rare or may not occur |
| Vaccine availability | Yes, vaccination of preschool children recommended; travelers to endemic regions; men who have sex with men | Yes, vaccination of infants recommended; individual with exposure risks; men who have sex with men | No | No | No | No |
| Control and prevention | Personal hygiene; proper sanitation | Preexposure vaccination; reduce exposure risk behaviors | Screening of blood/organ donors; reduce exposure risk behaviors | Preexposure or postexposure prophylaxis for HBV | Protection of water systems from fecal contamination | Unknown |

lifelong immunity against the virus. Symptoms range from mild, flulike symptoms to a more severe response that includes jaundice, extreme lethargy, nausea, fever, and joint pain. Any of these more severe symptoms may result in hospitalization. A second possible outcome from infection is chronic HBV infection, which occurs in 1% to 6% of infected adults (CDC, 1998b). These individuals are unable to rid their bodies of the virus and remain lifelong carriers of the hepatitis B surface antigen (HBsAg). As carriers, they are able to transmit the HBV to others. They may develop hepatic carcinoma or chronic active hepatitis. The signs and symptoms of chronic hepatitis B include anorexia, fatigue, abdominal discomfort, hepatomegaly, and jaundice.

Strategies for preventing HBV infection include immunization, prevention of nosocomial occupational exposure, and prevention of sexual and injection drug use exposure. Vaccination is recommended for persons with occupational risk, such as health care workers, and for children. The series of vaccines required for protection from HBV consists of three intramuscular injections, with the second and third doses administered 1 and 6 months after the first (CDC, 1991). All pregnant women should be tested for HBsAg, and if the mother is positive, newborns require hepatitis B immune globulin in addition to the hepatitis B vaccine at birth, and then at 1 and 6 months thereafter (CDC, 1996a). Hepatitis B immune globulin is given after exposure to provide passive immunity and thus prevent infection.

### OSHA Regulations

In 1992 the Occupational Safety and Health Administration (OSHA) released *Occupational Exposure to Bloodborne Pathogens* (OSHA 1992), the standard that mandates specific activities to protect workers from HBV and other bloodborne pathogens. Potential exposures for health care workers are needlestick injuries and mucous membrane splashes. The OSHA standard requires employers to identify the risk of blood exposure to various employees. If em-

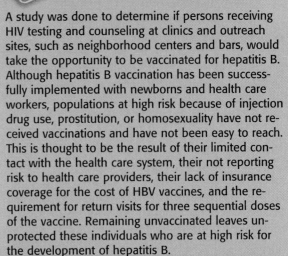

**Evidence-Based Practice**

A study was done to determine if persons receiving HIV testing and counseling at clinics and outreach sites, such as neighborhood centers and bars, would take the opportunity to be vaccinated for hepatitis B. Although hepatitis B vaccination has been successfully implemented with newborns and health care workers, populations at high risk because of injection drug use, prostitution, or homosexuality have not received vaccinations and have not been easy to reach. This is thought to be the result of their limited contact with the health care system, their not reporting risk to health care providers, their lack of insurance coverage for the cost of HBV vaccines, and the requirement for return visits for three sequential doses of the vaccine. Remaining unvaccinated leaves unprotected these individuals who are at high risk for the development of hepatitis B.

In this study, persons were tested for hepatitis B when they were tested for HIV, and if they did not already have immunity or if the test was negative for hepatitis B surface antigen, core antibody, or B surface antibody, they were offered the series of HBV vaccines. The rate of acceptance of the immunization was 51%, which is similar to the rate found in previous studies. However, the completion rate in this study was higher than previous studies, with 80% of those initially vaccinated returning for the complete series of HBV. Men who have sex with men (MSM) were more likely to return for all of the vaccines than heterosexuals. The authors believe that trust was a factor in the successful immunization of MSM, as the anonymous HIV testing services have been available since 1985. According to the authors, a similar trusting relationship has yet to be developed with injection drug users and sex workers.

**Nurse Use:** Nurses can offer programs such as an immunization program, along with an existing anonymous HIV testing program, to effectively reach high-risk adults.

Savage RB, Hussey MJ, Hurie MB: A successful approach to immunizing men who have sex with men against hepatitis B, *Public Health Nursing* 17(3):202-206, 2000.

ployees perform work that involves a potential exposure to others' body fluids, employers are mandated to offer the HBV vaccine to the employee at the employer's expense, and to offer annual educational programs on preventing HBV and HIV exposure in the workplace. Employees have the right to refuse the vaccine.

### Hepatitis C Virus

**Hepatitis C virus** (HCV) infection is the most common chronic bloodborne infection in the United States (CDC, 2002a). The hepatitis C virus is transmitted when blood or body fluids of an infected person enter an uninfected person. Those groups at highest risk include health care workers and emergency personnel who are accidentally exposed; infants who are born to infected mothers; and injection drug users who share needles or other drug use equipment. Others at risk include people who have sex with multiple partners, hemodialysis patients (from dialysis equipment shared with infected persons), and recipients of donor organs and blood products before 1992 (CDC, 2002a).

During the 1980s, HCV spread rapidly, resulting in approximately 230,000 new cases per year. Since 1989, the rate of new infections has declined to approximately 35,000 infections in 1999 (CDC, 2002b). It is estimated that there are 3.9 million people who are chronically infected with HCV living in the United States, and they are a source of HCV transmission to others (CDC, 2002a). Chronic liver disease from hepatitis C is the tenth leading cause of death among adults in the United States and is the most common reason for liver transplantation (CDC, 2001c).

The clinical signs of hepatitis C may be so mild that an infected individual does not seek medical attention. The incubation period ranges from 2 weeks to 6 months. Clients may experience fatigue and other nonspecific symptoms. Clients infected with HCV often present with an elevated level of the liver enzyme alanine aminotransferase (ALT), which may rise and fall during HCV infection. About 15% of infected persons will have spontaneous resolution of the infection, but most develop chronic liver disease. HCV infection may lead to cirrhosis or hepatocellular carcinoma (Chin, 2000; Lashley and Durham, 2002).

Primary prevention of HCV infection includes screening of blood products and donor organs and tissue; risk reduction counseling and services, including obtaining the sexual and injection drug use (IDU) history; and infection control practices. Secondary prevention strategies include testing of high-risk individuals, including those who seek HIV testing and counseling, and appropriate medical follow-up of infected clients. HCV testing should be offered to persons who received blood or an organ transplant before 1992; health care workers after exposure to blood or body fluids; children born to HCV-positive women; and persons who have ever injected drugs or been on dialysis. Routine testing for HCV is not recommended for health care workers, pregnant women, household contacts of HCV-positive persons, or the general population (CDC, 2002a).

## TUBERCULOSIS

**Tuberculosis** (TB) is a mycobacterial disease caused by *Mycobacterium tuberculosis*. Transmission is usually by exposure to the tubercle bacilli in airborne droplets from persons with pulmonary tuberculosis during talking, coughing, or sneezing. Common symptoms are cough, fever, hemoptysis, chest pains, fatigue, and weight loss. The incubation period is 4 to 12 weeks. The most critical period for development of clinical disease is the first 6 to 12 months after infection. About 5% of those initially infected may develop pulmonary tuberculosis or extrapulmonary involvement. The infection in about 95% of those initially

infected becomes latent and may be reactivated later in life. Reactivation of latent infections is common in older adults, immunocompromised persons; substance abusers; underweight and undernourished persons; and those with diabetes, silicosis, or gastrectomies (Chin, 2000).

## Epidemiology

The World Health Organization estimates that one third of the world's population is infected with TB, and it is the second leading cause of death worldwide among infectious diseases (CDC, 2001e). The incidence of tuberculosis in the United States showed a steady decline during the 1970s and early 1980s but increased between 1985 and 1992. This increase is believed to have been the result of the deterioration of community-oriented services for TB, the HIV epidemic, immigration from countries where TB is endemic, and the onset of multidrug-resistant TB. Since the peak of the resurgence in 1992, the total number of reported tuberculosis cases in the United States has been falling, although cases in foreign-born persons who reside in the United States have continued to rise. This overall decline has been attributed to improved community-oriented prevention and control programs at the state and local levels, resulting from increased federal funding to states in the mid 1990s (CDC, 2001e).

In 2000 the Institute of Medicine reported on the possibility of eradicating TB in the United States. Among their recommendations are that the United States participate in worldwide TB prevention and control efforts. The key to meeting this goal will be continued funding for prevention and control, because the problems that caused the resurgence of cases have not gone away. Table 39-4 displays the incidence of new cases in 1998 by ethnicity and sex.

### THE CUTTING EDGE

Tuberculosis, hepatitis B, and congenital syphilis have been identified by experts as diseases for which a strategy for elimination from the United States has been identified.

To accomplish this objective for TB, recommendations include the expansion of directly observed therapy (DOT) and the development of a safe and effective vaccine to prevent the development of TB in individuals who have been exposed to TB.

Centers for Disease Control and Prevention: Global disease elimination and eradication as public health strategies, *MMWR Morb Mortal Wkly Rep* 48(SU01):154, 1999c.

## Diagnosis and Treatment

TB screening tests include skin testing with purified protein derivative (PPD), followed by chest radiography for persons with a positive skin reaction and pulmonary symptoms. Persons who are immunosuppressed by drugs or

## HIV/AIDS, Hepatitis A, B, and C, Sexually Transmitted Diseases, and SARS

Jo-Ann Ackery, R.N., B.Sc.N., Toronto Public Health

### HIV/AIDS

Acquired immunodeficiency syndrome (AIDS) is a reportable disease in all provinces and territories in Canada. Physicians, hospitals, and laboratories are required under provincial legislation and regulations to report AIDS cases to the local public health department. The local health department transmits case data to the provincial ministry of health, which in turn, provides selected data to the Laboratory Centre for Disease Control (LCDC) at Health Canada in Ottawa.

In Canada the definition for AIDS is "a person who has an illness characterised by the following:

- One or more of the specified indicator diseases" (Canada does not include the definition of "CD4 T-lymphocyte count of less than 200/mL with documented HIV infection") and
- Either a positive test for HIV infection or absence of specified causes of underlying immunodeficiency" (Remis, 1995, pp. 1-2)

The first case of AIDS in Canada was reported in 1982, and by December 31, 2001, 18,026 cases had been reported. When adjustments are made for delays in reporting, the total number is estimated to be 19,310 (Health Canada, 2002c, p. 25). The number of reported AIDS cases has declined each year since 1994, probably as a result of improved antiretroviral treatments combined with drug prophylaxis regimens. The proportion of AIDS cases among women (relative to all reported AIDS cases in adults for whom sex and age are known) increased from 5.6% before 1992, peaked at 16.4% in 1999, and remained at 16% in 2001. However, there has been a steady increase in the proportion of adult female AIDS cases attributed to injection drug use, from 17.8% prior to 1996 to 34.9% in 2000.

Studies indicate that the prevalence of HIV among pregnant women in Canada is about 3 to 4 per 10,000, with large metropolitan areas having higher rates (Health Canada, 2002a, p 19). As of December 31, 2001, 208 pediatric AIDS cases (children age 0 to 14) had been reported since testing began, and 165 (79%) were attributed to perinatal transmission (Health Canada, 2002a, p. 24).

Of the cumulative total of 16,407 diagnoses of AIDS in male adults, 5% fell into the combined exposure category of men who have sex with men/injection drug users (MSM/IDU), and 77.9% were attributed to MSM (Health Canada, 2002a, p. 39). In 2000, an increase in the rate of new HIV infections among MSM has been observed in Toronto and Vancouver (Health Canada, 2002a, p. 39).

There is a lack of information regarding the HIV/AIDS epidemic among aboriginal people (First Nations, Inuit, Métis) because of variations between provinces in reporting ethnic status. The number of aboriginal AIDS cases was 437 by December 31, 2001. The proportion of these cases attributed to IDU increased from 10.3% prior to 1992 to 52.9% during 1997-2001. The proportion of

the country's AIDS cases attributed to aboriginal persons has increased from 1% before 1990 to 10% in 1999, although this group represents only 2.8% of the population. Aboriginal people are disproportionately affected by many social, economic, and behavioural factors (such as poverty) and are overrepresented in groups at high risk for HIV/AIDS (e.g., IDU, inmates in prison, persons with STDs) (Health Canada, 2002a, pp. 34-35).

Injection drug users account for 16% of cumulative positive adult HIV reports and 14.4% of adult AIDS cases up to December 31, 2001. Women, aboriginals, and street youths who inject drugs are at particular risk for HIV (Health Canada, 2002a). Programs such as needle exchange, methadone programs, peer counselors, and other risk reduction strategies can be employed to reach these groups.

HIV testing is available through confidential, nominal, or coded testing from physicians or clinics. Some provinces have legislated anonymous testing at designated sites. HIV is reportable in the three territories and in nine of the ten provinces. British Columbia has not yet made HIV reportable but is expected to do so by January 2003. HIV data are collected at the federal level by the reporting of confidential, nonnominal laboratory test data, contributed by the provinces and the territories. From 1985 to December 31, 2001, 50,259 individuals in Canada have been reported as testing positive for HIV (Health Canada, 2002c). However, a significant proportion of persons with risk factors have never been tested for HIV. The Bureau of HIV/AIDS, STD, and TB has estimated that by the end of 1999, there were 15,000 (or 30%) of HIV-infected Canadians who were not aware of their HIV infection (Health Canada, 2002a). Many provinces have guidelines or recommendations for physicians to encourage HIV testing during pregnancy; however, the choice remains with the woman.

### HEPATITIS A

The incidence of hepatitis A (HAV) in Canada has decreased from 8.78 per 100,000 in 1996 to 2.91 per 100,000 in 1999. The highest incidence in Canada is in British Columbia (8.43/100,000). HAV is preventable through immunization (Notifiable Diseases On-Line). In 2002, massive information and immunization campaigns were held in Vancouver, British Columbia, in Toronto, and in London, Ontario, because infected food-handlers potentially exposed large numbers of the public to hepatitis A.

### HEPATITIS B

The number of acute hepatitis B (HBV) cases in Canada has been estimated to be 2.3 per 100,000 (approximately 700 cases per year), a decrease from 2385 (incidence, 8.0/100,000) in 1996. The incidence is higher among males (3/100,000) than females (1.5/100,000). Major risk factors are IDU (34%), multiple heterosexual partners (24%), and sex with an HBV-infected partner (12%).

---

The views expressed in this box represent those of the writer and do not represent the views of the City of Toronto, Toronto Public Health.

> **BOX 39-3** **Nursing Interventions at the Primary, Secondary, and Tertiary Levels of Prevention**
>
> **PRIMARY PREVENTION**
> - Provide community education about prevention of communicable diseases to well populations.
> - Vaccinate for hepatitis A virus (HAV) or hepatitis B virus (HBV).
> - Provide community outreach for education and needle exchange.
>
> **SECONDARY PREVENTION**
> - Administer purified protein derivative (PPD).
> - Test and counsel for human immunodeficiency virus (HIV).
> - Notify partners and trace contacts.
>
> **TERTIARY PREVENTION**
> - Educate caregivers of persons with HIV about standard precautions.
> - Initiate directly observed therapy (DOT) for tuberculosis treatment.
> - Identify community resources for providing supportive care (e.g., funds for purchasing medications).
> - Set up support groups for persons with herpes simplex virus 2.

the types of relationships, the number of sexual partners and encounters, and the types of sexual behaviors practiced. The confidential nature of the information and how it will be used should be shared with the client to establish open communication and goal-directed interaction. Most clients feel uneasy disclosing such personal information. The nurse can ease this discomfort by remaining supportive and open during the interview to facilitate honesty about intimate activities. The nurse serves as a model for discussing sensitive information in a candid manner. When discussing precautions, direct and simple language should be used to describe specific behaviors. This encourages the client to openly discuss sexuality during this interaction and with future partners.

> **NURSING TIP**
>
> To be most effective, the nurse obtaining a client's sexual history should do the following:
> - Remain supportive and open to facilitate honesty
> - Use terms the client will understand (be prepared to suggest multiple terms)
> - Speak candidly so the client will feel comfortable talking
> - Ask questions in a nonthreatening and nonjudgmental manner
> - Acknowledge that many people are uneasy disclosing personal information

Nurses who are uncomfortable discussing topics such as sexual behavior or sexual orientation are likely to avoid assessing risk behaviors with the client. They will, consequently, be ineffective in identifying risks and in assisting the client in modifying them. It is important that nurses become adept at these skills to prevent and control STDs. Nurses can gain confidence in conducting sexual risk assessments by understanding their own values and feelings about sexuality and realizing that the purpose of the interaction is to improve the client's health. The nurse's comfort in discussing sexual behavior can be improved by using role-playing to practice assessments of sexual and injection drug use behavior, and by contracting with clients to make behavior changes.

Identifying the number of sexual and injection-drug-using partners and the number of contacts with these partners provides information about the client's risk. The chance of exposure decreases as the number of partners decreases, so people in mutually monogamous relationships are at low risk for acquiring STDs. This information can be obtained by asking, "How many sex (or drug) partners have you had over the past 6 months?" It is important to avoid basing assumptions about the sexual partner or partners on the client's sex, age, ethnicity, or any other factor. Stereotypes and assumptions about who people are and what they do are common problems that keep interviewers from asking the questions that lead to obtaining useful information. For example, it should not be taken for granted that if a man is homosexual, he always has more than one partner. Be aware also that the long incubation of HIV and the subclinical phase of many STDs lead some monogamous individuals to assume erroneously that they are not at risk.

> **DID YOU KNOW?**
>
> Assessing a client's risk of acquiring an STD should be done with all sexually active individuals. Such risk assessments should be included as baseline assessment data for those attending all clinics and those who receive school health, occupational health, public health, and home nursing services.

It is important to identify whether the person has sexual contact with men, women, or both. This information can be obtained by simply asking, "Do you have sex with men, women, or both?" This lets the client know that the nurse is open to hearing about these behaviors, and thus the nurse is more likely to obtain information that is relevant to sexual practices and risk. Women who are exclusively lesbian are at low risk for acquiring STDs, but bisexual women may transmit STDs between male and female partners. In addition, it is possible for men to have sexual contact with other men and not label themselves as homosexual. Therefore education to reduce risk that is aimed at homosexual men will not be heeded by men who do not see themselves as homosexual. In such situations the nurse can ask, "When was the last time you had sex with another man?"

Certain sexual practices are more likely to result in exposure to and transmission of STDs. Dangerous sexual activities include unprotected anal or vaginal intercourse, oral–anal contact, and insertion of finger or fist into the rectum. These practices introduce a high risk of transmission of enteric organisms or result in physical trauma during sexual encounters. The nurse can obtain information about sexual encounters by asking, "Can you tell me the kinds of sexual practices in which you engage? This will help determine what risks you may have and the type of tests we should do." Clients who engage in genital–anal, oral–anal, or oral–genital contact will need throat and rectal cultures for some STDs as well as cervical and urethral cultures.

Drug use is linked to STD transmission in several ways. Drugs such as alcohol put people at risk because they can lower inhibitions and impair judgment about engaging in risky behaviors. Addictions to drugs may cause individuals to acquire the drug or money to purchase the drug through sexual favors. This increases both the frequency of sexual contacts and the chances of contracting STDs. Thus the nurse should obtain information on the type and frequency of drug use and the presence of risk behaviors.

Another example of primary prevention is the administration of vaccines to prevent infection. Of the diseases presented here, hepatitis A and B both have vaccines available.

## Intervention

Interventions to prevent infection are aimed at preventing specific infections. These interventions can take several forms and include things such as education on how to prevent infection or the availability of vaccines. For example, on the basis of the information obtained in the sexual history and risk assessment just described, the nurse can identify specific education and counseling needs of the client. The nursing interventions focus on contracting with clients to change behavior and reduce their risk in regard to sexual practice.

### Sexual Behavior
Sexual abstinence is the best way to prevent STDs. However, for many people, sexual abstinence is not realistic and teaching about how to make sexual behavior safer is critical. Safer sexual behavior includes masturbation, dry kissing, touching, fantasy, and vaginal and oral sex with a condom.

If used correctly and consistently, condoms can prevent both pregnancy and STDs because they prevent the exchange of body fluids during sexual activity. Although the

---

**HOW TO   Use a Condom**

Correct use of a latex condom requires the following:

- Using a new condom with each act of intercourse.
- Carefully handling the condom to avoid damaging it with fingernails, teeth, or other sharp objects.
- Putting on the condom after the penis is erect and before any genital contact with the partner.
- Ensuring no air is trapped in the tip of the condom.
- Ensuring adequate lubrication during intercourse, possibly requiring use of exogenous lubricants.
- Using only water-based lubricants (e.g., K-Y Jelly or glycerin) with latex condoms; oil-based lubricants (e.g., petroleum jelly, shortening, mineral oil, massage oils, body lotions, or cooking oil) that can weaken latex should never be used.
- Holding the condom firmly against the base of the penis during withdrawal, and withdrawing while the penis is still erect to prevent slippage.
- Storage in a cool, dry place out of direct sunlight. Do not use after the expiration date. Condoms in damaged packages or condoms that show obvious signs of deterioration (e.g., brittleness, stickiness, or discoloration) should not be used regardless of their expiration date.

Modified from Centers for Disease Control and Prevention: Update: barrier protection against HIV infection and other sexually transmitted diseases, *MMWR Morb Mortal Wkly Rep* 42(30):520, 1993.

---

failure rate of condoms has been estimated to be 3.1%, this is believed to be related to incorrect use rather than condom failure (Novello et al, 1993). Thus information about proper use and how to communicate about them with a partner is also necessary. The nurse has many opportunities to convey this information during counseling. Instructions for the use of condoms are presented in the How To box.

Condom use may be viewed as inconvenient, messy, or decreasing sensation. Moreover, alcohol consumption may accompany sexual activity, which also may decrease condom use (Hale, 1996). The nurse can enable clients to become more skilled in discussing safer sex through role modeling and practicing communication skills through role play. Role-playing scenarios with partners who are resistant to condom use can help individuals prepare for situations before they occur.

Female condoms can also be a barrier to body fluid contact and therefore protect against pregnancy and STDs. The main advantage of the female condom is that its use is controlled by the woman. As it is made of polyurethane, it is also useful if a latex sensitivity develops to regular male condoms. Symptoms of latex allergy include penile, vaginal, or rectal itching or swelling after use of a male condom or diaphragm. The female condom consists of a sheath over two rings, with one closed end that fits over the cervix. The cost is about $3 per condom. Figure 39-3 provides instructions on its insertion.

---

**DID YOU KNOW?**

Most agency protocols recommend the use of latex condoms. Some may be lubricated with nonoxynol-9, a spermicide. If used frequently, nonoxynol-9 may result in genital lesions, which may provide openings for viruses to enter the body.

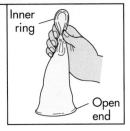

**1** Use your thumb and middle finger, and squeeze the ring toward the bottom so that it becomes thin and narrow. If you squeeze the inner ring near the top, when you insert it, your hand will be in the way.

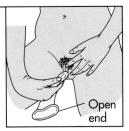

**2** Push the inner ring into your vaginal canal, behind your pubic bone. You will feel the female condom slide into place. IF you can feel the inner ring, or IF it causes any pain or discomfort, the ring is not up high enough near the cervix. Don't worry, you can't push it too far inside.

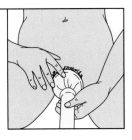

**3** Next, take your index finger, put it inside the condom, and push the condom up higher into the vagina. This way, the outer ring will be closer to the outside of your vagina. YES, it has to be on the outside of you, because HE has to go inside of the condom.

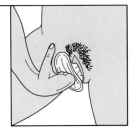

**4** The condom is in place. Be sure that:
- Your partner puts his penis inside of the female condom
- Use enough lubricant so the penis slips easily inside and out
- Use a new female condom for each sex act

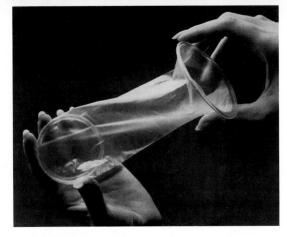

**Figure 39-3** Insertion and positioning of the female condom. *(Reproduced with permission of The Female Health Company, Chicago, Ill.)*

Clients should understand that it is important to know the risk behavior of their sexual partners, including a history of injection drug use and STDs, bisexuality, and any current symptoms. This is because each sexual partner is potentially exposed to all the STDs of all the persons with whom the other partner has been sexually active.

### Drug Use

Injection drug use is risky because the potential for injecting bloodborne pathogens, such as HIV and HBV, exists when needles and syringes are shared. During injection drug use, small quantities of drugs are repeatedly injected. Blood is withdrawn into the syringe and is then injected back into the user's vein. Individuals should be advised against using injectable drugs and sharing needles, syringes, or other drug paraphernalia. If equipment is shared, it should be in contact with full-strength bleach for 30 seconds, and then rinsed with water several times to prevent injecting bleach (CDC, 1994b). People who inject drugs are difficult to reach for health care services. Effective outreach programs include using community peers, increasing accessibility of drug treatment programs combined with

HIV testing and counseling, and long-term repeat contacts after completion of the program (CDC, 1990b).

> **WHAT DO YOU THINK?**
>
> Several healthcare experts have recommended that sterile needles be given to injection drug users as a way to prevent HIV. Others have said it supports drug use.

### Community Outreach

Because of the illegal nature of injectable drugs and the poverty associated with HIV, many people at risk have neither the inclination nor the resources to seek health care. Nurses may work to establish programs within communities because the opportunities for counseling on the prevention of HIV and other STDs are increased by bringing services into the neighborhoods of those at risk. Workers go into communities to disseminate information on safer sex, drug treatment programs, and discontinuation of drug use or safer drug use practices (e.g., using new needles and syringes with each injection). Some programs provide sterile needles and syringes, condoms, and literature about anonymous test sites.

### Community Education

Education of well populations about prevention of communicable diseases by a nurse educator is an example of primary prevention. Relevant information about modes of transmission, testing, availability of vaccines, and early symptoms can be provided to groups in the community. Providing accurate health information to large numbers of people is vital for preventing the spread of STDs. Nurses can provide educational sessions to community groups about HIV and other STDs. Such educational sessions are most effective in settings where groups normally meet and may include schools, businesses, and churches.

When addressing groups about HIV infection, it is important to discuss the number of people who are diagnosed with AIDS, the number infected with HIV, modes of transmission of the virus, how to prevent infection, common symptoms of illness, the need for a compassionate response to those afflicted, and available community resources. Teaching about other STDs can be incorporated into these presentations because the mode of transmission (sexual contact) is the same. Other information on these diseases can include the distribution, incidence, and consequences of the infection for individuals and society.

### Evaluation

Evaluation is based on whether risky behavior has changed to safe behavior and, ultimately, whether illness is prevented. Condom use is evaluated for consistency of use if the client is sexually active. Other behaviors, such as abstinence or monogamy, can be evaluated for their implementation. At the community level, behavioral surveys can be done to measure reported condom use and condom sales, and measures of disease incidence and prevalence can be calculated to evaluate the effectiveness of intervention.

## Secondary Prevention

Secondary prevention includes screening for diseases to ensure their early identification, treatment, and follow-up with contacts to prevent further spread. In general, client teaching and counseling should include education about preventing self-reinfection, managing symptoms, and preventing the infection of others.

### Testing and Counseling for HIV

The nurse should recommend that persons who have engaged in high-risk behavior be tested for HIV (Box 39-4). Individuals with the following characteristics are considered at risk and should be offered the HIV antibody test: those with a history of STDs (which are transmitted through the same behavior and may decrease immune functioning), multiple sex partners, or injection drug use;

---

**BOX 39-4  Who Should Be Advised to Receive HIV Testing and Counseling?**

- All clients in settings serving client populations at increased behavioral or clinical HIV risk
- All clients in settings with a >1% HIV prevalence
- Clients in communities with <1% HIV prevalence who have clinical signs or symptoms of HIV infection
- Clients who have a diagnosis of another sexually transmitted disease or bloodborne infection
- Clients who self-report HIV risk behavior or request an HIV test
- The following clients, regardless of setting prevalence or behavioral or clinical risk:
  - All pregnant women
  - All clients with possible acute occupational exposure
  - All clients with known sexual or needle-sharing exposure to an HIV-infected person

Modified from Centers for Disease Control and Prevention: Revised guidelines for HIV counseling, testing and referral. *MMWR Morb Mortal Wkly Rep* 50(RR-19), 2001f.

---

those who have intercourse without using a condom; those who have intercourse with someone who has another partner and those who have had sex with a prostitute; men with a history of homosexual or bisexual activity; those who have been a sexual partner to anyone in one of these groups; and those who underwent blood transfusion between January 1978 and March 1985.

If HIV infection is discovered before the onset of symptoms, early monitoring of the disease process and CD4+ lymphocyte counts or viral loads can be monitored. Additionally, prophylactic therapy with antibiotics or antiretroviral therapy may be started and may delay the onset of symptomatic illness. Thus testing enables clients to benefit from early detection and treatment, as well as risk-reduction education.

### HIV Test Counseling

Counseling directed toward understanding the meaning of the HIV antibody test is vital for clients. First, they must know that the antibody test is not diagnostic for AIDS but is indicative of HIV infection. Counseling involves the key activities of assessing risk, discussing risk behaviors and how to refrain from engaging in them, contracting between the client and the nurse to implement a risk reduction plan, and establishing the follow-up appointment to receive test results and posttest counseling.

#### Pretest Counseling

During pretest counseling, the nurse conducts the actual risk assessment, along with relevant teaching as described under Primary Prevention earlier in this chapter. Other activities include exploring how clients will cope with a positive test and assessing support systems. Asking clients to review how they have handled difficult situations in the past can determine how they might cope with learning they are HIV-positive. Also, during this time, the client is told who will have access to the test results. Although AIDS is reported nationally, the reporting of HIV infection varies among states.

Because there is no cure or vaccine available, preventing the transmission of HIV requires a risk assessment of the client's behavior and counseling on how to reduce identified risks. Sexually active individuals who have multiple partners must be encouraged to abstain, to enter a mutually monogamous relationship, or to use condoms. Injection drug users should be advised to enter a treatment program or discontinue drug use. If they continue to use drugs, they should be warned not to share needles, syringes, or any other drug paraphernalia.

### Posttest Counseling

Persons who have a negative test result are HIV negative, and they should be counseled about risk reduction activities to prevent any future transmission. It is important that the client understand that the test may not be truly negative, because it does not identify infections that may have been acquired within the several weeks before the test. As noted earlier, evidence of HIV antibody takes from 6 to 12 weeks. The client must be aware of the means of viral transmission and how to avoid infection.

Ideally, if pretest counseling was adequate, clients have contemplated the meaning of a positive test result. All clients who are antibody positive should be counseled about the need for reducing their risks and notifying partners. If the client is unwilling or hesitant to notify past partners, partner notification (or contact tracing, as will be described) is often done by the nurse. The client should visit a primary health care provider so physical evaluation can be performed and, if indicated, antiviral or other therapies begun. Box 39-5 describes the responsibilities of an individual who is HIV positive.

Psychosocial counseling is indicated when positive HIV test results precipitate acute anxiety, depression, or suicidal ideation. The client should be informed about available counseling services. The person should be cautioned to consider carefully who should be informed of the test results. Many individuals have told others about their HIV-positive test, only to experience isolation and discrimination. Plans for the future should be explored, and clients should be advised to avoid stress, drugs, and infections to maintain optimal health.

### Partner Notification/Contact Tracing

Partner notification, also known as contact tracing, is an example of a population-level intervention aimed at controlling communicable diseases. Partner notification programs usually occur in conjunction with reportable disease requirements and are carried out by most health depart-

> **BOX 39-5 Responsibilities of Persons Who Are HIV Infected**
>
> * Have regular medical evaluations and follow-ups.
> * Do not donate blood, plasma, body organs, other tissues, or sperm.
> * Take precautions against exchanging body fluids during sexual activity.
> * Inform sexual or injection drug–using partners of the potential exposure to HIV, or arrange for notification through the health department.
> * Inform health care providers of the HIV infection.
> * Consider the risk of perinatal transmission and follow up with contraceptive use.

ments. It is done by confidentially identifying and notifying exposed individuals of those found to have reportable diseases. This could result in, for example, family members and close contacts of individuals with TB being given a PPD test, which may be administered in the home.

Individuals diagnosed with a reportable STD are asked to provide the names and locations of their partners so that they can be informed of their exposure and obtain the necessary treatment. Clients may be encouraged to notify their partners and to encourage them to seek treatment. If the client agrees to do so, suggestions on how to tell partners and how to deal with possible reactions may be explored. In some instances, clients may feel more comfortable if the nurse notifies those who are exposed. If clients contact their partners about possible infection, the nurse contacts health care providers or clinics to verify examination of exposed partners.

If the client prefers not to participate in notifying partners, the nurse contacts them—often by a home visit—and counsels them to seek evaluation and treatment. The client is offered literature regarding treatment, risk reduction, and the clinic's location and hours of operation. The identity of the infected client who names sexual and injection drug–using partners cannot be revealed. Maintaining confidentiality is critical with all STDs but particularly with HIV, because discrimination may still occur.

## Tertiary Prevention

Tertiary prevention can apply to many of the chronic viral STDs and TB. For viral STDs, much of this effort focuses on managing symptoms and psychosocial support regarding future interpersonal relations. Many clients report feeling contaminated, and support groups may be available to help clients cope with chronic STDs.

### Observed Therapy

**Directly observed therapy** (DOT) programs for TB medication involve the nurse observing and documenting individual clients taking their TB drugs. When clients prematurely stop taking TB medications, there is a risk of the TB becoming resistant to the medications. This can affect an entire community of people who are susceptible to this airborne disease. Health professionals share in the responsibility of adhering to treatment, and DOT ensures that TB-infected clients have adequate medication. Thus DOT programs are aimed at the population level to prevent antibiotic resistance in the community, and to ensure effective treatment at the individual level. Many health departments have DOT home health programs to ensure adequate treatment. Directly observed treatment, short course (DOTS), is a variation applied in specific countries of the world to combat multidrug-resistant TB (CDC, 2001a).

The management of AIDS in the home may include monitoring physical status and referring the family to additional care services for maintaining the client in the home. Case management is important in all phases of HIV infection. It is especially important at this stage to ensure that clients have adequate services to meet their needs. This may include ensuring that medication can be obtained through identifying funding resources, maintaining infection control standards, reducing risk behaviors, identifying sources of respite care for caretakers, or referring clients for home or hospice care. Nursing interventions include teaching families about managing symptomatic illness by preventing deteriorating conditions such as diarrhea, skin breakdown, and inadequate nutrition.

## Standard Precautions

The importance of teaching caregivers about infection control in home care is vital. Concerns about the transmission of HIV may be expressed by clients, families, friends, and other groups. Whereas fear may be expressed by some, others who are caring for loved ones with HIV may not take adequate precautions such as glove wearing because of concern about appearing as though they do not want to touch a loved one. Others may believe myths that suggest they cannot be infected by someone they love.

Standard precautions must be taught to caregivers in the home setting. All blood and articles soiled with body fluids must be handled as if they were infectious or contaminated by bloodborne pathogens. Gloves should be worn whenever hands will be expected to touch nonintact skin, mucous membranes, blood, or other fluids. A mask, goggles, and gown should also be worn if there is potential for splashing or spraying of infectious material during any care. All protective equipment should be worn only once and then disposed of. If the skin or mucous membranes of the caregiver come in contact with body fluids, the skin should be washed with soap and water, and the mucous membranes should be flushed with water as soon as possible after the exposure. Thorough hand washing with soap and water—a major infection control measure—should be conducted whenever hands become contaminated and whenever gloves or other protective equipment (mask, gown) is removed. Soiled clothing or linen should be washed in a washing machine filled with hot water using bleach as an additive and dried on a hot-air cycle of a dryer.

## ▪ Practice Application

Yvonne Jackson is a 20-year-old woman who visits the Hopetown City Health Department's maternity clinic. Examination reveals she is at 14 weeks' gestation. She is single but has been in a steady relationship for the past 6 months with Phil. She states that she has no other children. The HIV test taken is a routine test taken during the initial prenatal visit. The results are positive.

Yvonne is shocked and emotionally distraught about the positive test results. Understanding that Yvonne will not be able to concentrate on all of the questions and information that need to be covered, the nurse prioritizes essential information to obtain and provide during this visit.

    **A.** List the relevant factors to consider on the basis of this information.

    **B.** What questions do you need to ask with regard to controlling the spread of HIV to others?

    **C.** What information is most important to give to Yvonne at this time?

    **D.** What follow-up does the nurse need to arrange for Yvonne?

**Answers are in the back of the book.**

## ▪ Key Points

- Nearly all communicable diseases discussed in this chapter are preventable because they are transmitted through specific, known behaviors.

- STDs are among the most serious public health problems in the United States. Not only is there an increased incidence of drug-resistant gonococcal infection, but other STDs, such as HPV (genital warts), HIV, and HSV (genital herpes), are associated with cancer.

- STDs affect certain groups in greater numbers. Factors associated with risk include being less than 25 years of age, being a member of a minority group, residing in an urban setting, being impoverished, and using crack cocaine.

- The increasing incidence, morbidity, and mortality of specific communicable diseases highlight the need for nurses to educate clients about ways to prevent communicable diseases.

- Many STDs do not produce symptoms in clients.

- Aside from death, the most serious complications caused by STDs are pelvic inflammatory disease, infertility, ectopic pregnancy, neonatal morbidity and mortality, and neoplasia.

- Hepatitis A is often silent in children, and children are a significant source of infection to others.

- The emergence of multidrug-resistant TB has prompted the use of directly observed therapy (DOT) in the United States and other countries to ensure adherence with drug treatment regimens.

- Early detection of communicable diseases is important because it results in early treatment and prevention of additional transmission to others. Treatment includes effective medications, stress reduction, and proper nutrition.
- Partner notification, or contact tracing, is done by identifying, contacting, and ensuring evaluation and treatment of persons exposed to sexual and injectable drug–using partners. Contact tracing is also conducted with TB and HAV.
- HIV infection has created an entirely new group of people needing health care. This rapidly growing population is straining a health care system that is already unable to meet the needs of many.
- Most of the care (both home and outpatient) that is provided for HIV is done within the community setting, which reduces direct health care costs but increases the need for financial support of home and community health services.

## Clinical Decision-Making Activities

1. Identify sources of TB treatment in your community. Is there a DOT program available through the health department or home health agency?
2. What is the rate of HAV infection in your community? How does this rate compare with the national average? Is HAV recommended for children in your community?

3. Identify the number of reported cases of AIDS and the number of reported cases of HIV infection within your state and locale (if reportable in your state). How are the cases distributed by age, sex, geographic location, and ethnicity?
4. Identify the location or locations of HIV testing services in your community. Are the test results anonymous or confidential? Describe how and to whom the results are reported.
5. Form small groups and role-play a nurse–client interaction involving risk assessment and counseling regarding safer sex and injection drug–using practices.

### Additional Resources

These related resources are found either in the appendix at the back of this book or on the book's website at **http://evolve.elsevier.com/Stanhope.**

**evolve Evolve Website**

STD Resources
WebLinks: Healthy People 2010

## References

Aral SO: The social context of syphilis persistence in the southeastern United States, *Sex Transm Dis* 23(1):9, 1996.

Brown ZA et al: The acquisition of herpes simplex virus during pregnancy, *N Engl J Med* 337(8):509, 1997.

Centers for Disease Control and Prevention: First 100,000 cases of acquired immunodeficiency syndrome: United States, *MMWR Morb Mortal Wkly Rep* 38:561, 1989.

Centers for Disease Control and Prevention: Nosocomial transmission of hepatitis B virus associated with a spring-loaded fingerstick device: California, *MMWR Morb Mortal Wkly Rep* 39(35):610, 1990a.

Centers for Disease Control and Prevention: Update: reducing HIV transmission in intravenous-drug users not in drug treatment—United States, *MMWR Morb Mortal Wkly Rep* 39(31):529, 1990b.

Centers for Disease Control and Prevention: Hepatitis B virus: a comprehensive strategy for eliminating transmission in the United States through standard childhood vaccination–ACIP, *MMWR Morb Mortal Wkly Rep* 40(RR-13):1, 1991.

Centers for Disease Control and Prevention: 1993 revised classification system for HIV infection and expanded surveillance case definition for AIDS among adolescents and adults, *MMWR Morb Mortal Wkly Rep* 41(RR-17), 1992.

Centers for Disease Control and Prevention: Update: barrier protection against HIV infection and other sexually transmitted diseases, *MMWR Morb Mortal Wkly Rep* 42(30):520, 1993.

Centers for Disease Control and Prevention: Human immunodeficiency virus transmission in household settings—United States, *MMWR Morb Mortal Wkly Rep* 43(347):353, 1994a.

Centers for Disease Control and Prevention: Knowledge and practices among injecting-drug users of bleach use for equipment disinfection—New York City, 1993, *MMWR Morb Mortal Wkly Rep* 43(24):439, 1994b.

Centers for Disease Control and Prevention: Prevention of perinatal hepatitis B through enhanced case management—Connecticut, 1994-1995 and United States, 1994, *MMWR Morb Mortal Wkly Rep* 45(27):584, 1996a.

Centers for Disease Control and Prevention: School-based HIV prevention education—United States, 1994, *MMWR Morb Mortal Wkly Rep* 45(35):760, 1996b.

Centers for Disease Control and Prevention: *Chlamydia trachomatis* genital infections—United States, 1995, *MMWR Morb Mortal Wkly Rep* 46(9):193, 1997a.

Centers for Disease Control and Prevention: CDC, HRSA work to implement CARE act provision, *HIV/AIDS Prevention,* March, Atlanta, 1997b.

Centers for Disease Control and Prevention: Nosocomial Hepatitis B virus infection associated with reusable fingerstick blood sampling devices—Ohio and New York City, *MMWR Morb Mortal Wkly Rep* 46(10):217, 1997c.

Centers for Disease Control and Prevention: Summary of notifiable diseases, 1996, *MMWR Morb Mortal Wkly Rep* 46(53), 1997d.

Centers for Disease Control and Prevention: AIDS among persons aged 50 years—United States, 1991-1996, *MMWR Morb Mortal Wkly Rep* 47(2):21, 1998a.

Centers for Disease Control and Prevention: 1998 guidelines for treatment of sexually transmitted diseases, *MMWR Morb Mortal Wkly Rep* 47(RR-1), 1998b.

Centers for Disease Control and Prevention: *The role of HIV surveillance as United States enters new era in the epidemic,* retrieved from http://www.cdc.gov/nchstp/od/surveillances.htm, January, 1998c.

Centers for Disease Control and Prevention: CDC guidelines for national human immunodeficiency virus case surveillance, including monitoring for human immunodeficiency virus and acquired immunodeficiency syndrome, *MMWR Morb Mortal Wkly Rep* 48 (RR-13), 1999a.

Centers for Disease Control and Prevention: Prevention of hepatitis A through active or passive immunization, *MMWR Morb Mortal Wkly Rep* 48(RR-12), 1999b.

Centers for Disease Control and Prevention: Global disease elimination and eradication as public health strategies, *MMWR Morb Mortal Wkly Rep* 48(SU01):154, 1999c.

Centers for Disease Control and Prevention: Fluoroquinolone-resistance in *Neisseria gonorrhoeae,* Hawaii, 1999, and decreased susceptibility to azithromycin in *N. gonorrhoeae,* Missouri, 1999, *MMWR Morb Mortal Wkly Rep* 49(37):835-837, 2000a.

Centers for Disease Control and Prevention: Missed opportunities for prevention of tuberculosis among persons with HIV infection—selected locations, United States, 1996-1997, *MMWR Morb Mortal Wkly Rep* 49(30):685, 2000b.

Centers for Disease Control and Prevention: Evaluation of a directly observed therapy short-course strategy for treating tuberculosis—Orel Oblast, Russian Federation, 1999-2000, *MMWR Morb Mortal Wkly Rep* 50(11):204-206, 2001a.

Centers for Disease Control and Prevention: *HIV/AIDS Surveillance Report* 13(1):12, 2001b.

Centers for Disease Control and Prevention: Prevalence of hepatitis C virus infection among clients of HIV counseling and testing sites—Connecticut, 1999, *MMWR Morb Mortal Wkly Rep* 50(27):577-581, 2001c.

Centers for Disease Control and Prevention: Revised recommendations for HIV screening of pregnant women, *MMWR Morb Mortal Wkly Rep* 50(RR-10):59-86, 2001d.

Centers for Disease Control and Prevention: World TB day—March 24, 2001, *MMWR Morb Mortal Wkly Rep* 50(1), 2001e.

Centers for Disease Control and Prevention: Revised guidelines for HIV counseling, testing, and referral, *MMWR Morb Mortal Wkly Rep* 50(RR-19), 2001f.

Centers for Disease Control and Prevention: Sexually transmitted diseases treatment guidelines 2002, *MMWR Morb Mortal Wkly Rep* 51(RR-6), 2002a.

Centers for Disease Control and Prevention: Summary of notifiable diseases—United States, 2000, *MMWR Morb Mortal Wkly Rep* 49(53), 2002b.

Chin J: *Control of communicable diseases manual,* Washington DC, 2000, American Public Health Association.

Corey L, Wald A: Genital herpes. In Holmes KK et al, editors: *Sexually transmitted diseases,* New York, 1999, McGraw-Hill.

Division of STD Prevention: *Sexually transmitted disease surveillance—2000,* Atlanta, 2001, CDC.

Fleming DT et al: Herpes simplex virus type 2 in the United States, 1976-1984, *N Engl J Med* 337(16):1105, 1997.

Hale PJ: Women's self-efficacy for the prevention of sexual risk behavior, *Res Nurs Health* 19:101, 1996.

Health Canada, Division of STD Prevention and Control, Bureau of HIV/AIDS STD and TB, Centre for Infectious Disease Prevention: *1998/1999 Canadian sexually transmitted diseases (STD) surveillance report,* Ottawa, 2000.

Health Canada: *Notifiable diseases online,* retrieved 2001 from http://cythera.ic.gc.ca/dsol/ndis/index_e.html, 2001a.

Health Canada, Population and Public Health Branch (Zhang J, Zou S, Giulivi A): Canada Communicable Disease Report, vol 27S3, *Hepatitis B in Canada,* Ottawa, 2001b.

Health Canada, Centre for Infectious Diseases Prevention and Control, *HIV/AIDS EPI updates,* Ottawa, 2002a.

Health Canada, Centre for Infectious Diseases Prevention and Control, Population and Public Health Branch: *STD EPI update, infectious syphilis in Canada,* Ottawa, 2002b.

Health Canada, Division of HIV/AIDS Epidemiology and Surveillance, Centre for Infectious Disease Prevention and Control, Population and Public Health Branch: *HIV and AIDS in Canada, surveillance report to December 31, 2001,* Ottawa, 2002c.

Hellinger F, Fleishman J: US AIDS treatment costs estimated at about 7 billion, *J Acquir Immune Defic Syndr* 24:182, 2000.

Herek GM, Capitanio JP, Widaman KF: HIV-related stigma and knowledge in the United States: prevalence and trends, 1991-1999, *Am J Public Health* 92(3):371-377, 2002.

Hook E, Handsfield H: Gonococcal infections in the adult. In Holmes KK et al, editors: *Sexually transmitted diseases,* New York, 1999, McGraw-Hill.

Institute of Medicine: *The hidden epidemic: confronting sexually transmitted diseases,* Washington, DC, 1997, National Academy Press.

Koutsky LA, Kiwiat NB: Genital human papillomavirus. In Holmes KK et al, editors: *Sexually transmitted diseases,* New York, 1999, McGraw-Hill.

Lashley FR, Durham JD: *Emerging infectious diseases,* New York, 2002, Springer.

Levy JA: *HIV and the pathogenesis of AIDS,* Washington, DC, 1998, ASM Press.

Musher DM: Early syphilis. In Holmes KK et al, editors: *Sexually transmitted diseases,* New York, 1999, McGraw-Hill.

Novello AC et al: Condom use for the prevention of sexual transmission of HIV infection, *JAMA* 269(22):2840, 1993.

Occupational Safety and Health Administration: Occupational exposure to bloodborne pathogens, Richmond, Va, 1992, Department of Labor and Industry.

Pantaleo G et al: Immunopathogenesis of human immunodeficiency virus infection. In DeVita VT, Hellman S, Rosenberg SA, editors: *AIDS: biology, diagnosis, treatment and prevention,* ed 4, Philadelphia, 1997, Lippincott-Raven.

Phillips I: Beta-lactamase producing, penicillin-resistant gonococcus, *Lancet* 2:656, 1976.

Remis R: *Guidelines for the surveillance of AIDS in Canada,* Laboratory Centre for Disease Control, Health Protection Branch, Ottawa, 1995, Health Canada.

Savage RB, Hussey MJ, Hurie MB: A successful approach to immunizing men who have sex with men against hepatitis B, *Public Health Nursing* 17(3):202-206, 2000.

U.S. Department of Health and Human Services: *Healthy people 2010: understanding and improving health,* ed 2, Washington, DC, 2000, U.S. Government Printing Office.

U.S. Department of Health and Human Services: HHS awards 923 million to ensure medical care, support services and prescription drugs for people with HIV/AIDS, retrieved April 10, 2002, at http://newsroom.hrsa.gov/releases/2002releases/TitleIIawards.htm.

U.S. Preventive Services Task Force: Screening for chlamydial infection: recommendations and rationale, *Am J Nurse Pract* 6(3):13, 2002.

Zenilman J et al: Penicillinase-producing *Neisseria gonorrhoeae* in Dade County, Florida: evidence of core-group transmitters and the impact of illicit antibiotics, *Sex Transm Dis* 15(1):45, 1988.

# Part 7

## Community-Oriented Nurses: Roles and Functions

At one time, the role of the public health nurse was primarily visiting clients at home and identifying cases of communicable disease. Over the decades, the role has become complex and now involves community-oriented practice. The role of the community health nurse is focused on improving the health of individuals and families through the delivery of personal health services, with an emphasis on primary prevention, health promotion, and health protection. Public health nursing practice emphasizes the delivery of services and interventions aimed at protecting entire populations from illness, disease, and injury. As the health care system has changed, the need for a comprehensive, population-focused public health system has become more evident. Nurses are able to provide care to individuals, families, and populations including aggregates and communities in a variety of settings and roles.

With increasing emphasis being placed on the community as the client, community-oriented nurses recognize that to address community health issues, they must be able to meet the needs of the individuals, families, and groups that are the nucleus of the community. In recent decades, the primary practice setting for the nurse was the hospital, but now nurses are caring for clients in many settings. Regardless of type of client, practice setting, specialty area of practice, or the functional role of the nurse, community-oriented nurses act as advocates for clients in meeting their needs through the health care system.

This section discusses the roles of manager, consultant, case manager, clinical nurse specialist, and nurse practitioner, with particular emphasis on the development of the advocacy role in community-oriented practice. Throughout the text, content is applicable to a variety of practice settings, including the more traditional public health practice arenas such as the health department. A few other practice settings with close association to community health nursing have been highlighted, such as school health, occupational health, home health, and congregational settings.

# Chapter 40

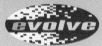

# Community-Oriented Nurse in Home Health and Hospice

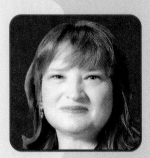

**Debra J. Giese, R.N., M.S.**
Debra J. Giese began in home care nursing in 1988, providing supplemental postpartum visits to mothers and newborns through a new managed care contract at the Milwaukee Visiting Nurses Association. By 1991, her career expanded to care for dying children and their families in hospice home care at Children's Hospital of Wisconsin. Debra received her master's degree in community mental health nursing at the University of Wisconsin Milwaukee in 1994. Since then, she has worked with student nurses in public health and as nursing director at Jefferson County Health Department in Louisville, Kentucky. Today, Debra is a doctoral student at the University of Kentucky and her research practice extends to the needs of foster care children, the concepts of attachment and loss, and primary prevention.

## Objectives

After reading this chapter, the student should be able to do the following:

1. Define home health and hospice care
2. Analyze the similarities and differences in the types of home health agencies
3. Discuss the educational requirements and competencies for a home health nurse
4. Relate the nursing process to standards of home health nursing practice
5. Identify the roles and functions of the interdisciplinary health care team
6. Examine the regulatory effects on home health care and nursing practice
7. Analyze the reimbursement mechanisms, issues, and trends relative to home health care

This chapter presents an important nursing specialty within community-oriented nursing: home health care and the related subspecialty of hospice nursing. Home health differs from other areas of health care in that health care providers practice in the client's environment. Home is a place where nurses have provided care for more than a century in the United States (see Chapter 2). Nurses provide family care within the context of the community environment.

The benefits of home care for the client and family are based on familiarity and being surrounded by family, friends, and favorite pets where love can be expressed and is interactional. The client may be empowered as choices involving food, treatments, medication schedules, and interaction with family and friends increase, leading to a feeling of security and well-being. Another benefit to home care is that it is more cost effective than institutional care (National Association of Home Care [NAHC], 2001).

The difficulty with home care includes privacy needs of the client and family, and the competence of the nurse. Some families may view having nurses, or professional

caregivers, in the house as an intrusion of privacy that can lead to a disruption of normal daily routine. Families also may need to make spatial adjustments in their home because of durable medical equipment needs. Nurses practice autonomously with little structure in the home setting; therefore competence and creativity are essential (Hanks and Smith, 1999; Snow, 2000). The home environment lacks many resources typically found in institutions, so it is also essential that nurses have good organi-

---

**NURSING TIP**

You have been asked to transfuse blood to a terminally ill leukemia client in the home immediately. No intravenous (IV) pump or pole will be available. You gather all needed and potentially needed supplies (being particularly aware of the possibility of a transfusion reaction) and go to the client's home. To make up for the lack of equipment, you titrate the IV drip rate to run over 2 hours and attach the blood bag to a clothes hanger, hanging it on the nearest drapery rod. How has this home care example demonstrated cost effectiveness, organizational skills, adaptability, and creativity?

---

*The author acknowledges the contribution of Dr. Linda Sawyer to this chapter in the fifth edition of this text.*

## Key Terms

**accreditation**, p. 978
**benchmarking**, p. 986
**client outcomes**, p. 986
**distributive care**, p. 970
**episodic care**, p. 970
**family caregiving**, p. 964
**hospice**, p. 975

**interdisciplinary collaboration**, p. 976
**intermittent care**, p. 979
**Outcome Based Quality Improvement**, p. 986
**Outcomes and Assessment Information Set**, p. 985
**palliative care**, p. 975

**regulation**, p. 979
**reimbursement system**, p. 979
**skilled nursing care**, p. 969
**telehealth**, p. 984
*See Glossary for definitions*

## Chapter Outline

Definition of Home Health Care
History of Home Health Care
Types of Home Health Care Agencies
*Official Agencies*
*Voluntary and Private Nonprofit Agencies*
*Combination Agencies*
*Hospital-Based Agencies*
*Proprietary Agencies*
Scope of Practice
*Contracting*
*Practice Functions of the Home-Health Nurse*
Standards of Home Health Nursing Practice
*Standards of Care*
*Standards of Professional Performance*

*Responsibilities of the Disciplines*
Hospice Care
*Home Care of the Dying Child*
Interdisciplinary Approach to Home Health and Hospice Care
Educational Requirements for Home Health Practice
*Certification*
Accountability and Quality Management
*Quality Control Mechanisms*
*Accreditation*
*Regulatory Mechanisms*
Financial Aspects of Home Health and Hospice Care
*Reimbursement Mechanisms*

*Cost Effectiveness*
*Hospice Reimbursement*
Effects of Legislation on Home Health Care Services
Legal and Ethical Issues
Trends in Home Health Care
*National Health Objectives*
Issues for the Twenty-first Century
*Access to Health Care*
*Technology and Telehealth*
*Health Insurance Portability and Accountability Act of 1996*
*Pediatric and Maternal–Child Home Care*
*Family Responsibility, Roles, and Functions*
*Measuring the Outcomes of Home Health Care*

zational skills, be adaptable to different settings, and demonstrate interpersonal savvy for working with the diverse needs of people in their homes.

When working in a client's home, the nurse is a guest and, to be effective, must earn the trust of the family. In this setting nurses have the opportunity to observe family life, a privilege usually reserved for family and friends. Family dynamics, lifestyle choices, communication patterns, coping strategies, responses to health and illness, and social, cultural, spiritual, and economic issues are but a few of the factors nurses assess when visiting in a family's home (Doherty and Hurley, 1994).

To provide effective, comprehensive care, nurses need to analyze the strength that clients gain from their neighborhoods—the social network that can support them when they are vulnerable and in crisis. Therefore nurses working in the home also need to gain the trust of communities by providing the needs of the clients they serve in that community with caring, honesty, competence, and ethical and cultural sensitivity (Doherty and Hurley, 1994).

The use of home health care continues to expand in response to increased demands for cost effectiveness, decreased hospital stays, consumer preferences, advanced and simplified technology, and proven quality of service.

## DEFINITION OF HOME HEALTH CARE

Home health care in today's society cannot be defined simply as "care at home." It includes an arrangement of disease prevention, health promotion, and episodic-illness–related services provided to people in their places of residence. Home health nursing, according to the American Nurses Association (ANA), "refers to the practice of nursing applied to a client with a health condition in the client's place of residence. . . . Home health nursing is a specialized area of nursing practice with its roots firmly placed in community health nursing" (ANA, 1999, p. 3). It involves the same primary preventive focus of care of aggregates of the community-oriented nurses. It also involves the secondary and tertiary prevention focuses of the care of individuals in collaboration with the family and other caregivers. The National Association of Home Care defines home health care as a broad spectrum of health and social services offered in the home environment to recovering, disabled, or chronically ill persons (NAHC, 2002).

Home health care involves the individual and family client, caregivers, multidisciplinary health care professionals, and goals to assist the client to return to an optimal level of health and independence. Differences in interpretation and actual delivery of home health care vary

---

**BOX 40-1 Levels of Prevention Applied to Home Care**

**PRIMARY PREVENTION**
The nurse implements the HANDS project (available at www.handsproject.org), visiting new mothers and babies to assess and provide counseling about at-risk problems of the new baby.

**SECONDARY PREVENTION**
The nurse provides counseling on diabetes diet and insulin injections to the newly diagnosed diabetic.

**TERTIARY PREVENTION**
The nurse provides direct care services to the stroke victim to avoid complications.

---

according to client needs and the provider and payer of these services.

It is essential to work with the family in the provision of care to an individual client. Family is defined by the individual and includes any caregiver or significant person who assists the client in need of care at home. **Family caregiving** includes assisting clients to meet their basic needs and providing direct care such as personal hygiene, meal preparation, medication administration, and treatments. Today, caregivers provide care in the home that was historically provided only in the hospital. Caregivers also provide maintenance care between the visits of the professional provider (Box 40-1).

A client's place of residence has its own uniqueness in terms of the location for providing care, depending on what the person calls home. Home may be a house, an apartment, a trailer, a boarding and care home, a shelter, a car, or a makeshift shelter under a bridge or in a cardboard box.

Client goals include health promotion, maintenance, and restoration. By maximizing the level of independence, home health nurses help their clients function at the best possible level without dependence. This assistance includes providing a combination of direct care and health education to enhance self-care, and linking the client with community services that provide limited assistance in the home. In addition, nurses contribute to the prevention of complications in chronically ill persons and help to minimize the effects of disability and illness.

---

**WHAT DO YOU THINK?**

Despite the current nursing shortage, increased client load, the complex technological needs of clients in the home, and reimbursement contracts so specific to secondary and tertiary care, it remains an ethical responsibility of the home-health nurse to promote health and primary prevention in the home and community.

---

The development of hospice home care programs has improved the care of terminally ill persons. If the client and family accept the hospice concept, most of their care can be handled comfortably at home instead of in the hospital. Reducing pain and suffering is possible through the use of medications and other measures that are closely supervised by nurses in the home.

In both home health and hospice, nurses continually assess the client's response to interventions, report their findings to the client's physician or other health care provider, and collaborate to modify the treatment plan as needed. Services can be tailored to any client need or problem. When the client's level of independence increases, the need for service decreases. Services are coordinated through an agency obligated to maintain quality care and to provide continuity. Thus the range of services provided in home health care is extensive. The strong connections of home health care to community-oriented nursing practice can be seen by briefly tracing the history of this nursing role. Many nurses believe home health nursing is community oriented, whereas many others believe that home health nursing is community-based nursing (see Chapter 1 or front cover for definitions). One of the interventions defined by the core functions of *assurance* for public health nurses is to provide essential services to those who need them. Therefore home personal health nursing is often a part of the practice of the community-oriented nurse.

## HISTORY OF HOME HEALTH CARE

Home health care began in the United States in the early 1800s. In these early years, nuns and religious sisters cared for the sick in the home. The Sisters of Charity of St. Joseph was established in Maryland in 1809. The first organized visiting nurse work was done by the Ladies' Benevolent Society of Charleston, South Carolina, founded in 1813. At first this society had a visiting committee of 16 ladies who were assigned a certain portion of the city in which to visit the sick. Later, nurses were hired by the "visitors" to provide nursing care to the sick at home. This society lasted well over 50 years, until the beginning of the Civil War, and was revived in 1902.

The precursor of modern home care, organized visiting nursing, was established in March 1877 when the women's branch of the New York City Mission sent trained nurses into the homes of the poor and the sick. The first home health nurse, Frances Root, was a member of the Bellevue Hospital Training School's first class. The establishment of the first visiting nurses association (VNA) in the United States occurred in 1885 when Elizabeth Marshall founded the Buffalo District Nursing Association. In 1886, Boston formed the Instructive Visiting Nursing Association. During this same period, Philadelphia's VNA established a pay service.

By 1890, some 13 years after the New York City Mission sent out its first nurse, 21 VNAs existed in the United States, most employing only one nurse each. These associations preceded the development, in 1893, of the Henry

Street Settlement, founded in New York by Lillian Wald. After 1894, the use of visiting nurses grew rapidly with the country's growing social consciousness (see Chapter 2).

As the demands on nurses visiting in the home increased, nurses began to question whether hospital training was enough for public health nurses. The demand for nurses experienced in providing care in the home greatly exceeded the supply of trained nurses. Community after community began nursing associations with untrained nurses. A few undergraduate programs affiliated with a VNA allowed students to leave the hospital for short periods of training in the community. The first postgraduate course in public health nursing was offered in 1906 by the Instructive District Nursing Association of Boston. Following these very simple training programs, Columbia University, in 1910, offered the first university course in public health nursing. This set a precedent for public health nursing education to be provided in universities.

In 1909, the Metropolitan Life Insurance Company began offering home nursing services to its millions of industrial policyholders in the United States and Canada. Initially, arrangements were made with Lillian Wald and the Henry Street Settlement to provide these nursing services. By 1912, Metropolitan was offering home nursing services from 589 nursing centers. These centers provided an opportunity to develop payment mechanisms based on the exact cost of visits to clients and to engage in a number of valuable health studies. Nurses collected data to project future health care needs of policyholders. Sixteen years later, John Hancock Mutual Life Insurance Company established a similar service for its policyholders.

Following the example of the Visiting Nurse Society of Philadelphia (the first to establish a pay service) and of the insurance companies, other nursing organizations began to charge for services. Charges were assessed either on an hourly basis, per visit, or by capitation to meet the needs of those who could pay for these services (see Chapter 5). The introduction of payment for services marked a change in the philosophy of home nursing services—from providing services only to the "worthy" poor to providing services to people who could afford to pay for the services.

The number of visiting nurses in the United States increased from 136 in 1902 to 3000 in 1912. With funding from both private and public sources, visiting nurses were employed by approximately 810 agencies, including VNAs, city and state boards of health and education, private clubs and societies, the tuberculosis leagues, hospitals and dispensaries, business concerns, settlements and day nurseries, churches, and charitable organizations.

Public health nursing continued to expand during the 1920s. Then came the dramatic crash of the stock market in October 1929 and the beginning of the financial depression in America. Public health nursing was greatly affected as the budgets of private agencies dwindled and reserve funds disappeared. At the same time, the socioeconomic problems experienced by clients and their families created more need for nursing service. When the country most needed accessible and comprehensive services, the quality could not be assured because of reduced staff size, elimination of educational programs, and limited supervision.

At this point, the federal government provided aid to the country and a new relationship between local communities and the state and federal governments developed. The Federal Emergency Relief Administration allocated federal funds to states so that nursing care could be given to the sick receiving federal relief. The Civil Works Administration provided funds for the use of nurses who were unemployed. These nurses worked primarily for official agencies and institutions. A large number of nurses found themselves working in public health without preparation or experience.

In the 1940s, hospitals began to take a more serious interest in home care because of the increased number of chronically ill clients being hospitalized. The Montefiore Hospital Home Care Program in New York began in 1947 and offered comprehensive nursing and social services. This service represented a change in the approach of home health from community-oriented nursing to community-based nursing, with follow-up of care moving from the hospital to the home. Before the enactment of Medicare in 1966, most agencies relied on public contributions and charity for their survival.

Home care reached a turning point with the passage of Medicare, which introduced regulations for home care practice as well as for reimbursement mechanisms. In 1967, a year after Medicare was enacted, there were 1753 Medicare-participating home health agencies in the United States. The majority of agencies were either VNAs or programs in public health departments. By 1980, there were 2924 home health agencies, an increase of about 48%. The Centers for Medicare and Medicaid Services (CMS), formerly known as the Health Care Financing Administration (HCFA), reported an increase in Medicare-certified home health agencies to 10,444 in 1997, and then a 31.5% decline to 7152 in 2000. This decrease can be directly attributed to changes in the Medicare home health reimbursement based on the Balanced Budget Act of 1997, which limited the amount spent per beneficiary (NAHC, 2001). As a result of cost containment strategies by the government, many smaller home health agencies could not survive. Today, there are over 20,000 total home health agencies in the United States, with approximately 12,848 of these being non-Medicare agencies.

Historically, the community-oriented nurses working in the home were social reformers, living in immigrant communities and providing nursing clinics, health education, and care for the sick. They provided for the nutritional

> **WHAT DO YOU THINK?**
>
> Throughout the history of home health nursing, these nurses have epitomized Florence Nightingale's philosophy that nurses are "messengers of health as well as ministers of disease" (Woodham-Smith, 1951).

needs of their communities as well as clothing, hygiene, and adequate shelter. They were responsible for developing needed programs and providing necessary services in communities, including prenatal care, postpartum visits to new mothers and babies, hot lunch school programs, preschool clinics, transportation services, summer camp programs, tuberculosis screening, blood typing, immunization for polio, and "sick room" equipment programs.

This combination of preventive services and illness care continued until the introduction of Medicare in 1966. The Medicare program emphasized an acute-disease–care payment program that influenced the services offered through home health and deleted all emphasis on illness prevention and health promotion. Some home health agencies continued to develop programs to benefit their communities, paying for them through their profits or through contributions. Today, a number of agencies are once again offering a combination of preventive and illness care services as a mechanism to decrease the long-term costs of health care. Several studies have been completed in recent years to show the importance of home health care with an emphasis on preventive services.

## TYPES OF HOME HEALTH CARE AGENCIES

Since the beginning of organized home care, many organizations have established programs to meet the home care needs of people. Home health agencies are divided into the following five general types based on administrative and organizational structures:

- Official
- Private and voluntary
- Combination
- Hospital based
- Proprietary

These types differ in organization and administration but are similar in terms of the standards they must meet for licensure, certification, and accreditation. Figure 40-1 shows the types of home health agencies. Table 40-1 lists the numbers and kinds of home health agencies, and Box 40-2 presents facts about home health agencies.

### Official Agencies

Official or public agencies include those agencies operated by the state, county, city, or other local government units, such as health departments. Most official agencies, in addition to having a home care component, also provide health education and disease prevention programs to people in the community.

Nurses employed in this setting also provide well-child clinics, immunizations, health education programs, and home visits for preventive health care. Official agencies are funded primarily by tax funds and are nonprofit. The home care services provided are reimbursed through Medicare, Medicaid, and private insurance companies. Official agencies offer more comprehensive services that include prevention services for two reasons: their primary objective is health promotion and disease prevention for

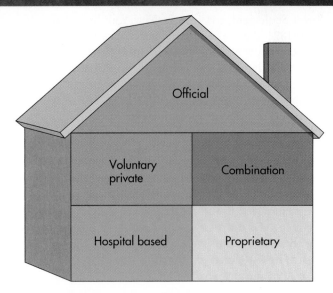

**Figure 40-1** Types of home health agencies.

the community, and additional public funding is available to allow them to provide the preventive services.

### Voluntary and Private Nonprofit Agencies

Voluntary and private agencies are grouped together as nonprofit home health agencies. Voluntary agencies are supported by charities such as United Way; by Medicare, Medicaid, and other third-party payers; and by client payments. The amount of financial assistance the voluntary agency receives depends on the community it serves. Traditionally, VNAs were the principal voluntary type of home health agency. With the arrival of Medicare in 1966, the private nonprofit agency emerged as an alternative agency to the public-supported program. These agencies included rehabilitation agencies, based in either rehabilitation facilities or skilled facilities.

Boards of directors that represent the communities they serve govern voluntary and private nonprofit agencies. These agencies are nongovernmental organizations and are exempt from federal income tax. Historically, voluntary agencies were responsible for the initial development of nursing in the home that was based on the client's need for service rather than the ability to pay.

### Combination Agencies

In some communities, to decrease cost and prevent duplication of services, official and voluntary home health agencies have merged into combination agencies to provide home health care. The services remain the same, and the board members either come from the two existing agencies or a new board is formed. The nurse may serve in several community-oriented nursing roles, as does the nurse in the official type of agency.

### Hospital-Based Agencies

Hospitals are frequently a primary site for health care services. In the 1970s, hospital-based agencies emerged in response to the recognized need for continuity of care from

## Table 40-1 Number and Kinds of Home Health Agencies

| YEAR | HOSPITAL | REHABILITATION HOSPITAL | SKILLED NURSING FACILITY | VISITING NURSE ASSOCIATION | COMBINATION AGENCY | PUBLIC | PROPRIETARY (NONPROFIT) | PRIVATE | OTHER | TOTAL |
|------|----------|-------------------------|--------------------------|----------------------------|--------------------|--------|-------------------------|---------|-------|-------|
| 1967 | 133 | 0 | 0 | 549 | 93 | 939 | 0 | 0 | 30 | 1753 |
| 1980 | 359 | 8 | 9 | 515 | 63 | 1260 | 186 | 484 | 40 | 2924 |
| 1990 | 1486 | 8 | 101 | 474 | 47 | 985 | 1884 | 710 | 0 | 5695 |
| 1996 | 2634 | 4 | 191 | 576 | 34 | 1177 | 4658 | 695 | 58 | 10,027 |
| 2000 | 2151 | 1 | 150 | 436 | 31 | 909 | 2863 | 560 | 56 | 7152 |

From Health Care Financing Administration, Center for Information Systems, Health Standards and Quality Bureau: Washington, DC, 2001, USDHHS, available at http://www.nahc.org.

### BOX 40-2 Home Health and Hospice Facts

- U.S. Medicare-certified agencies in 2002 totaled 6183 home health agencies and 2275 hospice agencies.
- Average cost per home visit: $138 in 2002.
- Medicare: $8.7 billion in 2000 for 90,729,921 visits to 2,496,793 clients.
- Medicaid: $17.6 billion in 1998 for 4,800,000 clients.

From Centers for Medicare and Medicaid: 2002 data compendium, available at: http://www.cms.gov/researchers/pubs/datacompendium/; Health Care Financing Administration Customer Information System, 2000; Outcomes Concept Systems: The quality management focus: key strategies for navigating the road ahead, 2002.

the acute care setting and also because of the high cost of institutionalization.

In 1983, implementation of the prospective payment system and diagnosis-related groups (DRGs) by the federal government caused a fundamental change in the attitudes of hospital personnel toward home care. Cost of care dictated earlier discharge of sicker clients to control profits. Increased liability risks, the desire for better client care, and the potential for several products and services increased the number of hospital-based home care agencies (Cassak, 1984).

Hospital-based agencies differ from other home health care agencies in that the already-established hospital board of directors is responsible for governing the agency. Moreover, clients of hospital-based home health care have access to existing inpatient services. Whether the agencies are official, voluntary, private nonprofit, or proprietary depends on the hospital structure. Regardless of the form they take, in most cases these agencies are a source of revenue for the hospital and may compete with community-based agencies. Hospital-based agencies outnumber all other types of Medicare-certified agencies except for proprietary agencies (NAHC, 1997).

## Proprietary Agencies

Agencies that are not eligible for income tax exemption are called proprietary (profit-making) agencies. Proprietary agencies can be licensed and certified for Medicare by the state licensing agency. The owner of the agency is responsible for governing. Reimbursement is primarily from third-party payers and individual clients if agencies do not accept Medicare. In recent years the number of Medicare-certified proprietary agencies increased significantly as hospitals began implementing quicker discharge of sicker patients (NAHC, 1997). Skilled nursing facilities that provide home health care may be proprietary agencies. These agencies are also freestanding in the community.

Although in 1995 home health care represented only 4% of all health care expenses (Levit et al, 1996), it was the fastest growing market in 1999. By 2002, the growth of home health care agencies declined because of a new reimbursement system introduced by CMS called Medicare Prospective Payment System (PPS).

Regardless of the type of home health agency existing in a community, the primary goal should be to provide quality home health care based on the community's health needs. Traditionally, most agencies were noncompetitive because of their humanitarian mission. Today, competition in home health care is on the rise as a result of the federal government's move to deregulate and deinstitutionalize health care. Competition could be a positive force in developing and maintaining quality home health programs. However, home health care is a business and can be profit producing, which requires strong utilization review and quality improvement mechanisms (see Chapter 22).

### WHAT DO YOU THINK?

If national competitive bidding for durable medical equipment is accepted, efficient health services and equipment will decrease in quality.

The changing environment in home health care has several implications for the community-oriented nurse. Clients are discharged from acute care at earlier stages of treatment, thereby needing a highly skilled level of care at home. Also, to survive in the competitive arena, agencies must continue to provide quality care and be cost effective without compromising accountability. These home care changes require that home health nurses, as both clinicians and managers, have highly developed administrative and case management skills (see Chapters 19 and 42).

## SCOPE OF PRACTICE

A common misconception of home health care is that it is a "custodial" type of nursing. It is important to remember that home health care nursing is part of community health nursing. Thus health promotion and disease prevention activities are a fundamental component of practice. Because home health care is often intermittent, a primary objective for the nurse is to facilitate self-care.

According to Orem (1995, p. 104), "Self-care is the practice of activities that individuals initiate and perform on their own behalf in maintaining life, health, and well-being." Home health nurses use this concept for all clients, regardless of the clients' abilities. For example, a client may be recuperating at home after suffering a cerebrovas-

cular accident (CVA, or stroke) and be unable to perform activities of daily living (ADLs) without assistance. Such clients can be instructed to perform these activities in a modified form. In this way they have some control over their life and self-care activities, and they can be taught to prevent possible losses in other self-care areas.

Family caregiving has become an area of concern for home care nursing research over the last 15 years. Although self-care is considered the ideal outcome of home health interventions, in reality many clients require assistance. Schumacher (1995) identified "family caregiving" as a negotiated and shifting combination of self-care and caregiving. Archbold et al. (1995) developed and tested a research-based intervention, the PREP System of Nursing Interventions, to increase the preparedness and competence of caregivers, identify strategies to enhance caregiving, and increase the ability to predict and control the situation. Innovative and cost-effective models of care and interventions are urgently needed in home health care for the next century (see the Evidence-Based Practice box).

A primary goal of home health care is to help prevent the occurrence of illness and to promote the client's well-

### Evidence-Based Practice

The authors developed a system of nursing interventions, named PREP, and pilot tested the interventions with 22 families. A quasi-experimental design was used, with 11 families randomly assigned to the control group and 11 to the experimental group. The PREP experimental group received care from one of three nurses over a 3- to 6-month period. The control group received standard home health care over the same time period. Effectiveness and acceptability of the intervention were evaluated through interviews at 2, 7, and 12 weeks after admission to PREP or standard home health and by a mailed survey at 8 to 12 months after completion of the study. Six dependent variables were measured: caregiver role strain, rewards of caregiving, caregiver depression, care effectiveness, hospital utilization, and cost for the care receiver.

The PREP system includes 10 key elements identified through previous research: systematic assessment, family focus, local knowledge of the family, cosmopolitan knowledge brought by nurses, blending of both local and cosmopolitan knowledge, family–nurse collaboration, individualized interventions, multiple strategies, therapeutic relationship, and early detection and intervention during difficult transitions.

PREP has three goals:
1. Increasing the preparedness and competence of caregivers through highly individualized interventions
2. Enriching caregiving through engaging in or modifying pleasurable and meaningful activities

3. Increasing the predictability in caregiving situations and the family's control over the environment

The PREP system was delivered through expanded home services, a PREP telephone advice line answered by nurses who knew the family, a "keep-in-touch" system of assessment contacts by telephone after home health discharge, and completion of PREP with a written summary of the family's strengths and progress, as well as a discussion with the family about their learning while on PREP.

There were no significant differences on the nine role-strain measures, rewards of caregiving, or the two depression scales between the experimental and control groups. The experimental group rated the PREP nurse as significantly more useful than the nurse or physical therapist in the control group. Caregivers in the experimental group perceived greater changes in preparedness for caregiving, enrichment, and predictability. Mean hospital costs were lower in the PREP group, although not significantly, but the number of hospitalizations in each group were equal. Additionally, the PREP system was acceptable to families. This pilot study supports the need for a larger evaluation of the PREP system.

**Nurse Use:** Home health nurses can use this study as a model to develop effective interventions and assess outcomes of interventions. Family-centered interventions may be the most effective in providing for long-term care in the future.

Archbold PG et al: The PREP system of nursing interventions: a pilot test with families caring for older members, *Res Nurs Health* 18:3, 1995.

being. In the home care setting, clients possess more control and determine their own health care needs. The effectiveness of service depends on the client's active involvement and understanding of plans established jointly by the client and nurse. The nurse facilitates the development of positive health behaviors for the individual who has had an episode of illness.

## Contracting

Contracting is a vital component of all nurse–client relationships. Constantly evolving legislative guidelines, third-party payer requirements, the high risk of liability, and the level of nurse autonomy require that contracting be used in the home care environment (see Chapter 25). Contracting is directly related to the nursing process (Figure 40-2).

## Practice Functions of the Home-Health Nurse

Home health nursing involves both direct and indirect functions. In performing these functions, the home health nurse assumes a variety of roles.

### Direct Care

Direct care refers to the actual physical aspects of nursing care—anything requiring physical contact and face-to-face interactions. In home health care, direct care activities include performing a physical assessment on the client, changing a dressing on a wound, giving medication by injection, inserting an indwelling catheter, or providing intravenous therapy. Direct care also involves teaching clients and family caregivers how to perform a certain procedure or task. By serving as a role model, the nurse helps the client and family develop positive health behaviors.

When in the home, nurses need to be aware of infection control guidelines for self-protection and to protect the client (see the How To box on infection control).

Nursing care is covered by Medicare and other third-party payers as long as the care being delivered is skilled care. To determine whether a service performed by the nurse is **skilled nursing care,** several factors are evaluated and must be adequately documented as follows. Some examples of skilled nursing services include the following:

- Observing and evaluating a client's health status and condition
- Providing direct care in administering treatments, rehabilitative exercises, medications, catheter insertion, colostomy irrigation, and wound care
- Helping the client and family develop positive coping behaviors
- Teaching the client and family to give treatments and medications when indicated
- Teaching the client and family to carry out the physician's orders such as treatments, therapeutic diets, and medication administration

> **HOW TO** **Determine If the Service Is "Skilled"**
>
> 1. Is the service complex, thereby requiring the knowledge and skill of a registered nurse?
> 2. Does the client's condition warrant skilled intervention?
> 3. Can this service be performed by a nonmedical person?
> 4. Does the service involve instructions and demonstrations by a registered nurse?

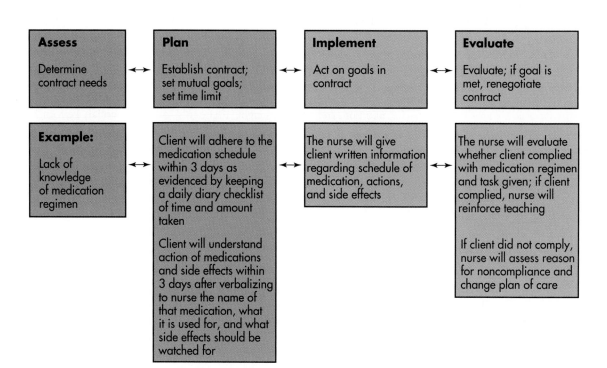

**Figure 40-2** Contracting in the nursing process.

- Reporting changes in the client's condition to the physician and arranging for medical follow-up as indicated
- Helping client and family identify resources that will help client attain a state of optimal functioning

### Indirect Care

Indirect care activities are those that a nurse does on behalf of clients to improve or coordinate care. These activities include consulting with other nurses and health providers in a multidisciplinary approach to care, organizing and participating in client care team conferences, advocating for clients with the health care system and insurers, supervising home health aides, obtaining results of diagnostic tests, and documenting care.

> **◖ DID YOU KNOW?**
>
> Home health agencies must provide nursing care as their primary service under Medicare.

### Episodic Versus Distributive Care

Although Medicare places an emphasis on episodic, or acute, care because of its limitations on benefits and requirements for skilled care, the home-health nurse cannot entirely separate primary, secondary, and tertiary prevention because of their interrelationship. These levels of prevention have been categorized into two levels of care: episodic and distributive.

**Episodic care** refers to the curative and restorative aspect of practice, or secondary and tertiary prevention, and **distributive care** refers to health maintenance and disease prevention, or primary prevention. A clinical example can illustrate the application of these two aspects in home health care.

Mr. Jones, 70 years old, was discharged from the hospital yesterday after heart surgery for coronary artery disease. Today he is admitted to home health services for skilled nursing, for an assessment of his cardiovascular status. Episodic care involves teaching Mr. and Mrs. Jones about medications, exercise, nutrition, and the signs and symptoms of possible postoperative cardiac problems. In addition, the home health nurse will provide direct care by assessing Mr. Jones's cardiovascular status and the healing of his incisions, and by helping him return to an optimal state of functioning. The Jones family's psychosocial adaptation and needs will also be addressed, and Mr. Jones's adjustment to his postsurgical status and his level of self-care will be assessed. All of this is episodic care.

In providing distributive care, the home-health nurse also teaches Mr. Jones how he can prevent an exacerbation of his condition by maintaining medical follow-up and adapting his lifestyle to increase his compliance with the programs set up for him. Primary prevention assessment strategies and counseling include environmental issues such as safety in the home and neighborhood, immunizations (e.g., influenza, pneumococcus), and reduction of stress factors.

### Nursing Roles in Home Health Care

Nurses wear many hats in home care, specifically in the roles of clinician, educator, researcher, administrator, and consultant. The experienced home health nurse, the nurse manager, or the administrator can fulfill these roles.

Home-health nurses in a staff position are clinicians who provide direct nursing care to clients and families. They are also educators because they teach clients and families the "how to" and "why" of self-care. Nurses also act as mentors, participating in the ongoing education of their colleagues, both formally, providing inservice education, and informally as team members. Additionally, they may teach classes to community groups regarding health education topics. The researcher role in home health care is increasingly important, as the efficacy, or quality, and cost effectiveness of care becomes mandated by Medicare and other payers. Home-health nurses often provide the data required for clinical or administrative changes to occur within their agency of employment. The home health care setting is filled with potential research areas. Research must be a priority in the future if quality and cost effectiveness are to be maintained. A home health administrator can be a nurse who has had advanced education with public health experience; requirements are stipulated by both federal and state rules and regulations. Finally, consultants may provide advice and counsel to staff and clients (see Chapter 42).

## STANDARDS OF HOME HEALTH NURSING PRACTICE

The home-health nurse practices in accordance with the Standards of Home Health Nursing Practice developed by the ANA (ANA, 1999). Periodically, the profession revises the scope of practice and standards of specialty practice to reflect the ongoing changes in the health care system and their effects on nursing care. The Standards of Home Health Nursing Practice were most recently revised in 1999. These latest standards have two parts: Standards of Care, which follow the six steps of the nursing process, and the eight Standards of Professional Performance. The Standards of Care are assessment, diagnosis, outcome identification, planning, implementation, and evaluation. The Standards of Professional Performance include quality of care, performance appraisal, education, collegiality, ethics, collaboration, research, and resource use. Both standards are discussed in detail in the following section.

### Standards of Care

#### Assessment

The home-health nurse is responsible for assessing the client and family during the initial home visit, as well as during all subsequent visits. This process establishes database information for the client and family, consisting of both subjective and objective data. Examples of subjective data include information that the client, family, and physi-

HOW TO    **Maintain Infection Control Standards for Home Care**

The practice of universal precautions means that all blood and body fluids are treated as potentially infectious. Universal precautions are implemented to prevent exposure and infection of caregivers. It is an important practice because many infections are subclinical.

- Use extreme care to prevent injuries when handling needles, scalpels, and razors. Do not recap, bend, break, or remove the needle from a syringe before disposal. Discard needles and syringes in puncture-resistant containers made of plastic or metal and dispose of them in a local landfill or as directed by your agency.

- Barrier precautions, such as gloves, masks, eye covering, and gowns, should be worn when contact with blood and body fluids is expected. Gloves must be worn when there may be contact with body fluids, mucous membranes, and nonintact skin, especially when drawing blood. Masks and eye covering are recommended when droplets or splashes of blood or other body fluids might occur. Wear gowns, aprons, or smocks to protect regular clothing from splashes of blood or body fluids.

- Hand hygiene is the single most important practice in preventing infections. Hand hygiene should be performed before and after providing client care and before and after preparing food, eating, feeding, or using the bathroom.

- Soiled dressings and perineal pads should be placed inside polyethylene garbage bags by using two bags to provide a double lining.

- Surfaces that may have been in contact with the human immunodeficiency virus (HIV) are easily decontaminated by common disinfectants such as Lysol. The virus is rapidly killed by household bleach. Surfaces can be disinfected with a solution of 1 part bleach to 10 parts water. This solution must be mixed daily to retain its disinfectant properties. Bathrooms and kitchens can be safely shared with persons infected with HIV, but towels, razors, and toothbrushes should not be shared. Household cleaning can be done in a regular manner unless there are spills of blood or body fluids. If a spill occurs, wear gloves and decontaminate the area by flooding the spill with a disinfectant, then use paper towels to remove visible debris and reapply disinfectant.

- Kitchen counters, dishes, and laundry should be cleaned in warm water and detergent after use. Bathrooms may be cleaned with a household disinfectant.

cians relate to the nurse by means of verbal communication. This information is obtained from direct questioning. An example of a database compiled by Medicare (NAHC, 2001) to assist with assessment and outcome measurement is known as the Outcomes and Assessment Information Set (OASIS) (found in Appendix C.3).

Objective data are obtained using a review-of-systems approach to physical examination, physical assessment skills, and direct observation. Assessment findings should be shared with clients, meanings explored, and a plan of care developed in partnership with clients and caregivers.

Data are recorded in the client's clinical home care record in the form of a flow sheet or assessment chart. It is during the assessment phase that the home-health nurse determines that other resources are needed, such as physical therapy, occupational therapy, speech therapy, home health aide, medical social services, Meals-on-Wheels, transportation assistance, or nutritional counseling. The family is included throughout the entire nursing process because they will assist in the implementation and evaluation of the plan of care.

## Diagnosis

From the baseline data obtained during the assessment phase, the home-health nurse develops nursing diagnoses for the problems identified. The Omaha System of classification of nursing diagnoses is one of the best approaches to nursing diagnosis in home health (see Chapter 9).

Diagnoses are validated with all who are involved: client, family, physician, and other providers. It is also well documented so that the plan of care and expected outcomes can be determined.

## Outcome Identification

Identifying appropriate client care and health outcomes is an important part of care. Outcomes that can be expected are to be specific to the client and the client's environment and are derived from the assessment and diagnosis. Outcomes are based on scientific evidence; are culturally sensitive; are mutually agreed on by all involved, including the client; can be measured; and are attainable. Outcomes are to be documented and provide direction for continuity of care.

## Planning

Nursing diagnoses give the home-health nurse the necessary information to develop short- and long-term goals with the client and family, and to formulate an individualized plan for interventions. This plan of care indicates expected client outcomes for each identified problem or nursing diagnosis. Goals focus on health promotion, maintenance, restoration, and the prevention of complications. The information is documented on the developed client care plan, which serves as a continuous resource for nurse accountability and as a means to promote continuity of care.

## Home Health Care in Canada

Barbara Mildon, R.N., M.N., C.H.E., Community Health Nurses Association of Canada (an associate group of the Canadian Nurses Association), and Saint Elizabeth Health Care

### HOME CARE AND THE HEALTH CARE SYSTEM

The responsibility for funding and administering health care in Canada belongs to the provincial and territorial governments. Nonetheless, the federal government provides provinces with some health care funding as long as the province adheres to the principles and service provisions prescribed in the Canada Health Act (CHA), the legislation that created and protects Canada's universal, publicly funded health care system. The CHA requires that hospital and physicians' services must be provided free of charge; however, it does not cover home care (or other health services such as medications or health promotion—disease prevention services). Although every province and territory has established a home care program, the eligibility criteria and the type and extent of services vary considerably. Since 1998, home care in Canada has gained increasing attention from governments at all levels, and from policymakers, as evidenced by conferences, policy initiatives, research studies, and home care demonstration projects (Sharkey, Larsen, and Mildon, in press). The establishment of a national program of funded home care has now been recommended in several major reports, including *The Health of Canadians—The Federal Role* (Standing Senate Committee on Social Affairs, vol 6 of the Kirby Report, 2002), *Quality End-of-Life Care: The Right of Every Canadian* (Standing Senate Committee on Social Affairs, Science and Technology 2000), and *Building on Values, The Future of Health Care in Canada,* the final report of the Romanow Commission (Commission on the Future of Health Care in Canada, 2002).

Research into the nature, costs, and benefits of home care has increased significantly in recent years, assisted by the establishment of research centers including the Home Care Evaluation and Research Centre of the University of Toronto. Many home care research reports have provided evidence of cost savings and/or the improved well-being of health system clients managed at home (e.g., Health Canada, 1999, 2002).

### SERVICES AVAILABLE FROM HOME CARE PROGRAMS

A survey of home care programs across Canada by the Canadian Home Care Association reveals a wide range of available services, although not all home care programs offer the full range. Services may include nursing care (including complex care such as intravenous therapy, chemotherapy administration, total parenteral nutrition administration, and so on), palliative care, mental health services, respiratory therapy, homemaking, personal care, physiotherapy, occupational therapy, speech therapy, respite care, oxygen therapy, laboratory services including blood and specimen collection, portable radiography and electrocardiography, transportation, nutrition counseling, and social work. In addition, many home care programs provide a case management function for clients and serve as the access point for long-term care placement. Home care programs may also offer information on and referral to community services such as Meals-on-Wheels and friendly visitor programs. The province of Quebec offers a provincewide 24-hour health information telephone service staffed by nurses that have access to the files of home care clients. New Brunswick and Ontario now provide all residents with access to a 24-hour telephone triage service that is staffed by registered nurses. The nurses utilize computer databases and algorithms as decision-making support tools in advising callers about health concerns or issues.

### ADMINISTRATION AND FUNDING OF HOME CARE PROGRAMS

In Canada, home care programs are usually administered by provincial health or social service departments or by local community/regional health boards. The department or board may employ staff to deliver the home care services or may contract out service delivery to external agencies. In addition, the federal government funds and operates two home care programs—one for Canadian Armed Forces veterans and another for Canada's First Nations populations. Home care expenditures in Canada have risen from 1.028 billion in 1990-91 to 2.096 billion in 1997-98 (Health Canada, 1998) and represent approximately 2.7% of the total health care spending in Canada (Thompson, 2000).

In Ontario, since 1996, home care programs have been administered by 43 locally situated Community Care Access Centres (CCACs). CCACs are not-for-profit, independent corporations accountable to the Ministry of Health through a board of directors. They receive funding from the provincial government intended to cover both the case management function performed by CCAC staff and the actual home care services. The CCACs have adopted a managed competition structure in which the services are provided by a variety of contractors selected through a request-for-proposal (RFP) process. Criteria for the successful RFP are based on the concept of best quality and best price.

## Implementation

Implementation of the plan occurs in three phases: before, during, and after the home visit, depending on plan requirements. It is the home-health nurse's responsibility to work with the client to facilitate return to an optimal level of functioning and health and to make certain that the client and family are active participants in the care. Instruction about diet, supervision of medications, and evaluation of diabetic management are examples of such actions.

## COST TO THE CLIENT

In general, professional services such as nursing, social work, physiotherapy, occupational therapy, and nutrition therapy are provided at no cost to the client. Some provinces charge a user fee for support services such as homemaking, personal care, and transportation. The user fee may be a set flat rate or established via a sliding scale based on income. In addition, because the number of hours of support service available is usually limited, clients may choose to purchase extra services. Some programs cover the full cost of supplies, equipment, and medications, whereas in others, clients pay some or all of such costs. Some programs offer clients a self-managed care option in which the client is given a sum of money with which to independently purchase services.

## TRENDS INFLUENCING HOME CARE

In Canada, six main trends have been identified as influencing home care:

- An aging population, with a preference to remain at home in the community, even in the face of physical or cognitive disabilities
- The movement toward the development and implementation of a national home care program to provide core services to all Canadians at no cost
- The shortage of nurses and other home care providers, particularly in jurisdictions where a disparity exists in wages and working conditions between health care sectors (e.g., home care versus institutional care)
- The growing availability of telemetry, digital photography, and remote wireless technology that supports remote assessment of client health status and needs (e.g., as related to complex wounds, cardiorespiratory function) by a specialized practitioner—which means that specialty services and practitioners in short supply are able to direct the care of a significantly higher number of clients, reduce cost and inconvenience related to client travel, and contribute to optimal health outcomes
- Ongoing concern over health system costs and the debate over the degree of privatization and for-profit health services within Canada's universal, publicly funded health care system
- The identification and utilization of standards of care, quality indicators, workload measurement systems, standardized assessment tools (e.g., the minimum data set used to assess functional status) and outcome monitoring processes that support best practices in client care, accreditation processes, optimal

utilization of scarce health human resources, and innovation in home care services

The events and initiatives described here emphasize the importance of the contribution of home care to Canada's health care system. The trends will continue to influence its evolution and the degree to which it realizes its full potential.

### References

Canadian Home Care Association: *Portrait of Canada: an overview of public home care programs,* Ottawa, 1998, Health Canada Publications (prepared by the Canadian Home Care Association in collaboration with l'Association des CLSC et des CHSLD du Quebec for Health Canada).

Commission on the Future of Health Care in Canada: *Building on values: the future of health care in Canada,* 2002, available on line at http://www.healthcarecommission.ca.

Health Canada: *Public home care expenditures in Canada, 1975–1976 to 1997-98, Fact Sheets,* Ottawa, 1998, Health Canada.

Health Canada: *Provincial and territorial home care programs: a synthesis for Canada,* Ottawa, 1999, Health Canada.

Health Canada: *Final report of the national evaluation of the cost-effectiveness of home care: a report prepared for the Health Transition Fund by Marcus Hollander and Neena Chappell,* 2002, available online at www.homecarestudy.com.

Sharkey S, Larsen L, Mildon B: An overview of home care in Canada: its past, present and potential, *Home Health Care Manag Pract* 2003 (in press).

Standing Senate Committee on Social Affairs, Science and Technology: *Quality end-of-life care: the right of every Canadian, final report,* Ottawa, 2000 (updated from *Of life and death* [1995]), available online at www.parl.gc.ca.

Standing Senate Committee on Social Affairs, Science and Technology: *The health of Canadians—the federal role: final report on the state of the health care system in Canada,* Ottawa, 2002, available online at www.parl.gc.ca.

Thompson LG: Clear goals, solid evidence, integrated systems, realistic roles, *Healthcare Papers* 1(4):60-66, 2000, available online at www.healthcarepapers.com.

*Canadian spelling is used.*

## Evaluation

Together, the client, family, and home-health nurse evaluate the client's status and progress toward achieving goals on an ongoing basis. During follow-up visits, previous goals may be replaced with new ones on the basis of the client's changing health status. The home-health nurse prepares the client and family for discharge as early as the initial visit. The short-term nature of the services is explained to the client and family. The frequency of visits and the duration of the service are decreased when the client is able to assume self-care or the family has learned how to care for the client. The nurse provides appropriate referral to other community resources if further assistance is needed upon termination of home care. If the nurse determines that the client or family will not be able to provide the needed care, the nurse must assist the client in making alternative plans for care. Plans may include the potential of moving toward long-term care within a facility or arranging for the employment of a caregiver in the home.

### DID YOU KNOW?

To avoid what is often referred to as the "home visit ritual" (i.e., visits that have no predetermined goal or outcome), the home-health nurse must establish both short- and long-term goals with clients and families. The goals provide for continuity of care and state the criteria for evaluating the client's condition and progress toward an optimum level of self-care.

## Standards of Professional Performance

### Quality of Care

Quality improvement activities are an important part of nursing care delivery. Nurses willingly participate in such activities as monitoring of care, seeing and analyzing opportunities for improving care, developing guidelines to improve care, collecting data, making recommendations, and implementing activities to enhance quality and to make changes in nursing practice. Results of these activities are used to make changes in health care delivery. According to the NAHC (2001), outcomes to determine quality indices in Medicare are taken from the OASIS-B1 database and integrated into Outcome Based Quality Improvement (OBQI). The OASIS-B1 and OBQI will be described in further detail later in this chapter.

### Performance Appraisal

Nurses, as described in Chapter 22, actively participate in quality management activities, including peer review—evaluation of oneself and the entire health team. Professional development is increasing in importance as home health care changes rapidly to meet society's health care needs.

### Education

Both the nurse and the employing agency are encouraged to endorse nursing participation in professional development, which includes continuing education and competence in home health nursing.

### Collegiality

The nurse shares expertise with others as appropriate and participates in the education and evaluation of students and other colleagues.

### Ethics

The *Code of Ethics for Nurses With Interpretive Statements* (ANA, 2001) is a guide for nurses facing ethical dilemmas.

It is the "profession's nonnegotiable ethical standard" (p. 5). The home-health nurse acts as a client advocate, maintaining client confidentiality, promoting informed consent, and making contacts to see that community resources are available to clients. Ethical conflicts and dilemmas are identified and resolved through formal agency mechanisms designed to address such issues. The nurse is responsible for building a trusting relationship with the family, determining whether the home is a safe and appropriate place to provide care for the particular client, and keeping current on research and ethical issues related to home care. The nurse acts in the area of professional obligations through political and social reform that affects client- and population-based care. The new client privacy guidelines from the Health Insurance Portability and Accountability Act of 1996 (HIPAA) require ethical conduct by the nurse, as just described.

### Collaboration

The nurse collaborates with the client, family, and health care team to formulate plans of care and goals and to identify and obtain needed services. The nurse initiates referrals and coordinates resources needed by clients.

### Research

Home-health nurses have a variety of opportunities to participate in research. All nurses should use appropriate research to improve practice. Although the home-health nurse may not have formal research training, the nurse may participate in research at some level if agency support and adequate resources are available. Knowing current research and integrating evidence-based practice into home care will elevate standards of practice and competence among nurses.

### Resource Use

The nurse uses appropriate agency and community resources, including delegating tasks to other caregivers, to provide good benefits and reasonable cost to the client. The nurse helps the client become an informed consumer to assist in empowerment and self-advocacy.

## Responsibilities of the Disciplines

The responsibilities and functions of the disciplines in home health care are dictated by Medicare regulations, professional organizations, and state licensing boards. Other specialized services can be provided in home health such as enterostomal therapy, podiatry, pharmaceutical therapy, nutrition counseling, intravenous therapy, respiratory therapy, and psychiatric or mental health nursing. Many of these services can be provided on a consulting basis, either in the form of staff education or through direct care. The multidisciplinary team may be composed of any or all of the following providers: physician, physical therapist, occupational therapist, social worker, home member, home health aide, and speech pathologist. Each client in the Medicare home care programs must be under the current care of a doctor of medicine, podiatry, or osteopathy to certify that the client has a medical problem. The physician must certify a plan of treatment for the home health agency before care is provided to the client.

Physicians in the community also serve in an advisory capacity to the home health agency by assisting in the development of home care policies and procedures relative to client care. Physician involvement in and acceptance of home health care is necessary if the benefits of home health care are to be recognized and appropriately used. The American Medical Association (AMA) in the early 1960s urged physicians to participate in home health programs, refer clients who would benefit from the services, and promote such programs in their communities. The *Physician Guide to Home Health Care* (AMA, 1979) explained the role and benefit of home health care for clients. Today, some physicians are making home visits to provide medical care.

The physical therapist (PT) provides maintenance, preventive, and restorative treatment for clients in the home. A PT provides direct and indirect care. Direct care activities include strengthening muscles, restoring mobility, controlling spasticity, gait training, and teaching active and passive resistive exercises. Indirect care activities of the PT include consulting with the staff and contributing to client care conferences by sharing skills and expertise. Physical therapy assistants may provide some therapy under the direction of a registered physical therapist. Assistants are high school graduates who have completed an approved assistants' program and have been licensed.

The occupational therapist (OT) helps clients achieve their optimal level of functioning by teaching them to develop and maintain the abilities to perform activities of daily living in their home. Occupational therapists focus most of their treatment on the client's upper extremities by helping to restore muscle strength and mobility for functional skills. This discipline is a valuable resource in assisting the client to become independent in self-care, the goal of all home health care professionals.

Speech pathologists assist people with communication problems related to speech, language, or hearing. Most clients receive direct care services, such as evaluation of speech and language ability, with specific plans being taught to the client and family for follow-up.

The social worker helps clients and families deal with social, emotional, and environmental factors that affect their well-being. Social workers assist directly by identifying and referring clients to appropriate community resources.

With the beginning of Medicare, the home health aide (HHA) became an important member of the home health care team. The home health nurse or physical therapist directly supervises the HHA. The role of the HHA is to help clients reach their level of independence by temporarily helping with personal hygiene and ADLs. Additional duties include light housekeeping, laundry, and meal preparation and shopping. The role of the homemaker (different from the HHA) helps with housekeeping chores.

## HOSPICE CARE

Historically, the word **hospice** referred to a place of refuge for travelers. The contemporary meaning refers to palliative care of the very ill and dying, offering both respite and comfort (Gurfolino and Dumas, 1994). Originating in nineteenth-century England, the earliest hospices first provided **palliative care** to terminally ill patients in hospitals and later extended the services into the homes. In 1970, the hospice movement in the United States gained momentum in response to awakened public interest generated by Dr. Elisabeth Kübler-Ross's work on death and dying (Kübler-Ross, 1969). Public-sponsored hospices, successful in meeting the special needs of the dying patient, attracted the attention of Congress. After evaluating a limited hospice benefit as a pilot, Congress enacted legislation in 1985 that provided coverage for hospice services under Medicare. Stringent controls and criteria for quality hospice care are imposed by both the CMS and the Joint Commission for Accreditation of Healthcare Organizations (JCAHO).

As a result of the hospice movement, persons with terminal diseases now have the option of dying at home with support services available. A variety of hospice care models in the United States use institutional services, home care service, or both. Those that use an existing hospital in conjunction with an established home health agency (hospital-based or contracted services) are probably the most cost efficient. Each organization contributes a portion of its resources to this concept of care. In addition to prescribed home care services, core services offered through hospice include volunteers, chaplain support, respite care, financial help with medicines and equipment, and bereavement support of the family after the client's death.

It should be noted that choosing hospice does not mean a client has chosen to die. Rather, one criterion for hospice is that the disease process or condition has progressed to the extent that further treatment cannot cure. It is the goal of hospice to increase the quality of remaining life. The hospice team is usually medically directed and nurse coordinated. Pain management, symptom control, and emotional support are primary areas of expertise offered.

A second criterion for hospice care is that death is expected within 6 months. Medicare covers this period; however, the client may survive longer than 6 months as a result of stability or improvement of the condition. At that time, the interdisciplinary hospice team reviews the case and determines whether to discharge the client or provide coverage through the hospice agency for the period after 6 months. Clients who are discharged can be readmitted when their condition changes. Hospice provides an on-call nurse who is available 24 hours a day to monitor changes in the client's condition and attend to the needs of the client and family. After the death of the client, hospice provides bereavement counseling and services for up to 1 year.

Hospice programs may be integrated with a home health, hospital, or skilled nursing agency, or they may be freestanding (Hospice Association of America, 2001). The philosophy of care is different for the terminally ill and requires that the multidisciplinary team have the knowledge, skill, compassion, and experience to work with the unique needs of this population. The primary goal is to help maintain the client's integrity and comfort. Palliative care, or care aimed at comfort rather than cure, is the objective. Nursing actions such as alleviating pain, encouraging the client, family, and friends to communicate with each other about essential sensitive issues related to death and dying, and coordinating care to ensure a comfortable, peaceful death contribute to palliative care.

Health care providers who work with the dying often experience unique stress. Staff stress must be identified and appropriately addressed to help in the delivery of quality care and to maintain the care provider's integrity. Some examples of stress experienced by hospice staff include the following: experience with multiple deaths in a short period of time and the inability to work through the past death events, friction experienced within the hospice team so that debriefing after a death cannot be accomplished, difficulty deciding how or when to set limits on involvement with clients and families, difficulty establishing realistic limitations as to what can be provided by hospice, and frustration when clients and caregivers do not follow the plan of care. The hospice nurse needs a firm foundation in home care skills, knowledge of community resources, the ability to function constructively as a team member, comfort with death and dying, and the mature ability to meet personal emotional needs as well as the emotional needs of the hospice client and family.

Not all terminal clients choose hospice care, and of those who do, not all are eligible for Medicare or covered by private insurance. If reimbursement becomes the primary admission criterion for hospice care, it will no longer be a real option for all terminal clients. The nurse who chooses hospice as a specialty area must be prepared to deal with these and other ethical issues. End-of-life care is of great concern to nursing, and many issues are also hotly debated by the public (e.g., client choice, available hospice services, reimbursement status, admission criteria, and assisted suicide) (see end-of-life information in Content Resources on the evolve website). The *Code of Ethics for Nurses With Interpretive Statements* (ANA, 2001) and involvement in a formal interdisciplinary ethics committee can assist nurses in resolving these dilemmas.

## Home Care of the Dying Child

In most situations, the terminally ill child desires to be home with his or her parents in familiar surroundings. It is in that secure place where families can provide the greatest comfort. The needs of the dying child and family are unique: society does not expect death to occur to the young or to precede that of the parent.

Knowledge of the child's physical, cognitive, psychosocial, and spiritual development will enable the nurse to provide appropriate pain management, assist the child and family to communicate with each other, advocate for their needs in the community, and refer to key players who can offer them assistance such as volunteers, counselors, or clergy.

Explaining death to children in terms they can understand can relieve them of the fear of the unknown. Providing answers about death to the child, siblings, family, and friends can best be accomplished during those teachable moments when the question regarding their condition or death is raised. Community interven-

tions, such as discussing death concepts and communication strategies to the dying child's classmates, can help these friends say good-bye and know the normalcy of the death process without fear. Assisting the dying child and family to prepare for the funeral service will give them a sense of mastery and control. The child can prepare special mementos that can be given to family and friends at the funeral and can assist the child and family to accept the death as inevitable while giving something of self to others. Last, bereavement telephone calls or visits by hospice staff continue for the family up to 1 year after the death of the child, at the 1-month, 3-month, 6-month, and 1-year anniversaries of the child's death and on holidays and the child's birthday. The family (including parents, grandparents, and siblings) can participate in community memorial services and support groups that are offered by the hospice program or other bereavement organizations.

## INTERDISCIPLINARY APPROACH TO HOME HEALTH AND HOSPICE CARE

**Interdisciplinary collaboration** is required in the home health and hospice settings. Its use is mandated for Medicare-certified home care agencies, and it is also inherent in the definitions of home health care. Without effective collaboration, there would be no continuity of care, and the client's home care program would be fragmented.

The collaborative process for home care directed toward secondary and tertiary prevention activities should begin in the hospital with the discharge planner and hospital nurse, who identify a client's need for home care and then review their observations and plans with the physician for approval and orders. The discharge planner then contacts the referral intake coordinator of the home care agency, specifying the services requested by the physician. If persons from several disciplines will be involved, the intake coordinator notifies the appropriate staff and monitors the interdisciplinary collaboration. Either the registered nurse or the physical therapist usually functions as the case manager to ensure that care is coordinated.

In home care, as in other health care settings, professionals may experience stress associated with changing roles and overlapping responsibilities. In collaborating, each home health care provider should carefully analyze the roles of all involved people to determine whether overlapping occurs, and then the team should adjust the plan of care accordingly. Professionals in home care are in a unique setting in which they can truly work together to accomplish the client's care goals.

> **NURSING TIP**
>
> Convene a family care conference to discuss issues with a client and family, develop a consistent team approach, and clarify roles and responsibilities.

In terms of legal accountability and compliance with federal regulations through a Medicare-approved home

**HOW TO  Use a Hospice Approach to Care in Any Setting**

The hospice philosophy of care means providing comfort measures to an individual prior to death. The circumstances of death vary. The individual may be any age, from infancy to the older adult. A nurse may be faced with the death of a single individual or of many people during a limited time. Death may occur in the individual's home, in a hospital setting, or in an uncontrolled setting such as the community. How does one adapt nursing care in any situation? What basic skills can professional caregivers use, that can be applied in any situation or setting? How do caregivers adapt to a hospice home death, inpatient death, or a sudden, unexpected death where, for example, many people have died as a result of a natural disaster or a terrorist act?

- Be prepared now. Consider your own philosophy of death so that you can assist others without distraction when that time comes. What do you have to do to develop your own philosophy of death, and how will that assist you to care for others? What do you believe about an afterlife? Is death the worst possible fate for all living beings?

- Different cultures vary in their beliefs and responses to death. Know the differences in cultural responses so that you can effectively help them in their time of need.

- Death events cannot be totally controlled—even in a hospice environment where the eventual death has been illustrated to family and friends and the dying individual prior to the death. Expect the unexpected and take cues from the client and the loved ones regarding their needs.

- Shock, disbelief, and crisis reactions occur even with prepared, hospice deaths. How can we caregivers assist family/friends during this time? Ask them what they need; provide them with the basics such as food or blankets; provide comfort; if it is not contraindicated, provide the family/friends with personal effects or mementos of the individual; give sensitive, caring support. Sit with them and listen. Sit with them in silence if that is what they need.

- In a disaster, when many people are affected, the philosophy of care is to provide the greatest good to the greatest number of people. In a triage situation, the needs of those with less severe injuries have priority over the needs of those who are closer to death (Mistovich, Hafen, and Karren, 2000). Responsibilities of caregivers and health professionals will be stretched to the maximum. How do we care for the needs of the dying? How do we attend to the responses of the public to their loved ones? Someone needs to be present to support them. A specified leader to a group of clients must delegate responsibility to a caregiver who can assist the dying and their loved ones.

- Your response and assistance during the untimely death of a loved one will be remembered either for the lack of caring or for the sensitive, kind support that you gave. This memory can delay or enhance the bereavement process that can bring closure or resolution to their loved one's death.

Mistovich J, Hafen B, Karren K: *Prehospital emergency care,* ed 6, Upper Saddle River, NJ, 2000, Prentice Hall.

health agency, it is the physician who must certify the plan of treatment for the client. However, in most instances, it is other health care professionals who evaluate the client's status, report the findings to the physician, and then, in collaboration with the physician, modify the plan of treatment for the client.

Medicare requires that interdisciplinary services be documented. Each professional must document the care provided to demonstrate accountability and provide continuity of care. Interdisciplinary collaboration and coordination through case conferences and contracts made between the caregivers must be documented in the clinical record. Quality improvement mechanisms such as chart audits and peer review verify the appropriate and effective use of collaboration.

Successful interdisciplinary functioning depends on numerous factors, including the knowledge, skills, and attitudes of each team member. Factors necessary for successful interdisciplinary team functioning are shown in Box 40-3. The plan of care should be implemented and reinforced by all involved disciplines. For example, nurses must reinforce the teaching by the physical therapist of the exercise regimen and gait training.

## EDUCATIONAL REQUIREMENTS FOR HOME HEALTH PRACTICE

Nurses come to home health from a variety of educational and practice backgrounds. Differences in both experience and educational preparation influence the contributions that nurses make to home health care. Home health nurses should be educated to function at a high level of competency so that they can be relied on not only by their professional colleagues but also by the community. A baccalaureate degree in nursing should be the minimum requirement for entry into professional practice in any community health setting. Nursing education has the responsibility to produce competent, skillful clinicians. A baccalaureate degree does not automatically mean a qualified, mature professional nurse. However, a quality education does lay the foundation for the development of such important characteristics, and the public deserves no less. Life experience, compassion, and awareness of self are factors that are necessary for the delivery of quality client care and professionalism.

In home health care, the nurse with a baccalaureate degree functions in the role of a generalist, providing skilled nursing and coordinating care for a variety of home health

---

**BOX 40-3** Factors for Interdisciplinary Functioning

**KNOWLEDGE**

1. Understand how the group process can be used to achieve group goals.
2. Understand problem solving.
3. Understand role theory.
4. Understand what other professionals do and how they see their roles.
5. Understand the conceptual differences between home care and practice versus institutional care and practices.

**SKILL**

1. Use principles of group process effectively.
2. Communicate clearly and accurately.
3. Communicate without using the profession's jargon.
4. Express self clearly and concisely in writing.

**ATTITUDE**

1. Feel confident in role as a professional.
2. Trust and respect other professionals.
3. Share tasks with other professionals.
4. Work effectively toward conflict resolution.
5. Be flexible.
6. Be "research-minded."
7. Be timely.

---

clients. The nurse with a master's degree is prepared for the advanced practice role as clinical specialist, nurse practitioner, researcher, administrator, or educator. As home care continues to develop its larger role in community health nursing, the need for specialized nurse clinicians will also increase to meet the highly technologic and complex care that has been moved from the hospital into the home setting. In managed care, more clinical specialists will be needed to provide case management and to develop programs to meet the needs of the population served by the managed care network. Nurse practitioners can be used to provide primary care to frail older adults and other homebound clients. Educational programs are increasing to prepare nurses for advanced practice roles in home health.

## Certification

Home-health nurses can seek certification as a generalist home-health nurse, home health clinical nurse specialist, nursing case manager, community health nurse, or clinical specialist in community health through the American Nurses Credentialing Center. The National Hospice Organization will certify hospice nurses. A baccalaureate degree in nursing is required for the generalist examination and a master's degree for the clinical specialist in home and community health nursing. Nurses must also demonstrate current practice. In a highly competitive health care environment, certification is expected to become more necessary to ensure the public of competence and quality.

## ACCOUNTABILITY AND QUALITY MANAGEMENT

### Quality Control Mechanisms

Since the beginning of Medicare, home health agencies have monitored the quality of care to their clients as a mandatory requirement for certification as a home health agency. All agencies are accountable to their clients, to their reimbursement sources, to themselves as health care providers, and to professional standards. Quality is demonstrated through evaluations reflecting that appropriate and needed care has been given to clients in a professional manner.

Clinical records are of great importance in assessing the quality of care. The care and services the client receives and any communication between the physicians and other home health providers must be documented. It is in the clinical record that nurses demonstrate that they are delivering quality care and are also identifying means to improve the quality of care. It is the legal method by which the quality of care can be assessed. This documentation also demonstrates the client's ongoing need for services and shows how the multiple disciplines arrange for continuity and comprehensive care. Documentation of nursing care is central to home care. The amount of documentation affects the home-health nurse more than the nurse in any other setting.

As an example, during the initial evaluation visit, the home-health nurse assesses the client and family's status. This information becomes a permanent part of the clinical record. Subsequent integrating of health services must be noted. Besides clinical notes of all home visits, progress notes must be sent to the client's physician, including the assessment of the client to verify the implementation of the plan of care.

Because individuals from outside the agency participate in the evaluation, the evaluation is viewed as an external means of monitoring the agency's performance. Evaluation requirements are listed in Box 40-4. Representatives from appropriate professional disciplines objectively report the findings of the review. It is the responsibility of the agency to plan and implement goals for the revision, modification, and correction of problems noted. From these reviews, the agency can maintain and improve care for the consumers in the community.

## Accreditation

**Accreditation** is a voluntary process; an agency chooses to participate. The accreditation decision is based on the data in a self-study, the report of a site visit team, and other relevant information. In the future, accreditation may become a requirement for licensure of all home health agencies. Today, home health agencies may be accredited through JCAHO or the Community Health Accreditation Program of the National League for Nursing (CHAP). Both organizations look at the organizational structure through which care is delivered, the process of care through home visits, and the out-

---

### BOX 40-4  Requirements for Agency Evaluation

1. The agency must have written policies requiring an overall evaluation of the agency's total program at least once a year by a group of professional personnel, agency staff, and consumers, or by professional people outside the agency working in conjunction with consumers.

2. The evaluation must consist of both an annual policy and an administrative review, and clinical record reviews must be done at least quarterly.

3. The evaluation will assess the extent to which the agency's program is appropriate, adequate, effective, and efficient in promoting client care.

4. Results are reported to and acted on by those responsible for the agency.

5. A written administrative record of the evaluation is maintained.

---

### BOX 40-5  Medicare Conditions of Participation

1. Definitions of home health agency terminology
2. Compliance with federal, state, and local laws
3. Organization, services, and administration
4. Group of professional personnel with advisory and evaluation function
5. Acceptance of clients, plan of treatment, and medical supervision
6. Services—skilled nursing, therapies, medical and social work, home health aide
7. Establishment and maintenance of clinical records
8. Evaluation of the agency's total program and behavior
9. Provision of oral and written Client Bill of Rights (see Box 40-6)
10. Confidentiality of medical records
11. Disclosure of ownership and management information
12. Compliance with accepted professional standards and principles
13. Qualification to provide outpatient physical or speech pathology services

U.S. Medicare and Medicaid Programs: Revision of conditions of participation for home health agencies and use of Outcome Assessment Information Set (OASIS): proposed rules, *Federal Register* 62(46):11003-11064, 1997.

---

comes of client care, focusing on improved health status. Performance improvement must be ongoing in the agency.

## Regulatory Mechanisms

Home health care is highly regulated when secondary and tertiary prevention are the goals. **Regulation** addresses the key aspects of home health care and is an important concern to the home-health nurse. The home-health nurse is responsible on a daily basis to practice within the guidelines set up by the regulatory agencies. The nurse interprets regulations to colleagues, clients, families, and the community.

CMS is accountable for overseeing the Medicare program, federal participation in the Medicaid program, and other health care quality improvement programs. CMS writes regulations that govern two components of health care: financing and quality improvement (Box 40-5).

Home health regulation is mostly carried out at the state level. State health departments license and certify home health agencies according to state licensing regulations and conditions of participation (CMS, 2002). These regulations serve as the basis for evaluation of each aspect of home health agencies.

Under Medicare regulations, a home health agency is defined as one that meets the following criteria:

- It primarily engages in providing skilled nursing and other therapeutic services.
- It has policies established by a group of professional personnel, including both physicians and nurses, to govern the services that it provides.
- It provides supervision of services by a physician or registered nurse.
- It maintains clinical records on all clients.
- It is licensed by state or local laws.
- It meets the conditions of participation.

Clients are accepted for treatment on the basis of a reasonable expectation that the client's medical, nursing, rehabilitation, and social needs can be met adequately by the agency in the client's place of residence.

Agencies must provide skilled nursing and at least one other service: physical, speech, or occupational therapy; or medical, social, or home health aide services. One service must be provided in its entirety by agency employees. The other services may be contracted. Clients are confined to home and require skilled nursing care on an **intermittent care** basis or speech therapy, physical therapy, or a continual need for occupational therapy.

The state agencies responsible for licensure and certification of home health agencies use these criteria in evaluating whether agencies are conforming to federal regulations. Refer to Chapter 22 for further discussion of quality management and regulatory control.

## FINANCIAL ASPECTS OF HOME HEALTH AND HOSPICE CARE

### Reimbursement Mechanisms

The **reimbursement system** for home health care is complicated and standardized. Before the federal government became involved, home health care was reimbursed either by clients who could pay for the service or by donations that subsidized care for those who could pay only a portion

**Table 40-2   Comparison of the Two Major Federally Supported Programs for Home Health Care**

| MEDICARE (TITLE XVIII) | MEDICAID (TITLE XIX) |
| --- | --- |
| Federal insurance program administered by Social Security Administration | Federal and state assistance program administered by the state |
| Age 65 and over or disabled | Income-based eligibility |
| Conditions of participation | Conditions of participation |
| Homebound status | Not necessarily homebound status |
| Intermittent service | Intermittent service |
| Skilled service | Not necessarily skilled service |
| Restorative program | Restorative with some custodial and maintenance |
| Physician certification | Physician certification |
| Therapies, medical, or social service | State option—therapist, medical, or social service |
| Pays rental and purchase | Pays purchase |
| Reimbursement—"reasonable cost" | Reimbursement—maximum allowed at state level |

or not at all. Now Medicare and Medicaid are the principal funding sources for home health care, with third-party health insurance providing another major source. Budgeted funds for public health from taxes cover preventive home care visits to the clients of the agency.

## Medicare

Medicare has the most standard payment system of all third-party payers and has traditionally set the criteria followed by other types of reimbursement. Reimbursement of home health services is handled through insurance companies under contract to the Social Security Administration.

Medicare does not cover services directed toward the prevention of illness or injury. This does not mean, however, that these activities cannot be performed. They must be done in conjunction with a "skilled" service. The following are examples of services that are reimbursable and covered under Medicare because they require skill, knowledge, and judgment on the part of the provider: observation and evaluation of physical status; teaching and training activities to client, family, or caregiver; therapeutic exercises (for restoration of or loss of function); insertion and irrigation of a catheter or tube; administration of intravenous and intramuscular medications and teaching of medication regimen; and complex wound care.

Medicare beneficiaries usually suffer from chronic conditions with multiple disease processes. Medicare beneficiaries rely on federal reimbursement criteria that definitely influence the providing of care. Medicare places an emphasis on episodic care because of its limitations in benefits and requirements for skilled care.

## Medicaid

Authorized by Title XIX of the Social Security Act, Medicaid provides health services to low-income persons. It is a medical assistance program for eligible people under Title XVI (Aid to Families with Dependent Children) or Title XVI (Supplemental Security Income) of the Social

Security Act. It is also available for those individuals whose income is not adequate to cover medical services and for disability coverage. Medicaid is administered by the states but is both state and federally funded. Providers are directly reimbursed by the state, which is also responsible for monitoring the operations and enforcing the regulations. Medicaid covers home health services, including skilled and unskilled services such as personal care. Needy children and some low-income older adults are eligible under Medicaid.

Table 40-2 compares Medicare with Medicaid. If a client has both Medicare and Medicaid or a private insurance plan, Medicare is used as the primary payment source provided the services being delivered to the client are *skilled*. After Medicare pays, then private insurance is used. When the client is no longer eligible for home care under Medicare, the Medicaid benefits can be used.

## Private Insurance

Third-party payers are represented by private insurance companies in which the person subscribes either individually or with a group such as an employer. Some states (e.g., Connecticut) have laws requiring that home health care be provided in health insurance coverage. Individuals under 65 years of age who need home care after surgery or a prolonged hospitalization use this benefit the most. This benefit can decrease a client's length of stay in the hospital and can assist in a faster return to the client's former level of functioning. Managed care organizations authorize a home health agency to provide a limited number of visits. In this environment, nurses must advocate for clients and provide good data to justify the need for care.

## Payment by Individuals

Some individuals may pay the home health agency directly. Individuals who do not meet their insurance coverage requirements and still want services pay either the agency charge or on a sliding scale, based on their financial status. For example, clients may not need skilled nursing service for assessment of their condition but may need the help of a home health aide to assist with personal hygiene needs. Some persons may pay for home health services that are needed or desired above and beyond the home health services offered by the Medicare program.

### Nursing Visit Charges

The Certified Medicare and Medicaid Service continuously gathers data regarding use of home care services by analyzing factors such as cost, frequency, duration of services, and number of visits. The federal government is interested in both continuing cost and quality of care.

## Cost Effectiveness

Refer to Chapter 5 for an in-depth discussion of the economics of health care and its impact on community-oriented nursing. Although public attention has focused on home health care as a cost-effective alternative to institutionalization in the last 15 years, the expansion of services and growth have resulted in greater scrutiny by CMS and other payers. Because of the increased number of home health agencies and limited capitation of direct and indirect costs, the federal government instituted a prospective payment system on October 1, 2000. This system prevents the abuse or fraudulent use of Medicare funding.

Nurses in many settings are not directly exposed to the financial aspects of health care. In home health, nurses must be "cost-conscious" so that they can interpret to clients what Medicare will or will not cover. It is often difficult for an older client to understand why Medicare will not pay for the nurse to make home visits to take their blood pressure if the client's condition remains stable. Medicare pays for services only if the client's condition remains unstable. The key words to remember for Medicare home health coverage are skilled, homebound, intermittent or part-time, and unstable.

Physician's case management frequently conflicts with Medicare guidelines. It should be noted that services or the frequency of services certified by a physician as being necessary for a particular Medicare client may not meet Medicare's guidelines of "reasonable and necessary" and therefore are not covered by Medicare. For example, a physician might order physical therapy for strengthening exercises for a postsurgical debilitated client. This is not a Medicare-approved physical therapy diagnosis, and therapy would not be provided. However, if skilled nursing is ordered for this same client and is "reasonable and necessary," during the skilled visit the nurse can instruct the family and client regarding a plan of rehabilitation that is developed by collaborating with the therapist.

## Hospice Reimbursement

One of the major issues confronting hospice care is the reimbursement structure in the health care delivery system. Initially, many hospices provided free services as a mission of ministering to the dying. Others accepted available payment from third-party payers for billable services. In November 1983, the federal government legislated a Medicare hospice benefit for reimbursement to Medicare hospice-certified agencies (Federal Register, 1984). Originally, the regulation was to be in effect through September 30, 1986, but additional legislation changed the hospice benefit to a permanent status in April 1986 (Public Health Law 99-272, 1986).

The hospice reimbursement benefit is optional for the Medicare-eligible client. Hospices may bill for skilled home care services under regular Medicare Part A benefits if the client does not want to use the hospice benefit. Responding to the perceived cost benefit potential of hospice care and the public demand for caring services during end of life, third-party payers are following Medicare's lead in providing hospice service options.

## EFFECTS OF LEGISLATION ON HOME HEALTH CARE SERVICES

The federal government plays a significant role in the delivery of home health care services. The information in this section is organized to present an overview of the historical development of the laws affecting home health. Congressional action can change federal legislation regarding home health care. After a law is enacted, the appropriate federal agency develops regulations to implement the law. For updated information concerning amendments, bills presented in Congress, or regulations, consult the *Federal Register* at your local library (or on the internet at http://www.access.gpo.gov/).

The Social Security Act of 1935 signaled the major entrance of the federal government into the area of social insurance. The Medicare program was enacted on July 30, 1965, as Title XVIII of the Social Security Act and became effective July 1, 1966. The program offers two coordinated insurance coverages: hospital insurance, referred to as Part A, and supplemental medical insurance, referred to as Part B. Each provides reimbursement for home health services. This legislation established requirements for client eligibility, reimbursement costs, and rules for physician and agency participation. Many changes in reimbursement have occurred since the programs began.

The Medicaid Community Care Act of 1981, Section 2176 of the Omnibus Reconciliation Act, recognized and supported the concept of community care as a viable alternative for clients requiring long-term care. States and providers of home health services were afforded the opportunity to develop their own plan and implement their own ideas without the burden of excessive federal regulations. There is a concern that the decrease in federal involvement will result in an increase in fraud and abuse in Medicare home care by some not-so-honest entrepreneurs.

The Patient Self-Determination Act: U.S. Code, 1990, part of the Omnibus Reconciliation Act of 1990 (Box 40-6), requires all health care agencies to provide written information to their clients about their rights and their options to refuse treatment, and to sign advance directives in compliance with state's laws. The clinical record must include whether the client has signed an advance directive, and either a copy of the directive or the contents of the directive.

---

**BOX 40-6   Client Bill of Rights**

1. Client has the right to be informed of his or her rights. The home health agency must protect and promote the exercise of these rights.

2. The Home Health Agency must provide the client with a written notice of the client's rights before furnishing care to the client or during the initial evaluation visit and before the initiation of treatment.

3. The Home Health Agency must maintain documentation showing that it has complied.

4. The client has the right to exercise his or her rights as a client of the agency.

5. The client's family or guardian may exercise the client's rights when the client has been judged incompetent.

6. The client has the right to have his or her property treated with respect.

7. The client has the right to voice grievances regarding treatment or care that is (or fails to be) furnished or regarding the lack of respect for property by anyone who is furnishing services on behalf of the agency, and must not be subjected to discrimination or reprisal for doing so.

8. The agency must investigate complaints made by a client or the client's family or guardian regarding treatment or care that is (or fails to be) furnished or regarding the lack of respect for the client's property by anyone furnishing services on behalf of the agency, and must document both the existence of the complaint and the resolution of the complaint.

9. The agency must inform and distribute information to the client, in advance, concerning the policies on advance directives, including a description of applicable state law.

10. The client has the right to confidentiality of clinical records.

11. The agency must advise the client of the agency's policies and procedures regarding disclosure of clinical records.

12. The client has the right to be advised, before care is initiated, of the extent to which payment for services may be expected from Medicare or other sources and the extent to which payment may be required from the client.

13. The client has the right to be advised of the availability of the toll-free home health agency hotline in the state, the purpose of the hotline, and the hours of operation.

From U.S. Congress: *Omnibus reconciliation act of 1990,* Washington, DC, 1990, U.S. Government Printing Office.

---

These documents communicate the client's wishes and take the form of either a living will or a durable power of attorney for health care. The goal of advance directives is to provide a mechanism for clients to make health care decisions while they are able. The directives can be changed at any time. The durable power of attorney names a person who will make health care decisions when the client is unable, whereas the living will indicates the client's decision to decline or stop treatment. States differ in the implementation of advance directives. An example of a living will from the state of Kentucky is presented in Appendix C.2.

## LEGAL AND ETHICAL ISSUES

In any health care system there is the potential for illegal and unethical actions. Much publicity has been given to Medicare fraud and abuse in the last decade. Exploiting the system has been partially caused by the increase in available federal money and the fee-for-service payment system. Examples of such practices include overuse of home health services when the client does not need them, inaccurate billing for services, excessive administrative staff, "kickbacks" for referrals, and billing of noncovered medical supplies. In 1977, the Medicare-Medicaid Anti-Fraud and Abuse Amendments (PL 95-142) were passed to deter such practices. During the late 1990s, the HCFA stepped up the enforcement of this act.

Home health nurses are confronted with multiple issues in everyday practice. Third-party payers have interpreted the definition of skilled care inconsistently over the years. The home-health nurse must abide by established federal regulations when delivering care to clients, even when the needs are greater than what is paid for. Frequency of visits poses another issue. Only intermittent visits are reimbursed. If the frequency increases, then full-time skilled services may be required. Continual reassessment of client and family needs is imperative to avoid inappropriate use and overuse of services. Home-health nurses must be knowledgeable about which medical supplies are covered. This information is readily available and nurses, as professionals, must work within regulatory guidelines and educate the community as to what should be and is actually covered.

Several stressors in home-health care affect nurses. Documentation is often overwhelming, but it is an essential part of client care. The home-health nurse must justify that care meets reimbursement and legal requirements and is necessary and appropriate. This accountability can be stressful. The role of the home health nurse is complex and continuously expanding, requiring ongoing education and excellent judgment. Home health care may be underused if the hospital orientation or physicians view home care as a burden because of the excess paperwork it entails.

Cost effectiveness, if not linked to quality, may raise ethical dilemmas for health care professionals. To exist in the competitive health care arena of today, home health care must be competitive. By properly organizing and using decision-making principles, home-health nurses do not have to sacrifice quality for cost effectiveness. In this environment, evidence-based nursing practice is essential.

> ### WHAT DO YOU THINK?
> If national competitive bidding for durable medical equipment is accepted, efficient health services and equipment will decrease in quality.

## TRENDS IN HOME HEALTH CARE

The 1970s began an era of regulation as the government assumed an important role in the financing of health care. Regulations have now been accused of jeopardizing the quality of care. In the 1980s, a different trend emerged—that of deregulation. In the 1990s, a more comprehensive restructuring of the health care system with more emphasis on home health care occurred, with more controls on the services allowed.

Health care providers and consumers are concerned about quality and cost-effective alternatives to institutional care. Home-health nurses can play a vital role in providing leadership to see that this realistic dream comes true. Quality care is provided in the home setting. The benefit of home health care is measurable in terms of evaluating client outcomes, as described earlier under Accountability and Quality Management.

The per visit cost of home health care is less than the per day cost of hospital care. It is assumed that greater self-care is a means to further cut health care costs. Home health care encourages the promotion of self-care. For home health care to thrive, nurses must continue to provide quality care while clarifying through research the contributions of home health care as a cost-effective part of the health care delivery system. Home health care should be seen as a primary means of delivering health care, not only as an alternative to institution care.

Competition in home health care is on the rise, resulting primarily from the actions by federal programs to deinstitutionalize and deregulate health care. Clients are being discharged in a more acute condition than previously. The increased level of acuity requires highly skilled clinicians in nursing. Administrators of home health agencies are being faced with "marketing" home health care to both consumers and payers. This task, although seemingly difficult, can be easy if accountability and quality are ensured in the agency.

### National Health Objectives

Because home-health nurses are working with clients and families in the home and community, they are in a position to promote the achievement of some of the key Healthy People 2010 objectives. The nurse can assess the client's status related to key objectives, identify available resources and gaps to meet client needs, and coordinate care with other providers and community agencies.

### Healthy People 2010 Objectives

The Healthy People 2010 box highlights the objectives the home-health nurse can assist the nation in meeting through their client case management activities. Clearly, these objectives relate to lifestyle issues. With appropriate health education and referral to community resources for assistance, numerous lives can be saved or prolonged and chronic disabilities reduced. In this way the nurse can contribute to meeting the national health objectives on a one-to-one client–provider level.

The overarching goals of the Healthy People 2010 objectives are to increase quality and years of healthy life and to eliminate health disparities between different segments of the population. The home-health nurse can be instrumental in assisting communities to set and meet these objectives by participating both in community planning activities and in the home health agency to identify which of the objectives the agency can work toward to meet their population needs.

## ISSUES FOR THE TWENTY-FIRST CENTURY

### Access to Health Care

There is no legal right to health care in the United States, and no recognized constitutional basis exists to solicit this right. The President's Commission for the Study of Ethical Problems in Medicine showed 34 million people were uninsured during some period of 1983 and determined that clients' inability to pay was a major detriment to obtaining health care services (President's Commission, 1983). The number of uninsured rose to 43.4 million by 1997 (U.S. Census Bureau, 1998), and many millions are estimated to be underinsured. A combination of inadequate health care funding, limited resources for private charitable care, and absence of legal recourse to obtain health care as a basic human right adversely affects the medically indigent and limits their access to home care. Additionally, welfare reform implemented in 1998 increased the numbers of persons who work in low-paying jobs and for small businesses, and the increasing costs of both health care and insurance have also contributed to the increased numbers of persons who lack access to health care.

Many home health agencies currently use endowment monies, have United Way funds, or have other charitable funds to provide indigent home health care. Some states have programs in which home health agencies agree to contribute a certain percentage of their time to provide indigent care. By the year 2000, 92% of all health care workers received their insurance through a managed care plan (CMS, 2002). Nursing is challenged to address access issues through clinical research, through public advocacy, and by devising cost-reducing strategies and models of care delivery.

### Technology and Telehealth

The incentives and pressures for early hospital discharge have created a transfer of technology from the hospital to

**Healthy People 2010** | **Examples of National Health Objectives for the Year 2010**

2-4  Increase the proportion of adults aged 18 years and older with arthritis who seek help in coping if they experience personal and emotional problems
3-1  Reduce the overall cancer death rate
3-11  Increase the proportion of women who receive a Pap test
3-12  Increase the proportion of adults who receive a colorectal cancer screening examination
3-13  Increase the proportion of women aged 40 years and older who have received a mammogram within the preceding 2 years
4-2  Reduce deaths from cardiovascular disease in persons with chronic kidney failure
4-7  Reduce kidney failure due to diabetes
5-1  Increase the proportion of persons with diabetes who receive formal diabetes education
5-2  Prevent diabetes
5-5  Reduce the diabetes death rate
5-7  Reduce deaths from cardiovascular disease in persons with diabetes
5-9  Reduce the frequency of foot ulcers in persons with diabetes
5-17  Increase the proportion of persons with diabetes who perform self-blood glucose monitoring at least once daily

6-3  Reduce the proportion of adults with disabilities who report feelings such as sadness, unhappiness, or depression that prevent them from being active
6-11  Reduce the proportion of people with disabilities who report not having the assistive devices and technology needed
12-6  Reduce hospitalizations of older adults with heart failure as the principal diagnosis
12-7  Reduce stroke deaths
12-8  Increase the proportion of adults who are aware of the early warning symptoms and signs of a stroke
12-10  Increase the proportion of adults with high blood pressure whose blood pressure is under control
14-5  Reduce invasive pneumococcal infections
15-13  Reduce deaths caused by unintentional injuries
15-14  Reduce nonfatal unintentional injuries
15-25  Reduce residential fire deaths
15-27  Reduce deaths from falls
15-28  Reduce hip fractures among older adults
24-10  Reduce deaths from chronic obstructive pulmonary disease (COPD) among adults
26-2  Reduce cirrhosis deaths

From U.S. Department of Health and Human Services: *Healthy people 2010: national health promotion and disease prevention objectives,* Washington, DC, 2000, U.S. Department of Health and Human Services.

the home care setting (Sheldon, 1994). At the same time, some technologies have been simplified and their reliability increased, allowing their safe use in the home. This trend is expected to continue. Parenteral nutrition, chemotherapy, intravenous therapy for hydration and antibiotics, intrathecal pain management, ventilators, apnea monitors, chest tubes, and skeletal traction are examples of current home care technologies. The home care nurse must be prepared to evaluate the cost and safety of technology for the home. Clients must be screened and meet specific admission criteria. All clients are not suited for home care, and it is up to the nurse to advocate for clients when home care is appropriate and when it is not appropriate. When appropriate, the nurse will become competent to use these technology skills in the home to maximize their performance, to reduce inherent liability risk, to increase client rehabilitation, and to use research to show that nursing is a vital member of this rapidly developing component of health care.

**Telehealth** is emerging as a viable and acceptable way to provide health care. Telehealth is defined as health information sent from one site to another by electronic communication (Thobaben, 1998). Examples of the uses of telehealth include telephone triage and advice, and telemonitoring equipment to measure vital signs, cardiac function, and point-of-care diagnostics. The WebTV and ViaTV phones are two examples of telecommunication devices that can be used to communicate between client and health care provider through the internet to transmit data, write e-mails, obtain medical information, and monitor or assess changes in condition (Finkelstein and Friedman, 2000).

**THE CUTTING EDGE**

In May 2002, a rice-sized silicon computer chip (12 by 2.1 mm), known as VeriChip, was surgically inserted into each shoulder of three family members. The VeriChip contains each individual's telephone number and medication list. This computer chip can provide emergency department personnel access to the client's health information with an external scanner.

## Health Insurance Portability and Accountability Act of 1996

In 1996, Congress recognized the importance of protecting the health care privacy of our citizens. All health care organizations were required to uphold the HIPAA federal privacy standards by April 14, 2003. The purpose of this legislation is to protect the client's private information through the electronic transfer of health records, allow the client's full access to his or her personal medical records, provide clear information (informed consent) specifying the medical use of the client's personal health information and records to allow the client to have control over that information, and ensure legal protection, with significant criminal and civic penalties to those individuals or agencies who do not comply with the privacy requirements. Although it will cost the health care industry a substantial amount to initiate these requirements, the cost savings, particularly as a result of the efficient use of electronic transfer of records, is expected to be over $29.9 billion dollars within 10 years (U.S. Department of Health and Human Services, 2002a).

Although the regulations will ensure the privacy of our citizens, they can impede access to health care delivery and prohibit needed research, particularly in public health, through its strict regulations. In March 2002, U.S. Department of Health and Human Services (USDHHS) Secretary Tommy G. Thompson proposed changes that clarify and strengthen the regulations while reducing obstacles to care. Although the HIPAA regulation also initially required all citizens to have a unique health identifier, this regulation has been postponed indefinitely (USDHHS, 2002a).

## Pediatric and Maternal–Child Home Care

Pediatric home care has changed tremendously over the past years, as more children are being treated outside the institutional environment. The family is the key to the successful managing of a child at home. A supportive and stable home environment for children can contribute to healing and maintenance of health. Policymakers in the United States are beginning to appreciate the relationship between home care and pediatrics. Legislation has been proposed to require that private insurance companies cover home care in employee benefit packages. New programs, resources, and options for funding are beginning to become available for care of children at home.

Specialized programs for the pediatric population are mandatory. Although infants have been treated in the home for years, the focus on high technology care requires evaluating key issues such as reimbursement, staff competence, and quality improvement. Pediatric needs range from an infant who needs observation and treatment with home phototherapy or a sleep monitor, to a child needing ventilator assistance and enteral feeding. Approximately 10 million children are disabled and institutionalized today because of terminal or chronic conditions. Pediatric home care in the future will continue to help parents care for their children at home if resources and interventions continue to be available.

Although maternal–child home care is not a new concept, there is a revitalized interest in expanding these home care services to reduce maternal and infant mortality and morbidity. The reemerging home care services target high-risk pregnant mothers and provide health education, short-term skilled nursing care, and anticipatory guidance. Recent research has demonstrated long-term positive health outcomes of prenatal and infant home visiting programs by nurses managing pregnancy-induced hy-

pertension, childhood injuries, and subsequent pregnancies among low-income women (Kitzman et al, 1997). Nursing interventions have reduced the use of welfare, child abuse and neglect, and criminal behavior for low-income, unmarried mothers for up to 15 years after the birth of the first child (Olds et al, 1997).

Home care of infants focuses on parent education about infant needs, parenting skills, instructions to improve growth and development outcomes, and skilled medical care. These programs are being shown to be cost effective. Programs to provide skilled home care to addicted mothers and infants include such services as family counseling, medical treatment, emotional support, methods to improve nutritional state and reduce infant irritability, and training in improving maternal–infant interaction (Struk, 1994). Some hospitals are developing programs that allow a nurse to provide continuity of care from hospital to home. A nurse who provides obstetric inpatient care may follow the mother and baby to the home to provide postpartum care. This trend requires that hospital nurses be well grounded in community-based nursing concepts.

## Family Responsibility, Roles, and Functions

The family plays an important role in the delivery of home health care. The term *family*, as discussed previously, refers to a caregiver responsible for the client's well-being. Women have traditionally been the caregivers for children and older adults in the United States. Now, however, women are less available to provide this care without assistance, because they are often working outside the home. At issue is whether home health care services should be used as a respite, or relief, type of care. Sometimes a family member is debilitated and unable to help the client without assistance. Should supportive services be paid by the federal government? On the other hand, some family members are capable of providing the needed care but are unwilling to do so. Who should pay for the service and who should provide the needed care?

Family responsibility is an issue that is difficult to resolve in this country. Assistance from social support systems helps in coping with the stress of caring for an ill family member. The goal is to maintain the client at home for as long as possible and to provide high-quality care. To do this, resources must be used appropriately and effectively. However, developing a public consensus to resolve these issues has been a problem.

## Measuring the Outcomes of Home Health Care

Included in the *Conditions of Participation* under Medicare, home health agencies must have a comprehensive, standardized patient assessment instrument for adults and non-maternity clients that drives care delivery and prospective payment (US Medicare and Medicaid Programs, 1997). This instrument, known as **Outcomes and Assessment Information Set** (OASIS), measures outcomes for quality improvement and client satisfaction with care. Funded by the CMS and the Robert Wood Johnson Foundation,

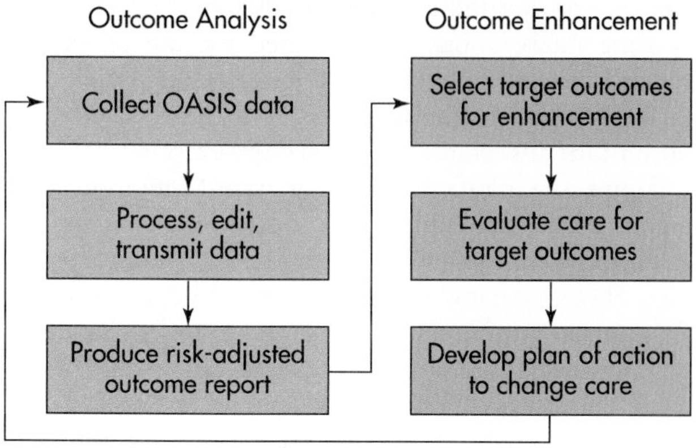

Outcome Analysis  Outcome Enhancement

Collect OASIS data | Select target outcomes for enhancement

Process, edit, transmit data | Evaluate care for target outcomes

Produce risk-adjusted outcome report | Develop plan of action to change care

**Figure 40-3** Two-stage QBQI framework. *(From U.S. Department of Health and Human Services and Centers for Medicare and Medicaid Services:* Outcome-based quality improvement (OBQI) implementation manual, *February 2002, pp 2.4, 2.10.)*

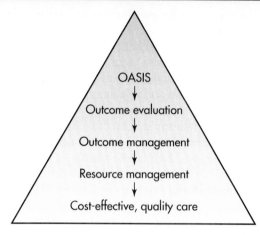

**Figure 40-4** The outcome paradigm. *(From U.S. Department of Health and Human Services and Centers for Medicare and Medicaid Services:* Outcome-based quality improvement (OBQI) implementation manual, *February 2002, pp 2.4, 2.10.)*

OASIS has undergone "12 years of research, development, and demonstration programs to design and test outcome measures for home care" (Center for Health Services and Policy Research, 1999, p. 1)

OASIS was revised and renamed in 1998 and is now OASIS-B1. Its database underwent another revision in August 2000 that includes changes in demographic and patient identifiers for greater accuracy in monitoring data. OASIS data are measured and reported to the CMS on the client's admission to home health care, after an episode of hospitalization, at the time of recertification, and on discharge from care. Data are submitted by each agency to a national databank, and agencies receive both results and comparisons with similar agencies to determine areas needing improvement. See Appendix B.3 for one part of this assessment.

Using the OASIS-B1 data, outcome analysis and improvement strategies can be accomplished through the **Outcome Based Quality Improvement** (OBQI) framework. Although not mandated by Medicare, the OBQI provides direction to improve client care. The OBQI is a two-stage framework that includes data analysis and outcome enhancement (Figure 40-3). The first stage, data analysis, enables an agency to compare its performance to a national sample, identify factors that may affect outcomes (through risk adjustment), and identify final outcomes that show improvement in or stabilizing of a client's condition. The second stage, known as outcome enhancement, involves the selection of specific **client outcomes** and then determining strategies to improve care (USDHHS and CMS, 2002). Figure 40-4 shows the OBQI outcome paradigm. The results of the OASIS and OBQI are the provision of cost-effective, quality care.

Accrediting organizations are also mandating the reporting of outcomes as a performance standard. JCAHO (1996) has revised the 1997 to 1998 standards for home health to focus more on performance improvement based on measurable data, including **benchmarking,** which

means comparing oneself with national standards and guidelines and with other agencies. Clinical guidelines, pathways, and clinical maps are other methods that agencies are using to standardize care and control costs.

These trends will have a great effect on the provision of home health care, the viability of agencies, and the role of home-health nurses in the future. Nursing research will be critical to demonstrate the cost effectiveness, as well as the quality, of the care provided by professional nurses. The future of home health nursing holds excitement, diversity, and opportunity.

## Practice Application

The home visit is the hallmark of home health nursing. When a nurse enters a client's home, she or he is a guest and must recognize that the services offered can be accepted or rejected. The first visit sets the stage for success or failure. The initial assessment of the client, the support system, and the environment is critical.

A. What strategies would the nurse consider to develop a trusting relationship during the first visit?
B. What would be the most important elements to assess in the home environment?
C. What is necessary for the nurse to include in the client contract?
D. How can the nurse assess preferred learning style?

**Answers are in the back of the book.**

## Key Points

- Home health care differs from other areas of health care in that the health care providers practice in the client's environment. This unique characteristic affects several components of nursing practice in the home care setting.

- Family, including any caregiver or significant person who takes the responsibility to assist the client in need of care at home, is an integral part of home health care.
- Home care reached a turning point with the arrival of Medicare, which provided regulations for home care practice and reimbursement mechanisms.
- Home health agencies are divided into the following five general types on the basis of the administrative and organizational structures: official, private and voluntary, combination, hospital based, and proprietary.
- Regardless of the type of home health agency in a community, the primary goal is to provide quality home health care to the community based on the health needs of people.
- Demonstration of professional competency is the foremost requirement for home-health care nurses.
- Home health care nursing is a division of community-oriented nursing. Thus health promotion activities are a fundamental component of practice.
- There are three accepted components of the concept of self-care: client education, client compliance, and self-help.
- Contracting is a vital component of all nurse–client relationships. Contracting refers to any working agreement, continuously renegotiable, between the nurse, client, and family.
- The home-health care nurse practices in accordance with the Standards of Home Health Nursing Practice developed by the American Nurses Association, Council of Community Health Nurses.
- Interdisciplinary collaboration is a required process in the home health care setting. Its use is mandated for Medicare-certified home care agencies, and it is also inherent in the definition of home health care.
- In home care, as in other care settings, professionals experience stress associated with changing roles and overlapping responsibilities. In collaborating, home health care providers should carefully analyze one another's roles to determine whether overlapping occurs and adjust the plan of care as needed.
- Since the advent of Medicare, home health agencies have monitored the quality of care to their clients as a mandatory requirement for certification as a home health agency. All agencies are accountable to clients and families, to their reimbursement sources, to themselves as a health care provider, and to professional standards.
- The home care nurse today faces many challenges. Ethical issues (reimbursement criteria and indigent care), role development (high technology and hospice nursing), and opportunities for research (quality of care and cost effectiveness) affect nursing practice in the home.
- The concept of home health care began in the 1800s with an emphasis on health promotion and disease prevention. With the advent of Medicare, the goal became episodic illness care. Today, home health is moving back to a greater emphasis on disease prevention and health promotion.
- With the development of managed care networks, home health agencies will be contracting with a group of health care organizations to provide care, or they will be purchased by a larger network and provide care only to the network's clients.
- Home care agencies may be accredited through the Joint Commission for Accreditation of Healthcare Organizations or the Community Health Accreditation Program.
- The Omnibus Reconciliation Act of 1990 introduced the home care client bill of rights and advance directives to empower clients with control over their own health care.

## Clinical Decision-Making Activities

1. Make a joint home visit with an experienced home health nurse to do the following:
   a. Evaluate the process and content of the nurse–client interaction to determine whether the visit was therapeutic or merely ritual and describe the process of the visit.
   b. Compare actual roles and functions with the Standards of Home Health Nursing Practice (ANA, 1999).
   c. Assess the level of skilled care the clients received and determine whether the care is needed and appropriate. Is it within the four questions asked in the section on practice functions? (See the How To box on p. 980.) Answer the questions in the How To box and relate your answers to the seven functions of skilled nursing care discussed on p. 980.
2. Make a joint home visit with another home health care professional and assess as in the preceding activity. Also, attend a client/family care conference meeting and write a summary of the process of the group. How has your attitude of an issue changed or not changed according to those expressed by various family members?
3. Review a client record. What client outcomes were met through home health care? What specific outcomes showed an improvement or a stabilizing condition?
4. Review your state's laws governing advance directives. Consider the legal and ethical advantages and disadvantages of having such directives. How would you write an advance directive for yourself?
5. Interview a nurse and determine how the client's bill of rights has affected practice. Do you think that the bill of rights is all-inclusive? What other rights do you think could or should be included?

**Additional Resources**

These related resources are found either in the appendix at the back of this book or on the book's website at **http://evolve.elsevier.com/Stanhope.**

**evolve** Evolve Website

Appendix C.2 The Living Will Directive

Appendix C.3 OASIS, Start of Care Assessment

Palliative Care

WebLinks: Healthy People 2010

## References

American Medical Association: *Physician guide to home health care,* Monroe, Wisc, 1979, AMA.

American Nurses Association: *The scope and standards of practice for home health nursing,* Washington, DC, 1999, ANA.

American Nurses Association: *Code of ethics for nurses with interpretive statements,* Kansas City, Mo, 2001, ANA.

Archbold PG et al: The PREP system of nursing interventions: a pilot test with families caring for older members, *Res Nurs Health* 18:3, 1995.

Canadian Home Care Association: *Portrait of Canada: an overview of public home care programs,* Ottawa, 1998, Health Canada Publications (prepared by the Canadian Home Care Association in collaboration with l'Association des CLSC et des CHSLD du Quebec for Health Canada).

Cassak D: Hospitals in home health care: an industry in transition, *Health Industry Today* 16:75, 1984.

Center for Health Services and Policy Research: *Medicare's OASIS: standardized outcome and assessment information set for home health care,* Denver, 1999.

Centers for Medicare and Medicaid Services: *Home health agency manual,* 2002, Baltimore, Md, CMS.

Centers for Medicare and Medicaid: 2002 data compendium, available at: http://www.cms.gov/researchers/pubs/datacompendium/; Health Care Financing Administration Customer Information System, 2000; Outcomes Concept Systems: The quality management focus: key strategies for navigating the road ahead, 2002.

Commission on the Future of Health Care in Canada: *Building on values: the future of health care in Canada,* 2002, available on line at http://www.health-carecommission.ca.

Doherty M, Hurley S: Suburban home care, *Nurs Clin North Am* 29(3):483, 1994.

Finkelstein J, Friedman R: Potential role of telecommunication technologies in the management of chronic health conditions, *Dis Manage Health Outcomes* 8(2):57-63, 2000.

Gurfolino V, Dumas V: Hospice nursing, *Nurs Clin North Am* 29(3):533, 1994.

Hanks C, Smith J: Implementing nurse home visitation programs, *Public Health Nurs* 16(4):235-245, 1999.

Health Canada: *Public home care expenditures in Canada, 1975-1976 to 1997-1998, Fact Sheets,* Ottawa, 1998, Health Canada.

Health Canada: *Provincial and territorial home care programs: a synthesis for Canada,* Ottawa, 1999, Health Canada.

Health Canada: *Final report of the national evaluation of the cost-effectiveness of home care: a report prepared for the Health Transition Fund by Marcus Hollander and Neena Chappell,* 2002, available online at www.homecarestudy.com.

Health Care Financing Administration: *Conditions of participation for home health agencies,* Subpart 1, Section 405.1229, *Evaluation,* Washington, DC, 1994, USDHHS.

Health Care Financing Administration, Center for Information Systems, Health Standards and Quality Bureau: Washington, DC, 2001, USDHHS, available at http://www.nahc.org.

Hospice Association of America: *Hospice facts and statistics,* Washington, DC, 2001, HAOA.

Joint Commission for Accreditation of Health Care Programs: 1997-1998 comprehensive for home care, Oakbrook Terrace, Ill, 1996, JCAHO.

Kitzman H et al: Effects of prenatal and infancy home visitation by nurses on pregnancy outcomes, childhood injuries, and repeated childbearing: a randomized, controlled trial, *JAMA* 278(8):644, 1997.

Kübler-Ross E: *On death and dying,* New York, 1969, McMillan.

Levit KR et al: National health expenditures, 1995, *Health Care Financing Review* 175, 1996.

Medicaid Program: Hospice care, *Federal Register* 48:560008-560036, Washington, DC, 1984, U.S. Government Printing Office.

Mistovich J, Hafen B, Karren K: *Prehospital emergency care,* ed 6, Upper Saddle River, NJ, 2000, Prentice Hall.

National Association of Home Care: *1997 national homecare and hospice directory,* ed 9, Washington, DC, 1997, NAHC.

National Association of Home Care: *Basic statistics about home care,* Washington, DC, 2001, NAHC.

National Association of Home Care: *A provider's guide to a Medicare home health certification process,* ed 3, Washington, DC, 2002, NAHC.

Olds DL et al: Long-term effects of home visitation on maternal life course and child abuse and neglect: fifteen year follow-up of randomized trial, *JAMA* 278(8):637, 1997.

Orem DE: *Nursing: concepts of practice,* ed 3, St Louis, Mo, 1995, Mosby.

Portnoy F, Dumas C: Nursing for the public good, *Nurs Clin North Am* 29(3):371, 1994.

President's Commission: *Securing access to health care,* Washington, DC, 1983, U.S. Government President's Office.

Public Health Law 99-272: *Omnibus Budget Reconciliation Act of 1985, Medicare and Medicaid Budget Reconciliation Amendments of 1985,* CIS-NO: Title IX, December, 1986.

Schumacher KL: Family caregiver role acquisition: role-making through situated interaction, *Sch Inq Nurs Pract* 9(3):211, 1995.

Sharkey S, Larsen L, Mildon B: An overview of home care in Canada: its past, present and potential, *Home Health Care Manag Pract* 2003 (in press).

Sheldon P: High technology in home care, *Nurse Clin North Am* 29(3):507, 1994.

Snow M: Competency: assuring competent RN infusion therapy in the home care setting, *Chart* 97(10):8, 2000.

Standing Senate Committee on Social Affairs, Science and Technology: *Quality end-of-life care: the right of every Canadian, final report,* Ottawa, 2000 (updated from *Of life and death* [1995]), available online at www.parl.gc.ca.

Standing Senate Committee on Social Affairs, Science and Technology: *The health of Canadians—the federal role: final report on the state of the health care system in Canada,* Ottawa, 2002, available online at www.parl.gc.ca.

Struk C: Women and children, *Nurs Clin North Am* 29(3):395, 1994.

Thobaben M: Health care technology issues in home care, *Home Care Provid* 3(5):244, 1998.

Thompson LG: Clear goals, solid evidence, integrated systems, realistic roles, *Healthcare Papers* 1(4):60-66, 2000, available online at www.healthcarepapers.com.

U.S. Census Bureau: *Population profile of the United States, 1997,* Washington, DC, 1998, U.S. Government Printing Office.

U.S. Congress: *Amendments to the Social Security Act: Medicare amendments,* Washington, DC: 1983, U.S. Government Printing Office.

U.S. Congress: *Omnibus reconciliation act of 1990,* Washington, DC, 1990, U.S. Government Printing Office.

U.S. Department of Health and Human Services: *Healthy people 2010: national health promotion and disease prevention objectives,* Washington, DC, 2000 U.S. Department of Health and Human Services.

U.S. Department of Health and Human Services: *HHS fact sheet: administrative simplification under HIPAA: national standards for transactions, security and privacy,* January 22, 2002a, Washington DC, USDHHS, Public Health Service, available at www.hhs.gov/news.

U.S. Department of Health and Human Services: *HHS news: HHS proposes changes that protect privacy, access to care: revisions would ensure federal privacy protections while removing obstacles to care,* March 21, 2002b, Washington, DC, USDHHS, Public Health Service, available at www.hhs.gov/news.

U.S. Department of Health and Human Services and Centers for Medicare and Medicaid Services: *Outcome-based quality improvement (OBQI) implementation manual,* February 2002, pp 2.4, 2.10.

U.S. Department of Health and Human Services and Health Care Financing Administration: *Outcome and assessment information set (OASIS) user's manual: implementing OASIS at a home health agency to improve patient outcomes,* Washington, DC, 2001, National Association for Home Care.

U.S. Medicare and Medicaid Programs: Revision of conditions of participation for home health agencies and use of Outcome Assessment Information Set (OASIS): proposed rules, *Federal Register* 62(46):11003-11064, 1997.

Woodham-Smith C: *Lonely crusader,* New York, 1951, McGraw-Hill.

# Chapter 41

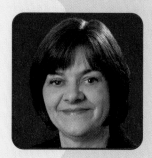 **http://evolve.elsevier.com/Stanhope**

# The Advanced Practice Nurse in the Community

**Molly A. Rose, R.N., Ph.D.**
Molly A. Rose is an associate professor at Thomas Jefferson University in Philadelphia, Pennsylvania, and is the coordinator of the graduate community health/public health nursing program entitled Community Systems Administration. She is a clinical nurse specialist in community health nursing and a family nurse practitioner. She has completed research in the areas of HIV and women, caregivers of children with HIV, HIV and the older adult, and health promotion and the older adult. Dr. Rose's roles in community/public health nursing have included the areas of home health, camp, and parish nursing; she was president of the board of directors of a free clinic for older adults; she was a VISTA nurse in the rural South; and she has been involved in homeless shelters, program planning and evaluation, school health, clinics for the underserved, and academia.

## Objectives

After reading this chapter, the student should be able to do the following:
1. Briefly discuss the historical development of the roles of the clinical nurse specialist and the nurse practitioner
2. Describe the educational requirements for community-oriented advanced practice nurses
3. Discuss credentialing mechanisms in nursing as they relate to the role of the advanced practice nurse
4. Compare and contrast the various role functions of community-oriented advanced practice nurses
5. Identify potential arenas of practice
6. Explore current issues and concerns related to practice
7. Identify five stressors that may affect nurses in expanded roles

This chapter explores the roles of the advanced practice nurse in community health. The advanced practice community-oriented nurse is a licensed professional nurse prepared at the master's level to take leadership roles in applying the nursing process and public health sciences to achieve specific health outcomes for the community; this nurse is often referred to as a public health or community health **clinical nurse specialist** (CNS). On the other hand, the advanced practice community-oriented nurse may be a **nurse practitioner** (NP) (Association of Community Health Nursing Educators, 2000). A nurse practitioner is generally a master's-prepared nurse who applies advanced practice nursing knowledge with physical, psychosocial, and environmental assessment skills to respond to common health and illness problems (American Association of Colleges of Nursing [AACN], 1996). The CNS and NP often work in similar settings. However, their client focuses differ. The NP's client is an individual or family, usually in a fixed setting. The CNS's clients may be individuals, families, groups at risk, or communities, but the ultimate goal is the health of the community as a whole (American Public Health Association, 1996; Gebbie and Hwang, 2000). Debate on the similarities in and differences between the two roles of CNS and NP has taken place over the past decade. The overlapping of their functions is becoming more evident, and future programs may prepare a blended "advanced practice nurse" (AACN, 1996; Dunn, 1997; Furlow, 1997; Lindeke, Canedy, and Day, 1997; Lyon, 2002; Pinelli, 1997; Quaal, 1999; Wright, 1997). Table 41-1 compares the functions of the CNS and the NP.

This chapter provides a history of the educational preparation of the advanced practice nurse. Functions in advanced practice and arenas for practice are discussed. Issues and concerns, role negotiation, and areas of role stress relative to the CNS and the NP in the community are also discussed.

## HISTORICAL PERSPECTIVE

Changes in the health care system and nursing have occurred in the past few decades because of a shift in societal demands and needs. Trends that have influenced the roles

## Key Terms

**administrator**, p. 996
**certification**, p. 992
**clinical nurse specialist**, p. 990
**clinician**, p. 993
**collaborative practice**, p. 1003
**consultant**, p. 996
**educator**, p. 995
**health maintenance organizations**, p. 1012

**Healthy People 2010**, p. 994
**independent practice**, p. 997
**institutional privileges**, p. 1002
**joint practice**, p. 997
**liability**, p. 1003
**nurse practitioner**, p. 990
**nursing centers**, p. 997
**parish nursing**, p. 997

**portfolios**, p. 1002
**prescriptive authority**, p. 1001
**primary health care**, p. 991
**professional isolation**, p. 1002
**protocols**, p. 994
**researcher**, p. 996
**third-party reimbursement**, p. 997
*See Glossary for definitions*

## Chapter Outline

Historical Perspective
Educational Preparation
Credentialing
Advanced Practice Roles
*Clinician*
*Educator*
*Administrator*
*Consultant*
*Researcher*

Arenas for Practice
*Private/Joint Practice*
*Independent Practice*
*Institutional Settings*
*Government*
*Other Arenas*
Issues and Concerns
*Legal Status*
*Reimbursement*

*Institutional Privileges*
*Employment and Role Negotiation*
Role Stress
*Professional Isolation*
*Liability*
*Collaborative Practice*
*Conflicting Expectations*
*Professional Responsibilities*
Trends in Advanced Practice Nursing

of the CNS and NP include a shift from institution-based health care to community-oriented health care, improvements in technology, self-care, cost-containment measures, accountability to the client, third-party reimbursement, and demands for making technology-related care more responsive to the client.

The CNS role began in the early 1960s and grew out of a need to improve client care. CNSs educate clients, communities, populations, families, and individuals; provide social and psychological support to clients; serve as role models to other nursing staff; consult with communities, nurses and staff in other disciplines; and conduct clinical nursing research (Cukr, 1996; Hemstrom et al, 2000).

In the United States during the 1960s, a shortage of physicians occurred, and there was an increasing tendency among physicians to specialize. The number of physicians who might have provided medical care to communities and families across the nation was reduced. As this trend continued, a serious gap in primary health care services developed. **Primary health care** includes both public health and primary care services.

The NP movement was begun in 1965 at the University of Colorado by Dr. Loretta Ford and Dr. Henry Silver. They determined that the morbidity among medically deprived children could be decreased by educating community-oriented nurses to provide well-child care to children of all ages. Nursing practice for these pediatric nurse practitioners included the identification, assessment, and management of common acute and chronic health problems, with appropriate referral of more complex problems to physicians (Silver, Ford, and Stearly, 1967). The priorities of the nursing profession have traditionally been to care for and support the well, the worried well, and the ill, offering physical care services previously provided only by physicians. Preparing nurses as primary health care providers was not only consistent with traditional nursing but also was responsive to society's critical need for primary health care services, including health promotion and illness prevention (Hooker and McCaig, 2001).

In 1965, the physician assistant (PA) role was initiated at Duke University. This program was intended to attract former military corpsmen for training as medical extenders

**Table 41-1** **Similarities and Differences in Functions Taught to Clinical Nurse Specialists (CNS) and Nurse Practitioner (NP)**

| FUNCTION | NP PROGRAM | CNS PROGRAM |
|---|---|---|
| Comprehensive assessment | Always | Often |
| Physiology and pharmacology | Almost always | Often |
| Diagnosis and management | Always | Often |
| Systems | Individual/family focus | More systems focused |
| Leadership | Usually | Usually |
| Program planning and evaluation | Less often | Always in community and public health CNS |
| Research | Generally | Generally |

(Fisher and Horowitz, 1977). Nurse practitioners are often combined into a single category with other nonphysician providers and are mistakenly portrayed as physician extenders. This misinterpretation of the intended role is addressed by one of the founders, Dr. Loretta Ford (1986).

As conceptualized, the nurse practitioner was always intended to be a nursing model focused on the promotion of health in daily living, on growth and development of children in families, and on the prevention of disease and disability. Nursing as a discipline and a profession evolved not because there was a shortage of physicians but because of societal needs. The early plans did not include preparing nurses to assume medical functions. The interests were in health promotion and disease prevention for aggregate populations in community settings, including underserved groups. These were the hallmarks of community-oriented nursing (Ford, 1986).

A report issued by the U.S. Department of Health, Education, and Welfare, *Extending the Scope of Nursing Practice* (1971), helped convince Congress of the value of NPs as primary health care providers. The Nurse Training Act of 1971 (PL 92-150) and the comprehensive Health Manpower Act of 1971 (PL 92-157) provided education monies for many NP and PA programs through the 1970s and into the 1980s. Similarly, in the 1970s, the concept of an expanded practice role for nurses was garnering interest in Canada. Canadian nurses saw the NP role as an opportunity to expand their scope of practice and perform the role in various settings largely outside tertiary care (Bajnok and Wright, 1993). The United Kingdom has a few advanced practice nurse programs but is continuing to explore the concept in relation to practice and curriculum development issues (Woods, 1997).

## EDUCATIONAL PREPARATION

Educational preparation for the public health and community health CNS includes a master's degree and is based on a synthesis of current knowledge and research in nursing, public health, and other scientific disciplines. In addition to performing the functions of the generalist in community-oriented nursing, the specialist possesses clinical experience

in interdisciplinary planning, organizing, community empowerment, delivering and evaluating service, political and legislative activities, and assuming a leadership role in interventions that have a positive effect on the health of the community. The public health and community health CNS's skills are based on knowledge of epidemiology, demography, biometry, community structure and organization, community development, management, program evaluation, and policy development (ACHNE, 2000).

In contrast to that of the CNS, educational preparation of the NP has not always been at the graduate level. Early NP programs were continuing education certificate programs, and the baccalaureate degree was not always a requirement. The recent trend, however, has been toward graduate education for NPs. The curriculum prepares NPs to perform a wide range of professional nursing functions including assessing and diagnosing, conducting physical examinations, ordering laboratory and other diagnostic tests, developing and implementing treatment plans for some acute and chronic illnesses, prescribing medications, monitoring client status, educating and counseling clients, and consulting and collaborating with and referring to other providers (AACN, 1996).

### WHAT DO YOU THINK?

CNS and NP preparation and functions continue to overlap, and future programs may begin to prepare advanced practice nurses who blend the skills of the clinical nurse specialist and the nurse practitioner.

## CREDENTIALING

Certification examinations for advanced practice nurses are offered by the American Nurses' Credentialing Center (ANCC). The purpose of professional certification is to confirm knowledge and expertise and provide recognition of professional achievement in a defined area of nursing. **Certification** is a means of assuring the public that nurses who claim to be competent at an advanced level have had their credentials verified through examination (ANCC, 2002). Although certification itself is not mandatory, many state boards of nursing require that nurses in advanced practice, particularly those in an NP role, be nationally certified to practice.

The American Nurses Association (ANA) began its certification program in 1973 and has offered NP certification examinations since 1976. The American Nurses Credentialing Center was opened in 1991 and offers certification in six NP and six CNS specialty areas. A nurse can also be certified as a generalist or as a BSN-prepared specialist in community health and 11 other specialty areas. Since 1985, the basic qualifications for certification as an NP have been a baccalaureate degree in nursing and successful completion of a formal NP program. As of 1992, a master's or higher degree in nursing is required for NP certification through the ANCC.

Examination topics for the NP certification examination include evaluating and promoting client wellness, assessing and managing client illness, nurse–client relationships, professionalism, and health policy and organizational issues (ANCC, 2002). The American Academy of Nurse Practitioners also has national competency-based certification examinations in two areas: family and adult nurse practitioners (American Academy of Nurse Practitioners, 2002).

The certification examination for CNSs in community health nursing was first offered in October 1990. Qualifications for this examination include a master's or higher degree in nursing with a specialization in community/public health nursing practice. Effective in 1998, eligibility requirements include holding a master's or higher degree in nursing with a specialization in community/public health nursing or holding a baccalaureate or higher degree in nursing and a master's degree in public health with a specialization in community/public health nursing. Examination topics for the community health CNS include public health sciences, community assessment process, program administration, trends and issues, theory, research, and the health care delivery system. Currently, there is not a certification examination specific to public health nurses (ANCC, 2002).

Certification for the community health CNS and NP is for 5 years. To maintain certification, the nurse must submit documentation of current RN licensure and meet a practice and continuing education requirement within the specialty area.

---

### ◖ DID YOU KNOW?

Two certification examinations are available for adult and family nurse practitioners (ANCC and Academy of Nurse Practitioners), and one certification examination is available for community health clinical nurse specialists (ANCC).

---

## ADVANCED PRACTICE ROLES

Advanced practice nurses holding a master's degree in nursing and specializing in public health nursing, community health nursing, or as a family nurse practitioner have many roles, some of which will be described here.

### Clinician

Most differences between the roles of the CNS and the NP are seen in clinical practice. Although the CNS's practice includes nursing directed at individuals, families, and groups, the primary responsibility is to take a leadership role in the overall assessment, planning, development, coordination, and evaluation of innovative programs to meet identified community health needs. The CNS provides the direction for community health care by identifying and documenting health needs and resources in a particular community and in collaborating with community-oriented nurse generalists, other health professionals, and consumers (ACHNE, 2000). Practicing within the role of **clinician,** the CNS is involved in conducting community assessments; identifying needs of populations at risk; and planning, implementing, and evaluating population-focused programs to achieve health goals, including health promotion and disease prevention activities.

The NP applies advanced practice nursing knowledge and physical, psychosocial, and environmental assessment skills to manage common health and illness problems of clients of all ages and both sexes. The NP's primary client is the individual and family. In the direct role of clinician, the NP assesses health risks and health and illness status, as well as the response to illness of individuals and families. The NP also diagnoses actual or potential health problems; decides on treatment plans jointly with clients; intervenes to promote health, to protect against disease, to treat illness, to manage chronic disease, and to limit disability; and evaluates with the client and other primary care team members how effective and comprehensive the nursing intervention may be in providing continuity of care (AACN, 1996).

Despite the setting of the community-oriented advanced practice nurse, the practice can be population focused. These interventions often include community assessment and analysis, case finding, an emphasis on prevention, and participation in public policy. An advanced practice nurse in the community may work in an agency or setting where the caseload consists of individuals who present themselves for services. The CNS goal would be to identify others in the community who may be at risk and in need of the services. Outreach activities can accomplish this while also trying to accomplish the goals and objectives of Healthy People 2010.

The ability of NPs to diagnose and treat has increased the provision of health care, teaching, and client compliance with treatment plans. The amount of physician involvement in the NP's practice is generally directed through state legislation (Pearson, 2002). Frequently, the

NP will use **protocols** or algorithms that have been previously agreed on by the physician and the NP. These documents, required by some states, serve as standing orders for the management of certain illnesses. Over the past few years, 48 state legislatures have broadened the authority of NPs to receive direct payment and write prescriptions (Pearson, 2002).

An important area for both CNSs and NPs to include in their advanced practice is health promotion/disease prevention. Within the past several decades, there has been a growing belief that the most effective way of dealing with major health problems is through prevention. This requires refocusing the health care system, identifying aggregates (populations) at risk, introducing risk reduction interventions, teaching people that they control their own health, and encouraging health promotion and disease prevention behaviors. It has been predicted that there will

be an even greater emphasis on community-focused care and that nursing will increasingly be viewed as the way to address many of the health care problems that plague society in this new millennium (Gebbie, 1997; Gebbie and Hwang, 2000; Hemstrom et al, 2000; Rains and Erickson, 1997). Both **Healthy People 2010**: National Health Promotion and Disease Prevention objectives (U.S. Department of Health and Human Services [USDHHS], 2001a) and Healthy People in Healthy Communities: A Community Planning Guide Using Healthy People 2010 (USDHHS, 2001b) are essential for CNSs and NPs in working toward the goal of a healthier nation (Gebbie, 1997; Rayella and Thompson, 2001). It is important that nurses and advanced practice nurses use the Put Prevention Into Practice (PPIP) program to help meet the two goals of Healthy People 2010: increasing quality and years of healthy life and eliminating health disparities

---

## Healthy People 2010 | Objectives Related to Each of the Leading Health Indicators for Population

**ACCESS TO CARE**

1-1 Increase the proportion of persons with health insurance

1-4.a Increase the proportion of persons of all ages who have a specific source of ongoing care

16-6.a Increase the proportion of pregnant women who receive early and adequate prenatal care beginning in first trimester of pregnancy

**IMMUNIZATION**

14-24.a Increase the proportion of young children who receive all vaccines that have been recommended for the universal administration for at least 5 years

14-29.a,b Increase the proportion of adults who are vaccinated annually against influenza and ever vaccinated against pneumococcal disease

**ENVIRONMENTAL QUALITY**

8-1.a Reduce the proportion of persons exposed to air that does not meet the U.S. Environmental Protection agency's (EPA's) health-based standards for harmful air pollutants (ozone)

27-10 Reduce the proportion of nonsmokers exposed to environmental tobacco smoke

**INJURY AND VIOLENCE**

15-15.a Reduce deaths caused by motor vehicles crashes (9 deaths per 100,000 population)

15-32 Reduce homicides

**MENTAL HEALTH**

18-9.b Increase the proportion of adults 18 years and older with recognized depression who received treatment

**RESPONSIBLE SEXUAL BEHAVIOR**

13-6.a Increase the proportion of sexually active persons who use condoms

25-11 Increase the proportion of adolescents who abstain from sexual intercourse or use condoms if currently sexually active

**SUBSTANCE ABUSE**

26-10.a Increase the proportion of adolescents not using alcohol or any illicit drugs during the past 30 years

26-10.b Reduce the proportion of adolescents reporting use of marijuana during the past 30 days

26-10.c Reduce the proportion of adults using any illicit drug during the past 30 days

**TOBACCO USE**

27-1.a Reduce cigarette smoking by adults

27-2.b Reduce cigarette use by adolescents in the past month

**OVERWEIGHT AND OBESITY**

19-2 Reduce the proportion of adults who are obese

19-3.c Reduce the proportion of children and adolescents aged 6 to 19 years who are overweight or obese

**PHYSICAL ACTIVITY**

22-2.a Increase the proportion of adults who engage regularly, preferably daily, in moderate physical activity for at least 30 minutes per day

22-7 Increase the proportion of adolescents who engage in vigorous physical activity that promotes cardiorespiratory fitness 3 or more days per week for 20 or more minutes per occasion

From U.S. Department of Health and Human Services: *Healthy people 2010: national health promotion and disease prevention objectives,* Washington, DC, 2000, U.S. Department of Health and Human Services.

(Melnickow, Kohatsu, and Chan, 2000; USDHHS, 2000). NPs and CNSs are especially involved in helping to meet the objectives related to the leading health indicators in the community (see the Healthy People 2010 box).

## Population-Focused Intervention

The following example illustrates population-focused intervention. A CNS was recently hired at a community hospital in the community health department. Traditionally, this department provided excellent health education and screening programs to individuals in the surrounding communities. However, outreach activities did not occur. After reviewing the data on attendance at community health events, the CNS developed and implemented a needs assessment in three neighboring communities not attending the events. In one neighborhood, consisting of 1800 apartments, 85% of the population were middle-income African Americans of all ages. The needs assessment revealed a strong interest in health promotion and disease prevention but nevertheless a lack of participation. The CNS developed a collaborative relationship with churches and community groups in the neighborhood. Health fairs and events were initiated (Box 41-1).

## Educator

Nurses in advanced practice function in several indirect nursing care roles. The **educator** role of the CNS and NP includes health education within a nursing framework (as opposed to health educators who may not have a nursing background) and professional nurse educator (faculty) roles.

The CNS identifies groups at risk within a community and implements, for example, health education interventions. The CNS and NP increase wellness and contribute to maintaining and promoting health by teaching the importance of good nutrition, physical exercise, stress management, and a healthy lifestyle. They provide education about disease processes and the importance of following treatment regimens. In addition, they provide anticipatory guidance and educate clients on the use of medications,

diet, birth control methods, and other therapeutic procedures (AACN, 1996). They also counsel clients, families, groups, and the community on the importance of assuming responsibility for their own health. This education may occur on an individual, family, or group level, in an institutional, ambulatory, or home setting, or it may occur in the community with vulnerable at-risk populations.

As professional nurse educators, the CNS and NP provide formal and informal teaching of staff nurses and undergraduate and graduate students in nursing and other disciplines (Figure 41-1). They also serve as role models by instructing (or being a preceptor to) students in advanced practice in the clinical setting.

---

### Evidence-Based Practice

Researchers reported on descriptive data related to encounters, number of visits, and other health variables for participants of a mobile health unit. The mobile health unit was implemented to increase access to nursing services, to improve and/or maintain functional status and health status, and to increase health promotion behaviors of rural older adult residents. Older adults who had difficulty obtaining health care because of illness, transportation problems, or financial factors were targeted for the mobile health care program. Of the 222 project participants, 1773 encounters were completed, with a mean number of visits per individual of 7.9.

**Nurse Use:** Participating older adults in the project demonstrated an increased number of breast and cervical cancer screenings; increased immunization rates for influenza, pneumonia, and tetanus; and decreased use of the emergency department.

Alexy BB, Elnitsky C: Rural mobile health unit: outcomes, *Public Health Nurs* 15(1):3, 1998.

---

### BOX 41-1 Levels of Prevention Related to Population-Focused CNS Activities

#### PRIMARY PREVENTION
Flu immunizations at churches; classes on breast self-examination; education on the need for early detection of breast cancer.

#### SECONDARY PREVENTION
"Men's Night Out" event with screenings for blood pressure, cholesterol (at neighborhood site); health fair at neighborhood sites with screenings

#### TERTIARY PREVENTION
Identified need and follow-up at clinics for groups with chronic diseases (diabetes, cancer, hypertension)

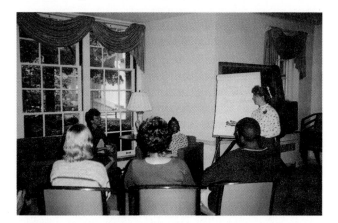

**Figure 41-1** A community health advanced practice nurse leads a training session for a group of congregational nurses.

## Administrator

The CNS and NP may function in administrative roles. As a health **administrator,** they may be responsible for all administrative matters within an agency setting. They may be responsible for and have direct or indirect authority and supervision over the organization's staff and client care. In this capacity, nurses in advanced practice serve as decision makers and problem solvers. They may also be involved in other business and management aspects such as supporting and managing personnel; budgeting; establishing quality control mechanisms; and program planning and influencing policies, public relations, and marketing (ACHNE, 2000; Lyon, 1996; Rankin and Chen, 2001).

## Consultant

Consultation is an important part of practice for CNSs and NPs. Consultation involves problem solving with an individual, family, or community to improve health care delivery. Steps of the consultation process include assessing the problem, determining the availability and feasibility of resources, proposing solutions, and assisting with implementing a solution, if appropriate (AACN, 1996) (see Chapter 42). The CNS and NP may serve as a formal or informal **consultant** to other nurses, providing them with information on improving client care. They may also consult with physicians and other health care providers or with organizations or schools to improve the health care of clients. For example, nurse consultants are often used at the district or state level of public health departments. CNSs and NPs work closely with nurse supervisors, other nurse practitioners, and staff public health nurses to develop programs and improve the services provided to clients at clinics and in the home. Nurse consultants in the public health arena may work with all other public health nurses or may work in departments as members of an interdisciplinary team such as maternal–child health, chronic diseases, or family planning.

> **NURSING TIP**
>
> Community-oriented clinical nurse specialists generally view the community as their client even when caring for individuals, families, and groups.

## Researcher

Improvement in nursing practice depends on the commitment of nurses to developing and refining knowledge through research. Practicing CNSs and NPs are in ideal positions to identify research nursing problems related to the communities they serve. They can apply their research findings to the community health practice setting.

All CNSs and most NPs are trained in the research process and, as **researchers,** can conduct their own investigations and collaborate with doctorate-prepared nurses, answering questions related to nursing practice and pri-

> **BOX 41-2  Example of a Healthy People 2010 Objective and Selected Advanced Practice Nursing Activities**
>
> **OBJECTIVE**
> Under Mental Health (objective 18-1): Reduce suicide rate to no more than six suicide deaths per 100,000 people.
>
> **ACTIVITIES**
> - Review recent literature and epidemiology of suicide.
> - Provide inservice education programs to groups of health professionals related to groups at risk for suicide and related assessment and screening tools for early detection and treatment of depression.
> - Become active in legislation activities related to firearm access.
> - Assess individual clients for depression and suicide risk.

mary health care. The acts of identifying, defining, and investigating clinical nursing problems and reporting findings encourages peer relationships with other professions and contributes to health care policy and decision making (Ingersoll, McIntosh, and Williams, 2000; Norris, 2001; Pope, 1997). For example, CNSs in administrative, consultant, or practitioner roles daily encounter situations that need further investigating (e.g., noncompliance with certain public health regimens or immunization schedules). They may anecdotally identify a trend that, if examined, could be dealt with through community-oriented strategies (Box 41-2). CNSs and NPs may collaborate with community-oriented nurses at all levels to develop the research design, collect and analyze the data, and determine the implications for further use of nursing interventions identified. It is important for these studies to be shared through nursing literature.

## ARENAS FOR PRACTICE

Positions for NPs and CNSs vary greatly in terms of scope of practice, degree of responsibility, power and authority, working conditions, creativity, and reward structure (Burgess and Misener, 1997). These factors and their effects on practice are influenced by nurse practice acts and other legislation (e.g., reimbursement and prescriptive privileges) that govern the legal practice in each state (Pearson, 2002). The following areas include traditional as well as alternative practice settings for CNSs and NPs.

## Private/Joint Practice

Research indicates that the opportunities for NPs in private practice settings increased throughout the 1980s. This trend is expected to continue (Safriet, 1992). In medical private practice settings, the NP may be the only professional nurse. Negotiating a role is important before entering into an employment contract in this situation. There must be clear communication between NPs and physicians so that there is mutual understanding and respect for each provider's role and the contribution each makes to the care of clients (Bartel and Buturusis, 2000; Steiger, Hagenstad, and Anderson, 1996). Currently, the CNS role in private/**joint practice** is not seen as frequently as that of the NP. This may change as health care continues to shift from primarily acute care settings such as hospitals to innovative models of community-oriented preventive care.

## Independent Practice

Nurses form an **independent practice** for several reasons, including personal or professional desire to break new ground for nursing and to meet health care needs within a community. It is important to investigate the state's nurse practice act to determine the limitations and the laws related to this arrangement. For example, NPs may provide a more comprehensive array of health services in states where they have legislative authority to prescribe drugs. Nurses in many states have successfully lobbied for **third-party reimbursement** for all RNs who provide direct care services to individual clients (Pearson, 1998). The independent practice option is more likely to be chosen by NPs and CNSs in states that have established legislation to provide for this nursing practice.

Another option for NPs and CNSs interested in independent practice is to contract with physicians or organizations to provide certain services for their clients or staff. Nurses need to define a service package and market it attractively. An example is providing a home visit to new parents after 2 weeks to assess the newborn, respond to parental concerns, and provide counseling and anticipatory guidance about nutrition, development, and immunization needs. This service may be marketed to pediatricians and family practice physicians who would offer or recommend the service to their clients as an option. An NP may negotiate with a local school board to provide preschool children with health examinations or physical assessments before the children participate in sports. Under a contract, CNSs may develop and implement health and safety programs on accident prevention and health promotion activities for small companies.

### Nursing Centers

**Nursing centers** or clinics, a type of joint practice developed by advanced practice nurses, provide opportunities for collaborative relationships for CNSs, NPs, baccalaureate-prepared nurses, other health care professionals, and community members (Jenkins and Torrisi, 1997). Primary health services may be provided by NPs, depending on state legislation. Community CNSs, along with nurses and nursing students, may identify aggregates at risk and work in partnership with the community to implement risk reduction activities (Hemstrom et al, 2000; Rankin and Chen, 2001; Reinhard et al, 1996). Nursing center models are discussed in more detail in Chapter 18.

### Parish Nursing

The **parish nursing** concept began in the late 1960s in the United States when increasing numbers of churches employed registered nurses to provide holistic, preventive health care to congregation members. The parish nurse functions as health educator, counselor, group facilitator, client advocate, and liaison to community resources (Magilvy and Brown, 1997).

Because these activities are complementary to the population-focused practice of community-oriented CNSs, parish nurses either have a strong public health background or work directly with both baccalaureate-prepared nurses and CNSs. Parish nurses positively affect client outcomes (Buijs and Olson, 2001; Hughes et al, 2001; Wallace et al, 2002). See Chapter 45 for further discussion about parish nursing.

---

**NURSING TIP**

The parish/congregational nurse role has been integrated into some nurses' volunteer activities.

---

## Institutional Settings

### Ambulatory/Outpatient Clinics

NPs and CNSs may be employed in the primary care unit of an institution (e.g., the ambulatory center or outpatient clinic). Ambulatory/outpatient facilities are cost effective and can improve the hospital's image in community service. Hospital clinics generally provide hospital referral, hospital follow-up care, and health maintenance and management for nonemergent problems. The population served is usually more culturally and economically diverse and represents a larger geographic area than that served by private practices. In these outpatient settings, NPs typically practice jointly with physicians to provide acute and chronic primary care. Hospital acute care outpatient services may include clinics for general medicine or family practice, or specialty-oriented clinics, such as pediatric, obstetric-gynecologic, and ear-nose-and-throat clinics. Outpatient clinics organized for chronic care may be problem-oriented (e.g., hypertension, diabetes, or acquired immunodeficiency syndrome [AIDS] clinics).

### Emergency Departments

Persons without access to health care, such as the medically uninsured and the homeless, often do not seek health care services until they become ill. Hospital emergency departments are increasingly used for nonemergent primary care. Although this is an inappropriate use of expensive health services, it is a result of the current system, which limits access to routine and preventive health care. Emergency department care is one of the most expensive services offered in health care today.

## The Community Health Clinical Nurse Specialist and the Family Nurse Practitioner in Canada

Maureen Cava, B.Sc.N., M.S., Toronto Public Health
Karen Wade, R.N., B.N., M.Sc.N., Toronto Public Health
Lianne Patricia Jeffs, R.N., M.Sc., Faculty of Nursing, University of Toronto

### ADVANCED NURSING PRACTICE IN CANADA

In Canada, *advanced nursing practice* (ANP) is an umbrella term that refers to an advanced level of practice, in which nurses use in-depth nursing knowledge and skill to meet the needs of their clients (individuals, families, groups, and populations). ANP nurses have a graduate degree in nursing with an advanced level of nursing practice, and they contribute to nursing knowledge and the development and advancement of the profession. For Canadian nurses specifically, it is the characteristics of the practice and the competencies the nurses demonstrate that determine whether they are in an ANP role, rather than their specific position or title (Canadian Nurses Association, 2002a).

In June 1999, the board of directors of the Canadian Nurses Association (CNA) approved the key elements of a national framework for ANP (CNA, 2002a). Core competencies for the ANP role include change agent, clinical expert, research, leadership, and collaboration. Each of the competencies draws from knowledge and experience that are substantive in depth, breadth, and range in one or more areas of nursing practice (CNA, 2002a).

Additional regulations and standards are not required for nurses in the ANP role, as they are practising within the scope of nursing as defined by their jurisdictions (CNA, 2002a). In some ANP roles, prescribing drugs may be within the scope of practice, and in these situations nurses need additional regulatory authority through registration in a special class and delegation of medical acts (CNA, 2002a). The CNA is currently working with many stakeholders to pursue a national regulatory framework for nurses requiring additional regulatory authority (CNA, 2002a).

### CLINICAL NURSE SPECIALIST IN CANADA

The CNA defines the clinical nurse specialist (CNS) as a registered nurse who holds a master's or doctoral degree in nursing with expertise in a clinical nursing specialty. An expert practitioner, the CNS provides direct care as well as education and consultation to clients and the health care team (CNA, 1993). The CNS role in Canada was implemented in the 1960s; however, formal educational programs did not develop until the late 1970s (Davies and Eng, 1995). The CNS practicing in the community has roles similar to those in the United States—practitioner, educator, consultant, researcher, and leader.

In Canada, the regulation of nursing practice is maintained through a registration/licensure system by examination. Currently, no special certification examination for the CNS exists. Nursing legislation and standards of practice across Canada rely on professional responsibility and accountability. All practitioners are thus responsible for their own actions and must not practice beyond their personal level of competence and preparation (Registered Nurses Association of British Columbia, 1998).

The CNS in Canada initially worked in acute care settings, such as hospitals, with a focus on secondary and tertiary prevention. The CNS working in the community brings expertise about disease prevention, health promotion, population health, group process, health education, healthy public policy, community assessment, program planning, and interdisciplinary models of care. The CNS also has knowledge and skills about complex com-

---

The views expressed in this box represent those of the writer and do not represent the views of the City of Toronto, Toronto Public Health.

---

Emergency services often require long waits for persons who have nonemergency problems. Fast-track/nonemergency sections of ERs have become commonplace to accommodate these situations. NPs in these settings see clients with nonemergent problems and provide the necessary treatment and appropriate counseling. CNSs may also help educate clients on the importance of health care and how to gain access to the preventive health care system. CNSs, with their knowledge of community health resources, can help ensure that psychosocial needs are assessed and met. CNSs can act as liaisons or go-betweens for community programs that serve the needs of special populations.

### Long-Term Care Facilities

In 2000, there were an estimated 35 million people aged 65 or older in the U.S., accounting for almost 13% of the total population. By 2030, it is projected that one in five people will be aged 65 or older (or 70 million people). The percentage of people 65 or older living in nursing home declined from 5.1% in 1990 to 4.5% in 2000 (Federal Interagency Forum on Aging-Related Statistics, 2000).

Gerontology is an increasingly important field of study, and many courses are available on health needs of older adults. NPs and CNSs with an interest in geriatrics need to continue their education in this area to increase their knowledge and skills specific to this at-risk aggregate. Many NPs and CNSs view long-term care facilities as exciting areas for practice and a way of increasing quality of care while containing costs for older adults and the disabled (Harrand and Bollstetter, 2000; Mezey, Fulmer, and Fairchild, 2000; Ryden et al, 2000). United States federal legislation provides reimbursement for NPs and CNSs to provide care to clients in Medicare-certified nursing homes

munity health issues and practise. The community CNS in Canada works in practice settings similar to those described in this chapter, which include community health centres, public health departments, occupational health settings, visiting nurses' agencies, home care agencies, community care access centres, parish nursing services, and community/population health services provided by hospitals (Deane, 1997).

## NURSE PRACTITIONER IN CANADA

For over four decades, nurse practitioners (NPs) have been an essential member of the primary health care team in Canada, particularly in Ontario (legislated as registered nurse in extended class). However, at this time, there is no public policy in Canada supporting a strategy for legislating and funding nurse practitioner services over the long term. A national coordinated framework to ensure effective integration of the NP role in the health care system is required (CNA, 2002a).

The nurse practitioner is a specialist in primary health care, whose scope of practice includes providing comprehensive health services encompassing health promotion, prevention of diseases and injuries, cure, rehabilitation, and services to clients of all ages in communities (Nurse Practitioners' Association of Ontario, 2002). Competency areas for the nurse practitioner in the community health care sector include health assessment and diagnosis; therapeutics (including pharmacologic, complementary, and counselling interventions); health promotion and disease prevention; family health; community development and planning; and team and centre responsibilities (College of Nurses of Ontario, 1998). Educational preparation for nurse practitioners in the community health care sector varies from province to province, and from baccalaureate-prepared to postbaccalaureate certificate to master's-prepared registered nurses.

Variation exists across Canada in the utilization of NPs in the community health care sector. Nurse practitioners practice autonomously, from initiating the care process and monitoring health outcomes to collaborating with other health care professionals in a variety of community health care environments (CNA, 2002b). These include, but are not limited to, community health centres, health services organizations, home care nursing, ambulatory care, specialty units and clinics, sexually transmitted disease clinics, medical services, family practice group and solo practices in partnership with physicians, underserviced areas in Canada, fast-track clinics in emergency departments, and other settings offering primary health care.

### References

Canadian Nurses Association: *Policy statement: clinical nurse specialist,* Ottawa, 1993, CNA.

Canadian Nurses Association: *Advanced nursing practice: a national framework,* Ottawa, 2002a, CNA.

Canadian Nurses Association: *The nurse practitioner position statement,* Ottawa, 2002b, CNA, available at www.cna_nurses.ca.

College of Nurses of Ontario: *A primer on the primary health care nurse practitioner,* Toronto, 1998, CNO, available at www.cno.org.

Davies B, Eng B: Implementation of the CNS role in Vancouver, British Columbia, Canada, *Clin Nurse Spec* 9(1):23, 1995.

Deane KA: CNS and NP: Should the roles be merged? *Can Nurse* 93(6):24, 1997.

Nurse Practitioners' Association of Ontario: *Role of primary health care and acute care nurse practitioners,* Toronto, 2002, NPAO, available at www.npao.org.

Registered Nurses Association of British Columbia: *Towards a definition of advanced nursing practice,* Vancouver, 1998, RNABC.

*Canadian spelling is used.*

and to recertify eligible clients for continued Medicare coverage. In long-term care facilities where clients are not ambulatory, NPs and CNSs may make regular nursing home rounds, assess the health status of clients, and provide care and counseling as appropriate. In long-term care facilities in which the residents are more ambulatory, NPs and CNSs also may provide health maintenance and other primary health care services to the nursing home clients.

## Industry

The Healthy People 2010 (USDHHS, 2001a) objectives include a section on occupational health and safety with goals to reduce work-related injuries and deaths. Thousands of new cases of disease and death occur each year from occupational exposures.

CNSs and NPs are increasingly useful in occupational health programs as business and industry seek ways to control their health care costs and to provide preventive and primary on-site care services. These services help reduce absences from work and increase productivity of workers. The CNS in an industrial setting assesses the health needs of the organization on the basis of claims data, cost–benefit health research, results of employee health screening, and the perceived needs of employee groups. With their advanced administrative and clinical skills, CNSs plan, implement, and evaluate companywide health programs (Lugo, 1997; Rogers and Livsey, 2000).

NPs in occupational settings generally practice independently, with physician consultation as needed. The health and welfare of the worker is the major concern. Responsibilities for maintaining employee health include direct nursing care for on-the-job injuries. Often clinical responsibility extends to monitoring work-related illnesses such as diabetes and hypertension. Employees may elect to see the NP for common problems and see a physician for more complicated problems. The role of the occupational health nurse is discussed in Chapter 44.

## Government

### U.S. Public Health Service

The U.S. Public Health Service operates the National Health Service Corps, which places health providers in federally designated areas with shortages of health workers, and the Indian Health Service, which provides health services to Native Americans.

During the 1970s, both the Corps and the Indian Health Service offered to pay to educate RNs to become nurse practitioners if they would promise to work for a designated period of time with the Public Health Service. These programs were discontinued during the 1980s when more emphasis was placed on physician recruitment. In 1988, Congress reauthorized two loan repayment programs for NPs' education—one with the Corps and one with the Indian Health Service. Depending on the needs of the area, an NP employed by the Public Health Service may be the only health care provider in the setting or may practice with a group of providers to serve a rural, an urban underserved, or a Native American population.

### Armed Services

The increased availability of physicians reduced the active recruitment of nurses to advanced degree programs by the armed forces during the 1980s. NPs are used in ambulatory clinics serving active duty and retired personnel and their dependents. CNSs use their skills with needs assessment and program planning/evaluation to develop programs aimed at improving the health of the aggregate military population.

### Public Health Departments

Public health departments are increasingly employing advanced practice nurses with master's degrees. These CNSs and NPs have administrative and clinical skills to work collaboratively with physicians and to manage and implement clinical services provided by the health departments. Home care and hospice services are nursing sections in many public health departments and require the services of community-oriented nurse clinical specialists.

Health departments also provide primary care services in well-child clinics, family planning clinics, and general adult primary health care clinics. A public health department may use NPs and CNSs, depending on the size of the department, the department's health priorities in the community, and financial constraints.

### Schools

School health nursing, discussed in Chapter 43, involves comprehensive assessment and management of care, with particular emphasis on health education, to promote healthy behaviors in children and their families. Innovative practice occurs in school nursing (Guajardo, Middleman, and Sansaricq, 2002; Karsting, 2002; McGhan et al, 2002; Proctor, 1997; Weiss, 2001). CNSs and NPs may be employed as school health nurses by school boards or county health departments to provide specific services to schools such as confirming that immunization status is current; performing hearing and vision screening; and providing many organizational, community assessment, and political functions. More progressive school systems employ an on-site nurse at each school within their jurisdiction. School-based health services may be staffed by CNSs and/or nurses prepared as school, pediatric, or family nurse practitioners. Services provided by these advanced nurse practitioners include not only basic health screening but also monitoring of children with chronic health problems and finding health care for children with limited access to medical care. These nurses work collaboratively with parents, community leaders, educators, and physicians to ensure that each child within the school community receives needed services. CNSs and NPs may be well suited to manage school health services if they meet specific criteria developed by individual states.

## Other Arenas

### Health Maintenance Organizations

**Health maintenance organizations** (HMOs) emphasize health promotion and disease prevention services to reduce health risks and avoid expensive medical care for the populations they serve. NPs may be employed in HMOs to provide cost-effective basic health care services. Recently, HMOs have been contracting with Medicare and Medicaid to provide services to enrollees. However, the ability of nurse practitioners to appear on panels as primary care providers varies by state. Nurse practitioners in the state of Maryland recently won legislative approval to serve as primary care providers for HMO clients, but the bill was vetoed by the governor (Pearson, 2002).

### Home Health Agencies

Major legislative changes in Medicare and third-party reimbursement for hospital services resulted in unprecedented growth in the home health care industry through the 1990s. Home health care is less expensive than extended hospital care and thus is an attractive option for third-party payers (Dick and Burns-Tisdale, 1996; Waszynski, Murakami, and Lewis, 2000). Additionally, equipment and drug companies are developing products for home use, physicians and hospitals are exploring the development of home services, and consumers are demanding more services. CNSs have traditionally been involved in home care in many capacities. Recently, NPs have entered the arena of home care nursing (Bakewell-Sachs et al, 2000).

Because of their knowledge and skills in the following areas, NPs and CNSs are well-qualified to provide home health care that yields positive outcomes for clients and their families:

- Public/community health principles
- Family and individual counseling skills

- Health education and strategies for adult learning
- Increased decision making

## Correctional Institutions

The organizational structure of prisons and jails has long been a barrier to providing or improving health care. Inmates are a population with health needs that can be met by CNSs and NPs.

CNSs are an asset within prison systems, planning and implementing coordinated health programs that include health education as well as health services. Where personnel resources are limited, CNSs provide counseling for inmates and their families to prepare prison clients for going back into the community upon their release. NPs often practice in on-site health clinics at prisons, providing both primary care services and health education programs (Blair, 2000; Crawford and Henderson-Nichol, 2000; Fogel and Belyea, 2001; Miller, 1999).

## ISSUES AND CONCERNS

### Legal Status

The legal authority of nurses in advanced practice is determined by each state's nurse practice act and, in some states, by additional rules and regulations for practice (Buppert, 1998). In the 1970s, regulations for the direct care role performed by NPs, including diagnosis and treatment, were less defined in state nursing laws than they are today, and the legal statutes of NPs were being questioned. Since 1971, when Idaho revised its nurse practice act to include the practice of NPs, other states have amended their nurse practice acts or revised their definitions of nursing to reflect the new nursing roles. CNSs and NPs in 41 states are regulated by their state boards of nursing through specific regulations. In Tennessee, NPs function under a broad nurse practice act but with no specific title protection, meaning that anyone can use the initials NP or CNS after their name. In six states (Alabama, Mississippi, North Carolina, Pennsylvania, South Dakota, and Virginia), NPs and CNSs are still regulated by both the state board of nursing and the board of medicine (Pearson, 2002).

Legislative authority to prescribe has changed dramatically in the last several years. By 2002, CNSs and NPs in all states (including the District of Columbia) had **prescriptive authority,** some with independent authority to prescribe and some dependent on physician collaboration (Pearson, 2002). Although legal problems and unresolved disputes still exist in a few states, tremendous gains have been made because of nurses' active involvement in the political and policy-making arenas (Lyon and Minarik, 2001).

## Reimbursement

The third-party reimbursement system in the United States, both public and private, is complicated. To practice independently or work collaboratively with physicians, NPs and CNSs need to be reimbursed adequately. Because states regulate the insurance industry, available third-party private reimbursement depends in large part on state statute. Advanced practice nurses want direct access to third-party payers. The most common mechanism through which NPs and CNSs get access to direct payment is through benefits-required laws. Laws also include the right to practice without being discriminated against by another provider or a health care agency (Pearson, 2002; Safriet, 1992).

The Rural Health Clinic Services Act of 1977 (PL 95-210) was the first breakthrough in third-party reimbursement for nurses in primary care roles (Table 41-2). The law authorized Medicare and Medicaid reimbursement to qualified rural clinics for services provided by NPs and PAs, regardless of the presence of a physician (Wasem, 1990). The intent of the act was to improve access to health care in some of the nation's underserved rural areas; however, its use from state to state has varied dramatically. Recent legislative changes to include the coverage of services by certified nurse midwives, clinical psychologists, and social workers, have improved the effectiveness of the Rural Health Clinic Services Act for reimbursement options.

In 1989, Congress mandated reimbursement for services furnished to needy Medicaid clients by a certified family nurse practitioner or certified pediatric nurse practitioner whether or not under the supervision of a physician. Presently, with the 1997 passing of the national reconciliation spending bill, NPs and CNSs can be directly reimbursed, regardless of geographic setting, at 85% of what a physician would have been paid (if the service is

| Table 41-2 | **Landmark U.S. Legislation for Advanced Practice Nurses** |
|---|---|
| 1977 | Rural Health Clinic Services Act authorized NP and PA services to be directly reimbursed when provided in a rural area. |
| 1989 | As part of Omnibus Budget Reconciliation Act (OBRA), Congress recognized NPs as direct providers of services to residents of nursing homes. |
| 1990 | Congress established a new Medicare benefit through the Federally Qualified Health Centers where services of NPs are directly reimbursed when provided in these centers. |
| 1997 | Passage of the national reconciliation spending bill. NPs and CNSs can now be directly reimbursed, regardless of geographic setting, at 85% of what the physician would have been paid (if the service is covered under Medicare part B). |

covered under Medicare part B) (Pearson, 1998). NPs and CNSs can now apply to be a Medicare provider. Once an NP/CNS has a provider number, he or she submits bills using the standard government form to the local Medicare insurance carrier agency for each visit or procedure (Buppert, 1998). This federal action also opened the door for an NP/CNS to get direct reimbursement from other third party payors. Every year, the Centers for Medicare and Medicaid Services (formerly known as Health Care Financing Administration) update Medicare reimbursement policy. In June 2001, a USDHHS Office of Inspector General report raised issues similar to those in a June 2000 American Medical Association petition, suggesting that the NP/CNS needed more stringent oversight of reimbursement claims. Nursing organizations, political groups, and coalitions have rallied to respond to these reports (Trossman, 2002).

## Institutional Privileges

Because of their direct care role, NPs in the community are more concerned than community-oriented CNSs about **institutional privileges.** It is often difficult for NPs to obtain hospital privileges within institutions where their clients are admitted. The traditional hospital nurse is automatically responsible to and governed by the department of nursing as a condition of employment. However, if an NP is employed in a private/joint practice with a physician, there is rarely a way for clinical privileges to be granted by the department of nursing because the nurse is not employed by the hospital. There are two reasons for providing a mechanism for community-based NPs to gain access to their hospital clients. First, if people are allowed to choose or purchase direct nursing care, access by NPs to hospital clients is necessary to deliver the care the client is paying for. Second, nursing must be accountable for and must regulate the practice of its practitioners. No other group can knowledgeably review or set the standards for nursing practice. Because the nursing department is responsible for writing and upholding nursing care standards within an institution, nurses should have the authority to grant or deny nursing privileges for all nurses within the setting, regardless of whether they are employed by the institution (Burgess and Misener, 1997). However, today when NPs apply for hospital privileges, they are usually received by physicians rather than their nurse peers.

State legislation and the role of the professional organization in encouraging institutional privileges are important. Legislative action, changes in nurse practice acts, Federal Trade Commission intervention, consumer demands, and pressures by nonphysicians will increase NPs' direct client access (Kelley, 1996; Safriet, 1992).

The changing economy and health care trends are altering the role of the traditional hospital. With competition for clients and nonhospital care increasing, hospitals are more willing to consider alternatives to the medical model. Efforts to obtain third-party reimbursement and institutional privileges for care provided by advanced practice nurses must continue.

## Employment and Role Negotiation

For NPs and CNSs to collaboratively provide comprehensive primary health care, they must understand and develop negotiating skills. Positive working relationships with health professionals, organizations, and clients require role negotiation, particularly when few guidelines exist for a role or a role is new and undeveloped. NPs and CNSs need to assess the internal politics of the organization as part of their role negotiation. Networking is another necessary skill. Forums, joint conferences, collaborative practice, and research provide opportunities to expand their functions (Kelley, 1996).

Because in some locations NPs and CNSs often seek employment, as opposed to being sought by employers, assertiveness is needed. Increased financial constraints and new health care legislation have reduced the number of job opportunities. NPs and CNSs should feel comfortable about marketing their skills. Marketing strategies should be designed to project an image that shows a nurse's individual achievement. In assessing and analyzing the needs of target markets, nurses must consider professional, institutional, and the target client groups' goals.

Methods of obtaining positions and negotiating future roles include providing portfolios of credentialed documents and samples of professional accomplishments such as audiovisual materials, program plans and evaluations conducted, client education packets, and history and physical assessment tools developed. **Portfolios** are folders that contain all of these documents to showcase the nurse's abilities. NPs and CNSs should keep current portfolios containing examples of their professional activities. Names, addresses, and telephone numbers of professional and personal references should be furnished in the portfolios (but only after the referring persons have granted permission).

## ROLE STRESS

Factors causing stress for advanced practice nurses include legal issues (as discussed previously), professional isolation, liability, collaborative practice, conflicting expectations, and professional responsibilities. NPs and CNSs should identify self-care strategies to cope with predictable stressors, some of which are discussed here.

## Professional Isolation

**Professional isolation** is a source of conflict for NPs and CNSs. Because they practice across all age-groups, NPs and CNSs are likely to be hired in remote practice employment sites. Rural communities unable to support a physician, for example, may find the NP an affordable and logical alternative for primary care services. The autonomy of practice in these sites attracts many NPs and CNSs, who may fail to consider the disadvantages of isolated practice. Long drives, long hours, lack of social and cultural activities, and lack of opportunity for professional development are often experienced by these rural practitioners. These sources of stress, which could lead to job dissatisfaction, can be reduced or eliminated by negotiating the employment contract to include educational and personal leaves.

## Liability

All nurses are liable for their actions. Because more legal action is appearing in the judicial system, specifically concerning NPs and CNSs, the importance of **liability** and/or malpractice insurance cannot be overemphasized. Although malpractice insurance may not be required to function as an NP or a CNS, most nurses carry their own liability insurance. It is in the best interest of NPs and CNSs to thoroughly investigate the coverage offered by different companies rather than to assume that the coverage is adequate. Practitioners who function without a physician on site are particularly vulnerable. The scope of the NP's and CNS's authority determines the liability standards applied. The limits of each practitioner's authority are legislated by individual states (Pearson, 2002).

## Collaborative Practice

The future of NPs and CNSs depends on whether they make a recognized difference in the health of families and communities, and on their ability to practice collaboratively with physicians. **Collaborative practice** defines a peer relationship with mutual trust and respect. Working out a collaborative practice takes a considerable amount of time and energy. Until such practice relationships evolve within joint practice situations, the quality health care that nursing and medicine can collaboratively provide will not be achieved. The arrangement demands the professional maturity to work together without territorial disputes, and the structure and philosophy of the organization must support joint practice as a mechanism for health care delivery. The growing pains of establishing such a practice produce stress for all involved; however, the results and benefits to clients and professionals are worth the effort.

Collaborative practice for CNSs and NPs involves more disciplines than just medicine. Advanced practice nurses work with baccalaureate-prepared nurses and other nurses, social workers, public health professionals, nutritionists, occupational and physical therapists, and community leaders and members to meet their goals for the health of individuals, families, groups, and communities. To work toward the Healthy People 2010 objectives, collaboration of multidisciplinary groups is essential. CNSs, NPs, and baccalaureate-prepared nurses can provide leadership in attaining this collaborative effort.

## Conflicting Expectations

Services provided by NPs and CNSs in health promotion and maintenance are often more time consuming and complex than just the management of clients' health problems. NPs and CNSs frequently experience conflict between their practice goals in health promotion and the need to see the number of clients required to maintain the clinic's financial goals. The problem becomes worse when the clinic administrator or physician views NPs or CNSs only as medical extenders and limits reimbursement to the nurse. A practice model that can assist nurses in including health promotion and maintenance activities as well as medical case management into each client visit uses (1) flexible scheduling, (2) health maintenance flow sheets, and (3) problem-oriented recording with nursing goals and plans prominently displayed in the health record. For CNSs, program planning and evaluation based on systematic needs assessments conducted with communities are methods to show the needs and benefits of health promotion/disease prevention. Being an educator and role model in carrying out Healthy People 2010 objectives will also emphasize the importance of health promotion and disease prevention in the health care system.

## Professional Responsibilities

Professional responsibilities contribute to role stress. Most states require NPs and CNSs in expanded roles to be nationally certified and to maintain certification. Recertification requires documentation of continuing education hours. Because there may not be many nurse practitioners in an area, continuing education may not be locally available and may require travel and lodging expenses in addition to time away from the practice site. Anticipating professional responsibilities and travel expenses in financial planning decreases these concerns. Negotiating with the employer for educational leave and expenses should be part of any contract.

Quality of client care, however, cannot be measured or ensured by continuing education or the nurse's credentials. Professional responsibility includes monitoring one's own practice according to standards established by the profession and protocols, if used, and a personal feeling of responsibility to the community. Continuous quality improvement is another professional responsibility for NPs and CNSs. This process should evaluate need, cost, and effectiveness of care in relation to client outcomes (Dever, 1997).

## TRENDS IN ADVANCED PRACTICE NURSING

On the basis of data provided by state board of nursing authorities in 2001, there were 94,283 NPs, 14,927 CNSs, 7399 certified nurse midwives, and 33,107 certified registered nurse anesthetists in the United States. These data show a continued increase in NPs and a decrease in CNSs. The loss of CNS positions in hospitals has occurred in financially stressed health care systems. Quality and cost of care have been adversely affected. Academics tended to emphasize NP programs as a result of the change. There has recently been an increased interest in CNSs (Munro, 2001) (see The Cutting Edge box). The need for NPs and CNSs is increasing, especially in light of health care reform, social changes, and complex specialized health problems (Lyon, 1996).

# THE CUTTING EDGE

There has been a decrease in the number of clinical nurse specialist programs in academia, but recently there has been an increased interest.

CNSs and NPs in collaboration with nurses, community agencies and members, and other disciplines have the potential to make an impact on health promotion and disease prevention at the individual, family, group, and community levels. Community-oriented CNSs and NPs are in excellent positions to use the Healthy People 2010 National Health Promotion and Disease Prevention objectives and the Healthy People in Healthy Communities model in planning their advanced practice nursing interventions. Other suggestions to increase the use of NPs and CNSs include continued reimbursement of services, admitting privileges by hospitals, and more collaborative systems (Miller, 1998).

## ■ Practice Application

### CASE 1: CLINICAL NURSE SPECIALIST

Martha Corley is a community health CNS who coordinates the after-care services for a community hospital's early discharge clients. Martha has worked with the nursing staff to develop a nursing history form to identify family and social supports available to clients who are likely to need nursing or supportive care for a limited time after discharge. With this and additional information from head nurses, Martha visits selected clients to begin discharge planning. She consults with each client and family to validate assessed needs. The physician is also consulted about medical therapies to be continued at home. Martha has access to nurses and other resources throughout the community that accept cases on contract. She outlines the initial care plan with nurse case managers assigned to the client and receives regular progress reports. An essential aspect of her practice is to evaluate outcomes of her interventions.

Which of the following is the best example of evaluation of Martha's nursing care?

A. Assessment of client and family satisfaction of her services
B. Reported medical complications of her caseload
C. Review of related literature about home care programs
D. Collected data on hospital readmissions of her clients

### CASE 2: FAMILY NURSE PRACTITIONER

Julie Andrews is a master's-level NP who practices with two board-certified family practice physicians in an urban of-

fice. Julie has her own appointment schedule and sees 12 to 20 adults and children on an average day. Although she sees some acutely ill clients, most of her appointments are for routine health maintenance visits. The two physicians also refer clients to Julie for management of stable chronic health problems such as hypertension and diabetes. She has received a number of referrals from Martha Corley (see case 1) of clients with hypertension and diabetes. Assignment of these clients to Julie by the physicians did not begin until Julie had been with the practice for about a year. During the first months of practice, Julie assessed the numbers and types of client problems seen in a typical week. She found that hypertension was the most frequent chronic problem. Julie reviewed a sample of records of clients with hypertension and found that many had recorded blood pressures indicating uncontrolled hypertension.

On the basis of this information, what advanced practice nursing intervention could Julie provide?

A. Continue to see the clients referred to her through the physicians and Martha.
B. Conduct an inservice education on the hypertension for the staff in the office.
C. Provide nurse practitioner visits for hypertensive clients and compare the outcomes to hypertension clients seen by the physicians in the office.
D. Provide care for all hypertensive clients in the office.

**Answers are in the back of the book.**

## ■ Key Points

- Changes in the health care system and nursing have occurred in the past few decades because of a shift in society's demands and needs.
- Trends such as a shift of health care from institution-based sites to the community, an increase in technology, self-care, cost-containment measures, accountability, third-party reimbursement, and demands for humanizing technical care have influenced the new roles of the CNS and NP.
- Educational preparation of the CNS has always been at the graduate level, whereas this has not been true of NP preparation; however, the trend is for the NP also to be prepared at the master's level.
- Specialty certification began through the ANA in 1976 for NPs, and through the ANCC in 1990 for community health CNSs.
- The roles of the NP and CNS are merging and many common features exist; however, controversy exists on this blending of roles.
- The major role functions of the NP and CNS in community health are clinician, consultant, administrator, researcher, and educator; typically, the NP spends a greater amount of time in direct care clinical activities and less time in indirect activities than the CNS.

- Major arenas for practice for NPs and CNSs in community health include private/joint practice, institutional settings, industry, government, public health agencies, schools, home health, HMOs, correctional health, nursing centers, and health ministry settings.
- Legal status, reimbursement, institutional privileges, and role negotiation are important issues and concerns to nurses who practice in an advanced role in community-oriented nursing.
- Major stressors for NPs and CNSs include professional isolation, liability, collaborative practice, conflicting expectations, and professional responsibilities.
- The use of Healthy People 2010 objectives is important in emphasizing health promotion and disease prevention in advanced practice nursing and in improving the health of the nation.

## Clinical Decision-Making Activities

1. Explore the development of the NP and CNS in the community. Give details about the differences in the roles.
2. Investigate graduate programs in community health within the state or region to determine the requirements for admission, the type of degree awarded, and whether or not NP and/or CNS preparation is available. Do the similarities and differences make sense to you? Why?
3. Review your state's nurse practice act and any rules and regulations governing advanced practice roles. Are rules different for NPs and CNSs? Give examples.
4. Negotiate a clinical observation experience with an NP and a CNS in community and public health, and compare and contrast their roles. Discuss the roles as you see them with the NP and CNS. When you consider your thoughts about the roles, have you considered what the CNS and NP have told you about their roles? How has their input changed your views?

## Additional Resources

These related resources are found either in the appendix at the back of this book or on the book's website at **http://evolve.elsevier.com/Stanhope.**

**evolve** **Evolve Website**

WebLinks: Healthy People 2010

## References

Alexy BB, Elnitsky C: Rural mobile health unit: outcomes, *Public Health Nurs* 15(1):3, 1998.

American Academy of Nurse Practitioners: *National competency-based certification examinations for adult and family nurse practitioner,* Austin, Tex, 2002, AANP.

American Association of Colleges of Nursing: *The essentials of master's education for advanced practice nursing,* Washington, DC, 1996, AACN.

American Nurses' Credentialing Center: *Advanced practice certification catalog,* Washington, DC, 2002, ANA.

American Public Health Association: *The definition and role of public health nursing practice in the delivery of health care,* Washington, DC, 1996, APHA, Public Health Nursing Section.

Association of Community Health Nursing Educators: *Graduate education for advanced practice in community/public health nursing,* Latham, NY, 2000, ACHNE.

Bajnok I, Wright J: Revisiting the role of the nurse practitioner in the 1990s: a Canadian perspective, *AACN Clin Issues Crit Care Nurs* 4(4):609, 1993.

Bakewell-Sachs S et al: Home care considerations for chronic and vulnerable populations, *Nurse Pract Forum* 11(1):65-72, 2000.

Bartel JC, Buturusis B: Clinical practice: new challenges for the advanced practice nurse, *Semin Nurse Manag* 8(4):182-187, 2000.

Blair P: Improving nursing practice in correctional settings, *J Nurs Law* 7(2):19-30, 2000.

Buijs R, Olson J: Parish nurses influencing determinants of health, *J Community Health Nurs* 18(1):13-23, 2001.

Buppert C: Reimbursement of nurse practitioner services, *Nurse Pract* 23(1):67, 1998.

Burgess SE, Misener TR: The professional portfolio: an APN job search marketing tool, *Clin Excellence Nurse Pract* 1(7):468, 1997.

Crawford M, Henderson-Nichol K: The health care needs of young offenders, *Professional Nurse* 16(8):1324, 2000.

Cukr PL: Viva la difference! The nation needs both types of advanced practice nurses: clinical nurse specialists and nurse practitioners, *Online J Iss Nurs* (Jun 15):1, 1996.

Dever GEA: *Improving outcomes in public health practice,* Gaithersburg, Md, 1997, Sage.

Dick KL, Burns-Tisdale S: Beth Israel home care: a model for practice. In Hickey JC, Ouimette RM, Venegoni SL: *Advanced practice nursing: changing roles and clinical applications,* Philadelphia, 1996, Lippincott-Raven.

Dunn L: A literature review of advanced clinical nursing practice in the USA, *J Adv Nurs* 25(4):814, 1997.

Federal Interagency Forum on Aging-Related Statistics: *Older Americans 2000: key indicators of well-being,* Federal Interagency Forum on Aging-Related Statistics, Washington, DC, 2000, U.S. Government Printing Office

Fisher DW, Horowitz SM: The physician's assistant: profile of a new health profession. In Bliss AA, Cohen ED, editors: *The new health professionals,* Germantown, Md, 1977, Aspen Systems.

Fogel CI, Belyea M: Psychological risk factors in pregnant inmates: a challenge for nurses, *MCN Am J Matern Child Nurs* 26(1):10-16, 2001.

Ford LC: Nurses, nurse practitioners: the evolution of primary care [book review], *Image J Nurs Scholar* 18:177, 1986.

Furlow L: Dear editor: CNS and NP, an argument for a single title, *Clin Nurse Spec* 11(1):29, 1997.

Gebbie KM: Using the vision of healthy people to build healthier communities, *Nurs Admin Q* 21(4):83, 1997.

Gebbie KM, Hwang I: Preparing currently employed public health nurses for changes in the health system, *Am J Public Health* 90(5):716-721, 2000.

Guajardo AD, Middleman AB, Sansaricq KM: School nurses identify barriers and solutions to implementing a school-based hepatitis B immunization program, *J School Health* 72(3):128-130, 2002.

Harrand AG, Bollstetter JJ: Developing a community-based reminiscence group for the elderly, *Clin Nurse Spec* 14(1):17-25, 2000.

Hemstrom M et al: The clinical nurse specialist in community health nursing: A solution for the 21st century, *Public Health Nurs* 17(5):386-391, 2000.

Hooker RS, McCaig LF: Use of physician assistants and nurse practitioners in primary care, 1995-1999, *Health Aff* 20(4):231-238, 2001.

Hughes CB et al: Primary care parish nursing: outcomes and implications, *Nurs Admin Quart* 26(1):45-59, 2001.

Ingersoll GL, McIntosh E, Williams M: Nurse-sensitive outcomes of advanced practice, *J Adv Nurs* 35(5):1272-1281, 2000.

Jenkins M, Torrisi D: Community partnership primary care case study: Abbottsford Community Health Center, *Nurse Pract Forum* 8(1):21, 1997.

Karsting KY: Adapting and using intensity measurement in school nursing, *J School Health* 72(2):83-84, 2002.

Kelley M: Primary care across clinical settings, *Nurs Clin North Am* 32(3):465, 1996.

Lindeke LL, Canedy BH, Day MM: A comparison of practice domains of clinical nurse specialists and nurse practitioners, *J Prof Nurs* 13(5):281, 1997.

Lugo NR: Nurse-managed corporate employee wellness centers, *Nurse Pract* 22(4):104, 1997.

Lyon BL: Meeting societal needs for CNS competencies: why the CNS and NP roles should not be blended in masters degree programs, *Online J Iss Nurs Adv Pract Nurs* (Jun 15)1, 1996.

Lyon BL: What to look for when analyzing clinical nurse specialist statutes and regulations, *Clin Nurse Spec* 16(1):33-34, 2002.

Lyon BL, Minarik PA: National Association of CNS model statutory and regulatory language governing CNS practice, *Clin Nurse Spec* 15(3):115-118, 2001.

Magilvy JK, Brown NJ: Parish nursing: advanced practice nursing model for healthier communities, *Adv Pract Nurs Q* 2(4):67, 1997.

McGhan SL et al: Developing a school asthma policy, *Public Health Nurs* 19(2):112-123, 2002.

Melnickow J, Kohatsu ND, Chan BKS: Put prevention into practice: a controlled evaluation, *Am J Public Health* 90(10):1622-1625, 2000.

Mezey M, Fulmer T, Fairchild S: Enhancing geriatric nursing scholarship: specialization versus generalization, *J Gerontol Nurs* 26(7):28-35, 2000.

Miller SK: Defining the acute in acute care nurse practitioner, *Clin Excellence Nurse Practit* 2(1):52-55, 1998.

Miller SK: Nurse practitioners in the county correctional facility setting: unique challenges and suggestions for effective health policy, *Clin Excellence Nurse Practit* 3(5):268-272, 1999.

Munro BH: Nursing practice: ethical decision-making—integral to the role of the advanced practice nurse, *Clin Nurse Spec* 15(1):6, 2001.

Norris AE: APNs: influencing practice through research, *Clin Nurse Spec* 15(2):58-59, 2001.

Pearson, LJ: Annual updates of how each state stands on legislative issues affecting advanced practice nursing, *Nurs Pract* 23(1):14, 1998.

Pearson LJ: Fourteenth annual legislative update, *Nurse Pract* 27(1):10-50, 2002

Pinelli JM: The clinical nurse specialist/nurse practitioner: oxymoron or match made in heaven? *Can J Nurs Admin* 10(1):85, 1997.

Pope RS: The role of nurse practitioners in research, *Nurse Pract Forum* 8(1):2, 1997.

Proctor SE: Nurses and nurse practitioners thinking differently about school nursing, *J School Nurs* 13(4):2, 1997.

Quaal SJ: CNS: role restructuring to advanced practice registered nurse, *Crit Care Nurs Q* 21(4):37-49, 1999.

Rains JW, Erickson GP: Putting prevention into practice, *J Prof Nurs* 13(2):124, 1997.

Rankin SH, Chen J: Nurse-managed centers: at the crossroads of education, practice and research, *Communic Nurs Res* 34(9):146, 2001.

Rayella PC, Thompson LS: Evolution of healthy communities: educational model of community partnership for health promotion, *Pol Polit Nurs Pract* 2(2):161-166, 2001.

Reinhard S et al: Promoting healthy communities through neighborhood nursing, *Nurs Outlook* 44(5):223, 1996.

Rogers B, Livsey K: Occupational health surveillance, screening, and prevention activities in occupational health nursing practice. *AAOHN J* 48(2):92-99, 2000.

Ryden MB et al: Value-added outcomes: the use of advance practice nurses in long-term care facilities, *Gerontologist* 40(6):654-662, 2000.

Safriet BJ: Health care dollars and regulatory sense: the role of advanced practice nursing, *Yale J Regul* 9:417, 1992.

Silver HK, Ford LC, Stearly SA: A program to increase health care for children: the pediatric nurse practitioner program, *Pediatrics* 39:756, 1967.

Steiger N, Hagenstad R, Anderson A: Budget development and implementation for the APN in independent practice, *Adv Pract Nurs Q* 2(1):41, 1996.

Trossman S: APRNs fight for their right to practice, *Am J Nurs* 102(1):63-65, 2002.

U.S. Department of Health and Human Services: *Healthy people 2010: national health promotion and disease prevention objectives,* Washington, DC, 2001a, U.S. Government Printing Office, available at www.health.gov/healthypeople/document.

U.S. Department of Health and Human Services: *Healthy people in healthy communities: a community planning guide using Healthy People 2010,* Washington, DC, 2001b, U.S. Government Printing Office, available at www.health.gov/Publications/ HealthyCommunities2001.

U.S. Department of Health and Human Services, Agency for Healthcare Research and Quality: *Putting prevention into practice,* Rockville, Md, 2000, available at www.ahrq.gov/ppip/ppipabou.html.

U.S. Department of Health, Education, and Welfare: *Extending the scope of nursing practice,* Washington, DC, 1971, U.S. Government Printing Office.

Wallace DC et al: Client perceptions of parish nursing, *Public Health Nurs* 19(2):128-135, 2002.

Wasem C: The Rural Health Clinic Services Act: a sleeping giant of reimbursement, *J Am Acad Nurs Pract* 2(2):85, 1990.

Waszynski CM, Murakami W, Lewis M: Community care management: APNs as care managers, *Care Manag J* 2(3):148-152, 2000.

Weiss M: Primary prevention works in grade school settings, *Nursingmatters* 12(3):6, 2001.

Woods LP: Conceptualizing advanced nursing practice: curriculum issues to consider in the educational preparation of advanced practice nurses in UK, *J Nurs* 25(4):820, 1997.

Wright KB: Advanced practice nursing: merging the clinical nurse specialist and nurse practitioner roles, *Gastroenterol Nurs* 20(2):57, 1997.

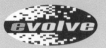
# Community-Oriented Nurse Leader and Consultant

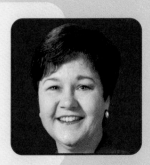

### Juliann G. Sebastian, A.R.N.P., Ph.D., F.A.A.N.

Juliann G. Sebastian developed an interest in public health and community-oriented nursing while in her B.S.N. program, where she provided care to underserved populations in rural Appalachia. Since that time, she has cared for a range of vulnerable populations across the life span and in a variety of settings. Her doctoral preparation was in administration, and she does research on communitywide systems of care delivery for underserved populations. She was a member of the inaugural cohort of Robert Wood Johnson Nurse Executive Fellows (1998-2001), during which time she focused on development of models of academic clinical nursing practice. Currently, she directs the academic clinical program of the College of Nursing at the University of Kentucky, in which faculty, staff, and students serve multiple vulnerable populations in community-based settings. As part of that role, she co-directs, with Dr. Marcia Stanhope, an integrated nurse-managed center that provides population-focused care to vulnerable populations such as homeless adults, uninsured children, families and adults, and high-risk adolescents.

## Objectives

After reading this chapter, the student should be able to do the following:

1. Explain why community-oriented nurses need effective leadership, management, and consultation skills in today's health care environment

2. Distinguish between nursing leadership, management, and consultation as they relate to community-oriented nursing

3. Explain how major trends in the health care environment influence the roles and functions of nurse leaders and consultants in community settings

4. Explain what is meant by partnership and how it is related to community-oriented nursing leadership and consultation

5. Give examples of ways that micro- and macro-level organizational theories are used in leadership, management, and consultation in community-oriented nursing

6. Distinguish between content and process theories of consultation and describe their applicability to community-oriented nursing practice

7. Apply the principles of process consultation in community-oriented nursing practice

8. Identify consultant and client responsibilities in the various phases of consultation

9. Describe the major competencies required to be effective in the nurse leader and consultant roles in community-oriented nursing

10. Understand key fiscal skills required by nurse leaders and consultants in community-oriented nursing

Community-oriented nurses have a responsibility to provide leadership in creating a new future for healthier communities. Members of the public ask whether better approaches to health care delivery might be developed that will ensure that all people around the world live in health-promoting communities and have access to quality health care, and to health promotion and illness prevention services. Increased attention to the public health infrastructure brought on by concerns about terrorism made community-oriented leadership more important to the professional and lay public (Piotrowski, 2002). Community-oriented nurses are relied on more and more to organize clinical services and manage resources and to help others perform these two functions (Koerner, 2000). They perform these functions in a variety of settings, including public health departments, community-based clin-

*Dr. Marcia Stanhope served as co-author of this chapter in the fourth and fifth editions. The author gratefully acknowledges her work.*

## Key Terms

**agency report card**, p. 1011
**alliances**, p. 1025
**budgets**, p. 1027
**business plan**, p. 1011
**capitated**, p. 1011
**coaching**, p. 1015
**coalition**, p. 1025
**conflict resolution**, p. 1033
**consultation**, p. 1012
**consultation contract**, p. 1022
**contracting**, p. 1032
**cost-effectiveness analysis**, p. 1037
**delegation**, p. 1027

**discounted fee for service**, p. 1011
**distribution effects**, p. 1030
**empowerment**, p. 1012
**enrollees**, p. 1011
**external consultant**, p. 1017
**generative leadership**, p. 1016
**informal structure**, p. 1016
**internal consultant**, p. 1017
**learning organizations**, p. 1016
**managed care**, p. 1010
**managed care organizations**, p. 1011
**negotiation**, p. 1022
**organically structured agencies**, p. 1016

**organizational structure**, p. 1016
**partnership**, p. 1009
**political skills**, p. 1039
**power dynamics**, p. 1033
**risk based**, p. 1011
**seamless system of care**, p. 1011
**servant leadership**, p. 1026
**service delivery networks**, p. 1011
**supervision**, p. 1025
**variance analysis**, p. 1036
**vertical integration**, p. 1011
*See Glossary for definitions*

## Chapter Outline

Major Trends and Issues
Definitions
Leadership and management
*Goals*
*Theories of Leadership and Management*
*Community-Oriented Nurse Manager Role*
Consultation
*Goal*

*Theories of Consultation*
*Process Consultation*
*Consultation Contract*
*Community-Oriented Nurse Consultant Role*
**Competencies for Community-Oriented**
   **Nursing Leadership, Management,**
   **and Consultation**

*Leadership Competencies*
*Interpersonal Competencies*
*Political Competencies and Power Dynamics*
*Organizational Competencies*
*Fiscal Competencies*

ics, schools, and managed care organizations. The roles of leader, manager, and consultant are important to the success of client outcomes that depend heavily on cost-effective, efficient delivery of care. Many aspects of health care continue to move from institutional settings to the community. In other cases, coordination of care across the community, including acute and long-term care settings, is important to promoting a healthy community. In these cases, community-oriented nurses need effective skills in communication, negotiation, and interdisciplinary collaboration. Community-oriented nurses, therefore, need good leading, managing, and consulting skills even if they do not have formal positions as managers or consultants.

Community-oriented nurses face two important challenges when using leadership and management skills. First, community-oriented nurses are accountable to the public as a whole. Because of this, they must focus attention not only on the populations that are served by their organizations but also on those that are not. Community-oriented nurses concern themselves with the total public, so their focus is always on the future and always on the interacting factors that influence the health of the public. Second, community-oriented nurses work with **partnerships** of community members and community organizations. Partnerships can be complex and require much time and

thoughtful attention. This requires special competencies of community-oriented nurses. For these reasons, this chapter examines the roles and functions of community-oriented nurse leaders, managers, and consultants in the early twenty-first century. It emphasizes nursing leadership in clinical practice, personnel management, and consulting with groups and individuals on a variety of issues affecting clinical nursing services in the community.

## MAJOR TRENDS AND ISSUES

The public health system in the United States is undergoing dramatic change, moving from a disorganized state to one that is focusing far more on the core public health functions of assessment, policy, and assurance (Institute of Medicine, 2003; Lasker and the Committee on Medicine and Public Health, 1997). Nurses make up the largest part of the public health workforce and are assuming leadership roles more than ever before. For example, most local programs of maternal–child health case management and direct services are carried out and/or supervised by community-oriented nurses, as are communicable disease programs and clinical preventive services. State directors of public health nursing are usually involved in developing policy, conducting quality assurance activities, and direct care practice. This means that nurses assume leadership roles at all levels in public and community health and need the skills necessary to improve the health care system to promote healthier communities.

Key changes occurring in health care today are highlighted in Table 42-1 (Hunter, 1998; Issel and Anderson,

### WHAT DO YOU THINK?

Consider the job redesign dilemma that Elizabeth Schaeffer faces in the following case:

Elizabeth Schaeffer, R.N., is the nurse manager of a mobile health clinic for migrant farmworkers. The clinic is owned by the local health department and is housed in a van that travels to migrant camps in a 10-county area providing outreach, case finding, and primary care services. The clinic employs two nurses, one social worker, one physical therapist, and two lay community health workers. The health department commissioner wants to increase efficiency by instituting cross-training, meaning that the workers can do each other's jobs. The commissioner asked Elizabeth whether it would be possible to train the nurses in the van to do certain physical therapy procedures, and to train the community health workers to do phlebotomy and run electrocardiograms. Elizabeth is concerned about the effects on quality of care and on employee morale if these jobs are redesigned. She is also concerned about whether these actions would be outside the nurses' scopes of practice. She also questions whether asking community health workers to take on these additional responsibilities would violate the nurse practice act in the state. She begins her analysis by reading the Standards for Public and Community Health Nursing Practice (Quad Council and ANA, 1999) and the standards for physical therapy services. What do you think Elizabeth should do next?

1996). Health care delivery is focusing on population care, with an emphasis on health rather than illness, and on cost containment, interdisciplinary care, information management, improved health outcomes, and privacy and security of personal health information. Job redesign, the kinds of responsibilities given to individual employees, the ways in which nurses are expected to interact with others, the amount and kind of reimbursement available from payers, new documentation requirements, and, finally, the way the present health system is organized, are all changes designed to make the system better. Management of change is a critical skill for nurses in this environment (McPhail, 1997).

Cost concerns have led to growth of managed care in both the private and public health care sectors. **Managed care** refers to integrating payment for services with delivery of services (Sullivan and Decker, 1997) and emphasizing cost-effective service delivery along a continuum of

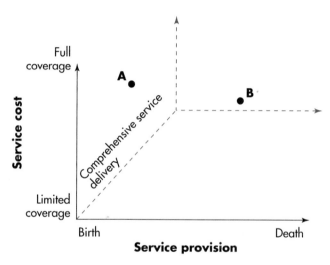

**Figure 42-1** Managed care service pathway.

### Table 42-1　Key Changes in Health Care Delivery

| OLD SYSTEM | NEW SYSTEM |
| --- | --- |
| Person-as-customer | Population-as-customer |
| Illness care | Wellness care |
| Revenue management | Cost management |
| Autonomy of professionals | Interdependence of professionals |
| Client as nonconsumer of cost and quality information | Client as consumer of cost and quality information |
| Clinical information availability | Clinical information privacy and security |
| Continuity of provider | Continuity of information |
| Emphasis on care processes* | Emphasis on outcomes of care* |
| Emphasis on clinical data confidentiality only† | Emphasis on privacy and security of personal health information (including confidentiality but broader)† |

Except for added material (see * and †), updated from Issel LM, Anderson RA: Take charge: managing six transformations in health care delivery, *Nurs Econ* 14(2):78, 1996.
*Hunter DJ: Public health management, *J Epidemiol Community Health* 52:342-343, 1998.
†New categories added.

care (Cohen and DeBack, 1999). In Figure 42-1, the person at point A may be a low-birth-weight infant requiring multiple costly services. By the time that individual is an adult (at point B) the extent and expense of his or her service needs may have declined if the care has been managed well. **Managed care organizations** (MCOs) may both pay for and provide services or they may pay for services and contract with selected health care providers to actually provide services for the **enrollees** in the MCO. Either way, a close connection exists between service payment and service delivery. In practice, this often means that someone functions as a gatekeeper and approves and monitors the delivery of services for individual enrollees.

Managed care organizations collect payment from enrollees, or clients, before services are delivered (usually on a periodic basis–e.g., monthly). Some MCOs are **capitated,** which means that clinical agencies receive a set payment for each MCO enrollee. Any costs over and above this amount are not reimbursed. Therefore MCOs have an incentive to keep their clients healthy, and when it is necessary to provide illness care, they prefer to provide the least expensive, most effective services. These types of contracts are considered to be **risk based,** which means that the clinical agency accepting the contract is at risk for the financial results of caring for the population. As a result, more health services are delivered in community settings, where costs are generally assumed to be lower. In other cases, MCOs reimburse health care providers on a **discounted fee-for-service** basis. This means that the MCO pays for the services that have been provided, but the MCO negotiates to pay less than the usual charge. The payment might be less than it costs the agency or clinician to provide the service.

Community-oriented nurse managers and consultants are being challenged to develop new, creative health programs focused on health promotion and disease prevention and to obtain payment from MCOs and other payers for their clients. Nurse managers and consultants must be able to anticipate the cost of providing nursing services to a certain population over a period of time and to develop a proposal (or a **business plan**) for a contract to provide the services. Because managed care organizations have an incentive to enroll the healthiest people, they may be less likely to actively recruit high-risk, disadvantaged groups. This suggests that the public health sector needs to monitor the health needs of vulnerable populations and ensure that these populations receive the health care services they require (Aday, 2001). In fact, public health nursing is returning to and focusing more attention on the core public health functions of community health assessment, policy making, and assurance of healthy communities.

The health system in some local areas has been reorganized to provide a full continuum of services in a **seamless system of care.** Large, vertically integrated systems are able to do this. **Vertical integration** means that the system owns all of the services that clients might need–for example, clinics, hospitals, laboratories, and home health agencies. In other cases, freestanding agencies collaborate and contract with one another to achieve seamlessness. The goal is to reduce fragmentation, which should be helpful for vulnerable populations, such as people who are homeless or abused, and populations with long-term care needs, such as frail older adults and their caregivers. Nurses traditionally focused on coordinating clients' care across agencies, but this new trend in the health care system places added emphasis on more relationships, such as alliances, agency partnerships, joint programs, and participation in **service delivery networks.** Nurse managers and consultants actively participate in these groups and need good political and negotiating skills to be effective.

Another important trend is related to the movement toward more partnerships between agencies and between health care providers and community members (Porter-O'Grady, 1999). The public has an increasing interest in becoming involved in planning for health services and in being active partners in their own care. It is critical for community members to take a partnership role in identifying community health needs and planning how to meet those needs. Nurse managers and consultants need to be able to listen well and collaborate with lay community members, whose goals are often different from those of health care professionals.

The public is increasingly using the internet, a wide variety of publications, and lay support groups to obtain health information. People need help deciding which information is good and how to best work with their health care providers to adapt information to their own health profiles. Those with low health literacy (see Chapter 31) need special help obtaining the health information necessary to be effective partners in health care (Committee on Communication for Behavior Change in the 21st Century, 2002).

One way of involving community members more actively is through continuous quality improvement programs. Continuous quality improvement includes quality assurance methods to make real improvements in nursing service delivery processes (Sullivan and Decker, 1997). This approach to quality emphasizes combining both formative and summative evaluation methods, actively including clients in the process, and identifying standards on which an agency's performance can be judged (Huang, 2002; Veazie et al, 2001). Continuous quality improvement is a process that focuses on systematically enhancing care delivery to improve outcomes (Sullivan and Decker, 1997). Such programs are also referred to as performance improvement programs. Managed care organizations often use **agency report cards** in selecting those agencies with which they will contract. An agency report card is a written listing of how the agency compares with others in the field on certain key indicators of quality, including morbidity and mortality measures, client satisfaction, and cost of care. Coalitions of business leaders may develop their own report card mechanism so they can provide insurance benefits to their employees using insurers that work with the best clinical agencies. The Leapfrog Group is an example of one such coalition (Wynd, 2002).

To know whether an agency is performing as expected, nurse managers and consultants must be familiar with their professional standards of care, the standards held by accrediting bodies, such as the Joint Commission on Accreditation of Healthcare Organizations, and guidelines for practice, such as those published by the federal Agency for Health Care Research and Quality, and by the U.S. Clinical Preventive Services Task Force (1996). Community-oriented nurse managers and consultants also need to know the purposes of clinical and management information systems and how to use these systems to link client outcomes with clinical and management processes. They need to be familiar with advances in use of computers in nursing practice and how to use minimum data sets and taxonomies for nursing diagnoses, interventions, and outcomes of nursing actions (Johnson and Maas, 1997; McCloskey and Bulechek, 1996).

A major trend in public health is a stronger focus on the public health infrastructure, or the capacity for implementing the core functions of public health and providing the essential services of public health. Public concern has grown because of fears of bioterrorism, and the resultant interest in infrastructure is likely to help other aspects of public health such as immunization production and delivery systems, food and water quality, and environmental health. Infrastructure refers to availability and training of personnel; adequacy of information systems and health, illness, and injury surveillance systems; policies, procedures, and funding for disaster preparedness and responsiveness; and "transorganizational" systems (Wright et al, 2000, p. 1204).

Finally, with the passage of the Health Insurance Portability and Accountability Act (HIPAA) in the United States in 1997 (Denker, 2002), new directions have been set in ensuring privacy and security of personal health information. As personal health information becomes more easily accessible through computerized medical records and electronic billing, the public has grown concerned about the privacy of that information. HIPAA resulted in the development of rules to protect the privacy and security of personal health information. Exceptions are in place for managing public health concerns such as disease outbreaks. However, the general trend is toward implementing precautions to prevent unnecessary access to another person's personal health information.

## DEFINITIONS

Nursing leadership refers to the influence that nurses exert on improving client health, whether clients are individuals, families, groups, or entire communities. Nursing management, on the other hand, refers to the ways nurses manage resources in providing clinical services. These resources might be people, as when a nurse coordinates an interdisciplinary team, or financial resources. An example of managing financial resources is when a nurse monitors the budget for an immunization program to make sure that personnel time, supplies, and equipment are being used efficiently. Nurses also manage time. For example, home health nurses must manage their time in order to provide

clients with direct and indirect nursing services, such as health education and making referrals (respectively). Leadership sets the direction, and management ensures that goals will be achieved. Nurses must possess strong leadership and management skills to be effective, whether or not they hold management positions.

**Consultation** has been described as a process in which the helper provides a set of activities that help the client perceive, understand, and act on events occurring in the client's environment. Caplan (1970) defined it as a process in which a specialist identifies ways to handle work problems involving the management of clients or the planning and implementing of programs. Consultation is moving away from a focus on only helping another solve a problem to focusing on creating change and developing innovations (McCutcheon and Perkin, 1996).

Management consultation refers to working directly with managers to solve problems or design new strategies to achieve organizational goals. Community-oriented nurses have a breadth of knowledge that makes them desirable consultants for colleagues both inside and outside the organizations in which they work. For example, a nurse working in a home health agency might be called on by a school nurse to give suggestions about the most effective way to intervene for a child using a respirator. Another example that occurs frequently is the informal consultation provided by nurses in the community, who help nurses working in hospitals make effective community referrals. At the population level, nurses who consult with a local health department about developing a program for obesity prevention in school-age children are focusing their efforts on a particular target population.

Consultation is closely linked with the ideas of **empowerment** and self-care. When consultants help clients identify and work through problems and learn new skills that clients see as most important, they are enabling clients to solve more of their own problems. This is very similar to the traditional nursing philosophy of helping people to solve their own problems, whether they are individuals, families, groups, or communities. Empowerment is consistent with Dorothea Orem's nursing theory of self-care (Orem, 1989), in which she states that the nurse's role is to promote clients' self-care abilities.

## LEADERSHIP AND MANAGEMENT
### Goals

The goals of community-oriented nursing leadership are as follow:

1. To work with others to ensure a healthy community
2. To serve as an advocate for vulnerable and high-risk populations
3. To participate in establishing public and organizational policies that promote a healthy living and working environment

One way community-oriented nurses achieve leadership goals is by participating in a Healthy Communities initiative at the local level. Working with others to develop policies for smoke-free public spaces is an example of promoting healthy living and working environments.

The goals of community-oriented nursing management are as follow:

1. To achieve agency and professional goals for client services and clinical outcomes
2. To help personnel perform their responsibilities effectively and efficiently
3. To develop new services that will enable the agency to respond to emerging community health needs

An example of how community-oriented nurses achieve management goals occurs when they develop plans for broad-based immunization clinics, such as smallpox vaccination clinics. Doing this in advance of confirmed bioterrorism is a way of preparing to meet an emerging community health need that achieves goals of protecting the public's health and helping personnel work effectively and efficiently. Examples of ways community-oriented nurse leaders and managers facilitate primary, secondary, and tertiary preventive services are found in Table 42-2.

## Theories of Leadership and Management

Leadership and management theories fall into two general categories: micro-level theories and macro-level theories. Community-oriented nurses use both micro- and macro-level theories to improve the health of the public and particular communities. Micro-level theories originate in psychology and help explain and predict individual behavior (e.g., motivation theories) and interpersonal issues (e.g., leadership theories, communication theories, and theories of group dynamics). Macro-level theories use a sociologic approach and explain issues at a broader, agency level. These theories (e.g., structural contingency, resource dependence, and institutional theories) focus on the best ways to organize work, on how to obtain the resources necessary to accomplish agency goals, on agency change, and on power dynamics.

## Intrapersonal/Interpersonal Theories Applied to Community-Oriented Nursing Leadership and Management

Many early management theories tried to predict how to encourage workers to be productive using micro-level approaches. In general, increasing productivity usually means increasing the numbers of billable activities in which one has engaged, such as numbers of patients seen, numbers of home visits provided, numbers of immunizations given. This approach sometimes worries community-oriented nurses, who grow concerned that seeing too many patients reduces the time necessary to provide good care. Another way of looking at productivity is in terms of outcomes. For example, a school nurse might report a reduction in student absenteeism that might be related to the newly initiated head lice program. The theories detailed in Table 42-3 are important to community-oriented nurses because the cost-containing and job-redesigning trends described earlier encourage productivity. It is still unclear how to best measure productivity in health care, and many ethical issues relate to decisions about increasing productivity.

Classical management theory says that the best way to increase worker productivity is to identify the most efficient way to do the task (usually through time and motion studies) and then assign a person to do that task repeatedly (Sullivan and Decker, 1997). If an agency is large enough to organize special teams of nurses, it might be able to increase productivity by doing this. For example, nurses on an intravenous therapy team in a visiting nurse agency are organized according to this theory because they specialize in tasks related to IV therapy. However, one must be aware that repeating the same task bores some individuals, whereas others enjoy the satisfaction of specializing in an area.

Neoclassical management theory, also known as the human relations approach (Sullivan and Decker, 1997), argues that managers should pay attention to workers' hu-

| Table 42-2 Examples of Levels of Prevention and Community-Oriented Nursing Leadership and Management | | |
|---|---|---|
| **LEVELS OF PREVENTION** | **NURSING LEADERSHIP (SETS GOALS)** | **NURSING MANAGEMENT (DIRECTS USE OF RESOURCES)** |
| Primary | Works with a community coalition to design a broad-based strategy for ensuring that the health and social needs of uninsured and underinsured populations are met | Develops policies and procedures for a referral program for referring low-income mothers and children for nutrition services |
| Secondary | Works with the local government and health department to design lead screening and abatement programs in high-risk census tracks | Designs protocols for lead screening program and hires staff to implement the program |
| Tertiary | Participates on a planning commission with local health department, hospitals, police, and political leaders to update a communitywide disaster response plan that accounts for bioterrorism | Serves as chair of a committee that organizes, staffs, and monitors the budget for a smallpox vaccination program |

man needs and group dynamics and foster cooperation to increase productivity. A nurse manager might consider identifying the types of clinical cases nurses are most interested in and assigning them only these types of clients. However, this could lead to inefficiency because nurses would not always be able to organize their work geographically and may spend more time than necessary in travel. Furthermore, many clients have multiple problems,

and nurses work with family groups as well as individuals, so it may be difficult to give assignments solely on the basis of clinical interests.

This emphasis on meeting human needs and encouraging cooperation led to the development of theories of motivation and leadership. Motivation theories can be categorized as need theories, cognitive theories, and social/ reinforcement theories. The most well known need theory is

### Table 42-3  Micro- and Macro-Level Organizational Theories Relevant to Nurse Managers

| AREA | THEORIES | MAJOR EMPHASIS |
|---|---|---|
| **Micro-Level Theories of Management and Leadership** | | |
| Management | Productivity enhancement | |
| | Classical management (Taylor, Fayol) | Skill is developed through repetition. |
| | Neoclassical management (Parker-Follet) | Focus is on workers' human needs and group dynamics. |
| | Motivation | |
| | Need theories | |
| | Basic human needs (Maslow) | People must fulfill lower-level needs before they can move on to higher-level needs. |
| | ERG theory (Alderfer) | Needs are categorized as existence, relatedness, and growth. |
| | Job redesign theory (Hackman and Oldham) | Jobs should be organized so they incorporate task identity, task variety, task significance, autonomy, and feedback in order to meet worker growth needs. |
| | Cognitive theories | |
| | Goal-setting theory (Locke) | People are more motivated to meet goals they have helped to set. |
| | Expectancy theory (Vroom) | People are more motivated to achieve outcomes they want and can reasonably expect. |
| | Social reinforcement theories | |
| | Reinforcement theory (Skinner) | Behavior is learned based on consequences of actions. |
| | Social learning theory (Bandura) | People learn from role models with whom they identify. They are most motivated when they feel confident in their ability to achieve a goal. |
| Leadership | Contingency theory (Fiedler, Blake, and Mouton) | The most effective leadership style depends on characteristics of the task, workers, and situation. |
| | Path-goal theory (House) | Leaders should facilitate goal achievement through helping to reduce barriers along the path. |
| T | Transformational leadership (Burns) | Leader encourages others to set new goals that are aligned with values. |
| **Macro-Level Organizational Theories** | | |
| Organizational structure | Structural contingency theory (Thompson; Burns, and Stalker) | The optimal organizational structure depends on characteristics of the work to be done, the skills of the workers, and the degree of uncertainty and change in the environment. |
| | Institutional theory (Meyer and Rowan; Scott) | Organizations are designed more in response to values, beliefs, and norms than as a result of rational planning. |
| Organizational effectiveness | Resource dependency theory (Pfeffer and Salancik) | Organizational activity is motivated by the need to acquire the resources necessary to survive. Power is a critical issue. |
| | Systems theory (Von Bertalanffy) | Organizations are interdependent; interorganizational relationships are key to success of individual groups and system-level outcomes. |

Maslow's theory of human needs (Maslow, 1970). Clayton Alderfer (1972) modified Maslow's work by proposing that people have only three basic needs: existence, relatedness, and growth needs. His theory became known as the ERG theory, and it said that people do not constantly strive to meet a higher-level need, as Maslow had stated, but often remain at a certain level. For example, nurses who are working in an understaffed, high-stress situation may function at the existence level until their situation changes.

Alderfer's theory was adapted by Hackman and Oldham (1976) to predict how to design jobs to increase worker productivity and job satisfaction. According to Hackman and Oldham's job redesign theory, persons with high growth needs are most productive and satisfied when their **jobs provide five elements: task variety, task identity, task significance, autonomy,** and **feedback.** A clinic nurse whose primary job responsibility is taking clients' vital signs and assigning them to examination rooms does not have a job that is high in either task variety or task identity. A nurse case manager who works with clients over a long period and helps them manage comprehensive health care needs has much higher task variety and identity.

Most nurses see their roles as high in task significance. Nurses have a great deal of clinical autonomy, which sometimes has challenges related to delegation of authority and supervision. Certain community health functions involve high levels of feedback; for example, working with children, families, and staff in school settings typically gives the nurse many opportunities for feedback from these groups.

If all five job design elements are high, the job is considered to possess job enrichment. This differs from job enlargement, in which only the three elements of task variety, task identity, and task significance are enhanced. People often do not find job enlargement to be motivating because they view it as simply adding tasks, whereas job enrichment increases individual responsibility, autonomy, and feedback. This is important for community-oriented nurse managers to know because many workers who are cross-trained or multiskilled may have had their jobs enlarged rather than enriched. Nurses who delegate tasks to others and supervise others should know whether these individuals are more motivated by existence, relatedness to colleagues, or growth needs, and attempt to meet their needs as much as possible. For example, nursing staff members in an adult day-care center who have high relatedness needs may appreciate opportunities to work together on center retreats and committees.

Cognitive theories explain that motivation results from a person's beliefs and expectations about what will occur as a result of their actions. For example, Locke's goal-setting theory (Latham and Locke, 1991) says that people are more motivated to achieve goals that they participate in setting, that are challenging, and for which they receive regular feedback. Combining this theory with Victor Vroom's (1964) expectancy theory, the nurse manager should identify each employee's goals and their expectations about which actions will lead to goal achievement and whether they believe themselves to be capable of these actions. In this way, the nurse manager can identify inaccurate perceptions (e.g., the perception that the nurse manager "plays favorites" may be incorrect) and ways to help workers achieve their own personal goals while achieving agency goals. Although some of these theories were developed many years ago, they have been supported by research and continue to be used in management practice today.

Social/reinforcement theories say that human motivation results from learning that occurs following a behavior. Reinforcement theory's basic premise is that behavior is conditioned by reinforcers applied after the behavior occurs. Reinforcers are often very effective ways of increasing productivity and improving worker morale. For example, the nurse manager of a mobile clinic who thanks staff for a job well done with notes or special acknowledgements is more likely to maintain a positive working environment.

A related theory is Albert Bandura's social learning theory (2001). Bandura says that people learn in part from role models and that confidence in one's ability to reach a goal is a key to motivation and the ability to sustain effort to achieve goals. Community-oriented nurses should be aware that they serve as role models for other staff and sometimes for lay workers as well. Nurses may wish to consciously use certain behaviors and work with staff to set achievable goals and develop strategies that are realistic to achieve the goal. In this way, they can combine strategies suggested by both cognitive and social/reinforcement motivation theories. For example, community-oriented nurses who are particularly skilled at conflict resolution or building coalitions can help others develop this skill through role modeling, goal setting, and coaching.

Good leadership skills are essential for nurse managers and consultants. Although many theories of leadership have been proposed, contingency, path–goal, and transformational leadership theories are especially relevant. Contingency leadership theory (Bond and Fiedler, 2001; Fiedler, 1967) states that the most effective leadership style is contingent (or dependent) on characteristics of the relationships between leaders and followers, the task, and the situation. The most effective leadership style depends on the degree of knowledge and maturity of group members (Hersey and Blanchard, 1996). Contingency theory says that individuals who are less familiar with the task or less self-directed will be more productive when the leader focuses on accomplishing the task through **coaching,** supervising, and follow-up. On the other hand, individuals who have technical expertise, are highly motivated, and are self-directed primarily need guidance, opportunity, and resources from the leader. In this case, the leader functions more as a facilitator and less as a supervisor. Contingency theory is particularly relevant to community-oriented nurses because so many of them work independently in clients' homes or in mobile clinics or other areas where supervision may be difficult. Contingency theory suggests that the nurse manager should know the level of skill, motivation, and maturity of the team members and adjust leadership style accordingly.

Path–goal theory (House, 1971) says that good leaders help others identify their goals and then develop ways to help them achieve those goals. In this way, leaders serve as facilitators who identify a path for achieving the goal and remove barriers along the path. This theory focuses on individual goals and meeting individual needs and is especially compatible with the role of the nurse consultant. A major goal in consultation is helping an individual, a program, a department, or an entire agency identify its needs and working with it to help it meet those needs.

Finally, transformational leadership incorporates the needs of both organizations and individuals. Transformational leadership is that form of leadership in which the leader motivates followers to achieve a vision that matches their values (Burns, 1978; Dunham-Taylor, 2000). Transformational leaders influence others to work toward achieving something new and as yet unimagined—essentially, a new dream. Whereas contingency and path–goal theories focus on identifying the best way to achieve a given goal, transformational leadership addresses the goal itself and the relationship of the goal to values. The transformational leader is able to transform, or change, the situation to one that differs from the status quo. Transformational leaders are sometimes found in **learning organizations,** or agencies that not only learn from past experience but also create new visions for their future (Sullivan and Decker, 1997). This form of leadership has been referred to as **generative leadership** ( Jaworski and Flowers, 1997) because it results in the generation of new ideas and new ways of working together. The nurse manager or consultant who recognizes opportunities for improving the health of the public and who works with others to design creative nursing programs is just one example of a transformational leader.

## Organizational Level Theories

The macro-level, or organizational-level, theories that are particularly relevant for public and community health nurse managers and leaders are structural contingency theory, institutional theory, resource dependence theory, and systems theory (see Table 42-3). Managers and consultants often ask which form of **organizational structure** will best promote the efficient achieving of organizational goals. Structural contingency theory predicts that the most effective structure depends on characteristics in the given situation (Thompson, 1967). This is a classical theory that continues to be relevant in today's world because it emphasizes an ecologic approach—that is, that the context in which people work matters when deciding how to organize the work. Organizational structure refers to the ways people in an agency organize themselves to accomplish the mission and goals of the agency. A picture is drawn of the organizational chart, which illustrates the formal lines of authority in the agency. Written documents define how the agency will operate and include the mission, vision, values, goals, philosophy, policies, procedures, and job descriptions. Together, all of these elements show what the agency is trying to accomplish and how employees at all levels will work together to accomplish it. Every agency has an **informal structure,** which is the way people actually work together; it includes informal communication patterns, informal sources of

power, and unwritten rules of conduct. Community-oriented nurse managers and consultants should be familiar with both formal and informal agency structures.

According to structural contingency theory, agencies should have more formal structures (1) when employees perform routine tasks that are not expected to vary a great deal, (2) when employees do not have high levels of professional education, and (3) when the industry or environment in which the agency operates is stable and not changing very much (Burns and Stalker, 1961). Typically, as an agency grows larger it becomes more highly structured, or formalized. This is often the case in large health departments, home health agencies, school districts, and ambulatory care clinics. On the other hand, organizations that accomplish their goals through the work of highly skilled professionals, that provide individual services that are expected to vary across clients, and that operate in a turbulent, rapidly changing environment are more likely to be successful if their structures are looser (Burns and Stalker, 1961), allowing employees latitude and autonomy in making decisions. **Organically structured agencies,** or loose organizations, are more likely to be decentralized, with much decision-making authority pushed down to the lowest level in the agency where employees have the information needed for making decisions. In the past, organic structures were most often seen in small agencies. Today, some health care organizations are moving toward more organic structures despite sometimes being very large. Individual units, departments, or programs often operate very autonomously. This places a great deal of authority and responsibility in the hands of nurse managers. In other cases, organizational leaders choose a more centralized approach, in part because these structures tend to be less costly. A health department with only a few major clinical departments will spend less on administrative overhead than one with numerous smaller clinical departments, each of which has its own managers and support staff.

Institutional theory focuses on how formal and informal values and norms affect agency activities. According to this theory, agency members are more likely to respond to widely shared values and norms of behavior than they are to formally written policies and procedures (Meyer and Rowan, 1977). For example, norms for treatment of substance abuse differ greatly from norms for treatment of severe mental illness (D'Aunno, Sutton, and Price, 1991). Addiction treatment groups tend to value dependence on a responsible professional and admit powerlessness over the addiction. Mental health professionals, on the other hand, value increasing individual self-reliance and increasing the client's self-control over health. When a community mental health center treats both types of clients, and particularly when treating dually diagnosed clients who are both drug dependent and severely mentally ill, treatment norms may conflict. In such a situation, the written policies and procedures are not good predictors of the actual treatment practices of individual providers (D'Aunno et al, 1991). Nurse managers and consultants must be aware of the powerful influence that values and norms play in agency work and understand the informal norms that exist.

Resource dependence theory (Pfeffer and Salancik, 1978) says that the primary motivator for organizational behavior is the desire to reduce uncertainty about getting the resources necessary to operate. These resources are usually financial but may also include key personnel, seats on influential community boards, or contracts with prestigious organizations. This theory is basically about power—keeping it and maintaining it. To be effective, community-oriented nurse managers and consultants must be able to accurately analyze power issues both within an agency and within the community. They must be able to predict the resource needs of the agency and how getting and maintaining those resources may affect power issues within the system. Examples of important resources include budgets, staff, space, equipment, and supplies. Agencies attempt to ensure that they have adequate resources to achieve their mission, vision, and goals.

Systems theory emphasizes the interdependence of agency players. Nurses often recognize interdependence of units within an agency but may be less aware of agency interdependence. Economists analyze how distribution of resources affects policies, which players in a system will be influenced by policies, and how they will be influenced. For example, if the federal government reduces money for health and human services, the clients of those services may be negatively affected. Employees of service agencies are also affected because agencies are likely to downsize to manage the reduced funding. Consequently, employees may either lose their jobs or experience wage cuts. Others likely to be affected include voluntary agencies and religious groups who might be expected to provide more services.

Roy's adaptation model of nursing has been extended to include nursing management (Roy, 2002). Roy argues that agencies are composed of interdependent systems. The role of nurse managers is to help the agency adapt to changing circumstances in the most effective way possible. Roy's model is particularly helpful for explaining and predicting how nurse managers and consultants can help agencies adapt to change. Nurse managers and consultants should analyze how well interdependent units function to achieve agency goals. Furthermore, nurse managers and consultants function as change agents because they foster agency adaptation.

Orlando's model of nursing offers suggestions that are especially appropriate for nursing leadership (Laurent, 2000). With Orlando's focus on including the client in every step of decision making about care, the process of care becomes more of a partnership. Likewise, by working with community members to identify community health needs and desirable policies and programs, the public health nurse is functioning as a leader and partner. For example, in one state, public health professionals partnered with the schools, the American Lung Association, and other community agencies to establish smoking cessation programs for adolescents (Dino et al, 2001).

## Community-Oriented Nurse Manager Role

First-line nurse managers may be team leaders or program directors (e.g., director of a satellite occupational health clinic or director of a small migrant health clinic), whereas mid-level or executive-level nurse managers may be division directors (including multiple programs or departments), local or state commissioners of health, or directors of large home health agencies with multiple offices. They function as coaches, facilitators, role models, evaluators, advocates, visionaries, community health program planners, teachers, and supervisors. Community-oriented nurse managers have ongoing responsibilities for the health of clients, groups, and communities, and for personnel and fiscal resources under their supervision.

## CONSULTATION

### Goal

The goal of consultation is to help clients empower themselves to take more responsibility, feel more secure, deal with their feelings and with others in interactions, and use flexible and creative problem-solving skills. The functions of a consultant differ from those of a manager because consultation is typically a temporary and voluntary relationship between a professional helper and a client. The similarities between consultants and managers are in their focus on empowerment and helping others develop. Consulting relationships are based on cooperation and respect between consultants and clients, who share equally in problem solving (Argyris, 1997).

The nurse's job responsibilities may include internal and external consultation. For example, a nurse may be employed to consult with other nurses in the agency about client care problems or, as an employee of the health department, may serve as a consultant to a local community retirement center about the public health care needs of its residents. If the nurse is an **internal consultant,** the nurse is employed on a full-time salaried basis by a community agency in which the consultation takes place. If the nurse is an **external consultant,** the nurse is employed temporarily on a contractual basis by the client. The client of the external nurse consultant may be a colleague, another health provider, or a community group or agency. The nature of the consultation relationship, whether it is internal or external, should not change the goal of consultation.

### Theories of Consultation

Several models of consultation have been developed. This chapter focuses on Edgar Schein's models because they are consistent with the nursing process and with nursing values of empowering clients and collaboratively working as partners with clients.

Purchase-of-expertise consultation (Figure 42-2) is defined as the purchase (hiring) of a professional helper by a client to provide expert information or service (Schein, 1969). Buyers may be individuals, groups, or agencies. In this model, the client defines the need for the consultant.

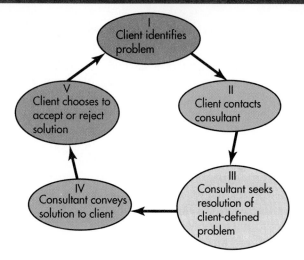

**Figure 42-2** The purchase-of-expertise consultation model.

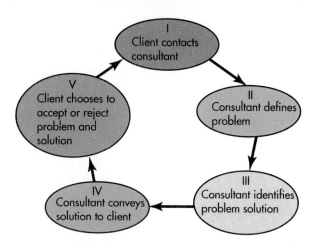

**Figure 42-3** The physician–client consultation model.

The need is defined as information the client seeks or an activity the client wants to implement. The advantage of this popular model is that the client does not have to spend time or energy in solving the identified problem, because that is the responsibility of the "expert consultant." The disadvantage is that the client may question the quality of the consultation if the client has identified the wrong problem or does not like the consultant's solution.

Although this model is often used, it may be unsatisfactory in effectively and efficiently identifying and solving client problems. Once the consultant has implemented steps to solve the problem, the client must live with the consequences of the changes. This model is likely to be effective by itself only when problems are simple and the client needs specific expert information (Rokwood, 1993).

Another popular consultative model is the physician–client model (Figure 42-3), in which the consultant is employed by the client to diagnose the problem and prescribe solutions without assistance from the client (Schein, 1969). Again, the major advantage of this model from the client's viewpoint is the limited time and energy required of the client. This model is often applied in nursing situations requiring consultation services. For example, the director of nursing at the public health department calls in a nurse consultant from the local university. Nurse productivity is poor, according to the director, and the nurse consultant is asked to diagnose what is wrong with the department. If the problem is found to be poor management rather than poor productivity by the staff, the administrator may be reluctant to accept the diagnosis. Because the client does not help diagnose the problem, the goals of consultation may not be met. The purchase-of-expertise and physician–client models are content models of consultation because they deal with the content (or nature) of the problem.

The process consultation model focuses on the process of problem solving and collaboration between consultant and the client (Rokwood, 1993). The major goal of the process model, as seen in Figure 42-4, is to help the client assess both the problem and the kind of help needed to solve it (Schein,

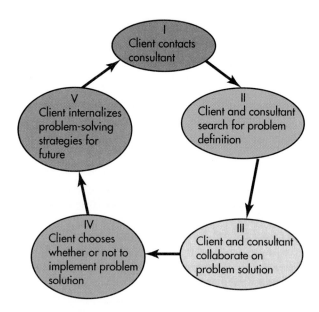

**Figure 42-4** The process consultation model.

1969). Process consultation includes assessing the underlying agency culture that influences the problem and its solution (Schein, 1990). Both consultant and client participate in the problem-solving steps that lead to changes or to actions for problem solution. The assumptions related to each of the three models are listed in Box 42-1.

Content and process consultation models do not need to be mutually exclusive (Rokwood, 1993; Schein, 1989). Instead, although consultants should emphasize process consultation, they should be willing to share their expert knowledge when appropriate. Because process consultation is collaborative, Schein (1989) recommends that consultants be willing to offer opinions and advice at all stages of the consultation process. Thus, although the major emphasis should be on process consultation, consultants may find it effective to integrate the two models at selected points, using both context and process.

## BOX 42-1 Assumptions of Schein's Consultation Models

### PURCHASE-OF-EXPERTISE MODEL

1. The client correctly diagnoses the problem.
2. The client correctly communicates the needs to the consultant.
3. The client correctly assesses the consultant's expertise to provide the information or perform the service.
4. The client knows the consequences of implementing the services suggested by the consultant.

### PHYSICIAN–CLIENT MODEL

1. The client is willing to reveal information needed by the consultant to make an appropriate diagnosis.
2. The consultant is able to get an accurate picture of the problem through observation.
3. The client accepts the diagnosis and the prescriptions offered by the consultant.

### PROCESS MODEL

1. Clients often do not know what the problem is and need assistance in problem diagnosis.
2. Clients are not aware of the services a consultant may offer and need assistance in finding proper help.
3. Clients want to improve situations and need guidance in identifying appropriate methods to reach goals.
4. Clients can be more effective if they learn how to diagnose their own strengths and limitations.
5. Consultants usually cannot spend enough time learning all variables that may help or hinder suggested courses of action, so they need to work with the client, who has intimate knowledge of the effects of proposed courses of action.
6. The client who learns to diagnose situation problems and who engages in decision making about alternative courses of action will be actively involved in implementing actions for problem resolution.
7. The consultant is an expert in problem diagnosis and in establishing an effective helping relationship and passes these skills to the client.

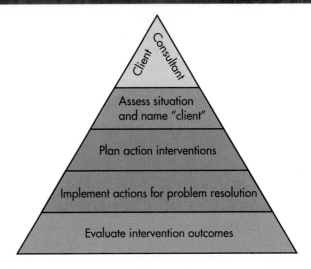

**Figure 42-5** Integration of the nursing process and the process model of consultation.

## Process Consultation

Process consultation involves a temporary relationship between client and consultant for the purpose of bringing about change. Consultation may be proactive or reactive. Proactive consultation is directed toward anticipating a future problem and taking steps to prevent it. Reactive consultation is directed toward curing an existing problem through therapeutic intervention. For example, a parent–teacher council developing a school-based family resource center contacts the nurse to assist with options for future nursing and health care for the students and their families. The board wishes to be proactive and plan for the needs of high-risk students and families. The administrator of a minimum-security prison has found that inmates are missing work for minor health problems and that health costs are skyrocketing. The nurse is asked to help explore solutions to the problem. Prison administration is reacting to an existing problem requiring immediate intervention.

The client is identified by determining who in the situation has the problem and needs to change. The following vignette illustrates this point:

Barry Henderson, R.N., has been asked by the pastor of his congregation to consult with the parish council regarding the po-

In the process model, the consultant is a resource person whose primary goal is to provide the client with choices for decision making. As shown in Figure 42-5, the process consultation model includes the same steps as the nursing process, establishing a nurse-client relationship based on trust to assess the problem, plan and implement actions, and evaluate the outcomes of nursing interventions. Nursing interventions may be described as direct client care or as consultation activities, depending on the goal of the intervention. The analysis and synthesis of the process consultation model by Blake and Mouton (1983) serves as the basis for the following discussion and application of this model.

### NURSING TIP

One of the most important decisions a nurse makes before accepting or writing a consultation contract is to identify the real client in the situation. It is not a good idea to prematurely accept the problem as presented by the person seeking the consultation. Sometimes the person is not a real client and defines the problem as he or she views it. Using the process model of consultation, the consultant can help define the real client and the real problem so as to develop workable solutions.

tential establishment of a health ministry. Barry decides that the consultation contract needs to include representatives of the parish council and parishioners themselves to find effective answers to the question. He realizes that time would be wasted and resistance to change would still be present if the focus were on only one group at a time. If he met separately with the parish council, they may decide such a program should include only one set of services. The parishioners may want either a different set of services, or to have services and programming organized in a very different manner. For example, the parish council may be especially interested in blood pressure screening, whereas the parishioners may be interested in wellness classes to keep the congregation healthy and home visiting for those who are ill. After spending much energy meeting with both groups separately, he would find that by being a messenger between the two groups rather than a facilitator for problem solving, the consultant role has been diluted. On the other hand, by meeting with both groups together, Barry could serve as a resource, helping them explore all viewpoints and alternatives for developing the new program. In this case, both the parish council and the parishioners are Barry's clients.

Once the client has been identified, the nurse must decide the best method(s) for intervening in the problem situation. Blake and Mouton (1983) describe five basic intervention modes or techniques that can be applied to the process consultation model: acceptant, catalytic, confrontation, prescriptive, and theory/principles (summarized in the How To box). The acceptant intervention mode involves clarifying emotional reactions so that more objective problem solving can begin. This intervention mode benefits the client by improving self-acceptance, emotional health, and the ability to objectively define and deal with problems. Two disadvantages exist with this intervention mode. Expressing emotions may only help the client accept the circumstances leading to the problem rather than taking actions to correct the problem, and the client's catharsis may be seen by others as hostile and aggressive (Blake and Mouton, 1983).

In the catalytic intervention mode, the consultant helps clients broaden their view of the situation by gaining additional information or by considering existing data (Blake and Mouton, 1983). The consultant helps the client clarify understanding of problems by increasing available information, breaking down barriers to communication by identifying ineffective communication patterns, and raising the awareness of all involved regarding the problem. The consultant is a facilitator providing the client with the information needed to solve a problem. Lack of information, however, may be the symptom, not the problem. The disadvantage of having the consultant improve information flow is that the client may rely on the facilitator for data rather than becoming efficient in finding solutions to future problems (Blake and Mouton, 1983; Caplan, 1970).

The confrontation intervention mode presents the client with facts that reveal the client's values and assumptions in ways that cannot be denied or disputed (Blake and Mouton, 1983). This intervention mode provides clients with an objective look at how their values and beliefs control their behavior. By looking at present behavior, the con-

sultant and client can examine alternative values to redirect behavior toward improved methods of problem solving. The disadvantage is that the client may not wish to participate in interactions that could be interpreted as criticism (Blake and Mouton, 1983). For example, a consultant may find that the staff nurses in a local ambulatory care clinic are going to resign their positions because they view the director's decisions as autocratic and uncompromising. On the second visit to the clinic, the consultant could confront the clinic director with these observations. The director may deny the behavior and point out evidence of having acted democratically. As a result of the confrontation, the director may regard the consultant's observations as personal or be willing to examine and analyze the differences between the perceived and the actual behavior.

The prescriptive intervention mode requires less collaboration between consultant and client because the consultant tells the client how to solve the problem (Blake and Mouton, 1983). This mode is best used along with other intervention modes, such as acceptant or catalytic. If clients do not participate in problem solution, they will not be able to solve future problems and may not follow the prescriptions offered. The advantage of the prescriptive intervention mode is its usefulness in situations where clients have lost confidence in their problem-solving ability or have given up in despair (Blake and Mouton, 1983). In the preceding example, the nurse consultant could decide that the best method of dealing with the problems between the staff and the director is to present a prescription for behavioral conduct to be implemented by the director and the staff. The consultant tells the group when and how follow-up evaluation will be done to look at the progress of both parties in solving their differences.

Use of the theory/principles intervention mode requires that the client learn theories, such as behavior theory, and their application to problem solving. This intervention mode introduces the theories after clients have shared their usual methods of problem solving. It also allows the client to apply the theories to problem situations while developing skills in problem diagnosis and solution. The major challenge with this mode is determining how to help clients learn practical ways to apply the theory (Blake and Mouton, 1983). This mode can be combined with another mode because consultation involves facilitating client learning (Evans, Reynolds, and Cockman, 1992). Evans et al (1992) explain that theory can be used to help clients better understand what the data are saying, better diagnose the problem, and generate more potentially effective decision alternatives. Before using this mode with the health department staff and director, the consultant may present a conference on leadership theories and principles and a discussion of the responsibilities in administrative decision making. The consultant may be able to show both parties how leadership styles should vary with the types of decisions to be made and with the people involved.

The choice of an intervention mode depends on the client and the problem. Blake and Mouton (1983) identified four categories of problems: power/authority, morale/

**HOW TO** **Apply Consultation Intervention Modes**

| Intervention mode | Definition | Client problems | Consultant actions |
|---|---|---|---|
| Acceptance | Consultant urges client to share feelings and move to more objective problem solving | • Low morale<br>• Feelings of powerlessness to change a situation | • Attempt to understand the client's feelings about the situation.<br>• Encourage the client to talk.<br>• Listen actively.<br>• Try to clarify the client's feelings and help the client to accept the feeling.<br>• Refrain from agreeing or disagreeing with the client's perception.<br>• Encourage the client to explore ways of dealing with the problems.<br>• Listen for more data to reveal the total scope of the problem. |
| Catalytic | Consultant broadens client's knowledge of problem by offering new data or clarifying existing data | • Standards are violated or changed<br>• Inability to meet goals or objectives | • Set a nonauthoritarian tone for the interaction by beginning the intervention with social conversation.<br>• Ask the client to describe the situation and use the description as a basis for the interaction.<br>• Suggest data-gathering techniques that may provide new information of interest to the client.<br>• Provide support to the client as the client attempts to accurately perceive the problem.<br>• Avoid specific suggestions.<br>• Encourage the client to make decisions about problem resolution. |
| Confrontation | Consultant presents clients with indisputable facts | • Additional insight needed<br>• Unwillingness to solve problem | • Continually question clients about their description of the situation.<br>• Present data and logic to test clients' chosen courses of action.<br>• Challenge clients' chosen courses of action.<br>• Probe for motives and causes of present situation.<br>• Provide own thought about situation without personally attacking client's values. |
| Prescriptive | Consultant tells client how to solve problem | • Inability to cope<br>• Needs immediate answer | • Probe for data about the client's situation.<br>• Act authoritatively.<br>• Control by telling the client how the problem is to be perceived.<br>• Tell the client the best solutions.<br>• Remind the client if he or she is procrastinating in implementing actions.<br>• Offer praise if the client does exactly what the consultant suggests. |
| Theory/principles | Consultant teaches how to solve problem using theories or principles | • Additional insight needed<br>• Lack of knowledge to solve problems | • Introduce theories for problem solving to the client.<br>• Use techniques to help the client internalize theories.<br>• Provide strategies for practical application of the theories, such as problem situations or critiques of application.<br>• Offer support when the theory is applied in the actual problem situation. |

cohesion, norms/standards, and goals/objectives. The power/authority problem results from questions about who has the right to supervise and who has the right to make decisions. The morale/cohesion problem occurs when the client has lost confidence in the ability to solve problems and feels powerless. The norms/standards problem occurs when group norms or professional or agency standards are violated or changed. Problems related to goals/objectives involve developing new goals, changing goals, or being unable to meet goals.

Several intervention modes may be used with each type of problem. The most common intervention for morale/cohesion or power/authority problems is the acceptant mode because the issue generally causes feelings that block decision making. The catalytic mode is the best choice with norms/standards and goals/objectives problems because it focuses on strengthening the client's perceptions of the most effective decision-making methods. The theory/principles intervention mode may be helpful regardless of the problem, especially when additional insights are needed. The prescriptive mode may not be helpful unless the client is unable to cope with the situation and needs immediate direction or answers to solve the problem (Blake and Mouton, 1983) or unless the problem is fairly straightforward (Rokwood, 1993).

## Consultation Contract

The consultation relationship is based on expectations. The consultant has expectations concerning time, money, resources, and the participation of the client in the process. Clients have expectations about what they will gain from the consultation relationship. Discussing the terms of a **consultation contract** makes expectations explicit, reduces the likelihood of violations of contract terms, and reduces the risk of additional demands being made on either party. Clients will want to know the type of content expertise the consultant has and the consultation processes, communication strategies, and types of feedback the consultant will provide (McCutcheon and Perkin, 1996). Areas to include in the written consultation contract are as follow:

1. Client and consultant goals
2. The identified problem
3. The consultant's resources
4. The time commitment
5. Limitations of the contract
6. Cost
7. Conditions under which the contract may be broken or renegotiated
8. Intervention modes to be used
9. Expected benefits for the client
10. Methods of data collection to be used
11. Client resources
12. Potential interventions
13. Evaluation methods to be used
14. Confidentiality

An example of a consultation contract appears in Figure 42-6.

Writing a contract for consultation relationships has a number of advantages. The contract terms assist the consultant in determining the number of hours that must be devoted to the interaction and in identifying needed resources and out-of-pocket expenses required to complete the interaction. **Negotiation** of the contract assists the client in identifying realistic expectations of the consultant and firmly establishes what the consultant will and will not do. The client has the opportunity during the negotiation to place limits on what the consultant can do, and the contract allows for future renegotiation of terms. Pricing methods for consultation services vary with the nature of the services. Consultants may price their services on the basis of the actual number of billable hours required to perform the service, or they may set a flat fee during the contract negotiation phase. Flat fees are more attractive to clients because they reduce uncertainty over the total cost of the consultation. They create an incentive for consultants to be efficient and to use an accurate method of estimating their services before the contract negotiation meeting.

Consultation involves seven phases:
1. Initial contact with the client
2. Definition of the relationship
3. Selection of a setting and approach
4. Collection of data and problem diagnosis
5. Intervention
6. Reduction of involvement and evaluation
7. Termination

The initial contact is made when the client or someone in a family, group, agency, or community communicates with the nurse about a potential problem that requires intervention. The communication may be a person-to-person contact during a home visit, may be written, or may occur by telephone. On initial contact, the client and the nurse have an exploratory meeting to define the problem, assess the nurse's interest and ability to help, and formulate future actions. If the nurse has little experience with the type of problem presented, the client may wish to seek assistance elsewhere. Also, if the nurse is quick to make decisions and has a directive approach, the client with a more laissez-faire attitude may have difficulty accepting the nurse's approach. The nurse may also conclude that the situation is not within the nurse's expertise and will want to recommend someone else to work with the client.

Next, the terms of the relationship are discussed. The nurse consultant finds out what the client expects to gain from the relationship and develops terms for the interaction. Finally, in the initial exploratory meeting, the setting for the consultation is decided, the time schedule is set, the goals of the interaction are established, and the mode of intervention is chosen.

When the terms of the contract are agreed on, the data gathering methods will be part of the agreement. Data gathering methods used by consultants include direct observation, individual and group interviews, use of questionnaires or surveys, and tape recordings. One particularly useful data gathering strategy is the focus group (Krueger and Casey, 2000). This is a group of eight to ten people who share a common characteristic, such as staff nurses in the same organization or community members

| | |
|---|---|
| Client Name: J. Hyde, Nurse Manager<br>Address: Residential Complex<br>Phone: 111-2222 | Consultant Name: P. Jones, Nursing Student<br>Address: College of Nursing<br>Phone: 333-4444 |

Estimated costs (external consultant only):      $500
(including phone, secretarial assistance, preparation, supplies, travel expenses, and consultant sessions)

Client problem definition:          Facility undergoing expansion: residents likely to need more assistance with health promotion and health monitoring. Average resident age is 72.3 yr. Residents have on avg. 2.5 chronic illnesses each. 10-15 miles from health facilities. Residents are becoming increasingly homebound.

Suggested intervention mode:      Catalytic/Prescriptive

Client goals:
A healthy resident population through accessible and ongoing health promotion and monitoring.

Scope of consultation (time and no. of sessions):
3 planning and data gathering sessions in 6 weeks; 3 evaluation sessions at 2- to 3-week intervals during data collection; final evaluation session.

Consultant resources (e.g., computer, secretary, library):
Computer to analyze data; library; assistance from faculty; staff to collect data (3 students).

Contract renegotiation and termination terms:
Renegotiation at 2- to 3-week evaluation conferences. Termination at final evaluation conference.

Client resources (e.g., records, secretary, copy):
Project records available to collect data; secretary type survey questionnaires; conference room for interviews; final report typing; supplies.

Anticipated client benefits:
Residential complex will have a plan for meeting health needs of residents. Residents will have increased access to health promotion and health monitoring services.

Contract limitations (e.g., who, what, when, how data will be shared):
Survey of residents' health needs, and perceptions of staff and administrators by CHN student. Report to nurse manager, facility manager, and college faculty.

Potential interventions (e.g., report shared with administration: meetings held with staff):
Meetings with staff and residents to obtain input on the problem and potential solutions. Review of resources to find the residential complex's ability to manage the problem itself.

Consultant goals:
Collect data as outlined.
Assess and define problem in collaboration with residents, staff, and administration. Identify resources for solving the problem. Develop a realistic method for solving the problem in collaboration with residents, staff, and administration.

Data collection methods:
Interviews:          Staff, nurse manager, facility manager, local health care providers
Surveys:          Residents
Focus groups:      Residents, staff and administrators, faculty
Phone:          N/A
Contract evaluation:
          At the end of 12 weeks will look at potential alternatives; choose one that is satisfactory to residents, staff, and administrators.

**Figure 42-6** Example of how to write a consultation contract.

## Evidence-Based Practice

This paper reports on the results of focus groups conducted to better understand the causes of under-immunization in children under 2 years of age. Developers of the Consortium for the Immunization of Norfolk's Children designed the study to accomplish three goals: (1) to identify barriers to childhood immunizations from the perspectives of mothers, (2) to supplement data already gathered in structured household interviews about barriers to childhood immunizations, and (3) to enable coalition participants to conduct a component of the community needs assessment. Six focus groups were conducted with mothers of preschool-age children. Study participants represented private, public, and military sectors of the economy, as well as parents who were homeless. The focus groups were conducted by trained moderators. Questions related to mothers' knowledge and attitudes about immunizations, positive and negative experiences in obtaining immunizations, barriers to obtaining immunizations, and suggestions for reducing barriers.

Focus group participants indicated they knew the importance of immunizations but found the process of obtaining both initial and subsequent immunizations to be confusing and complicated. They often did not know where to obtain immunizations, when to return for boosters, or that immunizations were free. They indicated that clinic hours were inconvenient and that public clinics were not "family friendly" (Butterfoss et al, 1997, p. 54). Participants felt that these clinics were uncomfortable and that staff were not always sensitive or responsive to them. They had difficulties with transportation, providing care for siblings, and scheduling appointments. Suggested strategies to overcome these barriers included implementing an immunization hotline, starting a media campaign in the local newspapers, and putting information on billboards and on bus and taxi boards. Focus group participants recommended providing immunizations in elementary schools, providing opportunities for walk-in clinic appointments, and considering a community van to transport parents and children to clinic appointments. Consortium members subsequently decided to institute an "adopt-a-clinic" program (Butterfoss et al, 1997, p. 54) to encourage local groups to improve the environments within public clinics (e.g., by adding fresh wallcoverings, furniture, play equipment).

**Nurse Use:** The nurse can more clearly define the health problem and find appropriate solutions to the problem by having a focus group that includes representatives of all persons affected by the problem and the solution.

Butterfoss FD et al: Use of focus group data for strategic planning by a community-based immunization coalition, *Fam Community Health* 20(3):49, 54, 1997.

living in the same neighborhood. Focus groups are led by one individual, who has prepared five or six open-ended questions to guide the discussion. A recorder takes thorough notes during the session. Focus group sessions are usually 1 hour in length and include refreshments. After the session, the leader and the recorder discuss their observations and impressions to capture all important data. The outcomes of focus group discussions can guide the development of written surveys (LoBiondo-Wood and Haber, 2002). The Evidence-Based Practice box illustrates how focus groups were used for strategic planning related to a community-based immunization program.

While data are being gathered and after the diagnosis has been finalized, the nurse actively engages in the chosen intervention mode. After fulfilling the terms of the contract, the nurse must disengage or reduce the amount of involvement with the client. Decreased contacts allow each side to evaluate the effectiveness of the intervention. During disengagement, the nurse reassures the client that future interactions are possible at the client's discretion. When the agreed-on period of disengagement has passed, the relationship is terminated. The nurse typically provides the client with a written summary of the findings and recommendations resulting from the interactions during the disengagement and termination phases (Ingersoll and Jones, 1992).

The consultation relationship involves responsibilities by both the nurse and the client. Although the contract defines the terms of the relationship, the client can assist in making the consultation process a success. Initially, the client must determine whether an internal or external consultant can best assist in solving the problem. An internal nurse consultant knows the agency and the values of the agency and the staff, is a team member, has expertise, and is probably committed to helping solve internal problems. The external nurse consultant brings new ideas and a broader regional or national perspective; has new or proven strategies to offer; can bring objectivity to the problem; and has a short-term, less expensive commitment to the agency. An example of a consultative intervention follows:

> *Intervention:* prescriptive
> *Client:* director of nursing
> *Consultant:* internal
> *Problem:* norms/standards

The client telephoned the state nurse consultant and requested a meeting at the local health unit. The purpose of the meeting was to review serious problems the local nursing staff was having in meeting program standards and requirements, as identified in a recent audit. The nurse consultant, Elizabeth, met with the client, Maggie, and reviewed her findings, sharing her analysis of the problems and contributing factors. The central problem was defined as inconsistent supervision of staff with a need for role clarification of supervisory responsibilities. Maggie was immobilized by the situation. Elizabeth directed Maggie to restructure the supervisory job descriptions to clearly reflect supervisory roles and expectations; she also recommended giving supervisors written performance evaluations and guidelines for improving staff performance. Elizabeth maintained contact with Maggie until termination of the consultation occurred and corrective action was completed.

## Community-Oriented Nurse Consultant Role

An agency whose delivery of care is similar to that of an official public health service will most likely employ a generalist nurse who provides traditional or nursing consultation for a broad range of community health activities (e.g., a community or public health nurse clinical specialist). A community health agency that provides a program approach to the delivery of community health services, such as family planning, maternity, child health, handicapped children's services, school health, or home health, will tend to employ specialist consultants. These consultants may have skills and training in specific clinical areas (e.g., a nurse with expertise in maternal and child health). Agencies providing primary health care require a consultant with both general knowledge of public health practice and specialized knowledge in a primary care clinical area. This is also a requirement in agencies involved in long-term and home health care.

The nurse consultant employed in an official health agency functions as an internal consultant to the employing agency. As a representative of the agency, the nurse provides nursing and consultation to colleagues, other disciplines, agency administration, and other health and human service agencies and/or community groups. Two primary roles of the internal consultant are resource person and facilitator.

With knowledge of available resources, the nurse consultant can identify gaps in service, identify the critical services provided by the health care delivery system, and promote services for meeting health or social needs of the population. The consultant facilitates staff nurse problem solving about individual client and family needs, health needs of a group of clients, or professional concerns and attitudes. The consultant may assist managers and administrators in solving problems about personnel, program needs, organizational goals, community relationships, and client population needs. The consultant also may facilitate communication across agencies by working with interagency **coalitions** or **alliances.**

A generalist nurse in an official public health agency is often required to function in a dual supervisor/consultant role. **Supervision** means decision making and implementing activities in an ongoing relationship, which is the opposite of consultation. Functions of the supervising role could replace the consultation role, and the staff could perceive the supervisor/consultant as being directly aligned with administration. Effective communication is vital.

The internal consultant as a representative of the employing agency has implied authority that may result in conflict between the consultant and the client. The amount of conflict depends on the centralizing or decentralizing of the public health agency and the degree of autonomy of the individual units in the organization. One way to decrease potential conflict is to clearly define the role the consultant is to assume. For example, in one state, the state health department has (centralized) jurisdiction over all the county health departments. The state has decided to decentralize by making all the county health departments autonomous in their delivery of health services. The state health department will continue to advise the county units about delivery of services but will not supervise the delivery of care. Nurses in the county units will have their own director, and the nurse consultants at the state level will be used as resource persons and facilitators.

Although the state health department was centralized and provided direct supervision to the counties for delivery of health care, the state family planning consultant was also responsible for supervising the county health department staff members who were responsible for delivery of family planning services. In the decentralized system, the supervisory functions are removed from the consultant's responsibilities, and the consultant facilitates the work of other nurses by offering advice and information that will assist them in understanding how to do their work.

The role of external nurse consultant also involves acting as a facilitator or a resource person. The external nurse consultant may represent the employing agency and provide information to the client for planning interagency programs to meet population needs. The external nurse consultant may serve as a resource to health educators, school personnel, psychologists, counselors, dentists, social workers, physicians, legislators, and probation officers, providing data about individual client, group, or community needs. The external consultant may be asked to serve as facilitator to an official agency board to solve problems about community health priorities or to serve as a facilitator or resource person to voluntary agencies, such as the American Red Cross or the American Heart Association.

Consultants from federal agencies are often used as external nurse consultants. The nurse consultant from the federal agency may come to the local or state agency to serve on request as facilitator or resource person helping with program planning, development, and implementation. The primary role function of this consultant is to serve as a resource person, although the consultant may facilitate movement toward identifying actual program objectives.

An example of a vital role community-oriented nurse consultants can play is in helping a community agency or a coalition conduct community needs assessments and develop strategic plans and associated action plans for achieving Healthy People 2010 goals (see the Healthy People 2010 box) (USDHHS, 2001a).

## COMPETENCIES FOR COMMUNITY-ORIENTED NURSING LEADERSHIP, MANAGEMENT, AND CONSULTATION

### Leadership Competencies

Community-oriented nurse managers and consultants need effective leadership, interpersonal, organizational, fiscal, and political competencies. Some competencies are similar to those required for leadership in other clinical areas, such as good communication skills and the ability to delegate ef-

**1-7** Increase the proportion of schools of medicine, schools of nursing, and other health professional training schools whose basic curriculum for health care providers includes the core competencies in health promotion and disease prevention

**7-7** Increase the proportion of health care organizations that provide patient and family education

**23-2** Increase the proportion of federal, tribal, state, and local health agencies that have made information available to the public in the past year on the leading health indicators, health status indicators, and priority data needs

**23-4** Increase the proportion of population-based Healthy People 2010 objectives for which national data area available for all population groups identified for the objective

**23-8** Increase the proportion of federal, tribal, state, and local agencies that incorporate specific competencies in the essential public health services into personnel systems

From U.S. Department of Health and Human Services: *Healthy people 2010: understanding and improving health,* ed 2, Washington DC, 2000, U.S. Government Printing Office.

---

**Table 42-4   Core Competencies for the Twenty-first–Century Leader**

| COMPETENCIES | KNOWLEDGE AND ABILITIES |
|---|---|
| Conceptual competencies | • Systems thinking<br>• Acclimatization to chaos<br>• Pattern recognition and synthesis<br>• Continuous learning |
| Participation competencies | • Involvement<br>• Empowerment<br>• Accountability |
| Interpersonal competencies | • Receptivity andsimilarity<br>• Immediacy and equality<br>• Facilitation<br>• Coaching |
| Leadership competencies | • Technical expertise<br>• Transformational style<br>• Interactive administering |

From Porter-O'Grady T, Wilson CK: *The leadership revolution in health care,* Gaithersburg, Md, 1995, Aspen.

---

fectively. Working in the community means being able to work with populations and groups. With health care focusing on improving the health of populations and mobilizing community action, community- oriented nurses need to build coalitions and partnerships and maintain working relationships with a variety of groups. Leadership essential to these roles involves identifying a vision and influencing others to achieve the vision, emphasizing that client needs are the basis for health services, empowering others, balancing attention to people and tasks, delegating tasks and managing time appropriately, and making decisions effectively. Increasingly, leaders must be smart, flexible, able to identify trends, and able to work comfortably with differ-

ent types of people and cultures (Lancaster, 1999). Table 42-4 identifies core competencies for nursing leaders in today's health care environment.

Nurse managers should be involved in developing agency-level vision, mission, and goal statements. The American Nurses Association (ANA) and the American Public Health Association, Public Health Nursing Section, both offer guidance in these areas.

## Servant Leadership

Effective nursing leaders understand the concept of **servant leadership.** Greenleaf (1998) points out that customers come first, and the leader's basic function is to serve customers. Expanded to the health care context, nurse managers and consultants need to remember that clients are the reason for their work, whether clients are individual clients in a primary care clinic; families in a home care caseload; aggregates, such as teachers and staff in a school setting; or entire communities. This means that basic organizational assumptions often must change. For example, the assumption of organizational hierarchy as a pyramid with clients at the bottom and administration at the top must be reversed. In a servant leadership context, administration is at the bottom of the pyramid and clients are at the top, with staff who work directly with clients located immediately below clients. This alteration in perspective is more than just a picture; it changes the leader's basic assumptions about work rules. For example, in a traditional bureaucracy, organizational efficiency is achieved by developing detailed rules governing how work is done. Often these rules do not match the needs of individual clients. If a single mother brings her three preschool children to a health department clinic for a checkup for her infant and must return at a different time to obtain immunizations for the 4- and 5-year-old children, her needs and the needs of her children have not been met. On the other hand, if the clinic is organized around family needs, as opposed to specializing in the needs of narrow age-groups, then all three of her children can be immunized in one visit and the client's needs have been met.

## Empowerment

Leaders provide empowerment by helping others empower themselves to make organizations more responsive to client needs. This means helping staff acquire the knowledge, skills, and authority to act on behalf of clients (Laurent, 2000). It means removing barriers to decision making and allowing staff nurses the authority to make client decisions in "real time," as needs demand, rather than requiring nurses to obtain numerous approvals. Empowerment is more than simply increasing workers' authority. It includes ensuring that they have the necessary information, knowledge, and skills to effectively make the decisions for which they are being empowered. For example, nurse managers who are responsible for preparing their own department or program **budgets** and for approving program spending must be given the opportunity to learn budgetary concepts. The concept of empowerment underpins the consulting process. Consultants assist others in identifying solutions to problems and, more important, in developing the ability to manage problems independently in the future.

## Balance Between People and Tasks

A key leadership skill for nurse managers and consultants is the ability to balance attention to people and to tasks (Hersey and Blanchard, 1996). This skill derives from contingency leadership theory and means that effective leaders do not focus all of their attention on simply getting the job done; if they do this, they may appear cold and uncaring and reduce staff morale. Similarly, effective leaders do not spend all of their time attending to workers' personal needs and problems. If they did this, the goals of the agency would never be met. Effective leaders must balance their focus, depending on the needs and skills of those with whom they work and on the demands of the situation. When time is a critical factor, such as in disasters or bioterrorism, effective leaders emphasize tasks, such as providing victim triage, meeting basic community needs for safe food and water, organizing shelter, and organizing and implementing mass immunization clinics. After the emergency has stabilized somewhat, they should attend to long-term mental health needs, such as shock, grief, and posttraumatic stress syndrome.

## Delegation

Effective leaders need to be able to manage time well and to delegate appropriately. For example, nurse consultants must be able to accurately predict the amount of time that will be required for each phase in the consulting process (McCutcheon and Perkin, 1996). The purposes of **delegation** include increasing agency efficiency, developing others' talents, and managing time well (Sullivan and Decker, 1997). Agency efficiency increases when tasks are assigned to the first level in the hierarchy where employees possess

---

> ### BOX 42-2   Time Management Tips
>
> - List goals for 5 years, 1 year, and daily.
> - Prioritize the goals.
> - Identify the tasks that must be performed to accomplish the goals.
> - Identify tasks that can be delegated.
> - Group the tasks in a meaningful way (e.g., geographically).
> - Plan strategies to minimize time-wasters. For example, plan office hours when people can find you in your office available to respond to questions.
> - Plan to work on tasks at times when you are at peak level of efficiency (e.g., plan tasks requiring mental alertness in the morning if you are more alert at that time).
> - Plan plenty of time to accomplish tasks with adequate transitional time between tasks.
> - Say no to tasks that are not essential to your position or your goals.
> - Take adequate breaks from work, including breaks during the day and vacations.
> - Maintain personal energy level through good health habits, including proper nutrition and adequate exercise and sleep.

the necessary skills and knowledge to complete the task and where the task is related to the goals of those positions. Delegation develops others' talents and can contribute to job satisfaction. Asking a community health nurse in a nursing clinic for the homeless to develop a booklet describing community resources for the homeless helps the staff nurse learn more about community resources, the gaps that exist in local resources, and where opportunities exist for interagency collaboration. The community health nurse is also likely to learn about visual presentation, layout and brochure design issues, and how to present material at the appropriate reading level. Finally, delegation is an important tool in time management. A school nurse may delegate locating resources for a screening clinic to the parent–teacher association, and the time saved can be spent on developing a teaching plan for volunteers who will help with the actual screening. Strategies for effective delegation and time management tips are listed in Box 42-2 and Table 42-5.

Delegation has become an increasingly important skill for nurses, whether they have official roles as managers or not. As more agencies increase their use of unlicensed assistive personnel and lay community workers, nurses are increasingly delegating selected aspects of practice to others and supervising the completing of those tasks. Two types of delegation occur in clinical practice. Direct delegation involves speaking to an individual personally and transferring responsibility for a task to that person (ANA 1996a). Indirect delegation results when an agency has policies and

**Table 42-5  Strategies for Effective Delegation**

| PROCESS STEP | PROCESS ACTIVITIES |
|---|---|
| Assessment | • Determine the work that is to be assigned.<br>• Assess the needs of the clients who will be affected.<br>• Evaluate the needs of the situation, including professional standards and agency policies.<br>• Identify relevant laws and regulations and what they say about delegation to various levels and categories of personnel. |
| Planning | • Determine who possesses the knowledge and skills to do the work safely and effectively.<br>• Develop assignments that allow people to function safely and to grow and develop.<br>• Identify the components of the tasks to be delegated.<br>• Develop realistic deadlines for completing the task.<br>• Determine the best process for delegation—when to ask for feedback, which resources are needed, the amount of supervision required. |
| Implementation | • Delegate without guilt.<br>• Communicate expectations clearly and succinctly and provide opportunities to ask questions.<br>• Explain any procedures or important elements of the task.<br>• Clarify tasks as necessary, listen to others' points of view, and communicate appreciation for others' efforts to provide quality service.<br>• Encourage staff to report any observation they feel is important, and emphasize the importance of quality and client satisfaction. |
| Evaluation | • Provide feedback at planned intervals.<br>• Seek out regular progress reports.<br>• Provide constructive criticism of behaviors, not personalities.<br>• Provide praise in public, constructive criticism in private. |

From Adams D: Teaching the process of delegation, *Semin Nurse Manag* 3(4):171, 1995.

procedures in place that stipulate the tasks that may be performed by someone other than the person who is accountable (ANA, 1996b). Sometimes nurses mistakenly think that they are not accountable for tasks that are indirectly delegated through agency policies (e.g., policies for cross-training). However, if nursing care has been delegated, then nurses are accountable for the safe and effective completion of that care.

When planning direct delegation, nurses should first decide when to delegate. The five factors that should be considered when deciding whether to delegate a task are as follow (Harrell, 1995):

1. The potential risk of harming the client
2. The complexity of the nursing task
3. The extent to which the task requires complex problem solving
4. The extent to which the outcome is predictable
5. The degree of interaction involved with the client

Generally, nurses should not delegate tasks that are high risk, complex, novel, or unpredictable, or that will result in nurses having limited contact with clients. Barriers to delegation include inadequate experience or education, lack of confidence, unclear role expectations, and lack of clarity about legal accountability (Harrell, 1995).

The first source of guidance for delegating tasks to unlicensed individuals is the state nurse practice act. The next source of assistance comes from specialty professional organizations. For example, the National Association of School Nurses, in collaboration with three other national

**BOX 42-3  Delegating Responsibility**

Nurse managers share responsibility for any tasks they delegate to others. The nurse manager delegates responsibility for a task but retains final accountability for the safe, effective outcome of the task (ANA, 1996a). It is critical, then, that nurse managers know that the individuals to whom they are delegating responsibility are both prepared and capable of effectively performing the tasks. Nurse managers should plan specific times to obtain progress reports on task completion. This will allow the opportunity to manage problems as they arise and to provide staff with helpful feedback or instruction if needed.

groups (Joint Task Force for the Management of Children With Special Needs, 1990), issued detailed guidelines about the school nurse's responsibility in delegation. In general, any task involving special knowledge from advanced education cannot be delegated to an unlicensed person. This includes assessment, data analysis, planning, monitoring, and evaluation (National Council on State Boards of Nursing, 1990). For example, a school nurse would assess a child with physical disabilities and develop a plan of care for that child. Selected aspects of that plan of care, such as assisting with feeding or emptying a catheter bag and recording output, could be delegated to an assistant, providing that person had received appropriate training and was competent to perform the task. This means that it is

**Table 42-6  Bernhard and Walsh's Decision-Making Model as Applied to Provision of Employee Wellness Services**

| DIMENSION | GOAL | SOLUTION #1: PROVIDE WELLNESS SERVICES USING CURRENT STAFF | | SOLUTION #2: CONTRACT FOR WELLNESS SERVICES WITH LOCAL CONSULTANTS | | SOLUTION #3: CONTRACT WITH LOCAL CONSULTANTS ONLY FOR EXERCISE PROGRAM | |
|---|---|---|---|---|---|---|---|
| Feasibility | Yes | Probably | 0.7 | Possibly | 0.3 | Likely | 0.8 |
| Risk | Low | Moderate | 0.1 | Low | 1.0 | Moderate | 0.2 |
| Cost | Low | Low | 1.0 | High | 0.0 | High | 0.3 |
| Quality | High | Fair | 0.5 | Excellent | 1.0 | Moderate | 0.5 |
| Certified instructor | Yes | No | 0.0 | Yes | 1.0 | Yes | 1.0 |
| Fully utilize staff | Yes | Yes | 1.0 | No | 0.0 | Partially | 0.5 |
| Consistent with company values | Yes | Yes | 1.0 | Maybe | 0.2 | Maybe | 0.4 |
| Totals | | | 4.3 | | 3.5 | | 3.7 |

Modified from Bernhard LA, Walsh M: *Leadership: the key to the professionalization of nursing,* ed 3, St Louis, Mo, 1995, Mosby. See text for further explanation.

not adequate that the nurse know the individual has been certified as a nursing assistant; the nurse also needs to know that the individual is competent to safely perform the delegated task. The nurse retains the legal accountability for safe client care. This responsibility may be shared with the person to whom one is delegating, but accountability is never transferred. Community-oriented nurse consultants may be asked to partner with schools to develop safe and appropriate health-related delegation policies (Truglio-Londrigan et al, 2002). Box 42-3 provides further information on delegation.

## Decision Making

Finally, a core leadership skill is the ability to make decisions effectively. Along with communication, decision-making skills have been found to be among the most important for nurse managers (Chase, 1994). This is a two-stage process in which nurse managers first must decide how much input they will seek from others and, second, must generate alternatives for the decision and choose among the alternatives. Including others in the decision-making process is beneficial in part because others may have information and ideas that would lead to a better decision, and also because others may support the decision more if they are involved in making it. However, participatory decision making is more time consuming than making decisions alone.

Choosing whether to include others in the decision-making process should be based on the extent to which the manager or consultant needs information and ideas from other people, the extent to which those affected are likely to support a decision they do not participate in making, and the extent to which time pressures are present. A decision tree can be used for selecting a leadership style that varies from a unilateral, independent decision process, to progressively more participative styles, with the most participative style involving delegating authority to a group that will be responsible for making the decision. Although many assume that autocratic decision making is not effective, in fact it may be both effective and efficient under certain circumstances, such as emergencies. In other situations, it may be better to seek input from others, individually or as a group, to seek suggestions for solutions from the group, or to simply turn a problem over to a group to solve on their own.

The next stage of the decision-making process is to generate alternative solutions and to choose among those solutions. Bernhard and Walsh (1995) developed a useful decision model for nurses. With this model, the nurse determines what characterizes a good decision in the case at hand and then determines what the goal is for that decision. For example, both risk and cost are important dimensions in most situations. The goal involves low cost and low risk to clients and staff. Other dimensions might be unique to the situation. Table 42-6 presents the process for deciding whether to develop an in-house wellness program for an occupational setting or to contract with a consulting group for that service. After identifying the key dimensions and goals, the nurse manager ranks each alternative according to how well it is likely to match the goals. For example, if an alternative poses no risk at all, then it completely matches the goal of low risk and receives a ranking of 1. If it poses moderate risk, the nurse might choose to give it a 0.5; if it poses a high level of risk, the nurse may give it a 0 because it does not match the goal at all. After rating each alternative along every dimension, the scores are added, and the alternative with the highest score is the one selected for implementation.

In this example, the occupational health nurse manager would choose to develop the wellness program in-house rather than using a consultant. The advantages of this model are that it allows for staff participation in identifying key dimensions and goals and brainstorming creative solutions; participants' values are built into the dimensions and goals; and it allows for both creative and logical thinking processes. This is a particularly helpful decision model for nurse consultants.

## Critical Thinking

Nurse managers and consultants must be adept at critical thinking. Critical thinking includes values, makes assumptions explicit, and encourages creativity and innovation (Tappen, Weiss, and Whitehead, 2001). It includes reflection about the connections between sociocultural and biophysiologic aspects of health status and services. Critical thinking may be fostered through the use of guided group discussions, in which group members are assisted to think about the connections just described and about the **distribution effects** that decisions may have on others. It is also fostered through activities to stimulate creativity, such as brainstorming, synectics (i.e., problem solving using creative thinking), and nominal group techniques (Sullivan and Decker, 1997). In the example of the occupational wellness program, the nurse manager would need to critically think about ways to increase program quality.

## Interpersonal Competencies

Nurse managers and consultants need effective interpersonal skills in communicating, motivating, appraisal and coaching, contracting, supervising, team building, and managing diversity.

### Communication

Good communication skills, including skills in the use of assertiveness techniques, are essential to being effective in managerial and consultation roles. Nurses have a particular challenge in communicating because many of those with whom they work may be in a different health profession or in a different field altogether. Nurses often communicate with lay workers. It is especially critical to listen carefully, to make underlying assumptions clear, and to speak in the other's language. This may mean avoiding the use of professional jargon and speaking in more commonly shared language or speaking in the listener's dominant language. It is increasingly important for public and community health nurses to be bilingual or multilingual, depending on the ethnic composition of the community. For example, a nurse manager working in a migrant clinic with a large Hispanic population should try to learn Spanish and to learn about the client population's culture.

Communication must be culturally competent to be effective. Because communication involves words, tone of voice, posture, eye contact, and space relationships, cultural norms often influence the meanings given to different aspects of body language. For example, whereas most advise direct eye contact when communicating, in some cultures this may be viewed as aggressive, especially when the eye contact is prolonged. Some cultures prefer the closer-space relationships that may make others feel they are being crowded. Other aspects of communication are important as well, such as the appropriate place for reprimands. It is never appropriate to reprimand or criticize in public, although public praise is usually an excellent idea. Nurse managers and consultants should be sensitive to the power of written communication and be aware that, although putting a message in writing is a good way to avoid confusion, it also may be seen as aggressive, distrustful, or a bid for power. On the other hand, managers and consultants must accurately doc-

---

## THE CUTTING EDGE

Agencies, localities, and professional organizations increasingly recognize the need for effective leadership in public health and community life. Public and community health nurses should watch for opportunities to participate in leadership development institutes or consider ongoing formal education through advanced public health nursing degree programs. Leadership development programs are available at various levels, with Leadership America representing the national level. Such programs introduce participants to the full range of leadership and quality-of-life issues in a community including health, education, politics, the arts, and business. This breadth of concerns is consistent with public and community health nurses' understanding that health results from the interaction of many facets of social and economic influences. Other leadership development opportunities are provided by professional organizations (e.g., Sigma Theta Tau, the International Honor Society for Nursing), continuing education, and local groups. Local and statewide public health groups provide leadership institutes focused on developing leadership for solving public health problems (Porter et al, 2002; Wright et al, 2000). Finally, master's degree programs in public health nursing provide systematic academic development of public and community health nursing leadership competencies and prepare nurses to sit for advanced practice nursing certification as community health nursing clinical specialists through the American Nurses Credentialing Center. Public and community health nurses should take advantage of opportunities such as these for lifelong learning and strengthening leadership skills.

Porter J et al: The Management Academy for Public Health: A new paradigm for public health management development, *J Public Health Manag Pract* 8(2):66-78, 2002; Wright K et al: Competency development in public health leadership, *Am J Public Health* 90(8):1202-1207, 2000.

ument their assessments and interventions (Ingersoll and Jones, 1992). The key is to make certain that the message that is communicated is the message that was intended. Effective communication skills are listed in Box 42-4.

### DID YOU KNOW?

Partnerships with community members and community agencies are essential to effective public and community health practice. Partnerships succeed when strong communication mechanisms are in place to ensure definition of needs and problems, timely problem resolution, and ongoing development of shared visions. Although some models of leadership imply that sharing a leader's personal vision is the key to success, in public and community health the development of shared visions and goals and the operational mechanisms to make those goals a reality is the key to success. Communication, the primary way to make this happen, can include regular advisory or coalition meetings, telephone calls, and clearly written policies and procedures.

## Motivating Others

One of the more difficult skills to master is motivating other people. In fact, one cannot ever really motivate others, because motivation is internal. However, the skillful manager can create a motivating environment, working to make certain that both individual and agency goals are met to the extent possible. Sometimes individual motivation may be low because employees do not believe they have the skills necessary to achieve their goals, or they believe that the system will not allow them to do so. The effective nurse manager identifies which perceptions are inaccurate and helps individuals develop plans for improving their personal capacities for achieving goals. Although adequate salaries are clearly important, it is not always possible to increase pay in the short run. Nurse managers possess other tools for increasing motivation, even when budgets are tight. One home health aide supervisor is known for the high level of morale among her staff and the unusually low level of turnover, despite low salaries. She makes a point of being available for discussion before the aides leave the agency in the morning and on their return in the afternoon. Also, she always puts a birthday card and small piece of candy in their mailboxes on their birthdays, and thanks them for a job well done. For the long-term good, public and community health nurse managers should work with others in the community to increase salaries if they are not competitive. Other keys to motivation are listed in Box 42-5.

### Appraisal and Coaching

Employee appraisal and coaching are closely related to motivation and individual development. The purpose of performance evaluation is to assist employees to more effectively meet the objectives of their roles and to help them

---

### BOX 42-4  Effective Communication Skills

- Listen actively.
- Restate the main points.
- Speak in the listener's language.
- Maintain culturally appropriate eye contact and body language.
- Provide an appropriate environment.
- Be aware of the power of written communication.
- Use simple, direct words.
- Use "I" statements and say how you feel.
- Provide frequent feedback.
- Reflect on the meaning of the message.

---

### BOX 42-5  Keys to Motivation

- Identify employee needs and goals.
- Identify employees' beliefs about their abilities to meet their goals.
- Discuss with employees their strengths and areas for future development.
- Discuss how the employees' goals and the organization's goals can be aligned.
- Jointly develop job-related goals with employees, including timetables with checkpoints.
- Provide frequent, regular feedback to employees.
- Identify with the employees their key reinforcers.
- Provide frequent thanks for a job well done and for progress toward goals.
- Facilitate the development of mentor–protégé relationship and role modeling.
- Provide opportunities for employees to learn new goal-related skills.
- Provide tangible signs of recognition, such as merit pay, employee of the month, special bonuses for achievements.

---

develop their potential in ways that facilitate achieving agency goals. Performance evaluation should not take place just before an annual appraisal interview is scheduled. It should be a regular part of the job, with the manager providing regular feedback on employee progress toward goals. Performance appraisal is particularly challenging for nurse managers because so many community health workers practice independently in the field. For example, nurse managers in home health must plan either to make visits with the nursing staff on a regular basis or to obtain other forms of input on employee performance, such as planning telephone or office conferences with staff.

Coaching involves "directing and closely supervising tasks, and explaining decisions, soliciting suggestions, and supporting progress" (Blanchard et al, 1985, pp. 30, 56, cited in Vestal, 1995, p. 73). With coaching, managers retain responsibility for decisions but request input and explain decisions. They support progress by helping the employee break the tasks into manageable parts, providing resources for accomplishing task and for acquiring the necessary skills, and praising task accomplishment. Coaching is most useful with people who may not yet be skillful in a particular area and who are not confident about their skills.

**Contracting** involves identifying expectations and responsibilities by both parties. Some contracts are informal, verbal agreements between individuals, whereas others (such as the consulting contract) are formal, written agreements.

## Supervision

Nurse managers who delegate tasks to others must supervise the completion of those tasks and build in mechanisms to make certain that the tasks are completed safely and effectively (ANA, 1996b). As stated earlier in the chapter, supervision means decision making and implementation of activities in an ongoing relationship. The ANA defines supervision as "the active process of directing, guiding, and influencing the outcomes of an individual's performance of an activity" (ANA, 1998, p. 9). Supervision may occur either on-site when the nurse manager is present and while the activity is being performed, or off site when the nurse manager "provides direction through various means of written and verbal communication" (ANA, 1998, p. 9). It is important for nurse managers to build effective means of providing off-site supervision because so many community health activities do not take place within a single agency (e.g., home health care occurs in individual homes, and school health services are provided in individual schools).

Handling criticism is a difficult skill that involves both the giving and the taking of criticism related to job performance. Nurse managers should provide constructive criticism as close as possible to the time they observe a problem with an employee's job performance. Constructive criticism focuses on the behaviors necessary to meet the job expectations and helps identify sources of problems, resources for managing problem behavior, and feedback. For example, if an employee is chronically tardy, the nurse manager should speak privately with the employee about the job expectation for promptness, identify why the employee is frequently tardy, establish a behavioral goal with time frames and consequences of achieving or not achieving the goal, and assist the employee to develop a plan for achieving the goal. The employee may simply be unaware of the importance of being punctual and can easily change the behavior. On the other hand, a behavior modification plan based on social learning theory may be useful to help change the behavior (Sullivan and Decker, 1997). Behavioral consequences may include both positive reinforcers, such as praise, and disciplinary measures, such as oral and written warnings, limited raises, suspension, and termination. Suspension and termination are normally used only with

problems related to safety, inability to perform job duties, breach of confidentiality, and illegal acts, and they are detailed in agency policies and procedures.

## Team Building

Finally, team building and managing diversity are group-level skills needed by nurse managers and consultants. Interdisciplinary teams increasingly are used to assess clients, plan client care or services, and manage quality improvement activities. Teams may include members of multiple health disciplines as, for example, with community health coalitions. They also may include people from other backgrounds, including lay community health workers. Nurse managers and consultants can facilitate team building by assisting the team to develop goals and ground rules, identifying who will fill various roles and determining how to share leadership, developing strategies for ongoing cooperation and recognition of contributions of each member, and resolving conflict. Key principles of an interactive team are listed in Table 42-7 (Coben et al, 1997).

## Managing Diversity

A key challenge to nurse managers is managing diversity in positive, growth-promoting ways that value diversity (Davidhizer, Dowd, and Newman, 1999). Because the demographic profile of the American workforce is changing so rapidly, the nature of the workplace is changing as well. Female and nonwhite groups are increasing the most rapidly in the workforce (American Association of Retired Persons, 1993), with projections that 25% of the workforce will be composed of African Americans, Hispanics, and Asian Americans by the year 2005 (Mancini, 1995). Nurse managers must understand cultural values and norms to communicate effectively and interpret behavior accurately. They must know how to prevent any form of racial, sexual, or ethnic harassment and ensure a positive and welcoming environment in the workplace.

---

**( DID YOU KNOW?**

When working with people from cultures different from their own, nurse managers and consultants are more likely to be effective if they take the time to learn as much as possible about the culture. This includes learning the language if possible. For example, nurses who are not Native Americans but who work with them should learn about the culture of the tribal groups with whom they are working. Similarly, nurse managers and consultants who work with immigrants should try to learn about the culture of that group. This helps clarify underlying beliefs, values, and assumptions that may influence managerial or consultative issues and improves communication effectiveness and the effectiveness of change processes. Nurses who are not Hispanic but work with many Spanish-speaking Hispanic persons will find it helpful to learn to speak conversational Spanish or at least hire a translator.

**Table 42-7   Guiding Principles of the Interactive Team**

| PRINCIPLE | DESCRIPTION | RESULT |
|---|---|---|
| Participation and leadership | All team members are viewed as equals, and their participation is encouraged and supported. | Team functions as a cohesive unit. |
| | Leadership role rotates and is assigned in turn to the individual having the greatest expertise for the situation. | Promotes equal distribution of leadership responsibilities. |
| Development of goals | Goals must be developed in a cooperative manner, with attention focused on meeting the needs of the client. Secondary focus should be placed on meeting the needs of all team members. | Teams functions as a cohesive unit. |
| Communication | Open communication among team members should be fostered and encouraged, with each member feeling comfortable expressing opinions and thoughts on any and all issues. | Effective team functioning |
| Decision making | Important decisions should be the joint responsibility of all team members. This should be accomplished through consensus. | Effective team functioning |
| Conflict resolution | Conflict must be dealt with openly in a productive manner, respectful of all viewpoints. Steps to resolve conflict should be designed when the team is first formed. | Effective team functioning |

From Coben SS et al: Meeting the challenge of consultation and collaboration: developing interactive teams, *J Learn Disabil* 30(4):430, 1997.

## Political Competencies and Power Dynamics

Political competencies include negotiation skills, **conflict resolution** skills, and skills in recognizing and managing **power dynamics.** Principled negotiation (Marriner-Tomey, 1996) involves bargaining based on the characteristics of the issues, rather than focusing on participant personalities. This form of negotiation emphasizes collaborative problem solving rather than rigid choice of a single position. It does not imply compromising values or goals but instead emphasizes development of mutually agreeable ways of achieving goals. Conflict resolution strategies can result in win–win, win–lose, or lose–lose outcomes. Strategies most likely to create win–win situations include collaboration, confronting problems directly, and ensuring that all parties have an adequate opportunity for input (Sullivan and Decker, 1997).

Community-oriented nurse managers and consultants must understand power dynamics. Because nurses possess altruistic values, they may believe that being powerful is not necessary. However, it is impossible to create health-promoting clinical services without some legitimacy in decision-making arenas. Nurse managers need power to ensure that working conditions are conducive to excellent clinical care. Power may originate in information, knowledge, position, or access to critical resources. Nurse managers who are knowledgeable about health care trends and issues, client needs, and clinical services are more likely to have expert power. Membership on community agency boards and advisory committees puts nurse managers in the position to influence service delivery.

Consultants' advice may be followed because of perceived expert power. The client feels that the consultant possesses superior knowledge or skills and is trustworthy and credible. Internal nurse consultants may have legitimate power resulting from their role in the organization. The external consultant has only assumed power, which may result in conflict for the consultant and the client. The client may not feel obligated to implement the recommendations. On the other hand, external consultants may possess referent power because of an affiliation with other well-known consultants or a national organization. The consultant's ability to persuade clients by offering reasons, new techniques, or methods of problem solving may establish the consultant's informational power.

## Organizational Competencies

Community-oriented nurse managers and consultants use organizational skills, such as planning, organizing, implementing and coordinating, monitoring and evaluating, improving quality, and managing fiscal resources.

### Planning

Planning includes prioritizing daily activities to achieve goals. It also includes long-range planning, such as working with nurses in a department to plan a new program. Because planning is primarily a cognitive activity, nurse managers and consultants may tend to lessen its importance and allow little time for adequate planning. However, planning is the basis for direct nursing services, so it is important to make adequate time for planning.

Several documents are available to help nurse managers and consultants plan nursing services. *Healthy People 2010: Understanding and Improving Health* (USDHHS, 2001a) defines the national health goals for the United States by the year 2010 and should be the basis for program planning. The 1998 Presidential Initiative on Racial and Ethnic Health outlines six targets for special efforts to reduce health disparities between racial and ethnic minority groups and the United States population as a whole (Hamburg, 1998). These areas of emphasis should be the special focus of community health programming until goals for eliminating health disparities across groups have been met.

Each community has different needs and strengths that should be incorporated into health planning. The Assessment Protocol for Excellence in Public Health (APEX-PH) (National Association of County Health Officials, 1991) gives detailed suggestions for maximizing a health department's ability to work with the community in meeting the year 2000 objectives. A Planned Approach to Community Health (PATCH) (Kreuter, 1992) provides guidelines for ways to work in partnership with the community to develop strategies for improving personal and community health.

### Collaboration

Nurses and consultants must collaborate with other disciplines to provide coordinated services for target populations requiring multiple services from diverse agencies. For example, high-risk students have problems that are not neatly categorized as health or education problems (Igoe, 2000). Therefore school nurses must work cooperatively with others to plan for comprehensive services. One model for doing this is the five-stage process for change (Figure 42-7), which is based on a partnership process built on trust (Melaville, Blank, and Asayesh, 1993). This model is made up of the following stages:

1. Organizing a group of people interested in the problem
2. Building trust and commitment to solving the problem
3. Developing a strategic plan for managing the problem
4. Taking action
5. Adapting the model to other situations and solidifying the program within the organizational structure

### Organizing

Organizing involves determining appropriate sequencing and timelines for the activities necessary to achieve goals and arranging for the appropriate people to carry out the plan. Flow sheets and timetables are helpful tools that allow nurse managers and consultants to visualize how tasks are organized and to identify gaps in the planning. Figure 42-8 illustrates a timetable for conducting a health fair.

**Figure 42-7** The five-stage process for change. *(From Melaville AI, Blank MJ, Asayesh G: Together we can: a guide for crafting a pro-family system of education and human services, Washington, DC, 1993, U.S. Government Printing Office.)*

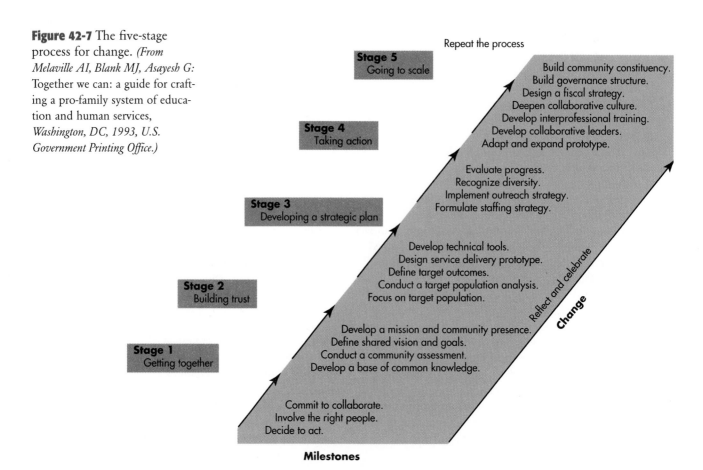

Repeat the process

**Stage 5** Going to scale

Build community constituency.
Build governance structure.
Design a fiscal strategy.
Deepen collaborative culture.
Develop interprofessional training.
Develop collaborative leaders.
Adapt and expand prototype.

**Stage 4** Taking action

Evaluate progress.
Recognize diversity.
Implement outreach strategy.
Formulate staffing strategy.

**Stage 3** Developing a strategic plan

Develop technical tools.
Design service delivery prototype.
Define target outcomes.
Conduct a target population analysis.
Focus on target population.

**Stage 2** Building trust

Develop a mission and community presence.
Define shared vision and goals.
Conduct a community assessment.
Develop a base of common knowledge.

**Stage 1** Getting together

Commit to collaborate.
Involve the right people.
Decide to act.

Reflect and celebrate

Change

**Milestones**

## Implementing

Implementing a plan includes not only following the timelines but also making certain that the relevant regulations are adhered to, that activities are appropriately documented, and that the work of all team members is coordinated. Nurse managers and consultants should give sufficient attention to the change process by helping those involved identify the need for change, keeping them informed, soliciting their input, and making modifications in the plan as necessary.

## Monitoring and Evaluating

Monitoring and evaluating are critical to community-oriented nursing services. Nurse managers should monitor nursing services on a regular basis and make improvements as soon as the need for improvements becomes apparent. Professional standards and the standards of various accrediting bodies guide the focus of monitoring and evaluating. The Joint Commission on Accreditation of Healthcare Organizations standards for home health and ambulatory care clinics provides detailed and explicit minimum standards that all such agencies should be expected to meet.

In addition to professional standards of practice available from the American Nurses Association and specialty nursing organizations, the Agency for Healthcare Research and Quality has published clinical guidelines for prevention and treatment of selected health problems, such as wound care, pain, and tobacco cessation. Although adhering to the clinical guidelines is voluntary, health professionals may need to justify not following them if client outcomes are poor. Managed care organizations are likely to use guidelines to standardize the process of care and needs for resources. One of the challenges for the nurse manager and consultant is keeping abreast of the numerous standards applicable to the practice setting and the changes in those standards.

One example of a guideline that is useful in making programmatic decisions is the concept of screening test sensitivity and specificity. When planning screening clinics, nurse managers must choose tests that are both sensitive and specific. A test is sensitive to a health problem when it is likely to detect all cases of the problem and not give false negatives. On the other hand, to be useful, a test must also be specific to that health problem and not give false positives. These concepts provide a useful decision-making tool for the nurse manager. Formulas for determining sensitivity and specificity, and guidelines for screening programs are in Box 42-6.

Finally, community-oriented nurse managers should evaluate and monitor changes in client health outcomes. Effective outcomes management programs can be used for ongoing planning and program improvements for target populations (Monson and Martin, 2002).

## Fiscal Competencies

### Forecast Costs

Finally, nurse managers must be skilled in the area of fiscal management. Nurse managers and consultants must be able to forecast the cost of nursing services. This is especially important in a managed care environment because the forecast should include risk rating of the likely health and illness experiences of a target population. Combining community health assessment skills, epidemiologic projections, and consultation are key steps in this process. After developing a profile of the anticipated health and illness experiences of a target population, the next step is anticipating the amount and kind of nursing resources needed by the population. These skills are basic to the development of proposals for managed care contracts.

| Activity | Month 1 | Month 2 | Month 3 | Month 4 |
|----------|---------|---------|---------|---------|
| Identify planning group | ●——→ | | | |
| Decide which displays to include | | ●——→ | | |
| Reserve location | | ●——→ | | |
| Invite exhibitors | | ●——→ | | |
| Develop referral policies for follow-up of screening tests | | ●————————→ | | |
| Arrange for publicity | | ●——————————————→ | | |
| Conduct the health fair | | | | ●→ |

**Figure 42-8** Sample timetable for conducting a health fair.

---

### BOX 42-6   Screening Test Sensitivity and Specificity

**DEFINITIONS**

Sensitivity = [number of true positives ÷ (number of true positives + number of false negatives)] × 100

Specificity = [number of true negatives ÷ (number of true negatives + number of false positives)] × 100

**CRITERIA FOR A SCREENING PROGRAM**

- Test has high sensitivity and specificity.
- Test meets acceptable standards of simplicity, cost, safety, and patient acceptability.
- Disease that is focus of screening should be sufficiently serious in terms of incidence, mortality, disability, discomfort, and financial cost.
- Evidence suggests that the test procedure detects the disease at a significantly earlier stage in its natural history than the stage in which the symptoms appear.
- A generally accepted treatment that is easier or more effective than treatment administered at the usual time of symptom presentation must be available.
- The available treatment is acceptable to patients as established by studies on compliance with treatment.
- Prevalence of the target disease should be high in the population to be screened.
- Follow-up diagnostic and treatment service must be available and accompanied by an adequate notification and referral service for those positive on screening.

Modified from Valanis B: *Epidemiology in health care*, ed 3, Stamford, Conn, 1999, Appleton & Lange.

---

### BOX 42-7   Components of the Expense Section of an Operating Budget

- Salaries
  - Direct salary costs
    - Staff
  - Indirect salary costs
    - Fringe benefits for staff
- Expenses
  - Direct expenses
    - Supplies
    - Equipment
    - Travel
  - Other
- Overhead
  - Administration
  - Depreciation
  - Ancillary services
  - Marketing
  - Other

Modified from Finkler SA, Kovner CT: *Financial management for nurse managers and executives*, Philadelphia, 2000, Saunders.

---

## Develop and Monitor Budgets

Nurse managers have taken on more responsibility for developing and monitoring their own department budgets as agencies have decentralized. They must be able to develop a justifiable budget and monitor how actual spending compares with planned spending. Box 42-7 lists the usual expenses to be included in an operating budget. It is helpful to obtain staff input when developing a budget in order to make financial projections as realistic as possible. Combining anticipated volume, revenues, and expenses allows the nurse manager to anticipate a breakeven point for new services (i.e., determining when a new program can be expected to be financially self-sufficient).

Table 42-8 shows a portion of a variance report. **Variance analysis** means identifying the variation between actual and planned results, determining the cause of the variation, and correcting problems when they exist. Spending more than anticipated is not always negative; it may simply indicate that client or service volume was higher than anticipated. This could, however, be of concern in an agency that is fully capitated and receives a set amount of money to see a client for usually a year, regardless of the cost of the services the client needs. Additional services do not bring in additional revenues. Nurses in fully capitated environments have more opportunity than ever before to focus on health promotion and illness prevention services.

Higher expenses than planned are not always under the control of the nurse manager. For example, if the prevailing wage increases because of changes in the labor market, an agency may spend more than expected on salaries. On the other hand, spending less than predicted does not always indicate that a program is running efficiently. It may be that client volume is down, or that staff are not providing adequate services.

In the example in Table 42-8, the nurse manager observes that more has been spent on salaries and supplies than originally budgeted, and less on travel. Is this desirable or undesirable? To analyze the variance, the nurse should ask if the prices for labor and supplies were higher than expected or if the agency has used more nursing time or supplies than planned (Finkler and Kovner, 2000). The answers to these questions will help determine whether the variance resulted from factors under the manager's control, such as inefficiency, or from factors outside of the manager's control, such as higher wages or higher prices than expected. The answers will also help determine whether the variance resulted from an increase in client volume or an alteration in case mix, with the agency serving sicker clients. Whether a client volume variance or case mix alteration is seen as desirable will depend partly on whether the agency is paid on

**Table 42-8 Variance Report**

| ITEM | EXPECTED BUDGET ($) | ACTUAL BUDGET ($) | VARIANCE ($) |
|---|---|---|---|
| Salaries | 40,000 | 42,000 | (2000) |
| Supplies | 750 | 1000 | (250) |
| Travel | 1000 | 600 | (400) |
| Total | 41,750 | 43,600 | (1850) |

**Table 42-9 Comparing Cost Effectiveness of Two Smoking Cessation Programs for 30 Employees**

| | INTERVENTION A | INTERVENTION B |
|---|---|---|
| **Direct Costs** | | |
| Development | | |
| Program design implementation (nurse, $22/hr) | $176 (8 hr) | $22 (1 hr) |
| Diary and pamphlet distribution | $44 (2 hr) | $44 (2 hr) |
| Operation | | |
| Program (nurse, $22/hr; 30 employees × 15 min/wk × 12 wk) | $1980 (90 hr/12 wk) | $88 (4 hr) |
| Diaries | $150 | $0 |
| Pamphlets | $15 | $15 |
| **Indirect Costs** | | |
| Employee time away ($12/hr) (30 employees × 15 min/wk × 12 wk) | $1080 (90 hr/12 wk) | $48 (4 hr) |
| **Total Costs** | | |
| Total costs | $3445 | $217 |
| 3-month quit rate | 15.90% | 8.90% |
| Number of employees quit | 4 | 2 |
| Annual health care costs for smoker ($228/yr) | $912 | $456 |
| Cost-effectiveness ratio for number of employees who quit | 861:1 | 108:1 |
| Cost-effectiveness ratio for health care costs of smokers | 3.7:1 | 0.47:1 |

From Mastroianni K, Machles D: What are consulting services worth? applying cost analysis techniques to evaluate effectiveness, *AAOHN J* 45(1):41, 1997.

a fee-for-service basis or on a capitated basis. In a capitated environment, higher volume will be viewed in a more positive light if the services are primary care health promotion services, and more negatively if the services are inpatient acute care services. On the other hand, in the traditional fee-for-service environment, there is a stronger incentive to prefer higher volume in the inpatient acute care areas.

## Conduct Cost-Effectiveness Analysis

Regardless of the type of reimbursement system in place, nurses should be able to conduct a **cost-effectiveness analysis** of their interventions. Such analyses are not measurements of the efficiency of a program (see Chapter 21 for a discussion of this distinction) but are comparisons of the money spent for the outcomes across two or more interventions. Cost-effectiveness analyses compare alterna-

tive approaches for achieving the same goals. The example in Table 42-9 shows the comparison costs and outcomes of two different approaches to smoking cessation in an occupational health site (Mastroianni and Machles, 1997). The total costs of intervention A, which includes weekly meetings with a nurse, diaries, and pamphlets, come to $3445. Intervention B does not include planned weekly meetings with the nurse; instead, employees may choose to meet with the nurse as they desire. This intervention also does not include diaries. The total cost of intervention B is $217.

The cost-effectiveness ratio for each intervention is calculated by dividing the total cost by the number of people who quit smoking (the outcome). Another approach is to divide the total cost by the total savings in health costs for clients who quit smoking. Using either approach, the ratio for intervention B is lower, which means that the costs to achieve the outcome were lower than for intervention A. Thus intervention B would be the preferred option.

## Practice Application

The nurse manager of a nursing clinic in a residential facility for frail older adults approached the local college of nursing for assistance with health promotion and health monitoring activities for the residents. The facility was undergoing renovation and was expected to more than triple its capacity by the time the renovation was completed. The nurse manager thought the health promotion activities that were already in place would be inadequate to serve the growing needs. Most of the residents were over 70 years of age and had several chronic illnesses each. The residential complex was 10 to 15 miles away from health care facilities.

Sheila, the nurse manager, supervised a staff of three nurses and one homemaker aide. She contracted with a local physical therapy firm for services as needed for the residents. Sheila had asked the staff if they thought they could realistically expand their services, and they suggested consultation. The staff commented that residents really needed nurses who could provide health monitoring and skilled nursing services in their apartments, because so many were increasingly homebound. Staff members were hesitant about expanding into home care themselves because they feared it would mean a cutback in the health promotion activities they were currently engaged in. They thought the needs, and the resources that would be required to meet the needs, should be evaluated before making any final decision.

What should the staff do to complete the evaluation of the problem?

A. Call a meeting of persons affected by the problem and decide on using an internal or external consultant to help evaluate the problem.
B. Write a contract and indicate how they want the evaluation to be done.
C. Develop a plan to implement home health services because the plan would include an analysis of needs and resources.
D. Continue with their health promotion activities and decide about home health services when more resources could be identified.

**Answer is in the back of the book.**

## Key Points

- Community-oriented nurse leaders, managers, and consultants should work with organizations, coalitions, and community groups to design local strategies that will help achieve the Healthy People 2010 goals.
- The goals of community-oriented nursing leadership and management are (1) to achieve organization and professional goals for client services and clinical outcomes, (2) to empower personnel to perform their responsibilities effectively and efficiently, (3) to develop new services that will enable the organization to respond to emerging community health needs, and (4) to work with others for a healthy community.
- Nurses use micro-level management theories to help them function in leadership roles, facilitate individual and group motivation, and foster effective group dynamics. Macro-level management theories provide direction for planning and organizing work, obtaining resources necessary to achieve organizational goals, and managing power dynamics.
- Nurse managers may be team leaders or program directors, directors of home health agencies or community-based clinics, or commissioners of health. They function as visionaries, coaches, facilitators, role models, evaluators, advocates, community health and program planners, and teachers. They have ongoing responsibilities for clients, groups, and community health and for personnel and fiscal resources under their direction.
- The goal of consultation is to stimulate clients to take responsibility, feel more secure, deal constructively with their feelings and with others in interaction, and internalize skills of a flexible and creative nature.
- Consultation models can be categorized as content or process models. Both purchase-of-expertise and physician–client models are content models. Purchase-of-expertise model consultation involves hiring an expert to provide information or service. In the physician–client model of consultation, the client hires the consultant to find the problem and offer solutions without background data or assistance from the client. Process model consultation helps the client assess both the problem and the kind of help needed to solve the problem.
- Five basic intervention modes or techniques applied to process consultation are acceptant, catalytic, confrontation, prescriptive, and theory/principles. The use of a particular intervention mode is based on the client and the problem. Four categories of problems are power/authority, morale/cohesion, norms/standards, and goals/objectives.
- Consultation involves seven basic phases: initial contact, definition of the relationship, selection of setting and approach, data collection and problem diagnosis, intervention, reduction of involvement and evaluation, and termination.
- Nurse consultants may function as internal consultants within an organization or external consultants outside the client organization.
- Nurse managers and consultants use a wide variety of skills, including leadership, interpersonal, organizational, and political skills. Leadership skills in-

clude abilities to influence others to work toward achieving a vision, empower others, balance attention to people and tasks, delegate tasks, manage time, and make decisions effectively.

- Interpersonal skills include communication, motivation, appraisal and coaching, contracting, team building, and diversity management skills.
- Organization skills include planning, organizing, and implementing community health nursing services, monitoring and evaluating services, quality improvement, and managing fiscal resources.
- **Political skills** are those used in negotiation and conflict management and managing power dynamics.
- Generally, both nurse managers and consultants must hold a baccalaureate degree in nursing or higher. Organizations employing nurses without this credential should help them obtain additional education in the areas of community or public health nursing, management theories and principles, and theories and principles of consultation.

## Clinical Decision-Making Activities

1. Discuss with your class members the implications that managed care has for nurse managers and consultants in community-based organizations and in the public health departments. What other implications can you think of in addition to those described in the text?

2. Draft a vision and mission statement for a nursing clinic with your classmates. Develop goals and objectives that follow the vision and mission you selected. What type of employees would you need to hire? List some of the policies and procedures you would need to have in such a clinic on the basis of your vision, mission goals, and objectives.

3. Have several class members obtain the vision, mission, and philosophy statements from several agencies in which students have community health clinical experiences. Compare these statements in terms of the agencies' target populations, basic values, and essential functions.

4. Interview one or more practicing public health staff nurses. Ask them to describe the activities of their jobs that could be categorized as consultation. During the interview, attempt to determine the following:
   a. How they define consultation
   b. The goals they are attempting to achieve with their consulting activities
   c. The model they seem to be applying in their consulting activities
   d. The intervention modes they use
   e. Whether their activities are of a generalist or a specialist nature and of an internal or external consultative nature
   f. The strengths and limitations they perceive in themselves regarding their consultative functions (e.g., education, experiential, organizational, relational, economic)

5. Interview one or more public health nurse consultants. During the interview, attempt to determine the answers to the preceding questions. Compare the responses of the two groups (consultants and staff nurses). Analyze the factors you think account for the similarities and differences.

## Additional Resources

These related resources are found either in the appendix at the back of this book or on the book's website at **http://evolve.elsevier.com/Stanhope.**

**evolve** **Evolve Website**

Appendix A.3 Declaration of Alma Alta
WebLinks: Healthy People 2010

## References

Adams D: Teaching the process of delegation, *Semin Nurse Manag* 3(4):171, 1995.

Aday LA: *At risk in America: the health and health care needs of vulnerable populations in the United States,* San Francisco, 2001, Jossey-Bass.

Alderfer CP: *Existence, relatedness, and growth: human needs in organizational settings,* New York, 1972, Free Press.

American Association of Retired Persons: *America's changing workforce,* Washington, DC, 1993, AARP.

American Nurses Association: *Scope and standards for nurse administrators,* Washington, DC, 1996a, ANA.

American Nurses Association: *Registered professional nurses and unlicensed assistive personnel,* ed 2, Washington, DC, 1996b, ANA.

Argyris C: Field theory as a basis for scholarly consulting, *J Soc Issues* 3(4):811, 1997.

Bandura A: Social cognitive theory: an agentic perspective, *Annu Rev Psychol* 52:1-26, 2001.

Bernhard LA, Walsh M: *Leadership: the key to the professionalization of nursing,* ed 3, St Louis, Mo, 1995, Mosby.

Blake R, Mouton J: *Consultation,* ed 2, Reading, Mass, 1983, Addison-Wesley.

Bond GE, Fiedler FE: The effects of leadership personality and stress on leader behavior: implications for nursing practice, *J Nurs Adm* 31(10):463-465, 2001.

Burns JM: *Leadership,* New York, 1978, Harper & Row.

Burns T, Stalker GM: *The management of innovation,* London, 1961, Tavistock.

Butterfoss FD et al: Use of focus group data for strategic planning by a community-based immunization coalition, *Fam Community Health* 20(3):49, 1997.

Caplan G: *The theory and practice of mental health consultation,* New York, 1970, Basic Books.

Chase L: Nurse manager competencies, *J Nurs Adm* 24(4S):56, 1994.

Coben SS et al: Meeting the challenge of consultation and collaboration: developing interactive teams, *J Learn Disabil* 30(4):427, 1997.

Cohen EL, DeBack V: *The outcomes mandate: case management in health care today,* St Louis, Mo, 1999, Mosby.

Committee on Communication for Behavior Change in the 21st Century: Improving the Health of Diverse Populations: 2002, *Speaking of health: Assessing health communication strategies for diverse populations,* Washington, DC, 2002, Institute of Medicine, National Academies Press.

D'Aunno T, Sutton RI, Price RH: Isomorphism and external support in conflicting institutional environments: a study of drug abuse treatment units, *Acad Manag J* 34:636, 1991.

Davidhizer R, Dowd S, Newman GJ: Managing diversity in the healthcare workplace, *Health Care Superv* 17(3):51-62, 1999.

Denker AL: What HIPAA means for your clinical practice, *Semin Nurse Manag* 10(2):85-89, 2002.

Dino GA, et al: Teen smoking cessation: making it work through school and community partnerships, *J Public Health Manag Pract* 7(2):71-80, 2001.

Dunham-Taylor J: Nurse executive transformational leadership found in participative organizations,. *J Nurs Adm* 30(5):241-250, 2000.

Essential Public Health Services Work Group: *Public health in America: the nation's health,* Washington, DC, 1994, U.S. Public Health Service.

Evans B, Reynolds P, Cockman P: Consulting and the process of learning, *J Eur Industr Train* 16(2):7, 1992.

Fiedler FE: *A theory of leadership effectiveness,* New York, 1967, McGraw-Hill.

Finkler SA, Kovner CT: *Financial management for nurse managers and executives,* Philadelphia, 2000, Saunders.

Greenleaf R: *The power of servant leadership: essays,* San Francisco, 1998, Berrett-Koehler.

Hackman JR, Oldham GR: Motivation through the design of work, *Organiz Behav Human Perform* 16:250, 1976.

Hamburg M: Eliminating racial and ethnic disparities in health: response to the Presidential initiative on race, *Public Health Rep* 113:372, 1998.

Harrell MS: Practical strategies for delegation and team building in a redesigned environment, *Semin Nurse Manag* 3(4):180, 1995.

Hersey P, Blanchard K: *Management of organizational behavior,* ed 7, Englewood Cliffs, NJ, 1996, Prentice Hall.

House RJ: A path-goal theory of leader effectiveness, *Adm Sci Q* 16:321, 1971.

Huang CL: Health promotion and partnerships: collaboration of a community health management center, county health bureau, and university nursing program, *J Nurs Res* 10(2):93-104, 2002.

Hunter DJ: Public health management, *J Epidemiol Community Health* 52:342-343, 1998.

Igoe JB: School nursing today, a search for new cheese, *J Sch Nurs* 16(5):9-15, 2000.

Ingersoll GL, Jones LS: The art of the consultation note, *Clin Nurse Spec* 6(4):218, 1992.

Institute of Medicine: *The future of the public's health,* Washington, DC, 2003, National Academies Press.

Issel LM, Anderson RA: Take charge: managing six transformations in health care delivery, *Nurs Econ* 14(2):78, 1996.

Jaworski J, Flowers BS: *Synchronicity: the inner path of leadership,* San Francisco, 1997, Berrett-Koehler.

Johnson M, Maas M, editors: *Iowa Outcomes Project: nursing outcomes classification (NOC),* St Louis, Mo, 1997, Mosby.

Joint Task Force for the Management of Children with Special Health Needs: *Guidelines for the delineation of roles and responsibilities for the safe delivery of specialized health care in the educational setting* [unpublished manuscript], Reston, Va, 1990, The Council for Exceptional Children.

Koerner JG: Nightingale II: nursing leaders remembering community, *Nurs Adm Q* 24(2):13-18, 2000.

Kreuter MW: PATCH: its origins, basic concepts, and links to contemporary public health policy, *J Health Educ* 23(3):134, 1992.

Krueger RA, Casey MA: Focus groups: a practical guide for applied research, ed 3, Thousand Oaks, Calif, 2000, Sage.

Lancaster J: Leading in times of change. In Lancaster J, editor: *Nursing issues in leading and managing change,* St Louis, Mo, 1999, Mosby.

Lasker RD and the Committee on Medicine and Public Health: *Medicine and public health: the power of collaboration,* New York, 1997, New York Management Academy of Medicine.

Latham GP, Locke E: Self-regulation through goal setting, *Organiz Behav Human Decision Processes* 50:212, 1991.

Laurent CL: A nursing theory for nursing leadership, *J Nurs Manag* 8(2):83-87, 2000.

LoBiondo-Wood G, Haber J: *Nursing research: methods, critical appraisal, and utilization,* ed 5, St Louis, Mo, 2002, Mosby.

Mancini M: Managing cultural diversity. In Vestal KW, editor: *Nursing management: concepts and issues,* Philadelphia, 1995, Lippincott.

Marriner-Tomey A: *A guide to nursing management and leadership,* ed 5, St Louis, Mo, 1996, Mosby.

Maslow A: *Motivation and personality,* New York, 1970, Harper & Row.

Mastroianni K, Machles D: What are consulting services worth? applying cost analysis techniques to evaluate effectiveness, *AAOHN J* 45(1):35, 1997.

McCloskey JC, Bulechek GM, editors: *Nursing interventions classification,* ed 2, St Louis, Mo, 1996, Mosby.

McCutcheon S, Perkin B: Effective consultation in nursing, *Can J Nurs Adm* 9(1):87, 1996.

McPhail G: Management of change: an essential skill for nursing in the 1990s, *J Nurs Manag* 5(4):199, 1997.

Melaville AI, Blank MJ, Asayesh G: *Together we can: a guide for crafting a pro-family system of education and human services,* Washington, DC, 1993, U.S. Government Printing Office.

Meyer JW, Rowan B: Institutionalized organizations: formal structure as myth and ceremony, *Am J Sociol* 83:340, 1977.

Monsen KA, Martin KS: Using an outcomes management program in a public health department, *Outcomes Manage,* 6(3):120-124, 2002.

National Association of County Health Officials: *APEX-PH: assessment protocol for excellence in public health,* Washington, DC, 1991, NACHO.

National Council on State Boards of Nursing: *Concept paper on delegation* [unpublished manuscript], Chicago, 1990, NCSBN.

Orem D: Nursing administration: a theoretical approach. In Henry B et al, editors: *Dimensions of nursing administration: theory, research, education, and practice,* Boston, 1989, Blackwell Scientific.

Pfeffer J, Salancik GR: *The external control of organizations: a resource dependence perspective,* New York, 1978, Harper & Row.

Piotrowski J: Public health priority no. 1: three new leaders vow to tackle bioterror, disease prevention and health education as public health gains heightened attention, *Mod Healthc* 32(29):6-7, 2002.

Porter J et al: The Management Academy for Public Health: A new paradigm for public health management development, *J Public Health Manag Pract* 8(2):66-78, 2002.

Porter-O'Grady T: Sustainable partnerships: the journey toward health care integration. In Cohen EL, DeBack V, editors: *The outcomes mandate: case management in health care today,* St Louis, Mo, 1999, Mosby.

Porter-O'Grady T, Wilson CK: *The leadership revolution in health care,* Gaithersburg, Md, 1995, Aspen.

Quad Council and American Nurses' Association: *Scope and standards of public health nursing practice,* Washington, DC, 1999, American Nurses' Publishing.

Rokwood GF: Edgar Schein's process versus content consultation models, *J Counsel Develop* 71:636, 1993.

Roy SC: The nurse theorists: 21st century updates—Callista Roy, interview by Jacqueline Fawcett, *Nurs Sci Q* 15(4):308-310, 2002.

Schein EH: *Process consultation: its role in organizational development,* Reading, Mass, 1969, Addison-Wesley.

Schein EH: Process consultation as a general model of helping, *Consult Psychol Bull* 41:3, 1989.

Schein EH: Organizational culture, *Am Psychol* 45:109, 1990.

Sheldon P, Bender M: High-technology in home care: an overview of intravenous therapy, *Nurs Clin North Am* 6(2):507, 1994.

Sullivan EJ, Decker PJ: *Effective leadership and management in nursing,* ed 4, Menlo Park, Calif, 1997, Addison-Wesley.

Tappen RM, Weiss SA, Whitehead DK: *Essentials of nursing leadership and management,* Philadelphia, 2001, Davis.

Thompson JD: *Organizations in action,* New York, 1967, McGraw-Hill.

Truglio-Londrigan M et al: A plan for the delegation of epinephrine administration in nonpublic schools to unlicensed assistive personnel, *Public Health Nurs* 19(6):412-422, 2002.

U.S. Clinical Preventive Services Task Force: *Guide to primary preventive services,* ed 2, Washington, DC, 1996, USDHHS.

U.S. Department of Health and Human Services: *Healthy people 2010: understanding and improving health,* ed 2, Washington, DC, 2001a, U.S. Government Printing Office.

U.S. Department of Health and Human Services: *Healthy people in healthy communities: a community planning guide using healthy people 2010,* Washington, DC, 2001b, U.S. Government Printing Office.

Valanis B: *Epidemiology in health care,* ed 3, Stamford, Conn, 1999, Appleton & Lange.

Veazie MA et al: Building community capacity in public health: the role of action-oriented partnerships, *J Public Health Manag Pract* 7(2):21-32, 2001.

Vestal KW: *Nursing management: concepts and issues,* Philadelphia, 1995, Lippincott.

Vroom VH: *Work and motivation,* New York, 1964, Wiley.

Wright K et al: Competency development in public health leadership, *Am J Public Health* 90(8):1202-1207, 2000.

Wynd C: Leapfrog Group jumps over nursing, *Nurs Manag* 33(12):20, 2002.

# Chapter 43

# Community-Oriented Nurse in the Schools

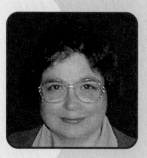

**Janet T. Ihlenfeld, R.N., Ph.D.**
Janet T. Ihlenfeld's practice is focused on child health and community health nursing. In her role as professor, she has supervised students studying well-child health care in day-care centers and in high schools. She has also contributed to several projects that developed innovative educational tools for child health undergraduate nurse education.

## Objectives

After reading this chapter, the student should be able to do the following:

1. Discuss professional standards expected of school nurses
2. Differentiate between the many roles and functions of school nurses
3. Describe the different variations of school health services and coordinated school health programs
4. Analyze the nursing care given in schools in terms of the primary, secondary, and tertiary levels of prevention
5. Anticipate future trends in school nursing

According to the U.S. Department of Health and Human Services (USDHHS), in 2001 there were over 53 million children who attended one of 117,000 schools every day (USDHHS, 2001, p. 2). These children need health care during their school day, and this is the job of the school nurse. There are approximately 47,600 school nurses in the public schools alone (Pfizer Pharmaceuticals, 2001).

It is commonly thought that school nurses only put bandages on cuts and soothe children with stomachaches. However, that is not their major role. School nurses give comprehensive nursing care to the children and the staff at the school. At the same time, they coordinate the health education program of the school and consult with school officials to help identify and care for other persons in the community.

The school nurse gives care not only to the children in the school building itself but in other settings where children are—for example, in juvenile detention centers, in preschools and day-care centers, during field trips, at sporting events, and in the children's homes (National Association of School Nurses, 2001).

The school nurse, therefore, must be flexible in giving nursing care, education, and help to those who need it. This chapter will discuss the history of nursing in the schools and the functions of school nurses today. In addition, the standards of practice for school nurses are discussed, as the nurse takes on a variety of roles. Different types of school health services are reviewed, including government-financed programs.

The primary, secondary, and tertiary levels of nursing care that nurses give to children in the schools are presented. The most common health problems that the school nurse finds in children are also discussed under their appropriate prevention levels. The chapter ends with a discussion of the ethical dilemmas that may arise for school nurses. The future of nursing in the schools is predicted for ever-changing communities.

## HISTORY OF SCHOOL NURSING

The history of school nursing began with the earliest efforts of nurses to care for people in the community. In the late 1800s in England, the Metropolitan Association of Nursing provided medical examinations for children in the schools of London. By 1892, nurses in London were responsible for checking the nutrition of the children in the schools (Ross, 1999). These ideas spread to the United States where, in 1897, nurses in New York City schools began to identify ill children. They then excluded these chil-

## Key Terms

**advanced practice nurse**, p. 1045
**American Academy of Pediatrics**, p. 1045
**Americans With Disabilities Act**, p. 1044
**case manager**, p. 1047
**Centers for Disease Control and Prevention**, p. 1048
**community outreach**, p. 1047
**consultant**, p. 1047
**counselor**, p. 1047
**crisis team**, p. 1057
**direct caregiver**, p. 1046
**do-not-resuscitate orders**, p. 1061
**emergency plan**, p. 1053

**full-service school-based health centers**, p. 1049
**health educator**, p. 1046
**individualized education plans**, p. 1044
**individualized health plans**, p. 1044
**National Association of School Nurses**, p. 1045
**PL 93-112 Section 504 of the Rehabilitation Act of 1973**, p. 1044
**PL 94-142 Education for All Handicapped Children Act**, p. 1044
**PL 105-17 Individuals With Disabilities Education Act**, p. 1044

**primary prevention**, p. 1049
**researcher**, p. 1048
**Safe Kids Campaign**, p. 1051
**school-based health centers**, p. 1049
**School Health Policies and Programs Study 2000**, p. 1046
**school-linked programs**, p. 1049
**secondary prevention**, p. 1049
**standard precautions**, p. 1053
**tertiary prevention**, p. 1050
*See Glossary for definitions*

## Chapter Outline

History of School Nursing
*Federal Legislation in the 1970s, 1980s, and 1990s*
Standards of Practice for School Nurses
Educational Credentials of School Nurses
Roles and Functions of School Nurses
*School Nurse Roles*

School Health Services
*Federal School Health Programs*
*School Health Policies and Program Study 2000*
*School-Based Health Programs*
*Full-Service School-Based Health Centers*
*Programs in England*
School Nurses and Healthy People 2010

The Levels of Prevention in the Schools
*Primary Prevention in the Schools*
*Secondary Prevention in the Schools*
*Tertiary Prevention in the Schools*
Controversies in School Nursing
Ethics in School Nursing
Future Trends in School Nursing

dren from classes so that other children would not be infected (Hawkins, Hayes, and Corliss, 1994). Health education was also important during this time. Many states had laws in the late 1800s mandating that nurses teach within the schools about the abuse of alcohol and narcotics (Veselak, 2001).

In the early 1900s in the United States, the main health problem in the community was the spread of infectious diseases. On October 2, 1902, in New York City, Lillian Wald's Henry Street Settlement nurses began going into homes and schools to assess children. These public health nurses were at first in only four schools caring for about 10,000 children. They made plans to identify children with lice and other infestations and those with infected wounds, tuberculosis, and other infectious diseases (Hawkins et al, 1994; Kalisch and Kalisch, 1995).

The need for school nurses was immediately recognized by the health care community. By 1910, Teachers College in New York City added a course on school nursing to their curriculum for nurses. By the 1920s, school nurse teachers were employed by most municipal health departments. As the years went by and communities struggled with serious economic issues and hardships during the Depression, school nurses continued to provide health care to children in the schools. In the 1940s, the nurses were mostly employed by the school districts directly. The nurses also provided home nursing, and health education for the children and their parents (Hawkins et al, 1994). In addition, school nurses became concerned with the condition of school buildings (Cromwell, 2001).

After World War II and into the 1950s, as a result of the increased use of immunizations and antibiotics, the number of children with communicable disease in the schools fell. School nurses then turned their attention to screening children for common health problems and for vision and hearing. School nurses were less likely to teach health concepts in the children's classrooms and more likely to consult with teachers about health education (Hawkins et al, 1994). However, there was an increased emphasis on employee health, and school nurses began screening teachers and other school staff for health problems (Veselak, 2001).

The 1960s saw an upsurge in the call for higher levels of education for school nurses. A position paper delivered at the 1960 American Nurses Association (ANA) convention called for the bachelor of science in nursing degree as the minimum educational preparation for school nurses. By 1970, the first school nurse practitioner program was begun at the University of Colorado. There, school nurses learned advanced concepts of school nursing practice to provide primary health care to children (Hawkins et al, 1994).

## Federal Legislation in the 1970s, 1980s, and 1990s

Community involvement in health in schools was a major thrust in the 1970s and 1980s. Counseling and mental health services were added to the responsibilities of school nurses, who began to directly teach children concepts of health. Children were no longer just being screened for illnesses (Hawkins et al, 1994). Because of federal laws that required schools to make accommodations for handicapped children, medically fragile children were attending schools, often for the first time. One of these laws, **PL 93-112 Section 504 of the Rehabilitation Act of 1973,** was an important step in helping all children enjoy a normal educational experience (Betz, 2001). This law was followed by **PL 94-142 Education for All Handicapped Children Act,** which required that children with disabilities have services provided for them in the schools.

Following the passage of the **Americans With Disabilities Act** in 1992, **PL 105-17 Individuals With Disabilities Education Act** (IDEA) passed in 1997. Both of these laws required that more children be allowed to attend schools. Schools had to make allowances for their special needs, which included ensuring that their school experience was in balance with their health care needs by developing **individualized education plans** (IEPs) and **individualized health plans** (IHPs). That meant that more children with human immunodeficiency virus (HIV), acquired immunodeficiency syndrome (AIDS), chronic illnesses, or mental health problems were in the classrooms and needed more attention from the school nurse (Betz,

### Table 43-1   Federal Legislation Affecting School Nursing

| LAW | EFFECT ON SCHOOL NURSES AND CHILDREN |
|---|---|
| 1973: PL 93-112, Section 504 of the Rehabilitation Act | Children cannot be excluded from schools due to a handicap. The school must provide health services that each child needs. |
| 1975: PL 94-142, Education for All Handicapped Children Act | All children should attend school in the least restrictive environment. Requires school district's committee on the handicapped to develop individualized education plans (IEPs) for children. |
| 1992: Americans with Disabilities Act | Persons with disabilities cannot be excluded from activities. |
| 1997: PL 105-17, Individuals with Disabilities Education Act (IDEA) | Educational services must be offered by the schools for all disabled children from birth through age 22 years. |

Compiled from Betz CL: Use of 504 plans for children and youth with disabilities: nursing application, *Pediatr Nurs* 27(4):347-352, 2001.

### Table 43-2   High Points in School Nursing History

| DECADE | MAJOR EVENTS IN SCHOOL NURSING |
|---|---|
| 1890s | English and American nurses are used in schools to examine children for infectious diseases and to teach about alcohol abuse. |
| 1900s | Henry Street Settlement in New York City sends nurses into schools and homes to investigate the children's overall health. |
| 1910s | School nursing course added to Teachers College nursing program. |
| 1920s and 1930s | School nurses are employed by community health departments. |
| 1940s | School districts employ school nurses. |
| 1950s | Children are screened in schools for common health problems. |
| 1960s | Educational preparation for school nurses is debated. |
| 1970s | School nurse practitioner programs begun. Increased emphasis put on mental health counseling in schools. |
| 1980s | Children with long-term illness or disabilities attend schools. |
| 1990s | School-based and school-linked clinics are started. Total family and community health care is offered. |
| 2000s | School nurses give comprehensive primary, secondary, and tertiary levels of nursing care. |

2001). Table 43-1 summarizes the effects of these laws on school nurses and schoolchildren.

Also during the 1990s, the responsibilities of the school nurse were extended to include the development of complete clinics and health care agency centers within or attached to the schools (Hawkins et al, 1994). These school-based clinics will be discussed later in this chapter. By 2002, some school nurses are responsible for several schools, and they give care under a variety of nursing roles. Table 43-2 gives the highlights of school nursing history over the last century.

## STANDARDS OF PRACTICE FOR SCHOOL NURSES

The professional body for school nurses is the **National Association of School Nurses** (NASN), headquartered in Maine. This association provides the general guidelines and support for all school nurses. It revised the standards of professional practice for school nurses in 2001. These standards require that all school nurses use the nursing process throughout their practice: assessment, analysis, planning, implementation, and evaluation.

In addition, the professional standards rely on nurses to give care based on 11 criteria (NASN, 2001). These criteria include the ability to do the following:

- Develop school health policies and procedures
- Evaluate their own nursing practice
- Keep up with nursing knowledge
- Interact with the interdisciplinary health care team
- Ensure confidentiality in providing health care
- Consult with others to give complete care
- Use research findings in practice
- Ensure the safety of children, including when delegating care to other school personnel
- Have good communication skills
- Manage a school health program effectively
- Teach others about wellness

In general, the NASN standards (Box 43-1) compare very well with those developed by the **American Academy**

of **Pediatrics** (AAP) regarding giving health care to students in the schools. The AAP (2001c) developed their own ideas about how nurses function in schools based on their assessment of school children's health needs. These guidelines are very similar to those written by the NASN. The AAP stated that school nurses should ensure the following:

- That children get the health care they need, including emergency care in the school
- That the nurse keeps track of the state-required vaccinations that children have received
- That the nurse carries out the required screening of the children based on state law
- That children with health problems are able to learn in the classroom

The AAP recommends that the nurse be the head of a health team that includes a physician (preferably a pediatrician), school counselors, the school psychologist, members of the school staff including the administrator, and teachers. The goal is for children to get complete health care in the schools.

## EDUCATIONAL CREDENTIALS OF SCHOOL NURSES

The NASN recommends that school nurses be registered nurses who also have bachelor's degrees in nursing and a special certification in school nursing (NASN, 2001). The AAP has the same recommendations (2001c). However, not all nurses have been educated this way. There are no general laws regarding the educational background of school nurses. School nurses in some states are required to be registered nurses, but licensed practical nurses are also seen in some schools. Box 43-2 gives the states that have laws regarding the education of school nurses. Only about half of all U.S. states require some form of additional study for school nurse specialty certification (Kolbe, Kann, and Brener, 2001).

---

**( DID YOU KNOW?**

The educational preparation for school nurses in the United States ranges from an associate's degree to a master's degree with certification credentials.

---

As an example of how the laws may be changing, in May 2001, the governor of Nevada signed a law requiring that a school nurse be a registered nurse with an endorsement in the specialty of school nursing from that state. In addition, that nurse must now be supervised by a chief nurse who oversees the school nurse programs in the school district. This standardized the school nursing programs in the state of Nevada for the first time. Before this, there were differences in educational levels between the school nurses in the urban areas and those in the rural areas of Nevada (Pro D, 2001).

School nurses in some schools may be **advanced practice nurses** who specialize in caring for children. They

---

**BOX 43-1  Summary of Major Concepts of NASN Standards**

- Give and evaluate appropriate up-to-date nursing care.
- Collaborate well with other health providers and school staff.
- Maintain school health office policies including privacy and safety of health records.
- Teach health promotion and maintenance to children, families, and communities.

Modified from National Association of School Nurses: *Scope and standards of professional school nursing practice.* Washington, DC, 2001, American Nurses.

---

**BOX 43-2** **States Mandating Educational Standards for School Nurses**

| | | |
|---|---|---|
| Arizona | Indiana | New York |
| California | Iowa | North Carolina |
| Colorado | Maine | Ohio |
| Delaware | Massachusetts | Oklahoma |
| District of | Michigan | Oregon |
| Columbia | Minnesota | Pennsylvania |
| Hawaii | Nevada | Rhode Island |
| Idaho | New Jersey | Vermont |
| Illinois | New Mexico | West Virginia |

Modified from Centers for Disease Control, National Center for Chronic Disease Prevention and Health Promotion, Adolescent and School Health: *SHPPS 2000: school health policies and programs study: state-level summaries, health services, Table 3-13*, states that require newly hired school nurses to have specific educational backgrounds, Washington, DC, CDC, 2000e, available at http://www.cdc.gov/nccdphp/dash/shpps/summaries/health_serv/table3_13.htm.

---

may be nurse practitioners who have specialized in child health nursing (pediatrics), in family nursing, or in the school nurse practitioner role. There may also be clinical nurse specialists in child health nursing or community health nursing who are school nurses. The higher the educational level of the school nurse, the better able that nurse is to give complete care to the children and their families. These advanced practice nurses may be certified by professional organizations such as the ANA or their own professional organization. Most hold master's degrees in nursing.

School nurses do not start their nursing careers in the schools. All have prior experience in nursing—most from working either in hospitals or communities. In addition, most have spent years working with children, so they are aware of their special health needs.

## ROLES AND FUNCTIONS OF SCHOOL NURSES

School nurses give care to children as direct caregivers, educators, counselors, consultants, and case managers. They must coordinate the health care of many students in their schools with the health care that the children receive from their own health care providers.

In Healthy People 2010, goal 7-4 is that there should be one nurse for every 750 children in each school (USDHHS, 2000). Most schools have not achieved this objective. In 1994, approximately 28% of the nation's schools met that standard. The **School Health Policies and Programs Study 2000** (SHPPS 2000, a study by the Centers for Disease Control and Prevention [CDC, 2000c]) found that by 2000 only Delaware, the District of Columbia, and Vermont required the 1 to 750 ratio. The new goal is that 50% of the country's elementary, middle, junior high, and senior high schools have this many nurses by 2010. Having fewer nurses in the schools means that the nurses

are expected to perform many different functions. It is therefore possible that they are unable to give the amount of comprehensive care that the students need.

---

**DID YOU KNOW?**

Many schools do not have a nurse in the building every day.

---

In 1999, Michigan did not mandate the use of nurses in the schools. A 1999 survey of school nurses in that state showed that 76% of them were performing their functions alone in the school, regardless of the number of children in the school. In addition, 56% had no support person at all to help them carry out their school health services. Their roles were the same as those of other school nurses: giving direct care, teaching health-related topics to children and staff, and creating policies and procedures related to health in the school. Seventy percent of the nurses were members of the individual educational planning committee of the schools, which made them important members of the school staff who made decisions about the educational and health care needs of the children (Periard, Knecht, and Birchmeier, 1999).

In contrast to Michigan, Massachusetts in 2001 set aside $7.4 million over 5 years to fund school health programs. These programs added a school nurse manager to the team to supervise all of the school nurses in a particular school district. This person works with the principals and other school officials. The manager also gives evaluations, feedback, and advice to the school nurses (Descoteaux, 2001).

## School Nurse Roles

### Direct Caregiver

The school nurse is expected to give immediate nursing care to the ill or injured child or school staff member. **Direct caregiver** is the traditional role of the school nurse.

Although most school nurses are in public or private schools and give care only during school hours, the nurse in a boarding school gives nursing care to children 24 hours a day and 7 days a week. In boarding schools, the children live at school and go home only for vacations. The nurse also lives at the school and may be on call all the time. The nurse in the boarding school is very important to the children because this nurse is the gatekeeper to their complete health care (Thackaberry, 2001). The nurse makes all of the health care decisions for the child and has a referral system to contact other health care providers, such as physicians and psychological counselors, if needed.

### Health Educator

The school nurse in the **health educator** role may be asked to teach children both one-on-one and in the classroom. The nurse uses different approaches to teach about health, such as teaching proper nutrition or safety information.

Many school nurses teach the older elementary girls and boys about the coming changes in their bodies as puberty arrives. Other school nurses may teach the health education classes that are required by the states to be included in the programs.

## Case Manager

The school nurse is expected to function as a **case manager,** helping to coordinate the health care for children with complex health problems. This may include the child who is disabled or chronically ill, who may be seen by a physical therapist, an occupational therapist, a speech therapist, or another health care provider during the school day. The nurse sets up the schedule for the child's visits so that those appointments do not unnecessarily impact negatively on the child's academic day.

## Consultant

The school nurse is the person who is best able to provide health information to school administrators, teachers, and parent–teacher groups. As a **consultant,** the school nurse can provide professional information about proposed changes in the school environment and their impact on the health of the children. The nurse can also recommend changes in the school's policies or engage community organizations to help make the children's schools healthier places.

## Counselor

The school nurse may be the person whom children trust to tell important secrets about their health. It is important that, as a **counselor,** the school nurse have a reputation as being a trustworthy person to whom the children can go if they are in trouble or when they need someone to talk to (Croghan, 1999). Nurses in this situation should tell children that if anything they reveal points out that they are in danger, the parents and school officials must be told. However, privacy and confidentiality, as in all health care, is important.

For example, in Queensland, Australia, in 2000, over 16,800 high school students went to the school nurse to discuss various health issues. Over 66% went to talk about mental health issues, such as depression, child abuse, violence, and suicide (Children Turn to School Nurses, 2001-2002).

In addition, the school nurse may be the person to help with grief counseling in the schools. (The school crisis team will be discussed later.)

## Community Outreach

When participating in **community outreach,** nurses can be involved in community health fairs or festivals in the schools, using that opportunity to teach others. They can be part of an influenza immunization program for the school staff and can promote a health education fair and do blood pressure screenings. They can initiate a liaison, coordinating with local health charities to provide education to the schools (Thackaberry, 2001).

In the community, school nurses may also be found in adult learning centers. A school nurse in Nashua, New Hampshire, works in an adult learning center where adults receive job training. High school dropouts can return to earn their general equivalency degree (GED) at that center. This nurse provides comprehensive health education programs to the adults at the school, including diet and nutrition classes. Because the people who come to the center range in age from infancy through adulthood, the nurse is able to give care to all age groups through health assessment and direct nursing care (Allers-Korostynski, 2000).

In London, England, a school nurse is in a community center to help teenagers who have dropped out of school or who have health problems. This nurse gives health care education related to substance abuse and teenage pregnancy during regular meetings at the center. The program has been successful and has expanded to monthly sessions (Duncan, 2000).

## Researcher

Little research has been done on nurses caring for children in the schools. The school nurse is responsible for making sure that the nursing care given is based on solid, evidence-

### Evidence-Based Practice

The vaccination of all children for hepatitis B (three doses) is recommended for all schoolchildren. Each state has its own requirements and method of vaccinating the children. This research surveyed school nurses in Houston, Texas, to obtain their opinions about the hepatitis vaccination program there. Fifth grade students ($n = 7288$) in 65 area elementary schools were to be vaccinated after receiving parental permission. After the vaccination program, the school nurses in each of the schools were sent questionnaires asking for their assessment of the program. Fifty-eight nurses returned their 13-item questionnaires. The nurses reported that getting parental consent for each of the three doses of the vaccine was their main problem. Other problems reported were lack of cooperation from the children, lack of school staff support, and finding that some parents did not see vaccination as necessary.

**Nurse Use:** The school nurses recommended that only one parental consent form be used for all three doses of the vaccine and that incentives be used to increase the rate of return of the signed parental consent forms. In addition, they recommended that increased education be done to help parents, children, teachers, and school staff understand the importance of vaccination against hepatitis B.

Guajardo AD, Middleman AB, Sansaricq KM: School nurses identify barriers and solutions to implementing a school-based hepatitis B immunization program, *J Sch Health* 72(3):128-130, 2002.

based practice. Therefore the school nurse, as an educator, is in the right position to do studies as a **researcher** that advance school nursing practice.

## SCHOOL HEALTH SERVICES

School health services vary in their scope. However, there are common parts to the programs (Duncan and Igoe, 1998).

### Federal School Health Programs

The federal government, through the coordination of the **Centers for Disease Control and Prevention,** has developed a plan that school health programs should follow (CDC, 2001) (Figure 43-1). This plan has eight parts:

- Health education
- Physical education
- Health services
- Nutrition services
- Counseling, psychological, and social services
- Healthy school environment
- Health promotion for staff
- Family/community involvement

This plan was originally developed in 1987 after the CDC began funding schools for HIV-prevention education programs. By 1992, this educational system was so successful that it was expanded to include school health programs to teach children prevention of other chronic illnesses. These include diseases caused in part by risk factors such as poor diet, lack of exercise, and smoking.

Then, in 1998, the government expanded the program again to include a more complete school health education program that included the parents and the community in the children's care. By 2001, 20 states have been funded for their school health programs by the CDC. The funding has paid for the development of health education plans of study, or curricula, which include policies, guidelines, and training for these health programs. The states then use these courses to teach the children. The schools are actively involved in helping the children practice problem solving, communication, and other life skills so they can reduce their risk factors.

According to the CDC, two states in particular have been very successful with these programs. West Virginia has developed a program called the Instructional Goals and Objectives for Health Education and Physical Education, which increased the ability of the children to pass the President's Physical Fitness Test. In Michigan, the Governor's Council on Physical Fitness, Health, and Sports developed an Exemplary Physical Education Curriculum project that made up educational materials and plans for children to achieve high physical fitness scores. All of these programs were paid for by the federal school health program funding (CDC, 2001).

### School Health Policies and Program Study 2000

After the CDC began funding educational programs about prevention of HIV in the schools in 1987, it was clear that there was a need to expand these programs. By 1992, the CDC began giving money to fund other school health programs that taught students about heart disease,

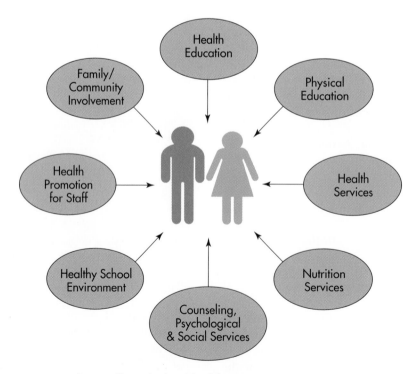

**Figure 43-1** The eight components of a coordinated school health program. *(From Centers for Disease Control and Prevention:* At a glance: school health programs: an investment in our nation's future 2001, *p 3, Washington, DC, 2001, CDC, available at http://www.cdc.gov/ nccdphp/dash/00binaries/ataglance.pdf.)*

cancer, stroke, diabetes, and substance abuse prevention (Kolbe et al, 2001). These programs have been evaluated by the School Health Policies and Programs Study 2000 (CDC 1999, 2001; USDHHS, 2001).

SHPPS 2000 looked at all eight parts of the school health program in all 50 states and the District of Columbia. The study found that only half of the states had the recommended one school nurse for every 750 students that was discussed earlier in this chapter. It also found that most school health programs had access to mental health counselors, but that the food in the schools' cafeteria tended to be high in salt and fat. Although most schools had rules forbidding weapons on the school grounds or use of tobacco, parental involvement in the school health programs was only about 50% (Kolbe et al, 2001).

## School-Based Health Programs

Because many schoolchildren may not receive health care services other than screening and first aid care from the school nurse, the U.S. government began funding **school-based health centers** (SBHCs) during the 1990s. These are family-centered, community-based clinics run within the schools. The program is called *Healthy Schools, Healthy Communities* (USDHHS, 1997).

These clinics give expanded health services, including mental health and dental care as well as the more traditional health care services (AAP, 2001a). The SBHCs can range in size from small to large. There are school clinics open to the community only during the school year and also health centers that are open 24 hours a day all year. An example of the more limited clinic is the SBHC in Gulfport, Mississippi, where 12 clinics are run in the schools by the local hospital during the school year months of August through May (Hospitals' Outreach, 2000).

Another example of a clinic is the **school-linked program,** which is coordinated by the school but has community ties (AAP, 2001a). An example of this is the *Collaborative Model for School Health* in Pitts County, North Carolina. The nurses employed by the local hospital in that area provide health care for children in kindergarten through fifth grade. There is collaboration between the county health department, the local university's nursing school, and other private health care providers to give primary, secondary, and tertiary nursing care. An evaluation of the program has shown that the children's school attendance and learning has increased as a result of the presence of more complete school health services (Farrior et al, 2000).

At a center in Texas, an urban SBHC is located in a school district where many of the children lack health insurance. The school nurses there are assisted by three part-time nurse practitioners and one community health nurse. The school nurse is responsible for the record keeping on the children's immunizations, does the screening, and gives the first aid to injured children. Then the school nurse refers children who need additional health care to the SBHC in the school. Parents like the program because

they trust the school nurse. They also like its location inside the school because everyone can receive health care without having to travel far to get to a clinic (Carpenter and Mueller, 2001).

## Full-Service School-Based Health Centers

Because the SBHCs have been so successful, in some areas they have grown into **full-service school-based health centers,** or FSSBHCs. These centers give care not only to students in a comprehensive health care setting but also to other persons in the community. They may provide social services, day care, job training, and educational counseling in addition to the medical and nursing care, mental health counseling, and dental care seen in smaller school-based centers (USDHHS, 2001).

For example, there are three different sites of federally funded FSSBHCs in Modesto, California, run by the Golden Valley Health Center. Each of these clinics is open 40 hours a week to provide health care for the children and families of migrant and seasonal farmworkers in the area. This program is successful because it provides health care in the school for entire families in an area where some families may not have access to health care. Because the building has separate entrances, the center can be open after the school day has ended, so it is used a great deal (USDHHS, 2001).

## Programs in England

School nurses in England have the same responsibilities as those in the United States. These nurses are also bound by their own laws regarding school nursing. In 1998, England prepared a national framework for school nurses to follow. It included the same general areas of health care that are familiar to U.S. nurses. This included giving care related to being healthy, promoting mental health, caring for children with chronic illnesses or complex needs, and caring for the community's health. Within these areas, the nurse gives care to the school population as the client (McRae, 2000).

## SCHOOL NURSES AND HEALTHY PEOPLE 2010

Many Healthy People 2010 objectives are directed toward the health of children. In addition, several point directly at the care that nurses give to children in the schools. The Healthy People 2010 box gives the objectives that involve school-age children. These objectives are concerned with the children with disabilities in the schools, the number of children with major health problems, and the ratio of nurses to children in the schools. Nurses can accomplish the goals using the three levels of prevention, as discussed next.

## THE LEVELS OF PREVENTION IN THE SCHOOLS

The three levels of prevention, primary, secondary, and tertiary, have always been a part of health care in the schools (Wold and Dagg, 2001). **Primary prevention** provides health promotion and education to prevent health problems in children. **Secondary prevention** includes the screening of

**Healthy People 2010** | Objectives Related to School Health and School Nursing

6-9 Increase the proportion of children and youth with disabilities who spend at least 80% of their time in regular education programs

7-2 Increase the proportion of middle, junior high, and senior high schools that provide comprehensive school health education to prevent health problems in the following areas: unintentional injury; violence; suicide; tobacco use and addiction; alcohol or other drug use; unintended pregnancy, HIV/AIDS, and STD infection; unhealthy dietary patterns; inadequate physical activity; and environmental health

7-4 Increase the proportion of the nation's elementary, middle, junior high, and senior high schools that have a nurse-to-student ratio of at least 1:750

9-11 Increase the proportion of young adults who have received formal instruction before turning age 18 years on reproductive health issues, including all of the following topics: birth control methods, safer sex to prevent HIV, prevention of sexually transmitted diseases, and abstinence

14-23 Maintain vaccination coverage levels for children in licensed day-care facilities and children in kindergarten through the first grade

14-24 Increase the proportion of young children who receive all vaccines that have been recommended for universal administration for at least 5 years

14-27 Increase routine vaccination coverage levels of adolescents

15-31 Increase the proportion of public and private schools that require use of appropriate head, face, eye, and mouth protection for students participating in school-sponsored sports

15-39 Reduce weapon carrying by adolescents on school property

16-23 Increase the proportion of territories and states that have service systems for children with special health care needs

21-13 Increase the proportion of school-based health centers with an oral health component

22-8 Increase the proportion of the nation's public and private schools that require daily physical education for all students

24-5 Reduce the number of school or work days missed by persons with asthma due to asthma

26-9 Increase the age and proportion of adolescents who remain alcohol and drug free

27-11 Increase smoke-free and tobacco-free environments in schools, including all school facilities, property, vehicles, and events

28-2 Increase the proportion of preschool children age 5 years and under who receive vision screening

28-4 Reduce blindness and visual impairment in children and adolescents age 17 years and under

From U.S. Department of Health and Human Services: *Healthy people 2010: understanding and improving health,* ed 2, Washington, DC, 2000, U.S. Government Printing Office.

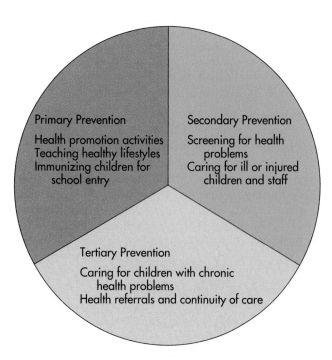

**Figure 43-2** Levels of prevention in schools.

children for various illnesses, monitoring their growth and development, and caring for them when they are ill or injured. **Tertiary prevention** in the schools is the continued care of children who need long-term health care services, along with education within the community (Figure 43-2).

## Primary Prevention in the Schools

Children need continued health services in the schools. The school nurse sees them on an almost daily basis and is the person who is usually given the role of teaching them about and promoting their health.

The school nurse may have the opportunity to go into the classroom to teach health promotion concepts—for example, hand-washing or tooth-brushing skills. They may spend time with the teachers, giving them the latest information on healthy lifestyles for children, or how to spot a child who may be ill or in need of counseling.

School nurses use the nursing process while they care for children in the schools. In their primary prevention efforts, they assess children and families to determine their level of knowledge about health issues. Finding out whether children are at risk for preventable problems is also done.

Then, the nurse analyzes the assessment findings. Plans are made to develop teaching plans or health promotion activities. Once these activities are implemented, the nurse can evaluate and revise the plan.

### NURSING TIP

To promote involvement of parents with the health of their 5-year-old children who are beginning school, some school nurses send out a questionnaire about the child's health to parents. The parents then meet with the nurse over coffee, return the questionnaire, and sign any needed health care consents. This also gives the nurse an opportunity to teach the parents about the child's health issues. This has greatly increased the communication between the nurse and the parents.

From: McRae J: School's back! *Nurs Times* 96(30):32-33, 2000.

The areas of primary prevention that the school nurse focuses on include prevention of childhood injuries, prevention of substance abuse behaviors, reducing the risk of the development of chronic diseases, and monitoring the immunization status of children.

### Prevention of Childhood Injuries

Injuries to children and teenagers are the leading cause of death in this age-group (Deal et al, 2000). The school nurse educates children, teachers, and parents about preventing injuries. Working with the national **Safe Kids Campaign,** the school nurse can give educational programs reminding children to use their seat belts or bicycle helmets to prevent injuries. Other classes can be on crossing the street, water safety, and fire safety. The school nurse, as the trusted person at school, is able to quickly give information to help prevent injuries from occurring, since most injuries are preventable (Rubsam, 2001).

School nurses also provide health promotion to prevent playground injuries. These number over 100,000 injuries to children per year. School nurses assess school playgrounds for equipment safety on the basis of the U.S. Consumer Product Safety Commission guidelines (Bernardo, Gardner, and Seibel, 2001).

School nurses also promote skateboard and scooter safety by providing health educational workshops to children and their families. Scooter and skateboard injuries numbered about 51,000 in 1999 (AAP, 2002).

These programs can be implemented by the nurse on a communitywide scale. Research has shown that once behaviors of children related to safety are taught, their effects spread quickly throughout the community. This makes the entire community safer (Klassen et al, 2000).

### Substance Abuse Prevention Education

Primary prevention interventions by the school nurse include educating children and adolescents about the effects of drugs and alcohol on their bodies. Preventing use and "saying no" to drugs has been part of the school health program for many years. Teenagers are taught by the school nurse to stay away from drugs: marijuana, cocaine, crack, heroin, alcohol.

There has been an increase in the use of "club drugs" such as LSD, ketamine, GHB, Rohypnol, and Ecstasy (MDMA). The school nurse can teach about the serious side effects of Ecstasy, especially that it causes a very high body temperature that can lead to death. Teaching the teenagers about the dangers of all drugs is the responsibility of the school nurse. In addition, the school nurse can teach parents and other members of the community about the latest drug fads, increasing everyone's awareness of these dangerous trends (Wood and Synovitz, 2001).

### Disease Prevention Education

The nurse has the opportunity to teach children healthy lifestyles to reduce their risk of disease later in life. For example, children can be taught ways to reduce their risk from getting heart disease. In one school program in North Carolina, teachers taught third and fourth graders about eating healthy foods, getting exercise, and preventing smoking (Harrell et al, 2001). The school nurse can then reinforce the teachers' educational plans or develop the program further for other age-groups to teach them how to take care of their heart.

Getting health promotion information to the parents of the children is often a challenge for the school nurse. In the West Seneca school district near Buffalo, New York, one of the district's school nurses has a column in the *District Newsletter* that is sent to all residents of the town. Each newsletter focuses on a different area of health promotion, which in March/April 2002 was on sun exposure and use of tanning booths (Krystofik, 2002a). In this way, the school nurse was able to promote the health of not only the schoolchildren but the community as well.

### Required Vaccinations for Schoolchildren

All states have laws that require that children receive immunizations, or vaccinations, against communicable diseases before they attend school (Boyer-Chuanroong and Deaver, 2000). School nurses must be up to date on the latest laws on immunizations for children in their own state.

For children entering kindergarten, these vaccinations include diphtheria, pertussis, and tetanus (the DPT series); measles, mumps, and rubella (the MMR series); polio; and others. Table 43-3 lists the mandated immunizations for school entry for each state. Chapter 26 has a more complete discussion of communicable diseases and immunizations in children.

The school nurse must keep a complete file of all of the children's vaccination records in order to meet the state's laws. These files should contain the student's name, date of birth, address, and telephone number, parents/guardians names, and contact information. It should also include their primary health care provider's name, telephone number, and

**Table 43-3** **Required Immunizations for School Entry: Elementary, Junior, and High Schools Combined**

| IMMUNIZATION | STATES REQUIRING THE IMMUNIZATION | IMMUNIZATION | STATES REQUIRING THE IMMUNIZATION |
|---|---|---|---|
| Diphtheria | All 50 states | Hepatitis B—cont'd | District of Columbia |
| Tetanus | All states except New York | | Florida |
| Polio | All 50 states | | Georgia |
| Measles | All states except North Carolina | | Hawaii |
| Chickenpox | Alabama | | Idaho |
| | Alaska | | Indiana |
| | Arkansas | | Iowa |
| | California | | Kentucky |
| | Colorado | | Louisiana |
| | Connecticut | | Maryland |
| | District of Columbia | | Massachusetts |
| | Florida | | Michigan |
| | Georgia | | Minnesota |
| | Louisiana | | Mississippi |
| | Maryland | | Missouri |
| | Massachusetts | | Nebraska |
| | Michigan | | Nevada |
| | Mississippi | | New Hampshire |
| | New York | | New York |
| | North Carolina | | North Dakota |
| | Oklahoma | | Ohio |
| | Rhode Island | | Oklahoma |
| | South Dakota | | Pennsylvania |
| | Virginia | | Rhode Island |
| Hepatitis B | Alaska | | South Carolina |
| | Arizona | | Texas |
| | Arkansas | | Utah |
| | California | | Virginia |
| | Colorado | | Washington |
| | Connecticut | | Wisconsin |
| | Delaware | | Wyoming |

From Centers for Disease Control, National Center for Chronic Disease Prevention and Health Promotion, Adolescent and School Health: *SHPPS 2000: School Health Policies and Programs Study—state-level summaries, health services, Table 3-5:* States that require specific immunizations for entry into each school level, by type of immunization. Washington, DC, CDC, 2000a, available at http://www.cdc.gov/nccdphp/dash/shpps/summaries/health_serv/table3_5.htm.

address. Most important, the information should include all the vaccinations with the dates the child received booster shots. This makes it easy for the school nurse to find out which children still need immunizations or boosters.

Because children are prevented from attending school if they have not had the required shots, the school nurse must make every effort to find missing data in the immunization record. The nurse must contact the parents to get the immunization history for the child. Written notes should be sent to each child's home at least 1 year before each new immunization is needed so that the parents have

time to get the child to their health care provider for the shots. If the parents or guardians do not speak English, these notes should be translated into the family's language (Boyer-Chuanroong and Deaver, 2000). If the parents have lost the information that gives the child's immunization history, the nurse should encourage them to contact their physician or nurse practitioner to get it.

Many problems with children not being immunized or having incomplete vaccination records may come up in families who have moved a great deal or who may not have a regular physician. The parents may have no idea whether the child has even received the shots. Families may also be without health care insurance to pay for the immunizations, or they may have insurance that does not pay for preventive care. In these cases, the parents have to pay for the immunizations, which can be expensive. Certain low-income families without health care insurance may qualify for federal programs that provide free immunizations to children. Each state has its own program, so school nurses should become familiar with what their state provides.

## Secondary Prevention in the Schools

Because secondary prevention involves caring for children when they need health care, this is the largest responsibility for the school nurse. This includes caring for ill or injured students and school employees. It also involves screening and assessing children, and referral to appropriate health agencies or providers. The school nurse uses the nursing process during secondary prevention activities. When an ill or injured child comes to the school's health office, the nurse must immediately assess the child for the degree of illness or injury.

> ### DID YOU KNOW?
>
> The health records of children in schools are to be kept private, just as they are in hospitals and other health agencies.

Children seek out the school nurse for a variety of different needs:
- Headaches
- Stomachaches
- Diarrhea
- Anxiety over being separated from the parents
- Cuts, bruises, or other injuries

In addition, children may seek reassurance from the school nurse or even appear to hide in the nurse's office. This may be due to harassment or bullying from other children in the school (Sweeney and Sweeney, 2000).

Once the assessment data are gathered, the nurse determines the course of action and follows it through the implementation and evaluation phases. This occurs for direct child health care as well as for screening children for other health problems. If assessment data identify a child as having a health problem, the school nurse continues to follow the nursing process to further care for that child.

### Nursing Care for Emergencies in the School

The school nurse cares for children who are injured or become ill in the schools. The school nurse should have an **emergency plan** in place so that a routine can be followed when emergencies occur. This plan should include making an assessment of the emergency and surveying the scene, treating the injured or ill children or teachers, and calling for backup help from the community's emergency medical units if needed.

The AAP has recommended that a plan be developed in the schools in case of an emergency when a child or staff member needs immediate care. The school nurse should make up this plan so that a staff member in the school, for example the principal or an athletic coach, can follow it in case the nurse is not in the building at the time of the emergency. The following recommendations are based on the AAP's guidelines (AAP, 2001b):
- The plan should include when to call 911 for local emergency personnel. It should include how to make arrangements to transfer a child to the hospital via ambulance in case more care is needed. If the nurse is not in the school at all times, the plan should have at least two different staff members responsible for determining if emergency care is needed. These persons should be educated by the school nurse on proper first aid techniques so that correct care is given until further help arrives.
- All staff in the schools should be taught **standard precautions.** These policies should be written into the emergency plan. Members of the athletic staff such as coaches and physical education teachers should also be up to date on emergency health procedures. If they are not, the school nurse should teach them about the policies and provide a means to review first aid procedures with them on a regular basis.
- Individualized emergency plans should be made for all students who may have a health problem that could result in an emergency situation in the school. This plan could be for the child with food allergies (e.g., to peanuts), one who has a sensitivity to insect bites that could result in anaphylactic shock, or those with chronic illnesses such as asthma, diabetes, or hemophilia.
- The children in the schools should be taught by the nurse basic first aid procedures, including standard precautions related to blood exposure. This lesson, depending on the age and grade level of the children, would allow the children to help in a playground accident while the adults are being summoned to the scene.

All emergency procedures should be written and easily accessible to anyone in the school. Research has shown that the nurse may not always be at the school and the emergency may have to be handled by a teacher, administrator, secretary, custodian, or coach (Sapien and Allen, 2001). Along with the procedures and an emergency manual written or obtained by the school nurse, there should be an injury or illness log for personnel to fill out so that there is an accurate record of what happened. Along with this form, there should be procedures for notifying the parents or legal guardians about the emergency, what was done for the child, and where the child was sent if transfer to a hospital or other medical agency was required.

Because the school nurse may have to give nursing care to a child or adult in respiratory or cardiac arrest, the nurse should have current certification in cardiopulmonary resuscitation (CPR). Other education in the area of emergency nursing would also be helpful to the school nurse, including pediatric advanced life support (PALS) or emergency nursing for pediatrics (ENPC) certification (Sapien and Allen, 2001).

## Emergency Equipment in the School Nurses' Office

The school nurse needs a great deal of equipment to deal with emergencies in the school. These needs are based on the guidelines of the AAP (AAP, 2001b). The health office should have basic items on hand (Box 43-3). Necessary equipment includes full oxygen tanks with oxygen masks of different kinds (bag-valve masks, resuscitation masks), splints for sprained or broken limbs, cervical spine collars to keep a child's head in proper alignment, and sterile dressings. Various sizes of these items are needed as children may be of different ages in the school. Another recommended item for the nurse's office includes an epinephrine autoinjector kit in case a child goes into anaphylactic shock after exposure to an allergen (AAP, 2001b; Sapien and Allen, 2001). This should be locked in a medication cabinet because there is a needle in the kit. Of course, gloves should also be available to meet standard precautions guidelines. A telephone should be available for calling emergency personnel and parents. Next to the telephone should be paper and pen so that instructions from the emergency personnel can be written down.

## Giving Medication in School

The school nurse, as part of secondary prevention, may be responsible for giving medications to children during the school day (McCarthy, Kelly, and Reed, 2000). These may include prescribed medications, medications that the parents have asked the school's nurse to give (such as cold remedies), or vitamins. In all instances, the nurse should develop a series of guidelines to help with the legal administration of medications in the school. Parents should be sure to tell the school nurse if the child is on any medications (AAP, 2001).

The prescribed drug should have the original prescription label on it and be in the original container so that

there are no errors. In addition, the AAP (1993) recommended that the physician inform the school nurse about possible side effects of the medication that may occur during the school day. If the physician does not contact the nurse first, the nurse should call the physician and ask. A current, signed parental consent form for giving the medication should also be in the student's file.

There should be a current medication (drug) book in the nurse's office so that it can be consulted for information. The nurse is responsible for giving the medication and is expected by state law to know its action, side effects, and implications. The school nurse should also have a means of contacting a pharmacist to ask questions regarding the medication if needed.

## Assessing and Screening Children at School

The AAP's Committee on School Health (AAP, 2000a) has developed guidelines for the school nurse to use when screening children in the schools. The plans are for the state-required screening of children as well as for more complete health examinations for children in the school.

Children should receive screening for vision, hearing, height and weight, oral health, tuberculosis, and scoliosis in the schools (CDC, 2000b). For each of these areas, the school nurse should keep a confidential record of all of the screening results for the children in the school. Each state has different laws regarding the screenings and the nurse should be aware of these laws. Table 43-4 gives the requirements for each of the states.

In addition, some children may not have a regular physician or other primary health care provider such as a nurse practitioner to give them health care. For these children, the AAP (2000a) has recommended that children have a physical and developmental examination in the school setting. This would include getting information on their language skills and their motor abilities. Also to be tested are their social abilities and their height and weight. As the children grow up, their level of physical growth should be noted as well as their sexual maturation. Dental assessments should also be made.

Physical examinations to play in a school sport are also given in the school. The school nurse would arrange for the sports physicals and help to monitor the examinations being done by the school's physician or nurse practitioner.

Screening for tuberculosis (TB) in schoolchildren is also done in several states. This can be a problem as the child has to have the Mantoux test or the TST test given to them first. Then they have to return to have the test site read by the nurse. If the site is positive, the child has been exposed to tuberculosis and needs further health screening. One study showed that it was more efficient to have the children screened for TB at the clinic and then have the school nurse read the test and send that information to the health clinic for follow-up (DeLago et al, 2001).

The school nurse can also screen children and adolescents for hypertension, or high blood pressure. One study in a city's middle high schools found that some teenagers

---

> ### BOX 43-3  Items for the Well-Stocked Nurse's Office
>
> - Gloves
> - Oxygen and oxygen masks
> - Suction machine
> - Sterile dressings
> - Splints
> - Bed or cot
> - Locked medication cabinet
> - Epinephrine autoinjector kit

## Table 43-4 States That Require Districts or Schools to Screen Students for Health Problems

| STATE | VISION | HEARING | HEIGHT AND WEIGHT | DENTAL | SCOLIOSIS | TUBERCULOSIS |
|---|---|---|---|---|---|---|
| Alabama | | | | | X | |
| Alaska | X | X | | | | X |
| Arizona | | X | | | | |
| Arkansas | X | X | | | X | |
| California | X | X | | | X | |
| Colorado | X | X | | | | |
| Connecticut | X | X | | | X | X |
| Delaware | X | X | | | X | |
| District of Columbia | X | X | X | X | X | X |
| Florida | X | X | X | | X | |
| Georgia | X | X | | X | X | |
| Hawaii | | | | | | X |
| Idaho | | | | | | |
| Illinois | X | X | | | | X |
| Indiana | | | | | | |
| Iowa | | | | | | |
| Kansas | X | | | X | | |
| Kentucky | X | X | X | | X | |
| Louisiana | X | X | | | | |
| Maine | X | X | | | X | |
| Maryland | X | X | | | X | |
| Massachusetts | X | X | X | | X | |
| Michigan | X | X | | | | |
| Minnesota | | | | | | |
| Mississippi | X | X | | | | |
| Missouri | X | X | | X | | |
| Montana | | | | | | |
| Nebraska | X | X | X | X | X | |
| Nevada | X | X | | | X | |
| New Hampshire | | | X | | | |
| New Jersey | X | X | X | | X | X |
| New Mexico | X | X | X | | | |
| New York | X | X | X | X | X | |
| North Carolina | | | | | | |
| North Dakota | | | | | | |
| Ohio | X | X | | | | |
| Oklahoma | | | | | | |
| Oregon | X | X | | | | |
| Pennsylvania | X | X | X | X | X | X |
| Rhode Island | X | X | X | X | X | |
| South Carolina | | | | | | |
| South Dakota | | | | | X | |
| Tennessee | X | X | | | | |

From Centers for Disease Control, National Center for Chronic Disease Prevention and Health Promotion, Adolescent and School Health: *SHPPS 2000, school health policies and programs study: health services, Table 3.9.* States that require districts or schools to screen students for health problems, by health problem. Washington, DC, CDC, 2000b, available at http://www.cdc.gov/nccdphp/dash/shpps/summaries/health_serv/table3_9.htm.

*Continued*

**Table 43-4  States That Require Districts or Schools to Screen Students for Health Problems—cont'd**

| STATE | VISION | HEARING | HEIGHT AND WEIGHT | DENTAL | SCOLIOSIS | TUBERCULOSIS |
|-------|--------|---------|-------------------|--------|-----------|--------------|
| Texas | X | X | | | | |
| Utah | X | X | | X | X | X |
| Vermont | X | X | X | | | |
| Virginia | X | X | | | | |
| Washington | X | X | | | X | |
| West Virginia | | X | | | X | X |
| Wisconsin | | | | | | |
| Wyoming | | | | | | |

From Centers for Disease Control, National Center for Chronic Disease Prevention and Health Promotion, Adolescent and School Health: *SHPPS 2000: school health policies and programs study, health services, Table 3.9.* States that require districts or schools to screen students for health problems, by health problem. Washington, DC, CDC, 2000b, available at http://www.cdc.gov/nccdphp/dash/shpps/summaries/health_serv/table3_9.htm.

had high blood pressure (Meininger et al, 2001). These teens can be taught techniques to reduce their blood pressure to reduce their risk of cardiovascular disease as they get older.

## Screening Children for Lice

School nurses also must screen children for lice infestation. According to one study, between 6 and 12 million cases of lice occur every year in the United States, and most are in school-age children. Lice are found most often in white middle-class children because of their oval hair shafts. Lice are more often seen in clean hair as well. Therefore, the suggestion that lice is associated with unclean homes in poverty areas is incorrect (Kirchofer, Price, and Telljohann, 2001). The school nurse needs to check children for lice because in many areas, children with lice are excluded from school. During the "lice check," the nurse must check the children's hair for both lice and nits (Ten Steps, 2000).

It is the responsibility of the school nurse to teach children, parents, and teachers how to prevent lice and treat cases of infestation. The nurse can do this by teaching children not to share combs and hats, and parents to completely treat the child with the anti-lice medications. Parents also need to be told to remove all nits from the head with a fine-toothed comb and to wash all bed linens and clothing (Kirchofer et al, 2001).

## Identification of Child Abuse or Neglect

The school nurse is mandated by state laws to report suspected cases of child abuse or neglect. These laws differ from state to state and the nurse should be aware of the particular requirements for reporting in each state.

When the nurse identifies a child who may be abused, or receives information from a teacher or other staff member that leads to the belief that a child has been abused, the nurse must contact the appropriate legal authorities as well as the school's principal. A confidential file should be made about the incident. However, the nurse should let the government authorities, usually the state or county child protection department, look into the suspected case. In all cases, the child should be protected from harm, and those who have no right to know that child abuse or neglect is suspected should not be given any information.

## Communicating With Health Care Providers

The school nurse often makes an assessment of a child that requires referral to the child's family physician or other health care provider. The findings from these assessments must be communicated accurately to the child's parent

---

**HOW TO  Develop Good Relationships With Families**

School nurses need to have good relationships with families. The nurse can make this possible by doing the following:

1. Being visible at school events
2. Sending home invitations for parents and guardians to call the nurse at any time
3. Inviting parents to visit the school health office
4. Calling parents or guardians to ask about ill children
5. Offering to help families cope with children who have long-term illnesses
6. Acting as a referral source for families with health care needs
7. Including parents and members of the community in health education activities

and the provider. The nurse must be able to get the information quickly and accurately to the child's parents.

One way to do this is to write a detailed report about the findings. This information can be given to the child to give to his or her parents. However, the child may lose the report before it gets to there. The information can be mailed to the parents, but this takes more time. Perhaps the best way is to telephone the parents, telling them that the child needs to see the physician or nurse practitioner and that the child will be bringing the information home that day. In this way, the parents can ask the child for the report and the child is aware that the parents expect it.

One state, Nebraska, developed a plan where the school nurse writes the health care problem information on a referral card for the parents to give to the child's physician. Then the physician can follow up on the problem and write information that the school nurse needs to know regarding the child's diagnosis, the plan of care, and special needs in the school for the child's care. This *School Nurse Referral Care Program* is one way to help the nurse know what was found in the health care appointment that the nurse recommended (Nebraska School Nurses Improve Communication, 2000).

## Efforts to Prevent Suicide

Suicide is the third leading cause of death in teenagers. Recommendations have been made about reducing the incidence of suicide in teenagers. A suicide prevention program developed in one school district, discussed below, contains ideas for the school nurse to use. Suicide prevention must be addressed by school nurses. Nurses can lead educational programs within the schools to emphasize coping strategies and stress management techniques for children and adolescents who have problems, and to teach about the risk factors. The school nurse can teach faculty members to look for the risk factors. The school nurse can also help organize a peer assistance program to help teenagers cope with school stresses (King, 2001).

If a student threatens suicide at school, the school nurse should intervene by ensuring the safety of the student and by removing him or her from the school situation immediately. While parents are being notified, the nurse should assess the child's suicide risk and refer the child or teenager to crisis intervention or mental health services.

In the unfortunate instance where a teenager who attended the school has committed suicide, the school nurse is called upon to help the school population, both students and teachers, cope with the death. Grief counseling should be set up and coordinated by the school nurse. In addition, further assessments should be made regarding the suicide potential among the deceased teenager's friends, as suicide clusters have been seen to occur.

## Violence at School

It has been estimated that over 1 million high school students carried guns to school in 1998 (AACAP, 2000a, 2000b). In the past several years, there have been school shootings by students against other students and teachers. This has happened in at least seven states and one foreign country. In each of these cases, a student or students brought firearms to school and used them resulting in injuries and deaths of students and teachers (Associated Press, 2002; Steger, 2000; Williams and Kalkenberg, 2002).

The school nurse may be able to help identify students who will act in this way. Furthermore, the nurse can provide health education classes to help children learn positive ways of dealing with conflict.

The mother of a murdered girl in Padukah, Kentucky, herself a registered nurse, stated that there are six characteristics that may help point out a student who may be thinking about such drastic violence (Steger, 2000):

- *Venting:* having mood swings
- *Vocalizing:* threatening others
- *Vandalizing:* damaging property
- *Victimizing:* sees themselves as a victim
- *Vying:* belonging to gangs
- *Viewing:* witnesses the abuse of others

By helping to identify the student who might be considering school violence or by teaching students and teachers about these warning signs in students, the school nurse may be able to help prevent violent actions through education and follow-up of children who need help.

## School Crisis Teams: Responding to Disasters

Events that occur in or near schools may cause a crisis for children, teachers, and staff. Possible crises include the death of a student or teacher due to accident, injury, homicide or suicide; an accident or fire in the school or community; or a disaster in the community that affects many children's families, such as a tornado, hurricane, or earthquake (Chemtob, Nakashima, and Hamada, 2002).

Schools should have crisis plans in place to help the children, teachers, parents, and community cope with the sudden event. **Crisis teams** should be in place to help everyone respond quickly to the crisis, to ensure the safety of the school, and to follow up on the effects of the crisis on the members of the school.

The crisis plan should include an administrative policy made either for the entire school district or, if the schools are large, for each individual school. The plan should include the names of the persons on the crisis team: the superintendent of the school district, the school nurse, the guidance counselor, the school psychologist or social worker, teachers, police or school security, clergy from the community, and parents.

The school nurse is involved with triaging injured people, working with the emergency medical personnel as they care for the injured or ill, and assessing the degree of shock, stress, or grieving in the children, teachers, parents, and others in or near the school. The school nurse is also there to be a counselor to help everyone cope with the emotional parts of this serious event (Starr, 2002) (Box 43-4).

The nurse can help the crisis team make a checklist for everyone to follow that tells what to do in every possible

---

**BOX 43-4    Dealing With a Disaster: Responsibilities of the School Nurse**

- Provide triage.
- Communicate with emergency medical personnel.
- Assess the school community for the presence of shock and stress.
- Recommend reduced television viewing of the disaster.
- Provide grief counseling.
- Communicate with the children, parents, and school personnel.
- Follow up with assessment of children for anxiety, depression, regression, and posttraumatic stress disorder.

---

Modified from Calarco C: Preparing for a crisis: crisis team development, *J Sch Nurs* 15(1):46-48, 1999; Starr NB: Helping children and families deal with the psychological aspects of disaster, *J Pediatr Health Care* 16(1):36-39, 2002.

---

**BOX 43-5    States That Require School Nurses to Participate in Individualized Education Plans for Students**

| | | |
|---|---|---|
| Alaska | Louisiana | Pennsylvania |
| Connecticut | Maryland | Rhode Island |
| Delaware | Massachusetts | Vermont |
| Florida | Missouri | West Virginia |
| Hawaii | New Mexico | Wisconsin |
| Illinois | Oregon | |

---

Compiled from Centers for Disease Control, National Center for Chronic Disease Prevention and Health Promotion, Adolescent and School Health: SHPPS 2000: *School Health Policies and Programs Study—state-level summaries, health services, Table 3-11*, States that require school nurses to participate in the development of individualized education plans (IEPs) or individualized health plans (IHPs), Washington, DC, CDC, 2000d, available at http://www.cdc.gov/nccdphp/dash/shpps/summaries/health_serv/table3_11.htm.

---

crisis situation. Then, at the end of the crisis, the crisis team should take time to counsel all of the people who helped in the crisis including the teachers, emergency personnel, and parents, as well as the children. That way everyone can talk about the crisis. The crisis plan should be reviewed every year to see what parts of the plan need updating (Calarco, 1999).

## Tertiary Prevention in the Schools

Using the nursing process, the school nurse gives nursing care related to tertiary prevention when working with children who have long-term or chronic illnesses or with special needs. The nurse participates in developing an individual education plan (IEP) for students with long-term health needs (Box 43-5).

For example, nurses must have information about children's medications to be given during school hours. They also need to know if the children need any therapy during the school day, such as physical or occupational therapy. If the child has a hearing or vision problem, the nurse may need to ask the teacher to seat the child in the best place in the classroom so the child can see or hear the teacher and other children better. If a child is in a wheelchair or uses crutches, the school building itself may need to be altered so that the child can get around the school and use the restrooms. It is the responsibility of the nurse to tell

---

**DID YOU KNOW?**

Children with disabilities who live in residential care facilities because of their long-term health needs go to school every day.

---

the school's administrators about any needs such as these (AAP, 2000a).

### Children With Asthma

Asthma is the leading cause of children being absent from school due to a chronic illness. Children may be hospitalized with an asthma attack or they may have just returned home from the hospital. Asthma can also be caused by allergic triggers that affect children in the school. Possible culprits are chalk dust from the blackboards, molds or mildew in the school, or dander from pets that live in some classrooms (Clearing the Air, 2001).

There may also be concerns about the quality of the air in the school building because many doors are shut. There are industrial arts classes and other sources of air pollution in the school (U.S. Environmental Protection Agency, 2000). The school nurse can keep track of the indoor air quality of the school so that school administrators have data about what can affect the children. Figure 43-3 contains the questions developed by the U.S. Environmental Protection Agency that the school nurse should answer regarding the air quality of the school.

The nurse uses tertiary prevention when helping children who have asthma. This includes administering, or helping them use, their inhalers or other asthma rescue medications. It also includes teaching the teachers, children, and parents about asthma and ways that can reduce the factors that the child may be allergic to in the classroom (Perry and Toole, 2000). Many schools have management programs in place to help children with asthma. As an example, the Buffalo Schools Asthma Alliance provides the latest information to school nurses on how to care for children with asthma in schools (Center for Asthma and Environmental Exposure, 1999).

# Health Officer/School Nurse

*This checklist discusses three major topic areas:*
Student Health Records Maintenance
Public Health and Personal Hygiene Education
Health Officer's Office

**Instructions:**
1. Read the IAQ *Backgrounder*.
2. Read each item on this Checklist.
3. Check the diamond(s) as appropriate or check the circle if you need additional help with an activity.
4. Return this checklist to the IAQ Coordinator and keep a copy for future reference.

Name: _____

Room or Area: _____

School: _____

Date Completed: _____

Signature: _____

### MAINTAIN STUDENT HEALTH RECORDS

There is evidence to suggest that children, pregnant women, and senior citizens are more likely to develop health problems from poor air quality than most adults. Indoor Air Quality (IAQ) problems are most likely to affect those with preexisting health conditions and those who are exposed to tobacco smoke. Student health records should include information about known allergies and other medically documented conditions, such as asthma, as well as any reported sensitivity to chemicals. Privacy considerations may limit the student health information that can be disclosed, but to the extent possible, information about students' potential sensitivity to IAQ problems should be provided to teachers. This is especially true for classes involving potential irritants (e.g., gaseous or particle emissions from art, science, industrial/vocational education sources). Health records and records of health-related complaints by students and staff are useful for evaluating potential IAQ-related complaints.

**Include information about sensitivities to IAQ problems in student health records**
• Allergies, including reports of chemical sensitivities.
• Asthma.
◇ Completed health records exist for each student.
◇ Health records are being updated.
O Need help obtaining information about student allergies and other health factors.

**Track health-related complaints by students and staff**
• Keep a log of health complaints that notes the symptoms, location and time of symptom onset, and exposure to pollutant sources.
• Watch for trends in health complaints, especially in timing or location of complaints.
◇ Have a comprehensive health complaint logging system.
◇ Developing a comprehensive health complaint logging system.
O Need help developing a comprehensive health complaint logging system.

**Recognize indicators that health problems may be IAQ**
• Complaints are associated with particular times of the day or week.
• Other occupants in the same area experience similar problems.

• The problem abates or ceases, either immediately or gradually, when an occupant leaves the building and recurs when the occupant returns.
• The school has recently been renovated or refurnished.
• The occupant has recently started working with new or different materials or equipment.
• New cleaning or pesticide products or practices have been introduced into the school.
• Smoking is allowed in the school.
• A new warm-blooded animal has been introduced into the classroom.
◇ Understand indicators of IAQ-related problems.
O Need help understanding indicators of IAQ-related problems.

### HEALTH AND HYGIENE EDUCATION

Schools are unique buildings from a public health perspective because they accommodate more people within a smaller area than most buildings. This proximity increases the potential for airborne contaminants (germs, odors, and constituents of personal products) to pass between students. Raising awareness about the effects of personal habits on the well-being of others can help reduce IAQ-related problems.

**Obtain *Indoor Air Quality: An Introduction for Health Professionals***
• Contact IAQ INFO, 800-438-4318.
◇ Already have this EPA guidance document.
◇ Guide is on order.
O Cannot obtain this guide.

**Inform students and staff about the importance of good hygiene in preventing the spread of airborne contagious diseases**
• Provide written materials to students (local public health agencies may have information suitable for older students).
• Provide individual instruction/counseling where necessary.
◇ Written materials and counseling available.
◇ Compiling information for counseling and distribution.
O Need help compiling information or implementing counseling program.

**Figure 43-3** Indoor air quality checklist. *(From U.S. Environmental Protection Agency:* Indoor air quality [IAQ] tools for schools: health officer/school nurse checklist, 2000, *available at http://www.epa.gov/iaq/schools/tfs/healthof.html.)*

*Continued*

**Provide information about IAQ and health**
- Help teachers develop activities that reduce exposure to indoor air pollutants for students with IAQ sensitivities, such as those with asthma or allergies (contact the American Lung Association [ALA], the National Association of School Nurses [NASN], or the Asthma and Allergy Foundation of America [AAFA]). Contact information is also available in the IAQ Coordinator's Guide.
- Collaborate with parent-teacher groups to offer family IAQ education programs.
- Conduct a workshop for teachers on health issues that covers IAQ.
◇ Have provided information to parents and staff.
◇ Developing information and education programs for parents and staff.
O Need help developing information and education program for parents and staff.

**Establish an information and counseling program regarding smoking**
- Provide free literature on smoking and secondhand smoke.
- Sponsor a quit-smoking program and similar counseling programs in collaboration with the ALA.
◇ "No Smoking" information and programs in place.
◇ "No Smoking" information and programs in planning.
O Need help with a "No Smoking" program.

**HEALTH OFFICER'S OFFICE**

Since the health office may be frequented by sick students and staff, it is important to take steps that can help prevent transmission of airborne diseases to uninfected students and staff (see your IAQ Coordinator for help with the following activities).

**Ensure that the ventilation system is properly operating**
- Ventilation system is operated when the area(s) is occupied.
- Provide an adequate amount of outdoor air to the area(s). There should be at least 15 cubic feet of outdoor air supplied per occupant.
- Air filters are clean and properly installed.
- Air removed from the area(s) does not circulate through the ventilation system into other occupied areas.
◇ Ventilation system operating adequately.
O Need help with ventilation-related activities.

☐ **No Problems to Report.** I have completed all the activities on this checklist, and I do not need help in any areas.

**Figure 43-3, cont'd** Indoor air quality checklist.Indoor air quality checklist. *(From U.S. Environmental Protection Agency:* Indoor air quality [IAQ] tools for schools: health officer/school nurse checklist, *2000, available at http://www.epa.gov/iaq/schools/tfs/healthof.html.)*

## Children With Diabetes Mellitus

New York State has estimated that in the year 2000, over 12,000 children attending school have diabetes. Ten percent to 20% have non–insulin-dependent diabetes, and the rest are diagnosed with insulin-dependent diabetes mellitus (New York Sate Department of Health, 2000). The school nurse must establish a plan of care for children with diabetes. This includes plans to monitor blood glucose and giving insulin or other medications during the school day. Special nutritional needs also need to be discussed (American Diabetes Association, 1999).

## Children Who Are Autistic

Because all children are expected to attend some school regardless of their illness, children with autism go to regular schools in most cases. Because a child with autism has severe communication problems, the school nurse gives help to the child, the teachers, and the parents so that the child's school day is pleasant. The nurse can give the child prescribed medications for mood or prevention of seizures. The nurse also is responsible for preparing the teachers about the communication problems that the child may have. The nurse may recommend the use of sign language, picture boards, or other types of communication devices that are used by the child. In addition, the nurse can teach the parents about autism. The nurse can also help parents work with others in the health care system so that the child can have a positive learning experience at school (Cade and Tidwell, 2001).

**HOW TO** **Help Injured Children Return to School After Long Absences**

This article discussed how a school nurse helped a sixth-grade boy who had received serious facial burns return to school. Enrique was afraid of how the children would respond to the pressure mask he wore to minimize future scarring. The nurse had a meeting with Enrique's mother and the school's principal and also contacted nurses from the hospitals' burn unit. The school nurse came up with the following plan:

1. The school nurse taught the boy's classmates about burns and their treatment.
2. The boy came to class with the nurse and showed his classmates his face without this pressure mask. He then put it back on.
3. Both Enrique and the nurse answered the children's questions.
4. Changes were made in his schedule so he could be out of the sun during the school day and during gym time.

The nurse found that Enrique's burns were soon forgotten and he was accepted by his friends.

From Carnes PF: Enrique and friends: a sixth-grader faces his classmates for the first time following a disfiguring accident, *Nursing 2000* 30(10):57-61, 2000.

**WHAT DO YOU THINK?**
Children with mental disabilities attend school. How would this affect other children in the classroom?

## Children With Special Needs in the Schools

Children who need urinary catheterization, dressing changes, peripheral or central line intravenous catheter maintenance, tracheotomy suctioning, gastrostomy or other tube feedings, or intravenous medication also attend schools. The nurse may supervise a health aide who is assigned to the child to care for complex nursing needs. In all these cases, the school nurse provides tertiary care to maintain the child's health. The nurse has the skills needed to assess the child's well-being. In addition, the nurse may have to teach another person in the school how to care for the child in case the nurse is not in the building when the child needs help. It is the responsibility of the school nurse to keep up with the latest health care information through inservice programs (Krystofik, 2002b).

Children with HIV or AIDS may also attend school. Because of privacy and confidentiality laws, the school nurse may not even know that the child attends the school. In these cases, the nurse may be aware of the child's HIV status either by direct notification from the parents or physician, or just by knowing that certain drugs the child is on during the school day are anti-HIV medications. In all cases, the nurse cannot release that information to anyone.

As part of regular health education in the school, the school nurse can provide education about HIV/AIDS prevention and risks, to the children, school employees, and community (AAP, 1998). The school nurse should also be part of the school health advisory committee to develop an HIV/AIDS health curriculum that teaches not only about HIV/AIDS prevention but also about the disease itself, so that children and families are not afraid to go to school with children who have the disease. Continuing education programs can be useful to teach the teachers and parents about the disease (AAP, 1998).

## Children With DNR Orders
## and the School Nurse

As part of tertiary prevention, the school nurse also maintains the health of children with terminal diseases who go to school. These children have been largely mainstreamed into the regular school population. The PL 92-142 Education for All Handicapped Children Act stated in 1975 that all children should go to school in the "least restrictive environment" (AAP, 2000b). Therefore, there may be children who have **do-not-resuscitate orders** (DNR orders) at school, and some may die at school. DNR orders are signed by the parents and the physician according to the state's law. Under law, the school nurse is bound to obey the DNR order; however, it is not clear how the schools view them.

The AAP's committees on school health and bioethics proposed a set of guidelines in 2000 to help school health providers and the schools decide what to do when a child with a DNR order attends the school. A formal request should be sent to the school and the school board from the physician regarding the written DNR order. The

school nurses should be involved in discussions regarding when to use the DNR order. The decision not to do anything for a dying child, and how to function if the child were to suddenly face death, is made in advance in discussions between the school nurse, the parents, the physician, and the school officials.

When a child dies in school, the nurse is responsible for helping the children who witnessed the death. The nurse becomes a grief counselor and helps the children and teachers cope with the death. Further education about death and dying given by the school nurse would also help the school community cope with death in the schools.

## Homebound Children

Even though the laws regarding disabled persons state that all children should go to school, some children cannot do so. Instead, they may be taught in the home or in another institutional setting such as the hospital. In these situations, the school nurse should be a liaison between the child's teacher, physician, school administrators, and parents regarding the child's needs. The nurse helps these individuals make up the child's IEP so that it is appropriate for the child and does not remove necessary learning from the plan. The child should be allowed to go to school when he or she is able. Then, the school nurse coordinates the child's health care needs and classes (AAP, 2000c).

## Pregnant Teenagers and Teenage Mothers
## at School

Many teenage girls who are pregnant attend school. Therefore, the school nurse may provide on-going care to the mother. Although this may appear to be primary prevention, it is tertiary prevention because adolescent pregnancies are considered to be at high-risk. This is discussed in more detail in Chapters 26 and 34.

## CONTROVERSIES IN SCHOOL NURSING

School nursing has evolved into a complex health care role, and some areas of the field still cause controversy—for example, birth control education and giving out birth control to students in the schools. A study carried out in South Carolina regarding whether school-based health clinics should provide contraception services found that the community wanted gynecologic health care available to the adolescents. However it was not to be given at the school-based center. They agreed that abstinence sex education could be provided in the schools, but they wanted all other services to be referred by the nurses to community agencies (Lindley, Reininger, and Saunders, 2001).

Differences of opinion exist about giving teenage girls emergency contraception. In Europe, France has voted to allow school nurses to give out "morning-after pills" to teenage girls who ask for them in junior high and senior high schools (French Distribute, 2002). Because there are differences in opinion relating to sex education and reproductive services in the schools, the school nurse should make an effort to communicate with the community,

**Table 43-5 On-line Resources for School Nurses**

| ORGANIZATION | INTERNET ADDRESS |
|---|---|
| The American Academy of Child and Adolescent Psychiatry | www.aacap.org |
| American Academy of Pediatrics | www.aap.org |
| National Association of School Nurses | www.nasn.org |
| Center for Health and Health Care in the Schools | www.healthinschools.org |

From Centers for Disease Control and Prevention: *At a glance. School health programs: an investment in our nation's future 2001.* Washington, DC, 2001, CDC, p 3, available at http://www.cdc.gov/nccdphp/dash/00binaries/ataglanc.pdf.

school board, teachers, parents, and students about what they think about different types of services in the schools.

## ETHICS IN SCHOOL NURSING

The school nurse may be faced with ethical issues in the schools. For example, a child may have a DNR order that the parents wish to be used if the child dies at school (see earlier), but following the DNR order may be against the nurse's personal beliefs. Perhaps a girl asks the nurse where she can get an abortion, and wishes to talk to the school nurse about how she feels, but the nurse is against abortions. Or a teenager asks for emergency contraception, which the nurse cannot condone (Roye and Johnsen, 2002). In these cases, the nurse must give nursing care to the student client and keep personal beliefs out of the discussion. However, if the nurse feels so strongly that he or she cannot work with the situation, then another school nurse should be called for help, or the student should be referred to other health providers who can give the care the student needs.

## FUTURE TRENDS IN SCHOOL NURSING

The future of school nursing is strong. The amount of health care being given in the schools is increasing. In the future, school nursing will entail telehealth and telecounseling to teach health education (Whitten et al, 2001). The internet will be used by school nurses to work with children and parents. On-line resources are listed in Table 43-5. The school nurse is responsible for keeping up with the latest changes in health care and health practice so that the health of children in the schools can be enhanced by new trends in health care.

## THE CUTTING EDGE

School nurses communicate with some families by using the internet.

From Whitten P et al: School-based telehealth: an empirical analysis of teacher, nurse, and administrator perceptions, *J Sch Health* 71(5):173-180, 2001.

## ■ Practice Application

Erin and Sandy, student nurses in their last semester of nursing school, were invited by their former high school to give a talk on nursing as a career at the school's career day. During their presentation, which included a multimedia PowerPoint video presentation on nursing, a student asked, "Why would I want to be a school nurse? Ours just sits in the office handing out bandages"

How should Erin and Sandy respond?

A. Talk about the many things that school nurses are responsible for.

B. Ask how other high school students in the room feel about this comment.

C. Use the classroom's intercom to ask the school nurse to come to the classroom.

D. Discuss the ways the school nurse prevents injuries from becoming infected.

Answer is in the back of the book.

## ■ Key Points

- School nurses provide health care for children and families.
- In the early 1900s, school nurses screened children for infectious diseases.
- By 2002, school nurses provided direct care, health education, counseling, case management, and community outreach.
- The National Association of School Nurses (NASN) is the professional organization for school nurses.
- School nurses have varying educational levels depending on state laws.
- The U.S. government supports school-based health centers, school-linked programs, and full-service school-based health centers.
- Healthy People 2010 has objectives to enhance the health of children in the schools.
- Primary prevention provides health promotion and education to prevent childhood injuries and substance abuse.

- The school nurse monitors the children for all of their state-mandated immunizations for school entry.
- Secondary prevention involves screening children for illnesses and providing direct nursing care.
- School nurses develop plans for emergency care in the schools.
- Giving medications to children in the school must be monitored carefully to prevent errors.
- School health nurses are mandated reporters to tell the authorities about suspected cases of child abuse and/or neglect.
- Tertiary prevention includes caring for children with long-term health needs, including asthma and disabling conditions.
- School nurses carry out catheterizations, suctioning, gastrostomy feedings, and other skills in the schools.
- Some ethical dilemmas in the schools are related to women's health care.
- Some nurses use the internet to help communicate with children and their families.

3. Arrange to visit an elementary school health office during screening activities. Observe the interaction between the nurse and the children. Describe how the nurse is using the nursing process during the screening process.
4. Organize a group of nursing students to volunteer at a school health fair. Develop a health education booth for the fair. Describe how the health information can be used by the children, families, and the community.
5. Attend the annual school board meeting that discusses the budget for the next year. Analyze the budget for health services. How will this be adequate to care for the children? What issues influence the budgetary process?
6. On the internet, focus on your state's health department. What trends do you see relating to health in the schools?

## Clinical Decision-Making Activities

1. For the state where you live, make a list of the immunizations required for children attending schools. Then contrast this to the immunizations you received when in school. How has this changed over the years?
2. Contact the nurse in your former high school. Interview the nurse, focusing on the major focus of the role. Describe what the nurse likes best and least about the role. What changes can be made to make the responsibilities easier?

## Additional Resources

These related resources are found either in the appendix at the back of this book or on the book's website at **http://evolve.elsevier.com/Stanhope.**

**evolve** Evolve Website

WebLinks: Healthy People 2010

## References

Allers-Korostynski M: Adult learning center: a unique adventure for a school nurse, *J Sch Nurs* 16(2):50-51, 2000.

American Academy of Child and Adolescent Psychiatry, Gaensbauer T, Wamboldt M: *Facts about gun violence,* 2000a, available at http://www.aacap.org/info_families/NationalFacts/coGunViol.htm.

American Academy of Child and Adolescent Psychiatry: *Policy statement, children and guns,* 2000b, available at http://www.aacap.org/publications/policy/polstgun.htm.

American Academy of Child and Adolescent Psychiatry: *Facts for families: psychiatric medications for children and adolescents, part III: questions to ask,* no. 51, 2001, available at http://www.aacap.org/publications/factsfam/medquest.htm.

American Academy of Pediatrics, Committee on Pediatric AIDS: Human immunodeficiency virus/acquired immunodeficiency syndrome education in schools, *Pediatrics* 101(5):933-935, 1998, available at http://www.aap.org/policy/Re9741.html

American Academy of Pediatrics, Committee on School Health: Guidelines for the administration of medication in school, *Pediatrics* 92(3):499-500, 1993 [reaffirmed 1997], available at http://www.aap.org/policy/04524.html.

American Academy of Pediatrics, Committee on Injury and Poison Prevention: Skateboard and scooter injuries, *Pediatrics* 109(3):542-543, 2002.

American Academy of Pediatrics, Committee on School Health: School health assessments, *Pediatrics* 105(4):875-877, 2000a.

American Academy of Pediatrics, Committee on School Health and Committee on Bioethics: Do not resuscitate orders in schools, *Pediatrics* 105(4):878-879, 2000b, available at http://www.aap.org/policy/re9842.html.

American Academy of Pediatrics, Committee on School Health: Home, hospital, and other non-school-based instruction for children and adolescents who are medically unable to attend school, *Pediatrics* 106(5):1154-1155, 2000c, available at http://www.aap.org/policy/re9956.html.

American Academy of Pediatrics, Committee on School Health: School health centers and other integrated school health services, *Pediatrics* 107(1):198-201, 2001a, available at http://www.aap.org/policy/re0030.html.

American Academy of Pediatrics, Committee on School Health: Guidelines for emergency medical care in school, *Pediatrics* 107(2):435-436, 2001b, available at http://www.aap.org/policy/re9954.html.

American Academy of Pediatrics, Committee on School Health: The role of the school nurse in providing school health services, *Pediatrics* 108(5):1231-1232, 2001c.

American Diabetes Association: Care of children with diabetes in the school and day care setting, *Diabetes Care* 22 (Suppl 1):S94-S97, 1999.

Associated Press: 18 slain in German school, *Buffalo News,* p A-1, April 26, 2002.

Bernardo LM, Gardner MJ, Seibel K: Playground injuries in children: a review and Pennsylvania trauma center experience, *J Soc Pediatr Nurs* 6(1):11-20, 2001.

Betz CL: Use of 504 plans for children and youth with disabilities: nursing application, *Pediatr Nurs* 27(4):347-352, 2001.

Boyer-Chuanroong L, Deaver P: Meeting the preteen vaccine law: a pilot program in urban middle schools, *J Sch Health* 70(2):39-44, 2000.

Cade M, Tidwell S: Autism and the school nurse, *J Sch Health* 71(3):96-100, 2001.

Calarco C: Preparing for a crisis: crisis team development, *J Sch Nurs* 15(1):46-48, 1999.

Carnes PF: Enrique and friends: a sixth-grader faces his classmates for the first time following a disfiguring accident, *Nursing* 30(10):57-61, 2000.

Carpenter LM, Mueller CS: Evaluating health care seeking behaviors of parents using a school-based health clinic, *J Sch Health* 71(10):497-499, 2001.

Center for Asthma and Environmental Exposure, Buffalo Schools Asthma Alliance: *Managing an asthma attack in school,* Buffalo, NY, 1999, State University of New York at Buffalo.

Centers for Disease Control and Prevention, Division of Adolescent and School Health: *At a glance. School health programs: an investment in our nation's future 1999,* Washington, DC, 1999, CDC, available at http://www.cdc.gov/nccd-php/dash/ataglanc1999.pdf.

Centers for Disease Control and Prevention, National Center for Chronic Disease Prevention and Health Promotion, Adolescent and School Health: *SHPPS 2000: School Health Policies and Programs Study: state-level summaries, health services, Table 3-5:* States that require specific immunizations for entry into each school level, by type of immunization, Washington, DC: CDC, 2000a, available at http://www.cdc.gov/nccdphp/dash/shpps/summaries/health_serv/table3_5.htm.

Centers for Disease Control and Prevention, National Center for Chronic Disease Prevention and Health Promotion, Adolescent and School Health: *SHPPS 2000, School Health Policies and Programs Study: Table 3.9,* States that require districts or schools to screen students for health problems, by health problem, Washington, DC, CDC, 2000b, available at http://www.cdc.gov/nccdphp/dash/shpps/summaries/health_serv/table3_9.htm.

Centers for Disease Control and Prevention, National Center for Chronic Disease Prevention and Health Promotion, Adolescent and School Health: *SHPPS 2000: School Health Policies and Programs Study: state-level summaries, health services, Table 3-10,* States that require specific student-to-nurse and school-to-nurse ratios, Washington, DC, CDC, 2000c, available at http://www.cdc.gov/nccdphp/dash/shpps/summaries/health_serv/table3_10.htm.

Centers for Disease Control and Prevention, National Center for Chronic Disease Prevention and Health Promotion, Adolescent and School Health: *SHPPS 2000: School Health Policies and Programs Study: state-level summaries, health services, Table 3-11,* States that require school nurses to participate in the development of individualized education plans (IEPs) or individualized health plans (IHPs), Washington, DC, CDC, 2000d, available at http://www.cdc.gov/nccdphp/dash/shpps/summaries/health_serv/table3_11.htm.

Centers for Disease Control and Prevention, National Center for Chronic Disease Prevention and Health Promotion, Adolescent and School Health: *SHPPS 2000: School Health Policies and Programs Study: state-level summaries, health services, Table 3-13,* States that require newly hired school nurses to have specific educational backgrounds, Washington, DC, CDC, 2000e, available at http://www.cdc.gov/nccdphp/dash/shpps/summaries/health_serv/table3_13.htm.

Centers for Disease Control and Prevention: *At a glance: School health programs—an investment in our nation's future 2001,* Washington, DC, 2001, CDC, available at http://www.cdc.gov/nccd-php/dash/00binaries/ataglanc.pdf.

Chemtob CM, Nakashima JP, Hamada RS: Psychosocial intervention for post-disaster trauma symptoms in elementary school children: a controlled community field study, *Arch Pediatr Adolesc Med* 156(3):211-216, 2002.

"Children turn to school nurses for advice," *Aust Nurs J* 9(6):15, 2001-2002.

"Clearing the air on asthma," *NEA Today* 19(8):34, 2001.

Croghan E: Do not underestimate the school nurse, *Nurs Times* 95(20):47, 1999.

Cromwell GE: The school nurse and her relationship to the school patrons, *J Sch Health* 71(8):390, 2001, reprinted from *J Sch Health* 19(5):142-143, 1946.

Deal LW et al: Unintentional injuries in childhood: analysis and recommendations, *Future Child* 10(1):4-22, 2000.

DeLago CW et al: Collaboration with school nurses: improving the effectiveness of tuberculosis screening, *Arch Pediatr Adolesc Med* 155(12):1369-1373, 2001.

Descoteaux A: The school nurse manager: a catalyst for innovation in school health programming, *J Sch Nurs* 17(6):296-299, 2001.

Duncan C: Health hang-out for East Enders, *Nurs Times* 96(30):33, 2000.

Duncan P, Igoe JB: School health services. In Marx E, Wooley SF, with Northrop D, editors, *Health is academic: a guide to coordinated school health programs,* pp 169-194, New York, 1998, Teachers College Press.

Farrior KC et al: A community pediatric prevention partnership: linking schools, providers, and tertiary care services, *J Sch Health* 70(3):79-83, 2000.

French pharmacies distribute morning-after pill to teenagers for free, *Associated Press Online,* 1/10/2002, available at http://nl.newsbank.com/nl-search/we/ Archives?p_action=list&p_topdoc=21.

Guajardo AD, Middleman AB, Sansaricq KM: School nurses identify barriers and solutions to implementing a school-based hepatitis B immunization program, *J Sch Health* 72(3):128-130, 2002.

Harrell JS et al: School-based interventions to improve the health of children with multiple cardiovascular risk factors. In Funk SG et al, editors: *Key aspects of preventing and managing chronic illness,* pp 71-83, New York, 2001, Springer.

Hawkins JW, Hayes ER, Corliss CP: School nursing in America—1902-1994: a return to public health nursing, *Public Health Nurs* 11(6):416-425, 1994.

Hospitals' outreach program offers more than a "school nurse," *AHA News* 36(10):6, 2000.

Kalisch PA, Kalisch BJ: *The advance of American nursing,* Philadelphia, 1995, Lippincott.

King KA: Developing a comprehensive school suicide prevention program, *J Sch Health* 71(4):132-137, 2001.

Kirchofer GM, Price JH, Telljohann SK: Primary grade teacher's knowledge and perceptions of head lice, *J Sch Health* 71(9):448-452, 2001.

Klassen TP et al: Community-based injury prevention interventions, *Future Child* 10(1):83-110, 2000.

Kolbe LJ, Kann L, Brener ND: Overview and summary of findings: School Health Policies and Programs Study 2000, *J Sch Health* 71(7):253-259, 2001.

Krystofik DA: Nurse's corner: too much sun is not a good thing, *Our Schools: West Seneca Central Schools Newsletter,* p 7, March/April 2002a.

Krystofik DA: Nurse's corner: staff development day provides day of professional growth for school nurses, *Our Schools: West Seneca Central Schools Newsletter,* p 7, March/April 2002b.

Lindley LL, Reininger BM, Saunders RP: Support for school-based reproductive health services among South Carolina voters, *J Sch Health* 71(2):66-72, 2001.

McCarthy AM, Kelly MW, Reed D: Medication administration practices of school nurses, *J Sch Health* 70(9):371-376, 2000.

McRae J: School's back! *Nurs Times* 96(30):32-33, 2000.

Meninger JC et al: Identification of high-risk adolescents for interventions to lower blood pressure. In Funk SG et al, editors, *Key aspects of preventing and managing chronic illness,* New York, 2001, Springer.

National Association of School Nurses: *Scope and standards of professional school nursing practice,* Washington, DC, 2001, American Nurses.

Nebraska school nurses improve communication: Providers, parents and nurses interact on students' health, *Nation's Health* 30(3):7, 2000.

New York Sate Department of Health: *Children with diabetes: a resource guide for families of children with diabetes,* Albany, NY, 2000, NYDOH.

Periard ME, Knecht LD, Birchmeier N: A state association surveys school nurses to identify current issues and role characteristics, *J Sch Nurs* 15(4):12-18, 1999.

Perry CS, Toole KA: Impact of school nurse case management on asthma control in school-aged children, *J Sch Health* 70(7):303-304, 2000.

Pfizer Pharmaceuticals: *Opportunities to care: the Pfizer guide to careers in nursing,* New York, 2001, Pfizer Pharmaceuticals Group.

Pro D: New school nurse law passed: AB #1 signed by governor—a school nurse's perspective on the legislative process, *Nev RNformation* 10(3):8, 2001.

Ross SK: The clinical nurse specialist's role in school health, *Clin Nurs Spec* 13(1):28-33, 1999.

Roye CF, Johnsen JRM: Adolescents and emergency contraception, *J Pediatr Health Care* 19(1):3-9, 2002.

Rubsam JM: Identification of risk factors and effective intervention strategies corresponding to the major causes of childhood death from injury, *J NY State Nurses Assoc* 32(2):4-8, 2001.

Sapien RE, Allen A: Emergency preparation in schools: a snapshot of a rural state, *Ped Emerg Care* 17(5):329-333, 2001.

Starr NB: Helping children and families deal with the psychological aspects of disaster, *J Pediatr Health Care* 16(1):36-39, 2002.

Steger S: Killed at school, *RN* 63(4):36-38, 2000.

Sweeney JF, Sweeney DD: Frequent visitors to the school nurse at two middle schools, *J Sch Health* 70(9):387-389, 2000.

"Ten steps to keep schools louse-free," *Dermatol Times* 21(5):42, 2000.

Thackaberry J: Who cares for the health of your school? *Independent School* 60(4):94-97, 2001.

U.S. Department of Health and Human Services: *Healthy People 2010: understanding and improving health,* ed 2, Washington, DC, 2000, U.S. Government Printing Office.

U.S. Department of Health and Human Services, Bureau of Primary Health Care, Health Resources and Services Administration: *Healthy schools, healthy communities, a success story,* 1997, available at http://www.bphc.hrsa.gov:80/ hshc/hshc2.htm.

U.S. Department of Health and Human Services, Center for School-Based Health, Bureau of Primary Health Care, Health Resources and Services Administration: *Beyond access to care for students, full service school-based health centers,* 2001, available at http://www. bphc.hrsa.gov:80/Center/students.htm.

U.S. Environmental Protection Agency: *Indoor air quality (IAQ) tools for schools: health officer/school nurse checklist,* 2000, available at http://www.epa.gov/iaq/ schools/tfs/healthof.html.

Veselak KE: Historical steps in the development of the modern school health program, *J Sch Health* 71(8):369-372, 2001 [reprinted from *J Sch Health* 9(7):262-269, 1959].

Whitten P et al: School-based telehealth: an empirical analysis of teacher, nurse, and administrator perceptions, *J Sch Health* 71(5):173-180, 2001.

Williams CJ, Kalkenberg P: Germany in shock after school bloodbath, *Buffalo News,* pp A-1, A-6, April 27, 2002.

Wold SJ, Dagg NV: School nursing: a framework for practice, *J Sch Health* 71(8):401-404, 2001 [reprinted from *J Sch Health* 48(2):111-114, 1978].

Wood R, Synovitz LB: Addressing the threats of MDMA (Ecstasy): implications for school health professionals, parents and community members, *J Sch Health* 71(1):38-41, 2001.

# Chapter 44

**evolve** http://evolve.elsevier.com/Stanhope

# Community-Oriented Nurse in Occupational Health

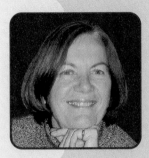

**Bonnie Rogers, Dr.P.H., C.O.H.N.-S., L.N.C.C., F.A.A.N.**

Bonnie Rogers is an associate professor of nursing and public health and director of the North Carolina Occupational Safety and Health Education and Research Center at the University of North Carolina, School of Public Health, Chapel Hill. She is certified in occupational health nursing and is a fellow in the American Academy of Nursing and the American Association of Occupational Health Nurses. In addition to managerial, consultant, and educator/research positions, Dr. Rogers has also practiced for many years as a public health nurse, occupational health nurse, and occupational health nurse practitioner. She has published more than 150 articles and book chapters and two books, including *Occupational Health Nursing Concepts and Practice* and *Occupational Health Nursing Guidelines for Primary Clinical Conditions*. Dr. Rogers is a strong advocate of occupational health research and serves as chairperson of the NIOSH National Occupational Research Agenda Liaison Committee. She has served on numerous Institute of Medicine committees, including the Nursing, Health and the Environment Committee and the Committee to Assess Training Needs for Occupational Safety and Health Personnel in the United States. Dr. Rogers is past president of the American Association of Occupational Health Nurses and recently completed several terms as an appointed member of the National Advisory Committee on Occupational Safety and Health. She is a consultant in occupational health and ethics.

## Objectives

After reading this chapter, the student should be able to do the following:
1. Describe the nursing role in occupational health
2. Describe current trends in the U.S. workforce
3. Describe examples of work-related illness and injuries
4. Use the epidemiologic model to explain work–health interactions
5. Cite at least three host factors associated with increased risk from an adverse response to hazardous workplace exposure
6. Explain one example each of biological, chemical, enviromechanical, physical, and psychosocial workplace hazards
7. Complete an occupational health history
8. Describe functions of OSHA and NIOSH
9. Describe an effective disaster plan

---

Many changes have occurred in the nature of work and workplace risks, the work environment, workforce composition and demographics, and health care delivery mechanisms. An analysis of the trends suggests that work–health interactions will continue to grow in importance, affecting how work is done, how hazards are controlled or minimized, and how health care is managed and integrated into workplace health delivery strategies. Although some workers may never face more than minor adverse health effects from exposures at work, such as occasional eyestrain resulting from poor office lighting, every industry has grappled with serious hazards (U.S. Department of Health and Human Services [USDHHS], National Institute for Occupational Safety and Health [NIOSH], 1996).

In America, work is viewed as important to one's life experiences, and most adults spend about one third of their time at work (Rogers, 1994). Work–when fulfilling, fairly compensated, healthy, and safe–can help build long and contented lives and strengthen families and commu-

nities. No work is completely risk free, and all health care professionals should have some basic knowledge about workforce populations, work and related hazards, and methods to control hazards and improve health.

Important developments are occurring in occupational health and safety programs designed to prevent and control work-related illness and injury and to create environments that foster and support health-promoting activities. Occupational health nurses have performed critical roles in planning and delivering worksite health and safety services, which must continue to grow as comprehensive and cost-effective services. In addition, the continuing increase in health care costs and the concern about health care quality have prompted the including of primary care and management of non–work-related health problems in the health services programs. In some settings, family services are also provided.

Health at work is an important issue for most individuals for whom the nurse provides care. As many individuals spend much time at work, the workplace has significant in-

## Key Terms

agents, p. 1075
environment, p. 1075
hazard communication standard, p. 1086
host, p. 1074
National Occupational Research Agenda,
   p. 1086

National Institute for Occupational Safety
   and Health, p. 1086
occupational health hazards, p. 1083
occupational health history, p. 1082
work–health interactions, p. 1073
workers' compensation, p. 1068

worksite walk-through, p. 1083
See Glossary for definitions


## Chapter Outline

Definition and Scope of Occupational Health
   Nursing
History and Evolution of Occupational Health
   Nursing
Roles and Professionalism in Occupational
   Health Nursing
Workers as a Population Aggregate
Characteristics of the Workforce
Characteristics of Work

Work–Health Interactions
Application of the Epidemiologic Model
Host
Agent
Environment
Organizational and Public Efforts to Promote
   Worker Health and Safety
On-site Occupational Health and Safety
   Programs

Nursing Care of Working Populations
Worker Assessment
Workplace Assessment
Healthy People 2010 Related to Occupational
   Health
Legislation Related to Occupational Health
Disaster Planning and Management

fluence on health and can be a primary site for the delivery of health promotion and illness prevention. The home, the clinic, the nursing home, and other community sites such as the workplace will become the dominant areas where health and illness care will be sought (Hall-Barrow, Hodges, and Brown, 2001).

This chapter describes the nurse's role in occupational health, working with employees and the workforce population. The focus is on the knowledge and skills needed to promote the health and safety of workers through occupational health programs, recognizing work-related health and safety and the principles for prevention and control of adverse work–health interactions. The prevalence and significance of the interactions between health and work underscore the importance of including principles of occupational health and safety in nursing practice. The types of interactions and the frequent use of the general health care system for identifying, treating, and preventing occupational illnesses and injuries require nurses to use this knowledge in all practice settings. The epidemiologic triad is used as the model for understanding these interactions, as well as risk factors, and effective nursing care for promoting health and safety among employed populations.

## DEFINITION AND SCOPE OF OCCUPATIONAL HEALTH NURSING

Adapted from the American Association of Occupational Health Nurses (AAOHN, 1999), occupational health nursing means the specialty practice that focuses on the promotion, prevention, and restoration of health within the context of a safe and healthy environment. It involves the prevention of adverse health effects from occupational and environmental hazards. It provides for and delivers occupational and environmental health and safety services to workers, worker populations, and community groups. It is an autonomous specialty, and nurses make independent nursing judgments in providing health care. Occupational health nurses work in traditional manufacturing, industry, service, healthcare facilities, construction sites, consulting, and government settings. Their scope of practice is broad and includes worker/workplace assessment and surveillance, primary care, case management, counseling, health promotion/protection, administration and management, research, legal/ethical monitoring, and a community orientation. The knowledge in occupational health and safety is applied to the workforce aggregate.

## HISTORY AND EVOLUTION OF OCCUPATIONAL HEALTH NURSING

Nursing care for workers began in 1888 and was called industrial nursing. A group of coal miners hired Betty Moulder, a graduate of the Blockley Hospital School of Nursing in Philadelphia (now Philadelphia General Hospital) to take care of their ailing co-workers and families (AAOHN, 1976). Ada Mayo Stewart, hired in 1885 by the Vermont Marble Company in Rutland, Vermont, is often considered the first industrial nurse. Riding a bicycle, Miss Stewart visited sick employees in their homes, provided emergency care, taught mothers how to care for their children, and taught healthy living habits (Felton, 1985). In the early days of occupational health nursing, the nurse's work was family centered and holistic.

Employee health services grew rapidly during the early 1900s as companies recognized that the provision of work-site health services led to a more productive workforce. At that time, workplace accidents were seen as an inevitable part of having a job. However, the public did not support this attitude, and a system for **workers' compensation** arose that remains today (McGrath, 1945).

Industrial nursing grew rapidly during the first half of the twentieth century. Educational courses were established, as were professional societies. By World War II there were approximately 4000 industrial nurses (Brown, 1981). The American Association of Industrial Nursing (AAIN) (now called the American Association of Occupational Health Nurses) was established as the first national nursing organization in 1942. The aim of the AAIN was to improve industrial nursing education and practice and to promote interdisciplinary collaborative efforts (Rogers, 1994).

Passage of several laws in the 1960s and 1970s to protect workers' safety and health led to an increased need for occupational health nurses. In particular, the passing of the landmark Occupational Safety and Health Act in 1970, which created the Occupational Safety and Health Administration (OSHA) and the National Institute for Occupational Safety and Health (NIOSH), discussed later in this chapter, resulted in a great need for nurses at the worksite to meet the demands of the many standards being implemented. The act focused primarily on education and research. In 1988, the first occupational health nurse was hired by OSHA to provide technical assistance in standards development, field consultation, and occupational health nursing expertise. In 1993, the Office of Occupational Health Nursing was established within the agency.

## ROLES AND PROFESSIONALISM IN OCCUPATIONAL HEALTH NURSING

As U.S. industry has shifted from agrarian (agriculture) to industrial to highly technologic processes, the role of the occupational health nurse has continued to change. The focus on work-related health problems now includes the spectrum of human responses to multiple, complex interactions of biopsychosocial factors that occur in community, home, and work environments. The customary role of the occupational health nurse has extended beyond emergency treatment and prevention of illness and injury to include the promotion and maintenance of health, overall risk management, and efforts to reduce health-related costs in businesses. The interdisciplinary nature of occupational health nursing has become more critical as occupational health and safety problems require more complex solutions. The occupational health nurse frequently collaborates closely with multiple disciplines and industry management, as well as with representatives of labor.

Occupational health nurses constitute the largest group of occupational health professionals. The most recent national survey of registered nurses indicates that there are approximately 33,000 licensed occupational health nurses (USDHHS, 1996). Occupational health nurses hold positions as nurse practitioners, clinical nurse specialists, managers, supervisors, consultants, educators, and researchers. Data also show that approximately 60% of occupational health nurses report that they are employed in single-managed occupational health nurse units in a variety of businesses. The occupational health nursing role requires the nurse adapt to an agency's needs as well as to the needs of specific groups of workers.

The professional organization for occupational health nurses is the American Association of Occupational Health Nurses (AAOHN). The AAOHN's mission is comprehensive. It supports the work of the occupational health nurse and advances the specialty. The AAOHN also does the following:

- Promotes the health and safety of workers
- Defines the scope of practice and sets the standards of occupational health nursing practice
- Develops the Code of Ethics for occupational health nurses with interpretive statements
- Promotes and provides continuing education in the specialty
- Advances the profession through supporting research
- Responds to and influences public policy issues related to occupational health and safety

The AAOHN Standards of Occupational and Environmental Health Nursing Practice and the Code of Ethics are shown in Boxes 44-1 and 44-2.

The AAOHN describes 10 job roles for occupational health nurses: clinician, case manager, coordinator, manager, nurse practitioner, corporate director, health promotion specialist, educator, consultant, and researcher (AAOHN, 1997). The majority of occupational health nurses work as solo clinicians, but increasingly, additional roles are being included in the specialty practice. In many companies, the occupational health nurse has assumed expanded responsibilities in job analysis, safety, and benefits management. Many occupational health nurses also work as independent contractors or have their own businesses providing occupational health and safety services to industry, as well as consultation. With the current changes in health care delivery and the movement toward managed care, occupational health nurses will need increased skills in primary care, health promotion, and disease prevention. The aim of the occupational health nurse will be to devote much attention to keeping workers and, in some cases, their families healthy and free from illness and worksite injuries. Specializing in the field is often a requirement.

Academic education in occupational health and safety is generally at the graduate level. Training grants from NIOSH support master's and doctoral education with emphases in occupational health nursing, industrial hygiene, occupational medicine, and safety. These programs are offered through Occupational Safety and Health Education and Research Centers throughout the country. A listing of these programs can be found in Box 44-3. Certification in

## BOX 44-1 American Association of Occupational Health Nurses: Standards of Occupational and Environmental Health Nursing Practice

**STANDARD I: ASSESSMENT**

The occupational and environmental health nurse systematically assesses the health status of the individual client or population and the environment.

**STANDARD II: DIAGNOSIS**

The occupational and environmental health nurse analyzes assessment data to formulate diagnoses.

**STANDARD III: OUTCOME IDENTIFICATION**

The occupational and environmental health nurse identifies outcomes specific to the client.

**STANDARD IV: PLANNING**

The occupational and environmental health nurse develops a goal-directed plan that is comprehensive and formulates interventions to attain expected outcomes.

**STANDARD V: IMPLEMENTATION**

The occupational and environmental health nurse implements interventions to attain desired outcomes identified in the plan.

**STANDARD VI: EVALUATION**

The occupational and environmental health nurse systematically and continuously evaluates responses to interventions and progress toward the achievement of desired outcomes.

**STANDARD VII: RESOURCE MANAGEMENT**

The occupational and environmental health nurse secures and manages the resources that support an occupational health and safety program.

**STANDARD VIII: PROFESSIONAL DEVELOPMENT**

The occupational and environmental health nurse assumes accountability for professional development to enhance professional growth and maintain competency.

**STANDARD IX: COLLABORATION**

The occupational and environmental health nurse collaborates with employees, management, other health care providers, professionals, and community representatives.

**STANDARD X: RESEARCH**

The occupational and environmental health nurse uses research findings in practice and contributes to the scientific base in occupational and environmental health nursing to improve practice and advance the profession.

**STANDARD XI: ETHICS**

The occupational and environmental health nurse uses an ethical framework as a guide for decision making in practice.

From American Association of Occupational Health Nurses: *Standards for occupational health nursing practice,* Atlanta, 1999, AAOHN.

## BOX 44-2 AAOHN Code of Ethics

- Occupational and environmental health nurses provide health care in the work environment with regard for human dignity and client rights, unrestricted by considerations of social or economic status, personal attributes, or the nature of the health status.
- Occupational and environmental health nurses promote collaboration with other health professionals and community health agencies in order to meet the health needs of the workforce.
- Occupational and environmental health nurses strive to safeguard employees' rights to privacy by protecting confidential information and releasing information only upon written consent of the employee or as required or permitted by law.
- Occupational and environmental health nurses strive to provide quality care and to safeguard clients from unethical and illegal actions.

- Occupational and environmental health nurses, licensed to provide health care services, accept obligations to society as professional and responsible members of the community.
- Occupational and environmental health nurses maintain individual competence in occupational health nursing practice, based on scientific knowledge, and recognize and accept responsibility for individual judgments and actions, while complying with appropriate laws and regulations (local, state, and federal) that impact the delivery of occupational and environmental health services.
- Occupational and environmental health nurses participate, as appropriate, in activities such as research that contribute to the ongoing development of the profession's body of knowledge while protecting the rights of subjects.

From American Association of Occupational Health Nurses: *Code of ethics,* 1999, AAOHN.

## THE CUTTING EDGE

Performance-based competencies in occupational and environmental health nursing have recently been developed and published by The American Association of Occupational Health Nursing.

occupational health nursing is provided by the American Board for Occupational Health Nurses (ABOHN) and is met through experience, continuing education, professional activities, and examination.

## WORKERS AS A POPULATION AGGREGATE

The population of the United States is expected to increase from approximately 272 million people in 1999 to an estimated 297 million people by the year 2010 (U.S. Bureau of the Census, 1999). By 2010, the U.S. population will be older. The greatest growth will be among people over age 65, with a reduction of the under-25-year-olds. This will be reflected in the workforce, with a decrease in the number of young job seekers. It is estimated that by the year 2010, 67% of the workforce will be between the ages of 25 and 54, and 17% will be older than 55 years of age (Institute of Medicine [IOM], 2000). The number of adults age 65 years and older will more than double between now and the year 2050. By that year, one in five Americans will be an older adult.

There were more than 3.9 million civilian wage and salary workers in the United States, employed in about 63,000 different worksites (Bureau of Labor Statistics [BLS], 2003). More than 91% of those who are able to work outside of the home do so for some portion of their lives (BLS, 1999). Neither of these statistics indicates the full number of individuals who have potentially been exposed to work-related health hazards. Although some individuals may currently be unemployed or retired, they continue to bear the health risks of past occupational exposures. The number of affected individuals may be even larger, as work-related illnesses are found among spouses, children, and neighbors of exposed workers.

Americans are employed in diverse industries that range in size from one to tens of thousands of employ-

---

### BOX 44-3 Directors NIOSH Education and Research Centers (ERCs)

**ALABAMA EDUCATION AND RESEARCH CENTER**
University of Alabama at Birmingham
School of Public Health
1665 University Blvd.
Birmingham, AL 35294-0022
(205) 934-6208
Fax: (205) 975-5444
R. Kent Oestenstad, Ph.D., Director
E-Mail: oestenk@uab.edu

**CALIFORNIA EDUCATION AND RESEARCH CENTER—NORTHERN**
University of California, Berkeley
School of Public Health
140 Warren
Berkeley, CA 94720-7360
(510) 642-0761
Fax: (510) 642-5815
Robert C. Spear, Ph.D., Director
E-Mail: spear@uclink4.berkeley.edu

**CALIFORNIA EDUCATION AND RESEARCH CENTER—SOUTHERN**
University of California
School of Public Health
650 Young Drive South
Los Angeles, CA 90095-1772
(310) 825-7152
Fax: (310) 206-9903
William C. Hinds, Sc.D., C.I.H., Director
E-Mail: whinds@ucla.edu

**CINCINNATI EDUCATION AND RESEARCH CENTER**
University of Cincinnati
Department of Environmental Health
P.O. Box 670056
Cincinnati, Ohio 45267-0056
(513) 558-1749
Fax: (513) 558-2772 or 4397
C. Scott Clark, Ph.D., P.E., C.I.H., Director
E-Mail: clarkcs@uc.edu

**HARVARD EDUCATION AND RESEARCH CENTER**
Harvard School of Public Health
Department of Environmental Health
665 Huntington Avenue
Boston, MA 02115
(617) 432-3323
Fax: (617) 432-0219
David C. Christiani, M.D., Director
E-Mail: dchris@hohp.harvard.edu

**ILLINOIS EDUCATION AND RESEARCH CENTER**
University of Illinois at Chicago
School of Public Health
2121 West Taylor St.
Chicago, IL 60612-7260
(312) 996-7469
Fax: (312) 413-9898
Lorraine M. Conroy, Sc.D., C.I.H., Director
E-Mail: lconroy@uic.edu

**BOX 44-3** **Directors NIOSH Education and Research Centers (ERCs)—cont'd**

**IOWA EDUCATION AND RESEARCH CENTER**
Heartland Center for Occupational Health and Safety
Department of Occupational and Environmental Health
100 Oakdale Campus—124 IREH
Iowa City, IA 52242-5000
(319) 335-4415
Fax: (319) 335-4225
Nancy L. Sprince, M.D., M.P.H., Director
E-Mail: nancy-sprince@uiowa.edu

**JOHNS HOPKINS EDUCATION AND RESEARCH CENTER**
Johns Hopkins University
School of Hygiene and Public Health
615 North Wolfe Street
Baltimore, MD 21205
(410) 955-4037
Fax: (410) 955-1811
Jacqueline Agnew, Ph.D., Director
E-Mail: jagnew@jhsph.edu

**MICHIGAN EDUCATION AND RESEARCH CENTER**
University of Michigan
School of Public Health
1420 Washington Heights
Ann Arbor, MI 48109-2029
(734) 936-0758
Fax: (734) 763-8095
Thomas G. Robins, M.D., Director
E-Mail: trobins@umich.edu

**MINNESOTA EDUCATION AND RESEARCH CENTER**
University of Minnesota
School of Public Health
Box 807 Mayo Memorial Building
Minneapolis, MN 55455
(612) 626-4855
Fax: (612) 626-0650
Ian A. Greaves, M.D., Director
E-Mail: igreaves@mail.eoh.umn.edu

**NEW YORK/NEW JERSEY EDUCATION AND RESEARCH CENTER**
Mt. Sinai School of Medicine
Department of Community and Preventive Medicine
P.O. Box 1057
One Gustave L. Levy Pl.
New York, NY 10029-6574
(212) 241-4804
Fax: (212) 996-0407
Philip J. Landrigan, M.D., M.Sc., Director
E-Mail: p_landrigan@smtplink.mssm.edu

**NORTH CAROLINA EDUCATION AND RESEARCH CENTER**
University of North Carolina
School of Public Health
Rosenau Hall, CB# 7469
Chapel Hill, NC 27599-7410
(919) 966-1765
Fax: (919) 966-9081
Bonnie Rogers, Dr.P.H., R.N., Director
E-Mail: rogersb@email.unc.edu

**SOUTH FLORIDA EDUCATION AND RESEARCH CENTER**
University of South Florida
College of Public Health
13201 Bruce B. Downs Blvd., MDC Box 56
Tampa, FL 33612-3805
(813) 974-6626
Fax: (813) 974-4986
Stuart M. Brooks, M.D., Director
E-Mail: sbrooks@com1.med.usf.edu

**TEXAS EDUCATION AND RESEARCH CENTER**
University of Texas Health Science
Center at Houston
School of Public Health
P.O. Box 20186
Houston, TX 77225-0186
(713) 500-9459
Fax: (713) 500-9442
George L. Delclos, M.D., Director
E-Mail: gdelclos@utsph.sph.uth.tmc.edu

**UTAH EDUCATION AND RESEARCH CENTER**
University of Utah
Rocky Mountain Center for Occupational
and Environmental Health
75 S. 2000 East
Salt Lake City, UT 84112
(801) 581-8719
Fax: (801) 581-7224
Royce Moser, Jr., M.D., M.P.H., Director
E-Mail: rmoser@rmcoeh.utah.edu

**WASHINGTON EDUCATION AND RESEARCH CENTER**
University of Washington
Department of Environmental Health
P.O. Box 357234
Seattle, WA 98195-7234
(206) 685-3221
Fax: (206) 543-9616
Michael S. Morgan, Sc.D., Director
E-Mail: mmorgan@u.washington.edu

ees. Types of industries include traditional manufacturing (e.g., automotive and appliances), service industries (e.g., banking, health care, and restaurants), agriculture, construction, and the newer high-technology firms, such as computer chip manufacturers. Approximately 95% of business organizations are considered small, employing fewer than 500 people (BLS, 1995). Although some industries are noted for the high degree of hazards associated with their work (e.g., manufacturing, mines, construction, and agriculture), no worksite is free of occupational health and safety hazards. The larger the company, the more likely it is that there will be health and safety programs for employees. Smaller companies are more apt to rely on external community resources to meet their needs for health and safety services.

## Characteristics of the Workforce

The U.S. workplace has been rapidly changing (BLS, 2003). Jobs in the economy continue to shift from manufacturing to service. Longer hours, compressed workweeks, shift work, reduced job security, and part-time and temporary work are realities of the modern workplace (IOM, 2000). New chemicals, materials, processes, and equipment are developed and marketed at an ever-increasing pace.

The workforce is also changing. As the U.S. workforce is expected to grow to approximately 155 million by the year 2010, it will become older and more racially diverse (IOM, 2000). By the year 2005, minorities are projected to be 28% of the workforce and women approximately 48% of the workforce (Figure 44-1). These changes are going to present new challenges to protecting worker safety and health.

The demographic trends in the U.S. workforce describe a changing population aggregate that has implications for the prevention services targeted to that group. Major changes in the working population are reflected in the increasing numbers of women, older individuals, and those with chronic illnesses who are part of the workforce. Because of changes in the economy, extension of life span, legislation, and society's acceptance of working women, the proportion of the employed population that these three groups represent will probably continue to grow.

In an era in which the demand for workers is expected to outstrip the available supply, businesses must be concerned about strategies to increase health status, employment longevity, and satisfaction of workers. For example, in the late 1990s while nearly 60% of all women were employed (representing 48% of the workforce), it was predicted that women would account for 67% of the increase in the labor force in the twenty-first century (BLS, 1997). These workers tended to be married, with children and aging parents for whom they were responsible. This aggregate of workers presents new issues for individual and family health promotion, such as child care and elder care, that can be addressed in the work environment. In 1990, more than half of the female labor force was concentrated in three areas: administrative support/clerical (26%), service (14%), and professional

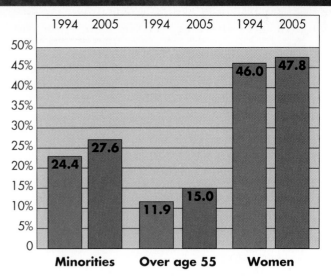

**Figure 44-1** Projected changes in civilian labor force 1994 to 2005. *(From Fullerton H: The 2005 labor force: growing, but slowly,* Monthly Labor Rev *118[11]:29, 1995.)*

specialty (14%). Twelve percent were employed in fields such as labor, transportation and moving, machine operation, precision products, crafts, farming, forestry, and fishing. In the male labor force, nearly 20% worked in precision production, crafts, or repair occupations, 13% in executive positions, 11% in professional specialty occupations, and 10% in sales. Other trends shaping the profile of the workforce include more education and mobility. Increasing mismatches between skills of workers and types of employment were seen in the 1990s. Future employment trends projected to 2008 are shown in Figure 44-2. Of the top 20 occupations (of 500 listed by the Bureau of Labor Statistics) projected to gain the largest number of jobs, or about 39% growth (8 million jobs), the five fastest growing include three computer-related occupations, personal care and home health, and medical assistants (BLS, 2000).

## Characteristics of Work

There has been a dramatic shift in the types of jobs held by workers. Following the evolution from an agrarian economy to a manufacturing society and then to a highly technologic workplace, the greatest proportion of paid employment is now in the occupations of service (e.g., health care, information processing, banking, and insurance), professional and technical positions (e.g., managers and computer specialists), and clerical work (e.g., word processors and secretaries). During the 1996 to 2000 period, service-providing industries accounted for virtually all of the job growth. Only construction added jobs in the goods-producing business sector, offsetting declines in manufacturing and mining. Health services, business services, social services, and engineering, management, and related services are expected to account for almost one of every two worker jobs (Table 44-1) (IOM, 2000).

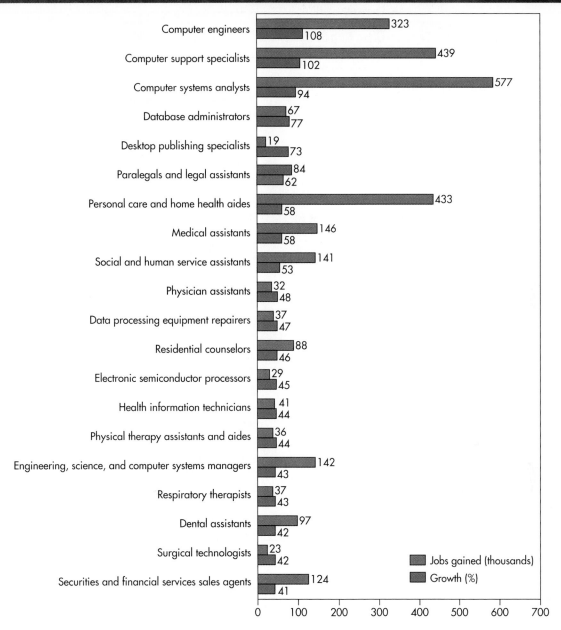

**Figure 44-2** Employment growth in the fastest growing occupations, projected for 1998-2008. *(From Bureau of Labor Statistics: A special issue: charting the projections, 1998-2008, Occupat Outlook Q 43(4):2-38, 2000.)*

This change in the nature of work has been accompanied by many new occupational hazards, such as complex chemicals, nonergonomic workstation design (requiring the adaptation of the workplace or work equipment to meet the employee's health and safety needs), and many issues related to work organization such as job stress, burnout, and exhaustion. In addition, the emerging of a global economy with free trade and multinational corporations presents new challenges for health and safety programs that are culturally relevant.

## Work–Health Interactions

The influence of work on health, or **work–health interactions,** is shown by statistics on illnesses, injuries, and deaths associated with employment. In 2001, 1.5 million reported work-related illnesses and injuries resulted in lost time from work. Of these, approximately 5% were severe enough to result in temporary or permanent disabilities that prevented the workers from returning to their usual jobs (BLS, 2003). Then occupations accounted for nearly one third of the 1.5 million injuries and illnesses involving days away from work in 2001 (Figure 44-3). Truck drivers, nonconstruction laborers, and nursing aides and orderlies were the top three occupations representing days away from work in 2001, with registered nurses being the tenth occupation with lost days from work.

Employers reported 6.3 work injuries and occupational illnesses per 100 workers in 1999. That same year,

**Table 44-1  Selected Job Categories, Exposures, and Associated Work-Related Diseases and Conditions**

| JOB CATEGORIES | EXPOSURES | WORK-RELATED DISEASES AND CONDITIONS |
|---|---|---|
| All workers | Workplace stress | Hypertension, mood disorders, cardiovascular disease |
| Agricultural workers | Pesticides, infectious agents, gases, sunlight | Pesticide poisoning, "farmer's lung," skin cancer |
| Anesthetists | Anesthetic gases | Reproductive effects, cancer |
| Automobile workers | Asbestos, plastics, lead, solvents | Asbestosis, dermatitis |
| Butchers | Vinyl plastic fumes | "Meat wrappers' asthma" |
| Caisson workers | Pressurized work environments | Caisson disease ("the bends") |
| Carpenters | Wood dust, wood preservatives, adhesives | Nasopharyngeal cancer, dermatitis |
| Cement workers | Cement dust, metals | Dermatitis, bronchitis |
| Ceramic workers | Talc, clays | Pneumoconiosis |
| Demolition workers | Asbestos, wood dust | Asbestosis |
| Drug manufacturers | Hormones, nitroglycerin, etc. | Reproductive effects |
| Dry cleaners | Solvents | Liver disease, dermatitis |
| Dye workers | Dyestuffs, metals, solvents | Bladder cancer, dermatitis |
| Embalmers | Formaldehyde, infectious agents | Dermatitis |
| Felt makers | Mercury, polycyclic hydrocarbons | Mercurialism |
| Foundry workers | Silica, molten metals | Silicosis |
| Glass workers | Heat, solvents, metal powders | Cataracts |
| Hospital workers | Infectious agents, cleansers, radiation | Infections, latex allergies, unintentional injuries |
| Insulators | Asbestos, fibrous glass | Asbestosis, lung cancer, mesothelioma |
| Jack-hammer operators | Vibration | Raynaud's phenomenon |
| Lathe operators | Metal dusts, cutting oils | Lung disease, cancer |
| Office computer workers | Repetitive wrist motion on computers | Tendonitis, carpal tunnel syndrome, tenosynovitis, eye strain |

occupational injuries alone cost billions in lost wages and lost productivity, administrative expenses, health care, and other costs (BLS, 2003). This figure does not include the cost of occupational diseases. These figures are often described as the "tip of the iceberg," because many work-related health problems go unreported. But even the recorded statistics are significant in describing the amount of human suffering, financial loss, and decreased productivity associated with workplace hazards.

The high number of work injuries and illnesses can be drastically reduced. In fact, significant progress has been made in improving worker protection since Congress passed the 1970 Occupational Safety and Health Act. For example, vinyl chloride–induced liver cancers and brown lung disease (byssinosis) from cotton dust exposure have been almost eliminated. Reproductive disorders associated with certain glycol ethers have been recognized and controlled. Fatal work injuries have declined substantially through the years. Notably, since 1970, fatal injury rates in coal miners have been reduced by more than 75%, and there has been a general downward trend in the prevalence of coal miner's pneumoconiosis (NIOSH, 2000).

The U.S. workplace is rapidly changing and becoming more diverse. Major changes are also occurring in the way work is organized, with increased shiftwork, reduced job security, and part-time and temporary work as realities of the modern workplace. As shown in Figure 44-4, the temporary help industry grew from less than 1 million in 1986 to nearly 3.9 million in 2001 (BLS, 2003). A self-report survey done in 1998 showed that over 21 million workers reported they worked at home (BLS, 1998b). In addition, new chemicals, materials, processes, and equipment (such as latex gloves in health care, and fermentation processes in biotechnology) continue to be developed and marketed at an accelerating pace.

## APPLICATION OF THE EPIDEMIOLOGIC MODEL

The epidemiologic triad can be used to understand the relationship between work and health (Figure 44-5) (Campos-Outcalt, 1994). With a focus on the health and safety of the employed population, the **host** is described as any susceptible human being. Because of the nature of work-related hazards, nurses must assume that all employed individuals

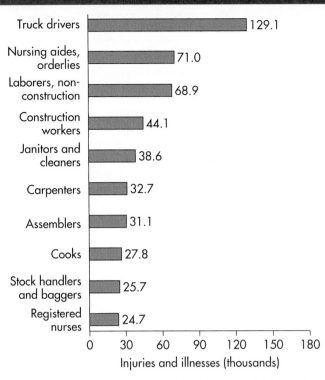

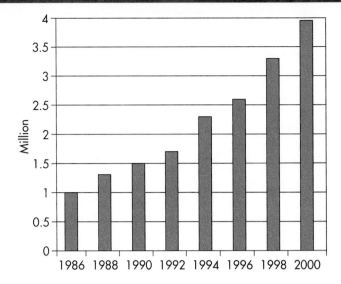

**Figure 44-4** Employment in personnel supply services, 1986 to 2000 (wage and salary workers in millions). *(From Bureau of Labor Statistics:* Career Guide, *Washington, DC, 2003, U.S. Department of Labor.)*

**Figure 44-3** Ten occupations with the most injuries and illnesses involving days away from work, 2001. Total number of injuries and illnesses involving days away from work was 1.5 million. *(From Bureau of Labor Statistics:* Lost work time injuries and illnesses, *Washington, DC, 2003, U.S. Department of Labor.)*

and groups are at risk of being exposed to occupational hazards. The **agents,** factors associated with illness and injury, are occupational exposures that are classified as biological, chemical, enviromechanical, physical, or psychosocial (Box 44-4). The third element, the **environment,** includes all external conditions that influence the interaction of the host and agents. These may be workplace conditions such as temperature extremes, crowding, shiftwork, and inflexible management styles. The basic principle of epidemiology is that health status interventions for restoring and promoting health are the result of complex interactions among these three elements. To understand these interactions and to design effective nursing strategies for dealing with them in a proactive manner, nurses must look at how each element influences the others.

## Host

Each worker represents a host within the worker population group. Certain host factors are associated with increased risk of adverse response to the hazards of the workplace. These include age, sex, health status, work practices, ethnicity, and lifestyle factors (Rogers, 2003). For example, the population group at greatest risk for experiencing work-related accidents with subsequent injuries is new workers with less than 1 year of experience on the current job. Thirty-one percent of nonfatal injuries and illnesses involving days away from work in

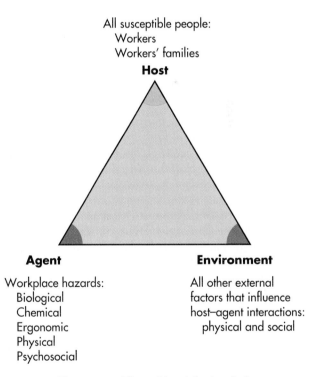

**Figure 44-5** The epidemiologic triad.

1997 occurred among new workers (the highest percentages were in mining [44%], agriculture, forestry, and fishing [43%], construction [41%], and wholesale and retail trade [34%]). Nearly two thirds of injury and illness cases with days away from work occurred among workers with 5 or fewer years of service with their employer. The host factors of age, sex, and work experience combine to increase this

---

**BOX 44-4    Categories of Work-Related Hazards**

**Biological and infectious hazards.** Infectious/biological agents, such as bacteria, viruses, fungi, or parasites, that may be transmitted via contact with infected patients or contaminated body secretions/fluids to other individuals

**Chemical hazards.** Various forms of chemicals, including medications, solutions, gases, vapors, aerosols, and particulate matter, that are potentially toxic or irritating to the body system

**Enviromechanical hazards.** Factors encountered in the work environment that cause or potentiate accidents,

injuries, strain, or discomfort (e.g., unsafe/inadequate equipment or lifting devices, slippery floors, workstation deficiencies)

**Physical hazards.** Agents within the work environment, such as radiation, electricity, extreme temperatures, and noise, that can cause tissue trauma

**Psychosocial hazards.** Factors and situations encountered or associated with one's job or work environment that create or potentiate stress, emotional strain, or interpersonal problems

From Rogers B: *Occupational health nursing: concepts and practice*, St Louis, Mo, 2003, Elsevier.

---

group's risk of injury because of characteristics such as risk taking, lack of knowledge, and lack of familiarity with the new job.

Older workers may be at increased risk in the workplace because of diminished sensory abilities, the effects of chronic illnesses, and delayed reaction times (Stine and Brown, 1996). A third population group that may be very susceptible to workplace exposure is women in their child-bearing years. The hormonal changes during these years (along with the increased stress of new roles and additional responsibilities) and transplacental exposures are host factors that may influence this group's response to potential toxins.

In addition to these host factors, there may be other, less well understood individual differences in responses to occupational hazard exposures. Even if employers maintain exposure levels below the level recommended by occupational health and safety standards, 15% to 20% of the population may have health reactions to the "safe" low-level exposures (Levy and Wegman, 2000). This group has been termed hypersusceptible. A number of host factors appear to be associated with this hypersusceptibility: light skin, malnutrition, compromised immune system, glucose-6-phosphate dehydrogenase deficiency, serum alpha-1-antitrypsin deficiency, chronic obstructive pulmonary disease, sickle cell trait, and hypertension. Individuals who have known hypersusceptibility to chemicals that are respiratory irritants, hemolytic chemicals, organic isocyanates, and carbon disulfide may also be hypersusceptible to other agents in the work environment (Levy and Wegman, 2000). Although this has prompted some industries to consider preplacement screening for such risk factors, the associations between these individual health markers and hypersusceptible response are speculative and require further research.

## Agent

Work-related hazards, or agents (see Box 44-4), present potential and actual risks to the health and safety of workers in the millions of business establishments in the United States. Any worksite commonly presents multiple and interacting exposures from all five categories of agents. Table

44-2 lists some of the more common workplace exposures, their known health effects, and the types of jobs associated with these hazards.

### Biological Agents

Biological agents are living organisms whose excretions or parts are capable of causing human disease, usually by an infectious process. Biological hazards are common in workplaces such as health care facilities and clinical laboratories where employees are potentially exposed to a variety of infectious agents, including viruses, fungi, and bacteria. Of particular concern in occupational health are infectious diseases transmitted by humans (e.g., from client to worker or from worker to worker) in a variety of work settings (USDHHS, NIOSH, 1996). Bloodborne and airborne pathogens represent a significant class of exposures for U.S. health care workers at risk. Occupational transmission of bloodborne pathogens (including the hepatitis B and C viruses and the human immunodeficiency virus [HIV]), occurs primarily by means of needlestick injuries but also through exposures to the eyes or mucous membranes (EPINet, 1999). The risk of hepatitis B virus infection following a single needlestick injury with a contaminated needle varies from 2% to greater than 40%, depending on the antigen status of the source person and the nature of the exposure. The risk of hepatitis C virus transmission depends on the same factors and ranges from 3.3% to 10%.

Transmission of tuberculosis (TB) within health care settings (especially multidrug-resistant TB) has reemerged as a major public health problem (USDHHS, NIOSH, 1996). Since 1989, outbreaks of this type of TB have been reported in hospitals, and some workers have developed active drug-resistant TB. In addition, among workers in health care, social service, and corrections facilities who work with populations at increased risk of TB, hundreds have experienced tuberculin skin test conversions. Reliable data are lacking on the extent of possible work-related TB transmission among other groups of workers at risk for exposure. Many workers in these settings were employed as maintenance workers, se-

**Table 44-2  Employment by Major Industry Divisions in 1988 and 1998 and Projected for 2010**

| INDUSTRY GROUP | 1988 | 1998 | 2010 |
|---|---|---|---|
| Total | 117.8 | 138.5 | 162.8 |
| Nonfarm wage and salary | 104.6 | 125.0 | 147.9 |
| Goods producing | 25.1 | 25.3 | 25.3 |
| Mining | 0.7 | 0.6 | 0.5 |
| Construction | 5.1 | 6.0 | 6.8 |
| Manufacturing | 19.3 | 18.7 | 18.1 |
| Service producing | 80.6 | 100.7 | 122.6 |
| Transportation, communication, and public utilities | 5.5 | 6.5 | 7.6 |
| Wholesale trade | 6.0 | 6.8 | 7.8 |
| Retail trade | 17.9 | 22.5 | 25.2 |
| Finance, insurance, and real estate | 6.6 | 7.3 | 8.2 |
| Services | 26.0 | 37.6 | 51.5 |
| Personnel supply services | 1.4 | 3.2 | 4.9 |
| Computer and data processing services | 0.7 | 1.6 | 2.8 |
| Health services | 7.1 | 9.8 | 11.7 |
| Offices of medical doctors | 1.2 | 1.8 | 2.8 |
| Offices of dentists | 0.5 | 0.6 | 0.7 |
| Offices of other health practitioners | 0.2 | 0.5 | 0.8 |
| Nursing and personal care facilities | 1.3 | 1.8 | 2.2 |
| Hospitals | 3.3 | 3.9 | 4.5 |
| Social services | 1.6 | 2.6 | 3.8 |
| Federal government | 3.0 | 2.7 | 2.6 |
| State and local governments (including public schools) | 14.4 | 17.2 | 19.7 |
| Agriculture* | 3.4 | 3.6 | 3.6 |
| Private household workers | 1.2 | 1.0 | 0.8 |
| Nonagricultural self-employed† | 8.7 | 9.0 | 10.5 |

Historical data are from the Bureau of Labor Statistics Survey of Nonfarm Employment, Hours, and Earnings, annual averages, selected years. Projections are by the Committee to Assess Training Needs for Occupational Safety and Health Personnel in the United States, Institute of Medicine, based on the Bureau of Labor Statistics' projections for 1996 to 2006.
Numbers of employees given in millions.
*Agriculture includes landscaping firms, which account for the increases in this sector, as the increases for landscaping firms more than offsets the declines in farm employment.
†This group also includes unpaid family workers.

curity guards, aides, or cleaning people, who were not well protected from inadvertent exposure. These included contaminated bed linen in the laundry, soiled equipment, and trash containing contaminated dressings or specimens (Centers for Disease Control and Prevention [CDC], 1999).

## Chemical Agents

Over 300 billion pounds of chemical agents are produced annually in the United States. Of the approximately 2 million known chemicals in existence, less than 0.1% have been adequately studied for their effects on humans. Of those chemicals that have been linked to carcinogens, approximately half test positive as animal carcinogens. Most chemicals have not been studied epidemiologically to determine the effects of exposure on humans (Levy and Wegman, 2000). As a consequence of general environmental contamination with chemicals from work, home, and community activities, a variety of chemicals have been found in the body tissues of the general population (Stine and Brown, 1996). These tissue loads may result in part from the accidental release of chemicals into the environment, such as that which occurred in Love Canal when chemicals leached out from buried industrial wastes (USDHHS, 2000).

In many workplaces, significant exposure to a daily, low-level dose of workplace chemicals may be below the exposure standards but may still carry a potentially chronic and perhaps cumulative assault on workers' health. Predicting human responses to such exposures is further complicated because multiple chemicals often combine and interact to create a new chemical agent. Human effects may be associated with the interaction of these agents rather than with a single chemical. Another concern about occupational exposure to chemicals is reproductive health effects. Workplace reproductive hazards have become important legal and scientific issues. Toxicity to male and female reproductive systems has been demonstrated from exposure to common agents such as lead, mercury, cadmium, nickel, and zinc, as well as in antineoplastic drugs. Since data for predicting human responses to many chemical agents are inadequate, workers should be assessed for all potential exposures and cautioned to work preventively with these agents. High-risk or vulnerable workers, such as those with latex allergy–a widely recognized health hazard, should be carefully screened and monitored for optimal health protection (NIOSH, 1997a). To accurately assess and evaluate the exposure and recommend changes for abatement, it is essential that the nurse have a good understanding of the basic principles of toxicology, including routes of exposure (inhalation, skin absorption, and ingestion), dose–response relationships, and differences in effects (i.e., acute versus chronic toxicity).

> ⟨ **DID YOU KNOW?**
>
> Only 0.1% of the nearly 2 million known chemicals produced have been tested for their effect on humans.

## Enviromechanical Agents

Enviromechanical agents are those that can potentially cause injury or illness in the workplace. They are related to the work process or to working conditions, and they can cause postural or other strains that can produce adverse health effects when certain tasks are performed repeatedly. Examples are repetitive motions, poor or unsafe workstation–worker fit, slippery floors, cluttered work areas, and lifting heavy loads. In 2001, sprains and strains were by far the most frequent disabling conditions, accounting for 669,000 of the cases (43.5%) of days away from work. Bruises accounted for 136,000 cases (9.0%), and cuts and lacerations accounted for another 114,000 cases (7.4%) (Figure 44-6). The back and shoulders were the body parts most often affected by disabling work incidents. Repeated trauma disorders accounted for 35% of the nonfatal occupational illnesses cases recorded in 2001. Included in this category are carpal tunnel syndrome (CTS) and tendonitis (BLS, 2003).

Severity of illness or injury can be estimated from the number of days away from work. Six days was the median number of days away from work for all types of injury and illness. CTS, fractures, amputations, tendonitis, and multiple injuries had median days away from work greater than the 6-day median for all injuries and illnesses combined (Figure 44-7). The most frequently reported upper-extremity musculoskeletal disorders affect the hand/wrist region.

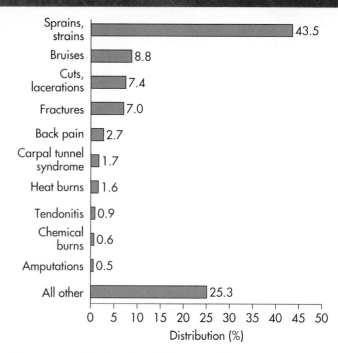

**Figure 44-6** Distribution of injury and illness cases with days away from work in private industry, by nature of injury or illness, 2001. Total number of injury and illness cases with days away from work was 1.5 million. *(From Bureau of Labor Statistics: Lost worktime injuries and illnesses, Washington, D.C., 2003, U.S. Department of Labor)*

In 2003, CTS, the most widely recognized condition, occurred in 26,000 full-time workers. This syndrome required the longest recuperation period of all conditions resulting in lost work days, with a median 25 days away from work (BLS, 2003).

Back pain/injury is one of the most common and significant musculoskeletal problems in the world (BLS, 2003). In 2001, back injuries and disorders accounted for 37% of all nonfatal occupational injuries and illnesses involving days away from work in the United States. Although the exact cost of back disorders is unknown, the estimates are staggering and in the billions per year. Regardless of the estimate used, the problem is large both in health and economic terms. Moreover, as many as 30% of U.S. workers are employed in jobs that routinely require them to perform activities that may increase risk of developing low back disorders. The research on these hazards, related human responses, and prevention is evolving. Injuries and illnesses related to this category of agents have been termed cumulative trauma, which composes the largest category of work-related illness and disability claims in the United States. The most productive strategy in preventing these exposures appears to be redesigning the workplace and the work machinery or processes.

## Physical Agents

Physical agents are those that produce adverse health effects through the transfer of physical energy. Commonly encountered physical agents in the workplace include tem-

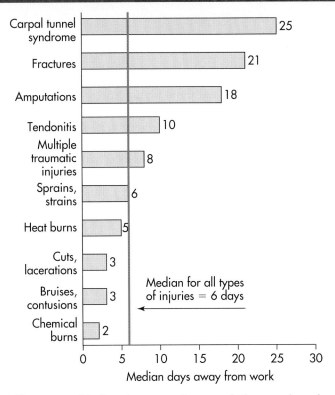

**Figure 44-7** Median days away from work due to selected types of nonfatal occupational injury or illness in private industry, 1997. *(From Bureau of Labor Statistics:* Career Guide, *Washington, DC, 2003, U.S. Department of Labor.)*

perature extremes, vibration, noise, laser, radiation, and lighting (Payling, 1994; Platt, 1993). For example, vibration, which accompanies the use of power tools and vehicles such as trucks, affects internal organs, supportive ligaments, the upper torso, and the shoulder–girdle structure. Localized effects are seen with handheld power tools; the most common is Raynaud's phenomenon. The control of worker exposure to these agents is usually accomplished through engineering strategies such as eliminating or containing the hazardous agent. In addition, workers must use preventive actions, such as practicing safe work habits and wearing personal protective equipment when needed. Examples of safe work habits include taking appropriate breaks from environments with temperature extremes and not eating or smoking in radiation-contaminated areas. Personal protective equipment includes hearing protection, eye guards, protective clothing, and devices for monitoring exposures to agents such as radiation.

## Psychosocial Agents

Psychosocial agents are conditions that create a threat to the psychological and/or social well-being of individuals and groups (Rogers, 2001). A psychosocial response to the work environment occurs as an employee acts selectively toward his environment in an attempt to achieve a harmonious relationship. When such a human attempt at adaptation to the environment fails, an adverse psychosocial re-

### Evidence-Based Practice

The authors of this study were interested in how organizations and the psychosocial environment of work affect morbidity and mortality, especially related to heart disease. The authors investigated previously established risk factors for heart disease in a sample of 2682 men from Kuopio, Finland.

Baseline assessments were completed of biological, behavioral, and psychosocial factors related to each participant. Also done were an assessment of the prevalence of current illnesses and an evaluation of each person's work environment, income, and education.

The study concluded that there were risks of mortality from a number of causes for men in low-income, high-demand jobs that had few resources to complete the job. Mortality also increased in all low-income jobs that had lots of resources regardless of the job demands. However, men in high-demand, low-income jobs with few resources were at greater risk for heart disease than other workers.

Considering all the factors related to the individual and the workplace, the authors thought that the results over time of the effects of poor working conditions and low income lead to feelings of hopelessness, depression, poor behavior, psychological risk profiles, higher levels of morbidity, and increased mortality risk.

**Nurse Use:** Because the low-income worker is at greater risk for mortality, occupational nurses can be aware of the organization of the workplace, the job demands, and the work environment on the population of low-income workers. Increasing the skills of the workers, creating a democratic work environment, and focusing on job satisfaction and economic rewards for enhancing worker skills are a few recommended interventions. Health education and counseling directed to the population, spending quality family time, and encouraging hobbies and recreational events can help.

Lynch J et al: Workplace conditions, socioeconomic status and the risk of mortality and acute myocardial infarction: the Kuopio ischemic heart disease risk factor study, *Am J Public Health* 87(4):617, 1997.

sponse may occur. Work-related stress or burnout has been defined as an important problem for many individuals (Parkes and Sparkes, 1998). Responses to negative interpersonal relationships, particularly those with authority figures in the workplace, are often the cause of vague health symptoms and increased absenteeism. Epidemiologic work in mental health has pointed to environmental variables such as these in the incidence of mental illness and emotional disorder (see the Evidence-Based Practice box).

The psychosocial environment includes characteristics of the work itself, as well as the interpersonal relationships required in the work setting and shiftwork. About 10% of U.S. workers do some form of shiftwork that has the potential to lead to a variety of psychological and physical problems including exhaustion, depression, anxiety, and gastrointestinal disturbance. Strategies to minimize the adverse effects of shiftwork, such as rotating shifts clockwise, are beneficial. Job characteristics such as low autonomy, poor job satisfaction, and limited control over the pace of work have been associated with an increased risk of heart disease among clerical and blue-collar workers.

Interpersonal relationships among employees and coworkers or bosses and managers are often sources of conflict and stress. Another aspect is organizational culture. This refers to the norms and patterns of behavior that are sanctioned within a particular organization. Such norms and patterns set guidelines for the types of work behaviors that will enable employees to succeed within a particular firm. Examples include following organizational norms for working overtime, expressing constructive dissatisfaction with management, and making work a top priority (USDHHS, NIOSH, 2002). These factors and the employee's response to them must be assessed if strategies for influencing the health and safety of workers are to be effective.

Nonfatal violence in the health care worker's workplace is a serious problem that is underreported. Much of the study of health care worker violence has been in psychiatric settings; however, reports in other areas such as the emergency department have been reported. Risk factors associated with this type of violence must be identified and strategies implemented to reduce the risk (USDHHS, NIOSH, 1996).

## Environment

Environmental factors influence the occurrence of host–agent interactions and may direct the course and outcome of those interactions. The physical environment involves the geologic and atmospheric structure of an area and the source of such elements as water, temperature, and radiation, which may serve as positive or negative stressors. Although aspects of the physical environment (e.g., heat, odor, ventilation) may influence the host–agent interaction, the social and psychological environment can be of equal importance (Whelton and Gordis, 2000).

New environmental problems continue to arise, such as an increase in industrial wastes and toxins and indoor and outdoor environmental pollution, which present opportunities for significant health threats to the working and general population. The social aspects of the environment encompass the economic and political forces affecting society and its health. This includes factors such as sanitation and hygiene practices, housing conditions, level and delivery of health care services, development and enforcement of health-related codes (e.g., occupational health and safety, pollution), employment conditions, population crowding, literacy, ethnic customs, extent of support for health-related research, and equal access to health care. In addition, addictive behaviors such as alcohol and substance abuse and various forms of

psychosocial stress may be an outgrowth of negative social environments.

Consider an employee who is working with a potentially toxic liquid. Providing education about safe work practices and fitting the employee with protective clothing may not be adequate if the work must occur in a very hot and humid environment. As the worker becomes uncomfortable in the hot clothing, protection may be compromised by rolling up a sleeve, taking off a glove, or wiping the face with a contaminated piece of clothing. If the norms in the workplace condone such work practices (e.g., "Everyone does it when it's too hot"), the interventions that address only the host and agent will be ineffective; strategies to address the environment itself must be considered, such as cooling fans or minimization of exposure through job rotation. The epidemiologic triad can be used as the basis for planning interventions to restore and promote the health of workers. These efforts are influenced by society and by organizational activities related to occupational health and safety (Rogers, 2003).

The occupational environment, within the context of the social environment, is represented by the workplace and work setting and the interactive effects of this environment on the worker. The nurse must consider the hazards and threats posed by this environment and the commitment of the employer to providing a safe and healthful workplace through use of preventive strategies and controls (e.g., engineering, substitution) (Rogers, 2003).

## ORGANIZATIONAL AND PUBLIC EFFORTS TO PROMOTE WORKER HEALTH AND SAFETY

Promotion of worker health and safety is the goal of occupational health and safety programs (Sofie, 2000). These programs are offered primarily by the employer at the workplace, but the range of services and the models for delivering them have been changing dramatically over the past few years. In addition to specific services, legislation at the federal and state levels has had a significant effect on efforts to provide a healthy and safe environment for all workers. Under the Occupational Safety and Health Act and because of increased public concern about worker health and safety, companies have recently been cited for not meeting minimal occupational health and safety standards. Criminal charges have been filed against business owners when preventable work-related deaths occurred. These events have redirected an emphasis on preventive occupational health and safety programming.

Unless they have OSHA-regulated exposures, business firms are not required to provide occupational health and safety services that meet any specified standards. With few exceptions, there is no legal recourse for specific services or level of personnel provided by employers to protect worker health and safety. Therefore the range of services offered and the qualifications of the providers of occupational health and safety vary widely across industries. An important stimulus for health and safety programs is avoiding cost that can be attributed to the effectiveness of prevention services, as well as the need to support occupational health and safety and health promotion at the worksite.

## On-Site Occupational Health and Safety Programs

Optimally, on-site occupational health and safety services are provided by a team of occupational health and safety professionals. The core members of this team are the occupational health nurse, occupational physician, industrial hygienist, and safety professional. In addition, more and more ergonomists are playing an important role in the occupational health and safety team. The largest group of health care professionals in business settings is occupational health nurses; therefore the most frequently seen model is that of the one-nurse unit. This nurse collaborates with a community physician or occupational medicine physician who provides consultation and accepts referrals when medical intervention is needed. The collaboration may occur primarily through telephone contact, or the physician may be under contract with the company to spend a certain amount of on-site time each week. As companies become larger, they are likely to hire additional nurses, safety professionals, industrial hygienists, and physicians, the latter usually on a part-time or consultant basis. An increasingly popular option is to contract some health, safety, and industrial hygiene work to external providers. The largest firms often have corporate occupational health and safety professionals who set policy and participate in company decision making at the corporate level. These professionals work with the nurses employed at the individual sites within the company. Depending on the needs of the company and the workers, additional professionals may be on the occupational health and safety team, including employee assistance counselors, physical therapists, health educators, physical fitness specialists, and toxicologists.

The services provided by on-site occupational health programs range from those focused only on work-related health and safety problems to a wide scope of services that includes primary health care (Box 44-5). In industries that have exposures regulated by law, certain programs are required, such as respiratory protection or hearing conservation. The ability of a company to offer additional programs depends on employee needs, management's attitudes and understanding about health and safety, acceptance by the workers, and the economic status of the company. A significant increase in the number of health promotion and employee assistance programs offered in industry has occurred over the past few years. Health promotion programs focus on lifestyle choices that cause risks to health (e.g., job stress, obesity, smoking, stress responses, or lack of exercise) (O'Donnell, 2002). Employee assistance programs are designed to address personal problems (e.g., marital/family issues, substance abuse, or financial difficulties) that affect the employee's productivity. As such efforts are cost effective for businesses, they should continue to increase.

Similar types of occupational health and safety programs are available on a contractual basis from community-

---

> **BOX 44-5** Scope of Services Provided Through an Occupational Health and Safety Program
>
> - Health/medical surveillance
> - Workplace monitoring/surveillance
> - Health assessments
>   - Preplacement
>   - Periodic, mandatory, voluntary
>   - Transfer
>   - Retirement/termination
>   - Executive
>   - Return to work
> - Health promotion
> - Health screening
> - Employee assistance programs
> - Case management
> - Primary health care for workers and dependents
> - Worker safety and health education related to occupational hazards
> - Job task analysis and design
> - Prenatal and postnatal care and support groups
> - Safety audits and accident prevention
> - Workers' compensation management
> - Risk management, loss control
> - Emergency preparedness
> - Preretirement counseling
> - Integrated health benefits programs

---

based providers. These may be offered by free-standing occupational health clinics, health maintenance organizations, hospitals, emergency clinics, and other health care organizations. In addition, consultants in each discipline work in the private sector (self-employed, in group practice, or in insurance companies) and in the public sector (in local and state health departments or departments of labor and industry). These services may be provided on site, delivered at a specific location in the community, or offered through a mobile van that visits companies. These multiple resources have increased the options for companies that need occupational health and safety services, and they have also broadened the employment opportunities for health and safety professionals.

## NURSING CARE OF WORKING POPULATIONS

The nurse is often the first health care provider seen by an individual with a work-related health problem. Consequently, nurses are in key positions to intervene with working populations at all levels of prevention. Prevention may be accomplished in the prepathogenesis period by measures designed to promote general optimal health, by protection against specific disease agents, or by the establishment of barriers against agents in the environment. These procedures have been termed *primary prevention.*

As soon as the disease is detectable, early in pathogenesis, secondary prevention may be accomplished by early diagnosis and prompt and adequate treatment. When the process of pathogenesis has progressed and the disease had advanced beyond its early stages, secondary prevention may be accomplished by means of adequate treatment to prevent sequelae and limit disability. Later, when defect and disability have been fixed, tertiary prevention may be accomplished by rehabilitation.

The occupational health nurse practices all levels of prevention (Rogers, 2003). Delivery of primary prevention services to employees is directed toward promoting health and averting a problem. In the occupational health setting, the purpose of health promotion is to maintain or enhance the well-being of individuals or groups of employees, and the company in general. This may include programs designed to enhance coping skills or good nutrition and knowledge about potential health hazards both in and outside of the workplace.

Health protection (i.e., taking primary prevention measures) is designed to eliminate or reduce the risk of disease in order to prevent the development of an illness or injury. Walk-throughs by the occupational health nurse and/or other team members to identify workplace hazards are aimed at health protection.

Specific protection programs or interventions often require active participation on the part of the employee. Participation in an immunization program, use of personal protective equipment, such as respirators or gloves, and smoking cessation are examples of specific health protection measures.

Secondary prevention occurs after a disease process has already begun. It is aimed at early detection, prompt treatment, and prevention of further limitations. For employees, early detection involves health surveillance and periodic screening to identify an illness at the earliest possible moment in its course, and elimination or modification of the hazard-producing situation. Interventions aimed at disability limitation are intended to prevent further harm or deterioration, and they include referral for counseling and treatment of an employee with an emotional or mental health problem whose work performance has deteriorated, and removal of workers from heavy metal exposure who manifest neurologic symptoms.

Tertiary prevention is intended to restore health as fully as possible and assist individuals to achieve their maximum level of functioning. Rehabilitation strategies such as return-to-work programs after a heart attack or limited duty programs after a cumulative trauma injury are examples of tertiary prevention.

## Worker Assessment

The initial step of assessment involves the traditional history and physical assessment, emphasizing exposure to occupational hazards and individual characteristics that may predispose the client to the increased health risk of certain jobs. The **occupational health history** is an indispensable component of the health assessment of individuals (Rogers, 2003). Because work is a part of life for most people, including an occupational health history into all routine nursing assessments is essential. Many workers in the United States do not have access to health care services in their workplaces. Yet it is not unusual to find health care providers in the community who have little or no knowledge about workplaces or expertise in occupation-related illnesses and injuries. Because of the large number of small businesses that do not have the resources for maintaining on-site health care, injured and ill workers are first seen in the public and private health care sector (e.g., in clinics, emergency rooms, physicians' offices, hospitals, health maintenance organizations, and ambulatory care centers). Nurses are often the first-line assessors of these individuals and perhaps the only contact for education about self-protection from workplace hazards.

Identifying workplace exposures as sources of health problems may influence the client's course of illness and rehabilitation and may also prevent similar illnesses among others with potential for exposure (Levy and Wegman, 2000). Including occupational health data into client assessments begins with recognizing the possible relationship between health and occupational factors. The next step is to integrate into the history-taking procedure some routine assessment questions that will provide the data necessary to confirm or rule out occupationally induced symptoms. Symptoms of hazardous workplace exposures may be indicated by vague complaints involving any body system. These complaints are often similar to common medical problems. Three points that occupational health histories should include are a list of current and past jobs the client has held; questions about exposures to specific agents and relationships between the symptoms and activities at work, their job titles, or history of exposures; and other factors that may influence the client's susceptibility to occupational agents (e.g., lifestyle history such as smoking, underlying illness, previous injury, or disabling condition).

Questions about the employee's occupational history can be included in existing assessment tools. The more complete the data collected, the more likely the nurse is to notice the influence of work–health interactions. All employees should be questioned about their employment history. To describe only a current status of "retired" or "housewife" may lead to the omission of needed data. The nurse should be aware that not all workers are well informed about the materials with which they work or about potential hazards. For this reason, the nurse must develop basic knowledge about all of the types of jobs held by clients and the possible hazards associated with them. Because there is an increased likelihood of multiple exposures from other environments, such as the home and the community, that may interact with workplace exposures, the nurse should extend the questioning to include this information.

Identifying work-related health problems should be an integrated focus of any assessment effort. A systematic approach for evaluating the potential for workplace exposures is the most effective intervention for detecting and preventing occupational health risks. Figure 44-8 shows one short assessment tool that can be incorporated into routine history taking. Similar questions can be included in the assessment of workers' spouses and dependents, who may receive secondhand or indirect exposure to occupational hazards.

During these health assessments, the nurse has the opportunity to teach about workplace hazards and prevention measures the worker can use. At the same time, the nurse is obtaining information that will be valuable in optimizing the fit between the job and the worker. Such assessments can be done during preplacement examinations before the client begins a job, on a periodic basis during employment, or when a work-related health problem or exposure becomes apparent. Work-related health assessments should also be conducted when an employee is being transferred to another job with different requirements and exposures. The goal of these assessments is to identify agent and host factors that could place the employee at risk and to determine prevention steps that can be taken to eliminate or minimize the exposure and potential health problem.

When the health data from such assessments are considered collectively, the nurse may determine some patterns in risk factors associated with the occurrence of work-related injuries and illnesses in a total population of workers. For example, a nurse practitioner in a clinic noted a dramatic increase in the number of dermatitis cases among her clients. When she looked at factors in common among these individuals, she determined that they all worked at a company with solvent exposure commonly associated with dermal irritations. She worked with the union and the company to assess the environment/agent exposure to the employees. This nursing intervention led to a safer work environment and a decrease in dermatitis in this population group. Such an approach can be used at the company, industry, and community levels. The initial collection of data and the questioning about workplace exposures are vital steps for any intervention.

## Workplace Assessment

The nurse may conduct a similar assessment of the workplace itself. The purpose of this assessment, known as a **worksite walk-through** or survey, is to become knowledgeable about the work processes and the materials, the requirements of various jobs, the presence of actual or potential hazards, and the work practices of employees (Rogers, 2003). Figure 44-9 shows a brief outline that can

be used to guide a worksite assessment. More complex surveys are performed by industrial hygienists and safety professionals when the purpose of the walk-through is environmental monitoring using sampling techniques or a safety audit. However, most occupational health nurses have developed expertise in these areas and include such tasks as part of their functions. For all health care providers who assess workers, this information makes an important database. In addition, for the on-site health care provider, worksite walk-throughs assist the professional in developing rapport with and being seen as a credible worker among the employees.

A worksite survey begins with an understanding of the type of work that occurs in the workplace. All business organizations are classified by the U.S. Department of Commerce with a numerical code, the Standard Industrial Classification (SIC) code. This code, usually a two- to four-digit number, indicates a company's product and, therefore, the possible types of **occupational health hazards** that may be associated with the processes and materials used by its employees. SIC codes are used to collect and report data on businesses. For example, illness and injury rates of one company are compared to the rates of other companies of similar size with the same SIC code to determine whether the company is having an excess of illness or injury. All OSHA and workers' compensation data are reported by the SIC code. In addition, by knowing the SIC code of a company, a health care professional can access reference books that describe the usual processes, materials, and byproducts of that kind of company.

The nurse will want to review the work processes and work areas by jobs or locations in the workplace. These preliminary data provide clues about what hazards may be present and an understanding of the types of jobs and health requirements that may be involved in a particular industry. A description of the work environment is next and provides an overall picture of general appearances, physical layout, and safety of the environment. Are safety signs posted and readable where needed? Is there clutter or dampness on the floor that could cause slips or falls?

A description of the employee group is necessary information to understand the demographics and the work distribution in the company. Knowing about shiftwork and productivity can be helpful in pinpointing potential stressors. Human resources management and corporate commitment to health and safety is needed to develop a supportive culture for effective and efficient programming. Assessing the status of policies and procedures and assessing opportunities for input into improving service are important to establish the organization's strength in occupational health and safety management. Gathering data about the incidence and prevalence of work-related illnesses and injuries and the cost patterns for these conditions provides useful epidemiologic trend data and helps to target high-cost areas. The types of occupational safety and health services and programs are important to know. This will show whether required programs are being offered and includes health promotion and disease prevention strategies.

**WHAT DO YOU THINK?**
There is an acceptable level of risk in any job.

## I. Present Job

A. What is your job title? _____

B. What do you do for a living? _____

C. How long have you had this job? _____

D. Describe the specific tasks of this job: _____
_____

E. What product or service is produced by the company where you work? _____
_____

F. Are you exposed to any of the following on your present job?

| Metals | Radiation | Stress |
|---|---|---|
| Vapors, gases | Vibration | Others: _____ |
| Dusts | Loud noise | |
| Solvents | Extreme heat or cold | |

G. Do you feel you have any health problems that may be associated with your work?
If yes, describe: _____
_____

H. How would you describe your satisfaction with your job? _____
_____

I. Have any of your co-workers complained of illness or injuries that they associate with their jobs?
If yes, describe: _____
_____

## II. All Past Work

Starting with your first job, please provide the following information:

| Job title | Years held | Description of work | Exposures | Injuries/Illnesses | Personal protection equipment used |
|---|---|---|---|---|---|
| | | | | | |
| | | | | | |
| | | | | | |
| | | | | | |
| | | | | | |

## III. Other Exposures

A. Do you have any hobbies which involve exposure to chemicals, metals, or any of the other agents mentioned before? If yes, describe: _____

B. Are any other members of your household exposed to any of the substances listed above? If yes, describe:
_____

C. Do you live near any factories, dump sites, or other sources of pollution? If yes, describe: _____
_____

**Figure 44-8** Occupational health history form.

Name of company: _____  Date: _____

Address: _____

Telephone: _____

Parent company (if any): _____

Location of corporate offices: _____

SIC code: _____

## The Work:

Major products: _____

Major processes and operations, raw materials, by-products: _____

_____

Type of jobs: _____

_____

Potential exposures: _____

_____

## Work Environment

General conditions: _____

Safety signs: _____

Physical environment: _____

## Worker Population

Employees

Total number: _____ Number in production: _____ Others: _____

% Full-time: _____ % Men: _____ % Women: _____

% First shift: _____ % Second shift: _____ % Third shift: _____

Age distribution: _____

% Unionized: _____ Names of unions: _____

## Human Resources Management

Corporate commitment to health

Personnel

Policies/procedures

Input/surveys/committees

Record keeping

## Health Data

Work-related illnesses, injuries, deaths per annum: _____

OSHA recordable: _____ Workers' compensation: _____

Other: _____ Most frequent complaints: _____

Average number of monthly calls to the health unit: _____

Absenteeism rate: _____

## Occupation Health and Safety Services

Examinations

Employee assistance

Treatment of illness/injury

Health education

Physical fitness, health promotion activities

Mandatory programs

Safety audits

Environmental monitoring

Health risk appraisal

Screenings

Health promotion

## Control Strategies

Engineering

Work practice

Administrative

Personal protective equipment

**Figure 44-9** Worksite assessment guide.

## HOW TO    Assess a Worker and the Workplace

Assessing the worker for a work-related problem is a critical practice element. You need to do the following:

- Complete general and occupational health history taking with emphasis on workplace exposure assessment, job hazard analysis, and list of previous jobs.
- Conduct a health assessment to identify agent and host factors that interact to place workers at risk.
- Identify patterns of risk associated with illness/injury.

Assessing the work environment is necessary to determine workplace exposures that create worker health risk. You need to do the following:

- Understand the work being done.
- Understand the work process.
- Evaluate the work-related hazards.
- Gather data about incidence/prevalence of work-related illness/injuries and related hazards.
- Examine prevention and control strategies in place for eliminating exposures.

Finally, examining control strategies that are effective in eliminating or reducing exposure is important in determining risk reduction. Control strategies follow a hierarchical approach. Engineering controls can reduce worker exposure by modifying the exposure source, such as putting needles in a puncture-proof container.

Work practice controls include good hygiene and proper waste disposal and housekeeping. Administrative controls reduce exposure through job rotation, workplace monitoring, and employee training and education. Finally, personal protective control is the last resort and requires the worker to actively engage in strategies for protection such as use of gloves, masks, and gowns to prevent exposures (Rogers, 2003).

The more information that can be collected before the walk-through, the more efficient the process of the survey will be. After the survey is conducted, the nurse can use the information with the aggregate health data to evaluate the effectiveness of the occupational health and safety program and to plan future programs.

## NURSING TIP

Both corporate culture and cost-effective programs are key factors in influencing the development of occupational health services.

## HEALTHY PEOPLE 2010 RELATED TO OCCUPATIONAL HEALTH

In an attempt to meet the goal of increasing the span of healthy life for Americans, health promotion and protection strategies are proposed to address the needs of large population groups such as the American workforce. As part of the Healthy People 2010 document, occupational safety and health objectives are identified to promote good health and well-being among workers, including the elimination and reduction of elements in occupational environments that cause death, injury, disease, or disability. In addition, this document promotes the minimizing of personal damage from existing occupationally related illness. These objectives are shown in the Healthy People 2010 box.

## LEGISLATION RELATED TO OCCUPATIONAL HEALTH

The occupational health and safety services provided by an employer are influenced by specific legislation at federal and state levels. Although the relationship between work and health has been known since the second century (Ramazzini, 1713), public policy that effectively controlled occupational hazards was not enacted until the 1960s. The Mine Safety and Health Act of 1968 was the first legislation that specifically required certain prevention programs for workers. This was followed by the Occupational Safety and Health Act of 1970, which established two agencies, the Occupational Safety and Health Administration and the National Institute for Occupational Safety and Health, each with discrete functions (Box 44-6) to carry out the act's purpose of ensuring "safe and healthful working conditions for working men and women" (PL 91-596, 1970).

In the context of the Occupational Safety and Health Act, OSHA, a federal agency within the U.S. Department of Labor, was created to develop and enforce workplace safety and health standards and regulations that regulate workers' exposure to potentially toxic substances, enforcing these at the federal and state levels. Specific standards and information about compliance can be obtained from federal, regional, and state OSHA offices, which can be found on the OSHA website (www.osha.gov).

The **National Institute for Occupational Safety and Health** (NIOSH) was established by the Occupational Safety and Health Act of 1970 and is part of the Centers for Disease Control and Prevention (CDC). In 1996, NIOSH and its partners unveiled the **National Occupational Research Agenda** (NORA), a framework to guide occupational safety and health research into the following decade. The NIOSH agency identifies, monitors, and educates about the incidence, prevalence, and prevention of work-related illnesses and injuries and examines potential hazards of new work technologies and practices (USDHHS, NIOSH, 1999). NORA (Box 44-7) identifies targeted research areas with the highest likelihood of reducing the still significant toll of workplace illness and injury.

Many standards have been established by OSHA and promulgated to protect worker health. One example is the **hazard communication standard.** This standard is based on the premise that while working to reduce and eliminate potentially toxic agents in the work environment, an important line of defense is to provide the work community with information about hazardous chemicals so as to min-

## Healthy People 2010 | Objectives Focusing on Occupational Health

20-1 Reduce deaths from work-related injuries
20-2 Reduce work-related injuries resulting in medical treatment, lost time from work, or restricted work activity
20-3 Reduce the rate of injury and illness cases involving days away from work due to overexertion or repetitive motion
20-4 Reduce pneumoconiosis deaths
20-5 Reduce deaths from work-related homicides
20-6 Reduce work-related assault
20-7 Reduce the number of persons who have elevated blood lead concentrations from work exposures

20-8 Reduce occupational skin diseases or disorders among full-time workers
20-9 Increase the proportion of worksites employing 50 or more persons that provide programs to prevent or reduce employee stress
20-10 Reduce occupational needlestick injuries among health care workers
20-11 Reduce new cases of work-related noise-induced hearing loss

From U.S. Department of Health and Human Services: *Healthy people 2010: national health promotion and disease prevention objectives,* Washington, DC, 2000, U.S. Government Printing Office.

### BOX 44-6 Functions of Federal Agencies Involved in Occupational Safety and Health

**OCCUPATIONAL SAFETY AND HEALTH ADMINISTRATION (OSHA)**

- Determines and sets standards and permissible exposure limits (PELs) for hazardous exposures in the workplace
- Enforces the occupational health standards (including the right of entry for inspection)
- Educates employees and employers about occupational health and safety
- Develops and maintains a database of work-related injuries, illnesses, and deaths
- Monitors compliance with occupational health and safety standards

**NATIONAL INSTITUTE FOR OCCUPATIONAL SAFETY AND HEALTH (NIOSH)**

- Conducts research and reviews findings to recommend exposure limits for occupational hazards to OSHA
- Identifies and researches occupational health and safety hazards
- Educates occupational health and safety professionals
- Distributes research findings relevant to occupational health and safety

From Centers for Disease Control and Prevention, U.S. Department of Health and Human Services, National Institute for Occupational Safety and Health: *National occupational research agenda,* publication No. 99-108, Washington, DC, 1999, U.S. Government Printing Office.

imize exposures. The hazard communication standard, which was first established in 1983, requires that all worksites with hazardous substances inventory their toxic agents, label them, and provide information sheets, called material safety data sheets (MSDSs), for each agent. In addition, the employer must have in place a hazard communication program that provides workers with education about these agents. This education must include agent identification, toxic effects, and protective measures. Numerous standards have been established by OSHA for specific chemicals and programs. A standard familiar to all health care professionals is the *bloodborne pathogens standard.*

Workers' compensation acts are important state laws that govern financial compensation to employees who suffer work-related health problems. These acts vary by state, and each state sets rules for the reimbursement of employees with occupational health problems for medical expenses and lost work time associated with the illness or injury. Workers'

compensation claims and the experience-based insurance premiums paid by industry have been important motivators for increasing the health and safety of the workplace.

**NURSING TIP**

NIOSH publications, many of which are free, are online at http://www.cdc.gov/niosh/homepage.html.

## DISASTER PLANNING AND MANAGEMENT

Although disaster planning and management have been functions of occupational health and safety programs, this is an area of legislation that affects businesses and health professionals. The legislation of the Superfund Amendment and Reauthorization Act (SARA) requires that written disaster plans be shared with key resources in the community,

---

**BOX 44-7**  **National Occupational Research Agenda (NORA) Priority Research Areas**

**DISEASE AND INJURY**
- Allergy and irritant dermatitis
- Asthma and chronic obstructive pulmonary disease
- Fertility and pregnancy abnormalities
- Hearing loss
- Infectious diseases
- Low back disorders
- Musculoskeletal disorders of the upper extremities
- Traumatic injuries

**WORK ENVIRONMENT AND WORKFORCE**
- Emerging technologies
- Indoor environment
- Mixed exposures
- Organization of work
- Special populations at risk

**RESEARCH TOOLS AND APPROACHES**
- Cancer research methods
- Control technology and personal protective equipment
- Exposure assessment methods
- Health services research
- Intervention effectiveness research
- Risk assessment methods
- Social and economic consequences of workplace illness and injury
- Surveillance research methods

From Centers for Disease Control and Prevention, U.S. Department of Health and Human Services, National Institute for Occupational Safety and Health, *National occupational research agenda*, publication No. 99-108, 1999.

---

such as fire departments and emergency departments. Concern about disasters, such as the terrorist attacks on the World Trade Center and Pentagon on September 11, 2001, the methyl isocyanate leak in Bhopal, India, or the community exposure to chemicals at Times Beach, Missouri, has mandated more attention to disaster planning.

The goals of a disaster plan are to prevent or minimize injuries and deaths of workers and residents, minimize property damage, provide effective triage, and facilitate necessary business activities. A disaster plan requires the cooperation of different personnel within the company and community. The nurse is often a key person on the disaster planning team, along with safety professionals, physicians, industrial hygienists, the fire chief, and company management. The potential for disaster (e.g., explosions, fires, leaks) must be identified, and this is best achieved by completing an exhaustive chemical and hazard inventory of the workplace. The material safety data sheets and plant blue-prints are critical for correctly identifying substances and work areas that may be hazardous. Worksite surveys are the first step to completing this inventory.

Effective disaster plans are designed by those with knowledge of the work processes and materials, the workers and workplace, and the resources in the community. Specific steps must be detailed for actions to be put in place by specific individuals in the event of a disaster. The written plan must be shared with all who will be involved. Employees should be prepared in first aid, cardiopulmonary resuscitation, and fire brigade procedures. Plans must be clear, specific, and comprehensive (i.e., covering all shifts and all work areas) and must include activities to be conducted within the worksite and those that require community resources. Transportation plans, fire response, and emergency response services should be coordinated with the agencies that would be involved in an actual disaster. The disaster plan, emergency and safety equipment, and the first response team's abilities should be tested at least annually with a drill. Practice results should be carefully evaluated, with changes made as needed.

Hospitals and other emergency services, such as fire departments, should be involved in developing the disaster plan and should receive a copy of the plan and a current hazard inventory. It is imperative that the plan and hazard inventory be periodically updated. The occupational health nurse or another company representative should provide emergency health care providers with updated clinical information on exposures and appropriate treatment. It should never be presumed that local services will have current information on substances used in industry. Representatives of these agencies should visit the worksite and accompany the nurse on a worksite walk-through so that they are familiar with the operations.

In disaster planning, the nurse is often assigned or assumes the responsibility for coordinating the planning and implementing efforts, working with appropriate key people within the company and in the community to develop a workable, comprehensive plan. Other tasks include providing ongoing communication to keep the plan current; planning the drills; educating the employees, management, and community providers; and assessing the equipment and services that may be used in a disaster.

In the event of a disaster, the nurse should play a key role in coordinating the response. Principles of triage may be used as the response team determines the extent of the disaster and the ability of the company and community to respond. Postdisaster nursing interventions are also critical. Examples include identifying the ongoing disaster-related health needs of workers and community residents, collecting epidemiologic data, and assessing the cause and the necessary steps to prevent a recurrence.

Occupational health nursing is a broad, dynamic specialty practice. The public health foundation provides the basis for practice supporting a health promotion and protection and prevention model. The occupational health nurse must have interdisciplinary skills and linkages to provide the most effective care and service. Occupational

## BOX 44-8  Levels of Prevention Applied to Occupational Health

**PRIMARY PREVENTION**

Nurses provide education of safety in the workplace to prevent injury.

**SECONDARY PREVENTION**

Nurse screens for hearing loss resulting from noise levels in the plant.

**TERTIARY PREVENTION**

Nurse works with chronic diabetic workers to ensure appropriate medication use and blood glucose screening to avoid lost work days.

health nurses are involved in all levels of prevention in their practice (Box 44-8).

## Practice Application

An insurance company recently renovated its claims processing office area and fitted the workstation with new computers. The company's occupational health nurse noticed an increase in visits to the health unit for complaints of headaches, stiff neck muscles, and visual disturbances consistent with computer usage.

To conduct a complete investigation of this problem, the nurse assessed the workers, the agent (computer), previously existing potential agents, and the work environment. Interventions focused on designing the health hazard out of the work process, if possible. In the present example, the first level of intervention was to refit the workstation for better worker use of the computer.

Minimizing the possible hazards of the agent involved recommendations for desks, chairs, and lighting designs that would accommodate the individual worker and allow shielding of the monitor. The nursing interventions included strengthening the resistance of the host by prescribing appropriate rest breaks, eye exercises, and relaxation strategies. Recognizing that previous cervical neck injury or impaired vision may increase the risk of adverse effects from computer work, the nurse would include assessment for these factors in employees' preplacement and periodic health examinations.

For the environmental concerns, the nurse educated the manager about the health risks of paced, externally controlled work expectations and recommended alternatives.

This case is an example of which of the following:

A. The application of the occupational health history
B. A worksite assessment or walk-through
C. A work–health interaction
D. The use of the epidemiologic triad in exploring occupational health problems

Answer is in the back of the book.

## Key Points

- Occupational health nursing is an autonomous practice specialty.
- The scope of occupational health nursing practice is broad, including worker and workplace assessment and surveillance, case management, health promotion, primary care, management/administration, business and finance skills, and research.
- The workforce and workplace are changing dramatically, requiring new knowledge and new occupational health services.
- The type of work has shifted from primarily manufacturing to service and technologic jobs.
- Workplace hazards include exposure to biological, chemical, enviromechanical, physical, and psychosocial agents.
- The Occupational Safety and Health Act of 1970 states that workers must have a safe and healthful work environment.
- The interdisciplinary occupational health team consists of the occupational health nurse, occupational medicine physician, industrial hygienist, and safety specialist.
- Work-related health problems must be investigated and control strategies implemented to reduce exposure.
- Control strategies include engineering, work practice, administration, and personal protective equipment.
- The Occupational Safety and Health Administration enforces workplace safety and health standards.
- The National Institute for Occupational Safety and Health is the education and research agency that provides grants to investigate the causes of workplace illness and injuries.
- Workers' Compensation Acts are important laws that govern financial compensation of employees who suffer work-related health problems.
- The occupational health nurse should play a key role in disaster planning and coordination.
- Academic education in occupational health nursing is generally at the graduate level.

## Clinical Decision-Making Activities

1. Arrange to visit a local industry to observe work processes and discuss working conditions. See if you can identify the work-related hazards and make recommendations for eliminating them.
2. Interview the occupational health nurse in an industry setting and ask questions about scope of practice, job functions, and contributions to the business. Compare and contrast what you have learned about this nurse role to that of the school health nurse.
3. Contact the American Association of Occupational Health Nurses and ask what the most pressing

trends are in the specialty. What are some of the complex issues related to these trends?

4. Obtain a proposed standard for the Occupational Safety and Health Administration, critique it, and submit your comments.

5. Attend a workers' compensation hearing, analyze the problem, and critique the outcome. How is your critique affected by what you thought the outcome should be?

**Additional Resources**

These related resources are found either in the appendix at the back of this book or on the book's website at **http://evolve.elsevier.com/Stanhope.**

## Appendix

Appendix I.3 Comprehensive Occupational and Environmental Health History

**evolve** Evolve Website

Appendix D.1 Immunization for Health Care Workers
WebLinks: Healthy People 2010

## References

American Association of Occupational Health Nurses: *The nurse in industry,* New York, 1976, AAOHN.

American Association of Occupational Health Nurses: *Guidelines for developing job descriptions in occupational and environmental health nursing,* Atlanta, 1997, AAOHN.

American Association of Occupational Health Nurses: *Standards for occupational health nursing practice,* Atlanta, 1999, AAOHN.

Brown M: *Occupational health nursing,* New York, 1981, MacMillan.

Bureau of Labor Statistics: *Handbook of labor statistics,* Washington, DC, 1995, U.S. Department of Labor.

Bureau of Labor Statistics: *Employment projections: 1997,* Washington, DC, 1997, U.S. Department of Labor.

Bureau of Labor Statistics: *Employment and wages, annual averages: BLS bulletin 2511* (December), Washington, DC, 1998a, U.S. Department of Labor.

Bureau of Labor Statistics: *Work at home in 1997, current population survey* [Press release 98-93]. Washington, DC, 1998b, U.S. Department of Labor.

Bureau of Labor Statistics: *Employment projections: 1998,* Washington, DC, 1998c, U.S. Department of Labor.

Bureau of Labor Statistics: *Employment projections: 1999,* Washington, DC, 1999, U.S. Department of Labor.

Bureau of Labor Statistics: A special issue: charting the projections—1998-2008, *Occupa Outlook Q* 43(4):2-38, 2000.

Bureau of Labor Statistics: *Handbook of labor statistics,* Washington, DC, 2003, U.S. Department of Labor.

Campos-Outcalt D: Occupational health epidemiology and objectives for the year 2000: primary care, *Clin Office Pract* 21(20):213, 1994.

Centers for Disease Control and Prevention: *Major TB guidelines,* retrieved June 29, 1999, from http://www.cdc.gov/nchstp/tb/pubs/mmwrhtml/maj_guide.htm.

Centers for Disease Control and Prevention, U.S. Department of Health and Human Services, National Institute for Occupational Safety and Health: *National occupational research agenda,* publication No. 99-108, 1999.

Centers for Disease Control and Prevention, U.S. Department of Health and Human Services, National Institute for Occupational Safety and Health: *National occupational research agenda,* publication No. 99-108, Washington, DC, 1999, U.S. Government Printing Office.

EPINet: *Exposure prevention information network data reports,* Charlottesville, 1999, University of Virginia, International Health Care Worker Safety Center.

Felton J: The genesis of American occupational health nursing, part 1, *Occupat Health Nurs* 33:615, 1985.

Fullerton H: The 2005 labor force: growing, but slowly, *Monthly Labor Rev* 118(11):29, 1995.

Hall-Barrow J, Hodges LC, Brown P: A collaborative model for employee health and nursing education: successful program, *AAOHN J* 49(9):429-436, 2001.

Institute of Medicine: *Safe work in the 21st century,* Washington, DC, 2000, National Academy Press.

Levy BS, Wegman DH: *Occupational health: recognizing and preventing occupational disease,* Philadelphia, 2000, Lippincott Williams & Wilkins.

Lynch J et al: Workplace conditions, socioeconomic status and the risk of mortality and acute myocardial infarction: the Kuopio ischemic heart disease risk factor study, *Am J Public Health* 87(4):617, 1997.

McGrath B: Fifty years of industrial nursing, *Public Health Nurs* 37:119, 1945.

National Institute for Occupational Safety and Health: *Latex allergy,* publication No. 97-135, Washington, DC, 1997a, U.S. Government Printing Office, available at www.cdc.gov/niosh/latexfs.html.

National Institute for Occupational Safety and Health: *Musculoskeletal disorders (MSDs) and workplace factors,* Washington, DC, 1997b, U.S. Government Printing Office, available at www.cdc.gov/niosh/ergtx1l.html.

National Institute for Occupational Safety and Health: *Workpalce injury/illness rates,* Washington, DC, 2000, U.S. Government Printing Office.

National Occupational Health and Safety Act of 1970: Public law No. 91-596.

O'Donnell M: *Health promotion in the workplace,* New York, 2002, Delmar.

Parkes KR, Sparkes TJ: *Organizational interventions to reduce work stress: are they effective? a review of the literature,* Oxford, UK: University of Oxford, Health and Safety Executive, Contract Research Report No. 193, 1998.

Payling K: A hazard we can no longer ignore: effects of excessive noise on well-being, *Prof Nurse* 9(6):418, 1994.

Platt J: Radon: its impact on the community and the role of the nurse, *AAOHN J* 41(11):547, 1993.

Ramazzini B: *De morbis artificum* [diseases of workers], 1713. [translated by Wright WC, Chicago, 1940, University of Chicago Press].

Rogers B: The role of the occupational health nurse. In McCunnery RM, Brandt-Rauf PW, editors: *A practical approach to occupational and environmental medicine,* Boston, 1994, Little, Brown.

Rogers B: Municipal healthcare workers: work-related hazards, *State Art Rev* 16(1):143-161, 2001.

Rogers B: *Occupational health nursing: concepts and practice,* St Louis, Mo, 2003, Elsevier.

Sepkowitz K: Tuberculosis and the health care worker: a historical perspective, *Ann Intern Med* 120(1):71, 1994.

Sofie JK. Creating a successful occupational safety and health program, *AAOHN J* 48:125-130, 2000.

Stine D, Brown T: *Principles of toxicology,* Boca Raton, Fla, 1996, Lewis.

U.S. Census Bureau: *Resident population of the United States: middle series projections, 2006-2010, by age and sex,* Washington, DC, 1999, U.S. Government Printing Office, available at www.census.gov/population/projections/nation/nas/npas0610.txt.

U.S. Department of Health and Human Services: *Data from the national sample survey of registered nurses,* Rockville, Md, 1996, Bureau of Health Professions.

U.S. Department of Health and Human Services: *Healthy people 2010: understanding and improving health,* ed 2, Washington, DC, 2000, U.S. Government Printing Office.

U.S. Department of Health and Human Services, National Institute for Occupational Safety and Health: *National occupational research agenda,* Cincinnati, Ohio, 1996, USDHHS.

U.S. Department of Health and Human Services, National Institute for Occupational Safety and Health: *The changing organization of work and the safety and health of working people,* publication No. 2002-116, Cincinnati, Ohio, 2002, USDHHS.

Whelton PK, Gordis L: Epidemiology of clinical medicine, *Epidemiol Rev* 22(1):140-144, 2000.

# Chapter 45

**evolve** http://evolve.elsevier.com/Stanhope

# Community-Oriented Nurse as Parish Nurse

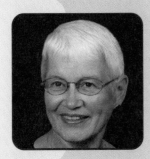

**Ruth D. Berry, R.N., M.S.N.**
Ruth D. Berry has been in public health nursing practice and faculty positions for several decades. She became Parish Nurse in a unique faculty practice collaborative arrangement with the University of Kentucky College of Nursing and Second Presbyterian Church, Lexington, Kentucky. She has served as Health Ministry–Parish Nurse Consultant for the Presbyterian Church–USA and continues to mentor new and continuing parish nurses on a regular basis. She and a colleague initiated parish nurse seminars, which continue to be held annually in Santa Fe, New Mexico. Ruth helped script the philosophy of parish nursing and develop a framework for educational preparation in parish nursing as a member of the International Parish Nurse Resource Center's 1993 Colloquium. She was invited to Keimyung University College of Nursing, Korea, for centennial celebration presentations on international trends and challenges in parish nursing. Ruth has been author and conference presenter for nurses and related health and healing professionals on parish nursing/health ministries both regionally and nationally.

## Objectives

After reading this chapter, the student should be able to do the following:

1. Describe the heritage of health and healing in faith communities
2. Describe models of parish nursing and current trends of the nursing specialty
3. Identify characteristics of the philosophy of parish nursing
4. Develop awareness of the community-oriented nurse's role as parish nurse in faith communities for health promotion and disease prevention
5. Examine the role of holistic health care for wellness in faith communities
6. Help faith communities include Healthy People 2010 guidelines in program planning
7. Collaborate with key partners to implement congregational health ministries relevant for the faith community
8. Use the nursing process in a faith community
9. Evaluate programs for healthy congregations throughout the life span
10. Examine the legal, ethical, and financial issues related to parish nursing

---

Parish nursing has long-established roots in the healing and health professions. Throughout historical accounts of nursing, caring for members of communities has been important. The earliest accounts of concern for others stem from communities of faith. Wholeness in health and being in "right" relationships with one's creator have sustained individuals and groups during times of illness, brokenness, and stress, and when cure was not possible (Chandler, 1999; Meisenhelder and Chandler, 2000; Rydholm, 1997; Solari-Twadell and McDermott, 1999). Today **parish nurses** help individuals, families, and congregations become more aware of the relationship of wholeness in body, mind, and spirit (McDermott, Solari-Twadell, and Mathews, 1998; Schank, Weis, and Matheus, 1996; Sellers and Haag, 1998; Solari-Twadell and

McDermott, 1999; Tuck, Pullen, and Wallace, 2001). Parish nurses balance knowledge and skill in the role and facilitate the faith community to become a caring congregation—a congregation that is a source of health and healing.

Parish nurses address universal health problems of individuals, families, and groups of all ages. The members of congregation populations experience birth, death, acute and chronic illness, stress, dependency concerns, challenges of life transitions, growth, and development; they also face decisions regarding healthy lifestyle choices. Congregational members live in communities that make decisions about policies for financing and managing health care and for keeping environments safe and communities healthy for present and future generations. Parish nurses encourage partnering with other community health

## Key Terms

**congregants**, p. 1106
**congregational model**, p. 1093
**faith communities**, p. 1093
**healing**, p. 1094
**health ministries**, p. 1093
**holistic care**, p. 1094

**holistic health center**, p. 1097
**institutional model**, p. 1094
**parish nurse coordinator**, p. 1099
**parish nurse**, p. 1092
**parish nursing**, p. 1093
**partnership**, p. 1097

**pastoral care staff**, p. 1094
**polity**, p. 1105
**wellness committee**, p. 1100
*See Glossary for definitions*

## Chapter Outline

Definitions in Parish Nursing
Heritage and Horizons
*Faith Communities*
*Health Care Delivery*
*Parish Nursing Community*
Parish Nursing Practice
*Characteristics of the Practice*

*Scope and Standards of Parish Nursing Practice*
*Educational Preparation of a Parish Nurse*
*Holistic Health Care*
*Functions of the Parish Nurse*
Issues in Parish Nursing Practice
*Professional Issues*
*Ethical Issues*

*Legal Issues*
*Financial Issues*
Healthy People 2010 Leading Health Indicators and Faith Communities
Population-Focused Parish Nursing: Faith Community and School

resources to arrive at creative responses to health issues and concerns.

Parish nursing continues to gain prominence as nurses reclaim their traditions of healing, acknowledge gaps in service delivery, and, along with the rise of nursing centers, affirm the independent functions of nursing. In 1998, the American Nurses Association (ANA) accepted *parish nursing* as the most recognized term for the practice of nurses working with congregations or faith communities. With the Health Ministries' Association (HMA), the ANA published the *Scope and Standards of Parish Nursing* (HMA and ANA, 1998). Although most parish nurses are in Protestant congregations, the concept is evident in most faith communities, including communities that serve diverse cultures. By the end of the twentieth century, parish nursing had expanded to most states in the United States. Parish nurses are also serving faith communities in South Korea, Canada, Australia, New Zealand, Swaziland, and Russia (Berry et al, 2000; Bondine, 1997; Culp, 1997; Developing, 2000; Granberg-Michaelson, 1997; Kucey, 1999; Lukits, 2000; McDermott et al, 1998; Olson, Simington, and Clark, 1998; Van Loon, 1996, 1998).

## DEFINITIONS IN PARISH NURSING

**Faith communities** are congregational communities that gather in churches, cathedrals, synagogues, temples, or mosques and acknowledge common faith traditions. **Parish nursing** is the most commonly used term for the professional advanced nurse practice role in this context. A parish nurse in a church has been referred to as congregational health minister, an emergency church nurse, a faith community nurse, or a health ministries nurse. Parish nurses respond to health and wellness needs within the context of populations of faith communities and are partners with the church in fulfilling the mission of health ministry.

The faith community includes persons throughout the life span. This includes active and less active members, as well as those confined to home or in nursing homes. Often, the church's mission also includes individuals and groups in the geographic community who are not designated church members. The services may be extended to those beyond the congregation. **Health ministries** are those activities and programs in faith communities organized around health and healing focuses to promote wholeness in health across the life span (Figure 45-1).

The services may be specifically planned or may be more informal. A professional or a lay person may provide them. These services include visiting the homebound, providing meals for families in crisis or when a family member returns home after hospitalization, prayer circles, volunteering in community care groups for people with acquired immunodeficiency syndrome (AIDS), serving "healthy heart" church suppers, or holding regular grief support groups (Figure 45-2). The parish nurse emphasizes the nursing discipline's spiritual dimension while incorporating physical, emotional, and social aspects of nursing with individuals, families, and congregational communities.

Parish nurse models that have been widely implemented include congregation-based and institution-based models. In the **congregational model,** the nurse is usually autonomous. The development of a parish nurse/health ministry program arises from the individual community of faith. The nurse is accountable to the congregation and its

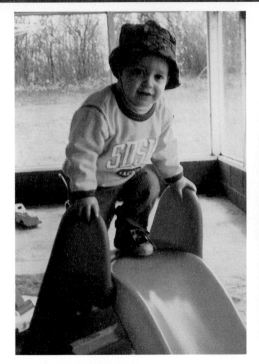
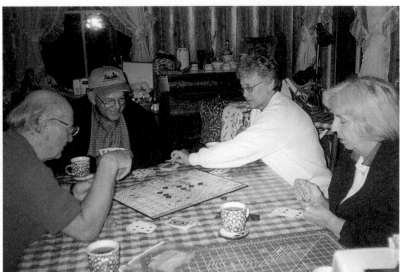

**Figure 45-1** Promoting healthy activities across the life span in church and community activities.

governing body. The **institutional model** includes greater collaboration and partnership; the nurse may be in a contractual relationship with hospitals, medical centers, long-term care establishments, or educational institutions. In either model, nurses work closely with professional health care members, **pastoral care staff,** and lay volunteers who represent various aspects of the life of the congregational community. To promote **healing,** the nurse builds on strengths to promote the connecting and integrating of inner spiritual knowing and healthy lifestyle choices to achieve optimal wellness in the many circumstances faced by individuals and families in life. Intentional and compassionate presence of a spiritually mature professional nurse in individual or group situations is vital. In this role, providing holistic care with congregation populations is important. **Holistic care** is concerned with the relationship between body, mind, and spirit in a constantly changing environment (Dossey, Keegan, and Guzzetta, 2000). The nurse and members of the congregation assess, plan, implement, and evaluate programs. The process of realizing holistic care is enhanced by an active wellness committee or health cabinet (Figure 45-3). These committees

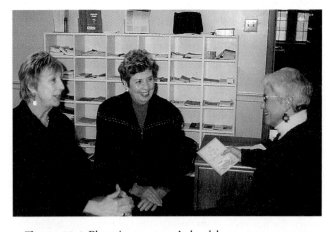

**Figure 45-2** Planning women's health support groups.

are most effective when members represent the broad spectrum of the life of the church. The parish nurse uses all the knowledge and skills of this specialty to give effective services. The outcome is a truly caring congregation that supports healthy, spiritually fulfilling lives. Resources for parish nursing can be found on this book's evolve website at http://evolve.elsevier.com/Stanhope.

## HERITAGE AND HORIZONS
### Faith Communities

In the roots of many faith communities are concerns for justice, mercy, and the need for spiritual and physical healing. The appeal for caring, the healing of diseases, and acknowl-

**DID YOU KNOW?**

Parish nurses are employed by senior living complexes and nursing homes to offer a spiritual focus to the nursing practice at various levels of living arrangements for older adults. At the same time, they serve one or more congregations in the community.

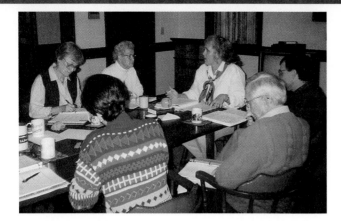

**Figure 45-3** Working with wellness committees promotes healthy programs and activities.

**Evidence-Based Practice**

The relationship between prayer and health outcomes was studied in a mail survey of a randomly selected population of members of a mainstream denomination in the United States. The study's purpose was to examine the relationship of prayer to eight categories of physical and mental health. Health status was measured by the Medical Outcomes Study Short-Form 36 Health Survey. The mail survey provided self-reports of health and resulted in an overall high level of functioning. Those persons who prayed more frequently scored lower in physical functioning and in the ability to carry out role activities and they scored higher in pain. However, these same persons also had significantly higher mental health scores than did those who prayed less. These persons of advanced age and poor physical health were praying more than younger healthy members. The study also reinforced other research that showed that persons pray more often as failing health accompanies aging. One explanation for increased prayer was that as the individual perceived increased vulnerability with the disabilities, increased efforts toward gaining strength and comfort were made. The study affirms the protective results of prayer on the persons' mental health.

**Nurse Use:** Parish nurses can be encouraged to continue to support members of faith communities in prayer, help them find the space and moments to pray during times of stress, illness, and grief, and encourage support groups to assist persons to enhance prayer and meditation practices.

Meisenhelder JB, Chandler EN: Prayer and health outcomes in church members, *Altern Ther Health Med* 6(4):56-60, 2000.

edging periods of illness and wellness is universal. Throughout a major portion of the twentieth century, religion played an important role in the lives of many in this country. More than half of the population prays daily. Eighty-five percent of clients state that they would like to have their health care provider pray with them, and at least 60% to 85% of the U.S. population indicate that they have some religious affiliation or an attachment to a house of worship (Centers for Disease Control and Prevention [CDC], 1999; Koenig, 2002; Matthews et al, 1998; Princeton Religion Research Center, 1996; Tuck et al, 2001). Researchers in the last decade of the twentieth century have become intrigued with relationships between spirituality and religion (Koenig et al, 1997; Matthews et al, 1998; Meisenhelder and Chandler, 2000; Oman and Reed; 1998; Oxman, Freeman, and Manheimer, 1995) (see the Evidence-Based Practice box about prayer and health outcomes). An important aspect of living out one's spirituality and religion is being a part of a community of faith from birth to death, throughout wellness and illness. Participating as individuals or as families, all benefit from associating with a supportive faith community or congregation.

The biblical account of Phoebe (Romans 16:1-2) exemplifies the tradition of health and healing within a congregation. Additionally, many Old Testament accounts and healing stories in the New Testament provide additional faith foundations (Psalms 106, 107, 113; Mark; Luke; Acts). The charge of the early church was to preach, teach, and heal. The church provided access to services such as shelter and food; the church tended to wounds and offered comfort and safety. So, too, nuns, deacons, deaconesses, the Gemeindeschwester or Fuersorgerin in Europe, and "emergency nurses" in African-American congregations are all examples of the healing professions serving in communities as they encounter more caring congregations.

The origins of wholeness and salvation are derived from similar concepts of Sodzo (Greek) and shalom, or wholeness. These terms and harmony in health are common to most faith communities and have a biblical base. Writings in Christian and Jewish sources address the individual and

community relationships with God as the source for a wise use of resources of self, environment, and one's community. Hygiene, health, and healing were a part of the Holiness Code of Leviticus. Throughout history, health existed at the center of the interaction between one's creator and mankind. The integration of faith and health within the caring community results in beneficial outcomes. Persons who encounter assaults with physical and emotional illness and who are able to call upon their faith beliefs and religious traditions are able to increase coping skills and realize spiritual growth. In a study of 100 older adults with cancer, there were higher levels of hope and positive moods in those who had high levels of intrinsic religiosity (Fehring, Miller, and Shaw, 1997). Coping skills, spiritual strengths, and practices such as prayer or meditation extend beyond the current situation and assist in future life challenges and total well-being.

Using strengths from earliest memories of faith traditions and previous learning experiences, as well as the ability to accept support from family and friends, help individuals and groups to interpret brokenness, disasters, joys, births, deaths, illness, and recovery. Encouraging growth in faith beliefs, and honoring traditions and rituals of the faith community bring individuals, families, and congregations in closer connection with their creator (Figure 45-4). The consolation of sacred liturgies, religious rituals, sacred space, and communal events aid the grieving and the healing process; they also affirm transcendent life (Achterberg Dossey, and Kolkmeier, 1994; Chandler, 1999; Woodward and Underwood, 1997; Wright, 1998). Additionally, recent studies show that support from members of groups that are meaningful to a person's total well-being aids in recovery and healing (Matthews et al, 1998; Oman and Reed, 1998).

Some of the major Protestant faith communities in the late nineteenth and early twentieth centuries used missionaries to develop multipurpose activities in communities, which included health activities and education along with religious messages. Hospitals were built in the United States and abroad, and underserved populations were targeted. As political and economic forces have changed through the years, so health ministry strategies of the churches have altered their approaches. Some churches have identified with community development efforts to help empower people to meet their needs for food, education, clean environments, social support, and primary health care. Churches have also recognized the need to increase awareness in several areas including one's personal responsibility for healthy choices; the escalating cost of health care and the need for cost containment; the in-

creasing numbers of the uninsured and underserved; the issues of domestic violence, substance abuse, and individuals with human immunodeficiency virus (HIV) infection and AIDS; and the ever-increasing dilemma of interpreting the complex changes within the health care delivery system. These efforts have been translated into a variety of position statements endorsed by the governing bodies of the faith communities.

The Presbyterian Church (U.S.A.) is cited as an example of a long-standing tradition of encouraging members to be good stewards or responsible managers of body, mind, the environment, and total resources. Studies in the late 1980s, the publication of essays titled "Health Care and Its Costs," and the meetings of the Task Force on Health Costs and Policies resulted in a 1988 policy statement, *Life Abundant: Values, Choices and Health Care* (Office of the General Assembly [OGA], 1988). Congregations were asked to responsibly model holistic and compassionate concern for health and the providing of care. Furthermore, the policy statement endorsed employing parish nurses or other health professionals as agents of the congregation's mission to encourage the role of "communities of health and healing" (OGA, 1988, p. 20).

The Presbyterian denomination's Health Network was formed in 1989. Nurses joined the efforts 2 years later, and annual parish nurse seminars have been held ever since. The seminars have been attended by nurses and clergy from many denominations and traditions. The seminars further implement the 1988 policy statement, increase

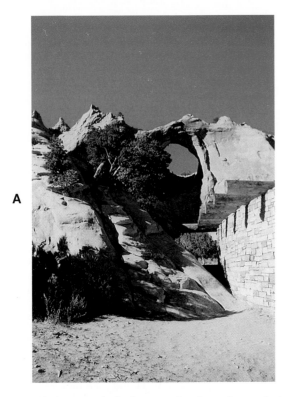

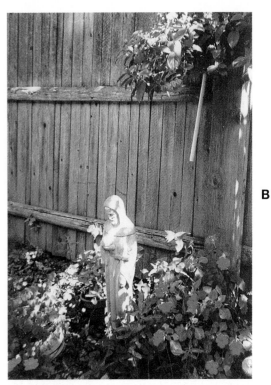

A

B

**Figure 45-4** Religious symbols, images, rituals, and sacred places are a significant part of a faith lifestyle and practice for many people. **A,** Native American. **B,** Judeo-Christian traditions.

awareness of the parish nurse concept, provide a forum for networking and support, provide nurturing for the nurse healers, encourage adequate education and skill preparation, and encourage implementation of parish nurse services in congregations or groups of congregations throughout the country.

The **holistic health centers** of the 1970s were a pivotal development that involved faith communities and highlighted the role of the nurse with the faith community in health and wellness promotion. The centers emphasized a comprehensive team approach to total health care. The health teams included family and clergy who emphasized personal responsibility for health and encouraged preventive health practices. The formulation of parish nursing in the early 1980s built on the strengths of these holistic health centers and focused on the nurse–clergy team working with individuals and their families. Nurses used their abilities to listen to the spoken and unspoken concerns of individuals and made assessments and judgments that were based on their knowledge of the health sciences and humanities (Figure 45-5). The attributes of the nurses were recognized by clergy and acute care institutions in the upper Midwest. By the mid 1980s, Lutheran General Hospital and the Reverend Granger Westberg embarked on a pilot project with six Chicago congregations that included four Protestant and two Roman Catholic communities (Solari-Twadell et al, 1994). Loyola University and Swedish Covenant Hospital were among the forerunners in revitalizing the nurse's role in the healing traditions; acknowledging the importance of body, mind, and spirit connections; incorporating education; and providing health promotion services within congregations.

## Health Care Delivery

Early chapters in Parts 1 and 2 of this text familiarize the reader with the historical, economic, social, political, environmental, and ethical trends in the past years. The health care delivery system is challenged to work within parameters of tighter financial constraints while also welcoming

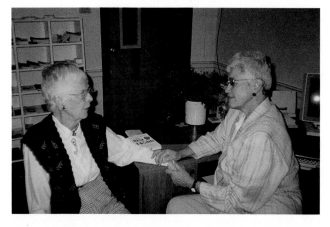

**Figure 45-5** A parish nurse provides support for spiritual and emotional needs as well as physical needs.

advanced technology and addressing new health concerns. The following are examples of issues that are important to this chapter. Hospitals discharge clients earlier and clients return to their homes sicker with few, if any, caregivers available. Caregivers are faced with the multiple tasks of coordinating employment, managing finances, maintaining former and ongoing family responsibilities, and learning new skills as a caregiver. Many diseases and conditions are indeed preventable, and health care costs need to be cut. Fragmented care and inadequate caregiver training and availability are problems for the disenfranchised, underserved, and the uninsured, as well as for the economically well situated and better-educated persons. Suburban and rural families are challenged to seek the best ways to meet the multiple demands of young children, teens, and aging parents. Consumer demand for involvement in health care decisions continues to increase, and society emphasizes individual responsibility for health. Simultaneously, consumers have increased interest in their own well-being and have expressed needs for more current health information to be available in a wider variety of formats (Loeb, O'Neill, and Gueldner, 2001; Swinney et al, 2001). These numerous interacting and overlapping forces are both a challenge and a burden for the population.

In addition to consumer interest and a heightened awareness of responsibility for one's own health, health care providers and managed care systems have found it financially advantageous for their participants to be healthy and remain out of the system. Thus with rising costs of care, scarce resources for populations, and the complex system demands on individuals and families to seek health care, the challenge for the consumer now is how to cope with these forces. In the twenty-first century, consumers and health care providers are still muddling through the complexity and fragmentation of the delivery system as it affects the young, old, and very old; the poor, middle-income, and well-to-do; persons of diverse ethnic origins; and those affected by disparities within society.

A primary focus of the community-oriented nurse in the last few decades has been to coordinate care and to link health care providers, groups, and community resources as the client tries to understand diverse health plans. Negotiating with individuals, agencies, and community partnerships within the complex maze of the broader health care environment demands a knowledgeable and seasoned professional. Nurses are aware of the necessity of collaborative practices and the formation of **partnerships** to care for groups and individuals throughout the age span. These nurses recognize the need for health promotion and disease prevention at all levels; they regularly assess the need to interpret care plans given to clients by health care providers. They advocate for healthy lifestyle choices in exercise, nutrition, substance use, and stress management. They realize that information and guidance must be available via media, in schools, workplaces, faith communities, and residential neighborhoods (Figure 45-6). Parish nurses

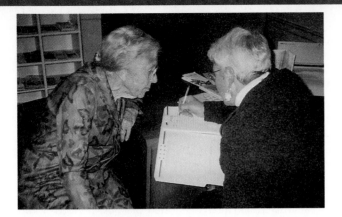

**Figure 45-6** Reviewing health plans with the "young" older adult.

share these and other important community-oriented nursing functions as they serve populations through faith communities.

## Parish Nursing Community

The beginnings of the parish nursing movement coincided with the recognition of more independent functioning of the nurse, the articulation and proliferation of advanced practice nursing roles, the growth of nursing centers, and technologic advances. Parish nurse services were one of the responses to assist with care coordination, to foster continuity of care, and to facilitate the assessment and planning for health and wellness of entire faith communities. As in the early history of the development of public health nursing in this country, parish nurses found that health promotion services were needed in underserved urban and rural areas (Baldwin et al, 2001; Wallace et al, 2002). Nurses identified gaps in the delivery of service. They found that congregants residing in communities that offered access to adequate health services also requested and benefited from health counseling and health promotion services at all levels of prevention.

The parish nurse services emphasized health promotion and disease prevention and provided the benefits of holistic care through the supportive, caring faith community. Nurses acknowledged the inner strength of persons and groups to increase healing. The nurses developed effective skills in negotiation, collaboration, and leadership. They also honed astute nonverbal and verbal communication skills. They embraced the vital role of families for healthy outcomes, and parish nurses knew that community support augmented the interventions chosen by individuals and families. Working with the congregation as the population group, parish nurses attempt to include in the wellness programs those persons who are less vocal or visible in the community of faith. The spiritual dimension of health was and is optimized by complementing the nursing role with pastoral care.

Gradually, nurses, other health care professionals and faith communities formed new and diverse health and faith partnerships. Arrangements with medical centers,

mental health centers, health care providers, and other parish nurses were formed. Coalitions of parish nurse networks were important as congregations developed into centers of support and caring. Parish nurses also began to affiliate with coalitions of inner city churches, networks of rural churches, individual hospitals, chaplaincy programs, and health departments. If the vision or mission of the congregation extends beyond its immediate membership, then those outside of the immediate faith community who would benefit from the services are also potential recipients. Nurses may then include arrangements with nearby community centers, visiting nurse associations, community health centers, or forms of neighborhood nursing such as those in the former block nurse programs. Current block nurse program options are discussed later in the chapter. Some parish nurses work with one or more congregation's and with one or more faith traditions.

Nurses in any of the arrangements consider the environment and population characteristics of congregations and the community. The strengths and assets of the congregation are the building blocks for services, and because faith communities traditionally value the talents and gifts of their members, efforts flourish within and beyond the faith community. Nurses address the identified needs for health promotion and disease prevention, and they understand the importance of the body–mind–spirit connection.

To support the parish nurse community, the International Parish Nurse Resource Center (IPNRC) was established. The center's mission is the promotion and development of quality parish nurse programs through research, education, and consultation (International Parish Nurse Resource Center, 1998). Establishment of the philosophy, mission, assumptions, and strategic purpose of the specialty were conceived with the guidance of the IPNRC. Additionally, core curricula as standard preparation for parish nurse and for parish nurse coordinator were endorsed (McDermott et al, 1998). The center has offered several faculty preparation seminars so that by the turn of the century, numerous basic curriculum programs of study can be offered across the country.

Throughout the years, the IPNRC has been vigilant in addressing emerging issues such as documentation accountability, certification for parish nurses, and accreditation concerns (related to the Joint Commission on Accreditation of Healthcare Organizations [JCAHO]) for parish nurses connected with institutional hospital systems. In January 2002, the IPNRC was transferred to Deaconness Parish Nurse Ministries in St. Louis, Missouri. Information about accessing the center can be found on this book's website at http://evolve.elsevier.com/Stanhope.

The development of programs of study for the new specialty paralleled the adoption of the ANA's *Scope and Standards of Practice of Parish Nursing Practice* (1998). The document was developed by parish nurses active in the interfaith Health Ministries' Association (HMA). Professional and lay persons in both health and faith disciplines concerned about health ministries comprise the HMA. Members of the parish nurse section include professional nurse members committed to improving the practice and developing statements of agreement related to parish nursing.

As advanced practice nurse, community-oriented nurse, and parish nurse practices increase in numbers and varieties of arrangements, evaluation of practice trends within the health care delivery system and the needs of society are necessary. Nursing must be accountable and responsive to those being served, as well as to those who provide opportunities to serve.

## PARISH NURSING PRACTICE
### Characteristics of the Practice

The goal of parish nursing is to develop and sustain health ministries within faith communities. Parish nursing is community-based and population-focused professional nursing practice with communities of faith to promote whole person health. Parish nursing is complemented by solid health ministry programs in congregations, and together they are able to offer comprehensive and in-depth services. The parish nurses are well aware of the beliefs, faith practices, and level of spiritual maturity of congregants served, and they link these with health and healing.

### NURSING TIP

Developing a keen sense of the value of the congregation within the geopolitical community and appreciating its associations within the local and wider community is beneficial.

Many parish nurses function in a part-time capacity. Some nurses are responsible for service with several congregations, whereas others engage in parish nursing as part of a full-time commitment in other capacities. Working in several arenas adds distinctive perspectives to a parish nurse service. Depending on the practice model, the nurse has a narrowly defined or a wider realm of responsibility. Parish nurse practices may be integrated into a health care facility or into practices that collaborate with related professional practice areas such as health departments or colleges of nursing. Hospital systems such as those in Charlotte (North Carolina), Chicago, St. Louis, and Hollywood (California) employ **parish nurse coordinators,** who facilitate different arrangements with several faith communities of varying backgrounds. Both rural and urban settings find these arrangements effective for facilitating health ministry programs (Chase-Ziolek, 1999). International programs also utilize coordinators with similar or different faith communities in rural and urban areas. Parish nurses may also have regional responsibilities that correspond to intermediate governing areas of the faith community. These regions may be clusters of churches or areas such as districts, synods, presbyteries, or jurisdictions. Practices in which several parish nurses are supervised by a coordina-

tor have built-in opportunities for sharing, partnering, and mentoring.

### THE CUTTING EDGE

Public health and religious leaders have joined a challenging new partnership in the Institute for Public Health and Faith Collaborations (IPHFC). The cooperative venture is between Centers for Disease Control and Prevention and the Association of Schools of Public Health and is based at Emory University, Decatur, Georgia (located between the CDC and the School of Public Health is Emory University's Nell H. Woodruff School of Nursing).

The Third Invitational Parish Nurse Educational Colloquium sponsored by the IPNRC affirmed assumptions of the practice of parish nursing (Solari-Twadell, McDermott, and Matheus, 2000). Those gathered affirmed that the client in parish nursing embraces individuals, families, congregations, and communities across the life span. The practice includes the full cultural and geographic community regardless of ethnicity, lifestyle, sex, sexual orientation, or creed. The nurse in the practice incorporates faith and health, and employs the nursing process in providing services to the faith community as well as to the community served by that faith community. Facilitating collaborative health ministries in the faith communities is an important component of the practice. Additionally, the group affirmed that while the curricula stem from a Judeo-Christian theological framework, parish nursing respects diverse traditions of faith communities and encourages adaptation of the programs to these faith traditions.

At the first IPNRC-sponsored colloquium, five characteristics identified as central to the philosophy of parish nursing (Solari-Twadell et al, 1994) were conceived by nursing educators and practitioners affiliated with early parish nurse efforts. These characteristics were foundational to the evolving practice; the curricula formed; the growth, replication, and enhancement of the practice; and the assumptions that followed.

The first characteristic, *spiritual dimension,* is central to the practice of parish nursing. Nursing incorporates the physical, psychological, social, and spiritual dimensions of clients into professional practice, and although parish nursing includes all four, it focuses on intentional and compassionate care, which stems from the spiritual dimension of all humankind. Second, the *roots of the role balance both knowledge and skills* of nursing, using nursing sciences, the humanities, and theology. The nurse combines nursing functions with pastoral care functions.

Visits in the office, home, hospital, or nursing home often involve prayer, and they may include a reference to scripture, symbols, sacraments, and liturgy of the faith community represented by the nurse. The values and beliefs of the faith community are integral to the supportive care given. Nurses also assist with services of worship, commemoration, baptism, healing, wholeness, funerals, and others as appropriate within the faith community.

The third characteristic is that the *focus of the specialty is the faith community and its ministry.* The faith community is the source of health and healing partnerships, which result in creative responses to health and health-related concerns. Partnerships may be among individuals, groups, and health care professionals within the congregation. Partnerships may also be among various congregations or community agencies, institutions, or individuals. Partnerships also evolve as the congregation visualizes its health-related mission beyond the walls, stones, and steeples of its own place of worship.

As in other areas of community-oriented nursing, parish nurse services *emphasize strengths of individuals, families, and communities.* Parish nurses endorse this fourth characteristic in their practice. As congregations realize the need for and care for one another, their individual and corporate relationship with their creator often is enhanced. This provides additional coping strength for future crisis situations within the family and community. Finally, *health, spiritual health, and healing* are considered an ongoing, dynamic process. Because spiritual health is central to well-being, influences are evident in the total individual and noted in a healthy congregation. Well-being and illness may occur simultaneously; spiritual healing or well-being can exist in the absence of cure. Faith communities that value individual and congregational health can move beyond their "congregational" boundaries to address health-related concerns in the geopolitical communities locally, nationally, and globally. Studying health care reform issues, domestic and youth violence, and safe environmental conditions in light of faith beliefs prepares members to participate in policy-making activities to promote the ethical principle of justice (see Chapter 6).

## Scope and Standards of Parish Nursing Practice

The nursing profession's minimal level of professional nursing practice delineated in the ANA's *Standards of Clinical Nursing Practice* (1998) was the foundation for developing the *Scope and Standards of Parish Nursing* (HMA and ANA, 1998). Nurses well-versed in the parish nursing practice field compiled a document that carefully reviewed specialties closely related to parish nursing such as public health nursing and holistic nursing. Specialty areas within professional nursing achieve a major milestone when the standards and scope common to that practice are recognized.

The unique practice of parish nursing and the minimum scope and standards of care for the independent practice of the profession guide the nurse's practice and relate to activities of "health promotion within the context of the client's values, beliefs and faith practices." The parish nurse's "client focus . . . is the faith community, including its family and individual members and the community it serves" (HMA and ANA, 1998, p. 3). Nurses en-

courage individuals, families, and entire faith communities to promote health and healing within the context of the faith community to arrive at wellness outcomes. As in other arenas of nursing, the client level is multidimensional. "The clients of a parish nurse represent the total life span of three client levels: the faith community and its families and individuals" (p. 17). Using the nursing process for assessment, program planning, and evaluation, the parish nurses target specified age-groups or health-related concerns.

The *Scope and Standards* delineate examples of the parish nurse's independent functions. These functions are in compliance with and reflect current nursing practice, client health promotion needs, professional standards, and the legal scope of professional nursing practice. Nurses function within the nurse practice act of their jurisdiction (i.e., their state). If dependent functions are practiced, parish nurses must be in compliance with the legal criteria of the jurisdiction's nurse practice act (ANA, 1998). For example, when influenza vaccine or immunization clinics are offered, appropriate arrangements are made to use nurses from a community cooperating agency (health department), or the parish nurse must have a contractual policy agreement with the cooperating agency to provide the immunizations. In addition to a narrative description and glossary of terms, the document outlines standards of care and standards of professional performance. In keeping with wise use of persons and materials, standards of professional performance elaborate on collaboration and resource use. The parish nurse collaborates with those who "share a commitment to promoting health" and "facilitates a health ministry that maximizes resources to achieve the desired health outcomes for all clients" (HMA and ANA, 1998, pp. 20, 22).

## Educational Preparation of a Parish Nurse

After successful completion of one of the standard courses and with a thorough grasp of the *Scope and Standards* of the practice, parish nurses adapt to local community needs. They work with the **wellness committee** in congregations to assess assets and areas of need in order to plan services that will arrive at outcomes congruent with goals established by the congregation and communities served.

The practice generally requires that parish nurses have a baccalaureate degree in nursing and hold a valid license in the state of practice. Three to 5 years' experience in professional nursing and evidence of a mature faith are beneficial.

Seminars have offered opportunities to raise awareness of the practice and have provided networking and nurturing support for nurses. The annual Westberg Symposium offered by the IPNRC offers comprehensive sessions and a forum for nurses to network, gain new knowledge, and stay abreast of current resources, trends, and issues in the practice.

Advanced practice opportunities also enrich a specialty practice. Master's-prepared nurses (with specialization in community-oriented nursing, holistic nursing, or mental health nursing) and nurse practitioners have found niches in parish nursing. Major universities have had creative arrangements for faculty and student clinical options at the undergraduate and graduate levels (Lough, 1999; Magilvy and Brown, 1997; Rouse, 2000; Tolley, 1998; Trofino, Hughes, and Hay, 2000). A 1500-member congregation in Florida employed a full-time master's-prepared nurse certified in holistic nursing by the American Holistic Nurses Association (AHNA). Faculty practice arrangements at the University of Kentucky (with a 1000-member congregation); collaborations between the Divinity School and nursing programs to form the Health and Nursing Ministries Program at Duke University; University of Colorado faculty arrangements offering opportunities for doctoral and master's-level students; and the pioneering Parish Health Nurse program at Georgetown University are notable.

Preparation and continuing education must continue to include the basics and enrichment courses in nursing practice, research, theology, and pastoral care. Additionally, the nurse needs updates in areas of public health, medicine, sociology, cultural diversity, and human growth and development across the life span. Improving collaboration, negotiation, and coordination skills, as well as consultation, leadership, management, and research skills, is essential. Parish nurses accept responsibility for ongoing professional education within nursing and pastoral care arenas (Louis and Alpert, 2000; Sellers and Haag, 1998; Solari-Twadell et al, 1994).

The challenge for the practice is to document trends, maintain and enhance quality of preparation and services offered, engage in evidence-based practice, use increased numbers of advanced practice nurses, network within professional organizations, and become involved in outcomes-oriented research. To remain at the cutting edge of the profession and recognize competency among practitioners, the specialty must pursue professional certification. Both the profession and consumers will increasingly demand credentialing, which is regularly updated as a mark of excellence. Although there are almost 5000 parish nurses in the country, the critical numbers of those salaried full-time and those energized to take the next step seriously have yet to be realized. The fitting approach to certification may well be addressed by the parish nurse section of the HMA, as they have had previous experience in working together on professional credibility issues. Currently, parish nurses may receive advanced credentialing in related areas such as community-oriented nursing and holistic nursing.

## Evidence-Based Practice

The study authors described the practice of parish nurses using the framework of the nursing minimum data set (NMDS). Nurses working in 22 faith communities used the standardized nursing classification system of the North American Nursing Diagnosis Association (NANDA) and the nursing intervention classification (NIC) to collect data. Nurses recorded nursing diagnoses and nursing interventions. The most frequently reported were those that emphasized health promotion and illness prevention. The identified diagnoses reflected the major focus of parish nursing as described in the literature of the practice: health-seeking behavior, knowledge deficit, individual management of therapeutic regimen, grieving, social isolation, and potential for enhanced spiritual well-being. The study also affirmed that the parish nurse functioned as educator, counselor, referral agent, and advocate/facilitator. The results of the study will be helpful in describing parish nurse practice in various settings and with different populations. Validation by a focus group of nurses also proved to be helpful, as the nurses shared experiences and elicited suggestions for changes in documentation.

**Nurse Use:** Further work will be needed to arrive at diagnoses and interventions and to refine and expand the classification system. Additionally, the practice will be described more fully as the nursing outcomes classification (NOC) of the parish nurse practice is documented and studied.

Coenen A et al: Describing parish nurse practice using the nursing minimum data set, *Public Health Nurs* 16(6): 412-416, 1999.

## NURSING TIP

The parish nurse benefits from several years of practice experience following the basic undergraduate preparation, because the nature of the position demands a seasoned professional.

## Holistic Health Care

Holistic health practice asks the nurse and client to embrace a commitment to optimal wellness, seek the meaning of wellness for the individual or situation, and consider options from an array of therapies. Harmony between the physical, emotional, psychological, and spiritual self is sought. In addition to sharing backgrounds and functions similar to those of community-oriented nursing, parish nursing also parallels and benefits from commonalities and distinct practices of holistic nursing. Holistic nurses acknowledge wholeness as an entirety that is more than all dimensions consolidated (Dossey, 1997; Dossey et al, 2000; Frisch et al, 2000). The holistic nursing practice views the nurse as "an instrument of healing and a facilitator in the healing process" (Frisch et al, 2000, p. xxvi). Like parish nursing, holistic nursing emphasizes wholeness of persons across the life span.

The AHNA had its beginnings in the early 1980s as did parish nursing, although roots of the practice also followed even earlier traditions. The philosophy of holistic nursing practice embraces concepts of presence, healing, and holism. The interconnectedness of body, mind, and spirit is basic to both holistic nursing and parish nursing. Strengths of the practitioners of holistic nursing are that they have formed an association of professionals, have established a core curriculum for the practice as well as standards of practice, and have established a route for certification. To become eligible for the certification examination in holistic nursing, a nurse first compiles and submits a portfolio that is a qualitative assessment of the nurse as a person and of the practice.

The current standards of holistic nursing practice were approved by the AHNA in 2000 and contain five core values. These standards provide guidelines for practice, education, and research. The standards are a guide for all professional nurses, and parish nurses will find them helpful in embracing more holistic practices and interventions. Nurses will be helped to more fully understand responses to life situations and will be guided in the individual nurse or client "journey towards wholeness and healing" (Frisch et al, 2000, p. xxi).

The nurse professional attains enrichment for self and persons or groups served, by studying and embracing holistic nursing principles, as these principles are challenges to "integrate self care, self responsibility, spirituality, and reflection in . . . lives" (Frisch et al, 2000, p. xxvi). Parish nurses have already utilized some of the interventions commonly used in holistic nursing, and additional exploration would enhance practice possibilities to promote wellness and healing for practitioner and client. Both parish nurses and holistic nurses share the skill of creating a healing environment (Chandler, 1999; Dossey et al, 2000; Quinn, 1992). Listening coupled with intentional compassion is basic to effective interventions. Selected interventions that are often used in both specialties of nursing are prayer, meditation, counseling, guided imagery, health promotion guidance, journaling, therapeutic touch, healing presence, and massage. Encouraging options for herbal medicine, manual healing, alternative systems of medical practices, and many other complementary caring and healing modalities facilitate the goal of healing (Dossey et al, 2000). Parish nurses interested in learning more about holistic nursing practice and interventions are advised to contact nearby university nursing faculty, teaching medical centers, or the AHNA.

## Functions of the Parish Nurse

Examples of parish nursing interventions have been cited throughout this chapter. This section summarizes and expands on some of the usual functions and describes activities. A primary independent function is that of *personal health counseling.* Parish nurses discuss health risk appraisals, plan for healthier lifestyles, and provide support and guidance related to numerous acute and chronic, actual and potential health problems and perform spiritual assessments. The personal health counseling function may be practiced individually or with groups; counseling may be in homes, hospitals, schools, places of work, or nursing homes, or at the faith community facility. Some nurses have designated offices, whereas others use space that is most conducive to the particular activity or client need.

The health and spiritual assessment as an intervention offers excellent opportunities for screening. Utilizing interventions of listening, presence, and support is paramount for the personal health counseling function and blends well with the functions of pastoral care and integrating faith and health discussed later. Counseling for physical, emotional, and mental health and wellness is paramount. Additionally, simple and flexible approaches to spiritual assessment are beneficial for both an initial assessment to guide overall interventions and also to perform periodic assessments as situations may dictate. As one of the trusted members of the pastoral staff, the parish nurse will find it helpful to develop ease in inquiring about a few important areas of a persons' spiritual journey. History of family relationships and past association with faith communities provide background information. Astutely employing the art of listening turns the basic nursing intervention into a most effective technique.

Compassionate, careful listening involves being still, reflecting, and being intentionally in the present. Being sensitive to the differing needs of personal spirituality during various points along life's journey is important to consider while guiding persons through the spiritual assessment. The nurse then also helps individuals share necessary information about spirituality needs with other health care providers.

Numerous instruments or tools are available for use in spiritual assessments (Carson and Koenig, 2002; Dossey et al, 2000; Koenig, 2002; Pulchalski and Romer, 2000; Silverman, 1997; Sulmasy, 1997). Puchalski and Romer (2000) provide a fairly simple spiritual assessment tool that was used to familiarize health care practitioners at George Washington University Medical Center. Its ease in use with persons from a wide variety of faith traditions as well as with those with no or unknown faith traditions lends itself to a compassionate presence for other health assessments and interventions. The inquiries include the following four areas: What is your faith tradition or belief? How important is this faith to you and what influence has it had in your life? What is your community of faith and how do you participate? and finally, How could the health care system/practitioner help you to address your spiritual needs? This instrument is one approach to spiritual assessment, and questions can be reordered to suit different situations. Also, it is an instrument that may be applied to many situations within all of professional nursing. Each nurse must guide the assessment to obtain the information needed to promote health and healing.

A second function of parish nursing is *health education.* Parish nurses publish information in congregation news bulletins, distribute information, and have available a variety of resources for the physical, mental, and spiritual health of the congregation. Classes are held to address identified needs, individual teaching is done as needed, and discussions are held for targeted meetings or support groups. Nurses deftly use a mix of classes, written material, resources, public media, or inclusion in clergy sermons to create awareness of a wide variety of concerns. Parish nurses strive to promote wholeness in health and create a fuller understanding of total physical, mental, and spiritual well-being. The health education function can be shared with a professional or trained lay volunteer or the wellness committee members.

An important function for nurses while striving to enhance the faith–health relationship is that of *pastoral care*. With the aid of spiritual assessments, and stressing the spiritual dimension of nursing practice, the nurse lends support during times of joy and sorrow, in health and illness, from birth to death, and in times of stress (Figure 45-7). The nurse identifies spiritual strengths that assist in healing and instill hope. Presence is utilized as a powerful intervention in pastoral care. The nurse may employ hymns, prayers, favorite scripture verses, psalms, pictures, church windows, candlelight, aromas, stories, or other images that are important for the individual or group to embrace the connectedness between faith, health, and well-being. (For practice implications, see the Evidence-Based Practice box about the use of prayer.) Additionally, combining prayer and other contemplative or spiritual practices is beneficial. "Creating sacred space and combining use of several senses can powerfully reinforce healing memories" (Chandler, 1999, p. 68).

As a *liaison* between resources in the faith community and the local community, the parish nurse creates awareness of those resources both in and beyond the congregation, helps individuals, families, and congregations create the appropriate resource match, and links these persons with the services. The *advocate* function of the parish nurse is used while negotiating and working as liaison; advocacy for issues of concern to the faith community and its members is also employed as a separate function. It may also be utilized with the function of facilitator.

As *facilitator*, the parish nurse links congregational needs to the establishment of support groups in some cases, or referral to support groups in other cases. The parish nurse also facilitates changes within the congregation to increase accessibility for the physically or mentally challenged. Arrangements for meals and services to those who are homebound can be made. Very often, the nurse also works with volunteer coordinators to train volunteers or ensures that interested persons acquire training to function as lay caregivers to meet congregational needs. Box 45-1 is an example of how the parish nurse works with other providers and community resources to meet the health needs of a client. Congregations are also keenly aware that more than half of the members of mainline churches are part of the growing population of older adults in the country. They also witness increasing numbers of persons who are either uninsured or underinsured, and they see that many families have childcare needs during working hours. These groups are members of or live near faith communities. To provide healthier living for these groups, food pantries, day-care for seniors, congregate meals, arrangements for preschool and latch-key children, tutoring, Meals-on-Wheels, visiting less-mobile members, and outreach for vulnerable populations are examples of valuable services. Not only does facilitating for those in and beyond the faith community benefit the recipients but also the partnering provides opportunities for the volunteers to serve and gain a feeling of worth.

Another important component of the facilitator role challenges the nurse to be the catalyst for beneficial and healthy partnerships that augment both members of the

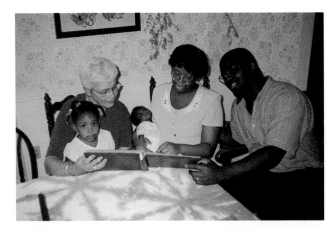

**Figure 45-7** A parish nurse visits with a family of the congregation in their home.

> **BOX 45-1 Parish Nursing as Healing Ministry: An Adult Daughter's Reflection**
>
> What a pleasure to be able to commend (parish nurse's) personal friendship and professional help! Without her support it would have been difficult, if not impossible, for my father to live at home during his last 6 years. But she had, along with his doctor, the sure feeling that it was the right thing for him and that it could be done. When the time came that he needed caregivers around the clock, she skillfully conveyed suggestions in such a way that the caregivers' cultural differences were not a barrier. She helped them grow as caregivers, appreciating their accomplishments, even to having a blackberry-picking "outing" at her home.
>
> My father in his earlier years had been a deacon and had loved visiting shut-ins. It brought him so much happiness that he in turn received his church's caring, healing ministry through his parish nurse. He attended church on Sundays beyond what one would expect of one in his 90s, and almost his last Sunday was the day he celebrated turning 96.
>
> Thank you, (parish nurse), for our "Mission Accomplished"!
>
> With permission, A.F.H.

partnership. Partnerships and facilitating healthier living for older adults are involved in community arrangements of the Elderberry Institute (at http://www.elderberry.org). For more than two decades, programs known as block nursing programs (BNP) and Living at Home (LAH) were known to community-oriented nurses, who welcomed the arrangements as reminiscent of early public health nursing and neighborhood nursing efforts. These efforts reappeared in 1981 as block nursing out of a need to address concerns arising in communities experiencing the social and political environmental changes of the decade. Nurses in Minnesota, spearheaded by Martinson and Jamieson and following examples of public health nursing pioneer Lillian Wald, combined their professional nursing experience, their keen knowledge of the neighborhood, and the belief that communities could pool their own resources to meet the needs of its residents. In the early St. Anthony Block Nursing program, residents received in-home support and health care with a mix of professionals and volunteers as caregivers (block companions). Residents from 6 to 85 years of age were served (Elderberry Institute, 2002; Martinson et al, 1985). One evaluation of the program indicated that 85% of the persons served were able to remain out of nursing homes.

Block nursing joined a program with a related mission to become the Living at Home and Block Nursing Program (LAH/BNP, Inc.) groups in 1987 in Minnesota. Ten years later, the Elderberry Institute was established to extend and support the LAH/BNP groups. Minnesota was joined by another state, Texas, in program development and community groups that focus on assisting communities in assessing the needs of their aging population and in creating locally owned and operated programs to meet those needs. By the end of 2001, there were 40 local programs in the two states commemorating the twentieth anniversary of the founding St. Anthony program. The Elderberry Institute provides technical assistance, training, and education for staff and volunteers and guides program operations for the new arrangements. The early block nurse programs were altered in accordance with changes in society and the local community; they have been replicated in Japan and Israel. Partnerships with hunger programs, and other community resources such as parish nurse services, keep these community groups viable. They strive to maintain a strong local citizen board. Parish nurses in communities not served by Elderberry Institute programs are encouraged to become familiar with similar elder care resources and community groups in their locales.

The strength of the foregoing program is in the demonstrated strong, collaborative, community partnerships. Community-oriented nurses as parish nurses can envision comprehensive, population-focused practices or implement programs at beginning levels as community-based practices to ensure seamless care for individuals and families. The continuing challenge for nurses, other health care providers, and the communities will be to garner government, foundation, and private funding and combine it

---

**BOX 45-2    A Sampling of Parish Nurse Interventions and Activities**

- Sharing the joys of a new member in the family; sharing sorrows of losses
- Anticipating changes in health status or in growth and development
- Being present for questions that seem difficult or unacceptable to ask the health care provider
- Explaining and assisting in considering choices when new living and care arrangements must be made
- Listening to the concerns of a youngster anticipating diagnostic procedures
- Praying with the spouse of a dying parishioner
- Helping individuals and families make decisions regarding advance directives in light of faith beliefs
- Helping teens consider options when overwhelmed with serious life issues
- Providing information, support, and prayer regarding advance directives
- Seeking community resources/opportunities for fitness and nutrition classes
- Working with the wellness committee to ensure that fellowship meals meet nutritional and spiritual needs of older adults
- Offering educational opportunities about health care legislation changes and its influence on the congregation and community
- Accompanying a faith community member to a 12-step meeting
- Participating in worship leadership with pastoral staff

From Berry R: A parish nurse. In Office of Resourcing Committees on Preparation for Ministry: *A day in the life of . . . : a kaleidoscope of specialized ministries,* Louisville, Ky, 1994, Presbyterian Church (USA), Distribution Management Service.

---

with support from volunteer activities, family involvement, and community groups to create the unique mix needed for the distinctiveness of each community. Nurses are asked to partner with community members where they live, work, attend school, and gather for worship; to closely partner with these same members to advocate for those who are powerless; to keenly identify health and health-related needs; to detect and address those needs to prevent costly use of the health care system; and to be closely aligned with those who can implement visionary policy that improves health care for community members across the life span.

Box 45-2 lists several selected activities of parish nurses (Berry, 1994). However, the creative implementing of the parish nurse concept by each individual nurse with a unique faith community will result in a wealth of possibilities to activate the functions. Healthy activities to be encouraged in congregations are numerous and the nurse often works with the congregation to stretch beyond its immediate borders to augment services in the community that promote health and wellness.

## ISSUES IN PARISH NURSING PRACTICE

Every new discipline or care area must be alert to issues of accountability to populations served, as well as to those who entrust the nurse with the responsibility to serve a designated population. Discussions of health promotion plans include the individual, the family, and the faith community. Additionally, negotiations with the pastoral staff, congregations, institutions, and the wider community may be involved in job description preparation or program planning. Issues such as privacy, confidentiality, group concerns, access, and record management must be discussed with the pastoral staff or the contracting agency at the outset of any parish nurse agreement. Because the role involves professional, legal, ethical, theological, and relational issues, the nurse will need to review, respect, and reflect on the parameters involved. Planning carefully with appropriate persons facilitates positive outcomes and avoids conflicts with individual and group rights and state regulations.

### Professional Issues

Annual and periodic evaluations of parish nurse practices, as well as assessments and evaluations of services needed, are certainly indicated. These evaluations include self, peer, congregational, and/or institutional evaluations. Professional appraisal is standard in nursing practice. The appraisals guide professional development as well as program development. Because the scope of parish nursing practice is broad and it focuses on the independent practice of the discipline, the nurse must consider a wide variety of issues such as position description, professional liability, professional educational and experiential preparation, collaborative agreements, and working with lay volunteers as well as practicing and retired professionals. Abiding by the professional nursing code is understood; however, the nurse must also know the **polity,** expectations, and mission of the particular faith community. The nurse also continually interprets the profession for the faith community.

The nurse must be knowledgeable about lines of authority and channels of communication in the congregation as well as in the collaborative institutions. Nurses need to become well acquainted with the personnel committees of the congregation. Personnel committees provide guidance and contribute to the evaluation. They also advocate for parish nurse services and raise awareness with the congregational staff members and programs.

Nurses in parishes advocate for well-being and thus are in unique positions to highlight justice issues in local and national legislation. As the faith community reflects on the implications of legislation for their congregation and

national faith community, the nurse contributes information to policymakers about the implications for health and well-being for the parish, for the local community, and globally. Active participation in political activities contributes to spiritual growth and healthy functioning.

### Ethical Issues

Issues evolve from client, faith community, and professional arenas. The nurse's interventions are guided by professional responsibilities that include the *Code for Nurses* (ANA, 1999), *Scope and Standards of Practice* (HMA and ANA, 1998), individual and group rights, statements of faith, polity, and doctrines of the faith community served. Professional and therapeutic relationships are maintained at all times; consulting and counseling with minors and individual members of the opposite sex are conducted using professional ethical principles. Policies about these issues are established at the outset of the practice in conjunction with the pastoral team, the wellness committee, the parish nurse, and the local congregation's governing or judicatory body.

As in other community health situations, the parish nurse, along with the client, identifies parameters of ethical concerns, plans ahead with clients to consider healthy options in making ethical decisions, and supports clients in their journey to choose alternatives that will strengthen coping skills and allow them to grow stronger in faith and health. "In addition, parish nurses ought to consider the virtue ethics, such as caring, forgiveness, and compassion, in their decision making" (HMA and ANA, 1998, p. 19).

Communities of faith strive to be caring communities and value the fellowship among its members. However, confidentiality is of utmost importance in parish nursing practice. The parish nurse values client confidentiality but at the same time delicately assists the client and client family at the appropriate time to "share" concerns with pastoral staff or fellow **congregants.** This sharing may gain valuable support to promote optimal healing. The nurse is often the staff member who helps the family to the stage of acceptance of a health concern. How much to share and when to share a concern is indeed a private affair and a part of the important journey of healing. A joyous event for one family may be a devastating event or even a depressing reminder of a past event for another family. The celebrations and joys of a healthy new infant one week may raise guilt and ambivalence for congregational members when, within a brief time, another family's long-awaited child dies at birth.

## Legal Issues

As an advocate of client and group rights, the nurse identifies and reports neglect, abuse, and illegal behaviors to the appropriate legal sources. The nurse appropriately refers members to pastoral or community resources if the scope of the problem is not within the realm of the professional nurse. Referral is also indicated if conflict between nurse and client is such that no further progress is possible. The parish nurse who has a positive relationship that values open dialogue with the pastoral team will be supported in efforts to select the most appropriate community resource for clients.

The nurse must personally and professionally abide by the parameters of the nurse practice act of the jurisdiction, maintain an active license of that state, and practice according to the scope and standards of practice. Additional legal concerns are those of institutional contractual agreements, records management, release of information, and volunteer liability. Resources would include the faith community's legal consultant, the faith community's national position statements, and guidelines of the health or university partner and those of the HMA and IPNRC (HMA, ANA, 1998; Solari-Twadell and McDermott, 1999; Solari-Twadell et al, 1994, 2000).

## Financial Issues

Innovative arrangements for variations of the basic models mentioned earlier call for sustained financial support. The nurse is called on to partner in finding funds and network-

ing with potential supporters. The nurse is accountable for money spent and for fundraising, whether the position is salaried or volunteer. Educational and promotional materials, equipment, travel time, continuing education, and malpractice insurance are selected areas that need to be included in the budget of the parish nurse. If these materials are not budget items, services may be limited, and this needs to be interpreted to the faith community.

## HEALTHY PEOPLE 2010 LEADING HEALTH INDICATORS AND FAITH COMMUNITIES

The 1990 health objectives (Healthy People 2000) and the current Healthy People 2010 indicators encourage communities to cooperatively lend support to individuals and families to attain an improved health status that can be passed on to future generations. Faith communities have long held a position of esteem in communities. Congregations are enduring, strong establishments that provide a safe place to gather and to care for and with their members, and they are able to offer forums for dialogue of critical issues. The Carter Center in Atlanta and the Park Ridge Center in Chicago have collaborated with health care professionals and leaders of faith traditions to identify roles of faith communities to address national health objectives and approaches to improving overall public health. By the beginning of the twentieth century, faith communities recognized the attainment of almost half of the 1990 objectives and affirmed the development of the goals and objectives of Healthy People 2000 (Marty, 1990).

Because faith communities are rooted in healing traditions and also hold issues of justice and mercy as a priority, the Healthy People 2010 goals to increase quality and years of healthy life and to eliminate health disparities can be readily addressed. Because values of health and faith institutions are closely aligned, evidences of partnering are becoming more prominent. The National Heart, Lung and Blood Institute, which urges partnerships with faith communities, has offered suggestions for program planning for several decades. Another national-level effort to strengthen the potential partnerships between faith communities and health care professionals is the Caucus on Public Health and the Faith Community of the American Public Health Association (APHA), formed in 1995. Health care professionals of many faiths are able to share research and voice their interest in holistically supporting their communities and clients.

Examples of congregational models addressing the specific objectives that encourage attainment of national health objectives are increasingly being documented (Berry, 1994; Marty, 1990; Magilvy and Brown, 1997; Weiss et al, 1997; Swinney et al, 2001). Specific national objectives dealing with nutrition; physical activity; use of tobacco, alcohol, and other drugs; immunization status; environmental health; and injury and violence are within the realm of the health education role of the parish nurse. Activities include age-appropriate discussions of preven-

## Healthy People 2010 | Objectives Related to Youths in Faith Communities

### OVERWEIGHT AND OBESITY

Overweight and Obesity: Priority—promote good nutrition and healthier weights

**19-3** Reduce the proportion of children and adolescents who are overweight and obese

**19-3.a** Reduce childhood obesity rates from 11% to 5%

### PHYSICAL ACTIVITY

Priority: promote daily physical activity

**22-7** Increase the proportion of adolescents who engage in vigorous physical activity that promotes cardiorespiratory fitness 3 or more days per week for 20 or more minutes per occasion

From U.S. Department of Health and Human Services: *Healthy people 2010: national health promotion and disease prevention objectives,* Washington, DC, 2000, U.S. Department of Health and Human Services.

---

tive activities with various groups, classes on the use and misuse of alcohol, tobacco, and other drugs, and discussions regarding responsible sexual behavior in the context of faith values.

Faith communities can be effective environments in which to address health promotion related to overweight, obesity, and sedentary lifestyle. The surgeon general's report (U.S. Department of Health and Human Services [USDHHS], 2001) and numerous newspaper, professional, and lay journal articles have noted drastic changes in the past two decades (CDC, 1999; Courtney, 2002; Covington et al, 2001; National Institutes of Health, 2000). Almost 97 million adults in the United States are overweight or obese. More alarming is that children and youths are following unhealthy patterns as well. The number of overweight and obese children has doubled. During the same period, the number of teens who are overweight has tripled. Parish nurses can be catalysts in affecting the indicators in the faith community as well as in the neighborhood and in the community. The national health indicators and specific objectives relating to the public health problems of obesity and sedentary lifestyle and suggestions for health promotion interventions in faith communities are presented in the Healthy People 2010 box. Additionally, the parish nurse in collaboration with the wellness committee of the faith communities in the area will find helpful suggestions from the U.S. Department of Health and Human Services (USDHHS), including *Healthy People in Healthy Communities: A Community Planning Guide Using Healthy People 2010* (USDHHS, 2000, 2001a).

Guiding faith communities to develop efforts that create healthy environments and promote healthy behaviors for all age-groups is helpful. See the How To box for an example of intervening with young families (see Figure 45-7). Alerting entire congregation communities to the benefits of health promotion to prevent the onset of chronic illness helps to minimize sickness visits to health care professionals, improve quality of life, and increase savings of scarce individual, government, and private insurance health care dollars. The nurse and the supportive faith community play major roles in caring for those families who are expe-

### HOW TO Intervene in Maternal and Infant Health

- Visit family immediately after the birth of a new infant to further assess parenting skills and parent–infant bonding, reinforce a holistic reflection of life transition, and plan for faith community support as indicated in those areas not addressed by family or other community agencies.

- Augment community prenatal classes or facilitate classes in faith community, stressing growth and development of prenatal and postnatal period, family transitions, and adequate health monitoring needed by parents, children, and new family members.

- Facilitate expectant parent support group to reinforce positive health during pregnancy; interpret plans negotiated with health care provider; promote spiritual reflection of family life transition to encourage connectedness with creator and beliefs of faith community; and provide emotional, social, community support to family.

riencing alterations of functional and emotional health because of chronic illness. Monitoring disabling physical functioning, encouraging adherence to treatment plans, interpreting rehabilitation programs, noting specific progress, offering day centers for mentally ill persons, and offering support from the entire faith community are selected approaches to address the two overall goals and objectives of Healthy People 2010.

Wellness committees and parish nurses with the faith community's input may regularly review the progress toward meeting the challenges set forth in Healthy People 2010, make comparisons between national and specific state data, and then assess the extent to which the specific congregation or groups of congregations are in need of risk reduction. Most advantageous for the faith community would be for the parish nurse, wellness committees, and other interested persons to engage in partnership activities with community efforts such as health fairs. Health fairs are effective strategies for health promotion

---

**BOX 45-3** **Levels of Prevention Related to Overweight, Obesity, and Physical Activity**

**PRIMARY PREVENTION**

- Hold classes on healthy eating, food pyramid appropriate for various age levels (elementary school, adolescents, new parents).
- Promote and encourage age-appropriate activities that include physical exercise in youth group meetings, retreats, trips, vacation church school, nursery programs.
- Encourage a variety of activities and discourage extended inactivity.
- Encourage healthy snacks and meals for youth outings and at educational hour, and parenting sessions.
- Write house-of-worship newsletter articles informing parents of need for adequate exercise and proper nutrition for healthy lifestyles in growing and adult years.
- Encourage parents to be proactive in school parenting councils as well as in neighborhood recreation leagues to ensure exercise programs and activities so that children/youths expend energy to promote proper weight maintenance and prevent fat accumulation.
- Encourage faith community leaders to sponsor a safe indoor/outdoor activity area for neighborhood or at-risk children.

**SECONDARY PREVENTION**

- Provide health assessment and counseling during home visits for health promotion initiated for other family members—for example, at visits after a hospitalization or a birth.

- Be available for health counseling for teens prior to and after youth activities.
- In schools associated with faith communities, assist with height and weight screening to identify young persons needing attention.

**TERTIARY PREVENTION**

- Collaborate closely with faith education teachers, youth ministers/counselors about sessions that deal with nutrition behavior change, exercise behavior modification with injury prevention guidelines, health problems of overweight young persons, and advantages of reduced weight, support, stress management, improved quality-of-life sessions.
- Follow up and monitor health care provider's plan of care for young persons who have been identified as overweight; support and encourage them to withstand peer ridicule during behavior changes.
- Assist in making choices for behavior change (suggest avoiding calorie-rich or nutritionally lacking foods during school meal and snack times; suggest possible paths for walking and bicycling; suggest courts and gyms available for more strenuous exercise).
- Discuss in youth groups and parenting groups the need for loving, caring friends and the support needed for long-term behavior modification programs that are life-long efforts.

---

efforts guided by the Healthy People 2010 framework. Dillon and Sternas (1997) describe steps to successfully plan, implement, and evaluate health fairs that support health promotion and disease prevention efforts. These and similar activities promote increased health of the entire community and they include persons of all ages, encourage enthusiasm, offer fellowship and leisure, and reduce duplication of effort.

As faith communities continue to address Healthy People 2010 indicators, a focus on eliminating health disparities among groups differing in racial/ethnic background, age, sex, income, disabilities, and geographic location would be most beneficial to overall community understanding and enhancement. Nurses working in collaboration with faith community wellness committees can be key members of efforts to address these justice and social righteousness issues (Box 45-3).

## POPULATION-FOCUSED PARISH NURSING: FAITH COMMUNITY AND SCHOOL

This chapter has stressed a population focus for parish nursing. In Christian traditions, the scriptural story of the Good Shepherd who cares for the whole flock and also for the lost, silent, or "out of bounds" individuals so that they

may again become a part of the flock is an effective parallel with population interests. In the previous section on national health objectives, numerous examples are given of the parish nurse as a catalyst who facilitates efforts to address health indicators and the related objectives. The entire faith community is considered; those who find it difficult to voice their concern or those on the margins are intentionally sought to become part of efforts to promote healthy behaviors and healthy environments.

Faith communities often work closely with other populations or environments closely aligned with the mission or outreach of the faith community (Boland, 1998; Brendtro and Leuning, 2000; Lough, 1999; Reusch and Gilmore, 1999; Tolley, 1998; Trofino et al, 2000). They may be closely related with an individual nursing home, a childcare or an adult day-care center, an immigrant community, at-risk populations, a preschool, or a local neighborhood, elementary, or high school. The example of the LAH/BNP programs working with older, less mobile, or frail populations was cited earlier in this chapter. In all of these situations, parish nurses use their best community-oriented nursing skills to collaborate with all key individuals and groups involved.

Using an elementary school as an example of another population associated with the faith community, the key

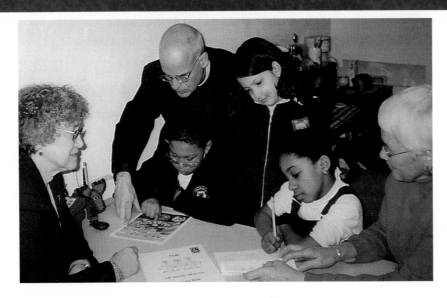

**Figure 45-8** Planning a healthy lifestyle curriculum with principal, clergy, and pupils in faith community school population.

players are brought to the table for discussions (Figure 45-8). The teachers, principal, clergy, parent–teacher group, staff, students, special education teachers, and recreation leaders are all potential participants. Assessing the school environment, programs, and population is advisable. The group would consider the abilities of the faculty, staff, pupils, and parents. It would assess the physical environment for safe and healthy activities, and the program for enrichment opportunities in music, art, physical education, dance. It would discuss health topics, curriculum appropriate for growth and development, healthy choice opportunities throughout the day's activities, opportunities for parents and pupils to learn skills for life-long learning, as well as other topics desired by the group. Suggestions can come from Healthy People 2010, state elementary school guidelines, and faith community school documents and guidelines. The agenda can be as comprehensive or as focused as the group wishes, but working within a timeline can be beneficial to see outcomes. The nurse would guide the group as it ascertains strengths and develops a plan for implementation of focused objectives and a plan for evaluating and reporting their efforts.

## Practice Application

The nursing process is a method that can be used to begin program planning and evaluation with faith communities. Such an approach can involve congregational members and parish nurses in a dynamic endeavor to jointly learn about the members' individual health status, as well as that of the faith community and the local and broader geographic community. Parish nurse programs are derived in various ways. Initially, the impetus for parish nursing may stem from an unmet health need within the congregation; from visions of a lay or health professions member concerned about caring within the congregation; or from discussions of a committee dealing with health and wellness issues.

Which of the following activities is most likely to increase the interest and involvement of the congregation's members?
A. Writing a contract for parish nurses services
B. Surveying the faith communities' environment
C. Gathering information on leaders and valued activities in the congregation through focus groups of pastoral staff
D. Assessing the needs of the congregational members through a survey
E. Holding a health fair

Answer is in the back of the book.

## Key Points

- Parish nurse services respond to health, healing, and wholeness within the context of the church. Although the emphasis is on health promotion and disease prevention throughout the life span, the spiritual dimension of nursing is central to the practice.
- Parish nursing has evolved from roots of healing traditions in faith communities; early public health nursing efforts working with individuals, families, and populations in the community; and more recently the independent practice of nursing.
- The parish nurse partners with the wellness committee and volunteers to plan programs and consider health-related concerns within faith communities.
- To promote a caring faith community, usual functions of the parish nurse include personal health counseling, health teaching, facilitating linkages and referrals to congregation and community resources, advocating and encouraging support resources, and providing pastoral care.
- Parish nurses collaborate to plan, implement, and evaluate health promotion activities considering the

faith community's beliefs, rituals, and polity. Healthy People 2010 leading indicators and objectives are effective frameworks for health ministry efforts of wellness committees and basic to partnering for programs.

- Nurses in congregational or institutional models enhance the health ministry programs of the faith communities if carefully chosen partnerships are formed within the congregation, with other congregations, and also with local health and social community agencies.
- Nurses working in the parish nursing specialty must seek to attain adequate educational and skill preparation to be accountable to those served and to those who have entrusted the nurse to serve.
- Nurses are encouraged to consider innovative approaches to creating caring communities. These may be in congregations as parish nurses; among several faith communities in a single locale or regionally; or in partnership with other community agencies or models such as block nursing.
- To sustain oneself as a parish nurse healer, the nurse takes heed to self-heal and self-nurture while supporting individuals, families, and congregation communities in their healing process.

## Clinical Decision-Making Activities

1. Contact the local council of churches to see if there is a parish nurse in your community. If so, make contact and arrange to spend a day with the nurse.
   a. Interview the nurse about the parish nurse role functions. Contrast the nurse's answers to what you learned in this chapter.
   b. Ask how the parish nurse standards of practice are integrated into the practice. How can you verify the answer?
2. Discuss with classmates the similarities and differences between home health care nursing and parish nursing. Review the content in this chapter and Chapter 40. Compare your answers.

3. Choose a Healthy People 2010 indicator to implement in a parish nursing setting. Discuss plans for implementing the objective and evaluating the outcomes. What data did you use to develop a plan for implementing? How did you choose your population?
4. Interview a clergy member of a local church, temple, or mosque in your area. Ask him or her to elaborate on traditions of health and healing connections within the tradition. Consider all points of view and think how you might be able to respond to a region's differences as a parish nurse.
5. Visit a senior citizen day-care center and speak with participants about important events in their lives. Did they refer to rituals from faith traditions? Ask them about their associations with faith communities during their lives. How does their answer help define the important events?
6. With classmates, interview a youth group leader and nurse in a local faith community about the concern of preventing risky sexual behavior among youths. What perspectives of this concern would the church staff need to consider? What help does the parish nurse or other health professional provide? How does this issue relate to growth and development within a community of faith? Be specific.

### Additional Resources

These related resources are found either in the appendix at the back of this book or on the book's website at **http://evolve.elsevier.com/Stanhope.**

**evolve** **Evolve Website**

Parish Nursing Resources
WebLinks: Healthy People 2010

## References

Achterberg J, Dossey B, Kolkmeier L: *Rituals of healing,* New York, 1994, Bantam Books.

American Nurses Association: *Standards of clinical nursing practice,* Washington, DC, 1998, ANA.

American Nurses Association: *Code for nurses with interpretive statements,* Washington, DC, 1999, ANA.

Baldwin KA et al: Perceived needs of urban African American church congregants, *Public Health Nurs* 18(5):295-303, 2001.

Berry R: A parish nurse. In Office of Resourcing Committees on Preparation for Ministry: *A day in the life of . . . : a kaleidoscope of specialized ministries,* Louisville, Ky, 1994, Presbyterian Church (USA), Distribution Management Service.

Berry R et al: Weaving international parish nurse experiences: sharing the story of Korea. In Solari-Twadell A, coordinator: *Weaving parish nursing into the new millennium,* proceedings of the 14th Annual Westberg Symposium, Itasca, Ill, 2000.

Boland CS: Parish nursing: addressing the significance of social support and spirituality for sustained health-promoting behaviors in the elderly, *J Holist Nurs* 16(3):355-368, 1998.

Bondine D: Parish nursing, *Perspectives* 21(2):8, 1997.

Brendtro MJ, Leuning C: Educational innovations—nurses in churches: a population-focused clinical option, *J Nurs Educ* 39(6):385-388, 2000.

Carson VB, Koenig HG: *Parish nursing: stories of services and health care,* Philadelphia, 2002, Templeton Foundation Press.

Centers for Disease Control and Prevention: *Engaging faith communities as partners in improving community health,* Atlanta, Ga, 1999, CDC.

Chandler E: Theology and ethics. In Weist WE, editor: *Healthcare and its costs: a challenge for the church,* Lanham, Md, 1988, University Press of America.

Chandler E: Spirituality, *Hospice J* 14(3):63-74, 1999.

Chase-Zoliek M: A comparison of urban versus rural experiences of nurses volunteering to promote health in churches, *Public Health Nurs* 16(4):270-279, 1999.

Coenen A et al: Describing parish nurse practice using the nursing minimum data set, *Public Health Nurs* 16(6):412-416, 1999.

Courtney A: Obesity a health issue with heavy costs to public, *Lexington Herald Leader,* January 14, 2002.

Covington CY et al: Kids on the move: preventing obesity among urban children, *Am J Nurs* 101(3):73-81, 2001.

Culp L: Health ministries: caring for body and soul, *Reg Nurse J* 9(3):8, 1997.

Developing parish nursing, Kai-Taiki: *Nursing New Zealand* 6(2):6, 2000.

Dillon DL, Sternas K: Designing a successful health fair to promote individual, family, and community health, *J Community Health Nurs* 14(1):1, 1997.

Dossey BM, editor: *Core curriculum for holistic nursing,* Gaithersburg, Md, 1997, Aspen.

Dossey BM, Keegan L, Guzzetta CE: *Holistic nursing: a handbook for practice,* ed 3, Gaithersburg, Md, 2000, Aspen.

Elderberry Institute: *Who we are,* retrieved March 15, 2002, from www.elderberry.org.

Fehring RJ, Miller JR, Shaw C: Spiritual well-being, religiosity, hope, depression, and other mood states in elderly people coping with cancer, *Oncol Nurs Forum* 24(4):663, 1997.

Frisch NC et al: AHNA standards of holistic nursing practice: guidelines for caring and healing, Gaithersburg, Md, 2000, Aspen.

Granberg-Michaelson K: Staying healthy: the spiritual dimension, *Contact* 155:3, 1997.

Health Ministries' Association, American Nurses Association: *Scope and standards of parish nursing practice,* Washington, DC, 1998, ANA.

International Parish Nurse Resource Center: "Role of parish nurse, mission and resources" [brochure], Park Ridge, Ill, 1998, IPNRC.

Koenig HG: *Spirituality and patient care,* Philadelphia, 2002, Templeton Foundation Press.

Koenig HG et al: Religious coping in the nursing home: a biopsychosocial model, *Int J Psychiatr Med* 27(4):365, 1997.

Kucey M: Worklife: professional practice and parish nurses, *Can Nurse* 95(1):51-52, 1999.

Lenehan G: Free clinics and parish nursing offer unique rewards, *J Emerg Nurs* 24:3, 1998.

Loeb SJ, O'Neill J, Gueldner SH: Health motivation: a determinant of older adults' attendance at health promotion programs, *J Community Health Nurs* 18(3):151-165, 2001.

Lough MA: An academic–community partnership: a model of service and education, *J Community Health Nurs* 16(3):137-149, 1999.

Louis M, Alpert P: Spirituality for nurses and their practice, *Nurs Leadersh Forum* 5(2):43-51, 2000.

Lukits A: Parish nurses fill gap in health care system, *Reg Nurse J* 12(4):10-12, 2000.

Magilvy JK, Brown NJ: Parish nursing: advanced practice nursing model for healthier communities, *Adv Pract Nurs Q* 2:67, 1997.

Martinson IM et al: The block nurse program, *J Community Health Nurs* 2(1):21, 1985.

Marty M, editor: *Healthy people 2000: a role for America's religious communities,* Chicago, 1990, Park Ridge Center.

Matthews DA et al: Religious commitment and health status, *Arch Fam Med* 7(2):118-124, 1998.

McDermott MA, Solari-Twadell PA, Mathews R: Promoting quality education for the parish nurse and parish nurse coordinator, *Nurs Health Care Perspect* 19(1):4, 1998.

Meisenhelder JB, Chandler EN: Prayer and health outcomes in church members, *Altern Ther Health Med* 6(4):56-60, 2000.

National Institutes of Health: *The practical guide: identification, evaluation, and treatment of overweight and obesity in adults,* NIH publicaton No. 00-4084. Rockville, Md, 2000, USDHHS.

Nouwen HJ: *The wounded healer,* New York, 1979, Image Books.

Office of the General Assembly: *Life abundant: values, choices, and health care,* Louisville, Ky, 1988, Presbyterian Distribution Services.

Olson J, Simington J, Clark M: Educating parish nurses, *Can Nurse* 94(8):40-44, 1998.

Oman D, Reed D: Religion and mortality among the community-dwelling elderly, *Am J Public Health* 88(10):1469, 1998.

Oxman TE, Freeman DH, Manheimer ED: Lack of social participation or religious strength and comfort as risk factors for death after cardiac surgery in the elderly, *Psychosom Med* 57(1):5, 1995.

Princeton Religion Research Center: *Religion in America,* Princeton, 1996, Gallup Poll.

Pulchalski CM, Romer AL: Taking a spiritual history allows clinicians to understand patients more fully, *J Palliat Med* 3(1):129-137, 2000.

Quinn JF: Holding sacred space: the nurse as healing environment, *Holist Nurs Pract* 6(4):26-36, 1992.

Reusch AC, Gilmore GD: Developing and implementing a healthy heart program for women in a parish setting, *Holist Nurs Pract* 13(4):9-18, 1999.

Rouse DP: Parish nursing as community-based pediatric clinical experience, *Nurse Educ* 25(1):8-11, 2000.

Rydholm L: Patient-focused care in parish nursing, *Holist Nurs Pract* 11(3):47, 1997.

Schank MJ, Weis D, Matheus R: Parish nursing: ministry of healing, *Geriatr Nurs* 17 (1):11-13, 1996.

Sellers SC, Haag BA: Spiritual nursing interventions, *J Holist Nurs* 16(3):338-354, 1998.

Silverman HD: Creating a spirituality curriculum for family practice residents, *Altern Ther Health Med* 3(6):54, 1997.

Solari-Twadell PA, McDermott MA, editors: *Parish nursing: promoting whole person health within faith communities,* Thousand Oaks, Calif, 1999, Sage.

Solari-Twadell PA, McDermott MA, Matheus R, editors: *Parish nursing education: preparation for parish nurse managers/coordinators: promoting congregational health, healing and wholeness for the twenty-first century,* Park Ridge, Ill, 2000, IPNRC, Advocate Health Care.

Solari-Twadell PA et al: *Assuring viability for the future: guideline development for parish nurse education programs,* Park Ridge, Ill, 1994, Lutheran General HealthSystem.

Sulmasy DP: *The healer's calling: a spirituality for physicians and other health professionals,* New York, 1997, Paulist Press.

Swinney J et al: Community assessment: a church community and the parish nurse, *Public Health Nurs* 18(1):40-44, 2001.

Tolley M: Experiencing the neighborhood: the parish as clinical site, *Oklahoma Nurse* 43(1):31, 1998.

Trofino J, Hughes CB, Hay KM: Primary care parish nursing: academic, service and parish partnerships, *Nurs Admin Q* 24(1):59-74, 2000.

Tuck I, Pullen L, Wallace D: Comparative study of the spiritual perspectives and interventions of mental health and parish nurses, *Issues Ment Health Nurs* 22(6):593-606, 2001.

U.S. Department of Health and Human Services: *Healthy people 2010* [CD-ROM], Rockville, Md, 2000, U.S. Government Printing Office, available at http://www.health.gov/healthypeople.

U.S. Department of Health and Human Services: *Healthy people in healthy communities: a community planning guide using healthy people 2010,* Rockville, Md, 2001a, Office of Disease Prevention and Health Promotion.

U.S. Department of Health and Human Services: *The surgeon general's call to action to prevent and decrease overweight and obesity,* Rockville, Md, 2001b, Public Health Service, available at http://www.surgeongeneral.gov/topics/obesity.

Van Loon A: International: Faith community nursing, *Int J Nurs Pract* 2(3):168, 1996.

Van Loon A: The development of faith community nursing programs as a response to changing Australian health policy, *Health Educ Behav* 25(6):790-799, 1998.

Wallace DC et al: Client perceptions of parish nursing, *Public Health Nurs* 19(2):128-135, 2002.

Woodward KL, Underwood A: The ritual solution, *Newsweek* 130(12):62, September 22, 1997.

Wright KB: Professional, ethical and legal implications for spiritual care in nursing, *Image J Nurs Scholarsh* 30(1):21-26, 1998.

# Public Health Nursing at the Local, State, and National Levels

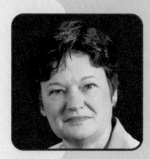

**Diane V. Downing, R.N., M.S.N.**

Diane V. Downing began practicing public health nursing in 1980 as a public health nurse with the Marion County Health Department in Indiana. She also worked at the local level as assistant commissioner for nursing and quality assurance in the New York City Department of Health. She has worked at the state level in Indiana as the Sudden Infant Death Syndrome project coordinator, as division director for local health standards and evaluation, and as division director for the Maternal and Child Health Division. At the national level, she worked as the director of the Policy and Research Division of the Public Health Foundation. She is currently public health program specialist with Arlington County Department of Human Services, Virginia.

## Objectives

After reading this chapter, the student should be able to do the following:

1. Define public health, public health nursing, and local, state, and national roles
2. Identify trends in public health nursing
3. Describe examples of public health nursing roles
4. Discuss emerging public health issues that affect public health nursing
5. Describe collaborative partnerships of public health nursing
6. Identify educational preparation of public health nurses and competencies necessary to practice
7. Explore team concepts in public health settings

All public health is partnerships. **Public health programs** are designed with the goal of improving a population's health status. They go beyond the administration of health care to include community health assessment, analysis of health statistics, public education, outreach, record keeping, professional education for providers, surveillance, compliance to regulations for some institutions/agencies and school systems, and follow-up of populations. Examples of follow-up care are for persons with active, untreated tuberculosis, pregnant women who have not kept prenatal visits, and underimmunized children. Public health programs are frequently implemented by the development of partnerships or coalitions with other providers, agencies, and groups in the location being served. Public health nurses are involved in these activities in various ways depending on the public health agency (local, state, or federal) and the identified needs.

Public health is not a branch of medicine; it is an organized community approach designed to prevent disease, promote health, and protect populations. It works across

*The author acknowledges the foundational work for this chapter by Mary Eure Fisher in the fifth edition of this book.*

many disciplines and is based on the scientific core of epidemiology (Institute of Medicine [IOM], 1988). Public health nurses work with multidisciplinary teams of people both within the public health areas and in other human services agencies. The health of communities is a shared responsibility that requires a variety of diverse and often nontraditional partnerships. A critical partnership that shapes public health nursing practice in the United States is the interaction of local, state, and federal public health agencies.

## ROLES OF LOCAL, STATE, AND FEDERAL PUBLIC HEALTH AGENCIES

In the United States, the local–state–federal partnership includes federal agencies, the state and territorial public health agencies, and the 3200 local public health agencies. The interaction of these agencies is critical to effectively leverage precious resources, financial and personnel, and to address the health of populations. Public health nurses working in all of these agencies work together to identify, develop, and implement interventions that will improve and maintain the nation's health.

**Federal public health agencies** develop regulations that implement policies formulated by Congress, provide

## Key Terms

**federal public health agencies**, p. 1114
**local public health agencies**, p. 1116
**public health**, p. 1117

**public health nursing**, p. 1117
**public health programs**, p. 1114
**state public health agency**, p. 1115

*See Glossary for definitions*

## Chapter Outline

Roles of Local, State, and Federal Public Health
    Agencies
History and Trends of Public Health
Scope, Standards, and Roles of Public Health
    Nursing

Issues and Trends in Public Health Nursing
Models of Public Health Nursing Practice
Education and Knowledge Requirements
    for Public Health Nurses

Certification for Public Health Nursing
National Health Objectives
Functions of Public Health Nurses

a significant amount of funding to state and territorial health agencies for public health activities, survey the nation's health status and health needs, set practices and standards, provide expertise that facilitates evidence-based practice, coordinate public health activities that cross state lines, and support health services research (IOM, 1988). The U.S. Department of Health and Human Services (USDHHS) and the Environmental Protection Agency (EPA) are the federal agencies that most influence public health activities at the state and local levels (see Chapter 3). The USDHHS includes the Centers for Disease Control and Prevention (CDC), the Health Resources and Services Administration (HRSA), the Agency for Healthcare, Research and Quality (AHRQ), and the Food and Drug Administration (FDA). The USDHHS is the agency that facilitates development of the nation's Healthy People Objectives (USDHHS, 2000).

Each of the states and territories has a single identified official **state public health agency** that is managed by a state health commissioner. The structure of state public health agencies varies. Some states require that the state health commissioner be a physician. A growing number of states do not limit the position to physicians but rather require specific public health experience. California, Maryland, Iowa, Washington, and Michigan are examples of states that focus on public health experience as a requirement for the state health commissioner position. Public health nurses have been appointed to the state health commissioner positions in a number of states. For example, public health nurses have been appointed to health commissioner positions in the states of California, Washington, and Michigan. The Association of State and Territorial Health Officials defines the state public health agency as the organizational unit of the state health officer, who works in partnership with other government agencies, private enterprises, and voluntary organizations to ensure that services essential to the public's health are provided for all populations. State public health agencies are responsible for monitoring health status and enforcing laws and regulations that protect and improve the public's health. These agencies receive funding from federal agencies for the implementation of public health interventions. Communicable disease programs, maternal and child health programs, chronic disease prevention programs, and injury prevention programs are examples. The agencies distribute federal and state funds to the local public health agencies to implement programs at the community level, and they provide oversight and consultation for local public health agencies. State health agencies also delegate some public health powers, such as the power to quarantine, to local health officers.

**Local public health agencies** have responsibilities that vary depending on the locality, but they are the agencies that are responsible for implementing and enforcing local, state, and federal public health codes and ordinances and providing essential public health programs to a community. The goal of the local public health department is to safeguard the public's health and to improve the community's health status. The health department's authority is delegated by the state for specific functions (Box 46-1). As with state health departments, some states require that local health directors be physicians, whereas others focus on public health experience. For example, public health nurses in Maryland, Washington, Wisconsin, and California hold local health director positions. The duties of local health departments vary depending on the state and local public health codes and ordinances and the responsibilities assigned by the state and local governments. Usually, the local public health department provides for the administration, regulatory oversight, public health, and environmental services for a geographic area.

The majority of local, state, and federal public health agencies will be involved in the following:

- Collecting and analyzing vital statistics (Chapter 11)
- Providing health education and information to the population served (Chapter 13)
- Receiving reports about and investigating and controlling communicable diseases (Chapters 38 and 39)
- Protecting the environment to reduce the risk to health (Chapter 10)
- Providing some health services to particular populations at risk or with limited access to care (local public health agencies, guided by state and federal policies and goals and community needs) (Chapters 24 to 30, 32 to 40, 43 to 45)
- Identifying public health problems for at-risk and high-risk populations

Public health nurses work for local, state, and federal agencies. They work in partnership with each other, other

public health staff, other governmental agencies, and the community to safeguard the public's health and to improve the community's health status. Public health agency staffs include physicians, nutritionists, environmental health professionals, health educators, and various laboratory workers, epidemiologists, health planners, and paraprofessional home visitors and outreach workers. Community-based organizations include the United Way, the American Red Cross, free clinics, Headstart programs, day-care centers, community health centers, hospitals, senior centers, advocacy groups, churches, academic institutions, and businesses. Other governmental agencies include the fire/emergency services department, law enforcement agencies, schools, parks and recreation departments, and elected officials. Changes in local, state, and federal governments affect public health services, and public health nursing has to develop strategies for dealing with these changes. To meet the changing needs of a community, public health nurses must identify new public health concerns and help develop programs to provide needed services.

## HISTORY AND TRENDS OF PUBLIC HEALTH

A person born today can expect to live 30 years longer than the person born in 1900. Medical care accounts for 5 years of that increase, but public health is responsible for the additional 25 years through prevention efforts brought about by changes in social policies, community actions, and individual and group behavior changes (USDHHS, 2000). Historically, public health nurses were valued by and important to society and functioned in an autonomous setting. They worked with populations and in settings that were not of interest to other health care disciplines or groups. Much public health service was delivered to the poor and to women and children, who did not have political power or voice. During the course of the twentieth century, public health responsibilities expanded beyond communicable disease prevention, occupational health, and environmental health programs to include reproductive health, chronic disease prevention, and injury prevention activities. As a result of Medicaid managed care, many public health agencies were no longer providing personal health care services. Public health agencies began to shift emphasis from a focus on primary health care services to a focus on core public health activities such as the investigation and control of diseases and injuries, community health assessment, community health planning, and involvement in environmental health activities. As the twentieth century came to a close, genetics, newly emerging communicable diseases, preventing bioterrorism and violence, and handling and disposal of hazardous waste were emerging as additional public health issues (CDC, 1999). The twenty-first-century public health nurse will be competent in areas such as epidemiology, analytic assessment skills, health status monitoring and surveillance, community mobilization, and risk communication.

---

**BOX 46-1** **Public Health Agency Functions**

Generally, local public health agencies perform the following functions:

- Provide and disseminate health information
- Provide leadership in health planning
- Provide essential public health and environmental services
- Collect statistics on births
- File a certificate for every birth or death in that area

Public health activities at the beginning of the twenty-first century were shaped by the September 11, 2001, airplane attacks of the World Trade Center, the Pentagon, and a field in Pennsylvania, in which thousands were murdered. However, public health nursing activities at the federal, state, and local levels were even more dramatically affected by a series of anthrax exposures that occurred shortly after the airplane attacks. In addition to anthrax exposures in Florida and New York, a month after the plane attacks, thousands of workers at the Brentwood Post Office and the Senate Building in Washington, D.C., were exposed to an especially virulent strain of anthrax from a contaminated letter. The anthrax exposures alerted policymakers to the weakening public health infrastructure required to respond to bioterrorism events. By the end of the twentieth century, resources for communicable disease services had decreased as surveillance and containment activities and protection of water and food supplies produced decreasing communicable disease rates. As society grappled with the upheaval created by the reality of a bioterrorism event, public health nurses learned to leverage existing authority and expertise to ensure that all critical issues threatening the public's health are addressed. Nurses are well positioned to actively participate in policy decisions that will ensure that a public health infrastructure able to prevent and respond to bioterrorism will be strengthened and maintained within the context of general communicable disease surveillance and response. Public health nurses are facing issues such as unprecedented influenza, tetanus, and childhood vaccine shortages and emerging infections that compete with bioterrorism activities for resources.

During the twentieth century, public health nurses were a major force in the nation, achieving immunization rates that accounted for the dramatic decrease in measles. In 1996, nearly 900,000 fewer cases of measles were reported than in 1941 (Turnock, 1997, p. 1). However, the general public was not informed about how this immunization activity was accomplished or about its effect on improving health and lowering health care cost. For public health services to receive adequate funding, it is necessary for the public and the government to be aware of the benefits provided to a community by public health nurses. Public health nurses must be at the table when issues are being discussed and decisions are being made to make certain that public health programs are provided for the populations at risk and that funds are available to cover those services. For example, the twenty-first-century public health nurse is working to develop a public health system able to monitor and detect suspicious trends and respond rapidly to prevent widespread exposure, whether the result of a deliberate or a natural epidemic. A prime example of emerging infectious diseases is the severe acute respiratory syndrome (SARS), caused by a virus, that brought illness and death to many in 2003. The disease spread quickly from China to other countries, being transported by airline passengers traveling internationally.

## SCOPE, STANDARDS, AND ROLES OF PUBLIC HEALTH NURSING

In 1920, C. E. A. Winslow defined **public health** as "the science and art of preventing disease, prolonging life and promoting health and efficiency through organized community effort" (Turnock, 1997, p. 9). This definition is still used in public health textbooks because it focuses on the relationship between social conditions and health across all levels of society. Reflecting Winslow's definition, the Public Health Nursing Section of the American Public Health Association defined **public health nursing** as "the practice of promoting and protecting the health of populations using knowledge from nursing, social and public health sciences" (1996, p. 1). Public health nursing is a specialty practice of nursing defined by scope of practice and not by practice setting (Quad Council of Public Health Nursing Organizations, 1999; APHA Public Health Nursing Section, 2001). Public health nursing practice focuses on the individuals, families, communities, and populations where public health nurses live, work, and play.

---

**WHAT DO YOU THINK?**

In this era of managed care, a critical question is whether public health will take a position as a community advocate or be a part of the medical marketplace and become just another commodity. Once, medicine was seen as a mission-driven, value-laden profession serving society for the common good, but now it is seen as a partner with managed care bargaining for roles and resources (Citrin, 1998, p. 351). What is the role of public health nurses in the twenty-first century?

---

**HOW TO** Implement the Core Public Health Functions in a Community: Essential Elements of the Public Health Role

- Conduct community assessments.
- Prevent and control epidemics.
- Provide a safe and healthy environment.
- Measure performance, effectiveness, and outcomes of health services.
- Promote healthy lifestyles.
- Provide laboratory testing.
- Provide targeted outreach to vulnerable populations and form partnerships.
- Provide personal health care services.
- Conduct research and create innovations (in programs).
- Mobilize the community for action.

From National Association of City and County Health Officials: *Blueprint for a healthy community: a guide for local health departments,* Washington, DC, 1994, NACCHO.

---

**BOX 46-2    Tenets of Public Health Nursing**

The Quad Council of Public Health Nursing Organizations (1999) identified the following eight tenets of public health nursing. These tenets, which distinguish public health nursing from other nursing specialties, are included in the *Scope and Standards of Public Health Nursing Practice* published by the American Nurses' Association.

1. Population-based assessment, policy development, and assurance processes are systematic and comprehensive.
2. All processes must include partnering with representatives of the people.
3. Primary prevention is given priority.
4. Intervention strategies are selected to create healthy environmental, social, and economic conditions in which people can thrive.
5. Public health nursing practice includes an obligation to actively reach out to all who might benefit from an intervention or service.
6. The dominant concern and obligation is for the greater good of all of the people or the population as a whole.
7. Stewardship and allocation of available resources supports the maximum population health benefit gain.
8. The health of the people is most effectively promoted and protected through collaboration with members of other professions and organizations.

---

From Quad Council of Public Health Nursing Organizations: *Scope and standards of public health nursing practice,* Washington, DC, 1999, pp 2-4, American Nurses Association.

---

Additional knowledge, skills, and aptitudes are necessary for a nurse to go beyond focusing on the health needs of the individual to focusing on the health needs of populations (see Chapters 1 and 15). This additional knowledge distinguishes the public health nurse from other nurses who are practicing in the community setting. Public health nursing practices arise from knowledge gained from the physical and social sciences, psychological and spiritual fields, environmental areas, political arena, epidemiology, economics, community organization, and life experience. Jan Wallinder's (1997, p. 77) explanation that "public health nurses define and redefine their roles as they live them" describes the essence of the spirit of commitment most practicing public health nurses experience. The Quad Council of Public Health Nursing Organizations identified eight tenets (Box 46-2) that distinguish the public health nursing specialty from other nursing specialties. Although other nurses may practice some or all of these eight tenets, they are not incorporated as a core foundation of the practice in other specialties. Public health nurses always adhere to all

eight tenets of public health nursing (Quad Council of Public Health Nursing Organizations, 1999).

A variety of settings and a diversity of perspectives are available to nurses interested in developing a career in public health nursing. Public health nurses working at the federal, state, and local levels integrate community involvement and knowledge about the entire population with clinical understandings of the health and illness experiences of individuals and families in the population. They translate and articulate the health and illness experiences of diverse, often vulnerable individuals and families in the population to health planners and policymakers, and they help members of the community voice their problems and aspirations. Public health nurses are knowledgeable about multiple strategies for intervention, from those applicable to the entire population, to those for the family and the individual. Public health nurses translate knowledge from the health and social sciences to individuals and population groups through targeted interventions, programs, and advocacy. Public health nurses are directly engaged in the interdisciplinary activities of the core public health functions of assessment, assurance, and policy development. In any setting, the role of public health nurses focuses on the prevention of illness, injury, or disability, and the promotion and maintenance of the health of populations (Public Health Nursing Section, 1996).

Public health nurses deliver services within the framework of ever-constricting resources coupled with emerging and complex public health issues. This requires the efficient, equitable, and evidence-based use of resources. The National Public Health Performance Standards Program (CDC, 2002), a federal, state, and local partnership, has developed evaluation instruments that can be used to collect and analyze data on the programs provided through state and local public health systems. The instruments link with the 10 essential services of public health that define the core functions of public health (see Chapter 1).

Public health nurses make a significant difference in improving the health of a community by monitoring and assessing critical health status indicators such as immunization levels, infant mortality rates, and communicable diseases. On the basis of their assessment and in partnership with the community, public health nurses advocate for evidence-based interventions to respond to negative health status indicators. Public health nurses provide the "linkage between epidemiologic data and clinical understanding of health and illness as it is experienced in peoples' lives" (Public Health Nursing Section, 1996).

Public health's shift from being the primary care provider of last resort to the development of partnerships to meet the health promotion and disease prevention needs of populations in a community has raised concerns about available health care for the uninsured and underinsured. The public health nurses' role in this ongoing shift in health care delivery is still being developed for many agencies. Public health nurses retain responsibility for ensuring that all populations have access to affordable, qual-

## Evidence-Based Practice

This descriptive study looked at a health department parenting project to see whether teen mothers' self-esteem, social support, and parenting competence improved while receiving case management services from public health nurses during the first 18 months of motherhood. A sample of 56 first-time teen mothers participated in the study; 45% were Hispanic and 44% were white. Public health nurses received special training in assessment of and intervention with teen mothers. The nurses provided assessments, interventions, referrals for medical care, vocational training and finances, and education in prenatal and postnatal care, diet, family planning, childcare and child health, and safe-baby environment. The nurses also arranged for transportation for mothers to keep appointments and encouraged the teens to stay in school. The nurses used home visits and phone calls to maintain contact with the mothers.

Data were collected at 6, 12, and 18 months using the Rosenberg self-esteem scale, the inventory of socially supportive behaviors by Barrera, and the parental sense of competency scale by Gibard. The study results indicated that mothers need special attention during the first months of parenting to enhance that self-esteem and to encourage better parenting. Social support was found to decrease as the child moved toward 18 months and the parents' competence in caring for the baby slightly increased.

**Nurse Use:** Teen pregnancy is a national concern because it usually results in less education and less future earning power for the teen mother. Early intervention to promote self-esteem and to encourage social support from family, friends, and agencies and competent parenting skills for the mother may make a difference for the health of the baby and the mother's ability to become a happy, healthy, productive adult.

Herrmann MM, Van Cleve L, Levisen L: Parenting, competence, social support, and self-esteem in teen mothers case managed by public health nurses, *Public Health Nurs* 15(6):432, 1998.

ity health care services. They accomplish this by advocating for legislation that promotes universal health care, such as increased funding for community health centers, and by forming partnerships with hospitals, free clinics, and other organizations to ensure health care for all populations in the community. Case management at the community level is a renewed effort in public health nursing. Through case management activities, public health nurses link populations with needed health care providers (see Chapter 19) (see the Evidence-Based Practice box).

Uninsured individuals seek services on a sliding payment scale from such sources as university or public hospital clinics or from a variety of free clinics. Public health nurses serve as a bridge between these populations and the resource needs for this at-risk group by approaching health care providers on behalf of individuals seeking medical/health services and keeping the needs of this population on the political agenda. Frequently, low-income populations or populations with multiple chronic illnesses lack the knowledge and skills to negotiate the complex health care system. This population needs education and training in identifying their problems, approaches to self-care, and illness prevention strategies and lifestyle choices that will have an effect on their health. The public health nurse understands barriers these populations confront, such as transportation issues, and difficulty understanding and following health care provider instructions.

Although vulnerable populations have always benefited from public health nursing services, the populations that are most acutely in need of public health nursing services have changed dramatically over the last couple of decades. Of particular concern are the number of young women and their partners who are substance abusers and have risky behaviors that put their pregnancy or children at high risk of injury or abuse. Public health nurses at the federal, state, and local levels have developed innovative, collaborative approaches to prepare staff to work effectively with this population.

## ISSUES AND TRENDS IN PUBLIC HEALTH NURSING

The discovery and development of antibiotics in the 1940s, coupled with immunization programs and improvements in sanitation, contributed to the decrease in infectious disease–related morbidity and mortality during the twentieth century (CDC, 1999). Twenty-first-century issues facing public health nursing include increasing rates of drug resistance to community-acquired pathogens, societal issues such as welfare reform, racial and ethnic disparities in health outcomes, behaviorally influenced issues (such as chronic diseases, violence in society, and substance abuse), and unequal access to health care. Public health nurses must keep abreast of the issues that affect all of society. Assessments need to be changed to include the factors that affect the populations that they serve.

For example, a major twenty-first-century public health challenge is emerging infections resulting from drug-resistant organisms. The widespread, often inappropriate, use of antimicrobial drugs has resulted in loss of effectiveness for some community-acquired infections such as gonorrhea, pneumococcal infections, and tuberculosis and increasing rates of drug resistance in community-acquired pathogens such as *Streptococcus pneumonia*, *Escherichia coli*, and *Salmonella* spp. (Goosens and Sprenger, 1998). Mainous et al (1997) report that clients and health care providers are responsible for the inappropriate use of antibiotics. The author reports that 79% of adults surveyed in Kentucky and Louisiana believed antibiotics were indicated and effective to treat an upper respiratory infection with discolored nasal discharge. The public health nurse can influence this trend by objecting to inappropriate use of antibiotics by providers and educating individuals, families, health care providers, and the community about the dangers of misuse and overuse of antibiotics.

> **NURSING TIP**
>
> Many of the epidemics of the future will be defined by social problems such as substance abuse and teen pregnancy.

Societal issues such as welfare reform will influence a population's ability to obtain preventive health services either because they lose government-sponsored health care coverage or because the low-wage jobs they take do not allow time off for health care. When childcare is an issue for the welfare mother returning to work, consideration must be given to effects on the individual, family, community, and population. Public health nurses assess the problem and determine what is wrong with a system that forces parents to go to work so they can be removed from welfare roles but that does not provide for childcare. The question to be answered by a nurse is "What will it take to change the system?"

Partnerships and collaboration among groups are much more powerful in making change than the individual client and public health nurse working alone. As another example, the depressed, nonfunctional mother in need of counseling is a significant public health concern because the mother's, children's, and family's needs are not being met. Frequently, the problem may not be obvious to the health professional who sees this woman for the first time. Public health nurses have special preparation to help them both identify the individual's problem and look at its effects on the broader community. In this example, the children may grow to be adults with mental health problems, and the community mental health services will need to be able to handle the increase in this population. Children may become violent adults, resulting in a need for more correction facilities. Mothers may need additional mental health services. Children may be absent from school often and may not be able to contribute to society. They may be nonproductive in the workplace because absence from school leads to lack of skills. Often, one problem of the single individual places great burdens on the community.

Healthy People 2010 includes objectives to address racial and ethnic disparities in health outcomes (CDC, 2000). The IOM (2002) reports that disparities in health care treatment account for some of the gaps in health outcomes between racial and ethnic groups. This report found that minorities receive lower-quality health care than white people, regardless of insurance status, income, and severity of the condition. Public health nurses work as case managers and at the policy level to promote equal access to health care including health literature and spoken services that reflect the community in which the services are being delivered (see Chapter 8). The public health nurse working directly as a case manager or in a clinic setting can promote ethnicity-friendly services by partnering with other community agencies such as interpreter services. Equal access to health care can be facilitated by identifying and alerting the community to gaps in services available in the community. For example, some communities may appear to have an adequate number of pediatricians to meet the community's needs. However, a community assessment may reveal that the community is home to a high number of children who rely on Medicaid as payment for services, or to families whose primary language is not English. Matching this information with the pediatrician population may reveal that none of the pediatricians accept Medicaid as payment for services, or they all deliver services in English only.

Population-focused public health nursing requires that public health nurses consider health, social, and environmental factors that influence the health of communities, families, and individuals. A public health nurse providing communicable disease control services for the homeless population or the refugee population will also work for policies that ensure affordable housing.

Some macro-level trends affecting public health today are as follows (Brownson and Kreuter, 1997):

- Changes in health care delivery systems
- Changing patterns in the racial and ethnic composition in the U.S. population
- The aging of the population
- Rapid development of information technologies
- Development of numerous and diverse health-related partnerships
- Educational needs and changes within the public health workforce

> **HOW TO** **Educate Nurses for Roles in Public Health: Curriculum Objectives for Public Health Nursing**
>
> The nurse should be able to do the following:
> - Articulate similarities and differences between individual-focused and population-focused nursing practice
> - Describe the history and current perspectives of public health nursing practice
> - Demonstrate skills used to apply key nursing contributions to public health practice (core functions and essential services) in a community
> - Apply principles and skills of population health to practice in the public health agency
> - Use current information and communication technology in all public health agencies
> - Communicate the benefits of public health and public health nursing practice

## MODELS OF PUBLIC HEALTH NURSING PRACTICE

In response to the IOM (1988) report that described public health in a state of disarray and the need for all federal public health agencies to work to identify core public health functions, public health nurses have worked to develop models of practice that will operationalize the role of public health nursing. This section will present examples of models that are receiving attention and use across the nation. These models also serve as examples of the important work that can be accomplished by local, state, and federal partnerships.

> ### WHAT DO YOU THINK?
>
> Changes have occurred in public health nursing (Frank, 1959, p. vii). Changes are occurring and will continue to occur in public health nursing. Public health nurses have to learn to function in an organization that must deal with many changes, as changes occur continually because of the many internal and external factors from people, programs, politics, and the unknown, as well as known local, state, and federal actions. Which skills help the public health nurse adapt to changes?

Washington State public health nursing directors (Public Health Nursing Directors, 1993) examined public health nursing interventions within the framework of individual, family, and community levels of service. They identified public health nursing activities within the core public health functions of assessment, policy development, and assurance. For example, under the core public health function of assessment, public health nurses analyze data and needs of specific populations at the community level of service. At the family level of service, they evaluate a family's assets and concerns, and at the individual level of service they identify individuals within the family in need of services (Public Health Nursing Directors, 1993).

In Virginia, a statewide committee led an examination of the role of public health nursing in the context of increasing public expectation of accountability and the shift of public health nursing emphasis from clinical services to population-focused services. Their work resulted in a document that identifies public health nursing roles within the framework of the core public health functions (see Chapter 1). The work identifies the educational needs of staff that would prepare them to function effectively in the changing public health arena. Essential elements of the role were identified. These essential elements are being implemented through multidisciplinary public health teams. The document includes a matrix that demonstrates the relationship of the public health functions defined by the essential elements to the public health nursing roles at the local level, as well as the role of the state in this responsibility (see Appendix J.1).

The Public Health Nursing Section of the Minnesota Department of Health (2001) developed a framework called the intervention model that defines public health nursing interventions by level of practice. Public health nurses deliver services within a framework of core interventions. The three levels of public health nursing practice are systems, community, and individual/family. The model identifies 17 population-based public health interventions delivered by public health nurses. It also identifies population-based interventions as those that do the following:

- Focus on entire populations possessing similar health concerns or characteristics
- Are guided by an assessment of health status
- Consider the broad determinants of health, such as housing, income, education, cultural values, and community capacity
- Consider all levels of prevention, with primary prevention a priority
- Consider all levels of practice (community, system, and individual/family) (see Appendix J.1)

## EDUCATION AND KNOWLEDGE REQUIREMENTS FOR PUBLIC HEALTH NURSES

The Public Health Nursing Section of the American Public Health Association (1996) states the educational preparation of public health nurses should be at least a baccalaureate degree, because "All public health nurses should have a background in the social and behavioral sciences, epidemiology, environmental health, current treatment modalities, and health care delivery options in order to fully understand health policy, research, and treatment choices and to translate this knowledge into the promotion of healthy populations" (Public Health Nursing Section, 1996).

The Council on Linkages Between Academia and Public Health Practice (2001) examined a decade of work to identify a list of core public health competencies that represent a set of skills, knowledge, and attitudes necessary for the broad practice of public health. They capture the crosscutting competencies necessary for all disciplines that work in public health, including public health nurses, physicians, environmental health specialists, health educators, and epidemiologists. The competencies are applied (at the three skill levels of *aware, knowledgeable, and proficient*) to three job categories of frontline staff, senior-level staff, and supervisory and management staff. A detailed list of core competencies by job category and skill level is available at http://www.TrainingFinder.org/competencies. In addition to having the core public health competencies, public health nurses have specialized competencies as described in the *Scope and Standards of Public Health Nursing Practice* (Quad Council, 1999). The core public health competencies are divided into the following eight domains. The content related to the domains can be found in the chapters noted.

1. Analytic assessment skills: Chapters 1, 9, 12, 14, 15, and 24-37
2. Basic public health sciences skills: Chapters 3, 6, 8, 10, 11, 16, 20-23, 38, and 39
3. Cultural competency skills: Chapters 4 and 7
4. Communication skills: Chapters 13 and 19
5. Community dimensions of practice skills: Chapters 15, 17, 18, and 40-46
6. Financial planning and management skills: Chapter 5
7. Leadership and systems thinking skills: Chapter 42
8. Policy development/program planning skills: Chapters 8 and 21

Many of these core public health competencies are provided by public health nurses who have learned these skills in the workplace while gaining knowledge through years of practice. Rapid changes in public health are providing a challenge to public health nurses in that there is neither the time nor the staff to provide as much on-the-job training as is needed to learn and upgrade skills and knowledge of staff. Nurses with baccalaureate or master's preparation are needed to provide a strong public health system (see Chapter 1).

## CERTIFICATION FOR PUBLIC HEALTH NURSING

Two levels of certification are available for nurses in public health nursing. Both are offered through the American Nurses' Credentialing Center. Although certification is voluntary, being recognized as competent in a specialty area says to clients and employers that the nurse has the knowledge and skills essential to public health nursing practice. The nurse who is certified focuses on a holistic approach to care of the total population, including the promotion and maintenance of health, health education,

case management, coordination, and the provision of continuity of care. To be eligible to take the certification examination at the generalist level, one must be a registered nurse and licensed in the United States or its territories, have a baccalaureate or higher degree in nursing or a related field, have at least 30 contact hours of continuing education applicable to the field in the past 3 years, and have practiced in the community health field a minimum of 1500 hours in the last 3 years. Nurses are examined on such topics as public health science; individual, family, and community as client; areas of practice; public health issues/problems; and professional issues. The clinical specialist in community-oriented nursing is discussed in Chapter 41.

## NATIONAL HEALTH OBJECTIVES

Since 1979, the U.S. surgeon general has worked with local, state, and federal agencies, the private sector, and the U.S. population to develop health objectives for the nation. These objectives are revisited every 10 years. In 2000, the USDHHS released *Healthy People 2010: Understanding and Improving Health*. These objectives will guide the work of public health nurses over the next decade. Healthy People 2010 includes the needs of the United States for a public health infrastructure (see the Healthy People 2010 box).

State health departments play a key role in implementing the Healthy People objectives. Examples of state Healthy People 2010 goals can be located on the Public Health Foundation website at www.phf.org. State health departments help set local goals using the Healthy People 2010 objectives as a framework. Knowing that public health departments do not have the resources to accomplish these goals independently, collaboration is essential to quality nursing practice and is encouraged at the local

---

### Healthy People 2010 | National Health Objectives Related to the Public Health Infrastructure

23-4 Increase the proportion of population-based Healthy People 2010 objectives for which national data are available for all population groups identified for the objective

23-6 Increase the proportion of population-based Healthy People 2010 objectives that are tracked regularly at the national level

23-7 Increase the proportion of population-based Healthy People 2010 objectives for which national data are released within 1 year of the end of data collection

23-8 Increase the proportion of federal, tribal, state, and local agencies that incorporate specific competencies in the essential public health services into personnel systems

23-9 Increase the proportion of schools for public health workers that integrate into their curricula specific content to develop competency in essential public health services for their employees

23-10 Increase the proportion of federal, tribal, state, and local agencies that provide continuing education to develop competency in essential public health services for their employees

23-11 Increase the proportion of state and local public health agencies that meet national performance standards for essential public health services

23-12 Increase the proportion of federal, tribal, state, and local public agencies that conduct or collaborate on population-based prevention research

From U.S. Department of Health and Human Services: *Healthy people 2010: understanding and improving health,* ed 2, Washington, DC, 2000, U.S. Government Printing Office.

level with existing groups. New partnerships are developed related to specific goals. Communities develop coalitions to address selected objectives, based on community needs, to include all of the local community stakeholders such as social services, mental health, education, recreation, government, and businesses. Membership varies from community to community depending on that community's formal and informal structure. The groups join the coalition for a variety of reasons. For example, businesses see the value of developing a productive workforce that will be of importance to them and the community in the future.

The Healthy People 2010 objectives are developed to achieve the two major goals of increasing quality and years of healthy life and eliminating health disparities (USDHHS, 2000). Public health nurses help clients identify unhealthy behaviors and then help them develop strategies to improve their health. Some of the behaviors addressed by public health nurses are tobacco use, physical activity, and obesity, all of which affect quality and years of healthy life. Public health nurses also organize the community to conduct community health assessments to identify where health disparities exist and to target interventions to address those disparities. For example, community health assessments may disclose that certain populations are at higher risk for asthma, diabetes, low immunization rates, high cigarette smoking behavior, or exposure to environmental hazards.

Some Healthy People 2010 communicable disease areas of focus are vaccine-preventable infectious diseases, emerging antimicrobial resistance, and human immunodeficiency virus (HIV), acquired immunodeficiency syndrome (AIDS), and sexually transmitted diseases. To help clients reduce their risk of acquiring a communicable disease, public health nurses provide clients with instructions on the use of barrier methods of contraception and information on the hazards of multiple sexual partners and street drug use. Getting a complete sexual history on all clients coming to the health department for services takes special skills but is essential to determine the behaviors that have brought the client to the local health department. Abstinence as a birth control method can be addressed with all populations. Education of young persons before they become sexually active has helped reduce the incidence of some sexually transmitted diseases in this population.

## FUNCTIONS OF PUBLIC HEALTH NURSES

Public health nurses have many functions depending on the needs and resources of an area. Advocate is one of the many roles of the public health nurse. As an advocate, the public health nurse collects, monitors, and analyzes data and discusses with the client which services are needed, whether the client is an individual, a family, a community, or a population. The public health nurse and the client then develop the most effective plan and approach to take, and the nurse helps the client implement the plan so that the client can become more independent in making decisions and getting the services needed. At the community and population levels, public health nurses promote healthy behaviors, safe water, air, and sanitation. They advocate for healthy policies that will develop healthy communities (see Chapter 17).

Legislation is a public health tool used to ensure the health of populations. Implemented with extreme concern for the balance between individual rights and community rights, public policy is a critical, but often uncomfortable function for the public health nurse. Examples of legislation that has successfully improved the health of populations are required immunizations for school entry, seat belt use, smoke-free environments, and bicycle and motorcycle helmet use.

Case manager is a major role for public health nurses. Public health nurses use the nursing process of assessing, planning, implementing, and evaluating outcomes to meet clients' needs. Clear and complex communications are frequently an important component of case management. Other health and social agency participants may not be familiar with the home and community living conditions that are known to the public health nurse. It is the nurse who has been there and seen the living conditions and who can tell the story for the client or assist the individual or family with the telling of their story. Case managers assist clients in identifying the services they need the most at the least cost. They also assist communities and populations in identifying services that will increase the overall community health status.

Public health nurses are a major referral resource. They maintain current information about health and social services available within the community. They know what resources will be acceptable to the client within the social and cultural norms for that group. The nurse educates clients to enable them to use the resources and to learn self-care. Nurses refer to other services in the area, and other services refer to the public health nurse for care or follow-up. For example, the mother and new baby may be referred to the public health nurse for postnatal care with postpartum home visit follow-up.

Assessment of literacy is a large part of public health nursing. Many individuals are limited in their ability to read, write, and communicate clearly. The public health nurse has to be culturally sensitive and aware of the specific areas of unique problems of clients, such as financial limitations that may in turn limit educational opportunities. Frequently, when a person goes to a physician's office, clinic, or hospital, they are clean and neatly dressed. The assumption is made that when they nod at the health care provider it means that they understand what has been said. This is frequently not the case, but the client is embarrassed to admit that he or she does not understand what has been said. Being illiterate does not mean a person is mentally slow. It is important for the public health nurse to follow up on the many contacts the individual or family has with medical, social, and legal services to clarify what is understood and to find an answer to the questions

## *Community Health Nursing in the Traditional Setting in Canada*

Karen Wade, R.N., B.N., M.Sc.N., Toronto Public Health
Maureen Cava, B.Sc.M.S., Toronto Public Health

### ORGANIZATION OF PUBLIC HEALTH SERVICES IN CANADA

A Canadian Public Health Association (CPHA, 1997) survey that assessed the status of provincially and territorially mandated public health services in Canada revealed that the organization of public health and its linkages with other health and nonhealth sectors varies considerably. Funding for public health services also varies. Programs and services that are integrated into comprehensive health organizations are usually funded through a health board. The legislative mandate for public health focuses primarily on health protection and control of communicable diseases. Other secondary acts and regulations include legislation regarding secondhand smoke, environmental contaminants, and health standards in public places (CPHA, 1997). In most provinces and territories, public health is the responsibility of the Ministry of Health or its equivalent. In several provinces, public health functions are the shared responsibility of ministries such as health, social services, seniors, children, and families.

### SCOPE OF PUBLIC HEALTH NURSING IN CANADA

In some areas of Canada, the terms *community health nurse* and *public health nurse* are used interchangeably. In others, the term *community health nurse* encompasses the specialty of public health nursing. In Canada, the focus of community/public health nursing practice is primarily health promotion, illness and injury prevention, health protection, and health maintenance (CPHA, 1990). The CPHA (1990) has taken the position that a baccalaureate degree in nursing is essential for community/public health nursing practice.

The CPHA defines community/public health nursing as "an art and a science that synthesizes knowledge from the public health sciences and professional nursing theories. Its goal is to promote and preserve the health of populations and is directed to communities, groups, families, and individuals across their life span, in a continuous rather than episodic process. . . . (They) work in collaboration with, among others, communities, families, individuals, other professionals, voluntary organizations, self-help groups, informal health care providers, governments, and the private sector" (1990, p. 3). Community/ public health nurses are proactive regarding social and health care trends; changing needs of communities; changes in policies and legislation that affect the health of communities, families, and individuals; and changes in the health care system (CPHA, 1990).

### KEY ACTIVITIES OF COMMUNITY/PUBLIC HEALTH NURSES IN CANADA

The CPHA (1990) identified 11 key activities of community/public health nurses in Canada (they are similar to the roles and functions of public health nurses in the United States):

*Care/service provider:* Assesses client's health status, and plans, implements, and evaluates care in partnership with the client; uses health promotion and illness and injury prevention strategies

*Communicator:* Uses effective communication skills (1) with individual clients, (2) to represent the views of individuals, groups, and communities, (3) to facilitate interagency and intersectoral cooperation, and (4) to strive for sufficient community resource allocation

*Community developer:* Applies knowledge of community assessment and community development models to facilitate public participation in identifying and decision making about health issues

*Consultant:* Provides expertise/information to clients, lay helpers, professionals, social and community

---

The views expressed in this box represent those of the writer and do not represent the views of the City of Toronto, Toronto Public Health.

---

that have not been asked by the client or answered by the services.

The public health nurse is an educator, teaching to the level of the client so that information received is information that can be used. Patience and repetitions over time are necessary to develop the trust and to enable the client to use the relationship with the nurse for more information. As educator, the public health nurse identifies community needs (e.g., playground safety, hand hygiene, pedestrian safety, safe-sex practices) and develops and implements educational activities aimed at changing behaviors over time.

Public health nurses are direct primary caregivers in many situations both in the clinic and in the community. Where the public health nurse provides primary care is determined by community assessment and is usually in response to an identified gap that the private sector is unable to respond to, coupled with an assessment of the impact of the gap in services on the health of the population. Examples include prenatal services for uninsured women, free or low-cost immunization services for targeted populations, directly observed therapy for patients with active tuberculosis, and treatment for sexually transmitted diseases.

agencies, professional associations, and all levels of government

*Educator:* Provides formal/informal presentations/ teaching and educational programs to individuals, groups, families, aggregates, and communities

*Facilitator:* Acts as a leader in developing a proactive approach to health issues and/or encouraging individuals or communities to take action on issues; acts as an enabler in supporting the community to participate in identifying and taking ownership of health issues; acts as an advocate for the disadvantaged

*Policy formulator:* Identifies the need for and participates in the development of and evaluation of policy conducive to health

*Researcher/evaluator:* Identifies and investigates key issues and approaches to community health; uses research/program evaluation findings to inform programming and to allocate resources

*Resource manager/planner/coordinator:* Involves communities in health services planning, priority setting, and allocation

*Social marketer:* Uses marketing techniques and skills to promote healthy living as well as health promotion programs

*Team member/collaborator:* Fosters team building as well as interdisciplinary, interagency, and intersectoral cooperation and collaboration

## THE FUTURE OF PUBLIC HEALTH NURSING IN CANADA

Canada is undergoing health system reform and health care restructuring. Although there is increased emphasis on health promotion and disease prevention, the determinants of health and community-based services (Reutter and Ford, 1998), the primary emphasis of the Canadian system is still on acute care. Moreover, there is increased emphasis on containing the costs of treatment (CPHA, 2001). Health systems reform and diminishing resources are leading to a reexamination of the roles and activities of public health nurses. Public health nurses in several Canadian provinces have identified that although they

are embracing multiple and broader roles (as just identified) and are increasingly working in partnership with others, there is an increased emphasis on service provision to high-risk families and groups (Chalmers, Bramadat, and Andrusyszen, 1998; Reutter and Ford, 1998).

Canadian community health nursing standards of practice are being developed by a national committee of community health nurses under the auspices of the Community Health Nurses Association of Canada (CHNAC), an interest group of the Canadian Nurses Association. These standards will support the certification of community health nursing as a specialty by the Canadian Nurses Association (CHNAC, 2002).

### References

Canadian Public Health Association: *Community health: public health nursing in Canada—preparation and practice,* Ottawa, 1990, CPHA.

Canadian Public Health Association: *Public health infrastructure in Canada,* Ottawa, 1997, CPHA.

Canadian Public Health Association: *The future of public health in Canada,* Canadian Public Health Association Board of Directors discussion paper, Ottawa, 2001, CPHA.

Chalmers KI, Bramadat IJ, Andrusyszen MA: The changing environment of community health practice and education: perceptions of staff nurses, administrators, and educators, *J Nurs Educ* 37(3):109-117, 1998.

Community Health Nurses Association of Canada: *Canadian community health nursing standards of practice,* April, 2002—draft for consultation, available at www.communityhealthnursescanada.org.

Reutter LI, Ford JS: Perceptions of changes in public health nursing practice: a Canadian perspective, *Int J Nurs Stud* 35:85-94, 1998.

*Canadian spelling is used.*

Public health nurses ensure that direct care services are available in the community for at-risk populations by working with the community to develop programs that will meet the needs of those populations. Currently, no system of outreach service in the medical models of care addresses the multiple needs of high-risk populations. High-risk populations frequently do not understand the medical, social, educational, or judicial system and the professional languages, codes of behavior, or expected outcomes of these services. Clients need a case manager, a health educator, an advocate, and a role model to enable them to benefit from these services and to teach them how

to avoid complex and expensive problems in the future. The local public health nurse fills these roles and many more for this population. These are examples of the difficult clinical issues that public health nurses face in making ethical and professional decisions.

The public health nurse's role is unique and essential in many situations. Access to homes gives the nurse information that usually cannot be gathered in the hospital or clinic setting. The public health nurse learns to ask intimate questions creatively and to seek information that will facilitate case management and provide the clinical and social care needed, including other community resources.

Careful attention must be paid to privacy and confidentiality in delivering public health nursing services. The credibility of the nurse and the agency depends on the professional handling of the public health information of each and every staff member.

---

**( DID YOU KNOW?**

It is important for public health nurses to practice confidentiality when they have knowledge about an individual, family, communicable disease outbreak, community-level problem, or any special knowledge obtained in the public health work setting.

---

When a disaster (see Chapter 20) occurs, public health nurses at the local, state, and federal levels have multiple roles in assessment, planning, implementing, and evaluating needs and resources for the different populations being served. Whether the disaster is local or national, small or large, natural or caused by humans, public health nurses are skilled professionals essential to the team. As a health care facility, the local public health department has a disaster plan, as well as a role in the local, regional, and state disaster plans. Public health nurses' roles include providing education that will prepare communities to cope with disasters, professional triage for local shelters, conducting enhanced communicable disease surveillance, working with environmental health specialists to ensure safe food and water for disaster victims and emergency workers, and serving on the local emergency planning committee. Their presence may be required in other regions of the state or country to provide official public health nursing duties in a time of crisis, such as a hurricane, that requires a lengthy period of recovery. Each governmental jurisdiction has an emergency plan. The public health agency is expected to provide planning and staffing during a disaster. These local emergency preparedness plans may be multigovernmental, which requires coordination between communities.

Essential and unique roles for public health nurses exist in the area of communicable disease control. Public health nursing skills are necessary for education, prevention, surveillance, and outbreak investigation. Public health nurses can find infected individuals; notify contacts; refer; administer treatments; educate the individual, family, community, professionals, and populations; act as advocates; and in general be state-of-the-art resources to reduce the rate of communicable disease in the community (see Chapters 38 and 39). The communicable disease role is one of the most important roles for public health nursing during disasters. During the September 11, 2001, airplane attacks, public health nurses at the federal, state, and local levels immediately implemented active enhanced surveillance activities. Information about communicable diseases seen at the local level was passed on to the state public health agency and finally to the CDC. At each step, the data were analyzed for evidence of unusual disease trends.

When October, 2001, alerts from the CDC began presenting information about a photo editor in Florida who had been hospitalized with inhalation anthrax, public health nurses and hospital infection control practitioners throughout the nation increased activity. Public health response to disasters requires that resources be redirected temporarily from other programs while maintaining programs that will prevent additional outbreaks. Therefore public health nurses not normally involved in communicable disease activities can be shifted to this function. The exposures resulting from the anthrax-tainted letters presented unprecedented public health challenges. The Washington, D.C., anthrax exposures resulted in thousands of possible work-related exposures, five cases of inhalation anthrax in the region, and two deaths over a period of months. Public health at the federal, state, and local levels was looked to for coordinated leadership and answers to a situation in which experience was limited and answers were uncertain.

Although communicable disease control is a core public health service, the role of public health as incident commander in a widespread public health emergency is a new role. Issues such as how to conduct mass treatment in response to a bioterrorism event; which jurisdiction is in charge; how to communicate uncertain information to the public; and who should take antibiotics for how long had to be rapidly resolved across jurisdictional and agency lines. The anthrax exposures are typical of the nature of public health emergencies. They unfold as the communicable disease moves through communities.

Public health nurses are essential partners in disaster drills. In Virginia, an electrical company has a nuclear plant that requires annual multijurisdictional disaster drills. These disaster planning and practice sessions are an opportunity for local public health nurses to get to know other agencies' representatives and to let them know what public health nursing can offer. Because public health nurses are out in the communities and have assessment skills, they are essential in evaluating how the disaster was handled and making suggestions about how future events might be managed. To be most effective as disaster responders, public health nurses have to be a part of the team *before* an emergency. Knowing what type of disaster is likely to occur in a community is essential for planning. Types of disasters vary from place to place, but there is a history of past events and how they were handled, as well as resources and training from regional, state, and federal agencies. Public health nurses can help educate the public about the individual responsibilities and preparations that can be in place both for the person and for the community. Box 46-3 presents additional examples of public health nurses' functions by level of prevention. Public health nurses at the local, state, and federal levels work in partnership to accomplish each function.

## BOX 46-3  Levels of Prevention Used in Public Health Nursing

### PRIMARY PREVENTION: THE PRIORITY FOCUS

- Partnering with the community to conduct a community health assessment to identify community assets and gaps
- Partnering with the community to develop programs in response to identified gaps
- Providing information about safe-sex practices
- Conducting contacting/tracing for individuals exposed to a patient with an active case of tuberculosis or a sexually transmitted disease
- Educating day-care centers and families about the dangers of lead-based paint
- Educating day-care centers, schools, and the general community about the importance of hand hygiene to prevent transmission of communicable diseases
- Inspecting day-care centers, nursing homes, and hospitals to ensure patient safety and quality of care
- Providing immunizations
- Advocating for issues such as mandatory seat belt legislation, smoke-free environments, and universal access to health care
- Providing no-charge infant car seats accompanied by classes in use of safety seats
- Identifying environmental hazards such as housing quality, playground safety, pedestrian safety, and product safety hazards, and working with the community and policymakers to mitigate the identified hazards
- Conducting ongoing disease surveillance for communicable diseases and implementing control measures when an outbreak is identified

### SECONDARY PREVENTION

- Identifying and treating patients in a sexually transmitted disease clinic
- Identifying and treating patients in a tuberculosis clinic
- Providing directly observed therapy (DOT) for patients with active tuberculosis
- Conducting lead screening activities for children
- Implementing screening programs for genetic disorders/metabolic deficiencies in newborns; breast, cervical, and testicular cancer; diabetes; hypertension; and sensory impairments in children, and ensuring follow-up services for patients with positive results

### TERTIARY PREVENTION

- Case management services that link patients with chronic illnesses to health care and community support services
- Case management services that link patients identified with serious mental illnesses to mental health and community support services

## ■ Practice Application

A retirement community in a small town reported to the local health department 24 cases of severe gastrointestinal illness that had occurred among residents and staff of the facility during the past 24 to 36 hours. It was determined that the ill clients became sick within a short, well-defined period, and most recovered within 24 hours without treatment. The communicable disease outbreak team, composed of public health nurses, public health physicians, and an environmental health specialist, was called to respond to this possible epidemic.

How should they respond to this situation? (Refer to Chapter 11 for help in answering this question.)

A. Call the Centers for Disease Control and Prevention and ask for help with surveillance.

B. Send all the ill persons in the retirement community to the hospital.

C. Evaluate the agent, host, and environment relationships to determine the cause of the problem.

D. Close the dining room and find another source to provide food to the residents.

Answer is in the back of the book.

## ■ Key Points

- Local public health departments are responsible for implementing and enforcing local, state, and federal public health codes and ordinances while providing essential public health services.
- The goal of the local health department is to safeguard the public's health and improve the community's health status.
- Public health nursing is the practice of promoting and protecting the health of populations using knowledge from nursing and social and public health sciences.
- Public health is based on the scientific core of epidemiology.
- Marketing of public health nursing is essential to inform both professionals and the public about the opportunities and challenges of populations in public health care.
- A driving force behind public health nursing changes is the economy and the increase in managed care.
- Public health nurses need ongoing education and training as public health changes.

- Some of the roles public health nurses function in are advocate, case manager, referral source, counselor, primary care provider, educator, outreach worker, and disaster responder.
- Public health nurses have an important role in helping with local disasters, including planning, staffing, and evaluating events.

## Clinical Decision-Making Activities

1. What are some of the various roles of the public health nurse in the local, state, and federal public health systems? Contrast the roles. Explain why they may be different from one another.
2. How can public health nurses prepare themselves for change? Illustrate what you mean.
3. What can today's public health nurses learn from the past practice of public health nurses? How can you verify your answer?
4. Describe collaborative partnerships that public health nurses have developed. How do partnerships help solve public health problems?
5. What are some external factors that have an effect on public health nursing? How can you deal with the complexities of these factors?
6. What are core functions used by public health nurses as they plan interventions? Do these functions make sense to you? Explain.

7. If you were a public health nurse for a day, what would you like to accomplish? Why? Is your answer supported by evidence? Be specific.
8. How would you determine the most pressing public health issue in your community? Gather several points of view from key leaders in the community.
9. Give an example of a policy change or an effect from the work of public health nurses. How did this policy make a difference in client health outcomes?

## Additional Resources

These related resources are found either in the appendix at the back of this book or on the book's website at **http://evolve.elsevier.com/Stanhope.**

### Appendixes

Appendix J.1 Examples of Public Health Nursing Roles and Implementing Public Health Functions

Appendix J.2 Public Health Guidelines for Practice

### *evolve* Evolve Website

WebLinks: Healthy People 2010

## References

American Public Health Association, Public Health Nursing Section: *Definition and role of public health nursing,* Washington, DC, 1996, APHA.

Brownson R, Kreuter M: Future trends affecting public health: challenges and opportunities, *J Public Health Manag Pract* 2(3):49, 1997.

Canadian Public Health Association: *Community health: public health nursing in Canada—preparation and practice,* Ottawa, 1990, CPHA.

Canadian Public Health Association: *Public health infrastructure in Canada,* Ottawa, 1997, CPHA.

Canadian Public Health Association: *The future of public health in Canada,* Canadian Public Health Association Board of Directors discussion paper, Ottawa, 2001, CPHA.

Centers for Disease Control and Prevention: 2002 achievements in public health, 1900-1999: control of infectious diseases, *MMWR Morb Mortal Wkly Rep* 48:621-629, 1999.

Centers for Disease Control and Prevention: National Public Health Performance Standards Program, local public health system performance assessment instrument, version: field test 5b, May 2000, Atlanta, Ga, CDC, available at http://www.phppo.cdc.gov/nphpsp/Partners.asp.

Centers for Disease Control and Prevention: National Public Health Performance Standards Program, state public health system performance assessment instrument, version: state tool, May 2002 (draft), Atlanta, Ga, CDC, available at http://www.phppo.cdc.gov/nphpsp/Partners.asp.

Chalmers KI, Bramadat IJ, Andrusyszen MA: The changing environment of community health practice and education: perceptions of staff nurses, administrators, and educators, *J Nurs Educ* 37(3):109-117, 1998.

Citrin T: Topics for our times: public health—community or commodity? reflections of healthy communities, *Am J Public Health* 88(3):351, 1998.

Community Health Nurses Association of Canada: *Canadian community health nursing standards of practice,* April, 2002—draft for consultation, available at www.communityhealthnursescanada.org.

Council on Linkages Between Academia and Public Health Practice: *Core competencies for public health professionals,* Washington, DC, 2001, Public Health Foundation.

Frank CM Sr: *Foundations of nursing,* ed 2, Philadelphia, 1959, Saunders.

Goosens H, Sprenger M: Community-acquired infections and bacterial resistance, *BMJ* 317:654-657, 1998.

Herrmann MM, Van Cleve L, Levisen L: Parenting, competence, social support, and self-esteem in teen mothers case managed by public health nurses, *Public Health Nurs* 15(6):432, 1998.

Institute of Medicine: *The future of public health,* Washington, DC, 1988, National Academy Press.

Institute of Medicine: *Unequal treatment: confronting racial and ethnic disparities in health care,* Washington, DC, 2002, National Academy Press.

Mainous A et al: Patient knowledge of upper respiratory infections: implications for antibiotic expectations and unnecessary utilization, *J Fam Pract* 45:75-83, 1997.

National Association of City and County Health Officials: *Blueprint for a healthy community: a guide for local health departments,* Washington, DC, 1994, NACCHO.

Public Health Nursing Directors of Washington: *Public health nursing within core public health functions,* Olympia, Wash, 1993, Washington State Department of Health.

Public Health Nursing Section, Minnesota Department of Health: *Public health interventions—applications for public health nursing practice,* St Paul, Minnesota, Department of Health, 2001, APHA.

Quad Council of Public Health Nursing Organizations: "The tenets of public health nursing," unpublished white paper, 1997.

Quad Council of Public Health Nursing Organizations: *Scope and standards of public health nursing practice,* Washington, DC, 1999, American Nurses' Association.

Reutter LI, Ford JS: Perceptions of changes in public health nursing practice: a Canadian perspective, *Int J Nurs Stud* 35:85-94, 1998.

Turnock BJ: *Public health: what it is and how it works,* Gaithersburg, Md, 1997, Aspen.

U.S. Department of Health and Human Services: *Healthy people 2010: understanding and improving health,* ed 2, Washington, DC, 2000, U.S. Government Printing Office.

Wallinder J: Supporting one another: the definition of PHN, *Public Health Nurs* 14(2):77, 1997.

# Answers to Practice Applications

## CHAPTER 1

C and G are population focused, looking at the needs of their subpopulation and planning programs to meet their needs. A, B, D, and F are likely to be practicing community health nursing if their focus is health protection, health promotion, and disease prevention of the individuals/families in their subpopulations. B and D are more likely to be practicing community-based nursing, caring for clients who are ill.

## CHAPTER 2

A. It is easier to use a population-focused approach to solving these problems. If you can show through a community needs assessment that these are problems for a large number of people in the community and are putting the community at risk for increased health problems, more costly health care, and less social and economic growth, then one can convince policymakers to establish programs directed at these problems. With limited health care dollars the emphasis is on the greatest good for the greatest number.

B. A historical approach will build understanding of the public policy elements limiting care of various populations, by exploring what attempts have been made in the past to innovate or reform services for these populations, determining what has limited these attempts, and identifying examples of programs or policies that have been successful.

## CHAPTER 3

The correct answer is D. The nurse's responsibility is to educate clients about appropriate health care resources in their community and to allow families to choose care based on their own unique needs and preferences.

## CHAPTER 4

A. Identify what experiences each nurse has had in dealing with similar public health problems. Find out what the other nurses see as important to do first. Avoid forcing the "Western view" on local people who may be comfortable with a non-Western approach.

B. Find out if the water is safe. Is there sufficient, safe food? Is there shelter? Do people need (have) clothes?

C. Deal first with injuries and illnesses, then move to teaching first aid and safe eating and drinking water practices. Also set up groups or other arenas for people to deal emotionally with the stress of the traumas experienced.

## CHAPTER 5

A. Agencies are reimbursed for visits either by private insurance or Medicare or by clients through self-pay.

B. The payment for the visit is determined by using a cost basis or a charge basis. Cost basis reflects the actual cost to the agency to deliver the service. Charge basis reflects the cost plus additional monies charged for the visit, which may include indigent care visits or profit to be paid to stockholders if the agency is a for-profit agency.

C. Nursing care costs, although they may be known, are usually not used alone to determine the costs of a visit. The visit cost includes money for lights, water, supplies, secretarial and administrative salaries and benefits, as well as nurse salaries and benefits.

D. There is rationing in all of health care. Home health visits are rationed by the criteria set by the federal government for Medicare clients, such as a limited number of visits per year, and by private insurance, which also limits the number of visits per year. The individual client who must pay out of pocket sets his or her own limits and self-rations the amount he or she may be willing to pay for home health visits.

## CHAPTER 6

A. 
1. Ann's job entailed the monitoring of federal money and the supervising of funded programs within her division.
2. The federal government had allocated considerable money to the state agency to subsidize pediatric primary care programs.
3. The pediatric primary care programs had never received a formal evaluation.
4. The director of the state agency was using considerable federal money targeted for the pediatric primary care program in his district to supplement home health care services for the indigent homebound elderly persons.

B. 
1. The first ethical issue involved the inappropriate allocation of federal funds.
2. The second ethical issue involved a statewide lack of accountability regarding the use of federal funds.
3. The third ethical issue involved the conflict that occurs when two equally indigent populations need primary care services but inadequate money is available to subsidize both.

C. 
1. Ann developed new policies for allocation of funds. In order for any agency within the state to receive funding from the Division of Primary Care, the agency had to follow the new policies.
2. Ann also initiated a task force to develop specific procedures for the policies she developed. The procedures and their implementation were reviewed by the task force monthly. Representatives from the federal government and all the state-funded primary care programs constituted the task force. The task force became a safety net for anyone misappropriating federal funds, thus ensuring accountability.
3. Periodic unannounced site visits to all agencies within the state were made by peer administrators from the 20 districts in the state health department.
4. Regarding the pediatric primary care program in his district, the director for the state agency would receive funds only if he submitted specified monthly reports to Ann about the pediatric program's performance.
5. The director for the state agency and his staff were given help regarding how to interpret the policies and follow the procedures.

6. As a result of Ann's initiatives, the director for the state agency followed the new guidelines, which ensured that the pediatric primary care program received all of the money the program was due. In addition, he sought new funding to assist the indigent homebound elderly persons with chronic illnesses in his district.

## CHAPTER 7

The correct answer is C. Jenny was serving as a cultural broker between the patient and the professional health care system and facilitated effective communication. She provided an opportunity for clarification of any misinformation regarding cancer treatment. The nurse also facilitated open communication with the father and his family.

## CHAPTER 8

A plan of action to influence the health department about its decision to close the prenatal clinic would include the following:

A. In the law library, the state register was reviewed to see if regulations for the block grants had been finalized.

B. State health statistics were checked, which included vital statistics providing the current infant and maternity mortality rates in the state, and compared to national statistics.

C. The literature was reviewed for research that would show the relationships between prenatal care, normal deliveries, and complications of pregnancy and delivery.

D. After discussion, the group met with the state nurses' association to create answers. Together the groups contacted their local senators and representatives and asked for a meeting to discuss the issue.

E. The legal aid society was contacted to find a lawyer interested in consulting with them in preparing written and oral testimony.

F. The testimony was presented to the state health department during the process of preparing the regulations for the block grants.

## CHAPTER 9

The correct answer is C. It is becoming increasingly important for nurses to collect standardized assessment data, document care using standardized intervention terms, and generate standardized outcomes of care. However, it is also essential that nurses use their critical thinking skills and judgment and an individualized approach as they apply all the steps of the nursing process.

## CHAPTER 10

Answers to the first case scenario:

A. You would include in your assessment a Denver II on Billy to determine the neurologic effects of the lead on his growth and development, an assessment of the population to find the total child population under 6 years of age who may benefit from screening, and a community assessment to find the number of older homes in the community that may have lead-based paint.

B. Prevention strategies would include assisting the parents in enrolling Billy in Headstart to stimulate his development, because of his altered growth and development state; a blood level screening program for children under 6 years of age in the community to determine other children who may need to be referred for treatment; and a communitywide lead poisoning prevention program that includes educational materials about where lead is found in home environments and how to test for it. The nurse can target parent group leaders, local newspapers, and the school system to distribute educational materials.

Answers to the second case scenario:

Possible responses to the problem are short-term alternate drinking water (bottled), long-term extension of water lines from a nearby municipality, monitoring and cleanup of the contaminated groundwater (including testing other wells), testing children for lead poisoning, and informing the community of the risks and remedies.

## CHAPTER 11

The correct answer is D. There is controversy about prostate cancer screening, and the experts disagree. The revised American Cancer Society guidelines recommend that prostate cancer screening be offered only after men are informed of their risk and benefits. Age recommendations for screening are 45 years and older in African-American men and 50 years and older in white men. Prostate cancer screening should be offered to men who have 10 years or more of life expectancy left.

Population risks include incontinence and impotence for some but not all forms of treatment for prostate cancer. Individual risks for Rob are increased due to his family history of prostate cancer, as well as personal lifestyle habits of smoking and consumption of a high-fat diet. It is believed that hereditary cancer is more aggressive than regular cancer.

Population benefits include increased survival rate when prostate cancer is detected in the early stages rather than the advanced stages, 100% vs. 31%. Personal benefits may include decreased psychologic stress from fear of dying from prostate cancer, especially with family history of father dying from prostate cancer.

Two loci have been identified for hereditary prostate cancer: one on chromosome 1 and one on chromosome x. However, additional research is needed before genetic testing for cancer susceptibility testing in high-risk men is available. High risk for cancer susceptibility testing is usually defined as having several family members with cancer and/or earlier age of onset than normal for the cancer. Cancer susceptibility testing is not appropriate for all persons with cancer, only persons in the high-risk group. Genetic testing is new, and there are many misconceptions. Community health nurses are often some of the first health professionals who come into contact with at-risk persons and/or who are asked questions by the public. Therefore it is critical that community health nurses know and understand the basic concepts of cancer susceptibility testing. In addition, community health nurses need to know referral sources for additional genetic information that include genetic counselors.

## CHAPTER 12

1. All—A-E.
2. EBP in nursing takes into account the best evidence from research findings and evidence from community knowledge and experience to make decisions that promote the health of the community in a culturally appropriate manner.

## CHAPTER 13

The correct answer is C. This community health education need will require in-depth planning to meet the needs of the community. If Kristi works with the local health department and presents both a community forum and informational brochures, she can reach more of the target audience either in person or through literature.

## CHAPTER 14

A. One useful approach is to organize evaluation efforts according to the client systems and the focuses of care. In the outreach program the targeted client systems are specific aggregates (indigent or vulnerable groups) and the community (rural county), and the focuses of care are health promotion and illness prevention. This strategy involves examining existing data for the client systems (e.g., population demographics and health statistics; data related to the focuses of care, such as clinic utilization patterns; and the amount and type of health education materials disseminated at different locations). In addition, focus groups can be organized, targeting neighborhood or clinic-related populations, to assess perceived needs, utilization, and self-reported behavior change.

B. Departments of health at the local and state levels are an excellent resource for vital statistics and health data. Extensive information is accessible on the internet from national, state, and local government agencies: census data and demographics, morbidity, mortality, and age-specific death rates. These community health indicators are available from the government documents section of many university libraries, the Centers for Disease Control and Prevention (CDC), and the National Centers for Health Statistics (NCHS). In addition, many local communities and community health systems publish health-related report cards with updated information about use of existing health services.

C. Successful community health promotion and illness prevention interventions are based on theories of individual and community level health behavior change and social learning. Health programs must be individualized to individuals and communities, culturally relevant, and designed to maximize active consumer participation to meet the needs of a specific population. It is essential to assess the clients' values, prior health-related behaviors, and health care utilization patterns to design effective interventions.

D. It is important to identify key informants in this rural community who are involved with the target population in a variety of institutional and community settings. These informants may include nurses, physicians, social workers, mental health personnel, community and religious leaders, teachers, and health program consumers.

E. Lay health promoters are generally informal leaders in the community. These individuals are trained to deliver health educational messages, written materials, and reminders about clinics and other cues to prompt citizen participation. Nurses can work with lay health promoters to solicit the involvement of concerned citizens, community leaders, and health professionals to participate in a community coalition to seek funding and support to ultimately sustain the program[MO1].

## CHAPTER 15

The correct answer is B. A high level of community motivation is critical for any community-focused intervention and will help to ensure active community involvement in the planning process and commitment to the intervention itself.

## CHAPTER 16

A. Nursing roles include coordination, referred, case management.

B. Liz might coordinate getting nutritious food for Ethyl by arranging for Meals-On-Wheels to deliver a hot meal daily and extra meals for the weekend to be delivered on Friday.

C. Because Ethyl is alone a lot, the Meals-On-Wheels driver can be taught to observe any unusual or out-of-the-ordinary behaviors. Should anything be noticed, the driver should call the Coordinating Assessment and Monitoring (CAM) Agency in the hospital emergency department.

C. Liz might also arrange through the Senior Center for their van to take Ethyl into town weekly to shop and/or visit the physician.

D. After the episode where Ethyl was found in her yard, Liz coordinated with her neighbor to organize a rotating system among other neighbors so that one person went by to see Ethyl daily.

D. A remote monitoring system was put into Ethyl's home so she can call the CAM whenever she feels not "up to par."

C. Liz can also arrange for Ethyl's sister, Suzanna, to call Ethyl each day to check on her.

D. The most significant outcome achieved by Liz's case management would be to arrange sufficient basic services to allow Ethyl to remain at home. These include the following:
- Coordination of food (both Meals-On-Wheels and grocery shopping)
- Organizing a team of people to regularly check on Ethyl both to determine her health status and also for stimulation and socialization
- Arranging transportation to get regular health care
- Ensuring that Ethyl knows how to use technology to communicate with others in her circle of support as well as health care providers, e.g., portable cellular phone, remote paging systems, etc.

## CHAPTER 17

The true statements are B, C, and D. These examples pertain to local communities and rely on participation, cooperation, equity, and the use of technology.

## CHAPTER 18

A. Possible short-term outcomes include (1) increased student participation in activities offered at the university and (2) positive student/parent feedback at the conclusion of the program.

B. One possible intermediate outcome would be increased high school graduation rates.

C. One possible long-term outcome would be participants will continue their education at the university level.

## CHAPTER 19

The correct sequence is C, B, A, D. The first piece of information (C) is essential to understanding the level, amount, and nature of services the client is eligible to receive. The client must be informed, her needs assessed, and her options discussed (B). Family care options must be understood to formulate resource possibilities for the client (A). Arrangement for a facility site visit may or may not be essential but may be preferred (D).

## CHAPTER 20

The correct answer is A. Sharing her feelings with a trained professional who is familiar with the devastating circumstances in which Paula is involved will be most helpful. Although calling home might be comforting, family members with no experience in disaster work would not be able to fully appreciate the stress that Paula is experiencing.

## CHAPTER 21

Eva would include all the steps in planning her project.

She contacted the pastor of the church who was planning to open the soup kitchen to discuss the issue (formulation and assessment). She found him most receptive to the idea of developing a solution to the health care needs of the homeless. In her assessment, Eva found that no other health services were available to the homeless in the community. She looked at national data to estimate needs and size of the population. She talked with the community health nursing faculty to discuss potential solutions to the problem. She talked to members of the homeless population to get their perceptions of their needs.

On completing her assessment, Eva conceptualized the solutions. Several solutions were possible: work with the health department, attempt to provide better care through the local medical center, or open a clinic on site at the soup kitchen where most of the people gathered so that transportation would not be a problem.

After considering the solutions, Eva detailed the plan looking at the resources needed for opening a clinic at the soup kitchen. She considered supplies, equipment, facilities, and acceptability to the clients. She also considered the time involved, the activities required to implement a program, and funding sources.

In evaluating the possibilities, Eva considered the cost, the client and community benefits, and acceptability to clients, self, faculty, and the church. Although it would have been easier for her to choose to work with the health department or the medical center, she knew that the solution most acceptable to the clients would be to have a clinic located at the soup kitchen. The clinic would be more accessible, transportation would not be needed, and health services through the clinic could possibly prevent more costly hospital and emergency care (value).

Eva presented her plan to the faculty and the church. She convinced them that it would not be a costly endeavor. She had nurses in the community who volunteered to help, she had a carpenter who would donate his time to build an examining room in the back of the soup kitchen, and she had equipment promised to her by community physicians. The client assessment indicated that a first-aid and health assessment clinic was what was needed most. With approval from all (implementation), Eva began the clinic in 1981, seeing 25 to 35 clients a week, 1 hour per day for 5 days per week.

Eva evaluated the relevance of the program via the needs assessment process. She tracked the progress of the program by keeping records of her activities. She kept track of the resources in relation to the number of persons served (efficiency) and used these data to convince the church and the college of nursing to fund the ongoing clinic operation after she graduated. A summative evaluation of the clinic was completed by the faculty at the end of 4 years. The program's impact was outstanding. The clinic had grown. The client demand was high; most of the health problems could be handled at the clinic, which eliminated the cost burden to the community for more expensive health care; and it was highly acceptable to the clients (effectiveness). This clinic began as a service to 25 people for 1 hour per day. Today this clinic is open all day, 5 days per week, has more than 900 clients per year, and provides for more than 5000 client visits per year. The success of this clinic shows the effect that one community health nursing student can have on a community.

## CHAPTER 22

A. Outcomes of parenting education should provide evidence that behavior change has occurred because of the educational intervention. Menaka might use the outcome measure of episodes of praising children. She could construct a questionnaire for clients of the nurses who attended her classes on teaching parenting skills and for clients of nurses who had not attended her classes as a control group. Question for client questionnaire: Each week, how many times do you use praise with your child/children for doing something well. A. 0; B. 1; C. 2; D. 3; E; 4 or more.

B. An increase in this measure over time would indicate that the nurses had provided quality instruction that had improved the praising behavior in the parent. The differences in responses between the clients of the nurses who were taught parenting skills and those who were not could be statistically analyzed for significant differences.

## CHAPTER 23

A. Several contributing factors should be considered, including each of the following:
- The group was unwilling to confront conflict when three members failed to carry out their expected parts.
- Member responsibilities may have been incompletely described when the agreement to work together was specified.
- Students showed a lack of commitment to the project purpose.

B. Lifestyle behavior changes are best sustained through continuing support from family and friends. As individuals develop healthier attitudes and behavior, a variety of family, school or work, and neighborhood supports is needed. Nurses, in partnership with important others in the community, must initiate, participate in, facilitate, and encourage formal and informal groupings within that community that advocate positive practices and contest norms that promoted or ignored risk-taking activities.

## CHAPTER 24

A. No. The idealized version never existed. There have always been stressors, which presented challenges for families. While not as prominent, there have always been differing family structures within U.S. society.

B. According to a report from the National Commission on Children, people are both discouraged and encouraged about the status of America's families. The contradictions in this report indicate a disparity between people's perceptions of their own families (healthy) and the perception of families outside their own (unhealthy or dysfunctional).

C. There are liberal people in our society who believe the definition of family should be and is expanding and should include two-parent, single-parent, remarried, gay, adoptive, foster, and many other alternative family forms. That is, families are what people define them to be and the govern-ment with its health and economic sanctions should be supportive of all family groups. However, there are conservative people who believe that the definition of families should remain limited to the blood, legal, and adoptive guidelines.

D. How we ourselves define family will influence how we live, how we provide nursing care to families, and what health and welfare programs we are willing to support in the society.

## CHAPTER 25

A. A home visit would allow for a more extensive assessment of the family within the four models of health: clinical, role-performance, adaptive, and eudaemonistic. The community health nurse phoned the home to make an appointment for a home visit. Amy's mother answered the phone and indicated that Amy was at school during the day. The nurse introduced herself and explained that the counselor at the high school had talked with Amy about the possibility of having a community health nurse from the health department help her to learn more about her pregnancy, labor and delivery, and caring for a new infant. Amy's mother sounded both relieved and enthusiastic about having the nurse visit. Although Amy was in school during the day, she could arrange to be at home so the nurse could meet her at the end of the agency working day. An appointment was made for later in the week to meet with Amy and her mother. At this point, the initiation and previsit phases of the home visit process were completed by the nurse.

B. At the first home visit, it became apparent that Amy and her mother were interested in continuing community health nursing service. During her visit with Amy and her mother, the nurse added to her assessment by exploring with them what they saw as problems and concerns. This is consistent with an approach focused on empowerment. Amy and her mother identified a number of questions and concerns. How could Amy finish her education and care for a child? What would labor and delivery be like? How could Amy and her boyfriend avoid unplanned pregnancies in the future? How could the family members be supportive and yet have their own needs met?

C. A second visit was scheduled to include Amy's boyfriend and father. During the second visit, additional areas related to clinical health of the family, in terms of acute or chronic conditions, were assessed using a family genogram. Because it was apparent that there was a potential conflict between individual and family development needs that had implications for the adaptive processes of the family, time was spent identifying both family needs and individual needs and how best to meet these needs.

D. A contract was negotiated to continue visiting with Amy, but the visits would occur at school during a study period. The focus would be on prenatal teaching on the nurse's part, with Amy agreeing to attend a group for pregnant students offered at the school. Visits also were arranged with Amy's mother to discuss her concerns. These approaches reflected acknowledgment of the family's abilities to be actively and competently involved in resolving problems they had identified. Over time, the contract was modified and expanded to include well-child supervision during the year following the birth of a healthy baby boy.

## CHAPTER 26

A. The correct answer is 3. John is dealing with issues of industry verses inferiority. Encouraging him to be a part of his plan is a strategy to give him control. Choosing a reward system and using concrete activities acknowledge his level of cognitive development.

B. The correct answer is 2. Parents set examples by adhering to healthy lifestyles. It would be appropriate for the nurse to also offer Mrs. D. information to help her stop smoking.

C. Peer involvement is very important to John. School-age children compare themselves to others to determine their own adequacy. He compares himself to his friends at school. He may be reluctant to use his inhalers at school because he sees himself as different than others.

D. He needs MMR#2. If he has not had chicken pox, he needs the varicella vaccine. He should also begin the hepatitis B series, although it is acceptable to wait until he is 11 or 12. If it is fall, he is an excellent candidate for the influenza vaccine (see Chapter 38).

## CHAPTER 27

Although all of these proposed interventions may be appropriate, ensuring Josie's safety is the primary concern. The correct response is C.

## CHAPTER 28

A. Lab test: CBC with differential, CD4+ T-cell count/percentage and CD4+/CD8+ ratio, HIV RNA viral load test, multichannel chemistry panel, urinalysis, TB test, and chest x-ray. Conduct a history and physical assessment: assess general appearance, including weight changes and muscle wasting; eye examination; skin assessment and breakdown, including swollen, tender lymph nodes, mouth lesions, painful swollen gums, skin rashes, and lesions; neurologic and genitourinary examination; and nutrition screen.

B. Hyperthermia, social isolation, risk for infection, fluid volume deficit, ineffective coping, body image disturbance, altered nutrition, altered health maintenance, and altered family processes.

C. Ensure adequate hydration and nutrition, control fever and replace fluid loss, facilitate the restoration of usual bowel patterns, and prevent skin breakdown.

D. There is no cure at this time; however, goals should focus on the quality of life. Antiviral therapy suppresses the replication of HIV infection in the body. Retrovir is an antiviral agent most frequently used to treat AIDS. Monitor and treat opportunistic infections such as *Pneumocystis carinii* pneumonia as they occur. Develop an achievable plan that integrates psychosocial and health care goals. Link John to the needed services, and continue to monitor/track the services for achievements.

E. Begin with the dietitian, social worker, and the clinical nurse specialist in HIV management at the local public health department. Community-based and national AIDS organizations that should be consulted for assistance include Aids for AIDS, Aids Service Center, HIV/AIDS Legal, Homeless Health Care, and Project New Hope.

F. Preservation and efficient use of energy. Enhanced self-esteem. Increased sense of personal control. Maintenance of supportive family structure. Anxiety decreased to manageable levels.

## CHAPTER 29

I. The correct answers are C, D, and E. First, the nurse completed a physical examination and administered the Mini-Mental Status Examination short form (to assess cognitive function) and found that Mrs. Eldridge had eight errors.

The medications, an antihypertensive and a diuretic, were verified with the physician and the pharmacist. One pill bottle did not have a label, and the pharmacist said the unknown medication was probably a sleeping pill because its description fit one that had been prescribed. The pharmacist said that the sleeping pill was an old prescription and had not been refilled in some time.

A meeting was arranged with the son at the health department after a neighbor agreed to stay with Mrs. Eldridge. After revealing what had been observed, the son was both shocked and saddened. He went on to say that he had had an uneasy feeling about his mother for the past couple of weeks but that he "just couldn't put a finger on what was going on." Because of Mrs. Eldridge's obvious cognitive impairment, the nurse asked for validation of what information she had been able to obtain. She learned that Mrs. Eldridge had been hypertensive for several years and had always been faithful about taking her

medications, keeping appointments, and eating a healthy diet. He went on to say that he had been dreading the day when he would have to look for a nursing home for his mother for an extended stay.

Mrs. Eldridge's son and nurse met again 2 weeks later at Mrs. Eldridge's home. The home and Mrs. Eldridge were clean, and Mrs. Eldridge apologized for not remembering the first meeting. It appeared that the sleeping pill, which she had taken to help with the sad feeling and insomnia that accompanied the anniversary of her husband's death, had caused Mrs. Eldridge's intellectual impairment. Mrs. Eldridge and her son had a frank discussion about her living arrangements, and both agreed she would stay in her apartment. Mrs. Eldridge also wished that should her health deteriorate to a point that all hope for recovery was lost, she be allowed to die a peaceful death. The nurse suggested that both mother and son discuss this issue and come to an agreement on the advance directive measure; both agreed.

II. The factors that make this situation difficult are as follows:
A. Mrs. Eldridge lives alone.
B. Mrs. Eldridge demonstrates problems with memory and self-care.
C. The nurse must balance Mrs. Eldridge's autonomy with the need to intervene for her safety.

## CHAPTER 30

The nurse planned to evaluate the safety of the home environment and to begin her assessment of the family's understanding of the situation and their concerns. She found that Joel's mother and grandmother were optimistic about the future and delighted to bring him home after such a long hospitalization. They recognized that he would probably suffer motor and visual impairments, yet they wanted to participate in a program to help him develop to his best potential.

The nurse also assessed knowledge of infant care and availability of infant care items. The nurse recommended the purchase of a cool mist humidifier. Because the family had been so involved in providing Joel's daily care in the nursery, they had become skilled in this area and no knowledge deficits were identified.

In planning for early intervention services, several factors were considered. Joel's family expressed a desire for developmental services. Joel's chronic lung disease made him susceptible to complications of respiratory tract infections, making it unwise to expose him to groups of young children. Lack of financial resources limited access to services. Later the community development center would serve as the main program.

During the week following Joel's discharge from the hospital, he was seen at the health department by the pediatrician and nurse to establish a baseline health appraisal. The DDT Denver II was administered using Joel's corrected age (birth age in weeks minus number of weeks premature). Results showed delays in all areas. Nutritional assessment showed that weight gain was only minimally acceptable but consistent with the growth demonstrated in the hospital.

The nurse planned to continue biweekly home visits with the physical therapist to develop further intervention techniques and establish goals in self-help, social, emotional, cognitive, and language skills. Periodic evaluations were performed by the multidisciplinary staff at the follow-up clinic. In collaboration with the physician and nutritionist, the nurse also planned a schedule of health appraisal, nutritional assessments, and family assessments to identify health problems and to guide well-child care.

## CHAPTER 31

The answer is D, gather data first. Assessment is the first step in the core functions of public health. It is best to fully understand multiple points of view about the issues and to have a firm knowledge of the legal, ethical, and health-related aspects of the problems before beginning to consider policy options. This also gives you time to work with the administrators of the migrant health clinic to obtain their input and support and to find out whether your actions should be affiliated officially with the clinic or if you need to function as an independent citizen.

# CHAPTER 32

The correct answer is C. An assessment may have revealed that Tonya did not have transportation and was also responsible for caring for some of the other children in the household. Advocating for support services to assist Tonya in providing for her children raises her self-esteem and opens the door for the nurse to assist Tonya in finding a way out of her situation.

# CHAPTER 33

A. Collection of a family database via meeting with the family at a comfortable time and place. In keeping in mind cultural needs, permission should be obtained from the male head of family.
  * Family composition: extended family, housing, education, work/vocation, financial resources, religious practices, ritual, recreation.
  * Family environment: housing, furnishings, living space; sleeping arrangements; bathroom facilities; food preparation arrangements; eating arrangement; adequate water, sewer, lights, ventilation, etc.; condition of yard; pets; transportation; provisions for emergencies; environmental hazards; family attitudes toward home, neighborhood, and community.
  * Goals for the future: type of home, neighborhood to live in.
  * Neighborhood: sociocultural characteristics; traffic patterns; street lighting; resources such as shopping, transportation, education, health and illness; environmental stressors such as noise, crime, substance abuse, crowding; environmental hazards: air quality, neighbors' attitudes; family involvement in neighborhood.
  * Family structure: organization; roles; socialization processes for roles; division of labor, authority, and power; values, beliefs, stresses related to family structure and roles.
  * Emotional, social coping: conflict, life changes, support systems.
  * Life satisfaction: What is going well in life? How happy are you?
  * Health behavior: present health status; perception of vulnerability to disease; perception of present health problems; potential health problems; belief about cause, cure, treatment; risk behaviors; health beliefs; self-care, health care resources.
B. Public health department, migrant health care centers, free clinics, emergency departments, client may be eligible for Medicaid, but eligibility and resources vary from state to state. Another issue is legality of their stay (are they legal?). Many states/clinics will want evidence of legal entry.
C. Potential barriers are lack of money for treatment or medication; language; need for male presence, which may inhibit client and provider; transportation to clinics; attitudes of health care workers; clinic times that are during prime work hours; fear of being unable to work; need for follow-up; fear of being reported if illegal; limitation of medical record and health history.

# CHAPTER 34

1. Develop a separate young father's program, and recruit a male program leader.
2. Develop a school-based child care center for students and teachers, and use the center as a service learning opportunity for teen program participants.
3. Design a presentation on violence—both intimate partner violence and child violence.
4. Recruit volunteer adult mentors to work closely with individual teens throughout their pregnancy.

# CHAPTER 35

A. The volunteer who delivers the meals.
B. Monitoring weight, mood, suicidal ideation, cognition, function, sleep, and side effects.
C. Screening for depression and referral and treatment of depression.
D. The nurse, community mental health center, primary care office, internet websites.

# CHAPTER 36

A. Consider Mr. Jones's readiness for change, educational needs regarding health effects of smoking, and risks to family members from sidestream smoke.
B. Consider support groups such as AA for Mr. Jones and Al-Anon for Anne and how this could be helpful. Is it realistic for Anne to stop her grandfather from drinking if he doesn't want to? What else would be helpful to know about his drinking (e.g., where he drinks, what his behavior is like when he is drinking, health risks related to drinking, effects of his drinking on her children), and how would this affect the interventions?
C. Is there evidence of Anne's concern about her children's health as a place to begin? If Anne is not ready to stop "cold turkey," what steps can she begin to take towards the ultimate goal of stopping? What local resources are available?
D. Consider Anne's knowledge of good parenting skills. Consider counseling needs—what stressors are Anne and her children dealing with in their family and environment? How does age affect the potential interventions? Which child is at greater risk? Consider school resources, day care possibilities, and community resources for recreational activities.
E. Consider what the local neighborhood can do to help as well as what community resources are available. Which community leaders might be helpful? Could Jane facilitate a meeting between the local neighbors and law enforcement to help establish helpful communication and relationships? What prevention and treatment programs are available and at what cost? Are legislators aware of the cost benefits of drug treatment compared with law enforcement?

# CHAPTER 37

A.    The nurse needs to listen carefully to the pain and anguish the daughter felt about hitting her mother. She can convey a nonjudgmental attitude and help the daughter and mother explore ways in which both of their needs could be more effectively met. She can provide information and resources to allow the daughter some respite from constant caretaking and a way to continue her own activities.
B.
  1. Assess the situation: Mrs. Smith felt stiff and seemed to have more joint pain from her arthritis in the mornings. With further assessment it became clear that, by late afternoon, her joints were more flexible and less painful.
  2. Discuss options with the family: When nurse, daughter, and client discussed their options, they decided that Mary would wash only her mother's anal area in the morning and put clean pads under her if indicated. Total hygienic care would be done in the late afternoon.
  3. Teach alternative approaches: Mrs. Jones demonstrated to Mary alternative ways to move, turn, and wash her mother to minimize the strain on her arthritic joints and to incorporate some effective exercise into the bath.
  4. Make appropriate referrals and coordinate services: On two mornings each week, a home health care aide was engaged to stay with Mrs. Smith. Mary could then do family shopping and errands and participate in activities in which she had previously been involved.
C.    Mrs. Jones will need to monitor the situation carefully for any further signs of abuse. Any further instance of violence must be discussed with the daughter and immediately reported. In a subsequent visit, the nurse evaluated the effectiveness of her teaching and learned that Mary and her mother were working much more cooperatively on Mrs. Smith's care.

# CHAPTER 38

1. The best answer is C. Trusted leaders provide an entry point into the community; they can help develop a plan that is best suited to meet perceived and actual needs.
2. The best answer is A. Trust in public health programs must be developed before a crisis situation occurs. The assistance of community leaders at the time of crisis is extremely helpful but will be more effective if word of mouth has already established that public health officials are not associated with immigration. An appeal for the safety of friends and family may sometimes be more effective than emphasizing the threat to the individual.
3. The best answer is probably a combination of A, B, C, and D and may depend on the literacy level of the community. Some immigrant groups are largely illiterate in their own language.
4. All of these options have possibilities, but the best answer is B because community leaders know best how to reach their members in a culturally appropriate manner. However, state-produced materials, if culturally and linguistically appropriate, are very helpful because they are already developed. An ongoing relationship with community representatives is necessary because disease control messages often need to be developed and delivered quickly.

# CHAPTER 39

A. Questions the nurse asks Yvonne seek information about past injection drug use and sexual partners. The nurse evaluates Yvonne's comfort in sharing the information with Phil as she explores what she believes Phil's response might be. The nurse offers to role-play the situation of Yvonne telling Phil about the possibility of his infection, risks, and the importance of testing for the HIV antibody. Rather than contacting other previous sexual and drug-using partners herself, Yvonne requests that health department staff contact them about being tested for possible infection. She gives the nurse the names and addresses of two additional drug-using partners.
B. The most immediate concerns for Yvonne are the need to seek ongoing care to monitor the HIV infection and to decide whether to continue the pregnancy. The nurse asks Yvonne whether she has a primary health care provider. The information given includes providing Yvonne a list of providers and counseling about the importance of establishing an ongoing relationship with a primary health care provider for follow-up of the HIV infection. She tells Yvonne that important information about her health may be identified that will help to determine her ability to carry and deliver the baby if she chooses to continue the pregnancy. Other important information includes the implications of the test results, such as how they may affect the infant's and mother's health.
C. The nurse explains that transmission to the fetus is possible during the pregnancy and she may have a greater chance of progressing from asymptomatic infection to symptomatic HIV disease but that medications would be given to try to prevent this from happening. The nurse explores possibilities with Yvonne about the decision regarding her ability to physically, emotionally, and financially cope with rearing a child that possibly may be ill. Family members and other potential resources are assessed. The need for Yvonne to tell health care providers or blood handlers about the HIV infection is reviewed. The nurse schedules a second appointment for follow-up counseling 1 week after the initial test results are given. She also gives Yvonne the telephone number of the local AIDS support group and arranges to make a home visit to her in 2 days.
D. At the follow-up home and clinic visits, specific information is given regarding infection control in the home and safer sexual relations. The nurse ensures that Yvonne is taking steps toward receiving prenatal care and medical care for the HIV infection. The nurse reviews information about how to maintain health and avoid stressors and contracts with

Yvonne to initiate home visits to provide reinforcement of adequate prenatal nutrition and teaching and to assess Yvonne's physical health as the pregnancy progresses.

# CHAPTER 40

A. 1. Respecting the family's customs and space, as well as sensitivity to the timing of questions, will help develop a trusting relationship.
2. Flexibility and keeping promises is even more important in the home.
3. Give the family a time range when making an appointment to allow for delays at other homes and for traffic.
4. Provide the client and family information about the referral, the purpose of your visit, what services are available, and how to contact the agency.
5. Deal first with the issue that is uppermost on the client's mind, not what is first on your agenda. This strategy will decrease client anxiety and improve the ability to understand and focus on what you need to tell them.
B. 1. Taking a detailed history.
2. Doing a physical assessment.
3. Walking through the important parts of the house (bedroom, bathroom, kitchen, and hallways) provides baseline data for forming the plan of care.
4. Listening to clients provides the most important clues to health status and effective teaching strategies.
5. Begin completing necessary forms. Some clients will not be able to complete all the forms and required information on the first visit because of pain or fatigue. Focus on the essentials and complete the rest on a second visit.
C. 1. Set short- and long-term goals with clients.
2. Have a plan for every visit to progress toward the goals.
3. Clients and families must be informed that home health services are time limited and that they need to learn to provide their own care.
4. Nurses need to set limits, model expected behaviors, and write in the behaviors of the client.
5. Develop principles to facilitate and encourage self-care.
6. Plan for modifying care to allow as much independence as possible.
7. Writing plans to teach client rather than do for the client.
D. 1. Understand adult learning principles.
2. Identify the characteristics that indicate client's preferred learning style by asking.

# CHAPTER 41

Case 1: The best method of evaluation would be D. Client outcome data on rehospitalization and/or medical complications are used to evaluate the service. Also evaluating the aftercare service and assessing client and family satisfaction by questionnaire and telephone is a useful evaluation approach.
Case 2: The most correct answer is C. After her assessment, Julie could negotiate with the physicians to randomly assign 30 hypertensive clients to her for follow-up care. Then at a later date (6 to 9 months later), she could compare blood pressure measurements in the two groups.

# CHAPTER 42

The correct answer is A. The nurse manager thus used a participative decision-making approach at the meeting, and the group decided to obtain external consultation through the local college of nursing.

The community health faculty member assigned Patricia, a community health student, to assess this community's request for consultation. Patricia met with the nurse manager and the manager of the residential complex to discuss the problem, assess her ability to help, and explore the client's expectations for herself and for the college of nursing. After careful consideration, Patricia and the nurse manager determined that a survey of residents' needs, community resources, and staff perceptions would assist them in planning the alternatives they could explore for providing additional health promotion and health monitoring to the residents.

With the approval of the community health faculty member, Patricia and her fellow students agreed to implement a health screening survey project and to collect data about the residential program, such as the physical facilities, the available equipment and supplies, and staff available to provide assistance with health screening and promotion activities. They collected data on existing relationships with community referral sources, including local home care programs, money available to support program expansion at the residential facility, and the attitudes of staff and residents toward expansion. Anticipated outcomes to be evaluated for the consultation included recommending to the management of the residential program that home care services be made more accessible for residents using one of several options. The facility might contract for such a program with the college of nursing, develop a service contract with the health department for a satellite home care agency on facility grounds, or provide space for a proprietary home care agency to operate within the facility.

At the evaluation conference, Patricia and her colleagues shared the results of their data collection. After careful consideration of the data, the nurse manager and the manager of the residential facility agreed that residents needed more access to home care and decided to develop a contract with the college of nursing for provision of home nursing services on site. This would enable the current staff to devote their energies to aggregate health promotion activities.

## CHAPTER 43

The correct answer is A. Use this opportunity to show how school nurses respond to the primary, secondary, and tertiary prevention health needs of children and families.

## CHAPTER 44

The correct answer is D. This is an example of how the epidemiologic triad can be used to assess clients and plan nursing care. It illustrates the usefulness of approaching occupational health problems with an epidemiologic perspective.

## CHAPTER 45

Regardless of the earliest beginnings, discussions; questions; eliciting statements of healthy and unhealthy events in the lives of the members; and surveying the physical, social, emotional, and spiritual environmental conditions of the faith community will begin to shape the path. Formation of a broadly representative wellness committee will help to plan the formal and informal assessment methods and careful documentation of activities and communication.

Building on strengths of the congregation, gathering information on leaders and valued activities in the congregation, and becoming informed regarding lines of authority and communication help to provide a foundation for the service. The best answer is D, planning a congregational survey. This increases interest and involvement of the members. Results assist in focusing a possible goal. If the majority of the congregation is over the age of 55 years, it would be helpful to assess areas such as needs for retirement planning, current health status and adequacy of health financing options, involvement in caregiving for parents as well as adult children, needs for involvement in meaningful volunteer activities, and ability to holistically engage in activities appropriate for the life stage. Assessment would also include the impact of the over-55 age-group on the remainder of the congregation and the surrounding community. Information regarding resources within the church and geopolitical community is helpful.

Organizing and implementing a health fair to address identified needs often is beneficial in creating awareness of health needs, pro-
viding information to act on identified health concerns, increasing visibility of the value of health and faith connection, and promoting interest for additional congregational members to become involved in the parish nurse/health ministry program. The greater the involvement by the members, the greater the ownership of the program by the total faith community. Evaluation of the activity will yield information regarding which areas or activities should be continued or reinforced, which need to change focus, and which should be omitted.

In addition to the group and population activities, the parish nurse meets regularly with the pastoral staff and coordinates with other committee chairs. Together, they identify individuals requiring further assessment or support; become aware of issues that need to be clarified, supported, or addressed; and determine individuals, groups, or issues that have not yet become a part of the parish nurse or congregational wellness program. Home visits, phone calls, and visits to hospitals or community agencies are also part of the parish nurse's weekly activities. Agendas might include advocacy and interpretation with a health care provider, monitoring dementia progress, supporting a new mother embarking on a "new" career at home, leading a support group, therapeutic touch, prayer, and visualization.

## CHAPTER 46

The team organized to develop the case definition, plan the interview questions and sampling, and organize the specimen collection. Interviews were used to determine characteristics of the illness and to attempt to identify the source by dietary recall and living arrangements. The dietary recall was focused on the food consumed during the three meals before illness onset. While the interviews were being conducted, an environmental investigation concentrated on food preparation, service, and storage, along with housekeeping procedures. The administrative staff of the retirement community kept a daily log documenting all interventions implemented to determine what effect the measures undertaken to stop the spread of illness may have actually had on controlling the spread of illness.

It was initially thought that the infectious agent was a "Norwalk-like" virus, classified under the heading of human caliciviruses (HCV). Specimen testing, however, confirmed the presence of a virus strain similar to the Mexican virus, also an HCV, but classified in a different genogroup than the Norwalk virus. Clinically, symptoms are indistinguishable. The outbreak was revealed to have been caused by a virus strain closely related to the Mexican virus. Fecal-oral spread through food contamination, close person-to-person contact, and possible respiratory spread were hypothesized for this highly contagious virus.

There is a great deal to be learned about the transmission from persons who are asymptomatic. A majority of the residents of the facility became ill even after the institutional precautions were implemented, such as closing the dining room and limiting contacts between residents, encouraging disinfection of common areas of the retirement community, and placing emphasis on personal hygiene and glove use by staff. Ill staff were told to stay home until at least 2 days after their symptoms subsided. Handwashing by the staff was emphasized using antibacterial soap and drying with paper towels. The use of disposable items was encouraged when possible. Due to the recent increase in gastrointestinal illness in older populations in the state and the fragile state of health of many of the residents, as a result of this investigation, recommendations for control measures during gastroenteritis outbreaks in institutions became incorporated into a checklist for long-term care facilities to increase the level of awareness of the importance of strict adherence to hygienic practices in institutional settings.

# Appendixes

**A** International/National Agendas for Health Care Delivery

  **A.1** Schedule of Clinical Preventive Services

  **A.2** Select Major Historical Events Depicting Financial Involvement of Federal Government in Health Care Delivery

  **A.3** Declaration of Alma Ata

The above appendixes are available on Evolve website at http://evolve.elsevier.com/Stanhope

**B** Community-Oriented Nursing Resources, p. A-2

  **B.1** Content Resources and Appendixes available on EVOLVE, p. A-2

**C** Contracts and Forms: Samples

  **C.1** Community-Oriented Health Record (COHR)

  **C.2** The Living Will Directive

  **C.3** OASIS—Start of Care Assessment

The above appendixes are available on Evolve website at http://evolve.elsevier.com/Stanhope

**D** Drug and Immunization Information

  **D.1** Immunizing Agents and Immunization Schedules for Health Care Workers

  **D.2** Herbs and Supplements Used for Children and Adolescents

The above appendixes are available on Evolve website at http://evolve.elsevier.com/Stanhope

**E** Screening Tools

  **E.1** Vision and Hearing Screening Procedures

  **E.2** Screening for Common Orthopedic Problems

The above appendixes are available on Evolve website at http://evolve.elsevier.com/Stanhope

**F** Health Risk Appraisal, p. A-61

  **F.1** Lifestyle Assessment Questionnaire, p. A-3

  **F.2** Healthier People Health Risk Appraisal, p. A-13

  **F.3** 1999 Youth Risk Behavior Survey, p. A-21

**G** Community Assessment Tools, p. A-27

  **G.1** Community-As-Partner Model, p. A-27

**H** Family Assessment Tools, p. A-29

  **H.1** Family Systems Stressor-Strength Inventory (FS³I)

  **H.2** Friedman Family Assessment Model (Short Form), p. A-29

  **H.3** Case Example of Family Assessment

Appendixes H.1 and H.3 are available on Evolve website at http://evolve.elsevier.com/Stanhope

**I** Individual Assessment Tools, p. A-31

  **I.1** Instrumental Activities of Daily Living (IADL) Scale, p. A-31

  **I.2** Comprehensive Older Persons' Evaluation, p. A-32

  **I.3** Comprehensive Occupational and Environmental Health History, p. A-35

**J** Essential Elements of Public Health Nursing, p. A-123

  **J.1** Examples of Public Health Nursing Roles and Implementing Public Health Functions, p. A-39

  **J.2** Public Health Guidelines for Practice, p. A-45

  **J.3** Quad Council Public Health Nursing Core Competencies and Skill Levels, p. A-47

# Appendix B

## Community-Oriented Nursing Resources

### Appendix B.1  Content Resources and Appendixes Available on Evolve

The following resources and appendixes can be found on this textbook's Evolve website at http://evolve.elsevier.com/Stanhope under Content Resources in their related chapter.

#### CHAPTERS 2, 3, 5, AND 8

**Appendix A.2**   Select Major Historical Events Depicting Financial Involvement of the Federal Government in Health Care Delivery

#### CHAPTERS 3 AND 4

**Appendix A.3**   Declaration of Alma Ata

#### CHAPTERS 5, 14, 18, AND 24 TO 30

**Appendix A.1**   Schedule of Clinical Preventive Services

#### CHAPTER 15

Community-Oriented Health Record (COHR) and forms

#### CHAPTERS 24 AND 25

**Appendix H.1**   Family Systems Stressor-Strength Inventory
**Appendix H.3**   Case Example of Family Assessment
List of Family Assessment Tools

#### CHAPTER 26

**Appendix E.1**   Vision and Hearing Screening Procedures
**Appendix E.2**   Screening for Common Orthopedic Problems
Accident Prevention in Children
Common Behaviors of the School-Age Child and Adolescent
Common Concerns and Problems of the First Year (Neonate and Infant)
Common Concerns and Problems of the Toddler and Preschool Years
Developmental Behaviors: School-Age Children
Developmental Characteristics: Summary for Children
Feeding and Nutrition Guidelines for Infants
Health Problems of the School-Age Child and Adolescent
Identification of "At Risk" Newborns
Immunization Schedule for Children and Adolescents: Range of Ages for Routine Immunizations
Immunization Schedule for Children Not Immunized in the First Year of Life
Immunizations for Specific At-Risk Populations
Immunizations: General Recommendations
Infant Reflexes
Infant Stimulation
Normal Variations and Minor Abnormalities in Newborn Physical Characteristics
Summary of Rules for Childhood Immunization
Tanner Stages of Puberty

#### CHAPTER 30

**Appendix C.2**   The Living Will Directive
Assessment Tools for Communities with Physically Compromised Members
Assessment Tools for Families with Physically Compromised Members
Assessment Tools for Physically Compromised Individuals

#### CHAPTER 33

Resources for the Nurse Working with Migrant Farmworkers

#### CHAPTER 36

Smoking Cessation Resources

#### CHAPTER 39

Resources on Sexually Transmitted Diseases

#### CHAPTER 40

**Appendix C.3**   OASIS: Start of Care Assessment
Palliative Care Information

#### CHAPTER 44

**Appendix D.1**   Immunizing Agents and Immunization Schedules for Health Care Workers

#### CHAPTER 45

Parish Nursing Resources

#### CHAPTER 46

**Appendix J.3**   Core Competencies and Skill Levels for Public Health Nursing

# Appendix F

## Health Risk Appraisal

### F.1 Lifestyle Assessment Questionnaire

## Purpose

This assessment tool and the analysis it provides are designed to help you discover how the choices you make each day affect your overall health.

By participating in this assessment process, you will also learn how you can make positive changes in your lifestyle, enabling you to reach a higher level of wellness.

Some of the questions are personal. While you may leave them blank, the more information you provide about your current lifestyle, the more accurately the LAQ can assess your current level of wellness and risk areas.

## Confidentiality

The National Wellness Institute, Inc. subscribes to the guidelines established by the Society of Prospective Medicine concerning confidentiality in the use of health risk appraisals and risk reduction systems. These guidelines specifically state that only the participant and health professionals authorized by the participant should receive copies of his/her own health risk appraisal results.

The National Wellness Institute, Inc. strongly encourages all users of the LAQ to strictly follow these guidelines and maintain the confidentiality of all answers.

## What is Wellness?

Wellness is an active process of becoming aware of and making choices toward a higher level of well-being. **Remember**, leading a wellness lifestyle requires your **active involvement**. As you gain more knowledge about what enhances your well-being, you are encouraged to use this information to make informed choices which lead to a healthier life.

## General Instructions

The enclosed answer sheet is for you to record your answers to the Lifestyle Assessment Questionnaire. Please make certain that you complete all of the information at the top of the answer sheet including your zip code, group code, and social security number. If a group code has not been provided for you, leave this item blank.

Your questionnaire will be scored by an optical mark reading instrument; therefore, please use only a No. 2 (soft) pencil for marking your responses. To assure the most accurate results, follow the instructions shown on the answer sheet. Only your answer sheet needs to be returned for scoring. You may keep this questionnaire.

*The Lifestyle Assessment Questionnaire was written by the National Wellness Institute, Inc.'s Cofounders; Dennis Elsenrath, Ed.D., Bill Hettler, M.D., and Fred Leafgren, Ph.D.*

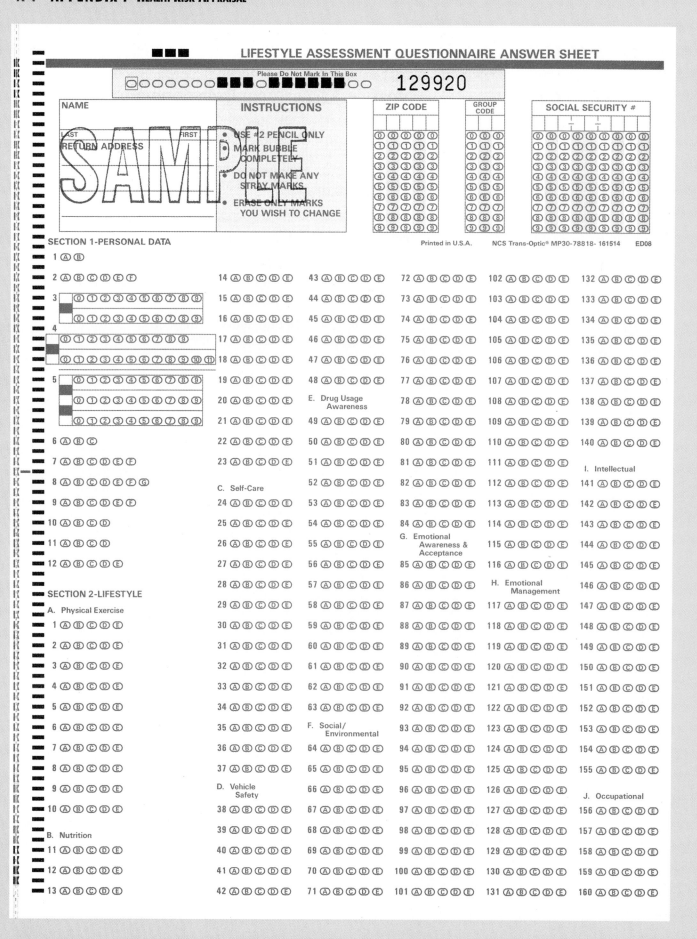

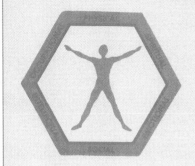

# Lifestyle Assessment Questionnaire™

## Answer Sheet

## SIDE 2

**J. Occupational (Cont.)**

**SECTION 3-HEALTH RISK APPRAISAL**

| | | | |
|---|---|---|---|
| 161 Ⓐ Ⓑ Ⓒ Ⓓ Ⓔ | 1 Ⓐ Ⓑ | 33 Ⓐ Ⓑ Ⓒ | 39 Ⓐ Ⓑ |
| 162 Ⓐ Ⓑ Ⓒ Ⓓ Ⓔ | 2 Ⓐ Ⓑ Ⓒ | 34 Ⓐ Ⓑ Ⓒ Ⓓ Ⓔ | 40 Ⓐ Ⓑ |
| 163 Ⓐ Ⓑ Ⓒ Ⓓ Ⓔ | 3 Ⓐ Ⓑ Ⓒ | 35 Ⓐ Ⓑ Ⓒ Ⓓ | 41 Ⓐ Ⓑ Ⓒ |
| 164 Ⓐ Ⓑ Ⓒ Ⓓ Ⓔ | 4 Ⓐ Ⓑ | 36 Ⓐ Ⓑ Ⓒ Ⓓ | 42 Ⓐ Ⓑ Ⓒ |
| 165 Ⓐ Ⓑ Ⓒ Ⓓ Ⓔ | 5a | 37 Ⓐ Ⓑ Ⓒ | |
| 166 Ⓐ Ⓑ Ⓒ Ⓓ Ⓔ | | 38 Ⓐ Ⓑ Ⓒ Ⓓ | |
| 167 Ⓐ Ⓑ Ⓒ Ⓓ Ⓔ | | | |
| 168 Ⓐ Ⓑ Ⓒ Ⓓ Ⓔ | 5b | 16 Ⓐ Ⓑ Ⓒ Ⓓ Ⓔ Ⓕ Ⓖ Ⓗ | |
| 169 Ⓐ Ⓑ Ⓒ Ⓓ Ⓔ | | 17 | **SECTION 4-TOPICS FOR PERSONAL GROWTH** |
| 170 Ⓐ Ⓑ Ⓒ Ⓓ Ⓔ | | | 1 ◯    23 ◯ |
| 171 Ⓐ Ⓑ Ⓒ Ⓓ Ⓔ | 6 Ⓐ Ⓑ Ⓒ | 18 Ⓐ Ⓑ Ⓒ Ⓓ | 2 ◯    24 ◯ |

Section 3 items with number fields (digits 0–9):

5a, 5b, 7, 8, 9, 10, 11, 13, 14a, 14b (double rows each)

15a, 15b, 17, 19, 20, 21, 22, 23, 25 (with digit fields)

**K. Spiritual**

| | | | |
|---|---|---|---|
| 172 Ⓐ Ⓑ Ⓒ Ⓓ Ⓔ | 7 | 19 | 5 ◯    27 ◯ |
| 173 Ⓐ Ⓑ Ⓒ Ⓓ Ⓔ | | 20 | 6 ◯    28 ◯ |
| 174 Ⓐ Ⓑ Ⓒ Ⓓ Ⓔ | 8 | | 7 ◯    29 ◯ |
| 175 Ⓐ Ⓑ Ⓒ Ⓓ Ⓔ | | 21 | 8 ◯    30 ◯ |
| 176 Ⓐ Ⓑ Ⓒ Ⓓ Ⓔ | | 22 | 9 ◯    31 ◯ |
| 177 Ⓐ Ⓑ Ⓒ Ⓓ Ⓔ | 9 | | 10 ◯    32 ◯ |
| 178 Ⓐ Ⓑ Ⓒ Ⓓ Ⓔ | | 23 | 11 ◯    33 ◯ |
| 179 Ⓐ Ⓑ Ⓒ Ⓓ Ⓔ | 10 | | 12 ◯    34 ◯ |
| 180 Ⓐ Ⓑ Ⓒ Ⓓ Ⓔ | | 24 Ⓐ Ⓑ Ⓒ Ⓓ Ⓔ | 13 ◯    35 ◯ |
| 181 Ⓐ Ⓑ Ⓒ Ⓓ Ⓔ | 11 | 25 | 14 ◯    36 ◯ |
| 182 Ⓐ Ⓑ Ⓒ Ⓓ Ⓔ | | | 15 ◯    37 ◯ |
| 183 Ⓐ Ⓑ Ⓒ Ⓓ Ⓔ | 12 Ⓐ Ⓑ Ⓒ | 26 Ⓐ Ⓑ Ⓒ | 16 ◯    38 ◯ |
| 184 Ⓐ Ⓑ Ⓒ Ⓓ Ⓔ | 13 | 27 Ⓐ Ⓑ Ⓒ Ⓓ Ⓔ | 17 ◯    39 ◯ |
| 185 Ⓐ Ⓑ Ⓒ Ⓓ Ⓔ | | 28 Ⓐ Ⓑ Ⓒ | 18 ◯    40 ◯ |
| | 14a | 29 Ⓐ Ⓑ Ⓒ Ⓓ Ⓔ | 19 ◯    41 ◯ |
| | | 30 Ⓐ Ⓑ Ⓒ Ⓓ Ⓔ | 20 ◯    42 ◯ |
| | 14b | 31 Ⓐ Ⓑ Ⓒ Ⓓ Ⓔ | 21 ◯    43 ◯ |
| | | 32 Ⓐ Ⓑ Ⓒ | 22 ◯ |

## Section 1: PERSONAL DATA

### INSTRUCTIONS:

*Please complete the following general information about yourself by marking your answers in the appropriate places on the LAQ answer sheet. Please take your time and read each question carefully.*

1. Sex
   a) male
   b) female
2. Race
   a) White
   b) Black
   c) Hispanic
   d) Asian
   e) American Indian
   f) other
3. Age
4. Height (feet and inches)
5. Weight (pounds)
6. Body frame size
   a) small
   b) medium
   c) large
7. Marital Status
   a) married
   b) widowed
   c) separated
   d) divorced
   e) single
   f) cohabiting
8. What was the total gross income of your household last year?
   a) under $12,000
   b) $12,000-$20,000
   c) $20,001-$30,000
   d) $30,001-$40,000
   e) $40,001-$50,000
   f) $50,001-$60,000
   g) over $60,000
9. What is the highest level of education you have completed?
   a) grade school or less
   b) some high school
   c) high school graduate
   d) some college or technical school
   e) college graduate
   f) postgraduate or professional degree
10. On the average day, how many hours do you watch television?
    a) 0 hours
    b) 1-3 hours
    c) 4-7 hours
    d) more than 8 hours
11. Where do you live?
    a) in the country
    b) in a city
    c) suburb
    d) small town
12. If you live in a city, suburb, or small town, what is the population?
    a) under 20,000
    b) 20,000-50,000
    c) 50,001-100,000
    d) 100,001-500,000
    e) over 500,000

## Section 2: LIFESTYLE

### INSTRUCTIONS:

*This section will help determine your level of wellness. It will also give you ideas for areas in which you might improve. Some questions touch on very personal subjects. Therefore, if you prefer to skip certain questions, you may. However, the more questions you answer, the more you will learn about your health and how to improve it.*

*Please respond to these statements using the following responses. If an item does not apply to you, do not mark it.*

A *Almost always (90% or more of the time)*
B *Very often (approximately 75% of the time)*
C *Often (approximately 50% of the time)*
D *Occasionally (approximately 25% of the time)*
E *Almost never (less than 10% of the time)*

### PHYSICAL EXERCISE

*Measures one's commitment to maintaining physical fitness.*

1. I exercise vigorously for at least 20 minutes three or more times per week.
2. I determine my activity level by monitoring my heart rate.
3. I stop exercising before I feel exhausted.
4. I exercise in a relaxed, calm, and joyful manner.
5. I stretch before exercising.
6. I stretch after exercising.
7. I walk or bike whenever possible.
8. I participate in a strenuous activity (tennis, running, brisk walking, water exercise, swimming, handball, basketball, etc.).
9. If I am not in shape, I avoid sporadic (once a week or less often), strenuous exercise.
10. After vigorous exercise, I "cool down" (very light exercise such as walking) for at least five minutes before sitting or lying down.

### NUTRITION

*Measures the degree to which one chooses foods that are consistent with the dietary goals of the United States as published by the Senate Select Committee on Nutrition and Human Needs.*

11. When choosing non-vegetable protein, I select lean cuts of meat, poultry, fish, and low-fat dairy products.
12. I maintain an appropriate weight for my height and frame.
13. I minimize salt intake.
14. I eat fruits and vegetables, fresh and uncooked.
15. I eat breakfast.
16. I intentionally include fiber in my diet on a daily basis.
17. I drink enough fluid to keep my urine light yellow.
18. I plan my diet to insure an adequate amount of vitamins and minerals.
19. I minimize foods in my diet that contain large amounts of refined flour (bleached white flour, typical store bread, cakes, etc.).
20. I minimize my intake of fats and oils including margarine and animal fats.

1

21. I include items from all four basic food groups in my diet each day (fruits and vegetables; milk group; breads and cereals; meat, fowl, fish or vegetable proteins).
22. To avoid unnecessary calories, I choose water as one of the beverages I drink.
23. I avoid adding sugar to my foods. I minimize my intake of pre-sweetened foods (sugarcoated cereals, syrups, chocolate milk, and most processed and fast foods).

## SELF-CARE

*Measures the behaviors which help one prevent or detect early illnesses.*

24. I use footgear of good quality designed for the activity or the job in which I participate.
25. I record immunizations to maintain up-to-date immunization records.
26. I examine my breasts or testes on a monthly basis.
27. I have my breasts or testes examined yearly by a physician.
28. I balance the type and amount of food I eat with exercise to maintain a healthy percent body fat.
29. I take action to minimize my exposure to tobacco smoke.
30. When I experience illness or injury, I take necessary steps to correct the problem.
31. I engage in activities which keep my blood pressure in a range which minimizes my chances of disease (e.g., stroke, heart attack, and kidney disease).
32. I brush my teeth after eating.
33. I floss my teeth after eating.
34. My resting pulse is 60 or less.
35. I get an adequate amount of sleep.
36. If I were to have sex, I would take action to prevent unplanned pregnancy.
37. If I were to have sex, I would take action to prevent giving and/or getting sexually transmitted disease.

## VEHICLE SAFETY

*Measures one's ability to minimize chances of injury or death in a vehicle accident.*

38. I do not operate vehicles while I am under the influence of alcohol or other drugs.
39. I do not ride with drivers who are under the influence of alcohol or other drugs.
40. I stay within the speed limit.
41. I practice defensive driving techniques.
42. When traffic lights change from green to yellow, I prepare to stop.
43. I maintain a safe driving distance between cars based on speed and road conditions.
44. Vehicles which I drive are maintained to assure safety.
45. Because they are safer, I use radial tires on cars that I drive.
46. When I ride a bicycle or motorcycle, I wear a helmet and have adequate lights/reflectors.
47. Children riding in my car are secured in an approved car seat or seat belt.
48. I use my seat belt while driving or riding in a vehicle.

## DRUG USAGE AND AWARENESS

*Measures the degree to which one functions without the unnecessary use of chemicals.*

49. I use prescription drugs and over-the-counter medications only when necessary.
50. If I consume alcohol, I limit my consumption to not more than one drink per hour and no more than two drinks per day.
51. I avoid the use of tobacco.
52. Because of the potentially harmful effects of caffeine (e.g., coffee, tea, cola, etc.), I limit my consumption.
53. I avoid the use of marijuana.
54. I avoid the use of hallucinogens (LSD, PCP, MDA, etc.).
55. I avoid the use of stimulants ("uppers"—e.g., cocaine, amphetamines, "pep pills," etc.).
56. I avoid the use of nonmedically prescribed depressants ("downers"—e.g., barbituates, quaaludes, minor tranquilizers, etc.).
57. I avoid using a combination of drugs unless under medical supervision.
58. I follow the instructions provided with any drug I take.
59. I avoid using drugs obtained from illegal sources.
60. I understand the expected effect of drugs I take.
61. I consider alternatives to drugs.
62. If I experience discomfort from stress or tension, I use relaxation techniques, exercise, and meditation instead of taking drugs.
63. I get clear directions for taking my medicine from my doctor or pharmacist.

## SOCIAL/ENVIRONMENTAL

*Measures the degree to which one contributes to the common welfare of the community. This emphasizes interdependence with others and nature.*

64. I conserve energy at home.
65. I consider energy conservation when choosing a mode of transportation.
66. My social ties with family are strong.
67. I contribute to the feeling of acceptance within my family.
68. I develop and maintain strong friendships.
69. I do my part to promote a clean environment (i.e., air, water, noise, etc.).
70. When I see a safety hazard, I take action (warn others or correct the problem).
71. I avoid unnecessary radiation.
72. I report criminal acts I observe.
73. I contribute time and/or money to community projects.
74. I actively seek to become acquainted with individuals in my community.
75. I use my creativity in constructive ways.
76. My behavior reflects fairness and justice.
77. When possible, I choose an environment which is free of **noise** pollution.
78. When possible, I choose an environment which is free of **air** pollution.
79. I participate in volunteer activities benefiting others.
80. I help others in need.
81. I beautify those parts of my environment under my control.

2

*Continued*

82. Because of limited resources, I do my part to conserve.

83. I recycle aluminum, glass, and paper products.

84. I involve myself with people who support a positive lifestyle.

## EMOTIONAL AWARENESS AND ACCEPTANCE

*Measures the degree to which one has an awareness and acceptance of one's feelings. This includes the degree to which one feels positive and enthusiastic about oneself and life.*

85. I have a good sense of humor.

86. I feel positive about myself.

87. I feel there is a satisfying amount of excitement in my life.

88. My emotional life is stable.

89. I am aware of my needs.

90. I trust and value my own judgment.

91. When I make mistakes, I learn from them.

92. I feel comfortable when complimented for jobs well done.

93. It is okay for me to cry.

94. I have feelings of sensitivity for others.

95. I feel enthusiastic about life.

96. I find it easy to laugh.

97. I am able to give love.

98. I am able to receive love.

99. I enjoy my life.

100. I have plenty of energy.

101. My sleep is restful.

102. I trust others.

103. I feel others trust me.

104. I accept my sexual desires.

105. I understand how I create my feelings.

106. At times, I can be both strong and sensitive.

107. I am aware when I feel angry.

108. I accept my anger.

109. I am aware when I feel sad.

110. I accept my sadness.

111. I am aware when I feel happy.

112. I accept my happiness.

113. I am aware when I feel frightened.

114. I accept my feelings of fear.

115. I am aware of my feelings about death.

116. I accept my feelings about death.

## EMOTIONAL MANAGEMENT

*Measures the degree to which one controls and expresses feelings, and engages in effective, related behaviors.*

117. I share my feelings with those with whom I am close.

118. I express my feelings of anger in appropriate ways.

119. I express my feelings of sadness in healthy ways.

120. I express my feelings of happiness in desirable ways.

121. I express my feelings of fear in appropriate ways.

122. I compliment myself for a job well done.

123. I accept constructive criticism without reacting defensively.

124. I set appropriate limits for myself.

125. I stay within the limits that I have set.

126. I recognize that I can have wide variations of feelings about the same person (such as loving someone even though you are angry with her/him at the moment).

127. I am able to develop close, intimate relationships.

128. I say "no" without feeling guilty.

129. I would feel comfortable seeking professional help to better understand and cope with my feelings.

130. I reduce feelings of failure by setting achievable goals.

131. I relax my body and mind without using drugs.

132. I can be alone without feeling lonely.

133. I am able to be spontaneous in expressing my feelings.

134. I accept responsibility for my actions.

135. I am willing to take the risks that come with making change.

136. I manage my feelings to avoid unnecessary suffering.

137. I make decisions with a minimum of stress and worry.

138. I accept the responsibility for creating my own feelings.

139. I can express my feelings about death.

140. I recognize grieving as a healthy response to loss.

## INTELLECTUAL

*Measures the degree to which one engages her/his mind in creative, stimulating mental activities, expanding knowledge, and improving skills.*

141. I read a newspaper daily.

142. I read twelve or more books yearly.

143. On the average, I read one or more national magazines per week.

144. When I watch TV, I choose programs with informational/educational value.

145. I visit a museum or art show at least three times yearly.

146. I attend lectures, workshops, and demonstrations at least three times yearly.

147. I regularly use some of my time participating in hobbies such as photography, gardening, woodworking, sewing, painting, baking, art, music, writing, pottery, etc.

148. I read about local, state, national, and international political/public issues.

149. I learn the meaning of new words.

150. I engage in some type of writing activity such as a regular journal, letter writing, preparation of papers or manuscripts, etc.

151. I am interested in understanding the views of others.

152. I share ideas, concepts, thoughts, or procedures with others.

153. I gather information to enable me to make decisions.

154. I listen to radio and/or TV news.

155. I think about ideas different than my own.

## OCCUPATIONAL

*Measures the satisfaction gained from one's work and the degree to which one is enriched by that work. Please answer these items from your primary frame of reference, (e.g., your job, student, homemaker, etc.).*

156. I enjoy my work.

78818 - 3/3

157. My work contributes to my personal needs.

158. I feel that my job in some way contributes to my well-being.

159. I cooperate with others in my work.

160. I take advantage of opportunities to learn new work-related skills.

161. My work is challenging.

162. I feel my job responsibilities are consistent with my values.

163. I find satisfaction from the work I do.

164. I find healthy ways of reducing excessive job-related stress.

165. I use recommended health and safety precautions.

166. I make recommendations for improving worksite health and safety.

167. I am satisfied with the degree of freedom I have in my job to exercise independent judgments.

168. I am satisfied with the amount of variety in my work.

169. I believe I am competent in my job.

170. My co-workers and supervisors respect me as a competent individual.

171. My communication with others in my work place is enriching for me.

## SPIRITUAL

*Measures one's ongoing involvement in seeking meaning and purpose in human existence. It includes an appreciation for the depth and expanse of life and natural forces that exist in the universe.*

172. I feel good about my spiritual life.

173. Prayer, meditation, and/or quiet personal reflection is/are important part(s) of my life.

174. I contemplate my purpose in life.

175. I reflect on the meaning of events in my life.

176. My values guide my daily life.

177. My values and beliefs help me to meet daily challenges.

178. I recognize that my spiritual growth is a lifelong process.

179. I am concerned about humanitarian issues.

180. I enjoy participating in discussions about spiritual values.

181. I feel a sense of compassion for others in need.

182. I seek spiritual knowledge.

183. My spiritual awareness occurs other than at times of crisis.

184. I believe in something greater or that I am part of something greater than myself.

185. I share my spiritual values.

# Section 3: HEALTH RISK APPRAISAL

## INSTRUCTIONS:

*This section is intended to help you identify the problems most likely to interfere with the quality of your life. It will also show you choices you can make to stay healthy and avoid the most common causes of death for a person your age and sex.*

*This Health Risk Appraisal is not a substitute for a checkup or physical exam that you get from a doctor or nurse. It only gives you some ideas for lowering your risk of getting sick or injured in the future. It is NOT designed for people who already have HEART DISEASE, CANCER, KIDNEY DISEASE, OR OTHER SERIOUS CONDITIONS. If you have any of these problems and you want a Health Risk Appraisal anyway, ask your doctor or nurse to read this section of the printout with you.*

**If you don't know or are unsure of an answer, please leave that item blank.**

1. Have you ever been told that you have diabetes (or sugar diabetes)?
   a. yes
   b. no

2. Does your natural mother, father, sister or brother have diabetes?
   a. yes
   b. no
   c. not sure

3. Did either of your natural parents die of a heart attack before age 60? (If your parents are younger than 60, mark no).
   a. yes, one of them
   b. yes, both of them
   c. no
   d. not sure

4. Are you now taking medicine for high blood pressure?
   a. yes
   b. no

5. What is your blood pressure now?
   a. _____ systolic (high number)
   b. _____ diastolic (low number)

6. If you *do not* know the number, select the answer that describes your blood pressure.
   a. high
   b. normal or low
   c. don't know

7. What is your TOTAL cholesterol level (based on a blood test)?
   _____ (mg/dl)

8. What is your High Density Lipoprotein (HDL) cholesterol level (based on a blood test)?
   _____ (mg/dl)

9. How many cigars do you usually smoke per day?
   _____

10. How many pipes of tobacco do you usually smoke per day? _____

11. How many times per day do you usually use smokeless tobacco (chewing tobacco, snuff, pouches, etc.)? _____

12. How would you describe your cigarette smoking habits?
    a. never smoked **Go to 15**
    b. used to smoke **Go to 14**
    c. still smoke **Go to 13**

4

*Continued*

13. How many cigarettes a day do you smoke?
    _____ cigarettes per day **Go to 15**

14. a. How many years has it been since you smoked cigarettes regularly?
       _____ years
    b. What was the average number of cigarettes per day that you smoked in the 2 years before you quit?
       _____ cigarettes per day

15. In the next 12 months, how many thousands of miles will you probably travel by each of the following?
    (NOTE: U.S. average = 10,000 miles)
    a. car, truck, or van: _____,000 miles
    b. motorcycle: _____,000 miles

16. On a typical day how do you USUALLY travel?
    (Check one only)
    a. walk
    b. bicycle
    c. motorcycle
    d. sub-compact or compact car
    e. mid-size or full-size car
    f. truck or van
    g. bus, subway, or train
    h. mostly stay home

17. What percent of the time do you usually buckle your safety belt when driving or riding?
    _____%

18. On the average, how close to the speed limit do you usually drive?
    a. within 5 mph of limit
    b. 6-10 mph over limit
    c. 11-15 mph over limit
    d. more than 15 mph over limit

19. How many times in the last month did you drive or ride when the driver had perhaps too much alcohol to drink?
    _____ times last month

20. When you drink alcoholic beverages, how many drinks do you consume in an average day? (If you *never* drink alcoholic beverages, write 0.)
    _____ alcoholic beverages/average day

21. On the average, how many days per week do you consume alcohol?
    _____ days/week

## (MEN GO TO QUESTION 31)

## WOMEN ONLY (QUESTIONS 22-30)

22. At what age did you have your first menstrual period?
    _____ years old

23. How old were you when your first child was born (if no children, write 0)?
    _____ years old

24. How long has it been since your last breast x-ray (mammogram)?
    a. less than 1 year ago
    b. 1 year ago
    c. 2 years ago
    d. 3 or more years ago
    e. never

25. How many women in your natural family (mother and sisters only) have had breast cancer?
    _____ women

26. Have you had a hysterectomy?
    a. yes
    b. no
    c. not sure

27. How long has it been since you had a pap smear test?
    a. less than 1 year ago
    b. 1 year ago
    c. 2 years ago
    d. 3 or more years ago
    e. never

28. How often do you examine your breasts for lumps?
    a. monthly
    b. once every few months
    c. rarely or never

29. About how long has it been since you had your breasts examined by a physician or nurse?
    a. less than 1 year ago
    b. 1 year ago
    c. 2 years ago
    d. 3 or more years ago
    e. never

30. About how long has it been since you had a rectal exam?
    a. less than 1 year ago
    b. 1 year ago
    c. 2 years ago
    d. 3 or more years ago
    e. never

## WOMEN GO TO QUESTION 35

## MEN ONLY (QUESTIONS 31-34)

31. About how long has it been since you had a rectal or prostate exam?
    a. less than 1 year ago
    b. 1 year ago
    c. 2 years ago
    d. 3 or more years ago
    e. never

32. Do you know how to properly examine your testes for lumps?
    a. yes
    b. no
    c. not sure

33. How often do you examine your testes for lumps?
    a. monthly
    b. once every few months
    c. rarely or never

34. About how long has it been since you had your testes examined by a physician or nurse?
    a. less than one year ago
    b. 1 year ago
    c. 2 years ago
    d. 3 or more years ago
    e. never

35. How many times in the last year did you witness or become involved in a violent fight or attack where there was a good chance of a serious injury to someone?
    a. 4 or more times
    b. 2 or 3 times
    c. 1 time or never
    d. not sure

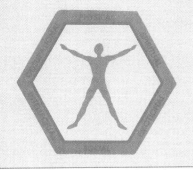

## Lifestyle Assessment Questionnaire™

## Answer Sheet

## SIDE 2

©1989, National Wellness Institute, Inc.  All rights reserved.

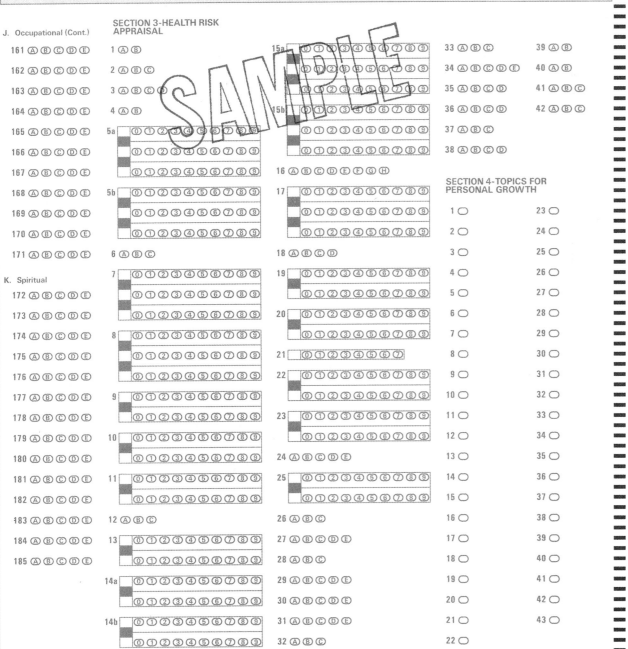

**J. Occupational (Cont.)**

**SECTION 3-HEALTH RISK APPRAISAL**

161 Ⓐ Ⓑ Ⓒ Ⓓ Ⓔ

162 Ⓐ Ⓑ Ⓒ Ⓓ Ⓔ

163 Ⓐ Ⓑ Ⓒ Ⓓ Ⓔ

164 Ⓐ Ⓑ Ⓒ Ⓓ Ⓔ

165 Ⓐ Ⓑ Ⓒ Ⓓ Ⓔ

166 Ⓐ Ⓑ Ⓒ Ⓓ Ⓔ

167 Ⓐ Ⓑ Ⓒ Ⓓ Ⓔ

168 Ⓐ Ⓑ Ⓒ Ⓓ Ⓔ

169 Ⓐ Ⓑ Ⓒ Ⓓ Ⓔ

170 Ⓐ Ⓑ Ⓒ Ⓓ Ⓔ

171 Ⓐ Ⓑ Ⓒ Ⓓ Ⓔ

**K. Spiritual**

172 Ⓐ Ⓑ Ⓒ Ⓓ Ⓔ

173 Ⓐ Ⓑ Ⓒ Ⓓ Ⓔ

174 Ⓐ Ⓑ Ⓒ Ⓓ Ⓔ

175 Ⓐ Ⓑ Ⓒ Ⓓ Ⓔ

176 Ⓐ Ⓑ Ⓒ Ⓓ Ⓔ

177 Ⓐ Ⓑ Ⓒ Ⓓ Ⓔ

178 Ⓐ Ⓑ Ⓒ Ⓓ Ⓔ

179 Ⓐ Ⓑ Ⓒ Ⓓ Ⓔ

180 Ⓐ Ⓑ Ⓒ Ⓓ Ⓔ

181 Ⓐ Ⓑ Ⓒ Ⓓ Ⓔ

182 Ⓐ Ⓑ Ⓒ Ⓓ Ⓔ

183 Ⓐ Ⓑ Ⓒ Ⓓ Ⓔ

184 Ⓐ Ⓑ Ⓒ Ⓓ Ⓔ

185 Ⓐ Ⓑ Ⓒ Ⓓ Ⓔ

1 Ⓐ Ⓑ
2 Ⓐ Ⓑ Ⓒ
3 Ⓐ Ⓑ Ⓒ
4 Ⓐ Ⓑ
5a
5b
6 Ⓐ Ⓑ Ⓒ
7
8
9
10
11
12 Ⓐ Ⓑ Ⓒ
13
14a
14b

15a
15b
16 Ⓐ Ⓑ Ⓒ Ⓓ Ⓔ Ⓕ Ⓖ Ⓗ
17
18 Ⓐ Ⓑ Ⓒ
19
20
21
22
23
24 Ⓐ Ⓑ Ⓒ Ⓓ Ⓔ
25
26 Ⓐ Ⓑ Ⓒ
27 Ⓐ Ⓑ Ⓒ Ⓓ Ⓔ
28 Ⓐ Ⓑ Ⓒ
29 Ⓐ Ⓑ Ⓒ Ⓓ Ⓔ
30 Ⓐ Ⓑ Ⓒ Ⓓ Ⓔ
31 Ⓐ Ⓑ Ⓒ Ⓓ Ⓔ
32 Ⓐ Ⓑ Ⓒ

33 Ⓐ Ⓑ Ⓒ Ⓓ
34 Ⓐ Ⓑ Ⓒ Ⓓ Ⓔ
35 Ⓐ Ⓑ Ⓒ Ⓓ
36 Ⓐ Ⓑ Ⓒ Ⓓ
37 Ⓐ Ⓑ Ⓒ
38 Ⓐ Ⓑ Ⓒ Ⓓ

39 Ⓐ Ⓑ
40 Ⓐ Ⓑ
41 Ⓐ Ⓑ Ⓒ
42 Ⓐ Ⓑ Ⓒ

**SECTION 4-TOPICS FOR PERSONAL GROWTH**

1 ○   23 ○
2 ○   24 ○
3 ○   25 ○
4 ○   26 ○
5 ○   27 ○
6 ○   28 ○
7 ○   29 ○
8 ○   30 ○
9 ○   31 ○
10 ○  32 ○
11 ○  33 ○
12 ○  34 ○
13 ○  35 ○
14 ○  36 ○
15 ○  37 ○
16 ○  38 ○
17 ○  39 ○
18 ○  40 ○
19 ○  41 ○
20 ○  42 ○
21 ○  43 ○
22 ○

*Continued*

ould you describe your

times do you engage
work which lasts at
ing and which is hard
eavier and your heart

terrain vehicle (ATV),
u wear a helmet?

**39.** Do you eat some food every day that is high in fiber, such as whole grain bread, cereal, fresh fruits, or vegetables?
  a. yes
  b. no

**40.** Do you eat foods every day that are high in cholesterol or fat, such as fatty meat, cheese, fried foods, or eggs?
  a. yes
  b. no

**41.** In general, how satisfied are you with your life?
  a. mostly satisfied
  b. partly satisfied
  c. not satisfied

**42.** Have you suffered a personal loss or misfortune in the past year that had a serious impact on your life? (For example, a job loss, disability, separation, jail term, or the death of someone close to you.)
  a. yes, 1 serious loss or misfortune
  b. yes, 2 or more
  c. no

## R PERSONAL GROWTH

reas in which you
onse to your selection
ovide you with
equests.

e information.

**20.** Spiritual or philosophical values
**21.** Communication skills
**22.** Automobile safety
**23.** Suicide thoughts or attempts
**24.** Substance abuse
**25.** Anxiety associated with public speaking, tests, writing, etc.
**26.** Enhancing relationships
**27.** Time-management skills
**28.** Death and dying
**29.** Learning skills (i.e., speed-reading, comprehension, etc.)
**30.** Financial management
**31.** Divorce
**32.** Alcoholism
**33.** Men's issues
**34.** Women's issues
**35.** Medical self-care
**36.** Dental self-care
**37.** Self-testes exam
**38.** Aging
**39.** Self-esteem
**40.** Premenstrual syndrome (PMS)
**41.** Osteoporosis
**42.** Recreation and leisure
**43.** Environmental issues

"no" without feeling

and pain
crowded rooms, etc.)
nning

**IMPORTANT—** If you have finished completing all sections of the LAQ, please make sure you have answered the questions in Section 1 requesting your sex, race, age, height and weight. Results cannot be generated for the Health Risk Appraisal section without this information.

*Continued*

## You and Your Lifestyle Are the Major Determinants for Joyful Living

**Major Causes of Death**

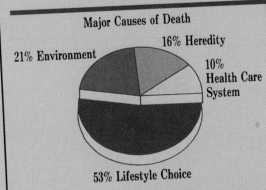

21% Environment
16% Heredity
10% Health Care System
53% Lifestyle Choice

The circle graph to the left indicates the factors which contribute to your enjoyment and quality of life. While medical professionals contribute to the quality of your life, this graph clearly shows that the majority of those factors which contribute to your well-being are controlled by you. As you make responsible, informed choices, your chances of improving your health and well-being increase.

## The LAQ's Role . . .

We believe this instrument is useful in helping individuals identify the most likely causes of death and disability. More importantly, it identifies those areas of self-improvement which will lead to higher levels of health and well-being.

The areas assessed in the LAQ emphasize the importance of creating a balance among the many different aspects of your lifestyle. Each of these areas affects one another and determines your overall wellness status. Also, each provides an opportunity for learning, making responsible decisions, and personal growth.

We invite you to use the information provided by the LAQ to your best advantage to increase your level of wellness.

## Words from the Past

Wellness is a term that has enjoyed growing popularity during the past several decades. Although the term was introduced relatively recently, the concept of prevention has been present for centuries. The following passages provide a brief glimpse of the wellness philosophy through the years. Wellness is a movement which has become a major part of modern culture and is the most important weapon available to combat lifestyle illnesses.

*"For many years, while engaged in the practice of medicine, the author of this volume has been more and more impressed with the idea that the causes of suffering, diseases, and premature deaths, which we witness around us on every hand, lie near our own doors . . . and that the men and women of today, are, at least, equally as responsible for existing suffering, as those who have gone before them, and often much more so. In fact, he feels satisfied that by far the greatest portion of all the suffering, disease, deformity, and premature deaths which occur are the direct result of either the violation of, or the want of compliance with the laws of our being; calamities, which, were the requisite knowledge possessed by the community, can and should be avoided."*
—JOHN ELLIS, M.D., 1859

*"It is universally admitted at the present time that preventive medicine is of far greater importance than curative medication, and many of the most eminent members of the profession are devoting themselves exclusively to this branch."*
—J. H. KELLOGG, M.D., 1902

*"To ward off disease or recover health, men as a rule find it easier to depend on the healers than to attempt the more difficult task of living wisely."*
—RENE DUBOS, Ph.D., 1959

*"It's what you do hour by hour, day by day, that largely determines the state of your health; whether you get sick, what you get sick with, and perhaps when you die."*
—LESTER BRESLOW, M.D., 1969

---

## AL DATA

general information about s in the appropriate places ke your time and read each

of your household

tion you have

gree

rs do you watch

town, what is the

## Section 2: LIFESTYLE

### INSTRUCTIONS:

*This section will help determine your level of wellness. It will also give you ideas for areas in which you might improve. Some questions touch on very personal subjects. Therefore, if you prefer to skip certain questions, you may. However, the more questions you answer, the more you will learn about your health and how to improve it.*

*Please respond to these statements using the following responses. If an item does not apply to you, do not mark it.*
A *Almost always (90% or more of the time)*
B *Very often (approximately 75% of the time)*
C *Often (approximately 50% of the time)*
D *Occasionally (approximately 25% of the time)*
E *Almost never (less than 10% of the time)*

### PHYSICAL EXERCISE
*Measures one's commitment to maintaining physical fitness.*

1. I exercise vigorously for at least 20 minutes three or more times per week.
2. I determine my activity level by monitoring my heart rate.
3. I stop exercising before I feel exhausted.
4. I exercise in a relaxed, calm, and joyful manner.
5. I stretch before exercising.
6. I stretch after exercising.
7. I walk or bike whenever possible.
8. I participate in a strenuous activity (tennis, running, brisk walking, water exercise, swimming, handball, basketball, etc.).
9. If I am not in shape, I avoid sporadic (once a week or less often), strenuous exercise.
10. After vigorous exercise, I "cool down" (very light exercise such as walking) for at least five minutes before sitting or lying down.

### NUTRITION
*Measures the degree to which one chooses foods that are consistent with the dietary goals of the United States as published by the Senate Select Committee on Nutrition and Human Needs.*

11. When choosing non-vegetable protein, I select lean cuts of meat, poultry, fish, and low-fat dairy products.
12. I maintain an appropriate weight for my height and frame.
13. I minimize salt intake.
14. I eat fruits and vegetables, fresh and uncooked.
15. I eat breakfast.
16. I intentionally include fiber in my diet on a daily basis.
17. I drink enough fluid to keep my urine light yellow.
18. I plan my diet to insure an adequate amount of vitamins and minerals.
19. I minimize foods in my diet that contain large amounts of refined flour (bleached white flour, typical store bread, cakes, etc.).
20. I minimize my intake of fats and oils including margarine and animal fats.

## F.2 Healthier People Health Risk Appraisal

Form C

### The HEALTHIER PEOPLE NETWORK, Inc.

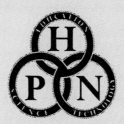

*. . . linking science, technology, & education to serve the public interest . . .*

**IDENTIFICATION NUMBER**

The health risk appraisal is an educational tool, showing you choices you can make to keep good health and avoid the most common causes of death (for a person of your age and sex). This health risk appraisal is **not** a substitute for a check-up or physical exam that you get from a doctor or nurse; however, it does provide some ideas for lowering your risk of getting sick or injured in the future. It is NOT designed for people who already have HEART DISEASE, CANCER, KIDNEY DISEASE, OR OTHER SERIOUS CONDITIONS; if you have any of these problems, please ask your health care provider to interpret the report for you.

**DIRECTIONS:**
To get the most accurate results, **answer as many questions as you can.** If you do not know the answer leave it blank.

*The following questions __must__ be completed or the computer program cannot process your questionnaire:*

*1. SEX    2. AGE    3. HEIGHT    4. WEIGHT    15. CIGARETTE SMOKING*

**Please write your answers in the boxes provided.**    ➥    (Examples:  ☒ or  98 )

| # | Question | Answer |
|---|----------|--------|
| 1. | **SEX** | 1 ☐ Male    2 ☐ Female |
| 2. | **AGE** | Years |
| 3. | **HEIGHT** (Without shoes) (No fractions) | Feet    Inches |
| 4. | **WEIGHT** (Without shoes) (No fractions) | Pounds |
| 5. | Body frame size | 1 ☐ Small  2 ☐ Medium  3 ☐ Large |
| 6. | Have you ever been told that you have diabetes (or sugar diabetes)? | 1 ☐ Yes    2 ☐ No |
| 7. | Are you now taking medicine for high blood pressure? | 1 ☐ Yes    2 ☐ No |
| 8. | What is your blood pressure now? | ___ / ___ <br> Systolic (High Number)/Diastolic (Low Number) |
| 9. | If you do **not** know the numbers, check the box that describes your blood pressure. | 1 ☐ High  2 ☐ Normal or Low  3 ☐ Don't Know |

© 1992 The Healthier People Network, Inc.

*Continued*

Form   C

| | |
|---|---|
| 10.  What is your TOTAL cholesterol level (based on a blood test)? | ☐ mg/dl |
| 11.  What is your HDL cholesterol (based on a blood test)? | ☐ mg/dl |
| 12.  How many cigars do you usually smoke per day? | ☐ cigars per day |
| 13.  How many pipes of tobacco do you usually smoke per day? | ☐ pipes per day |
| 14.  How many times per day do you usually use smokeless tobacco? (Chewing tobacco, snuff, pouches, etc.) | ☐ times per day |
| 15.  **CIGARETTE SMOKING**  How would you describe your cigarette smoking habits? | 1 ☐ Never smoked  ☛ Go to 18<br>2 ☐ Used to smoke  ☛ Go to 17<br>3 ☐ Still smoke  ☛ Go to 16 |
| 16.  **STILL SMOKE**  How many cigarettes a day do you smoke?  ☛ GO TO QUESTION 18 | ☐ cigarettes per day  ☛ Go to 18 |
| 17.  **USED TO SMOKE**  a. How many years has it been since you smoked cigarettes fairly regularly?  b. What was the average number of cigarettes per day that you smoked in the 2 years before you quit? | ☐ years<br>☐ cigarettes per day |
| 18.  In the next 12 months, how many thousands of miles will you probably travel by each of the following? (NOTE: U.S. average = 10,000 miles)  a. Car, truck, or van:  b. Motorcycle: | ☐ ,000 miles<br>☐ ,000 miles |
| 19.  On a typical day, how do you USUALLY travel?  (Check one only) | 1 ☐ Walk<br>2 ☐ Bicycle<br>3 ☐ Motorcycle<br>4 ☐ Sub-compact or compact car<br>5 ☐ Mid-size or full-size car<br>6 ☐ Truck or van<br>7 ☐ Bus, subway, or train<br>8 ☐ Mostly stay home |
| 20.  What percent of time do you usually buckle your safety belt when driving or riding? | ☐ % |
| 21.  On the average, how close to the speed limit do you usually drive? | 1 ☐ Within 5 mph of limit<br>2 ☐ 6-10 mph over limit<br>3 ☐ 11-15 mph over limit<br>4 ☐ More than 15 mph over limit |
| 22.  How many times in the last month did you drive or ride when the driver had perhaps too much alcohol to drink? | ☐ times last month |
| 23.  How many drinks of an alcoholic beverage do you have in a typical week?  ☛ *MEN GO TO QUESTION 33* | (Write the number of each type of drink)<br>☐ Bottles or cans of beer<br>☐ Glasses of wine<br>☐ Wine coolers<br>☐ Mixed drinks or shots of liquor |

Form C

## WOMEN ONLY

24. At what age did you have your first menstrual period?

[ ] years old

25. How old were you when your first child was born?

[ ] years old   (If no children, write 0)

26. How long has it been since your last breast x-ray (mammogram)?

1 □ Less than 1 year ago
2 □ 1 year ago
3 □ 2 years ago
4 □ 3 or more years ago
5 □ Never

27. How many women in your natural family (mother and sisters only) have had breast cancer?

[ ] Women

28 Have you had a hysterectomy operation?

1 □ Yes
2 □ No
3 □ Not sure

29. How long has it been since you had a pap smear test?

1 □ Less than 1 year ago
2 □ 1 year ago
3 □ 2 years ago
4 □ 3 or more years ago
5 □ Never

★30 How often do you examine your breasts for lumps?

1 □ Monthly
2 □ Once every few m
3 □ Rarely or never

★31 About how long has it been since you had your breasts examined by a physician or nurse?

1 □ Less than 1 year ago
2 □ 1 year ago
3 □ 2 years ago
4 □ 3 or more years ago
5 □ Never

★32. About how long has it been since you had a rectal exam?

1 □ Less than 1 year ago
2 □
3 □ 2 years ago
4 □   or more years ago
5 □ Never

☛ **WOMEN GO TO QUESTION 34**

## MEN ONLY

★33. About how long has it been since you had a rectal or prostate exam?

1 □ Less than 1 year ago
2 □ 1 year ago
3 □ 2 years ago
4 □ 3 or more years ago
5 □ Never

☛ **MEN CONTINUE ON QUES. 34**

★34. How many times in the last year did you witness or become involved in a violent fight or attack where there was a good chance of a serious injury to someone?

1 □ 4 or more times
2 □ 2 or 3 times
3 □ 1 time or never
4 □ Not sure

★35. Considering your age, how would you describe your overall physical health?

1 □ Excellent
2 □ Good
3 □ Fair
4 □ Poor

★ Questions with a star symbol are not used by the computer to calculate your risks; however, answering these questions may help you plan a more healthy lifestyle.

*Continued*

| | |
|---|---|
| ★36. In an average week, how many times do you engage in physical activity (exercise or work which lasts at least 20 minutes without stopping and which is hard enough to make you breathe heavier and your heart beat faster)? | 1 ☐ Less than 1 time per week<br>2 ☐ 1 or 2 times per week<br>3 ☐ At least 3 times per week |
| ★37. If you ride a motorcycle or all-terrain vehicle (ATV), what percent of the time do you wear a helmet? | 1 ☐ 75% to 100%<br>2 ☐ 25% to 74 %<br>3 ☐ Less than 25%<br>4 ☐ Does not apply to me |
| ★38. Do you eat some food every day that is high in fiber, such as whole grain bread, cereal, fresh fruits or vegetables? | 1 ☐ Yes          2 ☐ No |
| ★39. Do you eat foods every day that are high in cholesterol or fat, such as fatty meat, cheese, fried foods, or eggs? | 1 ☐ Yes          2 ☐ No |
| ★40. In general, how satisfied are you with your life? | 1 ☐ Mostly satisfied<br>2 ☐ Partly satisfied<br>3 ☐ Not satisfied |
| ★41. Have you suffered a personal loss or misfortune in the past year that had a serious impact on your life? (For example, a job loss, disability, separation, jail term, or the death of someone close to you.) | 1 ☐ Yes, 1 serious loss or misfortune<br>2 ☐ Yes, 2 or more<br>3 ☐ No |
| ★42a. Race | 1 ☐ Aleutian, Alaska native, Eskimo or American Indian<br>2 ☐ Asian<br>3 ☐ Black<br>4 ☐ Pacific Islander<br>5 ☐ White<br>6 ☐ Other<br>7 ☐ Don't know |
| ★42b. Are you of Hispanic origin, such as Mexican-American, Puerto Rican, or Cuban? | 1 ☐ Yes          2 ☐ No |
| ★43. What is the highest grade you completed in school? | 1 ☐ Grade school or less<br>2 ☐ Some high school<br>3 ☐ High school graduate<br>4 ☐ Some college<br>5 ☐ College graduate<br>6 ☐ Post graduate or professional degree |

Name _____

Address_____

City _____ State ___ ___ Zip ___ ___ ___ ___ ___

(Note: Name and address are optional, depending on how your report will be returned to you. If you wish to remain anonymous, copy your Identification Number onto a receipt form. You can then use this receipt to claim your computerized report.)

# The
# HEALTHIER PEOPLE NETWORK, Inc.

## Participant's Guide to Interpreting the
## HEALTH RISK APPRAISAL REPORT

Unhealthy habits lead to early death or chronic illness. Every year, 1.3 million people in the United States die prematurely from conditions which could be prevented or delayed. This Health Risk Appraisal may help you avoid becoming one of these statistics by giving you a picture of how your health risks relate to your particular characteristics and habits.

## WHAT IS A HEALTH RISK APPRAISAL?

The Health Risk Appraisal is an estimation of your risk of dying in the next ten years from each of 42 causes of death. The twelve most important of these are printed individually on your report. The others are grouped together and printed as "All Other". These risks are calculated by a computer program which compares your characteristics to national mortality statistics using equations developed by epidemiologists. This Health Risk Appraisal does not tell you how long you will live, nor does it diagnose or treat disease.

## RISK FACTORS

Most chronic diseases develop slowly in the presence of certain risk factors. Risk factors are either controllable or uncontrollable. Controllable risk factors include lifestyle habits that you can change such as smoking, exercise, diet, stress and weight. Uncontrollable risk factors include items such as your age and sex, and the health history of your family.

The Health Risk Appraisal uses both controllable and uncontrollable risk factors in calculating health risks. Your focus, however, should be on controllable risk factors.

To help you decide which controllable risk factors to concentrate on, the Health Risk Appraisal identifies your controllable risk factors for each cause of death. Your report gives you an idea of their relative importance by indicating the number of risk years you could gain by controlling these factors.

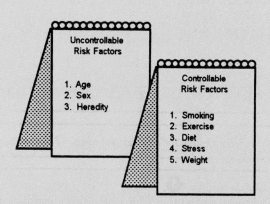

To identify your personal risks, to see what the numbers on your report mean, and to learn which risk factors you need to control, turn the page.

*Continued*

Page 2 of your report lists some **ROUTINE PREVENTIVE SERVICES** that are specific for people of your age and sex. The report also lists some **GENERAL RECOMMENDATIONS FOR EVERYONE**. For the 48 year old woman used in this example, the following messages were printed:

| ROUTINE PREVENTIVE SERVICES FOR WOMEN YOUR AGE | GENERAL RECOMMENDATIONS FOR EVERYONE |
|---|---|
| Blood Pressure and Cholesterol test<br>Pap Smear test<br>Breast cancer screening (check with your doctor or clinic)<br>Rectal exam (or Sigmoidoscopy)<br>Eye exam for glaucoma<br>Dental Exam<br>Tetanus-Diphtheria booster shot (every 10 years) | * Exercise briskly for 15-30 minutes at least three times a week.<br>* Use good eating habits by choosing a variety of foods that are low in fat and high in fiber.<br>* Learn to recognize and handle stress - get help if you need it. |

The standard report can also print health education messages.

## HEALTH RISK APPRAISAL LIMITS

Health Risk Appraisal is an educational tool. It does not take into consideration whether or not you already have a medical condition and it does not consider rare diseases and other health problems which are not fatal but can limit your enjoyment of life, such as arthritis.

Health Risk Appraisal does not predict when you will die or specifically what diseases you might get. It does tell you, however, your chances of getting a disease relative to a large group of people your age and sex, who answered the questionnaire just as you did.

Health Risk Appraisal does take into consideration lifestyle factors which account for a large number of premature deaths. When you become familiar with your particular risks, you can then do something about them!

## CHOOSING A HABIT TO WORK ON

Health Risk Appraisal is intended to encourage you to work on habits you can change by showing you which behaviors should have top priority. If you can't change the behavior that is at the top of your list (the one that would give the largest number of **RISK YEARS GAINED**), try to concentrate on changing the next highest one. You don't have to change your entire lifestyle overnight. In fact, trying to change too many habits at once is probably the quickest way to become discouraged and fail.

## MAKE A PLAN FOR CHANGING HABITS

Make a plan for changing the habit you choose as your first priority, write it down and keep it in sight. Be prepared for temptation! Observe the time, situation, or place that most often triggers your unhealthy habit and be ready to combat it when it appears. Let family and friends know of your goals and ask for their encouragement.

### REWARD YOURSELF

Rewards are an important part of changing behavior. Give yourself a reasonable reward when you accomplish your goal. Don't eat half a gallon of ice cream after losing 10 pounds! Choose a healthy and enjoyable reward and you'll be on the road to good health!

# F.3 1999 Youth Risk Behavior Survey*

This survey is about health behavior. It has been developed so you can tell us what you do that may affect your health. The information you give will be used to develop better health education for young people like yourself.

DO NOT write your name on this survey. The answers you give will be kept private. No one will know what you write. Answer the questions based on what you really do.

Completing the survey is voluntary. Whether or not you answer the questions will not affect your grade in this class. If you are not comfortable answering a question, just leave it blank.

The questions that ask about your background will be used only to describe the types of students completing this survey. The information will not be used to find out your name. No names will ever be reported.

Make sure to read every question. Fill in the ovals completely. When you are finished, follow the instructions of the person giving you the survey.

***Thank you very much for your help.***

DIRECTIONS
- Use a #2 pencil only.
- Make dark marks.
- Fill in a response like this: A B C D.
- To change your answer, erase completely.

1. How old are you?
   A. 12 years old or younger
   B. 13 years old
   C. 14 years old
   D. 15 years old
   E. 16 years old
   F. 17 years old
   G. 18 years old or older
2. What is your sex?
   A. Female          B. Male
3. In what grade are you?
   A. 9th grade          D. 12th grade
   B. 10th grade         E. Ungraded or other grade
   C. 11th grade
4. How do you describe yourself? **(Select one or more responses.)**
   A. American Indian or Alaska Native
   B. Asian
   C. Black or African American
   D. Hispanic or Latino
   E. Native Hawaiian or Other Pacific Islander
   F. White

*From Centers for Disease Control and Prevention, available at www.cdc.gov/mccdphp/dash/yrbs/survey99.htm, accessed Aug, 1999.*

5. How tall are you without your shoes on?

DIRECTIONS
Write your height in the shaded blank boxes. Fill in the matching oval below each number.

EXAMPLE

| HEIGHT | | HEIGHT | |
|---|---|---|---|
| FEET | INCHES | FEET | INCHES |
| 5 | 7 | | |
| ③ | ⓪ | ③ | ⓪ |
| ④ | ① | ④ | ① |
| ⑤ | ② | ⑤ | ② |
| ⑥ | ③ | ⑥ | ③ |
| ⑦ | ④ | ⑦ | ④ |
| | ⑤ | | ⑤ |
| | ⑥ | | ⑥ |
| | ⑦ | | ⑦ |
| | ⑧ | | ⑧ |
| | ⑨ | | ⑨ |
| | ⑩ | | ⑩ |
| | ⑪ | | ⑪ |

6. How much do you weigh without your shoes on?

Directions: Write your weight in the shaded blank boxes. Fill in the matching oval below each number.

EXAMPLE

| WEIGHT (LB) | | | WEIGHT (LB) | | |
|---|---|---|---|---|---|
| 1 | 5 | 2 | | | |
| ⓪ | ⓪ | ⓪ | ⓪ | ⓪ | ⓪ |
| ① | ① | ① | ① | ① | ① |
| ② | ② | ② | ② | ② | ② |
| ③ | ③ | ③ | ③ | ③ | ③ |
| | ④ | ④ | | ④ | ④ |
| | ⑤ | ⑤ | | ⑤ | ⑤ |
| | ⑥ | ⑥ | | ⑥ | ⑥ |
| | ⑦ | ⑦ | | ⑦ | ⑦ |
| | ⑧ | ⑧ | | ⑧ | ⑧ |
| | ⑨ | ⑨ | | ⑨ | ⑨ |

*Continued*

**The next five questions ask about personal safety.**

7. **When you rode a motorcycle** during the past 12 months, how often did you wear a helmet?
   A. I did not ride a motorcycle during the past 12 months
   B. Never wore a helmet
   C. Rarely wore a helmet
   D. Sometimes wore a helmet
   E. Most of the time wore a helmet
   F. Always wore a helmet

8. **When you rode a bicycle** during the past 12 months, how often did you wear a helmet?
   A. I did not ride a bicycle during the past 12 months
   B. Never wore a helmet
   C. Rarely wore a helmet
   D. Sometimes wore a helmet
   E. Most of the time wore a helmet
   F. Always wore a helmet

9. How often do you wear a seat belt when **riding** in a car driven by someone else?
   A. Never             D. Most of the time
   B. Rarely            E. Always
   C. Sometimes

10. During the past 30 days, how many times did you **ride** in a car or other vehicle **driven by someone who had been drinking alcohol?**
    A. 0 times           D. 4 or 5 times
    B. 1 time            E. 6 or more times
    C. 2 or 3 times

11. During the past 30 days, how many times did you **drive** a car or other vehicle **when you had been drinking alcohol?**
    A. 0 times           D. 4 or 5 times
    B. 1 time            E. 6 or more times
    C. 2 or 3 times

**The next 10 questions ask about violence-related behaviors.**

12. During the past 30 days, on how many days did you carry **a weapon** such as a gun, knife, or club?
    A. 0 days            D. 4 or 5 days
    B. 1 day             E. 6 or more days
    C. 2 or 3 days

13. During the past 30 days, on how many days did you carry a **gun?**
    A. 0 days            D. 4 or 5 days
    B. 1 day             E. 6 or more days
    C. 2 or 3 days

14. During the past 30 days, on how many days did you carry a weapon such as a gun, knife, or club **on school property?**
    A. 0 days            D. 4 or 5 days
    B. 1 day             E. 6 or more days
    C. 2 or 3 days

15. During the past 30 days, on how many days did you **not** go to school because you felt you would be unsafe at school or on your way to or from school?
    A. 0 days            D. 4 or 5 days
    B. 1 day             E. 6 or more days
    C. 2 or 3 days

16. During the past 12 months, how many times has someone threatened or injured you with a weapon such as a gun, knife, or club **on school property?**
    A. 0 times           E. 6 or 7 times
    B. 1 time            F. 8 or 9 times
    C. 2 or 3 times      G. 10 or 11 times
    D. 4 or 5 timesH. 12 or more times

17. During the past 12 months, how many times were you in a physical fight?
    A. 0 times           E. 6 or 7 times
    B. 1 time            F. 8 or 9 times
    C. 2 or 3 times      G. 10 or 11 times
    D. 4 or 5 timesH. 12 or more times

18. During the past 12 months, how many times were you in a physical fight in which you were injured and had to be treated by a doctor or nurse?
    A. 0 times           D. 4 or 5 times
    B. 1 time            E. 6 or more times
    C. 2 or 3 times

19. During the past 12 months, how many times were you in a physical fight **on school property?**
    A. 0 times           E. 6 or 7 times
    B. 1 time            F. 8 or 9 times
    C. 2 or 3 times      G. 10 or 11 times
    D. 4 or 5 timesH. 12 or more times

20. During the past 12 months, did your boyfriend or girlfriend ever hit, slap, or physically hurt you on purpose?
    A. Yes               B. No

21. Have you ever been forced to have sexual intercourse when you did not want to?
    A. Yes               B. No

**The next five questions ask about sad feelings and attempted suicide. Sometimes people feel so depressed about the future that they may consider attempting suicide, that is, taking some action to end their own life.**

22. During the past 12 months, did you ever feel so sad or hopeless almost every day for **two weeks or more in a row** that you stopped doing some usual activities.
    A. Yes               B. No

23. During the past 12 months, did you ever **seriously** consider attempting suicide?
    A. Yes               B. No

24. During the past 12 months, did you make a plan about how you would attempt suicide?
    A. Yes
    B. No

25. During the past 12 months, how many times did you actually attempt suicide?
    A. 0 times
    B. 1 time
    C. 2 or 3 times
    D. 4 or 5 times
    E. 6 or more times

26. **If you attempted suicide** during the past 12 months, did any attempt result in an injury, poisoning, or overdose that had to be treated by a doctor or nurse?
    A. **I did not attempt suicide** during the past 12 months
    B. Yes
    C. No

**The next 12 questions ask about tobacco use.**

27. Have you ever tried cigarette smoking, even one or two puffs?
    A. Yes                   B. No

28. How old were you when you smoked a whole cigarette for the first time?
    A. I have never smoked a whole cigarette
    B. 8 years old or younger
    C. 9 or 10 years old
    D. 11 or 12 years old
    E. 13 or 14 years old
    F. 15 or 16 years old
    G. 17 years old or older

29. During the past 30 days, on how many days did you smoke cigarettes?
    A. 0 days            E. 10 to 19 days
    B. 1 or 2 days       F. 20 to 29 days
    C. 3 to 5 days       G. All 30 days
    D. 6 to 9 days

30. During the past 30 days, on the days you smoked, how many cigarettes did you smoke **per day?**
    A. I did not smoke cigarettes during the past 30 days
    B. Less than 1 cigarette per day
    C. 1 cigarette per day
    D. 2 to 5 cigarettes per day
    E. 6 to 10 cigarettes per day
    F. 11 to 20 cigarettes per day
    G. More than 20 cigarettes per day

31. During the past 30 days, how did you **usually** get your own cigarettes? (Select only **one** response.)
    A. I did not smoke cigarettes during the past 30 days
    B. I bought them in a store such as a convenience store, supermarket, or gas station
    C. I bought them from a vending machine
    D. I gave someone else money to buy them for me
    E. I borrowed them from someone else
    F. I stole them
    G. I got them some other way

32. **When you bought cigarettes** in a store during the past 30 days, were you ever asked to show proof of age?
    A. I did not buy cigarettes in a store during the past 30 days
    B. Yes
    C. No

33. During the past 30 days, on how many days did you smoke cigarettes **on school property?**
    A. 0 days            E. 10 to 19 days
    B. 1 or 2 days       F. 20 to 29 days
    C. 3 to 5 days       G. All 30 days
    D. 6 to 9 days

34. Have you ever smoked cigarettes regularly, that is, at least one cigarette every day for 30 days?
    A. Yes                   B. No

35. Have you ever tried **to quit** smoking cigarettes?
    A. Yes                   B. No

36. During the past 30 days, on how many days did you use **chewing tobacco or snuff,** such as Redman, Levi Garrett, Beechnut, Skoal, Skoal Bandits, or Copenhagen?
    A. 0 days            E. 10 to 19 days
    B. 1 or 2 days       F. 20 to 29 days
    C. 3 to 5 days       G. All 30 days
    D. 6 to 9 days

37. During the past 30 days, on how many days did you use **chewing tobacco or snuff on school property?**
    A. 0 days            E. 10 to 19 days
    B. 1 or 2 days       F. 20 to 29 days
    C. 3 to 5 days       G. All 30 days
    D. 6 to 9 days

38. During the past 30 days, on how many days did you smoke **cigars, cigarillos, or little cigars?**
    A. 0 days            E. 10 to 19 days
    B. 1 or 2 days       F. 20 to 29 days
    C. 3 to 5 days       G. All 30 days
    D. 6 to 9 days

**The next five questions ask about drinking alcohol. This includes drinking beer, wine, wine coolers, and liquor such as rum, gin, vodka, or whiskey. For these questions, drinking alcohol does not include drinking a few sips of wine for religious purposes.**

39. During your life, on how many days have you had at least one drink of alcohol?
    A. 0 days            E. 20 to 39 days
    B. 1 or 2 days       F. 40 to 99 days
    C. 3 to 9 days       G. 100 or more days
    D. 10 to 19 days

40. How old were you when you had your first drink of alcohol other than a few sips?
    A. I have never had a drink of alcohol other than a few sips
    B. 8 years old or younger
    C. 9 or 10 years old
    D. 11 or 12 years old
    E. 13 or 14 years old
    F. 15 or 16 years old
    G. 17 years old or older

41. During the past 30 days, on how many days did you have at least one drink of alcohol?
    A. 0 days            E. 10 to 19 days
    B. 1 or 2 days       F. 20 to 29 days
    C. 3 to 5 days       G. All 30 days
    D. 6 to 9 days

*Continued*

42. During the past 30 days, on how many days did you have five or more drinks of alcohol in a row, that is, within a couple of hours?
    - A. 0 days
    - B. 1 day
    - C. 2 days
    - D. 3 to 5 days
    - E. 6 to 9 days
    - F. 10 to 19 days
    - G. 20 or more days

43. During the past 30 days, on how many days did you have at least one drink of alcohol **on school property?**
    - A. 0 days
    - B. 1 or 2 days
    - C. 3 to 5 days
    - D. 6 to 9 days
    - E. 10 to 19 days
    - F. 20 to 29 days
    - G. All 30 days

**The next four questions ask about marijuana use. Marijuana also is called grass or pot.**

44. During your life, how many times have you used marijuana?
    - A. 0 times
    - B. 1 or 2 times
    - C. 3 to 9 times
    - D. 10 to 19 times
    - E. 20 to 39 times
    - F. 40 to 99 times
    - G. 100 or more times

45. How old were you when you tried marijuana for the first time?
    - A. I have never tried marijuana
    - B. 8 years old or younger
    - C. 9 or 10 years old
    - D. 11 or 12 years old
    - E. 13 or 14 years old
    - F. 15 or 16 years old
    - G. 17 years old or older

46. During the past 30 days, how many times did you use marijuana?
    - A. 0 times
    - B. 1 or 2 times
    - C. 3 to 9 times
    - D. 10 to 19 times
    - E. 20 to 39 times
    - F. 40 or more times

47. During the past 30 days, how many times did you use marijuana **on school property?**
    - A. 0 times
    - B. 1 or 2 times
    - C. 3 to 9 times
    - D. 10 to 19 times
    - E. 20 to 39 times
    - F. 40 or more times

**The next nine questions ask about cocaine and other drugs.**

48. During your life, how many times have you used **any** form of cocaine, including powder, crack, or freebase?
    - A. 0 times
    - B. 1 or 2 times
    - C. 3 to 9 times
    - D. 10 to 19 times
    - E. 20 to 39 times
    - F. 40 or more times

49. During the past 30 days, how many times did you use **any** form of cocaine, including powder, crack, or freebase?
    - A. 0 times
    - B. 1 or 2 times
    - C. 3 to 9 times
    - D. 10 to 19 times
    - E. 20 to 39 times
    - F. 40 or more times

50. During your life, how many times have you sniffed glue, breathed the contents of aerosol spray cans, or inhaled any paints or sprays to get high?
    - A. 0 times
    - B. 1 or 2 times
    - C. 3 to 9 times
    - D. 10 to 19 times
    - E. 20 to 39 times
    - F. 40 or more times

51. During the past 30 days, how many times have you sniffed glue, breathed the contents of aerosol spray cans, or inhaled any paints or sprays to get high?
    - A. 0 times
    - B. 1 or 2 times
    - C. 3 to 9 times
    - D. 10 to 19 times
    - E. 20 to 39 times
    - F. 40 or more times

52. During your life, how many times have you used **heroin** (also called smack, junk, or China White)?
    - A. 0 times
    - B. 1 or 2 times
    - C. 3 to 9 times
    - D. 10 to 19 times
    - E. 20 to 39 times
    - F. 40 or more times

53. During your life, how many times have you used **methamphetamines** (also called speed, crystal, crank, or ice)?
    - A. 0 times
    - B. 1 or 2 times
    - C. 3 to 9 times
    - D. 10 to 19 times
    - E. 20 to 39 times
    - F. 40 or more times

54. During your life, how many times have you taken **steroid pills or shots** without a doctor's prescription?
    - A. 0 times
    - B. 1 or 2 times
    - C. 3 to 9 times
    - D. 10 to 19 times
    - E. 20 to 39 times
    - F. 40 or more times

55. During your life, how many times have you used a needle to inject any **illegal** drug into your body?
    - A. 0 times
    - B. 1 time
    - C. 2 or more times

56. During the past 12 months, has anyone offered, sold, or given you an illegal drug **on school property?**
    - A. Yes
    - B. No

**The next eight questions ask about sexual behavior.**

57. Have you ever had sexual intercourse?
    - A. Yes
    - B. No

58. How old were you when you had sexual intercourse for the first time?
    - A. I have never had sexual intercourse
    - B. 11 years old or younger
    - C. 12 years old
    - D. 13 years old
    - E. 14 years old
    - F. 15 years old
    - G. 16 years old
    - H. 17 years old or older

59. During your life, with how many people have you had sexual intercourse?
    - A. I have never had sexual intercourse
    - B. 1 person
    - C. 2 people
    - D. 3 people
    - E. 4 people
    - F. 5 people
    - G. 6 or more people

60. During the past 3 months, with how many people did you have sexual intercourse?
    A. I have never had sexual intercourse
    B. I have had sexual intercourse, but not during the past 3 months
    C. 1 person
    D. 2 people
    E. 3 people
    F. 4 people
    G. 5 people
    H. 6 or more people

61. Did you drink alcohol or use drugs before you had sexual intercourse the **last time?**
    A. I have never had sexual intercourse
    B. Yes
    C. No

62. The **last time** you had sexual intercourse, did you or your partner use a condom?
    A. I have never had sexual intercourse
    B. Yes
    C. No

63. The **last time** you had sexual intercourse, what one method did you or your partner use to **prevent pregnancy?** (Select only **one** response.)
    A. I have never had sexual intercourse
    B. No method was used to prevent pregnancy
    C. Birth control pills
    D. Condoms
    E. Depo-Provera (injectable birth control)
    F. Withdrawal
    G. Some other method
    H. Not sure

64. How many times have you been pregnant or gotten someone pregnant?
    A. 0 times          C. 2 or more times
    B. 1 time           D. Not sure

**The next seven questions ask about body weight.**

65. How do **you** describe your weight?
    A. Very underweight
    B. Slightly underweight
    C. About the right weight
    D. Slightly overweight
    E. Very overweight

66. Which of the following are you trying to do about your weight?
    A. **Lose** weight
    B. **Gain** weight
    C. **Stay** the same weight
    D. I am **not trying to do anything** about my weight

67. During the past 30 days, did you **exercise** to lose weight or to keep from gaining weight?
    A. Yes              B. No

68. During the past 30 days, did you **eat less food, fewer calories, or foods low in fat** to lose weight or to keep from gaining weight?
    A. Yes              B. No

69. During the past 30 days, did you **go without eating for 24 hours or more** (also called fasting) to lose weight or to keep from gaining weight?
    A. Yes              B. No

70. During the past 30 days, did you **take any diet pills, powders, or liquids** without a doctor's advice to lose weight or to keep from gaining weight? (Do not include meal replacement products such as Slim Fast.)
    A. Yes              B. No

71. During the past 30 days, did you **vomit or take laxatives** to lose weight or to keep from gaining weight?
    A. Yes              B. No

**The next seven questions ask about food you ate or drank during the past 7 days. Think about all the meals and snacks you had from the time you got up until you went to bed. Be sure to include food you ate at home, at school, at restaurants, or anywhere else.**

72. During the past 7 days, how many times did you drink **100% fruit juices** such as orange juice, apple juice, or grape juice? (Do **not** count punch, Kool-Aid, sports drinks, or other fruit-flavored drinks.)
    A. I did not drink 100% fruit juice during the past 7 days
    B. 1 to 3 times during the past 7 days
    C. 4 to 6 times during the past 7 days
    D. 1 time per day
    E. 2 times per day
    F. 3 times per day
    G. 4 or more times per day

73. During the past 7 days, how many times did you eat **fruit?** (Do **not** count fruit juice.)
    A. I did not eat fruit during the past 7 days
    B. 1 to 3 times during the past 7 days
    C. 4 to 6 times during the past 7 days
    D. 1 time per day
    E. 2 times per day
    F. 3 times per day
    G. 4 or more times per day

74. During the past 7 days, how many times did you eat **green salad?**
    A. I did not eat green salad during the past 7 days
    B. 1 to 3 times during the past 7 days
    C. 4 to 6 times during the past 7 days
    D. 1 time per day
    E. 2 times per day
    F. 3 times per day
    G. 4 or more times per day

75. During the past 7 days, how many times did you eat **potatoes?** (Do **not** count french fries, fried potatoes, or potato chips.)
    A. I did not eat potatoes during the past 7 days
    B. 1 to 3 times during the past 7 days
    C. 4 to 6 times during the past 7 days
    D. 1 time per day
    E. 2 times per day
    F. 3 times per day
    G. 4 or more times per day

*Continued*

76. During the past 7 days, how many times did you eat **carrots?**
    A. I did not eat carrots during the past 7 days
    B. 1 to 3 times during the past 7 days
    C. 4 to 6 times during the past 7 days
    D. 1 time per day
    E. 2 times per day
    F. 3 times per day
    G. 4 or more times per day

77. During the past 7 days, how many times did you eat **other vegetables?** (Do **not** count green salad, potatoes, or carrots.)
    A. I did not eat other vegetables during the past 7 days
    B. 1 to 3 times during the past 7 days
    C. 4 to 6 times during the past 7 days
    D. 1 time per day
    E. 2 times per day
    F. 3 times per day
    G. 4 or more times per day

78. During the past 7 days, how many **glasses of milk** did you drink? (Include the milk you drank in a glass or cup, from a carton, or with cereal. Count the half pint of milk served at school as equal to one glass.)
    A. I did not drink milk during the past 7 days
    B. 1 to 3 glasses during the past 7 days
    C. 4 to 6 glasses during the past 7 days
    D. 1 glass per day
    E. 2 glasses per day
    F. 3 glasses per day
    G. 4 or more glasses per day

**The next eight questions ask about physical activity.**

79. On how many of the past 7 days did you exercise or participate in physical activity for **at least 20** minutes **that made you sweat and breathe hard,** such as basketball, soccer, running, swimming laps, fast bicycling, fast dancing, or similar aerobic activities?
    A. 0 days          E. 4 days
    B. 1 day           F. 5 days
    C. 2 days          G. 6 days
    D. 3 days          H. 7 days

80. On how many of the past 7 days did you participate in physical activity for **at least 30** minutes that did **not** make you sweat or breathe hard, such as fast walking, slow bicycling, skating, pushing a lawn mower, or mopping floors?
    A. 0 days          E. 4 days
    B. 1 day           F. 5 days
    C. 2 days          G. 6 days
    D. 3 days          H. 7 days

81. On how many of the past 7 days did you do exercises to **strengthen or tone your muscles,** such as push-ups, sit-ups, or weight lifting?
    A. 0 days          E. 4 days
    B. 1 day           F. 5 days
    C. 2 days          G. 6 days
    D. 3 days          H. 7 days

82. On an average school day, how many hours do you watch TV?
    A. I do not watch TV on an average school day
    B. Less than 1 hour per day
    C. 1 hour per day
    D. 2 hours per day
    E. 3 hours per day
    F. 4 hours per day
    G. 5 or more hours per day

83. In an average week when you are in school, on how many days do you go to physical education (PE) classes?
    A. 0 days          D. 3 days
    B. 1 day           E. 4 days
    C. 2 days          F. 5 days

84. During an average physical education (PE) class, how many minutes do you spend actually exercising or playing sports?
    A. I do not take PE        C. 10 to 20 minutes
    B. Less than 10            D. 21 to 30 minutes
       minutes                E. More than 30 minutes

85. During the past 12 months, on how many sports teams did you play? (Include any teams run by your school or community groups.)
    A. 0 teams         C. 2 teams
    B. 1 team          D. 3 or more teams

86. During the past 12 months, how many times were you injured while exercising, playing sports, or being physically active and had to be treated by a doctor or nurse?
    A. 0 times         D. 3 times
    B. 1 time          E. 4 times
    C. 2 times         F. 5 or more times

**The next question asks about AIDS education.**

87. Have you ever been taught about AIDS or HIV infection in school?
    A. Yes
    B. No
    C. Not sure

**This is the end of the survey.**
**Thank you very much for your help.**

# Appendix G

## Community Assessment Tools

## G.1 Community-As-Partner Model

The community-as-partner model was developed to illustrate public health nursing as a synthesis of public health and nursing. The model, originally titled community-as-client, has evolved to incorporate the philosophy that nurses work with communities as partners. This is congruent with what was learned about how communities (and people, for that matter) change and grow best, that is, by full involvement and self-empowerment, not by imposed programs and structures.

The model's "heart" is the assessment wheel (Figure G-1), which depicts that the people actually are the community—the core elements. Without people there is no community, and it is the people (their demographics, values, beliefs, history) that is of interest to the public health nurse. Surrounding the people, and integral with them, are the identified eight subsystems of a community. These subsystems (physical environment, education, safety and transportation, politics and government, health and social services, communication, economics, and recreation) both affect and are affected by the people. To understand this interaction, one must understand each subsystem; therefore incorporate its assessment into assessment of the people.

The "wheel" (actually the entire community, including the people and subsystems) is shown with broken lines between each subsystem to show that these are not discrete, but that all subsystems affect each other. Within the community are lines of resistance, those "strengths" that defend against stressors (e.g., a school-based program to prevent teen violence); identifying strengths in the community is as important as identifying "problems." Surrounding the community are lines of defense, depicted in the model as "flexible" and "normal" to indicate that there are two types of defense: one is the usual (normal) "health" of a community and the other is more dynamic (flexible) and changes more rapidly. Two illustrations may assist in clarifying these lines. The flexible line of defense

Elizabeth T. Anderson, RN, FAAN, DrPH
*Professor and Chair, Department of Community Health and Gerontology*
*University of Texas School of Nursing at Galveston*
*University of Texas Medical Branch*
*Galveston, Texas*

may be a temporary response to a stressor. For instance, an environmental stressor such as flash flooding or a major fire may call into play resources from within the community and from surrounding areas; these resources are considered the flexible lines of defense. The normal line of defense is the usual level of health a community has reached over time. Examples of normal lines of defense include the immunization rate, adequate housing, or access to Meals-on-Wheels for shut-ins; all of these contribute to the health of the community.

Stressors affect the community and may be of the community or from outside the community. Either way, the community's response to stressors is mitigated by its overall health state, that is, by the strength of its lines of resistance and defense. Knowing these strengths is one purpose of the community assessment. In the analysis phase of the nursing process, the nurse will weigh the stressor and the degree of reaction it causes in order to describe a community nursing diagnosis that, in turn, will give direction to goals and interventions. One method for stating the community nursing diagnosis is to state the "problem" as the degree of reaction (from which the goal is derived) and the "as related to" as stressors ("causes" that help define needed interventions). Using this method, an example of a community nursing diagnosis might be as follows: High rate of tuberculosis (the problem, the degree of reaction) related to poor hygiene and sanitation, crowded living conditions, poverty, and consumption of raw milk (stressors) as manifested by open garbage, and poor ventilation; an average of 5.6 persons per household; and sale of raw milk for income (the "data" collected in your assessment).

Think for a moment how each subsystem contributes to the health of the community. The nurse can see how an inadequate infrastructure, such as modern sewage treatment or unemployment, can affect the health of all of the citizens.

Many models exist to provide a framework for assessing a community. This systems model gives one other way to describe a community. Working with the community is a vital and challenging task for nurses. Using a model wherein the community is viewed as a partner will help formulate community-focused interventions and promote the health of the entire community.

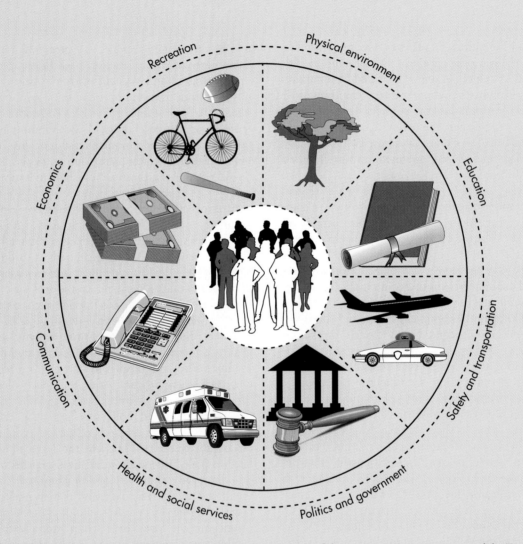

**Figure G-1** The community assessment wheel, the assessment segment of the community-as-partner model. *(From Anderson ET, McFarlane J:* Community-as-partner: theory and practice in nursing, *ed 3, Philadelphia, 2000, Lippincott Williams & Wilkins.)*

# Appendix H

## Family Assessment Tools

## H.2 Friedman Family Assessment Model (Short Form)

Before using the following guidelines in completing family assessments, two words of caution. First, not all areas included below will be germane for each of the families visited. The guidelines are comprehensive and allow depth when probing is necessary. The student should not feel that every subarea needs to be covered when the broad area of inquiry poses no problems to the family or concern to the health worker. Second, by virtue of the interdependence of the family system, one will find unavoidable redundancy. For the sake of efficiency, the assessor should try not to repeat data, but to refer the reader back to sections where this information has already been described.

### IDENTIFYING DATA

1. Family Name
2. Address and Phone
3. Family Composition (see table)
4. Type of Family Form
5. Cultural (Ethnic) Background
6. Religious Identification
7. Social Class Status
8. Family's Recreational or Leisure-time Activities

### DEVELOPMENTAL STAGE AND HISTORY OF FAMILY

9. Family's Present Developmental Stage
10. Extent of Developmental Tasks Fulfillment
11. Nuclear Family History
12. History of Family of Origin of Both Parents

### ENVIRONMENTAL DATA

13. Characteristics of Home
14. Characteristics of Neighborhood and Larger Community
15. Family's Geographic Mobility
16. Family's Associations and Transactions with Community
17. Family's Social Support Network (ecomap)

### FAMILY STRUCTURE

18. Communication Patterns
    *Extent of Functional and Dysfunctional Communication (types of recurring patterns)*
    *Extent of Emotional (Affective) Messages and How Expressed*
    *Characteristics of Communication Within Family Subsystems*
    *Extent of Congruent and Incongruent Messages*
    *Types of Dysfunctional Communication Processes Seen in Family*
    *Areas of Open and Closed Communication*
    *Familial and External Variables Affecting Communication*
19. Power Structure
    *Power Outcomes*
    *Decision-Making Process*
    *Power Bases*
    *Variables Affecting Family Power*
    *Overall Family System and Subsystem Power*
20. Role Structure
    *Formal Role Structure*
    *Informal Role Structure*
    *Analysis of Role Models (optional)*
    *Variables Affecting Role Structure*
21. Family Values
    *Compare the Family to American or Family's Reference Group Values and/or Identify Important Family Values and their Importance (Priority) in Family*
    *Congruence Between the Family's Values and the Family's Reference Group or Wider Community*
    *Congruence Between the Family's Values and Family Member's Values*
    *Variables Influencing Family Values*
    *Values Consciously or Unconsciously Held*
    *Presence of Value Conflicts in Family*
    *Effect of the Above Values and Value Conflicts on Health Status of Family*

## FAMILY FUNCTIONS

22. Affective Function
    *Family's Need-Response Patterns*
    *Mutual Nurturance, Closeness, and Identification*
    *Separateness and Connectedness*
23. Socialization Function
    *Family Child-Rearing Practices*
    *Adaptability of Child-Rearing Practices for Family Form and Family's Situation*
    *Who Is (Are) Socializing Agent(s) for Child(ren)?*
    *Value of Children in Family*
    *Cultural Beliefs That Influence Family's Child-Rearing Patterns*
    *Social Class Influence on Child-Rearing Patterns*
    *Estimation About Whether Family Is at Risk for Child Rearing Problems and, if so, Indication of High-Risk Factors*
    *Adequacy of Home Environment for Children's Needs to Play*
24. Health Care Function
    *Family's Health Beliefs, Values, and Behavior*
    *Family's Definitions of Health-Illness and Their Level of Knowledge*
    *Family's Perceived Health Status and Illness Susceptibility*
    *Family's Dietary Practices*
    *Adequacy of Family Diet (Recommended 24-hour food history record)*
    *Function of Mealtimes and Attitudes Toward Food and Mealtimes*
    *Shopping (and its Planning) Practices*
    *Person(s) Responsible for Planning, Shopping, and Preparation of Meals*
    *Sleep and Rest Habits*
    *Physical Activity and Recreation Practices (not covered earlier)*
    *Family's Drug Habits*
    *Family's Role in Self-Care Practices*
    *Medically Based Preventive Measures (physicals, eye and hearing tests, and immunizations)*
    *Dental Health Practices*
    *Family Health History (both general and specific diseases—environmentally and genetically related)*
    *Health Care Services Received*
    *Feelings and Perceptions Regarding Health Services*
    *Emergency Health Services*
    *Source of Payments for Health and Other Services*
    *Logistics of Receiving Care*

## FAMILY STRESS AND COPING

25. Short- and Long-term Familial Stressors and Strengths
26. Extent of Family's Ability to Respond, Based on Objective Appraisal of Stress-Producing Situations
27. Coping Strategies Utilized (present/past)
    *Differences in Family Members' Ways of Coping*
    *Family's Inner Coping Strategies*
    *Family's external coping strategies*
28. Dysfunctional Adaptive Strategies Utilized (present/past; extent of usage)

## FAMILY COMPOSITION FORM

| Name (Last, First) | Gender | Relationship | Date and Place of Birth | Occupation | Education |
|---|---|---|---|---|---|
| 1. (Father) | | | | | |
| 2. (Mother) | | | | | |
| 3. (Oldest child) | | | | | |
| 4. | | | | | |
| 5. | | | | | |
| 6. | | | | | |
| 7. | | | | | |
| 8. | | | | | |

*From Friedman MM, Bowden VR, Jones, EG: Family nursing: research, theory, and practice, ed 5, Stamford, Conn, 2003, Prentice Hall.*

# Appendix I

## Individual Assessment Tools

### I.1 Instrumental Activities of Daily Living (IADL) Scale

Name _____ Rated by _____ Date _____

| | |
|---|---|
| **1. Can you use the telephone**<br>without help, — 3<br>with some help, or — 2<br>are you completely unable to use the telephone? — 1 | **7. Can you do your own laundry**<br>without help, — 3<br>with some help, or — 2<br>are you completely unable to do any laundry at all? — 1 |
| **2. Can you get to places beyond walking distance**<br>without help, — 3<br>with some help, or — 2<br>are you completely unable to travel unless special arrangements are made? — 1 | **8a. Do you take medicines or use any medications?**<br>Yes (If yes, answer Question 8b.) — 1<br>No (If no, answer Question 8c.) — 2 |
| **3. Can you go shopping for groceries**<br>without help, — 3<br>with some help, or — 2<br>are you completely unable to do any shopping? — 1 | **8b. Do you take your own medicine**<br>without help (in the right doses at the right time), — 3<br>with some help (if someone prepares it for you and/or reminds you to take it), or — 2<br>are you completely unable to take your own medicine? — 1 |
| **4. Can you prepare your own meals**<br>without help, — 3<br>with some help, or — 2<br>are you completely unable to prepare any meals? — 1 | **8c. If you had to take medicine, could you do it**<br>without help (in the right doses at the right time), — 3<br>with some help (if someone prepared it for you and/or reminded you to take it), or — 2<br>would you be completely unable to take your own medicine? — 1 |
| **5. Can you do your own housework**<br>without help, — 3<br>with some help, or — 2<br>are you completely unable to do any housework? — 1 | **9. Can you manage your own money**<br>without help, — 3<br>with some help, or — 2<br>are you completely unable to manage money? — 1 |
| **6. Can you do your own handyman work**<br>without help, — 3<br>with some help, or — 2<br>are you completely unable to do any handyman work? — 1 | |

From Philadelphia Geriatric Center, Philadelphia, PA. Used with permission.

*Continued*

# I.2 Comprehensive Older Persons' Evaluation

---

Name (print): _____  Date of visit: _____

Chief complaint: _____

---

Today, I will ask you about your overall health and function and will be using a questionnaire to help me obtain this information. The first few questions are to check your memory.

**Preliminary Cognition Questionnaire:** Record if answer is correct with (+); if answer is incorrect with (−).

1. What is the date today? _____
2. What day of the week is it? _____
3. What is the name of this place? _____
4. What is your telephone number or room number?
   Record answer: _____
   If subject does not have phone, ask:
   What is your street address? _____
5. How old are you? Record answer: _____ _____
6. When were you born? Record answer from records if patient cannot answer: _____ _____
7. Who is the president of the United States now? _____

8. Who was the president just before him? _____
9. What was your mother's maiden name? _____
10. Subtract 3 from 20 and keep subtracting from each new number until you get all the way down _____
    Total errors: _____

If more than 4 errors, ask 11. If more than 6 errors, complete questionnaire for informant.

11. Do you think you would benefit from a legal guardian, someone who would be responsible for your legal and financial matters? Do you have a living will? Would you like one?
    a. no
    b. has functioning legal guardian for sole purpose of managing money — describe:
    c. has legal guardian
    d. yes

---

From Pearlman R: Development of a functional assessment questionnaire for geriatric patients: the comprehensive older persons evaluation, J *Chronic Disease* 40(56): 85S-94S, 1987.

### I.2 Comprehensive Older Persons' Evaluation—cont'd

**Demographic Section:**

1. Patient's race or ethnic background—record: _____
2. Patient's gender (circle)    male    female
3. How far did you go in school?
   a. post-graduate education
   b. four-year degree
   c. college or technical school
   d. high school complete
   e. high school incomplete
   f. 0-8 years

**Social Support Section:** Now there are a few questions about your family and friends.

4. Are you married, widowed, separated, divorced, or have you never been married?
   a. now married
   b. widowed
   c. separated
   d. divorced
   e. never married
5. Who lives with you? (circle all responses)
   a. spouse
   b. other relative or friend—specify: _____
   c. group living situation (non-health)
   d. lives alone
   e. nursing home, number of years: _____
6. Have you talked to any friends or relatives by phone during the last week?
   a. yes
   b. no
7. Are you satisfied by seeing your relatives and friends as often as you want to, or are you somewhat dissatisfied about how little you see them?
   a. satisfied—skip to #8
   b. dissatisfied—ask A
      A. Do you feel you would like to be involved in a Senior Citizens Center for social events, or perhaps meals?
         1. no
         2. is involved—describe: _____
         3. yes
8. Is there someone who would take care of you for as long as you needed if you were sick or disabled?
   a. yes—Skip to C
   b. no—Ask A
      A. Is there someone who would take care of you for a short time?
         1. yes—Skip to C
         2. no—Ask B
      B. Is there someone who could help you now and then?
         1. yes—Ask C
         2. no—Ask C
      C. Who would we call in case of an emergency? Record name and telephone: _____

**Financial Section:** The next few questions are about your finances and any problems you might have.

9. Do you own, or are you buying, your own home?
   a. yes—skip to #10
   b. no—ask A
      A. Do you feel you need assistance with housing?
         1. no
         2. has subsidized or other housing assistance
         3. yes—describe: _____
      B. What type of housing did you have prior to coming here?
10. Are you covered by private medical insurance, Medicare, Medicaid, or some disability plan? (Circle all that apply)
    a. private insurance—specify and skip to #11:
       _____
    b. Medicare
    c. Medicaid
    d. disability—specify and ask A:
       _____
    e. none
    f. other—specify: _____
       A. Do you feel you need additional assistance with your medical bills?
          1. no
          2. yes
11. Which of these statements best describes your financial situation?
    a. my bills are no problem to me—skip to #12
    b. my expenses make it difficult to meet my bills—ask A
    c. my expenses are so heavy that I cannot meet my bills—ask A
       A. Do you feel you need financial assistance such as: (circle all that apply)
          1. food stamps
          2. social security or disability payments
          3. assistance in paying your heating or electrical bills
          4. other financial assistance? describe: _____

**Psychological Health Section:** The next few questions are about how you feel about your life in general. There are no right or wrong answers, only what best applies to you. Please answer yes or no to each question.

12. Is your daily life full of things that keep you interested? _____
13. Have you, at times, very much wanted to leave home? _____
14. Does it seem that no one understands you? _____
15. Are you happy most of the time? _____
16. Do you feel weak all over much of the time? _____
17. Is your sleep fitful and disturbed? _____

*Continued.*

I.2   Comprehensive Older Persons' Evaluation—cont'd

18. Taking everything into consideration, how would you describe your satisfaction with your life in general at the present time?
    a. good
    b. fair
    c. poor
19. Do you feel you now need help with your mental health; for example, a counselor or psychiatrist?
    a. no
    b. has—specify: _____
    c. yes

**Physical Health Section:** The next few questions are about your health.

20. During the past month (30 days), how many days were you so sick that you couldn't do your usual activities, such as working around the house or visiting with friends?   _____
21. Relative to other people your age, how would you rate your overall health at the present time?
    a. excellent—skip to #22
    b. very good—skip to #22
    c. good—ask A
    d. fair—ask A
    e. poor—ask A
        A. Do you feel you need additional medical services such as a doctor, nurse, visiting nurse or physical therapy?
            1. doctor
            2. nurse
            3. visiting nurse
            4. physical therapy
            5. none
22. Do you use an aid for walking, such as a wheelchair, walker, cane or anything else? (circle aid usually used)
    a. wheelchair
    b. other—specify: _____
    c. visiting nurse
    d. walker
    e. none
23. How much do your health troubles stand in the way of your doing things you want to do?
    a. not at all—skip to #24
    b. a little—ask A
    c. a great deal—ask A
        A. Do you think you need assistance to do your daily activities; for example, do you need a live-in aide or choreworker?
            1. live-in aide
            2. choreworker
            3. has aide, choreworker or other assistance— describe:_____
            4. none needed

24. Have you had, or do you currently have, any of the following health problems? (if yes, place an "X" in appropriate box and describe; medical record information may be used to help complete this section.)

| | HX | Current | Describe |
|---|---|---|---|
| a. Arthritis or rheumatism? | | | |
| b. Lung or breathing problem? | | | |
| c. Hypertension? | | | |
| d. Heart trouble? | | | |
| e. Phlebitis or poor circulation problems in arms or legs? | | | |
| f. Diabetes or low blood sugar? | | | |
| g. Digestive ulcers? | | | |
| h. Other digestive problem? | | | |
| i. Cancer? | | | |
| j. Anemia? | | | |
| k. Effects of stroke? | | | |
| l. Other neurological problem? specify: _____ | | | |
| m. Thyroid or other glandular problem? specify: _____ | | | |
| n. Skin disorders such as pressure sores, leg ulcers, burns? | | | |
| o. Speech problem? | | | |
| p. Hearing problem? | | | |
| q. Vision or eye problem? | | | |
| r. Kidney or bladder problems, or incontinence? | | | |
| s. A problem of falls? | | | |
| t. Problem with eating or your weight? specify: _____ | | | |
| u. Problem with depression? specify: _____ | | | |
| v. Problem with your behavior? specify: _____ | | | |
| w. Problem with your sexual activity? | | | |
| x. Problem with alcohol? | | | |
| y. Problem with pain? | | | |
| z. Other health problems? specify: _____ | | | |

*Continued.*

I.2   Comprehensive Older Persons' Evaluation—cont'd

Immunizations: _____
_____
_____

25. What medications are you currently taking, or have been taking, in the last month? (May I see your medication bottles?) (If patient cannot list, ask categories a-r and note dosage and schedule, or obtain information from medical or pharmacy records and verify accuracy with the patient.)

Allergies: _____

|  | | Rx (Dosage and Schedule) |
|---|---|---|
| a. | Arthritis medication | _____ |
| b. | Pain medication | _____ |
| c. | Blood pressure medication | _____ |
| d. | Water pills or pills for fluid | _____ |
| e. | Medication for your heart | _____ |
| f. | Medication for your lungs | _____ |
| g. | Blood thinners | _____ |
| h. | Medication for your circulation | _____ |
| i. | Insulin or diabetes medication | _____ |
| j. | Seizure medication | _____ |
| k. | Thyroid pills | _____ |
| l. | Steroids | _____ |
| m. | Hormones | _____ |
| n. | Antibiotics | _____ |
| o. | Medicine for nerves or depression | _____ |
| p. | Prescription sleeping pills | _____ |
| q. | Other prescription drugs | _____ |
| r. | Other nonprescription drugs | _____ |

26. Many people have problems remembering to take their medications, especially ones they need to take on a regular basis. How often do you forget to take your medications? Would you say you forget often, sometimes, rarely, or never?
    a. never
    b. rarely
    c. sometimes
    d. often

**Activities of Daily Living:** The next set of questions asks whether you need help with any of the following activities of daily living.

27. I would like to know whether you can do these activities without any help at all, or if you need assistance to do them. Do you need help to: (If yes, describe, including patient needs.)

|  | | Yes | No | Describe (include needs) |
|---|---|---|---|---|
| a. | Use the telephone? | | | |
| b. | Get to places out of walking distance? (using transportation) | | | |
| c. | Shop for clothes and food? | | | |
| d. | Do your housework? | | | |
| e. | Handle your money? | | | |
| f. | Feed yourself? | | | |
| g. | Dress and undress yourself? | | | |
| h. | Take care of your appearance? | | | |
| i. | Get in and out of bed? | | | |
| j. | Take a bath or shower? | | | |
| k. | Prepare your meals? | | | |
| l. | Do you have any problem getting to the bathroom on time? | | | |

28. During the past six months, have you had any help with such things as shopping, housework, bathing, dressing and getting around?
    a. yes—specify: _____
    b. no

Signature of person completing the form:

_____

# I.3  Comprehensive Occupational and Environmental Health History

## WORK HISTORY

1. List your current and past longest held jobs, including the military:

| COMPANY | DATES EMPLOYED | JOB TITLE | KNOWN EXPOSURES |
|---|---|---|---|
| | | | |
| | | | |
| | | | |

*Continued*

2. Do you work full-time?     NO ___     YES ___     How many hours per week? ___

3. Do you work part-time?     NO ___     YES ___     How many hours per week? ___

4. Please describe any health problems or injuries that you have experienced in connection with your present or past jobs:

5. Have you ever had to change jobs due to health problems or injuries?     YES ___     NO ___
   If yes, describe:

Did any of your co-workers experience similar problems?

6. In what type of business do you currently work?

7. Describe your work (what you actually do):

8. Have you had any current or past exposure (through breathing or touching) to any of the following?

| | | | | |
|---|---|---|---|---|
| __ acids | __ chloroprene | __ phenol | __ beryllium | __ welding fumes |
| __ chlorinated naphthalenes | __ isocyanates | __ trichloroethylene | __ ethylene dibromide | __ carbon tetrachloride |
| __ halothane | __ perchloroethylene | __ asbestos | | ride |
| __ PBBs | __ TDI or MDI | __ cold (severe) | __ methylene chloride | __ fiberglass |
| __ styrene | __ ammonia | __ manganese | | __ noise (loud) |
| __ alcohols | __ chromates | __ phosgene | __ rock dust | __ solvents |
| __ chloroform | __ ketones | __ trinitrotoluene | __ vinyl chloride | __ x-rays |
| __ heat (severe) | __ pesticides | __ benzene | __ cadmium | |
| __ PCBs | __ toluene | __ dichlorobenzene | __ ethylene dichloride | |
| __ talc | __ arsenic | __ mercury | __ nickel | |
| __ alkalis | __ coal dust | __ radiation | __ silica powder | |
| | __ lead | __ vibration | | |

9. Did you receive any safety training about these agents? YES ___     NO ___

   Explain:

10. Are you involved in any work processes such as grinding, welding, soldering, or polishing that create dust, mists, or fumes? YES ___     NO ___
    If yes, describe:

11. Did you use any of the following personal protective equipment when exposed?

| | | |
|---|---|---|
| ___ boots | ___ respirator | ___ welding mask |
| ___ gloves | ___ sleeves | ___ glasses/goggles |
| ___ shield | ___ earplugs/muffs | |
| ___ coveralls | ___ safety shoes | |

12. Is your work environment generally clean? YES __ NO __
    If no, describe:

13. What ventilation systems are used in your workplace?

14. Do they seem to work? Are you aware of any chemical odors in your environment?
    If so, explain:

15. Where do you eat, smoke, and take your breaks when you are on the job?

16. Do you use a uniform or have clothing that you wear only to work? YES __ NO __

17. How is your work clothing laundered (at home, by employer, etc.)?

18. How often do you wash your hands at work and how do you wash them? (running water, special soaps, etc.)

19. Do you shower before leaving the work site? YES __ NO __

20. Do you have any physical symptoms associated with work? YES __ NO __
    If yes, describe:

21. Are other workers similarly affected? YES __ NO __

## HOME EXPOSURES

1. Which of the following do you have in your home?
   __ air-conditioner __ fireplace __ electric stove
   __ central heating (gas or oil?) __ air purifier __ woodstove

2. In approximately what year was your home built?

3. Have there been any recent renovations? YES __ NO __
   If yes, describe:

4. Have you recently installed new carpet, bought new furniture, or refinished existing furniture? YES __ NO __
   If yes, explain:

5. Do you use pesticides around your home or garden? YES __ NO __
   If yes, describe:

6. What household cleaners do you use? (List most common and any new products you use.)

7. List all hobbies done at your home:

*Continued*

8. Are any of the agents listed earlier for work exposures encountered in hobbies or recreational activities?
   YES __    NO __

9. Is any special protective equipment or ventilation used during hobbies? YES __    NO __ If yes, explain:

10. What are the occupations of other household members?

11. Do other household members have contact with any form of chemicals at work or during leisure activities?
    YES __    NO __
    If yes, explain:

12. Is anyone else in your home environment having symptoms similar to yours? YES __    NO __
    If yes, explain briefly:

## COMMUNITY EXPOSURES

1. Are any of the following located in your community?
   __ industrial plant       __ major source of air pollution      __ waste site
   __ landfill               __ toxic spill                        __ other_____

2. What is your source of drinking water?
   __ private well           __ public water source                __ other

3. Are neighbors experiencing any health problems similar to yours?   YES __    NO____
   If yes, explain:

## KEY OCCUPATIONAL AND ENVIRONMENTAL HEALTH QUESTIONS TO BE ASKED WITH ALL HISTORIES

1. What are your current and past longest held jobs?

2. Have you been exposed to any radiation or chemical liquids, dusts, mists, or fumes? YES __    NO __

3. Is there any relationship between current symptoms and activities at work or at home? YES __    NO __

From Pope AM, Snyder MA, Mood LH, editors: Nursing, health, and environment: strengthening the relationship to improve the public's health, *Washington, DC, 1995, National Academy Press.*

# Appendix J

## Essential Elements of Public Health Nursing

### J.1 Examples of Public Health Nursing Roles and Implementing Public Health Functions

This document is intended to clearly present the role of public health nurses in Virginia as members of the multidisciplinary public health team in a changing health care environment. The following matrices present the role of public health nursing in Virginia. The following definitions were used to develop these matrices.

Essential Element is taken from the National Association of City and County Health Officials' (NACCHO) Document "Blueprint for a Healthy Community." The following public health essential elements are used as a framework to present the role of public health nursing in Virginia:
• Conducting Community Assessments
• Preventing and Controlling Epidemics
• Providing a Safe and Healthy Environment
• Measuring Performance, Effectiveness, and Outcomes of Health Services
• Promoting Healthy Lifestyles

From National Association of City and County Health Officials: Blueprint for a healthy community: a guide for local health departments, Washington, DC, 1994, The Association.

• Providing Targeted Outreach and Forming Partnerships
• Providing Personal Health Care Services
• Conducting Research and Innovation
• Mobilizing the Community for Action

**Public Health Function** is defined as a broad public health activity needed to ensure a strong, flexible, accountable public health structure. It may require a multidisciplinary team to carry out.

**Public Health Nurse Role** is the activity the public health nurse is responsible for, either alone or as a member of a team, to accomplish the stated public health function. This can be the public health nurse at the local level or at the state level.

**State Role** is what public health nurses need from the state level to do their jobs (e.g., policy, aggregate data, training). This refers to any Central Office program or staff, not just nurses.

A process was implemented that would involve all public health nurses in Virginia. Although this lengthened the timeline to completion, it will ensure that the final document represents a consensus developed through creative open dialogue.

**ESSENTIAL ELEMENT 1: Conduct Community Assessment**—Systematically collect, assemble, analyze, and make available health-related data for the purpose of identifying and responding to community and state level public health concerns and conducting epidemiologic and other population-based studies.

| PUBLIC HEALTH FUNCTION | PHN ROLES | STATE ROLES |
|---|---|---|
| Develop frameworks, methodologies, and tools for standardizing data collection and analysis and reporting across all jurisdictions and providers. | • Provide, review, and comment on proposed methodologies and tools for data collection.<br>• Field test tools and methods. | • Collaborate with professional organizations and academic and governmental institutions to develop and test tools and methods.<br>• Provide educational opportunities in areas of and use of tools.<br>• Work with local level agencies to standardize definitions, data collected, etc. across jurisdictions and amongst all stakeholders (schools, community-based organizations, and private providers). |

## ESSENTIAL ELEMENT 1: Conduct Community Assessment—cont'd

| PUBLIC HEALTH FUNCTION | PHN ROLES | STATE ROLES |
|---|---|---|
| Collect and analyze data. | • Collaborate with the community to identify population-based needs and gaps in service.<br>• Analyze data and needs, knowledge, attitudes, and practices of specific populations.<br>• Identify patterns of diseases; illness and injury and develop or stimulate development of programs to respond to identified trends. | • Provide aggregated data to the local level in a timely and accurate manner.<br>• Provide census tract-level aggregated data to the local level.<br>• Provide national and state comparisons to be used with local data to obtain trends and assist localities in documenting need, progress, etc. to attain standard outcomes. |

## ESSENTIAL ELEMENT 2: Preventing and Controlling Epidemics—Monitoring disease trends and investigating and containing diseases and injuries.

| PUBLIC HEALTH FUNCTION | PHN ROLES | STATE ROLES |
|---|---|---|
| Develop programs that prevent, contain, and control the transmission of diseases and danger of injuries (including violence). | • Provide community-wide preventive measures in the form of health education and mobilization of community resources.<br>• Ensure isolation/containment measures when necessary.<br>• Ensure adequate preventive immunizations.<br>• Implement programs that control the transmission of diseases and danger of injuries during disasters. | • Work with local jurisdictions to develop tools such as videos, PSAs, and/or posters that local jurisdictions can use.<br>• Work with local jurisdictions to develop disaster plans for the control of the transmission of diseases and danger of injuries during disasters.<br>• Facilitate state-level partnerships that promote health, healthy lifestyles, and wellness (individual and family). |
| Develop regulatory guidelines for the prevention of targeted diseases. | • Implement regulatory measures.<br>• Implement OSHA Guidelines for Blood borne Pathogens and the Prevention of the Transmission of TB in Health Care Settings. | • In partnership with localities, develop regulatory guidelines.<br>• Serve as clearinghouse or source of information. |

## ESSENTIAL ELEMENT 3: Providing a Safe and Healthy Environment—Maintaining clean and safe air, water, food, and facilities both in the community and the home environment.

| PUBLIC HEALTH FUNCTION | PHN ROLES | STATE ROLES |
|---|---|---|
| Develop methods/tools for collection and analysis of health-related data (occurrence of mortality and morbidity relating to both communicable and chronic diseases, injury registries, sentinel event establishment, environmental quality, etc.). | • Provide reporting guidelines and consultation regarding disease prevention, diagnosis, treatment, and follow-up of cases/contacts to physicians and institutions (emergency department, university and secondary school student health, prisons, industries, etc.).<br>• Conduct/participate in community needs assessments to determine customer/provider knowledge deficits and perceptions of need.<br>• Provide education to individuals, providers, targeted populations, etc., in response to knowledge deficits, disease outbreaks, toxic waste emissions, etc.<br>• Provide individual follow-up/case management of communicable diseases that are transmitted by air, water, food and fomites (TB, hepatitis A, salmonella, and staphylococcus, etc.). | • Develop standard methodology and tools for collection and analysis of health-related data.<br>• Provide training in area of data collection and analysis.<br>• Evaluate activities and outcomes of interactions.<br>• Work in partnership with localities to develop program based on data analysis needs. |

**ESSENTIAL ELEMENT 3: Providing a Safe and Healthy Environment—cont'd**

| PUBLIC HEALTH FUNCTION | PHN ROLES | STATE ROLES |
| --- | --- | --- |
| Develop programs that promote a safe environment in the home. | • Provide childhood lead poisoning screenings and follow-up.<br>• Teach clients to inspect homes for safety violations and toxic substances and to practice safe behaviors; assist families to access/use available resources/safety devices.<br>• Assess/teach regarding safe food selection, preparation, and storage.<br>• Train/supervise volunteers/auxiliary personnel in performance of the above tasks<br>• Teach families that all men, women, and children have a right to a safe environment free of physical or mental abuse. | • Provide consultation and technical assistance to state/local organizations regarding laws and regulations that protect health and ensure safety.<br>• In partnership with localities, develop and evaluate educational programs. |
| Develop programs that promote a safe environment in the workplace. | • Provide consultation in implementation of OSHA regulations relating to occupational exposure to diseases.<br>• Provide educational program related to healthy lifestyles (smoking cessation, back protection, etc).<br>• Ensure provision of screenings for individuals to determine baselines and occurrence of infectious diseases and preventable deterioration of health and function: hearing, back soundness, lung capacity, RMS indicators, PPDs, etc.<br>• Assist in policy/practice development to address prevention of the above.<br>• Provide immunizations. | • Monitor and assist localities to implement prevention activities.<br>• Assist localities in developing and evaluating educational programs.<br>• Monitor outcomes of screening activities and evaluate interventions. |
| Develop programs that promote a safe environment in the school setting. | • Provide consultation on implementation of OSHA regulations relating to occupational exposure to diseases.<br>• Provide educational programs related to healthy lifestyles (smoking cessation, etc.).<br>• Ensure provision of screenings for students to determine baselines and occurrence of infectious disease and preventable deterioration of health and function.<br>• Assist in policy/practice development to address prevention of the above.<br>• Provide immunizations. | • Develop guidelines that ensure accountability in meeting standards set forth.<br>• Ensure that policy is developed to protect children in the school environment.<br>• Monitor immunization status of children and provide immunizations during outbreaks and evaluate activities. |
| Develop programs that promote a safe environment in the community. | • Identify population clusters exhibiting an unhealthy environment; provide consultation/group education regarding preventive measures.<br>• Participate in development of local disaster plans to ensure provision of safe water, food, air, and facilities.<br>• Respond in time of natural disasters such as floods, tornadoes, hurricanes.<br>• Participate in developing plans for shelter management during disasters, especially "Special Needs" shelters that may require nursing staff. | • In times of disaster, facilitate availability of resources across jurisdictions.<br>• Have a statewide plan.<br>• Ensure that localities have developed plans to protect the public in time of national and/or other disasters.<br>• Coordinate efforts statewide.<br>• Assist localities in responding.<br>• Evaluate efforts. |

*Continued*

## ESSENTIAL ELEMENT 3: Providing a Safe and Healthy Environment—cont'd

| PUBLIC HEALTH FUNCTION | PHN ROLES | STATE ROLES |
|---|---|---|
| Develop and issue standards that guide regulations, mandate, policy, and program development.<br>Develop protocols to ensure accountability of all health care providers, public and private.<br>Provide inservice training to all providers of health care services. | • Survey work sites, schools, institutions, etc. for compliance to regulations that protect health and ensure safety.<br>• Provide technical assistance, that is, interpretation, implementation, and evaluation processes.<br>• Share and implement knowledge gained in inservice training. | • Develop a systematic evaluation tool for collection of data to measure trends.<br>• Assist localities in developing standards to mandate accountability.<br>• Provide consultation/technical assistance to localities. |

## ESSENTIAL ELEMENT 4: Measuring Performance, Effectiveness, and Outcomes of Health Services—Monitoring health care providers and the health care system to identify gaps in service, deteriorating health status indicators, effectiveness of interventions, and accessibility and quality of personal and population-wide health services.

| PUBLIC HEALTH FUNCTION | PHN ROLES | STATE ROLES |
|---|---|---|
| Promote competency in public health issues throughout the health delivery system. | • Provide educational and technical assistance in areas such as case management and appropriate treatment and control of communicable diseases to the community. | • Develop appropriate regulatory, educational and technical assistance programs.<br>• Provide technical assistance and training to local health department for local forecasting and interpretation of data. |
| Collect data. | • Participate in data collection with a target population.<br>• Ensure that the data collection system supports the objectives of programs serving the community by participating in the design and operation of data collection systems.<br>• Collect data via surveys, polls, interviews, focus groups that will enable assessment of the community's perception of health status and understanding how the system works and how to obtain needs service. | • Work with localities (health districts, private providers, other state and local agencies) to develop standard data elements and definitions across jurisdictions and among all stakeholders, especially for consistency in coding of population-based data.<br>• Identify data collection and analytic issues related to monitoring the impact of health system changes such as costs and benefits of record linkage, strategies for ensuring confidentiality, and strategies for analyzing trends in health within a broader social and economic context.<br>• Advocate for uniform data collection from all managed care plans so that outcomes and health trends can be analyzed and tracked and sentinel events reported. |
| Analyze data to ensure accurate diagnosis of health status, identification of threats to health, and assessment of health service needs. | • Participate in a systematic approach to convert data into information that will identify gaps in service at the local and state level and will lead to action.<br>• Monitor health status indicators to identify emerging problems and facilitate community-wide response to identified problems.<br>• Facilitate data analysis as part of a local collaborative effort. | • Develop a systematic, integrated statewide approach to converting data into information that directs action.<br>• Ensure that resources, such as hardware and software to analyze data are available at the local level.<br>• Work with localities (health districts, private providers, other state and local agencies) to address issues related to variable access to technology, confidentiality issues.<br>• Educate and train currently employed public health nurses in areas of epidemiology and population-based services. |

| PUBLIC HEALTH FUNCTION | PHN ROLES | STATE ROLES |
| --- | --- | --- |
| Monitor health status indicators for the entire population and for specific population groups and/or geographic areas. | • Identify target populations that may be at risk for public health problems such as communicable diseases, unidentified and untreated chronic diseases.<br>• Conduct surveys or observe targeted populations such as preschools, child-care centers, high-risk census tracks to identify health status.<br>• Monitor health care utilization of vulnerable populations at the local and regional level. | • Develop methodology for identification, measurement, and analysis of key indicators of health care utilization of vulnerable populations. |
| Monitor and assess availability, cost-effectiveness, and outcomes of personal and population-based health services. | • Identify gaps in services (e.g., a neighborhood with deteriorating immunization rates may indicate lack of available primary care services).<br>• Ensure that all receive the same quality of care, including comprehensive preventive services.<br>• Monitor the impact of health system reforms on vulnerable populations.<br>• Evaluate the effectiveness and outcomes of care.<br>• Plan interventions based on the health of the overall population, not just for those in the health care system.<br>• Identify interventions that are effective and replicable. | • Develop analyses that demonstrate the cost effectiveness of investment in public health services.<br>• Develop protocols and technical assistance for ensuring accountability of Medicaid-managed care plans and other government-funded plans for service delivery and overall health status of their covered populations.<br>• Identify standard theoretical, methodological, and measurement issues that are specific to population subgroups for monitoring the impact of health system changes on vulnerable populations. |
| Disseminate information. | • Disseminate information to the public on community health status, including how to access and use services appropriately.<br>• Disseminate information to other health care providers regarding gaps in services or deteriorating health status indicators. | • Ensure a mechanism for public accountability of performance and outcomes through public dissemination of information and in particular ensure that underservice, a risk inherent in capitated plans, is measurable through available data.<br>• Ensure that information is provided to communities, local health departments, managed care plans, and other appropriate state agencies. |

**ESSENTIAL ELEMENT 5: Promoting Healthy Lifestyle**—Providing health education to individuals, families, and communities.

| PUBLIC HEALTH FUNCTION | PHN ROLES | STATE ROLES |
| --- | --- | --- |
| Promote informed decision making of residents about things that influence their health on a daily basis. | • Exert influence through contact with individuals and community groups.<br>• Accept and issue challenge of healthy lifestyles to all contacts.<br>• Reinforce and reward positive informed decisions made for healthy lifestyles. | • Develop and monitor standards or the changes to determine changes in behavior. |
| Promote effective use of media to encourage both personal and community responsibility for informed decision making. | • Be a resource for the community.<br>• Gather data and address findings as appropriate.<br>• Work with community groups to promote accurate information for healthy lifestyle through the media.<br>• Utilize current information and other agencies' resources to maximize information accessible to public. | • Assist localities to provide current information to community organizations and other state organizations.<br>• Serve as a resource for localities and work with media. |

## ESSENTIAL ELEMENT 5: Promoting Healthy Lifestyle—cont'd

| PUBLIC HEALTH FUNCTION | PHN ROLES | STATE ROLES |
|---|---|---|
| Develop a public awareness/marketing campaign to demonstrate the importance of public health to overall health improvement and its proper place in the health delivery system.<br><br>Develop public information and education systems/programs through partnerships. | • Provide education to special groups, for example, local politicians, school boards, PTAs, churches, civic groups, news media and regarding the benefits of preventive health.<br><br>• Provide educational sessions/ programs to public regarding components of healthy lifestyles.<br>• Access grants/other funding sources to promote healthy lifestyle decisions; (e.g., cervical and breast cancer prevention; bike helmets, hypertension).<br>• Provide/promote teaching for individual and families at every opportunity (home, clinic, community settings). | • Develop training activities to assist localities in marketing.<br><br>• Assist localities in developing and evaluating educational programs.<br>• Assist localities in funding.<br>• Hold regional/state training sessions.<br>• Evaluate outcomes and plan ongoing educational systems/program. |

## ESSENTIAL ELEMENT 6: Providing Targeted Outreach and Forming Partnerships—Ensuring access to services, including those that lead to self-sufficiency, for all vulnerable populations and ensuring the development of culturally appropriate care.

| PUBLIC HEALTH FUNCTION | PHN ROLES | STATE ROLES |
|---|---|---|
| Ensure accessibility to health services that will improve morbidity, decrease mortality, and improve health status outcomes. | • Provide family-centered case management services for high-risk and hard-to-reach populations that focus on linking families with needed services.<br>• Improve access to care by forming partnerships with appropriate community individuals and entities.<br>• Increase influence of cultural diversity on system design and on access to care, as well as on individual services rendered.<br>• Ensure that translation services are available for the non–English speaking population.<br>• Participate in ongoing community assessment to identify areas of concern and above needs for rules.<br>• Provide outreach services that focus on preventing epidemics and the spread of disease, such as tuberculosis and sexually transmitted diseases. | • Provide funds in cooperation with locality.<br>• Ensure policy development that includes case management and is culturally sensitive.<br>• Provide adequate ongoing continuing education for staff (especially in areas common to all localities).<br>• Participate in state-level contract development to ensure that contracts with health plans require and include incentives for health plans to offer and deliver preventive health services in the minimum benefits package.<br>• Educate financing officials about the roles of public health both in performing core public health services and in ensuring access to personal health services. |

## ESSENTIAL ELEMENT 7: Providing Personal Health Care Services—Provide targeted direct services to high-risk populations.

| PUBLIC HEALTH FUNCTION | PHN ROLES | STATE ROLES |
|---|---|---|
| Provide direct services for specific diseases that threaten the health of the community and develop programs that prevent, contain, and control the transmission of infectious diseases. | • Plan, develop, implement, and evaluate:<br>  • Sexually transmitted disease services<br>  • Communicable disease services<br>  • HIV/AIDS services<br>  • Tuberculosis control services<br>• Develop and implement guidelines for the prevention of the above targeted diseases. | • Establish standards/criteria for personal health care.<br>• Work with local health departments to assist in developing infrastructure and management techniques to facilitate record-keeping and appropriate financial monitoring and tracking systems, which enable local health departments to enter into contractual arrangements for preventive health and primary care services. |

| PUBLIC HEALTH FUNCTION | PHN ROLES | STATE ROLES |
|---|---|---|
| Provide health services, including preventive health services, to high-risk and vulnerable populations (e.g., the uninsured working poor), and in geographic areas where primary health care services are not readily accessible or available in a privatized setting. | •• Provide coordination, follow-up, referral, and case management as indicated.<br>• Integrate supportive services, such as counseling, social work, nutrition, into primary care services.<br>• Assess existing community medical capacity for referral and follow-up. | • Continue to work at the state and local level to build primary and preventive health services capacity, particularly in traditionally underserved areas, to ensure availability to providers and primary care sites essential to primary care access. |

**ESSENTIAL ELEMENT 8: Conducting Research and Innovation**–Discovering and applying improved health care delivery mechanisms and clinical interventions.

| PUBLIC HEALTH FUNCTION | PHN ROLES | STATE ROLES |
|---|---|---|
| Ensure ongoing prevention research relating to biomedical and behavioral aspects of health promotion and prevention of disease and injury. | • Develop outcome measures.<br>• Identify research priorities for target communities and develop and conduct scientific and operations research for health promotion and disease/injury prevention. | • Provide training in area of measuring program effectiveness. |
| Implement pilot or demonstration projects. | • Develop and implement linkages with academic centers, ensuring that clients and populations who participate in research projects benefit as a result of the research. | • Support evaluations and research that demonstrate the benefits of public health, as well as the consequences of failure to support public health interventions. |

**ESSENTIAL ELEMENT 9: Mobilizing the Community for Action**–Providing leadership and initiating collaboration.

| PUBLIC HEALTH FUNCTION | PHN ROLES | STATE ROLES |
|---|---|---|
| Provide leadership to stimulate development of networks or partnerships that will ensure the availability of comprehensive primary health care services to all regardless of ability to pay.<br><br>Initiate collaboration with other community organizations to ensure the leadership role in resolving a public health issue. | • Advocate for improved health.<br>• Disseminate of health information.<br>• Build coalitions.<br>• Make recommendations for policy implementation or revision.<br>• Facilitate resources that manage environmental risk and maintain and improve community health.<br>• Provide information for a community group working on impacting policy at the local, state, or federal level.<br>• Use results of community health assessments to stimulate the community to develop a plan to respond to identified gaps in service. | • Facilitate the establishment and enhancement of statewide high-quality, needed health services.<br>• Administer quality improvement programs.<br>• Use information-gathering techniques of assessment to assist policy/legislature activities to develop needed health services and functions that require statewide action or standards.<br>• Recommend programs to carry out policies. |

# J.2 Public Health Guidelines for Practice

## AMERICAN PUBLIC HEALTH ASSOCIATION DEFINITION OF PUBLIC HEALTH NURSING

Public health nursing is a systematic process by which:
1. The health and health care needs of a population are assessed in order to identify subpopulations, families, and individuals who would benefit from health promotion or who are at risk of illness, injury, disability, or premature death.
2. A plan for intervention is developed with the community to meet identified needs that takes into account available resources, the range of activities that contribute to health, and the prevention of illness, injury, disability, and premature death.
3. The plan is implemented effectively, efficiently, and equitably.
4. Evaluations are conducted to determine the extent to which the interventions have an impact on the health status of individuals and the population.
5. The results of the process are used to influence and direct the current delivery of care, deployment of

*From American Public Health Association:* The definition and role of public health nursing: a statement of APHA Public Health Nursing Section, *Washington, DC, 1996, The Association.*

health resources, and the development of local, regional, state, and national health policy and research to promote health and prevent disease.

This systematic process for public health nursing practice is based on and is consistent with (1) community strengths, needs, and expectations; (2) current scientific knowledge; (3) available resources, (4) accepted criteria and standards of nursing practice, (5) agency purpose, philosophy, and objectives, and (6) the participation, cooperation, and understanding of the population. Other services and organizations in the community are considered and planning is coordinated to maximize the effective use of resources and enhance outcomes.

The title "public health nurse" designates a nursing professional with educational preparation in public health and nursing science with a primary focus on population-level outcomes.

## Examples of activities of public health nurses

The activities of public health nurses include the following:

1. They provide essential input to interdisciplinary programs that monitor, anticipate, and respond to public health problems in population groups, regardless of which disease or public health threat is identified.
2. They evaluate health trends and risk factors of population groups and help determine priorities for targeted interventions.
3. They work with communities or specific population groups within the community to develop public policy and targeted health promotion and disease prevention activities.
4. They participate in assessing and evaluating health care services to ensure that people are informed of programs and services available and are assisted in the use of available services.
5. They provide health education, care management, and primary care to individuals and families who are members of vulnerable populations and high-risk groups.

## AMERICAN NURSES ASSOCIATION STANDARDS OF PUBLIC HEALTH NURSING PRACTICE

### Standards of care

**Standard I. Assessment:** The public health nurse assesses the health status of populations using data, community resources identification, input from the population, and professional judgment.

**Standard II. Diagnosis:** The public health nurse analyzes collected assessment data and partners with the people to attach meaning to that data and determine opportunities and needs.

**Standard III. Outcome Identification:** The public health nurse participates with other community partners to identify expected outcomes in the populations and their health status.

**Standard IV. Planning:** The public health nurse promotes and supports the development of programs, policies, and services that provide interventions that improve the health status of populations.

**Standard V. Assurance: Action Component of the Nursing Process for Public Health Nursing:** The public health nurse ensures access and availability of programs, policies, resources, and services to the population.

**Standard VI. Evaluation:** The public health nurse evaluates the health status of the population.

### Standards of professional performance

**Standard I. Quality of Care:** The public health nurse systematically evaluates the availability, accessibility, acceptability, quality, and effectiveness of nursing practice for the population.

**Standard II. Performance Appraisal:** The public health nurse evaluates his or her own nursing practice in relation to professional practice standards and relevant statutes and regulations.

**Standard III. Education:** The public health nurse acquires and maintains current knowledge and competency in public health nursing practice.

**Standard IV. Collegiality:** The public health nurse establishes collegial partnerships while interacting with health care practitioners and others and contributes to the professional development of peers, colleagues, and others.

**Standard V. Ethics:** The public health nurse applies ethical standards in advocating for health and social policy and delivery of public health programs to promote and preserve the health of the population.

**Standard VI. Collaboration:** The public health nurse collaborates with the representatives of the population and other health and human service professionals and organizations in providing for and promoting the health of the population.

**Standard VII. Research:** The public health nurse uses research findings in practice.

**Standard VIII. Resource Utilization:** The public health nurse considers safety, effectiveness, and cost in the planning and delivery of public health services when using available resources to ensure the maximum possible health benefit to the population.

*From American Nurses Association:* Scope and standards of public health nursing practice, *Washington DC, 1999, American Nurses Publishing.*

# J.3 Quad Council Public Health Nursing Core Competencies and Skill Levels

The Quad Council of Public Health Nursing Organizations is an alliance of the four national nursing organizations that address public health nursing issues: the Association of Community Health Nurse Educators (ACHNE), the American Nurses Association's Congress on Nursing Practice and Economics (ANA), the American Public Health Association–Public Health Nursing Section (APHA), and the Association of State and Territorial Directors of Nursing (ASTDN). In 2000, prompted in part by work on educating the public health workforce being done under the leadership of the Centers for Disease Control (CDC), the Quad Council began the development of a set of national public health nursing competencies.

The approach utilized by the Quad Council was to start with the Council on Linkages between Academia and Public Health Practice (COL) "Core Competencies for Public Health Professionals" and to determine their application to two levels of public health nursing practice: the staff nurse/generalist role and the manager/specialist/consultant role.

The "Quad Council PHN Competencies" document is designed for use with other documents. It complements the "Definition of Public Health Nursing" adopted by the APHA's Public Health Nursing Section in 1996 and the *Scope and Standards of Public Health Nursing* (Quad Council, 2000). Differentiating PHN competencies at the generalist and specialist levels will help to clarify the PHN specialty for both the discipline of nursing and the profession of public health. In addition, the ability to identify PHN competencies should facilitate collaboration among public health nurses and other public health professionals in education, practice, and research in order to improve the public's health.

In developing the competencies the Quad Council members concurred that the generalist level would reflect preparation at the baccalaureate level.

Further, the specialist level competencies described in this document reflect preparation at the master's level in community/public health nursing and/or public health.

The Quad Council determined that, although the Council on Linkages competencies were developed with the understanding that public health practice is population focused and public health nursing is also population focused, one of the unique contributions of public health nurses is the ability to apply these principles at the individual and family level *within the context of population-focused practice*.

These competencies can be found through the WebLinks on this book's evolve website at http://evolve.elsevier.com/Stanhope.

# Index

## A

Abbottsford & Schuylkill Falls Family
 Practice and Counseling Centers,
 mission and goals of, 418b
Aberdeen, Countess of, 36
Aboriginal population. *See also* Native
 Americans
Canadian, poverty of, 780
Abortion
 adolescents and, 810, 811b, 813, 815
 spontaneous, herpes simplex 2 infection and, 943
 women's right to, 654
Abuse. *See also* Child abuse; Family violence; Older adult abuse
 adolescent victims of, 809
 attitudes toward, 895
 development of patterns of, 881-882
 homicide and, 887
 intrafamilial, 606-607
 legal issues involving, 463
 of older adults, 709, 841. *See also*
 Older adult abuse and neglect
 of physically compromised individuals, 730-731
 factors affecting, 731f
 of prison population, 895-896
 of women with disabilities, 671
Academic nursing centers, 416-417
Acceptant intervention mode, 1020, 1021t
Access for physically compromised individuals, 729
Accidents
 children/adolescents in, 633-636
 male involvement in, 690-691
 nonfatal, for men, 690-691
 prevention of, client education about, 300
Accommodating, defined, 461b
Accommodation, Piaget's definition of, 626
Accountability
 in Canada, 140-141
 individual, 519
Accreditation
 defined, 522
 of home health care agencies, 978-979
Acetaminophen, water pollution by, 233
Acquired immunodeficiency syndrome.
 *See* AIDS
Action on Smoking and Health, contact
 information for, 869b
Action research, defined, 286
Active voice, use of, 303b
Activities of daily living, difficulty with,
 for physically compromised
 clients, 701, 723, 725
Acupuncture
 auricular, for treating drug withdrawal,
 866
 for children, 642
 theory of, 708b
ADA. *See* Americans with Disabilities
 Act
Addiction treatment, 867-868
Addicts, attitudes toward, 851
Administration. *See also* Community-oriented nurse manager
 advanced practice nurse roles in, 996
Adolescent health. *See* Child and adolescent health
Adolescent period, defined, 623

Adolescents
 abortion and, 810, 811, 811b, 813,
 815
 assessment of, 623-624, 624t
 ATOD risk of, 864
 causes of mortality in, 808
 as clients, 809-810
 coercive sex among, 813-814
 communicating with, 624
 confidentiality and, 634
 female, poverty and, 779
 health care of, 808-809
 health guidance for parents of, 623b
 homeless, health problems of, 786-789
 increasing resiliency of, strategies for,
 861
 injuries/accidents of, 634
 male, paternity and, 814-815
 migrant, 800-801
 in motor vehicle accidents, 692
 nutritional assessment in, 630
 physically compromised, 724-725
 pregnant. *See* Teen pregnancy
 seeking to become pregnant, 810
 sexual activity of
 in Canada, 816-817
 influences on, 813-814
 trends in, 810-811
 sexual victimization of, 813-814
 suicide prevention for, 1057
 tobacco use by, 639
 treatment of, without parental consent, 634
 vulnerable, evidence-based interventions for, 765b
Adoption
 adolescent peer attitudes toward, 813
 pregnant teenager and, 815, 818b
Adult Children of Alcoholics, 868
Adult day health, 710-711
Adults
 mental health of, Healthy People
 2010 objectives for, 840
 physically compromised. *See also*
 Physically compromised client
 community resources and, 729
 families of, 728
Advance medical directives, 709, 981-982
Advanced Dispensing System for prescription drugs, 867
Advanced nurse practitioner
 collaborative practice of, 1003
 liability of, 1003
 Medicaid reimbursement of, 1001-1002
 professional isolation of, 1002-1003
 professional responsibilities of, 1003
Advanced practice nurse, 990-1007
 in Canada, 998-999
 with child health specialization, 1045-1046
 as clinician, 993-995
 credentialing of, 992-993
 educational preparation of, 992
 in health and wellness centers, 415
 historical perspective on, 990-992
 institutional privileges of, 1002
 legal status of, 1001
 Medicare reimbursement of, 184
 in nursing centers, 427t
 practice application for, 1004

Advanced practice nurse—cont'd
 practice arenas for, 996-1001
 reimbursement of, 1001-1002
 role stress of, 1002-1003
 roles of, 993-996
 title protection legislation for, 186
Advanced practice nursing
 key points, 1004-1005
 trends in, 1003-1004
Advocacy. *See also* Consumer advocacy
 allocation and, 460
 in case management, 456-459
 components of, 143-144
 conceptual framework for, 144
 defined, 132b, 143
 for environmental health, 243-244
 ethical principles for, 145b
 ethics and, 143-145
 impact of, 460
 for men's health, 694
 for migrant farmworkers, 803
 nursing, 188-189
 *versus* nursing process, 459t
 practical framework for, 145
 process of, 457-459
 skill development in, 459-460
 skills required for, 456-457
AFDC. *See* Temporary Assistance for
 Needy Families
Affective disorders, 827-828
Affective domain, 301
 *versus* cognitive domain, 301t
Affirming, characteristics of, 458-459
Afghanistan
 health care problems in, 74
 war impacts in, 82
African Americans
 community services use by, 158
 cultural attitudes/practices of, 162t
 environmental control perspectives
 of, 165
 food preferences and nutrition-related
 risk factors of, 167t
 health indicators for, 269
 infant mortality rate for, 269
 mental health of, 842-844, 843b
 as percentage of U. S. population, 53
 in rural areas, health needs/problems
 of, 383t
African-American children
 injuries to, 633
 poverty and, 779, 779t
African-American nurses, 32-33
African-American women
 breast cancer in, 656-657, 667
 cancer in, mortality from, 666
 cardiovascular disease in, 664
 causes of death among, 659t-660t
 cigarette smoking by, 666-667
 colorectal cancer in, 667
 as heads-of-households, poverty of, 671
 overweight, 667
 prison/jail rate of, 670
 Sister to Sister program for, 750
African-Americans
 smoking-attributable morbidity and
 mortality in, 856
 social organization of, 164
 stereotyping of, 159
 time values of, 164
Age, teaching strategies and, 306-307
Ageism, defined, 703

Agencies, organically structured, 1016
Agency for Healthcare Research and
 Quality, 62, 177
 website for, 715
Agency report cards, 1011
Agency survey, definition, advantages/
 disadvantages of, 495t
Agent-host-environment interaction,
 261, 261f, 262b
Aggregate, defined, 10
Aging
 five Is of, 709
 influences on, 704-706
 myths of, 703
 theories of, 703-704
 biological, 703-704
 developmental, 704
 psychosocial, 704
Agriculture, health risks in, 382-383
Aid to Families of Dependent Children.
 *See also* Temporary Assistance for
 Needy Families
 immigrant eligibility for, 149
AIDS, 23, 74, 254, 903-904
 adult cases of, by exposure category,
 935f
 case management program for, 455
 children with, in schools, 1061
 defined, 934-935
 drug use and, in Canada, 853
 economic costs of, 933
 epidemiology and control of, 88-89
 in homeless persons, 786
 parasitic opportunistic infections associated with, 927
 political/social impact of, 932
 practice application for, 697
 prevention and control of, by PAHO,
 80
 risk management of, in Canada, 948
 in rural areas, 379
 social quarantine rejected for, 179
 in women, 667-668, 667t
 in women of childbearing age, 667-668
AIDS Drug Assistance Programs, 933
Aikenhead, Mary, 25
Air pollutants, child exposure to, 640
Air quality
 assessment of, 229-233, 232b
 criteria pollutants in, 232b
 indoor, assessment of, 229
 in schools, 1058, 1059f
Alameda County study, 330
Al-Anon, 868
Alateen, 868
Alcohol
 blood levels of, 854, 855f
 driving under the influence of,
 Canadian statistics on, 852
 physiologic effects of, 854
 tobacco, and other drug use, 848-873.
 *See also* Alcohol abuse; Drug
 abuse; Psychoactive drugs;
 Substance abuse; specific substances
Alcohol abuse
 addiction treatment for, 867-868
 assessment for, 863-864
 attitudes toward, 850-851
 biopsychosocial model of, 860
 brief interventions for, 868-869
 in Canada, 852-853

Alcohol abuse–cont'd
codependency and family involvement in, 865-866
criminal justice *versus* harm reduction models of, 851
definitions of, 851-854
detoxification and, 866-867
education about, 851
emotional reasons for, 850
enabling of, 866
evidence-based practice for, 856
4 H's of, 863
groups at risk for, 864-865
Healthy People 2010 objectives for, 861
historical perspective on, 848-850
key points, 871
myths about, 850-851
nurses' attitudes toward, 851
outcomes of, 870
paradigm shift in, 851
practice application for, 870-871
predisposing/contributing factors, 859-860
during pregnancy, 865
prevention of
community-based activities in, 860
evidence-based practice in, 862
by increasing youth resiliency, 861
primary, 860-863
secondary, 863-864
tertiary, 866-870
setting for, 859-860, 860
socioeconomic problems due to, 863
stages of change in, 870
tolerance to, 854
treatment of, 867-868
"just say no" model of, 862, 865
Alcohol use
accidents involving, 633
adolescent, 623
injuries/accidents and, 634
among adolescents, 809
by Canadian men, 685
by Canadian women, 660
disorders related to, 692-693
economic costs of, 854
male reproductive effects of, 692
by older adults, 864-865
during pregnancy, 663
prevalence of, 848
risk from, 606
Alcoholics Anonymous, 868
Alcoholism
defined, 854
in Native Americans, 154
recognition as disease, 585
Alderfer, Clayton, human needs theory of, 1014t, 1015
Al-Gasseer, Naeema, 176
Alliances, working with, 1025
Allocation, characteristics of, 460
Alma Ata conference, 73
and primary care in international health, 77
Alternative and complementary medicine for heart disease, 689b
Alternative healing, cultural variations in, 162t
Alternatives, generating, 459-460
Ambulatory care nurses in nursing centers, 428t
Ambulatory clinics, advanced practice nurses in, 997
Ambulatory payment classes, 121
American Academy of Pediatrics
emergency equipment recommendations of, for school nurses, 1054
on in-school administration of medications, 1054
school nursing standards of, 1045
screening guidelines of, 1054
American Association of Occupational Health Nurses
Code of Ethics of, 1069b
standards of, 1068, 1069b
training grants of, 1068-1069
American Birth Control League, 653
American Cancer Society, contact information for, 869b

American Geriatrics Society, website for, 715
American Health Security Act of 1993, 42
American Heart Association, contact information for, 869b
American Lung Association
contact information for, 869b
indoor air quality materials of, 229
American Medical Association, founding of, 25
American Medical Directors Association, website for, 715
American Nurses Association, 39
Code of Ethics of, 132, 140-143, 142b
*Metathesaurus* of, 206-207
nursing center defined by, 414b
in policy setting, 184
recommendations for health care reform, 125b
American Nurses Credentialing Center, 449, 993
American Public Health Association, 30
Code of Ethics of, 132
public health nursing defined by, 345
website for, 352b
American Red Cross, 29
disaster education by, 476
disaster mental health training by, 483
in disaster preparedness, 473, 477t
disaster response responsibilities of, 478t
disaster-related stress recommendations of, 484
home nursing course of, 35
American Urological Association Symposium Index, 689
Americans for Nonsmokers Rights, contact information for, 869b
Americans with Disabilities Act, 681-682
HIV/AIDS provisions of, 937
impact of, 711t
mental health provisions of, 831t, 832
provisions of, 737
school nursing provisions of, 1044, 1044t
Amphetamines, physiologic effects of, 857-858
Amplifying, characteristics of, 457-458
Andragogy
defined, 306
*versus* pedagogy, 307t
Anencephaly, folic acid for preventing, 662-663
Angina, symptoms of, 687
Anorexia, 668
Anthrax
bioterrorist threat of, 913, 916
syndromes due to, 916
Antibiotics
inappropriate use of, 942, 1119-1120
for viral disease, 902
water pollution by, 233
Antidepressants in smoking cessation, 868
Antismoking programs, 639-640
Anxiety
children's, about death, 727
of migrant farmworkers, 799
in women, 666
Anxiety disorders
characteristics of, 840
prevalence of, 828
APHA. *See* American Public Health Association
Appraisal, employee, 1031-1032
Appropriate technology in Healthy Cities movement, 399
Arenaviruses, bioterrorist threat of, 913
Armed forces, women in, 682
Armed services, advanced practice nurses in, 1000
Army Nurse Corps, 35
Arthritis in Lyme disease, 924
ASH, contact information for, 869b
Asian American women, causes of death among, 659t
Asian Americans, mental health of, 843-844

Asians
communication patterns of, 163
cultural attitudes/practices of, 162t
environmental control perspectives of, 165
food preferences and nutrition-related risk factors of, 167t
as percentage of U. S. population, 53
social organization of, 164f
stereotyping of, 158
Assault
by men, 691-692
prevalence of, 887
Assault victims, emergency response to, 896b
Assertive community treatment for mentally ill persons, 834
Assertiveness, defined, 461
Assessment
defined, 6, 20
ethics in, 139
surveys evaluating, 11
Assessment Protocol for Excellence in Public Health, 1034
Assessment tools
Assimilation, Piaget's definition of, 626
Assisted living for older adults, 713
Assisted suicide of people with disabilities, 737-738
Association of Community Health Nursing Educators, 9
Association of Occupational and Environmental Clinics, website for, 244
Assurance, 19
components of, 13
defined, 6, 20
ethics of, 139-140
Asthma
children with, 1058
practice application for, 648
increased incidence of, 228
medications for, promoting use by children, 735
nursing guide for, 638b
Asthma "friendliness," school survey for, 638b
Atherosclerosis
chelation therapy for, 708b
childhood onset of, 626
Athletes, physically impaired, 737
ATOD. *See* Alcohol, tobacco, and other drug use
Attack rate, defined, 259
Attention deficit disorder
with hyperactivity, 638-639
nursing guide for, 639b
Audit process, 527-528, 527f
concurrent *versus* retrospective, 527-528
Autism, children with, 1060
Autonomy
ethical issues in, 465
principle of, 135-136
respect for, 135b
Avian influenza virus, A (H5N10), 921
Avoiding, defined, 461b

**B**

Babesiosis, 924
Bacille Calmette-Gu_rin vaccine, 88
*Bacillus anthracis*, 913, 916
Back pain
chiropractic for, 708b
chronic, 725
work-related, 1078
Balanced Budget Act of 1997, 106
children's health coverage in, 68
impact of, 711t
Medicare and, 59
nursing involvement in, 187-188
provisions affecting vulnerable populations, 752
provisions of, 110t
Bandura, Albert, social learning theory of, 1014t, 1015
Basal cell carcinoma of skin, 690

Battered women, 885-887. *See also* Family violence; Intimate partner violence
nursing interventions for, 893-894
self-blame in, 886
Batterers
court-mandated interventions for, 889
programs for, 886
Behavior, problem, in children/adolescents, 638-639
Behavior in humanistic theory, 300
Behavior Risk Factor Surveillance System, 350, 353
Behavioral change
after community health education, 313-314
public health influences on, 3
Behavioral Risk Factor Surveillance System, 267
Behavioral risks in family health, 606-607
Behavioral theory, 298-299
Behaviors
family, 601b
target, 298
Beliefs, personal, about poverty, 775, 776
Benchmarking, 986
Beneficence, 135b
ethical issues in, 465
Benign prostatic hyperplasia, risk factors for, 689
Bereavement, stress following, 838
Bernoulli, Daniel, 251t
Best practices, 285
Betts, Virginia Trotter, 176
Bias, types of, 277
Bilateral organizations, 79
examples of, 80
Bill of Rights Act, 832
Bioethics
defined, 132b
influences of, 132
origins of, 131
Biofeedback for children, 643
Biological hazards, work-related, 1076b, 1076-1077
Biological risks, 600-601
Biomedical model, 319
Bioterrorism, 91-92, 255
with anthrax, 913, 916
potential agents of, 913
preparation for, 477
preparedness for, 178
response to, 479-480
threats of, 2
Bipolar illness, 827-828
Birth control
adolescents and, 809, 812-813
hormonal, 813t
legalization of, 653-654
Birth control movement, origins of, 653
Birth defects
fetal alcohol syndrome and, 865
rubella and, 919
Birth rate
among teens, 810
Canadian, 570
changes in, 567
U. S., 53
Bisexual women, health of, 670
Block grants, funding by, 172
Block nursing programs, 1104
Blood alcohol concentration
Canadian limits on, 853
CNS effects of, 854, 855f
Blood transfusions, in-home, nursing tip for, 962
Bloodborne Pathogen Standard, 178
Blue Cross/Blue Shield, 118
Board of directors, nursing center, 429
Board of nursing, 179
Boards of health (Canadian), 227
Body maintenance, components of, 694
Body mass index, 632
calculation of, 668
Body systems, age-related changes in, 705t
Bolton, Frances Payne, 35
Bolton Act of 1943, 35
*Borrelia burgdorferi*, 924

Botulism, 921
  bioterrorist threat of, 913
Boundaries, windshield survey of, 357t
Bovine spongiform encephalopathy, 904
Brain, age-related changes in, 705
Brain plasticity, implications of, 828
Brainstorming, 459
Brazil, World Bank projects in, 80
Breads/cereals, dietary guidelines for, in children/adolescents, 628t
Breast cancer
  ethnicity and, 667
  GIS study of, 271
  hormone replacement therapy and, 663
  teaching about, cultural issues in, 155
  in white *versus* African-American women, 656-657
Breast self-examinations, client education about, 299
Breastfeeding, advantages of, 626
Breckinridge, Mary, 33f
  Frontier Nursing Service and, 31, 32b
Brewster, Mary, 28b
Brief interventions for ATOD, 868-869
  FRAMES acronym for, 869, 869b
Brown, Esther Lucile, 39
Brucellosis, 926
Budget limits, defined, 99
Budgets, developing and monitoring, 1036-1037, 1036b
Buhler-Wilkerson, K., 34
Bulimia, 668
Bupropion HCl for smoking cessation, 868
Burr and Klein's family stress theory, 601-602, 602b
Bush, George W., 60
Business cycle, 101
Business plans, 1011
  for nursing centers, 430, 432

**C**
Cadet Nurses Corps, 35
Caffeine
  content in common substances, 858t
  sources and physiologic effects of, 857
Calcium, supplemental, for preventing osteoporosis, 663
California, Healthy Cities and Communities movement in, 402
*Campylobacterium* in food-borne illness, 921
Canada
  advanced practice nurses in, 998-999
  alcohol, tobacco, and other drug use in, 852-853
  community-oriented, population-focused practice in, 16-17
  community/public health nursing in, 16, 36, 1124-1125
  environmental health in, 225-227, 228f, 226-227
  ethics and community health nursing in, 140
  families in, 570-571
  family benefits in, 571
  federal health care initiatives in, 183
  government's health care role in, 182
  health care expenditures in, 52, 112
  health care in
    government roles in, 113
    for high-risk populations, 751
  health care system in, 83-84
  Healthy Cities and Communities movement in, 403
  home health care in, 972-973
  infectious disease risk in, 914-915, 948-949
  legislative process in, 182
  men's health in, 684-685
  NAFTA and, 75
  national health insurance in, 83
  nursing practice regulation in, 182-183
  political system of, 182
  population health leadership by, 77
  primary health care systems and transformation in, 66-67
  public health in, 24
  remote areas of

Canada—cont'd
  health issues in, 386-387
  infant mortality rate in, 748
  teen pregnancy in, 816-817
  women's health in, 660-661
Canada Health Act, 226
  ethics in, 141
Canadian Institute for Advanced Research, 77
Canadian Red Cross, 36-37
Canadian Tobacco Use Monitoring Survey, 852
Cancer
  in children, 235
  in men, 688-690, 695
    of prostate, 688-689
    of skin, 690
    testicular, 689-690
  in women, 666-667
Candidiasis, oral, AIDS-related, 935
Cannabinoids, 858
Cannabis. *See also* Marijuana
  economic uses of, 858
Capacity mapping of community strengths, 893
Capitation, 18-19, 122
  defined, 1011
Carcinogens, work-related exposure to, 1077-1078
Cardiovascular disease
  in homeless persons, 786
  hormone replacement therapy and, 664
  in men, 687-688
  prevention of, 263b
  risk of, 600-601
  web of causality for, 261-262, 262f
  in women, 664
    prevention of, 665b
Cardiovascular system, age-related changes in, 705t
CARE, 80
Care Home Health Services, 526
Care management, defined, 447
Care map tools, functions of, 453-454
Caregiver
  defined, 705
  health risks of, 841
  unpaid, 654
Caregiver burden, 654
Caregiving
  family. *See* Family caregiving
  school nurse's role in, 1046
*Carey v. Population Services*, 811b
Carnegie Foundation, 81
Carondelet Health, St. Mary's Hospital, 455
Carpal tunnel syndrome, work-related risk of, 1078
Carve outs, 750, 753
Case finding for vulnerable populations, 749
Case management, 446-469
  applications of, 456b
  concepts of, 448-455
  core components of, 451f
  definitions of, 447-448
  ensuring high-quality care in, 456
  ethical issues in, 465
  evidence-based practice in, 454
  forces affecting, 452f
  Healthy People 2010 objectives for, 448
  with homeless persons, 790
  key points for, 466
  knowledge domains for, 453, 453b
  legal issues in, 462-465
  in men's health, 694-695
  models of, 451f, 456
  nursing process in, 449-450, 450t
  practice application for, 465
  prevention in, 460b
  public health examples of, 455-456
  roles in, 452b
  skills required for, 456-462
  for vulnerable populations, 768-769, 769f
  websites for, 464b
Case management plans, 453

Case manager
  credentialing resources for, 464b
  knowledge and skill requisites of, 451, 453
  nurses as, 1123
  roles of, 448, 450-451, 452b
  school nurse as, 1047
  tools of, 453-455
Case registers, functions of, 509-510, 510b
Case-control studies, 274-275, 274f
Case-fatality rate, 259-260
  calculation of, 260t
Catalytic intervention mode, 1020, 1021t
Categorical funding, 178
Categorical programs, 174
Catholic Relief Services, 80
Cat-scratch disease, 926
Causality
  assessing, 277
  criteria for, 277b
  statistical associations of, 276
CBA. *See* Cost-benefit analysis
CEA. *See* Cost-effectiveness analysis
Center for Research on Women with Disabilities, 671
Center for Studying Health Systems Change, 52
Centers for Disease Control and Prevention, 177
  Disability and Health Team of, 724
  nosocomial infection prevention by, 928
  public health programs supported by, 352
  reportable disease list of, 908
  school health funding by, 1048-1049
  Task Force on Community Preventive Services of, 7
  universal precautions of, 928
  waterborne disease defined by, 923
Centers for Medicare and Medicaid Services, 52, 172, 177, 710
  conditions of participation of, 52-53
  cost-control efforts of, 58-59
Centers of Excellence for Women's Health (Canadian), 661
Cerebrovascular accident, case management of, 465
Certification
  of advanced practice nurses, 992-993
  defined, 522
  for public health nursing, 1122
Certified nurse midwives, 59
  training and certification of, 59
Cervical cancer
  herpes simplex 2 infection and, 943
  HPV infection and, 943-944
  teaching about, cultural issues in, 155
Cervical cap, uses and effectiveness of, 662t
Cestodes, diseases caused by, 927t
CfCs. *See* Conditions for coverage
Chadwick, Edwin, 253
Change agent roles, 367
Change partner roles, 367
Charge method, 121
Charter, defined, 522
Chelation therapy for atherosclerosis, 708b
Chemical hazards, work-related, 1076b, 1077-1078
Chemical Safety Information, Site Security and Fuels Regulatory Act, provisions of, 242b
Chemicals
  environmental, adverse effects of, 224-225
  synthetic, numbers introduced since WWII, 224
  toxic, adverse reproductive outcomes and, 236, 236t
Chengdu, China, Healthy Cities project in, 405
Chest pain, assessing, 687
Chewing tobacco, 856
Chickenpox
  required immunizations for, 1052t
  *versus* smallpox, 917

Child abuse and neglect, 882-885
  assessment of, 884
  in foster care, 883-884
  incidence of, 617
  indicators of, 884
  legislation addressing, 181
  mandatory reporting of, 892-893
  parents at risk for, evidence-based practice and, 13
  of physically compromised, 730
  prevalence of, 882
  prevention of, 572b
  risk factors for, 882-883, 883b
  screening for, in schools, 1056
  by teen parents, 821
Child and adolescent health, 616-651.
  *See also* Well-child care; specific age-groups
  acute illness in, 636-637
  advanced practice nursing specialization in, 1045-1046
  behavioral alterations in, 638-639
  chronic health problems in, 637-638
  community resources for, 645b
  community-oriented nurse and, 645, 647
  complementary/alternative medicine for, 641-644
  environmental health hazards affecting, 641
  Healthy People 2010 objectives for, 626, 645, 646-647
  home-based service programs for, 644-645
  homeless programs and, 645
  immunizations in, 630-631
  injuries and accidents in, 633-636
  key points in, 649
  nutrition and, 626-630
  obesity in, 632-633
  practice application in, 648
  promoting parental involvement in, 1051
  tobacco use by, 639-641
Child Health Insurance program, 617
Child Health Plus, 173
Child Labor Act, migrant children's exclusion from, 800
Childbearing women, poverty and, 779
Childbirth, maternal deaths in, 89-90
Childrearing
  practices of, and development of abusive patterns, 881-882
  stresses in, 563-564
Children
  AIDS in, 936
  asthma in, 1058
  autistic, 1060
  deaths of, firearm accidents as leading cause of, 889
  development of, 617-626
  with diabetes mellitus, 1060
  with disabilities, 1058
  disaster reactions of, 481, 481b
  dying, home care of, 976
  effects of parental cohabitation on, 567
  environmental health of, 235-236
  explaining death to, 976
  family status of, 564
  health of, in rural areas, 381-382
  hepatitis A in, 944
  HIV infection in, 937, 938
    immunizations for, 938
  home health care for, 985
  home-bound, 1061
  homeless, health problems of, 786-789
  injuries to
    preventing, 1051
    return to school after, 1060
  mental health of
    Healthy People 2010 objectives for, 839
    postdisaster, 485
  of migrant farmworkers, 800-801
  nutrition deficits in, 90-91
  physically compromised, 724-725
    community resources and, 729
    death anxiety in, 727
    families of, 726-728
    legal rights of, 737

Children–cont'd
  poverty and, 616, 779
    by ethnic group, 779t
  preventing substance abuse by, 1051
  required immunizations for,
    1051-1053, 1052t
  with special needs, in school, 1061
  status of, 616-617
  teaching, 306-307
  uninsured, study of, 437
  upbringing of, family violence and,
    881-882
Children's Bureau, 31
Chile, physician-nurse influence in, 78
China
  health care system in, 85
  Healthy Cities and Communities
    movement in, 405
  nursing's changing role in, 78
Chinese culture, health care issues in,
  157
CHIP. See Community Health
  Improvement Process
Chiropractic
  for back pain, 708b
  for children, 641-642
Chlamydia
  cause, symptoms, treatment, 942-943
  coinfection with gonorrhea, 938
  increased rates of, 938
  and increased risk of HIV infection,
    935
  risk management of, in Canada, 949
  summary of, 940t
Cholera
  mortality rate for, in 1853 study, 253t
  waterborne sources of, 925
Cholesterol, screening for, 265
Chronic illness
  after disasters, 485
  agencies pertaining to, 38
  in Canadian men, 684
  in Canadian women, 660
  in children, 724-725
  in children/adolescents, 637-641
  and costs of care, 111, 111t
  deaths due to, 253
  defined, 722
  disease management approach to,
    454-455
  focus on, 105
  in older adults, 109, 707-708, 708t
  rise of, 36-39
  in rural residents, 379
  in U.S. youth, 729
Church World Service, 80
Cigarette smoke, mainstream versus sidestream, 856
Cigarette smoking
  among adolescents, 809
  annual number of deaths due to, 855
  by Canadian men, 684-685
  cardiovascular disease and, 664
  cultural and gender differences in, 691
  deaths from, 320, 856f
  health care costs related to, 320
  lung cancer and, 666-667
  by men, 691
  physical compromise due to, 723
  in rural areas, 379
Cirrhosis, alcohol-related, 692
Cities. See Healthy Communities and
  Cities movement
CITYNET-Healthy Cities, 401-402
Civil immunity, 181
Civil Rights Act of 1964, title VII of, 654
Civil Works Administration, 33
  nursing service coverage by, 965
Civilian Health and Medical Program of
  the Uniformed Services, 117
Clarifying, characteristics of, 458
Clean Air Act, 229
  provisions of, 241b
Clean Water Act, provisions of, 241b
Cleveland Visiting Nurse Association, 30
Client. See also entries under Patient
  aggregate, in Neuman Systems Model,
    206
  defined, 198t
  identifying, 1019

Client Bill of Rights, 982b
Client outcomes. See Health outcomes
Client populations. See Populations
Client problem, defined, 207
Client satisfaction, 530, 539
  evidence-based practice and, 530
  tool domains and examples of, 534f
Client system in integrative model of
  health promotion, 321
Climate Change Plan for Canada, 227
Clinical nurse specialist, 990. See also
  Advanced practice nurse
  in Canada, 998-999
  as clinicians, 993-995
  credentialing of, 993
  versus nurse practitioners, 992t
  practice application for, 1004
Clinical practice, guidelines for, defined,
  526
Clinical preventive services, guidelines
  for, 327
Clinical specialist, in nursing centers,
  427t
Clinical trials, 276
  randomized, 285
Clinician, advance practice nurses as,
  993-995
Clinton, Bill, 62, 493, 748
Clitoris, excision of, 663-664
Clostridium botulinum, food intoxication
  due to, causal agents and charac-
  teristics, 922t
Clostridium perfringens, food intoxication
  due to, causal agents and charac-
  teristics, 922t
CMS. See Centers for Medicare and
  Medicaid Services
CNMs. See Certified nurse midwives
Coal miners, health needs/problems of,
  383t
Coalitions, working with, 1025
Cocaine, forms of, 857
Cocaine use, physiologic/emotional ef-
  fects of, 856-857
Code of Regulations, 188
Codependency
  in ATOD, 865-866
  defined, 866
Codes of ethics
  ANA, 132
  Canadian, 140
  defined, 132b
  ICN, 132
  Nightingale Pledge as, 131-132
Cognitive development, Piaget's theory
  of, 626, 627t
Cognitive domain, 301
  versus affective domain, 301t
Cognitive theories, 299
  of management, 1015
Cohabitation
  effects of, 568
  reasons for, 567-568
Cohesion, definition and traits promot-
  ing, 542
Cohort studies, 272-274, 273f
  prospective, 273
  retrospective, 274
Collaborating, defined, 461b
Collaboration
  defined, 421b
  factors influencing, 422t
  process of, 461-462, 462f
  skills in, 1034
  stages of, 463b
Colonias, diseases associated with, 75
Colorectal cancer, 666-667
Commodification, 81
Common law, 180
Common vehicle, defined, 906
Commons, windshield survey of, 357t
Communicable disease. See Infectious
  disease
Communication
  about environmental health risks,
    239-240
  with abusive families, 892
  with adolescents, 624
  cultural variations in, 162t, 165
  in groups

Communication–cont'd
  skills in, 550, 550b
  structure of, 546
  with legislators, 186b, 187
  in management/consultation,
    1030-1031
  skills in, 1031b
Communitarianism, 136-137
Community(ies)
  assessment of, by nursing centers,
    422-423
  as client, 342-373
  concepts of, 345t
  definitions of, 329, 342-344
  of geographic/political boundaries,
    34-3443
  group contributions to, 554-555
  Healthy People 2010 educational
    goals for, 297
  high-density, violence in, 877-878
  historical perspectives on, 328-329
  interdependence in, 344
  multilevel studies of, 330-331
  physically compromised clients and,
    728-729
  of place, 343
  poverty and, 782-783
  of problem ecology, 343
  recreational facilities in, effect on vio-
    lence levels, 878
  stressors in, 203, 204t, 205
  structure of, 203
  subgroup communication in, 203, 205
  subsystems of, 197-198
  as target of practice, 344. See also
    Community as client
  types of, 343-344, 344b
  typologies of, 343
  variables in, 203t
  violence in, assessing for, 891b
Community advocates in nursing centers, 429
Community as client
  assessment of, quick method for, 356
  evidence-based practice and, 351
  goals and means for, 346-352
  key points for, 371
  nursing process flow chart for, 354f
  nursing process in, 352-370
    assessment, 353-360
    diagnosis, 360
    evaluation, 369-370
    implementation, 366-368
    planning, 360-366
  personal safety and, 370-371
  practice application for, 371
Community assessment
  in program management, 494
  real-time, 494b
Community collaboration
  Healthy People 2010 goals and,
    419-421
  stakeholders in, 421b
Community competence, 347-349
  essential conditions of, 348t
Community development model, 286
Community form, definition, advan-
  tages/disadvantages of, 495t
Community groups. See Groups
Community Guide, 351-352
Community health. See also Public
  health
  assessment of, 329
    database for, 355t
    steps in, 355b
  components of, 349t
  defined, 347
  health risk factors and, 8b
  health status and, 8b
  in Healthy People 2010, 349-350
  levels of care in
    for coronary heart disease, 334t
    for failure to thrive, 333t
  planning for, 360, 362-366
  problems and strengths in, 356
  process characteristics of, 347-349
  promoting goals for, through groups,
    555-556
  quality of life and, 8b
  records in, 535

Community health. See also Public
  health–cont'd
  sociodemographic characteristics of,
    8b
  status characteristics of, 346-347, 347b
  strategies for improving, 351-352
    website information for, 352b
  structure characteristics of, 347
Community health clinics in China, 85
Community health education, 294-317.
    See also Learning
  affective domain in, 301, 301t
  appropriate materials for, 311
  client involvement in, 312
  client literacy and, 308-309
  cognitive domain in, 301, 301t
  educational plan in, 313
  educator effectiveness in, 302-306
  educator evaluation in, 313
  effective teaching in, 312b
  enhancement strategies for, 312b
  environmental realms in, 304b
  evidence-based practice in, 308
  goals and objectives for, 310-311, 312t
  Healthy People 2010 objectives for,
    296-298
  identifying need for, 310, 311b
  individualized, 311
  instruction events in, 302
  key points in, 315
  versus learning, 298
  learning barriers in, 307-310
  for nonnative English speakers, 304
  population considerations in, 306-307
  practice application for, 315
  principles of, 300-306
  process evaluation in, 313
  process of, 310-313
  product of, 313-315
  program development in, 294-295,
    295f
  psychomotor domain in, 301, 302t
Community Health Improvement
  Process, 7, 524, 525f
Community health nurse specialists, credentials for, 14
Community health nursing
  ANA quality assurance standards on,
    521
  in Canada, 36, 1124-1125
  versus community-based nursing,
    13-15
  defined, 14
  funding for, 31
  milestones in, 38t
Community health nursing practice
  defined, 15b
  law and, 181-182
Community health planning. See also
  Program management
  characteristics of, 491
Community health promotion, 318-339
  evidence-based practice in, 332
  examples of, 334-335
  health definitions and, 323-325
  historical perspective on, 322-323
  integrative model for, 321-322,
    333-335
    community models in, 329-330
    community perspectives in, 328-329
    health definitions in, 323-324
    health promotion definitions in,
      324-325
  integrative model of, 318-319
    client system in, 321
    foci of care in, 321-322
  key points in, 336
  multilevel interventions for, 319
  multilevel projects in, 331-332
  multilevel studies of, 330-331
  practice application for, 335
  prevention methods/risk reduction in,
    325-328
  and shift from illness management to
    wellness, 319-320
  shift from individual to population
    and multilevel interventions in,
    320-321
  through group work, 547-554

Community Health Promotion model in Healthy Cities movement, 399, 400f
Community health workers. See also Community-oriented nurse; Community-oriented nursing
  in nursing centers, 428t
  role of, 331
Community Mental Health and Mental Retardation Centers Construction Act, provisions of, 110t
Community mental health centers, 831
  patient rights and, 832
Community Mental Health Centers Act
  focus of, 831t
  implementation of, 752
  passage of, 831
  provisions affecting vulnerable populations, 752
Community models/frameworks, 329-330
Community nursing centers, 58
Community outreach, school nurse's role in, 1047
Community partnerships, 331-332, 350-351. See also Partnerships
  in management/consultation, 1031
  in nursing centers, 414
  in rural areas, 391-392
  for rural maternal-infant health, 381-382
Community practice, models of, 399-401
Community projects, multilevel, 331-332
Community resources. See also Resources
  for at-risk families, 613, 615
  for child and adolescent health, 645b
  for physically compromised adults, 729
Community Support Program, 828
  activities of, 833b
Community trials, 276
Community-as-client goals, 202-203
Community-as-partner model, 329, 359
Community-based health care
  cost containment and, 54
  effects of, 65, 68
Community-based nursing
  case management in, 455-456
  versus public health/community health nursing, 13-15
Community-based nursing practice, 345
  defined, 15b
Community-oriented nurse
  in comprehensive primary health care centers, 416
  in home health and hospice, 962-989. See also Home health; Hospice
  roles of, 24
  in schools. See School nursing
  types of, 344
Community-oriented nurse management. See also Leadership
  goals of, 1012-1013
  key points, 1038-1039
  levels of prevention and, 1013t
  practice application for, 1038
  theories of, 1014-1016, 1014t
    classic, 1013
    intrapersonal/interpersonal, 1013-1016
    neoclassical, 1013-1014
    organizational level, 1016-1017
Community-oriented nurse manager, 1008-1041. See also Consultation
  competencies of, 1025-1038
    fiscal, 1035-1038, 1035-1038
    interpersonal, 1030
    leadership, 1025-1030
    organizational, 1035-1038
    political/power dynamics, 1033
  role of, 1017
Community-oriented nursing
  epidemiologic concepts in, 261
  ethics in, 139-140
  focus of, 345-346
  functions of, 35-36
  goals of, 23

Community-oriented nursing—cont'd
  lack of funding for, 39
  new payment forms for, 41
  in rural areas, 388
  systems perspective of, 197-199
Community-oriented nursing diagnosis, 360
Community-oriented nursing practice
  competencies for, 193
  defined, 15b
  economics and future of, 125-126
Community-oriented primary health care, 391-392
Comparison groups, 268-269
Compassionate Investigational New Drug Program, 858
Competence, community, 347-349
  essential conditions of, 348t
Competing, defined, 461b
Complementary and alternative medicine
  for children/adolescents, 641-644
  heart disease symptoms due to, 688
  for older adults, 708, 708b
  for physically compromised clients, 733
  resources for, 644b
  safety of, 643
Comprehensive Environmental Response, Compensation, and Liability Act, provisions of, 241b
Comprehensive Health Planning Act, provisions of, 110t
Comprehensive primary health care centers, 416
Compromising, defined, 461b
Computed axial tomography, 828
Computers
  access to, 55
  health care applications of, 106
Concept, defined, 194
Conceptual models
  characteristics of, 196
  defined, 196t
  using, 196-197
Conceptual–theoretical–empirical structure, developing, 195-196
Conditions for coverage, 53
Conditions of participation, 53
Condoms
  correct use of, 952-953
  female, 952-953, 953f
  male adolescent use of, 812
  with nonoxynol-9, safety of, 952
  uses and effectiveness of, 662t
Confidentiality
  with adolescent clients, 634
  in community assessment, 359
  Health Insurance Portability and Accountability Act and, 1012
  legal issues involving, 463
Conflict, group, 549-551, 556-557
Conflict management
  in advocacy, 460-461
  behaviors used in, 461b
  in groups, example of, 550-551
  skills in, 1033
  violent, childhood exposure to, 881-882
Confounding, 277
Confrontation intervention mode, 1020, 1021t
Congenital defects. See Birth defects
Congenital rubella syndrome, 919
Consensus Conference on the Essentials of Public Health Nursing Practice and Education, 9, 14
Consensus in collaboration, 463b
Consequentialism, 134
Constituency, promoting self-determination for, 457
Constitutional law, community-oriented nursing and, 179
Consultants
  internal versus external, 1017
  school nurse as, 1047
Consultation. See also Community-oriented nurse manager
  community-oriented nurse's role in, 1025

Consultation. See also Community-oriented nurse manager—cont'd
  contracts for, 1022, 1023f, 1024
  defined, 1012
  defining real client in, 1019-1020
  focus groups in, evidence-based practice and, 1024
  goal of, 1017
  intervention modes of, applying, 1021t
  management, 1012
  process, 1020-1022, 1022
  theories of, 1017-1019
Consumer, influence of, 64
Consumer advocacy. See also Advocacy
  for mental health, 828
  for mentally ill persons, 832-833
  self-help organizations and, 833b
Consumer confidence report, 233
Consumer partnerships, 518
Consumer price index, 777
Consumer/Survivor Mental Health Research and Policy Work Group, activities of, 833b
Contact tracing for STDs, 950-951, 955
Contingency theory of leadership, 1015
Continuity theory of aging, 704
Contraception
  counseling about, 657, 662
  emergency
    for reducing pregnancy risk, 822-823
    for teenage girls, 1061
    uses and effectiveness of, 662t
  methods of, 662t
Contraceptive vaginal rings, adolescents' use of, 813t
Contracts
  consultation, 1022, 1023f, 1024
  contingency versus noncontingency, 611
  with families, 611-612, 611b
  health care, for vulnerable populations, 750
  for home health care, 969, 969f
  negotiation of, 1022, 1024
  nursing center, 434
  risk-based, 1011
  types of, 1032
Contributions, defined, 58
Cooperation
  defined, 461
  in Healthy Cities movement, 399
Coping strategies, Burr and Klein's framework for, 599, 600t
CoPs. See Conditions of participation
Core Functions Project, 7
Coronary heart disease
  Framingham study of, 330
  levels of care for, 334-335
  in men, 687-688
  prospective cohort study of, 273, 273f
Corporal punishment in school, 877
Correctional health, legal issues in, 182-183
Correctional institutions, advanced practice nurses in, 1001
Cost accounting studies, 510
Cost effectiveness analysis, 510-511, 511b
Cost effectiveness of nursing centers, 433
Cost efficiency analysis, 511-512, 511b
Cost shifting, defined, 52
Cost studies
  in program management, 510-512
  in program planning, 499
Cost-benefit analysis, 101-102, 510
Cost-effectiveness analysis, 101-102
  conducting, 1037, 1037t
  of home care agencies, 102
  procedure for, 103
Cost-utility analysis, 101-102
Cottage industry, health care system and, 18
Council on Linkages, 7
  competencies of, 9
Counseling
  adoption, for pregnant teenager, 816
  contraceptive, 657, 662

Counseling—cont'd
  preconceptual, 662-663
  pregnancy, for pregnant teenager, 816
Counselor, school nurse as, 1047
CPM. See Critical path method
CQI. See Total quality management/Continuous quality improvement
Craven, Florence Sarah Lees, 26
Credentialing
  for advanced practice nurses, 992-993
  defined, 521
  for school nurses, 1045-1046
  voluntary, 521-522
Creutzfeldt-Jakob disease, variant, 904
Crimean War, influence on nursing care, 26
Criminal justice model of drug abuse, 851
Crisis, family, characteristics of, 598-599
Crisis poverty, 784
Critical path method, 505, 508
Critical paths, functions of, 453
Critical theory, 299-300
Critical thinking, 1030
Cross-sectional studies, 275
Cross-tolerance, defined, 867
Cryptosporidiosis, 927
Cryptosporidium infection
  symptoms, transmission, and causes of emergence, 912t
  waterborne, 925
  waterborne illness due to, 923
CUA. See Cost-utility analysis
Cue logic, 578, 579-580
Cultural accommodation, 157
Cultural assessment, 160-161
Cultural awareness, 155, 156b
Cultural blindness, 159
Cultural competence, 153-158
  defined, 153
  developing, 154-158
    stages of, 154
    theoretical model of, 154-158, 155t
  dimensions of, 156-158
  inhibitors to, 158-160
  in management/consultation, 1030, 1032
Cultural conflict, 159-160
Cultural desire, 156
Cultural diversity, 148-169. See also Culture; Ethnicity; Race
  evidence-based practice in, 158
  immigrant issues and, 149-151
  key points in, 167-168
  managing, 1032
  mental health and, 842
  practice application in, 167
Cultural encounter, 156
Cultural groups, variations among, 161, 162t, 163-166
  factors influencing, 152b
Cultural imposition, 159
Cultural issues
  in health promotion, for vulnerable populations, 764, 766
  in migrant health care, 801-802
Cultural knowledge, 155-156
Cultural preservation, 157
Cultural relativism, 159
Cultural repatterning, 157
Cultural skill, 156
Culturally appropriate health care, 750
Culture
  definition and examples of, 152
  group, 544
  nutrition and, 166, 167t
  organizational elements of, 152
  socioeconomic status and, 166-167
  teaching strategies and, 307
  time orientation of, 164-165
Culture shock, 160
Cumulative risks, 747-748
Curing, defined, 707-708
Cyclospora, 904
  in food-borne illness, 921

**D**

d'Aiguillon, Duchess, 36
Dairy, dietary guidelines for, in children/adolescents, 628t

DALYs. *See* Disability-adjusted life-years
DARE, effectiveness of, 862-863
Data collection
    in combined Neuman-Omaha system, 213-214, 214b, 215t-216t, 217
    for community assessment, 353, 355
Data gathering, 353
Data generation, 355
Data sources, epidemiologic, 267
Database, composite, 356
Date rape, 880, 887
Day care, infectious disease spread in, 636-637
Deadbeat parents, 779-781
Death. *See also* Hospice care; Mortality rate
    causes of, 53, 253, 254f-255f, 903-904
        in adolescents, 808
        for Canadian men, 684
        for Canadian women, 660
        in men, 687-694
        in men *versus* women, 686-687, 686t
    of children, firearms as leading cause of, 889
    explaining to children, 976
    substance abuse-related, 848
    unexpected, family mental stress following, 838
Death rate
    as indicator of community health status, 347b
    public health influence on, 4
    for rural residents, 379
Decision making
    ethical, 132-134
        care ethics in, 138
        deontological, 135
        feminist ethics in, 138
        principlism in, 135
        process of, 134
        steps in, 133t
        virtue ethics in, 137b
    skills in, 1029-1030, 1029t
Decision trees, 497, 498f
Declaration of Alma Ata, 56
Defined contributions, 58
Defined health care, 58
*Definition and Role of Public Health Nursing in the Delivery of Health Care,* 8
Dehydration, diarrhea-related, 90
Deinstitutionalization
    advocacy efforts and, 832-833
    civil rights legislation and, 832
    goal and effects of, 832
    negative effects of, 785-789
Delano, Jane, 31
Delegation, skills in, 1027-1029, 1028b, 1028t
Demand, defined, 100
Demand management, defined, 448
Dementia, evidence-based practice and, 291
Demographics
    health care expenditures and, 107, 109
    shifts in, 148
Demography, health care, 53
Demonstrations, educational, 303b
Denial as addiction symptom, 864
Denmark, Healthy Cities and Communities movement in, 404
Dental disease in migrant farmworkers, 799
Deontology, 134-135
    defined, 132b
    origins of, 136
Department of Agriculture, health care functions of, 62-63, 178
Department of Commerce
    health care functions of, 62
    health data reports of, 174t
Department of Defense, health care functions of, 62, 177
Department of Health and Human Services. *See* U. S. Department of Health and Human Services
Department of Justice, health care functions of, 63, 178
Department of Labor
    health care functions of, 62, 177-178
    health data reports of, 174t

Depo-Provera, adolescents' use of, 813t
Depressants, physiologic effects of, 854
Depression
    in abuse victims, 886
    in impoverished women, 672
    in older adults, 705, 706t, 841
        practice application for, 844
    prevalence of, 828
    public health nursing during, 33-34
    in Russian immigrants, 91
    treatment options for, 840
    in women, 665-666
Detoxification
    defined, 866
    outpatient/home, 866
Deutsch, Naomi, 34
Developed countries
    defined, 73
    nurses' role in, 78
Developing countries. *See* Lesser-developed countries
Development
    defined, 617
    psychosocial, male, 682-683
Developmental Disabilities Assistance Act, 832
    focus of, 831b
Developmental disability. *See also* Physically compromised client
    defined, 730
    services for individuals with, 723-724
Developmental influences, health problems and, 561
Developmental issues for physically compromised child, 725
Developmental stifling, defined, 722
Developmental theory, 300
    of family, 576-577
Devil's advocate position, 553
Devolution, 172
Diabetes mellitus
    case study of, 580-581
    children with, 1060
    client education about, 300
    complications of, 665
    ethnic differences in, 269
    gestational, 665
    Healthy People 2010 objectives for, 154
    in Mexican Americans, 732
    prevention of, 324b, 500
    in women, 664-665
Diagnosis, dual, defined, 722
Diagnosis-related groups, 106, 116
    establishment of, 521
    impact of, 711t
Diaphragm, uses and effectiveness of, 662t
Diarrheal disease, 925-926
    causes of, 90
    in international health, 90
Diathesis-stress model of mental health care, 833
Diet. *See also* Nutrition
    high-fat, obesity and, 632
    in illness prevention, 604
    recommendations for, 630
Dietary deficiencies, 91
Dietary guidelines in childhood/adolescence, 628t
Differential vulnerability hypothesis, 748
Digital divide, 55
    defined, 52b
Digital rectal examination, 688
Dioxin, contamination with, 243
Diphtheria
    required immunizations for, 1052t
    tetanus, and acellular pertussis vaccine, 630
Directly observed therapy for TB medication, 88, 955-956
Disabilities. *See also* Physically compromised client
    causes of, 722-723, 722b, 723f
    children with, 1058
    defined, 721
    legislation pertaining to, 736-738, 736b
    in low-income people, 729, 730f
    severe, chronic, 720-721

Disabilities. *See also* Physically compromised client—cont'd
    women with, 670-671
    work, definition and economic impact of, 724
Disability and Health Team, 724
Disability-adjusted life-years, 86-87
    calculating, 86b
Disadvantaged populations, defined, 749
Disaster management, 470-489
    evidence-based practice in, 485
    occupational health nursing and, 1087-1089
    preparedness in, 473-478
        agencies involved in, 476, 477t
        community, 473-475
        future of, 477-478
        nurse's role in, 475-476
        Office of Homeland Security in, 478
        personal, 473
        professional, 473
    prevention levels in, 485b
    public health nurses' role in, 1126
    recovery in, 484-486
        nurse's role in, 484-486
    response in, 478-484
        agency involvement in, 478-479, 478t
        bioterrorism and, 479-480
        federal plan for, 479
        international, 484
        nurse's role in, 481-483
        and psychologic stress, 484
        shelter management in, 483
    stages of, 472
Disaster medical assistance teams, 479
Disaster workers, psychological stress of, 484
Disasters, 470-472
    at-risk populations in, 482
    community effects of, 480-481
    defining, 471-472
    effects and distribution of, 470-471
    evidence-based practice in, 485
    gathering information in, 483
    Healthy People 2010 objectives for, 472
    levels of, 478-579
    mitigation of, 472
    mock, 476
    natural *versus* man-made, 471
    school crisis teams for responding to, 1057-1058, 1058b
    types of, 472b
Disease. *See also* Illness
    *versus* infection, 906
    infectious. *See* Infectious disease
    natural history of, 262
    notifiable, in Canada, 914
    reportable, CDC list of, 908
Disease incidence as indicator of community health status, 347b
Disease management, 320
    components of, 454
    defined, 448
Disease prevention, 56. *See also* Prevention
    for children, 1051
    defined, 52b
    landmark initiatives in, 323b
    methods for, 325-328
    for older adults, 714-715
Disease self-management, definitions of, 325
Disenfranchisement of vulnerable populations, 759
Disengagement theory of aging, 704
Disorder, defined, 721
Disparities, health. *See* Health disparities
Distribution effects, 844
Distributive care, defined, 970
Distributive justice, 135b, 136
Distributive outcomes, 460
District nursing, 25-26
    in Sweden, 84
    in United Kingdom, 83
District nursing associations, 26
Diversity, managing, 1032

Divorce rate
    Canadian, 570-571
    changes in, 566
    ethnic differences in, 566
Dix, Dorothea Lynde, 830
DNR orders, 709
    children with, school nurse and, 1061
Doctors without Borders, 81
Doll, Richard, 252t
Domestic violence. *See* Child abuse and neglect; Family violence; Intimate partner violence; Older adult abuse and neglect
Do-not-resuscitate orders. *See* DNR orders
Dose-response relationship, 277b
DOT. *See* Directly observed treatment programs
Driving under the influence, Canadian statistics on, 852
Drowning, adolescent involvement in, 634
Drug abuse. *See also* Alcohol abuse; Alcohol use; Substance abuse
    adolescent, 623
        injuries/accidents and, 634
    annual cost per addict, 850f
    HIV/AIDS spread through, 67
    injection, HIV transmission by, 936
    by injection. *See* Injectable drug use
    prevention/treatment of, federal expenditures on, 850, 850f
    risk from, 606
    STD transmission and, 952
    treatment of, 850, 850f
Drug addiction
    defined, 853
    recognition as disease, 585
Drug dependence, defined, 853
Drug education, 861-863
Drug Strategy and Controlled Substances Programme (Canada), 852
Drug testing, appropriateness and types of, 864
Drug trade, profits from, 849
Drug treatment centers, closures of, 850
Drug users, attitudes toward, 932
Drug withdrawal, acupuncture for treating, 866
Drugs. *See also* Prescription drugs
    cross-tolerance of, 867
    definitions of, 851
    determining relative safety of, 862
    entry routes of, 224
    free, from pharmaceutical companies, 457
    "good" *versus* "bad," 850, 865
    illicit, overdoses/impurities of, 865
    war on, problems with, 849
Drunk drivers, accidents involving, 633
DTaP vaccine, 630
Dual diagnosis, defined, 722
Durable medical power of attorney, 709
Durable power of attorney, 982
Dying. *See* Death; Hospice care
d'Youville, Marguerite, 36

**E**

E-mail, health care providers and, 55
Early Periodic Screening and Developmental Testing, 174
Eating disorders. *See also* Obesity; Overweight
    Healthy People 2010 objectives for, 839
    in women, 666, 668
Ebola hemorrhagic fever, 904
Ebola virus, 74, 254
    characteristics of, 908
    symptoms, transmission, and causes of emergence, 912t
Ecologic fallacy, 275
Ecologic studies, 275
Ecomaps, 605f
    content of, 604-606
    developing, 588, 589f
Economic development, international health and, 81-82
Economic growth, defined, 101
Economic Opportunity Act, 41

Economic risks
  in family health, 604
  as predictors of health, 606
Economics, 98-129. *See also* Funding;
    Payment systems
  analysis tools for, 101-103
  defined, 98
  evidence-based practice in, 102
  factors affecting, 122-124
  and future of community-oriented
    nursing, 125-126
  health care
    factors influencing, 107-111
    trends in, 106-107
  key points in, 127
  practice application for, 126-127
  of primary prevention, 124-125
  principles of, 99-103
Ecstasy, physiologic effects of, 859
EDTA, heart disease symptoms due to,
    688
Education
  about nonviolence conflict resolution,
    877
  advanced practice nurse roles in, 995
  for clinical nurse specialists/nurse
    practitioners, 992
  drug, 861-863
  free appropriate public, right to, 737
  health status and, 757
  for home health practice, 977-978
  for teen parents, 821-822
Education for All Handicapped
    Children Act, school nursing pro-
    visions of, 1044, 1044t
Educational programs, clear, guidelines
    for, 303b
Educators
  case managers as, 452b
  effective, 302-306
  evaluation of, 313
  guiding principles for, 303b
  learning barriers associated with,
    307-308
  in nursing centers, 428-429
  public health nurses as, 1124
Effectiveness
  defined, 102
  *versus* efficiency, 101b
Efficiency
  defined, 100-102
  *versus* effectiveness, 101b
Egalitarianism, 136
Ego development, Erikson's stages of,
    625t
Ehrlichiosis, 904, 924
Eidemiologic triangle, 905, 905f
*Eisenstad v. Baird,* 811b
El Salvador, Healthy Cities and
    Communities movement in, 405
Elder abuse. *See* Older adult abuse
Elderberry Institute, 1104
Elimination
  infant, 620t
  neonatal, 619t
  of toddlers/preschoolers, 621t
Elizabethan poor laws, 24, 25, 775
Emergencies, in-school, nursing care for,
    1053-1054
Emergency departments
  advanced practice nurses in, 997-998
  educating about family violence, 895
  nonurgent use of, 59
Emergency housing, 788
Emergency Maternity and Infant Care
    Act of 1943, 35
Emergency Planning and Community
    Right-to-Know Act, provisions
    of, 242b
Emergency plans, 1053
Emergency support functions, 479
Emotional abuse
  characteristics of, 884
  of older adults, 888
Empirical indicators, defined, 196, 196t
Empiricism, 299t
  defined, 298
Employee assistance programs, 864
Employees. *See also* Workers
  appraisal of, 1031-1032

Employers
  discrimination by, against persons
    with disabilities, 737
  influence of, 64
  insurance provided by, 118-119
Employment, by industry divisions,
    1077t
Employment Insurance Act (Canadian),
    571
Empowerment
  assumptions of, 612
  consultation and, 1012
  of families, 612-613
  of vulnerable populations, 764, 766
Enabling
  defined, 866
  loose health care eligibility as, 756-757
Enabling legislation, 118
Enabling services in nursing centers,
    415-416
Encephalitis, equine, 924
Encephalopathy, bovine spongiform,
    904
Endemic, defined, 907
England
  Elizabethan poor laws in, 24, 25, 775
  school nursing in, 1049
*Entamoeba*
  in traveler's diarrhea, 926
  waterborne illness due to, 923
Entropy, defined, 197
Enviromechanical hazards, work-related,
    1078, 1078f
Environment
  defined, 198t
  family, 601b
  Healthy People 2010 objectives for,
    994
  in Neuman Systems Model, 201
  physical, 601b
  rural, 385
Environment Canada, 226
Environmental control, cultural varia-
    tions in attitudes toward, 165
Environmental epidemiology, 225-227
Environmental hazards, work-related,
    1076b, 1080
Environmental health, 222-247
  advocacy in, 243-244
  assessment of, 228-235
  in Canada, 225-227, 228f, 226-227
  Chadwick's study of, 253
  of children, 235-236
  components of, 222
  evidence-based practice in, 225
  government agencies involved in,
    244b
  in health care industry, 243-244
  Healthy People 2010 objectives for,
    223
  historical context of, 222-224
  key points in, 245-246
  nurse competencies in, 223b
  nurse roles in, 244-245
  nursing process applied to, 229
  organizations involved with, 244b
  practice application for, 245
  precautionary principle in,
    236-237
  and reduction of environmental
    health risks, 237-243
  referral sources for, 244
  sciences pertaining to, 224-228
Environmental health assessment,
    228-236
  of air quality, 229, 232b
  of environmental exposure history,
    228-229, 230b
  of food, 233
  of lead exposure, 231
  resources for, 232b-233b
  of water quality, 224, 233
  websites for, 232-233b
Environmental health hazards
  for children, 640t
    prevention strategies for, 642t
  in disasters, 485-486
  in rural areas, 382-384
Environmental justice, 243
Environmental monitoring, 242

Environmental protection
  governmental, 240-243
    agencies involved in, 240
  laws pertaining to, 241b
Environmental Protection Agency
  Envirofacts section of website, 233
  indoor air quality materials of, 229
Environmental quality, Healthy People
    2010 goals for, 420
Environmental regulations
  compliance with, 242
  enforcement of, 242
Environmental risks, assessment of, in
    family health, 604-606
Environmental standards, types of, 242
Enzyme-linked immunosorbent assay for
    HIV testing, 937
Epidemics
  defined, 258, 907
  modern-day, 2
  point, 270
  in U. S. history, 24
Epidemiologic triangle, 261-262, 261f,
    262b
  components of, 225-227, 225f
Epidemiology, 225-227, 248-283
  analytic, 271-275
  attack rate in, 259
  basic concepts in, 255-265
  bias in studies in, 277
  case-control studies in, 274-275, 274f
  causality in, 276-277
  cohort studies in, 272-274
    prospective, 273
    retrospective, 274
  in community-oriented nursing,
    278-279
  comparison groups in, 268-269
  contributions of, 248-249
  cross-sectional studies in, 275
  cyclical patterns in, 270-271
  data sources for, 267
  definitions and descriptions of,
    250-251
  descriptive, 269-271
    *versus* analytic, 250-251
  ecologic studies in, 275
  environmental, 225-227
  epidemiologic triangle in, 261-262,
    261f, 262b
  event-related clusters in, 271
  experimental studies in, 275-276
  geographic patterns in, 270
  Healthy People 2010 objectives for,
    250
  historical perspectives on, 251-255
  incidence measures in, 256-258
  incidence *versus* prevalence in, 258-259
  key points in, 280
  methods in, 267-269
  milestones in, 251t-252t
  morbidity and mortality measures in,
    255-256
  mortality rate in, 259-261, 260t
  personal characteristics in, 269
  of point epidemics, 270
  popular, 278-279
  practice application in, 279-280
  prevalence proportion in, 258
  preventive interventions in, 262-265,
    263b, 264f
  process in, 251
  rate adjustment in, 267-268
  risk calculation in, 257-258
  screening in, 265-267, 265b, 266t
  secular trends in, 270
  study design comparisons in, 272t
Episodic care, defined, 970
Equifinality, defined, 196f
Equine encephalitis, 924
Equity in Healthy Cities movement, 399
ERG theory, 1014t, 1015
Erikson, Erik
  developmental theory of, 624
  for men, 682
  for older adults, 704
  ego development stages of, 625t
*Escherichia coli*
  in fast-food hamburgers, 921
  resistant strains of, 254-255
  in traveler's diarrhea, 926

*Escherichia coli* 0157:H7, 904
  causes and symptoms of, 923
  symptoms, transmission, and causes
    of emergence, 912t
  waterborne illness due to, 923
Estradiol, water pollution by, 233
Ethical dilemma, defined, 132, 132b
Ethical issues
  in case management, 465
  defined, 132
  in home health/hospice care, 982-983
  in parish nursing, 1105-1106
Ethics, 130-147. *See also* Codes of ethics;
    Decision making, ethical
  advocacy and, 143-145
  ANA Code of, 140-143
  in Canadian community health nurs-
    ing, 140
  of care, 137-138
  and core community-oriented nursing
    functions, 139-140
  decision making and, 132-134
  definitions, theories, and principles
    of, 134-137
  environmental health risks and, 240
  evidence-based practice in, 134
  feminist, 138
  history of, 131-132
  key points in, 145-146
  key terms in, 132, 132b
  open-mindedness in, 133
  practice application for, 145
  principles of, 135b
  in public health, 142-145
  in school nursing, 1062
  virtue, 137
Ethnicity
  and cancer in women, 666
  definition and examples of, 153
  health disparities and, 748-749
  and HIV/AIDS in women, 667-668
  life expectancy and, 656
  windshield survey of, 357t
Ethnocentrism, 159
Ethylenediamine triacetic acid, heart dis-
    ease symptoms due to, 688
European Healthy Cities Networks, 404-
    405
European Healthy Cities Project, 397
Evaluation
  in community health nursing, 305-306
  defined, 207, 369, 491
  formative/process, 491
  short- *versus* long-term, after commu-
    nity health education, 314-315,
    314b
  skills in, 1035
  summative/impact, 491
Evening primrose oil for children, 643
Evidence
  defined, 287
  experimental, 277b
Evidence-based practice, 284-293. *See
    also under* specific subject head-
    ings
  barriers to, 286
  and core public health functions, 291,
    292t
  current perspectives on, 287-288
  definitions of, 285-286
  future perspectives on, 288
  and Healthy People 2010 objectives,
    288, 290
  history of, 284-285
  implementation of, 286
  individual differences and, 287
  key points for, 292
  nursing applications of, 290-291
  in nursing centers, 434-436
  practice application of, 291-292
  in prevention, 289b
  resources for, 289b
  situated perspective in, 287
  University of Maryland model of,
    434f
Executive branch of government, 171
Exercise
  by Canadian men, 685
  by Canadian women, 661
  client education about, 300
  health benefits of, 606

Exercise–cont'd
  Healthy People 2010 objectives for, 994
  inadequate, in children/adolescents, 632
  lack of, in U. S., 318
  for physically compromised clients, 743
Expectancy theory, 1014t, 1015
Experimental evidence, 277b
Experimental technology, legal issues involving, 463
Exposure, health problems due to, in homeless persons, 786
Extrapolation, 224

**F**

Failure-to-thrive, levels of care for, 334
Faith communities
  defined, 1093
  heritage of, 1094-1099
Faith-Based Initiative Center, 60
Fallacies, ecologic, 275
Family(ies), 562-593
  abusive, 606-607
    communication with, 892
    emphasizing strengths of, 893
  births and, 567
  Canadian, 570-571
    government benefits for, 571
  challenges of working with, 563, 565
  of children with chronic health problems, 637-638
  children's status in, 564
  as client, 573
  cohabitation of, 566-567
  as component of society, 573
  as context, 573
  contracting with, 611-612, 611b
  corporal punishment in, 877
  cultural variations in, 162t
  definitions of, 568-569, 601b
  demographics of, 565-568
  developing relationships with, in school nursing, 1056
  divorce in, 566
  dysfunctional, 572, 572b
  empowering, 612-613
  functions of, 568
  grandparents as, 568
  health traditions of, 564b
  healthy, 572, 572b
    characteristics of, 572b
  Healthy People 2010 objectives for, 565
  homeless, programs for, 645
  homicide in, 887
  idealization of, 594
  influence on adolescent sexual behavior, 814
  keystone issues of, 580-581, 580f, 581f
  life cycle changes in, 599t
  life experiences of, 568, 569f
  low-income
    in Canada, 571
    resources for, 606
  marriage/remarriage in, 566
  normative versus nonnormative life events in, 601
  as percentage of U. S. households, 53
  percentage owning guns, 635
  of physically compromised individuals, 726-728, 727f
  role of
    in health concepts, 561
    in home health care, 985
  setting appointments with, 579
  single-parent, 563, 567
    economic status of, 757
  single-woman-headed, poverty rate for, 782
  stories of, 578, 579
  structure of, 568-569, 569b
  of substance abusers, codependency of, 865-866
  as system, 573
  of teen parents, 822
  two-income, 563, 564
Family and Medical Leave Act, 654, 682

Family assessment intervention model, 583, 584f
  assumptions of, 585b
Family caregiving
  in home care nursing research, 968
  for older adults, 710
  responsibilities of, 964
Family crisis, characteristics of, 598-599
Family demographics, defined, 565-566
Family health, 569, 572
  defined, 597
  early emphases in, 596
  example of, from Neuman Systems Model, 597
  legal issues in, 181
Family health risks, 594-615
  appraisal of, 600-607
    for biological/age-related factors, 600-602
    for environmental factors, 602, 604-606
    for lifestyle factors, 606-607
  community resources and, 615
  concepts in, 596-599
  early approaches to, 596
  evidence-based practice and, 608
  key points in, 613-614
  nursing interventions for, 599-607
  policies affecting, 595
  practice application for, 613-614
  prevention strategies and, 612b
  reducing, 607-615
    by empowering families, 612-613
    with family contracting, 611-612
    with home visits, 607-611
Family Individual Family Service Plans, 737
Family leave legislation, 588
Family nursing
  approaches to, 573, 574f, 575f
  assessment in, 583-586
    models of, 583-585
  barriers to, 582-583
  defined, 562
  evidence-based practice in, 602
  key points in, 590-591
  outcome present-state testing model of, 578-582
  practice applications in, 590
  and social/family policy changes, 586, 588-590
  theoretical frameworks for, 573, 575-578, 575f
  theory base for, 562
Family planning
  Healthy People 2010 objectives for, 812
  male involvement in, 695
Family policy
  at-risk families and, 613
  changes in, 586, 588-590
  influences of, 595
Family resilience, defined, 572
Family stress theory, Burr and Klein's, 601-602, 602b
Family systems, stressor, strength inventory, 583-584
Family violence, 881-882. See also Child abuse and neglect; Intimate partner violence; Older adult abuse and neglect
  attitudes toward, 895
  child witnesses of, 882-883
  against children, 882-883
  development of, 881-882
  against female partners, 885-887
  forced sex and, 880
  health professional education about, 895
  media education about, 877
  against older adults, 887-888
  organized religion and, 877
  during pregnancy, 887
  screening for, 894-895
  screening women for, 889
  stress and, 882
  types of, 882
  women at risk for, 894-895
FAPE. See Free appropriate public education

Farm residency, defined, 376b
Farmers, health needs/problems of, 383t
Farmworkers
  migrant. See Migrant farmworkers
  seasonal, 795
Farr, William, 252t
Fast food, nutritional quality of, 632
Fat, dietary, for children, 629
Fathers, adolescent, 814-815
Feasibility studies for nursing centers, 432
Federal Bureau of Prisons, health care functions of, 178
Federal Emergency Management Agency, 473, 478
Federal Emergency Relief Administration, 33
  nursing service coverage by, 965
Federal income guidelines, 777
Federal Insecticide, Fungicide, and Rodenticide Act, provisions of, 241b
Federal poverty level, defined, 754
Federal Rehabilitation Act of 1973, 737
Federal Response Plan, 479
  purpose of, 479b
Federally qualified health centers, 416
Federation of Planned Parenthood, 653
Feedback
  in community health nursing, 305-306
  providing, 302
Feeding, infant, 626
Fee-for-service reimbursement, 121-122
  discounted, 1011
Female genital mutilation, 663-664
Female householder families, poverty of, 671
Female partner abuse, nursing interventions for, 893-894
Feminist ethics, 138
Feminists, defined, 138
FERA. See Federal Emergency Relief Administration
Fetal alcohol syndrome, 663
  in Canada, 853
  as cause of birth defects/mental retardation, 865
Fiber, dietary, for children, 630
Field Guide to Health Planning: Assessment Protocol for Excellence in Public Health, A, 351, 352b
Filipinos, spatial preferences of, 163
Filoviruses, bioterrorist threat of, 913
Fiscal competencies, 1035-1038
Fish, mercury-contaminated, 222, 236, 243
FITNE study, 212, 213
Five Day Plan to Stop Smoking, contact information for, 869b
Five Is, 709
5H club, 771
Fliedner, Theodor, 25
Fluoride, supplemental, for formula-fed infants, 629
Flynn, Beverly, 176
Focus groups
  for defining health problems, 1024
  definition, advantages/disadvantages of, 495t
Food, Drug, and Cosmetic Act, provisions of, 110t
Food and Drug Administration, health care functions of, 63
Food infection, 921
Food intoxication
  causal agents and characteristics, 922t
  examples of, 921
Food poisoning. See Food-borne illness
Food Quality Protection Act, 236
  provisions of, 242b
Food safety, 3
  assessment of, 233
  rules for, 922-923, 923b
Food-borne Disease Outbreak Surveillance System, 921
Food-borne illness, 921-924
  in travelers, 925
Ford, Loretta, 991, 992
Ford Foundation, 81
Forensic nursing, 880, 896-897

Formative evaluation, 491
Foster care
  for abused children, 883-884
  policies affecting, 589
Foundation for a Smoke-Free America, contact information for, 869b
Fractures
  fragility, 725
  hip, 725
Frameworks, 194-219
  community, 329-330
  Donabedian, 498
  key points for, 217-218
  Neuman Systems Model, 198-199, 200f, 201-203, 204f, 205-206
  Omaha System Model, 206-213
  organizational, of nursing centers, 426
  practice application for, 217
Framing
  of family client stories, 580-581
  in OPT model, 578
Framingham Heart study, 330
Frankel, Lee, 28b
  funding efforts of, 31
Fraud, legal issues involving, 463
Free appropriate public education, right to, 737
Freeman, Ruth, 40b
Friedan, Betty, 654
Friedman family assessment model, 584-585, 585b
Frontier, defined, 376b
Frontier Nursing Service, establishment of, 31, 32b
Frost, Wade Hampton, 252t
Fruits, dietary guidelines for, in children/adolescents, 628t
Fry, Elizabeth, 25
Functional limitations, defined, 721
Funding, 111-121
  for Canadian health care, 112-113
  categorical, 178
  for community-oriented nursing, 39
  federal, for public health, 34-35
  government, 173
  for international health, 78-79
  for nursing centers, 433-434
  private, 117-121
    through employment programs, 118-119
    through health insurance, 118
    through managed care, 119-120
    through medical savings accounts, 120-121
  program, 512
  public, 112-113, 115-118
    through Medicaid, 115t, 116-117, 117f
    through Medicare, 115-116, 115t, 116f
    through military agencies and IHS, 117
    through public health agencies, 117
  for public health nursing, 31

**G**

Gamblers Anonymous, 868
Gangs, youth, 634
  violence of, 878
Gardner, Mary, 30
Garlic for reducing LDLs, 689b
Gastrointestinal system, age-related changes in, 705t
Gastrointestinal virus in children, home management of, 636b
Gatekeepers, role of, 547b
GBD. See Global burden of disease
Gebbie, K., 12-13
Gender
  in health problems, 56
  in mortality/morbidity rates, 269
General systems theory, 197
Generative leadership, 1016
Genetic testing, 256
Genital herpes. See Herpes simplex 2 infection (genital)
Genital mutilation, female, 663-664
Genital warts. See also Human papillomavirus infection
  summary of, 941t

Genitourinary system, age-related changes in, 705t
Genograms, 603f
  development of, 586, 586f
  interpretive categories for, 588b
  interviewing for, 588b
  symbols for, 587f-588f
Gentrification, negative consequences of, 785
Geographic information systems, epidemiologic applications of, 271
Geographic patterns, epidemiologic, 270
Geriatric Assessment and Intervention Team, 710
Geriatric Resource Nurse model, 714
Geriatrics, defined, 703
Germ theory, 252
German measles, characteristics and immunization, 919-920
Gerontological nursing
  community-based models for, 710-714
    adult day health in, 710-711
    assisted living in, 713
    home health in, 711-712
    hospice in, 712
    long-term care in, 713-714
    nursing roles in, 710
    rehabilitation in, 714
    senior centers in, 710
  defined, 703
Gerontological Nursing Interventions Research Center, website for, 715
Gerontology, defined, 703
Gestational diabetes mellitus, 665
Giardia
  in traveler's diarrhea, 926
  in waterborne disease, 925
  waterborne illness due to, 923
Gilden, Robyn, 233
Gilligan, C., 137-138
Global burden of disease, 86-87
Goals
  defined, 199t
  establishing, for infant malnutrition, 363-364, 364t
Goal-setting theory, 1014t, 1015
Gold standard, 285
Gonorrhea
  antibiotic-resistant, 942
  cause, symptoms, treatment, 938
  coinfection with chlamydia, 938
  and increased risk of HIV infection, 935
  risk management of, in Canada, 949
  summary of, 940t
Government
  advanced practice nurses in, 1000
  Canadian, health care functions of, 182
  initiatives of. See also Legislation
    Canadian, for women, 661
    local, in diaster preparedness, 477t
    services for at-risk families, 613
    trends and shifts in roles of, 172-173
    U. S. See U. S. government
Grandmothers as primary caregivers, evidence-based practice and, 604
Grandparents as heads of households, 568
Grant writing, guidelines for, 512
Grants, funding from, 433-434
Graunt, John, 251t
Great Depression, public health nursing during, 33-34
Grey Nuns of Montreal, 36
Griswold v. Connecticut, 653-654, 811b
Gross domestic product
  defined, 101
  versus gross national product, 107
Gross national product
  defined, 101
  versus gross domestic product, 107
Group approaches, 540-559
Group culture, 544
Groups
  beginning interactions in, 549, 550b
  cohesion of, 542–544, 542f
  conflicts in, 556-557
  contribution to community life, 554-555
  definitions of, 541-542

Groups–cont'd
  effectiveness of
    evaluating, 552
      team building for, 552-554
    evaluation of, 551-552
    evidence-based practice with, 553
    examples of, 541-542
    formal versus informal, 554
    Healthy People 2010 goals for, 552
    key points for, 557
    leader directiveness in, 554
    leadership in, 545-546, 545b
    member interactions in, 541
    minority dissent in, 553
    neighborhood/regional activist, 555
    nominal, defined, 358
    norms in, 544-545, 544f
    positive versus negative health influences of, 547
    practice application for, 556-557
    in promoting community health goals, 555-556
    promoting individual health through, 547-554
    purposes of, 542
    recruitment by, 542
    structure of, 546-547
    task and maintenance functions of, 542-543
Growth, defined, 617
Growth and development
  adolescent, 625t
  infant, 620t
  neonatal, 619t
  neonatal to adolescent, 617-624
  of toddlers/preschoolers, 621t
Growth hormones, 623
Growth spurt, adolescent, 623
Gugulipid for reducing LDLs, 689b
Guide to Clinical Preventive Services, 7, 526
Guide to Disability Rights Law, A, 736-737
Guidelines for Adolescent Preventative Services, 623, 624b
Gun control legislation, 635, 889
Gun violence, reducing
  among children and adolescents, 634-635
  safety measures in, 889
Guns, ownership of, 634-635
  among adolescents, 809
Gynecologic age of adolescents, 819

H

Hackman and Oldham job redesign theory, 1015
Haemophilus influenzae type B vaccine in Canada, 914
Haitian culture, health care issues in, 158
Halfway houses, 867-868
Hallucinogens, mental and physiologic effects of, 859
Hamburger, E. coli contamination of, 921, 923
Handgun control, 889
Handicap, defined, 722
Hantavirus, 254
  symptoms, transmission, and causes of emergence, 912t
Hantavirus pulmonary syndrome, 904
  characteristics of, 908
Harm reduction model of drug abuse, 851
Hartford Institute for Geriatric Nursing, website for, 715
Hawes, Bessie M., 33
Hazard communication standard, 234, 1086-1087
Head Start Program, 645
  for migrant children, 800
Heads-of-household, women as, 671
Healing
  biblical accounts of, 1113
  defined, 707
  nontraditional, 151
Healing ministries, parish nursing as, 1103b
Health
  biomedical model of, 319
  definitions of, 52b, 199t, 249-250, 323-324

Health–cont'd
  determinants of, 601b
  disease versus health paradigms of, 320
  historical perspectives on, 322b
  holistic view of, 322
  perceptions of, cultural variations in, 162t
  rural definition of, 385
Health agencies, federal, 176-177
Health and wellness centers, 415-416
Health behaviors
  factors affecting, 595
  group influences on, 547
  Kulbok's model of, 324-325
  Milio's propositions for improving, 329b
  motivation for, 596
Health beliefs/practices of migrant farmworkers, 801-802
Health Canada, 226
  website for, 852
Health care
  access to, 52, 97, 123
    Healthy People 2010 goals for, 420
    home care and, 984-985
    by vulnerable populations, 748-749
  adolescent, 808-809
  aging population and, 2
  Canadian, government roles in, 115
  carve outs in, 753
  changes in, 1011
  community-oriented/community-based, 14
  comprehensive services in, 750
  congressional actions pertaining to, 171-172
  consumption of, as community health indicator, 8b
  controlling costs of, 122
  costs of, 42
  culturally/linguistically appropriate, 750
  environmental health risks associated with, 232b
  evaluation of, historical development of, 492-493, 492t
  expenditures for, 54, 106-107
    1980-2002, 107t
    1980 to 2010, 114t
    in Canada, 112
    changes in, 108b
    demographics affecting, 107, 109
    distribution of, 108f
    factors affecting, 107, 109, 110t, 111
    by health condition, 111t
    for older adults, 109t
    projections for, 108t
  government's role in, 172-173
  for immigrants, 151, 796-798
  international. See International health care
  local government responsibilities for, 63-64, 64b
  managed. See Managed health care
  migrant farmworker opinions on, 797
  national objectives for, 595
  nursing models of, 413, 414
  primary. See Primary health care
  pyramid of, 7, 7f
  reimbursement for. See Health insurance; Reimbursement
  resource allocation in, 122-124
  rural access to, 380-381
  social mandate for, 447
  state responsibilities for, 63
  wrap-around services in, 749
Health care access, barriers to, 752
Health care delivery
  economics of. See Economics
  parish nursing and, 1097-1098. See also Parish nursing
  population-focused approach to, 341. See also Population-focused practice
Health Care Financing Administration. See also Centers for Medicare and Medicaid Services
  creation of, 172
  renaming of, 710
Health care industry, environmental threats in, 243-244

Health care insurance. See Health insurance
Health care markets, 99
Health care needs, rural, 383t
Health care planning, historical development of, 492-493, 492t
Health care policies, social Darwinism reflected in, 756
Health care practices
  of Canadian men, 684
  of Canadian women, 660
Health care practitioners, payments to, 121-122
Health care rationing, 123
Health care reform, 97
  in Canada, 66
  in Clinton administration, 493
  Community Health Improvement Process in, 524, 525f
  Democratic versus Republican positions on, 172
  failure of, 1
  in Latin America, 80
  recommendations for, 125b
  support for, 42-43
Health care settings, Healthy People 2010 educational goals for, 297
Health care system, 50-71. See also Primary health care; Public health care
  in Canada, 83-84
  changes in, 1010t
  in China, 85
  consumer influence on, 64
  demographic trends in, 53
  economic trends in, 54
  employer influence on, 64
  health workforce trends in, 54
  integrated, 18
  key points for, 68-69
  legislative influences on, 64-65
  MCO influences on, 64
  in Mexico, 85-86
  organization of, 55-64
  practice application for, 68
  primary, 55-56
  priorities in, 3
  seamless, 1011
  social trends in, 53-54
  in Sweden, 84-85
  technologic trends in, 54-55
  transformation of, 64-65
  trends affecting, 53-55
  U. S., 51-53
    access to, 52
    context of, 103, 105-106
    cost of, 51-52
    quality of, 52-53
  in United Kingdom, 83
Health Care Without Harm, 244
Health centers, federally qualified, 416
Health changes
  after community health education, 313-314
  groups for, 548-549
    established, 548
    selected membership, 548-549
  strategies for, groups in, 551
Health commodification, 81
Health concerns of Canadian women, 660
Health departments
  growth of, 105
  local, 63-64, 64b, 178
  state, 63, 63b, 178
Health disparities
  eliminating, 349
  health care areas affected by, 749
  in vulnerable populations, 747-749, 760
Health economics, defined, 98
Health education. See also Community health education
  in needs assessment, 496
  in parish nursing, 1102-1103
  school nurse's role in, 1046-1047
  for vulnerable populations, 764, 766
Health events
  determinants of, 250-251
  distribution of, 250

Health fairs, 304b
organizing, 297
Health field concept, 759
Health for All by the Year 2000, 72
Health for All in the 21st Century, 72
objectives of, 74
as strategic process, 74-75
WHO's commitment to, 74-75
Health history, occupational, 1082-1083, 1084f-1085f
Health indicators, leading, Healthy People 2010 objectives for, 420, 994
Health information, privacy and security of, 1012
Health insurance. *See also* Medicaid; Medicare
for addiction treatment, 850
changing role of, 105
cost of, 119
evolution of, 118
extending coverage by, 3
for home health/hospice care, 980
lack of, 52, 123, 437, 438, 616-617
effects on vulnerable populations, 753
for mental illness, 837
national, in Canada, 83
and noncoverage of community-oriented nursing, 39
policy challenges for, 590
quality of care and, 52
reform of, 3
in rural areas, 378, 379
in Sweden, 84-85
universal coverage by, 19
visiting nursing service coverage by, 965
Health Insurance Portability and Accountability Act, 119
home health care provisions of, 984-985
impact of, 711t
nursing centers and, 435
privacy/security provisions of, 1012
provisions of, 110t, 172
Health interventions
defined, 207
epidemiologic basis for, 279
spectrum of, 264-265, 264f
Health literacy, health status and, 757
Health maintenance, 325. *See also* Holistic health care; Well-child care; Wellness
Health Maintenance Organization Act, provisions of, 110t
Health maintenance organizations, 59
advanced practice nurses in, 1000
characteristics of, 58
enrollment in, 119-120
Health Manpower Act of 1971, 992
Health ministries, defined, 1093
*Health Objectives for the Nation,* 11
Health of Canada's Communities, 386
Health outcomes. *See also* entries under outcomes
in home health care, 985-986
homelessness and, 785
prayer and, evidence-based practice and, 1095
for vulnerable populations, 760-761
Health Plan Employer Data and Information Set, 518
Health Planning and Resource Development Act, 110t
Health policy. *See* Policy entries
Health problems
chronic, in children/adolescents, 637-641
focus groups for defining, 1024
nurse's role in, 367
quantifying, 259
Health professional shortage areas, 380-381
Health professionals, multidisciplinary, in nursing centers, 429
Health program planning
population-level model of, 496-498
process of, 495, 496t

Health promotion, 56. *See also* Community health promotion
ATOD and, 860-861
client education about, 300
for coronary heart disease, 334t
definitions of, 52b, 324-325
for failure to thrive, 333t
in Healthy Cities movement, 399
Healthy People 2010 goals for, 600
*versus* illness prevention/health maintenance, 325
landmark initiatives in, 323b
methods of, 319
for migrant farmworkers, 802
for older adults, 714-715
for physically compromised individuals, 731-733
recommendations for, 125b
for vulnerable populations, 766
culturally/linguistically appropriate, 764, 766
WHO definition of, 324
Health records, children's, confidentiality of, 1053
Health Resources and Services Administration, 60, 176-177
community health status indicators of, 350
Health resources for at-risk families, 613
Health risk appraisal, 326, 327b
advantages and disadvantages of, 327-328
Health risks. *See also* Risk entries
accumulated, 598
community health and, 348-349
defined, 598
and development of outcomes, 597-598
environmental
communication about, 239-242
in environmental standards, 242
ethics and, 240
nursing interventions for, 239
outrage factors and, 238b
preventive strategies for, 238b
reducing, 237-242, 237b
in rural areas, 382-384
family. *See* Family health risks
occupational. *See also* Occupational health risks
in rural areas, 382-384
reducing, 595
of vulnerable populations, 758-759
Health Sector Reform Program, Mexican, 85
Health Security Act of 1993, 172
Health services
brokering, 768-769
rural patterns of use, 380, 380t
Health services delivery
developmental framework for, 103, 104f
tracer method for evaluating, 509
Health status
assessments of, 11
Canadian primary care and, 66
as characteristic of community health, 346-347, 347b
as community health indicator, 8b
environmental interface with, 13
homelessness and, 785-789
as indicator of community health, 349t
male
cultural differences in, 687
in U. S., 681-682
poor, by household income, 756-757, 756f
poverty and, 778-783
of rural residents, 378-379
socioeconomic factors affecting, 123, 756-758
of vulnerable populations, 758
*Health: United States,* 173
Health values of migrant workers, 801-802
Health workforce
ethnic makeup of, 148
in primary care, 59-60

Health workforce—cont'd
shortages in, 65
trends in, 54
Healthier People Network, health risk appraisal instrument of, 327
Healthier People Questionnaire, 326
Healthy Cities initiative, 352
Healthy Communities and Cities movement, 341, 396-411, 503
action research and, 401, 403
in Canada, 403
characteristics of, 398
in China, 405
community-oriented nursing implications of, 407-408
in El Salvador, 405
European networks of, 404-405
evidence-based practice in, 401
future of, 406-407
Healthy People 2010 objectives for, 408-409
history of, 397-398
in Latin America, 406
models of, 399-401
in Nepal, 405
origins and focus of, 396-397
physically compromised clients and, 734
in Poland, 404
process for, 398
requirements of, 734
in Russia, 403-404
terms pertaining to, 398-399
in U. S., 401-403
in Venezuela, 405-406
Healthy People 2000, 13
Healthy People 2010, 12
access to care goals of, 786
adolescent sexuality objectives of, 812
ATOD use objectives of, 861
child health objectives of, 626, 645, 646-647, 646t
child/adolescent nutrition objectives of, 633
communicable disease objectives of, 904
and community as partner, 348
community collaboration and, 419-421
community health in, 349-350
community health strategies in, 351
community partnerships and, 350-351
development of, 43
disaster management objectives of, 472
educational objectives of, 296-298
environmental health objectives of, 222
epidemiology objectives of, 250
evidence-based practice objectives and, 288, 290
focus areas of, 176b, 503
goals of, 175, 1026
related to access to care, 124
group work goals of, 552
gun violence reduction goals of, 635
health initiatives contributing to, 323
health objectives of, 56, 57t, 202
health promotion goals of, 600
healthy community strategies of, 328b
healthy lifestyles in, 318
home health care and, 984, 985
immunization objectives of, 907
influenza vaccine objectives of, 921
leading health indicators of, 420, 994
parish nursing and, 1106-1108
Lyme disease objectives of, 924
men's health objectives of, 680, 694, 695
mental health objectives of, 837-844
migrant farmworker objectives of, 803
national health objectives in, 503
as national health policy guidance, 174-175
Nigerian applications of, 75
in nursing center development, 419
nursing centers and, 412
objectives of, 1122-1123
for reducing diabetes, 154

Healthy People 2010—cont'd
occupational health objectives of, 1086-1087
older adult objectives of, 714, 716
physically compromised client objectives of, 733-734
program planning objectives of, 502
on public health infrastructure and workforce, 141
quality assurance objectives of, 520
quality management goals in, 524
racial/ethnic health care disparities in, 1120
rural health objectives of, 390-391
school nursing objectives and, 1049, 1050
STD objectives of, 932
teen pregnancy goals of, 812
tobacco use objectives of, 320, 640
vaccine-preventable disease objectives of, 919
vulnerable population objectives of, 766-767, 768
website for, 350
website summary of, 42
women's health objectives of, 57, 646
women's reproductive health objectives of, 657
Healthy People in Healthy Communities, 328
Healthy People reports, 11, 42
recommendations of, 125b
Heart disease
complementary and alternative therapies for, 689b
in men, 687-688, 695
rates of, for men *versus* women, 687t
Heavy metals
children's absorption of, 235
children's exposure to, 640
Hebert, Marie Rollet, 36
*Helicobacter pylori* in peptic ulcer disease, 906
Helplessness, learned, 309
in abused women, 886
Hemp, economic uses of, 858
Henry Street Settlement, 28b, 29, 30, 965, 1043
Hepatitis
sexually transmitted, 944
waterborne sources of, 925
Hepatitis A infection
cause, symptoms, prevention/treatment, 944
immune globulin recommendations for, 946b
profile of, 945t
risk management of, in Canada, 948
Hepatitis B infection
cause, symptoms, prevention/treatment, 944, 946
elimination strategy for, 947
immunizations for, evidence-based practice and, 1047
profile of, 945t
required immunizations for, 1052t
risk management of, in Canada, 948-949
work-related exposure to, 1076
Hepatitis C infection
profile of, 945t
risk management of, in Canada, 949
work-related exposure to, 1076
Hepatitis D infection, profile of, 945t
Hepatitis E infection, profile of, 945t
Hepatitis G infection, profile of, 945t
Herbal remedies
contraindicated, for children, 643b
for improving memory, 836
prevalence of, 641
Herbicides, child exposure to, 640
Herd immunity, 906
Heroin use, physiologic effects of, 855
Herpes simplex 2 infection (genital), 943f
cause, symptoms, treatment, 942-943
increased rates of, 938
summary of, 941t
Hill, A. Bradford, 252t

Hill-Burton Act
  amendments to, 110t
  impact of, 711t
  provisions affecting vulnerable populations, 751
  provisions of, 110t
Hip fractures in older adults, 725
Hispanic American women, causes of death among, 659t
Hispanic Americans
  cultural attitudes/practices of, 162t
  environmental control perspectives of, 165
  food preferences and nutrition-related risk factors of, 167t
  mental health of, 843
  as percentage of U. S. population, 53
  social organization of, 164f
  spatial preferences of, 163
  time values of, 164
Hispanic children, poverty of, 779, 779t
Hispanic culture, health care issues in, 157
Hispanic women
  as heads-of-households, poverty of, 671
  overweight, 668
  prison/jail rate of, 670
HIV infection, 23, 254, 932-938
  case management of, 455
  children with, in schools, 1061
  in community, 937-938
  drug use and, in Canada, 853
  economic costs of, 933
  epidemiology of, 936, 936t
  manhood stereotypes and, 693
  in men, 693-694, 695
  in migrant farmworkers, 799
  natural history of, 933-935
  opportunistic infections associated with, 908
  patient responsibilities and, 955, 955b
  perinatal/pediatric, 937
  persons at risk for, 256
  prevention of, 693-694, 694b
  resources for, 938
  risk management of, in Canada, 948
  risk reduction program for, 332
  by sex and race/ethnicity, 936t
  standard precautions for, 956
  summary of, 940t-941t
  surveillance of, 936-937
  symptoms, transmission, and causes of emergence, 912t
  testing and counseling for, 954-955, 954b
  testing for, 937
  transmission of, 935-936, 935b
    perinatal, 936
  tuberculosis associated with, 87, 88
  in women, 667-668, 667t
  work-related exposure to, 1076
HIV testing, 935, 937
Hodgkin's lymphoma in children, adult sequelae of, 725
Holistic health care
  defined, 1094
  parish nursing and, 1101-1102
Holistic health centers, faith communities' involvement in, 1097
Home, safety measures in, 889
Home care, legal issues in, 181-182
Home care agencies, cost-effectiveness analysis of, 102
Home Care Client Satisfaction instrument, 526
Home health aide, role in home care, 975
Home health care
  access issues in, 984-985
  accountability/quality management of, 978-979
  advanced practice nurses in, 1000-1001
  agency accreditation for, 978-979
  in Canada, 972-973
  for children, 985
  client goals in, 964
  contracting for, 969, 969f
  cost effectiveness of, 981

Home health care—cont'd
  definition of, 963-964
  direct, 969-970
  educational requirements for, 977-978
  episodic versus distributive, 970
  facts about, 967b
  family's role in, 985
  financial aspects of, 979-981
  growth of, 64
  Health Insurance Portability and Accountability Act and, 984-985
  Healthy People 2010 objectives for, 984
  history of, 964-966
  indirect, 970
  infection control standards for, 971
  key points, 986-987
  legal/ethical issues in, 982-983
  legislation pertaining to, 981-982
  Medicare conditions of participation for, 979b
  Medicare versus Medicaid programs for, 980t
  nursing process in, 970-974
  nursing roles in, 970
  for older adults, 711-712
  outcomes of, 971, 985-986
  practice application for, 996
  professional standards in, 974-975
  quality improvement programs in, 524, 526
  regulatory mechanisms for, 979-980
  reimbursement mechanisms for, 979-981
  responsibilities of disciplines in, 974-975
  scope of practice, 968-975
  standards of practice, 970-974
  stresses in, 984
  technology/telehealth issues in, 983-984
  trends in, 984
  types of agencies, 966-968
Home Health Care Classification, 207, 207t
Home health nursing
  certification of, 978
  classification of, 346
Home safety, evaluation of, 713f
Home visits, 607-611. See also Home health care; Visiting nurse associations
  advantages/disadvantages of, 607
  phases and activities of, 608t
  process of, 607-611
  purpose of, 607
  reasons for, 610, 610b
  voluntary versus required, 609
Home-based service programs, 644-645
Homeland Security, Office of, 478
Homeless child syndrome, 645
Homeless families, programs for, 645
Homeless persons
  case management for, 790
  with children, 788
  children/adolescents, 787-788
  health care for, private funding of, 788-789
  health problems of, 785-787, 786t
  older adults, 787
  pregnancy women as, 787
Homeless women, support systems of, 672
Homelessness, 774-793
  at-risk populations and, 787
  in Canada, 780-781
  causes of, 785
  clients' perceptions of, 783
  concept of, 783-785
  demographics of, 758
  evidence-based practice for, 783
  federal programs for, 788
  health care and
    nurse's role in, 789-790
    practice application for, 790
  health effects of, 785-789
  heath status and, 758
  key points, 790-791
  prevalence of, 783-784, 785
  prevention of, 788

Homelessness—cont'd
  profile of, 785b
  of women, 671
Homeopathy for children, 642
Homicide, 878-879
  abused women and, 886
  adolescent, 634
  in families, 887
  as leading cause of death, 878
  perpetrators of, 877-878
  in rural areas, 379
Homophobia in rural areas, 379
Homosexuals, attitudes toward, 932
Hookworm, control of, 30
Hopelessness of vulnerable populations, 760
Horizontal transmission of disease, 906
Hormone replacement therapy
  cardiovascular disease and, 664
  controversy over, 663
  health risks associated with, 672
  osteoporosis and, 663
Hospice care, 975-976
  for dying children, 975-976
  facts about, 967b
  financial aspects of, 979-981
  health care provider stress in, 976
  at home, 964
  interdisciplinary approach to, 976-977
  legal issues in, 181-182
  Medicare coverage of, 975
  for older adults, 712
  philosophy of, applications of, 977
  reimbursement for, 979-980, 981
Hospital Construction and Facilities Act, impact of, 711t
Hospitals
  acute care facilities of, downsizing of, 54
  growth of, 105
  home health agencies in, 967
  home nursing programs of, 965
  psychiatric, 830-831
Hot flashes, alternative therapies for, 672-673
Households
  single-parent, percentage of children in, 616
  women-headed, poverty of, 671
    by ethnicity/race, 669f
Housing
  emergency, 788
  low-income, 788
  migrant farmworker opinions on, 797
  for migrant farmworkers, 795-796
  windshield survey of, 357t
Housing Assistance Council, 796
Huang for treating obesity, 689b
Human capital, 124
  defined, 754
Human genome project, 582
Human immunodeficiency virus. See HIV infection
Human papillomavirus infection
  characteristics of, 943-944
  summary of, 941t
  symptoms, transmission, and causes of emergence, 912t
Human Population Laboratory study, 330
Human relations theory of management, 1013-1014
Humanistic theory, 300
  of aging, 704
Hyde Amendment, 654
Hydrophobia. See Rabies
Hypertension
  prevention of, 500
  screening for, in schoolchildren, 1054, 1056
Hypotheses, testing of, 197

I

I PREPARE pneumonic, 229, 230b
Identity, sexual, in women with disabilities, 671
Illicit drugs, overdoses/impurities of, 865
Illness. See also Disease
  acute, in children/adolescents, 636-637
  chronic. See Chronic illness

Illness—cont'd
  food-borne, 233, 921-924
  socioeconomic status and, 123
  vaccine-preventable, Healthy People 2010 objectives for, 919
  waterborne, 921-924
  versus wellness emphasis, 319-321
Illness care
  for coronary heart disease, 334t
  for failure to thrive, 333t
Illness prevention
  client education about, 294, 295b
  studies contributing to, 331
Illness-focused nursing care, shift from, to health-focused care, 414, 415f
Immigrants. See also Migrant farmworkers; Migrant health care
  benefit eligibilities of, 149-150
  community's role with, 151
  definitions of, 151
  environmental conditions of, 26-27
  family conflicts of, 151
  health care for, 151, 796-798
  health issues of, 149-151
  illegal, practice application for, 769
  language barriers of, 151
  legal, 149
  nontraditional healing practices of, 151
  numbers of, by country of birth, 150t
  risk factors for, 151
  Russian, health issues of, 564b
  undocumented, 149
    denial of preventive health care to, 911
Immigration
  demographics of, 53
  economic impacts of, 150-151
  legislation restricting, 752
Immigration and Nationality Act, 149
Immigration Reform and Control Act, 149
Immune globulin for hepatitis A, 946b
Immune system, age-related changes in, 705t
Immunity
  acquired, 906
  civil, 181
  herd, 906
  natural, 906
  sovereign, 181
Immunizations. See also Vaccines
  active versus passive, 906
  Canadian regulations for, 915
  for children/adolescents, 630-631
    barriers to, 630-631
    contraindications to, 631
    legislation for, 631
    recommendations for, 631
    schedule for, 918
  cost of, 630
  Healthy People 2010 objectives for, 420, 994
  for hepatitis, 945t, 946
  for hepatitis B, evidence-based practice and, 946, 1047
  for HIV-infected children, 938
  for immigrant children, 564
  for influenza, 920-921
  for measles, 918-919
  parental education about, evidence-based practice and, 918
  for pertussis, 920
  policies on, after 9/11, 589-590
  preschool, PERT for, 507f
  against rabies, 926
  for rubella, 919-920
  for school children, 1051-1053, 1052t
  theory of, 631
  WHO program on, 87
Immunocompromised patients, parasitic opportunistic infections in, 927
Impact evaluation, 491
Impairment, defined, 721
Implementation
  components of, 366
  factors influencing, 366-368
  mechanisms of, 368
  skills in, 1035

*Improving Health in the Community: A Role for Performance Monitoring,* 7
Incest, patterns and long-term implications of, 885
Incidence
  measures of, 256-258
  *versus* prevalence, 258-259
Incidence proportion, 256
Incidence rate, 256
Independent practice, advanced practice nurses in, 997
India, health promotion in, 78
Indian Health Service, 117
Indiana University School of Nursing, Healthy Cities project and, 401-402
Indicators approach, definition, advantages/disadvantages of, 495t
Individualized education plans, 1044
Individualized health plans, 1044
Individuals with Disabilities Education Act, 737
  school nursing provisions of, 1044, 1044t
Indoor air quality, assessment of, 229
Industrial nursing, 1067-1068. *See also* Occupational health nursing
Industry, advanced practice nurses in, 999-1000
Infant care by teen parents, 820-821
Infant feeding, 626
  supplements to, 626, 629
Infant formula, iron supplements for, 626, 629
Infant mortality rate
  for African Americans, 269
  calculation of, 260t
  Canadian, for infants in remote areas, 748
  ethnic differences in, 686
  in health professional shortage areas, 381t
  in U.K., 83
  in U. S., 83, 617
Infants
  abuse risk for, evidence-based practice for, 730
  assessment of, 618-619
  developmental levels of, intervention activities for assessing, 365t
  developmentally delayed, practice application for, 738
  HIV infection in, 937
  home health care for, 985
  injuries/accidents in, 633-634
  low-birth-weight
    in health professional shortage areas, 381t
    of teen mothers, 819-820
  malnutrition in, 819
    problem analysis of, 358t
    problem prioritizing for, 362t
    progress notes on, 369t
    risk of, 360
  nutritional assessment in, 626, 628t, 629
  physically compromised, 724-725
    legal rights of, 737
  rickets risk in, prevention strategies for, 629, 629b
  SIDS in, 637
  syphilis in, 942
Infection
  *versus* disease, 906
  in infants/children, 636
  in older adults, 710
  opportunistic
    HIV/AIDS-related, 908, 935
    from parasites, 927
Infectious disease, 902-931
  advances in management of, 105
  agent factors in, 905, 905b
  as agents of bioterrorism, 913, 916-917
  in American colonial period, 24
  in Canada, 914-915
  communicable period of, 906-907
  control of, 913
  cyclical patterns in, 270-272
  in day-care centers, 636-637
    evidence-based practice for, 637

Infectious disease—cont'd
  decline of, 1119
  development of, 906-907
  drug-resistant forms of, 1119-1120
  economic cost of, 905
  elimination/eradication of, 911
  emerging forms of, 908-910, 910t, 911f, 912t
  endemic, 907
  environmental factors in, 906
  epidemic, 907
  epidemiologic triangle in, 905, 905f
  food- and waterborne, 921-924
  Healthy People 2010 objectives for, 904
  historical/current perspectives on, 903-904
  host factors in, 905-906
  immunizations against, 87
  incubation period of, 906
  key points, 929
  in lesser-developed countries, 86
  nationally notifiable, 909b
  new, 254-255
  new forms of, 1119
  nosocomial, 928
  pandemic, 907
  parasitic, 926-928
  practice application for, 928-929
  prevention of, 910-913, 913
    primary, 950-954
    secondary, 954-955
    tertiary, 955-956
  public health influence on, 3
  public health nurses' role in, 1126
  reportable, 908
  resistance to, 906
  spectrum of, 907
  surveillance of, 907-908
  threats of, 2
  transmission of, 905-907
  in travelers, 925-926
  uncontrolled, 23
  universal precautions for, 928
  vaccine-preventable, 917-921
    in Canada, 914-915
  vector-borne, 924-925
  waterborne, 923-924
  from zoonoses, 926
Infectious disease risk, 932-959
  for AIDS, 948
  Canadian management of
    for gonorrhea, 949
    for SARS, 949
    for syphilis, 949
  for chlamydia, 949
  from hepatitis, 944-950
  for hepatitis A, 948
  for hepatitis B, 948-949
  for hepatitis C, 949
  for HIV, 932-938, 948
  key points, 956-957
  nurse's role in, 950-956
  practice application for, 956
  for STDs, 938-944
    chlamydia, 942-943
    gonorrhea, 938, 942
    herpes simplex virus 2, 943
    human papillomavirus, 943-944
    syphilis, 942
  for tuberculosis, 947, 950
  work-related, 1076
Infectious hazards, work-related, 1076b
Infectiousness, defined, 906
Inflation, 101
Influenza, characteristics and immunization, 920-921
Influenza vaccine in Canada, 914-915
Influenza viruses, types of, 920
Informant interviews, 355
Information exchange process in advocacy, 457-458
Information management in Omaha System, 208
Inhalants, categories of, 859
Injectable drug use
  community outreach about, 953-954
  identifying, in sexual partners, 952
  infectious disease risk and, 953
Injectable drug users, risks of, 865

Injuries
  alcohol-related, prevention of, 693b
  in children/adolescents, 623, 633-636, 634t
    preventing, 636b, 1051
  fatal, for men, 690
  Healthy People 2010 objectives for, 420, 994
  to men, 695
  to migrant children, 800
  to migrant farmworkers, 798
  needlestick, 1076
Insecticides, leukemia and, 222
Institute for Public Health and Faith Collaborations, 1099
Institute of Medicine, public health report of, 7, 42
Institutional privileges of nurse practitioners, 1002
Institutional theory, 1014t, 1016-1017
Institutionalization in mental health care, 830-831
Instruction
  effective, 312b
  events of, 302
Instructive District Nursing Association, 27
Instructive Visiting Nursing Association, 964, 965
Instrumental activities of daily living, difficulty in performing, 701
Insurance. *See also* Health insurance
  worker's compensation, 681-682
Integrated systems, 18
Integration, horizontal *versus* vertical, 106
Integrative model for health promotion. *See* Community health promotion, integrative model for
Integrative outcomes, 460
Integrity, defined, 139
Intellectual capacity, aging and, 705
Intellectual impairment, three Ds of, 709
Intensity, 111
Interactionist theory of family, 577-578
Inter-African Committee, objectives of, 664b
Interagency Council on the Homeless, 788
Interdependence, 344
Interdisciplinary theory of family, 577-578
International Conference on Primary Health Care, 73
International Congress of Nursing on nursing preparedness for terrorism, 92
International cooperation in Healthy Cities movement, 398
International Council of Nurses, Code of Ethics of, 132
International health care, 72-95
  in border areas, 76
  economic development and, 81-82
  evidence-based practice in, 76, 91
  health care systems in, 82-86
  key points in, 92-93
  major health problems in, 86-92
  major organizations in, 78-81
  nursing and, 78
  organizations for, classification of, 79
  population health's role in, 76-77
  practice application for, 92
  primary health care in, 77-78
International Red Cross, 81
Internet
  access to, 55
  in community health education, 310
  health care applications of, 106
  for health information, 1011
    assessing quality of, 310
  school nursing resources on, 1062t
Interpersonal relationships, work-related, 1079-1080
Interpersonal theories of leadership/management, 1013-1016
Interpreters, selecting and using, 163, 164
Interpretivism, 299t
  defined, 298

Intervention activities
  for determining infants' developmental levels, 364, 365t
  implementation and evaluation of, 367t
  for implementing outreach programs for at-risk infants, 366t
Interventions. *See also* Health interventions
  community health, evaluating, 369-370
  modes for, in consultation, 1021t
Interviews
  informant, 355
  oral history, 41
Intimate partner violence, 885-887. *See also* Family violence
  assessing for, 891
  attitudes toward, 895
  nursing interventions for, 893-894
  during pregnancy, safety behaviors for preventing, 887
  as process, 886-887
  sexual, 887
  signs of, 885-887
  during teen pregnancy, 817-818
Intrauterine device, uses and effectiveness of, 662t
Iowa Nursing Interventions Classification, 207t
Iowa Nursing Outcomes Classification, 207t
Irish Sisters of Charity, 25
Iron, supplemental, for non-breast-fed infants, 626, 629
Iron deficiency, 91
  during teen pregnancy, 819-820
Isolation
  legal basis for, 179
  professional, of advanced nurse practitioners, 1002-1003
  social
    family violence and, 882
    health status and, 758
Isoniazid, TB bacillus resistance to, 88
Isosporiasis, 927

**J**

Japan, health promotion in, 78
Jargon, avoiding, 303
JCAH. *See* Joint Commission on Accreditation of Hospitals
Jenner, Edward, 251t
Job redesign theory, 1014t
John Hancock Mutual Life Insurance Company, 965
Johnson, Lyndon Baines, 39, 778
Joint Commission on Accreditation of Health Care Organizations, 105
Joint Commission on Accreditation of Hospitals, nursing service standards of, 521
Joint practice, advanced practice nurses in, 997
Judicial branch of government, 171
Judicial bypass, 811b
Judicial law, 180
Junk food, prevalence of, 632
"Just say no" model of drug use prevention, 862, 865
Justice
  distributive, 135b, 136
  environmental, 243
  ethical issues in, 465
  libertarian view of, 136
  social, defined, 750

**K**

Kennedy, John F., 654, 778, 796
Kerr-Mills Act, 778
Key informants, definition, advantages/disadvantages of, 495t
Keystone family issues, 580-581, 580f, 581f
Kickbusch, Ilona, 397
Knowledge manager, 288
Koch, Robert, 252t
Kohlberg, Lawrence, moral development theory of, 683
Kosovo Women's Health Promotion Project, 74

**L**

La Salle Neighborhood Nursing Center
  evidence-based practice in, 437
  mission and goals of, 417b
  Youth Opportunities Initiative of, 441
Labor organizations
  in diaster preparedness, 477t
  disaster response responsibilities of, 478t
Lac Courte Oreilles Indians, evidence-based assessment of, 12
LaCrosse virus, 924
Ladies' Benevolent Society, 24
LaLonde, M., 323, 323f
LaLonde Report, 77
Latex allergy, symptoms of, 952
Latin America, health care reform in, 80
Latin American network of Healthy Cities, 406
Law. See also Legislation; Policy
  common, 180
  community health practice and, 181-183
  constitutional, community-oriented nursing and, 179
  environmental, 241b
  judicial, 180
  nursing practice and, 180-181
Lay advisors in community interventions, 368
Lead
  assessing levels of, 231
  health effects of, 222
  reducing levels of, 226
Lead poisoning
  community partnership for reducing, 332
  practice application in, 245
  preventing, 237, 238b
Leadership. See also Community-oriented nurse management; Community-oriented nurse manager
  behaviors of, examples of, 545b
  competencies needed for, 1025-1032, 1026t
  critical thinking skills in, 1030
  decision-making skills in, 1029-1030, 1029t
  delegation skills in, 1027-1029, 1028b, 1028t
  empowerment role of, 1027
  and finding people-task balance, 1027
  group, 545-546
  in group work teams, 553-554
  public health, 519
  servant, 1026-1027
  styles of, 546
  theories of, 1013-1016, 1014t
  time management skills in, 1027b
Leading health indicators, Healthy People 2010 objectives for, 420, 994
Learned helplessness, 309
  in abused women, 886
Learners, learning barriers related to, 308-309
Learning
  barriers to, 307-309
    educator-related, 307-308
    learner-related, 308-309
  versus education, 298
  facilitation of, versus teaching, 306b
  formats for, examples of, 304b
  nature of, 300
  participatory, 305
  philosophical perspectives of, 298, 299t
  readiness for, 300
  selecting formats for, 303-314
  theories of, 298-300, 299t
    behavioral, 298-299
    cognitive, 299
    critical, 299-300
    developmental, 300
    humanistic, 300
    social learning, 300
Learning contracts, developing, 305
Learning environment, effective, 304
Learning experience, organizing, 304-305

Learning organizations, transformational leadership in, 1016
Lectures, educational, 304b
Legal issues
  in case management, 462-465
  in home health/hospice care, 982-983
  in parish nursing, 1106
Legionella pneumophila, symptoms, transmission, and causes of emergence, 912t
Legionnaires' disease, 254, 904
Legislation. See also Law; Policy
  for advanced practice nurses, 1001, 1001t
  affecting school nursing, 1044-1045, 1044t
  affecting vulnerable populations, 751-753, 751b
  Canadian
    for health care, 112
    for national health, 83-84
    process of, 183
  for clients with disabilities, 736-738, 736b
  community-oriented nursing and, 179-180
  distribution effects of, 752
  enabling, 118
  for family policy, 586, 588
  gun control, 635
  for health care planning, 493
  health care-related, 64-65
  for home health services, 981-982
  for homeless, 783, 788
  immigration-related, 149
  men's health care, war and, 682
  for mental health services, 831-832, 831t
  occupational health-related, 1086-1087
  older adult-related, 710, 711t
  process of, 184, 185f, 186, 186b
  public health-related, 1123
  re technology/cost controls, 110t
  tips for involvement in, 187b
Legislative branch of government, 171
Legislative process, Canadian, 182
Legislators, communication with, 186b
Lesbians, health of, 670
Lesser-developed countries
  communicable disease in, 86
  defined, 74
  disasters in, 470-471
  health problems of, 74
  maternal and women's health in, 89
  nurses' role in, 78
Leukemia
  childhood, 235
    adult sequelae of, 725
  insecticide exposure and, 222
Liability
  of advanced nurse practitioners, 1003
  in case management, 462
Liberal democratic theory, 136
Libertarianism, 136
Liberty Mutual Insurance Company, case management and, 455
Lice, screening children for, 1056
Licensure, definition and process of, 522
Life, quality of, as community health indicator, 8b
Life care planning, 455
Life events
  health risks and, 598
  normative versus nonnormative, 598, 601
Life expectancy
  by country, 683t
  ethnic differences in, 686
  gender differences in, 701
  increases in, 109
  male versus female, 686
  for men, 683, 686
    in Canada, 684
  public health influence on, 3
  shifts in, 700
  for women, 656-657, 657t
    Canadian, 660
    by country, 657t
Life review, functions of, 704
Life-event risks, 601

Lifestyle Assessment Questionnaire, 327
Lifestyle risks in family health, 606-607
Lifestyles
  of Canadian men, 684-685
  of Canadian women, 660-661
  family, goals for, 632-633
  habits of, affecting morbidity/mortality, 596
  health care system and, 54
  health-promoting, 335
  healthy
    in Healthy People 2010 objectives, 318
    for vulnerable populations, 766
  of vulnerable populations, 763
Limitations, functional, defined, 721
Lind, James, 251t
Linguistic issues in health promotion for vulnerable populations, 764, 766
Linguistically appropriate health care, 750
Lipids, screening for, 265
Listening, compassionate, 1102
Listeria in food-borne illness, 921
Listeriosis, 926
Literacy
  assessment of, 1123-1124
  level of, health education and, 308-309
  U. S. survey of, 308
Litigation, malpractice, 530
Liver cancer, case study of, 581-582
Liver disease, alcohol-related, 692
Liverpool Relief Society, 26
Living wills, 709, 982
Local government
  in disaster preparedness, 477t
  disaster response responsibilities of, 478t
  health departments of, 178
Locke's goal-setting theory, 1014t, 1015
Loeb, Mrs. Solomon, 28b
Longitudinal studies, 273
Long-term care facilities
  advanced practice nurses in, 998-999
  for older adults, 713-714
Louis, Pierre Charles-Alexandre, 251t
Low back pain, chronic, 725
Low-birth-weight infants
  in health professional shortage areas, 381t
  of teen mothers, 819
Low-income housing, 788
Lundeen model, 414
Lung cancer
  deaths due to, 639
  from sidestream smoke, 856
  in women, 666-667
Lyme disease, 254, 904
  cause, clinical symptoms, treatment, 924
  symptoms, transmission, and causes of emergence, 912t

**M**

MacLeod, Charlotte, 36
Macroeconomic theory, 101
Mad cow disease, 904
Maintenance function, defined, 542-543
Maintenance norms, 544
Maintenance specialists, role of, 547b
Malaria
  cause, symptoms, prevention, 925
  epidemiology and control of, 89
Malignant melanoma, 690
Malnutrition, infant
  problem analysis of, 358t
  problem prioritizing for, 362t
  progress notes on, 369t
  risk of, 360
Malpractice, defined, 180
Malpractice litigation, 530
  legislative response to increased incidence of, 521
Managed care
  in community mental health, 829-830
  defined, 1010-1011
  and disincentives to serve vulnerable populations, 753
  financial arrangements for, 119-120

Managed care—cont'd
  Medicare, 58-59
  in mental health care, 837
  quality of, 52
  types of, 120b
  for vulnerable populations, 750
Managed care organizations
  agency report cards of, 1011
  capitated, 1011
  characteristics of, 58
  defined, 52b
  enrollees in, 1011
  health care influences of, 64
  nurses as managers in, 1009
  pathways in, 1010f
  reimbursement by, discounted fee-for-service, 1011
  roles of, 518
  unfulfilled expectations for, 518
Managed health care
  population-focused, 2
  regionalizing, 64
Management, theories of, 1013-1016, 1014t
Managers, nurses as. See Community-oriented nurse manager
Mance, Jeanne, 36
Man-made disasters, 471
Marburg virus, symptoms, transmission, and causes of emergence, 912t
Marginalization of vulnerable populations, 759-760
Marihuana Tax Act of 1937, 858
Marijuana use
  among adolescents, 809
  in Canada, 852-853
  incidence and physiologic effects of, 858-859
  medical, 858-859
  tolerance of, 858
Marine Hospital Service, 24
Marital rape, 880, 887
Market, defined, 99
Market model of health care reimbursement, 755
Marriage
  Canadian, 570-571
  dual-career, 566
  interracial, 566
  trends in, 566
Mary Augustine, Sister, 25
Maryknoll Missionaries, 80
Maslow, Abraham, 704
Maslow's theory of human needs, 1014t, 1014-1015
Mass media in community interventions, 368
Massachusetts, Healthy Cities and Communities movement in, 402
Massage therapy for children, 643, 644t
Maternal and women's health in international health, 89-90
Maternal-child care, home health services for, 985
Maternal-infant health in rural areas, 381, 381t
Maternity and Infancy Act, 31
MAUT. See Multi-attribute utility technique
Maximum contaminant level, 240
McIver, Pearl, 34
McKinney Homeless Assistance Act
  provisions affecting vulnerable populations, 751
  provisions of, 783, 788
MCOs. See Managed care organizations
MDMA, physiologic effects of, 859
Mead, George Herbert, 577
Means testing, 111
Measle, mumps, and rubella vaccine, 914
Measles
  characteristics and immunization, 918-919
  required immunizations for, 1052t
Media
  poverty discourses of, 776
  violence in, 877
  windshield survey of, 357t

Mediating structures, small groups as, 368
Medicaid, 5. *See also* Centers for Medicaid and Medicare Services
  for abortions, 654
  advanced nurse practitioner reimbursement by, 1001-1002
  AIDS/HIV costs to, 933
  disadvantages of, 751
    for minority groups, 751
  expenditures for, 117f
  funding for, 173
  home health care requirements for, *versus* Medicare requirements, 980t
  for home health/hospice care, 980
  immigrant eligibility for, 149, 151
  for improving health care access, 123
  and increasing health care expenditures, 107
  legal issues in, 181
  *versus* Medicare, 15t
  passage of, 105
  provisions and financing of, 116-117
  Title XIX of, 110t
  for vulnerable populations, 750
Medicaid Community Care Act of 1981, 981
Medical assistants in nursing centers, 428t
Medical care system, effectiveness of, 193
Medical jargon, avoiding, 303
Medical savings accounts, 120-121
Medical technology, defined, 103
Medically indigent population, 755
Medically underserved populations, 391-392
Medicare, 5. *See also* Centers for Medicaid and Medicare Services
  AIDS/HIV costs to, 933
  ANA support of, 39
  costs of, 115-116
  funding for, 173
  home health care requirements for, 979b
    *versus* Medicaid requirements, 980t
  home health payments by, 965
  for home health/hospice care, 980
  hospice coverage by, 975
  and increasing health care expenditures, 107
  and interdisciplinary home care/hospice services, 976-977
  legal issues in, 181
  means testing for, 111
  *versus* Medicaid, 115t
  men's participation in, 681
  Part A, 115
  Part B, 115
  passage of, 105
  provisions and financing of, 115-116
  for reimbursing advanced practice nurses, 184
  for reimbursing nurse practitioners, 1001, 1001t
  and responsibilities of disciplines in home care, 974-975
  Title XVIII of, 110t
  for vulnerable populations, 750
  women enrolled in, health status of, 672
Medicare managed care, 58-59
Medications. *See also* Drugs; Prescription drugs
  administering, in schools, 1054
Medicin San Frontieres, 81
Melatonin for children, 643
Memory
  age-related impairment of, 705
  herbal remedies for improving, 836
Men
  causes of death of, 686t, 687-694
  development of, 682-683
    moral, 682-683
    psychosocial, 682-683
  health resources use by, 681
  life expectancies of
    by country, 683t
    *versus* female, 701
  minority, unemployment rate for, 876

Meningitis, TB, 87
Meningococcal disease in Canada, 914
Menopausal symptoms, alternative therapies for, 672-673, 673b
Menopause, effects of, 663
Men's health, 680-699
  in Canada, 684-685
  cultural differences in, 687
  definitions of, 680-681
  hotline/website for, 681
  mortality and, 683, 686
  needs in, 696t
  nurse's role in, 694-695
  practices of, 694
  status of, in U. S., 681-682
  *versus* women's, 686-687
Men's health nurse practitioner, 695
Mental disorders, severe, characteristics of, 827-828
Mental health
  of adolescents, 809
  after disasters, 485
    evidence-based practice and, 485
  cultural diversity in perceptions of, 842
  *Healthy People 2010* objectives for, 420, 994
  of men, 695
  of migrant farmworkers, 799
  in rural areas, 382
  of women, 665-666
Mental health care, 826-847
  current/future perspectives on, 837
  deficiencies in, 837
  deinstitutionalization and, 832-833
  evolution of, 830-832
  factors affecting, 826
  frameworks for, 833-835
  historical perspective on, 830
  key points, 844-845
  national objectives for, 837-844
  nurse's role in, 835-837
  practice application for, 844
  psychiatric hospitals in, 830-831
  reform in, 831
  relapse management in, 833
  systems of, 829-830
    managed care, 829-830
Mental health centers, community, 830
Mental Health Planning Act, 832
Mental health problems *versus* mental illness, 828
Mental health services
  federal legislation for, 831-832, 831t
  state systems of, 832
Mental Health Study Act
  focus of, 831t
  passage of, 831
Mental Health Systems Act, repeal of, 832
Mental hygiene movement, 831-832
Mental illness
  consumer advocacy and, 828
  co-occurrence of, 840
  diagnostic technology in, 828-829
  impacts of, 828
  information/help resources for, 842b
  managed care coverage of, 829-830
  *versus* mental health problems, 828
  neurobiology of, 828-829
  prevention of, 834-835, 835b
  scope of, 827-828
  serious, *Healthy People 2010* objectives for, 840-841
Mental problems, information/help resources for, 842b
Mental retardation, fetal alcohol syndrome and, 865
Mercury
  in fish, 222, 236, 243
  toxic effects of, 236, 236t
Mercy Corps International, 74
Messages, clarity of, 302-303
Metaparadigm, defined, 195, 196, 196t
*Metathesaurus,* 206-207
Methadone, mechanisms of action of, 867
Methamphetamines, 857-858
Methyl mercury in fish, 222, 236, 243

Metropolitan areas, subclassifications of, 376
Metropolitan county, defined, 376b
Metropolitan Life Insurance Company
  nursing services offered by, 965
  visiting nurse program of, 31
Mexican Americans, diabetes in, 732
Mexican immigrants, health values of, 801-802
Mexican National Academy of Medicine, 76
Mexico
  health care system in, 85-86
  NAFTA and, 75-76
  population health applications in, 77
  primary health care services in, 77-78
Microeconomic theory, 99
Microprocessors, health care applications of, 55
Microsporidiosis, 927
Midwives
  certified nurse, 59
  nurse, 31, 32b
Migrant Clinicians' Network, 802
Migrant farmworkers
  assessment of, 803
  child/adolescent, 800-801
  culture and lifestyles of, 794
  defined, 795
  ethnicity of, 795
  health care access of, 796-797
  health of, 796
  housing of, 795-796
  income of, 796, 797
  lifestyles of, 795-796
  occupational/environmental health problems of, 798-800
  political advocates for, 803
  in rural areas, health needs/problems of, 383t
  testimonies of, 797b
  undocumented, 795
Migrant Head Start Program, 800
Migrant Health Act, 796
Migrant health care, 798-807
  cultural considerations in, 801-802
  evidence-based practice in, 802
  health promotion/illness prevention for, 802
  key points, 804
  nurse's role in, 802-804
  office of, 796
  practice application for, 804
Milbank Memorial Fund, 81
Milio, Nancy, 41
Mine Safety and Health Act of 1968, 1086
Minnesota, outcomes of care in, documentation of, 519
Minnesota Heart Health program, 330-331
Minorities. *See also* Women of color; specific groups
  diabetes in, 664-665
  health disparities of, 748-749
  Medicaid for, disadvantages of, 751
  mental health of, 842
  in rural areas, 377, 382
  unemployment rate for, 876
Missionaries, health activities of, 1096
Mobilizing for Action through Planning and Partnerships, 351, 352b
Model State Emergency Health Powers Act, 173
Models, function of, 196-197
Moderation Management, 854
Moller-Murphy Symptom Management Assessment Tool, 834-835
Mongolian spots, 165
Monitoring
  environmental, 242
  skills in, 1035
Montefiore Hospital Home Care Program, 965
Moral development
  male, 682-683
  stages of, 683b
Morality, 131
  defined, 132b
Morbidity, measures of, 255-256F

Mortality
  causes of, 36
  early, factors contributing to, 4
  female, causes of, in U. S., 658t
  measures of, 255-256F
Mortality rate. *See also* Death
  changes in, 53-54
  female, 656-657
  male, 686
  maternal, 89-90
  types and calculation of, 259-261, 260f
Mothers
  single, 567
    economic status of, 756-757
    practice application for, 613-614
  teenage
    evidence-based practice and, 1119
    gestational weight gain recommendations for, 820t
    infant interactions with, 821
    in school, 1061
  working, in Canada, 571
Motivation
  in cognitive theory, 1015
  for health behaviors, 596
  keys to, 1030-1031, 1031b
  level of, health education and, 309
Motor vehicle accidents
  adolescent involvement in, 634, 692
  child/adolescent mortality from, 633
Moulder, Betty, 1067
Multi-attribute utility technique, 505, 507t, 508
  steps in, 509b
Multi-City Action Plans, 404-405
Multilateral organizations, 79-80
Music therapy for children, 643
*Mycobacterium tuberculosis,* 947
Myocardial infarction, symptoms of, 687

**N**

Nar-Anon, 868
Narcotics Anonymous, 868
National Alliance for the Mentally Ill, 828
  activities of, 833b
National Assessment of Adult Literacy, 308
National Association of County Health Officials, website for, 352b
National Association of Psychiatric Survivors, activities of, 833b
National Association of School Nurses, standards of, 1045, 1045b
National Campaign to Prevent Teen Pregnancy, 822
National Cancer Institute, contact information for, 869b
National Center for Chronic Disease Prevention and Health Promotion, website for, 352b
National Center for Nursing Research, 42, 62
  establishment of, 193
National Center on Birth Defects and Developmental Disabilities, 724
National Childhood Vaccine Injury Act, 631
National Committee for Quality Assurance, 52
National Environmental Education Act, provisions of, 242b
National Environmental Policy Act, provisions of, 241b
National Family Caregiver Support Program, impact of, 711t
National Guidelines Clearinghouse, website for, 526, 715
National Health and Nutrition Examination Survey, 267
National Health Circle for Colored People, 32-33
National Health Interview Survey, 267
National Health Planning and Resource Development Act, 493
National Health Planning and Resource Development Act, provisions affecting vulnerable populations, 752

National Health Planning and Resource Development Act, provisions of, 110t
National Health Planning and Resource Development Act of 1974, provisions affecting vulnerable populations, 752
National Health Quality Improvement Act of 1986, 521
National Health Service Corps, 60
National Hospital Discharge Survey, 267
National Institute for Occupational Safety and Health, 1086
  Education and Research Centers of, 1070b-1071b
  functions of, 1087b
National Institute of Mental Health, 828
National Institute of Nursing Research, 177
  establishment of, 193
  funding by, 173
National Institute on Alcohol Abuse and Alcoholism, recommendations of, 854
National Institutes of Health, 177
  epidemiology initiatives of, 252t
National League for Nursing, 39
  Accrediting Commission of, 522
National Library of Medicine, toxicology databases of, 225
National Mental Health Act
  focus of, 831t
  passage of, 831
National Mental Health Association, activities of, 833b
National Mental Health Consumers' Association, activities of, 833b
National Migrant Resource Program, 796
National Nosocomial Infection Surveillance, 928
National Nursing Centers Consortium, 440, 440b
National Occupational Research Agenda, 1086, 1088b
National Organization for Public Health Nursing, 30
National Organization for Women, 654
National Women's Health Network, 654
Native Alaskans
  health indicators for, 269
  in rural areas, health needs/problems of, 383t
Native American children, injuries to, 633
Native American women, causes of death among, 659t
Native Americans
  alcoholism of, 154
  cultural attitudes/practices of, 162t
  environmental control perspectives of, 165
  evidence-based assessment of, 12
  food preferences and nutrition-related risk factors of, 167t
  health indicators for, 269
  mental health of, 844
  in rural areas, health needs/problems of, 383t
  stereotyping of, 158
Natural disasters, 23, 471
Nature. See also Environment
  cultural attitudes toward, 165
Naturopathy
  for children, 642
  theory of, 708b
Navy Nurse Corps, 35
Near poor, 777
Needle Stick Safety and Prevention Act, 178
Needlestick injuries, 1076
Needs assessment
  population, 494-495
  in program management, 494-495
  steps in, 496f
  tools for, 495t
Negentropy, defined, 196f
Neglect, older adult, 709, 841. See also Older adult abuse and neglect
Negligent referrals in case management, 463

Negotiation
  contract, 1022, 1024
  process of, 460-461
Neighborhood poverty, 777
Neisseria gonorrhoeae, 938, 940t. See also Gonorrhea
Nematodes, diseases caused by, 927t
Neonatal period, defined, 618, 619t
Neonate
  assessment of, 618
  cultural variations in, 165
  herpes simplex 2 infection in, 943
  immunity in, 631
  infections in, 636
Nepal, Healthy Cities and Communities movement in, 405
Net positive value, 101-102
Neuman, Betty, Health Care Systems Model of, 583
Neuman Systems Model, 195, 198-199, 200f, 201-203, 204f, 205-206
  case study using, 597
  community applications of, 202-203, 205
  for community outcomes, 205-206
  environment in, 201
  flexible line of defense in, 199
  health promotion in, 202
  individual and community applications of, 205-206
  lines of resistance in, 201
  normal line of defense in, 199, 205
  Omaha System merger with, 212-217
  prevention in, 201-202
Neural tube defects, folic acid for preventing, 662-663
Neurobiological disorders, Moller-Murphy Symptom Management Assessment Tool for, 834-835
Neuromuscular system, age-related changes in, 705t
Neurotoxicity, failure to test for, 236
Neurotoxins, health effects of, 222
Nevirapine for AIDS, 88-89
New Jersey, case management methods in, 455
New York City, public health services in, 24
Newborn. See Neonate
Newman, Diana, 213
NGOs. See Nongovernmental organizations
Nicotine replacement therapy, 868
Nicotine use
  physiologic effects of, 855-856
  tolerance of, 855
Nigeria, Healthy People 2010 goals and, 75
Nightingale, Florence, 25-26, 322, 965
  and environmental health issues, 222-223
  role in setting standards of care, 520
  values of, 131
Nightingale Tracker, 212, 213
903, guidelines for in-school use of, 1053
No Place Like Home: A History of Nursing and Home Care in the United States, 34
Noddings, N., 138
Nominal groups, defined, 358
Nonfarm residency, defined, 376b
Nongonococcal urethritis, 943
Nongovernmental organizations, 79
  examples of, 80-81
  web pages of, 81
Non-Hodgkin's lymphoma in children, adult sequelae of, 725
Nonmaleficence, 135b
  ethical issues in, 465
Nonmetropolitan statistical area, defined, 376b
Nonrelational propositions, 194
Norms
  defined, 544-545
  functions of, 544
North American Free Trade Agreement
  Canadian concerns about, 75
  health impacts of, 75, 76f

North American Nursing Diagnosis Association, 207, 207t
  community-level diagnoses of, 360
  individual focus of, 360
North Karelia study, 330
Nosocomial infections, 928
Notifiable disease, Canadian list of, 914
NPs. See Nurse practitioners
Nuclear magnetic resonance, 636-637
Nurse managers. See Community-oriented nurse manager
Nurse practice acts, state, 179
Nurse practitioners. See also Advanced practice nurse
  in Canada, 999
  versus clinical nurse specialists, 992t
  as clinicians, 993-995
  credentialing of, 993
  educational preparation of, 990
  historical perspective on, 991
  institutional privileges of, 1002
  Medicare reimbursement of, 1001, 1001t
  in nursing centers, 427t
  origins of, 41, 59
  practice application for, 1004
  protocols for, 994
Nurse Training Act of 1971, 992
Nurse-client relationship with migrant farmworkers, 802-804
Nurse-midwives
  introduction of, 31, 32b
  in nursing centers, 427t
Nurses
  in Canadian primary health care system, 67
  in China, 85
  in environmental health, 243-244
  minority, increasing number of, 54
  need for, 54
  in nursing centers, 440-441
  shortage of, 105
  state board examiners of, 63
  in Swedish health delivery system, 84-85
Nursing
  boards of, 179
  district, 25-26
  in international health, 78, 176
  Roy's adaptation model of, 1017
  systems theory models of, 197-198
  transcultural, standards for, 155
Nursing advocacy, 188-189
Nursing assessment, cultural, 160-161
Nursing audit method, 521
Nursing care
  culturally competent, 153-154
  ethic of, 137-138
Nursing centers, 412-445, 419-424
  academic, 416-417
  advanced practice nurses in, 997
  ANA definition of, 414b
  business aspects of, 430-434
  business plans for, 432
  collaboration in, 420-421, 421b, 422t
  community assessment by, 422-423
  for comprehensive primary health care, 416
  defined, 413-414
  development of, essentials in, 431b
  developmental foundations of, 419-424, 424t-425t
  education and research in, 436-438
  essential technology and information systems in, 435-436
  evidence-based practice in, 434-436, 437
  evolution of, 424t-425t
  examples of, 417, 418b
  feasibility studies for, 432
  funding for, 433-434
  future of, 438-441
  for health and wellness, 415-416
  Health Insurance Portability and Accountability Act and, 435
  Healthy People 2010 and, 412, 419
  historical perspective on, 423-424
  key points for, 441-442
  national/regional organizations of, 440

Nursing centers–cont'd
  not-for-profit versus proprietary, 417
  organizational frameworks of, 426
  organizational partners of, 430
  populations using, 417
  practice application of, 441
  program evaluation in, 437-438
  quality improvement in, 435
  quality indications for, 435
  reimbursement mechanisms of, 414-415, 415b
  research in, template for, 439b
  for special care, 416
  staffing of, 427t-428t
  start-up/sustainability of, 430
  strategic plans for, 432-433
  student orientation of, 428
  team approach in, 424, 426-430
  types of, 414-419
Nursing Council on National Defense, 35
Nursing diagnosis
  community-oriented, 360
  defined, 207
Nursing education
  in China, 85
  development of, 105
  in institutions of higher learning, 131
  Nightingale model of, 25
  for public health nursing, 39-41
Nursing goals, defined, 199t
Nursing interventions. See also Interventions
  defined, 207
  multilevel, by nursing centers, 423
  in nursing centers, 414
  telehealth, 453, 454
Nursing knowledge, structure of, 194-195
Nursing minimum data set, 1101
Nursing models of care, 413, 414
Nursing organizations, consolidations of, 39
Nursing practice
  classification systems for, 207t
  defined, 179
  law and, 180-181
  in Omaha System, 208
  in remote Canadian areas, 387
  in rural areas, 385-389, 385b
  preparation for, 389
  research on, 388-389
  targets of, 344
Nursing process
  versus advocacy, 459t
  case management and, 449-450, 450t
  concepts of, 207-208
  flow sheet of, 370f
  versus problem-solving and medical diagnostic process, 208t
Nursing research. See also Research
  in nursing centers, template for, 439b
  WHO priorities for, 436, 438b
Nursing services
  forecasting costs of, 1035
  reimbursement for, 122
Nursing skills for rural areas, 383t
Nursing theory
  language of, 195-196, 196t
  mid-range, defined, 196t
Nursing's Agenda for Health Care Reform, 125b
Nursing's Agenda for the Future, 189
Nursing-sensitive Outcomes Classification, 360
Nutrition. See also Diet
  adolescent, 625t
  assessment of
    in adolescents, 630
    in childhood, 629-630
    in infants, 626, 628t, 629
  community partnership for improving, 332
  culture and, 166, 167t
  factors influencing, 626
  in illness prevention, 604
  infant, 620t
  in international health, 90-91
  neonatal, 619t
  for older adults, 710

Nutrition—cont'd
  for physically compromised clients, 732
  during teen pregnancy, 819, 820t, of toddlers/preschoolers, 621t
Nutritional supplements for older adults, 704
Nutting, Mary Adelaide, 30

O

Oaxaca, migration-health study of, 76
Obesity. See also Eating disorders; Overweight
  in Canadians, 684
  in children/adolescents, 632-633
    management guidelines for, 632b
  client education about, 300
  defined, 668
  Healthy People 2010 objectives for, 420, 994
  medical/psychosocial consequences of, 632
  physical and psychologic effects of, 668
  in U. S., 318
Objectives, establishing, for infant malnutrition, 363-364, 364t
O'Brien, Mary, 236-237
Occupational health, legal issues in, 181
Occupational health and safety programs
  advanced practice nurses in, 999-1001
  on-site, 1081, 1081b
Occupational health history, 1082, 1084f-1085f
Occupational health nursing, 1066-1091. See also Work; Workers
  AAOHN code of ethics for, 1069b
  AAOHN standards for, 1069b
  definition and scope of, 1067
  in disaster management, 1087-1089
  epidemiologic model in, 1074-1080
  Healthy People 2010 objectives and, 1087
  history and evolution of, 1067-1068
  key points, 1089
  legislation related to, 1086-1087
  nursing care and, 1081-1086
  and organizational/public efforts to promote worker health, 1081
  origins of, 29
  practice application for, 1089
  roles and professionalism in, 1068-1070
Occupational health risks
  for Canadian men, 685
  of migrant farmworkers, 798-800
  in rural areas, 382-384
Occupational injuries, fatal, for men, 690
Occupational Safety and Health Act
  passage of, 1068
  positive impacts of, 1074
  provisions of, 241b
Occupational Safety and Health Administration, 176
  creation of, 1068
  functions of, 177-178, 1087b
Occupational therapist, role in home care, 975
Office of Children's Environmental Health (Canada), 226
Office of Emergency Management, 474
Office of Homeland Security, 178-179, 478
Office of Migrant health, 796
Office of Women's Health, 655
Office on Smoking and Health, contact information for, 869b
Office on Women's Health, 655
Ojibwa Indians, evidence-based assessment of, 12
Older adult abuse and neglect, 841, 887-888
  identifying, 888
  practice application for, 717
  precipitating factors in, 888-889
  types of, 709, 888
Older adults, 700-719. See also Aging
  ATOD risk of, 864-865
  body system changes in, 705t

Older adults—cont'd
  care options for, 712b
  community-based nursing models for, 710-714
  definitions of, 703
  demographics of, 700-703
  and difficulty in performing ADLs, 701
  with disabilities, percentage of, 703f
  disaster reactions of, 481
  ethical and legal issues of, 709-710
  evidence-based resources for, 715b
  family caregiving for, 710
  functional assessment of, 707, 707f
  health assessment of, 706-707
  health concerns of, 707-710
  health expenditures for, 109t
  health promotion, disease prevention for, 714-717
  health status of, 758
  home safety evaluation for, 713f
  homeless, 788
  infection risk of, 710
  key points, 718
  mental health of, 841-842
  over 65
    in 1990 and 2000, 702f
    living arrangements of, 702f
  as percentage of population, 53, 109
  physically compromised, abuse of, 730
  policies affecting, 589
  in poverty, 782
  practice application for, 717
  subgroups of, 700
Older American Resources and Services, functional assessment of, 707
Older Americans Act of 1965, impact of, 711t
Older Americans Act of 1972
  impact of, 711t
  Title V of, 711t
Older women, health of, 672
Omaha System, 206-213
  definitions in, 207
  description of, 208-209
  intervention scheme of, 209, 210b, 211b
  Neuman Systems Model merger with, 213-217
  Nightingale Tracker in, 212, 213
  nurse/administrator needs and, 206
  nursing process concepts in, 207-208
  practice and education applications of, 212
  prevention in, 216b
  problem classification scheme of, 209, 210b, 211b
  problem rating scale of, 209-210, 212t
  theoretical framework of, 208
Omnibus Budget Reconciliation Act
  impact of, 711t
  mental health focus of, 831t
  nurse practitioner provisions of, 1001t
  provisions of, 110t
Omnibus Budget Reconciliation Act of 1981, provisions of, 110t
Omnibus Budget Reconciliation Act of 1987, older adult rights in, 709
Omnibus Reconciliation Act of 1989, provisions of, 110t
Open space, windshield survey of, 357t
Opioids, tolerance to, 855
Opportunistic infections, HIV/AIDS-related, 908, 935
Oral contraceptives, uses and effectiveness of, 662t
Oral histories, conducting interviews for, 41
Organizational frameworks of nursing centers, 426
Organizational skills for managers/consultants, 1033-1035
Organizational theories, 1016-1017
  of management, 1016-1017
Organized religion, family violence and, 877
Organizing, skills in, 1034
Organophosphate pesticides, migrant farmworker exposure to, 798-799
Orlando's model of nursing, 1017

Osteoporosis, incidence, causes, prevention of, 663
Ottawa Charter for Health Promotion, 396-397
  health promotion defined by, 324
Outcome Based Quality Improvement, 986, 986f
Outcome present-state testing model, 578-579
  case study using, 581-582
Outcomes
  case management criteria for, 454
  distributive, 460
  health risk and, 597-598
  integrative, 460
  nursing center data on, 434-436
Outcomes and Assessment Information Set, 985-986, 986f
Outpatient clinics, advanced practice nurses in, 997
Outreach to vulnerable populations, 749
Overeaters Anonymous, 868
Overweight. See also Obesity
  in children/adolescents, prevalence of, 632t
  defined, 632, 668
  Healthy People 2010 objectives for, 420, 994
Oxfam, 80

P

Pacific Islanders, mental health of, 843-844
PAHO. See Pan American Health Organization
Palliative care, history of, 975
Pan American Health Organization, 176
  functions and organization of, 79-80
  Healthy Cities project and, 406
Pandemic, defined, 907
Parasitic diseases, 926-927
  control and prevention of, 927-928
  examples of, 927t
  intestinal, 927
  opportunistic, 927
Parental consent laws, 811b
Parental notification laws, 811b
Parenting style, influence on adolescent sexual behavior, 814
Parents. See also Family(ies); Fathers; Mothers
  abusive
    characteristics of, 885
    identifying, 883
  of adolescents, health guidance guidelines for, 623b
  and adolescents' decisions about reproductive health care, 811b
  consent of, for adolescent health treatments, 634
  deadbeat, 779-781
  immunization education for, evidence-based practice and, 918
  involvement in child health, 1051
  and risk of child abuse, evidence-based practice and, 13
  single, children living with, 616
  by teen parents, 820-821
Parish nurse, functions of, 1102-1105
Parish nursing, 1092-1113. See also Faith communities
  advanced practice nurses in, 997
  characteristics of, 1099-1105
  community of, 1098-1099
  definitions pertaining to, 1093-1094
  ethical issues in, 1105-1106
  Healthy People 2010 leading indicators and, 1106-1108
  key points, 1109-1110
  models of, 1093-1094
  population-focused, 1108-1109
  practice application for, 1109
  preparation for, 1100-1101
  professional issues in, 1105
  roles in, 1092-1093
  scope and standards of, 1100
  spiritual assessments and, 1103
Participant observation, 355
Partner notification about STDs, 950-951, 955
Partner pressure, influences of, 813-814

Partnerships. See also Community partnerships
  characteristics of, 350b
  consumer, 518
  as goals of community health practice, 346
  health care, 1011-1012
  parish nursing and, 1097-1098
PAs. See Physician assistants
Pasteur, Louis, 252
Pathfinder Fund, 81
Path-goal theory of leadership, 1015-1016
Pathogens, drug-resistant, 1119-1120
Patient education about men's health, 694
Patient Protection Act, elements of, 126b
Patient Safety Act of 1997, 186
Patient Self-Determination Act, 981
  impact of, 711t
  provisions of, 709
Patients' bill of rights, 53
Pawtucket Heart Health program, 330
Payment systems, 121-122
  for health care organizations, 121
  for health care practitioners, 121-122
  for nursing services, 122
PCP. See Pneumocystis carinii pneumonia
Peacemakers, role of, 547b
Pedagogy
  versus andragogy, 307t
  defined, 306
Peer pressure
  anticipatory guidance about, 809
  influences of, 813
Pelvic inflammatory disease as complication of gonorrhea, 942
Pennsylvania Hospital, founding of, 24
Peptic ulcer disease, Helicobacter pylori in, 906
Permitting process in environmental protection, 240, 242
Persistent bioaccumulative toxins, 243
Persistent organic pollutants, 243
Person, defined, 198t
Personal Responsibility and Work Opportunity Reconciliation Act, 655
  provisions of, 812
Personal Responsibility and Work Opportunity Reconciliation Act of 1996, 779
Personal safety in community practice, 370-371
PERT. See Program evaluation review technique
Pertussis, characteristics and immunization, 920
Pertussis vaccine in Canada, 914
Pest Management Regulatory Agency (Canada), 226
Pesticide exposure
  of children, 640
  migrant farmworker opinions on, 797
  in migrant farmworkers, 798-799
  symptoms of, 799
Pew Charitable Trusts, health promotion recommendations of, 125b
Pharmaceutical companies, free drug programs of, 457
Pharmaceuticals, health commodification of, 81
PHC. See Primary health care
Philanthropic organizations, 79
  examples of, 81
Philosophy, defined, 196t
Physical activity, Healthy People 2010 goals for, 420
Physical environment, 601b
Physical hazards, work-related, 1076b, 1078-1079
Physical therapist, role in home care, 975
Physically compromised client, 720-743. See also Disabilities
  abuse of, 730-733
  abuse risk of
    evidence-based practice for, 730
    factors affecting, 731f
  assisted suicide of, 737-738
  attitudinal barriers for, 734-735

Physically compromised client–cont'd
  cope of problem of, 722-724
  cultural implications for, 728
  definitions/concepts of, 720-722
  and difficulty performing ADLs, 723
  facilities access for, 729
  health care for, impediments to, 733t
  healthy cities movement and, 734-735
  Healthy People 2010 objectives for,
    733-734
  key points, 738
  legislation affecting, 736-738
  low-income, 729
  nurse's role with, 735-736
  practice application for, 738
  prevention interventions for, 732b
  social implications for, 725
  states with highest percentage of, 723
  stresses of, 724-729
    for adults, 725
    for community, 728-729
    for family, 726-728
    in infancy through adolescence,
      724-725
  workplace discrimination against, 737
Physician assistants
  origins of, 59, 991-992
  training and functions of, 59-60
Physician Leadership on Natural Drug
    Policy, 850
Physician-client consultation model,
    1018, 1018f, 1019b
Physicians
  payments to, 121-122
  role in home care, 975
Piaget, Jean, cognitive development the-
    ory of, 626, 627t
Pinel, Philippe, 830
Plague, 924
  bioterrorist threat of, 913
Planned Approach to Community Health,
    351, 352b, 1033-1034
Planning. See also Program management
  case management, 453
  defined, 491
  life care, 455
  program, budgeting system and, 505-
    506, 506b, 507t
  skills in, 1033-1035
  strategic, 493-494
  in nursing centers, 420-421
Plasmodium, drug resistance of, 925
Playgrounds, safety on, 635-636, 635b
Pneumocystis carinii pneumonia, 927
  AIDS-related, 935
  symptoms, transmission, and causes
    of emergence, 912t
Point epidemics, 270
Poland, Healthy Cities and
    Communities movement in, 404
Police power, 179
  health care and, 172
Policy. See also Law; Legislation
  in effecting social change, 368
  ethics in development of, 139
  family. See Family policy
  nurse's role in, 184-189
Policy development
  defined, 6, 20
  example of, 12-13
Policy setting
  government, 17-174
  nurse's role in, 184-189
Polio, required immunizations for, 1052t
Politics, windshield survey of, 357t
Pollutants
  air. See also Air quality
    child exposure to, 640
  entry routes of, 224
  persistent organic, 243
  website for identifying, 230
Pollution
  point versus nonpoint sources of, 235
  risk assessment for, 234-235
  three R's for reducing, 238b
Pollution Prevention Act, provisions of,
    242b
Polysubstance use/abuse, 861-863
Poor, near, 777
Poor laws, Elizabethan, 24, 25, 775

Popular epidemiology, 278-279
Population(s)
  aging of, 2
  boundaries for, 496
  defined, 10, 20
  disadvantaged, defined, 748-749
  estimated increases in, by age cohort,
    109, 109t
  medically underserved, 391-392
  rural, characteristics of, 377-378
  size/distribution of, in program plan-
    ning, 496
  special, 561
  U. S., 53
  vulnerable. See Vulnerable populations
Population groups, priority, defined, 748
Population growth, patterns of, 376-377
Population health, 76-77
  Canadian leadership in, 77
  determinants of, 77
Population management, activities of,
    446
Population needs assessment, 494-495
Population-focused practice, 1120
  for advanced practice nurses, 995
  benefits to nurses, 16
  in community health promotion,
    320-321
  community-oriented, in Canada,
    16-17
  defined, 20
  emphasis on, 5
  establishing leadership in a, 18-19
  free-living populations and, 13
  increasing influence of, 65
  managed care and, 2
  nursing roles redefined in, 17-18
  in parish nursing, 1108-1109
  practice application for, 19
  versus practice focused on individuals,
    9-10
  in prevention of early deaths, 4
  problem definition in, 10
  rebirth of, 346
Positive predictive value, 266-267
Positron emission tomography, 829
Posttraumatic stress disorder in rape sur-
    vivors, 880
Pott, Percival, 251t
Poverty, 774-793
  in Canada, 780-781
    initiatives for, 781
  children living in, 616
  community and, 782-783
  concept of, 775-776
  crisis, 784
  cultural attitudes toward, 776
  defining, 777-778
  environmental perspectives on, 778
  federal definition of, 754, 756
  global, 755
  health care and, practice application
    for, 790
  health status and, 756-758, 778-783
  key points, 790-791
  media discourses about, 776
  neighborhood, 777
  of older adults, 782
  persistent, 777
  personal beliefs about, 775
  physically compromised individuals
    in, 729, 730f
  political dimensions of, 777-778
  populations affected by, 756-758
  public attitudes toward, 775-776
  testing values and beliefs about, 776
  threshold model of, 754
  types of, 755b
  War on, 778
  women living in, 671-672
Poverty level, federal, defined, 754
Poverty rates, U. S., 782
Poverty thresholds, 777
  by family size, 777t
Power dynamics, managing, 1033
Power of attorney, durable medical, 709
PPD test, procedure for, 950
PPM. See Program planning method
PPOs. See Preferred provider organiza-
    tions

Practice guidelines, evidence-based, 526
Pragmatism, 299t
  defined, 298
Prayer, health outcomes and, evidence-
    based practice and, 1113
Precautionary principle, Wingspread
    statement on, 236-237, 237b
Preconceptual counseling, 662-663
Preferred provider organizations, 119
  characteristics of, 58
Pregnancy
  abuse during, 887
    safety behaviors for preventing, 887
  alcohol use during, 663
  drug use during, 867
  homelessness during, 787
  substance use during, 663
  teen. See Teen pregnancy
  unintended, 662
    campaign for reducing, 654, 654b
Pregnancy Risk Assessment Monitoring
    System, 267
Prejudice. See also Bias; Cultural compe-
    tence
  defined, 159
  forms of, 160b
Prematurity in teen pregnancy, 819
Prenatal care
  access to, 663
  for pregnant teenager, 810, 818-819
PREP interventions, evidence-based
    practice and, 968
Presbyterian Church, health focus of,
    1096-1097
Preschool period, defined, 619
Preschoolers
  assessment of, 619-620, 621t
  injuries/accidents of, 634
Prescription drugs
  Advanced Dispensing System for, 867
  increased use of, by older adults,
    864-865
  reduced co-payments for, 59
  regulation of, 110t
Prescriptive intervention mode, 1022
Presidential Initiative on Race, 748
President's Commission on Mental
    Health, focus of, 831t
President's Commission on the Status of
    Women, 654
Prevalence proportion
  definition and calculation of, 258
  versus incidence, 258-259
Prevention. See also Disease prevention
  versus bedside care, 34
  in case management, 460b
  client education about, 294, 295b
  of communicable disease, 27
  of coronary heart disease, 334t
  of diabetes, 324b
  in disaster management, 485b
  environmentally related, 238b
  in epidemiology, 262-265
  evidence-based practice in, 289b
  of failure to thrive, 333t
  in Healthy Cities project, 407b
  impact of, 13
  levels of, 10, 10b
    cultural variations and, 165b
    in Neuman Systems Model, 201-202
  primary
    defined, 52b
    economics of, 124-125, 124b
  in public health care system, levels of,
    64b
  in rural environments, 388, 388b
  secondary, defined, 52b
  tertiary, defined, 52b
Preventive programs, population-based,
    contributions of, 3-4
Preventive services, clinical, guidelines
    of, 327
Primary care
  in Canada, 66-67
  defined, 52b
  delivery system for, 58-59
  integration with public health, 65, 68
  practice guidelines for, 526
  versus primary health care, 58t
  workforce for, 59-60

Primary care generalists, 56
Primary care system, 56
Primary health care, 50, 55-56
  in Canada, 66-67
  in China, 85
  defined, 52b, 55
  in Healthy Cities movement, 398
  integration into nursing center model,
    419b
  in international health, 77-78
  versus primary care, 58t
  types of, 991
  workforce for, 56
Primary health care centers, comprehen-
    sive, 416
Primary health care movement, 56
Primary nursing care, in-home, 714
Primary prevention
  defined, 52b
  economics of, 124-125
Principlism, 135
  defined, 132b
Prioritizing, problem, for infant malnu-
    trition, 360, 362-363, 362b, 362t
Priority population groups, defined, 748
Prison population, violence and, 895-896
Private practice, advanced practice
    nurses in, 996-997
Private voluntary organizations, 79
  examples of, 80-81
  web pages of, 81
Probability, determining, 364
Problem analysis
  for community assessment, 356, 358
  of infant malnutrition, 358t
Problem correlates, 358
Problem prioritizing for infant malnutri-
    tion, 360, 362-363, 362b, 362t
Problem-purpose-expansion method,
    459-460
Problem-solving
  in advocacy, 459
  in ethical decision making, 132
  linear, 580
  solution ranking in, 497,498f
Process
  as characteristic of community health,
    346-347, 347b
  as indicator of community health,
    349t
Process consultation, 1019-1020, 1021t,
    1022
Process consultation model, 1018f,
    1019b, 1019f
Process evaluation, 491
Professional negligence, defined, 180
Professional Review Organization, estab-
    lishment of, 521, 529
Professional Standards Review
    Organization
  enabling legislation for, 521
  establishment of, 529
Progestins, uses and effectiveness of,
    662t
Program evaluation, 498-505
  defined, 498
  evidence-based practice in, 500
  objective formulation in, 501-502
  process of, 501-502, 501f
  sources of, 502-503
  steps in, 500-501, 500f, 504
Program evaluation review technique,
    505, 506-508, 507t
  objectives of, 507b
  for preschool immunization program,
    507f
Program management, 490-515
  advanced planning and evaluation
    models in, 505-510
  benefits of, 493-494
  components of, 490
  cost studies in, 510-512
  definitions and goals in, 491-492
  evaluation in, 498-505
  funding for, 512
  historical overview of, 492-493
  key points in, 513
  need assessment in, 494-495
  planning process in, 495-498
  practice application for, 512-513

Program of All-Inclusive Care for the Elderly, 714
Program planning
  comparison of methods, 507t
  stakeholder perspectives on, 496-497
Program planning method, 505, 506, 507t
Program planning model for community as client, 358
Programs
  developing plans for, 499
  *versus* projects, 491
Prohibition
  attitudes toward, 851
  negative effects of, 849
Project DARE, effectiveness of, 862-863
Proportion, defined, 255-256
Proportionate mortality rate, calculation of, 260-261, 260t
Prospective payment system
  impact of, 711t
  purpose of, 116
Prospective reimbursement, 121
Prostate cancer, 688-689
  screening for, 265
Prostate-specific antigen for assessing prostate, 688
Protection and Advocacy for Mentally Ill Individuals Act, 832
  focus of, 831t
Protein, dietary guidelines for, in children/adolescents, 628t
Protocols, NP use of, 994
Protozoans, diseases caused by, 927t
PSRO. *See* Professional Standards Review Organization
Psychiatric hospitals, 830-831
Psychoactive drugs, 854-859 *See also* specific drugs
  depressants, 854-855
  hallucinogens, 859
  historical overview of, 849
  stimulants, 855-856
  uses and classification of, 854
Psychomotor learning, 301-302
  levels of, 302t
Psychopharmacology
  controversies over, 829
  impacts of, 829
Psychosocial hazards, work-related, 1076b, 1079-1080
Ptomaine poisoning, 921
Puberty, defined, 623
Public assistance, numbers receiving, 778
Public education, free appropriate, right to, 737
Public health. *See also* Community health
  advocacy in, 143-145
  best-practice programs in, 353
  in Canada, 24
  case management in, 455-456
  in China, 85
  in colonial period and new republic, 24-25
  core functions of, 7, 193
    EBP interventions and, 291
  defined, 6, 52b, 1117
  in 18th and 19th centuries, 25
  ethical practice of, 144b
  federal role in, 30
  funding of, 117
  historical measures for providing, 24
  history and trends of, 1116-1117
  history of, 22-49
  increasing federal action for, 34-35
  integration with primary care, 65, 68
  milestones of, 24, 25t
  prevention levels in, 10
  records in, 535
  TQM/CQI in, 524-530
  U. S. policies on, 24
Public Health Act of 1831 (Canada), 36
Public health agencies, roles of, 1114-1116
Public health care
  Canadian, 67
  contributions of, 3-5
  definitions in, 6-7

Public health care–cont'd
  national health expenditures for, 4-5
  nurses' participation in, 5-6
  vision and mission of, 4f
  for vulnerable populations, 760-761
Public Health Code of Ethics, 145
Public health departments, advanced practice nurses in, 1000
Public health education in nursing centers, 415
Public health nurse. *See also* Community-oriented nursing
  evolving roles of, 971
Public health nurses
  in Canada, 37
  functions of, 1123-1124
  in nursing centers, 427t
  roles of, 13-14
Public health nursing
  African-American nurses in, 32-33
  barriers to specializing in, 18-19
  in Canada, 16-17, 36
  certification for, 1122
  characteristics of, 8-13
  *versus* community-based nursing, 13-15
  competencies of, 9b
  core public health functions and, 11-13
  curriculum objectives in, 1120
  defined, 9, 15b, 1117
  educational preparation for, 9, 18b, 39-41, 1121-1122
    in Canada, 17
  evidence-based practice of, 12, 13, 34
  funding for, 31
  graduate level preparation for, 18
  history of, 1, 22-49, 965
    1600 to 1865, 25b
    1866 to 1945, 38t
    1946 to 2000, 44t
    1970s to present, 41-44
  key points in, 45-46
  at local, state, and national levels, 1114-1130. *See also* Public health agencies
  Nightingale's influence on, 26
  in official health agencies, 30-31
  origin of term, 28b
  population-focused practice of. *See* Population-focused practice
  practice application for, 65
  preparation areas in, 10b
  primary features of, 9
  professional changes in, 41
  psychologic focus in, 39
  roles in, 15-18
  scope of, 14, 1117-1119
  specialization in, 2-21, 14, 15f, 38
  standards and roles of, 1117-1119
  tenets of, 1118b
  types of, 14
  during World War I, 31
  during World War II, 35-36
  between world wars, 33-34
Public health nursing specialists, defined, 20
Public health professionals
  competencies for, 344b
  core competencies of, 7
Public Health Service, establishment of, 24, 172
Public Health Service Act, migrant health provisions of, 796
Public health services, Canadian, 1124
Public health system
  changes in, 1009-1012
  organization of, 60-62
Public policy
  on environmental health, 641
  in Healthy Cities movement, 399
  influencing, 31
Pulmonary disease in men, 691
Purchase-of-expertise consultation model, 1017-1018, 1018f, 1019b
Purified protein derivative test, procedure for, 950
Put Prevention into Practice program, 327, 714

**Q**

Q fever, 924
QUAD Council, 7
  establishment of, 521
  skill levels defined by, 9
Quality assurance/quality improvement, 498-499
  functions of, 519-520
  Healthy People 2010 goals for, 520
  historical perspective on, 520
  models for, 526, 531-533, 531f
    evaluation, interpretation, action, 533
    outcome of, 532-533
    process for, 532
    structure of, 530, 532
  in nursing centers, 435
  in TQM/CQI, 526-527
  traditional, *versus* TQM, 527, 527b
Quality care, components of, 523
Quality Care Task Force of the National Nursing Centers Consortium, guidelines of, 435
Quality control, 526
  in home health care, 978-979
Quality evaluation, sentinel method of, 530
Quality indicators, for nursing centers, 435, 436t
Quality management, 516-539
  abbreviations used in, 518b
  approaches to, 521-524
  client satisfaction and, 530
  in community and public settings, 524-530
  definitions and goals of, 519-520
  evaluative studies in, 529-530
  Healthy People 2010 goals for, 520
  historical development of, 520-521
  key points for, 536
  model program of, 531–534
  practice application for, 535
  prevention in, 534b
  records of, 535
Quality of adjusted life years in cost-effectiveness analysis, 102
Quality of care, 52-53
Quality of life
  attitudes toward, 54
  as community health indicator, 8b
Quarantine, legal basis for, 179

**R**

Rabies, cause, symptoms, prevention, 926
Race
  definition and examples of, 152
  diminishing importance of, 152
  economic/health status and, 756, 757f
  health disparities and, 748-749
  life expectancy and, 656
  in mortality/morbidity rates, 269
  windshield survey of, 357t
Racism
  defined, 159
  forms of, 160b
  in rural areas, 379
Ranchers. *See also* Farmers; Farmworkers
  health needs/problems of, 383t
Rape, 887-889
  attitudes toward, 880
  date/marital, 887
  marital, 887
  pornography and, 880
  prevalence of, 887
  prevention of, 887-888
  statutory, enforcment of laws pertaining to, 814
  underreporting of, 887
  victims *versus* survivors of, 880-889
Rate, defined, 256
Rathbone, William, 26
Ratio as risk approximation, 258
Rational Recovery, 868
Rawls, John, 136
Raynaud's phenomenon, work-related, 1079
Readiness to learn, 300
Reality norms, 544
Real-time community assessment, 494b
Recognition, defined, 522-523

Records, requirements and types of, 535
Referrals, negligent, in case management, 463
Refugee Act of 1980, 149
Regional Nursing Centers Consortium, 440
Registered nurses, defined, 179
Regulations, defined, 179
Regulatory action, 186-188
Rehabilitation Act of 1973, school nursing provisions of, 1044, 1044t
Rehabilitation services
  for older adults, 714
  origins of, 737
Reimbursement
  fee-for-service, 1011
  for home health/hospice care, 979-981
  in nursing centers, 414-415, 415b
  policies for, 755-756
  prospective, 121
  retrospective, 121
Reinforcement theory, 1014t
Reinforcers, uses of, 298
Relapse management in mental health care, 833, 834
Relaxation therapy for children, 643
Reliability, 265-266
Relief, international, for disasters, 484
Relief Nursing Service, 33
Religion
  organized, family violence and, 877
  windshield survey of, 357t
Religious organizations, projects of, 80-81
Reminiscence, functions of, 704
Report cards, agency, 1024
Reportable diseases, CDC list of, 908
Reproductive health, 657, 662-665
  discussing with adolescents, 810
  policies affecting, 589
Reproductive health care, adolescents and, 810
  in Canada, 816
Reproductive outcomes, adverse, environmental agents implicated in, 236t
Research. *See also* Nursing research
  action, defined, 286
  advanced practice nurse roles in, 996
  in nursing centers, 428-429, 436-437
  on rural nursing practice, 388-389
  school nurse's role in, 1047-1048
Resilience, defined, 754
Resource Conservation and Recovery Act, provisions of, 241b
Resource dependency theory, 1014t, 1017
Resources. *See also* Community resources
  on case manager credentialing, 464b
  on complementary and alternative medicine, 644b
  for environmental health assessment, 232b-233b
  on evidence-based practice, 289b
  on HIV, 938
  Internet, on school nursing, 1062t
  for low-income families, 606
  on men's health, 681
  on migrant health care, 681
  on older adults, 715b
  on smoking cessation, 869b
  for vulnerable populations, 767-768
Respiratory disease in homeless persons, 786
Respiratory system, age-related changes in, 705t
Respite care for caregivers, 711
Retrospective reimbursement, 121
Rheumatoid arthritis in Lyme disease, 924
Rich-poor gap, increases in, 755
Rickets in infants, prevention strategies for, 629, 629b
*Rickettsia rickettsii*, 924
Rifampin, TB bacillus resistance to, 88
Right to Know, 228, 233-234
Risk. *See also* Health risks
  calculating, 257-258
  cumulative, 747

Risk—cont'd
defined, 239b, 256, 596
epidemiologic definition of, 746
Risk assessment, 325-326
environmental, 234-235
steps in, 326
Risk Factor Update Project, 326
Risk factors
for coronary heart disease, 330
as indicator of community health status, 347b
for violence, assessing, 889, 890f, 891b
Risk management, functions of, 528
Risk marker, defined, 748
Risk reduction, methods for, 325-328
Risk sharing arrangements, 454
Risk taking
adolescent, 634, 809
male, 686
Risk-based contracts, 1011
Robb, Isabel Hampton, 243
Robert Wood Johnson Foundation, primary care workforce initiatives of, 54
Rockefeller Sanitary Commission, 30
Rockerfeller Foundation, 81
Rocky Mountain spotted fever, cause, clinical symptoms, treatment, 924
Roe v. Wade, 654
Rogers, Carl, 704
Role modeling with abuse victims, 893
Role negotiation in community assessment, 359
Role structure, group, 546
Roosevelt, Franklin D., 701
Root, Frances, 26, 964
Rotavirus vaccine, recall of, 631
Roy's adaptation model of nursing, 1017
Rubella, characteristics and immunization, 919-920
Rules of transformation, 601
Rural, defined, 376b
Rural environments, 374-395
Canadian, 386-387
community partnership for improving health service in, 331-332
evidence-based practice in, 385
future perspectives for, 389-391
health care delivery issues and barriers, 384-385
health outreach in, 335
health status in, 378-384
versus urban health status, 390b
Healthy People 2010 objectives for, 390-391
historical overview of, 374-375
key points for, 393
nursing care in, 385-389
nursing practice in, preparation for, 389
population characteristics of, 377-378, 378t
practice application for, 392-393
prevention in, 388, 388b
professional-community-client partnerships in, 391-392
public health in, 29, 30
research on, 388-389
terms pertaining to, 375-377, 376b
urban continuum with, 376-377
Rural Health Clinic Services Act of 1977, 1001, 1001t
Rural life, characteristics of, 384b
Rurality, definitions of, 375-376
Rural-urban continuum, 376-377, 377f
Rush, Benjamin, 830
Russia
Healthy Cities and Communities movement in, 403-404
immigrants from, health issues of, 564
Ryan White Comprehensive AIDS Resource Emergency Act, 933
provisions of, 110t

S

Safe Drinking Water Act, provisions of, 241b
Safe Kids Campaign, 1051

Safety
adolescent, 625t
of complementary and alternative medicine, 643
drug, 862
food, 3, 233, 922-923, 923b
home, evaluation of, 713f
infant, 620t
neonatal, 619t
personal, in community practice, 370-371
playground, 635-636, 635b
sports, guide to, 623b
of toddlers/preschoolers, 621t
Safety fairs, 634
Safety measures
home, 889
for preventing violence during pregnancy, 887
for reducing gun violence, 889
Safety net providers, 123
St. Louis virus, 924
Salk, Jonas, 252t
Sallmon, Marla, 176
Salmonella
in food-borne illness, 921
in waterborne illness, 923
Salmonella typhimurium, epidemiologic study of, 279
Salmonellosis, 926
causes and symptoms of, 923
Salvation Army in disaster management, 476
Sanger, Margaret, 653
Sanitation
in American colonial period, 24
lack of access to, 79
SARS. See Severe acute respiratory syndrome
Satisfaction surveys, 530
Scheme, Piaget's definition of, 626
Schiff, Jacob, 28b
Schizophrenia
antipsychotic drugs for, 829
caregiving for, evidence-based practice for, 841
School crisis teams, 1057-1058, 1058b
School Health Policies and Programs Study 2000, 1046, 1049
School health programs
federal, 1048
legal issues in, 181
School nurse practitioner, first program for, 1043-1045
School nursing, 29-30, 1042-1065
controversies in, 1061-1062
credentials for, 1045-1046
developing family relationships in, 1056
emergency care in, 1053-1054
in England, 1049
ethics in, 1062
first inclusion in curriculum, 1043
Healthy People 2010 and, 1049
history of, 1042-1045
key points, 1062-1063
legislation on, 1044-1045, 1044t
online resources for, 1062t
practice application for, 1062
practice standards in, 1045
prevention in, 1049-1061
primary, 1050-1053
secondary, 1053-1058
tertiary, 1058, 1060-1061
roles/functions in, 1046-1047
services provided by, 1048-1049
states mandating standards for, 1045b
trends in, 1062
School-age children
assessment of, 622-624, 622t
injuries/accidents of, 634
nutritional assessment in, 629-630
School-age period, defined, 622
School-based health centers, 1049
School-linked programs, 1049
Schools
advanced practice nurses in, 1000
air quality in, 1058, 1059f-1060f
asthma "friendliness" of, 638b

Schools—cont'd
Healthy People 2010 educational goals for, 297
injured child's return to, 1060
and physically compromised children, 727
physically compromised students and, 729
preventing violence in, 1057
"sick," 642b
violence associated with, 877
Scope and Standards of Public Health Nursing Practice, 9
Scope of practice, legal definition of, 180
Screening
epidemiologic, 265-267, 265b, 266t
lipid, 265
literacy, 309
negative predictive value of, 266-267
positive predictive value of, 266-267
prostate, 265
reliability of, 265-266
of schoolchildren, 1054, 1055t-1056t, 1056
states requiring, 1055t-1056t
sensitivity and specificity in, 266, 1035, 1036b
validity of, 266-267
Seat belt safety programs, 634
Seat belts, child/adolescent use of, 633
Seattle, Chief, 236
Secondary prevention, defined, 52b
Secondhand smoke, deaths due to, 639
Secular trends, epidemiologic, 270
Security. See also Safety
home, improving, 889
Selective serotonin reuptake inhibitors, 829
Self-care
cultural variations in, 162t
definitions of, 325
neglect of, 322
Self-care movement, 322-323
Self-efficacy, defined, 309
Self-esteem of abuse victims, 886
Self-help groups, tension between leaders and members of, 545-546
Self-help organizations for mentally ill persons, 833b
Self-management of chronic illness in older adults, 708
Senior centers, services of, 710
Sensitivity, test, 266
Sensors, applications of, 55
Sensory system, age-related changes in, 705t, 841
September 11, 2001
bioterrorism threat and, 178, 255
community response to, 480
immunization policies after, 589-590
and Model State Emergency Health Powers Act, 172-173
psychological effects of, 481, 481B
response to, 479
stress following, 828
Sequencing, 305
Servant leadership, 1026-1027
Service centers, windshield survey of, 357f
Service delivery networks, 1011
Settlement houses, 27. See also Henry Street Settlement
Severe acute respiratory syndrome, 904
characteristics of, 907
risk management of, in Canada, 949
website for, 907
Sex education, controversy over, 1061-1062
Sexual abuse, 882. See also Child abuse and neglect; Intimate partner violence; Rape
assessment of, 884-885
of intimate partner, 887
during teen pregnancy, 817-818
Sexual activity, adolescent, 812-813
in Canada, 816-817
coercive, 813-814
family influences on, 814

Sexual assault
assessing for, 887, 889
on intimate partner, 887
on men, 692
in prisons, 895-896
Sexual assault examination, training in, 880
Sexual behavior
adolescent
in Canada, 816
trends in, 810-811
discussing, 952-953
responsible, Healthy People 2010 objectives for, 420, 994
Sexual contact, HIV/AIDS spread through, 67
Sexual debut, 812
age at, and use of birth control, 813
Sexual history, 950-951
Sexual identity in women with disabilities, 671
Sexual orientation, discussing, 952
Sexual practices, high-risk, 952
Sexual victimization of adolescents, 813-814
Sexually transmitted diseases
co-infection of, 932
community education about, 954
Healthy People 2010 objectives for, 812, 934
new forms of, 932
partner notification about, 950-951
rape and, 880
sexual practices conducive to, 952-953
teen pregnancy and, 810b
Shattuck, Lemuel, 252t
Shattuck Report, 25
Shelters, disaster, 383
Sheppard-Towner Act, provisions of, 174
Sheppard-Towner Program, 31
Shigella, waterborne illness due to, 923
"Sick" schools, 642b
SIDS. See Sudden infant death syndrome
Silver, Henry, 991
Silver Spring Community Health Center, 414
Single photon emission computed tomography, 829
Sister to Sister, services of, 749
Sisters of Charity of St. Joseph, 964
Situated perspective, defined, 287
Skilled nursing care in home health care, 969-970
Skilled nursing facilities, Medicare payments to, 116
Skin, age-related changes in, 705t
Skin cancer, 690
Skinner, B. F., reinforcement theory of, 1014t
Sleep
infant, 620t
neonatal, 619t
of toddlers/preschoolers, 621t
Sleep patterns, adolescent, 625t
Sleet (Scales), Jessie, 32
Smallpox
bioterrorist threat of, 913, 916-917
versus chickenpox, 917
U. S. vulnerability to, 178
Smith, Claudia, 228
Smoke, secondhand, deaths due to, 639
SmokEnders, contact information for, 869b
Smoking. See Cigarette smoking; Tobacco use
Smoking cessation programs, 868
resources for, 869b
Smoking prevention programs, 639-640
Smoking reduction programs, 332
Snow, John, 252t
cholera study of, 253, 253t, 255
Social change
early versus late adopters of, 368
health policy and, 367-368
nurse's role in, 367-368
Social Darwinism, defined, 756
Social environment, family, 601b

Social isolation
  family violence and, 882
  health status and, 758
Social justice, defined, 750
Social learning theory, 300, 1014t
Social mandate of Healthy People 2010, 447
Social organization, cultural variations in, 164
Social policy, 588-589
Social risks in family health, 602, 604
Social Security
  federal expenses for, 109
  funding for, 173
Social Security Act, 34-35, 778
  1965 amendments to, 41, 105
  1983 amendments to, 106
  amendments to, 110t
  impact of, 711t
  Medicaid amendments to, 116, 122, 778
  Medicare amendments to, 115-116, 751, 778, 981-982
    impact of, 711t
  provisions affecting vulnerable populations, 751
  provisions of, 110t
  PSRO amendments of, 521
  Title XIX of, 105, 116. See also Medicaid
    impact of, 711t
  Title XVIII of, 105, 115. See also Medicare
    impact of, 711t
  Title XX of, impact of, 711t
  Title XXI of, 751
Social welfare, American ideas of, 24
Social workers
  in nursing centers, 428t
  role in home care, 975
Social/reinforcement theories of management, 1015
Socioeconomic resources, vulnerability and, 754-756
Socioeconomic status
  culture and, 166-167
  health status and, 123
  and incidence of diabetes, 665
  injury incidence and, 633
  obesity and, 668
  in rural areas, 377-378
Socioeconomic status gradient, defined, 754-755
South Africa, health promotion in, 78
Sovereign immunity, 181
Space, cultural variations in attitudes toward, 163-164
Special care centers, 416
Specificity, test, 266
Speech pathologist, role in home care, 975
Speizer, Frank, 252t
Spermicides, vaginal, uses and effectiveness of, 662t
Spina bifida, folic acid for preventing, 662-663
Spiritual assessments, 1103
Sports, disabled persons' participation in, 737
Sports safety, guide to, 623b
Spouse abuse, 885-887
SPPICEES mnemonic, 714
Squamous cell carcinoma of skin, 690
Staff review committees, 527
Stakeholders
  in community collaboration, 421
  defined, 420
  perspectives of, 496-497
Standard metropolitan statistical area, defined, 376b
Standard precautions
  for HIV infection, 956
  school staff training in, 1053
Stanford Heart Disease Prevention program, 330
Stanton, Elizabeth Cady, 653
Staphylococcus aureus
  food intoxication due to, 922t
  vancomycin-resistant, 904

State Child Health Improvement Act, provisions of, 172
State Child Health Insurance Program, 173
  funding for, 173
  and increasing health care expenditures, 107
  legislation authorizing, 751
State government
  in disaster preparedness, 474
  health departments of, 63, 63b, 178
  nurse practice acts of, 179
Statutory rape, enforcment of laws pertaining to, 814
Stereotyping, 158-159
Sterilization, surgical, 662t
Stewart, Ada Mayo, 29, 1067
Stewart B. McKinney Homeless Assistance Act, provisions of, 788
Stewart B. McKinney Homeless Assistance Act of 1988, provisions affecting vulnerable populations, 751
Stewart B. McKinney Homeless Assistance Act of 1994, provisions of, 783
Stewart Machine Co. v. David, 172
Stimulants, 855-856
  physiologic effects of, 855
Stories, family, 578, 579
Strategic planning, 493-494
  in nursing centers, 420-421
Strategic plans for nursing centers, 432-433
Street people. See also Homeless families; Homeless persons; Homeless women; Homelessness
  windshield survey of, 357t
Strength and balance training, evidence-based practice and, 291
Streptomycin for TB, 88
Stress
  of advanced practice nurses, 1002-1003
  after natural disasters, 485
  age-related vulnerability to, 758
  chronic, in vulnerable populations, 760
  in disaster workers, 484
  family, Burr and Klein's theory of, 601-602, 602b
  family violence and, 882
  public health burden of, 828
  work-related, 1079-1080
Stress reactions, delayed, 484
Stressors, community, 203, 204t, 205
Stroke, 695
Structural contingency theory, 1014t, 1015
Structure
  as characteristic of community health, 346-347, 347b
  as indicator of community health, 349t
Structure-function theory of family, 573, 575
Structure-process-outcome evaluation, 508-509
Stunting, 91
Subpopulations, defined, 10
Substance abuse. See also Alcohol abuse; Drug abuse
  defined, 852
  health and economic effects of, 848
  Healthy People 2010 objectives for, 420, 944
  by men, 695
  during pregnancy, 663
  preventing, through child education, 1051
  risk from, 606
  during teen pregnancy, 819
Suburban, defined, 376b
Sudden infant death syndrome, 637
Suicide
  adolescent, 634
  assisted, of people with disabilities, 737-738
  case-control study of, 274
  handguns used in, 889

Suicide-cont'd
  incidence of, 881
  male, 691
  prevention of, 881
  risk factors for, 691t
  in rural areas, 379
  in young people, Healthy People 2010 objectives for preventing, 839
Suicide prevention in schools, 1057
Suicide risk in older adults, practice application for, 844
Summative evaluation, 491
Superfund Amendments and Reauthorization Act, provisions of, 241b
Supervision
  defined, 1025
  skills in, 1032
Supplements to infant feeding, 626, 629
Supply, defined, 100
Supply-and-demand curve, 100, 100f
Support groups
  for substance abusers, 868
  in violence prevention, 892
Supporting, characteristics of, 458
Surgeon General's Report on Health Promotion and Disease Prevention, 596
Surgery, advances in, 105
Surveillance, 267
  infectious disease, 907-908, 907b
Surveys
  data from, 353
  definition, advantages/disadvantages of, 495t
Sweatshops, environmental conditions of, 26-27
Sweden, health care system in, 84-85
Syphilis
  cause, symptoms, treatment, 942
  congenital, 942
    elimination strategy for, 947
  risk management of, in Canada, 949
  summary of, 941t
Systematic review
  defined, 286
  steps in, 286
Systems models, 197-199
  Neuman's, 198-199, 200f, 201-203, 204f, 205-206
  Omaha, 206-213
Systems theory, 1014t, 1017
  case study in, 581-582
  of family, 575-576
  in mental health care, 833

T

Taliban, conditions under, 74, 82
TANE. See Temporary Assistance for Needy Families
Target behaviors, 298
Targets of practice, 344
Task Force on Community Preventive Services, 7
Task function, defined, 542-543
Task norms, 544
Task specialists, role of, 547b
Tax Equity and Fiscal Responsibility Act
  impact of, 711t
  provisions affecting vulnerable populations, 752
  provisions of, 110t
Teaching, effective, 312b
Team approach
  in groups, 552-554
  in nursing centers, 424, 426
  principles of, 1032, 1033t
TEAM MED project, 205-206
Technology
  appropriate, in Healthy Cities movement, 399
  in community health education, 309-310
  and costs of care, 111
  experimental, legal issues involving, 463
  in home care setting, 983-984
  influence on health care system, 64-65
  intensity of use of, 103
  limitations of, 81
  medical, defined, 103

Technology-cont'd
  trends in, 54-55
  in U. S. health care system, 103, 105-106
Technology and information systems for nursing centers, 435-436
Teen mothers
  evidence-based practice and, 1119
  gestational weight gain recommendations for, 820t
  gynecologic age of, 819
  promoting interactions with baby, 821
  in school, 1061
Teen parenting
  infant care and, 820-821
  schooling and educational needs and, 821-822
Teen pregnancy, 617, 808-825. See also Adolescents
  adoption counseling and, 818b
  background factors in, 811-814
  in Canada, 816-817
  community-based interventions for, 822-823
  in developed countries, 810-811
  early identification of, 815-816
  evidence-based practice and, 818
  home-based interventions for, 822
  incidence of, 810
  key points, 823-824
  low-birth-weight infants/preterm delivery and, 819-820
  and mother's gynecologic age, 819
  nutrition during, 819, 820t
  practice application for, 823
  prenatal care for, 818-819
  preventing, 815b, 822-823
    with emergency contraception, 823
  repeat, 821
  sexual abuse during, 818
  special issues in, 816-822
  state expenditures for, 808
  STDs and, 810b
  testing for, 815
  trends in, 810-811
  violence during, 817-818
  vitamin and mineral requirements during, 820t
  weight gain during, 819
  young men and, 814-815
Telehealth, 453, 454
  in home care setting, 983-984
Telemetry, remote, 55
Television, violence on, 622
Temporary Assistance for Needy Families, 655, 777, 778. See also Aid to Families of Dependent Children
Terrorists, precautions against, 477b
Tertiary prevention, defined, 52b
Testicular cancer, 689-690
Testicular self-examination, 689, 689f, 690
Tetanus, required immunizations for, 1052t
Thematic instrument for measuring death anxiety in children, 727
Theory, definitions of, 196
Theory/principles intervention mode, 1022
Thimerosol, safety of, 631
Thinking, critical, 1030
Thioacetazone, 88
Third World First, 80
Third-party payers, 121
  and use of evidence-based practice, 287
Third-party payment, 124
Thompson, Tommy G., 985
Thought patterns, changing, 299
Three Ds, 709
Threshold model of poverty, 7546
Tick-borne disease, 924-925
TIMDAC. See Thematic instrument for measuring death anxiety in children
Time
  cultural variations in attitudes toward, 164
  perceptions of, cultural variations in, 162t

Time management skills, 1027b
Tobacco smoke, exposure to, by smokers and nonsmokers, 224
Tobacco use
  among adolescents, 809
  by Canadian women, 660
  cancer and, 666-667
  in children/adolescents, 639-641
  evidence-based practice for, 639
  Healthy People 2010 objectives for, 320, 420, 994
  by men, 691, 695
  physical compromise due to, 723
  risk from, 606
Toddlers
  assessment of, 619-620, 621t
  defined, 619
  injuries/accidents of, 634
  physically compromised, legal rights of, 737
Tolerance
  to alcohol, 854
  to marijuana, 858
  to nicotine, 855
  to opioids, 855
Total quality management/continuous quality improvement, 516-517
  in community and public health settings, 524-530
  definitions of, 519
  Deming's guidelines for, 523
  optimal organizational structure for, 523-524
  quality assurance/quality improvement in, 526-527
  tools of, 523
  *versus* traditional management, 527, 527t
Touch, cultural attitudes toward, 162t
Town and Country Nursing Service, 29
Toxic Substances Control Act, provisions of, 241b
Toxic waste, popular epidemiology of, 278-279
Toxicants, developmental, 235
Toxicology, 224-225
  defined, 224
  NLM databases on, 225
*Toxoplasma* in food-borne illness, 921
Toxoplasmosis, 926
TQM. *See* Total quality management
Tracer method, 509, 529
Transcultural nursing, standards for, 155
Transdermal contraceptive patch, adolescent use of, 813t
Transformation, rules of, 601
Transformational leadership theory, 1014t, 1016
Transfusions. *See* Blood transfusions
Transitions, family, 601
Transmission, disease, modes of, 906
Transportation
  for migrant farmworkers, 797
  windshield survey of, 357t
Trauma in homeless persons, 786
Travel
  diseases associated with, 925-926
  health assessment and, 82
  international, risks of, 74
Treatments, experimental, legal issues involving, 463
Trematodes, diseases caused by, 927t
*Treponema pallidum*, 941t
Triage, defined, 482-483
TriCare Prime, 177
TriCare Standard, 177
Trust building, 463b
Tuberculosis
  in Canada, 914
  control of, 87-88
  diagnosis and treatment of, 947, 950
  directly observed therapy for, 955-956
  elimination strategy for, 947
  epidemiology of, 87-88, 947
  in immunosuppressed persons, 935
  in migrant farmworkers, 799
  mortality from, 28-29
  resistant strains of, 254-255
  screening for, in schoolchildren, 1054
  work-related exposure to, 1076

Tularemia, 924
  bioterrorist threat of, 913
Turning Point, website for, 493
Tuskegee Syphilis Study, 159
Typhoid fever, control of, 30-31

**U**

Uganda, health promotion in, 78
Unemployment, stress and violence associated with, 876
UNICEF. *See* United Nations Children's Fund
U. S. Agency for International Development, 80
U. S. Bureau of Primary Care, funding from, 433-434
U. S. Consumer Product Safety commission, playground safety guidelines of, 635
U. S. Department of Health and Human Services
  Agency for Health Care Research and Quality of, 62
  assessment projects of, 11
  creation of, 172
  Division of Nursing of, 60-61
  divisions of, 176-177
  epidemiology initiatives of, 252t
  functions and organization of, 60-62
  health data reports of, 174t
  mission and goals of, 60
  National Center for Nursing Research of, 62
  Office on Women's Health of, 655
  organization of, 61f
  primary care workforce initiatives of, 54
  public health nursing requirements of, 9
  regional offices of, 62t
U. S. government
  community health-related agencies of, 176-178
  in community-oriented nursing regulation, 179-180
  in disaster preparedness, 473
  environmental protection role of, 240-243
  health care data analysis by, 173, 174t
  health care functions/structures of, nursing impacts of, 178-179
  health care funding by, 173
  health care policy setting by, 173-174
  health care structures/functions of, 173-174
  public health policies of, 24
  role in Healthy People 2010, 174-175
  structure of, 171-174
  trends in, 172-173
U. S. Preventive Health Services Task Force, 265
  *Guide of,* 7
  recommendations for women's health, 673-674
U. S. Public Health Service
  advanced practice nurses in, 1000
  Core Functions Project of, 7
  funding from, 433-434
  national health objectives of, 323
  role of, 30
United Kingdom
  health care system in, 83
  infant mortality rate in, 83
United Nations
  health data reports of, 174t
  structure of, 175
United Nations Children's Fund
  Alma Ata conference of, 73
  functions and organization of, 79
United Nations Fund for Population Activities, 90
United States
  demographics of, 53
  health care expenses in, 98
  health goals in, 596
  Healthy Cities and Communities movement in, 401-402
  homelessness in, 783
  infant mortality rate in, 83
  public health history of, 24-25

Universal precautions, 928
  in home care, 971
University of Akron, Center for Nursing, nursing center, mission and goals of, 418b
University of Maryland, School of Nursing, Clinical Enterprise, mission and goals of, 418b
University of Michigan Community Family Health Center, mission and goals of, 418b
University of Virginia, self-learning modules for geriatric care, 714
Urban, defined, 376b
Urban areas. *See also* Healthy Communities and Cities movement
  world population living in, 398
Urbanization
  and spread of disease, 24
  and women in work force, 26
Urethritis, nongonococcal, 943
Utilitarianism, 134
  defined, 132b
  origins of, 136
Utility, defined, 99
Utilization management, defined, 447-448
Utilization review, purpose and types of, 528

**V**

Vaccine information statements, 631
Vaccines. *See also* Immunizations
  adverse reactions to, 631
  diseases prevented by, 917-921
  DTaP, 630
  fear of, 631
Vaccines for Children, 631
Vaginal spermicides, uses and effectiveness of, 662t
Validity, 266-267
Values
  changing, 54
  defined, 132b
  illuminating, 459
  in quality assurance programs, 532
Vancomycin, resistance to, 904
Variance, defined, 454
Variance analysis, 1036, 1037t
Vectors, disease, 906
Vegetables, dietary guidelines for, in children/adolescents, 628t
Venezuela, Healthy Cities and Communities movement in, 405-406
Veracity, ethical issues in, 465
VeriChip, 984
Verifying, characteristics of, 458
Vertical transmission of disease, 906
Veterans' Administration, 117
Veterans' health benefits, eligibility for, 682
Viagra, cost of, 111
*Vibrio*, waterborne illness due to, 923
*Vibrio parahemolyticus,* food intoxication due to, 922t
Victimization, sexual, of adolescents, 813-814
Victims, abuse, role modeling with, 893
Victorian Order of Nurses, 36
Videotapes, producing, for health education, 303
Vietnamese, time values of, 164-165
Violence, 874-901. *See also* Child abuse and neglect; Family violence; Gun violence; Intimate partner violence; Older adult abuse and neglect; Sexual abuse
  adolescent victims of, 623
  assaultive, by men, 691-692
  community sanctions against, 889
  defined, 875-876
  ethnic/racial differences in, economic factors in, 876
  in families, 881-889
  forensic nursing and, 896-897
  Healthy People 2010 objectives for reducing, 420, 876, 994
  against individuals or oneself, 877-878

Violence–cont'd
  as innate *versus* learned behavior, 874-875
  interventions for, 889-895
    primary, 889-892
    secondary, 892
    tertiary, 892-895
  intimate partner, during teen pregnancy, 817-818
  intrafamilial, 606-607
  key points, 897
  in media, 877
  population density and, 877-878
  practice application pertaining to, 897
  prevention of, 891b
    community services in, 893b
    health care provider training for, 892
    individual/family strategies for, 891-892
    for men, 695
    in schools, 1057
    strategies for, 891b
  prison population and, 895-896
  risk factors for, assessing, 889, 890f, 891b
  in schools, 877
  social and community factors in, 876-878
  sociocultural factors in, 691-692
  during teen pregnancy, 817-818
  teenage victims of, 617
  toward women with disabilities, 671
  TV, 622
  victims of, role modeling with, 893
  in workplace, 1080
  youth, preventing culture of, 839
Viral disease, inappropriate antibiotic use for, 902
Virginia Garcia Migrant Clinic, evidence-based practice and, 802
Virtue ethics, 137, 137b
Visiting nurse associations
  establishment of, 26
  history of, 964
  lack of funding for, 39
Visiting Nurse Service of New York City, 27
Visiting Nurse Society of Philadelphia, 37-38
Visiting nurses, origins of, 27
*Visiting Nursing in the United States,* 28
Vitamin C for hypertension, 689b
Vitamin D, supplemental
  for preventing osteoporosis, 663
  for at risk infants, 629
Voluntary organizations in disaster preparedness, 477t, 478t
Volunteer Organizations Active in Disasters, 476
Vroom, Victor, expectancy theory of, 1014t, 1015
Vulnerability, 746-773
  cycle of, 760
  defined, 746-747
  factors contributing to, 754-760
    health risk, 758-759
    health status, 758
    marginalization, 759-760
    poverty, 756-758
    socioeconomic, 754-756
  outcomes of, 760
Vulnerable populations, 748-749
  assessment of, 761-763
    biological issues in, 762
    environmental issues in, 763
    guidelines for, 762b
    lifestyle issues in, 763
    for physical health, 761-762
    psychologic issues in, 762-763
    socioeconomic considerations in, 761
  carve outs for, 750
  community-oriented nursing approaches to, 760-761
  empowerment of, 764, 766
  evidence-based practice for, 768
  examples of, 748
  as financial risks, 750

Vulnerable populations–cont'd
 health and social services coordination for, 766
 health care delivery models for,
  644-645
 health care for, effective, 750
 health care trends for, 749-751
 health disparities of, 748-749
 health education for, 764, 766
 health risks of, 758-759
 health status of, 758
 Healthy People 2010 goals for,
  766-767
 insurance coverage for, 753
 intervention evaluations for, 769
 interventions for, principles of, 765b
 key points for, 770
 and lack of health insurance, 753
 legislation for, 751-753, 751b
 marginalization of, 759-760
 planning/implementing care for,
  763-764, 765b, 766
 policies affecting, 751-753
 poverty of, 756-758
 practice application for, 769
 preventive interventions for, 766, 767b
 research/practice conceptual model
  for, 755f
 resources for, 767-768
 social dynamics and outcomes for,
  754f
 socioeconomic resources of, 754-758

**W**

W. K. Kellogg Foundation, 80
 health care support from, 65
Waivers for vulnerable clients, 750
Wald, Lillian, 19, 27, 28b, 29, 29b, 34,
  40b, 965, 1043
 Children's Bureau and, 31
 and environmental health issues, 223
 and founding of National
  Organization for Public Health
  Nursing, 30
 funding efforts of, 31
 school nursing initiative of, 29
Wallinder, Jan, 1118
War
 health care and, 82
 health effects of, 74
 men's health care legislation and, 682
 neurologic/psychologic mental health
  disorders and, 830
War on Drugs, problems with, 849
War on Poverty, 778
Warts, genital. See also Human papillomavirus
 summary of, 941t
Water quality, assessment of, 233
Waterborne disease, 923-924
 agents causing, 923-924
 CDC definition of, 923
 of travelers, 925
Waters, Yssabella, 28
Weapons. See also Gun violence; Guns
 adolescent use of, 634
Web of causality, 261
 for cardiovascular disease, 261-262,
  262f
Weight control. See also Obesity;
  Overweight
 client education about, 300
 in women, 668-669
Weir Report on Nursing Education, 37
Welcome Home Ministries, 670b
Welfare. See also Aid to Families of
  Dependent Children; Temporary
  Assistance for Needy Families

Welfare–cont'd
 numbers receiving, 778
 political debate over, 778
Welfare reform, 778, 1120
 effects on childbearing women, 779
 and immigrant access to health care,
  797
 teen pregnancy/nonmarital births and,
  812
Well-child care
 by chiropractors, 642
 guidelines for, 618t
 origins of, 27, 27f
Wellness
 components of, 715
 versus illness emphasis, 319-321
Wellness committees of faith communities, 1100-1102
Wellness interventions, community partnership for, 332
Wellness inventories, 327
Wellness programs for older adults,
  714-715
Wellness-illness continuum, 717f
West Africa, WHO-World Bank projects
  in, 80
West Nile virus, 2, 23, 904, 924
 characteristics of, 908, 910
 symptoms, transmission, and causes
  of emergence, 912t
Whelan, Linda Tarr, 176
White children, poverty rate of, 779t
White women
 breast cancer in, 656-657, 667
 cardiovascular disease in, 664
 causes of death among, 659t
 cigarette smoking by, 666-667
 health of, versus women of color,
  669-670
 prison/jail rate of, 670
WHO. See World Health Organization
Whooping cough, characteristics and immunization, 920
Wife abuse, 885-887. See also Family violence; Intimate partner violence;
  Rape
Williams, Carolyn, 176
Williams v. Metro Home Health Care
  Agency, et al., 180-181
Windshield surveys, 355-356, 357t
Winslow, C. E. A., 1117
Women
 in armed services, 682
 battered, 885-887
 Canadian, in poverty, 780
 causes of death of, 658t-659t, 686t
 childbearing, poverty and, 779
 with disabilities, 670-671
 families headed by, poverty rate of, by
  ethnicity/race, 669f
 head-of-household, poverty of, 671
 Healthy People 2010 objectives for, 57
 homeless, 671
  support systems of, 672
 impoverished, 671-672
 incarcerated
  health of, 670
  outside transition programs for,
   670b
 life expectancies of
  by country, 683t
  versus male, 701
 life expectancy/mortality rates of,
  656-657, 657t
 migrant, 797
 morbidity in, 657
 nutrition deficits in, 90-91
 older. See Older women

Women–cont'd
 pregnant, homeless, 787
 prevention checklist for, 673b
 at risk, for family violence, 894-895
 rural, support network for, 666
 UN conferences on, 175
 U. S.
  age projections for, 673t
  causes of death among, 658t
  ethnic/racial distribution of, 669f
  in work force, 26
Women, Infants, and Children's program, 174, 645
 health care cost savings from, 604
 for homeless persons with children,
  788
Women for Sobriety, 868
Women of color
 health of, versus white women's
  health, 669-670
 older, illness and disability in, 672
Women to Women Project, 666
Women's health, 652-679
 alternative/complementary therapies
  for, 672-673
 in Canada, 660-661
 definitions of, 652-653
 disparities in
  for impoverished women, 671-672
  for incarcerated women, 670
  for lesbians, 670
  for older women, 672
  for women of color, 669-670
  for women with disabilities, 670-671
 historical perspectives on, 653-654
 international, 89-90
 key points for, 674-675
 policies and legislation for, 654-655
 practice application for, 674
 reproductive, 657, 662-665
 in Russian Healthy Cities project, 403
 U. S. Preventive Services recommendations for, 673-674
Women's health care, high-quality,
  means for providing, 658
Women's Health Equity Act, 655
Women's health issues
 cancer, 666-667
 cardiovascular disease, 664
 diabetes mellitus, 664-665
 genital mutilation, 663-664
 HIV/AIDS, 667-668
 menopause, 663
 mental health, 665-666
 osteoporosis, 663
 weight control, 668-669
Women's Health Leadership, 555
Women's health movement, origins of,
  653
Women's Health Strategy (Canadian), 661
Women's Health Time Capsule, 655
Work. See also Occupational health
 categories of
  exposures and diseases related to,
   1074t
  most injuries/illness associated
   with, 1075f
 characteristics of, 1072-1073, 1073f
 hazards related to, categories of,
  1076b
 health issues related to, 1066-1067,
  1073-1074, 1075f, 1074t, 1074,
  1075f
 stress and violence associated with,
  876
Work disability, definition and economic impact of, 724

Work ethic, changing attitudes toward,
  54
Workers. See also Employees
 aggregate characteristics of, 1070,
  1070, 1072, 1073f
 assessment of, 1082-1083
 health and safety of, epidemiologic
  model of, 1074-1080, 1075f
 nursing care of, 1081-1086
Workers' compensation
 migrant farmworker access to, 798
 origins of, 1068
Workers' Compensation Act, 681-682
Workers' compensation acts, 1087
Workforce. See Health workforce
Workplace
 assessment of, 1083-1084, 1084f-
  1085f, 1086
 discrimination in, against persons
  with disabilities, 737
 health risks in, for Canadian men, 685
 Healthy People 2010 educational
  goals for, 297
 toxic exposures in, 238-239, 238b
Works Progress Administration, 33
Worksite walk-through, 1083
World Bank
 functions and organization of, 80
 projects of, 80
World Health Organization
 Alma Ata conference of, 73
 community defined by, 342-343
 establishment and goals of, 176-177
 European Healthy Cities Project of,
  397
 examples of projects of, 79
 functions and organization of, 79
 health care indicators of, 56
 health data reports of, 174t
 health defined by, 323-324
 health promotion definition of, 324
 Healthy Cities initiative of, 352
 holistic health policies of, 75
 maternal mortality and, 90
 in nursing center development, 419
 nursing research priorities of, 436,
  438b
 proposals for banning female genital
  mutilation, 664
World War I, public health nursing during, 31
World War II
 neurologic/psychiatric mental health
  disorders after, 830
 public health nursing during, 35-36
Worldview, defined, 197
Wrap-around services, 749

**Y**

Yemen, World Bank projects in, 80
Youth Behavioral Health Risk Appraisal,
  598
Youth gangs, 634
 violence of, 878
Youth Opportunities Initiative, 441
Youth Risk Behavior Surveillance
  System, 809
Youth violence, preventing culture of,
  839

**Z**

Zoning, windshield survey of, 357t
Zoonoses, transmission and types of,
  926